Cardiac Pacing and Electrophysiology

THIRD EDITION

Nabil EL-Sherif, M.D.
Professor of Medicine and Physiology
and Director of Electrophysiology
State University of New York
Health Science Center
Chief, Division of Cardiology
Veterans Administration Medical Center
Brooklyn, New York

Philip Samet, M.D.
Professor of Medicine
University of Miami
School of Medicine
Chief, Division of Cardiology
Mount Sinai Hospital
Miami Beach, Florida

1991
W.B. SAUNDERS COMPANY
Harcourt Brace Jovanovich, Inc.
Philadelphia London Toronto Montreal Sydney Tokyo

In memory of my wife
Laila,
and what she gave me,
many years of happiness
and Tarek, Yasir, Khalid,
and Mona.

NABIL EL-SHERIF

In memory of Phyllis, my wife,
confidante, and friend
and all that she gave me—
many years of happiness
and Nettie, Joan, and Jerry.
And to Carole, my new source
of inspiration and strength.

PHILIP SAMET

CONTRIBUTORS

S. AADDAJ, M.S.
Electronic Technician, Hôpital Jean Rostand, Ivry, France
Catheter Ablation Techniques for Ventricular Tachycardia

MASOOD AKHTAR, M.D.
Professor of Medicine and Associate Chief, Cardiovascular Disease Section, Sinai Samaritan Medical Center, Mount Sinai Campus, Milwaukee, Wisconsin
Supraventricular Tachycardias: Clinical Characteristics, Diagnosis, and Management

M. ALDAKAR, M.D.
Staff Member, Hôpital Jean Rostand, Ivry, France
Catheter Ablation Techniques for Ventricular Tachycardia

EARL BAKKEN, B.E.E., Dr.H.C.
Founder, Consultant, Director, Bakken Society Fellow, Medtronic, Inc., Minneapolis, Minnesota
The Future of Electrical Devices in the Chronic Treatment of Tachyarrhythmias

S. SERGE BAROLD, M.D.
Professor of Medicine, University of Rochester School of Medicine and Dentistry, Rochester, New York; Chief, Cardiology Division, The Genesee Hospital, Rochester, New York
Interference in Cardiac Pacemakers: Exogenous Sources; Interference in Cardiac Pacemakers: Endogenous Sources

ERIC BERGER, M.D.
Clinical Assistant Professor of Medicine, Brown University Program in Medicine, Providence, Rhode Island; Co-director, Electrophysiology Laboratory, Division of Cardiology, Department of Medicine, Rhode Island Hospital, Providence, Rhode Island
Management of the Patient with Sudden Cardiac Arrest

ALAN D. BERNSTEIN, Eng.Sc.D., F.A.C.C.
Director of Technical Research, Department of Surgery, and Technical Director, Pacemaker Center, Newark Beth Israel Medical Center, Newark, New Jersey
Classification of Cardiac Pacemakers

J. THOMAS BIGGER, Jr., M.D.
Professor of Medicine and of Pharmacology, College of Physicians and Surgeons, Columbia University, New York, New York; Director, Arrhythmia Control Unit, Columbia-Presbyterian Medical Center, New York, New York
Risk Stratification for Arrhythmic Death After Myocardial Infarction

PIERRE BIRKUI, M.D.
   Faculty Staff, University of Paris, Paris, France; Lariboisière Hospital, Paris, France
   Multiprogrammability of Modern Cardiac Pacemakers

JOSEPH BORBOLA, M.D.
   Chief of Electrophysiology, Hungarian Institute of Cardiology, Budapest, Hungary
   Electrophysiologic Evaluation of Syncope of Unexplained Origin

MARTIN BORGGREFE, M.D.
   Director of Electrophysiology Department of the Cardiology Division of the Westfälische Wilhelms-Universität, Münster, Germany
   Ventricular Late Potentials: Clinical Aspects

MOHAMED BOUTJDIR, Ph.D.
   Research Associate, Cardiology Research Program, State University of New York Research Foundation, Brooklyn, New York
   Electrophysiology of Ventricular Arrhythmias in Myocardial Ischemia and Infarction

NANCY A. BRANYAS, M.D.
   Fellow in Cardiology, Washington University School of Medicine, St. Louis, Missouri
   The Pre-excitation Syndrome

GÜNTER BREITHARDT, M.D., F.E.S.C.
   Professor of Medicine (Cardiology) and Head, Department of Internal Medicine and Cardiology, Westfälische Wilhelms-Universität, Münster, Germany
   Ventricular Late Potentials: Clinical Aspects

DAVID BUCKLES, Ph.D.
   Instructor in Pediatric Cardiology, Medical University of South Carolina, Charleston, South Carolina; Computer Scientist, South Carolina Children's Heart Center, Medical University Children's Hospital, Charleston, South Carolina
   Tachycardia in Infants

ALFRED E. BUXTON, M.D.
   Associate Professor of Medicine, University of Pennsylvania School of Medicine, Philadelphia, Pennsylvania; Director, Electrophysiology Laboratory, University of Pennsylvania, Philadelphia, Pennsylvania
   The Automatic Implantable Cardioverter Defibrillator (AICD): Follow-Up and Complications

MICHAEL E. CAIN, M.D.
   Associate Professor of Medicine, Washington University School of Medicine, St. Louis, Missouri; Director, Clinical Electrophysiology Laboratory, Barnes Hospital, St. Louis, Missouri
   The Pre-excitation Syndrome

A. JOHN CAMM, M.D.
   Professor of Clinical Cardiology and Head of Department, Department of Cardiological Sciences, St. George's Hospital Medical School, Lon-

don, England; Honorary Consultant Cardiologist, St. George's Hospital, London, England
Rate-Responsive Pacing: Technical and Clinical Aspects

A. CANSELL, Ph.D.
Electronic Engineer, Société Odam, Wissembourg, France
Catheter Ablation Techniques for Ventricular Tachycardia

EDWARD B. CAREF, M.A.
Research Associate, Cardiology Division, State University of New York, Research Foundation and Veterans Administration Medical Center, Brooklyn, New York
The High-Resolution Electrocardiogram: Technical and Basic Aspects

MARK D. CARLSON, M.D.
Assistant Professor of Medicine, Case Western Reserve University School of Medicine, Cleveland, Ohio; Staff Physician, University Hospitals of Cleveland, Cleveland, Ohio
Atrial Flutter: Basic and Clinical Aspects

AGUSTIN CASTELLANOS, M.D.
Professor of Medicine, University of Miami School of Medicine, Miami, Florida; Director, Clinical Electrophysiology, Jackson Memorial Medical Center, Miami, Florida
Electrocardiography of Dual-Chamber Pacemakers

PENG-SHENG CHEN, M.D.
Assistant Professor in Residence, University of California, San Diego, California; Attending Staff, Medicine (Cardiology), UCSD Medical Center and Veterans Hospital, San Diego, California
Ventricular Defibrillation: Basic Concepts

PHILIPPE COUMEL, M.D.
Professor of Cardiology, Hôpital Lariboisière, Paris, France
Repetitive Monomorphic Ventricular Tachycardia

JAMES L. COX, M.D.
Professor of Surgery and Chief, Division of Cardiothoracic Surgery, Washington University School of Medicine, St. Louis, Missouri; Cardiothoracic Surgeon-in-Charge, Barnes Hospital, St. Louis, Missouri
Surgical Management of Cardiac Arrhythmias

WILLIAM CRAELIUS, M.D., Ph.D.
Assistant Professor of Medicine, State University of New York Health Science Center, Brooklyn, New York; Director of Computerized Electrocardiography, Cardiology Section, Veterans Administration Medical Center, Brooklyn, New York
The High-Resolution Electrocardiogram: Technical and Basic Aspects

FRED A. CRAWFORD, M.D.
Professor and Chairman of Surgery and Professor of Pediatrics, Medical University of South Carolina, Charleston, South Carolina; Director, Cardiothoracic Surgery, Medical University Hospital, Charleston, South Carolina
Tachycardia in Infants

PABLO DENES, M.D.
Professor of Medicine, University of Minnesota School of Medicine, St. Paul, Minnesota; Chief of Cardiology, St. Paul-Ramsey Medical Center, St. Paul, Minnesota
Electrophysiologic Evaluation of Syncope of Unexplained Origin

A. ROBERT DENNISS, M.D., B.S., B.Sc.(Med.), M.Sc., F.R.A.C.P.
Clinical Lecturer in Medicine, University of Sydney, Sydney, Australia; Cardiologist, Westmead Hospital, Sydney, Australia
Role of Programmed Stimulation and the Signal-Averaged Electrocardiogram

KARL P. DRESDNER, Jr., Ph.D.
Assistant Professor of Pharmacology, College of Physicians and Surgeons, Columbia University, New York, New York
Cellular Mechanisms of Cardiac Arrhythmias

ED DUFFIN, Ph.D.
Bakken Fellow, Medtronic, Inc., Minneapolis, Minnesota
The Future of Electrical Devices in the Chronic Treatment of Tachyarrhythmias

NABIL EL-SHERIF, M.D.
Professor of Medicine and Physiology and Director of Clinical Electrophysiology Program, State University of New York Health Science Center, Brooklyn, New York; Chief, Division of Cardiology, Veterans Administration Medical Center, Brooklyn, New York
Electrophysiology of Ventricular Arrhythmias in Myocardial Ischemia and Infarction; Atrioventricular and Intraventricular Conduction Disorders: Clinical Aspects; Complex Ventricular Arrhythmias and Nonsustained Ventricular Tachycardia: Risk Stratification and Management; The High-Resolution Electrocardiogram: Technical and Basic Aspects; Electrocardiography of Single-Chamber Pacemakers; Antitachycardia Pacing: Electrophysiologic Mechanisms

RODNEY H. FALK, M.D., M.R.C.P. (U.K.)
Associate Professor of Medicine; Boston University School of Medicine, Boston, Massachusetts; Director of Clinical Cardiology, Boston City Hospital, Boston, Massachusetts
Noninvasive External Cardiac Pacing

MICHAEL D. FALKOFF, M.D.
Associate Professor of Medicine, University of Rochester, Cardiology Division-Genesee Hospital, Rochester, New York; Director of Electrophysiology, Genesee Hospital, Rochester, New York
Interference in Cardiac Pacemakers: Exogenous Sources; Interference in Cardiac Pacemakers: Endogenous Sources

BELINDA FLORES, R.N., M.N.
Clinical Nurse Specialist, Hospital of the University of Pennsylvania, Philadelphia, Pennsylvania
The Automatic Implantable Cardioverter Defibrillator (AICD): Follow-Up and Complications

G. FONTAINE, M.D.
Director of the Department of Pacing and Clinical Electrophysiology, Hôpital Jean Rostand, Ivry, France
Catheter Ablation Techniques for Ventricular Tachycardia

JOHN M. FONTAINE, M.D.
Assistant Professor of Medicine, State University of New York Health Science Center at Brooklyn, New York; Director of Clinical Electrophysiology Labs, Brooklyn Veterans Administration Medical Center, Brooklyn, New York
Electrocardiography of Single-Chamber Pacemakers

R. FRANK, M.D.
Member of the Staff and Associate Professor of Cardiology, Hôpital Jean Rostand, Ivry, France
Catheter Ablation Techniques for Ventricular Tachycardia

DAVID W. FRAZIER, M.D.
Medical Resident, Duke University Medical Center, Durham, North Carolina
Ventricular Defibrillation: Basic Concepts

ROGER A. FREEDMAN, M.D.
Assistant Professor of Internal Medicine (Cardiology), University of Utah School of Medicine, Salt Lake City, Utah; Assistant Professor of Internal Medicine (Cardiology), University of Utah Medical Center, Salt Lake City, Utah
Sustained Ventricular Tachycardia: Clinical Aspects

CHRISTIAN FUNCK-BRENTANO, M.D.
Chef de Clinique, Assistant des Hôpitaux, Unité de Pharmacologie Clinique, Hôpital Saint-Antoine, Paris, France
Current Antiarrhythmic Agents: Clinical Pharmacology

ELI S. GANG, M.D.
Associate Professor of Clinical Medicine, UCLA School of Medicine, Los Angeles, California; Attending Physician, Cedars-Sinai Medical Center, Los Angeles, California
Normal and Abnormal Sinus Node Function

HASAN GARAN, M.D.
Associate Professor of Medicine, Harvard Medical School, Boston, Massachusetts; Co-director, Cardiac Arrhythmia Service, Department of Cardiology, Massachusetts General Hospital, Boston, Massachusetts
Management of the Patient With Sudden Cardiac Arrest

PAUL C. GILLETTE, M.D.
Professor of Pediatrics and Surgery, Medical University of South Carolina, Charleston, South Carolina; Director, South Carolina Children's Heart Center, Medical University Children's Hospital, Charleston, South Carolina
Tachycardia in Infants

WILLIAM B. GOUGH, M.D.
Assistant Professor of Medicine, State University of New York Health Science Center at Brooklyn, Brooklyn, New York; Supervisory Cardiovascular Physiologist, Veterans Administration Medical Center, Brooklyn, New York
Electrophysiology of Ventricular Arrhythmias in Myocardial Ischemia and Infarction; Antitachycardia Pacing: Electrophysiologic Mechanisms

Y. GROSGOGEAT, M.D.
> Professor of Medicine and Chief of the Cardiology Department, Hôpital Jean Rostand, Ivry, France
> Catheter Ablation Techniques for Ventricular Tachycardia

GERARD M. GUIRAUDON, M.D.
> Professor of Surgery, University of Western Ontario, London, Ontario, Canada; Staff Surgeon, University Hospital, London, Ontario, Canada
> Pacemaker Implantation Techniques

MOH'D. A. HABBAB, M.D.
> Clinical Electrophysiology Fellow, State University of New York Health Science Center, Brooklyn, New York; Consultant, Cardiology Department, Riyadh Armed Forces Hospital, Riyadh, Saudi Arabia
> Atrioventricular and Intraventricular Conduction Disorders: Clinical Aspects

MICHAEL S. HANNA, M.D.
> Instructor and Fellow, Cardiology Unit, University of Rochester School of Medicine and Dentistry, Rochester, New York; Assistant Attending, Strong Memorial Hospital, Rochester, New York
> Cellular Mechanisms of Cardiac Arrhythmias

MARK HAROLD, B.S.
> Electrophysiology Technologist, South Carolina Children's Heart Center, Medical University Children's Hospital, Charleston, South Carolina
> Tachycardia in Infants

ROBERT A. HEINLE, M.D.
> Clinical Associate Professor of Medicine, University of Rochester School of Medicine and Dentistry, Rochester, New York; Senior Attending Staff, The Genesee Hospital, Rochester, New York
> Interference in Cardiac Pacemakers: Exogenous Sources; Interference in Cardiac Pacemakers: Endogenous Sources

RAPHAEL HENKIN, Ph.D.
> Research Associate, Cardiology Section, Veterans Administration Medical Center, Brooklyn, New York
> The High-Resolution Electrocardiogram: Technical and Basic Aspects

RICHARD W. HENTHORN, M.D.
> Assistant Professor, Case Western Reserve University School of Medicine, Cleveland, Ohio; Staff Physician, University Hospitals of Cleveland, Cleveland, Ohio
> Atrial Flutter: Basic and Clinical Aspects

VINZENZ HOMBACH, M.D., F.E.S.C.
> Professor of Medicine (Cardiology) and Head, Department of Internal Medicine IV, University of Ulm, Ulm, West Germany
> The High-Resolution Electrocardiogram: Clinical Aspects

RAYMOND E. IDEKER, M.D.
> Professor of Pathology, Associate Professor of Medicine, Duke University Medical Center, Durham, North Carolina
> Ventricular Defibrillation: Basic Concepts

ROGER P. JAVIER, M.D.
    Assistant Professor of Medicine, University of Miami School of Medicine, Miami Beach, Florida; Co-Director, Cardiac Catheterization Laboratory, Mount Sinai Medical Center, Miami Beach, Florida
    Indications for Cardiac Pacing in Bradyarrhythmias

MOHAMMAD JAZAYERI, M.D.
    Sinai Samaritan Medical Center, Mount Sinai Campus, Milwaukee, Wisconsin; Assistant Professor of Medicine, Sinai Samaritan Medical Center, Mount Sinai Campus, Milwaukee, Wisconsin
    Supraventricular Tachycardias: Clinical Characteristics, Diagnosis, and Management

JAY L. JORDAN, M.D.
    Assistant Clinical Professor of Medicine, University of California at Los Angeles, Los Angeles, California; Attending Physician, Cedars-Sinai Medical Center, Los Angeles, California
    Normal and Abnormal Sinus Node Function

HRAYR S. KARAGUEUZIAN, M.Sc., M.Phil., Ph.D.
    Associate Professor (Adj.) of Medicine, UCLA School of Medicine, Los Angeles, California; Director, Cardiac Electrophysiology Research, Division of Cardiology, Cedars-Sinai Medical Center, Los Angeles, California
    Normal and Abnormal Sinus Node Function

GEORGE KELEN, M.D.
    Assistant Professor of Clinical Medicine, State University of New York Health Science Center, Brooklyn, New York; Cardiology Consultant, St. Vincent Medical Center, Staten Island, New York
    The High-Resolution Electrocardiogram: Technical and Basic Aspects

GEORGE J. KLEIN, M.D.
    Professor of Medicine, University of Western Ontario, London, Ontario, Canada; Staff Cardiologist, University Hospital, London, Ontario, Canada
    Pacemaker Implantation Techniques

CHU-PAK LAU, M.D., M.R.C.P.
    Lecturer in Cardiology, University of Hong Kong, Hong Kong; Cardiac Physician, University Medical Unit, Queen Mary Hospital, Hong Kong
    Rate-Responsive Pacing: Technical and Clinical Aspects

BRUCE D. LINDSAY, M.D.
    Assistant Professor of Medicine, Washington University School of Medicine, St. Louis, Missouri
    The Pre-excitation Syndrome

RICHARD M. LUCERI, M.D.
    Assistant Professor of Clinical Medicine, Division of Cardiology, University of Miami School of Medicine, Ft. Lauderdale, Florida; Director, Interventional Cardiac Arrhythmia Center, Holy Cross Hospital, Ft. Lauderdale, Florida
    Electrocardiography of Dual-Chamber Pacemakers

WILLIAM J. MANDEL, M.D., F.A.C.C., F.A.C.P.
Professor of Medicine (Adjunct), UCLA School of Medicine, Los Angeles, California; Director, Clinical Electrophysiology, Cedars Sinai Medical Center, Los Angeles, California
Normal and Abnormal Sinus Node Function

FRANCIS E. MARCHLINSKI, M.D.
Associate Professor of Medicine, University of Pennsylvania School of Medicine, Philadelphia, Pennsylvania; Co-Director, Electrophysiology Laboratory, Director of Arrhythmia Evaluation Center, Hospital of the University of Pennsylvania, Philadelphia, Pennsylvania
The Automatic Implantable Cardioverter Defibrillator (AICD): Follow-Up and Complications

ANTONI MARTINEZ-RUBIO, M.D.
Resident of the Department of Cardiology of the Westfälische Wilhelms-Universität, Münster, Germany
Ventricular Late Potentials: Clinical Aspects

JAY W. MASON, M.D.
Professor of Internal Medicine, Chief of Cardiology, University of Utah School of Medicine, Salt Lake City, Utah; Professor of Internal Medicine, Chief, Division of Cardiology, University of Utah Medical Center, Salt Lake City, Utah
Sustained Ventricular Tachycardia: Clinical Aspects

RAHUL MEHRA, Ph.D.
Senior Staff Scientist, Medtronic, Inc., Minneapolis, Minnesota
The High-Resolution Electrocardiogram: Technical and Basic Aspects

WILLIAM M. MILES, M.D.
Staff Physician, Roudebush VAMC Research Associate, Krannert Institute of Cardiology, Indianapolis, Indiana; Associate Professor of Medicine, Indiana University School of Medicine, Indianapolis, Indiana
Cardioversion and Defibrillation: Clinical Aspects

M. MIROWSKI, M.D.
Professor of Medicine, The Johns Hopkins University School of Medicine, Baltimore, Maryland; Director, Coronary Care Unit, Sinai Hospital of Baltimore, Baltimore, Maryland
The Automatic Implantable Cardioverter Defibrillator (AICD): Clinical Experience

FRED MORADY, M.D.
Professor of Medicine, University of Michigan, Ann Arbor, Michigan; Director, Cardiac Electrophysiology Laboratory, University of Michigan Medical Center, Ann Arbor, Michigan
Catheter Ablation Techniques for Supraventricular Tachyarrhythmias

MORTON M. MOWER, M.D.
Associate Professor of Medicine, The Johns Hopkins University School of Medicine, Baltimore, Maryland
The Automatic Implantable Cardioverter Defibrillator (AICD): Clinical Experience

JACQUES MUGICA, M.D.
>Chief of Medicine of the Department of Cardiac Stimulation, Surgical Center of Val d'Or Saint Cloud, Paris, France
>Multiprogrammability of Modern Cardiac Pacemakers

LING S. ONG, M.D.
>Research Fellow, Department of Cardiological Sciences, St. George Hospital Medical School, London, England
>Interference in Cardiac Pacemakers: Exogenous Sources; Interference in Cardiac Pacemakers: Endogenous Sources

C. THOMAS PETER, M.D.
>Professor of Medicine in Residence, UCLA Medical School, Los Angeles, California; Staff Cardiologist, Cedars-Sinai Medical Center, Los Angeles, California; Director, ECG and Electrophysiology and Regional Arrhythmia Center, Los Angeles, California
>Normal and Abnormal Sinus Node Function

PHILIP J. PODRID, M.D.
>Associate Professor of Medicine, Boston University School of Medicine, Boston, Massachusetts; Director of Arrhythmia Service, University Hospital, Boston, Massachusetts
>Evaluation of Arrhythmia Utilizing Noninvasive Techniques: Ambulatory Monitoring and Exercise Testing

MARK RESTIVO, Ph.D.
>Research Associate, Cardiology Division, State University of New York Research Foundation and Veterans Administration Medical Center, Brooklyn, New York
>Electrophysiology of Ventricular Arrhythmias in Myocardial Ischemia and Infarction; The High-Resolution Electrocardiogram: Technical and Basic Aspects; Antitachycardia Pacing: Electrophysiologic Mechanisms

DAVID A. RICHARDS, M.D., B.S., B.Sc.(Med.), F.R.A.C.P., F.A.C.C.
>Clinical Lecturer in Medicine, University of Sydney, Australia; Cardiologist, Westmead Hospital, Sydney, Australia
>Role of Programmed Stimulation and the Signal-Averaged Electrocardiogram

DAN M. RODEN, M.D.
>Associate Professor, Departments of Medicine and Pharmacology, Vanderbilt University School of Medicine, Nashville, Tennessee; Director, Arrhythmia Service, Vanderbilt University Hospital, Nashville, Tennessee
>The Long QT Syndrome and Torsades de Pointes: Basic and Clinical Aspects

MICHAEL R. ROSEN, M.D.
>Professor of Pharmacology and Pediatrics, Columbia University College of Physicians and Surgeons, New York, New York
>Antiarrhythmic Drugs

BERTRAND A. ROSS, M.D.
>Assistant Professor of Pediatrics, Children's Hospital of the King's Daughters, Norfolk, Virginia
>Tachycardia in Infants

DAVID L. ROSS, M.B., B.S., F.R.A.C.P., F.A.C.C.
Clinical Lecturer in Medicine, University of Sydney, Sydney, Australia; Cardiologist, Westmead Hospital, Sydney, Australia
Role of Programmed Stimulation and the Signal-Averaged Electrocardiogram

JEREMY N. RUSKIN, M.D.
Associate Professor of Medicine, Harvard Medical School, Boston, Massachusetts; Director, Cardiac Arrhythmia Service, Department of Cardiology, Massachusetts General Hospital, Boston, Massachusetts
Management of the Patient with Sudden Cardiac Arrest

SANJEEV SAKSENA, M.D., F.A.C.C.
Clinical Associate Professor of Medicine, University of Medicine and Dentistry of New Jersey—NJ Medical School, Newark, New Jersey; Director, Arrhythmia Service, Eastern Heart Institute, General Hospital Center at Passaic, Passaic, New Jersey
Hemodynamic Effects of Cardiac Arrhythmias and Pacemakers

PHILIP SAMET, M.D.
Chief, Division of Cardiology, Mt. Sinai Hospital, Miami Beach, Florida
Indications for Cardiac Pacing in Bradyarrhythmias

ARJUN D. SHARMA, M.D.
Associate Professor of Medicine and Assistant Professor of Pharmacology, University of Western Ontario, London, Ontario, Canada; Staff Cardiologist, University Hospital, London, Ontario, Canada
Pacemaker Implantation Techniques

NITARO SHIBATA, M.D.
Professor of Cardiology, The Heart Institute of Japan, Tokyo Women's Medical College, Tokyo, Japan
Ventricular Defibrillation: Basic Concepts

KONRAD K. STEINBACH, M.D., F.E.S.C., F.A.C.C.
Professor of Medicine (Cardiology), University of Vienna, Vienna, Austria; 3rd Medical and Cardiac Department, Ludwig Bolttman Institute for Arrhythmia Research, Wilhelminenspital, Vienna, Austria
Pacemaker Follow-up

JONATHAN S. STEINBERG, M.D.
Assistant Professor of Clinical Medicine, College of Physicians and Surgeons, Columbia University, New York, New York; Assistant Attending Physician in the Medicine Service, The Presbyterian Hospital, New York, New York
Risk Stratification for Arrhythmic Death After Myocardial Infarction

ANTHONY S. L. TANG, M.D.
Assistant Professor of Medicine, University of Ottawa, Ottawa, Ontario, Canada; Attending Staff, Ottawa Civic Hospital, Ottawa, Ontario, Canada
Ventricular Defibrillation: Basic Concepts

PETER P. TARJAN, Ph.D.
Professor and Chairman, Department of Biomedical Engineering, University of Miami, Coral Gables, Florida
Engineering Aspects of Modern Cardiac Pacing

PATRICK TCHOU, M.D.
Sinai Samaritan Medical Center, Mount Sinai Campus, Milwaukee, Wisconsin; Director of Cardiac Electrophysiology Lab, Milwaukee, Wisconsin
Supraventricular Tachycardias: Clinical Characteristics, Diagnosis, and Management

ALFONSO O. TOLENTINO, M.D.
Clinical Instructor in Cardiology, Mount Sinai Medical Center, Miami Beach, Florida
Indications for Cardiac Pacing in Bradyarrhythmias

J. TONET, M.D.
Member of the Staff, Hôpital Jean Rostand, Ivry, France
Catheter Ablation Techniques for Ventricular Tachycardia

GIOIA TURITTO, M.D.
Cardiac Electrophysiology Fellow, Cardiology Division, State University of New York Health Science Center, Brooklyn, New York
Complex Ventricular Arrhythmias and Nonsustained Ventricular Tachycardia: Risk Stratification and Management

SHANTHA URSELL, M.D.
Assistant Professor, State University of New York Health Science Center at Brooklyn, Brooklyn, New York; Director of Coronary Care Unit, State University of New York Health Science Center, Brooklyn, New York
Atrioventricular and Intraventricular Conduction Disorders: Clinical Aspects; Electrocardiography of Single-Chamber Pacemakers

JOHN B. UTHER, M.D., B.S., B.Sc.(Med.), F.R.A.C.P.
Clinical Lecturer in Medicine, University of Sydney, Australia; Head of Cardiology Unit, Westmead Hospital, Sydney, Australia
Role of Programmed Stimulation and the Signal-Averaged Electrocardiogram

ENRICO P. VELTRI, M.D.
Assistant Professor of Medicine, The Johns Hopkins University School of Medicine, Baltimore, Maryland; Chief, Division of Cardiology, Sinai Hospital of Baltimore, Baltimore, Maryland
The Automatic Implantable Cardioverter Defibrillator (AICD): Clinical Experience

RICHARD L. VERRIER, Ph.D.
Professor of Pharmacology, Georgetown University School of Medicine, Washington, D.C.
Neurogenic Aspects of Cardiac Arrhythmias

ALBERT L. WALDO, M.D.
The Walter H. Pritchard Professor of Cardiology and Professor of Medicine, Case Western Reserve University School of Medicine,

Cleveland, Ohio; Director, Adult Cardiac Electrophysiology and Staff Physician, University Hospitals of Cleveland, Cleveland, Ohio
Atrial Flutter: Basic and Clinical Aspects

JAMES N. WEISS, M.D.

Professor of Medicine, UCLA School of Medicine, Los Angeles, California; Division of Cardiology, UCLA Center for the Health Sciences, Los Angeles, California
Biochemical and Metabolic Aspects of Arrhythmias

J. MARCUS WHARTON, M.D.

Assistant Professor of Medicine, Duke University Medical Center, Durham, North Carolina; Director of Clinical Cardiac Electrophysiology, Duke University Hospitals, Duke University Medical Center, Durham, North Carolina
Ventricular Defibrillation: Basic Concepts

ANDREW L. WIT, Ph.D.

Professor of Pharmacology, College of Physicians and Surgeons, Columbia University, New York, New York
Cellular Mechanisms of Cardiac Arrhythmias

RAYMOND L. WOOSLEY, M.D.

Professor of Pharmacology and Medicine and Chairman, Department of Pharmacology, Georgetown University Medical Center, Washington, D.C.; Attending Staff, Georgetown University Hospital, Washington, D.C.
Current Antiarrhythmic Agents: Clinical Pharmacology

CHRISTOPHER R. C. WYNDHAM, M.D.

Clinical Professor of Medicine, Southwestern Medical School of University of Texas at Dallas, Dallas, Texas; Director of Electrophysiology, Director of Electrocardiography, Presbyterian Hospital of Dallas, Dallas, Texas
Antitachycardia Pacing: Clinical Aspects

RAYMOND YEE, M.D.

Assistant Professor, University of Western Ontario, London, Ontario, Canada; Staff Cardiologist, University Hospital, London, Ontario, Canada
Pacemaker Implantation Techniques

VICKI ZEIGLER, B.S.N.

Coordinator, Pacemaker and Dysrhythmia Surveillance Center, Medical University Children's Hospital, Charleston, South Carolina
Tachycardia in Infants

DOUGLAS P. ZIPES, M.D.

Professor of Medicine, Indiana School of Medicine, Indianapolis, Indiana; Attending Staff, University Hospital, Indianapolis, Indiana
Cardioversion and Defibrillation: Clinical Aspects

PREFACE

The objectives of the present edition diverge somewhat from those of the previous one. In 1980, the second edition of *Cardiac Pacing* dealt primarily with pacemaker devices, although some aspects of basic and clinical electrophysiology were also included. During the past decade, steady progress has occurred in the field of cardiac electrophysiology, including spectacular advances in the physiology and molecular biology of ion channels. This provides a more rational basis for the management of cardiac arrhythmias. Besides prevention, the three current approaches to the management of cardiac arrhythmias are pharmacologic therapy, surgical and ablative procedures, and the use of electrical devices. Starting with the title of the third edition, which was appropriately changed to *Cardiac Pacing and Electrophysiology*, the overall organization of the book reflects the significant changes in the field. The first four chapters discuss cellular mechanisms and biochemical, metabolic, and neurogenic aspects of cardiac arrhythmias. Clinical and electrocardiographic manifestations of various cardiac arrhythmias and diagnostic procedures such as programmed electrical stimulation and noninvasive techniques, including high resolution electrocardiography, are discussed in detail in the following chapters. Because of the paramount significance of sudden cardiac death, the current progress in this area is outlined in more than one chapter. The second half of the book is devoted to the management of cardiac arrhythmias. Pharmacologic therapy, surgical approaches, and the relatively new technique of catheter ablation are presented. Finally, the role of electrical devices is presented in great detail, commensurate with the rapid expansion that has occurred in this area. Standard topics in cardiac pacing have been updated to reflect the state of the art. In addition, recent advances in such areas as rate-responsive and physiologic pacing, multiprogrammability, electrophysiologic basis, clinical indications, and future directions of implantable automatic antitachycardia and defibrillator devices have been amply reviewed.

This book was made possible because of collaborative efforts of a large number of basic and clinical scientists who have particular interests and extensive experience in their respective subjects. It is intended to provide an authoritative up-to-date reference on cardiac pacing and electrophysiology. Although certain aspects of this broad field may be underrepresented, it is hoped that what is included here is of interest and will prove valuable to medical students, primary care physicians, and cardiovascular specialists.

NABIL EL-SHERIF, M.D.
PHILIP SAMET, M.D.

CONTENTS

1 Cellular Mechanisms of Cardiac Arrhythmias 1
   Michael S. Hanna, Karl P. Dresdner, Jr., and Andrew L. Wit

2 Electrophysiology of Ventricular Arrhythmias
   in Myocardial Ischemia and Infarction 18
   Nabil El-Sherif, William B. Gough, Mark Restivo and Mohamed Boutjdir

3 Biochemical and Metabolic Aspects of
   Arrhythmias 57
   James N. Weiss

4 Neurogenic Aspects of Cardiac Arrhythmias 77
   Richard L. Verrier

5 Evaluation of Arrhythmia Utilizing Noninvasive
   Techniques: Ambulatory Monitoring
   and Exercise Testing 93
   Philip J. Podrid

6 Normal and Abnormal Sinus Node Function 114
   Jay L. Jordan, Hrayr S. Karagueuzian, Eli S. Gang, C. Thomas Peter and
   William J. Mandel

7 Atrioventricular and Intraventricular Conduction
   Disorders: Clinical Aspects 140
   Shantha Ursell, Moh'd. A. Habbab and Nabil El-Sherif

8 Supraventricular Tachycardias:
   Clinical Characteristics, Diagnosis,
   and Management 170
   Masood Akhtar, Patrick Tchou and Mohammad Jazayeri

9 Atrial Flutter: Basic and Clinical Aspects 184
   Albert L. Waldo, Mark D. Carlson and Richard W. Henthorn

10 The Pre-excitation Syndrome 190
   Bruce D. Lindsay, Nancy A. Branyas and Michael E. Cain

11 Complex Ventricular Arrhythmias and
   Nonsustained Ventricular Tachycardia:
   Risk Stratification and Management 217
   Gioia Turitto and Nabil El-Sherif

12 Repetitive Monomorphic Ventricular
Tachycardia 233
Philippe Coumel

13 Sustained Ventricular Tachycardia:
Clinical Aspects 247
Roger A. Freedman and Jay W. Mason

14 The Long QT Syndrome and Torsades
de Pointes: Basic and Clinical Aspects 265
Dan M. Roden

15 Tachycardia in Infants 285
Paul C. Gillette, Fred A. Crawford, Bertrand A. Ross,
Vicki Zeigler, David Buckles and Mark Harold

16 Electrophysiologic Evaluation of Syncope of
Unexplained Origin 293
Joseph Borbola and Pablo Denes

17 Risk Stratification for Arrhythmic Death After
Myocardial Infarction 303
   A. AN OVERVIEW 303
     J. Thomas Bigger, Jr., and Jonathan S. Steinberg
   B. ROLE OF PROGRAMMED STIMULATION AND THE
     SIGNAL-AVERAGED ELECTROCARDIOGRAM 323
     A. Robert Denniss, David A. Richards, David L. Ross and
     John B. Uther

18 Management of the Patient with Sudden
Cardiac Arrest 333
Eric Berger, Hasan Garan and Jeremy N. Ruskin

19 The High-Resolution Electrocardiogram:
Technical and Basic Aspects 349
Nabil El-Sherif, Mark Restivo, William Craelius, Rahul Mehra, Raphael Henkin,
Edward B. Caref and George Kelen

20 The High-Resolution Electrocardiogram:
Clinical Aspects 372
Vinzenz Hombach

21 Ventricular Late Potentials: Clinical Aspects 387
Gunter Breithardt, Martin Borggrefe and Antoni Martinez-Rubio

22 Antiarrhythmic Drugs 401
Michael R. Rosen

23 Current Antiarrhythmic Agents: Clinical
Pharmacology 409
Christian Funck-Brentano and Raymond L. Woosley

24	Surgical Management of Cardiac Arrhythmias	436
	James L. Cox	
25	Catheter Ablation Techniques for Supraventricular Tachyarrhythmias	453
	Fred Morady	
26	Catheter Ablation Techniques for Ventricular Tachycardia	471
	G. Fontaine, A. Cansell, R. Frank, J. Tonet, S. Aaddaj, M. Aldakar and Y. Grosgogeat	
27	Engineering Aspects of Modern Cardiac Pacing	484
	Peter P. Tarjan	
28	Classification of Cardiac Pacemakers	494
	Alan D. Bernstein	
29	Multiprogrammability of Modern Cardiac Pacemakers	504
	Jacques Mugica and Pierre Birkui	
30	Rate-Responsive Pacing: Technical and Clinical Aspects	524
	Chu-Pak Lau and A. John Camm	
31	Hemodynamic Effects of Cardiac Arrhythmias and Pacemakers	545
	Sanjeev Saksena	
32	Pacemaker Implantation Techniques	561
	Arjun D. Sharma, Gerard M. Guiraudon, George J. Klein and Raymond Yee	
33	Electrocardiography of Single-Chamber Pacemakers	568
	John M. Fontaine, Shantha Ursell and Nabil El-Sherif	
34	Electrocardiography of Dual-Chamber Pacemakers	599
	Richard M. Luceri and Agustin Castellanos	
35	Interference in Cardiac Pacemakers: Exogenous Sources	608
	S. Serge Barold, Michael D. Falkoff, Ling S. Ong and Robert A. Heinle	
36	Interference in Cardiac Pacemakers: Endogenous Sources	634
	S. Serge Barold, Michael D. Falkoff, Ling S. Ong and Robert A. Heinle	

37 Indications for Cardiac Pacing in Bradyarrhythmias 652
Alfonso O. Tolentino, Roger P. Javier and Philip Samet

38 Pacemaker Follow-Up 662
Konrad K. Steinbach

39 Noninvasive External Cardiac Pacing 675
Rodney H. Falk

40 Antitachycardia Pacing: Electrophysiologic Mechanisms 685
Mark Restivo, William B. Gough and Nabil El-Sherif

41 Antitachycardia Pacing: Clinical Aspects 706
Christopher R. C. Wyndham

42 Ventricular Defibrillation: Basic Concepts 713
Raymond E. Ideker, Anthony S. L. Tang, David W. Frazier, Nitaro Shibata, Peng-Sheng Chen and J. Marcus Wharton

43 Cardioversion and Defibrillation: Clinical Aspects 727
William M. Miles and Douglas P. Zipes

44 The Automatic Implantable Cardioverter Defibrillator (AICD): Clinical Experience 737
Enrico P. Veltri, Morton M. Mower and M. Mirowski

45 The Automatic Implantable Cardioverter Defibrillator (AICD): Follow-Up and Complications 743
Francis E. Marchlinski, Alfred E. Buxton and Belinda Flores

46 The Future of Electrical Devices in the Chronic Treatment of Tachyarrhythmias 759
Ed Duffin and Earl Bakken

Index 765

1

Cellular Mechanisms of Cardiac Arrhythmias

Michael S. Hanna
Karl P. Dresdner, Jr.
Andrew L. Wit

The purpose of this chapter is to review the normal cellular electrophysiology that is responsible for impulse initiation and propagation in the heart and to describe the pathophysiology of the abnormal mechanisms that give rise to arrhythmias. In the past 40 years, since Coraboeuf and Weidman[1] first recorded cardiac action potentials, technical advances have had a profound impact on our understanding of cellular electrophysiology. Factors contributing to this understanding include the development of microelectrode studies[1,2] and the voltage clamp technique,[3,4] advances in biochemistry and membrane physiology, the use of computerized mapping studies,[5,6] the capability for disaggregating and isolating single cardiac cells,[7,8] and the recent introduction of patch clamp techniques to record from single cells and even single ion channels.[9–11] The development of animal models of relevant disease states such as ischemia[12,13] has led to insights into the pathophysiology of arrhythmias, the mechanisms of antiarrhythmic drug action, and the design of strategies for treatment intervention. The material in this chapter is derived largely from these sources, which form the basis of our understanding of the electrical properties of cardiac cells.

Description of Some Normal Electrophysiologic Properties

THE RESTING MEMBRANE POTENTIAL

Cardiac cells have an electrical potential difference across their surface membranes. This transmembrane potential gradient, or *membrane potential,* is a fundamental property of all cells. In cardiac cells, the membrane potential is intimately involved in the process of excitation and in the conduction of impulses. Some cardiac cells, such as atrial and ventricular muscle cells, remain at a stable, negative membrane potential until excited. This stable potential is called the *resting membrane potential* (V_r). Other cardiac cell types, such as those in the sinoatrial node, in the NH region of the AV node, and in Purkinje fibers, reach a maximum negative potential after excitation and then gradually depolarize over time until they reach a threshold potential and are re-excited. The most negative membrane potential of these "pacemaker" cells is termed the "maximum diastolic potential" (Fig. 1–1).

Origin of the Resting Membrane Potential

In the late nineteenth century, the work of Ringer[14] on the role of ions in maintaining excitability in frog heart and the studies by Nernst[15] of electrochemistry provided a foundation for understanding the origin of the resting membrane potential.[16] By the early twentieth century, Julius Bernstein[17] speculated that the resting membrane potential was the result of the cell membrane's high permeability to potassium at rest. Excitation, he believed, resulted from a nonspecific increase in the membrane's permeability to other ions. Further insights into the mechanism of the resting membrane potential developed over the next fifty years in studies done on squid giant axon. In particular, the work of Cole and Curtis[18] and of Hodgkin and Huxley[19] provided notable advancements in our knowledge of both the resting membrane potential and the action potential. The important findings arising from these seminal investigations included the observation that whereas the resting membrane potential in squid axon is primarily related to intracellular potassium concen-

---

Supported in part by Program Project Grant HL31393 from the Heart, Lung, and Blood Institute of the National Institutes of Health.

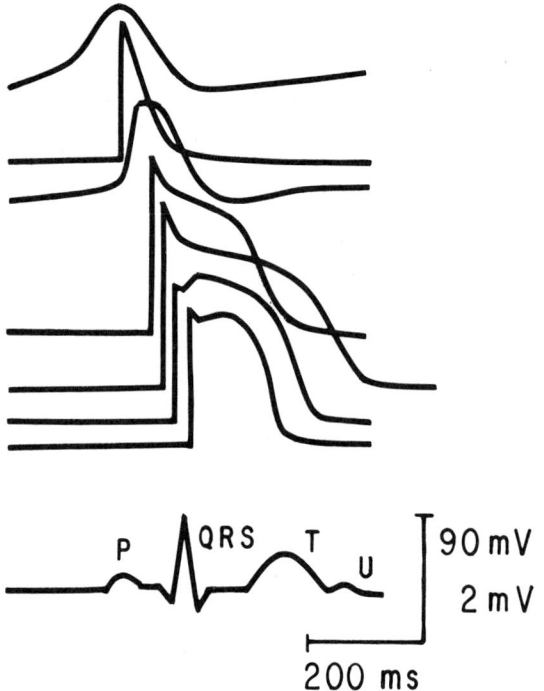

FIGURE 1-1
Transmembrane potentials in atrial and ventricular tissues during normal sinus rhythm. The traces from top to bottom are of sinoatrial nodal cell, atrial muscle cell, atrioventricular nodal cell, His bundle cell, free-running Purkinje fiber, subendocardial ventricular muscle cell, and epicardial ventricular muscle cell. The lowermost trace is of the body surface ECG. Vertical scale is 2 mV for ECG and 90 mV for transmembrane potentials. (Reprinted by permission from Dangman KH, Boyden PA: In Fox PP (ed.): Canine and Feline Cardiology, pp. 269-287. New York, Churchill & Livingstone, Publishers, 1988.)

tration and to the membrane potassium conductance, other ions (especially sodium) make small but significant contributions. The model which emerges from these and other studies contains two important concepts: first, that intracellular ion concentrations are carefully regulated by energy requiring active transport processes in the cell, and second, that discrete channels exist in the cell membrane that are *selectively permeable* to different ions. In the discussion that follows, we shall examine these concepts in detail.

A Hypothetical Cellular Model

The resting membrane potential in cardiac cells arises from the selective permeability of the cell membrane to different ions. These ions—potassium (K^+), sodium (Na^+), calcium (Ca^{2+}) and chloride (Cl^-)—are maintained at concentrations inside the cell that differ from their extracellular concentrations by the Na^+-K^+ pump and other active transport pumps. Consider the following model of a hypothetical cell. Note that, as a simplification, free ion concentration level rather than ion activity level will be used in this model. The model cell is situated in a physiologic bathing solution very much like plasma. For the moment we will concern ourselves with only two ions—Na^+ and K^+—and we will assume that the associated anion, Cl^-, can passively cross the membrane in either direction. Initially the cell will be in equilibrium with the extracellular solution; that is, the concentrations of the three ions will be the same inside and outside the cell (Fig. 1-2, Panel A).

Now let us introduce an ion cotransport pump. Assume that this pump will transport two K^+ ions into the cell for every two Na^+ ions it transports out per enzymatic cycle. Thus, the pump is electroneutral—it does not transport an excess of charged species in either direction. Also assume, for the moment, that the cell membrane has no passive permeability to Na^+ or K^+ ions—they may only cross the membrane via the pump, although Cl^- can still passively distribute itself across the membrane. Assume, moreover, that the pump will run until $[Na^+]_i$ inside the cell falls to some predetermined value—say 10 mM—and then shuts itself off. What then happens when we turn on the pump? As Na^+ and K^+ ions are transported across the membrane, $[Na^+]_i$ falls and $[K^+]_i$ rises. If the bathing reservoir is large enough, the small amount of ions transported from the cell should not alter the extracellular ion concentrations. Eventually, the pump lowers $[Na^+]_i$ to 10 mM, and the pump rate becomes small. This state of the model is presented in Figure 1-2B. The $[K^+]_i$ is now 144 mM, Na_i^+ is 10 mM, and Cl^- is unchanged. The electric potential across the membrane is still zero because the net transport process is electroneutral. However, a considerable concentration gradient across the cell membrane has occurred.

What would happen if the cell membrane were to become permeable to both K^+ and Na^+? Suppose, for example, that the membrane became selectively permeable to both Na^+ and K^+, and that the membrane permeability of K^+ was 10 times greater than that of Na^+. In this case, K^+ would leave the cell and Na^+ would enter the cell down their respective concentration gradients. K^+ efflux from the cell would exceed Na^+ influx into the cell, with a net loss of positive charge. *This would make the inside membrane of the cell more negative than the outside of the cell membrane* (Fig. 1-2C). Therefore, the cell would have a membrane potential due to the transmembrane ion concentration gradients and selective permeability of the membrane to different ions. Let us now explore the theory of the resting potential that is based on the concept of *equilibrium potential*. The net cellular efflux of K^+ would be zero when the membrane potential became sufficiently negative that a positive charge could no longer leave the cell. This value of resting potential is also known as an electrochemical equilibrium potential, because the outward-directed K^+ chemical concentration gradient is balanced by an inward-directed electrical potential gradient caused by transmembrane charge imbalance.

Thermodynamically, the transmembrane K^+ concentration gradient is the chemical potential for K^+, $\Delta M_c(K^+)$:

$$\Delta M_c(K^+) = RT \ln [K^+]_o/[K^+]_i \quad (1)$$

where $[K^+]_o$ is the potassium concentration outside the

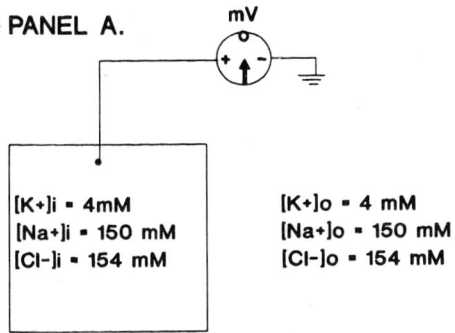

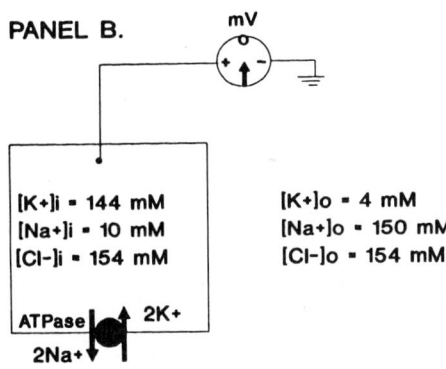

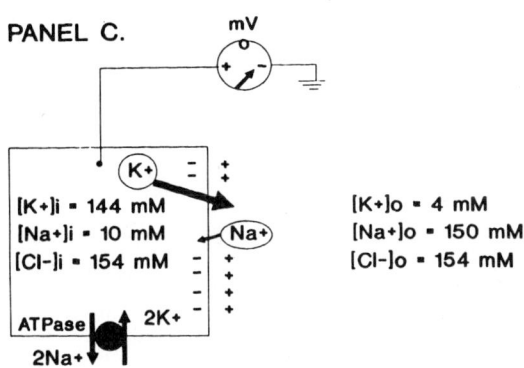

FIGURE 1–2
Panel A shows a model for the generation of the resting potential. Initially the intracellular and extracellular concentrations are the same. The model only considers Na$^+$, K$^+$, and Cl$^-$. The resting membrane potential would be 0 mV and is referenced to the extracellular space, which is ground by convention.

Panel B shows the same model as in A, except that now a hypothetical ATP-energized *electroneutral* Na/K pump has been added. Note that there is an infinite reserve of extracellular ions such that only intracellular composition is altered by the Na/K pump. At steady state, cytoplasmic K$^+$ is concentrated, whereas cytoplasmic Na$^+$ is pumped to a low level. This model lacks ion channels, and thus there is 0 mV of resting membrane potential.

Panel C shows the same model as in B, except that now the cell membrane contains a pathway for K$^+$ to diffuse out of the cell and a pathway for Na$^+$ to diffuse into the cell. Also, the membrane permeability to K$^+$ is much larger than to Na$^+$. There is thus a finite steady-state net loss of positive charges from the cell that creates a resting membrane potential that is negative on the inside of the cell membrane. The voltmeter indicates this membrane polarization. In all three panels, Cl$^-$ is not assumed to play an electrogenic role.

cell, $[K^+]_i$ is the potassium concentration inside the cell, R is the gas constant, and T is the temperature in Kelvin. The transmembrane electrical gradient for K$^+$, $\Delta M_e(K^+)$, is:

$$\Delta M_e(K^+) = ZFE \quad (2)$$

where Z is the valence, F is Faraday's constant, and E is the electric field strength. When electrochemical equilibrium exists, the electrical gradient is equal and opposite to the chemical concentration gradient:

$$\Delta M_e(K^+) = \Delta M_c(K^+) \quad (3)$$

Thus,

$$ZFE = RT \ln [K^+]_o/[K^+]_i \quad (4)$$

The electric field or membrane potential at equilibrium is the potassium equilibrium potential, E_K:

$$E_K = (RT/ZF) \ln [K^+]_o/[K^+]_i \quad (5)$$

This is simply the Nernst equation for K$^+$. For a typical cardiac cell, $[K^+]_i$ is about 150 mM and $[K^+]_o$ is about 4 mM. At a temperature of 37°C (310 K), and for Z = +1, the cardiac cell membrane potassium equilibrium potential is calculated as follows:

$$E_K = [(8,314 \text{ mV-C/mole/K}) (310 \text{ K})/(96,480 \text{ C/mole})]$$
$$\ln [K^+]_o/[K^+]_i$$
$$= 26.7 \text{ mV} \ln [K^+]_o/[K^+]_i = -96.8 \text{ mV} \quad (6)$$

Thus, at a membrane potential of −96.8, passive membrane potassium ion flux would be zero, at "equilibrium." The outward concentration gradient of potassium is balanced by the inward electrical gradient.

The actual resting membrane potential of cardiac cells is positive to E_K by 2 to 17 mV due to effects of other ions on the membrane potential.[20] This indicates that the membrane potential in a cardiac cell is close to the potassium equilibrium potential. However, the membrane potential is positive to the potassium equilibrium potential; thus K$^+$ passively diffuses from the cell down its electrochemical gradient. This continual K$^+$ efflux generates a background, resting membrane K$^+$ current that helps to stabilize the resting potential from small depolarizing membrane currents.

In most types of heart cells (e.g., Purkinje, atrial and ventricular muscle), as noted, the resting membrane potential is slightly positive to E_K, because the membrane permeability to K$^+$ is much larger than that for ions such as Na$^+$. Nonetheless, the small contribution made by Na$^+$ and other ions to the resting potential is important. The most practical relation for steady-state membrane potential is the Goldman-Hodgkin-Katz equation.[21,22] This equation uses permeability factors (P_K, P_{Na}, and P_{Cl}) for K$^+$, Na$^+$ and Cl$^-$, respectively, and assumes that the ions electrodiffuse independently and instantaneously across a homogeneous membrane. The electric field drop across this membrane is assumed also to be linear. The general voltage equation for the resting potential (E_r) is as follows:

$$E_r = (RT/F) \ln \frac{P_K [K^+]_o + P_{Na} [Na^+]_o + P_{Cl} [Cl^-]_o}{P_K [K^+]_i + P_{Na} [Na^+]_i + P_{Cl} [Cl^-]_i} \quad (7)$$

In the preceding equation, the contributions of different ions are "weighted" by their respective concentrations and permeabilities. Note that when the Na^+ permeability and Cl^- permeability are negligible, the above equation reduces to the K^+ equilibrium potential, E_K.

In Table 1–1, typical values of cardiac cell K^+, Na^+, H^+, Ca^{2+}, and Mg^{2+} activity are listed for intracellular and extracellular fluid. Ion activity is presented because these values are directly obtained from ion-sensitive microelectrode measurements.[23] The free ion concentration can be calculated easily from the ion activity. In mammalian saline solutions, the monovalent cation activity is about 0.75 of the value of free monovalent cation concentration. The divalent cation activity is about 0.3 of the value of free divalent cation concentration. Table 1–1 also gives the several cation transmembrane equilibrium potentials for cardiac cells, using Equations 1–6 (Nernst equation). Note that the typical cardiac cell resting potential for atrial muscle, ventricular muscle, and Purkinje fibers occurs between -80 and -90 mV. This is close to E_K, but not near E_{Na}, E_H, E_{Ca}, or E_{Mg}. As discussed, this occurs because resting membrane permeability to K^+ is much larger than it is for other cations.

In summary, the historical development of ideas concerning the resting membrane potential has been traced, beginning with the Bernstein hypothesis that membrane potential resulted from a high resting membrane permeability to potassium. By including the basic concept of electrodiffusion according to Nernst, the importance of selective membrane ion permeability and active membrane ion transport became evident. The general formulation of the Goldman-Hodgkin-Katz constant field equation was then used to model the resting potential (see Equation 7). The role of active transport will now be presented.

Na^+-K^+ ATPase

The Na^+-K^+ ATPase is an energy-requiring active transport pump spanning the cell membrane, which hydrolyzes one molecule of ATP while pumping out three Na^+ for every two K^+ ions pumped into the cell. This topic will be briefly reviewed here. For a more complete discussion of this pump, the reader is referred to recent excellent reviews.[24–27] Much of our knowledge of the Na^+-K^+ pump has been obtained from studies on noncardiac tissues, and therefore, extrapolation to cardiac tissues must be made with care. In addition, much is not known about the bioenergetics, stoichiometry, and changes in pump function that occur when cells become diseased.

The Na^+-K^+ pump is believed to be composed of two subunits: an alpha subunit (MW = 100,000d) and a beta subunit (MW = 400,000d). The alpha subunit spans the membrane and can bind cardiac glycosides. It is also phosphorylated by ATP. Normally, the cardiac Na^+-K^+ ATPase transports 3 Na^+ ions out of, while bringing 2 K^+ ions into, the cell per enzyme cycle, using as energy the hydrolysis of 1 molecule of ATP to ADP and P_i. Other modes of exchange (Na^+–Na^+, K^+–K^+) have also been described.[24] The direct consequence of the Na^+-K^+ pump activity is a large transmembrane concentration gradient for Na^+ and K^+ (see Table 1–1). The rate-limiting substrate for the Na^+-K^+ pump activity in cardiac tissue is normally intracellular Na^+. When the pump is inhibited by cardiac glycosides, $[Na^+]_i$ rises from its normal level of about 8 to 10 mM and is held in the range of 25 to 30 mM.[28] An Na^+/Ca^{2+} exchanger has been shown to prevent further elevation of intracellular Na^+ under these conditions.[28, 29] A number of important electrophysiologic phenomena are sensitive to $[Na^+]_i$. Some of these phenomena will be discussed below.

The electrogenic current produced by the Na^+-K^+ pump has important electrophysiologic consequences.[30] Since 3 Na^+ ions are extruded for every 2 K^+ ions pumped in across the cell membrane, each pump cycle results in the net loss of a positive charge. Thus, *electrogenic pump current* will contribute to the resting membrane potential. The magnitude of this contribution has been estimated in several studies, but results are conflicting. Part of the problem in interpreting these studies lies in their methodology. Most of the studies were performed in multicellular preparations, utilizing a cardiac glycoside to inhibit the pump while simultaneously measuring membrane potential.[31–34] Unfortunately, this method, by causing pump inhibition, produces a rise in K^+ concentration in the restricted extracellular spaces outside the cell, $[K^+]_e$. This accumulation of potassium can depolarize the cells and cause an overestimation of the role of the Na/K ATPase in determining the resting membrane potential. Recent studies have addressed this problem.

Eisner and Lederer[35] studied Purkinje fibers using rubidium-containing solutions, which tend to minimize the effects of extracellular concentration changes on membrane potential. They found that a depolarization of 3 to 4 mV accompanied pump inhibition. Hill et

TABLE 1–1
Typical Cardiac Cell Cation Activity Values and $E_{(ion)}$*

Ion	Extracellular Activity (mM)	Intracellular Activity (mM)	Equilibrium Potential (mV)	Reference No.
K^+	3.0	112	$E_K = -97$	20, 23, 66, 80
Na^+	113	7.0	$E_{Na} = +74$	23, 29, 66, 82
H^+	4.0×10^{-5}	10×10^{-5}	$E_H = -25$	23, 108
Ca^{2+}	0.6	3×10^{-5}	$E_{Ca} = +132$	23, 38, 39, 82
Mg^{2+}	0.3	0.3	$E_{Mg} = 0$	23, 109

*Ion activity is calculated from the free ion concentration times the cation activity coefficient (typically 0.75 for monovalent cations and 0.30 for divalent cations). $E_{(ion)}$ is the cell transmembrane equilibrium potential calculated from the Nernst equation at 37° C (see Equations 1–6 in text). Values are for quiescent cells at their resting potential.

al.[36] approached the $[K^+]_e$ accumulation problem in a different way. They monitored membrane potential, intracellular Na^+ concentration, and extracellular potassium concentration. The Na^+-K^+ pump of feline Purkinje fibers was inhibited with a high concentration of ouabain, and a 3-mV resting potential depolarization was observed before an increase in $[K^+]_e$ was apparent. Once $[K^+]_e$ began to increase, the magnitude of membrane potential depolarization was as predicted from the increase in $[K^+]_e$. This experiment suggested that the Na^+-K^+ electrogenic pump current contributes about 3 to 4 mV to the resting membrane potential.

Although small, this hyperpolarizing Na pump current has important electrophysiologic effects. Consider, for example, its effect on pacemaker activity in the heart. Certain cardiac tissues, such as the SA node, AV node, and His-Purkinje system, are able to initiate impulses and thus serve a pacemaker function. This property of *automaticity* (see below) is prevented by applying rapid electrical stimulation for several minutes to excite the tissue at a rate faster than its intrinsic pacemaker. The suppression of intrinsic automaticity by rapid "drive" is termed "overdrive suppression." Postdrive, the tissue ceases its pacemaker activity or beats more slowly for up to several minutes. The mechanism is as follows: during rapid stimulation, Na^+ influx into the cell increases because of the frequent openings of Na^+ channels during the action potential. As Na^+ enters the cell, the intracellular Na^+ concentration rises and activates the Na^+-K^+ pump. The pump acts to extrude Na^+ from, and to transport K^+ into, the cell. This produces a hyperpolarizing electrogenic pump current. This hyperpolarizing current drives the cell membrane potential away from its threshold potential and the cell becomes quiescent.[37] The sensitivity of cardiac tissue to overdrive suppression is frequently observed in the intact heart where the fastest pacemaker, such as the SA node, overdrives slower, subsidiary pacemakers. When the SA node is inhibited suddenly by selective vagal stimulation, there is a significant delay in the automatic firing of the alternative pacemakers such as the free-running Purkinje fibers. When Na^+-K^+ pump function is inhibited by cardiac glycosides, the overdrive suppression phenomenon in Purkinje fibers is diminished.

Electrogenic pump current also plays a role in action potential repolarization. Hyperpolarizing Na pump current accelerates the return of depolarized cells to the resting membrane potential. One of the earliest changes noted in cardiac cells after application of a cardiac glycoside is a lengthening of the action potential duration. Gadsby and Cranefield[34] were able to abolish this lengthening in action potential duration in cardiac glycoside treated Purkinje fibers by injecting a hyperpolarizing current equal to that expected from the Na^+-K^+ pump.

In summary, the Na^+-K^+ pump is a major ion transport mechanism in cardiac tissues. The pump is electrogenic, and this property has important effects on resting membrane potential and action potential duration. The major function of the Na^+-K^+ pump is the active transport of Na^+ and K^+ across the cell membrane. The ionic gradient produced by this transport is a fundamental requisite of the resting membrane potential. Also, the Na^+ gradient is a source of potential energy to be harnessed by other important ion transport systems. In the next section we will examine, as an example, sodium-dependent calcium homeostasis.

Calcium

Up to this point, our discussion of the resting membrane potential has centered largely on consideration of two ions, Na^+ and K^+. In our discussion of the Goldman-Hodgkin-Katz constant field equation (see Equation 7), we noted that these two ions are sufficient to reasonably approximate the resting membrane potential under physiologic conditions. Other ions, such as calcium, make relatively small contributions to the resting membrane potential. Nevertheless, the importance of calcium in normal cardiac physiology has been known since the time of Ringer.[14] Calcium is intimately involved in excitation-contraction coupling, in the function of pacemaker cells, and in the autonomic regulation of the heart. The permeability or conductance of certain ion channels in cardiac cells is calcium-dependent, and calcium functions as an important "second messenger" in many cell types. Moreover, calcium overload during ischemia and reperfusion may also be a factor in early cell death. The mammalian myocardial cell has evolved an elaborate system to release and sequester calcium during the cardiac cycle. During diastole, free calcium in the cytosol is maintained at a very low concentration of about 100 nanomolar.[38, 39] Since the extracellular concentration of calcium is about 2 mM, there is a large concentration gradient of calcium across the cell membrane. Despite this gradient, changes in extracellular calcium over a fairly wide range have minimal effect on resting membrane potential.[40] When the Goldman-Hodgkin-Katz constant field equation is corrected for the contribution of calcium, the correction amounts to about 0.5 mV of depolarization.[25]

Among the most important roles of calcium in the cardiac myocyte is its role in excitation-contraction coupling. This process, in which the electrical depolarization of the cell is accompanied by the mechanical cross-linking of actin and myosin proteins, is mediated by calcium. During diastole, the intracellular calcium concentration free in the cytosol remains around 100 nanomolar. During the action potential, however, calcium enters the cell down its concentration gradient through specific voltage-sensitive channels. In mammalian cardiac myocytes, large amounts of calcium are also released from the sarcoplasmic reticulum (SR). It has been proposed that calcium entering via channels on the cell membrane is a "trigger" for the larger calcium release from the calcium pool stored in the SR.[41] During repolarization, calcium is sequestered from the cytosol by a number of active transport processes. These include (1) an ATP-dependent, calmodulin-insensitive Ca^{2+} pump on the SR; (2) an energy-requiring active transport pump on the mitochondria; (3) an ATP-dependent, calmodulin-sensitive Ca^{2+} pump on the cell membrane; and (4) an Na^+-Ca^{2+} exchange mechanism that counter-transports Ca^{2+} and Na^+ across the cell membrane (a similar mechanism may also function in mitochondria). The Ca^{2+} channels on the cell membrane also are involved in the regulation of intracellular Ca^{2+} activity. Two types of Ca^{2+} channels have been identified in mammalian cardiac myocytes.[42] The two types of Ca^{2+} channels exhibit different voltage sensitivity and different sensitivities to Ca^{2+} antagonists such as verapamil and nifedipine. Finally, it should be noted that intracellular proteins such as calmodulin buffer intracellular calcium. This may have important implications concerning the response of the myocyte during acidosis and ischemia.

Na^+-Ca^{2+} Exchange

Having discussed in general terms the role of calcium in the cardiac myocyte, let us now turn to the Na^+-Ca^{2+} exchange mechanisms. This counter-transporter is important for several reasons. First, it is believed to play a central role in the regulation of Ca^{2+} during the normal cardiac cycle;[29] second, it may be prototypic of other exchange mechanisms (such as Na^+-H^+ exchange) that are poorly understood; and, third, it may be important in a number of electrophysiologic phenomena that occur during disease states, such as ischemia and digitalis toxicity.

Our knowledge of Na^+-Ca^{2+} exchange is less developed than that of the Na^+-K^+ pump. Whereas, in the latter, specific inhibitors (e.g., cardiac glycosides) exist to help elucidate pump effects, no such specific inhibitor of Na^+-Ca^{2+} exchange has been described. Also, although Na^+-K^+ ATPase has been harvested from tissues (e.g., kidney, shark rectal gland), to date this has not been done satisfactorily with the Na^+-Ca^{2+} exchanger. The resultant constraint to study the exchanger in situ in the presence of other interfering calcium currents has made this a limitation. Despite these difficulties, a consensus of evidence has emerged regarding some of the basic properties of the Na^+-Ca^{2+} exchanger. First, in mammalian systems, it is now widely believed that the exchanger transports 3 Na^+ ions for each Ca^{2+} ion per transport cycle. This implies that the exchanger is electrogenic and is voltage-sensitive. Assuming (a) equilibrium conditions, (b) physiologic concentrations of Na^+ and Ca^{2+} in the cytoplasm and extracellular space, and (c) a stoichiometry of 3 Na^+:1 Ca^{2+}, then the equilibrium potential for Na/Ca exchange, $E_{(Na/Ca)}$ can be predicted as follows:[43]

$$E_{(Na/Ca)} = 3 E_{Na} - 2 E_{Ca} \quad (8)$$

where $E_{Na} = (RT/ZF) \ln [Na^+]_o/[Na^+]_i = +74$ mV and
where $E_{Ca} = (RT/ZF) \ln [Ca^{2+}]_o/[Ca^{2+}]_i = +132$ (see Table 1–1)

Then, *at equilibrium,*

$$E_{(Na/Ca)} = 3(+74 \text{ mV}) - 2(+132) = -42 \text{ mV}$$

Thus, assuming that the above analysis is applicable, the reversal potential for the Na^+-Ca^{2+} exchanger is predicted to be positive to the resting membrane potential, and negative to the action potential plateau. During diastole, Na/Ca exchange would pump Ca^{2+} out of the cell and bring Na+ into the cell. The energy would be the inward Na^+ electrochemical gradient created by the Na^+-K^+ pump. Thus, Na/Ca exchange would help to lower intracellular Ca^{2+} during diastole. During the action potential, the Na/Ca exchange process would, in this generalized model, operate in the reverse mode. Ca^{2+} would be transported into the cell, while Na^+ would be extruded from the cell. This Ca^{2+} uptake would aid replenishment of intracellular Ca^{2+} stores and assist the subsequent contraction.[44] This description of Na/Ca exchange assumes constant cytoplasmic Ca^{2+} during the cardiac cycle and assumes equilibrium conditions. These assumptions are tenuous but allow some insight into this complex Na^+-Ca^{2+} exchange process and its role in cellular Ca^{2+} and Na^+ homeostasis.

Another important area in which the Na^+-Ca^{2+} exchanger may play an important role is in mediating the inotropic effects of cardiac glycosides. In the presence of digitalis, the Na^+-K^+ pump is inhibited. The resultant rise in Na^+_i alters the activity of the Na-Ca exchanger, favoring increased "reverse mode" exchange; that is, 3 Na^+ *out* for 1 Ca^{2+} *in*. This buffers the rise in intracellular Na^+ brought about by Na^+-K^+ pump inhibition but raises the level of $[Ca^{2+}]_i$. The increased $[Ca^{2+}]_i$ produces an increase in inotropy.

As we shall discuss later, Na/K ATPase pump inhibition may cause intracellular Ca^{2+} to rise to a pathologic level in cytoplasm and inside intracellular organelles that store Ca^{2+}, such as the SR and mitochondria. During cytoplasmic calcium intoxication, which causes the SR to release Ca^{2+} during early diastole, nonselective cation and/or anion channels on the cell membrane may be opened by the extra $[Ca^{2+}]_i$.[45] This may cause membrane depolarization following the action potential known as an *afterdepolarization*.[46] This mechanism is not understood, but it clearly has an important role in the genesis of certain arrhythmias.[46]

Summary: The Basis of Resting Potential

In the preceding discussion, we have developed the concepts of the resting membrane potential and of cellular homeostasis. As we have seen, the cell maintains both an electrical and concentration gradient across its surface membrane. The active transport exemplified by the Na^+-K^+ pump maintains the concentration gradient. The cell membrane ion channels have selective permeability and generate steady-state currents. The sum of these currents produces zero net current at the resting potential, as predicted fairly well by the Goldman-Hodgkin-Katz equation. The large resting potassium conductance of the cell membrane plays a major role in determining the resting membrane potential, as was first postulated nearly a century ago by Bernstein. Other ions such as sodium also help determine the level of the resting membrane potential, as does the electrogenic properties of certain ion transport pumps. Finally, we have discussed the mechanisms by which normal and abnormal impulses may arise or be suppressed in the cardiac cell. Next, the cellular mechanisms that become active during the cardiac action potential and some of the basic cellular mechanisms of cardiac arrhythmias will be presented.

Electrophysiology of the Normal Heart with Particular Attention to Regional Action Potentials and Normal Conduction Pathway

It is commonly acknowledged that cardiac arrhythmias arise from critical alterations in cellular electrophysiology. First, the basic electrophysiologic mechanisms that may cause cardiac arrhythmias will be reviewed in relation to the temporal appearance of the clinical surface ECG deflections: P, QRS, and T, which are generated by the normal electrical activity of the heart.[47] The propagating cardiac impulse produces regional cardiac action potentials. These can be measured with intracellular 3-M KCl–filled microelectrodes (see Fig. 1–1).

The different action potentials of the heart will be described in the order in which they occur during normal sinus rhythm. We will also describe how conduction velocity depends upon the changes in active membrane current flow produced by the various action potentials. The rate of conduction of excitation is complex in multicellular tissue, but simplified models such as the uniform cable model predict surprisingly well the effects of known variables (membrane capacitance, extracellular resistance, intracellular resistance, cable dimensions, and active membrane ionic currents) on impulse conduction velocity. We emphasize that the regional differences in cardiac action potentials have a complex basis and complex effects. We will present these concepts in a generalized form for the purposes of this review.

The earliest deflection observed on the ECG, the P wave, is produced by membrane depolarization, conduction, and repolarization in the atrium. The atrial tissue is normally excited by the pacemaker cells firing action potentials in the sinoatrial node (SAN). Let us examine the electrophysiology of the SAN.

SINOATRIAL NODE ACTION POTENTIAL

The total mass of the SAN is too small to generate a detectable deflection in the body's surface ECG. SAN cells spontaneously fire slow-response action potentials (see Fig. 1–1). Cells slowly depolarize from a diastolic potential between -60 mV and -70 mV to a threshold potential near -35 mV to -50 mV, where opening of membrane Ca^{2+} and Na^+ channels cause a slow-response action potential to fire.[48] The rate of slow-response depolarization rarely exceeds 50 volts per second, whereas the rate is several hundred volts per second in well polarized cells of other cardiac regions. The automaticity of SAN cells is increased by extracellular $[Ca^{2+}]$. This indicates that membrane inward Ca^{2+} current becomes more significant at higher $[Ca^{2+}]_o$. The slope of phase-4 (diastolic) depolarization is markedly increased by sympathetic stimulation; threshold is attained sooner, and this then increases the heart rate. An increase in parasympathetic tone from the vagus nerve has the opposite effect.[49]

The phase-4 depolarization of SAN cells is thought to be a complex process. The postulated mechanism involves a number of inward and outward membrane currents: (1) an inward Na^+ current activated following hyperpolarization (I_f), (2) a background outward K^+ current (I_{K1}), (3) an inward $Na+$ "window" current, (4) an inward L-type Ca^{2+} window current, (5) an inward T-Ca^{2+} channel current, and (6) an outward electrogenic Na/K ATPase current.[50]

The slow-response potential depolarizes the cell to at least 0 mV. SAN cells repolarize without an early phase of rapid repolarization (phase 1) and without a plateau phase (phase 2), features of cardiac cells with more negative diastolic potentials. Thus the SAN action potential has a rounded upstroke and a slow triangular phase of repolarization. The SAN action potential propagates slowly from the SAN to nearby atrial cells. The actual site of SAN cells that are the pacemaker for the heart at a given time may shift to another location in the SAN in response to changes in physiologic stimuli.

ATRIAL MUSCLE ACTION POTENTIAL AND CONDUCTION

Normal atrial cells have well polarized diastolic membrane potentials of -75 mV to -90 mV. The first phase of the atrial action potential (phase 0) is characterized by a rapid depolarization (100–200 V/s) with a large amplitude ($+100$ mV to $+110$ mV), which is caused by a large inward Na^+ current lasting several milliseconds (see Fig. 1–1). A strong Na^+ current can be activated if the initial membrane potential is negative to -70 mV. The main purpose of this current is to quickly discharge the cell membrane's capacitance. During phase 0, the depolarization effectively activates voltage-dependent L-type Ca^{2+} current, which is needed for normal activation of myocardial contraction. The atrial action potential has a relatively short duration because the plateau phase is brief and repolarization is rapid. The short atrial action potential duration allows early repolarization and rapid recovery of fast Na^+ channel excitability. The next action potential can occur soon after the first. This gives atria the ability to fire action potentials at a very rapid rate.

ATRIOVENTRICULAR NODE ACTION POTENTIAL AND CONDUCTION

On the ECG, the time between the peak of the P wave and the start of the QRS complex is partly due to slow conduction of action potentials through the atrioventricular node (AVN). The AVN has a complicated cellular structure. AVN cells lack transverse cell-to-cell electrical coupling and are small in size.[51] The basis for the slow conduction through AVN is not completely understood.[51] We know, however, that the slow conduction in the AVN delays excitation in the ventricles for 100–120 ms after atrial excitation (See Fig. 1–1).

In the most automatic AVN cells, the action potential closely resembles the automatic SAN action potential but has a slower rate of phase-4 depolarization.[52] Thus ionic current flow during AVN and SAN action potentials may be similar. The normal phase-4 depolarization of the AVN cells may not be seen because the atrial action potentials excite AVN cells before the AVN pacemaker cells can spontaneously depolarize and fire.[53]

An important function of the AVN is to serve as a low-pass filter. The AVN prevents a high frequency of impulses from being conducted into the ventricles.[51] The conduction time through the AVN is prolonged at increased atrial rates of excitation, and then only some of the atrial beats may be conducted. The mechanism of atrial rate-dependent AVN block of conduction is not fully understood, but one important factor is the postrepolarization refractoriness (PRR) of the slow-response AVN action potentials (see section on PRR below for further details).

CARDIAC PURKINJE FIBER ACTION POTENTIAL AND CONDUCTION

The total mass of Purkinje fibers in the heart is too small and too dispersed to generate a measureable deflection on the surface ECG. AVN excitation is conducted to the His bundle. The His bundle splits into two bundle branches of cardiac Purkinje fibers, which transmit excitation rapidly to the ventricles. The Purkinje fibers fan out into the ventricular endocardium, forming a layer (several cells thick) of subendocardial Purkinje fibers.

Only a small proportion of the subendocardial Purkinje fibers are actually in contact with the subadjacent subendocardial ventricular muscle cells.[54] Thus the subendocardial Purkinje cells may conduct excitation rapidly without continually transmitting excitation to the underlying muscle cells. Conduction would be slower if there was extensive endocardial contact with the underlying ventricular cells.[54] Instead, contact with underlying muscle occurs occasionally via a small number of well-dispersed nexal junctions, between the deepest subendocardial Purkinje and most superficial subendocardial ventricular muscle layer.[54]

Cardiac Purkinje fibers conduct excitation rapidly at several meters per second. They have the most negative diastolic membrane potentials (-85 mV to -95 mV), the most rapid rates of phase-0 depolarization (400–700 V/s) and the largest-amplitude upstrokes ($+110$ mV to $+130$ mV) in the heart. The rapid conduction of the Purkinje fiber action potential requires the rapid depolarizing Na^+ current (during phase 0), the numerous low-resistance electrical contacts to other Purkinje cells, and the relatively large cellular radius compared to other cardiac cells. Conduction velocity has been shown to be proportional to the square root of the fiber radius.[55]

The normal Purkinje fiber action potential has less phase-4 depolarization than AVN and SAN cells and is normally overdrive-suppressed by the faster SAN or AVN automaticity. Purkinje fiber phase-4 depolarization occurs at a level of membrane potential 30 mV more negative than that for the SAN and AVN cells. Therefore, different membrane currents may be active during the Purkinje fiber phase-4 depolarization than during the AVN and SAN phase-4 depolarization. However, evidence suggests that I_f, I_{K1}, steady-state inward Na^+ window current, and outward Na-K ATPase current may be responsible.[50]

The rapid phase-0 depolarization of the His bundle and Purkinje fibers terminates as a spike. This is due to the coexistence of a rapid brief repolarizing current (phase 1) called the transient outward current (I_{to}).[56] I_{to} may also contribute to the notch in the action potential that precedes the plateau phase when diastole is prolonged. Slow inward Ca^{2+} current (L-type) is also active during the outward I_{to} current.[56]

The long action potential duration of the Purkinje fibers is partially caused by the long plateau phase (see Fig. 1–1), which is maintained by a balance of inward and outward membrane currents. The plateau is abbreviated by low concentrations of TTX (tetrodotoxin), a specific blocker of the fast Na^+ channel.[57] Thus an important plateau current is the steady-state Na^+ window current. This Na^+ window current is the inward Na^+ current that exists due to fast Na^+ channels that do not inactivate during the action potential.[57]

The repolarization of the Purkinje fiber action potential (phase 3) occurs as a phase of rapid repolarization that brings the transmembrane potential back to the maximum diastolic potential. It occurs when the membrane current during the plateau becomes sufficiently outward. This occurs due to a gradual increase in time-dependent outward plateau I_K current.[58] An additional factor may be the transient accumulation of extracellular cleft $[K^+]$ during phases 2 and 3, which can increase membrane K^+ conductance and thus increase repolarizing K^+ currents.[59] At higher heart rates, the duration of the action potential decreases. The rate of Na-K ATPase transport is increased because the steady-state intracellular Na^+ activity is raised from the increased action potential frequency. The duration of both phase 2 and phase 3 and the magnitude of outward electrogenic current from Na-K ATPase transport have been temporally correlated.[60]

VENTRICULAR MUSCLE ACTION POTENTIAL AND CONDUCTION

The subendocardial ventricular cells are the first muscle cells to depolarize. Deeper wall and epicardial ventricular muscle cells have a shorter action potential duration and are normally activated in the canine heart about 40 ms after endocardial activation (see Fig. 1–1).[61] The longer duration of the subendocardial muscle and Purkinje cells may prevent retrograde excitation. The rapid coordinated wave of depolarization in the ventricles produces a large ECG deflection, the QRS complex. Ventricular muscle cells have a maximum diastolic potential between −83 mV and −90 mV and normally have no automaticity.[61] There is a rapid phase 0, caused by fast inward Na^+ current, which depolarizes the cell membrane at a rate of 100 to 200 V/s with an upstroke amplitude of about +100 mV. Ventricular cells have a brief phase of partial repolarization during phase 1, due to a transient outward current.[62]

The plateau potential (phase 2) of the ventricular cell is not flat like that of the Purkinje cell. It may be dome-shaped or rounded, reflecting a balance between large inward Ca^{2+} window currents, inward Na^+ window currents, and a gradual increase in I_K outward current.[62, 63]

Phase 3 repolarization occurs when outward current flow produced by I_K and the Na-K ATPase exceeds the inward currents of the plateau. The peak of the T wave (caused by ventricular repolarization) of the ECG begins when action potential repolarization is under way. The ECG interval from Q to the peak of T is a useful estimate of the average duration of a ventricular cell action potential.

Effects of Abnormal Cardiac Cell Electrophysiology on Cardiac Action Potentials and on Conduction

Cardiac disease such as atrial or ventricular hypertrophy, cardiac muscle dilation, viral infection, and myocardial ischemia/infarction can alter the cardiac action potential. Fundamental changes in the transmembrane potentials have been recorded by using intracellular microelectrodes to study the transmembrane potentials of isolated diseased tissue preparations[63–69] or diseased single cardiac myocytes.[70] The changes in the action potential that may occur from disease are: (1) reduction of maximum diastolic potential (MDP), (2) alterations in normal phase-4 depolarization, (3) appearance of abnormal automaticity, (4) slowing of phase-0 upstroke, (5) alterations in duration of plateau phase 2, (6) production of early afterdepolarizations (EADs) during phase 2, (7) slowing of phase-3 repolarization, and (8) production of delayed afterdepolarizations (DADs) during diastole soon after repolarization of an action potential. Let us review some of these changes.

REDUCTION OF MAXIMUM DIASTOLIC POTENTIAL (MDP) CAUSES DEPRESSION OF THE FAST NA+ CURRENT AND SLOWING OF CONDUCTION

Reduction of the MDP has numerous predictable effects. Ionic membrane currents are sensitive to the membrane potential. The most important effect is the slowing of conduction velocity and block of the action potential upstroke when the MDP is decreased. MDP reduction may also cause changes in phase-4 depolarization, and alterations in action potential duration. Reduction of MDP also may help cause three kinds of abnormal impulse initiation: (1) abnormal automaticity, (2) early afterdepolarizations, and (3) delayed afterdepolarizations.

Inactivation of the Fast Na+ Channel by MDP Reduction

The fast Na^+ current becomes inactivated as a function of MDP depolarization (Fig. 1–3).[69, 71] Studies of normal cells given a premature excitatory impulse during late phase-3 repolarization show that the resulting action potential fires from a reduced membrane potential and consequently has a slow phase-0 upstroke (Fig. 1–4). The rate of conduction of the cardiac impulse through the atrium, Purkinje fibers, and ventricle is markedly slowed when the upstroke velocity of phase 0 is decreased by MDP reduction. This observation has popularized the term *depressed fast-response action potential*. The observation of this effect in atrial, Purkinje, and ventricular cells, which are depolarized by 10 to 25 mV from normal values, is explained by the partial inactivation of the cell's Na^+ channels caused by the membrane's depolarization. This effect of MDP depolarization is similar to the effect that can occur when cardiac cells are excited to fire an action potential late in phase 3. In this case the action potential can have a depressed upstroke if the fast Na^+ channels are still partially inactivated from membrane depolarization.[70] In diseased hearts in which cells may have MDPs reduced to between −60 mV and −75 mV, the action potentials have a slowed phase-0 upstroke from partial fast Na^+ channel inactivation.[63–65, 72]

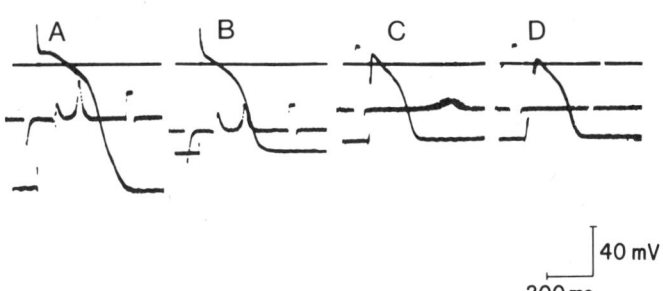

FIGURE 1–3
Records of changes in the transmembrane action potential of a canine Purkinje fiber caused by a gradual increase in the extracellular potassium ion concentration (left to right, from 2.7 mM to 10 mM KCl). The top line is the zero potential line. The horizontal trace inside the action potentials is the derivative (dV/dT) of the transmembrane potential (note square calibration pulses equal to 200 V/s). In trace A, maximum diastolic potential (MDP) is −92 mV, and dV/dT is 322 V/s. In trace B, action potential is beginning to change as 10 mM KCl washes into extracellular space. MDP is −66 mV, and consequently dV/dT is decreased to 200 V/s. In trace C, the action potential has lost its phase 0 spike and action potential duration is shortened. MDP is −58 mV, and dV/dT is very depressed, only 26 V/s. In trace D, MDP is only −55 mV, and dV/dT is less than 5 V/s. (Reprinted by permission from Dangman KH, Boyden PA: In Fox PP (ed.): Canine and Feline Cardiology, pp. 269–287. New York, Churchill & Livingstone, Publishers, 1988.)

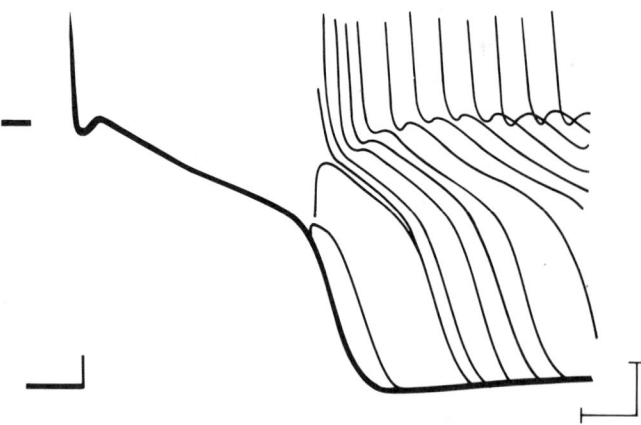

FIGURE 1-4
Records of a sheep Purkinje fiber action potential, showing the phenomenon of voltage-dependent refractoriness. During early phase 3 repolarization, the premature action potential has low amplitude and a slow upstroke, since its fast Na^+ channels have not recovered from voltage-dependent inactivation. As fiber repolarizes the premature action potential amplitude and upstroke velocity increase. Once the action potential has fully repolarized, the next action potential has a normal upstroke velocity, amplitude, and action potential plateau. Calibration bars at lower right are 20 mV for vertical bar, and 100 ms for horizontal bar. (Reprinted by permission from Dangman KH, Boyden PA: In Fox PP (ed.): Canine and Feline Cardiology, pp. 269–287. New York, Churchill & Livingstone, Publishers, 1988.)

If a premature impulse encounters cells during phase-1 to early phase-3 repolarization, then no action potential can be excited.[71] This depolarized period of the action potential is known as the *absolute refractory period*. It helps to explain why cells with an MDP reduced to about −60 mV in diseased cardiac cells *cannot* fire a fast-response action potential.[62, 72] The fast Na^+ current is inactivated by the reduction in MDP. Severe MDP depolarization can cause unidirectional or bidirectional block of action potential conduction in tissue.[72]

Inactivation of the L-Type Ca^{2+} Channel by MDP Reduction

The L-type Ca^{2+} current, like the fast Na^+ current, may be inactivated by MDP reduction.[62] However, when cells are depolarized to between −35 mV and −55 mV, slow-response Ca^{2+}/Na^+ action potentials may fire from atrial, Purkinje, and ventricular cells.[68, 73–76] The action potential may look like an SAN or AVN action potential. The upstroke velocity of the slow-response action potential may be less than 10 V/s, and conduction velocity may be very slow, less than 0.05 meters/s.[74] The slow-response action potential is noticeably increased by sympathetic stimulation (or increased intracellular cyclic AMP) and is suppressed by parasympathetic stimulation.[48, 49, 51]

An important factor controlling the repetition frequency of slow-response action potentials is post-repolarization refractoriness (Fig. 1–5).[77] The recovery of the Ca^{2+} channel from inactivation is slowed when the diastolic membrane potential is more depolarized.

Factors that reduce the repolarizing K^+ current (I_K) can prolong the plateau (phase 2) and repolarization (phase 3) of the action potential, and permit partial recovery of the Ca^{2+} channels during late phase 3.[78] This Ca^{2+} channel recovery may allow a slow-response action potential to occur during the plateau of a prolonged-action potential. This is termed an early afterdepolarization (see below for details).

The rate of rise and duration of the slow-response action potential depends on the magnitude of the slow inward current.[78] Strong electrical stimuli evoke increased inward Ca^{2+} current, which increases the upstroke velocity and the amplitude of the action potential. A reduction in the inward Ca^{2+} current may abbreviate the duration of the plateau phase of the fast-response action potential as well (Fig. 1–6).[63] This may cause an earlier repolarization of the action potential. The shorter action potential has a shorter absolute and relative refractory period. An earlier re-excitation of the cell is possible if an appropriate stimulus occurs.

Changes in Normal Automaticity Due to MDP Reduction

The rate of phase-4 depolarization is increased by a moderate reduction in MDP, which can be caused by increased membrane conductance to Na^+ and Ca^{2+}.

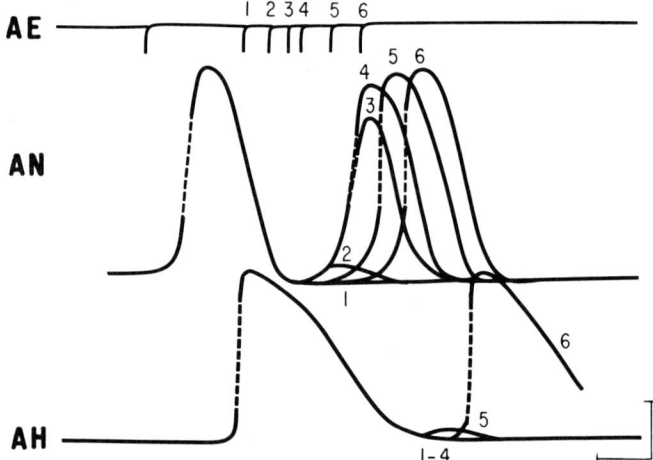

FIGURE 1–5
Traces shown are from an atrial endocardial surface electrogram (AE) and transmembrane potential records of rabbit atrioventricular node proximal region (AN) and distal region (AH). Following the first excitation, the subsequent excitations labeled in each trace 1 through 6 are an example of time-dependent refractoriness. The only premature beat to propagate from AE to AN to AH is no. 6. Earlier premature excitations 3–6 propagate from the atrium to proximal node but fail to excite distal node region AH. The earliest premature nos. 1 and 2 excite the atrium but do not excite even the proximal AV node. Thus, early additional impulses enter refractory tissue in the AV node, whereas later impulses encounter nonrefractory tissue. This is what is meant by time-dependent refractoriness. Lower calibration bar is 25 mV in the vertical scale and 50 ms in the horizontal scale. (Reprinted by permission from Dangman KH, Boyden PA: In Fox PP (ed.): Canine and Feline Cardiology, pp. 269–287. New York, Churchill & Livingstone, Publishers, 1988.)

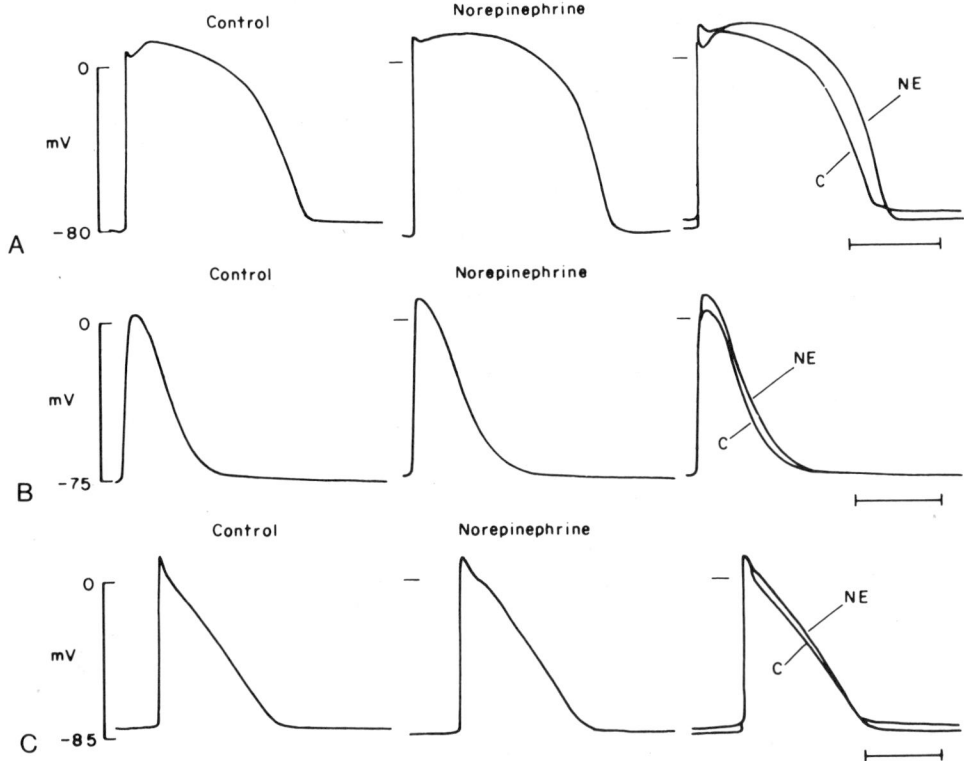

FIGURE 1-6
Records of canine epicardial muscle transmembrane potentials from normal (A), 5-day-old infarct (B), and 14-day-old infarct (C) tissue. Left-hand column of action potentials was obtained in normal Tyrode's solution. Center column of action potentials occurred after 31.3 micromolar norepinephrine. Right-hand column presents these action potentials superimposed. Note vertical mV axis and zero potential marks; horizontal mark is 100 ms. The plateau of the infarct-zone action potentials is clearly diminished, and this abbreviates the action potential duration (APD). The reduced APD was only slightly increased by catecholamines. Thus, in 5- to 14-day-old epicardial infarcts, decreases in Ca^{2+} current may markedly decrease APD. (Reprinted by permission from Boyden PA, Gardener PI, Wit AL: J Mol Cell Cardiol 20:525, 1988.)

Alternatively, a reduction in MDP caused by increased $[K^+]_o$, such as occurs during ischemia, will *decrease* phase-4 depolarization. The elevation in $[K^+]_o$ increases membrane K^+ conductance, which tends to drive the cells back towards E_K as was described earlier. If cells are depolarized to -40 mV to -60 mV by reduction of background K^+ current, (I_{K1}), abnormal automaticity may occur. Effects of I_{K1} reduction have been studied by using $[Ba^{2+}]_o$ to block I_{K1} (Fig. 1-7).[72] I_{K1} may be also reduced during myocardial ischemia by production of lysophosphatidylcholine or other lipid metabolites.[79]

Changes in Repolarization Due to MDP Reduction

MDP reduction alters outward K^+ currents that repolarize the action potential. Depolarization increases the driving force (MDP-E_K) for outward K^+ current produced by I_{K1}, the background K^+ current at the resting potential. I_{K1} may increase with MDP depolarization until the MDP is negative to -50 mV.[62] Depolarization also increases the steady-state I_K current.[62] These increases in outward K^+ current may reduce the action potential duration (APD) and thereby may reduce the period of depolarization available to activate inward plateau currents. The net effect will be to decrease APD.

Possible Primary and Secondary MDP Reduction

MDP reduction can arise due to (1) increased membrane Na^+ permeability; (2) reduced K^+ membrane permeability and (3) decreased potassium equilibrium potential (E_K) (from reduced $[K^+]_i$ and/or increased $[K^+]_o$)[80]; (4) Na-K ATPase inhibition[36]; and (5) increased $[Ca^{2+}]_i$.[45] A prolonged change in (MDP-E_K) due to depolarization will increase $[K^+]$ in the cardiac extracellular space and should reduce $[K^+]_i$.[81] Thus MDP reduction can decrease E_K and MDP further by stimulating additional cell K^+ loss. A second mechanism involves Ca^{2+}. In ventricular muscle, membrane depolarization increases free intracellular $[Ca^{2+}]$ and reduces intracellular $[Na^+]$.[82] In ischemic cells, the postulated increase in $[Ca^{2+}]_i$ may secondarily increase a nonspecific inward cation current, causing further MDP depolarization.[83] The reduction in $[Na^+]_i$ after MDP reduction slows active K^+ transport by the Na-K ATPase, and may cause a secondary decrease in E_K.

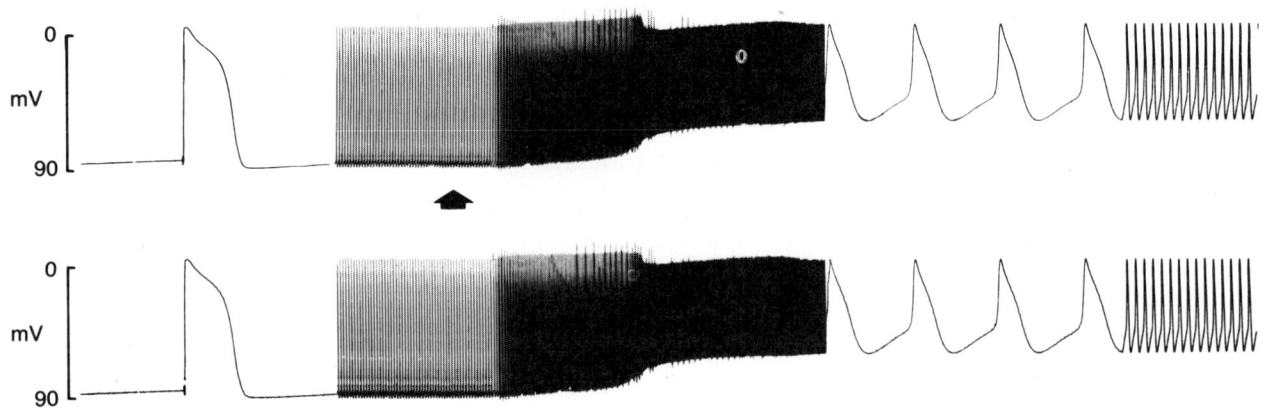

FIGURE 1–7
Records of action potentials in two separate canine cardiac Purkinje fibers, before and after exposure to 0.5 mM Ba^{2+}. The extracellular Ba^{2+} is known to cause a voltage- and time-dependent inhibition of cardiac K$^+$ currents, particularly the background inward rectifier, I_{K1}. At the arrow, Ba^{2+} was introduced. Ba^{2+} converted the fast-action potential with normal automaticity to an abnormally automatic, slow response type action potential. There was reduced diastolic membrane potential, increased phase 4 depolarization, and a slow-response action potential. Top trace is timer markers (1 per second). (Reprinted with permission from Hoffman BF, Dangman KH: In: Normal and Abnormal Conduction in the Heart, pp. 429–448. Mt. Kisco, NY, Futura Publishing, 1985.)

ABNORMAL ACTION POTENTIAL DURATION (APD) AND REFRACTORINESS

APD can be used to estimate the normal cell's absolute and relative refractoriness to the next action potential. However, in depolarized cardiac cells, only depressed fast-response or slow-response action potentials occur. These depressed action potentials require additional time for full recovery of excitability. Thus changes in both APD and in post-repolarization refractoriness can influence membrane excitability, resulting in slowed conduction and eventually in conduction block. Conduction block is frequently encountered at rapid heart rates in depolarized tissues.[72, 78]

Abnormal Impulse Initiation

Three kinds of abnormal cardiac impulse initiation are known: (1) abnormal automaticity, (2) early afterdepolarizations (EADs), and (3) delayed afterdepolarizations (DADs). These three types of abnormal impulse initiation may be seen in single cardiac cells as well as in cardiac tissue and thus reflect altered membrane currents.

ABNORMAL AUTOMATICITY

Abnormal automaticity is an abnormal spontaneous depolarization of cardiac cells that have a slightly depolarized MDP. It occurs in atrial, Purkinje, and ventricular cells when the MDP is reduced to -60 mV to -40 mV by infarction,[64–66, 68] drug toxicity,[84, 85] or stretch.[86] At these potentials there is little or no fast Na$^+$ channel activity. Rather, the upstroke of the abnormal action potential is mediated by Ca^{2+} current, since it is blocked by nifedipine.[87] Overdrive pacing will suppress abnormal automaticity only if the train of action potentials brings sufficient Na$^+$ into the cell to increase the activity of the electrogenic Na-K ATPase current.[88] The cellular mechanisms of abnormal automaticity are not well understood.[88]

Early Afterdepolarizations (EADs) During the Action Potential Plateau

EADs appear as a spontaneous single or a burst of slow-response or depressed fast-response action potentials arising during phase-3 repolarization of the action potential. In slowly beating Purkinje fibers in which cesium was experimentally used to block I_K, the action potential could be prolonged and could initiate slow Ca^{2+} action potentials during phase-3 repolarization (Fig. 1–8).[73] TTX-sensitive Na$^+$ window current can also contribute to EADs caused by quinidine.[89] In

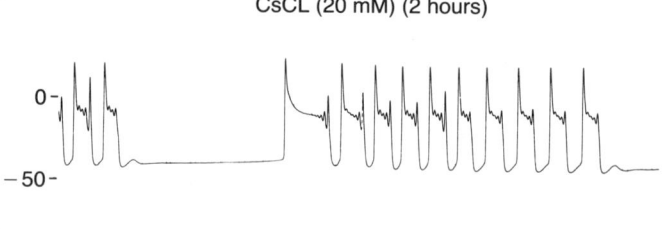

FIGURE 1–8
Transmembrane action potential records of a slowly firing cesium-depolarized (20 mM) Purkinje fiber illustrates the phenomena of both early (EAD) and delayed afterdepolarizations (DAD). EADs can be seen occurring during late phase 2/early phase 3 repolarization, and are promoted when phase 2 is prolonged by Cs$^+$. A DAD is seen after phase 3 is completed. (Reprinted by permission from Hoffman BF, Rosen MR: Circ Res 49:1, 1981.)

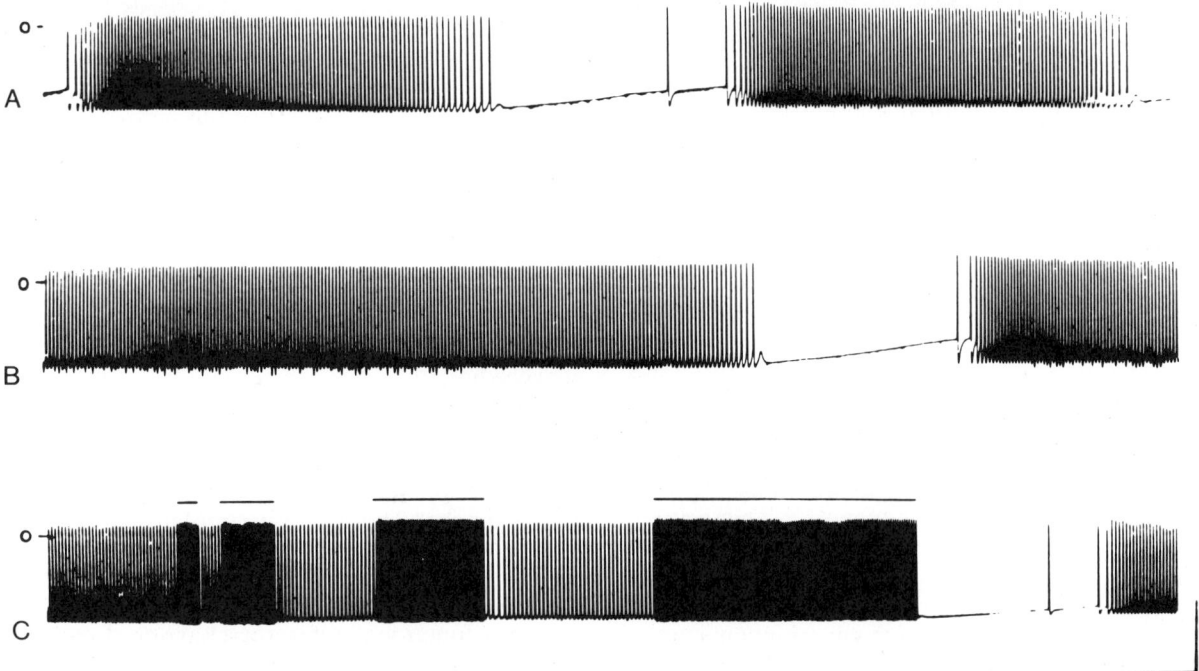

FIGURE 1-9
Transmembrane action potentials were measured in a depolarized region of canine epicardial muscle surviving 24 hours after infarction. The isolated tissue was exposed to 0.3 micromolar epinephrine and developed a triggered arrhythmia.

In A, the spontaneous train of action potentials shows an early acceleration in rate; the maximum diastolic potential (MDP) hyperpolarized, and there was slowing of the spontaneous rate followed by termination of the action potentials. The last action potential was accompanied by a delayed afterdepolarization (DAD). There was then a period of quiescence and slow MDP depolarization (lasting less than 1 minute). The triggered arrhythmia then spontaneously resumed.

B shows a continuation of the record in A. The train was longer lasting before spontaneous termination and there was a larger DAD. There was spontaneous overdrive suppression.

Panel C shows more of the same experiment. The effect of overdrive pacing at a cycle length of 300 ms was studied. Three attempts of brief pacing did not stop the triggered activity, but 36 s of overdrive pacing stopped the activity. Vertical scale = 60 mV, horizontal scale = 10 s. (Reprinted by permission of the American Heart Association, Inc., from Dangman KH, Dresdner KP, Zaim S: Circulation 78:1020, 1988.)

diseased cells, I_K may be decreased, and prolongation of the action potential may occur. In electrically isolated or partially uncoupled cells, EADs may occur and, as ectopic foci, may initiate extrasystoles. Catecholamines, hypoxia, and hypercapnia can induce EADs.[90-92] Some drugs (e.g., sotalol, N-acetyl procainamide, cibenzoline) that prolong repolarization can induce EADs.[73, 93]

Delayed Afterdepolarizations (DADs)

DADs occur after an action potential has completely repolarized back to the MDP. For an excellent recent, detailed review, see Cranefield and Aronson.[46] The DAD is a membrane oscillation that may reach the threshold for the slow Ca^{2+} or fast Na^+ channel and then fire an action potential. Once a single DAD has initiated an action potential, the process may repeat itself, resulting in a spontaneous, repetitive train of action potentials called *triggering*.[46] Pacing at a higher frequency typically causes the DAD to occur earlier following repolarization.[68, 78, 94] Pacing, catecholamines, or increased $[Ca^{2+}]_o$ increases the DAD amplitude.[46, 68] Increased cellular $[Ca^{2+}]_o$ is an essential aspect of this abnormal process. Ca^{2+} may become overloaded in the sarcoplasmic reticulum. This can help cause DADs in the atrium,[95] Purkinje fibers,[96] and ventricular muscle (see Fig. 1-9).[68] DADs have been observed at a wide range of MDPs.[95]

The mechanism of the DAD is complex and controversial. Na/Ca exchange or a nonselective Ca^{2+}-activated cation conductance are possible candidates for the inward current that causes the DAD.[45, 95, 96] In both cases, the major inward current charge carrier may be Na^+. The termination of a train of triggered action potentials may be spontaneous or may be facilitated by increased activity of the Na-K ATPase.[97, 98] In Figure 1-9A and B, triggered activity in an epicardial muscle cell surviving in a 24-hour infarct can be seen to terminate spontaneously with a subthreshold DAD. Figure 1-9C shows the effect of pacing overdrive of an epicardial muscle cell surviving in a 24-hour infarct.

Abnormalities in Cardiac Impulse Conduction

Whereas abnormal impulse initiation can arise from an abnormal property of a single cardiac cell, abnormal impulse conduction occurs when there is multicellular tissue of a certain mass in combination with cellular abnormalities. Conduction can be slowed, blocked, or reentrant.[78]

ABNORMAL CONDUCTION AND TISSUE ANISOTROPY

Several factors influence normal and abnormal action potential conduction in cardiac tissues. To propagate cardiac excitation, the tissue must fire action potentials when excited by depolarizing current from nearby action potentials. This depolarizing current can spread excitation only a few millimeters ahead in cardiac tissue. This is because intercellular current flow dissipates across the cell membrane. Depolarized cells with higher membrane conductance should dissipate intercellular current flow more quickly. There is also dissipation of intercellular current due to cytoplasmic current flowing to cells electrically coupled in the axial and transverse directions. After point stimulation, the spread of axial conduction is observed to be 2 to 3 times faster than transverse conduction.[55] This asymmetry in conduction rate is attributed to the lower axial versus transverse resistance of the cell-to-cell connections and has come to be known as *anisotropy*. It has been found that infarction causes edema and connective tissue formation that can spread apart surviving cardiac cells.[99] This may reduce cell-to-cell connections and slow conduction. In the extreme case, conduction may become so slow in the transverse direction as to appear as a pseudoblock.[100] Recent studies of healed infarcts with epicardial bipolar electrograms have shown the presence of highly fractionated electrogram deflections. Cells had normal action potentials, but conduction was greatly slowed due to a paucity of cell-to-cell connections.[99] Thus a reduction in cytoplasmic current flow can cause slowed conduction and block.[100]

REENTRANT ARRHYTHMIAS

Reentrant arrhythmias arise from alterations in normal electrophysiology of multicellular cardiac tissues.[101] Normally, the impulse initiated in the sinoatrial node propagates to the ventricles and ultimately encounters tissue that is completely refractory. Thus normal sinus excitatory impulses die out in the ventricular epicardium. However, if a portion of the tissue has not become refractory for some reason, then the excitatory impulse does not die out, but continues to propagate for a longer period of time. A portion of the tissue can become available for further excitation, if the myocardium (1) recovers from the action potential more quickly than normal (this reduces the relative refractory period); (2) conducts excitation more slowly than normal (this increases the time for partial recovery of excitability); or (3) is blocked from excitation initially (this prevents a portion of tissue from becoming refractory, and this may allow the tissue to become excited by a different impulse). Decreases in refractory period occur when the APD decreases, as in the atria during vagal stimulation. Thus atrial fibrillation is more easily induced during vagal stimulation.[102] Local catecholamine release can stimulate slow inward Ca^+ current. This can increase slow-response action potentials. These action potentials can conduct very slowly in depolarized tissue.[74] Tissue regions may become blocked to conduction in one direction. Impulses may propagate around the block and re-excite the region by propagation in the opposite direction.

The most basic models of reentry involve (1) slow conduction, (2) unidirectional block, and (3) a "pathway" of conduction that functions as a "long loop." The loop may be an anatomic one[103, 104] or functional one.[100, 105] The pathway may remain fixed or vary. Random pathways of reentry are most often associated with atrial and ventricular fibrillation, whereas a fixed pathway may cause other types of arrhythmias such as tachycardias.[106]

One important form of functional reentry, described originally by Allessie et al.[105] and known as the *leading circle* mechanism, involves a central region that remains functionally refractory due to continued impulse bombardment. The impulse circulates in tissue that is in a relative state of refractoriness. Therefore, the impulse activates action potentials from a decreased MDP. Such a mechanism thus causes slow conduction around a functional refractory barrier. Leading circle reentry may occur during atrial flutters or tachycardia.

Conditions for reentry may vary greatly, provided that the above three conditions hold. Slow conduction may be caused, for example, by reduced MDP, reduced longitudinal or axial resistance due to fibrosis, increased intracellular Ca^{2+}, or cellular acidosis. Unidirectional block may occur as a premature impulse moves into regions of increasing refractoriness, while conduction in the opposite direction would improve. Asymmetry of unidirectional conduction can lead to unidirectional block. This can involve anatomic factors (such as decreasing cell diameter) that decrease intercellular current flow in one direction while increasing it in the other direction. For these asymmetries in conduction to lead to unidirectional block, the action potentials are typically depressed. TTX has been shown to be an effective blocker in animal models of fibrillation involving depressed fast-response action potentials.[107] As a depressed response propagates, its amplitude and upstroke velocity may then decrease. Block may occur as an extinction of depolarizing axial intercellular and extracellular current evolves.

Conclusion

Basic cellular mechanisms of cardiac arrhythmias can be understood as the result of altered cellular electrophysiology. In some cases, the arrhythmias may be studied in a single cardiac cell. More complex arrhythmias require a syncytium of cardiac cells. Arrhythmias involve abnormalities in impulse initiation and in conduction. We have described in general terms the mechanisms that create alterations in cellular electrophysiology and thus suggested ways that cardiac arrhythmias may be produced.

References

1. Coraboeuf E, Weidman S: Potential de repos et potentials d'action de muscle cardiaque, mesurés à l'aide d'électrodes intense. C R Soc Biol 143:1329, 1949.

2. Ling G, Gerard RW: The normal membrane potential of frog sartorius fibers. J Comp Physiol 34:383, 1949.
3. Deck K, Kern R, Trautwein W: Voltage clamp technique in mammalian cardiac fibers. Pflugers Arch 280:50, 1964.
4. Hecht HH, Hutter OF, Lywood DW: Voltage-current relation of short Purkinje fibers in sodium-deficient solution. J Physiol 116:497, 1964.
5. El-Sherif N, Mehra R, Gough WB, et al.: Ventricular activation pattern of spontaneous and induced rhythms in canine one-day-old myocardial infarction. Evidence for focal and reentrant mechanism. Circ Res 51:152, 1982.
6. Wit AL, Allessie MA, Bonke FIM, et al.: Electrophysiologic mapping to determine the mechanism of experimental ventricular tachycardia initiated by premature impulses. Am J Cardiol 49:166, 1982.
7. Kono T: Roles of collagenases and other proteolytic enzymes in the dispersion of animal tissues. Biochim Biophys Acta 178:397, 1969.
8. Berry MN, Friend DS, Sheur J: Morphology and metabolism of intact muscle cells isolated from adult rat heart. Circ Res 26:679, 1970.
9. Hamill OP, Martz A, Neher E, et al.: Improved patch clamp techniques for high resolution current recording from cells and cell-free membrane patches. Pflugers Arch 391:85, 1981.
10. Lee KS, Weeks TA, Kao RL, et al.: Sodium current in single heart muscle cells. Nature 278:269, 1979.
11. Neher E, Sakmann B: Single channel currents recorded from membrane of denervated frog muscle fibers. Nature 260:799, 1976.
12. Harris AS, Rojas AG: Initiation of ventricular fibrillation due to coronary occlusion. Exp Med Surg 1:105, 1945.
13. Fozzard HA: Validity of myocardial infarction models. Circ Res 51/52(III):131, 1975.
14. Ringer S: Concerning the influence exerted by each of the constituents of the blood on the contraction of the ventricle. J Physiol 3:380, 1880–1882.
15. Nernst W: Zur Kinetik der losung befindlichen Korper: Theorie der diffusion. Z phys Chem ii:613, 1888.
16. Hille B: Ionic Channels of Excitable Membranes. Sunderland, Mass., Sinauer, 1984.
17. Bernstein J: Untersuchungen zur thermodynamik der bioelectrischen Strome. Erster Thail. Pflugers Arch 82:521, 1902.
18. Cole KS, Curtis HJ: Electric impedance of the squid giant axon during activity. J Gen Physiol 22:649, 1939.
19. Hodgkin AL, Huxley AF: A quantitative description of membrane current and its application to conduction and excitation in nerves. J Physiol 117:500, 1952.
20. Dangman KH, Dresdner KP, Mischler RE: Transmembrane action potentials and intracellular potassium activity of baboon cardiac tissues. Cardiovasc Res 32(3):204, 1988.
21. Goldman DE: Potential, impedance and rectification in membranes. J Gen Physiol 27:37, 1943.
22. Hodgkin AL, Katz B: The effect of sodium ions on the electrical activity of the giant axon of the squid. J Physiol 108:37, 1949.
23. Ammann D: Ion Selective Microelectrodes—Principles, Design and Application. New York, Springer-Verlag, 1986.
24. Eisner DA: The Na-K pump in cardiac muscle. In Fozzard HA, et al. (eds.): Handbook of Physiology, The Heart & Cardiovascular System, pp. 489–507. New York, Raven Press, 1986.
25. Sperlakis N: Origin of the cardiac resting potential. In Berne RM, et al. (eds.): Handbook of Physiology, The Cardiovascular System, Vol I pp. 187–267. Washington, D.C., American Physiological Society, 1979.
26. Glynn IM: The Na^+-K^+ transporting adenosine triphosphatase. In Matrinosi, AN (ed.): The Enzymes of Biological Membranes, pp. 35–114. New York, Plenum, 1985.
27. Jorgensen PL: Mechanism of the Na^+-K^+ pump. Protein structure and conformation of the pure Na^+-K^+ ATPase. Biochim Biophys Acta 694:27, 1982.
28. Deitmar JW, Ellis D: The intracellular sodium activity of cardiac Purkinje fibers during inhibition and reactivation of the Na-K pump. J Physiol 284:241, 1978.
29. Deitmar JW, Ellis D: Changes in the intracellular sodium activity of sheep heart Purkinje fibers produced by calcium and other divalent cations. J Physiol 277:437, 1978.
30. Vassalle M: Contribution of the Na^+/K^+ pump to the membrane potential. Experientia 43:1135, 1987.
31. Thomas RC: Electrogenic sodium pump in nerve and muscle cells. Physiol Rev 52:563, 1972.
32. Isenberg G, Trautwein W: The effect of dihydroouabain and lithium ions on the outward current in cardiac Purkinje fibers. Pflugers Arch 350:41, 1974.
33. Cohen I, Daut J, Noble D: An analysis of the actions of low concentrations of ouabain on membrane currents in Purkinje fibers. J Physiol 260:45, 1976.
34. Gadsby DC, Cranefield PF: Direct measurement of changes in sodium pump current in canine cardiac Purkinje fibres. Proc Natl Acad Sci 76:1783, 1979.
35. Eisner DA, Lederer WJ: Characterization of the electrogenic sodium pump in cardiac Purkinje fibers. J Physiol 294:279, 1979.
36. Hill JA, Trantham JL, Browning DJ, et al.: An upper limit for the electrogenic Na-K pump contribution to maximum diastolic potential in feline cardiac Purkinje fibers in steady state. Can J Physiol Pharmacol 64:641, 1986.
37. Vassalle M: Electrogenic suppression of automaticity in sheep and dog Purkinje fibers. Circ Res 27:361, 1970.
38. Sheu SS, Sharma VK, Banerjee SP: Measurements of cytoplasmic free calcium concentration in isolated rat ventricular myocytes with Quin 2. Circ Res 55:830, 1984.
39. Lee CO, Uhm DY, Dresdner K: Sodium-calcium exchange in rabbit heart muscle cells: Direct measurement of sarcoplasmic Ca^{+2} activity. Science 209:699, 1980.
40. Sperlakis N: The electrical properties of embryonic heart muscle cells. In DeMello WC (ed.): Electrical Phenomena in the Heart, pp. 1–61. New York, Academic Press, 1972.
41. Fabiato A: Simulated calcium current can both cause calcium loading in and trigger calcium release from the sarcoplasmic reticulum of a skinned cardiac Purkinje cell. J Gen Physiol 85:291, 1985.
42. Tseng GN, Boyden PB: Heterogeneous properties of calcium currents in isolated canine Purkinje and ventricular cells. (Submitted for publication).
43. Sheu SS, Blaustein MP: Sodium/calcium exchange and regulation of cell calcium and contractility in cardiac muscle, with a note about vascular smooth muscle. In Fozzard HA, et al. (eds.): The Heart and Cardiovascular System, pp. 509–535. New York, Raven Press, 1986.
44. Fabiato A: Calcium-induced release of calcium from cardiac sarcoplasmic reticulum. Am J Physiol 245:C1, 1983.
45. Colquhoun D, Neher E, Reuter H, et al.: Inward current activated by intracellular Ca^{++} in cultured cardiac cells. Nature 294:752, 1981.
46. Cranefield P, Aronson R.: Cardiac Arrhythmias: The Role of Triggered Activity and Other Mechanisms. Mt. Kisco, Futura Publishing Co., 1988.
47. Noble D: The Initiation of the Heartbeat, 2nd Ed. Oxford, Clarendon Press, 1979.
48. Noma A, Irisawa H: Membrane currents in the rabbit sinoatrial node cell. Pflugers Arch 364:45, 1976.
49. Difrancesco D, Tromba C: Muscarinic control of the hyperpolarization-activated current (I_f) in rabbit sino-atrial node myocytes. J Physiol 405:493, 1988.
50. Gintant GA, Cohen IS: Advances in cardiac cellular electrophysiology: Implications for automaticity and therapeutics. Ann Rev Pharmacol Toxicol 28:61, 1988.
51. Meijler FL, Janse MJ: Morphology and electrophysiology of the mammalian atrioventricular node. Pharmacol Rev 68(2):608, 1988.
52. Billete J, Janse M, Capelle FJL, et al.: Cycle-length dependent properties of AV node activation in rabbit hearts. Am J Physiol 231:1129, 1976.
53. Billete J: Atrioventricular nodal activation during premature stimulation of the atrium. Am J Physiol 252:H163, 1987.
54. Joyner RW: Modulation of repolarization by electrotonic interactions. Jpn Heart J 27(suppl):167, 1986.
55. Clerc L: Directional differences of impulse spread in trabecular muscle from mammalian heart. J Physiol 255:335, 1976.
56. Siegelbaum SA, Tsien RW: Calcium-activated transient outward current in calf cardiac Purkinje fibers. J Physiol 299:485, 1980.

57. Gintant GA, Datyner N, Cohen IS: Slow inactivation of a tetrodotoxin-sensitive current in canine cardiac Purkinje fibers. Biophys J 45:509, 1984.
58. Gintant GA, Datyner N, Cohen IS: Gating of delayed rectification in acutely isolated canine cardiac Purkinje fibers: Evidence for a single voltage-gated conductance. Biophys J 48:1059, 1986.
59. Kline RP, Kupersmith J: Effects of extracellular potassium accumulation and sodium pump activation on automatic canine Purkinje fibers. J Physiol 324:507, 1982.
60. Gadsby DC, Wit AL: Electrophysiological characterization of cardiac cells and the genesis of cardiac arrhythmias. In Cardiac Pharmacology, Chapter 10. New York, Academic Press, 1981.
61. Hoffman BF, Cranefield PF: Electrophysiology of the Heart. New York, Futura Publishing Co., 1960.
62. Tseng GT, Robinson RB, Hoffman BF: Passive properties and membrane currents of canine ventricular myocytes. J Gen Physiol 90:671, 1987.
63. Boyden PA, Gardener PI, Wit AL: Action potentials of cardiac muscle in healing infarcts: Response to norepinephrine and caffeine. J Mol Cell Cardiol 20:525, 1988.
64. Friedman PL, Stewart JR, Wit AL: Survival of subendocardial Purkinje fibers after extensive myocardial infarction in dogs. In vitro and in vivo correlations. Circ Res 33:597, 1973a.
65. Friedman PL, Stewart JR, Wit AL: Spontaneous and induced cardiac arrhythmias in subendocardial Purkinje fibers surviving extensive myocardial infarction in dogs. Circ Res 33:612, 1973b.
66. Dresdner KP, Kline RP, Wit AL: Intracellular K^+ activity, intracellular Na^+ activity and maximum diastolic potential of canine subendocardial Purkinje cells from one-day-old infarcts. Circ Res 60(10):122, 1987.
67. Ursell PC, Gardener PI, Albalba A, et al.: Structural and electrophysiological changes in the epicardial border zone of canine myocardial infarcts during infarct healing. Circ Res 56:436, 1985.
68. Dangman KH, Dresdner KP, Zaim S: Automatic and triggered impulse initiation in canine subepicardial ventricular muscle cells from border zones of 24-hour transmural infarcts. New mechanisms for malignant cardiac arrhythmias? Circulation 78:1020, 1988.
69. Downar E, Janse MJ, Durrer D: The effect of acute coronary occlusion on subepicardial transmembrane potentials in the intact porcine heart. Circulation 56:217, 1977.
70. Boyden PA, Albalba A, Dresdner KP: Electrophysiology and ultrastructure of canine subendocardial Purkinje cells isolated from control and 24 hour infarcted hearts. Circ Res (in press, 1989).
71. Weidman S: The effect of the cardiac membrane potential on the rapid availability of the sodium-carrying system. J Physiol 127:213, 1955.
72. Wit AL: Electrophysiological mechanisms of ventricular tachycardia caused by myocardial ischemia and infarction in experimental animals. In Josephson M (ed.): Ventricular Tachycardia, Mechanism & Management, pp. 33–95. New York, Futura Publishers, 1982.
73. Hoffman BF, Dangman KH: Are arrhythmias caused by automatic impulse generation? In Antonio Paes de Carvallo (ed.): Normal and Abnormal Conduction in the Heart, pp. 429–448. Mt. Kisco, NY, Futura Publishing Co., 1985.
74. Cranefield PF: The Slow Response and Cardiac Arrhythmias. Mt. Kisco, NY, Futura Publishing Co., 1975.
75. Katzung BG, Morganstern JA: Effects of extracellular potassium on ventricular automaticity and evidence for a pacemaker current in mammalian ventricular myocardium. Circ Res 40:105, 1977.
76. Surawicz B, Imanishi S: Automatic activity in depolarized guinea pig ventricular myocardium: Characteristics and mechanisms. Circ Res 39:751, 1976.
77. Mendez C, Moe GK: Some characteristics of transmembrane potentials of AV nodal cells during propagation of premature beats. Circ Res 19:993, 1966.
78. Wit AL: Cellular electrophysiological mechanisms of cardiac arrhythmias. In Singh BN (ed.): Control of Cardiac Arrhythmias by Lengthening Repolarization, pp. 1–32. Mt. Kisco, NY, Futura Publishing Co., 1988.
79. Kiyosue T, Arita M: Effect of lysophosphatidylcholine on resting membrane conductance of isolated guinea pig ventricular cells. Pflugers Arch 406:296, 1986.
80. Hanna MS, Dresdner KP, Kline RP, et al.: Characterization of transmembrane potential and intracellular potassium activity in the epicardial border zone 24 hours after myocardial infarction. Circulation 76(Suppl IV):IV, 1987.
81. Kline R, Cohen I: Extracellular $[K^+]$ fluctuations in voltage-clamped canine cardiac Purkinje fibers. Biophys J 46:663, 1984.
82. Sheu SS, Fozzard HA: Transmembrane Na^+ and Ca^{++} electrochemical gradients in cardiac muscle and their relationship to force development. J Gen Physiol 80:325, 1982.
83. Lee HC, Mohabir R, Smith N, et al.: Effect of ischemia on calcium-dependent fluorescent transients in rabbit hearts containing indo 1—Correlations with monophasic action potentials and contraction. Circulation 78:1047, 1988.
84. Dangman KH, Boyden PA: Cellular mechanisms of cardiac arrhythmias, Chapter 13. In Fox PP (ed.): Canine and Feline Cardiology, pp. 269–287. New York, Churchill & Livingstone Publishers, 1988.
85. Rosen MR, Danilo P: Effects of TTX, lidocaine, verapamil, and AHR 2666 on ouabain-induced delayed-after-depolarizations in canine cardiac Purkinje fibers. Circ Res 46:121, 1980.
86. Deck KA: Andergungen des Rhyepotentials und der Kabileigenschaften von Purkinje-faden bei der Dehnung. Pflugers Arch 280:131, 1964.
87. Dangman KH, Hoffman BF: Effects of nifedipine on electrical activity of cardiac cells. Am J Cardiol 46:1059, 1980.
88. Dangman KH, Hoffman BF: Studies on overdrive stimulation of canine cardiac Purkinje fibers: Maximum diastolic potential as a determinant of the response. JACC 2:1183, 1983.
89. Nattel S, Quantz MA: Pharmacological response of quinidine induced early afterdepolarizations in canine cardiac Purkinje fibers: insights into underlying mechanisms. Cardiovasc Res 22:808, 1988.
90. Trautwein W, Gottstein V, Dudel J. Der Aktionsstrom der Myokandfaser im Sauerstoffmangel. Pflugers Arch 260:40, 1954.
91. Corabouef E, Boistel J: L'Action des taux élevés de gaz carbonique sur le tissu cardiaque étudiée a l'aide de microélectrodes intracellulaires. Compt Rend Soc Biol (Paris) 147:654, 1953.
92. Brooks C McC, Hoffman PF, Suckling EE, et al.: In Excitability of the Heart. New York, Grune & Stratton, 1955.
93. Strauss HC, Bigger JT, Hoffman BF: Electrophysiological and beta-receptor blocking effects of MJ 1999 on dog and rabbit cardiac tissues. Circ Res 26:661, 1970.
94. Henning B, Kline R, Siegel MS, et al.: Triggered activity in atrial fibers of canine coronary sinus: role of extracellular potassium accumulation and depletion. J Physiol 383:191, 1987.
95. Tseng GN, Wit AL: Characteristics of a transient inward current that causes delayed after depolarizations in atrial cells of the canine coronary sinus. J Mol Cell Cardiol 19:1105, 1987.
96. January CT, Fozzard HA: Delayed-after-depolarizations in heart muscle. Mechanisms and relevance. Pharmacol Rev 40:219, 1988.
97. Moak JP, Rosen MR: Induction and termination of triggered activity by pacing in isolated canine Purkinje fibers. Circulation 69:149, 1984.
98. Wit AL, Gadsby DC, Cranefield PF: Electrogenic sodium extrusion can stop triggered activity in the canine coronary sinus. Circ Res 49:1029, 1981.
99. Gardener PL, Ursell PC, Fenoglio JJ, et al.: Electrophysiologic and anatomic basis for fractionated electrograms recorded from healed myocardial infarcts. Circulation 72(3):596, 1985.
100. Dillon SM, Allessie MA, Ursell PC, et al.: Influences of anisotropic tissue structure on reentrant circuits in the epicardial border zone of subacute canine infarcts. Circ Res 63:182, 1988.
101. Wit AL, Cranefield PF: Reentrant excitation as a cause of cardiac arrhythmias. Am J Physiol 4(1):H1, 1978.
102. Coumel P, Attuel P, Lavalle J, et al.: Syndrome d'arythmie auriculaire d'origine vagale. Arch Mal Coeur 71:645, 1978.
103. Boyden PA, Hoffman BF: The effects on atrial electrophysiology and structure of surgically induced atrial enlargement in dogs. Circ Res 49:1319, 1981.
104. Frame LH, Page RL, Hoffman BF: Atrial reentry around an

anatomic barrier with a partially refractory excitable gap—A canine model of atrial flutter. Circ Res 58:495, 1986.
105. Allessie MA, Bonke FIM, Schopman FJG: Circus movement in rabbit atrial muscle as a mechanism of tachycardia. III. The "leading circle" concept: A new model of circus movement in cardiac tissue without the involvement of an anatomical obstacle. Circ Res 41:9, 1977.
106. Hoffman BF, Rosen MR: Cellular mechanisms for cardiac arrhythmias. Circ Res 49:1, 1981.
107. Duff HJ, Sheldon RS, Cannon NJ: Tetrodotoxin: Sodium channel specific anti-arrhythmic activity. Cardiovasc Res 22:800, 1988.
108. Dresdner KP, Kline RP, Wit AL: Intracellular pH and maximum diastolic potential of canine subendocardial Purkinje cells from one-day-old infarcts. Circ Res (in press, 1989).
109. Blatter LA, McGuigan JAS: Free intracellular concentrations in ferret ventricular muscle measured with ion selective microelectrodes. Q J Exp Physiol 71:466, 1986.

2

Electrophysiology of Ventricular Arrhythmias in Myocardial Ischemia and Infarction

Nabil El-Sherif
William B. Gough
Mark Restivo
Mohamed Boutjdir

Ventricular tachycardia and ventricular fibrillation are serious complications of myocardial infarction and ischemic heart disease, the most prevalent forms of heart disease in the United States. Different electrophysiologic mechanisms may give rise to ventricular arrhythmias in myocardial ischemia and infarction. A better understanding of these mechanisms will provide a basis for improved management. More precise information is difficult to obtain from clinical electrophysiologic studies because of the limitations of the experimental protocols and techniques that can be utilized. This information could be obtained, however, from successful extrapolations from experimental studies on appropriate animal models to humans. In this chapter the electrophysiologic mechanisms of ventricular arrhythmias in myocardial ischemia and infarction are reviewed.

Classification

Following coronary artery occlusion, the area that was originally perfused becomes ischemic. Due to diffusion and collateral circulation, irreversible cell damage spreads from the central zone into the border zone.[1,2] Most infarctions will have one or more areas of necrosis surrounded by ischemic border zones. Purkinje and ventricular muscle fibers in the ischemic zone develop abnormal electrophysiologic properties and generate ventricular arrhythmias at various stages following infarction. Since the classic experiments on the dog heart by Harris,[3] it is known that ventricular arrhythmias after coronary artery occlusion occur in two distinct phases.

The first phase corresponds to the acute phase of ischemia and lasts until 15 to 30 minutes after coronary occlusion; the second starts 4 to 8 hours after occlusion and lasts 24 to 48 hours. The early phase of ventricular arrhythmias is more serious, can degenerate into rapid ventricular tachycardia and ventricular fibrillation, and has been attributed to reentrant excitation in ischemic myocardium.[4-9]

The second phase, which is more benign, consists of spontaneous multiform ventricular rhythms having about the same rate as the sinus rhythm and represents ectopic discharge from electrophysiologically abnormal Purkinje fibers.[7, 10-13] It is not known whether such a distinct bimodal distribution of arrhythmias occurs in other animals, including humans.[14] Furthermore, El-Sherif and associates[15-17] have shown that during the second phase of spontaneous ventricular rhythms, as well as following the subsidence of this phase, fast ventricular tachyarrhythmias and ventricular fibrillation could be induced by programmed electrical stim-

---

Cardiology Division, Department of Medicine, State University of New York, Health Science Center and Veterans Administration Medical Center, Brooklyn, New York

Supported by National Institutes of Health Grants HL36680 and HL31341 and the Veterans Administration Medical Research Funds.

ulation of the heart. These tachyarrhythmias, similar to those in the first phase, were attributed to reentrant excitation in ischemic myocardial border zones. Other investigators have shown that ventricular tachyarrhythmias can also be induced by programmed electrical stimulation in the chronic phase of canine myocardial infarction.[18–21]

Ventricular Arrhythmias in the Early Phase of Myocardial Ischemia

CHANGES IN TRANSMEMBRANE ACTION POTENTIALS

Transmembrane action potentials from intact canine and porcine hearts have been recorded during global and regional ischemia.[22–34] Within minutes of coronary artery occlusion, the cells in the center of the ischemic zone show progressive decrease in resting membrane potential, action potential amplitude, duration, and upstroke velocity (Fig. 2–1). In the first 1 to 3 minutes of ischemia, the refractory period changes concomitantly with the changes in action potential duration. After a brief initial shortening, the refractory period begins to lengthen even though action potential duration continues to shorten.[23] El-Sherif and colleagues[25] and Lazzara and coworkers[26] used the term "postrepolarization refractoriness" to indicate that at certain stages of ischemia the membrane may remain inexcitable even when it has been completely repolarized. Such increases in refractory period could exceed the basic cycle length, at which point 2:1 responses occur[23] (see Fig. 2–1). The marked dependence of recovery of excitability on the resting potential in partially depolarized ischemic myocardial cells is probably the most important determinant for the occurrence of slow conduction and conduction block in the acute phase of ischemia.[24] Since the recovery of excitability becomes markedly time-dependent, the basic heart rate and the coupling interval of premature beats have a crucial influence on local excitability in cell groups exhibiting a critical range of resting membrane potential.[24]

CONDUCTION DISORDERS

Conduction velocity remains fairly constant during the first 2 minutes of ischemia and then rapidly decreases thereafter.[27] There are two main reasons for the decline in conduction velocity: (1) the decrease in amplitude and upstroke velocity of the action potential and (2) the increase in extracellular and intracellular resistance. The contribution of changes in resistances has been calculated according to linear cable theory.[28] The predicted overall effect was a decrease in conduction velocity by 12% after 10 minutes and by 23% after 30 minutes. This indicates that, in intact hearts, in which conduction velocity decreases to approximately 50% of the control value within 4 to 5 minutes, the contribution of the changes in action potential upstroke

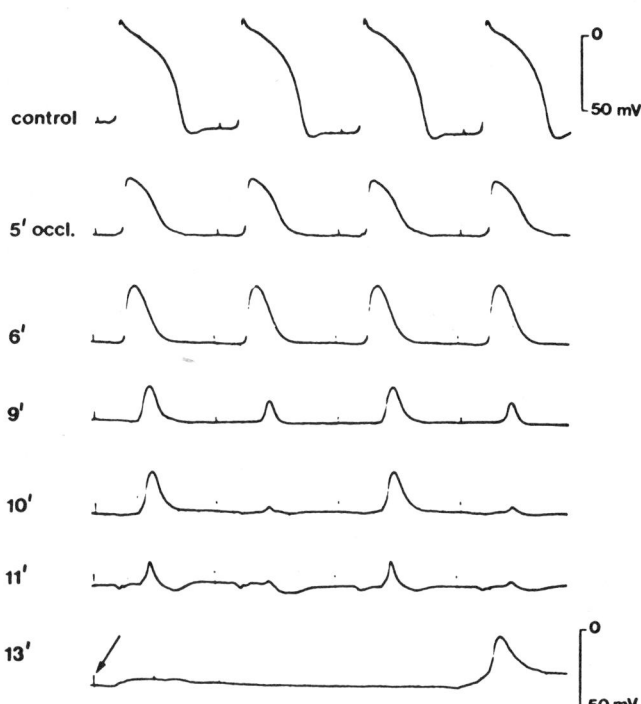

FIGURE 2–1
Transmembrane action potential recorded from the subepicardium of the left ventricle of an in situ pig heart before and after occlusion of the proximal left anterior descending artery. The figure shows the typical time course and character of changes which occur in subepicardial cells in the center of an ischemic region. The heart was paced at a basic cycle length of 390 ms. After 5 minutes of occlusion, the action potential was reduced in amplitude and duration, and upstroke velocity was decreased. The interval between stimulus artifact and beginning of action potential upstroke is increased. One minute later the plateau disappeared and the other changes were accentuated. At 9 minutes, an alternation in amplitude appeared which evolved into 2:1 responses. These responses degenerated further into small spikes that disappeared altogether by 13 minutes of ischemia. In the bottom trace, the last pacer artifact is indicated by an arrow. It produced no response, but after a pause of 1170 ms an action potential was produced by a sinus escape. This illustrates the tachycardia-dependent nature of the response of ischemic cells. (Reprinted by permission of the American Heart Association, Inc., from Downer E, Janse MJ, Durrer D: Circulation 56:217, 1977.)

characteristics is more important. The depressed upstroke of ischemic action potentials is the result of a depressed fast Na^+ current, and these action potentials are abolished at resting potentials positive to -60 mV[27] and by lidocaine.[29]

Conduction disorders in the ischemic myocardium have been demonstrated in extracellular recordings and have been correlated with the occurrence of ventricular tachyarrhythmias.[4–8] Fractionation of bipolar electrograms into multiple asynchronous spikes has been recorded and has been interpreted to suggest marked desynchronization of activation within the area of the recording. The occurrence of continuous electrical activity that bridges the diastolic interval between the sinus beat and the ectopic beat as well as between consecutive ectopic beats was taken as an indication that reentrant excitation is the underlying electrophysiologic mechanism for the ventricular arrhythmias.[15–17] The fractionation is most commonly seen when a composite electrode that averages the recording from multiple close bipolar electrodes is utilized.[15–17] It is also seen in recordings obtained from a bipolar electrode catheter with wide interpolar distance.[8]

The electrode catheter was originally utilized for intracardiac recordings from canine septal myocardium during acute ischemia following ligation of the anterior septal artery. In this study, conduction disorders in the ischemic septal myocardium were tachycardia-dependent and the onset of ventricular tachyarrhythmias was characteristically associated with a Wenckebach pattern of conduction delay (Fig. 2–2).[8] The electrode catheter recording technique was later adopted to record fractionated electrical activity in the diastolic interval from the left ventricular cavity in patients with chronic ischemic heart disease and ventricular tachyarrhythmias.[30]

MAPPING STUDIES

Multiple simultaneous electrograms and a multiplexer recording system have been utilized to construct iso-

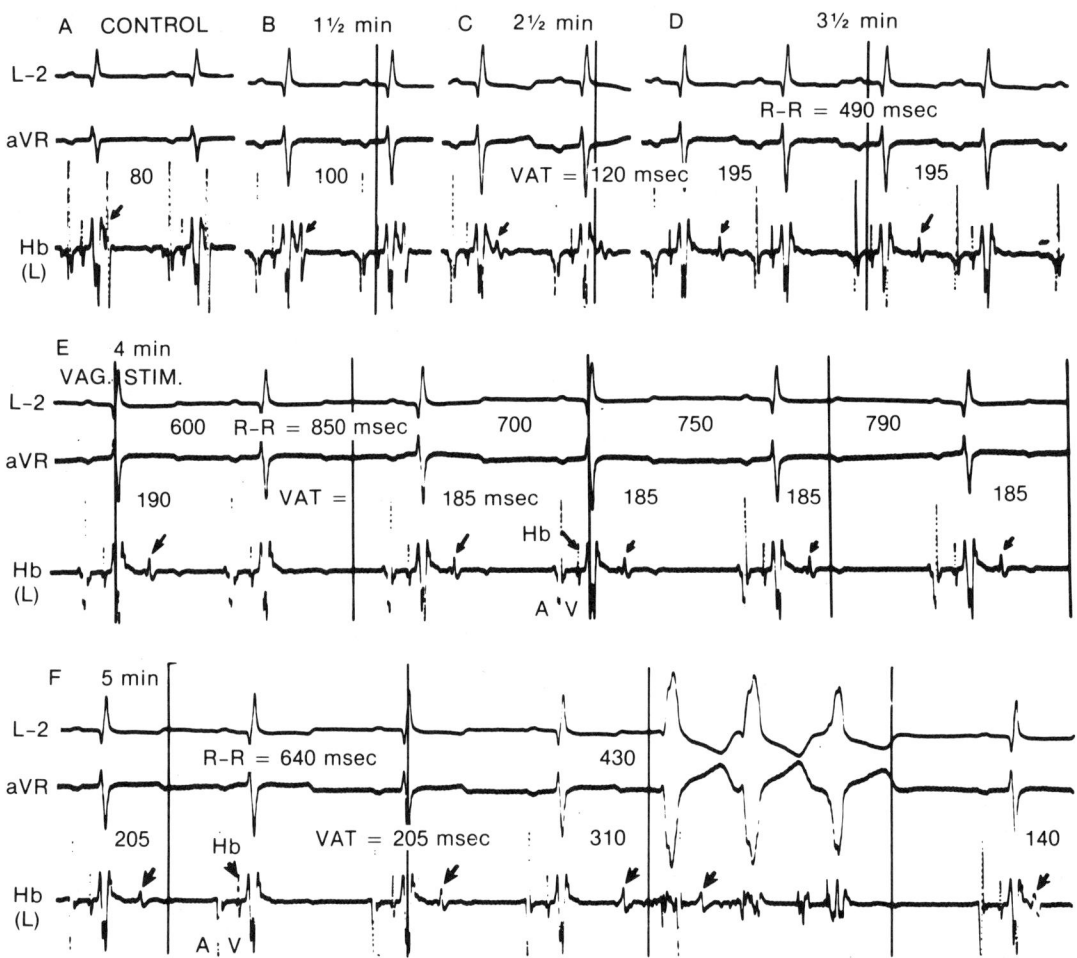

FIGURE 2–2
Electrode catheter recording of the septal myocardium following acute ligation of the anterior septal artery in the dog. Traces (from top to bottom) are ECG leads II and aVR and an electrode catheter recording of the His bundle from the left side, Hb (L). During control, the Hb (L) recording illustrated a discrete sharp biphasic deflection at the end of the ventricular complex that represented activation of septal myocardium (arrows). Following ligation, there was progressive delay in the inscription of the septal potential, with a marked decrease in the amplitude of the potential and an increase in its duration. At 3½ minutes following ligation, the ventricular activation time (VAT) measured from the onset of the ventricular complex to the delayed septal potential increased to 195 ms and the potential was inscribed every other beat, suggesting the occurrence of 2:1 conduction block to this area of septal myocardium.

Vagal stimulation applied in E slowed the heart rate and resulted in 1:1 conduction of the septal potential. This illustrates the tachycardia-dependent nature of conduction in ischemic myocardium. In F, 5 minutes after occlusion a short ventricular rhythm developed. The onset of the ventricular rhythm was characteristically associated with a Wenckebach pattern of conduction delay of the septal potential. Fractionated electrical activity preceded the onset of the first ectopic beat and bridged at least part of the diastolic interval between consecutive ectopic beats. This suggests that reentrant excitation is the underlying electrophysiologic mechanism of the ectopic rhythm. Note that the last ectopic beat was not followed by delayed diastolic activity.

(Reprinted by permission of the American Heart Association, Inc., from El-Sherif N, Scherlag BJ, Lazzara R: Circulation 51:1003, 1975.)

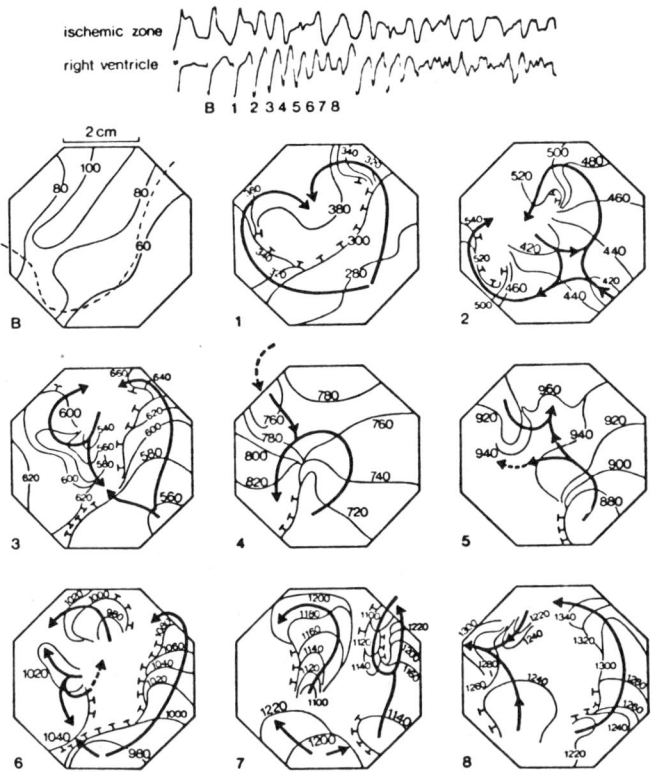

FIGURE 2-3
Electrograms recorded from ischemic epicardium and normal right ventricle during a run of ventricular tachycardia that degenerated into ventricular fibrillation 3½ min following left anterior descending artery occlusion in an isolated pig heart. Epicardial isochronal activation maps of the basic beat (B) and first eight ectopic beats are shown. The isochrones separate areas activated within the same 20-ms interval. Numbers are in milliseconds. The interrupted line in the activation map of the basic beat is the ischemic border zone.
During the first ectopic beat, earliest activity emerged at 280 ms in the normal zone and was blocked inside the border of the ischemic zone (bars indicate conduction block). The activation wavefront conducted slowly around both ends of the arc of block, coalesced, and then returned to reactivate sites proximal to the arc of the block and to initiate the first reentrant cycle. A figure-eight reentrant activation pattern continued during the second ectopic beat, and each of the two synchronous wavefronts had a diameter of about 1 cm. Following this, the activation pattern became irregular with fragmentation of wavefronts. Circus movements usually were not completed, and whenever they were, their diameter was small (see the circuit in beat 7 with a diameter of 0.5 cm). (Reprinted by permission from Janse MJ, Van Cappelle FJL, Morsink H, et al.: Circ Res 47:151, 1980.)

chronal maps of ventricular activation during acute ischemia.[9] This technique has allowed the demonstration of circus movements around areas of conduction block having a diameter of 1 to 2 cm on the epicardial surface of the ischemic zone during ventricular tachycardia occurring between 2 and 10 minutes after coronary occlusion. The localization, revolution time, and size of the circus movements changed from beat to beat. Ventricular tachycardia, which could terminate spontaneously or degenerate into ventricular fibrillation, was characterized by the presence of basically one fairly large circus movement. During ventricular fibrillation, reentrant circuits were multiple, were seldom completed, and had small diameters, on the order of 0.5 cm (Fig. 2-3).[9]

Other studies that have utilized tridimensional mapping techniques with improved spatial resolution have shown that during early ischemia in the cat heart, 76% of all ventricular premature beats occurred through intramural reentry in which a sinus beat was delayed in midmyocardial and subendocardial areas, giving rise to reexcitation in the subendocardium.[31] In 24% of cases, initiation of the first beat of ventricular tachycardia arose in either the subendocardium or subepicardium by a non-reentrant mechanism, as evidenced by the lack of intervening electrical activity between the end of the preceding sinus beat and the initiation of the ectopic beat. Ventricular tachycardia could be initiated, maintained, or terminated by either reentrant or non-reentrant mechanisms. Micro reentry or reflection[12] involving a small myocardial region could not be ruled out, and the nature of the non-reentrant ectopic activity was not determined. Janse and associates[33] have proposed that injury currents flowing between ischemic and nonischemic myocardium could initiate premature beats, either by directly stimulating the nonischemic myocardium at the end of the refractory period or by enhancing the amplitude of delayed afterdepolarizations.

IONIC AND METABOLIC CHANGES ASSOCIATED WITH ISCHEMIA

A number of new techniques, including ion-selective electrodes, nuclear magnetic resonance, and voltage- and ion-sensitive dyes, have improved our understanding of intracellular and extracellular ionic changes associated with acute ischemia. Acute coronary occlusion is associated with a loss of intracellular K^+, an increase of intracellular Na^+ and Ca^+ and of extracellular K^+, and both intracellular and extracellular acidosis.[34-45]

Since the experiments of Harris and colleagues,[34] cellular K^+ loss and extracellular K^+ accumulation has been considered to be a major determinant of the electrophysiologic changes that underlie the early phase of malignant ventricular arrhythmias following acute myocardial ischemia. However, the depolarization and depressed action potential characteristics of ischemic cardiac cells cannot be attributed solely to changes in K^+. Ischemic action potentials can be simulated in vitro by a combination of high K^+, hypoxia, and acidosis.[46] Other components of ischemia, particularly amphipathic lipid metabolites, free radicals, and locally accumulating catecholamines, may play a significant role in ischemic injury, and electrophysiologic alterations associated with ischemia.

Mechanisms of Ischemia-Induced Increase of Extracellular K^+

Following coronary occlusion, an increase in extracellular K^+ occurs in a triphasic fashion. An initial rapidly rising phase, lasting 1 to 15 minutes, is followed by a plateau phase that lasts approximately 20 to 30 minutes. The K^+ level may actually decrease during this plateau phase. A third phase then follows during which K^+ rises slowly but continuously. This third, slowly rising phase denotes irreversibility and loss of membrane integrity.[47] The major part of increase of extracellular K^+ during the first few minutes of ischemia is attributed to a net efflux of K^+ from the intracellular compartment.[41] The net cellular K^+ loss can result from at least four different mechanisms: (1) a decrease in K^+ influx due to reduced Na^+/K^+ pump, (2) an increase of K^+ efflux as a consequence of intracellular acidosis, (3) an increase of K^+ efflux through Ca^{2+}-activated K^+ channels, and (4) an increase of K^+ efflux by opening of ATP-dependent K^+ channels.

Both in hypoxic cardiac muscle[48] and in ischemic myocardium experiments,[39,41] the preponderance of evidence suggests that Na^+/K^+ pump activity is only partially suppressed during the first few minutes of ischemia and that active K^+ influx is still maintained. On the other hand, some studies have shown a close relationship between cellular K^+ loss and the development of intracellular acidosis.[49-52] The abrupt decrease of PO_2 within the cell will accelerate anaerobic energy metabolism, forming weak acids such as lactic acid and inorganic phosphate.[52] Buffering of protons by intracellular proteins will lead to a decrease of fixed impermeant negative charges and to an increase in activity of more permeant anions. An outward movement of anions and cations is expected qualitatively from an increase of intracellular permeant anions.[41,49] The resulting release of K^+, lactate, and inorganic phosphate into venous affluent following reduction of coronary blood flow[50,51] suggests an interrelationship between these ionic movements.

Recent studies using more sensitive intracellular Ca^{2+} indicators have suggested that ischemia causes a rapid (within 90 seconds) increase in both systolic and diastolic Ca^{2+}.[44] The early increase of intracellular Ca^{2+} may be mediated by accumulation of acid metabolites[53] or by release of ATP into extracellular space.[54] The increase of intracellular Ca^{2+} can lead to opening of Ca^{2+}-activated K^+ channels and therefore can explain the early rise of extracellular K^+ following ischemia. Furthermore, increased intracellular Ca^{2+} can depolarize cardiac cells by means of a Ca^{2+}-activated inward current. Such current can flow either through Na^+–Ca^{2+} exchange[55] or through Ca^{2+}-activated cation channels[56] that have been described in cardiac cells. It has been suggested that the protective effects of Ca^{2+} channel blockers during ischemia may be related to this mechanism.[32]

ATP-sensitive K^+ channels have been reported in cardiac muscle.[57] It has been suggested that ischemia may result in opening of these channels, resulting in increased K^+ efflux and accumulation of extracellular K^+.[57-59] Glyburide, a second-generation hypoglycemic sulfonylurea and a potent blocker of the ATP-sensitive K^+ channels[60,61] was recently shown to significantly reduce the rise of extracellular K^+ and intramyocardial conduction delay during the early phase of acute ischemia (Fig. 2–4).[62] However, the effects of glyburide may not be solely related to direct suppression of ATP-sensitive K^+ channels. The critical level of ATP that completely suppresses ATP-sensitive K^+ channels in excised membrane patches from heart is much lower than the concentration of ATP during ischemia except at a very late stage.[57]

Weiss and Lamp[63] have suggested that glycolysis may be more effective than oxidative phosphorylation in preventing ATP-sensitive K^+ channels from opening. It is possible that the effects of glyburide can be explained by an indirect metabolic effect on glycolysis. Glyburide was shown to promote glycolysis by stimulation of phosphofructokinase flux and transport of glucose into the cells as well as to stimulate pyruvate oxidation by the heart.[64]

The amelioration of increased extracellular K^+ may also be attributed to the effects of glyburide-induced insulin release, which is known to promote the movement of K^+ intracellularly.[65] Although no study has specifically addressed the effects of insulin on the initial rise of extracellular K^+ following ischemia, several studies have shown that an insulin-glucose-K^+ solution[66] administered as early as 30 minutes following ligation can improve the metabolic and electrical manifestations of ischemic myocardial damage.[67,68]

Role of Amphipathic Lipid Metabolites

Several fatty acid and phospholipid metabolites including long-chain acylcarnitines and lysophosphatidylcholine (LPC) have been shown to accumulate in ischemic myocardium in amounts that are capable of eliciting

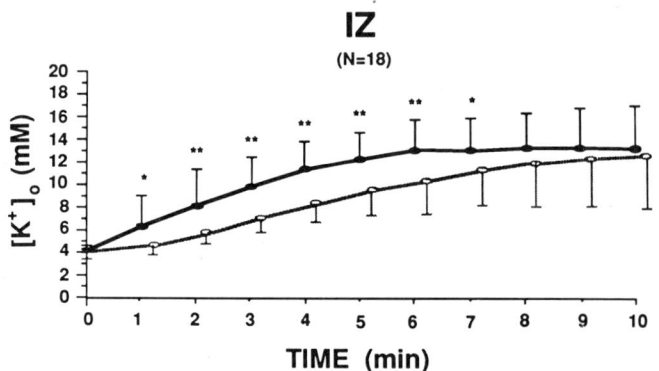

FIGURE 2–4
Time course of changes of extracellular potassium concentration, $[K^+]_o$, in mM during a 10-min period of left anterior descending coronary artery ligation in 10 dogs (control ischemia (CI), closed circles) and 10 minutes of ischemia following the administration of 0.15 mg/kg of glyburide (glyburide + ischemia (G + I), open circles). K^+-sensitive electrodes were introduced to record from mid-myocardial regions in the ischemic zone (IZ). There was a rapid rise of $[K^+]_o$ during CI, reaching a maximum mean peak at 6 minutes of 13.0 ± 2.6 mM. This was followed by a relatively steady level of $[K^+]_o$ for the remaining 4 minutes of occlusion. During G + I there was a significant reduction of the magnitude of rise of $[K^+]_o$ in the IZ during the first 7 minutes of occlusion. The reduction in mean $[K^+]_o$ continued at 8 to 10 minutes of occlusion but failed to reach statistical significance (* = p <0.01; ** = p <0.0001).

electrophysiologic changes in vitro.[69–73] The mechanism of the deleterious electrophysiologic effects of those metabolites likely involves their accumulation in the sarcolemma with subsequent disruption of membrane protein function.[73]

During myocardial ischemia, LPC increases substantially in both venous[69] and lymphatic[72] drainage, from ischemic tissue. This increase occurs within minutes of the onset of ischemia and is believed to represent an accumulation of metabolite in the extracellular space. LPC has been reported to depress several ionic membrane currents. LPC depresses the fast inward current[74,75] and decreases the slow inward current and the time-independent background current.[76] The reduction of resting membrane potential elicited by LPC in ventricular muscle may be due to the decrease in outward K^+ conductance.[76] LPC also increases intracellular Ca^{2+}, probably from intracellular stores[77,78] and has been shown to induce delayed afterdepolarizations in canine Purkinje fibers.[79] It is possible that LPC-induced delayed afterdepolarizations and triggered rhythm may contribute to arrhythmias in the early phase of myocardial ischemia[31] and reperfusion.[80]

In contrast to LPC, long-chain acylcarnitines are not found extracellularly until irreversible cell damage has occurred. However, 10 minutes of severe hypoxia has resulted in a four- to fivefold increase in the total cellular long-chain acylcarnitine fraction with a more than 70-fold increase in the sarcolemma.[81] The electrophysiologic derangements accompanying hypoxia (namely, a decrease in upstroke velocity, resting membrane potential, and action potential duration) paralleled the sarcolemmal accumulation of long-chain acylcarnitines.[81] Insertion of exogenous or endogenous long-chain acylcarnitines into the sarcolemma increased the number of alpha-adrenergic receptors.[82] When animals were pretreated with sodium-2-[5-(4-chlorophenyl)-pentyl]-oxirane-2-carboxylate (POCA), an inhibitor of carnitine acyltransferase I, the drug inhibited the ischemia-induced increase in long-chain acylcarnitines, LPC, and malignant ventricular arrhythmias.[83]

Role of Free Radicals

There is growing evidence that reactive oxygen metabolites such as the superoxide (O_2^-), hydrogen peroxide (H_2O_2), and hydroxyl (OH) radicals are important mediators of ischemic and, particularly, reperfusion myocardial damage.[84–87] Much of the support for this hypothesis stems from experimental observations in which a variety of interventions known to be capable of limiting free radical–producing reactions or enhancing endogenous antioxidant capacity (pretreatment or the addition of allopurinol, antioxidant enzymes [superoxide dismutase, catalase, peroxidase], or organic antioxidants [ascorbate, methionine]) have been shown to limit ischemic injury or reduce the vulnerability of the heart to reperfusion arrhythmias.[88–92] The mechanism of damage induced by oxygen free radicals may include injury to phospholipid proteins and nucleic acids[93] as well as inhibition of sarcolemmal Na^+/K^+-ATPase activity and of Ca^{2+}-ATPase activity of sarcoplasmic reticulum.[94–97] It has been suggested that oxygen free radicals may be able to promote thiol-disulfide interchange in the carrier protein.[98] If this were to occur during early reperfusion, free radicals might be the initiating cause of Ca^{2+} uptake in which the cells may be Na^+ loaded and depolarized.

In almost all studies of oxygen free radicals and ischemic injury, the association between the observed protection and the manipulation of free radicals was indirect and as such could have been circumstantial.[87] One reason is the ultrashort half-life of oxygen free radicals, which would make direct evaluation very difficult. The recent technique of electron spin resonance by which free radicals can be definitely identified and measured has confirmed that reperfusion, after a brief period of ischemia, does indeed result in a sudden burst of radical production.[99,100]

REPERFUSION ARRHYTHMIAS

Sudden release of coronary artery occlusion is known to be a potent arrhythmogenic stimulus, often leading to ventricular fibrillation.[101–103] The incidence and severity of reperfusion arrhythmias seem to correlate with the duration of occlusion before release[101] and the amount of myocardium at risk.[104] Other variables, such as heart rate and reperfusion blood flow, also influence outcome.[103,105] The electrophysiologic mechanisms underlying reperfusion arrhythmias have not been fully elucidated. Some studies have demonstrated a significant electrophysiologic role for alpha-adrenergic stimulation during both coronary occlusion and reperfusion linked to a change in density of alpha-adrenergic receptors in ischemic myocardium.[106,107] Nonspecific alpha-adrenergic blockade with phentolamine and specific alpha-adrenergic blockade with prazosin were found to decrease ventricular arrhythmias associated with coronary occlusion and/or reperfusion in a number of animal models.[107–112]

Some insight into the electrophysiologic mechanisms of reperfusion arrhythmias was provided by in vitro models of ischemia and reperfusion. Ferrier et al.[113] exposed an in vitro preparation of both ventricular muscle and Purkinje fibers to conditions simulating ischemia (hypoxia, acidosis, elevated lactate, and zero metabolic substrate for 40 minutes), and then superfusion with normal Tyrode's solution was reinstituted. Exposure to ischemic solution resulted in depressed excitability and progressive conduction block between muscle and Purkinje tissue. Return to normal Tyrode's solution resulted in a sequence of responses in the Purkinje fibers: prompt hyperpolarization, progressive depolarization to unresponsiveness, and final repolarization to control values. The depolarization phase was accompanied by oscillatory afterpotentials that initiated extrasystoles. The appearance of oscillatory afterpotentials during the reperfusion phase was accompanied by aftercontractions. Hayashi and coworkers[114] exposed isolated guinea pig papillary muscles to hypoxia (30 to 60 min) followed by reoxygenation (30 min) and showed that arrhythmia activity following reinstitution of oxygenated superfusion was characterized by aftercontractions and delayed afterdepolarizations arising from ventricular myocardium.

Recent studies that reexamined the Ferrier's reperfusion model suggest that the elevations of intracellular Na^+ and Ca^{2+} at the end of the ischemic phase are prime determinants of the changes that follow the onset of reperfusion.[115] The dramatic increase in resting tension argues for an increase in myofilament sensitivity to Ca^{2+} as the pH rises in addition to an increase in cytosolic Ca^{2+}, probably resulting from Ca^{2+} release from sarcoplasmic reticulum. The increase in intracellular free Ca^{2+} concentration could, in turn, activate a nonselective cation channel, leading to an inward current and membrane depolarization. This Ca^{2+}-activated cation channel may be involved also in development of triggered arrhythmias.[116]

Triggered Ventricular Rhythms in the Subacute Phase of Myocardial Infarction

Approximately 4 to 8 hours following coronary artery occlusion, spontaneous ventricular rhythms develop. The spontaneous multiform activity peaks 1 to 2 days post-infarction and usually subsides by the third day.[3] These rhythms arise from surviving subendocardial Purkinje fibers overlying the infarction.[7, 10, 12, 13] In vitro studies of these surviving subendocardial Purkinje fibers have suggested that two mechanisms may be responsible for the activity: (1) abnormal automaticity[11, 117] and (2) triggered activity.[118] However, the preponderance of evidence favors the second mechanism.

TRIGGERED ACTIVITY STUDIED IN VITRO

Delayed afterdepolarizations (DADs) giving rise to triggered activity were recorded in depolarized ischemic Purkinje fibers from a 1-day-old canine infarction.[118] The amplitude and rate of rise of the DADs were a function of both the cycle length (Fig. 2–5A) and the number of impulses in a stimulated train. A critically timed premature impulse may be followed by a DAD that triggers activity (Fig. 2–5B). However, in contrast to other preparations demonstrating triggered activity, one stimulated action potential during quiescence was often able to generate a suprathreshold DAD, which in turn initiated triggered activity (Fig. 2–6). The ease of inducing triggered activity in ischemic Purkinje fibers may explain the persistence of multiform ventricular rhythms in vivo in 1-day-old canine infarctions.[118] When triggered activity was initiated by normal automaticity in Purkinje fibers, a subthreshold DAD reached threshold and initiated an action potential. The result was extrasystolic groupings (i.e., bigeminal and trigeminal rhythms) or sustained triggered activity (Fig. 2–7). Entrance and exit block around sites of triggered activity is not uncommon in ischemic subendocardial preparations. The presence of entrance block around a site of triggered activity that is able to exit, at least intermittently, to the rest of the preparation (or the ventricles) can result in a parasystolic rhythm (Fig. 2–8).

Abnormally automatic or triggered activity had only been described to occur in Purkinje fibers until the report of Dangman and colleagues.[119] They studied epicardium surviving 1 day of ischemia and reported seeing sustained activity (in three of 12 preparations, averaging a maximum diastolic potential of −64 mV) and triggered activity arising from DADs (in two of the above three preparations). After the addition of 1 to 10 μM catecholamine to the superfusate, subthreshold DADs and nonsustained triggered activity were recorded in the other nine preparations. Therefore, it appears that ischemia has the capacity to render ventricular muscle spontaneous, as well as Purkinje fibers.

Effects of Overdrive Pacing

The effects of overdrive pacing on the sustained activity occurring 24 hours post-infarction have been studied in vitro in order to establish whether one might be able to differentiate the mechanism responsible for the sustained activity based on its response to overdrive pacing.

In Purkinje fibers that survived 24 hours of ischemia and in which nonsustained triggered activity had been recorded before it became sustained, rapid pacing at short cycle lengths terminated the sustained activity in about one half the preparations studied. The termination occurred immediately following the last overdriven beat or after a brief period of rhythmic activity (Fig. 2–9).[118] Dangman and Hoffman[120] found that the results of overdrive depended largely on the level of the resting or maximum diastolic potential of surviving fibers, although the rate and the length of the stimulus train were also important. Preparations with a high potential (more negative than −70 mV; "normal automaticity") were suppressed by overdrive pacing, whereas fibers with a low diastolic potential (less negative than −60 mV; "abnormal automaticity") were seldom suppressed and, in fact, showed acceleration after fast pacing rates. Rapid overdrive pacing of fibers that had an intermediate range of diastolic potential produced overdrive suppression. LeMarec and coworkers[121] reported that while 1 to 10 beats of overdrive only reset the sustained rhythm, 1 minute of overdrive pacing at a cycle length of 400 ms or less consistently caused transient hyperpolarization and slowing but not complete overdrive suppression. The studied fibers had an average maximum diastolic potential of −64 mV, the intermediate range of Dangman and Hoffman.[120] They classified their recorded response as indicative of abnormal automaticity. If sustained activity were due to triggered activity, they would have expected overdrive acceleration, a property observed by Dangman and Hoffman in preparations with a diastolic potential less negative than −60 mV.

These results and expectations are in sharp contrast to results in a preparation that has long been considered the prototypical model of triggered activity: the

FIGURE 2–5
Triggered activity arising from delayed afterdepolarizations in endocardial preparations obtained from 1-day-old canine infarction. A and B are transmembrane recordings from Purkinje cells in the ischemic zone from two different preparations.

In A, the preparation was stimulated at cycle lengths of 2000 ms, 1200 ms, and 1000 ms. Reduction of the cycle length of stimulation resulted in an increase of the amplitude of the afterdepolarization that reached threshold and initiated a run of triggered activity in the lower recording. The triggered rhythm terminated following a subthreshold delayed afterdepolarization.

In B, the effect of premature stimulation on the amplitude of the delayed afterdepolarization is demonstrated. The preparation was paced at a basic cycle length of 2500 ms. The coupling interval of the premature stimulus was shortened from 1500 ms to 1200 ms to 1000 ms. This resulted in an increase of the amplitude of the afterdepolarization that reached threshold following the short coupling interval and initiated a triggered rhythm. The rhythm terminated following a subthreshold afterdepolarization.

S = the timing of stimulation; T = time scale, representing 1-s intervals. (Reprinted by permission from El-Sherif N, Gough WB, Zeiler RH, Mehra R: Circ Res 52:566, 1983.)

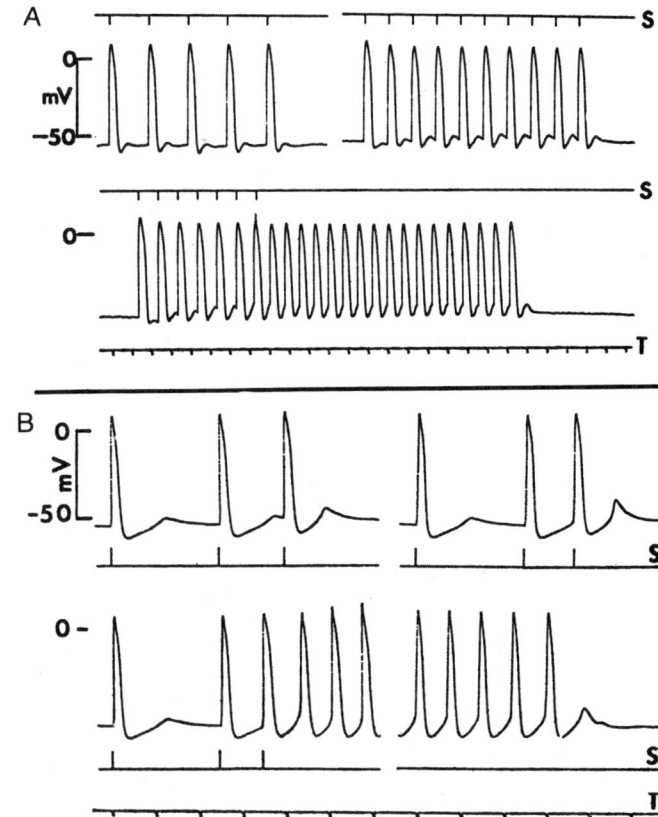

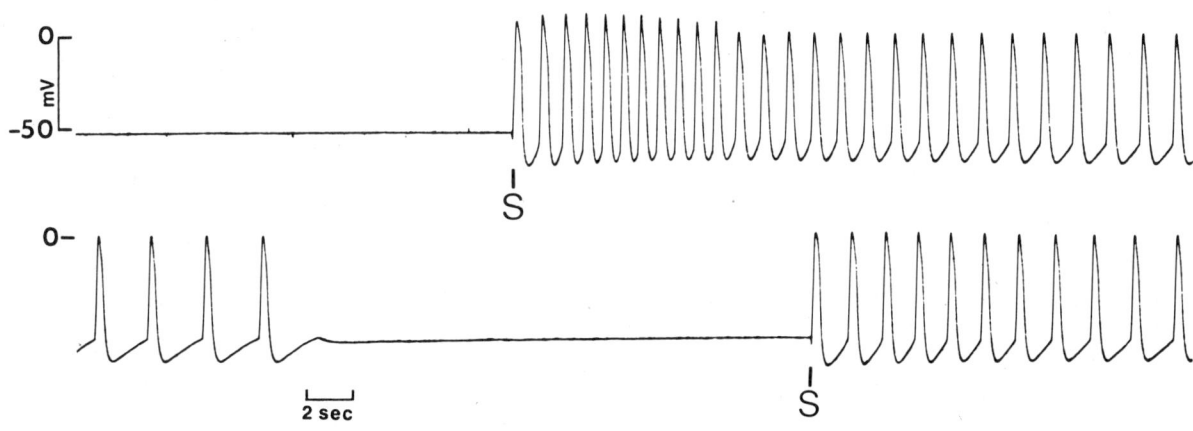

FIGURE 2–6
Initiation of triggered activity by a single stimulated action potential. Transmembrane recordings are from a Purkinje cell in the ischemic zone of an endocardial preparation from 1-day-old canine infarction. The depolarized cell (resting membrane potential, −53 mV) was quiescent. A single stimulated action potential initiated a run of triggered activity. In the bottom tracing, the activity slowed gradually and terminated following a subthreshold afterdepolarization. Following another quiescent period, triggered activity was again initiated by a single stimulated action potential.

digitalis-toxic Purkinje fiber. Overdrive pacing at a cycle length less than 300 ms was shown to terminate sustained rhythmic activity 89% of the time in the ouabain-toxic Purkinje preparation.[122] In 74% of these cases, the triggered activity persisted for 1 to 10 beats after the last paced beat (so-called afterbeats). These results in the digitalis-toxic preparation are similar to what we observed in ischemic tissue.[118]

In summary, the observations made in the above studies have been used to suggest criteria by which to differentiate whether a sustained rhythm is due to abnormal automaticity or to triggered activity. If it responds to overdrive pacing with no suppression[120] or acceleration,[121] it would be abnormal automaticity; if overdrive pacing produces suppression[120, 122] or acceleration,[121] then it could be triggered activity. However, inconsistency prohibits strict classification based on these criteria. As Cranefield and Aronson[123] concluded from review of overdrive studies, the results "are consistent with the assumption that the so-called

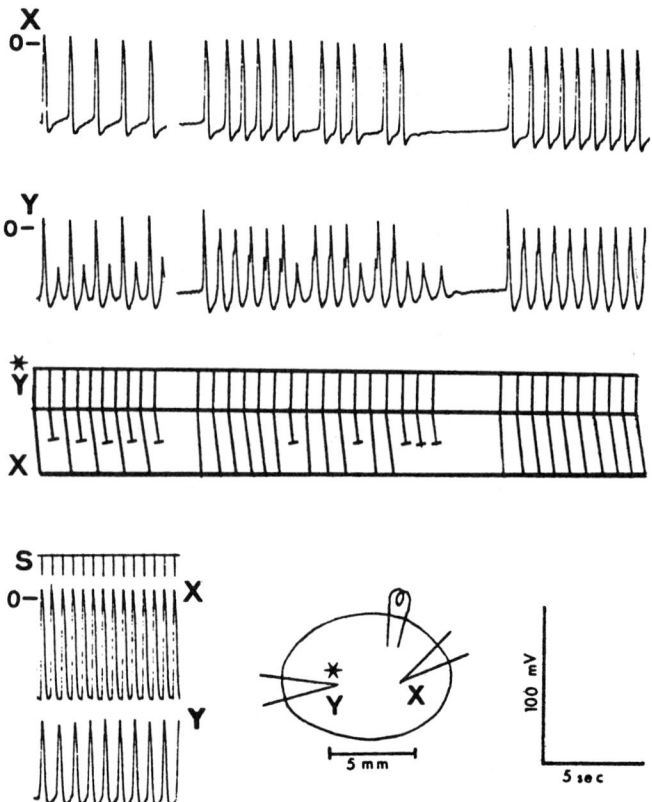

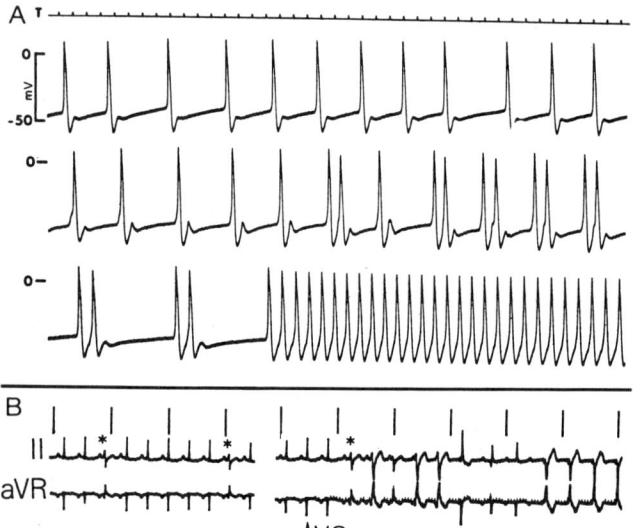

FIGURE 2–7
Extrasystolic rhythm due to triggered activity arising from delayed afterdepolarizations. A, Transmembrane recording from a Purkinje fiber in the ischemic zone of an endocardial preparation from a 1-day-old canine infarction. The upper tracing shows a background slow automatic rhythm. Each automatic action potential is followed by a low-amplitude delayed afterdepolarization. In the middle tracing, the amplitude of the delayed afterdepolarization gradually increased, reached threshold, and triggered a single action potential, resulting in a trigeminal rhythm followed by a bigeminal rhythm. In the lower tracing, a sustained triggered activity occurred when the subthreshold afterdepolarization that followed the single triggered action potential reached threshold potential. (Modified from El-Sherif N, Gough WB, Zeiler RH, Mehra R: Circ Res 52:566, 1983.)

B, Electrocardiographic tracing obtained from a dog 1 day following ligation of the left anterior descending artery. The tracing shows sinus tachycardia and extrasystolic ventricular ectopic beats with late fixed coupling (marked by *). Slight slowing of the sinus rhythm by vagal stimulation (VS) revealed the presence of a multiform ventricular rhythm. The extrasystolic beats and the multiform ventricular rhythm may be the result of triggered activity arising from delayed afterdepolarizations in ischemic Purkinje fibers surviving the infarct.

FIGURE 2–8
Intermittent parasystolic rhythm due to a triggered pacemaker, showing both entrance and exit block. Transmembrane recordings are from two Purkinje fibers (X and Y) in the ischemic zone of an endocardial preparation from a 1-day-old canine infarction (see schematic drawing). The recordings show intermittent triggered activity arising from delayed afterdepolarizations. The focus of triggered activity was probably located close to the Y recording (asterisk), and a varying degree of conduction delay and/or block occurred between the two sites. The Y recording showed electrotonic depolarizations that corresponded to the rhythmic discharge of the ectopic focus. Conduction delays between the two sites resulted in an electrotonic depolarization, followed by a second, larger upstroke in the Y recording. When conduction block occurred, the Y recording revealed only an electrotonic depolarization. In contrast to the Y recording, which could reveal the rhythmic activity of the ectopic focus, the X recording, a few millimeters distant from the ectopic focus, showed only delayed conducted action potentials. Each series of triggered activity was initiated by an action potential that was probably generated by background slow Purkinje automaticity arising from a different site in the preparation. The exit block between the focus of triggered activity and the rest of the preparation varied from 2:1 block (top left tracing) to Wenckebach periodicity (top middle tracing) to first-degree block (top right tracing). There was also a a period of repetitive conduction block at the end of the middle series of triggered activity.

Diagrammatic illustration of the conduction pattern from the ectopic focus is shown at the bottom of the upper tracings. The tracing at the lower left corner shows that when the preparation was stimulated (S) at a rate faster than the ectopic focus, entrance block was present. Besides the intermittence of the triggered activity and the varying degree of exit block, the tracings also show that there was a gradual slowing of the frequency of discharge between each new series of triggered activity. All these factors combined can make it very difficult to diagnose parasystolic rhythms in clinical records based on mathematical manipulation of interectopic intervals of manifest ectopic discharge.

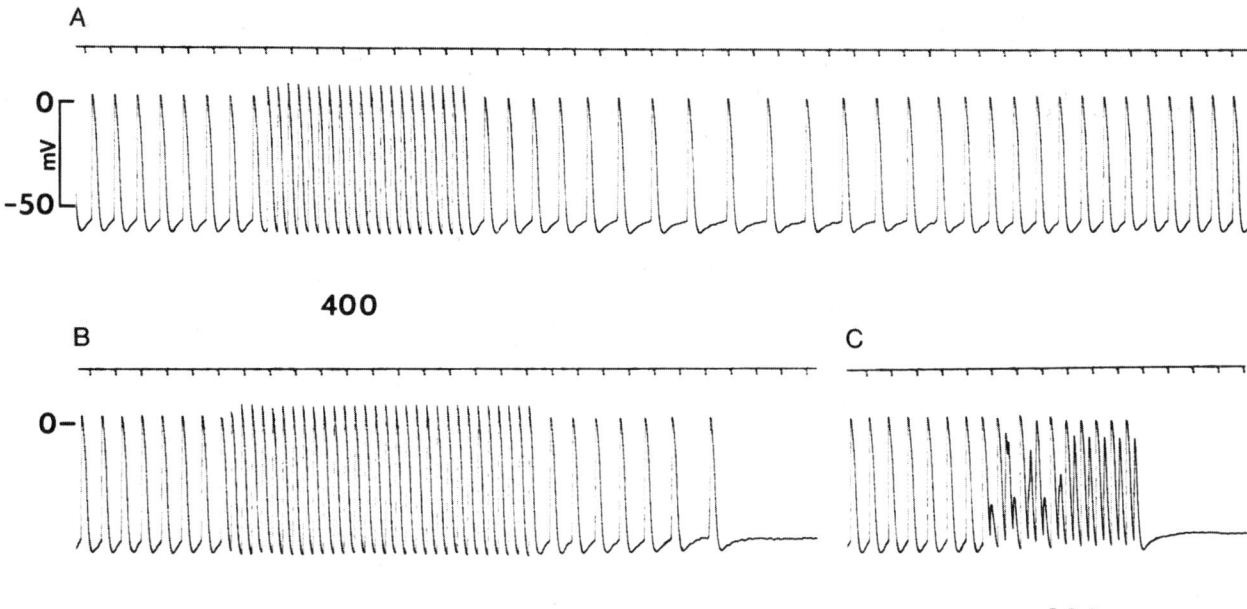

FIGURE 2–9
Termination of sustained triggered activity by a train of fast stimulation. Transmembrane recordings from a Purkinje cell in the ischemic zone of a small endocardial preparation.

A, A train of 20 stimulated impulses at a cycle length of 400 ms was followed by transient slowing of the rate of triggered rhythm before it returned to the prestimulation level. B, A longer train of stimulation (30 impulses) at a cycle length of 400 ms caused triggered activity to terminate during the slowing phase. C, Triggered activity was reinitiated, and a train of 20 stimulated impulses at a cycle length of 300 ms was immediately followed by quiescence. The time scale (T) designates 1-s intervals.

(Reprinted by permission from El-Sherif N, Gough WB, Zeiler RH, Mehra R: Circ Res 52:566, 1983.)

'abnormal automaticity' of Purkinje fibers is in fact triggered activity. . . ."

Dependence of Triggered Activity on Diastolic Potentials

Rhythmic activity in ischemic endocardial preparations is initiated in depolarized ischemic Purkinje fibers having a maximum diastolic potential averaging −59 ± 9 mV.[118] Superfusion of an ischemic preparation causes a recovery of the reduced diastolic potential toward normal resting potentials.[12, 124] During this recovery, sustained activity gives way to nonsustained activity and subthreshold DADs. At potentials between −80 mV and −85 mV, triggered activity and DADs were no longer observed.[118] Therefore, it appeared that sustained and nonsustained activity were dependent on membrane potential.

Dresdner and associates[124] have shown that intracellular K^+ activity was reduced after 24 hours of ischemia by 50.4 mM from 112 ± 19.8 mM. This K^+ loss was accompanied by a loss of the K^+ equilibrium potential. However, the loss of K^+ activity accounted for only about one half the reduction in the diastolic potential and, therefore, additional factors must be considered. The intracellular Na^+ activity of these ischemic Purkinje fibers was elevated to 15.6 ± 6.9 from 9.4 ± 2.6 ($p < 0.005$). Thus, the large loss of K^+ was not matched by an equivalent gain of Na^+. This gain of intracellular Na^+ would produce an elevation or overload of intracellular Ca^{2+}. During prolonged superfusion in vitro, both K^+ activity and the K^+-equilibrium potential returned toward normal, thereby providing an explanation for the improved diastolic potentials measured after significant superfusion.[13] The Na^+ activity decreased as the maximum diastolic potential became more negative. Partial inhibition of the Na^+-K^+ pump was measured during ischemia and may account for part of the K^+ loss and consequent depolarization.[125]

The apparent dependence of sustained activity on membrane potential was studied indirectly by LeMarec and colleagues[121] in Purkinje fibers from infarcts at 1 to 4 days. They too observed the improvement of diastolic potentials during the course of superfusion. They did not frequently record subthreshold DADs at 24 hours, but they did record subthreshold DADs more frequently at 48 to 96 hours after infarction, a time during which the maximum diastolic or resting potentials were increasing. DADs were observed especially on the second day, but rarely on the fourth day. They concluded that as time post-infarction increased and diastolic potentials returned to normal, there was a loss of abnormal automaticity, and a transient phase of triggered activity occurred.

Recordings of sustained triggered activity and abnormal automaticity would have the same appearance in a transmembrane recording. The dependence of this activity on the magnitude of diastolic potential was studied directly by the application of constant depolarizing or hyperpolarizing current.[126] This was similar to Ferrier's study[127] on the digitalis-toxic Purkinje fiber.

During sustained activity (maximum diastolic potential −61 ± 7 mV) hyperpolarizing current decreased the DADs, rendered them subthreshold, and terminated triggered activity (Fig. 2–10). During the quiescence caused by constant hyperpolarizing current, a stimulated train of action potentials produced DADs. Decreasing the current permitted augmented DADs. In quiescent preparations (resting potential −68 ± 7 mV), a train of stimulated action potentials was followed by subthreshold DADs. Depolarizing current increased the DAD amplitude. Sufficient depolarization caused triggered activity to occur (Fig. 2–11). To exclude depolarization-induced automaticity, constant currents were applied without a previous train of stimuli. Neither DADs nor triggered activity was evoked.

The main finding of this study was that in ischemic Purkinje fibers, 1 day post-infarction, there is a graded response of DADs to depolarizing currents and depolarized diastolic potentials.[126] On this basis, one can consider that the transition from nonsustained triggered activity to a sustained rhythm can be due to an enhancement of the abnormal DAD accompanying depolarization post-infarction. Similarly, a sustained rhythm can become nonsustained as a consequence of repolarization accompanying recovery from ischemia. The transition from threshold to subthreshold and vice versa can be only a 1-mV change in diastolic potential. One need not invoke a separate, intrinsically oscillatory mechanism, such as abnormal automaticity, to explain the existence of sustained versus nonsustained rhythms in the same heart or isolated preparation 1 day post-infarction. In addition, the DADs may become sufficiently suprathreshold that interventions such as overdrive pacing,[121] changes in temperature,[121, 128] or pharmacologic inhibitors[121, 129] may be unable to render these DADs subthreshold and thereby will not terminate the sustained triggered activity. Caution must be applied when concluding that such interventions might differentially distinguish sustained triggered activity from abnormal automaticity.

Ionic Mechanisms

The ionic mechanisms that produce DADs have not been studied with voltage clamp or patch clamp techniques in ischemic Purkinje fibers. The basic hypothesis for the mechanism by which charge is carried by the transient inward current that causes the DAD is derived from studies of Purkinje and ventricular muscle cells that have been overloaded with Ca^{2+} in a variety of ways. As recently reviewed,[130] there are two proposed mechanisms. The first mechanism, originally proposed by Kass and Tsien,[131] was a nonspecific cation channel, activated by a phasic rise in intracellular Ca^{2+}, which had significant permeability to Na^+, K^+ and Ca^{2+}. The inward current was thought to be carried predominantly by Na^+ with some Ca^{2+} contribution. The second proposed mechanism for transient inward current is the electrogenic Na^+-Ca^{2+} exchange pump driven by the transmembrane electrochemical gradient for Na^+ and Ca^{2+}.[132, 133] The stoichiometry for charge translocation is 3 Na^+ to 1 Ca^{2+}. Ca^{2+} overload produces a phasic release of Ca^{2+} from the sarcoplasmic reticulum into the myoplasm. This produces a transient decrease in the transmembrane Ca^{2+} gradient, which in turn facilitates Ca^{2+} extrusion and Na^+ entry by the exchanger. The electrogenicity of the exchange produces a transient inward current.

Clues to the mechanism that may be operative in ischemic Purkinje fibers have been derived by varying ionic concentrations and using specific inhibitors. An elevation of extracellular K^+ from 4 mM to 6 mM

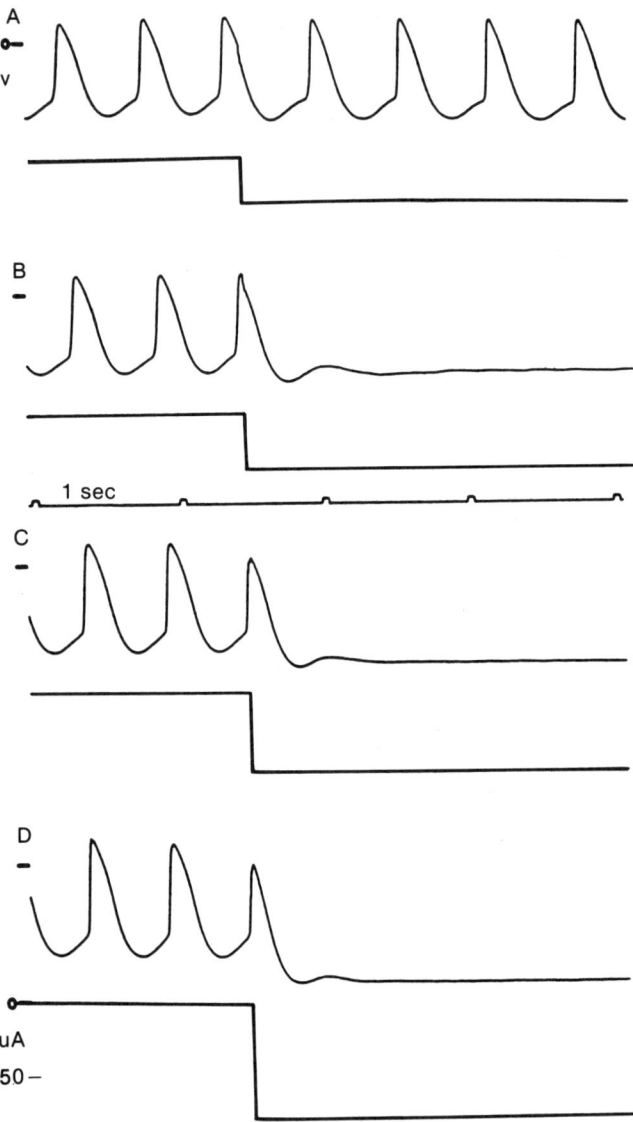

FIGURE 2–10
Effects of intermittent hyperpolarizing current during sustained activity from a canine endocardial preparation 1 day post-infarction. Hyperpolarizing current was initiated during an action potential.

A, Hyperpolarizing current prolonged the cycle length of sustained activity. B–D, Further graded increases in hyperpolarizing current produced a graded attenuation of subthreshold delayed afterdepolarizations. Calibration for transmembrane potential is shown in A, and calibration for current is shown in D. Time calibration separates B and C.

(Reprinted by permission from Gough WB, El-Sherif N: Am J Physiol 257:H770–H777, 1989.)

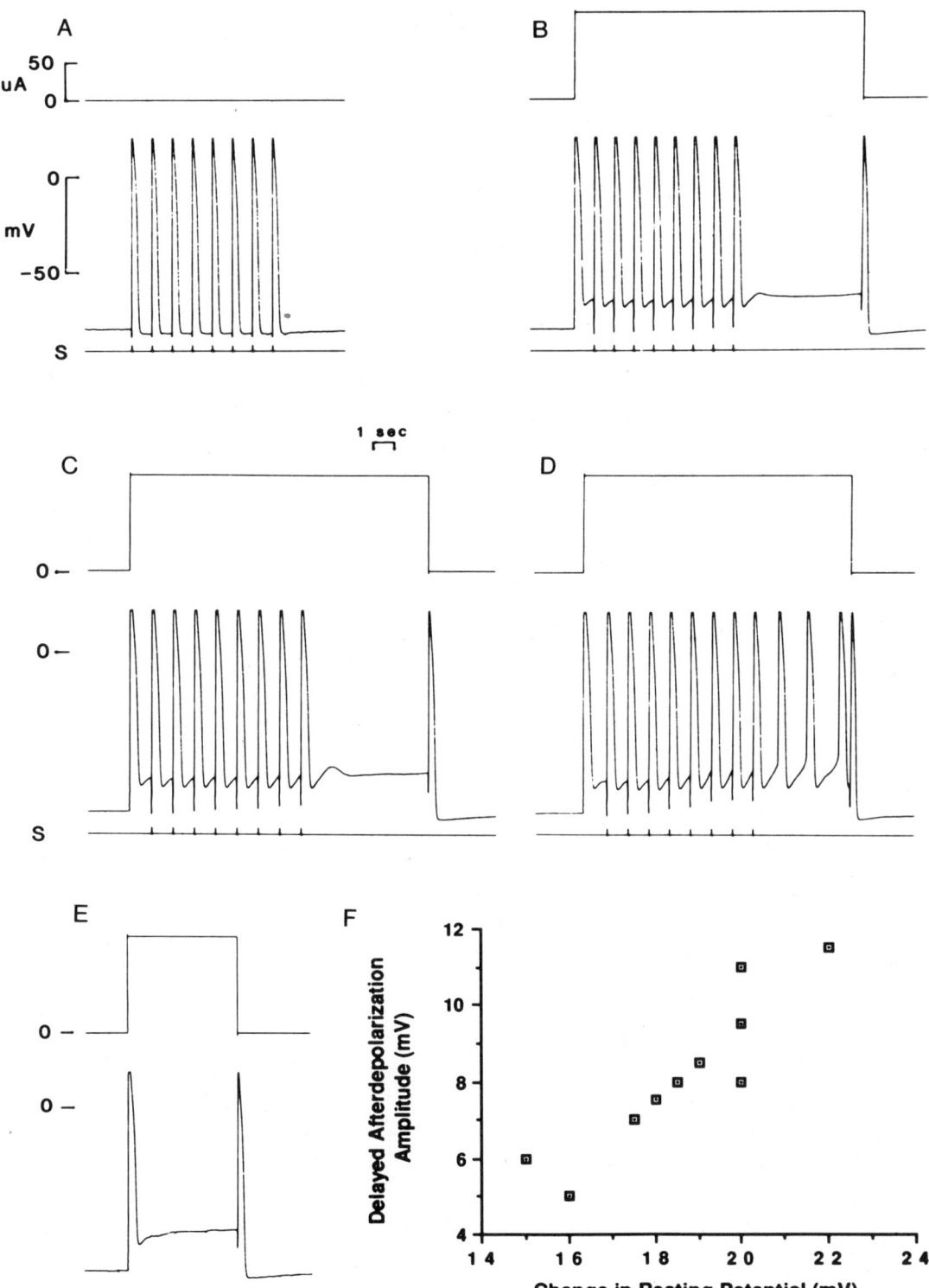

FIGURE 2–11
Effects of long depolarizing current on delayed afterdepolarization. Recordings were obtained from a canine endocardial preparation 1 day post-infarction.

A, Control. A train of 8 paced beats (cycle length = 1 s) produced no measurable delayed afterdepolarization. B and C, During long graded depolarizing current pulses initiated before stimulation, delayed afterdepolarization gradually increased in amplitude. D, Delayed afterdepolarization following the eighth beat induced triggered activity that ceased as soon as current was terminated. E, Depolarizing current equal in amplitude to that used in D produced neither a delayed afterdepolarization nor depolarization-induced automaticity. F, Amplitude of delayed afterdepolarization after the eighth driven beat is plotted as a function of change in resting potential.

(Reprinted by permission from Gough WB, El-Sherif N: Am J Physiol 257:H770–H777, 1989.)

caused suppression of DADs.[134] Therefore, the DAD is not dependent on a slight elevation of extracellular K^+. Reduction of extracellular Na^+ caused an initial enhancement of the DAD and a more rapid sustained activity. Reduced Na^+ caused a loading of the cell with Ca^{2+} and this could enhance a phasic release of Ca^{2+}. Later, triggered activity was suppressed (Fig. 2–12). Elevation of extracellular Ca^{2+} increased the amplitude of subthreshold DADs and enhanced their ability to trigger activity.[118]

The effects of ionic blockers may be direct as well as indirect. Tetrodotoxin has been shown to suppress DADs.[135] It may directly block the transient inward current or it may reduce the Na^+ inward current during the upstroke of the action potential, thereby reducing intracellular Na^+. A decreased intracellular Na^+ reduces intracellular Ca^{2+} thereby, reducing the amount of phasic Ca^{2+} release. Ca^{2+} channel blockers have been shown to reduce the rate of depolarization and amplitude of the DAD.[136] This could be a direct effect on the DAD or an indirect effect on the upstroke of the action potential that is initiated at reduced diastolic potentials. Less Ca^{2+} entering the myoplasm during the action potential would reduce the Ca^{2+} overload of the cell and, thereby, the amplitude of the DAD. Caffeine, at high concentrations (10 mM), and ryanodine, at micromolar concentrations, have been shown to reduce phasic Ca^{2+} release from the sarcoplasmic reticulum.[137] We have shown that both these agents suppress sustained triggered activity, thereby implying that this activity in ischemic fibers requires a phasic release of Ca^{2+}. When the release of Ca^{2+} from the sarcoplasmic reticulum is inhibited neither sustained nor nonsustained triggered activity occur (Fig. 2–13).

The Na^+-Ca^{2+} exchanger has been reported to be inhibited by the anthracycline antibiotic doxorubicin.[138] It successfully suppressed DADs and triggered activity both in digitalis-toxic Purkinje fibers and in 1-day ischemic subendocardial Purkinje fibers.[129] However, abnormal automaticity or sustained rhythms were not suppressed by doxorubicin in either of these preparations. Thus, the evidence, direct and indirect, suggests that Ca^{2+} overload is fundamental to the genesis of the DAD and that the Na^+-Ca^{2+} exchanger or a nonspecific cation channel may be an integral aspect of the ion-carrying mechanism underlying the DAD.

Role of Lysophosphatidylcholine

It seems clear from the studies of Dresdner and associates[124] that ischemia causes more changes intracellularly than a loss of K^+ and a gain of Na^+. One possibility is that a nonionic moiety produced during ischemia has significant effects on the membrane. A likely candidate for this is lysophosphatidylcholine (LPC), which has been shown to accumulate during acute ischemia and to permit the induction of DADs in normal Purkinje fibers.[79] When Tyrode's solution was recirculated and reoxygenated while it superfused an ischemic preparation manifesting sustained triggered activity, the triggered activity was maintained, and elevated levels of LPC (up to 5 μM) were measured in the superfusate after several hours.[139] In identical recirculation experiments that used normal tissue, there was no elevation of LPC, no reduction of the resting potentials, and no enhanced rhythmic activity. Therefore, such nonionic moieties may play an important role in the maintenance of reduced diastolic potentials and DADs.

Actions of Antiarrhythmic Agents

The effects of antiarrhythmic drugs on sustained triggered activity has been studied both in vitro and in vivo. Before triggered activity was suggested to exist, Allen et al.[140] reported that spontaneous activity 1-day post-infarction in subendocardial Purkinje fibers was significantly slowed by 20 μM lidocaine in three of four preparations, whereas it stopped activity in the fourth. In similar preparations showing sustained activity, LeMarec and colleagues[121] measured no significant effect on the cycle length with 5 μg/ml. However, when subthreshold DADs were present, lidocaine reduced their amplitude and prevented the induction of triggered activity, similar to its effects in digitalis-toxic Purkinje fibers.[141]

Ethmozin was first shown to suppress ventricular arrhythmias occurring one day post-infarction.[142] Ethmozin slows but does not abolish normal automaticity by its reduction of threshold potential. It abolishes barium-induced automaticity, terminating it with a subthreshold DAD.[143] Sustained activity, 24 hours post-infarction, was terminated with ethmozin. The termination occurred with a subthreshold DAD. During subsequent washout of ethmozin the quiescent preparation responded with subthreshold DADs and then triggered activity. Ethmozin decreased the amplitude of subthreshold DADs and abolished nonsustained triggered activity in these fibers.[143] The combination of lidocaine and ethmozin was used to construct a test by which sustained triggered activity could be differentiated from abnormal automaticity. If sustained activity was suppressed by ethmozin, it had to be either triggered activity or abnormal automaticity.[121] If it was suppressed by lidocaine, it was either normal automaticity or triggered activity. Therefore, if a preparation responded to both ethmozin and lidocaine, the underlying mechanism was concluded to be triggered activity. The problem faced by this matrix is that the level of lidocaine is crucial, because elevated lidocaine will suppress even abnormal automaticity.[140] If, as our recent study[126] suggests, there is a voltage-dependence of the DAD, then when it is raised to suprathreshold amplitudes that maintain a sustained rhythm, the level of lidocaine necessary to render it subthreshold may be in the same concentration range as that required to suppress abnormal automaticity.

Ca^{2+} channel blockers were shown to inhibit triggered activity either by directly suppressing DADs or by inducing exit block around sites of triggered activity (Fig. 2–14).[118, 136, 144] Ouabain at a concentration that has no toxic effect on normal Purkinje fibers may enhance arrhythmias in ischemic Purkinje fibers by increasing the magnitude of DAD and enhancing trig-

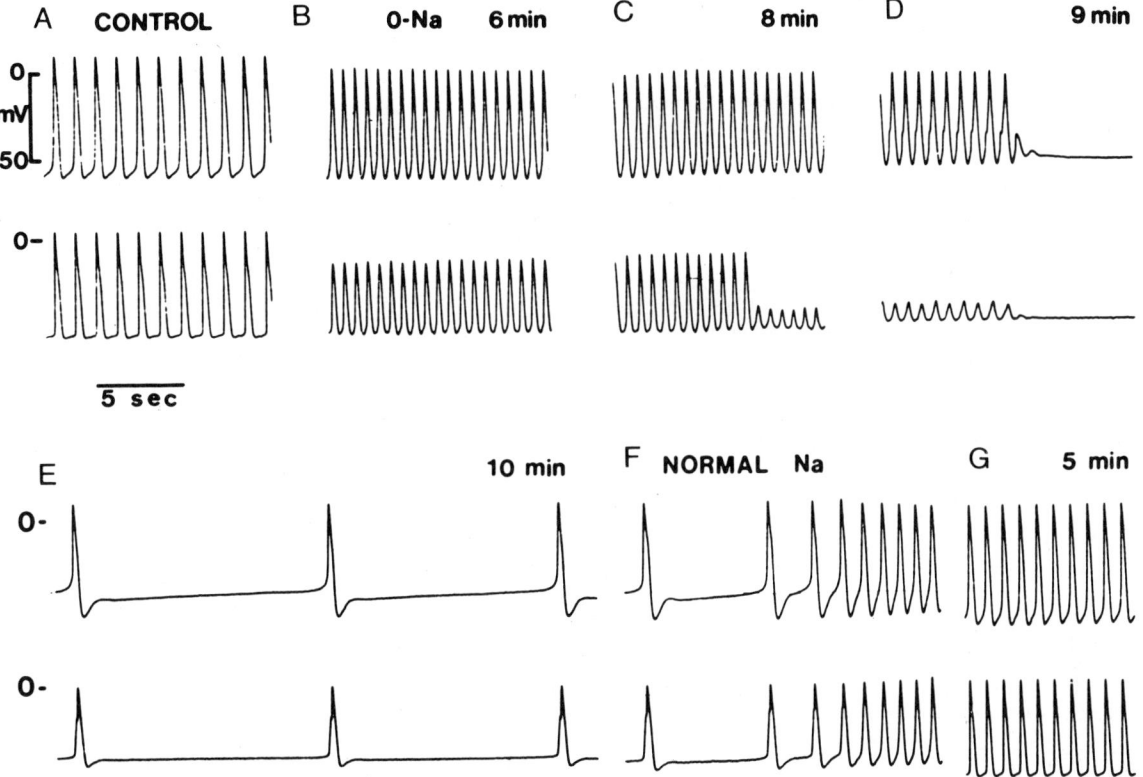

FIGURE 2–12
Effects of reduction of extracellular sodium (Na⁺) on triggered activity in 1-day-old canine infarction. Transmembrane action potential recordings were obtained from two Purkinje fibers in a 5 × 10 mm endocardial preparation from the ischemic region.

A, During control recording in normal Tyrode's solution, both fibers, separated by a distance of 3 mm, showed triggered activity at a cycle length of 1200 ms. B and C, Sodium chloride in the Tyrode's solution was replaced by choline chloride. This resulted in initial significant acceleration of the rate of triggered activity to a cycle length of 690 ms before the activity finally terminated in D. Note the occurrence of conduction block at the site of the lower recording with the recording showing electrotonic potentials synchronous with the action potentials in the upper recording. When activity terminated at the site of the upper recording, the preparation became quiescent and triggered activity could not be initiated. E, Very slow background automaticity. F and G, Return to normal Tyrode's solution. Triggered activity was reinitiated by the slow background automaticity similar to that shown in Figure 2–7.

FIGURE 2–13
Effects of 10^{-7} M ryanodine on sustained rhythmic activity of subendocardial Purkinje fibers from 1-day-old canine infarction. Left panel shows sustained rhythmic activity recorded during control. Ten minutes after superfusion with ryanodine, the rate of sustained rhythmic activity slowed, and the activity terminated with a subthreshold delayed afterdepolarization (middle panel). After 30 minutes of superfusion with ryanodine, stimulated trains failed to induce delayed afterdepolarizations or rhythmic activity (right panel). The time scale represents 1-s intervals.

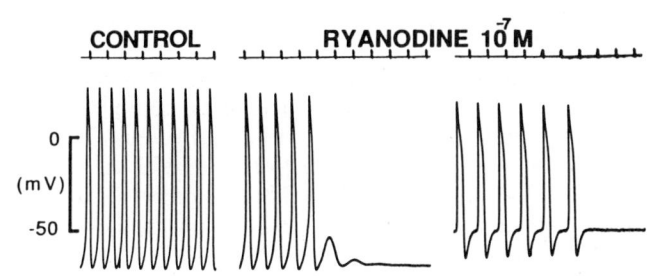

Electrophysiology of Ventricular Arrhythmias in Myocardial Ischemia and Infarction   31

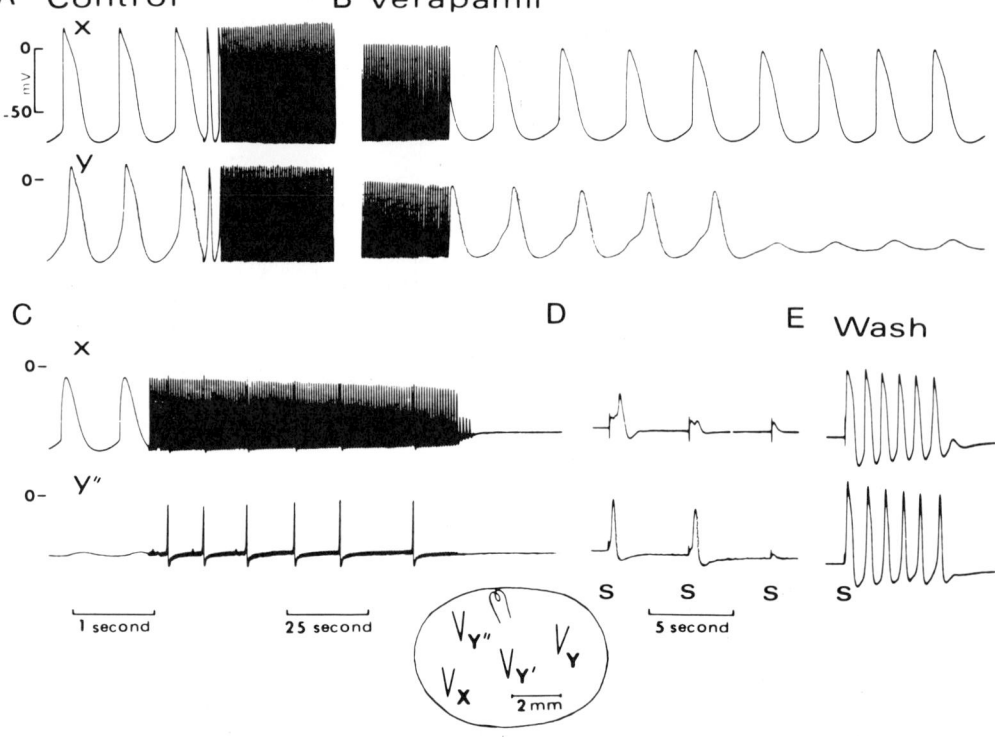

FIGURE 2–14
Induction of exit block from site of triggered activity by verapamil. Simultaneous transmembrane recordings from different Purkinje fibers in a small infarcted preparation from a 1-day-old canine infarction.

A, Control triggered activity. Exploring the preparation showed that the earliest activity was recorded close to site X, whereas the rest of the preparation was activated 20–60 ms later. B, Ten minutes of superfusion with verapamil (2.2×10^{-6} M) resulted in slowing of the rate of rhythmic activity, depression of action potentials, and increased delay between X and Y before complete conduction block developed. The microelectrode at Y then was moved to two new sites (Y' and Y"). Both sites showed low-amplitude electrotonic potentials simultaneous with action potentials at X. This suggested the rhythmic activity originated from a site close to X and that exit block developed between this site and the rest of the preparation.

C, Five minutes later, the action potential at X showed a gradual decrease in amplitude and maximum diastolic potential before the activity spontaneously terminated, at which time the preparation became quiescent. D, The preparation was stimulated (S) and a Wenckebach-type conduction block developed. E, Ten minutes of washout of verapamil resulted in improvement of the stimulated action potential and reinitiation of a triggered rhythm.

(Reprinted by permission from El-Sherif N, Gough WB, Zeiler RH, Mehra R: Cir Res 52:566, 1983.)

gered activity.[145] It was postulated that the common action of ischemia and digitalis in causing an increase in intracellular Ca^{2+} may work synergistically to cause DAD and triggered activity in Purkinje fibers. This may represent the mechanism responsible for increased susceptibility to digitalis toxicity in patients with ischemic heart disease.

The increased sensitivity of ischemic Purkinje fibers to the toxic effects of type III antiarrhythmic drugs was first shown in a study of clofilium.[146] During the course of in vitro superfusion, triggered activity ceased as the maximum diastolic potential improved. To these recovering Purkinje fibers, resting potential of -77 ± 5 mV, clofilium produced oscillatory early afterdepolarizations at concentrations that had no such effect on normal Purkinje fibers (resting potential of -86 ± 3 mV) (Fig. 2–15). These early afterdepolarizations were able to trigger activity in adjacent myocardium (Fig. 2–16). This preferential sensitivity of ischemic fibers to type III drugs was also observed with D-sotalol and bretylium.[147] The mechanism of this differential sensitivity may be due to the differences arising from the reduced maximum diastolic potential in ischemic Purkinje fibers. Snyders and Katzung[148] have reported that clofilium inhibits outward plateau current (i_K) in isolated myocytes, and Carmeliet[149] has measured similar changes due to sotalol. Dresdner and coworkers[124] have shown that these Purkinje fibers have reduced intracellular K and a reduced K equilibrium potential. These conditions could reduce i_K permeability and driving force to magnitudes that might support oscillations at plateau potentials.

TRIGGERED ACTIVITY STUDIED IN VIVO

Studies to demonstrate or disprove in vivo the occurrence of triggered rhythms post-infarction have relied on being able to record the initiation or termination of such triggered rhythms. During a sustained rhythm, interventions have been tried that had successfully suppressed triggered activity in vitro. The first approach[150] suppressed the sustained ventricular rhythms with the Ca^{2+} channel blocker verapamil, after beta-adrenergic blockade. These spontaneous ventric-

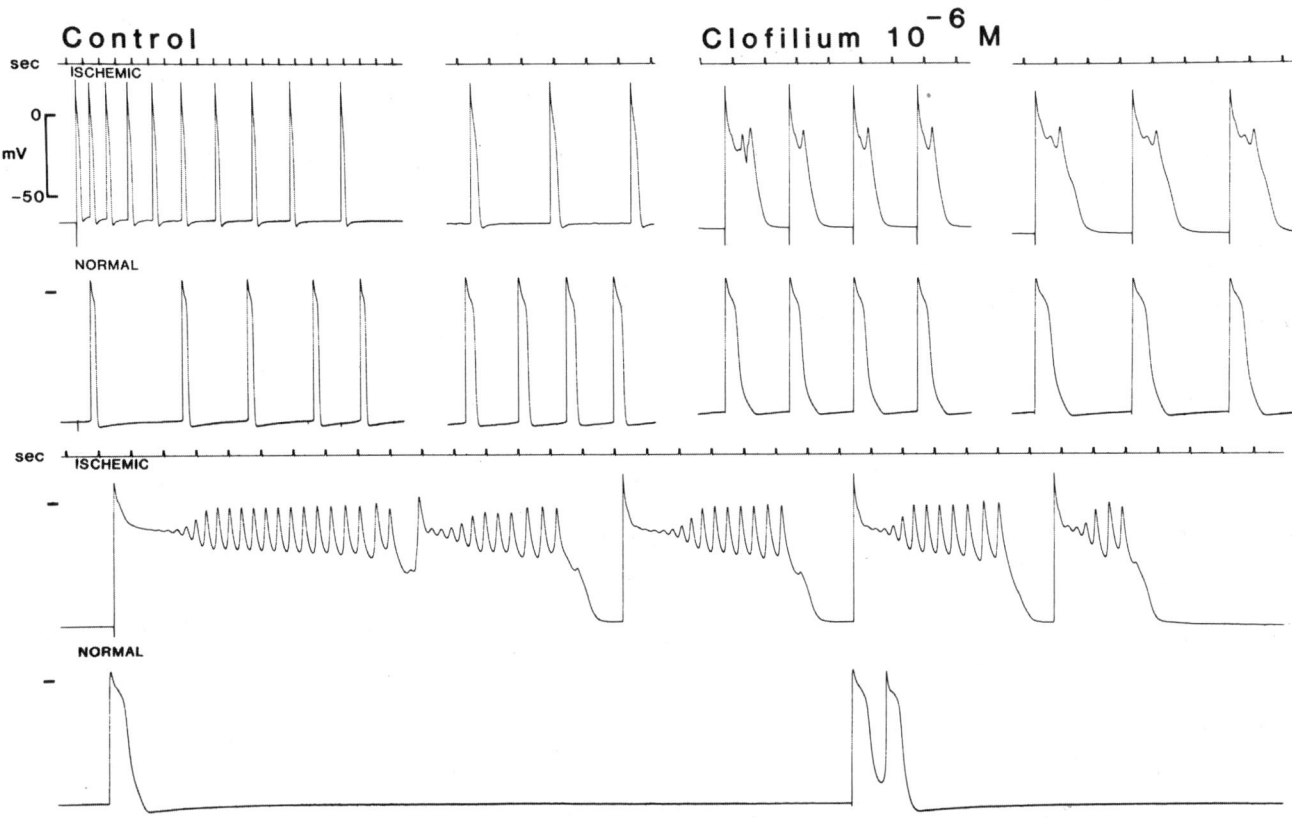

FIGURE 2–15
Transmembrane action potentials recorded from normal Purkinje fiber and ischemic subendocardial Purkinje fiber 1 day after infarction, demonstrating triggered activity from early afterdepolarizations in the ischemic fiber when perfused with clofilium. Under control conditions, in Tyrode's solution both fibers showed diastolic depolarization. In the ischemic preparation, triggered activity from delayed afterdepolarizations was observed. One stimulus evoked an action potential that was followed by a delayed afterdepolarization, which in turn initiated spontaneous action potential formation. The triggered activity started with a cycle length of 900 ms and gradually increased to a cycle length of approximately 3 s. After further superfusion, only a slow pacemaker activity persisted at a cycle length of 2.5 s.

After introducing clofilium into the perfusatae at 10^{-6} M and pacing at a cycle length of 2 s, early afterdepolarizations (EADs) occurred during the plateau of the action potential of the ischemic Purkinje fiber at a coupling interval of 500 ms. The normal action potential was prolonged only in phases 2 and 3 and showed no early or delayed afterpotentials. At a driven cycle length of 3 s, repolarization of the ischemic cell was more prolonged and was accompanied by EADs.

When the preparation was permitted to remain quiescent for periods of >30 s (bottom tracing) EADs developed in the ischemic fiber at a low membrane potential (in the range of −15 to −35 mV) and continued with a cycle length of 300 to 500 ms, thereby extending the duration of the action potential to beyond 10 s. Generally, the membrane potential of the nadir of the EADs became progressively greater during the plateau until repolarization was completed or reexcitation occurred. The normal Purkinje fiber showed slowing of late phase 3 repolarization consistent with EADs at high membrane potential that gave rise to a single triggered action potential.

(Reprinted by permission of the American College of Cardiology from Gough WB, El-Sherif N: J Am Coll Cardiol 11:431, 1986.)

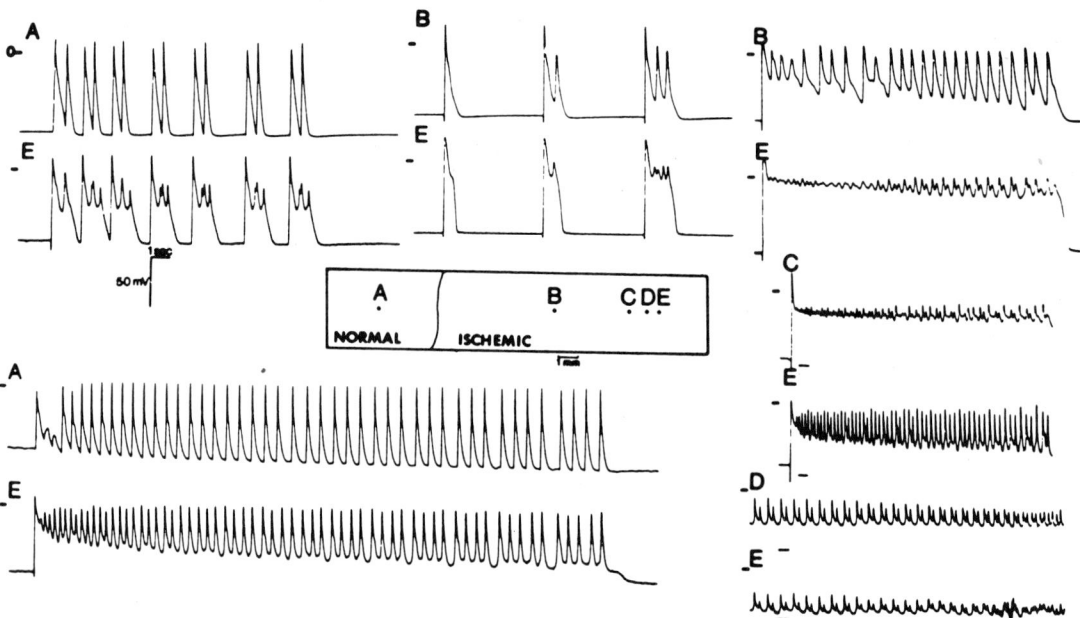

FIGURE 2–16
In vitro recordings from a canine endocardial preparation 1 day post-infarction. Transmembrane potentials were recorded from a normal site in the basal papillary muscle (site A) and the adjacent ischemic sites (sites B to E) during superfusion of 10^{-6} M clofilium, illustrating the ability of clofilium-induced EADs in ischemic endocardium to trigger activity in adjacent normal tissue.

Simultaneous records from site A (normal) and site E (ischemic) show that not all EAD-induced triggered activity in the ischemic region produced 1:1 activity in the normal area. A single stimulus to the ischemic area produced a rapid succession of action potentials, with up to three EADs (500 ms cycle length) in each. No more than one of these EADs was accompanied by activity in normal tissue. The resultant rhythm in the normal tissue was a bigeminal rhythm that became quiescent when the ischemic area became quiescent. After a pause of >1 minute, a single stimulus to the ischemic area produced an action potential 30 seconds long at site E (lower left). Activity at site A resembled aborted premature action potentials for two beats and then a sustained burst of activity (600 ms cycle length). The relation of EAD-induced triggered activity (cycle lengths as short as 250 ms) at site E to activity at site A soon resembled varying degrees of Wenckebach conduction, terminating finally when conduction was 5:4.

The transmission of EADs from one area of the ischemic region to other areas within the ischemic region was not homogeneous. To determine the distance over which there was synchrony of activity in the ischemic area, activity separated by 1.5 mm (sites C and E) and 0.5 mm (sites D and E) were studied. The closest resemblance to synchrony was observed between sites D and E (lower right). This record includes only plateau activity, and not the entire action potential.

The horizontal bar to the left of each recording is 0 mV. Note the compressed time scale in pair C and E and pair D and E. The horizontal bar beneath each record represents 1 second. (Reprinted by permission of the American College of Cardiology from Gough WB, El-Sherif N: J Am Coll Cardiol 11:431, 1988.)

ular rhythms were later shown to be modulated by adrenergic stimulation,[151] and so it is not surprising that beta-adrenergic blockade plus a Ca^{2+} channel blocker were necessary to successfully suppress these arrhythmias. Once the sustained rhythm was suppressed, it could be reinitiated by one or more stimulated beats (Fig. 2–17). Isochronal mapping studies excluded a circus movement reentry and showed a focal origin of activity from the Purkinje fibers that had survived the infarct.[152] Either intravenous catecholamines or intravenous Ca^{2+} enhanced the ability to induce triggered ventricular rhythms. The assumption was that the rhythm induced after Ca^{2+} channel blockade had the same mechanism as it did before the blockade.

The ability to record DADs in vivo was accomplished by Hariman and colleagues,[153] using the same technique they had used to record diastolic potentials in the sinus node—namely, the high-gain, low-pass filtered electrogram. Using a small apical infarction and multiple electrodes, the point of earliest activation was recorded to have a negative diastolic slope and an upstroke preceding each ventricular complex. Upon termination of a nonsustained rhythm, multiple rhythmic, slow, negative diastolic potentials were recorded before the quiescence. These potentials were consistent with subthreshold DADs (Fig. 2–18).

Evidence from Overdrive Pacing In Vivo

The development of ventricular rhythms beginning two hours after ligation up until 24 hours has been studied in the presence of AV block.[154] Nonsustained bursts of ventricular activity gave way to more sustained tachycardias. Accompanying an increase in the rate of the tachycardia was a decline in its response to overdrive pacing. While some dogs did not respond to overdrive pacing with immediate suppression, others responded with acceleration and then suppression, leading to the conclusion that triggered rhythms were present.

LeMarec and coworkers[121] applied pacing protocols in vivo to conscious dogs 1 day post-infarction. Pacing for 1 to 10 beats or for a minute of rapid overdrive rate did not cause a significant suppression or enhance-

FIGURE 2–17
Effect of propranolol and verapamil on spontaneous ventricular rhythms in 1-day-old canine infarction. *A*, Control electrocardiographic and arterial pressure recordings. A multiform ventricular rhythm (rate, 120/min) in the first half of the recording was gradually overdriven by a slightly faster sinus rhythm (rate, 125/min). Mean arterial pressure was 100 mm Hg during the control ventricular rhythm and increased to 120 mm Hg during the sinus rhythm. *B* was obtained 4 minutes following the administration of 1 mg/kg propranolol and 0.4 mg/kg verapamil. Mean arterial pressure decreased to 95 mm Hg (5% lower than control). The sinus rhythm was suppressed by vagal stimulation in order to be able to monitor the changes in the ventricular rhythm. The rate of the spontaneous ventricular rhythm gradually decreased to 105/min before it abruptly terminated, resulting in cardiac asystole. The asystolic period was terminated after 10 seconds by resumption of the sinus rhythm when vagal stimulation (VS) was turned off.

The recording in *C* was obtained a few seconds later and shows that the rate of the sinus rhythm was slower (100/min), compared with control, and the PR interval was significantly increased. A ventricular rhythm was reinitiated at a slightly faster rate of 104/min.

D was obtained 3 minutes later. The heart was again controlled by the sinus rhythm, and when this was suppressed by vagal stimulation (arrow) a single ventricular ectopic beat occurred. The asystolic interval that followed was terminated after 8 seconds by the introduction of two successive ventricular paced beats at a cycle length of 420 ms that reinitiated a ventricular rhythm at a rate of 75/min. S refers to the timing of ventricular stimulation. The heavy time lines represent 1-s intervals.

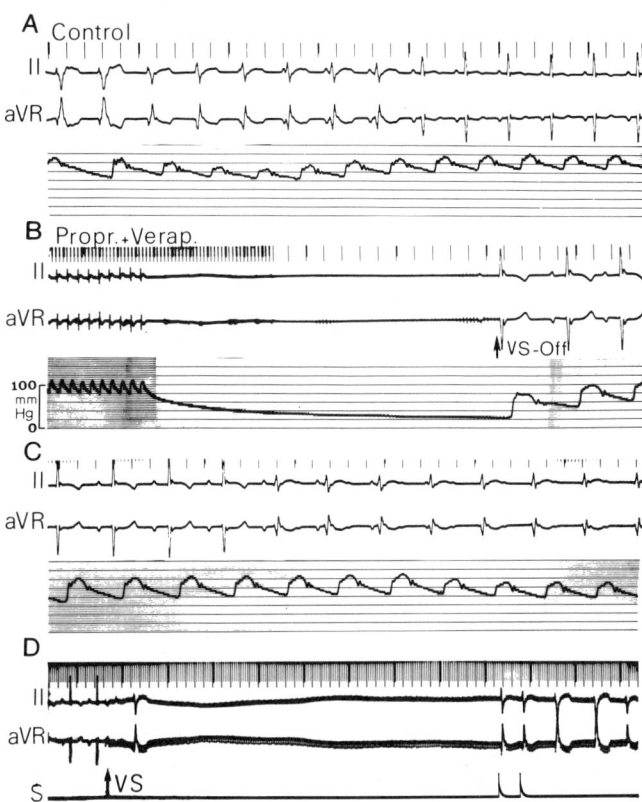

ment of the sustained rhythm. They expected that a triggered rhythm would show either acceleration or suppression and therefore concluded that none of the hearts acted as if a triggered rhythm were present. However, to further test whether the in situ heart might show triggered rhythms, dogs at 2 to 4 days post-infarction were studied. Triggered rhythms were induced in three of eight animals. Malafatto and Rosen[155] showed that in two of seven hearts studied 24 hours post-infarction, overdrive pacing during a sinus rhythm elicited a burst of accelerated ventricular tachycardia suggestive of a triggered rhythm. When these workers wished to validate a new in vivo model of triggered atrial activity, they used the results of their studies in the dog, 24 to 72 hours post-infarction, as a standard of triggered activity in vivo.

The results of these studies suggest that in vivo triggered rhythms exist post-infarction in the ventricles. Triggered rhythms are easier to elucidate at times later than 1 day post-infarction, if no antagonistic drugs are to be used. However, the possibility still remains that the same mechanism that supports nonsustained triggered activity is present at such a magnitude at 1 day post-infarction that it is not easily suppressed with overdrive protocols. There may be no precise response of sustained activity to overdrive pacing alone that permits differentiation of the underlying mechanism. The assumption is that, in ischemic tissue, abnormal automaticity and triggered activity are distinct entities, whereas in fact they may be a continuous manifestation of the same mechanism.

Reentrant Ventricular Rhythms in the Subacute Phase of Myocardial Infarction

In 1977, El-Sherif and associates[15–17] made the observation that in dogs that survived the initial stage of myocardial infarction arrhythmias, and that were studied 3 to 5 days post-infarction, reentrant ventricular rhythms occurred spontaneously but were more commonly induced by programmed electrical stimulation. The anatomic and electrophysiologic substrates for the reentrant rhythms were later characterized in a series of reports.[152, 156–164] These studies have shown that reentrant excitation occurred around zones (arcs) of functional conduction block. The arcs were attributed to ischemia-induced spatially nonhomogeneous lengthening of refractoriness. Sustained reentrant tachycardia was found to have a figure-eight activation pattern whereby clockwise and counterclockwise wavefronts were oriented around two separate arcs of functional conduction block. The two circulating wavefronts coalesced into a common wavefront that conducted slowly between the two arcs of block. Using reversible cooling, reentrant excitation could be successfully terminated only from localized areas along the common reentrant wavefront.[158]

ANATOMIC AND ELECTROPHYSIOLOGIC SUBSTRATES OF REENTRANT EXCITATION

After left anterior descending coronary artery ligation in dogs, blood flow is reduced more in the subendo-

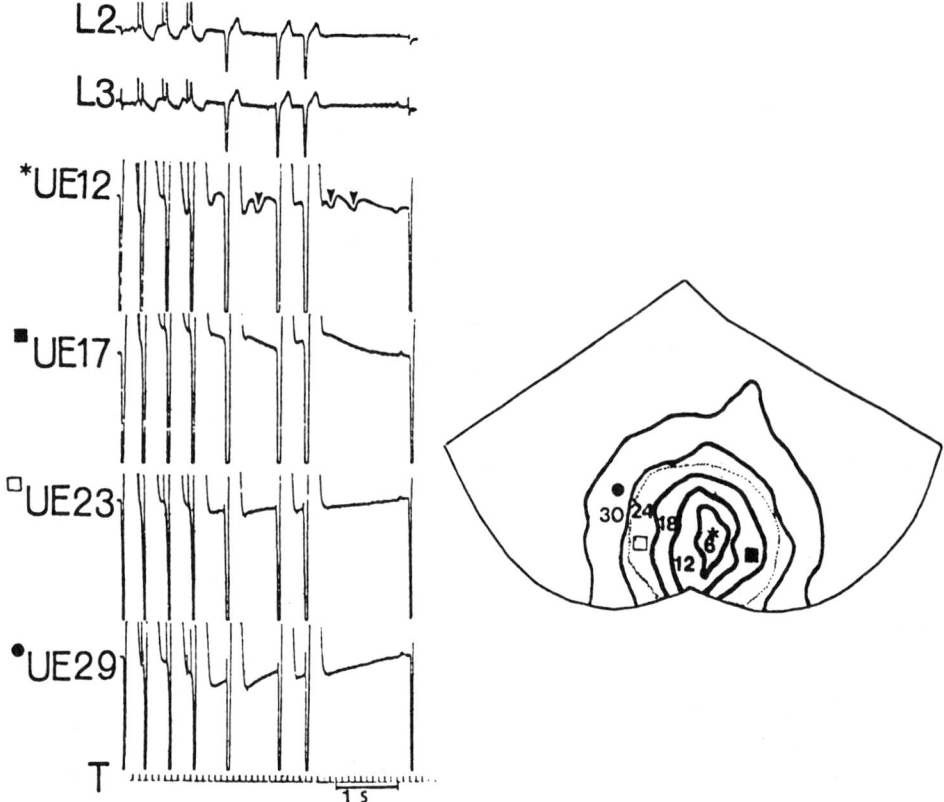

FIGURE 2–18
Recordings obtained from a dog 1 day following the creation of a small apical myocardial infarction by ligation of multiple distal branches of the left anterior and circumflex coronary arteries. The surface electrocardiographic leads show three stimulated ventricular beats at a cycle length of 400 ms followed by three spontaneous ventricular beats. Four unipolar electrograms (UE) recorded with high amplifications are displayed.

The diagram on the right shows the locations of the electrodes on the endocardial surface of the heart. The infarction is indicated by the dotted line. Numbers in the diagram indicate 6-ms isochrones. Negative-going diastolic slopes preceded the major ventricular deflections in the area of the earliest activation (UE 12 and 17). Positive-going slopes preceded the major ventricular deflection in unipolar electrograms recorded from areas remote to the area of earliest activity (UE 23 and 29). Note that slow negative-going potentials (arrowheads) were recorded from the area of earliest activity during the long diastolic interval between the first and second spontaneous beats and following the third beat. These potentials may represent subthreshold delayed afterdepolarizations that failed to propagate.

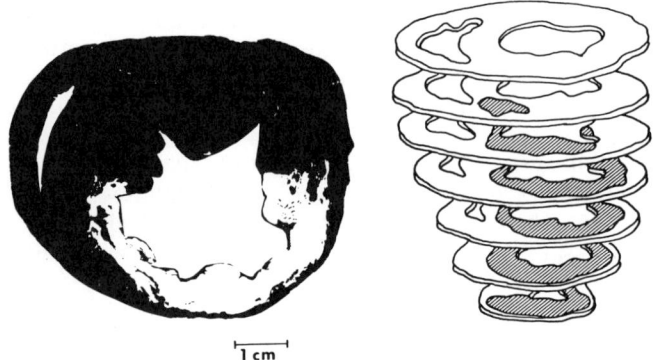

FIGURE 2–19
Anatomic characteristics of the infarction 4 days post-ligation of the left anterior descending coronary artery in the dog. On the right is a composite drawing of sections stained with nitro-blue tetrazolium. The shaded area represents necrotic tissue. The infarction is localized to the anteroseptal region and extends to the endocardial surface. A layer of surviving epicardium of varying thickness is present in all the sections. On the left is a photograph of the fourth section from the top. The dark-stained zone represents normal myocardium; the necrotic areas are unstained.

cardium, and resistance to flow in the infarcted tissue causes a redistribution of flow in the epicardial layers. Combined with the enlargement of collateral vessels, this results in sufficient flow to the epicardium that it usually survives.[165] Although the geometry of the infarction varies in different experiments, pathologic studies consistently reveal a layer of surviving epicardial tissue overlying the core of necrotic myocardium (Fig. 2–19). The epicardial layer varies in thickness from a few cells to a few millimeters, as verified histologically. The surviving epicardial layer is generally wedge-shaped, with more depth at the border than at the central portion of the infarction. Although the surviving epicardial layer looks intact on microscopic examination, this layer has a reduced myocardial blood flow.[165]

Intracellular recordings from the surviving "ischemic" epicardial layer show cells with variable degrees of partial depolarization, reduced action potential amplitude, and decreased upstroke velocity.[166–168] Full recovery of responsiveness frequently outlasts the action potential duration, reflecting the presence of postrepolarization refractoriness.[166, 167] In these cells, premature stimuli could elicit graded responses over a wide range of coupling intervals. Slowed conduction, Wenckebach periodicity, and 2:1 or higher degrees of conduction block could be easily induced by fast pacing or premature stimulation (Fig. 2–20). Isochronal mapping studies have shown that both the arcs of functional conduction block and the slow activation wavefronts of the reentrant circuit develop in the surviving electrophysiologically abnormal epicardial layer overlying the infarction.

The ionic changes induced by ischemia that explain abnormal transmembrane action potentials of myocardial cells in the subacute phase of myocardial infarction have not been fully explored. Some studies suggest that ischemic transmembrane action potentials may be generated by a depressed fast Na^+ channel. This was based on experiments that showed that ischemic cells are sensitive to the depressant effect of the fast channel blocker tetrodotoxin (TTX), but not to the slow channel blocker methoxyverapamil (D600) (Fig. 2–21).[166, 167] The fast channel may be depressed in ischemia for various reasons. This can only be partly explained by cellular depolarization, because the depression is usually out of proportion to the degree of depolarization of the resting potential.[168] The Na^+-K^+ pump may be depressed in surviving ischemic myocardial cells, leading to intracellular Na^+ loading.[169] This can diminish the electrochemical driving force for the inward Na^+ current.

Ultrastructural changes of the sarcolemmal membrane, as well as the effects of products released by ischemia, including lysophosphoglycerides,[170] have been implicated. Abnormal membrane properties of ischemic myocardial cells may not be the only cause for slowed conduction and block in the surviving ischemic epicardial layer. Electrical uncoupling and increase of extracellular resistance after ischemia have also been suggested.[171] Ischemia-induced increase in intracellular Ca^{2+} and low pH may increase the resistance of the gap junctions of the intercalated disc.[172]

Another factor that was considered by some authors is the anisotropic structure of the surviving epicardial layer.[173, 174] The epicardial muscle fibers are closely packed together and arranged parallel to each other in a direction generally perpendicular to the left anterior descending artery. Conduction in the direction along the long axis of myocardial fibers is more rapid than in the transverse direction.[175–178] The slower conduction in the transverse direction is due to higher axial resistivity, which may be partly explained by fewer and shorter intercalated discs in a side-to-side direction.[176] The normal uniform anisotropic conduction properties of the epicardial layer may be altered further following ischemia.

It was suggested that the site of conduction block of premature stimuli in the ischemic epicardial layer may be determined by its anisotropic properties (i.e., premature stimuli block along the long axis of epicardial muscle fibers).[178] We have shown that functional conduction block of premature stimuli in the ischemic epicardial layer is due to abrupt and discrete change in refractoriness. The spatially nonuniform refractory distribution occurs both along and across fiber direction, the same as the arcs of conduction block.[179]

EPICARDIAL ACTIVATION PATTERNS OF REENTRANT EXCITATION INDUCED BY PREMATURE STIMULATION

One to five days post-infarction in the canine heart, reentrant rhythms could be induced by the introduction of one or more premature stimuli (S_2S_3) during regular cardiac pacing (S_1) at relatively long cycle lengths (Fig. 2–22). Isochronal activation maps during S_1 usually show relatively fast conduction over the epicardial surface of the infarction. In a few dogs, however, areas of conduction block and slow conduction could be seen during S_1. In some of these areas, myocardial necrosis was seen to extend to the epicardial surface or within a few cell layers from the surface. The introduction of S_2 results in the development of an arc of unidirectional conduction block forcing the activation wavefront to travel around the two ends of the arc. The arc of conduction block is functional in nature and does not exist during S_1 stimulation.

The length of the arc of conduction block and the degree of slow conduction distal to the arc are crucial factors for the creation of a reentrant circuit. A premature beat that successfully initiates reentry results in a longer arc of conduction block and/or slower conduction compared with one that fails to induce reentry. When a single premature stimulus (S_2) fails to initiate reentry, the introduction of a second premature stimulus (S_3) may be necessary. S_3 usually results in a longer arc of conduction block and/or slower conduction around the arc. The slower activation wavefront travels around a longer more circuitous route, thus providing more time for refractoriness to expire along the proximal side of the arc of unidirectional block. Reexcitation of this site will initiate reentry. The beat that initiates the first reentrant cycle, whether it is an S_2 or an S_3, results in a continuous arc of conduction

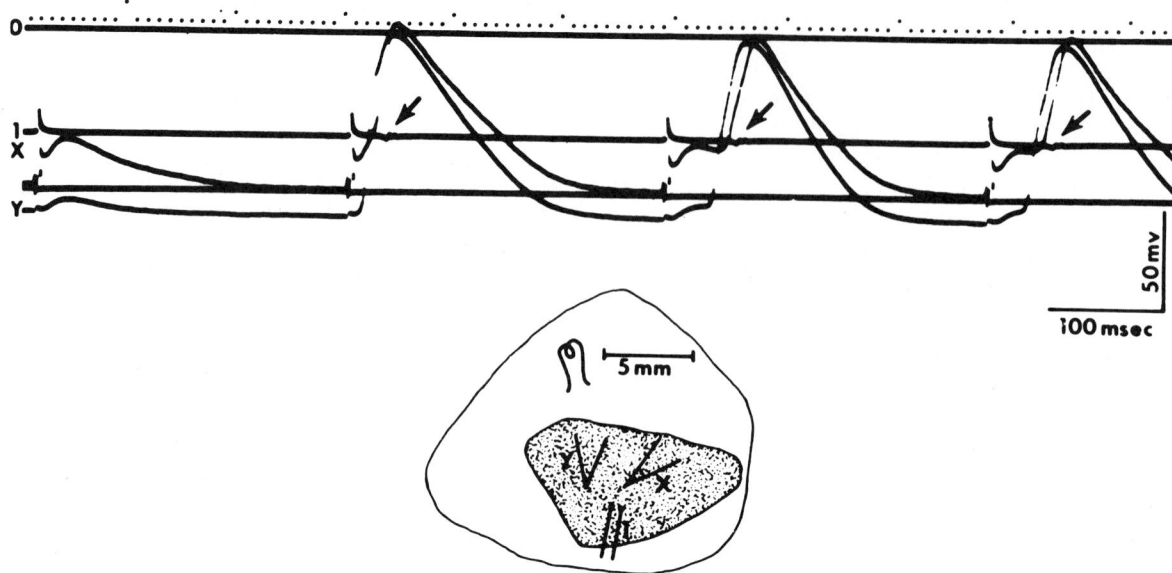

FIGURE 2–20
Recordings from a dog with 3-day old infarction illustrating action potential characteristics in ischemic epicardium. The sketch of the preparation shows two intracellular recordings (X and Y) and a close bipolar recording (I) from the infarction zone (hatched area). Ischemic cells had decreased upstroke velocity, reduced action potential amplitude, and a variable degree of partial depolarization. The two cells were recorded 5 mm apart in the infarction zone, but showed significant difference in their resting potential. The resting potential of the Y cell was only slightly reduced (−80 mV), but it still had a poor action potential. The preparation was stimulated at a cycle length of 290 ms, which resulted in a Wenckebach-like conduction pattern. Note that the pacing cycle length exceeded the action potential duration of the two cells, suggesting that refractoriness extended beyond the completion of the action potential (i.e., postrepolarization refractoriness). (Reprinted by permission of the American Heart Association, Inc., from El-Sherif N, Lazzara R: Circulation 6:605, 1979.)

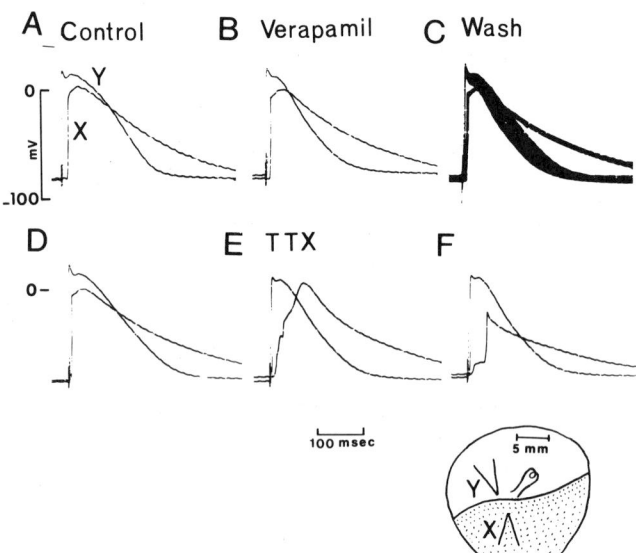

FIGURE 2–21
Action potential recordings of an ischemic (X) and normal (Y) myocardial cells from an epicardial preparation from a 3-day-old canine infarction, comparing the effects of tetrodotoxin (TTX) and verapamil. The resting potential of the ischemic cell was similar to that of the normal cell at −82 mV. However, the ischemic cell had a reduced action potential amplitude, decreased upstroke velocity, and a prolonged action potential duration.

Verapamil (1×10^{-6} g/ml) had no significant effect on the ischemic cell but resulted in acceleration of the early repolarization phase of the normal cell. On the other hand, TTX (1×10^{-6} g/ml) resulted in marked depression of the ischemic action potential with fractionation of the upstroke and, later, abbreviation of the action potential due to loss of the large amplitude hump on the plateau. This was associated with evidence of conduction delay and block in the ischemic zone.

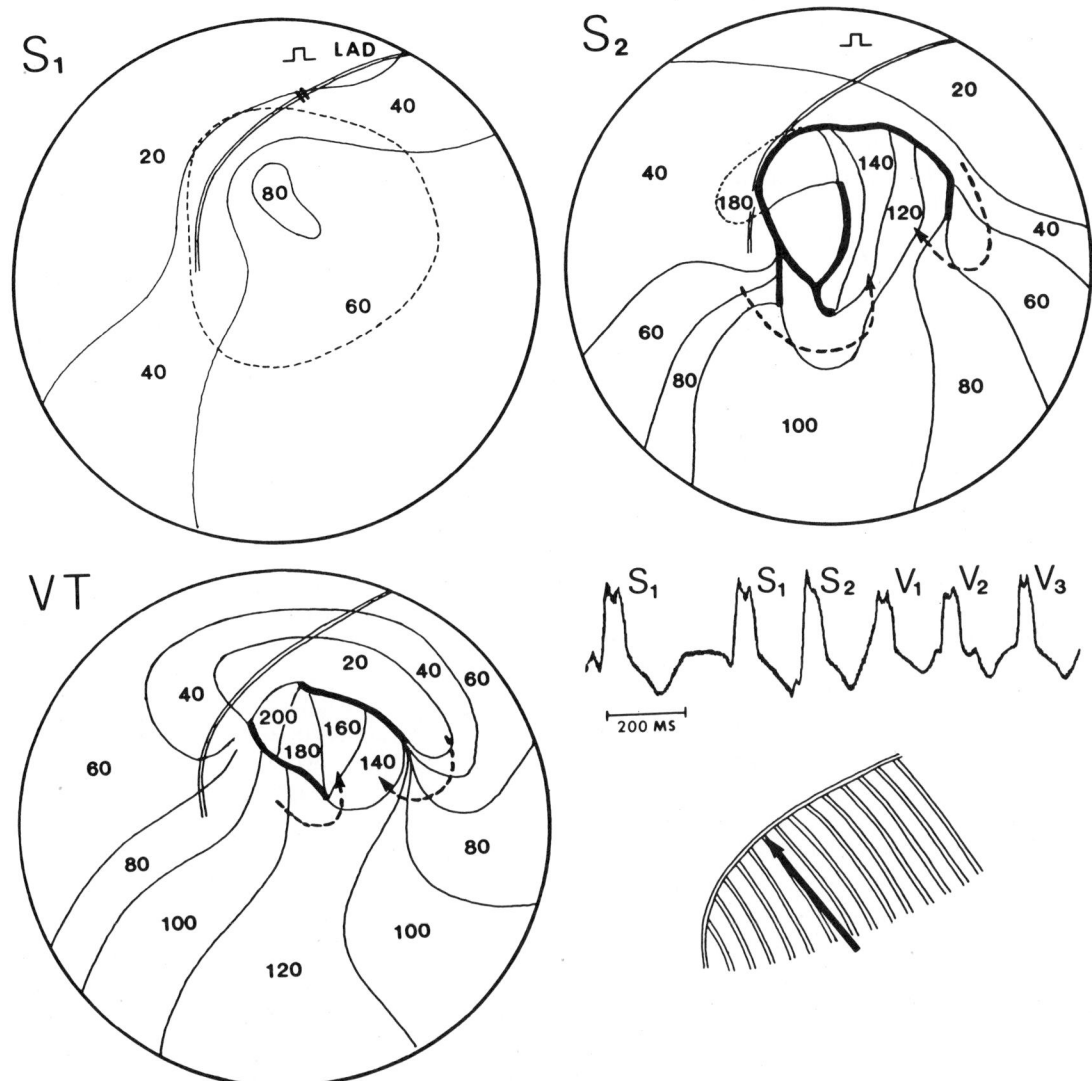

FIGURE 2–22
Epicardial isochronal activation maps during a basic ventricular stimulated beat (S_1), initiation of reentry by a single premature stimulus (S_2), and sustained monomorphic reentrant ventricular tachycardia (VT). A representative electrocardiogram is shown in the lower right panel. The recordings were obtained from a dog 4 days post-ligation of the left anterior descending artery (LAD). Site of ligation is represented by a double bar.

In this and subsequent maps, epicardial activation is displayed as if the heart is viewed from the apex located at the center of the circular map. The perimeter of the circle represents the AV junction. The outline of the epicardial ischemic zone is represented by the dotted line. Activation isochrones are drawn at 20-ms intervals. Arcs of functional conduction block are represented by heavy solid lines and are depicted to separate contiguous areas that are activated at least 40 ms apart.

During S_1 the epicardial surface was activated within 80 ms with the latest isochrone located in the center of the ischemic zone. S_2 resulted in a long continuous arc of conduction block within the border of the ischemic zone. The activation wavefront circulated around both ends of the arc of block and coalesced at the 100-ms isochrone. The common wavefront advanced within the arc of block before reactivating an area on the other side of the arc at the 180-ms isochrone to initiate the first reentrant cycle.

During sustained VT, the reentrant circuit had a figure-eight activation pattern in the form of a clockwise and counterclockwise wavefront around two separate arcs of functional conduction block. The two wavefronts joined into a common wavefront that conducted between the two arcs of block. The sites of the two arcs of block during sustained VT were different to a varying degree from the site of the arc of block during the initiation of reentry by S_2 stimulation.

The lower right panel illustrates the orientation of myocardial fibers in the surviving ischemic epicardial layer perpendicular to the direction of the LAD. The arrow represents the longitudinal axis of propagation of the slow common reentrant wavefront during a sustained figure-eight activation pattern, which is oriented parallel to fiber orientation and perpendicular to the nearby LAD segment.

block. The activation front circulates around both ends of the arc of block and rejoins on the distal side of the arc of block before breaking through the arc to reactivate an area proximal to the block. This results in splitting of the initial single arc of block into two separate arcs.

Subsequent reentrant activation continues with a figure-eight activation pattern, whereby two circulating wavefronts advance in clockwise and counterclockwise directions, respectively, around two arcs of conduction block. During a monomorphic reentrant tachycardia, the two arcs of block and the two circulating wavefronts remain fairly stable. The two arcs of functional conduction block are usually oriented parallel to the long axis of the epicardial muscle fibers.[174, 180] On the other hand, during a pleomorphic reentrant rhythm, both arcs of block and the circulating wavefronts can change their geometric configurations while maintaining their synchrony. Reentrant activation spontaneously terminates when the leading edge of both reentrant wavefronts encounters refractory tissue and fails to conduct. This results in coalescence of the two arcs of block into a single arc and termination of reentrant activation.[157]

The majority of reentrant circuits in the canine post-infarction model develop in the surviving epicardial layer and may be viewed as having an essentially two-dimensional configuration. However, some reentrant circuits were identified in intramyocardial[160] and subendocardial[152] locations. The latter location is of special interest because it may be comparable to reentrant circuits described in the surviving subendocardial muscle layer in the heart of patients with chronic myocardial infarction.[181, 182] This underscores the fact that, depending on the particular anatomic features of the infarction and the geometrical configuration of ischemic surviving myocardium, reentrant circuits could be located in epicardial, subendocardial, or intramyocardial zones.[21, 160, 183]

"SPONTANEOUS" REENTRANT EXCITATION VERSUS REENTRANT EXCITATION INDUCED BY PREMATURE STIMULATION

Conduction delay and conduction block in ischemic myocardium are characteristically tachycardia-dependent, meaning that conduction worsens at faster but not necessarily fast rates and improves at relatively slow rates.[15, 16] In dogs 1 to 5 days post-infarction, reentrant excitation commonly develops following a premature beat that interrupts an otherwise regular cardiac rhythm with a critically short cycle length. The regular rhythm can be either a sinus rhythm or paced atrial or ventricular rhythms.[16] For reentry to occur during regular cardiac rhythm, the heart rate should be within the relatively narrow critical range of rates during which conduction in a potentially reentrant pathway shows a Wenckebach-like pattern.[15] During a Wenckebach-like conduction cycle, a beat-to-beat increment in the length of the arc of conduction block and/or the degree of conduction delay will occur until the activation wavefront is sufficiently delayed for certain parts of the myocardium proximal to the arc of block to recover excitability and become reexcited by the delayed activation front. A Wenckebach-like conduction sequence may be the initiating mechanism for repetitive reentrant excitation (e.g., a reentrant tachycardia) or may result in a single reentrant cycle in a repetitive pattern, giving rise to a reentrant extrasystolic rhythm[160] (Fig. 2–23).

Figure 2–23

Isochronal maps of reentrant trigeminal rhythm. The figure illustrates epicardial activation maps as well as selected electrographic recordings from a dog 4 days post-infarction in which a reentrant trigeminal rhythm developed during sinus tachycardia.

During sinus rhythm at a cycle length of 325 ms, there was a consistent small arc of functional conduction block near the apical region of the infarct and relatively slow activation of nearby myocardial zones (map 1). The activation pattern, however, was constant in successive beats reflecting a 1:1 conduction pattern. Spontaneous shortening of the sinus cycle length to 305 ms resulted in the development of a single reentrant beat following every second sinus beat.

During the reentrant trigeminal rhythm, the epicardial activation map of the first sinus beat showed the development of a longer arc of functional conduction block compared with the one during sinus rhythm at a cycle length of 325 ms (map 2). The activation front circulated around both ends of the arc of block but was not sufficiently delayed on the distal side of the arc of block.

On the other hand, the activation map of the second sinus beat showed some lengthening of the arc of block at one end, but more characteristically a much slower conduction of the two activation fronts circulating around both ends of the arc of block (map 3). The degree of conduction delay was sufficient for refractoriness to expire at two separate sites on the proximal side of the arc, resulting in two simultaneous breakthroughs close to the ends of the arc, thus initiating reentrant excitation.

The leading edge of the two reentrant wavefronts coalesced but failed to conduct to the central part of the epicardial surface of the infarct—that is, to areas that were showing slow conduction during the preceding cycle. This limited the reentrant process to a single cycle (map 4). It also resulted in recovery of those myocardial zones in the central part of the infarct, allowing the next sinus beat to conduct with a lesser degree of conduction delay, thus perpetuating the reentrant trigeminal rhythm.

Analysis of the two electrograms recorded from each of the two reentrant pathways (pair B and C and pair D and E, respectively) shows a characteristic 3:2 Wenckebach-like conduction pattern. The figure illustrates the complexity of conduction patterns in ischemic myocardium and the presence of a zone of dissociated conduction. This is represented by site F, which was showing a 2:1 conduction pattern during the 3:2 Wenckebach cycle and reentrant trigeminal rhythm described above.

(Reprinted by permission of the American College of Cardiology from El-Sherif N, Gough WB, Zeiler RH, Hariman R: J Am Coll Cardiol 6:124, 1985.)

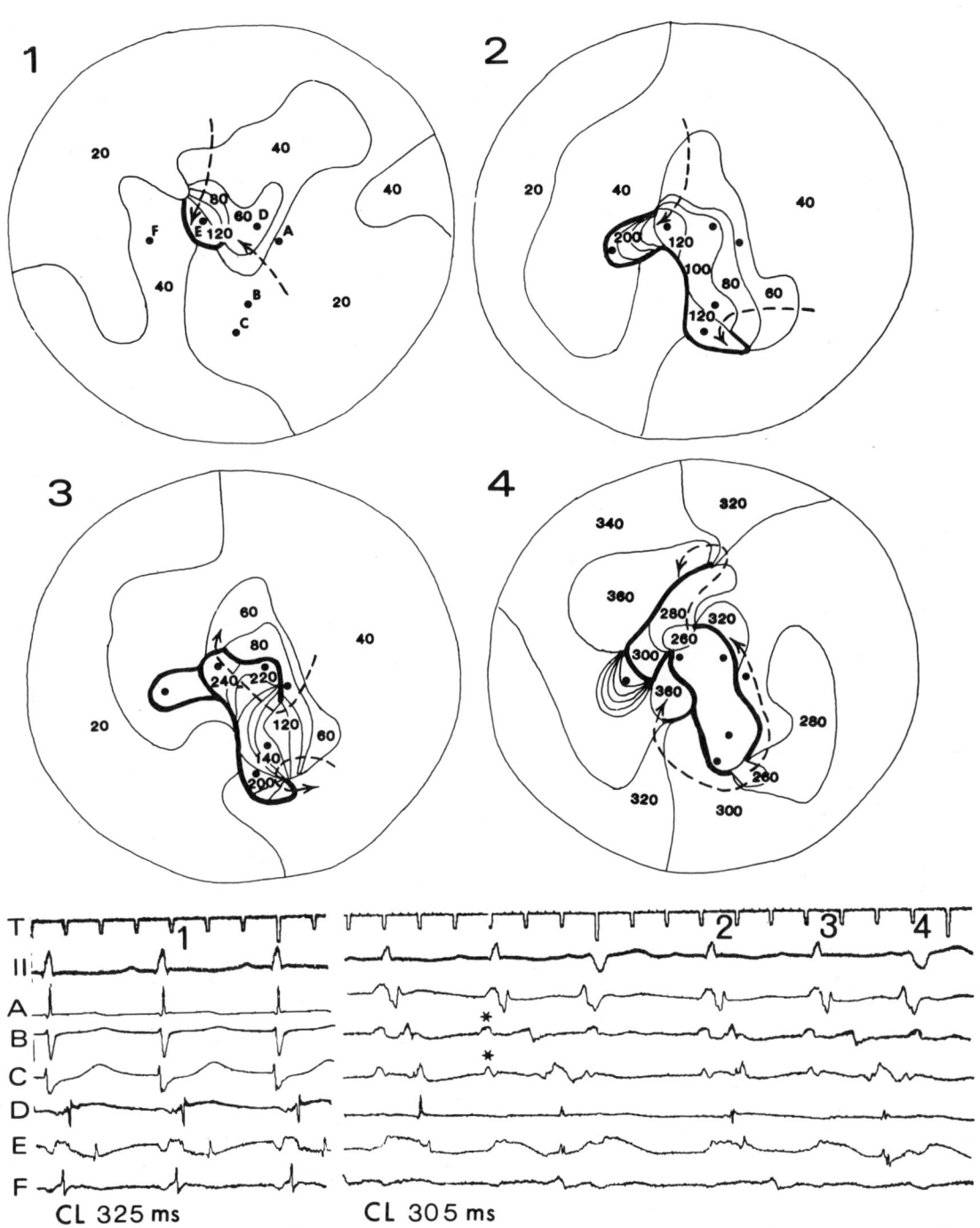

FIGURE 2–23 *See legend on opposite page*

Electrophysiology of Ventricular Arrhythmias in Myocardial Ischemia and Infarction 41

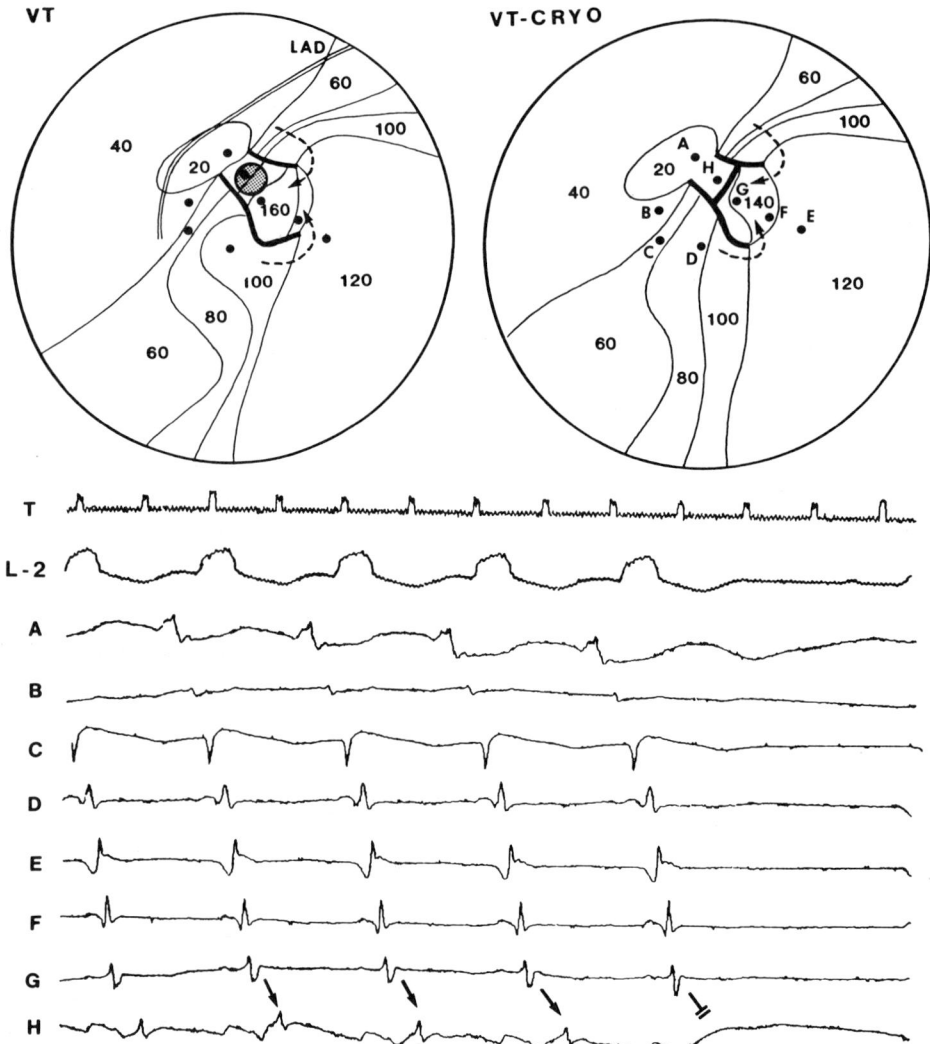

FIGURE 2–24
Interruption of a figure-eight reentrant tachycardia in the epicardial layer overlying 4-day-old canine infarction by cryothermal techniques. The control activation map is shown on the left (VT) and the map of the last reentrant beat prior to termination on the right (VT-CRYO). Selected epicardial electrograms are shown on the bottom. The position of the cryoprobe is represented by the shaded circle.

The reentrant circuit was interrupted by reversible cooling of the distal part of the common reentrant wavefront (site H). During control, the conduction time between the proximal electrode site G and the more distal site H was 33 ms. Prior to termination of the tachycardia, an incremental beat-to-beat increase of the conduction time between sites G and H occurred, associated with equal increases in the tachycardia cycle length. When conduction block developed between the two sites, the reentrant circuit was terminated, and electrogram H recorded an electrotonic potential but no local activation potential. This is represented on the isochronal map by an arc of conduction block (heavy solid line) that joins the two separate arcs of conduction block into one.

INTERRUPTION OF FIGURE-EIGHT REENTRANT CIRCUIT

As established by Mines,[184, 185] the criteria for proving the presence of circulating excitation are:

1. An area of unidirectional block must be demonstrated.
2. The movement of the excitatory wave should be observed to progress through the pathway, to return to its point of origin, and then to again follow the same pathway.
3. The best test for circulating excitation is to cut through the ring at one point. If impulses continue to arise in the cut ring, circus movement as cause can be ruled out.

El-Sherif et al. used reversible cooling and/or cryoablation of localized areas of the epicardial surface of the reentrant circuit to fulfill Mines's criteria for proving the presence of circulating excitation and to identify the critical site along the reentrant pathway at which interruption of reentrant activation could be successfully accomplished.[158]

These studies demonstrated that a figure-eight reentrant activation could be successfully interrupted when cooling or cryoablation was applied to the part of the common reentrant pathway immediately proximal to the zone of earliest reactivation (Fig. 2–24). At this site, the common reentrant wavefront is usually narrow and is surrounded on each side by an arc of functional conduction block. On the other hand, localized cooling to the site of earliest reactivation commonly failed to interrupt reentry. The common reentrant wavefront usually broke through the arc of functional conduction block and reactivated other sites close to the original reactivation site without necessarily changing the overall reentrant activation pattern.

ROLE OF SPATIAL NONHOMOGENEOUS LENGTHENING OF REFRACTORINESS IN THE INITIATION OF REENTRY

In the surviving ischemic epicardial layer, refractoriness was found to be prolonged in a spatially nonuniform manner.[162] The pattern of refractoriness resembled concentric rings of isorefractoriness which increased in a monotonic fashion from the normal zone toward the center of the ischemic zone (Fig. 2–25). The disparity of refractoriness per unit of distance was more marked along the septal border of the ischemic zone, resulting in more crowded refractory isochrones. The arc of functional conduction block induced by premature stimulation was found to occur along the steep gradient of refractoriness. The length and location of the arc depended on the degree of prematurity of the extrastimulus (S_1–S_2 interval).

When a single extrastimulus (S_2) failed to induce reentry, there were fewer adjacent sites with disparate refractoriness and hence a shorter arc of conduction block. The circulating wavefront reached the distal side of the arc of block before refractoriness expired proximal to the arc. The introduction of a second extrastimulus (S_3) could further shorten refractoriness in normal and ischemic zones by 10 to 40 ms. If shortening of refractoriness at some border zones occurred differentially (i.e., more in the normal than in the ischemic zones), this could result in lengthening of the arc of block. The longer arc of block would force the circulating wave to travel a longer pathway, reaching the distal side of the arc after expiration of refractoriness in areas proximal to the arc. These areas could then be reexcited to initiate reentry. When reentrant excitation was confined to a single beat, this was again explained by failure of refractoriness to shorten further in the central zone of the ischemic layer, resulting in conduction block in this zone and termination of reentry. Differential shortening of refractoriness in successive short cardiac cycles could thus modify the initial changes of refractoriness due to ischemia and could explain both the induction of reentry by multiple premature stimuli and the spontaneous termination of reentrant excitation.

The correlation of activation and refractory isochronal maps shown in Figure 2–25 was obtained from epicardial sites that were spaced 5 to 10 mm apart. Because of the relatively lower density of measurements of activation and refractoriness, several isochrones may have to be interpolated. From these studies a refractory gradient of 20 ms/cm was suggested as a threshold for the occurrence of functional conduction block. However, a higher resolution of both activation and refractory measurements would be necessary to discern (1) whether functional conduction block occurs abruptly or is preceded by decremental conduction, (2) whether the spatially disparate refractory gradient is due to gradual (albeit steep) increase in refractoriness or due to abrupt and discontinuous jumps of refractoriness, and (3) whether the line of functional conduction block would correlate with the abrupt change in refractoriness at the high resolution level.

Figure 2–26 was obtained from an experiment in which a high-density electrode plaque (a 1-mm interelectrode distance) was utilized to obtain activation and refractory measurements at sites of functional conduction block during premature stimulation. Functional conduction block was found to occur abruptly (within a 1-mm distance) and the activation wavefront prior to block did not show decremental conduction. The site of conduction block correlated with an abrupt increase of refractoriness of 10 to 85 ms over a 1-mm distance. Electrograms obtained 1 mm distal to the site of conduction block usually revealed an electrotonic deflection synchronous with the activation potential proximal to block. It was sometimes possible to demonstrate that the amplitude of the electrotonic deflection diminished with distance from the site of bock (Fig. 2–27).

The role of differential refractoriness and fiber orientation in the formation of the arc of functional conduction block was examined utilizing high-resolution activation and refractory maps generated at 1-mm intervals in the area of the arc of functional block.[179] Abrupt increase in refractoriness was found both along

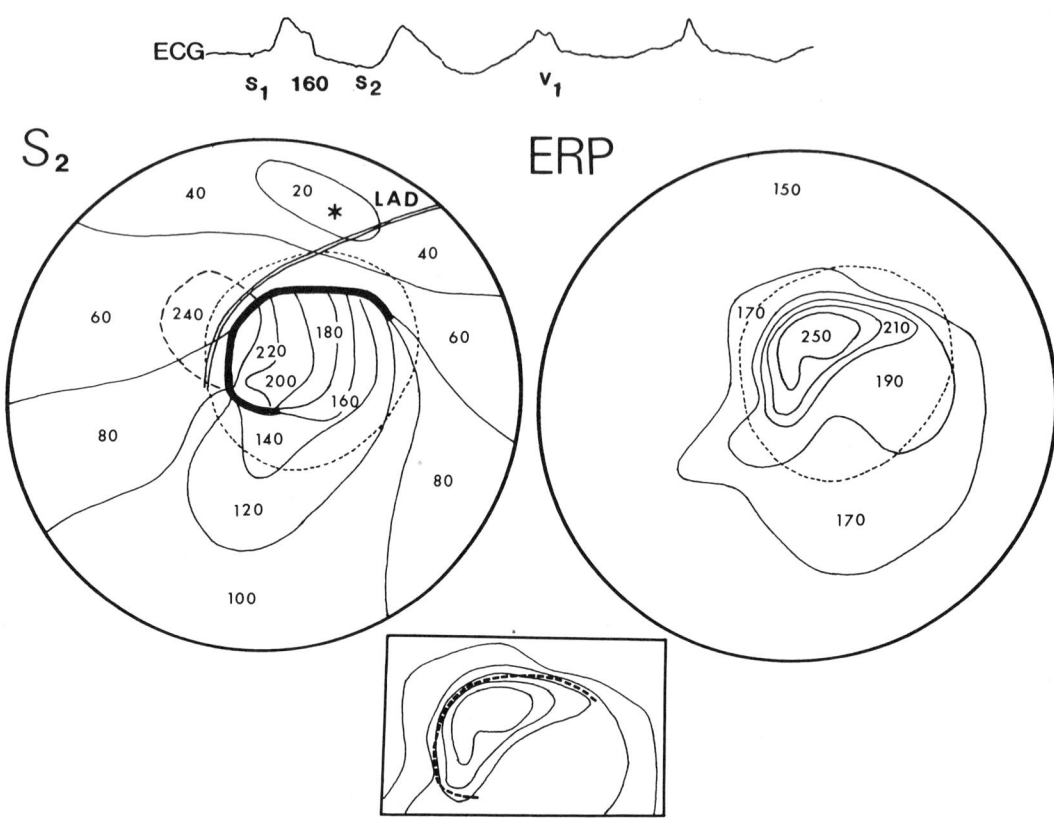

FIGURE 2–25
Correlation of isochronal maps of reentrant activation and refractory distribution in the epicardial surface from a 4-day-old canine infarction. The electrocardiogram at the top shows that a single premature stimulus (S_1) at a coupling interval of 160 ms initiated a reentrant rhythm. The epicardial activation map of S_2 is shown on the left; the refractory map of S_1 as encountered by S_2 is shown on the right and labeled ERP (effective refractory period). Both maps were drawn at 20-ms isochrones. The border of the ischemic zone is outlined on both maps by the dotted line.

The refractory map shows a nonuniform refractory distribution with ERPs of 150 to 170 ms located in the normal right and left ventricular epicardium, whereas the longest ERP of 250 msec was located in the center of the ischemic region. The dispersion of refractoriness was 100 ms, with concentric isochrones of refractoriness producing a graded increase in ERP going from the border zone toward the center of the ischemic zone. The steepest dispersion of refractoriness occurred inside the septal and basal borders of the infarction. The arc of functional conduction block encountered by S_2 developed between adjacent sites of short and long refractoriness with the sites of longer refractoriness being distal to the arc of block. This is shown in the inset at the bottom of the figure, in which the arc of block (represented by a heavy dotted line) was superimposed on the refractory isochronal map. Note that both disparate refractoriness and the functional arc of conduction block occurred parallel as well as perpendicular to the long axis of epicardial muscle fibers.

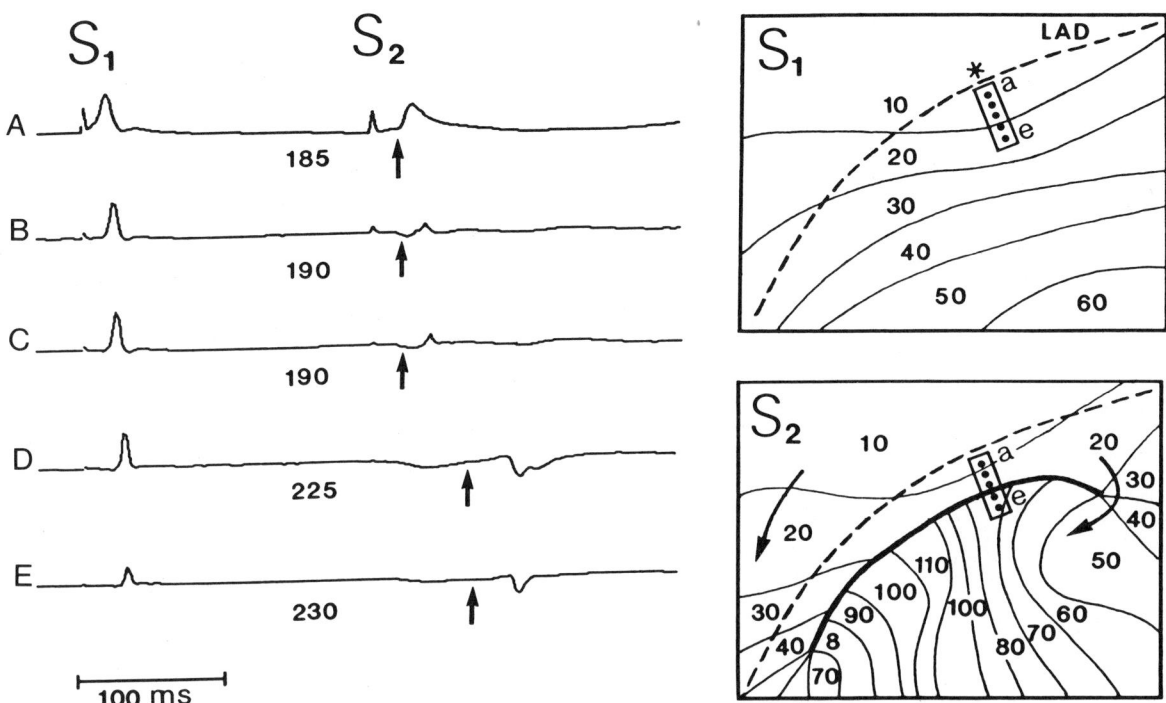

FIGURE 2–26
High-resolution determination of spatial refractory gradients and their relationship to the arc of functional conduction block from a 4-day-old canine infarction. A high-density bipolar electrode plaque with 1-mm interelectrode spacing was positioned on the epicardial surface at the site of the arc of block induced by premature stimulation (S_2), as determined from an earlier low-resolution sock electrode array. The plaque was oriented with the electrode rows perpendicular to the arc. The figure illustratres five bipolar electrograms recorded successively at distance of 1 mm (a to e). The values of the effective refractory period in milliseconds at each site are shown. The arrows indicate the end of the effective refractory period relative to S_1 activation at each site. The S_1 and S_2 activation maps are shown on the right. The asterisk on the S_1 map denotes the site of stimulation.

During S_1, sites a to e were activated sequentially within a 12-ms interval (conduction velocity of 42 cm/s). During S_2, conduction between sites a and c was relatively slow compared with S_1. Conduction block developed abruptly between sites c and d. Sites d and e were activated 65 ms later by the wavefront that circulated in a clockwise direction around one end of the arc of block. The site of conduction block coincided with a 35-ms abrupt increase in the effective refractory period between sites c and d. Note that the arc of block was parallel to the left anterior descending artery (LAD), represented by the dashed line.

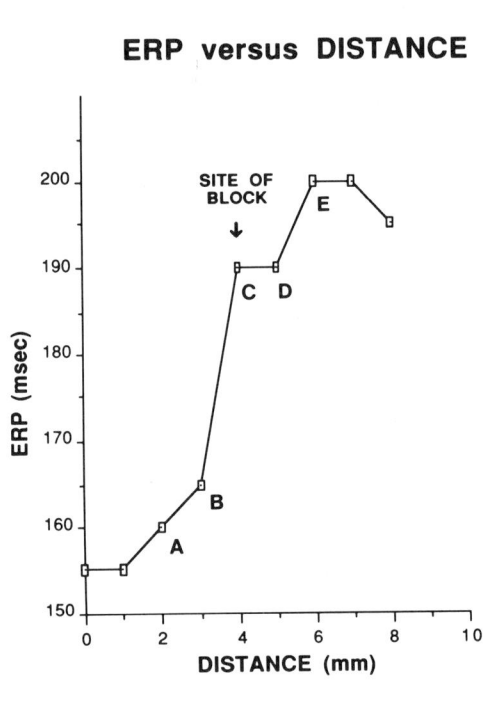 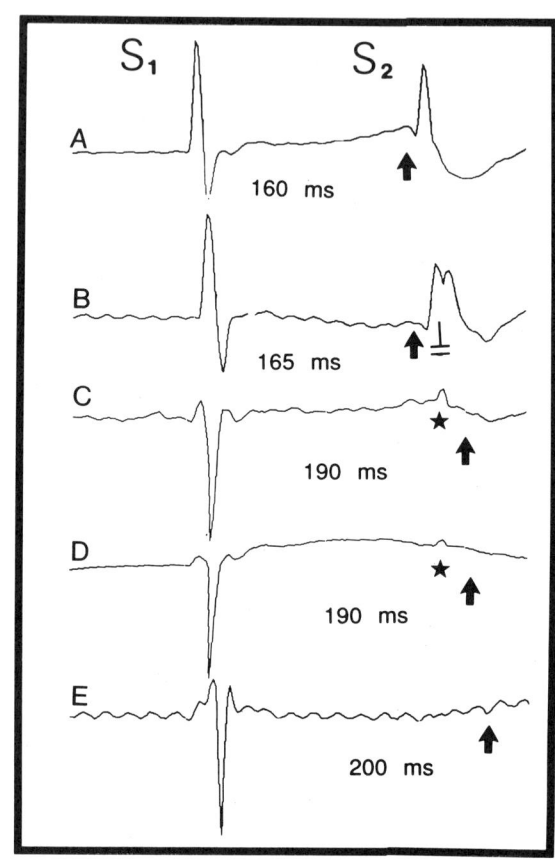

FIGURE 2-27
Illustration of five successive bipolar electrograms (A to E) recorded at distance of 1 mm across an arc of functional conduction block induced by S_2 stimulation (right panel). The layout of the high-density plaque is similar to that shown in Figure 2-26, but the recordings were obtained from a different experiment. The effective refractory period (ERP) at each site is shown; the arrows indicate the end of the ERP relative to S_1 activation. Abrupt conduction block occurred during S_2 stimulation between sites B and C and coincided with an abrupt increase of 25 ms in ERP. The asterisks indicate the electrotonic deflection recorded in electrograms C and D distal to block. The amplitude of the electrotonic deflection diminished with distance from site of block.

A graph illustrating the distribution of ERP across an 8-mm distance is shown on the left.

the fiber axis (27 ± 9 ms/mm) and across the fiber axis (14 ± 7 ms/mm). Although the difference along the fiber axis was greater, the arc of functional conduction block occurred in both orientations in which there was an abrupt change in refractoriness. The study suggests that in the ischemic ventricle, an arc of functional block occurs as a consequence of differentially graded refractoriness and can be independent of fiber orientation.

EFFECTS OF MODIFICATION OF THE SPATIAL PATTERN OF RECOVERY TIME ON THE INITIATION OF REENTRY

Further evidence of the role of spatially nonhomogeneous distribution of refractoriness in the formation of the arc of functional conduction block was obtained from experiments in which the initiation of reentry could be prevented by changing the activation pattern of the basic stimulated beat (S_1).[164] The spatial patterning of recovery time depended on the activation pattern of the basic beat, in addition to the spatially nonhomogeneous refractory distribution induced by ischemia. The dispersion of recovery time could be modified by stimulation at two ventricular sites during the basic beat. The arc of conduction block could be modified or abolished entirely by appropriate selection of the secondary stimulation site in the ischemic zone and the temporal sequencing of the paired stimuli (Fig. 2–28). Asynchronous dual stimulation, with preexcitation of an appropriate site in the ischemic zone, was frequently successful in preventing the initiation of reentry by a fixed coupled premature stimulus. In all instances that resulted in the prevention of reentry, the secondary site was distal to the arc of block that formed following the control S_2 stimulation. The secondary site should be in an area of long refractoriness that activated late during the basic beat. Properly applied dual stimulation differentially peels back recovery time in the ischemic zone.

Successful dual stimulation depended on the reduction of two factors: (1) the spatial gradient of recovery time and (2) the dispersion of recovery time across the arc. The former determines the extent and location of the continuous arc of conduction block; the latter determines whether areas distal to block are recovered during the premature stimulation. Reducing the difference in activation time across the arc of block to a value less than the effective refractory period of the premature stimulus (ERP_2) proximal to the arc is the mechanism by which dual S_1 stimulation can prevent the initiation of reentry.

SUSTAINED REENTRY ORIENTS AROUND CONTINUOUS ARCS OF FUNCTIONAL CONDUCTION BLOCK

We and others[174, 180] have shown that during sustained figure-eight monomorphic reentrant tachycardia, the two arcs of functional conduction block around which the reentrant wavefronts circulate are usually oriented parallel to the long axis of the epicardial muscle fibers. Some authors have suggested that these areas represent apparent or pseudo-block and are in fact due to very slow and possibly discontinuous conduction across the myocardial fibers.[174] In this case, reentrant activation may be oriented around a small central region of functional block rather than a long line of block. Electrograms recorded from these sites had long duration and were fractionated, a characteristic that was shown to result from activation transverse to the myocardial fiber long axis.[186] These conclusions, however, were based on relatively low resolution recordings (3.5-mm interelectrode distance).[174]

We have analyzed close bipolar electrograms obtained at high resolution (1-mm interelectrode distance) from sites of the arcs of block during sustained stable reentry. Electrograms recorded at each side of the line of block showed two distinct deflections; one represented local activation, and the second an electrotonus corresponding to activation recorded a 1-mm distance away. Both deflections were separated by a variable isoelectric period that correlated with the isochronal difference across the arc. In recordings obtained from the center of the arc, local activation and electrotonus were separated by 90 to 110 ms. This interval successively decreased toward both ends of the arc (Fig. 2–29). These observations provide evidence that circus movement reentry was sustained around a continuous arc of abrupt functional conduction block (7 to 25 mm long) and not very slow conduction across fibers.

Although refractoriness could not be measured during sustained reentry, the electrogram configurations reflecting conduction block were similar to those obtained during functional conduction block induced by premature stimulation across a refractory gradient (see Figs. 2–25 and 2–26). This suggests that disparate refractoriness along the line of block rather than anisotropic properties of the epicardial layer may be responsible for sustained reentrant excitation.

MECHANISM OF ACTION OF ANTIARRHYTHMIC AGENTS

Despite extensive studies directed at the cellular mechanisms of antiarrhythmic drugs, direct experimental evidence about their mode of action in ischemia-related reentrant arrhythmias remains scarce, and the proposed mechanisms of action remain largely inferential. Several electropharmacologic studies have been reported on ventricular arrhythmias in the canine subacute myocardial infarction phase.

El-Sherif and coworkers have studied the effects of lidocaine,[187] diphenylhydantoin,[188] and procainamide[189] on reentrant ventricular arrhythmias in the 3- to 5-day old canine post-infarction model. Utilizing composite electrode recordings from the ischemic epicardial layer, the investigators suggested that these drugs prolong refractoriness of potentially reentrant pathways and further depress slow conduction in the ischemic zone. Their antiarrhythmic action was attributed to conduction block of the reentrant pathway. Cobbe and associates[190, 191] studied the effects of D-sotalol and

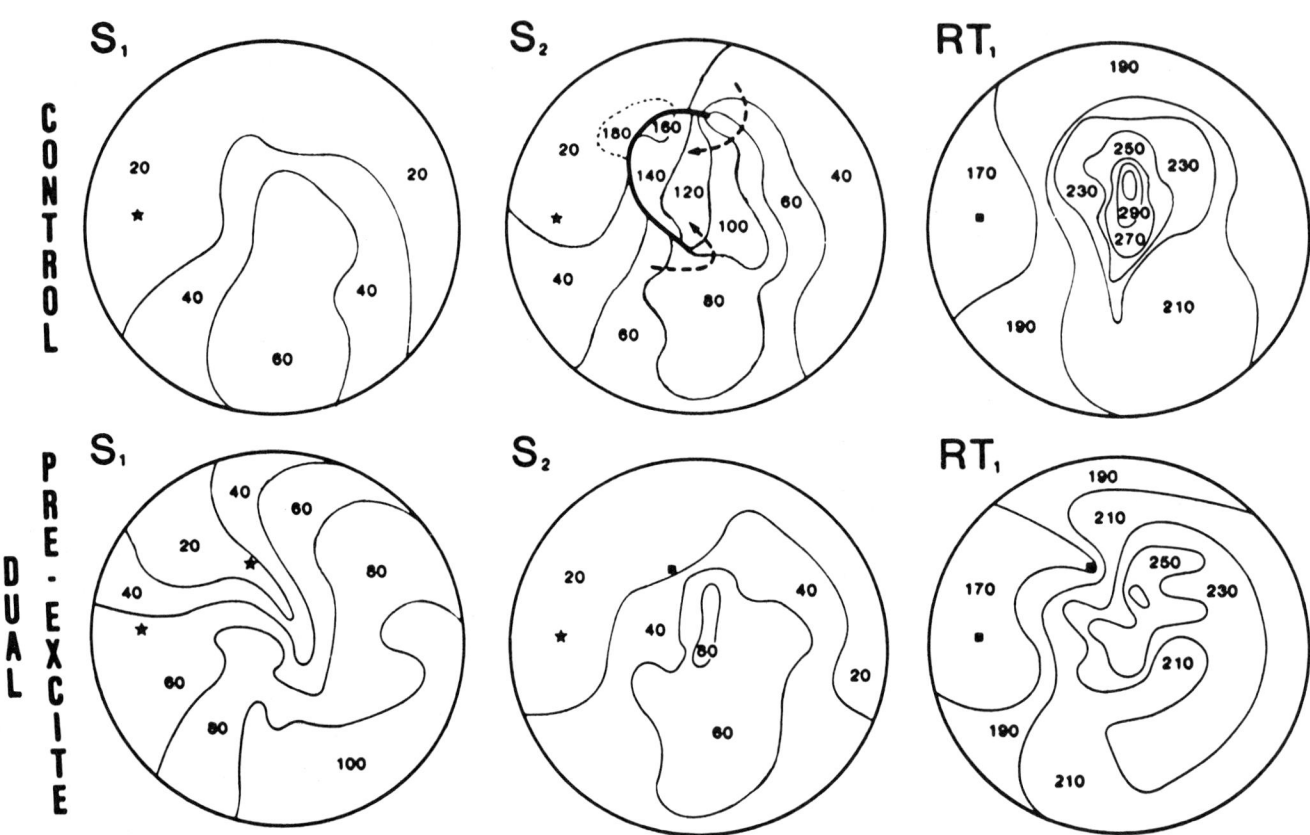

FIGURE 2–28
Abolition of the arc of functional conduction block by dual S_1 stimulation. *Control* (top): S_1 activation occurred within 60 ms. A gradient of recovery time (RT_1) between the 190- and 230-ms isochrones supported the formation of an arc of block during S_2. *Dual asynchronous stimulation* (bottom): The two sites of stimulation, one from the right ventricle (as in control) and one from the ischemic zone distal to the arc of block, are represented by asterisks. When the dual ischemic site was preexcited by 40 ms, no two adjacent sites differed in recovery time by more than 20 ms. A zone of graded recovery time that could support functional conduction block was not present. An arc of conduction block did not form.

In this experiment, the recovery time was computed by the sum of the activation time (stimulus artifact to response during S_1) plus the effective refractory period at each site.

(Reprinted by permission of the American Heart Association, Inc., from Restivo M, Gough WB, El-Sherif N: Circulation 77:429, 1988.)

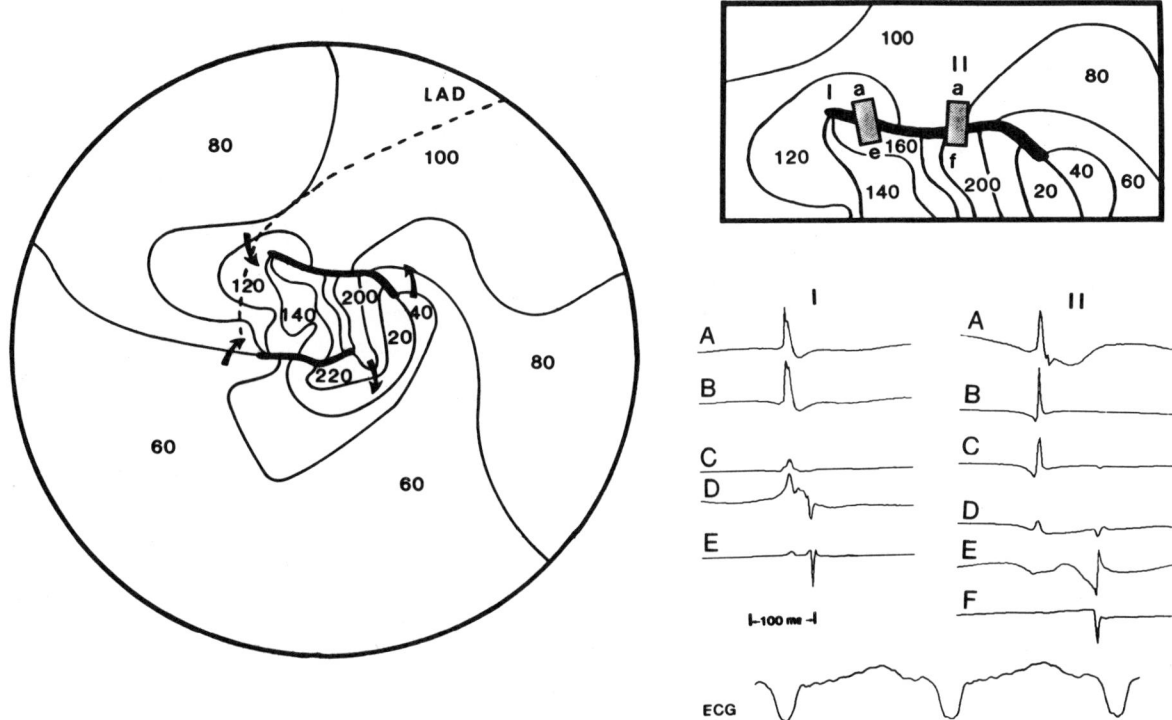

FIGURE 2–29
High-resolution recordings of activation across one of the two arcs of functional conduction block around which sustained figure-eight reentrant activation occurred. The left panel illustrates the epicardial activation pattern during a figure-eight reentrant tachycardia as obtained from a sock electrode array with 5- to 10-mm interelectrode distance. A high-density electrode plaque (1-mm interelectrode distance) was positioned at two locations across the upper arc of block. Shown on the right are an expanded map of the counterclockwise circuit around the upper arc of block and the electrograms along one row of bipolar electrodes at each location.

Plaque location II was situated near the center of the arc of block. Conduction between sites A and C during the left to right wavefront on the upper side of the arc was fast. Conduction block probably occurred between sites C and D. Similarly, conduction between sites F and E during the returning wavefront on the distal side of the arc was fast, and conduction block probably occurred between sites E and D. The two deflections recorded at site D were separated by an isoelectric interval of 85 ms, which corresponded to isochronal activation difference across the site of 81 to 100 ms. Both deflections most probably represented electrotonic potentials. It is possible, however, that one of the deflections, but not both, represented an activation potential. Electrograms C and E both show small deflections synchronous with the two potentials in electrogram D. These may reflect gradual diminution of the amplitude of the electrotonus with distance from site of block at D.

Plaque location I was obtained close to the septal end of the arc of block. A difference between proximal and distal activation potentials of 30 ms corresponded to an isochronal difference of 21 to 40 ms. Conduction block during the right to left wavefront on the proximal side of the arc of block probably occurred between sites D and E; an electrotonic deflection can be seen in electrogram E. Conduction block during the returning wavefront on the distal side of the arc of block appeared to have occurred between sites D and C. This interpretation suggests, however, that both deflections at site D represented activation potential. This could be possible only if the arc of conduction block was situated between the two poles of electrode D.

disopyramide in the same animal model, also using composite electrode recordings, and suggested a similar mechanism of action. Other investigators have studied the effects of disopyramide,[192] lidocaine,[193] procainamide,[194] timolol, and propranolol[195] in a canine occlusion-reperfusion model and reported essentially similar results. However, in all of these studies assessment of conduction was based either on recordings from a few sites or on composite electrode recordings. Also, assessment of refractoriness was limited.

The only study that attempted to investigate the effects of the antiarrhythmic agent lidocaine in acute myocardial ischemia, utilizing more detailed analysis of ventricular activation maps, was that of Cardinal and colleagues.[29] These authors reported that lidocaine in high concentration reduced the incidence of ventricular fibrillation occurring during occlusion by preventing the fractionation of wavefronts into multiple wavelets and microreentrant circuits. They proposed that lidocaine abolished reentry by converting areas of unidirectional block and slow conduction into areas of total block. This was attributed to the effects of lidocaine in depressing both the active generator properties (fast inward current) and the excitability of membranes in the ischemic zone.

Mehra and colleagues[196] have investigated the mechanism of lidocaine action on reentrant rhythms in the 3- to 5-day-old canine post-infarction model by analysis of activation, refractory, and excitability maps before and after lidocaine infusion (4 mg/kg + 50 µg/kg/min intravenously). Lidocaine was found to have the following effects:

1. It prolonged the effective refractory period at most sites in the ischemic zone and increased excitability threshold with some sites becoming inexcitable.
2. Effective refractory periods and excitability threshold of normal myocardium were not significantly altered.
3. For the premature beat, the conduction time from the normal to ischemic zone was consistently prolonged.
4. In a majority of experiments, lidocaine was able to prevent reentrant rhythms induced by premature beats with long coupling intervals but not at short coupling intervals; in other words, it significantly decreased the zone of reentry.

The common reentrant wavefront following premature beats with long coupling intervals was blocked in the ischemic zone, where effective refractory periods were prolonged and excitability threshold had increased (Fig. 2–30). Premature stimuli at short coupling intervals, however, showed further increase of conduction delay within the ischemic zone, and the delayed reentrant wavefront could still reexcite normal myocardium. Correlation of post-lidocaine activation, refractory, and excitability maps suggested that the increased conduction delay and conduction block of the premature beat following lidocaine administration generally occurred at ischemic sites that showed increased nonuniform refractory distribution and decreased excitability. The study clearly illustrated the potential significance of the correlation of activation, refractory, and excitability maps for understanding the mechanism of action of antiarrhythmic drugs on reentrant rhythms.

Conclusion

The progress that has been made in the last two decades toward understanding of the electrophysiologic alterations and the mechanisms of ischemia-related ventricular arrhythmias reflects the heightened aware-

---

FIGURE 2–30
Mechanism of antiarrhythmic action of lidocaine on reentrant ventricular rhythms in a dog with 4-day-old infarction. Control recordings are shown on the left panel, and post-lidocaine results are shown on the right. Arranged from top to bottom are the isochronal activation map, labeled S_2; the isorefractory map, labeled ERP_1 (effective refractory period); and the excitability map, labeled Excit. The epicardial maps are displayed as if the ventricles were folded out after a cut was made from crux to apex. The top left and right borders represent the right and left atrioventricular junctions. The two curvilinear surfaces on the right and left are contiguous and extend from the posterior base to the apex of the heart. The isochrones for the S_2 and ERP_1 maps are drawn at 20-ms intervals, and for the Excit. map at 1 mA.

During control, the reentry zone following S_2 stimulation was 80 ms (S_1–S_2 intervals of 160 to 240 ms). The figure shows that an S_1–S_2 interval of 175 ms induced a reentrant rhythm. The S_2 map shows the development of two arcs of block inside the upper and apical borders of the ischemic zone. The two circulating wavefronts around the upper arc of block coalesced and then re-excited normal myocardial zones on the upper septal border of the ischemic zone, initiating a reentrant rhythm. Comparison of control S_2 and ERP_1 maps shows that the arcs of block developed at areas with nonuniform refractory distribution (crowded refractory isochrones). The control Excit. map shows one inexcitable site (shaded area) and a significant increase of the excitability threshold in the central part of the ischemic zone. However, there was no correlation between the excitability threshold and the lengthening of ERP.

Following lidocaine administration, the reentry zone of S_2 was markedly reduced but not totally abolished. Only S_1–S_2 intervals of 160 to 170 ms could induce reentry. The figure shows that an S_1–S_2 interval of 175 ms failed to initiate a reentrant rhythm. The post-lidocaine S_2 map shows that both the clockwise and counterclockwise wavefronts blocked at the center of the ischemic zone. Evidence of slowed conduction preceding conduction block was manifested by the counterclockwise wavefront. The post-lidocaine ERP_1 shows no significant change in refractoriness in normal zones and nonuniform lengthening of refractoriness in the ischemic zone. The post-lidocaine Excit. map shows increase of excitability threshold in the ischemic zone, with many sites becoming inexcitable.

Correlation of post-lidocaine (S_2), refractory (ERP_1), and excitability (Excit.) maps suggests that the increased conduction delay and conduction block of the premature beat following lidocaine administration generally occurred at ischemic sites that showed increased nonuniform refractory distribution and decreased excitability.

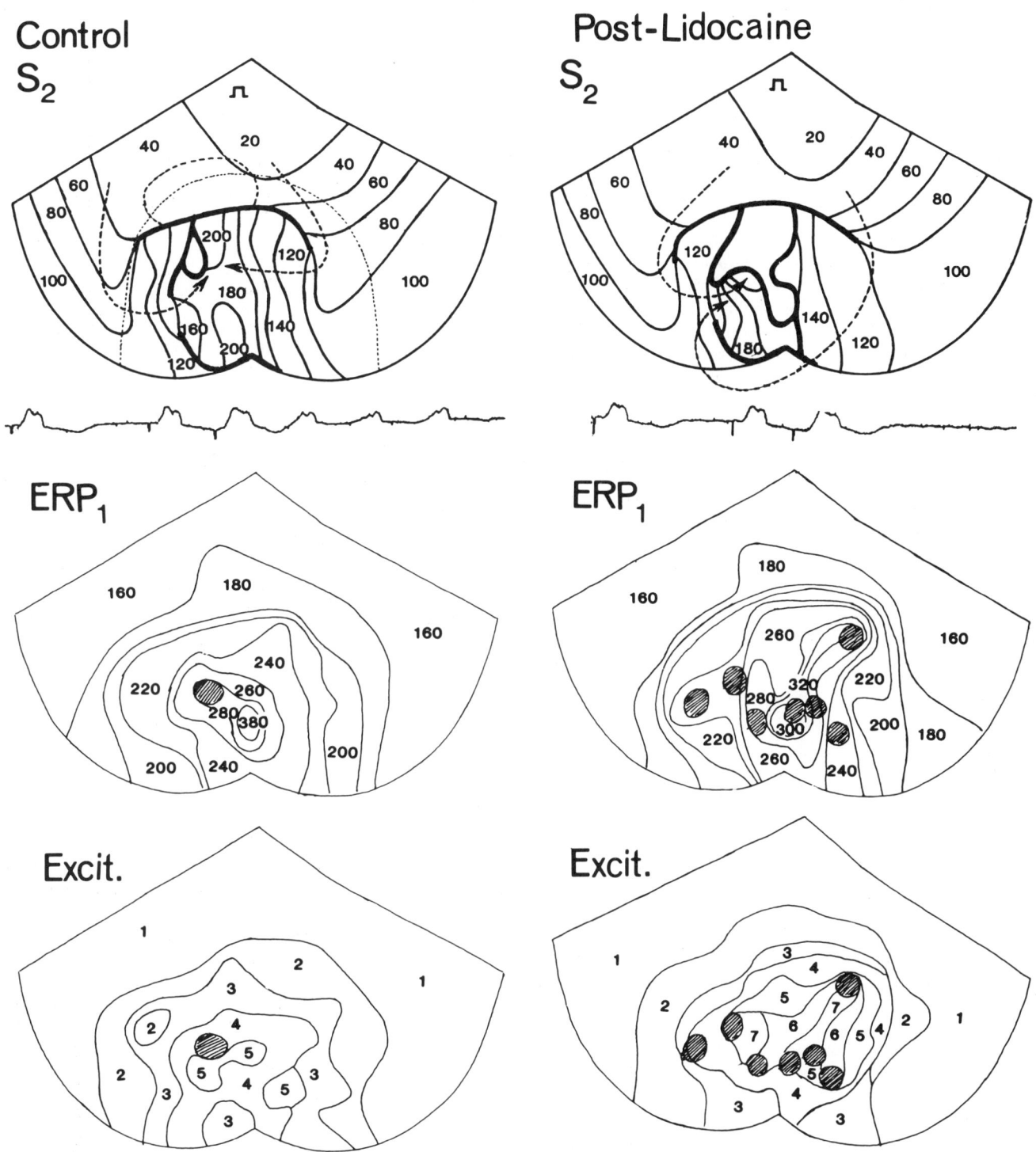

FIGURE 2–30 See legend on opposite page

ness of the revelance and serious nature of this clinical entity. Experimental studies of post-infarction ventricular arrhythmias have usually been conducted in dogs following one- or two-stage occlusion of one or more coronary arteries, although other animal species have also been utilized. A perfect animal model of myocardial infarction that faithfully reproduces the arrhythmias that might occur in humans does not exist. Most experimental models create a combination of localized myocardial ischemia and infarction in previously normal hearts. However, in humans the majority of ischemia and infarction occurs in hearts with preexisting coronary atherosclerosis. Furthermore, a reliable animal model for spontaneous ventricular tachycardia and ventricular fibrillation is not available, even though these arrhythmias are common in human infarction.

In spite of these and other limitations much progress has been made. There is now convincing evidence that reentrant excitation in ischemic myocardium underlies the spontaneous and often lethal ventricular tachyarrhythmias seen in the acute phase of myocardial infarction as well as in ventricular tachyarrhythmias induced by programmed stimulation in the subacute and, possibly, chronic phases. The role of nonreentrant mechanisms, possibly triggered activity in post-occlusion and, particularly, in reperfusion ventricular arrhythmias, is undergoing much investigation.

Triggered activity arising from delayed afterdepolarizations in ischemic Purkinje fibers, and possibly abnormal automaticity in ischemic depolarized cardiac cells, may explain some of the spontaneous multiform ventricular rhythms seen in the subacute phase of myocardial infarction and perhaps in the chronic phase as well. Delineation of the role of the autonomic system and new antiarrhythmic approaches that take advantage of recent understanding of the ionic and biochemical changes associated with ischemia are two promising areas of investigation. With the advent of new and sophisticated techniques applicable to both human and animal studies, the future holds promise for improved clinical management of post-infarction lethal ventricular arrhythmias.

References

1. Reimer KA, Low JE, Rasmussen MM, Jennings RB: The wavefront phenomenon of ischemic cell death. 1. Myocardial infarct size vs. duration of coronary occlusion in dogs. Circulation 56:786, 1977.
2. Fenoglio JJ, Karagueuzian HS, Friedman PL, et al.: Time course of infarct growth toward the endocardium after coronary occlusion. Am J Physiol 236:H356, 1979.
3. Harris AS: Late development of ventricular ectopic rhythms following experimental coronary occlusion. Circulation 1:1318, 1950.
4. Durrer D, Van Damm RTH, Freud GE, Janse MJ: Reentry and ventricular arrhythmias in local ischemia and infarction of the intact dog heart. Koninkl Med Akad Wetenschap Proc Ser Cx 74:321, 1971.
5. Waldo AL, Kaiser GA: A study of ventricular arrhythmias associated with acute myocardial infarction in the canine heart. Circulation 47:1122, 1973.
6. Boineau JP, Cox JL: Slow ventricular activation in acute myocardial infarction. A source of reentrant premature ventricular contractions. Circulation 48:703, 1973.
7. Scherlag BJ, El-Sherif N, Hope RR, Lazzara R: Characterization and localization of ventricular arrhythmias due to myocardial ischemia and infarction. Circ Res 35:372, 1974.
8. El-Sherif N, Scherlag BJ, Lazzara R: Electrode catheter recordings during malignant ventricular arrhythmias following experimental acute myocardial ischemia. Evidence for reentry due to local conduction delay and block in ischemic myocardium. Circulation 51:1003, 1975.
9. Janse MJ, Van Cappelle FJL, Morsink H, et al.: Flow of "injury" current and patterns of excitation during early ventricular arrhythmias in acute regional myocardial ischemia in isolated porcine and canine hearts. Evidence for two different arrhythmogenic mechanisms. Circ Res 47:151, 1980.
10. Friedman PL, Stewart JR, Fenoglio JJ, Wit AL: Survival of subendocardial Purkinje fibers after extensive myocardial infarction in dogs. In vitro and in vivo correlations. Circ Res 33:597, 1973.
11. Friedman PL, Stewart JR, Wit AL: Spontaneous and induced cardiac arrhythmias in subendocardial Purkinje fibers surviving extensive myocardial infarction in dogs. Circ Res 33:612, 1973.
12. Lazzara R, El-Sherif N, Scherlag BJ: Electrophysiologic properties of canine Purkinje cells in one-day-old myocardial infarction. Circ Res 33:722, 1973.
13. Horowitz LN, Spear JF, Moore EN: Subendocardial origin of ventricular arrhythmias in 24-hour-old experimental myocardial infarction. Circulation 53:56, 1976.
14. Bigger JT, Dresdale RJ, Heissenbuttel RH, et al.: Ventricular arrhythmias in ischemic heart disease: Mechanism, prevalence, significance, and management. Prog Cardiovasc Dis 19:255, 1977.
15. El-Sherif N, Scherlag BJ, Lazzara R, Hope RR: Reentrant ventricular arrhythmias in the late myocardial infarction period. 1. Conduction characteristics in the infarction zone. Circulation 55:686, 1977.
16. El-Sherif N, Hope RR, Scherlag BJ, Lazzara R: Reentrant ventricular arrhythmias in the late myocardial infarction period. 2. Patterns of initiation and termination of reentry. Circulation 55:702, 1977.
17. El-Sherif N, Lazzara R, Hope RR, Scherlag BJ: Reentrant ventricular arrhythmias in the late myocardial infarction period. 3. Manifest and concealed extrasystolic grouping. Circulation 56:225, 1977.
18. Michelson EL, Spear JF, Moore EN: Electrophysiologic and anatomic correlates of sustained ventricular tachyarrhythmias in a model of chronic myocardial infarction. Am J Cardiol 45:583, 1980.
19. Garan H, Fallon JT, Ruskin JN: Sustained ventricular tachycardia in recent canine myocardial infarction. Circulation 62:980, 1980.
20. Garan H, Ruskin J: Localized Reentry. Mechanism of induced sustained ventricular tachycardia in canine model of recent myocardial infarction. J Clin Invest 74:377, 1984.
21. Garan H, Fallon JT, Rosenthal S, Ruskin JN: Endocardial, intramural, and epicardial activation patterns during sustained monomorphic ventricular tachycardia in late canine myocardial infarction. Circ Res 60:879, 1987.
22. Kardesh M, Hogencamp CE, Bing RJ: The effect of complete ischemia on the intracellular electrical activity of the whole mammalian heart. Circ Res 6:715, 1958.
23. Downar E, Janse MJ, Durrer D: The effect of acute coronary artery occlusion on subepicardial transmembrane potentials in the intact porcine heart. Circulation 56:217, 1977.
24. Janse MJ, Kleber AG: Electrophysiologic changes and ventricular arrhythmias in the early phase of myocardial ischemia. Circ Res 49:1064, 1981.
25. El-Sherif N, Scherlag BJ, Lazzara R, Samet P: The pathophysiology of tachycardia- and bradycardia-dependent block in the canine proximal His-Purkinje system following acute myocardial ischemia. Am J Cardiol 34:529, 1974.
26. Lazzara R, El-Sherif N, Scherlag BJ: Disorders of cellular electrophysiology produced by ischemia of the canine His bundle. Circ Res 36:444, 1975.
27. Kleber AG, Janse MJ, Wilms-Schopman FJG, et al.: Changes in conduction velocity during acute ischemia in ventricular myocardium of the isolated porcine heart. Circulation 73:189, 1986.

28. Kleber AG, Riegger CB, Janse MJ: Electrical uncoupling and increase of extracellular resistance after induction of ischemia in isolated arterially perfused rabbit papillary muscle. Circ Res 61:271, 1987.
29. Cardinal R, Janse MJ, Van Eden I, et al.: The effects of lidocaine on intracellular and extracellular potentials, activation and ventricular arrhythmias during acute regional ischemia in isolated porcine heart. Circ Res 49:792, 1981.
30. Josephson ME, Horowitz LN, Farshidi A: Continuous local electrical activity. A mechanism of recurrent ventricular tachycardia. Circulation 57:659, 1978.
31. Pogwizd SM, Corr PB: Reentrant and nonreentrant mechanisms contribute to arrhythmogenesis during early myocardial ischemia: Results using three-dimensional mapping. Circ Res 61:352, 1987.
32. Antzelevitch C, Jalife J, Moe GK: Characteristics of reflection as a mechanism of reentrant arrhythmias and its relationship to parasystole. Circulation 61:182, 1980.
33. Janse MJ, van Capelle FJL: Electrotonic interactions across an inexcitable region as a cause of ectopic activity in acute regional myocardial ischemia. A study in intact porcine and canine hearts and computer models. Circ Res 50:527, 1982.
34. Harris AS, Bisteni A, Russel RA, et al.: Excitatory factors in ventricular tachycardia resulting from myocardial ischemia: Potassium a major excitant. Science 119:200, 1954.
35. Garlick PB, Radda GK, Seely PJ: Studies of acidosis in the ischemic heart by phosphorus nuclear magnetic resonance. Biophys J 184:547, 1979.
36. Hill JL, Gettes LS: Effect of acute coronary artery occlusion on local myocardial extracellular K^+ activity in swine. Circulation 61:768, 1980.
37. Hirche JH, Franz CHR, Schramm M: Myocardial extracellular K^+ and H^+ increase and nonadrenaline release as possible cause of early arrhythmias following acute coronary artery occlusion in pigs. J Mol Cell Cardiol 12:579, 1980.
38. Weiss J, Shine KI: Extracellular potassium accumulation during myocardial ischemia: Implications for arrhythmogenesis. J Mol Cell Cardiol 13:699, 1981.
39. Kleber AG: Resting membrane potential, extracellular potassium activity and intracellular sodium activity during acute global ischemia in isolated perfused guinea pig heart muscle. Circ Res 52:442, 1983.
40. Fleet WF, Johnson TA, Graebner CA, Gettes LS: Effect of serial brief ischemic episodes on extracellular K^+, pH and activation in the pig. Circulation 72:922, 1985.
41. Kleber AG: Extracellular potassium accumulation in acute myocardial ischemia. J Mol Cell Cardiol 16:389, 1986.
42. Kleber AG, Riegger CB, Janse MJ: Extracellular K^+ and H^+ shifts in early ischemia: mechanisms and relation to changes in impulse propagation. J Mol Cell Cardiol 19(Suppl V):35, 1987.
43. Steenbergen C, Murphy EA, Levy L, London RE: Elevation in cytosolic free calcium concentration early in myocardial ischemia in perfused rat heart. Circ Res 60:700, 1987.
44. Lee H-C, Mohabir R, Smith N, et al.: Effect of ischemia on calcium-dependent fluorescence transients in rabbit hearts containing Indo 1. Correlation with monophasic action potentials and contraction. Circ Res 78:1047, 1988.
45. Coronel R, Fiolet JWT, Wilms-Schopman FJG, et al.: Distribution of extracellular potassium and its relation to electrophysiologic changes during acute myocardial ischemia in the isolated perfused porcine heart. Circulation 77:1125, 1988.
46. Morena H, Janse MJ, Fiolet JWT, et al.: Comparison of the effects of regional ischemia, hypoxia, hyperkalemia, and acidosis on intracellular and extracellular potentials and metabolism in the isolated porcine heart. Circ Res 46:624, 1980.
47. Gettes LS: Effect of ischemia on cardiac electrophysiology. In Fozzard HA, Haber E, Jennings RB, et al. (eds.): The Heart and Cardiovascular System, pp. 1317–1342. New York, Raven Press, 1986.
48. Rau E, Shine K, Langer G: Potassium exchange and mechanical performance in anoxic mammalian myocardium. Am J Physiol 232:H85, 1977.
49. Boyle PJ, Conway EJ: Potassium accumulation in muscle and associated changes. J Physiol 267:1001, 1941.
50. Case RB: Ion alterations during myocardial ischemia. Cardiology 56:245, 1971/1972.
51. Mathar PP, Case RB: Phosphate loss during reversible myocardial ischemia. J Mol Cell Cardiol 5:375, 1973.
52. Opie LH: Metabolic regulation in ischemia and hypoxia. Circ Res 38(Suppl I):152, 1976.
53. Bers DM, Ellis D: Intracellular calcium and sodium activity in sheep heart Purkinje fibers. Effects of changes in external sodium and intracellular pH. Pflugers Arch 393:171, 1982.
54. Sharma VK, Sheu SS: Micromolar extracellular ATP increases intracellular calcium concentration in isolated rat ventricular myocytes. Biophys J 49:351A, 1986.
55. Mullins LJ: The generation of electric currents in cardiac fibers by Na/Ca exchange. Am J Physiol 237:C103, 1979.
56. Coloquhoun D, Neher E, Reuter H, Stevens CF: Inward current channels activated by intracellular Ca^{++} in cultured cardiac cells. Nature 294:742, 1981.
57. Noma A: ATP-regulated K channels in cardiac muscle. Nature 305:147, 1983.
58. Trube G, Hescheler J: Inward-rectifying channels in isolated patches of the heart cell membrane: ATP-dependence and comparison with cell attached patches. Pflugers Arch 401:178, 1984.
59. Kakei M, Noma A, Shibasaki T: Properties of adenosine triphosphate regulated potassium. J Physiol (Lond) 363:441, 1985.
60. Lazdunski M: The antidiabetic sulphonylurea glibenclamide is a potent blocker of the ATP modulated K^+ channel in insulin secreting cells. Biochem Biophys Res Commun 6:21, 1987.
61. de Weilli J, Schmid-Antomarchi H, Fosset M, Lazdunski M: ATP-sensitive K^+ channels that are blocked by hypoglycemia-inducing sulfonylureas in insulin-secreting cells are activated by galanin, a hyperglycemia-inducing hormone. Proc Natl Acad Sci USA 85:1312, 1988.
62. Bekheit S, Restivo M, Henkin R, et al.: Effects of glyburide on ischemia-induced changes in extracellular potassium and local myocardial activation: A novel antiarrhythmic mechanism (Abstract). J Am Coll Cardiol 13(Suppl A):142A, 1989.
63. Weiss TN, Lamp ST; Glycolysis preferentially inhibits ATP sensitive channels in isolated guinea pig cardiac myocytes. Science 238:67, 1987.
64. Schaeffer SW, Tan BH, Hozutturi M: Effect of glyburide on myocardial metabolism and function. Am J Med 79:48, 1985.
65. Andres R, Baltzan MA, Cader G, Zieler KL: Effects of insulin on carbohydrate metabolism and on potassium in the forearm of man. J Clin Invest 41:108, 1962.
66. Sodi-Pallares D, Testelli MR, Fishleder BL, et al.: Effects of an intravenous infusion of a potassium-glucose-insulin solution on the electrocardiographic signs of myocardial infarction. Am J Cardiol 9:166, 1965.
67. Maroko PR, Libby P, Sobel BE, et al.: Shell WE, Covel JW, Braunwald E: Effect of glucose-insulin-potassium infusion on myocardial infarction following experimental coronary artery occlusion. Circulation 45:1160, 1972.
68. Dalby AJ, Bricknell OL, Opie LH: Effect of glucose-insulin-potassium infusions on epicardial ECG changes and on myocardial metabolic changes after coronary artery ligation in dogs. Cardiovasc Res 15:588, 1981.
69. Snyder DW, Crafford WA Jr, Glashow JL, et al.: Lysophosphoglycerides in ischemic myocardium effluents and potentiation of their arrhythmogenic effects. Am J Physiol 241:H700, 1981.
70. Corr PB, Snyder DW, Cain ME, et al.: Electrophysiological effects of amphiphiles on canine Purkinje fibers: Implications for dysrhythmia secondary to ischemia. Circ Res 49:354, 1981.
71. Corr PB, Gross RW, Sobel BE: Amphipathic metabolites and membrane dysfunction in ischemic myocardium. Circ Res 55:135, 1984.
72. Akita H, Creer MH, Yamaha KA, et al.: The electrophysiological effects of intracellular lysophosphoglycerides and their accumulation in cardiac lymph with myocardial ischemia in dogs. J Clin Invest 78:271, 1986.
73. Corr PB, Dobmeyer DJ: Amphipathic and lipid metabolites and arrhythmogenesis: A perspective. In Rosen MR, Palti Y (eds.): Lethal Arrhythmias Infarction Resulting from Myocardial Ischemia and Infarction, pp. 91–104. Boston/Dordrecht/Lancaster, Kluwer Academic Pub., 1989.
74. Corr PB, Cain ME, Witkowski FX, et al.: Potential arrhyth-

mogenic electrophysiological derangements in canine Purkinje fibers induced by lysophosphoglycerides. Circ Res 44:822, 1979.
75. Arnsdorf MF, Sawicki GJ: The effects of lysophosphatidylcholine, a toxic metabolite of ischemia, on the components of cardiac excitability in sheep Purkinje fibers. Circ Res 49:16, 1981.
76. Clarkson CW, Ten Eick RE: On the mechanism of lysophosphatidylcholine-induced depolarization of cat ventricular myocardium. Circ Res 52:543, 1983.
77. Sedlis SP, Corr PB, Sobel BE, et al.: Lysophosphatidylcholine potentiates Ca^{++} accumulation in rat and cardiac myocytes. Am J Physiol 244:H32, 1983.
78. Sedlis SP, Sequeria JM, Ahumada GC, El-Sherif N: Effects of lysophosphatidylcholine on cultured heart cells: Correlation of rate of uptake and accumulation with cell injury. J Lab Clin Med 112:745, 1988.
79. Pogwizd SM, Onufer JR, Kramer JB, et al.: Induction of delayed afterdepolarizations and triggered activity in canine Purkinje fibers by lysophosphoglycerides. Circ Res 59:416, 1986.
80. Pogwizd SM, Corr PB: Electrophysiologic mechanisms underlying arrhythmias due to reperfusion of ischemic myocardium. Circulation 76:404, 1987.
81. Knabb MT, Saffitz JE, Corr PB, Sobel BE: The dependence of electrophysiologic derangements on accumulation of endogenous long-chain acylcarnitine in hypoxic neonatal rat myocytes. Circ Res 58:230, 1986.
82. Heathers GP, Yamada KA, Kanter EM, Corr PB: Long-chain acylcarnitines mediate the hypoxia induced increase in $alpha_1$-adrenergic receptors on adult canine myocytes. Circ Res 61:735, 1987.
83. Creer MH, Sobel BE, Saffitz JE, et al.: Prevention of accumulation of acylcarnitine, lysophosphatides and ventricular fibrillation by inhibition of carnitine acyltransferase I in ischemic hearts. Circulation 76(Suppl IV):IV-111, 1987.
84. Werns SW, Shea MJ, Lucchesi BR: Free radicals and myocardial injury: pharmacologic implications. Circulation 75:1, 1986.
85. Thompson JA, Hess ML: The oxygen free radical system: A fundamental mechanism in the production of myocardial necrosis. Prog Cardiovasc Dis 28:449, 1986.
86. Das D, Engelman RM, Rousou JA, et al.: Pathophysiology of superoxide radical as potential mediator of reperfusion injury in pig heart. Basic Res Cardiol 81:155, 1986.
87. Hearse DJ: Myocardial ischemia and reperfusion: A possible role for free radicals? In Rice-Evans C (ed.): Free Radicals, Oxidant Stress and Drug Action, pp. 13–42. London, Richelieu Press, 1987.
88. Manning AS, Coltart DJ, Hearse DJ: Ischemia and reperfusion induced arrhythmias in the rat: Effects of xanthine oxidase inhibition with allopurinol. Circ Res 55:545, 1984.
89. Burton KP: Superoxide dismutase enhances recovery following myocardial ischemia. Am J Physiol 248:H637, 1986.
90. Gross GJ, Farbo NE, Hardman HF, Warltier DC: Beneficial action of superoxide dismutase and catalase in stunned myocardium of dogs. Am J Physiol 250:H372, 1986.
91. Przyklenk K, Kloner RA: Superoxide dismutase plus catalase improve contractile function in the canine model of "stunned myocardium." Circ Res 58:148, 1986.
92. Badylak SF, Simmons A, Turek J, Babbs CF: Protection from reperfusion injury in the isolated rat heart by post-ischemic diferroxantine and oxypurinol administration. Cardiovasc Res 21:500, 1987.
93. Hammond B, Hess ML: The oxygen free radical system: Potential mediator of myocardial injury. J Am Coll Cardiol 6:215, 1985.
94. Kim MS, Akera T: O_2 free radicals: Cause of ischemia-reperfusion injury to cardiac Na^+-K^+ ATPase. Am J Physiol 252:H252, 1987.
95. Kramer JH, Mak IT, Weglicki WB: Differential sensitivity of canine cardiac sarcolemmal and microsomal enzymes to inhibition by free radical–induced lipid peroxidation. Circ Res 55:120, 1984.
96. Rowe GT, Manson NH, Caplan M, Hess ML: Hydrogen peroxide and hydroxyl radical mediation of activated leukocyte depression of cardiac sarcoplasmic reticulum. Circ Res 53:584, 1983.
97. Kaneko M, Blamish RE, Dhalla NS: Depression of heart sarcolemmal Ca^{2+} pump activity by oxygen free radicals. Am J Physiol 259:H368, 1989.
98. Reeves JP, Bailey CA, Hale CC: Redox modification of sodium-calcium exchange activity in cardiac sarcolemmal vesicles. J Biol Chem 261:4948, 1986.
99. Garlick PB, Davies MJ, Hearse DJ, Slater TF: Direct detection of free radicals in the reperfused rat heart using electron spin resonance spectroscopy. Circ Res 61:757, 1987.
100. Zweier JL, Flaherty JT, Weisfeldt ML: Direct measurement of free radical generation following reperfusion of ischemic myocardium. Proc Natl Acad Sci USA 84:1404, 1987.
101. Balke CW, Kaplinsky E, Michelson EL, et al.: Reperfusion ventricular tachyarrhythmias: Correlation with antecedent coronary artery occlusion tachyarrhythmias and duration of myocardial ischemia. Am Heart J 101:444, 1981.
102. Penny WJ, Sheridan DJ: Arrhythmias and cellular electrophysiological changes during myocardial ischemia and reperfusion. Cardiovasc Res 17:363, 1983.
103. Manning AS, Hearse DJ: Reperfusion-induced arrhythmias: mechanisms and prevention. J Mol Cell Cardiol 16:497, 1984.
104. Austin M, Wenger TL, Harrell FE Jr, et al.: Effect of myocardium at risk on outcome after coronary artery occlusion and release. Am J Physiol 243:H340, 1982.
105. Lederman SN, Wenger TL, Harrell FE Jr, Strauss HC: Effects of different paced heart rates on canine coronary occlusion and reperfusion arrhythmias. Am Heart J 113:1365, 1987.
106. Sheridan DJ, Penkoske PA, Sobel BE, Corr PB: Alpha-adrenergic contributions to dysrhythmias during myocardial ischemia and reperfusion in cats. J Clin Invest 65:161, 1980.
107. Corr PB, Shayman JA, Kramer JB, Kipnis RJ: Increased alpha-adrenergic receptors in ischemic cat myocardium: A potential mediator of electrophysiological derangements. J Clin Invest 67:1232, 1981.
108. Stewart JR, Burmeister WE, Burmeister J, Lucchesi BR: Electrophysiologic and antiarrhythmic effects of phentolamine in experimental coronary artery occlusion and reperfusion in the dog. J Cardiovasc Pharmacol 2:77, 1980.
109. Thandroyen FT, Worthington MG, Higginson LM, et al.: The effect of alpha- and beta-adrenoreceptor antagonist agents on reperfusion ventricular fibrillation and metabolic status in the isolated perfused rat heart. J Am Coll Cardiol 1:1056, 1983.
110. Benfey BG, Elfellah MS, Ogilvie RI, Varma DR: Antiarrhythmic effects of prazosin and propranolol during coronary artery occlusion and reperfusion in dogs and pigs. Br J Pharmacol 82:717, 1984.
111. Kane KA, Parratt JR, Williams FM: An investigation into the characteristics of reperfusion-induced arrhythmias in the anesthetized rat and their susceptibility to arrhythmogenic agents. Br J Pharmacol 82:349, 1984.
112. Wilber DJ, Lynch JJ, Montgomery DG, Lucchesi BR: Alpha-adrenergic influences in canine ischemic sudden death: Effects of $alpha_1$-adrenoceptor blockade with prazosin. J Cardiovasc Pharmacol 10:96, 1987.
113. Ferrier GR, Moffat MP, Lukas A: Possible mechanisms of ventricular arrhythmias elicited by ischemia followed by reperfusion: studies on isolated canine ventricular tissue. Circ Res 56:184, 1985.
114. Hayashi H, Ponnambalam C, McDonald TF: Arrhythmic activity in reoxygenated guinea pig papillary muscles and ventricular cells. Circ Res 61:124, 1987.
115. Yee R, Brown KK, Bolster DE, Strauss HC: The relationship between ionic perturbations and electrophysiologic changes in a canine Purkinje fiber model of ischemia and reperfusion. J Clin Invest 82:225, 1988.
116. Hill JA, Coronado R, Strauss HC: Reconstitution and characterization of a calcium-activated channel from heart. Circ Res 62:411, 1988.
117. Hoffman BF, Rosen MR: Cellular mechanisms of cardiac arrhythmias. Circ Res 49:1, 1981.
118. El-Sherif N, Gough WB, Zeiler RH, Mehra R: Triggered ventricular rhythms in one-day-old myocardial infarction in the dog. Circ Res 52:566, 1983.
119. Dangman KH, Dresdner KP, Zaim S: Automatic and triggered impulse initiation in canine subepicardial ventricular muscle cells from border zone of 24-hour transmural infarcts. Circulation 78:102, 1988.

120. Dangman KH, Hoffman BF: Studies on overdrive stimulation of canine cardiac Purkinje fibers: Maximal diastolic potential as a determinant of the response. J Am Coll Cardiol 2:1183, 1983.
121. LeMarec H, Dangman KH, Danilo P, Rosen MR: An evaluation of automaticity and triggered activity in canine heart one to four days after myocardial infarction. Circulation 71:1124, 1985.
122. Moak JP, Rosen MR: Induction and termination of triggered activity by pacing in isolated canine Purkinje fibers. Circulation 69:149, 1984.
123. Cranefield PF, Aronson RS: Cardiac Arrhythmias: The Role of Triggered Activity and Other Mechanisms, p. 441. Mount Kisco, NY, Futura Publishing Co., 1988.
124. Dresdner P, Kline RP, Wit AL: Intracellular K^+ activity, intracellular Na^+ activity and maximum diastolic potential in canine subendocardial Purkinje fibers from one-day-old infarcts. Circ Res 60:122, 1987.
125. Dresdner KP, Hannah NS, Kline RP, Wit AL: Na^+/K^+ pump failure in canine cardiac Purkinje fibers surviving an infarct (Abstract). Circulation 78:II-414, 1988.
126. Gough WB, El-Sherif N: Dependence of delayed afterdepolarizations on diastolic potentials in ischemic Purkinje fibers. Am J Physiol 257: H770–H777, 1989.
127. Ferrier GR: Effects of transmembrane potential on oscillatory afterpotentials induced by acetylstrophanthidin in canine ventricular tissues. J Pharmacol Exp Ther 215:332, 1980.
128. Mugelli A, Cerbai E, Amerini S, Visentin S: The role of temperature on the development of oscillatory afterpotentials and triggered activity. J Mol Cell Cardiol 18:1313, 1986.
129. Le Marec H, Spinelli W, Rosen MR: The effects of doxorubicin on ventricular tachycardia. Circ Res 74:881, 1986.
130. January CP, Fozzard HA: Delayed afterdepolarizations in heart muscles: mechanisms and relevance. Pharmacol Rev 30:219, 1988.
131. Kass R, Tsien RW, Weingart R: Ionic basis of transient inward current induced by strophanthidin in cardiac Purkinje fibers. J Physiol 281:208, 1978.
132. Nobel D: The surprising heart: A review of recent progress in cardiac electrophysiology. J Physiol 353:1, 1984.
133. Arlock P, Katzung BG: Effects of sodium substitute on transient inward current and tension in guinea pig and ferret papillary muscle. J Physiol 360:105, 1985.
134. Gough WB, Zeiler RH, El-Sherif N: Basis for reduced transmembrane potentials associated with triggered activity in ischemic subendocardial Purkinje fibers (Abstract). Circulation 66:II-156, 1982.
135. El-Sherif N, Zeiler RH, Gough WB: Effects of catecholamines, verapamil and tetrodotoxin in triggered automaticity in canine ischemic Purkinje fibers (Abstract). Circulation 62:III-281, 1980.
136. Gough WB, Zeiler RH, El-Sherif N: Effects of diltiazem on triggered activity in canine one-day-old infarction. Cardiovasc Res 18:339, 1984.
137. Boutjdir M, El-Sherif N, Gough WB: The effects of caffeine and ryanodine on delayed afterdepolarizations and sustained rhythmic activity in one-day-old infarction of the dog. Circulation. In press.
138. Carioni P, Vallani F, Carfoli E: The cardiotoxic antibiotic doxorubicin inhibits Na^+/Ca^{++} exchange of dog heart sarcolemmal vesicles. FEBS Lett 30:184, 1981.
139. Zeiler RH, Sequeria JM, Henkin R, et al.: Lysophosphatidyl choline: Putative agent for maintained triggered activity in ischemic cardiac Purkinje fibers (Abstract). J Am Coll Cardiol 9:252A, 1987.
140. Allen JD, Brennan FJ, Wit AL: Actions of lidocaine on transmembrane potentials of subendocardial Purkinje fibers surviving in infarcted canine hearts. Circ Res 43:470, 1978.
141. Rosen MR, Danilo P: Effects of tetrodotoxin, lidocaine, verapamil, AHR266 on ouabain-induced delayed afterdepolarizations in canine Purkinje fibers. Circ Res 46:117, 1980.
142. Danilo P, Langan WB, Rosen MR, Hoffman BF: Effects of the phenothiazine analog, EN-313, on ventricular arrhythmias in the dog. Eur J Pharmacol 45:127, 1977.
143. Dangman KH, Hoffman DF: Antiarrhythmic effects of automaticity and abolition of triggering. J Pharmacol Exp Ther 227:578, 1983.
144. Gough WB, Zeiler RH, El-Sherif N: Effects of nifedipine on triggered activity in one-day-old myocardial infarction in dogs. Am J Cardiol 53:303, 1984.
145. Hariman RJ, Zeiler RH, Gough WB, El-Sherif N: Enhancement of triggered activity in ischemic Purkinje fibers by ouabain: A mechanism of increased susceptibility to digitalis toxicity in myocardial infarction. J Am Coll Cardiol 5:672, 1985.
146. Gough WB, Hu D, El-Sherif N: Effects of clofilium on ischemic subendocardial Purkinje fibers one day post-infarction. J Am Coll Cardiol 11:431, 1988.
147. Gough WB, El-Sherif N: The differential response of normal and ischemic Purkinje fibers, to clofilium, d-sotalol, and bretylium. Cardiovasc Res, 23:554, 1989.
148. Synders DJ, Katzung BG: Clofilium reduces the plateau potassium current in isolated cardiac myocytes. Circulation 72:III-233, 1985.
149. Carmeliet E: Electrophysiologic and voltage clamp analysis of the effects of sotalol on isolated cardiac muscle and Purkinje fibers. J Pharmacol Exp Ther 232:817, 1985.
150. El-Sherif N, Gough WB, Zeiler RH, Mehra R: Ventricular rhythms in one-day-old canine infarction are due to triggered activity (Abstract). Circulation 66:II-357, 1982.
151. Martins JB: Autonomic control of ventricular tachycardia: Sympathetic neural influence on spontaneous tachycardia 24 hours after coronary occlusion. Circulation 72:933, 1985.
152. El-Sherif N, Mehra R, Gough WB, Zeiler RH: Ventricular activation patterns of spontaneous and induced ventricular rhythms in canine one-day-old myocardial infarction. Evidence for focal and reentrant mechanisms. Circ Res 51:152, 1982.
153. Hariman RJ, Holtzman R, Gough WB, et al.: In vivo demonstration of delayed afterdepolarization as a cause of ventricular rhythms in one-day-old infarction (Abstract). J Am Coll Cardiol 3:478, 1984.
154. Rosenshtraukh LV, Urtaler F, Anjukhousky EP, et al.: Serial production of controlled periods of temporary heart block used to unmask and assess latent ventricular automaticity during experimental acute myocardial infarction. J Am Coll Cardiol 8:95A, 1986.
155. Malfatto G, Rosen TS, Rosen MR: The response to overdrive pacing of triggered atrial and ventricular arrhythmias in the canine heart. Circulation 77:1139, 1988.
156. El-Sherif N, Smith RA, Evans K: Canine ventricular arrhythmias in the late myocardial infarction period. 8. Epicardial mapping of reentrant circuits. Circ Res 49:255, 1981.
157. Mehra R, Zeiler RH, Gough WB, El-Sherif N: Reentrant ventricular arrhythmias in the late myocardial infarction period. 9. Electrophysiologic-anatomic correlation of reentrant circuits. Circulation 67:11, 1983.
158. El-Sherif N, Mehra R, Gough WB, Zeiler RH: Reentrant ventricular arrhythmias in the late myocardial infarction period. Interruption of reentrant circuits by cryothermal techniques. Circulation 8:644, 1983.
159. El-Sherif N, Mehra R, Gough WB, Zeiler RH: Reentrant ventricular arrhythmias in the late myocardial infarction period. 11. Burst pacing versus multiple premature stimulation in the induction of reentry. J Am Coll Cardiol 4:295, 1984.
160. El-Sherif N, Gough WB, Zeiler RH, Hariman R: Reentrant ventricular arrhythmias in the late myocardial infarction period. 12. Spontaneous versus induced reentry and intramural versus epicardial circuit. J Am Coll Cardiol 6:124, 1985.
161. El-Sherif N: The figure-8 model of reentrant excitation in the canine postinfarction heart. In Zipes DP, Jalife J (eds.): Cardiac Electrophysiology and Arrhythmias, pp. 365–378. Orlando, Grune & Stratton, 1985.
162. Gough WB, Mehra R, Restivo M, et al.: Reentrant ventricular arrhythmia in the late myocardial infarction period in the dog. 13. Correlation of activation and refractory maps. Circ Res 57:432, 1985.
163. El-Sherif N, Gough WB, Restivo M: Reentrant ventricular arrhythmias in the late myocardial infarction period. 14. Mechanisms of resetting, entrainment, acceleration, or termination of reentrant tachycardia by programmed electrical stimulation. Pace 10:341, 1987.
164. Restivo M, Gough WB, El-Sherif N: Reentrant ventricular rhythms in the late myocardial infarction period: Prevention of reentry by dual stimulation during basic rhythm. Circulation 77:429, 1988.

165. Hirzel HO, Nelson GR, Sonnenblick EH, Kirk ES: Redistribution of collateral blood flow from necrotic to surviving myocardium following coronary occlusion in the dog. Circ Res 39:214, 1976.
166. El-Sherif N, Lazzara R: Reentrant ventricular arrhythmias in the late myocardial infarction period. 7. Effects of verapamil and D-600 and role of the "slow channel." Circulation 60:605, 1979.
167. Lazzara R, Scherlag BJ: The role of the slow current in the generation of arrhythmias in ischemic myocardium. In Zipes DP, Bailey JC, Elharrar V (eds.): The Slow Inward Current and Cardiac Arrhythmias, pp. 399–416. The Hague, Martinus Nijhoff, 1980.
168. Ursell PC, Gardner PI, Albala A, et al.: Structural and electrophysiological changes in the epicardial border zone of canine myocardial infarcts during infarct healing. Circ Res 56:436, 1985.
169. Schwartz A, Wood JM, Allen JC, et al.: Biochemical and morphologic correlates of cardiac ischemia. I. Membrane system. Am J Cardiol 32:46, 1973.
170. Sobel BE, Corr PB, Robinson AK, et al.: Accumulation of lysophosphoglycerides with arrhythmogenic properties in ischemic myocardium. J Clin Invest 62:546, 1978.
171. Spear JF, Michelson EL, Moore EN: Reduced space constant in slowly conducting regions of chronically infarcted canine myocardium. Circ Res 52:176, 1983.
172. Page E, Shibata Y: Permeable junctions between cardiac cells. Annu Rev Physiol 43:431, 1981.
173. Wit AL, Dillon S, Ursell PC: Influences of anisotropic tissue structure on reentrant ventricular tachycardia. In Brugada P, Wellens HJJ (eds.): Cardiac Arrhythmias. Where to Go From Here? (pp. 27–50). Mount Kisco, NY, Futura Publishing Co., 1987.
174. Dillon S, Allessie MA, Ursell PC, Wit AL: Influences of anisotropic tissue structure on reentrant circuits in the epicardial border zone of subacute canine infarcts. Circ Res 63:182, 1988.
175. Clerc L: Directional differences of impulse spread in trabecular muscle from mammalian heart. J Physiol (Lond) 255:335, 1976.
176. Spach M, Miller WT, Geselowitz DB, et al.: The discontinuous nature of propagation in normal canine cardiac muscle: Evidence for recurrent discontinuities of intracellular resistance that affect the membrane currents. Circ Res 48:39, 1981.
177. Spach MS, Miller WT, Dolber PC, et al.: The functional role of structural complexities in the propagation of depolarization in the atrium of the dog: Cardiac conduction disturbances due to discontinuities of effective axial resistivity. Circ Res 50:175, 1982.
178. Spach MS, Kootsey JM: The nature of electrical propagation in cardiac muscle. Am J Physiol 13:H3, 1983.
179. Restivo M, Gough WB, Wu K-M, et al.: Role of abrupt changes in refractoriness and fiber orientation in the formation of functional conduction block (Abstract). Circulation 76:IV-241, 1987.
180. Cardinal R, Vermeulen M, Shenasa M, et al.: Anisotropic conduction and functional dissociation of ischemic tissue during reentrant ventricular tachycardia in canine myocardial infarction. Circulation 77:1162, 1988.
181. Fenoglio JJ, Pham TD, Harken AH, et al.: Recurrent sustained ventricular tachycardia: Structure and ultrastructure of subendocardial regions where tachycardia originates. Circulation 68:518, 1983.
182. Harris L, Downar E, Mickleborough L, et al.: Activation sequence of ventricular tachycardia: Endocardial and epicardial mapping studies in the human ventricle. J Am Coll Cardiol 10:1040, 1987.
183. Kramer JB, Saffitz JE, Witkowski FX, Corr PB: Intramural reentry as a mechanism of ventricular tachycardia during evolving canine myocardial infarction. Circ Res 56:736, 1985.
184. Mines GR: On dynamic equilibrium in heart. J Physiol (Lond) 46:350, 1913.
185. Mines GR: On circulating excitations in heart muscles and their possible relation to tachycardia and fibrillation. Trans R Soc Can (ser 3, sect IV):43, 1914.
186. Spach MS, Dolber PC: Relating extracellular potentials and their derivatives to anisotropic propagation at a microscopic level in human cardiac muscle: Evidence for uncoupling of side-to-side fiber connections with increasing age. Circ Res 56:356, 1986.
187. El-Sherif N, Scherlag BJ, Lazzara R, Hope RR: Reentrant ventricular arrhythmias in the late myocardial infarction period. 4. Mechanism of action of lidocaine. Circulation 56:395, 1977.
188. El-Sherif N, Lazzara R: Reentrant ventricular arrhythmias in the late myocardial infarction period. 5. Mechanism of action of diphenylhydantoin. Circulation 57:465, 1977.
189. El-Sherif N: Electrophysiologic basis of procainamide therapeutic and toxic effects on ischemia-related reentrant ventricular arrhythmias (Abstract). Am J Cardiol 43:429, 1979.
190. Cobbe SM, Hoffman E, Ritzenhoff A, et al.: Action of sotalol on potential reentrant pathways and ventricular tachyarrhythmias in conscious dogs in the late post-myocardial infarction phase. Circulation 68:865, 1983.
191. Cobbe SM, Hoffman E, Ritzenhoff A, et al.: Action of disopyramide on potential reentrant pathways and ventricular tachyarrhythmias in conscious dogs in the late postmyocardial infarction phase. Am J Cardiol 53:1712, 1984.
192. Patterson E, Gibson JK, Lucchesi BR: Electrophysiologic effects of disopyramide phosphate on reentrant ventricular arrhythmia in conscious dogs after myocardial infarction. Am J Cardiol 46:792, 1980.
193. Patterson E, Gibson JK, Lucchesi BR: Electrophysiological action of lidocaine in a canine model of chronic myocardial ischemic damage. J Cardiovasc Pharmacol 4:925, 1982.
194. Michelson EL, Spear JF, Moore EN: Effects of procainamide on strength interval relations in normal and chronically infarcted canine myocardium. Am J Cardiol 47:1223, 1981.
195. Gang ES, Bigger JT, Uhl EW: Effects of timolol and propranolol in inducible sustained ventricular tachyarrhythmias in dogs with subacute myocardial infarction. Am J Cardiol 53:275, 1984.
196. Mehra R, Gough WB, Zeiler RH, El-Sherif N: Mechanism of lidocaine action on reentrant ventricular rhythms in the canine ischemic heart (Abstract). J Am Coll Cardiol 2:542, 1984.

3

Biochemical and Metabolic Aspects of Arrhythmias

James N. Weiss

Coronary artery disease is the most common cause of death in Western civilization today, and ventricular arrhythmias are the leading cause of mortality from coronary artery disease. Sustained ventricular arrhythmias in humans have been most extensively studied in the setting of chronic myocardial infarction. Each year in the United States about 15,000 people who have survived a previous myocardial infarction develop an episode of sustained ventricular tachycardia or fibrillation unassociated with a new infarction.[87] These arrhythmias can usually be reproduced by programmed ventricular stimulation in the clinical electrophysiology laboratory, which has provided the opportunity to study their behavior in response to pacing and drugs. Insights into the mechanisms responsible for these arrhythmias gained from both human and animal studies have led to the design of rational strategies for effective clinical management of this problem. Antiarrhythmic drug therapy, pacemakers, surgery, and catheter ablation techniques are viable therapeutic options.

In contrast to chronic myocardial infarction, sustained ventricular arrhythmias in the setting of acute myocardial ischemia and infarction pose a much greater clinical management problem, both in terms of magnitude and in the design of effective therapy. Over 1 million people in the United States suffer an acute myocardial infarction annually, with an overall mortality of approximately 50%. Most of these deaths are due to ventricular tachyarrhythmias, especially in the 60% of deaths (approximately 300,000 per year) that occur too suddenly for the patient to reach a hospital.[27] Thus the strategies for control of ventricular arrhythmias in association with chronic myocardial infarction are inapplicable in the majority (and much greater number) of patients who develop lethal ventricular arrhythmias during acute myocardial infarction and ischemia. Moreover, even though the mechanism (reentry) is probably the same in most cases of sustained ventricular arrhythmias associated with chronic and acute myocardial infarction, the pathophysiology is markedly different. In chronic infarction, scarring and fibrosis interfere with normal propagation of the cardiac impulse at the border zone of the infarct, causing slow conduction and altered refractoriness, the substrate for reentry, in these regions. Action potentials of individual cells are often normal in appearance. Alterations in the cable properties of the tissue from disruption of normal cell-to-cell connections, however, appear to be a major factor responsible for conduction abnormalities.[86] These conduction abnormalities typically remain stable over long periods of time, accounting for the ability of programmed stimulation to induce the same ventricular tachycardia time after time.

In contrast, during acute myocardial ischemia the conditions that promote sustained ventricular tachycardia are constantly changing as the process of cell death evolves. Action potential configuration is markedly abnormal and electrophysiologic properties of the ischemic tissue change continuously as byproducts of impaired metabolism accumulate, due to lack of washout, and exert toxic electrophysiologic effects. In this sense, a broader spectrum of biochemical and metabolic factors is more important in the genesis of arrhythmias during acute myocardial ischemia and infarction than in the setting of chronic myocardial infarction. The following discussion, therefore, will focus on the electrophysiologic derangements that occur during acute myocardial ischemia and during other conditions in which cellular metabolism is acutely impaired. Studies in this field have illuminated many of the relationships between function and metabolism in heart, although many uncertainties still exist.

Supported by NHBLI grants HL28746, HL36729, and Research Career Development Award HL01890; American Heart Association Grant-in-Aid 83-262; and Laubisch Endowment.

Basal Energy Utilization in the Heart

Figure 3–1 illustrates the proportion of metabolic energy used by various functions of the heart under basal conditions.[25] Tension development accounts for the largest proportion, about 60%. Forty percent of this energy is required to maintain tension within the cell (internal tension) and does not appear as external work. The other 20% is used to pump blood (external tension) and, excluding a component lost to heat, defines the overall mechanical efficiency of the heart as a pump. Fifteen percent of energy is dedicated to pumping the cytosolic Ca^{2+} that activated contraction during the previous systole into the sarcoplasmic reticulum, an internal storage site of Ca^{2+} that is released during the subsequent contraction. A Ca^{2+}-ATPase associated with the sarcoplasmic reticulum mediates this process. About 20% of metabolic energy is used to maintain essential cellular functions not directly related to electrical or contractile functions, such as protein synthesis and replacement of structural components. Electrical activity of the heart consumes less than 5% of total energy, primarily to fuel the Na^+-K^+ pump in order to maintain the ionic gradients essential to normal electrophysiologic function.

In the normally perfused heart, fatty acids are the preferred substrate for high-energy phosphate synthesis and account for over 60% of total adenosine triphosphate (ATP) production, with glucose metabolism accounting for the remainder.[55] Aerobic (oxidative) metabolism therefore supplies over 90% of the metabolic energy of the heart under basal conditions, and anaerobic metabolism of glucose to pyruvate via glycolysis provides less than 10%. Anaerobic glycolysis is intrinsically a much less efficient system for producing ATP than oxidative metabolism. One glucose molecule generates only 2 ATP molecules in the net process of being degraded to 2 pyruvate molecules via anaerobic glycolysis, whereas the pyruvate molecules subsequently yield 34 ATP molecules during oxidation in the mitochondria through the tricarboxylic acid cycle. This assumes great significance during myocardial ischemia, when anaerobic glycolysis becomes the predominant pathway for ATP synthesis, and is a partial explanation for the exquisite sensitivity of the heart to oxygen deprivation.

The other factor that accounts for the sensitivity of the heart to reduced blood flow is its high resting oxygen extraction. Roughly 75% of the oxygen delivered to the heart is extracted by the coronary arteries, a nearly maximal amount compared to the 20–25% extracted by most other tissues (with the exception of the kidneys). The only way in which the heart can increase oxygen consumption is by increasing oxygen delivery. In order to match supply and demand, sensitive feedback mechanisms regulate coronary blood flow according to metabolic needs.[6,85] As cardiac work increases, ATP is degraded to adenosine diphosphate (ADP) and adenosine monophosphate (AMP). AMP is subsequently dephosphorylated to adenosine by 5'-nucleotidase. Adenosine is a potent vasodilator that increases coronary blood flow in proportion to oxygen requirements. Through this mechanism, and possibly through other undefined mechanisms as well,[56] basal cardiac oxygen consumption of approximately 9 ml/100 g/min[25] can be increased manyfold during exercise and other states demanding a high cardiac output.

Although ATP is the ultimate source of energy exchange for most energy-dependent processes in the heart, other high-energy phosphate compounds play an important role. In particular, creatine phosphate acts as a buffer system which prevents marked changes in ATP levels from occurring during the transition from one workload state to another.[10,43] Figure 3–2 schematically illustrates the creatine phosphate shuttle in the heart. ATP generated inside the mitochondria is impermeable to the inner mitochondrial membrane. To reach the cytoplasm, ATP first binds to the enzyme

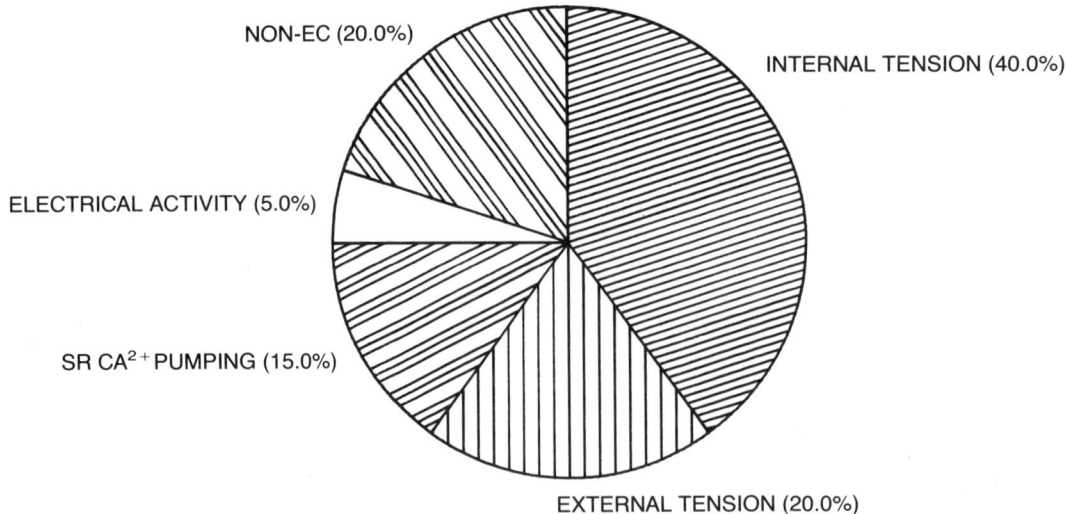

FIGURE 3–1
Basal energy utilization of the heart. Non-EC refers to energy utilization unrelated to excitation or contraction (e.g., protein synthesis). SR = sarcoplasmic reticulum.

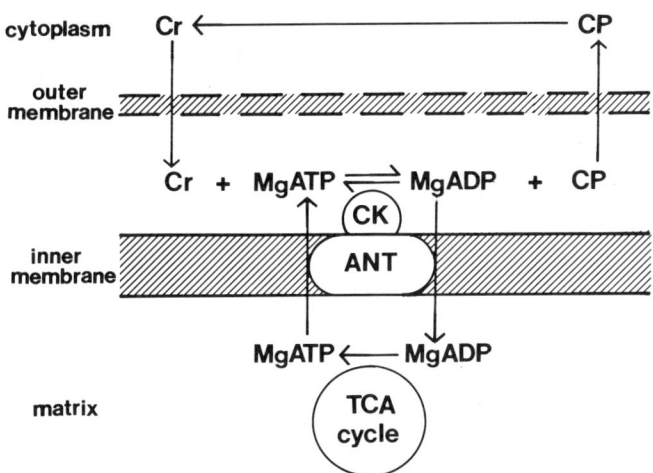

FIGURE 3–2
Schematic illustration of the creatine phosphate shuttle in heart. See text for description. Cr = creatine; CP = creatine phosphate; CK = creatine kinase; ANT = adenine nucleotide translocase.

adenine nucleotide translocase located on the mitochondrial inner membrane and is transported to mitochondrial creatine kinase, also associated with the inner membrane. Creatine kinase catalyzes the phosphorylation of creatine to creatine phosphate, converting ATP to ADP in the process. ADP is then returned to the inner mitochondrial matrix by adenine nucleotide translocase where it can be rephosphorylated. Creatine phosphate diffuses into the cytoplasm, where it can be converted to ATP by the reverse reaction with cytoplasmic creatine kinase. Thus the creatine kinase reaction "shuttles" ATP from sites of production (in the mitochondria) to sites of utilization (in the cytoplasm), and acts as a mechanism for buffering intracellular ATP levels during transitions to new workload states.[10] A major advantage of using the creatine kinase reaction to transfer energy is that the amount of free energy released when ATP is hydrolyzed can be maximized.[50] The free energy of ATP hydrolysis is proportional to $\log([ATP]/[ADP] \times [P_i])$, where P_i is inorganic phosphate. To maximize the free energy available from ATP, a low intracellular ADP concentration is necessary. In the absence of the creatine kinase shuttle, ADP generated at the site of ATP utilization would have to diffuse back to a mitochondrion to be rephosphorylated. Under these conditions the ability to resynthesize ATP would be limited by the rate of ADP diffusion, which is directly related to [ADP]. Thus although a low [ADP] would maximize the free-energy release from ATP hydrolysis, the ATP synthetic capability would be severely limited by suboptimal diffusion of ADP. The creatine kinase shuttle obviates this dilemma, since creatine phosphate can be present in millimolar concentrations in order to achieve rapid diffusion throughout the cell, yet [ADP] can be maintained at a very low level (approximately 30 μM)[11] because it needs only to diffuse to the nearest creatine kinase molecule to be rephosphorylated to ATP. In the case of the myofilaments, it has been suggested that creatine kinase bound to myosin generates ATP locally that is utilized preferentially over cytoplasmic ATP to support contractile function.[9,90] Some reports have suggested that sarcolemmal membrane-bound creatine kinase may be preferentially utilized to generate ATP for membrane functions such as the Na^+-K^+ pump,[28] although others have not been able to confirm this result.[73] The creatine kinase shuttle appears to be mainly used to facilitate mitochondrial ATP transport. There is no evidence that other ATP-generating metabolic pathways (e.g., glycolysis) utilize the shuttle in an obligatory fashion, although ATP from any source participates in the cytoplasmic creatine kinase reaction.

Energy Utilization During Acute Myocardial Ischemia

When coronary blood flow ceases, glycolysis becomes the predominant metabolic pathway for production of high-energy phosphates in ischemic myocardium. Although the rate of glycolysis accelerates manyfold during the first few minutes of ischemia, it cannot adequately meet the demand for energy. Within seconds the levels of creatine phosphate begin to plummet, as it is rapidly consumed to rephosphorylate ADP by the creatine kinase reaction. This buffering effect of creatine kinase is effective in retarding the decline in ATP, and after 10 minutes of ischemia total cellular ATP has only fallen by one third.[36] However, creatine phosphate levels are severely depleted at this point. Glycolysis accelerates during the first 1 to 3 minutes of ischemia but then is progressively inhibited by the build-up of lactic acid and NADH and the fall in intracellular pH.[78]

Despite the relatively slow fall in total cellular ATP concentration during acute ischemia, cardiac function begins to deteriorate almost immediately. However, all cardiac functions do not fail at the same time or in the order proportionate to the percentage of myocardial energy they consume.[58] The earliest two abnormalities, beginning within seconds of the onset of ischemia, are a loss of cellular K^+ [38,39,53,83,93,100] and a decrease in the rate of relaxation of tension.[83] The mechanisms of cellular K^+ loss during ischemia are discussed in detail later in this chapter. The reduced rate of relaxation during ischemia results in a loss of compliance of the ventricular muscle, which can be detected in humans as an early manifestation of angina by hemodynamic or echocardiographic techniques.[5,23] Relaxation of cardiac muscle is an energy-dependent process mediated by a Ca^{2+}-ATPase that pumps Ca^{2+} from the cytoplasm into the sarcoplasmic reticulum against a large concentration gradient. It has been hypothesized that during ischemia the free energy released when ATP is hydrolyzed falls rapidly below the level required by the Ca^{2+}-ATPase to pump Ca^{2+} into the sarcoplasmic reticulum.[49] The free energy of ATP hydrolysis will decrease dramatically as ADP and inorganic phosphate (P_i) levels rise despite little change in [ATP]. The rise in [P_i] resulting from breakdown of creatine phosphate and ATP has other important consequences and is a leading candidate to explain the loss of systolic force development that begins after 60 to 90 seconds of ischemia in isolated hearts,[83] and more rapidly in in vivo hearts following coronary occlusion.[57] Elevated intracellular [P_i] depresses systolic tension by reducing the sensitivity of the contractile proteins to Ca^{2+}.[69] Factors that also contribute to the decline in the force of contraction during acute ischemia include intracellular acidosis[42, 51] and mechanical factors related to collapse of the vascular space.[2] Other potential factors are reduced Ca^{2+} release from the sarcoplasmic reticulum as a result of impaired Ca^{2+} sequestration, depletion of ATP at critical sites regulating Ca^{2+} homeostasis, and a decline in transmembrane Ca^{2+} flux.

After active systolic tension development has ceased completely (within 5 minutes after the onset of ischemia), abnormalities in diastolic tension worsen. After 7 to 10 minutes of ischemia in isolated hearts, relaxation becomes incomplete and resting diastolic tension increases.[83] After 20 minutes, full contracture is present. The mechanism of the increase in diastolic tension is not yet clear but could be explained by an increase in diastolic intracellular [Ca^{2+}] above the threshold for activation of the myofilaments[64] or a rigor state induced by ATP depletion.[35] However, total cellular ATP levels are not depleted enough to induce rigor after this duration of ischemia unless a critical compartmentalized pool of ATP is involved.

The final function to fail during ischemia is the Na^+-K^+ pump. Teleologically this is reasonable, since without the maintenance of normal cellular ionic gradients, coordinated electromechanical activity is not possible. Evidence from isolated heart preparations has shown that despite the markedly increased K^+ efflux during ischemia, radioisotopically measured K^+ influx does not decrease for at least 45 minutes.[84] It was later demonstrated, using ion selective microelectrodes, that intracellular [Na^+] did not increase for at least 15 minutes after the onset of ischemia.[53]

Figure 3–3 illustrates the time course of some of the changes in cardiac function during acute ischemia in an isolated arterially perfused rabbit interventricular septum. Note the immediate deterioration in active tension development and the accumulation of extracellular K^+ measured with an intramyocardial K^+-sensitive electrode. The action potential gradually shortened during ischemia, although only modestly during the first 10 minutes, and the preparation became inexcitable after 33 minutes. Conduction velocity also decreased gradually, as can be inferred from the increase in the interval between the stimulus artifact and the action potential upstroke.

Arrhythmogenesis During Acute Myocardial Ischemia

Electrophysiologic alterations during acute ischemia include depolarization of the resting membrane potential, a decrease in the maximal rate of rise of the action potential upstroke ($\dot{V}_{max}$), decreased excitability, shortening of action potential duration, altered refractoriness including post-repolarization refractoriness, and abnormal automaticity. These changes lead to slow conduction and the possibility of unidirectional conduction block, the basis for reentry. Arrhythmias during acute myocardial ischemia occur in several phases.[31] Following coronary occlusion in the dog, there is a high incidence of premature ventricular beats (PVBs), ventricular tachycardia, and ventricular fibrillation for 20 to 30 minutes, after which the frequency of arrhythmias declines as the ischemic ventricular muscle becomes inexcitable. After a hiatus of 6 to 8 hours, ventricular arrhythmias return and may persist for several days. These later-phase arrhythmias are thought to result from abnormal automaticity in the subendocardial Purkinje fibers overlying the area of infarct,[21, 101] and they can trigger ventricular tachycardia and fibrillation. These fibers probably receive enough oxygen and nutrients from intracavitary blood to remain viable but have abnormal electrical activity. The later-phase arrhythmias form the rationale for electrocardiographic monitoring of patients for 72 hours fol-

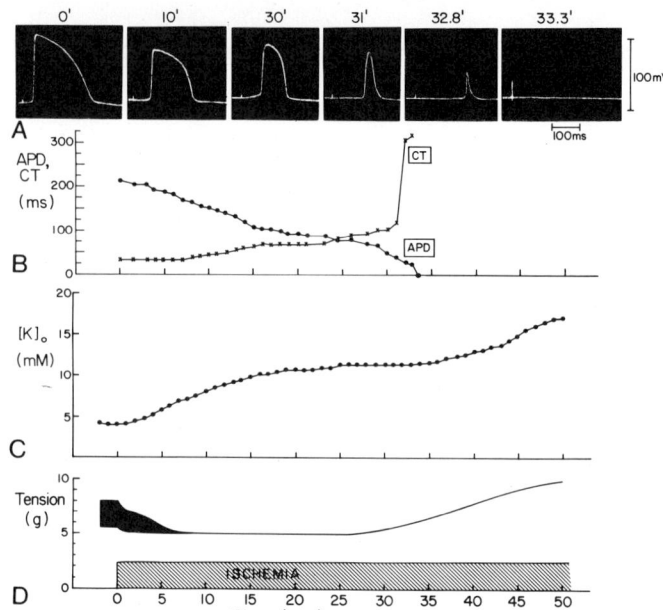

FIGURE 3–3
Changes in action potential duration, conduction time, [K^+]$_o$, and tension during a 50-minute period of global ischemia in an isolated rabbit interventricular septum. A shows representative action potentials recorded at various times after the onset of ischemia, from which action potential duration and conduction time from the site of stimulation to recording site have been measured and plotted in B below. C shows the change in [K^+]$_o$ measured with an intramyocardial K^+ sensitive electrode, showing the triphasic pattern of [K^+]$_o$ accumulation. D shows changes in the peak systolic and diastolic tension during the ischemic period. The development of contracture coincides with the secondary rise in [K^+]$_o$. APD = action potential duration; CT = conduction time. (Reprinted by permission from Weiss J, Shine KI: Am J Physiol 243:H318, 1982. Copyright American Physiological Society.)

lowing myocardial infarction. In contrast, the early-phase arrhythmias are responsible for the majority of deaths outside of the hospital in patients with acute myocardial infarction.

The mechanisms that commonly initiate ventricular tachycardia and fibrillation during the early phase of acute myocardial ischemia have been elegantly demonstrated in the studies of Janse and coworkers.[44] Following coronary occlusion in pigs, they found that the first beat initiating ventricular tachycardia or fibrillation typically arose from nonischemic tissue near the ischemic border zone. Excitation of this site was induced by injury currents flowing between the depolarized ischemic tissue and fully repolarized nonischemic tissue that were of sufficient magnitude to depolarize the normal tissue to its threshold during diastole. This PVB often acted as the trigger, causing reentry within the ischemic zone leading to ventricular tachycardia and fibrillation. Figure 3–4 illustrates an example of reentrant ventricular tachycardia during acute ischemia in an isolated rabbit ventricle that is consistent with this mechanism. The left ventricle was cut open along the posterior interventricular groove and pinned down as a sheet. Electrical activity at 128 points over the surface of the heart was recorded every 4 ms with a laser-scanning system after staining the preparation with the membrane potential–sensitive dye WW 781.[67] Seven minutes after the left ventricular free-wall was made ischemic (with perfusion of the interventricular septum maintained) a 3-beat run of ventricular tachycardia occurred. Activation maps of these 3 beats using 10-ms isochrome lines are shown in Figure 3–4B. The first beat originated in the nonischemic septum and propagated rapidly to the ischemic left ventricular free-wall, where it encountered refractory tissue at the base but conducted slowly around the apex. The slow conduction around the apex allowed the refractory tissue at the base to recover excitability before arrival of the impulse, which then reentered the nonischemic tissue to initiate the second beat of ventricular tachycardia. The impulse circulated one additional time before encountering refractory tissue at the apex, terminating the tachycardia.

Factors Causing Electrophysiologic Alterations During Acute Ischemia

The electrophysiologic abnormalities during acute myocardial ischemia that lead to arrhythmias such as shown in Figure 3–4 may arise from two sources: (1) direct effects of energy depletion and (2) secondary effects of a variety of by-products of metabolic inhibition that accumulate in the cellular environment because of the lack of washout. The first factor has generally been held to be less important, since most electrical activity is generated by ions flowing passively down their electrochemical gradients. Although ionic gradients must be maintained by energy-consuming processes, as discussed above, the Na^+-K^+ pump does not appear to be functionally compromised until relatively late in ischemia. However, recently it has been recognized that some ionic currents in heart are directly sensitive to cellular energy status, such as the Ca^{2+} channel (which requires phosphorylation to function)[71] and the ATP-sensitive K^+ channel.[70, 89]

Table 3–1 lists various sequelae of metabolic inhibition that have been implicated as causes of electrophysiologic abnormalities during acute ischemia. Most of these factors are thought to impair normal electrical activity by affecting the ionic currents that generate the action potential. However, certain factors may also alter the cell-to-cell connections that form the low-resistance pathways through which the action potential is propagated. For example, elevated intracellular $[H^+]$ and $[Ca^{2+}]$ are both known to increase internal resistance through these pathways and may contribute the reduced space constant of ventricular muscle and slowing of conduction velocity during acute ischemia.[1] Although there has been much interest recently in arrhythmogenicity due to altered passive electrical properties of the myocardium, the relative importance of this factor during acute ischemia is difficult to assess because of the prominent changes in ionic currents, which also alter propagation of the cardiac impulse.

EXTRACELLULAR K^+ ACCUMULATION

Extracellular K^+ ($[K^+]_o$) accumulation resulting from the increased K^+ efflux and lack of washout is a major factor contributing to the electrophysiologic abnormalities of acute ischemia. $[K^+]_o$ increases by as much as 12 mEq/L in the central ischemic zone during the first 10 minutes following coronary occlusion[38, 39, 100] and is largely responsible for depolarization of the resting membrane potential.[53, 96] The resulting inactivation of the fast Na^+ current reduces $\dot{V}_{max}$ of the action potential upstroke, which slows conduction velocity through the ischemic tissue. By depolarizing the membrane, elevated $[K^+]_o$ also shortens action potential duration and alters refractoriness of the ischemic tissue. Infusion of KCl into the coronary arteries of dogs has been shown to cause VPBs, ventricular tachycardia, and ventricular fibrillation.[32]

The mechanism of $[K^+]_o$ accumulation during acute myocardial ischemia is still controversial. It is well established that net K^+ loss results primarily from an increase in K^+ efflux rather than from a decrease in K^+ influx. This has been demonstrated by radioisotopic techniques[84] and with ion-selective electrodes.[53, 93] Kleber[53] used intracellular Na^+-selective microelectrodes to show that intracellular $[Na^+]$ did not increase for at least 15 minutes after the onset of ischemia, as would have been expected if Na^+-K^+ pump inhibition were the cause of net K^+ loss. Other studies have shown that in isolated sarcolemmal vesicles maximal Na^+-K^+ ATPase activity is depressed after durations of ischemia as short as 10 minutes.[8] However, this depression of maximal function does not appear to encroach upon maintenance of adequate Na^+-K^+ pump function until late ischemia, possibly as long as 45 minutes.[84]

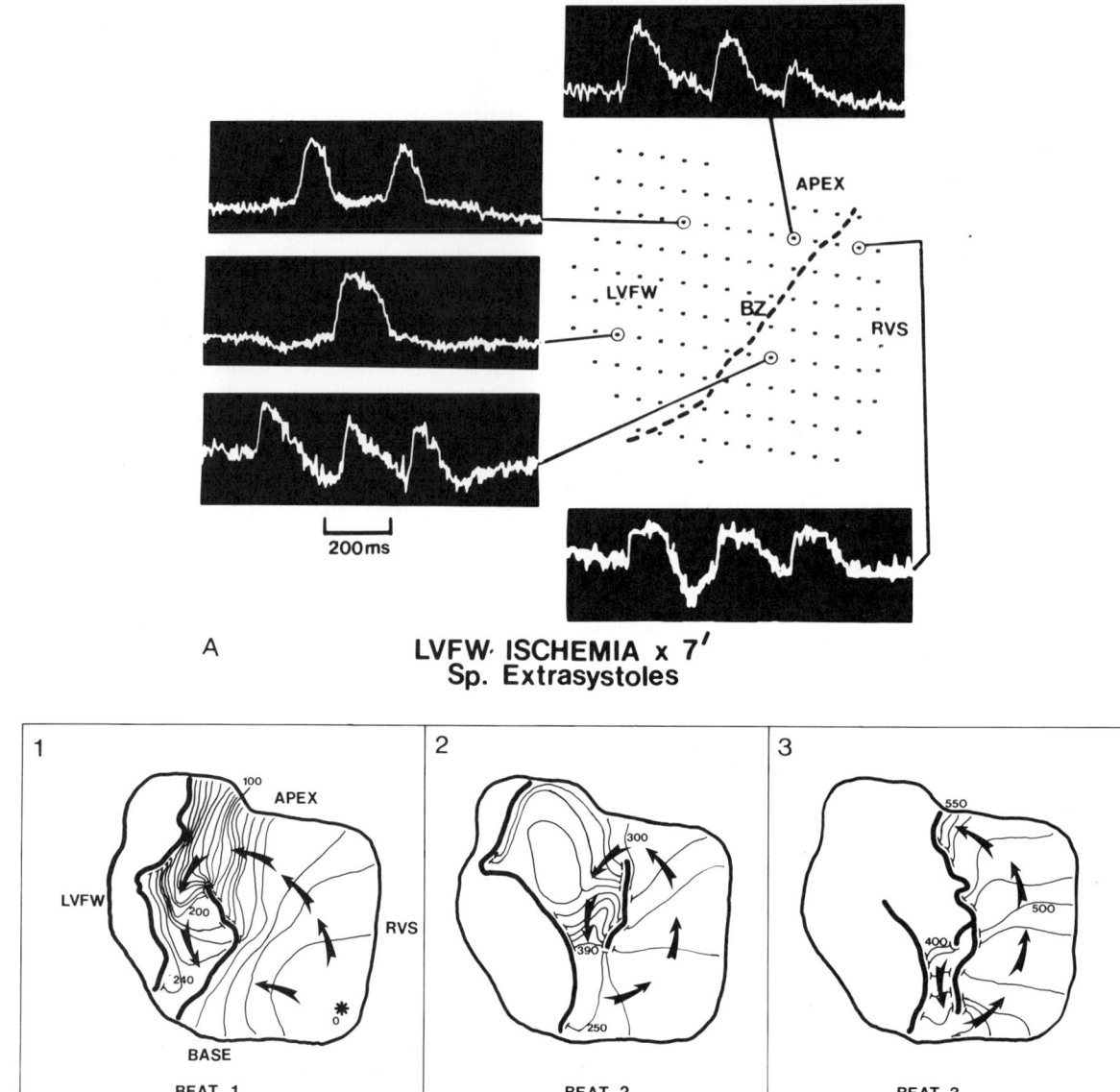

FIGURE 3–4
Activation mapping of a 3-beat run of reentrant ventricular tachycardia during regional ischemia in an isolated rabbit ventricle. A, Electrical activity was measured over the surface of an arterially perfused isolated rabbit ventricle with the membrane potential–sensitive dye WW 781, using a computer-controlled acousto-optical device directed laser beam to scan 128 sites (indicated by dots) every 4 ms. Optically measured action potentials from representative sites are shown during a 3-beat run of ventricular tachycardia that occurred 7 minutes after coronary flow to the left ventricular free-wall (LVFW) was stopped. Flow to the interventricular septum (RVS) was maintained. The border zone (BZ) between the two vascular beds is indicated by the dashed line. B, Activation maps (1–3) of each of the three ventricular tachycardia beats reconstructed from the timing of the action potential upstroke at all 128 sites. Isochrome lines are 10 ms apart. Asterisk indicates the earliest site of activation of the first beat (time zero). Arrows show the direction of impulse spread for the beat 1 (0–240 ms), beat 2 (250–390 ms) and beat 3 (400–550 ms). Zones of block are indicated by the heavy lines. This experiment was performed at the University of Pennsylvania in collaboration with Drs. S. Dillon and M. Morad. (Reprinted by permission from Weiss JN: Metabolic effects of ischemia: What are the implications for arrhythmogenesis and the treatment of arrhythmias? In Brugada P, Wellens HJJ (eds.): Cardiac Arrhythmias: Where to Go from Here?, pp. 83–104. New York, Futura Publishing Co., 1987.)

Two mechanisms have been postulated to account for the marked increase in K^+ efflux which begins within 30 seconds of the onset of ischemia: an increase in membrane K^+ conductance or K^+ efflux passively linked to anion (lactate and P_i) efflux. A third factor that may contribute to the elevation of $[K^+]_o$ during ischemia is free water loss from the extracellular space, which acts to concentrate extracellular K^+.[45] During ischemia, intracellular osmolarity increases due to the generation of lactate, P_i and other small molecules, causing intracellular edema and, conversely, extracellular dehydration. Although this mechanism may exaggerate the magnitude of $[K^+]_o$ achieved during ischemia it cannot be the full explanation since marked

TABLE 3–1
Factors Contributing to Electrophysiologic Abnormalities During Acute Ischemia

Elevated extracellular [K+]
Intracellular acidosis
Lactate accumulation
Catecholamine release
Elevated intracellular cyclic adenosine monophosphate
Lysophospholipid accumulation
Fatty acid ester accumulation
Free fatty acid accumulation
Free radicals

cellular K^+ loss also occurs acutely during hypoxia and exposure to metabolic inhibitors, when extracellular fluid shifts are not as significant.[75, 95] The hypothesis that cellular K^+ loss during ischemia may be due to anion-coupled K^+ efflux was based on the observation that the time course of lactate and P_i loss during low flow ischemia was similar to that of K^+ loss and that it quantitatively exceeded K^+ loss on a mole-to-mole basis by a factor of approximately 3.[54, 65] It was postulated that when anions such as lactate and P_i diffuse across the sarcolemma, they must be accompanied by an equal and opposite charge movement and that K^+, the most prevalent intracellular cation, might serve this purpose. It should be noted that this mechanism would not involve a change in membrane K^+ conductance. Gaspardone[24] showed that the efflux of certain anions such as chloride and 5,5-dimethyl-2,4-oxazolidione (DMO) caused an associated increase in K^+ efflux. However, both lactate and P_i are much more membrane-permeable as undissociated (hydrogenated) molecules than as charged anions, and it is possible that H^+ is the dominant charge-balancing cation during their efflux.

To test whether anion-coupled K^+ loss is a feasible explanation for cellular K^+ loss during ischemia, we exposed rabbit interventricular septa to glucose-free substrate prior to ischemia in order to deplete glycogen stores and reduce lactate production during the subsequent ischemic period. Net lactate, P_i, and K^+ loss were measured by collecting the perfusate during the first minute of reperfusion after 10 minutes of ischemia. As shown in Figure 3–5, exposure to glucose-free perfusate prior to ischemia reduced net lactate loss during ischemia and did not change P_i loss, but significantly increased K^+ loss. Thus, by this maneuver, anion and K^+ loss were dissociated during ischemia, suggesting that a simple relationship between the two does not exist. More compelling evidence that anion-coupled K^+ loss is not likely to be of major importance during ischemia comes from studies of K^+ loss during hypoxia and exposure to metabolic inhibitors. For example, marked K^+ loss occurred during selective inhibition of glycolysis despite a decrease in lactate efflux and maintenance of normal cellular high-energy phosphate levels.[95] Recently we have investigated the effects of elevating extracellular lactate to 30 mM during hypoxia in isolated rabbit interventricular septa.[99] Intracellular potential, venous lactate and P_i, tissue lactate and water, and the extracellular space were measured, from which the concentrations of intracellular and extracellular lactate during hypoxia were calculated. Net and unidirectional fluxes of lactate ion were then calculated from the Goldman-Hodgkin-Katz equations, assuming simple electrochemical diffusion. Neither net K^+ loss nor unidirectional K^+ efflux (measured by ^{42}K uptake and washout techniques, respectively) were affected by the presence of 30-mM exogenous lactate during hypoxia in a manner consistent with the predicted changes in net and unidirectional lactate ion fluxes. These findings suggest that during hypoxia, anion-coupled K^+ loss via simple electrodiffusion is not an important cause of increased K^+ efflux.

The remaining possible mechanism to account for increased K^+ efflux during myocardial ischemia is an increase in membrane K^+ conductance. Several observations are consistent with this mechanism. As shown in Figure 3–6, during acute ischemia the difference between the resting membrane potential (E_m) and the K^+ equilibrium potential (E_K) progressively decreased,[53, 96] indicating an increase in membrane K^+ conductance relative to that of other ions influencing the resting membrane potential. If the heart remained quiescent during ischemia the rate of $[K^+]_o$ accumulation was markedly reduced, consistent with the reduced driving force ($E_m - E_K$) for K^+ efflux in the absence of intermittent depolarization.[76, 96] The effects of heart

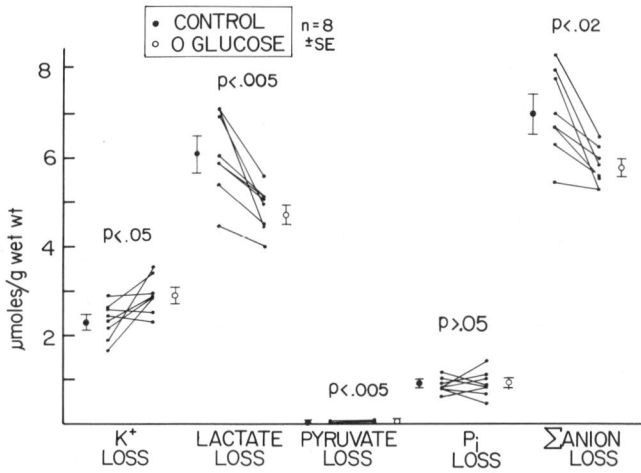

FIGURE 3–5
The effect of pre-exposure to substrate-free perfusate on K^+ vs. anion loss during ischemia. Net loss of K^+, lactate, pyruvate, inorganic phosphate, and the sum of the latter three anions are compared during two sequential 10-minute periods of ischemia in eight isolated rabbit septa. One period of ischemia (0 glucose) was preceded by a 10-minute exposure to glucose-free perfusate immediately prior to ischemia; the other ischemic period (CONTROL) served as the control. The order was reversed in half of the experiments. Lines connect the values obtained from individual preparations, with the mean and standard deviations of each group shown alongside. Paired T-tests were used to assess statistical significance. (Reprinted by permission from Weiss JN: Metabolic effects of ischemia: What are the implications for arrhythmogenesis and the treatment of arrhythmias? In Brugada P, Wellens HJJ (eds.): Cardiac Arrhythmias: Where to Go from Here?, pp. 83–104. New York, Futura Publishing Co., 1987. Copyright Futura Publishing Company, Inc.)

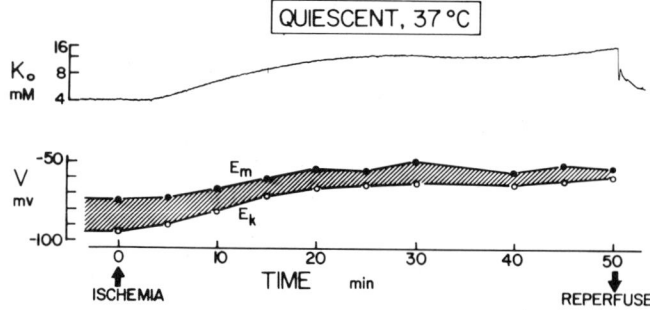

FIGURE 3–6
Changes in $[K^+]_o$, resting membrane potential (E_m), and the calculated K^+ equilibrium potential (E_k) during a 50-minute period of global ischemia in a quiescent rabbit septum. The difference between E_m and E_k progressively decreased during the ischemic period. (Reprinted by permission from Weiss J, Shine KI: Am J Physiol 250:H982, 1986. Copyright American Physiological Society.)

rate on $[K^+]_o$ accumulation during ischemia were also consistent with an increased membrane K^+ conductance.[96] Figure 3–7A shows that the rate of $[K^+]_o$ accumulation was different when a rabbit septal preparation was paced at 75 bpm compared to 150 bpm. However, if $[K^+]_o$ accumulation occurs primarily when the driving force for K^+ efflux is large, i.e. during systole, then the cumulative time spent in systole rather than the total duration of ischemia might correlate better with the level of $[K^+]_o$ accumulation. To estimate the cumulative time spent in systole, intracellular potential was measured during ischemia and the action potential duration integrated. Figure 3–7B shows that the level of $[K^+]_o$ for a given cumulative duration of systole was nearly identical at the two heart rates.

Although there is no direct evidence that membrane K^+ conductance increases during ischemia, membrane K^+ conductance is clearly altered by hypoxia and exposure to metabolic inhibitors. Voltage-clamped cat papillary muscles developed an increase in background K^+ currents during hypoxia.[17, 91] Similar effects were seen in isolated cardiac myocytes exposed to metabolic inhibitors.[41] Figures 3–8 and 3–12 show examples of the effects of inhibiting both glycolytic and mitochondrial metabolism on single cardiac myocytes isolated enzymatically from guinea pig ventricles. Exposure to metabolic inhibitors caused transient action potential prolongation followed by marked shortening leading to inexcitability (see Fig. 3–12). Under voltage clamp conditions, the current-voltage relations in Figure 3–8 show that metabolic inhibitors activated a large outward (repolarizing) current with a reversal potential near E_K, indicative of K^+ current.

Further insight into the nature of metabolically-sensitive K^+ currents was obtained from patch clamp experiments by Noma[70] and by Trube.[89] The patch clamp technique[30] is a method for studying currents through individual ionic channels in membranes, illustrated in Figure 3–9. A fire-polished glass electrode with a tip diameter of 1 to 5 μ is filled with an appropriate solution and brought into contact with the surface membrane of an isolated cell. Gentle suction is applied to form a high resistance seal (>10^{10} ohms)

between the electrode and a patch of membrane. The membrane patch can be studied in this configuration (cell-attached patch) or the electrode can be withdrawn to excise the patch. In the latter case, the cytoplasmic surface of the excised membrane patch faces the bath and is referred to as an excised inside-out patch. If the voltage (E_m) across the membrane patch is held constant, the current flow (I_m) through the membrane will be inversely proportional to the resistance (R_m) of the membrane patch by Ohm's law, $I_m = E_m/R_m$. If no ion channels are open in the membrane patch, R_m is very high and I_m is very small. When a channel opens, however, R_m falls and I_m must increase to keep E_m constant. If a second channel opens at the same time, twice as much current is required to hold E_m constant.

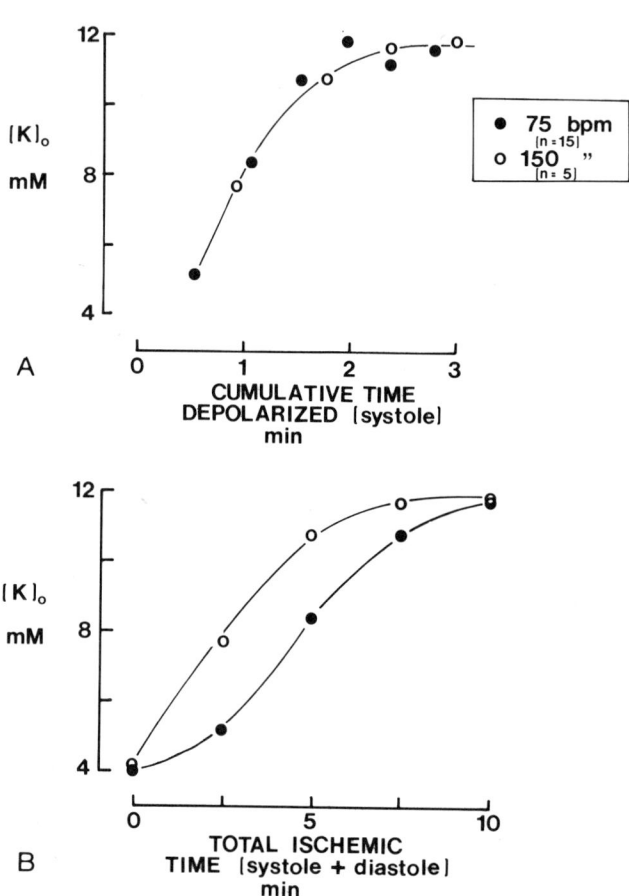

FIGURE 3–7
The level of $[K^+]_o$ accumulation plotted as a function of either the cumulative time spent depolarized during ischemia (A) or the total duration of ischemia (B) at two different heart rates: 75 beats per minute (bpm) (closed circles) and 150 bpm (open circles) in isolated rabbit interventricular septa. At each heart rate the action potential duration was measured during ischemia and summed over time to estimate the total time spent depolarized (systole) after various total durations (systole + diastole) of ischemia. Intracellular potential was recorded with floating glass microelectrodes, and $[K^+]_o$ with extracellular valinomycin K^+-selective electrodes. (Reprinted by permission from Weiss JN: Metabolic effects of ischemia: What are the implications for arrhythmogenesis and the treatment of arrhythmias? In Brugada P, Wellens HJJ (eds.): Cardiac Arrhythmias: Where to Go from Here?, pp. 83–104. New York, Futura Publishing Co., 1987. Copyright Futura Publishing Company, Inc.)

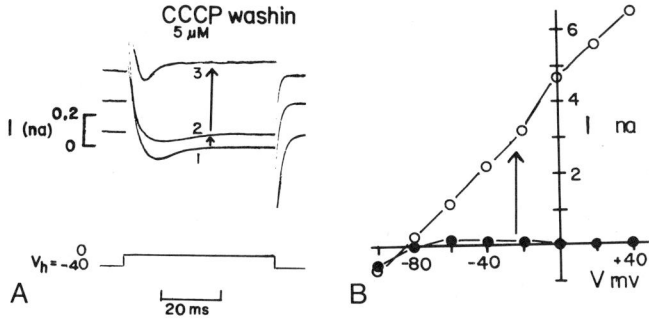

FIGURE 3–8
Effects of metabolic inhibition on ionic currents in a voltage-clamped single guinea pig ventricular myocyte. A shows superimposed 50-ms voltage clamps applied every 5 s from a holding membrane potential of −40 to 0 mV. About 5 minutes after the mitochondrial inhibitor CCCP (5 μm) + the glycolytic inhibitor 2-deoxyglucose (20 mM) were washed in, the current became progressively more outward (upward direction) with each successive clamp (labeled 1–3). B shows the current-voltage relations under control conditions (solid circles) and after 5-min exposure to the metabolic inhibitors (open circles). Note that the direction of the latter current reverses near E_K, and is very large (outward) at positive membrane potentials compared to the control. (Reprinted by permission from Weiss JN: Metabolic effects of ischemia: What are the implications for arrhythmogenesis and the treatment of arrhythmias? In Brugada P, Wellens HJJ (eds.): Cardiac Arrhythmias: Where to Go from Here?, pp. 83–104. New York, Futura Publishing Co., 1987. Copyright Futura Publishing Company, Inc.)

Figure 3–10 shows an example of single K^+ channel currents measured in an excised inside-out patch from a guinea pig ventricular myocyte. The bath and electrode solutions contained predominantly K^+ in order to detect only K^+ channels. When the bath solution contained 2 mM ATP, no K^+ channels were observed to open. However, when ATP was removed from the bath, openings of at least five individual K^+ channels were superimposed at times. Readmission of ATP to the bath solution caused all the channels to close.

The discovery of the ATP-sensitive K^+ channel, which opens only when cytoplasmic [ATP] falls below a critical level, would seem to be a natural candidate for the increased K^+ efflux during ischemia except for one problem: the concentration of ATP necessary to completely prevent the ATP-sensitive channel from opening in excised patches is about 0.2 mM.[70] Total cellular ATP concentration, however, is 3 to 4 mM in the normal myocardium and, as discussed previously, has fallen only modestly (to 2–3 mM) during ischemia at a time when K^+ efflux is markedly increased. Unless ATP in the vicinity of ATP-sensitive K^+ channels is depleted more rapidly than total cellular levels of ATP (i.e. ATP is compartmentalized), or the sensitivity of the channels to ATP is markedly reduced by sequelae of ischemia, it is unlikely that activation of ATP-sensitive K^+ channels could occur early enough to account for increased K^+ efflux during ischemia. Evidence for the first possibility will be discussed in the last section of this chapter. Regarding the second possibility, it has been shown in noncardiac cells that ADP significantly increases the concentration of ATP required to suppress ATP-sensitive K^+ channels.[66, 77]

The prominent contribution that $[K^+]_o$ accumulation makes to the electrophysiologic alterations of acute ischemia has two important consequences. The development of arrhythmias is initially facilitated by the alterations in conduction velocity and refractoriness resulting from membrane depolarization. However, progressive membrane depolarization and activation of ATP-sensitive K^+ channels, which are time-independent and antagonize the inward currents responsible for the upstroke of the action potential, eventually lead to inexcitability in the ischemic region, an antiarrhythmic event responsible for the end of the first phase of arrhythmias.[31] Thus the net effect of cellular K^+ loss during ischemia might be viewed as protective, initially facilitating arrhythmias during a relatively short time window (approximately 20 to 30 minutes), and subsequently preventing them by inducing inexcit-

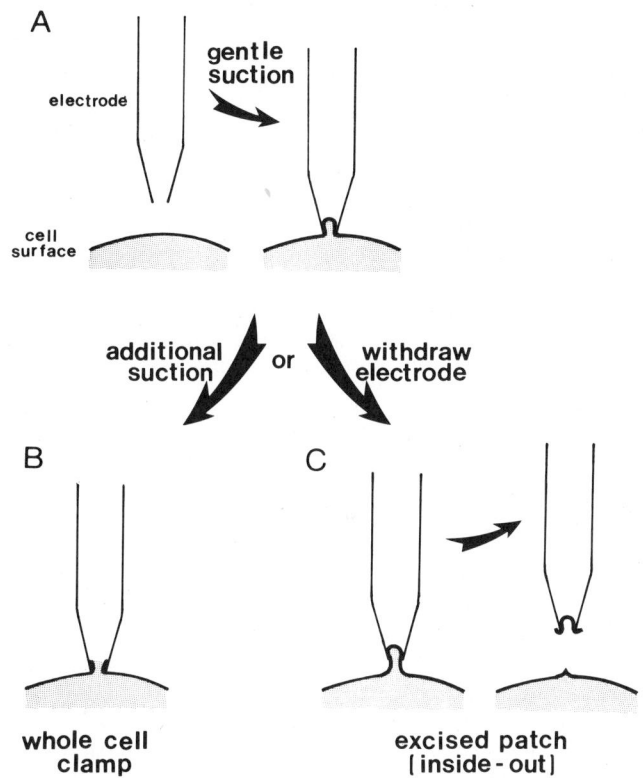

FIGURE 3–9
The tight gigaseal patch clamp technique. A, The patch electrode (tip diameter 1–5 μm) is brought into contact with the surface membrane of the cell and light suction applied to form a high resistance seal (>10¹⁰ ohms) between the bath and the electrode. B, Additional suction can be applied after the initial seal to rupture the membrane patch in the tip of the electrode in order to voltage clamp the whole cell or record the action potential. C, Alternatively, after the initial seal is formed, the electrode can be withdrawn from the cell, excising a patch of membrane in the tip of the electrode. In this configuration (inside-out patch) the surface of the membrane previously facing the cytoplasm now faces the bath. (Reprinted by permission from Weiss JN: Metabolic effects of ischemia: What are the implications for arrhythmogenesis and the treatment of arrhythmias? In Brugada P, Wellens HJJ (eds.): Cardiac Arrhythmias: Where to Go from Here?, pp. 83–104. New York, Futura Publishing Co., 1987. Copyright Futura Publishing Company, Inc.)

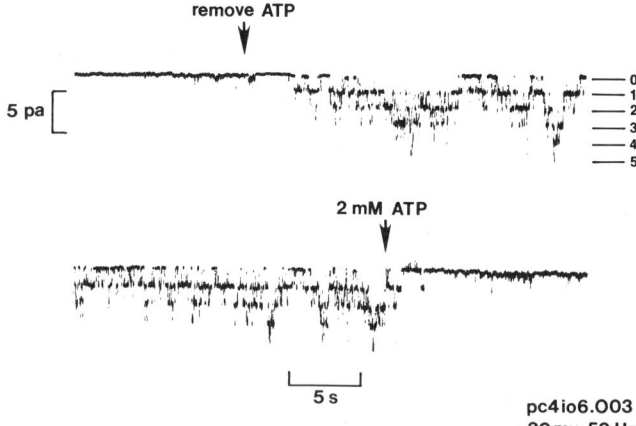

FIGURE 3-10
Single-channel current recording of the ATP-sensitive K^+ channel. An inside-out membrane patch was excised from a guinea pig ventricular myocyte (see Fig. 3-9) and voltage-clamped to a potential of -30 mV (bath relative to inside of electrode). With 2 mM ATP in the bath (facing the cytoplasmic surface of the membrane patch) no channel openings were detected (i.e., the current required to clamp the potential difference across the membrane at -30 mV was constant). When ATP was removed from the bath, however, 5 levels of current steps (right upper tracing) were observed, indicating openings of at least 5 separate ionic channels. Replacing ATP (at arrow) promptly suppressed openings of these channels. The electrode and bath solutions contained, respectively (in mM): 150 KCl, 5 HEPES, pH 7.3, and 150 KCl, 5 HEPES, 2 EGTA, 0.5 $CaCl_2$, 2 $MgCl_2$, with or without 2 MgATP, pH 7.1. Current tracings were filtered at 50 Hz. Inward current is downward. (Reprinted by permission from Weiss JN: Metabolic effects of ischemia: What are the implications for arrhythmogenesis and the treatment of arrhythmias? In Brugada P, Wellens HJJ (eds.): Cardiac Arrhythmias: Where to Go from Here?, pp. 83–104. New York, Futura Publishing Co., 1987. Copyright Futura Publishing Company, Inc.)

ability. In the absence of the marked increase in K^+ efflux during ischemia, it might be anticipated that membrane depolarization would be a much more drawn-out process related to gradual rundown of the Na^+-K^+ pump. In this situation the heart would be potentially susceptible to lethal reentrant arrhythmias over a much longer period of time. This argument may also be relevant to other factors listed in Table 3-1, several of which potentiate the electrophysiologic effects of hyperkalemia.

INTRACELLULAR ACIDOSIS AND LACTATE ACCUMULATION

The intracellular acidosis of ischemia is difficult to simulate in intact myocardium, but extracellularly applied acidosis typically caused action potential prolongation in ventricular muscle.[68, 94] In the presence of hyperkalemia, however, acidosis shortened action potential duration. Membrane depolarization has been reported in Purkinje fibers exposed to acidosis.[59] Voltage clamp studies have shown that both the fast sodium current and slow inward current are depressed by acidosis.[14] In isolated internally dialyzed single ventricular myocytes, the Ca^{2+} current was much more sensitive to intracellular acidosis than extracellular acidosis.[40] Intracellular acidification also activated a time-independent K^+ current causing shortening of the action potential plateau.[81] Intracellular acidosis causes an increase in intercellular resistivity which reduced conduction velocity.[92] The effects of hyperkalemia are significantly potentiated by acidosis.[47, 68, 94] Lactate, which may accumulate intracellularly to concentrations greater than 25 mM during ischemia,[78] has been shown to cause action potential duration shortening independent of its effect on pH.[80]

CATECHOLAMINE RELEASE AND ELEVATED CYCLIC AMP LEVELS

Catecholamines may accumulate significantly in the ischemic tissue and produce a number of pro-arrhythmic effects. By elevating intracellular cyclic AMP levels, catecholamines increase the Ca^{2+} current, facilitating slow-response action potentials in partially depolarized ischemic tissue. Tissue cyclic AMP levels correlate with the development of arrhythmias during ischemia.[74] Catecholamines facilitate the development of delayed afterdepolarizations and triggered automaticity, although their role in arrhythmogenesis during the early phases of ischemia is uncertain. Catecholamines also enhance nontriggered automaticity and may generate PVBs that subsequently trigger reentry. Secondary effects of catecholamines include stimulation of lipolysis, which may contribute to the generation of free fatty acids and related cardiotoxic lipid compounds (see below). Auto-oxidation of catecholamines is also a source of free radical production.

INTRACELLULAR CA^{2+} OVERLOAD

The issue of how quickly and to what extent intracellular Ca^{2+} levels rise during the first 10 minutes of ischemia is still controversial,[60, 64] but significant elevations in $[Ca^{2+}]_i$ probably occur coincident with the rise in diastolic tension.[83] During reperfusion, Ca^{2+} overload is a major complication and may be an important arrhythmogenic factor in this setting. Elevated intracellular Ca^{2+} may activate a transient inward current, I_{TI}, which is a cause of delayed afterdepolarizations and triggered automaticity. Activation of nonselective Ca^{2+}-activated cationic channels[16] and Na^+-Ca^{2+} exchange[82] have both been implicated as causes of I_{TI}. High intracellular Ca^{2+} activates phospholipase A_2, which results in the production of lysophosphoglycerides (see below).

LYSOPHOSPHOGLYCERIDES, FATTY ACID ESTERS, AND FREE FATTY ACIDS

Intracellular phospholipases are activated early during acute ischemia and act on phospholipids to generate lysophospholipids such as lysophosphatidyl choline (LPC). These compounds can increase adenylate cylase activity, which leads to further elevations in intracellular cyclic AMP levels, augmenting the Ca^{2+} current and the slow response in partially depolarized tissue.

More important, LPC has prominent direct effects in isolated cardiac muscle including cellular depolarization mediated by a decrease in membrane K^+ conductance[15] and changes in $\dot{V}_{max}$, excitability, and refractoriness due to changes in both active and passive membrane properties (for review see Corr[19]). These effects are potentiated by acidosis. Inhibition of fatty acid metabolism during ischemia leads to the accumulation of fatty acid esters, such as long-chain acyl carnitines, which have been shown to cause similar electrophysiologic abnormalities in isolated tissues. Long-chain acyl carnitines and acyl coA also may interfere with the Na^+-K^+ pump and with the function of intracellular membranes as well.[19] Both lysophosphoglycerides and fatty acid esters are thought to modify membrane function by inserting into the membrane and altering the interactions between phospholipids and integral membrane proteins. In higher concentrations, both groups of compounds have a detergent effect that disrupts membranes. There is still some controversy over whether lysophosphoglycerides and fatty acid esters accumulate rapidly enough during acute ischemia to cause the earliest electrophysiologic alterations.[18, 52] LPC also causes membrane depolarization by decreasing K^+ conductance.[15] As discussed previously, however, there is indirect but convincing evidence that membrane K^+ conductance increases during ischemia. This inconsistency does not exclude a major role for lysophosphoglycerides and fatty acid esters as causes of the electrophysiologic alterations of acute ischemia but merely emphasizes that multiple factors play a role, and the role of individual factors may change dramatically over the course of time. Free fatty acids are also elevated during acute ischemia and have depressant electrophysiologic effects on cardiac muscle.[19]

FREE RADICALS

Oxygen-derived free radicals generated during ischemia and reperfusion have recently received a great deal of attention (for review, see Thompson[88]). Approximately 5% of normal mitochondrial oxygen consumption involves the formation of the superoxide free radical $\cdot O_2^-$, which is normally dismuted by endogenous superoxide dismutase to form hydrogen peroxide. Alternatively, $\cdot O_2^-$ can react with hydrogen peroxide and a metal chelate such as Fe^{2+} by the Fenton reaction to form the hydroxyl free radical, $\cdot OH^-$, which causes lipid peroxidation and is very cytotoxic. Hydrogen peroxide can also react with Fe^{2+} by the Haber-Weiss reaction to form $\cdot OH^-$. Under normal conditions, endogenous catalase and glutathione peroxidase rapidly degrade hydrogen peroxide, preventing $\cdot OH^-$ accumulation. During ischemia, however, the endogenous free radical scavenging activities of superoxide dismutase and catalase may become impaired. Xanthine oxidase may also be activated during ischemia, in association with rises in intracellular $[Ca^{2+}]$. Hypoxanthine, a byproduct of adenine nucleotide degradation that accumulates during ischemia, is a substrate for xanthine oxidase and a potent source of $\cdot O_2^-$.

Xanthine oxidase is present in endothelial cells and, in some species (but not in humans), in the myocardium as well. Leukocytes generate hydrogen peroxide as part of their cytotoxic arsenal, which may be important during the inflammatory response to ischemia. It has been shown that the levels of oxygen-derived free radicals are elevated during acute ischemia and reperfusion,[102] although whether the concentrations of the free radical species achieved are sufficient to cause cytotoxicity is unknown. However, free radical scavengers have been shown in many, but not all, studies to improve recovery of cardiac function and reduce the incidence and severity of reperfusion arrhythmias following ischemia.[7, 88] Free radical–generating systems have also been shown to impair the ability of the sarcoplasmic reticulum to pump Ca^{2+} [88] and to induce electrophysiologic abnormalities in intact heart[26, 72] and isolated myocytes.[4] Figure 3–11 shows that many of the effects of ischemia on cardiac function can be mimicked by exposure of the heart to a free radical–generating system such as hydrogen peroxide. In the isolated arterially perfused rabbit interventricular septum, exposure to 1 mM hydrogen peroxide caused an immediate increase in K^+ efflux, followed by action potential shortening, loss of systolic tension, and progressive contracture.[26] Similar effects were seen with xanthine plus xanthine oxidase, and could be prevented

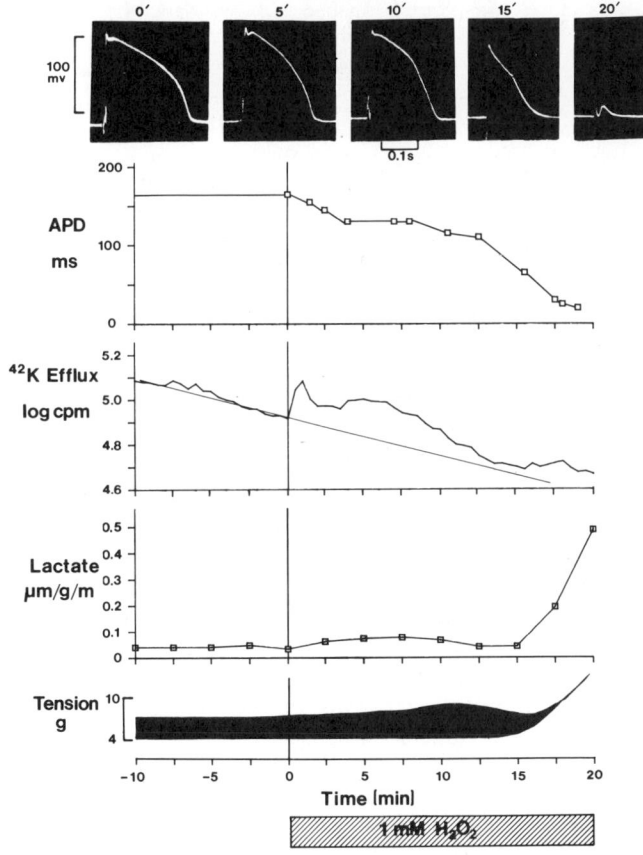

FIGURE 3–11
Effects of 1 mM hydrogen peroxide on the action potential, action potential duration (APD), $^{42}K^+$ efflux, venous lactate, and tension in an isolated arterially perfused rabbit interventricular septum.

by inclusion of the free radical scavengers superoxide dismutase and catalase.[26]

Further insights into the mechanism of free radical–induced cardiac dysfunction were obtained from voltage clamp experiments in single ventricular myocytes.[26, 97] Figure 3–12 compares the effects of 1 mM hydrogen peroxide and metabolic inhibitors on the action potential and current-voltage relations in two representative myocytes. Both interventions caused transient action potential lengthening followed by progressive shortening leading to inexcitability. The current-voltage relations were similar, showing activation of a large outward current consistent with the ATP-sensitive K^+ channel. Xanthine plus xanthine oxidase produced similar changes, which were markedly delayed if the free radical scavengers superoxide dismutase and catalase were included.[26] Thus, free radicals appeared to cause the same alterations in K^+ currents as metabolic inhibition, raising the possibility that free radicals either directly activated K^+ channels or indirectly activated the channels by themselves inhibiting metabolism. To resolve this question, patch clamp experiments were performed to examine directly the effects of hydrogen peroxide on ATP-sensitive K^+ channels. Single-channel currents of ATP-sensitive K^+ channels were recorded from cell-attached patches in cells that had been permeabilized by brief exposure of one end of the cell to saponin, a membrane detergent, as illustrated in Figure 3–13. Under these conditions the cytoplasm was dialyzed by the solution in the bath. If ATP was removed from the bath solution, ATP-sensitive K^+ channels opened and could be recorded in the cell-attached patch (Fig. 3–14).[48] Also, the metabolic machinery in these permeabilized cells remained intact.[99] If, instead of ATP, the bath solution contained the substrates necessary for mitochondrial ATP production, the cell was able to generate ATP endogenously and the ATP-sensitive K^+ channels closed (Fig. 3–14A). In the presence of the mitochondrial inhibitor FCCP, however, the channels reopened. Substrates for the ATP-producing steps of glycolysis were also effective in suppressing ATP-sensitive K^+ channels (Fig. 3–14B), even in the presence of a mitochondrial inhibitor (Fig. 3–14C). Creatine phosphate alone had no effect but was effective in suppressing ATP-sensitive channels once ADP was included, allowing creatine kinase to generate ATP (Fig. 3–14C). In cell-attached patches on permeabilized cells, 1 mM hydrogen peroxide did not increase the threshold concentration of ATP necessary to prevent ATP-sensitive K^+ channels from opening (about 0.5 mM). However, hydrogen peroxide completely and irreversibly prevented the ability of both glycolytic and mitochondrial substrates to suppress ATP-sensitive K^+ channels.[26] These findings suggest that free radicals directly damage the metabolic machinery of cells. Thus many, although not necessarily all, of the effects of free radicals on cardiac function may be attributed to a direct effect on cellular metabolism, which would account for the similarities with ischemia. Furthermore, these findings suggest that the large burst of free radical generation during reperfusion[102] may be an important cause of irreversible damage to the heart by virtue of the irreversible effects on cellular metabolism. Despite these intriguing possibilities, however, it remains a matter of speculation at this time whether free radicals accumulate in sufficient quantity to contribute significantly to the electrophysiologic abnormalities of acute ischemia and reperfusion.

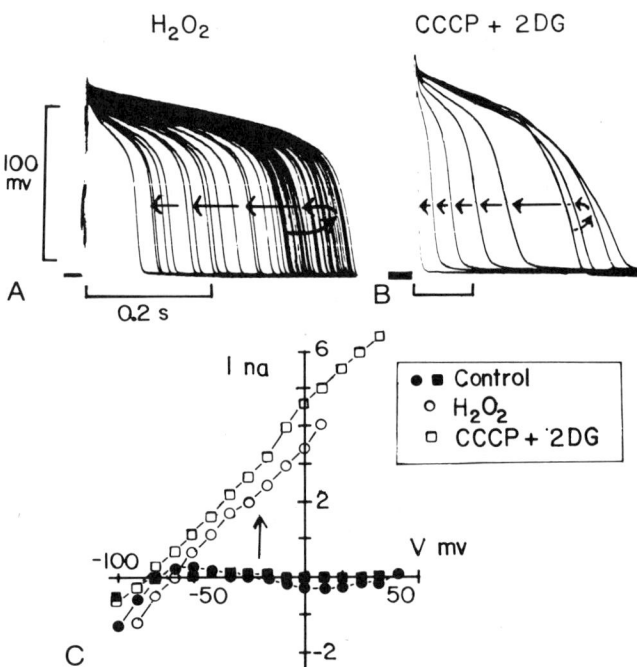

FIGURE 3–12
Comparison of the effects of hydrogen peroxide vs. metabolic inhibitors on the action potential and current-voltage relations in single guinea pig ventricular myocytes, using the patch clamp technique (whole cell clamp configuration shown in Fig. 3–9B). A, Tracing of superimposed action potentials shows that in response to 1 mM hydrogen peroxide (H_2O_2) the action potential duration was transiently prolonged and then shortened progressively until the cell became inexcitable. This effect was almost identical to that produced by exposure to the combination of 5 μm of the mitochondrial inhibitor CCCP and 20 mM of the glycolytic inhibitor 2-deoxyglucose (2DG) shown in B. The current-voltage relations under both conditions are shown in C (50-ms clamp duration, holding potential −40 mV). (Reprinted by permission from Weiss JN: Metabolic effects of ischemia: What are the implications for arrhythmogenesis and the treatment of arrhythmias? In Brugada P, Wellens HJJ (eds.): Cardiac Arrhythmias: Where to Go from Here?, pp. 83–104. New York, Futura Publishing Co., 1987. Copyright Futura Publishing Company, Inc.)

SUMMARY

The complexity of the ischemic environment, in which the concentrations of the various factors listed in Table 3–1 are continuously changing, precludes a quantitatively accurate assessment of the contribution of each individual factor to the electrophysiologic alterations during the early phase of acute myocardial ischemia. Even if each factor could be accurately quantified, its effects are so markedly influenced by interactions with the other factors that it is unlikely the precise pathophysiology could be unravelled. Despite these limita-

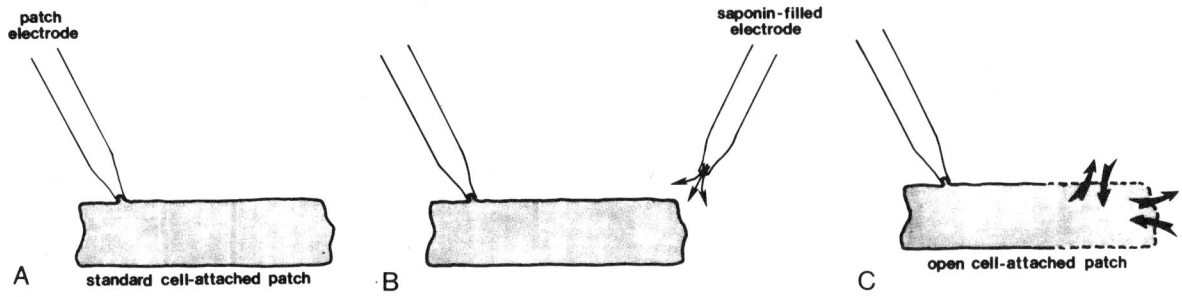

FIGURE 3–13
Technique for permeabilizing a cell in which single-channel currents are being recorded from a cell-attached patch. A, A standard cell-attached patch is formed at one end of an isolated myocyte. B, The other end of the cell is exposed briefly to a stream of solution containing 0.1% saponin delivered from a second electrode, positioned as shown using positive pressure. C, Once the membrane at the other end of the cell is disrupted, detected by a slight swelling of the cell, the saponin-containing electrode is removed. Single-channel currents can be recorded from the cell-attached patch on the now permeabilized cell.

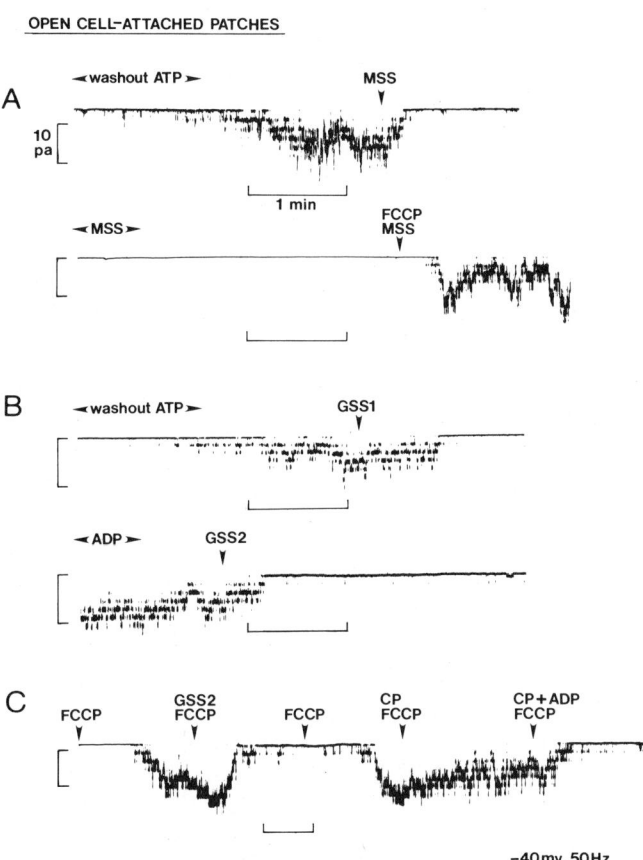

FIGURE 3–14
Effects of metabolic substrates on ATP-sensitive K^+ channels recorded from a cell-attached patch on a permeabilized guinea pig ventricular myocyte. See text for description of traces. Patch electrode contained (in mM) 150 KCl, 5 HEPES, pH 7.3; the bath contained 150 KCl, 5 HEPES, 2 EGTA, 0.5 $CaCl_2$, 2 $MgCl_2$, pH 7.1 to which various substrates were added. Mitochondrial substrates (MSS) including (in mM) 2 pyruvate, glutamate, and creatine, 1 K_2HPO_4, and 0.5 ADP. Glycolytic substrates included (in mM) either 2 fructose-1,6-diphosphate, 1 NAD and K_2HPO_4, and 0.5 ADP (GSS1); or 2 phosphoenolpyruvate and 0.5 ADP (GSS2). CP = creatine phosphate (2 mM). The patch electrode was held at +40 mV throughout (equivalent to a membrane potential of −40 mV). Inward current is downward. Filter setting is 50 Hz. (Reprinted by permission from Weiss JN, Lamp ST: Science, 238:67, 1987. Copyright 1987 by the AAAS.)

tions, much useful information about the pathophysiology of arrhythmogenesis during the early phase of acute myocardial ischemia has been gained by studying the effects of perfusate that has been modified to simulate various components of the ischemic environment.

Is Metabolism Compartmentalized in Heart?

It was noted previously that prominent changes in cardiac function during myocardial ischemia occur well before total cellular levels of high-energy phosphates, particularly ATP, are severely depleted. Much attention has therefore been paid to secondary effects of ischemia, such as those listed in Table 3–1, in order to account for early onset of severe cardiac dysfunction during ischemia. Another possible factor that could contribute to the discrepancy between high-energy phosphate levels and electromechanical dysfunction during ischemia is compartmentation of cardiac metabolism. According to this hypothesis, total cellular high-energy phosphate content, which represents the average cellular content, may not accurately reflect the true levels of high energy phosphates in critical subcellular compartments which preferentially supply energy for specific cardiac functions. Gudbjarnason and colleagues[29] were the first to suggest that during ischemia ATP might become "trapped" in mitochondria due to a breakdown of the creatine phosphate shuttle mechanism, so that total cellular ATP content overestimated the cytosolic ATP available for energy needs of the heart. Consistent with this mechanism, subsequent studies have indicated that adenine nucleotide translocase activity (see Fig. 3–2) is inhibited during ischemia, possibly by accumulated long-chain acyl coA.[19] Other investigators, however, have argued that this form of compartmentation is unlikely.[3]

There is evidence from several studies suggesting that ATP produced by anaerobic glycolysis may be used preferentially to support membrane function during ischemia and metabolic inhibition. McDonald and

MacLeod[63] found that during hypoxia, shortening of the action potential duration could be reversed by raising glucose to supraphysiologic levels (50 mM). Several investigators reported that during low-flow ischemia, concomitant inhibition of glycolysis resulted in much poorer recovery upon reperfusion than concomitant inhibition of oxidative phosphorylation despite identical total cellular levels of high-energy phosphates under both conditions.[12, 13] The development of ischemic contracture was found to occur at much higher tissue ATP levels when ATP originated from oxidative phosphorylation than anaerobic glycolysis,[61] consistent with the observation that glycogenolytic enzyme complexes are bound to sarcoplasmic reticulum in heart.[22] In cultured neonatal myocytes, exposure to phospholipases, whose activation during ischemia has been implicated as a mechanism of damage, caused much more severe cellular enzyme loss when glycolysis was selectively inhibited than when oxidative metabolism was selectively inhibited.[37] Again, total cellular high-energy phosphate levels were similar under both conditions. Cultured neonatal myocytes were also shown to manifest different electromechanical responses to selective inhibition of glycolysis and oxidative metabolism.[33, 34] Selective inhibition of glycolysis caused membrane depolarization and depressed $^{42}K^+$ uptake, but only modest suppression of contractility. Conversely, selective inhibition of oxidative metabolism caused severe depression of contractility but mild effects on membrane function. These findings are consistent with the hypothesis that high-energy phosphates generated by glycolysis and oxidative metabolism are preferentially utilized for different purposes in the heart: glycolysis for support of membrane functions (including sarcoplasmic reticulum), and oxidative phosphorylation for support of contractile function.

Figure 3–15 shows the results of experiments designed to test this hypothesis in the intact adult rabbit heart.[95] $[K^+]_o$ and tension were monitored in isolated arterially perfused rabbit interventricular septa during exposure to agents that selectively inhibited either glycolysis or oxidative phosphorylation. Selective inhibition of glycolysis resulted in a mild loss of developed tension and in marked extracellular K^+ accumulation. In contrast, selective inhibition of oxidative phosphorylation caused marked suppression of tension and only modest extracellular K^+ accumulation. Despite the marked abnormalities in cardiac function, tissue levels of high-energy phosphates remained normal during inhibition of glycolysis, and the dosage of mitochondrial inhibitors were chosen so that tissue high-energy phosphates also remained normal (Fig. 3–15B). Thus, during selective inhibition of glycolysis, oxidative metabolism was capable of maintaining normal total cellular levels of high-energy phosphates; yet these high-energy phosphates could not be effectively utilized to prevent cellular K^+ loss from the cell. Conversely, during mild selective suppression of oxidative metabolism, glycolytic high-energy phosphate production increased to maintain normal total cellular high-energy phosphate levels, but the glycolytically generated high-energy phosphates were not effectively

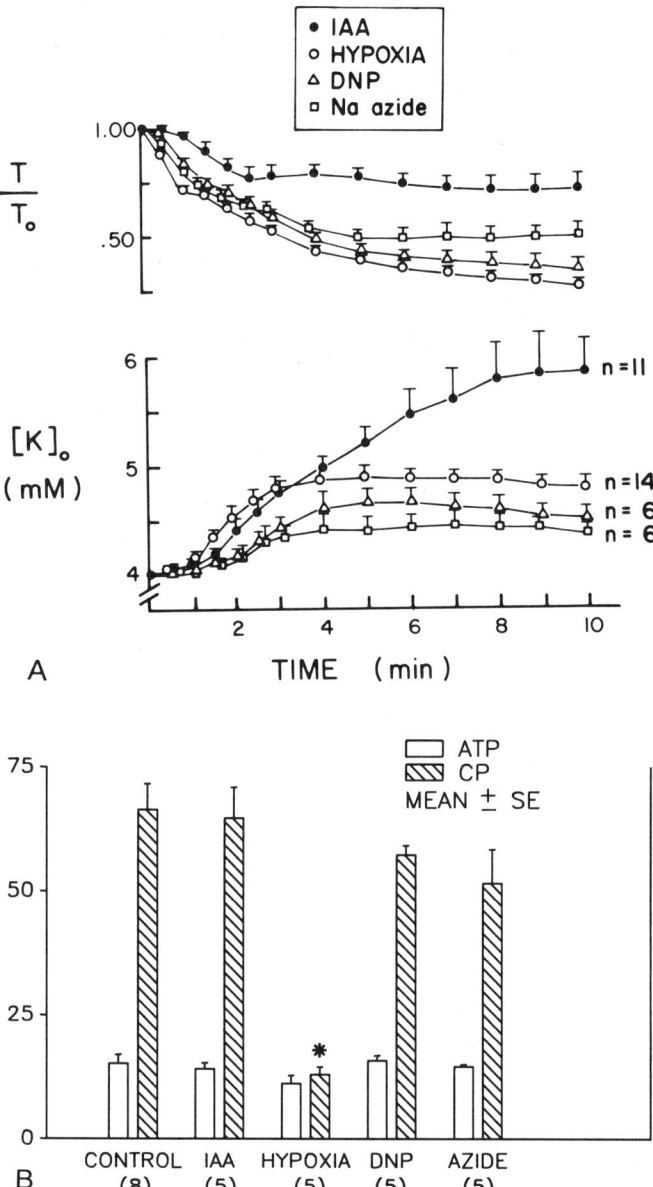

FIGURE 3–15

A. Comparison of the effects of selective inhibition of glycolytic versus oxidative metabolism on $[K^+]_o$ accumulation and tension (T/T_o) in isolated arterially perfused rabbit interventricular septa. Glycolysis was inhibited by adding 1 mM iodoacetate (IAA) to glucose-free perfusate containing pyruvate as substrate for oxidative metabolism (solid circles). Oxidative metabolism was inhibited with either hypoxia (open circles), 0.01 mM dinitrophenol (DNP) (triangles), or 1 mM Na azide (squares) with glucose present as substrate for glycolysis. Values are mean ± SE. (Reprinted by permission from Weiss JN: Metabolic effects of ischemia: What are the implications for arrhythmogenesis and the treatment of arrhythmias? In Brugada P, Wellens HJJ (eds.): Cardiac Arrhythmias: Where to Go from Here?, pp. 83–104. New York, Futura Publishing Co., 1987. Copyright Futura Publishing Company, Inc.)

utilized to prevent severe loss of tension. The preference for glycolytic versus oxidatively derived ATP was only partial, since simultaneous inhibition of both glycolysis and oxidative phosphorylation had much more severe effects on $[K^+]_o$ accumulation and tension development than did selective inhibition of either pathway alone.

Figure 3–16 shows a hypothetical scheme that might account for the experimental results described above. Oxidative phosphorylation in the mitochondria generates ATP, which is transported via the creatine phosphate shuttle to the cytoplasm in the form of creatine phosphate. The dense packing of mitochondria in the vicinity of the myofilaments preferentially favors conversion of mitochondrially generated creatine phosphate to ATP by myosin-bound creatine kinase.[9, 90] Conversely, glycolytic enzymes may be bound to the sarcolemmal membrane or intracellular structures and convert ADP to ATP locally near ion pumps or channels, favoring their utilization at those sites. Glycogenolytic enzyme complexes, for example, have been shown to be bound to the sarcoplasmic reticulum,[22] perhaps explaining the greater effectiveness of glycolytic than of oxidatively generated ATP at preventing contracture during ischemia.[61] It is often argued that the rate of diffusion of ATP in the cytoplasm would be too rapid to permit the existence of significant inhomogeneities in ATP levels at different locations within the cell, assuming that diffusion rates in the cytoplasm are equivalent to those in free solution. However, many processes compete for ATP once it is generated in the cell, which may limit the distance ATP can functionally travel before it is consumed. It is interesting that in internally dialyzed single cells under patch clamp conditions, inclusion of up to 15 mM MgATP in the internal dialysate (patch electrode solution) delayed but did not prevent activation of ATP-sensitive K$^+$ channels when the cells were exposed to metabolic inhibitors. Following exposure to 0.1 μM FCCP and 10 mM 2-deoxyglucose, the time until the cell became inexcitable due to activation of the ATP-sensitive K$^+$ current (an indicator of local [ATP] at the sarcolemmal membrane) was 7.2 ± 2.2 minutes in six cells with no MgATP in the internal dialysate, and 11.2 ± 3.0 minutes in six cells with 15 mM MgATP in the internal dialysate (S. Ji, J. Weiss, unpublished observations). This observation suggests that the rate of ATP diffusion in the cytoplasm is functionally much slower than the rate calculated for diffusion through free solution.

Although Figure 3–16 provides an attractive scheme to account for the experimental observations described above, there are many uncertainties in attributing directly changes in function of multicellular cardiac preparations to inhibition of specific metabolic pathways. In particular, metabolic inhibitors may not be completely specific (e.g. iodoacetate). Also, selective inhibition of glycolysis and oxidative phosphorylation have different effects on secondary factors such as intracellular pH and lactate, which may alter tension development and other functions.

To circumvent some of these problems, we attempted to study the relationship between specific metabolic pathways and cardiac function under more rigorous conditions. Using the patch clamp technique in isolated ventricular myocytes, we investigated the relationship between glycolysis versus oxidative phosphorylation in the regulation of ATP-sensitive K$^+$ channels.[98] Recall from Figure 3–14 that in permeabilized single cells, substrates for glycolytic or mitochondrial (oxidative) ATP production were equally effective in suppressing ATP-sensitive K$^+$ channels in cell-attached patches. Under these nonbeating conditions, the rate of ATP consumption in the cells was intrinsically low compared to that in the intact working heart, in which many cellular processes compete simultaneously for the ATP produced. To simulate the high level of intrinsic ATP consumption in the intact working heart, we exposed the permeabilized cells to an exogenous ATP-consuming system consisting of hexokinase and 2-deoxyglucose:

$$\text{2-deoxyglucose} + \text{ATP} \xrightarrow{\text{hexokinase}} \text{2-deoxyglucose-6-phosphate} + \text{ADP}$$

In the presence of ATP, hexokinase catalyzes the phosphorylation of 2-deoxyglucose, degrading ATP to ADP in the process. Figure 3–17A shows single-channel recordings of K$^+$ channels in a cell-attached patch on a permeabilized cell. In the presence of mitochondrial substrates (MSS) and hexokinase (HK) without 2-deoxyglucose (2-DG), only occasional openings of a normal, inwardly rectifying (I_{K1}) channel were observed, indicating that the mitochondria were generating sufficient ATP to keep ATP-sensitive K$^+$ channels in the patch closed (as in Fig. 3–14). At the first arrow, the mitochondrial substrates were removed and 2-deoxyglucose was added to the hexokinase. Multiple ATP-sensitive K$^+$ channels opened as cellular ATP was depleted. Readmission of the mitochondrial substrates in the presence of both hexokinase and 2-deoxyglucose (second arrow) now resulted in only a transient, partial suppression of ATP-sensitive K$^+$ channel activity, presumably because ATP generated by the mitochondria was being degraded by the hexokinase/2-deoxyglucose reaction before it could reach ATP-sensitive K$^+$ channels in the patch. However, glycolytic substrates remained effective at suppressing ATP-sensitive K$^+$ channels in the presence of hexoki-

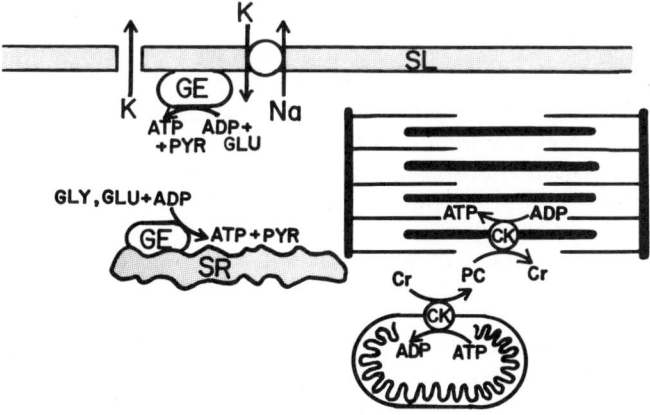

FIGURE 3–16
Hypothetical representation of compartmentation of glycolytic and oxidative metabolism in heart. SL = sarcolemma; SR = sarcoplasmic reticulum; GE = glycolytic enzymes; GLU = glucose; GLY = glycogen; PYR = pyruvate; Cr = creatine; PC = creatine phosphate; CK = creatine kinase.

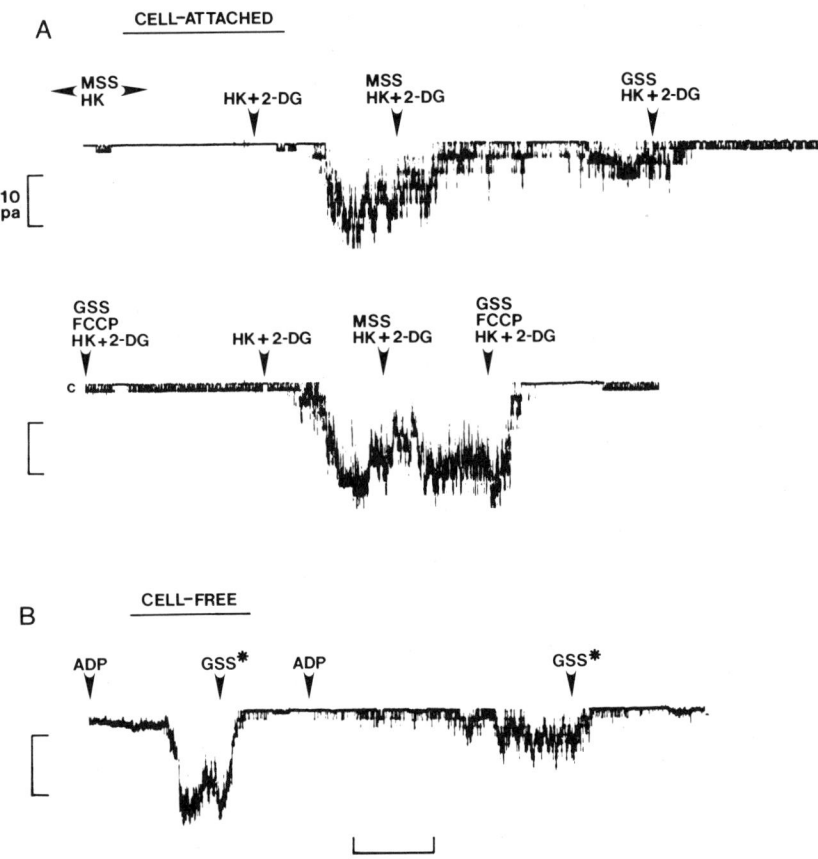

FIGURE 3–17
A, Effects of glycolytic substrates (GSS) vs. mitochondrial substrates (MSS) on ATP-sensitive K⁺ channels recorded from a cell-attached patch on a permeabilized ventricular myocyte in the presence of hexokinase (HK, 10 IU/mL) and 2-deoxyglucose (2-DG, 10 mM). See text for description of traces. Patch electrode and bath solutions are the same as in Figure 3–14 (GSS = GSS1) except for the absence of creatine in MSS. FCCP (1 µM) is a mitochondrial uncoupler. B, Effect of glycolytic substrates (GSS*) on ATP-sensitive K⁺ channels in an excised inside-out membrane patch. Patch electrode solution is the same as in Figure 3–14. Bath solution contained (in mM) 150 KCl, 5 HEPES, 2 EGTA, 0.5 CaCl$_2$, 2 MgCl$_2$ and either 0.5 mM ADP or GSS* which consisted of (in mM) 2 glyceraldehyde-3-phosphate dehydrogenase and phosphoenolpyruvate, 1 NAD and K$_2$HPO$_4$, 0.5 ADP, and 2 IU/ml glyceraldehyde-3-phosphate dehydrogenase. In both A and B the patch electrode potential was +40 mV throughout. Filter setting was 50 Hz. (Reprinted by permission of the publisher from Weiss JN, Lamp ST: Glycolysis and the metabolic regulation of cardiac ATP-sensitive K⁺ channels. In Ross A (ed.): Biology of Isolated Adult Cardiac Myocytes, pp. 418–421. New York, Elsevier Science Publishing Co., 1988. Copyright 1988 by Elsevier Science Publishing Company, Inc.)

nase and 2-deoxyglucose (third arrow), even after 1 µM FCCP (a mitochondrial inhibitor) was added (fourth arrow). Note that I_{K1} channels remained active in the presence of glycolytic substrates. The findings were reproducible. In 15 permeabilized cells, the average current through ATP-sensitive K⁺ channels with hexokinase and 2-deoxyglucose present fell to 81 ± 35% (SD) of the control value when mitochondrial substrates were added and fell to 34 ± 29% when glycolytic substrates and FCCP were added ($p < 0.005$; paired T-test). Inclusion of creatine with the mitochondrial substrates in 11 of these cells in order to facilitate mitochondrial energy transfer by the creatine phosphate shuttle did not improve their effectiveness at suppressing ATP-sensitive K⁺ channels. In all 15 cells, mitochondrial substrates had completely suppressed ATP-sensitive K⁺ channels when hexokinase without 2-deoxyglucose was present.

One possible explanation for the preferential use of glycolytic ATP by ATP-sensitive K⁺ channels is that key glycolytic enzymes bound to the sarcolemma or cytoskeleton in the immediate vicinity of ATP-sensitive K⁺ channels might provide a local source of ATP, as suggested in Figure 3–16. It is conceivable that if a membrane patch containing ATP-sensitive K⁺ channels was completely isolated from the cell to form an excised inside-out patch (as in Fig. 3–9), the patch may retain these glycolytic enzymes. Furthermore, if the enzymes remained functional and were provided with the appropriate glycolytic substrates, they might be capable of generating sufficient ATP to suppress ATP-sensitive K⁺ channels in the excised patch in the absence of exogenous ATP. In seven out of 38 excised inside-out patches, this was the case. Figure 3–17B shows an example. At the beginning of the trace, replacement of 2 mM ATP with 0.5 mM ADP caused multiple ATP-sensitive K⁺ channels to open. Addition of the glycolytic substrates promptly and reversibly caused ATP-sensitive K⁺ channels in the patch to close. In no patches did combinations of glycolytic substrates missing an essential component necessary for ATP production suppress ATP-sensitive K⁺ channels. These findings are consistent with the hypothesis that glycolytic enzymes associated with the ATP-producing steps of glycolysis (phosphoglycerate kinase or pyruvate kinase) were bound to the sarcolemma or cytoskeleton in the immediate vicinity of ATP-sensitive K⁺ channels. The ineffectiveness of glycolytic substrates in the majority (31 of 38) of patches may be related to loss of enzyme functionality during patch excision or a patch geometry that did not allow ATP generated locally by the glycolytic enzymes to accumulate sufficiently to suppress ATP-sensitive K⁺ channels.

The findings in single cells provide evidence that glycolytic enzymes bound to the sarcolemmal membrane act as a preferential source of ATP for ATP-sensitive K⁺ channels when the rate of cellular ATP consumption is increased by hexokinase and 2-deoxyglucose. To test the relevance of the above findings to the intact beating heart, the effects of inhibiting glycolysis on K⁺ efflux in isolated rabbit interventricular septa were investigated. Figure 3–18 shows that replacing glucose in the arterial perfusate with 2-deoxyglucose (to inhibit glycolysis) and pyruvate (as substrate for oxidative phosphorylation) resulted in an immediate increase in the rate of ^{42}K⁺ efflux without significantly affecting tension. The increased rate of ^{42}K⁺ efflux did not reverse when glucose was readmitted, possibly due to the intracellular accumulation of 2-deoxyglucose-6-phosphate. Subsequent exposure to iodoacetate (a more potent glycolytic inhibitor) and pyruvate caused a further dramatic and irreversible increase in ^{42}K⁺ efflux rate. We have previously shown that total cellular levels of creatine phosphate and ATP remain normal under these conditions.[95] Furthermore, glyburide, a specific blocker of ATP-sensitive K⁺ channels, prevented the increase in ^{42}K⁺ efflux induced by either method of selectively inhibiting glycolysis.[98a] These findings suggest that cardiac ATP-sensitive K⁺ channels can be activated by inhibiting glycolysis even though total cellular high energy phsophate levels remain normal.

To return briefly to the mechanism of ischemia-induced cellular K⁺ loss, increased K⁺ efflux during ischemia begins at a time when glycolysis is accelerating. If glycolysis is a preferential source ATP for ATP-sensitive K⁺ channels in heart, then it seems improbable that activation of these channels could be responsible for the early increase in K⁺ efflux. Whether there is a solution to this dilemma is unknown, but it is possible to speculate. For example it is conceivable that the global increase in cellular glycolytic flux during early ischemia may actually deplete the levels of substrates available to a component of membrane-bound glycolytic enzymes specifically associated with ATP-sensitive K⁺ channels. Reduced ATP production via these critical enzymes, combined with local accumulation of ADP, might then cause the associated ATP-sensitive K⁺ channels to open despite the overall increase in cellular glycolytic flux. The source of glycolytic substrate (exogenous glucose versus glycogen) may be important in this regard. During total ischemia, exogenous glucose utilization is reduced and glycogen rapidly becomes the main source of substrate for glycolysis. If ATP-sensitive K⁺ channels are associated with key glycolytic enzymes, but not with the full glycogenolytic enzyme complex, the ability of ATP derived from glycogenolysis to suppress ATP-sensitive K⁺ channels may be suboptimal. We have recently obtained evidence suggesting that the source of glycolytic substrate (exogenous glucose vs. glycogen) may be an important determinant of the severity of cardiac dysfunction during hypoxia.[79] Other results consistent with this possibility have also been previously reported. Dennis and coworkers[20] found that during low flow ischemia, the incidence of reperfusion arrhythmias was much higher when conditions were arranged to increase the contribution of glycogenolysis, as opposed to exogenous glucose utilization, to total glycolytic flux. In vascular smooth muscle Lynch[71a] has demonstrated that exogenous glucose and glycogen are preferentially utilized for different purposes. Further studies are needed to resolve these issues in heart.

Conclusions

In this chapter I have attempted to describe the various biochemical and metabolic factors that contribute to the development of arrhythmias in the setting of acute myocardial ischemia, some in more detail than others. I have also tried to impart to the reader a broad perspective (albeit not necessarily universally shared) of mechanisms by which cardiac metabolism is involved in the regulation of cardiac function. The clinical importance of understanding these mechanisms is immense. Arrhythmias during acute myocardial ischemia remain the leading cause of mortality from coronary artery disease.

Despite the effort that has gone into elucidating the pathophysiology of ischemic arrhythmogenesis, the impact on the clinical management of this problem is severely limited by the fact that the majority of deaths occur outside of a hospital. Because of this limitation, prevention of atherosclerosis and early detection and treatment of coronary artery disease will continue to have the greatest impact on cardiovascular mortality. In concert with these efforts, elucidation of the basic mechanisms relating cardiac metabolism and function will play a crucial role in improving methods for implementing these strategies and refining the in-hospital and paramedic-assisted management of acute myocardial ischemia.

The current use of free radical scavengers as a

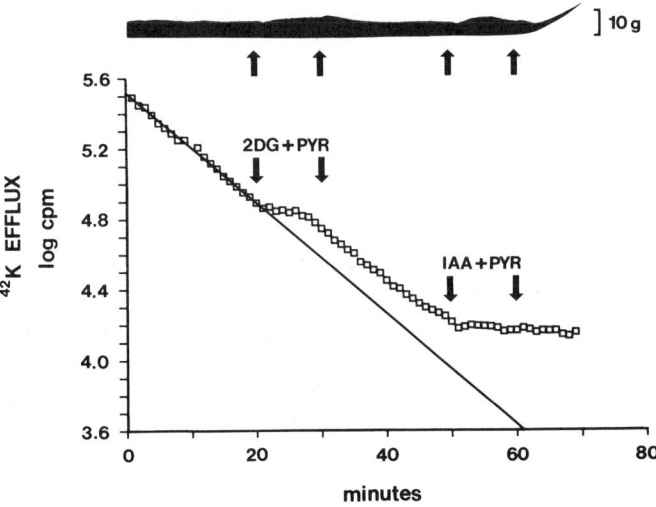

FIGURE 3–18
Effect of selectively inhibiting glycolysis on ^{42}K⁺ efflux in an isolated arterially perfused rabbit interventricular septum. Tension is shown in tracing above the graph. (Reprinted by permission of the publisher from Weiss JN, Lamp ST: Glycolysis and the metabolic regulation of cardiac ATP-sensitive K⁺ channels. In Ross A (ed.): Biology of Isolated Adult Cardiac Myocytes, pp. 418–421. New York, Elsevier Science Publishing Co., 1988. Copyright 1988 by Elsevier Science Publishing Co., Inc.)

standard component of cardioplegic solutions during cardiopulmonary bypass surgery at many centers is an example of a clinical application motivated by such insights from basic investigation. The issue of compartmentation of metabolic energy in heart, although still controversial, also has broad clinical implications. If it is true that metabolic pathways such as glycolysis and oxidative phosphorylation preferentially supply high-energy phosphates for specific cardiac functions, then interventions designed to preserve myocardium during acute myocardial infarction or cardiopulmonary bypass surgery must take into consideration not only total cellular high-energy phosphate levels but also the sources from which the high-energy phosphates are derived. The potential for manipulating a specific metabolic pathway to achieve a desired outcome could be an exciting approach in the design of new therapeutic strategies in these clinical settings. Understanding the mechanisms of ischemic arrhythmogenesis in greater detail may also suggest new approaches for reducing the risk of sudden death from myocardial infarction in the out-of-hospital setting.

Acknowledgments

I would like to express my appreciation to Kenneth Shine, Glenn Langer, Richard Weiss, Martin Morad, Alan Brady, Steven Dillon, Scott Lamp, Joshua Goldhaber, Sen Ji, Eva Runnman, and Bradley Hiltbrand for their generous help, advice, and collaboration in parts of the work described in this chapter.

References

1. Akiyama T: Electrical uncoupling across the ischemic border of in situ pig porcine hearts. Circulation (Suppl 3) 62:344, 1980.
2. Apstein CS, Ahn J, Brent BN, et al.: Ischemic "pump" failure: evidence for a mechanical, non-metabolic, initial cause. Circulation (Suppl. 2) 59:114, 1979.
3. Altschuld RA, Brierley GP: Interaction between creatine kinase of heart mitochondria and oxidative phosphorylation. J Mol Cell Cardiol 9:875, 1977.
4. Barrington PL, Meier CF, Dickens BF, et al.: Free radical scavengers protect canine myocytes from free radical-induced changes in the action potential. Circulation (Suppl. 3) 72:228, 1985.
5. Barry WH, Brooker JZ, Alderman EL, et al.: Changes in diastolic stiffness and tone of the left ventricle during angina pectoris. Circulation 49:255, 1974.
6. Berne RM, Knabb RM, Ely SW, et al.: Adenosine in the regulation of blood flow; a brief overview. Fed Proc 42:3136, 1983.
7. Bernier M, Hearse DJ, Manning AS: Reperfusion-induced arrhythmias and oxygen-derived free radicals. Circ Res 58:331, 1986.
8. Bersohn MM, Philipson KD, Fukushima JY: Sodium-calcium exchange and sarcolemmal enzymes in ischemic rabbit hearts. Am J Physiol 242:C288, 1982.
9. Bessman SP, Geiger PJ: Transport of energy in muscle: the phosphorylcreatine shuttle. Science 211:448, 1981.
10. Bittl JA, Balschi JA, Ingwall JS: Effects of norepinephrine infusion on myocardial high energy phosphate content and turnover in the living rat. J Clin Invest 79:1852, 1987a.
11. Bittl JA, DeLayre J, Ingwall JS: Rate equation for creatine kinase predicts the in vivo reaction velocity: ^{31}P NMR surface coil studies in brain, heart and skeletal muscle of the living rat. Biochem 26:6083, 1987b.
12. Bricknell OL, Opie LH: Effects of substrates on tissue metabolic changes in the isolated rat heart during underperfusion and on release of lactate dehydrogenase and arrhythmias during reperfusion. Circ Res 43:102, 1978.
13. Bricknell OL, Daries PS, Opie LH: A relationship between adenosine triphosphate, glycolysis and ischemic contracture in the isolated rat heart. J Mol Cell Cardiol 13:941, 1981.
14. Chesnais JM, Coraboeuf E, Sauviat MP, et al.: Sensitivity to H, Li, and Mg ions of the slow inward sodium current in frog atrial fibres. J Mol Cell Cardiol 7:627, 1975.
15. Clarkson CW, Ten Eick RE: On the mechanism of lysophosphatidyl choline-induced depolarization of cat ventricular myocardium. Circ Res 52:543, 1983.
16. Colquhoun D, Neher E, Reuter H, et al.: Inward current channels activated by intracellular Ca in cultured cardiac cells. Nature 294:752, 1981.
17. Conrad CH, Mark RG, Bing OL: Outward current and repolarization in hypoxic rat myocardium. Am J Physiol 244:H341, 1983.
18. Corr PB, Gross RW, Sobel BE: Arrhythmogenic amphiphilic lipids and the myocardial cell membrane. J Mol Cell Cardiol 14:619, 1982.
19. Corr PB, Gross RW, Sobel BE: Amphipathic metabolites and membrane dysfunction in ischemic myocardium. Circ Res 55:135, 1984.
20. Dennis SC, Hearse DJ, Coltart DJ: Metabolic effects of substrates on the isolated guinea-pig heart in relation to arrhythmias during reperfusion. Cardiovasc Res 16:209, 1982.
21. El-Sherif N, Scherlag BJ, Lazzara R: Electrode catheter recordings during malignant ventricular arrhythmia following experimental acute myocardial ischemia. Circulation 51:1003, 1975.
22. Entman ML, Kanike K, Goldstein MA, et al.: Association of glycogenolysis with cardiac sarcoplasmic reticulum. J Biol Chem 251:3140, 1976.
23. Fogelman AM, Abbasi AS, Pearce ML, et al.: Echocardiographic study of the abnormal motion of the posterior left ventricular wall during angina pectoris. Circulation 46:905, 1972.
24. Gaspardone A, Shine KI, Seabrooke SR, et al.: Potassium loss from rabbit myocardium during hypoxia: evidence for passive efflux linked to anion extrusion. J Mol Cell Cardiol 18:389, 1986.
25. Gibbs CL, Chapman JB: Cardiac energetics. In Berne RM, Sperelakis N, Geiger S (eds.): Handbook of Physiology, The Cardiovascular System, pp. 775–804. Bethesda, Md., American Physiological Society, 1979.
26. Goldhaber JI, Ji S, Lamp ST, et al.: Effects of exogenous free radicals on electromechanical function and metabolism in isolated rabbit and guinea pig ventricle. J Clin Invest In press.
27. Goldman L, Cook F, Hashimoto B, et al.: Evidence that hospital care for acute myocardial infarction has not contributed to the decline in coronary mortality between 1973–1974 and 1978–1979. Circulation 65:936, 1982.
28. Grosse R, Spitzer E, Kupriyanov VV, et al.: Coordinate interplay between (Na^+-K^+)-ATPase and creatine phosphokinase optimizes (Na^+-K^+)-antiport across the membrane of vesicles formed from the plasma membrane of cardiac muscle cell. Biochim Biophys Acta 603:142, 1980.
29. Gudbjarnason S, Mathes P, Ravens KG: Functional compartmentation of ATP and creatine phosphate in heart muscle. J Mol Cell Cardiol 1:325, 1970.
30. Hamill OP, Marty A, Neher E, et al.: Improved patch clamp for high resolution recording from cells and cell-free membrane patches. Pflügers Arch 391:85, 1981.
31. Harris AS, Rojas AG: The initiation of ventricular fibrillation due to coronary occlusion. Exp Med Surg 1:105, 1943.
32. Harris AS, Bisteni A, Russell RA, et al.: Excitatory factors in ventricular tachycardia resulting from myocardial ischemia: potassium a major excitant. Science 119:200, 1954.
33. Hasin Y, Barry WH: Myocardial metabolic inhibition and membrane potential, contraction, and potassium uptake. Am J Physiol 247:H322, 1984A.
34. Hasin Y, Doorey A, Barry WH: Electrophysiologic and mechanical effects of metabolic inhibition of high energy phosphate production in culture chick embryo ventricular cells. J Mol Cell Cardiol 16:1009, 1984B.

35. Hearse DJ, Garlick PB, Humphrey SM: Ischemic contracture of the myocardium: mechanisms and prevention. Am J Cardiol 39:986, 1977.
36. Hearse DJ: Oxygen deprivation and early myocardial contractile failure: a reassessment of the possible role of adenosine triphosphate. Am J Cardiol 44:1115, 1979.
37. Higgins TJC, Bailey PJ, Allsopp D: Interrelationship between cellular metabolic status and susceptibility of heart cells to attack by phospholipase. J Molec Cell Cardiol 14:645, 1982.
38. Hill JL, Gettes LS: Effect of acute coronary artery occlusion on local myocardial extracellular K^+ activity in swine. Circulation 61:768, 1980.
39. Hirche HJ, Franz CHR, Bos L, et al.: Myocardial extracellular K^+ and H^+ increase and noradrenaline release as possible cause of early arrhythmias following acute coronary artery occlusion in pigs. J Mol Cell Cardiol 12:579, 1980.
40. Irasawa H, Sato R: Intra- and extracellular effects of proton on the calcium current of isolated guinea pig ventricular cells. Circ Res 59:348, 1986.
41. Isenberg G, Vereecke J, Van der Heyden G, et al.: The shortening of the action potential by DNP in guinea-pig ventricular myocytes is mediated by an increase of a time-independent K conductance. Pflügers Arch 397:251, 1983.
42. Jacobus WE, Pores IH, Lucas SK, et al.: Intracellular acidosis and contractility in the normal and ischemic heart as examined by ^{31}P-NMR. J Mol Cell Cardiol (Suppl. 3) 14:13, 1982.
43. Jacobus WE: Respiratory control and the integration of heart high-energy phosphate metabolism by mitochondrial creatine kinase. Ann Rev Physiol 47:707, 1985.
44. Janse MJ, Van Capelle FJL, Morsink H, et al.: Flow of "injury" current and patterns of excitation during early ventricular arrhythmias in acute regional myocardial ischemia in isolated porcine and canine hearts. Circ Res 47:151, 1980.
45. Jennings RB, Steenbergen C: Nucleotide metabolism and cellular damage in myocardial ischemia. Ann Rev Physiol 47:727, 1985.
46. Ji S, Weiss JN: Electrophysiological effects of free radicals in isolated cardiac myocytes. Clin Res In press.
47. Kagiyama Y, Hill JL, Gettes LS: The effect of acidosis on potassium induced conduction changes. Circulation (Suppl. 3) 62:56, 1980.
48. Kakei M, Noma A, Shibasaki T: Properties of adenosine triphosphate-regulated K^+ channels in guinea pig ventricular cells. J Physiol 363:441, 1985.
49. Kammermeier H, Schmidt P, Jüngling E: Free energy change of ATP-hydrolysis: a causal factor of early hypoxic failure of the myocardium? J Mol Cell Cardiol 14:267, 1982.
50. Kammermeier H: Why do cells need phosphocreatine and a phosphocreatine shuttle? J Mol Cell Cardiol 19:115, 1987.
51. Katz AM, Hecht HH: The early "pump" failure of the ischemic heart. Am J Med 47:497, 1969.
52. Katz AM: Membrane-derived lipids and the pathogenesis of ischemic myocardial damage. J Mol Cell Cardiol 14:627, 1982.
53. Kleber A: Resting membrane potential, extracellular K^+ activity, and intracellular Na^+ activity during global ischemia in isolated perfused guinea pig hearts. Circ Res 52:442, 1983.
54. Kleber AG: Extracellular potassium accumulation in acute myocardial ischemia. J Mol Cell Cardiol 16:389, 1984.
55. Kobayashi K, Neely JR: Control of maximum rates of glycolysis in rat cardiac muscle. Circ Res 44:166, 1979.
56. Kroll K, Feigl EO: Adenosine is unimportant in controlling coronary blood flow in unstressed dog hearts. Am J Physiol 249:H1176, 1985.
57. Kübler W, Katz AM: Mechanism of early "pump" failure of the ischemic heart: possible role of adenosine triphosphate depletion and inorganic phosphate accumulation. Am J Cardiol 40:467, 1977.
58. Langer GA, Weiss JN, Schelbert HR: Cardiac ischemia. Part I—Metabolic and physiologic responses. West J Med 146:713, 1987.
59. Lauer MR, Rusy BF, Davis LD: H^+-induced depolarization in canine cardiac Purkinje fibers. Am J Physiol 247:H312, 1984.
60. Lee HC, Smith N, Mohabir R, et al.: Cytosolic calcium transients from the beating heart. Proc Nat Acad Sci 84:7793, 1987.
61. Lipasti JA, Nevalainen J, Alanen KA, et al.: Anaerobic glycolysis and the development of ischemic contracture in isolated rat heart. Cardiovasc Res 43:145, 1984.
62. Lynch RM, Paul RJ: Compartmentation of glycolytic and glycogenolytic metabolism in vascular smooth muscle. Science 222:1344, 1983.
63. McDonald TF, MacLeod DP: Metabolism and the electrical activity of anoxic ventricular muscle. J Physiol 229:559, 1973.
64. Marban E, Kitakaze M, Kusuoka H, et al.: Intracellular free calcium concentration measured with ^{19}F NMR spectroscopy in intact ferret hearts. Proc Nat Acad Sci 84:6005, 1987.
65. Mathur PP, Case RB: Phosphate loss during reversible myocardial ischemia. J Mol Cell Cardiol 5:375, 1973.
66. Misler S, Falke LC, Gillis K, et al.: A metabolite-regulated potassium channel in rat pancreatic B cells. Proc Natl Acad Sci 83:7119, 1986.
67. Morad M, Dillon S, Weiss J: An acousto-optical steered laser scanning system for the measurement of action potential spread in intact heart. In Deweer P, Salzburg BM (eds.): Optical methods in Cellular Physiology, pp. 211–226. New York, John Wiley and Sons, 1986.
68. Moreno H, Janse MJ, Fiolet JWT, et al.: Comparison of the effects of regional ischemia, hypoxia, hyperkalemia, and acidosis on intracellular and extracellular potentials and metabolism in the isolated porcine heart. Circ Res 46:634, 1980.
69. Nosek TM, Fender KY, Godt RE: It is diprotonated inorganic phosphate that depresses force in skinned skeletal muscle fibers. Science 236:191, 1987.
70. Noma A: ATP regulated K^+ channels in cardiac muscle. Nature 305:147, 1983.
71. Osterrieder W, Brum G, Hescheler J, et al.: Injection of catalytic subunits of cyclic AMP-dependent protein kinase into cardiac myocytes modulates Ca^{2+} current. Nature 298:576, 1982.
71a. Lynch RM, Paul RJ: Compartmentation of glycolytic and glycogenolytic metabolism in vascular smooth muscle. Science 222:1344, 1983.
72. Pallandi RT, Perry MA, Campbell TJ: Proarrhythmic effects of an oxygen-derived free radical generating system on action potentials recorded from guinea pig ventricular myocardium: a possible cause of reperfusion-induced arrhythmias. Circ Res 61:50, 1987.
73. Philipson KD, Nishimoto AY: ATP produced by myocardial sarcolemmal-bound creatine kinase is not preferentially used by the Na^+ pump. Biochem Biophys Res Comm 124(3):696, 1984.
74. Podzuweit T, Dalby AG, Cherry GW, et al.: Tissue levels of cyclic AMP in ischemic and non-ischemic myocardium following coronary artery ligation. J Mol Cell Cardiol 10:81, 1978.
75. Rau EE, Shine KI, Langer GA: Potassium exchange and mechanical performance in anoxic mammalian myocardium. Am J Physiol 232:H85, 1977.
76. Rau EE, Langer GA: Dissociation of energetic state and potassium loss from anoxic myocardium. Am J Physiol 235:H537, 1978.
77. Ribalet B, Ciani S: Regulation by cell metabolism and adenine nucleotides of a K^+ channel in insulin-secreting B cells (RIN m5F). Proc Natl Acad Sci 84:1721, 1987.
78. Rovetto MJ, Whitmer JT, Neely JR: Comparison of the effects of anoxia and whole heart ischemia on carbohydrate utilization in isolated working rat hearts. Circ Res 32:699, 1973.
79. Runnman E, Weiss JN: Exogenous glucose is superior to glycogenolysis at preserving cardiac function during hypoxia. Circulation 78(Suppl II):498, 1988.
80. Saman S, Opie LH: Mechanism of reduction of action potential duration of ventricular myocardium by exogenous lactate. J Mol Cell Cardiol 16:659, 1984.
81. Sato R, Noma A, Kurachi Y, et al.: Effects of intracellular acidification on membrane currents in ventricular cells of the guinea pig. Circ Res 57:553, 1985.
82. Shimoni Y, Giles W: Separation of Na-Ca exchange and transient inward currents in heart cells. Am J Physiol 253:H1330, 1987.
83. Shine KI, Douglas AM, Ricchiuti NV: Ischemia in isolated ventricular septa: mechanical events. Am J Physiol 231:1225, 1976.
84. Shine KI, Douglas AM, Ricchiuti NV: ^{42}K exchange during myocardial ischemia. Am J Physiol 232:H564, 1977.

85. Sparks HV, Bardenheuer H: Regulation of adenosine formation by the heart. Circ Res 58:193, 1986.
86. Spear JF, Michelson EN, Moore EN: Reduced space constant in slowly conducting regions of chronically infarcted canine myocardium. Circ Res 53:176, 1983.
87. Stevenson WG, Linssen GCM, Havenith MG, et al.: Late death after myocardial infarction: mechanisms, etiologies, and implications for sudden death. *In* Bruguda P, Wellens HJJ (eds.): Cardiac arrhythmias: where to go from here?, pp. 367–376. New York, Futura Publishing Company, Inc., 1987.
88. Thompson JA, Hess ML: The oxygen free radical system: a fundamental mechanism in the production of myocardial necrosis. Prog Cardiovasc Dis 28:449, 1986.
89. Trube G, Hescheler J: Inward-rectifying channels in isolated patches of heart cell membrane: ATP dependence and comparison with cell-attached patches. Pflügers Arch 401:178, 1984.
90. Ventura-Clapier R, Vassort G: Role of myofibrillar creatine kinase in the relaxation of rigor tension in skinned cardiac muscle. Pflügers Arch 404:157, 1985.
91. Vleugels A, Vereecke J, Carmeliet E: Ionic currents during hypoxia in voltage-clamped cat ventricular muscle. Circ Res 47:501, 1980.
92. Weingart R, Reber W: Influence of internal pH on r_i of Purkinje fibers from mammalian heart. Experientia 35:929, 1979.
93. Weiss J, Shine KI: Extracellular K^+ accumulation during myocardial ischemia in isolated rabbit heart. Am J Physiol 242:H619, 1982A.
94. Weiss J, Shine KI: $[K^+]_o$ accumulation and electrophysiological alterations during early myocardial ischemia. Am J Physiol 243:H318, 1982B.
95. Weiss J, Hiltbrand B: Functional compartmentation of glycolytic vs. oxidative metabolism in isolated rabbit heart. J Clin Invest 75:436, 1985.
96. Weiss J, Shine KI: The effect of heart rate on $[K^+]_o$ accumulation during myocardial ischemia. Am J Physiol 250:H982, 1986a.
97. Weiss J, Runnman E, Morad M: Hydrogen peroxide activates large outward K^+ currents in isolated ventricular myocytes from Cavia Bobaya (guinea pig) and Mus Rattus (rat). Mt Desert Is Biol Bull 26:51, 1986b.
98. Weiss JN, Lamp ST: Glycolysis preferentially inhibits ATP-sensitive K^+ channels in isolated guinea pig cardiac myocytes. Science 238:67, 1987a.
98a. Weiss JN, Lamp ST: Cardiac ATP-sensitive K^+ channels: evidence for preferential regulation by glycolysis. J Gen Physiol In press.
99. Weiss JN, Lamp ST, Shine KI: Cellular K^+ loss and anion efflux during myocardial ischemia and metabolic inhibition. Am J Physiol 256:H1165, 1989.
100. Wiegand V, Guggi M, Meesmann W, et al.: Extracellular potassium activity changes in the canine myocardium after acute coronary occlusion and the influence of beta-blockade. Cardiovasc Res 13:297, 1979.
101. Wit AL, Bigger JT: Possible electrophysiological mechanisms for lethal arrhythmias accompanying myocardial ischemia and infarction. Circulation (Suppl. 3) 51–52:96, 1975.
102. Zweier JL, Flaherty JT, Weisfeldt ML: Direct measurement of free radical generation following reperfusion of ischemic myocardium. Proc Natl Acad Sci 84:1404, 1987.

4

Neurogenic Aspects of Cardiac Arrhythmias

Richard L. Verrier

During the past few years there has been remarkable progress in elucidating the role of neural factors in the genesis of cardiac arrhythmias. As a result, it has been suggested that a new discipline has emerged, namely neurocardiology.[69, 101] The scope of the field is broad, ranging from studies of single cells to those involving whole organisms under conditions of changing behavioral states. The objectives of this chapter are to review the literature on neurocardiology and to provide a view of this field's horizons.

The Sympathetic Nervous System and Cardiac Arrhythmias

Several lines of evidence implicate primary involvement of adrenergic factors in arrhythmogenesis. Specifically, it has been shown that electrical stimulation of neural structures such as the posterior hypothalamus[147] or the stellate ganglia[45, 146] augments susceptibility to ventricular fibrillation. Infusion of epinephrine[49] or norepinephrine[116] also enhances predisposition to arrhythmia.

A close temporal relationship between sympathetic neural activity and vulnerability to ventricular fibrillation has been observed in the setting of acute coronary artery occlusion.[74] Within 2 minutes of left anterior descending coronary artery occlusion, the ventricular fibrillation threshold was found to be significantly decreased, corresponding to the period of maximal activation of cardiac sympathetic preganglionic fibers (Fig. 4–1). There was a concomitant reduction in coronary sinus blood flow, and oxygen tension decreased significantly. These changes persisted for 5 to 6 minutes and then returned to control levels despite continued obstruction of the coronary vessel. A transient decrease in ventricular fibrillation threshold also occurred during reperfusion but was not accompanied by increases in sympathetic neural discharge.

Bilateral stellectomy prevented the change in ventricular fibrillation threshold associated with coronary artery occlusion but had no influence on coronary sinus oxygen tension or blood flow. These observations suggest that enhanced cardiac sympathetic neural activity contributes to the development of arrhythmias during coronary artery obstruction. During reflow, stellectomy actually augments rather than reduces vulnerability to ventricular fibrillation.

The basis for the profibrillatory influence of sympathetic denervation during reperfusion is unclear. One possibility is that the ablation of adrenergic inputs augments the reactive hyperemic response and thereby increases the release of ischemic washout products. This is in accordance with the findings that a sympathetic alpha-receptor–mediated coronary vasoconstrictor influence operates in both the normal and ischemic heart.[11, 95] Schwartz and Stone[129] found that stellectomy increased the hyperemic response following coronary artery occlusion, as shown by an enhancement in repayment of flow debt, a factor that has been implicated in reperfusion-induced vulnerability to fibrillation.[133]

ADRENERGIC RECEPTOR SUBTYPES

It is well established that beta-adrenergic receptors play an important role in cardiac arrhythmogenesis. In support of this view it has been shown that beta-adrenergic blocking drugs such as propranolol,[20, 62] practolol,[33, 44] and metoprolol[10] afford significant protection against ventricular fibrillation during acute coronary artery occlusion. The protective influence of these agents appears to be due primarily to their adrenergic receptor blocking properties rather than to their membrane-stabilizing actions.[33, 44] Practolol has been shown to be superior to propranolol in protecting against

---

Supported by Grants HL-32905, HL-33567, and HL-35138 from the National Heart, Lung, and Blood Institute, National Institutes of Health, Bethesda, MD.

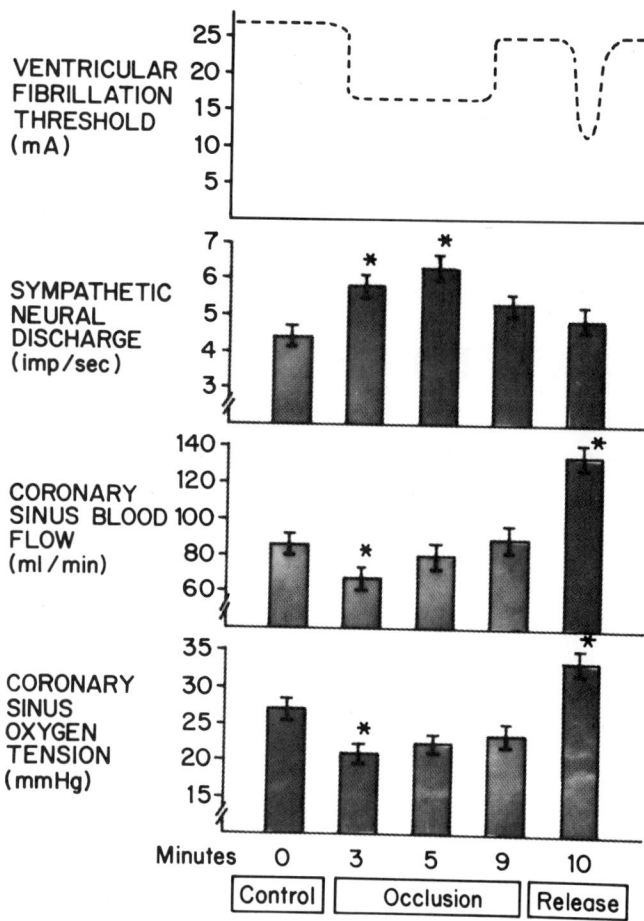

FIGURE 4—1
Effects of a 10-minute period of left anterior descending coronary artery occlusion and release on sympathetic neural activity, coronary sinus blood flow, and coronary sinus oxygen tension. A schematic representation of the time course of changes in ventricular fibrillation threshold is also displayed. Left anterior descending coronary artery occlusion resulted in a consistent activation of sympathetic preganglionic fibers that corresponds to the period of maximal increase in vulnerability to ventricular fibrillation. The concomitant changes in coronary sinus blood flow and reperfusion are also displayed. * = p <0.05 compared with control period. (Reprinted by permission of the C. V. Mosby Co. from Lombardi F, Verrier RL, Lown B: Am Heart J 105:958, 1983.)

ventricular fibrillation during coronary artery ligation.[111] Pearle and coworkers[111] suggested that part of the beneficial effect of beta-adrenergic blockade by a noncardioselective agent such as propranolol may be obviated by its potential vasoconstrictor effect, which is due to its inhibition of beta$_2$-receptor–mediated vascular smooth muscle relaxation. Indeed, there have been a number of patients with Prinzmetal's variant angina in whom the condition was aggravated by propranolol.[163] In these cases, it is reasonable to suggest that the drug provoked inappropriate vasoconstriction, an effect which would not be anticipated in response to cardioselective agents.

The possibility that intrinsic sympathomimetic activity might contribute to differences in the effects of beta-adrenergic blocking drugs on myocardial excitable properties has been investigated in our laboratory.[118]

The effects of three agents with differing degrees of intrinsic sympathomimetic activity were explored. Intravenous propranolol (0.5 mg/kg), oxyprenolol (0.5 mg/kg), and pindolol (0.05 mg/kg) were administered in anesthetized dogs. The effects of these drugs on ventricular vulnerability were studied over a 2-hour interval. Propranolol and oxyprenolol raised the ventricular fibrillation threshold by 42% and 56%, respectively (Fig. 4–2). In contrast, pindolol resulted in an elevation of only 25%. After endogenous norepinephrine stores were depleted with reserpine, pindolol injection actually decreased the ventricular fibrillation threshold. This effect was subsequently reversed by propranolol. These findings indicate that intrinsic sympathomimetic activity of beta-adrenergic blocking agents alters their net effect on myocardial excitability and vulnerability.

The specific influence of beta$_2$-adrenergic receptor stimulation and blockade on cardiac electrophysiologic properties was recently explored in anesthetized dogs by Hohnloser in our laboratory.[50] Selective beta$_2$-adrenergic receptor activation with salbutamol did not alter myocardial excitability but lowered serum potassium concentration. Excitability, refractoriness, and ventricular fibrillation threshold were also not altered after administration of 100 or 200 mcg/kg of the selective beta$_2$-antagonist ICI 118,551. However, at a dose of 500 mcg/kg, ventricular refractoriness and the fibrillation threshold increased. These alterations appear to be due to blockade of beta$_1$-adrenergic receptors rather than to membrane-stabilizing effects, since in catecholamine-depleted animals even the highest dose of ICI 118,551 did not alter myocardial electrical properties. Based on these findings, it was concluded that beta$_2$-adrenergic receptors do not influence electrophysiologic properties of the canine myocardium (Fig. 4–3). Beta$_2$-adrenergic receptor stimulation is also without effect on automaticity in sheep Purkinje fibers.[99] The influence of beta$_2$-adrenergic receptor stim-

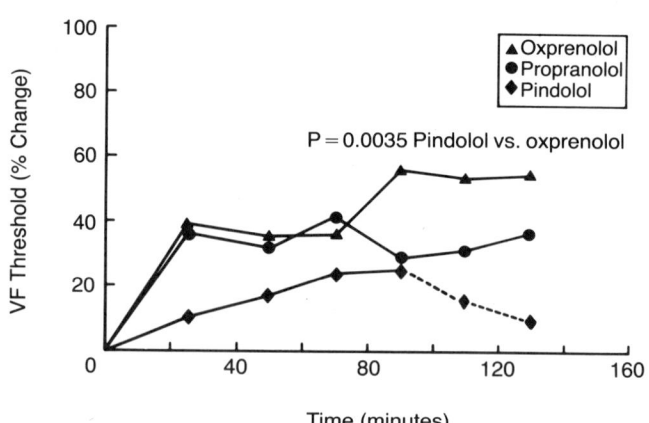

FIGURE 4—2
Differential effects of oxyprenolol (triangles), propranolol (circles) and pindolol (diamonds) on the ventricular fibrillation threshold. The intrinsic sympathomimetic activity of pindolol lessened its antifibrillatory action. (Reprinted by permission of the American College of Cardiology from Raeder EA, Verrier RL, Lown B: J Am Coll Cardiol 1:1442, 1983.)

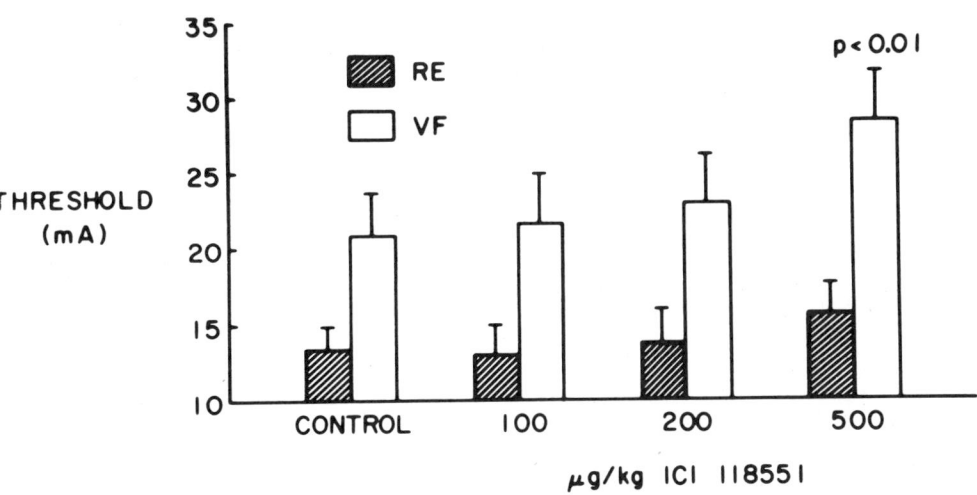

FIGURE 4–3
Effects of ICI 118551 on the thresholds for repetitive extrasystoles (RE) and ventricular fibrillation (VF). The ratio between these thresholds was diminished by the highest drug concentration from 0.64 to 0.52 (p <0.02). (Reprinted by permission of the C. V. Mosby Co. from Hohnloser SH, Verrier RL, Lown B: Am Heart J 113:1066, 1987.)

ulation and blockade on cardiac electrophysiologic properties in humans remains to be explored.

ROLE OF ALPHA-ADRENERGIC RECEPTORS

In the normal heart, alpha-adrenergic receptor stimulation or blockade does not appear to influence ventricular electrical stability.[66, 145] Specifically, it has been shown that intravenous administration of the alpha-adrenergic agonists phenylephrine[145] or methoxamine[66] is without effect on the vulnerable period threshold when the pressor response is controlled to prevent the reflex changes in autonomic tone. It has also been demonstrated that beta-adrenergic blockade completely abolishes the reduction in the ventricular fibrillation threshold produced by posterior hypothalamic or stellate ganglion stimulation.[147, 149] If alpha-adrenergic receptors were involved in the regulation of vulnerability in the normal heart, some component of the effect of sympathetic stimulation would have persisted after beta-adrenergic blockade. Finally, injection of the alpha-adrenergic blocking agent phenoxybenzamine does not alter the threshold for fibrillation.[151]

These observations are consistent with the recent findings of Martins,[85] who demonstrated that alpha-adrenergic stimulation with phenylephrine has no effect on ventricular refractoriness in dogs that had undergone sino-aortic denervation. At high doses a prolongation of Purkinje relative refractory period was observed. The physiologic significance of the latter finding, however, remains unclear.

Investigations of the role of alpha-adrenergic receptors in the setting of myocardial ischemia and infarction have yielded inconsistent results.[20, 25, 130, 134, 142] Several years ago we found that induction of alpha-adrenergic blockade with phentolamine reduced vulnerability to ventricular fibrillation during myocardial ischemia but not during reperfusion.[20] This is at variance with the findings of Sheridan and coworkers[134] and Stewart and colleagues,[142] who demonstrated an antiarrhythmic effect of alpha-adrenergic blocking agents on release-reperfusion. Although there are many possible explanations for the discrepancies, two considerations deserve particular emphasis. The first is that the pharmacologic agents employed may have influenced cardiac electrical properties through extra-adrenergic actions. Phentolamine in high doses, for example, is capable of exerting nonspecific membrane-stabilizing influences that could alter susceptibility to arrhythmias.[121] It is noteworthy in this context that stellectomy, which markedly reduces alpha- as well as beta-adrenergic receptor input, actually increases rather than decreases vulnerability to ventricular fibrillation during release-reperfusion.[74]

A principle that has been espoused by Corr and colleagues[25] is that kinetic properties of alpha-adrenergic receptors may be altered by prolonged ischemia and that this may in turn alter their influence on myocardial electrical stability. These investigators have demonstrated that the idioventricular rate can be increased during reperfusion by regional infusion of methoxamine, an alpha-agonist, into the reperfused zone.[134] Thus, alpha$_1$-adrenergic stimulation appears to produce electrophysiologic derangements during ischemia and reperfusion but it does not influence normal tissue. Recent studies involving x-ray microprobe analysis also suggest that alpha-adrenergic mechanisms may mediate a significant component of the increase in intracellular calcium during reperfusion (Fig. 4–4).[132] This surmise is based on in vivo studies using microelectrodes and membrane patches obtained from cultured myocytes. Specifically, an inward current has been described that is activated by increased cytosolic calcium.[17] Alpha-adrenergic stimulation has been shown to enhance this inward current by increasing cytosolic calcium during ischemia or reperfusion. Corr and coworkers[25] have suggested that the inward current may contribute to slowing of depolarization, which in turn would conduce to the development of delayed after-depolarizations and triggered activity.

ROLE OF CYCLIC NUCLEOTIDES

Cyclic nucleotides have increasingly been implicated as mediating factors in the arrhythmogenic influence of catecholamines.[24, 105, 106, 159] Opie and coworkers have

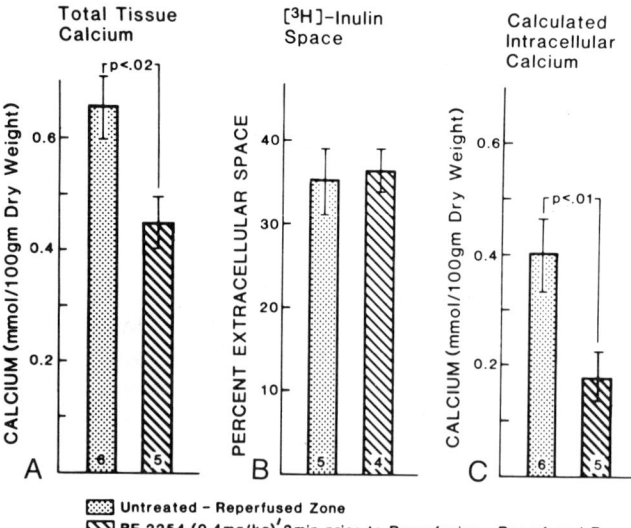

FIGURE 4—4
Effects of alpha$_1$-adrenergic blockade with BE-2254 given intravenously 2 minutes prior to reperfusion and after a 35-minute interval of ischemia on the total tissue calcium (A), the ^{3}H-inulin space (B), and the calculated intracellular calcium (C). Values represent means ± SEM in the reperfused zone in either untreated control animals or animals with alpha$_1$-adrenergic blockade. Although total tissue calcium was reduced by alpha$_1$-adrenergic blockade, it was still elevated over that seen in control tissue (0.3 mmole/100g dry weight). The increase in total tissue calcium in the presence of alpha$_1$-adrenergic blockade was due to a maintained increase in inulin space that was 24% in nonischemic tissue and likely reflects movement into irreversibly injured cells. However, alpha$_1$-adrenergic blockade with BE-2254 completely prevented the increase in intracellular calcium. These results were verified with pyroantimonate precipitation of calcium and electron microscopic X-ray microprobe analysis. (Reprinted by permission of the American Society for Clinical Investigation from Sharma AD, Saffitz JE, Lee BI, et al.: J Clin Invest 72:802, 1983.)

shown that in the isolated perfused rat heart the fibrillation threshold decreased as the tissue cAMP content increased. The influences of beta$_1$-receptor stimulation and of phosphodiesterase inhibition could be due to alterations in the intracellular level of cAMP. The effect of exogenous dibutyryl cAMP in decreasing the ventricular fibrillation threshold was not attributable to activation of adenyl cyclase, since the effect was still evident in the presence of the beta$_1$-specific blocker atenolol.[80] Moreover, the effect of exogenous dibutyryl cAMP was substantially increased by the addition of the phosphodiesterase inhibitor theophylline.[106]

Although these observations suggest that cAMP is capable of influencing vulnerability to ventricular fibrillation, its role in this regard as the second messenger of the effects of catecholamines on vulnerability will require further substantiation.

Sympathetic-Parasympathetic Interactions

This topic has been the subject of intense investigation over the past decade. The prevailing view is that the influences of vagus nerve activity on ventricular vulnerability are contingent on the level of pre-existing cardiac sympathetic tone.[26, 65, 78, 91, 116] This viewpoint is based on the observation that when sympathetic tone to the heart is augmented by thoracotomy,[65] sympathetic nerve stimulation,[65] or catecholamine infusion,[91, 116] simultaneous vagal activation exerts a salutary effect on ventricular vulnerability. Vagus nerve stimulation is without effect on ventricular vulnerability when adrenergic input to the heart is interrupted by beta-adrenergic blockade.[65]

Parasympathetic influences on ventricular vulnerability appear to be due to activation of muscarinic receptors, because vagally mediated changes in vulnerability are prevented by atropine administration.[116] The diminution of adrenergic effects by muscarinic activation has both a physiologic and a cellular basis. Muscarinic agents have been shown both to inhibit the release of norepinephrine from sympathetic nerve endings[72, 73] and to blunt the response to norepinephrine at receptor sites by cyclic nucleotide interactions.[158, 159]

In a recent study we examined whether alterations in serum potassium associated with catecholamine release might be a factor influencing sympathetic-parasympathetic interactions.[49] This issue seemed particularly relevant in light of clinical[7, 18, 103] and experimental[1, 48] evidence linking hypokalemia to the genesis of cardiac arrhythmias. This question was studied in chloralose-anesthetized dogs under conditions of changing autonomic nervous system activity. Epinephrine (1.0 mcg/kg/min) was infused intravenously to produce a brief rise and subsequent prolonged decline in serum potassium concentration (Fig. 4–5). This effect was accompanied by a decline in ventricular fibrillation threshold when baroreceptor activation was prevented by controlled exsanguination. After pretreatment with the beta$_1$-adrenergic blocking agent metoprolol (0.5 mg/kg), epinephrine did not alter vulnerability to ventricular fibrillation but still elicited hypokalemia. In contrast, selective beta$_2$-adrenergic blockade with ICI 118,551 (100 mcg/kg) abolished the epinephrine-induced fall in serum potassium concentration but was without influence on ventricular vulnerability. Muscarinic receptor activation by methacholine (3.0 mg/kg/min) had no effect on serum potassium concentration but significantly increased the ventricular fibrillation threshold. When methacholine and epinephrine were administered simultaneously, the decline in serum potassium concentration persisted, but the increase in ventricular vulnerability was completely annulled. Based on these observations, it was concluded that in the normal canine myocardium epinephrine produces an increase in vulnerability that is mediated through beta$_1$-adrenergic receptors and that the beta$_2$-receptor–mediated hypokalemia is uncoupled from epinephrine's electrophysiologic effects. Parasympathetic nervous system activation does not influence serum potassium concentrations but opposes the effects of epinephrine on susceptibility to ventricular fibrillation.

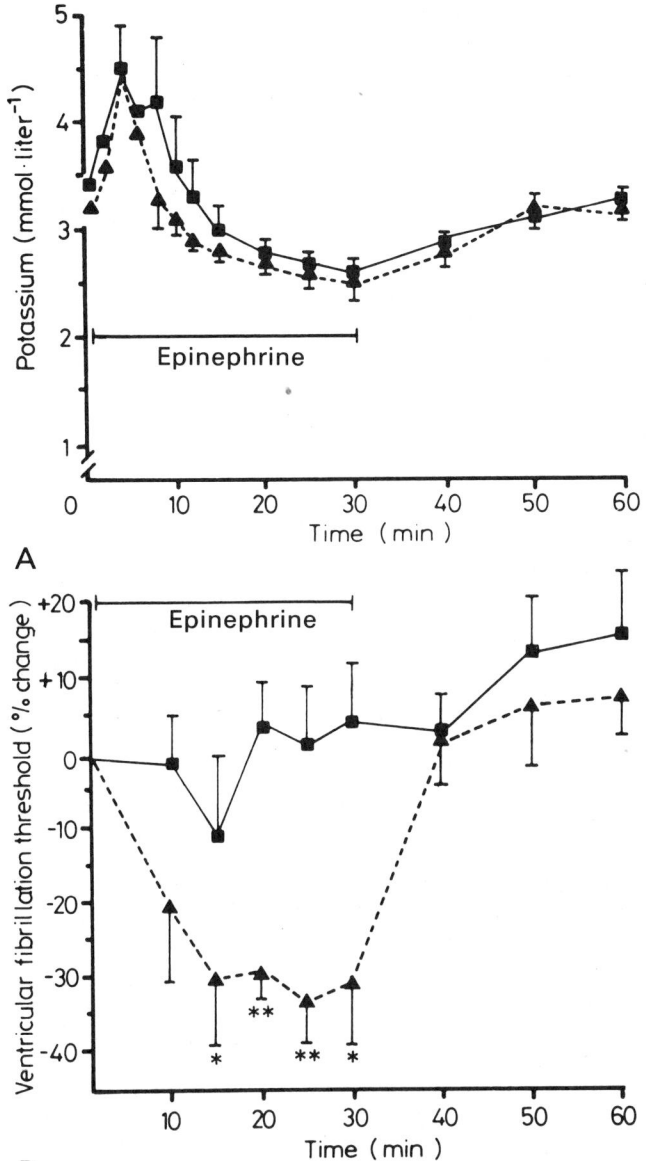

FIGURE 4–5
Influence of epinephrine on (A) serum potassium and (B) ventricular fibrillation threshold while blood pressure was controlled (triangles) and not controlled (squares). Blood pressure control did not alter the catecholamine induced changes in serum potassium. Epinephrine infusion produced a sustained decrease in threshold only during concomitant blood pressure control. Values are means ± SEM from six dogs. * = p<0.05; ** = p <0.01. (Reprinted by permission of the British Medical Association from Hohnloser SH, Verrier RL, Lown B: Cardiovasc Res 20:891, 1986.)

PARASYMPATHETIC INFLUENCES IN THE ISCHEMIC AND INFARCTED HEART

In a landmark study, Kent and Epstein[58, 59] found that vagus nerve stimulation significantly increased the ventricular fibrillation threshold and decreased susceptibility to fibrillation in the ischemic canine heart. Subsequently, Corr, Gillis, and colleagues[22, 23] found that the presence of intact vagi protected against ventricular fibrillation in chloralose-anesthetized cats during ligation of the left anterior descending coronary artery but was not beneficial during right coronary artery obstruction. Yoon and coworkers[165] and James et al.[53] were unable to demonstrate any effect of vagus nerve stimulation on ventricular fibrillation threshold during occlusion of the left anterior descending coronary artery in the canine heart. In a subsequent study, Corr and coworkers[24] found that cholinergic stimulation may actually exacerbate rather than ameliorate the arrhythmias that occur during reperfusion of the ischemic myocardium.

Our investigations indicate that intense cholinergic stimulation by electrical stimulation of the decentralized vagi or by direct muscarinic enhancement with methacholine affords only partial protection during myocardial ischemia in dogs whose heart rate is maintained constant by pacing.[148, 150] No salutary influence of parasympathetic stimulation, however, was noted following reperfusion (Fig. 4–6).[150]

The differing effects of vagus nerve activation on susceptibility to arrhythmia during ischemia and reperfusion have been confirmed and extended in recent investigations by Schwartz and coworkers.[131, 167] They have found that vagus nerve stimulation in cats reduces the incidence of ventricular fibrillation during occlusion but not during release-reperfusion. However, vagus nerve stimulation did lessen the occurrence of ventricular tachycardia during reperfusion, an effect that was completely rate-dependent. They proposed that enhancement of vagal tone may be beneficial in preventing excessive elevations in heart rate associated with increased sympathetic drive to the heart and thereby preserve jeopardized myocardial tissue from advancing ischemia. These investigators have also demonstrated an antifibrillatory effect of vagus nerve stimulation in the conscious dog.[131]

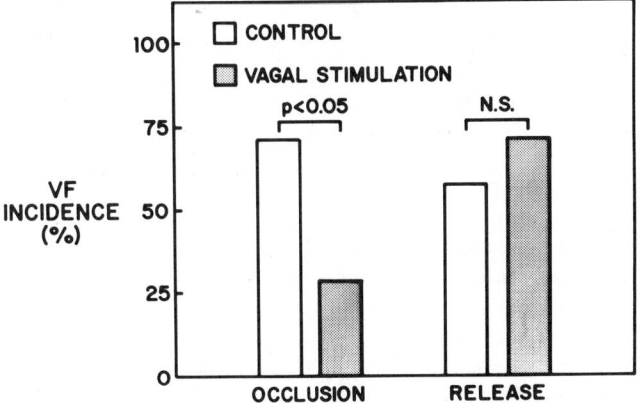

FIGURE 4–6
Influence of vagal stimulation on the incidence of ventricular fibrillation during a 10-minute period of left anterior descending coronary artery occlusion followed by abrupt release. Stimulation of the vagus nerve conferred significant protection against ventricular fibrillation (VF) during occlusion. There was no protection, however, during reperfusion. A constant heart rate was maintained by ventricular pacing at 200 beats per minute. (Reprinted by permission of Raven Press, Publishers, from Verrier RL, Hohnloser SH: In Hearse DJ, Manning AS, Janse MJ (eds.): Life-Threatening Arrhythmias During Ischemia and Infarction, pp. 153–168. New York, Raven Press, 1987.)

The role of the vagus nerve in the setting of acute myocardial infarction is also a subject of extensive investigation. In their classic studies, the Belfast group[160] demonstrated that in patients who were admitted to intensive care within 4 hours of onset of the attack, bradycardia was remarkably frequent. With diaphragmatic infarction, 61% of patients who were reached within 1 hour of onset of symptoms exhibited some bradycardia; these arrhythmias were short-lasting. When patients were accessed within 30 minutes of acute myocardial infarction, signs of autonomic imbalance were detected in 92% of 68 cases.[160] In 41 of these (55%), there were signs of excessive vagal activity, whereas in 27 (36%) there was sympathetic nervous system overactivity. Elevated parasympathetic activity was indicated by heart rates of 60 beats per minute or less, presence of atrioventricular block, or transient hypotension not caused by excessive bradycardia.

In canine experiments, Kerzner and colleagues[61] demonstrated that vagus nerve stimulation does not completely suppress the arrhythmias associated with myocardial infarction. In fact, it has been found that enhanced vagus nerve activity or acetylcholine infusion precipitates ventricular tachycardia during the quiescent, arrhythmia-free phase of myocardial infarction in dogs. This effect was completely rate-dependent. Thus, the antiarrhythmic effects of vagus nerve activity may be augmented or reversed by its profound influence on heart rate in the setting of acute myocardial infarction.[31, 61]

The net effect of neural activation on heart rhythm during infarction may be further complicated by necrotic changes in afferent and efferent sympathetic and vagal pathways within the ventricles.[166] In an elegant series of studies, Zipes and coworkers[3–5, 84] have demonstrated that sympathetic efferent fibers en route to the ventricle cross at the AV groove and travel in the superficial subepicardium in a base-to-apex direction and penetrate the myocardium to innervate the endocardium (Fig. 4–7). Sympathetic afferent fibers also appear to course through the superficial subepicardium in an apex-to-base direction and to traverse superficially at the atrioventricular groove. In comparison, vagal efferent fibers cross superficially at the AV groove, but then penetrate the myocardium, coursing intramyocardially or subendocardially in a base-to-apex direction and penetrating upward to innervate the epicardium. Vagal afferent fibers distribute nerve endings to the superficial epicardium, but traverse intramurally or subendocardially in an apex-to-base direction, emerging superficially to cross at the AV groove. Zipes and colleagues[166] have proposed that myocardial infarction can result in functionally denervated areas within the ventricle. They have shown that zones apical to the infarction fail to exhibit afferent reflexes in response to bradykinin or nicotine. Moreover, refractoriness of the affected areas is not altered by vagus nerve or stellate ganglion stimulation. There is a significant reduction of tissue norepinephrine levels, and the affected zone exhibits supersensitivity to infused norepinephrine or isoproterenol.[52] Taken in sum, these investigators suggest that selective myocardial damage

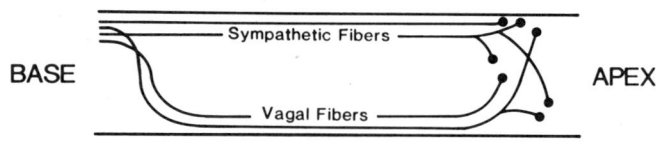

FIGURE 4–7
Schematic representation of the functional pathway of afferent and efferent sympathetic and vagal innervation to the ventricle according to Zipes and coworkers. Afferent pathways course apex-to-base, while efferent pathways travel base-to-apex. Solid circles indicate nerve endings. (Reprinted by permission of Grune & Stratton, Inc., from Zipes DP, Barber MJ, Takahashi N, et al.: In Zipes DP, Jalife DJ (eds.): Cardiac Electrophysiology and Arrhythmias, pp. 181–189. Orlando, FL, Grune & Stratton, Inc., 1985.)

to the epicardium or endocardium may preferentially interrupt one or the other limb of the autonomic nervous system, and this in turn may predispose to the genesis of some ventricular arrhythmias.

The current view of the influence of vagus nerve activity on cardiac arrhythmogenesis is summarized in Table 4–1.

Role of Alterations in Myocardial Perfusion

Coronary artery spasm has been increasingly implicated in the provocation of transient myocardial ischemia. Decreases in coronary blood flow independent of systemic hemodynamic effects have been observed not only in variant angina[15, 46, 103] but also in classic and unstable angina.[27, 46, 81, 86, 88] Deanfield and coworkers[27] reported recurrent episodes of ST-segment depression during ambulatory monitoring in patients with stable angina. These were not associated with changes in heart rate and were shown to result in myocardial ischemia. The authors concluded that transient primary impairments in coronary artery blood flow rather than increased myocardial metabolic demand were the underlying basis for myocardial ischemia. There is also evidence that diverse stimuli can lead to coronary

TABLE 4–1.
Sympathetic-Parasympathetic Interactions and Myocardial Electrical Stability

Vagal tone increases myocardial electrical stability and protects against ventricular fibrillation during myocardial ischemia.

This effect is indirect and is due to antagonism of adrenergic influences.

The basis for parasympathetic-sympathetic interactions is:
  Inhibition of norepinephrine release from nerve endings.
  Attenuation of response to catecholamines at receptor sites.

Beneficial effects of vagal activity may be vitiated if profound bradycardia and hypotension ensue.

Myocardial infarction may alter autonomic influences by damaging neural fibers.

vasoconstriction, including cold exposure,[60, 97, 98, 119, 120] exercise,[27, 46, 81, 164] myocardial infarction,[87, 104] and verbal conditioning.[79] The precise mechanisms responsible for inappropriate coronary vasoconstriction are unclear, but several studies indicate a central role of the sympathetic nervous system.[11, 32, 83, 95, 107, 114, 123, 144, 152-154]

The cold pressor test has been employed as a nonpharmacologic means for eliciting coronary artery spasm.[60, 97, 98, 119, 120] Mudge and coworkers[97] have demonstrated that hand immersion in cold water produces coronary vasoconstriction, ST-segment elevation, and chest pain in patients with coronary disease but not in normal individuals. The constrictor response is prevented by alpha-adrenergic blockade with phentolamine[97] but augmented by beta-adrenergic blockade with propranolol.[60] Potentiation of the coronary vasoconstrictor response to propranolol is believed to be the result of unopposed alpha-adrenergic vasomotor tone.[60]

Intracoronary platelet aggregation may constitute yet another important mechanism whereby neural factors predispose the heart to arrhythmias by impairing myocardial perfusion. The induction of platelet aggregation with adenosine diphosphate causes both myocardial infarction and lethal arrhythmias in animals.[41] Pathologic studies in patients who died suddenly have shown that the occurrence of platelet microthrombi and platelet aggregates is considerably greater than in those whose death was not sudden.[40, 56, 126]

Recent advances have facilitated investigation of the role of platelet aggregation in ventricular electrical stability. Folts and colleagues[34] have found that a critical coronary artery stenosis may induce a gradual decline of coronary blood flow over 5 to 10 minutes, followed by an abrupt recovery of flow to the initial level. These effects lead to ST-segment elevation and reduce the vulnerable period threshold for ventricular fibrillation.[67] Persuasive evidence implicates aggregation and disaggregation of platelets as a basis for these phenomena.[34, 35, 67] Specifically, antiplatelet drugs, including aspirin, sulfinpyrazone, and prostacyclin, have been shown to prevent the cyclical changes in coronary blood flow and the concomitant electrophysiologic alterations.[67] Furthermore, Folts and coworkers[34, 35] have been able to capture platelet plugs distal to the stenosis. It has been demonstrated that infused catecholamines frequently induce flow changes in unresponsive animals.[36] It was unknown, however, whether spontaneous fluctuations in autonomic nervous system activity could alter the pattern of cyclic coronary blood flow changes during partial stenosis.

To explore this issue, we examined the effects of bilateral vagotomy and stellectomy in chloralose-anesthetized dogs during partial stenosis of the left circumflex coronary artery.[117] Vagotomy decreased the frequency of coronary blood flow oscillations but not the magnitude of the flow changes. Bilateral cervical stellectomy reduced both the frequency of coronary blood flow changes and their magnitude (Fig. 4-8). In animals in which cyclical coronary blood flow changes were reduced or abolished by decentralizing the stellate ganglia, electrical stimulation of the main body of the

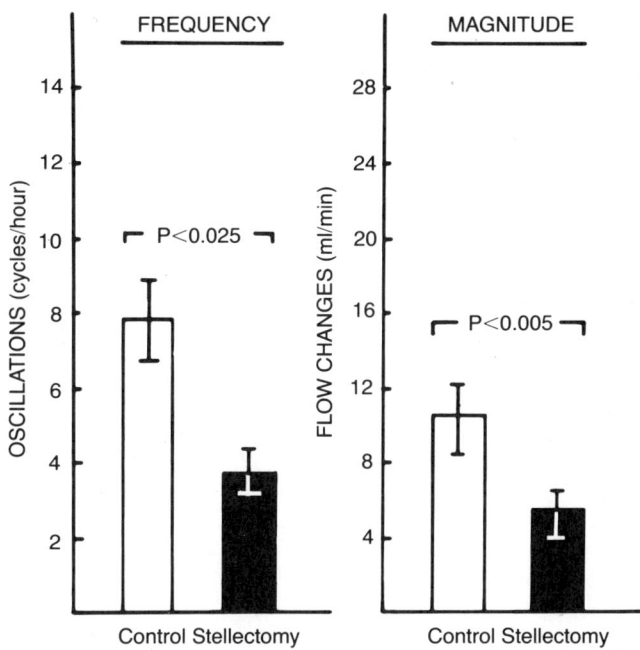

FIGURE 4-8
Influence of bilateral stellectomy on spontaneous oscillations of coronary blood flow during partial stenosis in nine dogs. (Reprinted with permission of the C. V. Mosby Co. from Raeder EA, Verrier RL, Lown B: Am Heart J 104:249, 1982.)

left ganglion restored the oscillation. Infusion of epinephrine also elicited the coronary blood flow changes. Blockade of muscarinic receptors by atropine resulted in a significant attenuation of flow changes, but this may have been partly due to a direct effect of atropine on platelets.

Alterations in platelet function may also provide an important mechanism whereby behavioral stress predisposes to cardiac arrhythmias. Haft and Fani[42] demonstrated that stress induces intracoronary aggregation of platelets in rats following heat and electric shock stress. Examination of the hearts revealed partial or total occlusion of coronary vessels by platelet thrombi and fibrin deposits. Corley and coworkers[21] found that, following shock avoidance stress in monkeys, there was myofibrillar degeneration, myocytolysis, and fuchsinophilia. Similar cardiac pathology has resulted from electric shock, intense light and sound, and audiopresentation to rats of a rat-cat fight.[115]

Collectively, these studies point to an important link between alterations in myocardial perfusion and neurally induced arrhythmias. The availability of these biological models and the evolution of improved imaging techniques are likely to expedite progress in defining neurocardiac interactions in the next few years.

Behavioral Stress and Cardiac Arrhythmias

Notable advances have been made in the past few years in characterizing the role of behavioral stress in the precipitation of cardiac arrhythmias. This is largely attributable to the development of relevant biobehavioral models and to the availability of quantitative methods for assessing myocardial electrical stability in conscious animals. Classic and instrumental aversive conditioning has been found to decrease electrical stability even in the normal heart.[75, 92, 153, 155] During evolving myocardial ischemia or infarction, stress states can trigger major arrhythmias, including ventricular fibrillation.[19] Natural emotions have also been shown to be capable of altering the propensity for fibrillation. Notably, elicitation of an angerlike state has been shown to decrease the vulnerable period threshold by 40 to 50%.[153, 154] Adrenergic factors appear to constitute the major effector component. This is bolstered by the observation that pharmacologic or surgical sympathectomy significantly blunts the arrhythmogenic influence of diverse types of stress.

Vagal influences also appear to play a role in modulating vulnerability during behavioral stress. This view is based on the observations of DeSilva in our laboratory,[28] that enhancing cardiac vagal tone by administration of morphine to dogs in a stressful environment increases the vulnerable period threshold to the levels observed in a nonstressful setting. When vagal efferent activity was blocked by atropine, a major portion of morphine's protective effect was abolished. Administration of morphine in the tranquil setting, in which cardiac adrenergic input was low, failed to alter the vulnerable period threshold. These findings indicate that central activation of the vagi by morphine protects against vulnerability during stress and that this protective action is due to antagonism of the fibrillatory influence of enhanced adrenergic input to the heart.

POST-STRESS ISCHEMIA

The concept that the deleterious effects of stress on the heart may be delayed is well established in the clinical literature.[13, 70, 82] With respect to exercise, for example, it is not uncommon to observe serious arrhythmias, including closely coupled extrasystoles, tachycardias, and fibrillation, in the period immediately following a stress test.[55] It has been suggested that the state of heightened vulnerability may be due in part to the fact that catecholamines are markedly elevated following an exercise challenge.[30] Electrocardiographic abnormalities have also been reported to occur after emotional arousal. McLaughlin and colleagues[82] described the case of a 34-year-old man who first experienced angina pectoris 3 to 4 minutes after sexual intercourse. Upon subsequent study using thallium-201 imaging, it was found that this individual experienced regional myocardial ischemia not during but following the exercise stress test. Although intriguing, such cases are isolated and have eluded systematic investigation.

We therefore undertook to examine the post-stress state in the experimental laboratory. The specific objective was to define the effects of sympathetic nervous system activation on myocardial perfusion in the normal and compromised coronary circulation in dogs. Our studies reveal that after induction of the angerlike state, there is a progressive increase in coronary vascular resistance that develops within 2 to 3 minutes and persists for 10 to 15 minutes after the anger episode (Fig. 4–9). The vasoconstrictor state lingers after heart rate and blood pressure have returned to control levels, indicating primary coronary vasoconstriction. In some animals the response is so intense as to obstruct flow completely in the affected vessel. The presence of myocardial ischemia is indicated by significant ST segment changes. Although this phenomenon, which we termed "delayed myocardial ischemia," is not fully understood, activation of the sympathetic nervous system is likely to be involved.[154] This is supported by the finding that the delayed myocardial ischemic response to anger can be abolished by bilateral stellectomy.[157] The phenomenon can also be elicited following stimulation of the left or right stellate ganglion in anesthetized animals.[43] Since the induction of delayed ischemia can be prevented by intravenous injection of prazosin, it appears that stimulation of alpha$_1$-adrenergic receptors within the coronary vasculature is involved (Fig. 4–10).

The basis for the delayed nature of the response remained an enigma. However, a clue was provided by the finding that there is a close temporal association between the onset of ischemia and the return of coronary arterial blood pressure to the control level following anger or sympathetic stimulation. The experimental interventions were carried out in order to define the role of pressure in delayed ischemia.[108] The first involved preventing the hypertensive response to stellate stimulation by controlled exsanguination. When this procedure was carried out, the coronary vasoconstrictor response was not delayed but occurred during stimulation. A series of interventions designed to raise arterial blood pressure was next performed. These entailed stimulating the left stellate ganglion without blood pressure regulation and allowing the delayed coronary vasoconstriction to occur. Thereafter, systemic blood pressure was raised to the stimulation level by occluding the aorta with a snare. Increasing arterial blood pressure in this manner consistently returned coronary arterial flow and intracoronary pressure to the control values. In contrast, elevating systemic pressure by restimulating the stellate ganglion failed to restore flow through the coronary artery.[108]

These findings are in accord with those of Gerova and colleagues.[39] Using sonomicrometers, they found that stellate stimulation decreased coronary vessel diameter only when the hypertensive response was prevented by regulated exsanguination. They also demonstrated that the vasoconstrictor response to nerve excitation could be abolished by intravenous administration of phentolamine. Thus, it appears that alpha-adrenergic receptor activation was the mechanism responsible for the increase in coronary vascular tone.

Our current view is that delayed myocardial ischemia results from an interplay between adrenergic and hemodynamic factors and that this interaction is the likely basis for the delayed nature of the ischemic response. The following hypothesis is proposed to account for

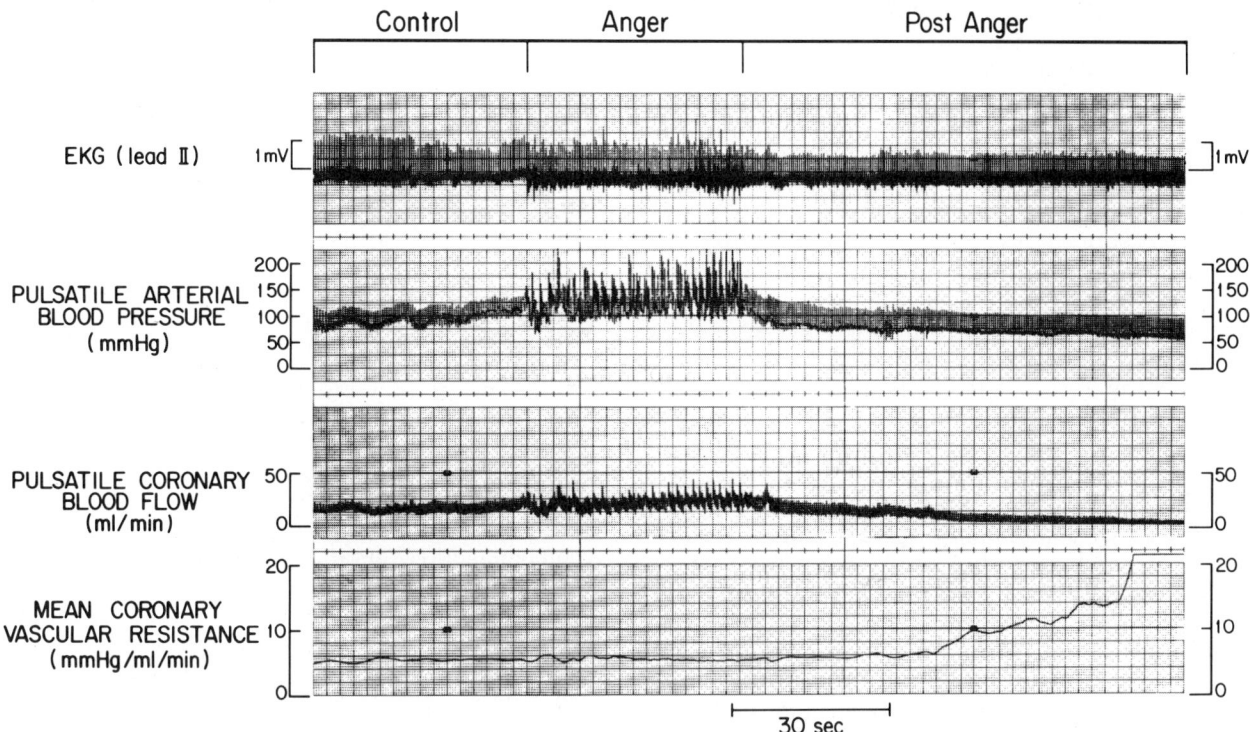

FIGURE 4–9
Effects on coronary hemodynamic function of inducing an angerlike state in a dog with coronary artery stenosis. During the stress (Anger) state, coronary arterial blood flow increased significantly and coronary vascular resistance was reduced. During the post-stress (Post Anger) recovery period, there was pronounced coronary vasoconstriction, evidenced by a fall in coronary arterial blood flow and an increase in coronary vascular resistance. These changes occurred when heart rate and arterial blood pressure returned to pre-stress (Control) levels, a response that suggests primary coronary vasoconstriction. (Reprinted by permission of the American Heart Association, Inc., from Verrier RL, Hagestad EL, Lown B: Circulation 75:249, 1987.)

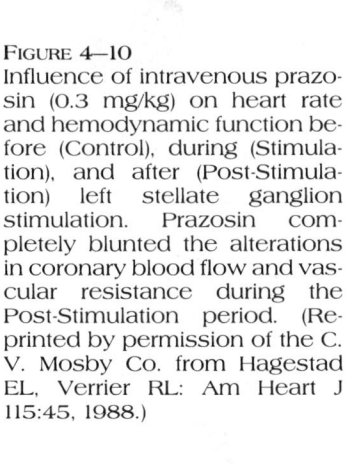

FIGURE 4–10
Influence of intravenous prazosin (0.3 mg/kg) on heart rate and hemodynamic function before (Control), during (Stimulation), and after (Post-Stimulation) left stellate ganglion stimulation. Prazosin completely blunted the alterations in coronary blood flow and vascular resistance during the Post-Stimulation period. (Reprinted by permission of the C. V. Mosby Co. from Hagestad EL, Verrier RL: Am Heart J 115:45, 1988.)

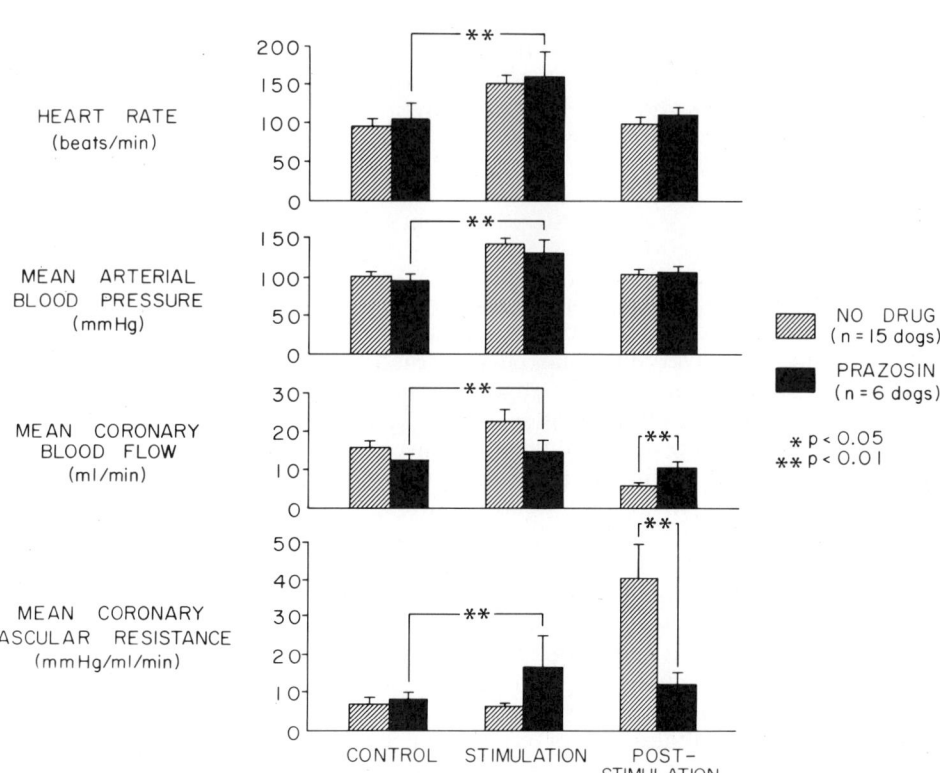

the available data.[43, 108, 109, 154] During activation of the sympathetic nervous system, arterial blood pressure increases in response to either behavioral stress or direct excitation of the stellate ganglia, thereby opposing the vasoconstrictor influence of alpha-adrenergic receptor stimulation on vascular smooth muscle. The net result is that coronary vascular resistance remains unaltered. However, during the post-excitation phase, systemic pressure returns abruptly to the control level, thereby lessening distending pressure within the coronary vessel. We hypothesized that the dissipation of catecholamines is delayed and thus the adrenergic vasoconstrictor influence predominates over the passive distending force. The imbalance leads to a decrease in coronary diameter and to an increase in vascular resistance. This formulation is analogous to that proposed by Masuda and Levy[90] to account for a delayed recovery of heart rate and contractility following cessation of sympathetic nerve stimulation. Our findings are summarized in Table 4–2.

These findings indicate that several characteristics of the post-stress state are conducive to myocardial ischemia and arrhythmias. These include relatively elevated catecholamine levels and reduced coronary distending pressure in the face of lingering neurohumorally mediated vasoconstrictor drive. These factors may be responsible for the delayed onset of ischemia following cessation of exercise or intense emotional arousal. This hazardous coexistence of enhanced neurogenic activity and inadequate coronary distending pressure may also occur under clinical conditions such as heart failure or hemorrhage. Schwartz and coworkers[128] have postulated that the markedly elevated sympathetic tone and concomitantly low coronary distending pressure may be responsible for the occurrence of coronary insufficiency and myocardial ischemia during hemorrhage.[89] Clearly, experimental modeling of these conditions and those associated with the post-stress state could lead to important new insights into the pathophysiology of coronary artery disease.

Sleep

Despite considerable progress in defining the influence of stress on myocardial perfusion and ventricular electrical stability, relatively little has been learned about the effects of sleep on cardiac arrhythmogenesis. Because sleep is a precisely integrated neurophysiologic state, its study could provide valuable insights into the linkage between the brain and the heart.

Clinical studies indicate that sleep suppresses ventricular arrhythmias.[9, 29, 76, 96, 112, 113, 122, 140, 161] Lown and coworkers[76] found that 45 of 54 subjects undergoing 24-hour ambulatory monitoring exhibited significant reduction in ventricular ectopic activity during sleep. When sleep stages were monitored, these investigators noted reduction of ventricular premature beats during all stages except rapid eye movement (REM) sleep.[29] The most marked abatement of arrhythmia was observed during slow wave sleep (stages 3 and 4). The

TABLE 4–2
Delayed Myocardial Ischemia

1. The ischemic state ensues 2 to 3 minutes following provocation of stress.*
2. Delayed ischemia can be prevented by stellectomy and induced by sympathetic stimulation. The latter effect can be blocked by alpha$_1$-adrenergic blockade.†
3. The interaction between coronary distending pressure and adrenergic factors appears to be responsible for the delayed nature of the response.‡
4. These findings carry important clinical implications, as they may help to explain the occurrence of myocardial ischemia in response to hemorrhage and heart failure. Under such conditions, the neurally induced rise in intravascular pressure may not be adequate to offset the coronary vasoconstrictor influence.

*Verrier RL, et al.[154]
†Hagestad EL, Verrier RL.[43]
‡Papageorgiou P, et al.[108, 109]

change in ventricular ectopic activity was not correlated with alterations in heart rate, which remained relatively constant during the various sleep stages. The frequency of ventricular premature beats was similar during the awake and REM periods. Pickering and colleagues[112, 113] and others[9, 161] reported results comparable to those of Lown and colleagues.[29, 76] A beneficial effect of sleep on myocardial electrical stability is also suggested by the infrequency of sudden cardiac death during sleep, although it comprises about one third of the diurnal cycle.[38, 100] Ventricular tachycardia and fibrillation, however, have been noted to occur in association with violent or frightening dreams.[77, 137] Nevertheless, it remains highly inferential that when sudden death does occur in the night, it is during REM sleep.

Only a few experimental studies have been conducted to define the effects of sleep on susceptibility to cardiac arrhythmias. Skinner and coworkers[135] have examined the influence of sleep stage on the incidence of ventricular arrhythmias during left anterior descending coronary artery occlusion in pigs. They found an increase in arrhythmias compared with the awake state in the period of the early sleep cycle during which transitional and slow wave sleep alternate. This was the case in the acutely infarcted as well as in the recently infarcted pig heart. The greatest increase in ventricular arrhythmias was observed during sustained periods of slow wave sleep. Later, when rapid eye movement sleep prevailed, the arrhythmia incidence abruptly decreased. Acute coronary artery occlusion performed after the inception of slow wave sleep reduced the latency in onset of ventricular fibrillation compared with that observed during the awake state. Coronary occlusion during REM sleep resulted in the opposite effect, namely, a delay in the development of ventricular fibrillation.

Skinner and colleagues[135] reached some unanticipated conclusions: (1) slow wave sleep, but not REM sleep, has a deleterious influence on the ischemic heart; (2) REM sleep may be beneficial, because it delays the development of ventricular fibrillation during coronary artery coclusion; and (3) the heart rate changes during sleep do not correlate with the effects of slow wave or

REM sleep on cardiac rhythm. It is curious that in pigs with coronary artery occlusion, arrhythmia was reduced not only during REM sleep but also during wakefulness. These investigators refer to the work of Baust and Bohnert in cats,[6] which indicates that reduction in sympathetic tone accounted for the slow tonic heart rates during REM sleep, whereas during slow wave sleep, bradycardia was due to increased parasympathetic tone. However, increased sympathetic tone is considered a characteristic of the awake state.

Snyder, Hobson and Goldfrank[141] and others[2, 16] have demonstrated that heart rate and arterial blood pressure are higher during wakefulness than during sleep. There may in fact be hemodynamic concomitants, as well as coronary artery flow changes, linked to neural alterations during sleep stages that influence the electrically unstable ischemic heart.

Recently we have obtained data that suggest that alterations in vagal tone may modulate cardiac electrophysiologic properties during sleep.[37] Specifically, the effects of REM and slow wave sleep on ventricular refractoriness were studied in chronically instrumented cats. Electrodes were implanted to record electrooculograms, electromyograms, and electroencephalograms for sleep stage determination. A right ventricular catheter was employed for cardiac electrical testing using the single stimulus technique. Both REM and slow wave sleep significantly increased the effective refractory period. This effect was independent of alterations in heart rate, as this variable was maintained fixed by pacing. These alterations were not prevented by bilateral stellectomy. However, when the muscarinic blocking agent atropine methylnitrate was administered, the sleep-induced changes were obviated. These results suggest that the electrophysiologic changes during sleep are mediated through fluctuations in cardiac vagal tone.

INFLUENCE OF SLEEP ON MYOCARDIAL PERFUSION

Clinical studies indicate that phasic changes in coronary blood flow occur throughout the diurnal cycle.[27, 63] In particular, Deanfield and coworkers[27] have found during 24-hour Holter monitoring in patients with stable angina that ST segments fluctuate substantially during day and night. Studies that correlate the ST-segment variation with the sleep stage would be of considerable interest.

The potential value of such investigations is underscored by a report by King and colleagues,[63] who explored the effects of sleep on the occurrence of Prinzmetal's variant angina. In an individual with angiographically documented coronary artery spasm, they found that the episodes of nocturnal chest pain accompanied by ST-segment elevation occurred primarily during the REM stage of sleep. The factors responsible for the episodes of nocturnal angina, however, were not defined.

In animal experiments, Vatner and coworkers[143] have observed that in the nocturnal period, when baboons were apparently asleep, coronary artery blood flow fluctuated by as much as twofold. The periodic fluctuations in blood flow were not coupled to changes in heart rate or arterial blood pressure and occurred while the animals remained motionless with eyes closed. Since the baboons were not instrumented for sleep recording, no data were obtained regarding sleep stage nor was the mechanism for the coronary blood flow surge defined.

We addressed the issue of sleep-induced coronary blood flow changes in a recent series of experiments carried out in chronically instrumented dogs.[64a] The animals were studied during natural sleep and the cycles were divided into 1-minute periods of quiet wakefulness, slow wave sleep, or REM sleep. Our preliminary findings indicate that during slow wave sleep there are moderate but significant reductions in heart rate and coronary blood flow and increases in coronary vascular resistance. In REM sleep, the coronary blood flow baseline is moderately elevated compared with slow wave sleep, and there are striking, episodic surges in flow. Coronary vascular resistance is reduced correspondingly. Heart rate and mean arterial pressure are also elevated during the flow surges, indicating that an increase in cardiac metabolic activity may be the basis for the coronary vasodilation. Since bilateral stellectomy prevented the surges in coronary blood flow, this effect does not appear to be due to nonspecific effects of somatic activity or respiratory fluctuations; rather, the changes appear to be the direct result of enhanced adrenergic discharge. In a recent study, we have demonstrated that in the presence of coronary stenosis, the phasic increases in sympathetic discharge during REM sleep result in a decrease rather than an increase in coronary arterial blood flow.[64b]

Final Comments

The main objective of this chapter was to provide a perspective on the literature that could be subsumed under the rubric of neurocardiology. Irrespective of whether or not this term is adopted into the medical literature, the fact remains that there have been major advances over the past few years in our understanding of neurocardiac interactions. As a result of the important conceptual and methodological foundations that have been established, we can anticipate significant progress in both the experimental and clinical sectors. Some promising avenues of research are indicated in Table 4–3.

Specifically, the application of state-of-the-art mapping techniques for the electrophysiologic study of tachyarrhythmias during nerve stimulation, particularly in conscious animals, could provide insights into mechanisms at the cardiac level.[12, 54, 68, 162] The relationship of anatomically inhomogeneous sympathetic and parasympathetic innervation to electrophysiologic function remains to be elucidated. Also, investigation of the effects of stress in animals with "mottled" infarcts should provide useful information.[57, 93, 94, 110] Indeed, postinfarction arrhythmias represent a substantial clin-

TABLE 4–3
Future Directions for Study of Neurocardiac Interactions

Research Focus	Research Approaches
Cardiac electrophysiologic mechanisms	Use of mapping techniques to define electrophysiologic processes responsible for stress related arrhythmias
Myocardial perfusion	Use of advanced imaging methods to determine mechanisms involved in stress-induced coronary artery spasm; also, application of platelet antibodies to characterize the role of platelets in the observed perfusion deficits
Baroreceptor function	Assessment of baroreceptor gain as an indicator of susceptibility to life-threatening arrhythmias[8, 71]
Central nervous system mapping	Application of lesioning and neurochemical techniques to delineate arrhythmogenic centers in the brain; also, pharmacologic study of the role of neurotransmitters in behaviorally induced arrhythmias
Behavior	Modeling of relevant states such as anxiety, panic, depression, and sleep

ical management problem that could benefit from further investigation. There is an additional important rationale for exploring the effects of stress in the infarcted myocardium—namely, as Inoue and Zipes[52] have shown, there may be necrotic damage to the heart's nerve supply which leads to catecholamine supersensitivity. This could be an important factor in neurally induced arrhythmia.

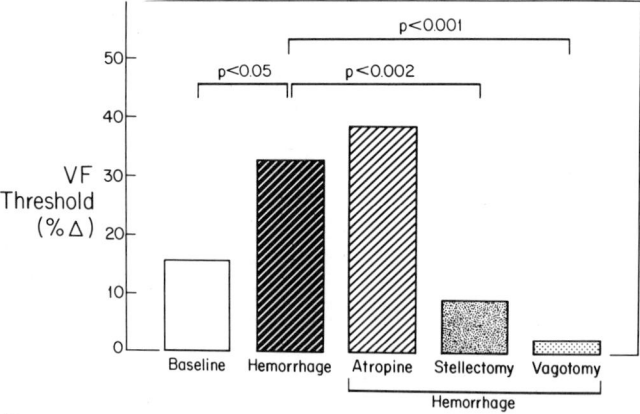

FIGURE 4–11
Comparison of the effect of fentanyl on ventricular fibrillation (VF) threshold during differing autonomic interventions. Hemorrhage significantly increased the antifibrillatory effect of fentanyl. Muscarinic blockade with atropine did not alter the drug's action, whereas stellectomy significantly reduced it. Bilateral cervical vagotomy abolished the effect of fentanyl completely. Values are percentage changes in ventricular fibrillation threshold after administration of fentanyl. (Reprinted by permission of the C. V. Mosby Co. from Saini V, Carr DB, Hagestad EL, et al.: Am Heart J 115:598, 1988.)

It is important to explore the role of myocardial perfusion as an intermediary mechanism in the genesis of arrhythmias. This will require consideration of the effects on platelet aggregability and coronary hemodynamic function. In both areas there have been many new exciting advances, clinically and experimentally, that could accelerate progress in the study of neural modulation of heart rhythm.

The neurohumoral component of brain-heart interactions remains largely unexplored. Pituitary secretion of beta-endorphin as well as the other neuromodulatory hormones may play a role in the dynamic control of cardiac electrophysiologic properties (Fig. 4–11).[14, 124] The recent discoveries of circulating peptides with significant cardiovascular effects (atrial natriuretic factor, gamma-mSH, enkephalins)[14, 51, 124, 125] add another promising dimension to the study of neurocardiac interactions. The roles of the thalamic gating system and amygdala and hypothalamic control centers in stress-induced vulnerability need to be defined.[136, 138, 139] A number of innovative techniques including reversible cryogenic blockade[136] and localized neuroinjection will be helpful in the pursuit of this objective.[139]

Finally, there is a need to continue diversification of the behavioral models. Some specific states deserving further study include anxiety, panic, depression, and sleep.[47, 127] Exploration of this avenue could lead to heuristic models for investigation of psychotropic as well as cardiovascular drugs.

References

1. Armitage AK, Burn JH, Gunning AJ: Ventricular fibrillation and ion transport. Circ Res 5:98, 1957.
2. Baccelli G, Guazzi M, Mancia G, Zanchetti A: Neural and non-neural mechanisms influencing circulation during sleep. Nature 223:184, 1969.
3. Barber MJ, Mueller TM, Henry DP, et al.: Transmural myocardial infarction in the dog produces sympathectomy in non-infarcted myocardium. Circulation 67:787, 1983.
4. Barber MJ, Mueller TM, Davies BG, et al.: Phenol topically applied to canine left ventricular epicardium interrupts sympathetic but not vagal afferents. Circ Res 55:532, 1984.
5. Barber MJ, Mueller TM, Davies BG, et al.: Interruption of sympathetic and vagal-mediated afferent responses by transmural myocardial infarction. Circulation 72:623, 1985.
6. Baust W, Bohnert B: The regulation of heart rate during sleep. Exp Brain Res 7:169, 1969.
7. Beck OA, Hochrein H: Serumkaliumspiegel und Herzrhythmusstorungen beim akuten Myokardinfarkt. Z Kardiol 66:187, 1977.
8. Billman GE, Schwartz PJ, Stone HL: The effects of daily exercise on susceptibility to sudden cardiac death. Circulation 69:1182, 1984.
9. Brodsky M, Wu D, Denes P, et al.: Arrhythmias documented by 24-hour continuous electrocardiographic monitoring in 50 male medical students without apparent heart disease. Am J Cardiol 39:390, 1977.
10. Brodsky MA, Verrier RL, Lown B: Effects of beta blockade with and without coronary dilators on vulnerability to ventricular fibrillation during coronary occlusion and reperfusion (Abstract). Circulation 66:II333, 1982.
11. Buffington CW, Feigl EO: Adrenergic coronary vasoconstriction in the presence of coronary stenosis in the dog. Circ Res 48:416, 1981.
12. Burgess MJ: Ventricular repolarization and electrocardiographic T wave form and arrhythmia vulnerability. In Levy MN, Vassalle M (eds.): Excitation and Neural Control of the

Heart, pp. 181–202. Bethesda, MD; American Physiological Society, 1982.
13. Caplin JL, Banim SO: Chest pain and electrocardiographic ST-segment elevation occurring in the recovery phase after exercise in a patient with normal coronary arteries. Clin Cardiol 8:228, 1985.
14. Carr DB, Saini V, Verrier RL: Opioids and cardiovascular function: Neuromodulation of ventricular ectopy. In Kulbertus HE (ed.): Neurocardiology, pp. 223–245. Mt. Kisco, Futura Publishing Co., 1988.
15. Chierchia S, Brunelli C, Simonetti I, et al.: Sequence of events in angina at rest: Primary reduction in coronary flow. Circulation 61:759, 1980.
16. Coccagna G, Mantovani M, Brignani F, et al.: Arterial pressure changes during spontaneous sleep in man. Electroencephalogr Clin Neurophysiol 31:277, 1971.
17. Colquhoun D, Neher E, Reuter H, et al.: Inward current channels activated by intracellular Ca^{2+} in cultured cardiac cells. Nature 294:752, 1981.
18. Cooper WD, Kuan P, Reuben SR, et al.: Cardiac arrhythmias following acute myocardial infarction: Associations with the serum potassium level and prior diuretic therapy. Eur Heart J 5:464, 1984.
19. Corbalan R, Verrier RL, Lown B: Psychological stress and ventricular arrhythmias during myocardial infarction in the conscious dog. Am J Cardiol 34:692, 1974.
20. Corbalan R, Verrier RL, Lown B: Differing mechanisms for ventricular vulnerability during coronary artery occlusion and release. Am Heart J 92:223, 1976.
21. Corley KC, Shiel FO, Mauck HP, et al.: Myocardial degeneration and cardiac arrest in squirrel monkey: physiological and psychological correlates. Psychophysiology 14:322, 1977.
22. Corr PB, Gillis RA: Role of the vagus nerves in the cardiovascular changes induced by coronary occlusion. Circulation 49:86, 1974.
23. Corr PB, Pearle DL, Gillis RA: Coronary occlusion site as a determinant of the cardiac rhythm effects of atropine and vagotomy. Am Heart J 92:741, 1976.
24. Corr PB, Penkoske PA, Sobel BE: Adrenergic influences on arrhythmias due to coronary occlusion and reperfusion. Br Heart J 40:62, 1978.
25. Corr PB, Yamada KA, Witkowski FX: Mechanisms controlling cardiac autonomic function and their relation to arrhythmogenesis. In Fozzard HA, Haber E, Jennings RB, et al. (eds.): The Heart and Cardiovascular System, pp. 1343–1403. New York, Raven Press, 1986.
26. Danilo P Jr., Rosen MR, Hordof AJ: Effects of acetylcholine on the ventricular specialized conducting system of neonatal and adult dogs. Circ Res 43:777, 1978.
27. Deanfield JE, Maseri A, Selwyn AP, et al.: Myocardial ischaemia during daily life in patients with stable angina: Its relation to symptoms and heart rate changes. Lancet 2:753, 1983.
28. DeSilva RA, Verrier RL, Lown B: The effects of psychological stress and vagal stimulation with morphine on vulnerability to ventricular fibrillation (VF) in the conscious dog. Am Heart J 95:197, 1978.
29. DeSilva RA: Central nervous system risk factors for sudden cardiac death. Ann NY Acad Sci 382:143, 1982.
30. Dimsdale JE, Hartley LH, Guiney T, et al.: Postexercise peril. Plasma catecholamines and exercise. JAMA 251:630, 1984.
31. El-Sherif N: Reentrant ventricular arrhythmias in the late myocardial infarction period: 6. Effect of the autonomic system. Circulation 58:103, 1978.
32. Feigl EO: Coronary physiology. Physiol Rev 63:1–205, 1983.
33. Fitzgerald JD: The role of beta-adrenergic blockade in acute myocardial ischaemia. In Oliver MF, Julian DG, Donald KW (eds.): Effect of Acute Ischaemia on Myocardial Function, pp. 321–351. Baltimore, Williams & Wilkins Co., 1972.
34. Folts JD, Crowell EB, Rowe GG: Platelet aggregation in partially obstructed vessels and its elimination with aspirin. Circulation 54:365, 1976.
35. Folts JD, Gallagher K, Rowe GG: Blood flow reductions in stenosed canine coronary arteries: vasospasm or platelet aggregation? Circulation 65:248, 1982.
36. Folts JD: Experimental arterial platelet thrombosis, platelet inhibitors, and their possible clinical relevance. Cardiovasc Rev Rep 3:370, 1982.
37. Francis GC, Hagestad EL, Verrier RL: Influence of sleep stage on ventricular refractoriness (Abstract). Physiologist 29:163, 1986.
38. Friedman M, Manwaring JH, Rosenman RH, et al.: Instantaneous and sudden deaths. Clinical and pathological differentiation in coronary artery disease. JAMA 225:1319, 1973.
39. Gerova M, Barta E, Gero J: Sympathetic control of major coronary artery diameter in the dog. Circ Res 44:459, 1979.
40. Haerem JW: Platelet aggregates and mural microthrombi in the early stages of acute, fatal coronary disease. Thromb Res 5:243, 1974.
41. Haft JI, Gershengorn K, Kranz PD, et al.: Protection against epinephrine-induced myocardial necrosis by drugs that inhibit platelet aggregation. Am J Cardiol 30:838, 1972.
42. Haft JI, Fani K: Intravascular platelet aggregation in the heart induced by stress. Circulation 47:353, 1973.
43. Hagestad EL, Verrier RL: Delayed myocardial ischemia following the cessation of sympathetic stimulation. Am Heart J 115:45, 1988.
44. Hai HA, Temte JV, Lown B: Changes in ventricular fibrillation threshold during coronary artery occlusion and release induced by beta adrenergic blockade (Abstract). Am J Cardiol 37:140, 1976.
45. Han J, Garcia de Jalon P, Moe GK: Adrenergic effects on ventricular vulnerability. Circ Res 14:516, 1964.
46. Hillis LD, Braunwald E: Coronary-artery spasm. N Engl J Med 299:695, 1978.
47. Hobson JA: What is a behavioral state? In Ferrendelli JA (ed.): Aspects of Behavioral Neurobiology, pp. 1–15. Bethesda, MD; Society for Neuroscience, 1978.
48. Hohnloser SH, Verrier RL, Lown B, et al.: Effect of hypokalemia on susceptibility to ventricular fibrillation in the normal and ischemic canine heart. Am Heart J 112:32, 1986.
49. Hohnloser SH, Verrier RL, Lown B: Effects of adrenergic and muscarinic receptor stimulation on serum potassium concentrations and myocardial electrical stability. Cardiovasc Res 20:891, 1986.
50. Hohnloser SH, Verrier RL, Lown B: Influence of $beta_2$-adrenoceptor stimulation and blockade on cardiac electrophysiologic properties and serum potassium concentration in the anesthetized dog. Am Heart J 113:1066, 1987.
51. Holtz J, Sommer O, Bassenge E: Sympatho-adrenal activity inhibited by atrial natriuretic factor (alpha-ANF) at physiological release rates in conscious dogs (Abstract). Circulation 74:II425, 1986.
52. Inoue H, Zipes DP: Results of sympathetic denervation in the canine heart: supersensitivity that may be arrhythmogenic. Circulation 75:877, 1987.
53. James RGG, Arnold JMO, Allen JD, et al.: The effects of heart rate, myocardial ischemia and vagal stimulation on the threshold for ventricular fibrillation. Circulation 55:311, 1977.
54. Janse MJ, Wilms-Schopman F, Wilensky RJ, et al.: Role of the subendocardium in arrhythmogenesis during acute ischemia. In Zipes DP, Jalife J (eds.): Cardiac Electrophysiology and Arrhythmias, pp. 353–362. Orlando, FL; Grune & Stratton, 1985.
55. Jelinek MV, Lown B: Exercise stress testing for exposure of cardiac arrhythmias. Prog Cardiovasc Dis 16:497, 1974.
56. Jorgensen L, Haerem JW, Chandler AB, et al.: The pathology of acute coronary death. Acta Anaesthesiol Scand (Suppl) 29:193, 1968.
57. Karagueuzian HS, Fenoglio JJ Jr., Weiss MG, et al.: Protracted ventricular tachycardia induced by premature stimulation of the canine heart after coronary artery occlusion and reperfusion. Circ Res 44:833, 1979.
58. Kent KM, Smith ER, Redwood DR, et al.: Electrical stability of acutely ischemic myocardium. Influences of heart rate and vagal stimulation. Circulation 47:291, 1973.
59. Kent KM, Epstein SE, Cooper T, et al.: Cholinergic innervation of the canine and human ventricular conducting system: Anatomic and electrophysiologic correlations. Circulation 50:948, 1974.
60. Kern MJ, Ganz P, Horowitz JD, et al.: Potentiation of coronary vasoconstriction by beta-adrenergic blockade in patients with coronary artery disease. Circulation 67:1178, 1983.
61. Kerzner J, Wolf M, Kosowsky BD, et al.: Ventricular ectopic

rhythms following vagal stimulation in dogs with acute myocardial infarction. Circulation 47:44, 1973.
62. Khan MI, Hamilton JT, Manning GW: Protective effect of beta adrenoreceptor blockade in experimental coronary occlusion in conscious dogs. Am J Cardiol 30:832, 1972.
63. King MJ, Zir LM, Kaltman AJ, et al.: Variant angina associated with angiographically demonstrated coronary artery spasm and REM sleep. Am J Med Sci 265:419, 1973.
64. Kirby DA, Verrier RL: Differential effects of rapid eye movement and slow wave sleep on coronary hemodynamic function (Abstract). Soc Neurosci Abstr 13:740, 1987.
64a. Kirby DA, Verrier RL: Differential effects of sleep stage on coronary hemodynamic function. Am J Physiol 256:H1378–H1383, 1989.
64b. Kirby DA, Verrier RL: Differential effects of sleep stage on coronary hemodynamic function during stenosis. Physiol Behav 45:1017, 1989.
65. Kolman BS, Verrier RL, Lown B: The effect of vagus nerve stimulation upon vulnerability of the canine ventricle: Role of sympathetic-parasympathetic interactions. Circulation 52:578, 1975.
66. Kowey PR, Verrier RL, Lown B: Effect of alpha-adrenergic receptor stimulation on ventricular electrical properties in the normal canine heart. Am Heart J 105:366, 1983.
67. Kowey PR, Verrier RL, Lown B, et al.: Influence of intracoronary platelet aggregation on ventricular electrical properties during partial coronary artery stenosis. Am J Cardiol 51:596, 1983.
68. Kramer JB, Saffitz JE, Witkowski FX, et al.: Intramural reentry as a mechanism of ventricular tachycardia during evolving canine myocardial infarction. Circ Res 56:736, 1985.
69. Kulbertus HE, Franck G (eds.): Neurocardiology. Mt. Kisco, Futura Publishing Co., 1988.
70. Lahiri A, Subramanian B, Millar-Craig M, et al.: Exercise-induced S-T segment elevation in variant angina. Am J Cardiol 45:887, 1980.
71. La Rovere MT, Specchia G, Mazzoleni C, et al.: Baroreflex sensitivity in post-myocardial infarction patients: Correlation with physical training and prognosis (Abstract). Circulation 74:II514, 1986.
72. Levy MN, Blattberg B: Effect of vagal stimulation on the overflow of norepinephrine into the coronary sinus during cardiac sympathetic nerve stimulation in the dog. Circ Res 38:81, 1976.
73. Loffelholz K, Muscholl E: A muscarinic inhibition of the noradrenaline release evoked by postganglionic sympathetic nerve stimulation. Naunyn-Schmiedebergs Arch Pharmacol 265:1, 1969.
74. Lombardi F, Verrier RL, Lown B: Relationship between sympathetic neural activity, coronary dynamics, and vulnerability to ventricular fibrillation during myocardial ischemia and reperfusion. Am Heart J 105:958, 1983.
75. Lown B, Verrier RL, Corbalan R: Psychologic stress and threshold for repetitive ventricular response. Science 182:834, 1973.
76. Lown B, Tykocinski M, Garfein A, et al.: Sleep and ventricular premature beats. Circulation 48:691, 1973.
77. Lown B, Temte JV, Reich P, et al.: Basis for recurring ventricular fibrillation in the absence of coronary heart disease and its management. N Engl J Med 294:623, 1976.
78. Lown B, Verrier RL: Neural activity and ventricular fibrillation. N Engl J Med 294:1165, 1976.
79. Lown B: Verbal conditioning of angina pectoris during exercise testing. Am J Cardiol 40:630, 1977.
80. Lubbe WF, Podzuweit T, Daries PS, et al.: The role of cyclic adenosine monophosphate in adrenergic effects on ventricular vulnerability to fibrillation in the isolated perfused rat heart. J Clin Invest 61:1260, 1978.
81. Luchi RJ, Chahine RA, Raizner AE: Coronary artery spasm. Ann Intern Med 91:441, 1979.
82. McLaughlin PR, Doherty PW, Martin RP, et al.: Myocardial imaging in a patient with reproducible variant angina. Am J Cardiol 39:126, 1977.
83. Mark AL, Abboud FM, Schmid PG, et al.: Differences in direct effects of adrenergic stimuli on coronary, cutaneous, and muscular vessels. J Clin Invest 51:279, 1972.
84. Martins JB, Zipes DP: Epicardial phenol interrupts refractory period responses to sympathetic but not vagal stimulation in canine left ventricular epicardium and endocardium. Circ Res 47:33, 1980.
85. Martins JB: Phenylephrine prolongs relative refractory period of Purkinje network in intact dog heart (Abstract). Circulation 74:II30, 1986.
86. Maseri A, Severi S, De Nes M, et al.: "Variant" angina: one aspect of a continuous spectrum of vasospastic myocardial ischemia. Pathogenetic mechanisms, estimated incidence and clinical and coronary arteriographic findings in 138 patients. Am J Cardiol 42:1019, 1978.
87. Maseri A, L'Abbate A, Baroldi G, et al.: Coronary vasospasm as a possible cause of myocardial infarction. A conclusion derived from the study of "preinfarction" angina. N Engl J Med 299:1271, 1978.
88. Maseri A, L'Abbate A, Chierchia S, et al.: Significance of spasm in the pathogenesis of ischemic heart disease. Am J Cardiol 44:788, 1979.
89. Master AM, Dack S, Horn H, et al.: Acute coronary insufficiency due to acute hemorrhage: An analysis of one hundred and three cases. Circulation 1:1302, 1950.
90. Masuda Y, Levy MN: Heart rate modulates the disposition of neurally released norepinephrine in cardiac tissues. Circ Res 57:19, 1985.
91. Matta RJ, Verrier RL, Lown B: Repetitive extrasystole as an index of vulnerability to ventricular fibrillation. Am J Physiol 230:1469, 1976.
92. Matta RJ, Lawler JE, Lown B: Ventricular electrical instability in the conscious dog. Effects of psychologic stress and beta adrenergic blockade. Am J Cardiol 38:594, 1976.
93. Michelson EL, Spear JF, Moore EN: Electrophysiologic and anatomic correlates of sustained ventricular tachyarrhythmias in a model of chronic myocardial infarction. Am J Cardiol 45:584, 1980.
94. Michelson EL: Recent advances in antiarrhythmic drug research: Studies in chronic canine myocardial infarction–ventricular tachyarrhythmia models. PACE 5:90, 1982.
95. Mohrman DE, Feigl EO: Competition between sympathetic vasoconstriction and metabolic vasodilation in the canine coronary circulation. Circ Res 42:79, 1978.
96. Monti JM, Folle LE, Peluffo C, et al.: The incidence of premature contractions in coronary patients during the sleep-awake cycle. Cardiology 60:257, 1975.
97. Mudge GH Jr., Grossman W, Mills RM Jr, et al.: Reflex increase in coronary vascular resistance in patients with ischemic heart disease. N Engl J Med 295:1333, 1976.
98. Mudge GH Jr., Goldberg S, Gunther S, et al.: Comparison of metabolic and vasoconstrictor stimuli on coronary vascular resistance in man. Circulation 59:544, 1979.
99. Mugelli A, Amerini S, DeBonfioli Cavalcabo P, et al.: Electrophysiological effects mediated by stimulation of cardiac beta$_2$-adrenoceptors with tulbuterol. Cardiovasc Drug Ther 1:101, 1987.
100. Myers A, Dewar HA: Circumstances attending 100 sudden deaths from coronary artery disease with coroners' necropsies. Br Heart J 37:1133, 1975.
101. Natelson BH: Neurocardiology. An interdisciplinary area for the 80s. Arch Neurol 42:178, 1985.
102. Nordrehaug JE, Johannessen K, von der Lippe G: Serum potassium concentration as a risk factor of ventricular arrhythmias early in acute myocardial infarction. Circulation 71:645, 1985.
103. Oliva PB, Potts DE, Pluss RG: Coronary arterial spasm in Prinzmetal angina: Documentation by coronary arteriography. N Engl J Med 288:745, 1973.
104. Oliva PB, Breckinridge JC: Arteriographic evidence of coronary arterial spasm in acute myocardial infarction. Circulation 56:366, 1977.
105. Opie LH, Muller CA, Lubbe WF: Cyclic A.M.P. and arrhythmias revisited. Lancet 2:921, 1978.
106. Opie LH: Basis for cardiovascular therapy with beta-blocking agents. Am J Cardiol 52:2D, 1983.
107. Orlick AE, Ricci DR, Alderman EL, et al.: Effects of alpha adrenergic blockade upon coronary hemodynamics. J Clin Invest 62:459, 1978.

108. Papageorgiou P, Hagestad EL, Verrier RL: Coronary distending pressure and delayed myocardial ischemia. Am Heart J, 116:59, 1988.
109. Papageorgiou P, Verrier RL, Hagestad EL: Interaction between neural and hemodynamic factors in delayed myocardial ischemia (Abstract). Fed Proc 46:641, 1987.
110. Patterson E, Holland K, Eller BT, et al.: Ventricular fibrillation resulting from ischemia at a site remote from previous myocardial infarction. A conscious canine model of sudden coronary death. Am J Cardiol 50:1414, 1982.
111. Pearle DL, Williford D, Gillis RA: Superiority of practolol versus propranolol in protection against ventricular fibrillation induced by coronary occlusion. Am J Cardiol 42:960, 1978.
112. Pickering TG, Goulding L, Cobern BA: Diurnal variations in ventricular ectopic beats and heart rate. Cardiovasc Med 2:1013, 1977.
113. Pickering TG, Johnston J, Honour AJ: Comparison of the effects of sleep, exercise and autonomic drugs on ventricular extrasystoles, using ambulatory monitoring of electrocardiogram and electroencephalogram. Am J Med 65:575, 1978.
114. Pitt B, Elliot EC, Gregg DE: Adrenergic receptor activity in the coronary arteries of the unanesthetized dog. Circ Res 21:75, 1967.
115. Raab W: Emotional and sensory stress factors in myocardial pathology. Am Heart J 72:538, 1966.
116. Rabinowitz SH, Verrier RL, Lown B: Muscarinic effects of vagosympathetic trunk stimulation on the repetitive extrasystole (RE) threshold. Circulation 53:622, 1976.
117. Raeder EA, Verrier RL, Lown B: Influence of the autonomic nervous system on coronary blood flow during partial stenosis. Am Heart J 104:249, 1982.
118. Raeder EA, Verrier RL, Lown B: Intrinsic sympathomimetic activity and the effects of beta-adrenergic blocking drugs on vulnerability to ventricular fibrillation. J Am Coll Cardiol 1:1442, 1983.
119. Raizner AE, Chahine RA, Ishimori T, et al.: Provocation of coronary artery spasm by the cold pressor test. Hemodynamic, arteriographic and quantitative angiographic observations. Circulation 62:925, 1980.
120. Ricci DR, Orlick AE, Cipriano PR, et al.: Altered adrenergic activity in coronary arterial spasm: Insight into mechanism based on study of coronary hemodynamics and the electrocardiogram. Am J Cardiol 43:1073, 1979.
121. Rosen MR, Gelband H, Hoffman BF: Effects of phentolamine on electrophysiologic properties of isolated canine Purkinje fibers. J Pharmacol Exp Ther 179:586, 1971.
122. Rosenblatt G, Hartmann E, Zwilling GR: Cardiac irritability during sleep and dreaming. J Psychosom Res 17:129, 1973.
123. Ross G: Adrenergic responses of the coronary vessels. Circ Res 39:461, 1976.
124. Saini V, Carr DB, Hagestad EL, et al.: Antifibrillatory mechanism of the narcotic agonist fentanyl. Am Heart J 115:598, 1988.
125. Sander GE, Giles TD, Kastin AJ, et al.: Cardiopulmonary pharmacology of enkephalins in the conscious dog. Peptides 2:403, 1981.
126. Schwartz CJ, Gerrity RG: Anatomical pathology of sudden unexpected cardiac death. Circulation 52:III18, 1975.
127. Schwartz GE, Weinberger DA, Singer JA: Cardiovascular differentiation of happiness, sadness, anger, and fear following imagery and exercise. Psychosom Med 43:343, 1981.
128. Schwartz JS, Carlyle PF, Cohn JN: Effect of coronary arterial pressure on coronary stenosis resistance. Circulation 61:70, 1980.
129. Schwartz PJ, Stone HL: Tonic influence of the sympathetic nervous system on myocardial reactive hyperemia and on coronary blood flow distribution in dogs. Circ Res 41:51, 1977.
130. Schwartz PJ, Vanoli E, Zaza A, et al.: The effect of antiarrhythmic drugs on life-threatening arrhythmias induced by the interaction between acute myocardial ischemia and sympathetic hyperactivity. Am Heart J 109:937, 1985.
131. Schwartz PJ, Stramba-Badiale M: Parasympathetic nervous system and malignant arrhythmias. In Kulbertus HE, Franck G (eds.): Neurocardiology, pp. 179–200. Mt. Kisco, Futura Publishing Co., 1988.
132. Sharma AD, Saffitz JE, Lee BI, et al.: Alpha-adrenergic-mediated accumulation of calcium in reperfused myocardium. J Clin Invest 72:802, 1983.
133. Sheehan FH, Epstein SE: Determinants of arrhythmic death due to coronary spasm: Effect of preexisting coronary artery stenosis on the incidence of reperfusion arrhythmia. Circulation 65:259, 1982.
134. Sheridan DJ, Penkoske PA, Sobel BE, et al.: Alpha adrenergic contributions to dysrhythmia during myocardial ischemia and reperfusion in cats. J Clin Invest 65:161, 1980.
135. Skinner JE, Mohr DN, Kellaway P: Sleep-stage regulation of ventricular arrhythmias in the unanesthetized pig. Circ Res 37:342, 1975.
136. Skinner JE, Reed JC: Blockade of frontocortical-brain stem pathway prevents ventricular fibrillation of ischemic heart. Am J Physiol 240:H156, 1981.
137. Skinner JE, Verrier RL: Task force report on sudden cardiac death and arrhythmias. In Smith OA, Galosy RA, Weiss SM (eds.): Circulation, Neurobiology, and Behavior, pp. 309–316. New York, Elsevier Science Publishing Co., 1982.
138. Skinner JE: Regulation of cardiac vulnerability by the cerebral defense system. J Am Coll Cardiol 5:88B, 1985.
139. Smith OA, DeVito JL: Central neural integration for the control of autonomic responses associated with emotion. Ann Rev Neurosci 7:43, 1984.
140. Smith R, Johnson L, Rothfeld D, et al.: Sleep and cardiac arrhythmias. Arch Intern Med 130:751, 1972.
141. Snyder F, Hobson JA, Goldfrank F: Blood pressure changes during human sleep. Science 142:1313, 1963.
142. Stewart JR, Burmeister WE, Burmeister J, et al.: Electrophysiologic and antiarrhythmic effects of phentolamine in experimental coronary artery occlusion and reperfusion in the dog. J Cardiovasc Pharmacol 2:77, 1980.
143. Vatner SF, Franklin D, Higgins CB, et al.: Coronary dynamics in unrestrained conscious baboons. Am J Physiol 221:1396, 1971.
144. Vatner SF, Higgins CB, Braunwald E: Effects of norepinephrine on coronary circulation and left ventricular dynamics in the conscious dog. Circ Res 34:812, 1974.
145. Verrier RL, Calvert A, Lown B, et al.: Effect of acute blood pressure elevation on the ventricular fibrillation threshold. Am J Physiol 226:893, 1974.
146. Verrier RL, Thompson P, Lown B: Ventricular vulnerability during sympathetic stimulation: Role of heart rate and blood pressure. Cardiovasc Res 8:602, 1974.
147. Verrier RL, Calvert A, Lown B: Effect of posterior hypothalamic stimulation on ventricular fibrillation threshold. Am J Physiol 228:923, 1975.
148. Verrier RL, Brooks WW, Lown B: Effect of cholinergic stimulation on vulnerability to ventricular fibrillation during myocardial ischemia and reperfusion (Abstract). Am J Cardiol 41:366, 1978.
149. Verrier RL, Lown B: Influence of neural activity on ventricular electrical stability during acute myocardial ischemia and infarction. In Sandøe E, Julian DG, Bell JW (eds.): Management of Ventricular Tachycardia: Role of Mexiletine, pp. 133–150. Amsterdam, Excerpta Medica (Internat. Congress Series No. 458), 1978.
150. Verrier RL, Lown B: Sympathetic-parasympathetic interactions and ventricular electrical stability. In Schwartz PJ, Brown AM, Malliani A, Zanchetti A (eds.): Neural Mechanisms in Cardiac Arrhythmias, pp. 75–85 New York, Raven Press, 1978.
151. Verrier RL: Neural factors and ventricular electrical instability. In Kulbertus HE, Wellens HJJ (eds.): Sudden Death, pp. 137–155. The Hague, Martinus Nijhoff, 1980.
152. Verrier RL, Raeder E, Lown B: Use of calcium channel blockers after myocardial infarction: Potential cardioprotective mechanisms. In Kulbertus HE, Wellens HJJ (eds.): The First Year After a Myocardial Infarction, pp. 341–352. Mt. Kisco, Futura Publishing Co., 1983.
153. Verrier RL, Lown B: Behavioral stress and cardiac arrhythmias. Annu Rev Physiol 46:155, 1984.
154. Verrier RL, Hagestad EL, Lown B: Delayed myocardial ischemia induced by anger. Circulation 75:249, 1987.
155. Verrier RL: Mechanisms of behaviorally induced arrhythmias. Circulation (Suppl I, Circulation Monograph #6) 76:I48, 1987.
156. Verrier RL, Hohnloser SH: How is the nervous system impli-

cated in the genesis of cardiac arrhythmias? *In* Hearse DJ, Manning AS, Janse MJ (eds.): Life-Threatening Arrhythmias During Ischemia and Infarction, pp. 153–168. New York, Raven Press, 1987.
157. Verrier RL, Kirby DA, Papageorgiou P: Plasma catecholamine and anger-induced delayed myocardial ischemia. Circulation 78:II555, 1988.
158. Watanabe AM, Besch HR Jr: Interaction between cyclic adenosine monophosphate and cyclic guanosine monophosphate in guinea pig ventricular myocardium. Circ Res 37:309, 1975.
159. Watanabe AM, Lindemann JP, Jones LR, et al.: Biochemical mechanisms mediating neural control of the heart. *In* Abboud FM, Fozzard HA, Gilmore JP, Reis DJ (eds.): Disturbances in Neurogenic Control of the Circulation, pp. 189–203. Bethesda, MD; American Physiological Society, 1981.
160. Webb SW, Adgey AAJ, Pantridge JF: Autonomic disturbance at onset of acute myocardial infarction. Br Med J 3:89, 1972.
161. Winkle RA, Lopes MG, Fitzgerald JW, et al.: Arrhythmias in patients with mitral valve prolapse. Circulation 52:73, 1975.
162. Wit AL, Josephson ME: Fractionated electrograms and continuous electrical activity: fact or artifact. *In* Zipes DP, Jalife J (eds.): Cardiac Electrophysiology and Arrhythmias, pp. 343–351. Orlando, FL; Grune & Stratton, 1985.
163. Yasue H: Beta-adrenergic blockade and coronary arterial spasm. *In* Sandøe E, Julian DG, Bell JW (eds.): Management of Ventricular Tachycardia—Role of Mexiletine, pp. 305–313. Amsterdam, Excerpta Medica, 1978.
164. Yasue H, Omote S, Takizawa A, Nagao M, et al.: Exertional angina pectoris caused by coronary arterial spasm: Effects of various drugs. Am J Cardiol 43:647, 1979.
165. Yoon MS, Han J, Tse WW, et al.: Effects of vagal stimulation, atropine, and propranolol on fibrillation threshold of normal and ischemic ventricles. Am Heart J 93:60, 1977.
166. Zipes DP, Barber MJ, Takahashi N, et al.: Recent observations on autonomic innervation of the heart. *In* Zipes DP, Jalife J (eds.): Cardiac Electrophysiology and Arrhythmias, pp. 181–189. Orlando, FL; Grune & Stratton, 1985.
167. Zuanetti G, De Ferrari GM, Priori SG, et al.: Protective effect of vagal stimulation on reperfusion arrhythmias in cats. Circ Res 61:429, 1987.

5

Evaluation of Arrhythmia Utilizing Noninvasive Techniques: Ambulatory Monitoring and Exercise Testing

Philip J. Podrid

Ambulatory monitoring and exercise testing are widely available tools for evaluating patients with and without cardiac disease. For patients with unexplained symptoms suggesting arrhythmia, such techniques are important for documenting the presence and nature of the rhythm disturbance. Increasing reliance is being placed on such techniques for evaluating patients with heart disease in an attempt to identify those at risk for experiencing a serious sustained ventricular tachyarrhythmia or sudden cardiac death. More important, these noninvasive methods have become an accepted approach to evaluate the effect of antiarrhythmic agents and to select an agent for long-term suppression of arrhythmia. This chapter will review the prevalence of arrhythmia in different patient populations, which has been documented with monitoring and exercise testing; the prognostic significance of ventricular arrhythmia in these different groups of patients; the usefulness of noninvasive methods for drug selection and their role for documenting aggravation of arrhythmia; the long-term results of patients managed noninvasively; and the strengths and weaknesses of this approach to drug selection.

Prevalence of Arrhythmia on Ambulatory Monitoring

The use of ambulatory monitoring has resulted in a better understanding of the prevalence of arrhythmia in different populations (Table 5–1) and has helped clarify its importance. Prior to the use of extended ambulatory monitoring, it had been reported that ventricular arrhythmia was rarely present in normal patients. In a study by Averill and Lamb,[1] ventricular arrhythmia was observed in only 0.8% of 67,375 normal subjects. Hiss and Lamb[2] reported the prevalence to be 0.6% in a study that involved 122,043 normal subjects. In the Tecumseh Study, Chiang and coworkers[3] reported a 5% prevalence. However, these studies were limited, since they utilized only ECG recordings that provide only 1 minute of information. Therefore, the apparent infrequent occurrence of ventricular arrhythmia in the normal population reflected an inadequate period of observation. Hinkle and coworkers[4] performed 6 hours of monitoring in 301 normal men and reported that 62% had ventricular

TABLE 5–1
Prevalence of Ventricular Arrhythmias in Different Populations

Population	Screening	Prevalence of VEA (%)
Normals	ECG	0.6–0.8
Normals	Monitoring	50–80
CAD	Monitoring	80–90
Post-MI	Monitoring	40–80
Congestive cardiomyopathy	Monitoring	80–90
Hypertrophic cardiomyopathy	Monitoring	40–50
MV prolapse	Monitoring	50–100
Sudden death survivors	Monitoring	100

VEA = ventricular ectopic activity; CAD = coronary artery disease; Post-MI = post–myocardial infarction; MV = mitral valve.

arrhythmia. In a study of 50 normal male medical students who underwent 24-hour monitoring, Brodsky and coworkers[5] reported that ventricular arrhythmia was present in 50%. In a follow-up study, 50 normal female medical students underwent 24-hour ambulatory monitoring, and the same prevalence of ventricular arrhythmia was observed.[6] Kostis et al.[7] reported that in a group of 100 patients with normal coronaries, as documented by cardiac catheterization, ventricular arrhythmia was present in 39%. In a report from the Framingham Heart Study,[8] 40% of 179 normal patients had ventricular premature beats (VPBs), whereas complex forms occurred in 12%. It is notable that among 61 patients with mitral valve prolapse, the prevalence of each form of ventricular arrhythmia was equivalent. As reported by Fleg and Kennedy,[9] ventricular arrhythmia was present in 80% of 98 elderly (ages 60–85), normal individuals. In this study, the absence of heart disease was confirmed by maximal exercise testing and thallium scanning. A similar prevalence of ventricular arrhythmia was reported by Glassen and colleagues[10] in a group of 13 patients between the ages of 60 and 84. Thus it appears that when extended ambulatory monitoring is used, 40 to 80% of patients will have documented VPBs. The prevalence of VPBs is directly related to age, and they are present in almost all patients over age 65.

While simple VPBs are common in the normal population, their density is usually low. In the study of Kostis et al.[7] only 4% of patients had more than 100 VPBs per 24 hours, while in the study of Brodsky and coworkers[5] only 2% of subjects had more than 50 VPBs per 24 hours. Sobotka and coworkers[6] observed more than 50 VPBs per 24 hours in 6% of normal subjects. Complex or repetitive arrhythmia is uncommon in normal subjects, being observed in approximately 2%.

The prevalence of VPBs is higher in patients who have underlying structural heart disease. In a study of 100 men with coronary artery disease, Ryan and coworkers[11] reported that 88% had VPBs, while 40% had repetitive forms. A similar prevalence was reported by Calvert and coworkers.[12] The prevalence of VPBs and repetitive forms is the same in patients with acute myocardial infarction.[13, 14]

Ventricular arrhythmia also is commonly present in patients with idiopathic dilated cardiomyopathy. Several studies have reported that the prevalence of frequent VPBs in this population is 70 to 95% while runs of nonsustained ventricular tachycardia occur in 50 to 80% of such patients.[15–19] Patients with hypertrophic cardiomyopathy also have a high prevalence of VPBs. Savage and colleagues[20] reported that 50% of 100 patients had multiform or repetitive VPBs, whereas 19% had runs of nonsustained VT. McKenna and coworkers[21] reported that 43% of patients with hypertrophic cardiomyopathy had multiform or repetitive VPBs and that 26% had runs of nonsustained VT. It may be concluded that in patients with underlying heart disease, frequent VPBs are commonly documented when 24-hour monitoring is used and that 20 to 30% will also have runs of nonsustained VT.

Patients who have been resuscitated from out-of-hospital sudden cardiac death represent a special subset of those with heart disease. The prevalence of VPBs in such patients has been reported by some authors to be 100%, and repetitive forms and runs of VT have been found in 75 to 80% of such patients.[22] In contrast, other authors have reported a much lower prevalence of ventricular arrhythmia.[23] The disparity may be related to a difference in referral patterns.

One of the important problems in establishing the prevalence of ventricular arrhythmia in patients with and without heart disease is related to the hourly and daily spontaneous variability of VPBs. Winkle[24] reported that there was marked variability in the hourly frequency of all forms of VPBs in patients referred for management of arrhythmia. In this study, half-hour periods were analyzed and it was observed that in many patients the spontaneous changes in VPB frequency mimicked drug efficacy or arrhythmia aggravation. In a recent study, Raeder and coworkers[25] reported a circadian rhythm of VPB frequency during a 24-hour period (Fig. 5–1). The density of VPBs was greatest in the early morning, decreased during the day, and reached the lowest level during the sleeping hours. Morganroth and colleagues[26] reported a significant variability in the daily presence and frequency of VPBs in a group of patients with heart disease who had never experienced sustained ventricular tachyarrhythmia. While the variability was great, the changes in VPB density were indirectly related to the hourly

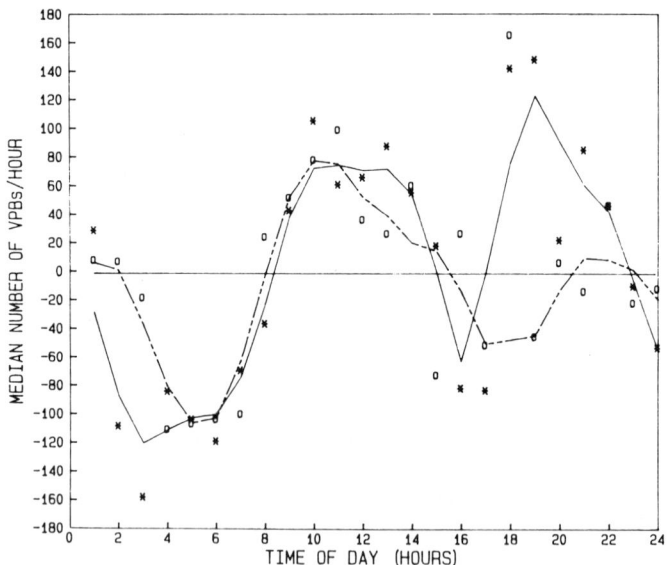

FIGURE 5–1
Diurnal variation of ventricular ectopic activity in a study of 48-hour ambulatory monitoring was performed on 92 patients. The frequency of ventricular premature beats (VPBs) was reproducibly present each day. However, the hourly frequency of VPBs showed wide spontaneous changes, demonstrating circadian variability. The frequency of VPBs decreased, reaching the lowest density at 4 to 6 A.M. Thereafter, the frequency increased, peaking mid-morning followed by a gradual decrease. * = median number of VPBs/hour on day 1; O = median number of VPBs/hour on day 2.

frequency of arrhythmia. Thus, in patients with a high density of VPBs (>300 VPBs/hour) variability was less marked and the daily hourly frequency was more reproducible. These authors reported the same relationship when repetitive forms were analyzed.[27] Pratt et al.[28] performed ambulatory monitoring in 27 patients who were entered in a drug study. After an average of 12 months, drug treatment was discontinued; then, after an appropriate washout period, ambulatory monitoring was repeated. In over one third of patients there was a significant reduction or elimination of all forms of arrhythmia, suggesting that there is often a marked change in the occurrence of arrhythmia, not only during brief periods of observation but after a prolonged period. When the second placebo period was compared to the first, there was a 50% decrease in VPBs, a 65% reduction in couplets, and an 83% decrease in runs of VT. In the studies by Raeder et al.[25] and Hohnloser and coworkers[29] involving 92 patients with a history of serious ventricular tachyarrhythmia who underwent two 24-hour periods of ambulatory monitoring, there was a high degree of reproducibility in the daily frequency of VPBs (R = 0.84), couplets (R = 0.81), runs of VT (R = 0.80), and number of VT beats (R = 0.76). Therefore, random changes in VPB density are less marked among patients who have experienced a sustained ventricular tachyarrhythmia. We[30] reported that the frequency of all forms of VPBs was highly reproducible in a group of 100 patients with serious arrhythmia who underwent 2 days of ambulatory monitoring.

Atrial arrhythmias are also commonly observed during ambulatory monitoring, although their frequency is more variable than that of ventricular arrhythmia. It is therefore difficult to establish their prevalence. Hinkle and colleagues[4] reported that 76% of normal subjects had a variety of supraventricular arrhythmias. In the study by Brodsky and coworkers,[5] 56% of normal male medical students had atrial premature beats although, as with VPBs, they were infrequent in most. In the study of normal women, Sobotka and coworkers[6] reported infrequent atrial premature beats in 64% of subjects. In the Framingham study,[8] atrial arrhythmia was observed in 17% of normal subjects who underwent 24-hour ambulatory monitoring, whereas 25% of those with mitral valve prolapse had such arrhythmia. As with VPBs, the prevalence of atrial arrhythmia increases with age. For example, in the Framingham study[31] the 22-year incidence of atrial fibrillation was 2.6/1000 patients in those subjects 25 to 34 years of age; in those between 35 and 44 years of age, the incidence was 19.7/1000. The incidence in patients 45 to 54 and 55 to 64 years of age was 26/1000 and 32/1000, respectively.

Additionally, the prevalence of atrial arrhythmia, including supraventricular tachyarrhythmias, is related to the presence of heart disease, especially when accompanied by atrial enlargement, as is the case with valvular heart disease or congestive heart failure. In a study of patients with hypertrophic cardiomyopathy, McKenna and coworkers[21] reported that 46% of patients had supraventricular tachycardia or atrial fibrillation on 24-hour ambulatory monitoring. However, the actual prevalence in patients with this or other conditions is uncertain, largely because of the highly random nature of this arrhythmia which is often brief and without symptoms and is infrequently reported in monitoring.

Relationship Between Arrhythmia Exposed on Ambulatory Monitoring and the Risk of Sudden Cardiac Death

Although ambulatory monitoring is a useful method for demonstrating ventricular arrhythmia, it remains uncertain which arrhythmia places the patient at risk for sudden death. It is now well established that the mechanism for sudden cardiac death is ventricular fibrillation. In several studies involving a total of 61 patients who experienced sudden cardiac arrest while undergoing ambulatory monitoring,[32-36] the most frequent mechanism was VT or ventricular fibrillation (VF). In 57 (89%) of these patients, the mechanism was VT/VF; a bradyarrhythmia was the mechanism in the other four patients (11%). In each patient there was a significant increase in VPBs and complex forms documented minutes to hours prior to the terminal event. Observations in the coronary care unit have also documented these same findings. The myocardium is rendered unstable as a result of some underlying cardiac disease. In rare cases, there is primary electrical instability that is not associated with any structural cardiac abnormality. Although there is no clinically useful measure of this underlying myocardial instability, it has been proposed that the presence of certain types of premature beats are indirect markers for this abnormality.

A number of studies have reported an association between the presence of VPBs and the risk of sudden cardiac death in patients with underlying coronary heart disease. Chiang and coworkers[3,38] reported on 5129 patients without symptoms or other evidence of heart disease and found that VPBs was present in 264 individuals (5.1%) during a routine recording. The prevalence of VPBs increased with age and was correlated with the subsequent documentation of heart disease. Thus, in individuals over age 30, 158/1000 with VPBs had coronary artery disease, whereas this diagnosis was established in only 50/1000 persons without VPBs. The incidence of sudden cardiac death was 61/1000 in subjects with VPBs and 10/1000 in those without VPBs (p <0.01).

A similar relationship between VPBs and sudden death was reported by Rodstein et al.[39] in a study involving 712 persons. Rabkin and coworkers[40] from the Manitoba study reported on 401 subjects who had VPBs but who were free of heart disease. After a follow-up of 10.8 years, 13.5% developed coronary heart disease, and among the clinical problems caused by coronary disease, sudden death had the strongest association with VPBs. In the study of Hinkle and colleagues[4, 41] involving 301 men monitored for 6 hours, 76% had supraventricular arrhythmia and 62% had ventricular arrhythmias. These authors reported that ventricular ectopy was significantly associated with the presence of coronary heart disease and the occurrence of sudden cardiac death.

The relationship between VPBs, the development of heart disease, and the occurrence of sudden death in an asymptomatic population is still uncertain. However, the association between ventricular arrhythmia and sudden death is better established in those with a recent myocardial infarction (MI) (Table 5–2). Among 2035 survivors of an acute myocardial infarction, 235 (11.5%) had VPBs on a resting electrocardiogram.[42] After a 3-year follow-up, sudden death occurred in 21.7% of those with VPBs and in 11.4% of those without VPBs. Kotler and coworker[43] utilized 12-hour ambulatory monitoring in 160 survivors of an acute MI and documented VPBs in 80%. After a follow-up period of 30 to 54 months, 13.8% of patients with frequent or repetitive VPBs died suddenly. In contrast, sudden death occurred in only 3% of those with absent or infrequent VPBs. Vismara and coworkers[44] performed 10-hour ambulatory monitoring in 64 patients 11 days after an acute MI. Complex or repetitive VPBs were present in 27 patients, 22 had single VPBs, and 15 patients had no VPBs. During a 26-month follow-up of these three groups, the incidence of sudden death was 30%, 18%, and 0%, respectively. In this study, the occurrence of VT or VF in the immediate post-MI period was not associated with sudden death or other arrhythmia during the recovery period.

In a large study involving 1734 men with a recent MI, Ruberman et al.[45] performed 1-hour sedentary monitoring. After an average follow-up of 24 months, the presence of complex or repetitive arrhythmia enhanced the risk of sudden death threefold, whereas any other VPB, regardless of frequency, was not associated with an enhanced risk. In this study, the 3-year sudden death mortality was 15.5% in those with complex arrhythmia, compared to 4.2% in those with other VPBs and 4.3% in those without arrhythmias.

Although each of these studies confirms that complex or repetitive arrhythmia is associated with an increased risk of sudden death, the most definitive studies are those in which 24-hour ambulatory monitoring was used. In such studies, the presence and frequency of arrhythmia is better defined and patients are grouped more accurately. Rappaport and Remedios[46] performed 24-hour ambulatory monitoring in 139 men within 3 weeks of an acute MI (Fig. 5–2). After an 11-month follow-up, the presence of VT on the monitor was associated with a sudden death mortality of 34%; in contrast, mortality was 6% in patients without VT. Bigger and coworkers[47] reported results from the multicenter post-infarction research study in which 820 patients underwent 24-hour monitoring 11 days after an acute MI. Nonsustained VT was present in 92 patients, and survival in this group after 3 years was 67%. In contrast, survival was 85% among the 728 patients without VT on monitoring (p <0.001). These authors concluded that runs of nonsustained VT documented on ambulatory monitoring were an independent risk factor for sudden death, increasing the risk of dying twofold. Similar results were reported by Mukharji and coworkers,[48] based on the MiLis study of 867 patients. The presence of nonsustained VT had a strong relationship to subsequent sudden cardiac death.

In the studies discussed above, the presence of nonsustained VT recorded on 24-hour ambulatory monitoring performed in the immediate post-MI period was an independent risk factor for subsequent sudden death. However, several other studies reported that left ventricular function was also an important independent factor. The first report of this relationship was that of Schulze and coworkers.[49] In this study, ambulatory monitoring was performed in 81 patients within 3 weeks of an acute MI. Additionally, a radionuclide ventriculogram was obtained, and patients were subdivided into those with a left ventricular ejection fraction (LVEF) of ≥ 40% or <40%. After a 9-month follow-up, eight patients died, and each had complex repetitive ventricular arrhythmia and LVEF ≤40%. There was no death in any other subgroup. In the study of Ruberman and colleagues[45, 50] the presence of congestive heart failure (CHF), which was based on clinical grounds, was an independent predictor of sudden death. Thus, in those patients without CHF or complex arrhythmia, the incidence of sudden death was 3%. In contrast, the presence of complex arrhythmia increased the rate of sudden death to 7%. The incidence of sudden death was 12% in patients with

TABLE 5–2
Ventricular Arrhythmia after Myocardial Infarction

Study	No. of Patients	Duration of Monitoring (hours)	Follow-up (months)	Sudden Death (%)	
				No Complex VEA*	Complex VEA*
Bigger	820	24	12	12 (6, 22)	36 (12, 35)
Kotler	160	6	36	20	60
Moss	978	6	36	4	15
Mukharji	388	24	14	3 (2, 7)	16 (7, 25)
Rappaport	139	24	12	6	34
Ruberman	1739	1	42	8 (3, 7)	25 (12, 22)
Vismara	64	10	26	11	30
Schultz	81	24	7	0 (0, 0)	28 (0, 28)

*Numbers in parentheses refer to breakdown of percentage with LV intact function, LV dysfunction, respectively.
VEA = ventricular ectopic activity; LV = left ventricular.

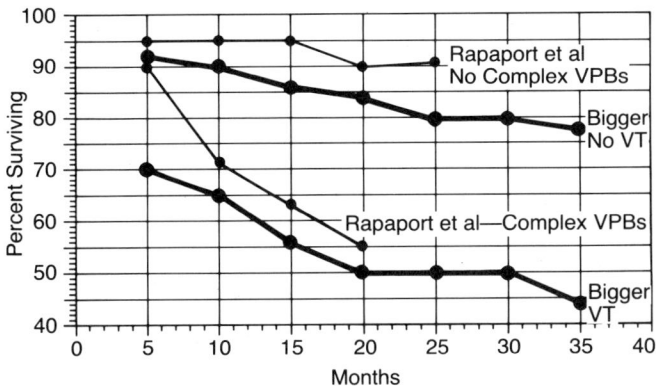

FIGURE 5–2
Role of complex ventricular premature beats (VPBs) or ventricular tachycardia (VT) in patients post–myocardial infarction. In two studies, Rappaport et al. and Bigger utilized 24-hour ambulatory monitoring for establishing the presence of ventricular arrhythmia. In both studies, the presence of complex arrhythmia enhanced the risk of sudden death after myocardial infarction.

CHF but with no complex arrhythmia. The incidence of sudden death was highest (22%) in those patients who had both CHF and complex arrhythmia. Similar results were reported by the MiLis group.[48] In patients with LVEF >40%, the incidence of sudden death after 1 year was 2% when no repetitive arrhythmia was present, but it was 7% when such arrhythmia was documented on 24-hour ambulatory monitoring. In contrast, the incidence of sudden death in patients with LVEF <40% was 7% when repetitive forms are absent, and 25% when repetitive forms were documented on monitoring.

In the report of Bigger et al.[47, 51] on the multicenter post-infarction trial, patients with LVEF <30% were compared to those with LVEF >30%. The 3-year sudden death mortality in those with LVEF >30% was 6% in the absence of nonsustained VT, and 12% with nonsustained VT. Among those with LVEF <30%, the sudden death mortality was 22% and 35%, respectively ($p < 0.001$).

In addition to the association between arrhythmia, LV function, and sudden death, other factors of importance that can be obtained from 24-hour ambulatory monitoring are heart rate, and hourly changes in heart rate (Table 5–3). In the multicenter postinfarction trial, Kleiger and coworkers[52] examined changes in R-R intervals (or heart rate) observed during the 24-hour period of ambulatory monitoring; patients were subdivided based on heart rate variability. When the standard deviation of R-R interval changes was >100 ms, during the day the sudden death mortality after 3 years was 10%. When the change in R-R intervals averaged 50 to 100 ms, the incidence of sudden death was 16%, and among patients with <50 ms difference of R-R intervals, the sudden death rate was 40%. When the presence of ventricular arrhythmia was also considered, the changes in standard deviation of R-R intervals continued to be an independent risk factor. Thus, the presence of runs of VT increased the mortality to 15%, 21%, and 50%, respectively, in those with changes in standard deviation of R-R interval of >100 ms, 50–100 ms and <50 ms, compared to 7%, 11%, and 26% when VT was absent.

The association between ventricular arrhythmia documented on ambulatory monitoring and the risk of sudden death has also been reported for patients with a congestive cardiomyopathy (Table 5–4). In a study by Follansbee et al.,[53] 9 of 19 patients with cardiomyopathy and CHF died suddenly. The occurrence of nonsustained VT was of prognostic significance, whereas no other arrhythmia regardless of frequency was important. Meineitz and coworkers[54] reported on 74 patients with idiopathic dilated cardiomyopathy, of whom 49% had runs of nonsustained VT on ambulatory monitoring. In this study there was no correlation between the type and frequency of ventricular arrhythmia and the degree of left ventricular impairment. However, patients who died suddenly had a significantly greater density of arrhythmia, and demonstrated runs of VT, compared to those who survived or to those dying of CHF in whom VT was absent ($p < 0.01$). Holmes and colleagues[55] reported that complex arrhythmia, particularly runs of nonsustained VT, represented an independent risk factor for sudden death. In their group of 31 patients, 9 had simple VPBs and 22 had repetitive forms. Hemodynamic parameters were comparable in these two groups. However, after a 25-month follow-up, 13 of 22 patients (59%) with repetitive arrhythmia died suddenly; in contrast, only 1 of 9 patients (11%) with simple VPBs died ($p < 0.025$). Chakko and Gheorghiade[18] studied 43 patients with dilated cardiomyopathy, of whom 20 received empiric antiarrhythmic therapy. During a 16-month follow-up there were 10 sudden deaths (23%) and, as in other studies, nonsustained VT was an independent risk factor. In a study of 69 patients with dilated cardiomyopathy, Unverferth and coworkers[56] reported that 24 patients (35%) died suddenly after 1 year. Univariate and multivariate analyses of prognostic factors for sudden death indicated that ventricular arrhythmia was an independent predictor ($p < 0.007$), as was the presence of a left ventricular conduction delay and elevated right atrial pressure.

In contrast to these studies, there have been others in which complex or repetitive ventricular arrhythmia were not associated with sudden death in patients with dilated cardiomyopathy. Von Olshausen et al.[17] obtained 24-hour ambulatory monitoring in 90 patients but found that the documentation of ventricular arrhythmia was of little help in identifying the patient at

TABLE 5–3
Mortality Related to Changes of Standard Deviation of R-R Interval (ms)

	Percent Mortality of		
	<50	50–100	>100
Runs of VT on monitor	50	21	15
No VT present	26	11	7
EF ≥40%	17	9	7
EF = 30–40%	39	20	13
EF ≤30%	49	26	22

VT = ventricular tachycardia; EF = ejection fraction.

TABLE 5-4
Relationship Between Ventricular Arrhythmia and Survival in Patients with Congestive Heart Failure

Study	No. of Patients	Follow-up (months)	Relationship to SCD
Huang	35	34	No
Wilson	77	12	No
Meineitz	74	11	Yes
Von Olshausen	60	12	No
Holmes	43	14	Yes
Chakko	43	16	Yes
Unverferth	61	12	Yes
Costanzo-Nordin	55	16	No
Follansbee	19	19	Yes

SCD = sudden cardiac death.

risk for sudden death. In a study by Huang and coworkers[57] that involved 35 patients with dilated cardiomyopathy, the presence of runs of VT was not associated with clinical or hemodynamic parameters nor was any ventricular arrhythmia predictive of outcome. Wilson and colleagues[15] reported on 77 patients with congestive cardiomyopathy in whom the average annual mortality was 20%. Neither total cardiac mortality nor sudden death was related to the presence of any type of ventricular arrhythmia. The only variable of prognostic significance was the functional class reflecting LV function. A study by Costanzo-Nordin[58] involving 55 patients failed to document any relationship between runs of VT and prognosis. As in other studies, the occurrence of VT was not associated with hemodynamic measurements or the severity of left ventricular dysfunction.

Patients with hypertrophic cardiomyopathy are another group in whom the risk of sudden death is high, and several reports have documented the prognostic importance of ventricular arrhythmia exposed on ambulatory monitoring studies. In the study by Savage and coworkers,[20] 100 patients with hypertrophic cardiomyopathy underwent 24-hour ambulatory monitoring. Within a 4-month period, two patients had sudden cardiac death, and both had had runs of VT on monitoring. The authors concluded that monitoring was of use for identifying the patient with hypertrophic cardiomyopathy who is at increased risk for a serious ventricular tachyarrhythmia. McKenna and colleagues[21] also observed that ambulatory monitoring was useful for exposing potentially serious ventricular arrhythmia in patients with hypertrophic cardiomyopathy. As in studies of patients with idiopathic congestive cardiomyopathy, the presence of VT was not related to hemodynamic measurements. Maron and coworkers[59] obtained 24-hour monitoring in 99 patients with hypertrophic cardiomyopathy. The presence of runs of VT on monitoring was associated with an 8.6% annual mortality, whereas the mortality was 1% per year in patients who did not have VT but who had any other type of ventricular arrhythmia (p <0.02).

In conclusion, the role of ambulatory monitoring for identifying the patient at an increased risk of sudden cardiac death appears to be related to the nature of the underlying heart disease. In normal subjects, ventricular arrhythmia, regardless of type, is not associated with an increased risk. In patients with chronic coronary artery disease, the presence of any type of ventricular arrhythmia increases the risk twofold, whereas in those with a recent MI, the presence of runs of nonsustained VT enhances the risk of sudden death two- to fivefold. Other variables of independent importance are left ventricular function and heart rate. While these factors may help identify a patient who is at higher risk, it must be remembered that the majority of patients with such findings survive. While ambulatory monitoring helps to identify a high-risk patient, there are other factors, as yet undefined, that may be important for subsetting even further such high-risk patients. In patients with hypertrophic cardiomyopathy, ambulatory monitoring is helpful in predicting outcome and identifying patients at high risk. As with post-MI patients, runs of VT are of prognostic significance. However, the role of ambulatory monitoring in those with dilated cardiomyopathy remains controversial. All forms of ventricular arrhythmia, including runs of VT, are common in this group of patients, and cardiac mortality is high. A substantial number of these patients die suddenly; however, the association between sudden death and the presence of nonsustained VT in ambulatory monitoring remains unclear, as studies are contradictory.

Role of Exercise Testing for Exposing Arrhythmias

Although extended ambulatory monitoring is the technique most often utilized to document rhythm disorders, exercise testing is another useful tool for inducing arrhythmias that may be transient and can elude detection even with prolonged periods of ambulatory monitoring. It has been reported that in more than 10% of patients with a history of serious arrhythmia, ambulatory monitoring for up to 48 hours failed to expose any significant arrhythmia, while potentially serious arrhythmia was exposed with exercise testing.[60] It may be concluded that exercise testing is a useful adjunctive method for exposing arrhythmia and is complementary to ambulatory monitoring.

Three theoretic mechanisms have been proposed to explain the occurrence of arrhythmia: (1) enhanced automaticity; (2) triggered automaticity; and (3) reentry.[61] Enhanced automaticity results from an increase in the rate of spontaneous depolarization of the myocardial tissue. This may be a normal physiologic increase in firing rate, such as during exercise when sinus node discharge rate is enhanced and heart rate increased, or it may occur in abnormal or diseased tissue, resulting in the augmentation of ectopic foci causing abnormal rhythm disturbances. Triggered automaticity, due to delayed afterpotentials, is caused by the continued influx of calcium ions at the conclusion of action potential repolarization. This ionic flux causes subthreshold oscillations of the membrane potential. If these "triggered" oscillations are of sufficient amplitude, a spontaneous action potential may be generated, causing a nonsustained or sustained arrhythmia. The last mechanism is reentry, resulting from a continuous circus movement of electrical activity around a physiologic circuit. This reentrant circuit is formed by tissues that are proximally and distally joined but that have different electrophysiologic characteristics, especially different conduction and refractory properties.

Regardless of the actual mechanism responsible for clinical arrhythmia, exercise testing results in a number of important physiologic changes that can affect any of these mechanisms and trigger arrhythmia. These changes include alterations in serum electrolytes, pH, sympathetic tone, circulating catecholamines, and the degree of ischemia, which may be responsible for activating one of these mechanisms, thus causing arrhythmia. Since arrhythmia potentially can be triggered by a variety of diverse factors, it is important to utilize a number of approaches for the evaluation of arrhythmia and particularly to establish the effect of antiarrhythmic drugs. One such important technique is exercise testing, which produces a number of important physiologic changes that can affect the myocardium and serve to initiate arrhythmia.

Exercise results in a reduction of vagal tone, a marked augmentation of sympathetic neural inputs to the heart, and an increase in circulating catecholamines (Fig. 5–3).[62] Catecholamines and the sympathetic nervous system enhance automaticity by increasing the slope or rate of rise of phase 4 spontaneous depolarization. As the slope of phase 4 increases, the time to reach the membrane threshold potential is shortened and the firing rate of the tissue is augmented. When normal pacemaker tissue is involved, this produces sinus tachycardia. However, if abnormal or ectopic atrial or ventricular foci become activated and fire at a faster rate, arrhythmias may develop. Enhanced sympathetic activity and catecholamines will also augment the flux of calcium ions into the myocardial cell, increasing the amplitude of delayed afterpotentials. If the amplitude of these afterpotentials is sufficient to reach threshold potential, an arrhythmia can be generated. An increase of sympathetic tone and circulating catecholamines will enhance conduction velocity and shorten the refractory period of atrial and ventricular tissue. Such changes, especially when superimposed upon underlying inhomogeneity, which is present when the myocardium has been damaged by some disease state, may predispose to arrhythmia. Additional changes in pH, O_2 and electrolytes that occur during exercise may further alter these properties. Finally, exercise testing increases the heart rate, blood pressure (or afterload), and myocardial inotropy, all of which increase the oxygen demands of the myocardium. In the presence of coronary artery disease, this may cause ischemia and often myocardial dysfunction, leading to increased wall stretch and tension, which are additional triggers for arrhythmia.

Incidence of Arrhythmias During Exercise (Table 5–5)

Although ventricular and supraventricular arrhythmias commonly occur during exercise testing, the documentation of ectopic activity requires continuous monitoring of rhythm.[63] Furthermore, the prevalence of different types of arrhythmias is related to the type and extent of heart disease.

Supraventricular arrhythmia is commonly provoked by exercise, but the actual frequency is uncertain since such arrhythmias have only infrequently been evaluated or documented. Similar to ambulatory monitoring, supraventricular premature beats are the most commonly observed type of supraventricular arrhythmia. In a study of 248 normal subjects who underwent 1385 two-step exercise tests, Beard and Owen[64] reported that supraventricular premature beats occurred in 34 tests (3.5%). Masters[65] reported that atrial premature beats were induced in 4.8% of 600 patients undergoing exercise. Although the prevalence of atrial premature beats is low, these studies did not employ

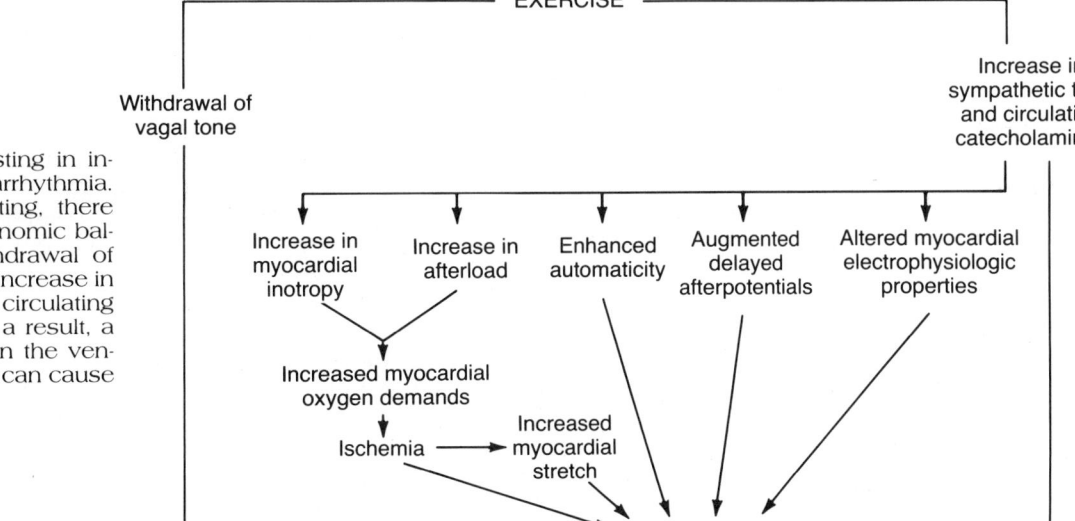

FIGURE 5–3
Role of exercise testing in inducing ventricular arrhythmia. During exercise testing, there are changes in autonomic balance—primarily withdrawal of vagal inputs and an increase in sympathetic tone and circulating catecholamines. As a result, a number of effects on the ventricular myocardium can cause arrhythmia.

TABLE 5-5
Prevalence of Arrhythmia During Exercise Testing

Study	No. of Tests	% Arrhythmia				
		APBs	SVT	AF	VPBs*	Complex VBPs*
Beard	1385	2.5	0.1	—	8.0	0.3
Master	600	4.8	—	0.3	18.3	0.3
Jelenik	1000	17.7	2.2	1.1	5.0	—
McHenry	650	10.0	—	—	50.0	22.0
Whinnery	60	27.0	—	—	50.0	15.0
Gooch	713	—	2.8	0.3	—	—
Graboys	300	—	0.8	0.1	—	—
Poblete	120	—	—	—	62.0	31.0
Ryan	100	—	—	—	55.0	20.0

*In patients with heart disease.
APBs = atrial premature beats; SVT = sustained ventricular tachycardia; AF = atrial fibrillation; VPBs = ventricular premature beats.

continuous ECG recording. In a study by Jelinek and Lown,[66] 625 patients underwent 1000 exercise tests during which the ECG was continuously recorded; supraventricular premature beats occurred in 177 patients (17.7%). McHenry and coworkers[67] reported that the prevalence of supraventricular arrhythmia was related to age; in their study, 6% of those 25 to 34 years of age had supraventricular arrhythmia, whereas arrhythmia occurred in 14% of those 45 to 54 years of age. An association with age was also reported by Whinnery,[68] who reported an incidence of supraventricular arrhythmia of 10%, 40%, and 31%, respectively, in patients without heart disease, those with cardiac problems, and those with other medical problems.

While atrial premature beats are common, a sustained supraventricular arrhythmia is infrequently induced by exercise testing, although the incidence also seems to depend upon the population under evaluation. Beard and Owen[64] observed only two cases of sustained arrhythmia in 1385 tests; Masters[65] reported that only two of 600 patients had atrial fibrillation. McHenry and coworkers[67] reported a 2.2% incidence of sustained supraventricular arrhythmia, similar to the studies of Gooch and McConnell[69] and Jelinek and Lown.[66] In a report by Graboys and Wright,[70] who reviewed 3000 patients, sustained supraventricular tachyarrhythmia was induced in 29 (1%). However, these 29 patients represented 14% of the 207 patients referred for management of atrial arrhythmia.

In conclusion, supraventricular premature beats are provoked by exercise in approximately 4 to 5% of healthy persons, and they are induced more frequently in those with heart disease. Sustained supraventricular tachyarrhythmias are less commonly observed during exercise.

As with atrial arrhythmia, the prevalence of ventricular arrhythmias exposed during exercise depends on the method for monitoring and the patient population studied. When intermittent recordings are obtained, VPBs are observed in 44% of tests; with continuous recordings, they are present in 62% of tests. More important, continuous monitoring increases the exposure of repetitive arrhythmia sixfold.[63] Using intermittent recording, Beard and Owen[64] observed VPBs in 18.3% of patients. Whinnery[68] reported VPBs in 5% of healthy patients, whereas VPBs were observed in 50% of those with heart disease. When continuous monitoring is used, VPBs are present in 3.4% of normal individuals and in up to 55% of patients with heart disease.[66,67]

The occurrence of repetitive forms (couplets or runs of VT) during exercise testing is also dependent on the population of patients studied. In normal men, Beard and Owen,[64] Whinnery,[68] and Poblete et al.[71] did not observe any repetitive arrhythmias; however, with continuous recording, McHenry and coworkers[67] reported that these forms were induced in 6% of normal subjects, but that repetitive forms occurred in 15 to 31% of those with heart disease.

Patients with a history of a sustained ventricular tachyarrhythmia often have a high density of arrhythmia exposed during exercise testing. VPBs are induced in all such patients, and approximately 75% will have repetitive forms.[62,63] The frequency of inducing sustained VT or VF is unknown. It is rare to see such arrhythmia induced in normal subjects or in those with heart disease who have no history of a sustained tachyarrhythmia, although the prevalence has not been reported. The provocation of sustained VT or VF in those with a history of such arrhythmia is more common, but the prevalence is not well established.

In conclusion, VPBs are commonly provoked during exercise testing, and the prevalence is related to the presence of heart disease. They occur in 20 to 30% of normal subjects, and repetitive forms are provoked in 4 to 5%. VPBs are present in 60 to 70% of patients with heart disease, and repetitive forms are observed in 20%. All patients with a history of a sustained ventricular tachyarrhythmia have VPBs with exercise, and 75% have repetitive forms.

Significance of Exercise-Induced Ventricular Arrhythmias

While the prognostic importance of VPBs, particularly repetitive forms, documented in ambulatory monitoring has been well established, the meaning of ventricular arrhythmia induced by an exercise test remains unclear. As indicated, all forms of arrhythmia occur frequently during exercise. Repetitive forms, uncommonly induced in normal individuals, occur more commonly in patients with heart disease, but their prognostic significance is uncertain. Weld and coworkers[72] reported a threefold increase in mortality among post-MI patients who had exercise-induced VPBs, compared to those patients without VPBs (12% vs. 4%). Although some studies reported that ventricular arrhythmia provoked by exercise is associated with an increased mortality, other parameters, such as exercise duration and ST-segment shifts, also are important, and it is unclear if arrhythmia is an independent factor.

The prognostic importance of exercise-induced ventricular arrhythmia in patients with coronary artery disease who have not had a recent MI is also unclear. In a study by Udall and Ellestad,[73] patients with coronary artery disease who had VPBs during exercise had an increased risk of sudden death, especially when significant ST-segment depression was also present. Califf and coworkers[74] reported on 1293 patients with coronary artery disease who underwent exercise testing within 6 weeks of cardiac catheterization. After a 3-year follow-up, the mortality in the group of patients without VPBs during exercise testing was 10%, compared to a 17% mortality in those with repetitive arrhythmias. In the same study, these workers reported no mortality after a 3-year follow-up among 620 patients without coronary artery disease who had any type of VPBs, including repetitive forms.

Safety of Exercise Testing in Patients with Ventricular Arrhythmia

Several studies have reported the safety of exercise testing in patients with coronary artery disease, but safety data in those presenting with a history of serious ventricular tachyarrhythmias are sparse. Irving and Bruce[75] surveyed more than 10,000 exercise tests carried out in over 50 centers adhering to the same protocol; Only five patients experienced VF (0.47%). In a survey of 50,000 bicycle ergometries, Atterhog and coworkers[76] reported only two major complications resulting in death (0.024%). However, neither study reported the risk of inducing other serious ventricular tachyarrhythmias, nor did they specify the risk of a major complication in those with a history of serious arrhythmia. Young and colleagues[77] reviewed 1377 exercise tests in 263 patients with a history of VT or VF. A sustained ventricular tachyarrhythmia necessitating an intervention occurred in 24 patients (9.1%) and involved 31 tests (2.3%). This included sustained VT in 22 tests and VF in 9. Additionally, a cardiac arrest due to severe bradycardia occurred in one patient. There was no association between any clinical parameter and the risk of experiencing a serious arrhythmia during exercise testing. Interestingly, the majority of these arrhythmic complications occurred during antiarrhythmic drug therapy rather than during baseline control studies. In contrast, it was observed that among a general population of 3444 patients with coronary artery disease who did not have a history of a serious arrhythmia, there were only four patients who had VT or VF (0.12%) during 8221 tests (0.051), an incidence similar to that reported by others.

Use of Noninvasive Techniques as a Guide to Antiarrhythmic Drug Therapy

Ambulatory monitoring and exercise testing serve an important role, not only for documenting the presence of ventricular arrhythmia and identifying the patient at risk but also as a method for selecting an effective antiarrhythmic drug for long-term therapy. At the present time two approaches are available for evaluating the effect of an antiarrhythmic drug: (1) noninvasive techniques and (2) invasive electrophysiologic testing.[30] Noninvasive techniques, utilizing both ambulatory monitoring and exercise testing, depend on the suppression of spontaneous ventricular arrhythmia for defining drug efficacy. Invasive electrophysiologic testing utilizes the induction of the clinical arrhythmia with drug efficacy defined as failure to reinduce the arrhythmia.

Noninvasive techniques are the preferred method for drug evaluation in patients with symptomatic arrhythmia and in those patients with heart disease who have complex arrhythmia, particularly runs of nonsustained VT, who are at high risk for sudden cardiac death and for whom drug therapy may be important for preventing a fatal outcome. For those patients who have experienced hemodynamically unstable VT or VF and for whom antiarrhythmic drug therapy is necessary, electrophysiologic testing is mandatory when spontaneous ventricular arrhythmia is absent on ambulatory monitoring and exercise testing. There is a controversy about the approach to therapy in patients with a history of VT or VF, who manifest a high density of spontaneous ventricular arrhythmia, especially runs of nonsustained VT that is reproducibly present. Both invasive and noninvasive techniques have been successfully applied to this group of patients. In this section we will review the usefulness of noninvasive techniques (i.e., ambulatory monitoring and exercise testing) for judging the effect of an antiarrhythmic drug and for selecting an agent that is effective, safe, and well tolerated.

Unfortunately there are no helpful guidelines for the selection of an effective antiarrhythmic agent for any individual patient. The only way to be certain of drug effect on arrhythmia is by its administration with an invasive or noninvasive evaluation (Fig. 5–4). Since there are now eight orally effective antiarrhythmic agents available for use in the United States,[78] the identification of an effective and safe drug for an individual can be a time-consuming, frustrating, and costly process. A systematic approach to drug evaluation is therefore essential for management.

Noninvasive methods for drug testing are based on the suppression of spontaneously occurring ventricular arrhythmia, especially repetitive forms. As indicated previously, such repetitive arrhythmia, particularly runs of VT, represents an independent risk factor for sudden death in patients with heart disease, as it is a possible marker for underlying electrical instability of the myocardium.[79] Repetitive arrhythmia such as nonsustained VT results from a reentrant mechanism similar to that responsible for sustained VT. However, if reentry is self-terminating, the VT is nonsustained. The nonsustained runs indicate an active reentrant circuit that, given the appropriate conditions, is capable of generating sustained VT, which may degenerate into VF. Alternatively, it is possible that repetitive arrhyth-

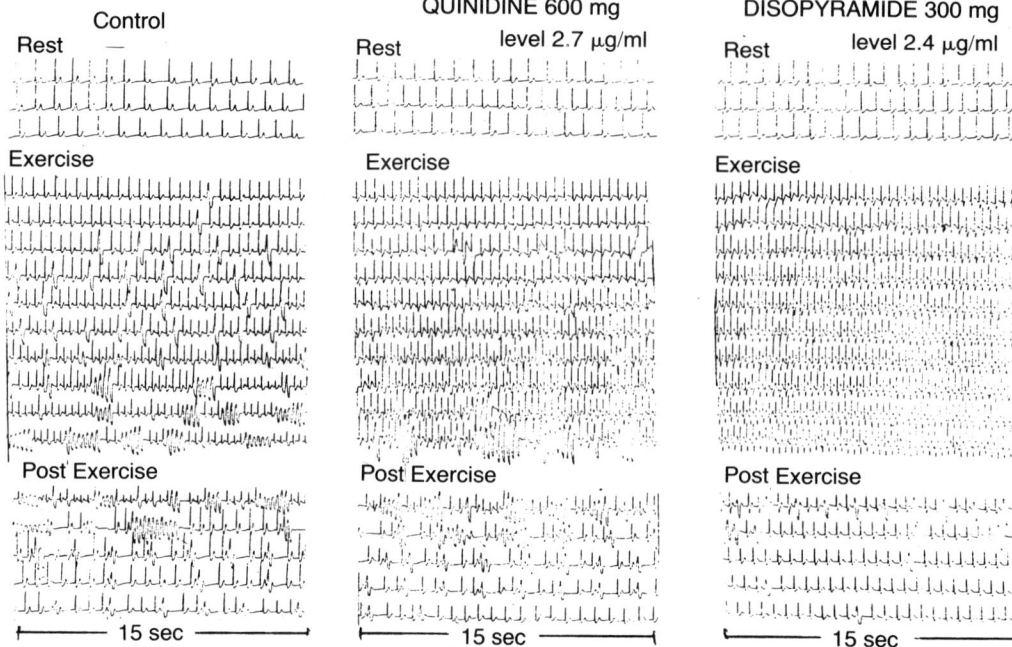

FIGURE 5–4
Results of quinidine and disopyramide therapy in the same patient. Although quinidine and disopyramide are in the same subclass and have the same electrophysiologic effects, the clinical response to these drugs varies. Response to one drug does not predict the effect of the other. In this patient, frequent runs of nonsustained ventricular tachycardia were induced by exercise testing. Disopyramide completely abolished arrhythmia, whereas quinidine was ineffective.

mia is only an epiphenomenon resulting from a mechanism different from that causing sustained VT and is not an indicator of an active circuit. Such spontaneous arrhythmia may, however, be a trigger for sustained arrhythmia if the appropriate substrate exists. A number of animal and human studies have confirmed that an appropriately timed VPB or series of sequential VPBs may penetrate a reentrant circuit, activate it, and induce a sustained reentrant ventricular tachycardia.[80, 81] As the frequency of spontaneous arrhythmia increases, the likelihood of triggering a sustained arrhythmia is augmented.

Whether VPBs and runs of VT represent markers for reentry or are triggers for a sustained tachyarrhythmia, the goal of antiarrhythmic therapy is the suppression of this spontaneously occurring arrhythmia. Once arrhythmia is documented and categorized, utilizing monitoring and exercise testing, antiarrhythmic drugs are administered for suppression. The theory on which therapy is based is that elimination of repetitive forms indicates (1) inactivation of the reentrant circuit, which is therefore no longer capable of generating or sustaining a tachyarrhythmia or alternatively (2), that the triggers for a tachyarrhythmia are abolished.

Prior to testing individual antiarrhythmic drugs, it is essential to establish the type and frequency of spontaneous arrhythmia present during a drug-free, baseline state. All antiarrhythmic drugs are discontinued and after an appropriate "washout" period, generally 5 half-lives of the previous drug, the baseline arrhythmia is evaluated. The patient undergoes 48 hours of ambulatory monitoring and performs an exercise test on a motorized treadmill. For those patients not able to exercise on the treadmill, bicycle ergometry is performed. During these baseline studies, the type, frequency, and reproducibility of spontaneous arrhythmia is established. Classification of the arrhythmia is based on the Lown grading system (Table 5–6).[37, 82]

Using the Lown grading system, an arrhythmia equation for both monitoring and exercise testing can be developed (Table 5–7). This equation provides a simple shorthand for indicating the type and frequency of arrhythmia present and permits a simple method for determining the results of an intervention.

Once the baseline type, density, and reproducibility of arrhythmia is established, a decision is made about the approach to use for drug evaluation.[79] If the spontaneous arrhythmia is of high density and is reproducibly present each day, noninvasive methods can be used. An adequate density of arrhythmia is defined as grade 2 VPBs for more than 50% of the hours monitored each day and repetitive arrhythmia during more than 30% of the hours monitored each day.

Evaluation of the effect of the antiarrhythmic drug

TABLE 5–6
Lown Grading System

Grade 0	No VPBs
Grade 1A	<30 VPBs/hour and <1/minute
Grade 1B	<30 VPBs/hour and occasionally >1/minute
Grade 2	>30 VPBs/hour
Grade 3	Multiform VPBs
Grade 4A	Couplets
Grade 4B	Runs of VT (>3 repetitive VPBs)
Grade 5	Early R on T VPBs (early cycle)

VPBs = ventricular premature beats; VT = ventricular tachycardia; R on T VPBs = early cycle.

TABLE 5–7
Arrhythmia Equation for Ambulatory Monitoring and Exercise Testing

Ambulatory Monitoring: $0^5, 1A^4, 1B^2, 2^{13}_{750}, 3^{17}_{4}, 4A^{21}_{40}, 4B^{17}_{7,9(240)}$

Grade	Explanation
0^5	Ventricular premature beats (VPBs) for 5 hours during the day
$1A^4$	Infrequenty VPBs (<30/hour + <1/min) present for 4 hours
$1B^2$	Infrequent VPBs (<30 VPBs/hour and occasionally >1/min) present for 2 hours
2^{13}_{750}	Frequent VPBS (>30/hour) present during each of 13 hours— total of 750 VPBs
3^{17}_{4}	17 hours during which multiform VPBs are present—up to 4 forms/hour
$4A^{21}_{40}$	Couplets occurred during 21 hours—up to 40/hour
Grade $4B^{17}_{7,9(240)}$	Runs of ventricular tachycardia (VT) present for 17 hours; 7 runs/hour, 9 beats in length, at rates of 240

Exercise Testing:

$R(3) = 2^{15}, 4A^2$

$E(6:30) = 2^{77}, 3^3, 4A^{12}, 4B^4_{5,200}$

$R(10) = 2^{169}, 3^4, 4A^{13}, 4B^{16}_{7,180}$

Period	Explanation
R = rest (3 min)	15 VPBs, 2 couplets
E = exercise (6½ min)	77 VPBs of 3 forms 12 couplets 4 runs of VT—maximum of 5 beats at rate of 200
R = recovery (10 min)	169 VPBs of 4 forms 13 couplets 16 runs of VT—maximum of 7 beats at rate of 180

on suppression of ventricular arrhythmia involves two types of testing, acute and maintenance.[82, 83] In acute drug testing, a single large dose of the antiarrhythmic drug is orally administered as a screen for drug effect, permitting identification of those agents that are of potential benefit (Fig. 5–5). Drugs tested in this fashion are those that are rapidly absorbed, achieve peak levels within 2 hours after drug administration, have no important active metabolites, and are rapidly cleared after the single dose so that, by the following day, the drug has been completely eliminated and arrhythmia returns to baseline, permitting another drug test.

On the morning of the acute drug test the patient undergoes a brief (30-minute) period of continuous monitoring by trendscription to document the type and frequency of arrhythmia present, for comparison with that present after drug administration. A brief period of exercise on a bicycle ergometer permits the patient to perform a level of work similar to that of routine daily activities. An ECG is recorded for measurement of P-R, QRS, and Q-T intervals. At the conclusion of this period, the patient receives a large dose of drug, which is approximately one half the usual daily dose used clinically and is adequate to bring the blood level into the therapeutic range within 2 hours. Continuous ECG monitoring by trendscription is performed for 3 hours after administration of the drug, and each hour bicycle exercise is repeated, an ECG for intervals recorded and blood drawn for drug levels.

At the conclusion of a series of acute drug tests, the agent (or combination of drugs) that appears to be the most effective is administered for 3 to 4 days, using a regular dosing schedule. Drugs with active metabolites, those slowly absorbed, or those with a long half-life requiring several days to achieve peak levels are not tested acutely but are evaluated only after a short period of maintenance therapy. This brief period of maintenance therapy permits drug levels to become steady-state and provides an opportunity to observe for toxic drug reactions.

At the end of this period of therapy, monitoring and exercise testing are repeated, and the results of both methods are used to define drug effect (Fig. 5–6). We have observed that 15% of patients deemed controlled on the basis of ambulatory monitoring continue to have complex arrhythmia during exercise testing. Therefore, arrhythmia must be suppressed with both methods before the drug is considered to be effective.

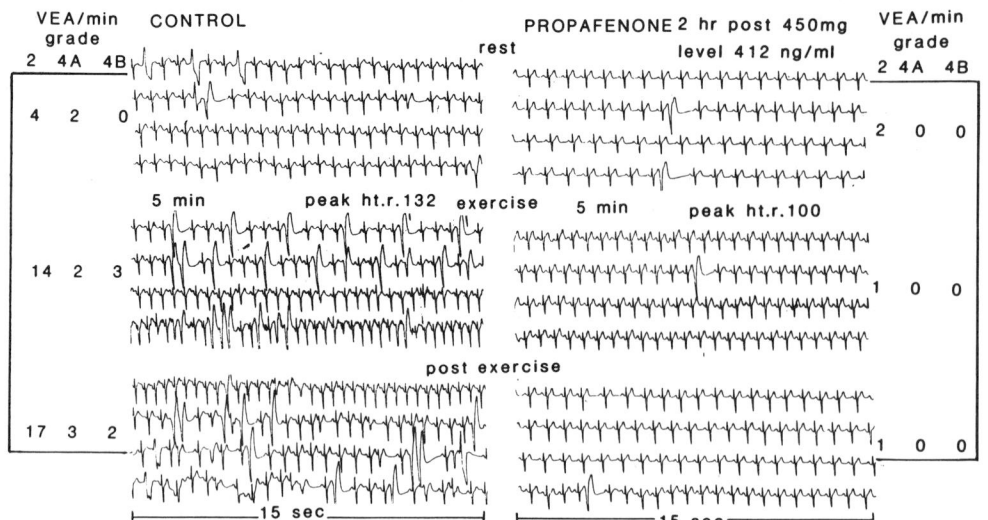

FIGURE 5–5
Acute drug testing with propafenone. In control, the patient had occasional ventricular premature beats (VPBs) at rest, whereas with exercise VPB frequency increased and couplets and runs of ventricular tachycardia were induced. Two hours after the patient received propafenone, VPBs were markedly reduced and no repetitive forms were present.

If arrhythmia is well controlled, the patient is discharged with follow-up every 3 to 6 months.

The criteria for defining drug efficacy when noninvasive methods (acute drug testing and monitoring and exercise testing) are utilized, include the following:

1. Total elimination of runs of VT
2. Reduction of ≥90% in couplets
3. Decrease of ≥50% in VPBs

Use of Drug Combinations

Although antiarrhythmic drugs are the cornerstone of arrhythmia management, each agent administered alone is effective in only 40 to 60% of patients.[85–89] Often, side effects further limit the usefulness of these drugs. In patients with a high density of spontaneous arrhythmia documented on monitoring or exercise testing, drugs administered as monotherapy often produce only partial suppression of arrhythmia. In some patients, a drug will be effective, but the dose necessary produces serious or disturbing side effects. In such situations, the combined use of antiarrhythmic drugs will often enhance arrhythmia control when single agents are not completely effective and may permit the use of lower doses of these drugs, reducing the occurrence of side effects. It should be emphasized, however, that each drug should first be evaluated individually with monitoring and exercise testing and that every combination is a new drug, which must also be fully evaluated.

One drug combination frequently administered is a membrane active drug and a beta blocking agent (Fig. 5–7). The rationale for the use of this combination is based on the electrophysiologic effects of these drugs. While the membrane-active agents reduce membrane conductivity, prolong membrane refractoriness, and reduce its excitability and decrease automaticity, cat-

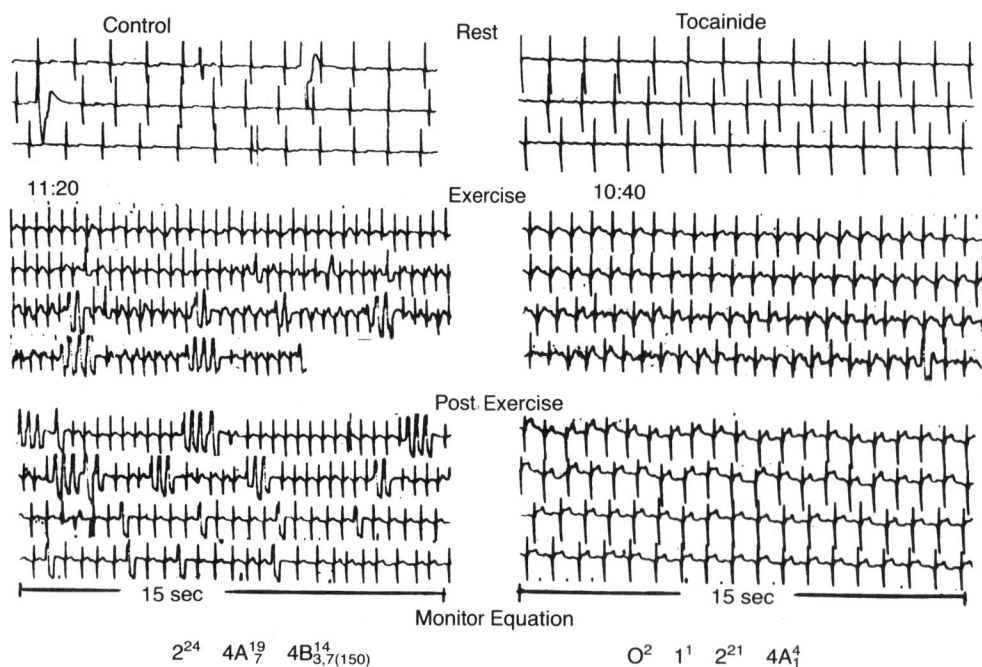

FIGURE 5–6
Maintenance therapy with tocainide. During baseline studies, runs of ventricular tachycardia (VT) were induced by exercise. On ambulatory monitoring the patient had frequent ventricular premature beats (VPBs) for 24 hours (2^{24}); couplets were present for 19 hours, with as many as 7 per hour ($4A_7^{19}$); and runs of VT occurred during 14 hours, with up to 3 runs/hour, 7 beats in length, and at a rate of 150 ($4B_{3,7(150)}^{14}$). During therapy with tocainide, arrhythmia was abolished with exercise. Ambulatory monitoring for 24 hours demonstrated no VPBs for 2 hours (0^2); infrequent VPBs for 1 hour (1^1); frequent VPBs for 21 hours (2^{21}); and 4 couplets during the day ($4A_1^4$).

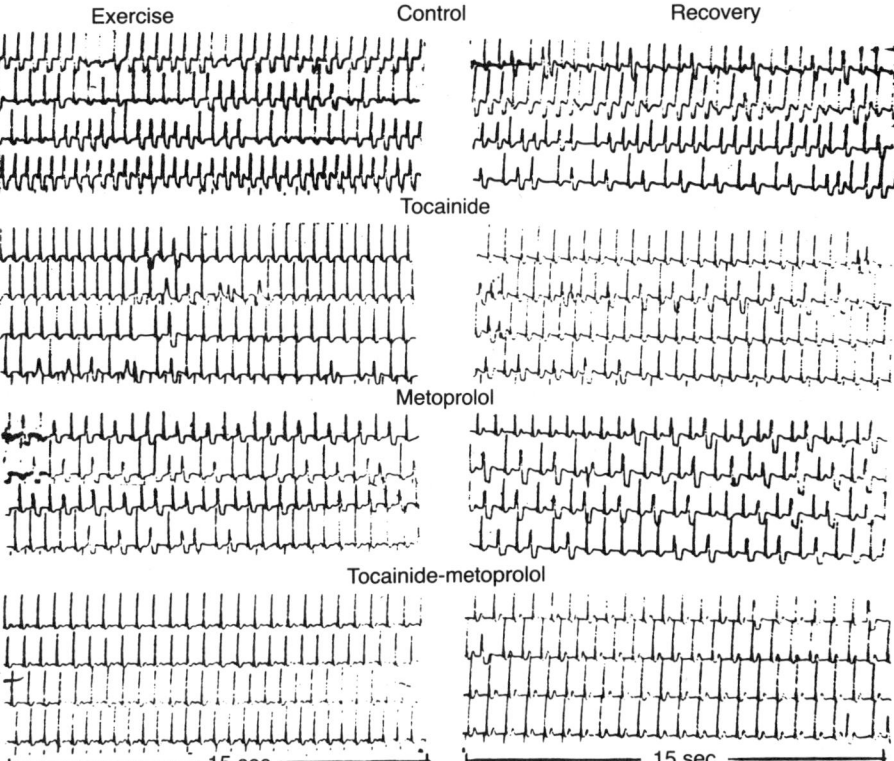

FIGURE 5–7
Combination therapy with a membrane drug (tocainide) and a beta blocker (metoprolol). During baseline evaluation, the patient had frequent ventricular premature beats (VPBs) and runs of ventricular tachycardia (VT). Monotherapy with tocainide and metoprolol reduced the frequency of arrhythmia. However, with the combination, arrhythmia was abolished.

echolamines produce opposite effects (i.e., they enhance conduction velocity, reduce membrane refractoriness, and increase its excitability and augment automaticity). Therefore, catecholamines may reverse the beneficial effects of the antiarrhythmic drugs. Beta blockers, by preventing these catecholamine-mediated effects on the heart, may potentiate the antiarrhythmic effects of the membrane drug. In a study by Hirsowitz and coworkers,[90] 51 patients with an incomplete response to monotherapy with a membrane-active agent received a beta blocker in combination with the membrane drug. As evaluated by ambulatory monitoring, the combination produced a significant reduction in VPBs (52%), couplets (21%), and runs of VT (43%), compared to the results of monotherapy (p <0.05). As expected, arrhythmia suppression evaluated with exercise testing was more impressive and VPBs, couplets, and runs of VT were reduced by 65%, 86%, and 83%, respectively (p <0.001). Of note, beta blockers administered as sole agents had no significant effect on arrhythmias. Although a large number of drugs were used in this study, there are other studies utilizing drug combinations with some individual drugs. Bigger[91] reviewed experience with mexiletine in the United States and reported that the overall response rate to mexiletine used as monotherapy was 14%, whereas 30% of patients responded when propranolol was administered in combination. Using ambulatory monitoring, Deedwania and coworkers[92] reported that nadolol administered to 18 patients in combination with procainamide or quinidine resulted in a further, significant reduction of ventricular arrhythmia, compared to monotherapy. The reduction in VPBs was 19% with monotherapy and 92% during combination therapy. Therapy was considered effective in only 29% of patients receiving either quinidine or procainamide alone, whereas 63% of patients responded to the combination of either drug with nadolol.

There have also been reports of the combined use of two membrane-active agents. Duff and coworkers[93] administered quinidine and mexiletine individually to 17 patients and reported that quinidine therapy resulted in a 59% reduction in VPBs and a 35% reduction in VT, whereas with mexiletine the decrease was 65% and 41%, respectively. The incidence of side effects was 82% for mexiletine and 65% during quinidine therapy. When combination therapy was used, VPBs were reduced by 86% and runs of VT by 94%. Significantly, side effects were reported in only 6% of patients during combination therapy, a result of lower doses. Similar results have been reported with other drug combinations. Klein and Marcus[94] administered propafenone to 30 patients who had only a partial response (20% VPB suppression) to either quinidine or procainamide. They reported improved antiarrhythmic efficacy, with an 80% VPB reduction. Although a similar degree of response could be achieved with monotherapy with propafenone, the dose necessary was higher compared to that used in combination (730 mg vs. 480 mg).

AGGRAVATION OF ARRHYTHMIA

Although each of the available and investigational antiarrhythmic drugs are effective for suppressing ventricular arrhythmia, all have the potential for aggravating the very arrhythmia being treated (Fig. 5–8).[95] The definition of aggravation proposed by Velebit and

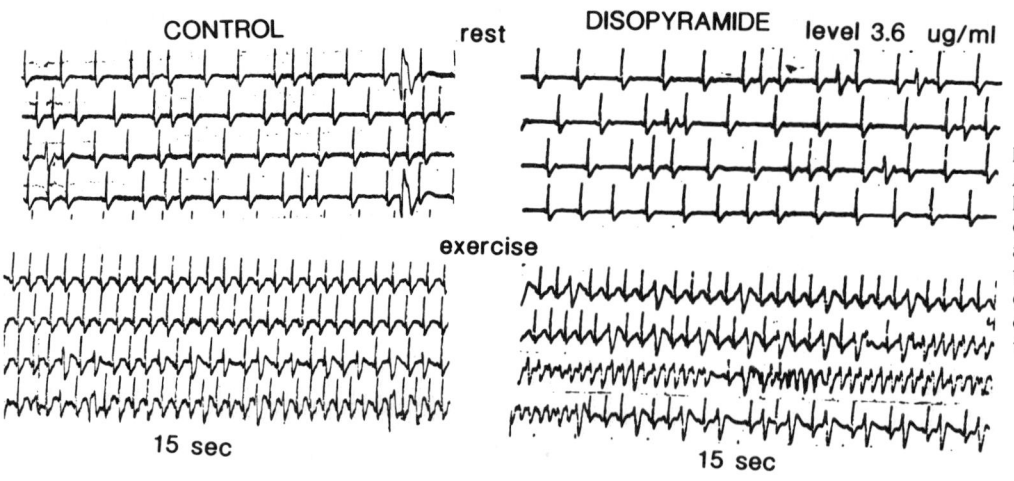

FIGURE 5–8
Aggravation of arrhythmia. During control, the patient had occasional VPBs both at rest and with exercise. During therapy with disopyramide, exercise induced several runs of polymorphic ventricular tachycardia.

coworkers[96] when noninvasive ambulatory monitoring and exercise testing are used for assessment, includes:

1. A fourfold increase in the frequency of VPBs compared to baseline, or
2. A tenfold increase in the number of repetitive forms (couplets or runs of VT), or
3. The occurrence of sustained ventricular tachyarrhythmia not present during the control period

One of the concerns in defining aggravation of arrhythmia has been the random variability of arrhythmia frequency. Since it has been reported that variability is indirectly related to VPB density, Morganroth and Horowitz[97] have proposed criteria for aggravation based on the baseline number of VPBs hourly. Thus, when the density of VPBs was 10 to 50 per hour, a tenfold increase was necessary to define aggravation. In contrast, when the density was 51 to 100 per hour, aggravation was a fivefold increase; when the density was 101 to 300 per hour, a fourfold increase was necessary; and when VPBs per hour were >300, a threefold increase in VPBs defined aggravation. In a review of almost 1300 noninvasive studies involving single-drug therapy, arrhythmia aggravation, as defined by the criteria of Velebit and coworkers[96] occurred in 9% of tests. Although the incidence varied from 6 to 19%, each drug was associated with this toxic side effect (Table 5–8).

In the first report of this complication,[96] it did not appear as if there were any factors that predicted the patient at risk. However, in a recent report of arrhythmia aggravation, this issue was addressed using a retrospective analysis.[98] Patients who had arrhythmia aggravation were compared to those who did not experience this complication during drug testing. Age, sex, nature and/or extent of the underlying heart disease, baseline ECG intervals, ECG interval changes due to drug, density of spontaneous arrhythmia on monitoring and exercise testing, and drug dose or blood level did not predict the patient at risk. The only factors that were related to arrhythmia aggravation were the nature of the presenting arrhythmia and left ventricular function. Thus patients presenting with sustained VT or VF were more likely to experience arrhythmia aggravation compared to those with NSVT or VPBs (odds ratio 3.9, p <0.01). The average LVEF in those with aggravation was 37%, compared to 43% in those without this complication (p = 0.08), but this was not statistically significant. However, the group of patients with LVEF <35% had a greater likelihood of aggravating compared to those in whom LVEF was >35% (odds ratio 2.5, p = 0.04). Of importance was the observation that aggravation with one drug did not predict aggravation with another agent, even of the same class or subclass. Finally, exercise testing played an important role in exposing this complication. In one third of cases, the worsening of arrhythmia was provoked by exercise testing, often at a time when 24-hour ambulatory monitoring demonstrated good control and even abolition of arrhythmia.

In conclusion, aggravation is a serious complication of antiarrhythmic drug therapy. Although it occurs more commonly in patients who have a history of a sustained ventricular tachyarrhythmia, especially when the LVEF is severely depressed, no other parameter is of help for predicting the patient at risk for this toxic side effect. Careful and systematic use of these drugs, employing monitoring and exercise testing performed before and during therapy, are essential to expose this potentially serious side effect.

Will Antiarrhythmic Drugs Prevent Sudden Death?

Many trials of antiarrhythmic drugs in different patient populations have been reported in the literature. These can be divided into those in which drug therapy was empiric, not guided by arrhythmia suppression, and those in which drug therapy was individualized, guided by the suppression of arrhythmia as evaluated by ambulatory monitoring and exercise testing.

RESULTS OF NON-GUIDED THERAPY

A number of studies have evaluated the role of antiarrhythmic drugs for preventing sudden death (Table 5–

TABLE 5-8
Aggravation of Arrhythmia by Antiarrhythmic Drugs

Drug	No. of Patients	No. with Aggravation	%
Disopyramide	102	6	6
Encainide	102	15	15
Ethmozine	82	9	11
Flecainide	26	3	12
Indecainide	16	3	19
Lorcainide	120	9	8
Mexiletine	350	23	7
Procainamide	55	5	9
Propafenone	124	10	8
Quinidine	180	20	15
Tocainide	180	14	8
Overall	1287	117	9

9). However, each of these studies has involved patients with a recent MI. There are as yet no data available about drug therapy in other groups of patients. The earliest studies in which antiarrhythmic drug therapy was compared to placebo involved the use of intravenous lidocaine. In one study by Morgensen[99] 79 patients were randomized and in another study by Bennett and coworkers,[100] 612 patients were randomized to lidocaine or placebo therapy. Neither study demonstrated a difference in outcome in the lidocaine-treated group. Lie and coworkers,[101] however, reported that compared to placebo lidocaine significantly reduced mortality and the occurrence of VF among 212 patients (10% vs. 0%, $p < 0.05$). In these studies, lidocaine was administered for only several days after the acute event, and therefore the effect of drugs on long-term outcome was not evaluated. Ryden and colleagues[102] reported on long-term tocainide treatment. Campbell et al.[103] and Chamberlain and coworkers[104] studied the effects of mexiletine therapy. However, total cardiac and arrhythmic mortality was not affected by drug therapy in any of these studies. In a recent protocol using mexiletine, the IMPACT Group[105] reported that the drug did not reduce the 1-year sudden death mortality of 630 post-MI patients randomized to drug or placebo (mortality 7.6% for mexiletine vs. 4.8% for placebo; $p = NS$). Negative results were also reported by Hugenholtz et al.,[106] who administered aprindine or placebo to 193 patients (mortality 7.3% vs. 9.3%; $p = NS$) and by Gottlieb and coworkers,[107] who used aprindine or placebo in 143 patients (mortality 17.8% vs. 22.2%; $p = NS$).

There have been several studies of quinidine therapy in post-MI patients, but duration of therapy was limited to only 3 to 15 days, and in none of these studies was a beneficial effect from therapy observed.[108, 109] Two large studies with phenytoin in which follow-up was 1 to 2 years likewise reported that there was no benefit from this drug in preventing sudden death.[110, 111] A study by Zainel and coworkers[112] involving disopyramide reported a significant reduction in mortality after 3 weeks of therapy (26.7% vs. 3.3%; $p < 0.105$); however, Jennings and colleagues[113] reported no benefit from disopyramide after a 1-year follow-up. Two studies in which procainamide was administered reported an improved survival in those receiving the drug compared to those on placebo. In a 3-week study, Koch Weser et al.[114] reported no mortality in those receiving procainamide compared to 6.1% in those on placebo ($p < 0.05$). Kosowsky and coworkers,[115] in a study of procainamide therapy for 1 year, reported a mortality of 10.3% in patients receiving placebo compared to 3.7% in those on procainamide ($p < 0.05$). However, in many patients side effects necessitated drug discontinuation, and therefore the number of patients receiving long-term therapy was small.

Although most of the above studies failed to demonstrate any benefit from antiarrhythmic drug therapy, the results are questionable because of the following shortcomings:

1. A small number of patients were involved. Since the endpoints were total cardiac or sudden death, which are relatively low-frequency events, it would be

TABLE 5-9
Randomized Trials of Antiarrhythmic Drugs in Post–Myocardial Infarction Patients

Study	Drug	No. of Patients	Duration of Therapy	% Mortality or VF		
				Control	Drug	P
Morgensen	Lidocaine	79	days	11.0	12.0	NS
Bennett	Lidocaine	610	days	7.0	16.0	NS
Lie	Lidocaine	212	days	10.0	0	<0.05
Ryden	Tocainide	112	6 months	8.9	8.9	NS
Campbell	Mexiletine	97	4 years	1.8	2.3	NS
Chamberlain	Mexiletine	344	1 year	11.6	13.2	NS
IMPACT	Mexiletine	630	1 year	4.8	7.6	NS
Hugenholtz	Aprindine	193	1 year	9.3	7.3	NS
Gottlieb	Aprindine	143	1 year	22.2	17.8	NS
Jones	Quinidine	103	3 days	12.4	8.9	NS
Holmberg	Quinidine	104	15 days	7.2	10.7	NS
Jennings	Disopyramide	95	1 year	10.2	4.3	NS
Zainel	Disopyramide	60	3 weeks	26.7	3.3	<0.05
Koch Weser	Procainamide	70	3 weeks	6.1	0	<0.05
Kosowsky	Procainamide	78	1 year	10.3	3.7	<0.05
Collaborative	Phenytoin	560	1 year	11.0	9.4	NS
Peter	Phenytoin	150	2 years	18.0	24.0	NS

VF = ventricular fibrillation; NS = not significant.

necessary to study a larger number of patients before any benefit could be seen.

2. Duration of therapy was brief in many of these studies, often involving only days to weeks. Therefore, it was not possible to establish the effect of the drug on long-term survival.

3. These studies were double-blinded, with patients randomized to drug or placebo without attention to the presence of arrhythmia. Moreover, its type, frequency, and reproducibility were not established. Often, baseline ambulatory monitoring was not performed prior to entry, and the only types of evaluation were analysis ECG rhythm strips or observation of bedside monitors.

4. The effect of the drug on ventricular arrhythmias was not evaluated. Follow-up ambulatory monitoring during therapy was not performed and the degree of suppression of arrhythmia by the drug was not determined. Usually, fixed drug doses were administered, and even when arrhythmia persisted there was no attempt to titrate the dose to arrhythmia suppression. Therapy was continued even if arrhythmia persisted. Therefore, these trials did not address the issue of whether suppression of spontaneously occurring ventricular arrhythmia will prolong life.

5. Each of the antiarrhythmia drugs can aggravate arrhythmia, and this was not considered or addressed in these studies. It is possible that this complication resulted in the death of some patients negating any beneficial drug effect.

As a result of these many problems and limitations, the NIH initiated the cardiac arrhythmia pilot study (CAPS) to be followed by the cardiac arrhythmia suppression trial, or CAST,[116] which will randomize 4000 post-MI patients with ventricular arrhythmia to therapy with placebo or an antiarrhythmic drug, with drug and dose selection guided by arrhythmia suppression as evaluated with ambulatory monitoring. Unlike previous trials, there is an attempt to suppress arrhythmia in this study.

RESULTS OF GUIDED THERAPY

Many data have been published about which arrhythmia places the patient at a higher risk for sudden death; however, it remains uncertain if this risk can be altered and whether survival can be improved by antiarrhythmic drug therapy. The post-MI antiarrhythmic drug trials have been disappointing, as no drug reduced mortality. The many recognized problems with these studies preclude any meaningful interpretation since the results therefore are not definitive. The most serious limitations concern inadequate documentation of the type and frequency of baseline arrhythmia, failure to treat the patient by administering a drug at an appropriate dose based on arrhythmia suppression, and continuation of therapy even when arrhythmia persisted. Often ambulatory monitoring was not used to evaluate therapy.

The goal of antiarrhythmic drug therapy is the suppression of arrhythmia, and it has been established that therapy must be individualized for each patient, guided by an assessment of the effect of drug on arrhythmia. Therefore, baseline and repeat monitoring and exercise testing are essential to judge the results of therapy when based on the suppression of spontaneous arrhythmia.

Although there are no appropriately performed placebo-drug comparative trials, data are available that strongly suggest that these agents do have a beneficial effect on prolongation of life. These studies involve patients presenting with serious ventricular arrhythmia (sustained VT or VF) who received therapy with these agents. While none of these studies are placebo-controlled, they usually have involved patients with recurrent VT or VF refractory to previous drug therapy. The recurrence rate in such patients receiving either no therapy or only empiric therapy is reported to be high,[117] and therefore it is possible to establish the effect of therapy guided by arrhythmia suppression.

Graboys and coworkers[83] reported on 123 patients with a history of out-of-hospital sudden death due to sustained VT or VF. In these patients drug therapy was guided noninvasively, the goal of therapy being the elimination of runs of nonsustained VT and ≥90% reduction in couplets on both ambulatory monitoring and exercise testing. In 98 patients, an effective drug was identified and arrhythmia was suppressed. The remaining 25 patients had continued runs of nonsustained VT despite the most effective drug selected. The mean follow-up for the entire group was 29.6 months, during which time there were 23 sudden deaths (8.2% annually). When the data were analyzed based on the response to therapy, the annual sudden death mortality was 2.3% in those patients controlled by antiarrhythmic drugs, whereas in the nonresponders there was a 43.6% annual sudden death rate (Fig. 5–9). There were no clinical differences between drug responders or those in whom drugs were not completely effective. Similar results were reported by Vlay and coworkers,[118] who studied 59 patients surviving an episode of out-of-hospital sudden death. Of the 52 patients who had ambulatory monitoring before discharge, 33 patients demonstrated no runs of VT and 19 patients had persistent runs of VT. There were no clinically significant differences between these two groups. After a follow-up of 700 days, 82% of those who responded to antiarrhythmic drugs remained alive and free of symptoms and recurrence. In contrast, only 42% of those with continued runs of VT were free of recurrence ($p < 0.002$). These authors calculated that the sensitivity and specificity of ambulatory monitoring was 100% and 68%, respectively, with a predictive accuracy of 73%.

In a noncontrolled and nonrandomized study by Hoffman et al.,[119] 50 patients with chronic stable coronary artery disease and runs of VT received antiarrhythmic drugs. Arrhythmia was suppressed in 39 patients and persisted in 11. After a follow-up of 16 months, there was a significantly better outcome in the drug responders (7% yearly mortality vs. 36%; $p < 0.005$). There was only 1 sudden death in the 39 responders, compared to 3 in the nonresponders (p <0.05).

Although there are no other studies reporting the long-term outcome of patients responding to drug compared to nonresponders, several studies evaluating individual drugs noninvasively have reported the long-term outcome. In a group of 313 patients undergoing in-hospital evaluation with mexiletine, Stein et al.[120] discharged 107 patients who responded to the drug and were free of side effects. After an average follow-up of 23 months, the annual sudden death mortality was 3.6%. A similar patient population receiving tocainide was studied by Hohnloser and coworkers.[121] They reported that 73 patients responding to tocainide, based on noninvasive methods, were discharged on this drug. After a 26-month follow-up, the recurrence rate of sudden death was 4.3% annually. Tordjman and colleagues[122] noninvasively evaluated encainide therapy in patients with serious ventricular arrhythmia. Among 48 patients discharged on encainide and followed for 25 months, arrhythmia recurrence was 6% per year. In a report by Cueni and Podrid,[123] 35 patients were discharged on propafenone, and after a follow-up of 23 months one patient died suddenly and four had a nonfatal recurrence.

It can be concluded that survival can be improved when the response to antiarrhythmic drugs is assessed noninvasively and when an agent that eliminates runs of nonsustained VT on monitoring and exercise testing and that is well tolerated is selected for long-term therapy. Noninvasive methods therefore are a reliable method for drug evaluation and selection.

ADVANTAGES AND LIMITATIONS OF NONINVASIVE TECHNIQUES FOR DRUG SELECTION

There are a number of important reasons for preferring noninvasive methods as a guide for selection of an effective antiarrhythmic drug to be administered for long-term suppression of arrhythmia. Monitoring and exercise testing procedures are widely available, easy to perform, without risk, and relatively inexpensive. Noninvasive techniques can be performed in most centers without the need to refer the patient to a specialized institution that has an electrophysiology laboratory. The tests can be repeated as frequently as the clinical situation warrants and can be performed in outpatients without the need for hospitalization. Therefore, if side effects occur that necessitate change of dose or drug, noninvasive testing can be repeated readily and simply without hospitalization. Finally, since the follow-up of patients with arrhythmia usually involves repeated outpatient monitoring and exercise testing, it is important to have baseline data available for comparison. Patients undergoing electrophysiologic testing for drug selection are also followed long-term with noninvasive methods, making a control evaluation mandatory. If long-term drug efficacy is determined noninvasively, why not select a drug based on noninvasive methods?

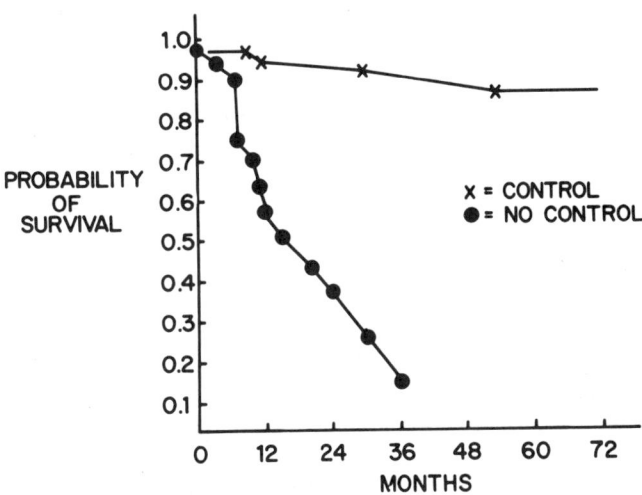

FIGURE 5—9
Results of antiarrhythmic drug therapy in 123 survivors of sudden death. Among 98 patients responding to antiarrhythmic drugs (control group) there was a 2.3% annual mortality. In contrast, the mortality among the 25 nonresponders to drug ("no control" group) was 43% per year. (with permission from Am J Cardiol). (Reprinted with permission from Graboys TB, Lown B, Podrid PJ, et al: Am J Cardiol 49:127, 1982).

Despite the many advantages offered by noninvasive techniques, several important limitations to the use of these techniques include:

1. Monitoring and exercise testing for arrhythmia management can be used only in patients who manifest a high density of spontaneous ventricular arrhythmia, since drug efficacy is defined by a certain percentage of reduction in VPBs. Therefore, when spontaneous arrhythmia is infrequent or absent, establishing drug effect is unreliable or even impossible with noninvasive methods.

2. Some patients demonstrate wide hour-to-hour or day-to-day variability in the presence and complexity of ventricular arrhythmia.[24-26] When such spontaneous changes in arrhythmia density are marked, it becomes difficult to distinguish between the effect of the drug and that which is attributed to random variability. Although it is well established that spontaneous changes in VPB frequency are common, it must be emphasized that the studies reporting this problem have involved patients with frequent VPBs who have not experienced serious ventricular arrhythmia. It has been observed that patients with a history of serious arrhythmia have a stable and high level of arrhythmia that is reproducible from day to day.[30] Moreover, it has been reported that random variability is related to the density of VPBs.[26] As the hourly frequency of VPBs increases, variability decreases. It has been proposed that criteria for drug efficacy should be related to the baseline level of VPBs. Concerns about VPB variability are diminished when the criteria for efficacy include elimination of certain forms in addition to a percent reduction in VPBs and when exercise testing is also used as a method for evaluating drug response. Similar concerns exist about the reproducibility of

arrhythmia during exercise testing. As with monitoring, it has been reported that there is lack of reproducibility in the type and density of arrhythmia when two sequential exercise tests are performed.[124] However, as with the studies of ambulatory monitoring, the patients reported were those with frequent but benign VPBs who had never experienced a sustained ventricular tachyarrhythmia. It has been observed that in patients with serious arrhythmia exercise testing does reproducibly induce arrhythmia.[30]

3. The current technology for automatic ambulatory monitoring often does not provide accurate VPB counts. More important, there may be failure to recognize complex VPBs, especially repetitive forms and runs of VT. Although the use of a technician-interactive system improves the ability to identify these forms, this remains a limitation.

4. While the use of exercise testing and ambulatory monitoring will expose ventricular arrhythmia and document their density, complexity, and reproducibility, it remains unclear what arrhythmias are associated with an increased risk for sudden death in different groups of patients. Noninvasive methods do not provide any estimate of risk. The presence of VT on monitoring in patients who have had a recent MI defines this group as having an increased risk of sudden death during a 1-year follow-up; yet the majority of these patients do not experience serious arrhythmia. Thus, when used for prognostic purposes Holter monitoring is not specific and the predictive accuracy is low. Moreover, potentially serious arrhythmia may be fleeting and difficult to document on ambulatory monitoring, making this technique insensitive. In some studies of post-MI patients, it is the frequency of VPBs that imparts risk; in other studies, the presence of runs of VT is of prognostic importance. In patients with coronary disease but without a recent MI, in patients with a cardiomyopathy, and in normal individuals, it is unclear what, if any, arrhythmia is important. Therefore, in some groups of patients noninvasive techniques provide only limited prognostic data.

5. The endpoints during drug therapy for defining efficacy are unclear. Certain forms of arrhythmia place the patient at risk, but it is uncertain what degree of arrhythmia suppression is necessary to define drug efficacy and protect the patient. Although drug effect may be a statistically significant reduction of VPBs, this may not correlate with protection from recurrence. Total elimination of arrhythmia may no doubt prevent a recurrence, but this endpoint is generally unachievable.

It has been reported that suppression of certain forms (primarily runs of VT) will prevent a recurrence of a serious sustained tachyarrhythmia; however, it is not clear whether complete abolition is essential or if only a percentage reduction is necessary. It is unclear what degree of suppression is important and the definitions of drug efficacy thus vary greatly.

In conclusion, ambulatory monitoring and exercise testing are valuable tools for evaluating arrhythmia in patients with and without heart disease. These noninvasive methods are important for determining the etiology of symptoms and for establishing prognosis in certain patient groups and identifying a high-risk group. Noninvasive methods also are an important and reliable way to select an effective antiarrhythmic drug.

References

1. Averill KH, Lamb LE: Electrocardiographic findings in 67,375 asymptomatic patients. 1. Incidence of abnormalities. Am J Cardiol 6:76, 1960.
2. Hiss RG, Lamb LE: Electrocardiographic findings in 122,043 individuals. Circulation 25:947, 1962.
3. Chiang BN, Perlman LV, Ostrander LD, et al.: Relationship of premature systoles to coronary heart disease and sudden death in the Tecumseh epidemiologic study. Ann Int Med 70:1159, 1969.
4. Hinkle L, Carver ST, Stevens M: The frequency of asymptomatic disturbances of cardiac rhythm and conduction in middle-aged men. Am J Cardiol 24:629, 1969.
5. Brodsky M, Wu D, Denes P, et al.: Arrhythmias documented by 24-hour continuous electrocardiographic monitoring in 50 male medical students without apparent heart disease. Am J Cardiol 39:390, 1977.
6. Sobotka PA, Mayer JH, Bauernfeind RA, et al.: Arrhythmias documented by 24-hour continuous ambulatory electrocardiographic monitoring in young women without apparent heart disease. Am Heart J 101:753, 1981.
7. Kostis JB, McCrone K, Moreyra AE, et al.: Premature ventricular complexes in the absence of identifiable heart disease. Circulation 63:1351, 1981.
8. Savage DD, Levy D, Garrison RJ, et al.: Mitral valve prolapse in the general population. III. Dysrhythmias: The Framingham Study. Am Heart J 106:582, 1983.
9. Fleg J, Kennedy H: Cardiac arrhythmias in a healthy elderly population. Chest 81:302, 1982.
10. Glasser S, Clark P, Applebaum H: Occurrence of frequent complex arrhythmias detected by ambulatory monitoring. Chest 75:565, 1979.
11. Ryan M, Lown B, Horn H: Comparison of ventricular ectopic activity during 24-hour monitoring and exercise testing in patients with coronary heart disease. N Engl J Med 292:224, 1975.
12. Calvert A, Lown B, Gorlin R: Ventricular premature beats and anatomically defined coronary heart disease. Am J Cardiol 39:627, 1977.
13. Moss AJ, Davis HT, DeCamilla J, et al.: Ventricular ectopic beats and their relation to sudden and nonsudden cardiac death after myocardial infarction. Circulation 60:998, 1979.
14. Bigger JT, Weld FM, Rolnitsky LM: Prevalence, characteristics and significance of ventricular tachycardia (three or more complexes) detected with ambulatory electrocardiographic monitoring in the late hospital phase of acute myocardial infarction. Am J Cardiol 48:815, 1981.
15. Wilson JR, Schwartz S, St. John Sutton M, et al.: Prognosis in severe heart failure: relation to hemodynamic measurements and ventricular ectopic activity. J Am Coll Cardiol 2:403, 1983.
16. Maskin CS, Siskind SJ, LeJeintel TH: High prevalence of nonsustained ventricular tachycardia in severe congestive heart failure. Am Heart J 107:896, 1984.
17. Von Olshausen K, Schaefer A, Mehmel HC, et al.: Ventricular arrhythmias in idiopathic dilated cardiomyopathy. Br Heart J 51:195, 1984.
18. Chakko CS, Gheorghiade M: Ventricular arrhythmias in severe heart failure: Incidence, significance and effectiveness of antiarrhythmic therapy. Am Heart J 109:497, 1985.
19. Neri R, Mestroni L, Salvi A, et al.: Ventricular arrhythmias in dilated cardiomyopathy: Efficacy of amiodarone. Am Heart J 113:707, 1987.
20. Savage DD, Serdes S, Maron BJ, et al.: Prevalence of arrhythmias during 24-hour electrocardiographic monitoring and exercise testing in patients with obstructive and nonobstructive hypertrophic cardiomyopathy. Circulation 59:866, 1979.

21. McKenna WJ, Chetty S, Oakley CM, et al.: Arrhythmia in hypertrophic cardiomyopathy: Exercise and 48-hour ambulatory electrocardiographic assessment with and without beta adrenergic blocking therapy. Am J Cardiol 45:1, 1980.
22. Lown B, Podrid PJ, DeSilva RA, et al.: Sudden cardiac death: Management of the patient at risk. Curr Prob Cardiol 4(12):1, 1980.
23. Venditti FJ, Kuchar D, Kelly PA, et al.: Holter vs. programmed stimulation in sustained ventricular arrhythmias. Frequency of adequate baseline holter data. Circulation 76(Suppl 4):IV-84, 1987.
24. Winkle RA: Spontaneous variability of ectopies frequently mimics antiarrhythmic drug effect. Circulation 57:1116, 1978.
25. Raeder EA, Hohnloser S, Graboys TB, et al.: Spontaneous variability and circadian distribution of ectopic activity in patients with malignant ventricular arrhythmia. J Am Coll Cardiol 12:656, 1988.
26. Morganroth J, Michelson EL, Horowitz LN, et al.: Limitations of routine long term electrocardiographic monitoring to assess ventricular ectopic frequency. Circulation 58:408, 1978.
27. Michelson EL, Morganroth J: Spontaneous variability of complex ventricular arrhythmias detected by long-term electrocardiographic recordings. Circulation 61:690, 1980.
28. Pratt CM, Delcos G, Wierman AM, et al.: The changing baseline of complex ventricular arrhythmias; a new consideration in assessing long term antiarrhythmic drug therapy. N Engl J Med 313:1444, 1985.
29. Hohnloser SH, Raeder EA, Podrid PJ, et al.: Predictors of antiarrhythmic drug efficacy in patients with malignant ventricular tachyarrhythmias. Am Heart J 114:1, 1987.
30. Podrid PJ: Treatment of ventricular arrhythmia. Noninvasive vs. invasive approach—applications and limitations. Chest 88:121, 1985.
31. Kannel WB, Abbott RD, Savage DD, et al.: Epidemiologic features of chronic atrial fibrillation. The Framingham Study. N Engl J Med 306:1018, 1982.
32. Milner PG, Platia EV, Reid PR, et al.: Ambulatory electrocardiographic recordings at the time of fatal cardiac arrest. Am J Cardiol 56:588, 1985.
33. Pandis FP, Morganroth J: Sudden death in hospitalized patients: Cardiac rhythm disturbances detected by ambulatory electrocardiographic monitoring. J Am Coll Cardiol 2:798, 1983.
34. Pratt CM, Frances MJ, Luck JC, et al.: Analysis of ambulatory electrocardiograms in 15 patients during spontaneous ventricular fibrillation with special reference to preceding arrhythmic events. J Am Coll Cardiol 2:789, 1983.
35. Gradman AH, Bell PA, DeBush RF: Sudden death during ambulatory monitoring. Clinical and electrocardiographic correlations. Report of a case. Circulation 55:210, 1977.
36. Lewis BH, Antman EM, Graboys TB: Detailed analysis of 24 hour ambulatory electrocardiographic recordings during ventricular fibrillation or Torsade de Pointes. J Am Coll Cardiol 2:426, 1985.
37. Lown B, Wolf M: Approaches to sudden death from coronary heart disease. Circulation 44:130, 1971.
38. Chiang BN, Perlman LV, Fulton M, et al.: Predisposing factors in sudden cardiac death in Tecumseh, Michigan. A prospective study. Circulation 41:31, 1970.
39. Rodstein M, Wollock L, Gubner RS: Mortality study of the significance of extrasystoles in an insured population. Circulation 44:617, 1971.
40. Rabkin SW, Mathewson FAL, Tate RB: Relationship of ventricular ectopy in men without apparent heart disease to occurrence of ischemic heart disease and sudden death. Am Heart J 101:135, 1981.
41. Hinkle L, Carver ST, Argyros DL: The prognostic significance of ventricular premature contractions in healthy people and in people with coronary disease. Acta Cardiol 43:15, 1974.
42. Coronary Drug Project Research Group. Prognostic importance of premature beats following myocardial infarction. Experience in the coronary drug project. JAMA 223:1116, 1973.
43. Kotler MN, Tabatznik B, Mower M, et al.: Prognostic significance of ventricular ectopic beats with respect to sudden death in the late post-infarction period. Circulation 470:959, 1973.
44. Vismara LA, Amsterdam EA, Mason DT: Relation of ventricular arrhythmias in the late hospital phase of acute myocardial infarction to sudden death after hospital discharge. Am J Med 59:6, 1975.
45. Ruberman W, Weinblatt E, Goldberg JD, et al.: Ventricular premature beats after myocardial infarction. N Engl J Med 297:750, 1977.
46. Rappaport E, Remedios P: The high-risk patient after recovery from myocardial infarction: Recognition and management. J Am Coll Cardiol 1:391, 1983.
47. Bigger JT, Fleiss JL, Kleiger R, et al.: The relationship between ventricular arrhythmias, left ventricular dysfunction, and mortality in the two years after myocardial infarction. Circulation 69:250, 1984.
48. Mukharji J, Rude PE, Poole K, et al.: Risk factors for sudden death following acute myocardial infarction: Two-year followup. Am J Cardiol 54:31, 1984.
49. Schulze RA, Strauss HW, Pitt B: Sudden death in the year following myocardial infarction. Relation to ventricular premature contractions in the late hospital phase of left ventricular ejection fraction. Am J Med 62:192, 1977.
50. Ruberman W, Weinblatt C, Goldberg JD: Ventricular premature complexes and sudden death after myocardial infarction. Circulation 64:297, 1981.
51. Bigger JT, Fleiss JL, Rolnitzky LM, et al.: Prevalence, characteristics and significance of ventricular tachycardia detected by 24-hour continuous electrocardiographic recordings in the late hospital phase of acute myocardial infarction. Am J Cardiol 58:1151, 1986.
52. Kleiger RE, Miller JP, Bigger JT, et al.: Decreased heart rate variability and its association with increased mortality after acute myocardial infarction. Am J Cardiol 59:256, 1987.
53. Follansbee WD, Michelson EL, Morganroth J: Unsustained ventricular tachycardia in ambulatory patients. Characteristics associated with sudden cardiac death. Ann Int Med 92:741, 1980.
54. Meineitz T, Hofmann J, Kasper W, et al.: Significance of ventricular arrhythmias in idiopathic dilated cardiomyopathy. Am J Cardiol 53:902, 1984.
55. Holmes J, Kubo SJ, Cody RJ, et al.: Arrhythmias in ischemic and nonischemic dilated cardiomyopathy: Prediction of mortality by ambulatory electrocardiography. Am J Cardiol 55:146, 1985.
56. Unverferth DV, Magorien RD, Moeschberger ML, et al.: Factors influencing the one-year mortality of dilated cardiomyopathy. Am J Cardiol 54:147, 1984.
57. Huang SK, Messer JV, Denes P: Significance of ventricular tachycardia in idiopathic dilated cardiomyopathy: observations in 35 patients. Am J Cardiol 51:507, 1983.
58. Costanzo-Nordin MR, O'Connell JB, Engelmeier RS, et al.: Ventricular tachycardia in dilated cardiomyopathy: A variable independent of hemodynamics, morphology and prognosis (Abstract). J Am Coll Cardiol 3:594, 1984.
59. Maron BJ, Savage DD, Wolfson JK, et al.: Prognostic significance of 24-hour ambulatory electrocardiographic monitoring in patients with hypertrophic cardiomyopathy: A prospective study. Am J Cardiol 48:252, 1981.
60. Graboys TB: Limitations of ambulatory ECG recording to assess therapy in the individual patient. In Wenger NK, Mock MB, Ringqvist I (eds): Ambulatory Electrocardiographic Recording, pp. 367–377. Chicago, Year Book Med Publishers, 1981.
61. Cranfield PT, Wit AL, Hoffman BF: Genesis of cardiac arrhythmias. Circulation 47:190, 1973.
62. Podrid PJ, Graboys TB: Exercise stress testing in the management of cardiac rhythm disorders. Med Clin North Am 68:1139, 1984.
63. Antmann ES, Graboys TB, Lown B: Comparison of continuous to intermittent electrocardiographic monitoring during exercise testing for exposure of cardiac arrhythmias. JAMA 241:2802, 1979.
64. Beard EF, Owen CA: Cardiac arrhythmias during exercise stress testing in healthy men. Aerospace Med 44:286, 1973.
65. Masters AM: Cardiac arrhythmias elicited by the two-step exercise test. Am J Cardiol 32:766, 1973.

66. Jelinek MV, Lown B: Exercise testing for exposure of cardiac arrhythmia. Prog Cardiovasc Dis 16:497, 1974.
67. McHenry PL, Fisch C, Jordan JW: Cardiac arrhythmias observed during maximal exercise testing in clinically normal men. Am J Cardiol 29:331, 1978.
68. Whinnery JE: Dysrhythmia comparison in apparently healthy males during and after treadmill and accelerated stress test. Am Heart J 105:732, 1983.
69. Gooch AS, McConnell D: Analysis of transient arrhythmia and conduction disturbances occurring during submaximal treadmill exercise testing. Prog Cardiovasc Dis 13:293, 1970.
70. Graboys TB, Wright RF: Provocation of supraventricular tachycardia during exercise stress testing. Cardiovasc Rev Rep 1:57, 1980.
71. Poblete PF, Kennedy HC, Cavales DG: Detection of ventricular ectopy in patients with coronary heart disease and normal subjects by exercise testing and ambulatory electrocardiography. Chest 74:402, 1978.
72. Wild FM, Chu KL, Bigger JT, et al.: Risk stratification with low-level exercise test two weeks after myocardial infarction. Circulation 64:306, 1981.
73. Udall JA, Ellestad MJ: Predictive complications of ventricular premature contractions associated with treadmill stress testing. Circulation 56:985, 1977.
74. Califf RM, McKinnis RA, McNeer JF, et al.: Prognostic value of ventricular arrhythmias associated with treadmill exercise testing in patients studied with cardiac catheterization for suspected ischemic heart disease. J Am Coll Cardiol 2L1060, 1983.
75. Irving J, Bruce R: Exertional hypotension and post exertional ventricular fibrillation in stress testing. Am J Cardiol 39:849, 1977.
76. Atterhog J, Jonsson B, Samuelson R: Exercise testing: A prospective study of complication rates. Am Heart J 98:572, 1979.
77. Young D, Lampert S, Graboys TB, et al.: Safety of maximal exercise testing in patients at high risk for ventricular arrhythmia. Circulation 70:184, 1984.
78. Podrid PJ: New and investigational antiarrhythmic drugs. Prim Cardiol 11(10):139, 1985.
79. Lown B: Sudden cardiac death: The major challenge confronting contemporary cardiology. Am J Cardiol 43:313, 1979.
80. Allessie MA, Binke FIM, Schopman FJG: Arcus movement in rabbit atrial muscle as a mechanism of tachycardia. III. The "leading circle" concept. Circ Res 41:9, 1977.
81. Willins HJJ, Lie KI, Duren DR: Observations of mechanisms of ventricular tachycardia in man. Circulation 54:237, 1976.
82. Podrid PJ, Lown B, Graboys TB, et al.: Use of short-term drug testing as part of a systematic approach for evaluation of antiarrhythmic drugs. Circulation 73(Suppl 2):81, 1986.
83. Graboys TB, Lown B, Podrid PJ, et al.: Long-term survival of patients with malignant ventricular arrhythmias treated with antiarrhythmic drugs. Am J Cardiol 50:437, 1982.
84. Gaughan CE, Lown B, Lanigan J, et al.: Acute oral testing for determining antiarrhythmic drug efficacy. I. Quinidine. Am J Cardiol 38:677, 1976.
85. Podrid PJ, Lown B: Mexiletine for ventricular arrhythmias. Am J Cardiol 47:895, 1981.
86. Podrid PJ, Lown B: Propafenone—a new drug for ventricular arrhythmias. J Am Coll Cardiol 4:117, 1984.
87. Podrid PJ, Lown B: Tocainide therapy for refractory symptomatic ventricular arrhythmia. Am J Cardiol 49:127, 1982.
88. Chesnie B, Lampert S, Podrid P, et al.: Lorcainide for refractory ventricular arrhythmias. J Am Coll Cardiol 3:1531, 1984.
89. Hession M, Lampert S, Podrid PJ, et al.: Ethmozine therapy in patients with complex arrhythmia. Am J Cardiol 60:59F, 1987.
90. Hirsowitz G, Podrid PJ, Lampert S, et al.: The role of beta blocking agents as adjunct therapy to membrane stabilizing drugs in malignant ventricular arrhythmia. Am Heart J 111:852, 1986.
91. Bigger JT: Interaction of mexiletine with other cardiovascular drugs. Am Heart J 107:1079, 1984.
92. Deedwania PL, Olukotun AY, Kupersmith J, et al.: Beta blockers in combination with class 1 antiarrhythmic agents. Am J Cardiol 60:21D, 1987.
93. Duff HJ, Roden D, Primm RK, et al.: Mexiletine in the treatment of resistant ventricular arrhythmias. Enhancement of efficacy and reduction of dose-related side effects by combination with quinidine. Circulation 67:1124, 1983.
94. Klein RC, Marcus FI: Efficacy of propafenone when used in combination antiarrhythmic therapy. J Electrophysiol 1:575, 1987.
95. Podrid PJ, Lampert S, Graboys TB, et al.: Aggravation of arrhythmia by antiarrhythmic drugs. Incidence and predictors. Am J Cardiol 59:38E, 1982.
96. Velebit V, Podrid PJ, Cohen B, et al.: Aggravation and provocation of ventricular arrhythmias by antiarrhythmic drugs. Circulation 65:886, 1982.
97. Morganroth J, Horowitz LN: Flecainide: Its proarrhythmic effect and expected changes in the surface electrocardiogram. Am J Cardiol 58:893, 1984.
98. Slater W, Lampert S, Podrid PJ, et al.: Clinical predictors of arrhythmia worsening by antiarrhythmic drugs. Am J Cardiol (in press 1988).
99. Morgensen L: Ventricular tachyarrhythmias and lignocaine prophylaxis in acute myocardial infarction. Acta Med Scand 513(Suppl):1, 1970.
100. Bennett MA, Wilner JM, Pentecoste BC: Controlled trial of lignocaine in prophylaxis of ventricular arrhythmias complicating myocardial infarction. Lancet 2:909, 1970.
101. Lie KJ, Wellens HJ, Van Champell FS, et al.: Lidocaine in the prevention of primary ventricular fibrillation. A double-blind randomized study of 212 consecutive patients. N Engl J Med 2291:1324, 1974.
102. Ryden L, Amman D, Conradson TB, et al.: Prophylaxis of ventricular tachyarrhythmias with intravenous and oral tocainide in patients with and recovering from acute myocardial infarction. Am Heart J 100:1006, 1980.
103. Campbell RWF, Achuff SC, Pottage A, et al.: Mexiletine in the prophylaxis of ventricular arrhythmias during acute myocardial infarction. J Cardiovasc Pharmacol 1:43, 1979.
104. Chamberlain DR, Julian DG, Boyle DM, et al.: Oral mexiletine in high-risk patients after myocardial infarction. Lancet 2:1224, 1980.
105. IMPACT Research Group. International mexiletine and placebo antiarrhythmic coronary trials: Report on arrhythmia and other findings. J Am Coll Cardiol 4:1148, 1984.
106. Hugenholtz PG, Hagemeijer F, Lubsen J, et al.: One-year followup in patients with persistent ventricular dysrhythmias after myocardial infarction treated with aprindine or placebo. In Sandoe E, Julian DG, Bell JW (eds.): Management of Ventricular Tachycardia Role of Mexiletine, pp. 572–604. Amsterdam, Excerpta Medica, 1978.
107. Gottleib S, Achuff SC, Millets EO, et al.: Prophylactic antiarrhythmic therapy of high-risk survivors of myocardial infarction. Lower mortality at 1 month but not at 1 year. Circulation 75:792, 1987.
108. Jones DT, Kostuk WJ, Gunton RW: Prophylactic quinidine for the prevention of arrhythmias after acute myocardial infarction. Am J Cardiol 33:655, 1974.
109. Holmberg S, Bergman H: Prophylactic quinidine treatment in myocardial infarction. Acta Med Scand 181:297, 1967.
110. Collaborative Group. Phenytoin after recovery from myocardial infarction. Controlled trial in 568 patients. Lancet 2:1055, 1971.
111. Peter T, Ross D, Duffield A, et al.: Effect on survival after myocardial infarction of long-term treatment with phenytoin. Br Heart J 42:1356, 1978.
112. Zainel N, Griffiths JW, Carmichael DJS, et al: Oral disopyramide for the prevention of arrhythmias in patients with acute myocardial infarction admitted to open wards. Lancet 2:887, 1977.
113. Jennings G, Jones MBA, Besterman EMM, et al.: Oral disopyramide in prophylaxis of arrhythmias following myocardial infarction. Lancet 1:51, 1976.
114. Koch Weser J, Klein SW, Foo-Canto LL, et al.: Antiarrhythmic prophylaxis with procainamide on acute myocardial infarction. N Engl J Med 281:1253, 1969.
115. Kosowsky BD, Taylor J, Lown B, Ritchie RF: Long term use of procainamide following acute myocardial infarction. Circulation 47:1204, 1973.

116. CAPS Investigators. The cardiac arrhythmia pilot study. Am J Cardiol 57:91, 1986.
117. Schaffer WA, Cobb LA: Recurrent ventricular fibrillation and modes of death in survivors of out-of-hospital ventricular fibrillation. N Engl J Med 293:259, 1975.
118. Vlay SC, Rackman CH, Reid PR: Prognostic assessment of ventricular tachycardia and ventricular fibrillation with ambulatory monitoring. Am J Cardiol 54:87, 1984.
119. Hoffmann A, Schutz E, White R, et al.: Suppression of high-grade ventricular ectopic activity by antiarrhythmic drug treatment as a marker for survival in patients with chronic coronary artery disease. Am Heart J 107:1103, 1984.
120. Stein J, Podrid PJ, Lampert S, et al.: Long-term mexiletine for ventricular arrhythmias. Am Heart J 107:1091, 1984.
121. Hohnloser SH, Long HW, Raeder EA, et al.: Short- and long-term tocainide therapy for malignant ventricular tachyarrhythmias. Circulation 73:143, 1986.
122. Tordjman T, Podrid PJ, Raeder E, et al.: Encainide for malignant ventricular arrhythmias. Am J Cardiol 58:87C, 1986.
123. Cueni L, Podrid PJ: Propafenone therapy in patients with serious ventricular arrhythmia—Noninvasive evaluation of efficacy. J Electrophysiol 1:548, 1987.
124. Sheps DS, Ernst JC, Briese FR, et al.: Decreased frequency of exercise induced ventricular ectopic activity in the second of two consecutive treadmill tests. Circulation 55:892, 1977.

6

Normal and Abnormal Sinus Node Function

Jay L. Jordan
Hrayr S. Karagueuzian
Eli S. Gang
C. Thomas Peter
William J. Mandel

NORMAL ANATOMY

The sinus node is a highly organized cluster of specialized cells located in the area of the junction between the superior vena cava and right atrium.[1] Crescent shaped, it varies in length from 9 to 15 mm and has a central body (5-mm wide and 1.5- to 2-mm thick) and tapering ends. A perinodal zone of unique cell type surrounding the sinus node of the rabbit has been identified. These perinodal fibers have electrophysiologic characteristics distinct from those of the sinus node and normal atrial tissue and may represent a buffer zone through which electrical activity must pass on its way out of or into the sinus node.

The vascular supply to the mammalian sinus node region comes from a central artery that does not appear to terminate in the sinus node. A rich supply of collateral vessels, densest centrally and sparser peripherally, is a constant feature. In humans, a single sinus node artery originates from the proximal 2 to 3 cm of the right coronary artery in 55%, and from the proximal 1 cm of the left circumflex artery in 45%.

SINOATRIAL NODE ELECTROGENESIS

The phenomenon of spontaneous phase-4 depolarization is the electrophysiologic characteristic that distinguishes pacemaker cells from all other cells in the body. Emergence of the sinus node as the dominant cardiac pacemakers is due to two basic electrophysiologic properties of the sinus node pacemaker cells: (1) the low level of the resting or maximum diastolic membrane potential (-60 mV) and (2) the rapid rate of rise of phase-4 diastolic depolarization. Extensive microelectrode studies using voltage-clamp indicate that sinoatrial pacemaker current is not a single pure current.

A time-dependent decay of potassium current (IK) superimposed on activation of the fast inward current if (also known as ip and ih) and on the slow inward (isi) current has been implicated in pacemaking.[2,3] A dominant role of IK decay has been ascribed to the true pacemaker cells with isi (carried mainly by calcium ions) contributing only to the last third of the pacemaker depolarization and to the upstroke. The contribution of if current (carried mainly by sodium ions) appears to be in perinodal cells where the maximum diastolic potential is more negative than that of the true nodal (central) cells.[2]

The rate of spontaneous depolarization of a pacemaker cell is determined by the level of maximum diastolic potential, the rate or slope of phase-4 depolarization, the level of the threshold potential, the rate of rise and amplitude of phase 0, and duration of the action potential (Fig. 6–1). Thus, slowing of the rate of spontaneous sinus node discharge may be due to an increased maximum diastolic potential, a reduced slope of diastolic depolarization, a threshold potential less negative than normal, a reduced slope and amplitude of phase 0, or a prolonged duration of the action potential.

An apparent slowing of sinus node automaticity,

Supported in part by ECHO Research Fund of Cedars-Sinai Medical Center. H. S. Karagueuzian is the recipient of Research Career Development Award No. HL 01293-05, National Heart, Lung, and Blood Institute, Bethesda, Md.

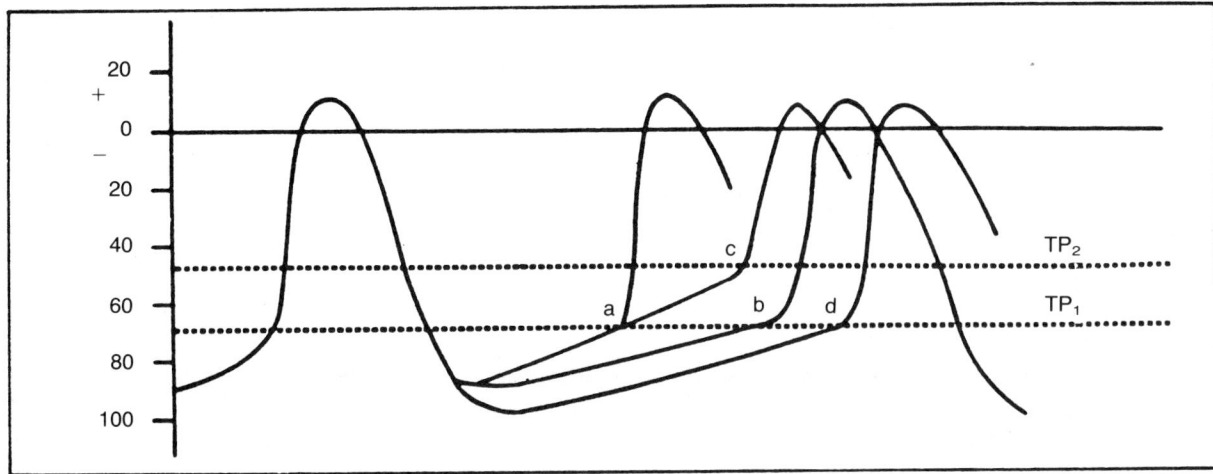

FIGURE 6–1
A typical sinus node action potential is seen on this graph. An indication of action potential voltage in millivolts is shown on the vertical axis. Points a and b identify different frequencies of sinus node depolarization dependent on the slope of phase 4 depolarization. In action potentials b and d, with equal slopes of phase 4 deplorization, maximum diastolic potential in b is greater (more negative than in d); therefore, the rate of discharge of the sinus node pacemaker in d is slower than in b. Another feature that will alter the rate of discharge of the sinus node is the threshold potential. At points, a, b, and d, the threshold potential is approximately −70 mV; at point c, the threshold potential is approximately −48 mV. This upward shift in the threshold potential (i.e., to less negative) results in a slowing in the rate of discharge when points a and c are compared.

manifesting itself electrocardiographically in a manner indistinguishable from abnormalities of sinus node pacemaker function, may result from slowing of conduction through the sinoatrial junction. Depression of sinoatrial conduction by verapamil in isolated rabbit sinus node preparations suggests that the slow channel plays a significant role in determining the conduction properties of the perinodal zone.[4]

EXTRINSIC FACTORS MODIFYING ELECTROPHYSIOLOGIC CHARACTERISTICS OF THE SINUS NODE

The Role of the Autonomic Nervous System

The mechanisms of initiating spontaneous phase-4 depolarization and the determinants of the rate of spontaneous depolarization are intrinsic properties of the pacemaker cell. Similarly, sinoatrial conduction time is a function of the intrinsic electrophysiologic properties of the sinoatrial junction. However, the characteristics of these intrinsic properties can be modified by parasympathetic and sympathetic influences.

Vagal stimulation or acetylcholine slows the sinus rate and intranodal conduction velocity and lengthens the effective and relative refractory period of the sinus node.[5] Corresponding changes in the sinus node action potential include increased negativity of the maximum diastolic potential and reduced slope of phase-4 diastolic depolarization.[6,7] In contrast, sympathetic stimulation or catecholamine infusion increases the spontaneous sinus node discharge rate, primarily because the rate of phase-4 depolarization is increased.[7,8] Sinoatrial conduction time is shortened by sympathetic stimulation.

During simultaneous stimulation of the sympathetic and parasympathetic systems, deceleration of sinus rate due to cholinergic stimulation predominates over the acceleratory effects of sympathetic stimulation. MacKary and coworkers[9] determined that when acetylcholine is added to a sinus node preparation, either alone or in combination with epinephrine, pacemaker shift occurs from the superior part of the sinus node to the inferior portion. Pacemaker cells in the inferior portion demonstrate deceleration due to acetylcholine, which is enhanced in the presence of epinephrine. Thus, functional inhomogeneity of the sinus node would seem to explain, in part, the predominance of the effect of cholinergic stimulation over that of sympathetic stimulation.

The Role of the Endocrine System

Sinus node cells isolated from the hearts of thyrotoxic rabbits have an increased rate of diastolic depolarization and a decreased action potential duration. In contrast, sinus node cells isolated from hypothyroid rabbits have a decreased rate of diastolic depolarization and an increased action potential duration.[10]

The Role of the Sinus Node Artery

The sinus node artery is larger than anticipated from knowledge of the extent of the area that it supplies. This disproportionately large size is considered by James and Nadeau to be of physiologic importance.[11,12] Based on predictable responses of the sinus rate to stretch[13,14] and the special arrangement of the sinus node cells around the sinus node artery, James suggests that the distention and collapse of this vessel play an important role in regulating sinus rate. Collapse of the artery results in an increase in tension on pacemaker cells (stretch) because of the relationship between the cells and the artery through the attachment of collagen to both the nodal cells and the arterial wall. Collapse of the artery thereby increases sinus rate. Distention of the artery has the opposite effect, leading to relaxation of the nodal cells and slowing of the heart rate. The precise intrinsic electrophysiologic properties of the sinus node that are modified by stretch and, therefore, by sinus node artery perfusion pressure have not yet been clearly defined.

Other Extrinsic Factors

Hypothermia depresses sinus automaticity by increasing the negativity of the maximum diastolic membrane potential, an effect mediated through inhibition of the sodium pump, resulting in accumulation of intracellular sodium. Hypothermia also reverses the acceleratory effect of increased extracellular calcium concentration and therefore may retard conductance through the slow channel.[15, 16] Conversely, hyperthermia in the isolated preparation and fever in humans increases sinus rate.[15]

Sinus Node Dysfunction

DEFINITION

The sick sinus syndrome is a descriptive term coined by Lown[17] and popularized by Ferrer[18] referring to a constellation of signs, symptoms, and electrocardiographic criteria defining sinus node dysfunction in a clinical setting. The syndrome is characterized by syncope or other manifestations of cerebral dysfunction in association with sinus bradycardia, sinus arrest, sinoatrial block, alternating bradyarrhythmias and tachyarrhythmias, or carotid hypersensitivity. However, clinical signs and symptoms result from failure of escape pacemaker function, not from sinus node malfunction per se. Thus, the sick sinus syndrome may represent a generalized disorder of the specialized conduction system of the heart, sinus node dysfunction being only one aspect.

INCIDENCE

The incidence of sinus node dysfunction in the general population is unknown. Limited information suggests that in cardiac patients the incidence of sinus node dysfunction is approximately 3 in 5000.[19] Between 6.3% and 24% of all patients with permanent pacemakers followed in pacemaker clinics worldwide have evidence of sinus node disease.[20-26] With increasing clinical awareness of the sick sinus syndrome and more liberal criteria for pacemaker insertion in general, in recent years abnormalities of sinus node function may have been the primary indication for permanent pacing in as many as 50% of permanently paced patients. Men and women appear to be equally affected by disturbances of sinus node function.[27] In terms of age, there seems to be a bimodal distribution of incidence of sinus node dysfunction, with peaks occurring in the third and fourth decades of life and again in the seventh (Fig. 6–2). The majority of patients in the older age group have coexisting hypertensive heart disease or coronary artery disease,[27-29] although many exceptions to this association have been cited.

ETIOLOGY

Many etiologic factors have been implicated in the development of abnormalities of sinus node function.[30-34] The most frequent anatomic findings in patients with the sick sinus syndrome are coronary atherosclerosis, atrial amyloidosis and diffuse fibrosis. Although sinus node dysfunction is characteristically thought of as a disease of the aged, the precise anatomic concomitants of the aging process responsible for sinus node dysfunction in the elderly have not been elucidated. The syndrome has also been described in association with other infiltrative disorders; collagen vascular disease; infectious processes including diphtheria, rheumatic fever, and viral myocarditis; as a familial pattern; and pericardial disease. Drug-induced abnormalities of sinus node function have been recognized with increasing frequency. However, perhaps the most common form of the sick sinus syndrome is the idiopathic variety.

Special consideration should be given to sinus node dysfunction in the setting of acute myocardial infarction. Sinus bradycardia is a common clinical manifestation of acute inferior and lateral myocardial infarction, and even sinus arrest has occasionally been reported.[35-37] Whether these manifestations of sinus node dysfunction are the consequence of ischemia to the sinus node per se or reflect local autonomic neural effects or edematous changes in surrounding tissue is speculative.[38, 39] Although the majority of patients demonstrate only transient depression of sinus node func-

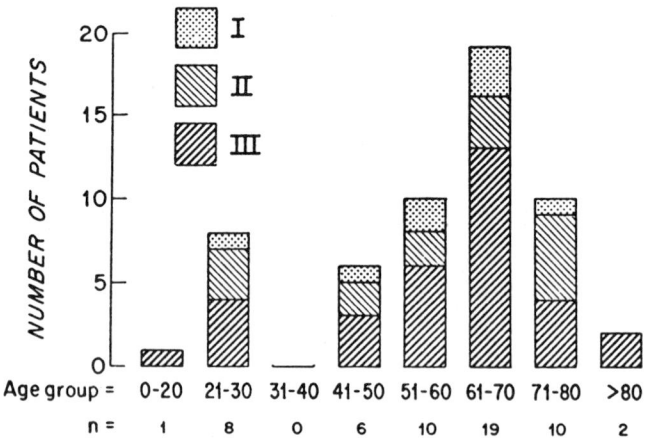

FIGURE 6–2
This figure demonstrates the age of onset of sinus node dysfunction in a group of sinus node dysfunction patients. Note the bimodal distribution of the patient population, with the vast majority being over 50 years of age. However, a small subgroup of patients are below the age of 30. (Reproduced by permission of the American Heart Association, Inc., from Rubenstein, JJ, et al.: Clinical spectrum of the sick sinus syndrome. Circulation 46:5, 1972.)

tion during the acute stage of the infarct, a small number will develop evidence of permanent sinus node dysfunction. Unfortunately, no long-term follow-up study of a large population of these patients has been reported that would allow a statement on the incidence of permanent sinus node dysfunction following an acute myocardial infarction. Experimental occlusion of the sinus node artery in dogs has resulted in variable degrees of sinus node dysfunction, ranging from profound slowing to no response whatsoever.[40-42] The variability in response has been attributed to differences in extent of collaterals and the occasional multiplicity of sinus node arteries in canine hearts.[43, 44]

ELECTROCARDIOGRAPHIC MANIFESTATIONS OF SINUS NODE DYSFUNCTION

Regular sinus rhythm is the normal rhythm of the heart. The normal rate of impulse formation by the sinus node in the adult is conventionally accepted as 60 to 100 beats/min. Sinus rhythm has a frontal-plane P vector oriented to the left and inferior generally between +30° and +60° (Fig. 6–3). A regular sinus rhythm with a rate over 100 defines sinus tachycardia. Sinus tachycardia rarely exceeds 160 beats per minute (bpm) in the adult; however, in the young adult, the normal sinus node is capable of discharging at rates over 180 bpm under the influence of maximum physiologic or pharmacologic stimulation. The maximum rate at which the sinoatrial junction is normally able to conduct sinus impulses is unknown. A regular sinus rhythm with a rate less than 60 bpm defines sinus bradycardia, perhaps the commonest electrocardiographic manifestation of sinus node dysfunction.

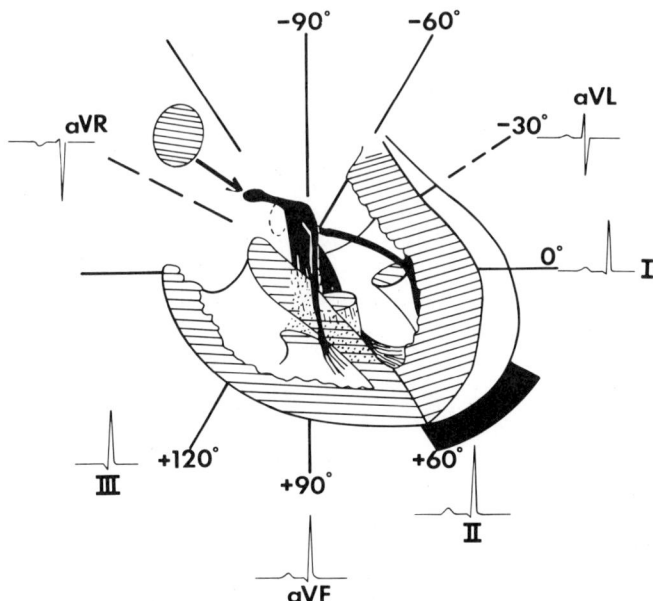

FIGURE 6–3
This diagram illustrates the normal P wave activation. Note that the normal P wave vector is between +30° and +60° in the frontal plane, leading to an isoelectric P wave in lead III and a negative P wave in lead aVR.

Sinus Arrhythmia

In sinus arrhythmia, the pacemaker is the sinus node but the rhythm is irregular. The definition of sinus arrhythmia has not been standardized; some authorities consider sinus arrhythmia to be present when the difference between the shortest P-P interval and the longest P-P interval is greater than 120 ms.[45] Other criteria defining sinus arrhythmia include variations in sinus cycle length of 10% or more[46] and variations in P-P intervals of 160 ms or greater.[47]

Sinus rate varies normally with the phases of respiration, increasing with expiration. It is not possible to distinguish irregularity of sinus impulse formation from variable conduction velocities through the sinoatrial junction on the surface electrocardiogram. In the setting of advanced AV block, variations in ventricular rate are often accompanied by parallel variations in sinus rate. This arrhythmia is termed *ventriculophasic arrhythmia* and may be related to variations in coronary flow or to alterations in autonomic tone.

Sinus Arrest

Alternatively designated *sinus pauses* or *atrial standstill*, sinus arrest denotes a cessation of sinus node impulse formation. Criteria for minimum duration of a pause that would qualify it as an arrest of sinus activity have not been established. Characteristically, the pause is not an exact multiple of the normal P-P interval.

Typically, the period of sinus arrest in patients with SSS is terminated by a sinus beat (Fig. 6–4). Escape pacemakers often fail to assume dominance of the cardiac rhythm despite markedly prolonged durations of sinus arrest.

Sinoatrial Exit Block

Sinoatrial exit block denotes failure of the sinus node impulse to conduct normally to the atrium. The site of block may be within the sinus node itself or within the sinoatrial junction. First-degree sinoatrial block describes an abnormal prolongation of the sinoatrial conduction time. Nonetheless, in this situation each spontaneously generated nodal impulse does arrive at the atrium, albeit the arrival is delayed. First-degree sinoatrial block cannot be recognized on the surface electrocardiogram.

Second-degree sinoatrial block is characterized by periodic failure of the sinus node impulse to conduct to the atrium, which is manifested as periodic absence of a P wave on the surface electrocardiogram. Sinoatrial Wenckebach periodicity results from progressive delay of sinoatrial conduction in the face of regular sinus node pacemaker activity. Electrocardiographically, this phenomenon is manifested as a progressive shortening of the P-P interval preceding the dropped P wave (Fig. 6–5).

Advanced second-degree sinoatrial block occurs when there is a regular interruption of anterograde sinoatrial conduction not preceded by progressive pro-

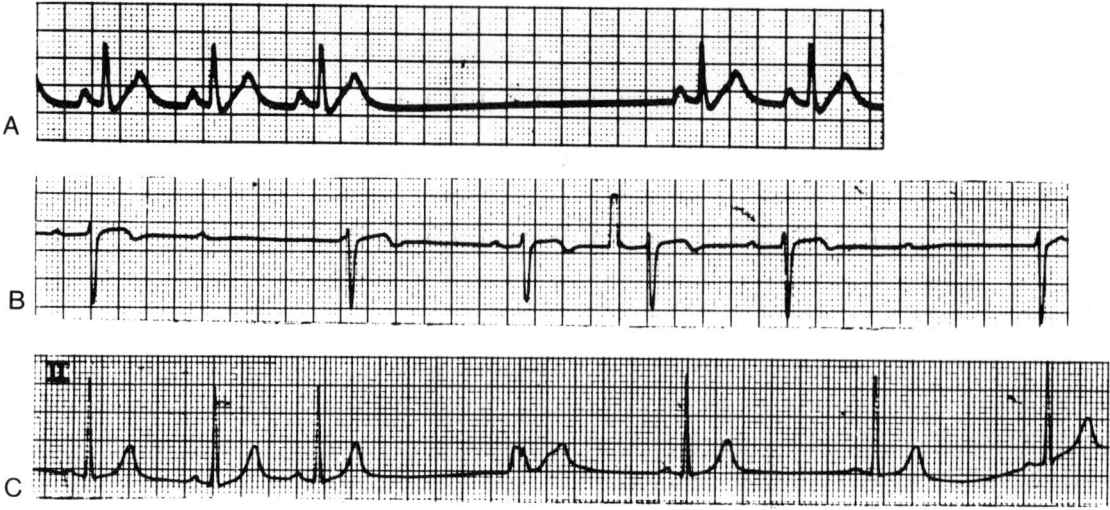

FIGURE 6–4
In A, an episode of sinus arrest occurs in which the P-P cycle of the long pause is not a multiple of basic sinus cycle length. There is no escape complex present. In B, during an episode of AV block probably of the Wenckebach type, junctional escape complexes are noted. In C, during a sinus arrhythmia, a ventricular escape complex is noted.

longation of sinoatrial conduction. Absence of a P wave on the surface electrocardiogram associated with second-degree sinoatrial block can be distinguished from that observed with sinus arrest; characteristically, the pause between P waves in the former circumstance is an exact multiple of the normal P-P interval (Fig. 6–6).

Third-degree or complete sinoatrial block cannot be distinguished from prolonged sinus arrest on the surface electrocardiogram. P waves are absent in both circumstances. Irrespective of the etiology, advanced SA block (or profound SA arrest) invariably is associated with significant clinical symptoms.

The Bradycardia-Tachycardia Syndrome

A frequent electrocardiographic manifestation of sinus node dysfunction is a pattern of slow sinus or subsidiary rhythms alternating with tachyarrhythmias, typically supraventricular in origin (Fig. 6–7). In keeping with the high incidence of atrial disease in patients with the sick sinus syndrome, atrial fibrillation is probably the supraventricular tachycardia most frequently observed in this setting. However, atrial flutter, accelerated AV junctional rhythms, and reentrant AV junctional tachycardias are also observed. Although less frequently encountered, ventricular tachycardia also may occur.[48, 49]

Abrupt spontaneous termination of a tachycardia episode is often accompanied by exaggerated suppression of sinus and subsidiary pacemaker activity in patients with SSS. Electrocardiogram abnormalities and central nervous system symptoms may become manifest only during this post-tachycardia period, sinus node dysfunction being otherwise occult in many patients with SSS.

Sinus Node Reentry

A supraventricular tachyarrhythmia unique to patients with the sick sinus syndrome is sinus node reentry tachycardia. Although some evidence suggests that sinus node reentry is a genuine phenomenon, certain investigators continue to doubt that the sinus node itself is involved in a tachycardia circuit.[50–56] Nonetheless, to qualify as a sinus node reentrant tachycardia, a supraventricular rhythm must meet certain criteria. It is usually initiated by premature atrial depolarizations occurring early in diastole; P waves during the tachyarrhythmia must have the same configuration as P waves during normal sinus rhythm; the rate of the tachyarrhythmia is characteristically slow (100 to 120

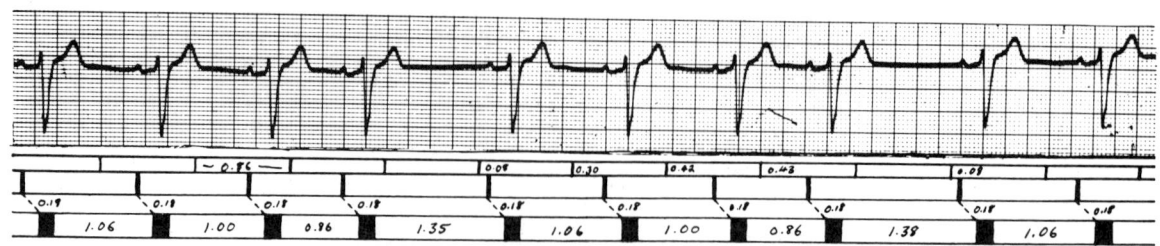

FIGURE 6–5
This electrocardiogram rhythm strip demonstrates repetitive group beating with fixed PR relationships but abbreviated R-R relationships followed by a pause. The laddergram below the tracing identifies that SA Wenckebach phenomenon occurs due to progressive delay at the SA junction. (Reproduced by permission from Greenwood RJ, Finkelstein D, Monheit R: Sinoatrial heart block with Wenckebach phenomenon. Am J Cardiol 8:141, 1961.)

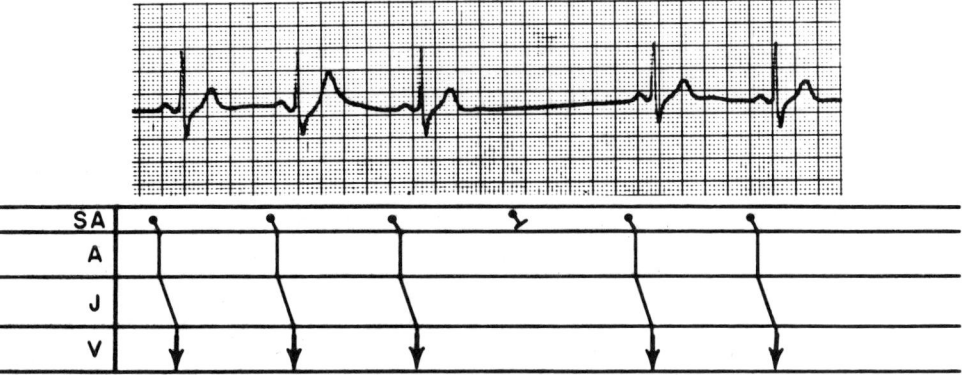

FIGURE 6–6
This rhythm strip and its accompanying laddergram identify the etiology of the pause seen on the rhythm strip. The P-P interval encompassing the pause is twice the normal sinus cycle length, showing that paroxysmal second-degree SA block occurs with delay at the SA junction.

bpm); and the duration of the arrhythmia is often brief (Fig. 6–8).[57, 58]

MECHANISMS OF SINUS NODE DYSFUNCTION IN THE SICK SINUS SYNDROME

Evaluation of sinus node function must take into account that its normal function depends on a balanced interaction between intact intrinsic electrophysiologic properties of pacemaker automaticity and sinoatrial conduction and factors extrinsic to the sinoatrial region. Thus, not only must the integrity of intrinsic electrophysiologic determinants of sinoatrial function be tested, but the integrity of the autonomic nervous system, the endocrine system, and the sinus node blood supply must also be evaluated. These extrinsic elements exert profound modifying influences on instrinsic electrophysiologic mechanisms of the sinus node and perinodal structures; dysfunction at any one of these sites may become clinically manifest as the sick sinus syndrome. Furthermore, although each component of this complex network of factors, on which normal sinus function depends, may be intact, the interaction between them may be abnormal. Possible disturbances of reflex feedback mechanisms should therefore be considered and explored.

CLINICAL AND LABORATORY EVALUATION OF SINUS NODE FUNCTION

The sick sinus syndrome must be included in the differential diagnosis of the patient with a clinical history of palpitations, vague neurologic complaints of intermittent dizziness and lightheadedness, or symptoms related to hypotension and reduced cardiac output (e.g., syncope). However, the intermittency of symptoms and electrocardiographic features may frustrate efforts to document a cause-and-effect relationship between clinical presentation and electrophysiologic events. Invasive electrophysiologic studies should be reserved for those patients in whom the diagnosis of sinus node dysfunction is in question.[59] Furthermore, the diagnostic situation in which the studies are performed should be optimized to enhance the probability that symptoms and electrocardiographic abnormalities will occur at that time.

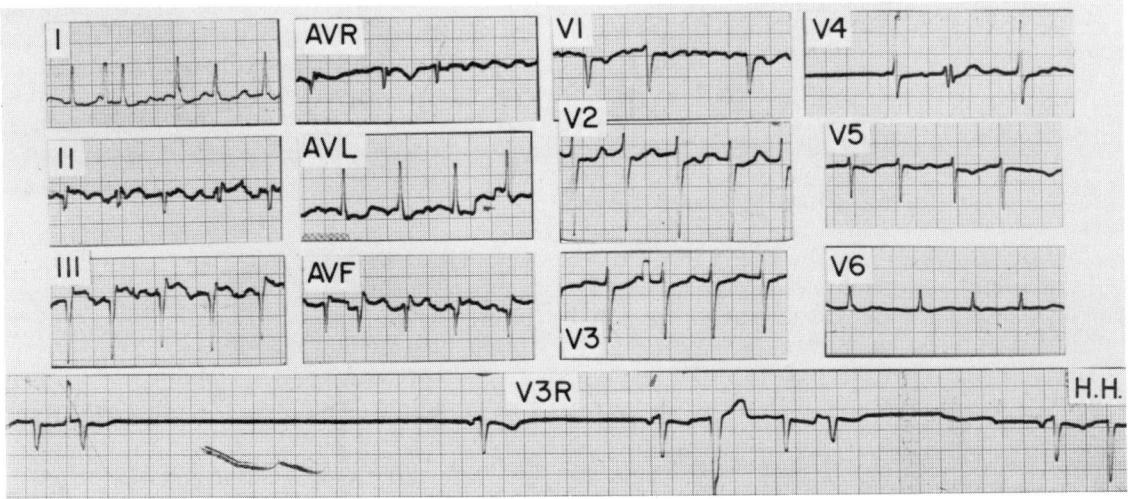

FIGURE 6–7
This standard electrocardiogram was obtained from a patient with a history of palpitations and dizziness. The 12-lead electrocardiogram identifies the presence of atrial fibrillation with a moderately rapid ventricular rate. During the rhythm strip (V3R), atrial fibrillation terminates spontaneously with a very pronounced pause followed by a sinus escape complex. This tracing is typical of episodes of bradycardia-tachycardia.

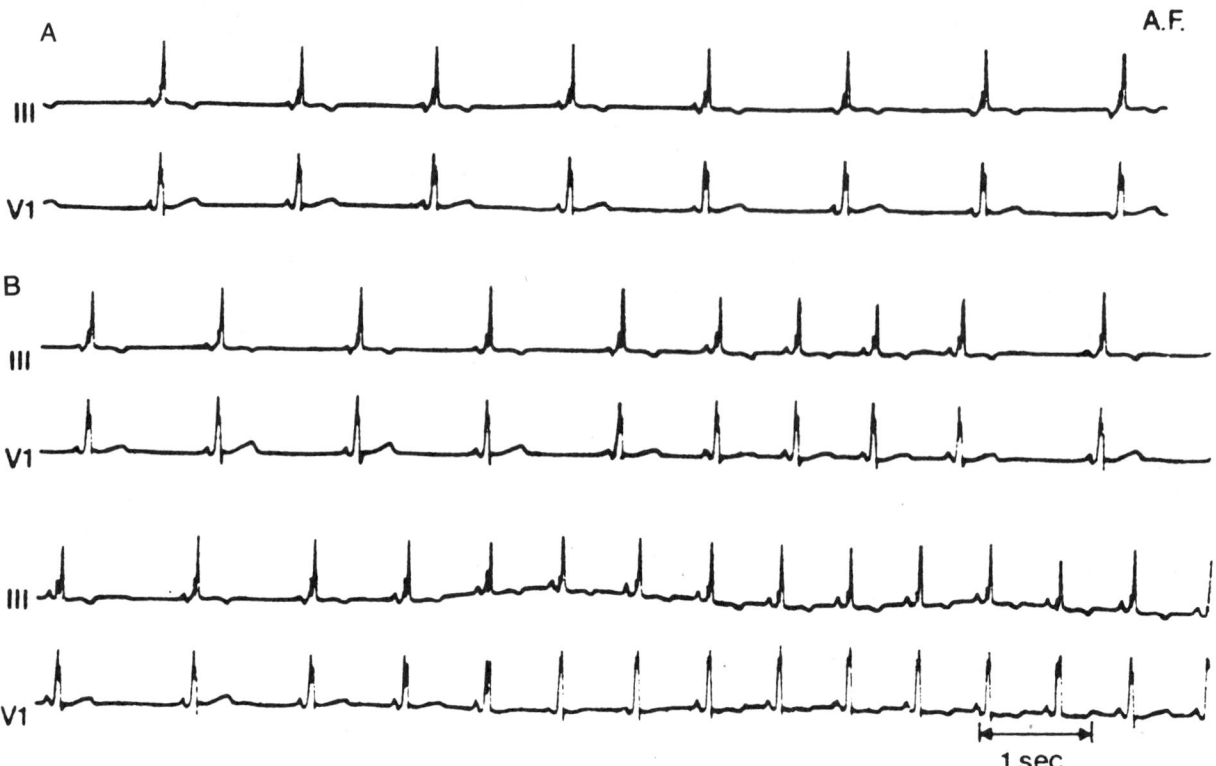

FIGURE 6–8
A, In the upper panel, sinus rhythm is interrupted by a short burst of accelerated sinus rate. In the lower panel, a more sustained episode of sinus rhythm acceleration is noted. B, In these tracings, from a different patient, termination of an episode of "sinus" tachycardia is seen, with the prompt restoration of sinus rhythm at a rate of approximately 65 beats per minute. Note the lack of change in P wave morphology in the various surface electrocardiographic leads during the burst of more rapid sinus rhythm. The episodes in both A and B are typical of paroxysmal sinus node reentry. (Reproduced by permission from Curry PVL, Krinkler DM: Paroxysmal reciprocating sinus tachycardia. In Kulbertus HE (ed.): Re-entrant Arrhythmias: Mechanisms and Treatment, p. 39. Baltimore, University Park Press, 1976.)

Electrocardiogram Monitoring

EXERCISE TESTING

Exercise testing assesses the ability of the sinus node to accelerate in response to internal physiologic chronotropic stimuli. Although a patient may have no evidence of sinus node dysfunction on the resting electrocardiogram, abnormal sinus node responses to stress may be uncovered by treadmill testing. Established norms for sinus node rate response for standard stress testing protocols for age and sex are available.[60, 61]

Exercise testing could potentially allow distinction between patients with the sick sinus syndrome and other groups of patients with slow resting or exercise heart rates.[62] For example, age-matched "healthy" patients with autonomic chronotropic incompetence secondary to myocardial disease will have lower oxygen consumption for any given heart rate during exercise because of the inability to increase cardiac output by increasing stroke volume. Also, these patients usually will not be able to reach as high a peak oxygen consumption as patients with the sick sinus syndrome with normal myocardial function.[62, 63]

In contrast to patients with abnormal sinus function, otherwise normal individuals with sinus node dysfunction as a consequence of heightened vagal tone would be expected to have normal heart rate responses to exercise.[64] Specifically, exercise is vagolytic, eliminating parasympathetic influences on sinus node function in all groups of patients. This explains the lack of effect on the maximum heart rate achieved during exercise by atropine administration.

As attractive as exercise testing may appear for distinguishing patients with sick sinus from other groups of individuals with slow heart rates, the sensitivity of the method is less than perfect. Some patients with sick sinus will demonstrate normal heart rate responses to exercise.

Holter Monitoring

Ambulatory monitoring with a Holter device is possibly a more useful physiologic technique than exercise testing for assessing sinus node function if performed during normal daily activities.[65] The intermittent occurrence of both bradyarrhythmias and tachyarrhythmias in patients with the sick sinus syndrome frequently is missed on a routine resting electrocardiogram. Furthermore, ambulatory monitoring can be diagnostic of many cases of the sick sinus syndrome if the simultaneous occurrence of symptoms and sinus dysrhythmia is documented. More recent technical advances have enabled a patient to carry a device to be used only when symptoms occur, transmitting an electrocardiogram to a central station by telephone or recording the electrocardiogram on a portable recorder.

Testing the Sinus Node–Autonomic Nervous System Axis

TESTS OF SINUS NODE RESPONSIVENESS TO AUTONOMIC ACTIVITY

The signs, symptoms, and electrocardiographic features of the sick sinus syndrome may be secondary to sinus node overresponsiveness or underresponsiveness to appropriate autonomic activity. Arguss and co-workers[64] have demonstrated that the slowing of the sinus rate with age may be, in part, secondary to increased parasympathetic tone. Other investigators have shown that in some patients sinoatrial block may be mediated by abnormal autonomic tone.[66, 67] Furthermore, it has been demonstrated that sinus arrhythmia is often produced primarily by periodic alterations in parasympathetic efferent cardiac activity.[68] Finally, patients with myocardial dysfunction have been shown to have profound abnormalities of parasympathetic and sympathetic control of heart rate.

The importance of the autonomic nervous system to intrinsic sinus node function has led some investigators to recommend that heart rate response to sympathomimetic (isoproterenol), sympatholytic (propranolol), vagotonic (bethanechol or edrophonium), and vagolytic (atropine) drugs be employed routinely in the clinical evaluation of patients with the sick sinus syndrome.[73] Unfortunately, no standardized or systematic protocols have been described for administration of these agents to evaluate heart rate response. Furthermore, before abnormalities of heart rate response to these agents can be quantified, dose-response curves in healthy subjects must be described for comparative purposes. In general, it might be anticipated that patients with intrinsic sinus node dysfunction may exhibit all, some, or various combinations of the following responses: (1) a blunted heart rate acceleration with isoproterenol administration, suggesting sinus node unresponsiveness to appropriate beta-adrenergic stimulation; (2) a blunted acceleration response to atropine, suggesting that sinus node dysfunction is not due to oversensitivity to parasympathetic tone; (3) an exaggerated response to atropine, indicating that oversensitivity to parasympathetic tone or increased parasympathetic tone are etiologic factors; and (4) an exaggerated slowing response to bethanechol or edrophonium, indicating oversensitivity to parasympathetic stimulation.

Subset of Testing the Sinus Node Autonomic Nervous System Axis

Having excluded the possibility that the sinus node responds inappropriately to changes in the autonomic environment with the above pharmacologic tests, it is then necessary to verify that the autonomic nervous system is itself intact. A characteristic clinical presentation of patients with the sick sinus syndrome may result from primary dysfunction of the autonomic nervous system. To test this possibility, autonomic activity should be provoked mechanically or pharmacologically. Carotid massage, the Valsalva maneuver, or phenylephrine-induced hypertension should normally produce slowing of the heart rate by reflex responses of the autonomic nervous system.[70–74] In contrast, lowering the blood pressure by titrated nitroprusside infusion should normally result in a reflex increase in heart rate.[74–78] In addition, heart rate changes induced by rapid positional changes should also be studied. Regrettably, blood pressure–heart rate response curves are not available for healthy subjects.

Recently, Dighton[79] suggested that persons with symptomatic sinus bradycardia are more likely to have an abnormal sinus rate response to autonomic stimulation and inhibition than are asymptomatic patients.

Intrinsic Heart Rate Determination

The intrinsic heart rate (IHR) is defined as the rate of spontaneous sinus node depolarization independent of the effects of the autonomic nervous system. The significance of the IHR is that its value theoretically depends only on intrinsic electrophysiologic mechanisms of sinus node automaticity. Complete autonomic blockade can be achieved with a modification of the protocol of Jose.[80–86] Propranolol (0.2 mg/kg) is administered intravenously at a rate of 1 mg/min to obtain a dose-response curve of heart rate response to beta blockade. Ten minutes later, atropine sulfate (0.04 mg/kg) is administered intravenously over 2 minutes. The resultant sinus rate is the observed IHR (IHR_o).

With the technique of intrinsic heart rate determination, patients with the sick sinus syndrome with intrinsic sinus node dysfunction can be distinguished from patients with disturbed autonomic regulation of sinus node function. An abnormal IHR_o reflects an abnormality of one or more intrinsic properties. In contrast, when the heart rate is normal after autonomic blockade, it follows that disturbed autonomic regulation is the most likely underlying mechanism responsible for the manifestations of sinus node dysfunction.

Normal values of intrinsic heart rate can be determined using the linear regression equation derived by Jose, relating predicted IHR (IHR_p) to age.[80]

$$IHR_p = 118.1 - (0.57 \times age)$$

For young individuals (under 45 years), the 95% confidence limit of IHR_p is $\pm 14\%$; for older individuals (over 45 years), the 95% confidence limit of IHR_p is $\pm 18\%$. An IHR_o falling within two standard deviations (SD) of the predicted IHR is considered indicative of normal sinus node function. Conversely, an IHR_o falling below and outside the 95% confidence limit of IHR_p is considered to be compatible with abnormal intrinsic sinus node function.

A comparative measure of intrinsic sinus node function also has been derived.[81] The ratio of IHR_o to the lowest it could be and still be normal (i.e., $IHR_o/IHR_p - 2SD$) represents a quantitative measure of the integrity of intrinsic sinus node function. By this method a ratio of 1 or greater indicates normal sinus node function.

Autonomic influences on intrinsic electrophysiologic properties of the sinus node vary from moment to moment depending on a host of internal and external stimuli and inhibitors. Moreover, autonomic influences can either mask or exaggerate abnormalities of intrinsic electrophysiologic properties, contributing to the evanescent quality of electrocardiographic features of the sick sinus syndrome. On the other hand, the intrinsic heart rate has been shown to be stable on repeated determinations over extended periods.

The magnitude and direction of autonomic tone at any point can be semiquantitated in humans by using the technique of IHR determination. The percentage of a person's resting heart rate (RHR) attributable to negative or positive autonomic chronotropic influences on intrinsic electrophysiologic mechanisms of sinus node automaticity can be determined by the following formula[81]:

$$(RHR/IHR - 1.00) \times 100$$

If a person's RHR is less than his or her IHR, the resultant value will be negative, indicating that net negative autonomic chronotropy is present. When the RHR is greater than the IHR, net positive autonomic chronotropy is present and the value will be positive.

Atrial Overdrive (Sinus Node Recovery Time)

In 1884, Gaskell reported that termination of rapid cardiac rhythms in the turtle heart resulted in a delay of return of spontaneous pacemaker activity.[82] Subsequent clinical reports emphasized this phenomenon in ventricular pacemakers.[83–85] Using these clinical observations, Lange[86] systematically studied overdrive suppression of the sinus node in the laboratory. With the use of transvenous pacing catheters, overdrive suppression evolved into a means of evaluating sinus node function in humans.[87]

Until recently, "suppression" of sinus node pacemaker automaticity by atrial overdrive pacing was considered a phenomenon that could be of value in unmasking occult sinus node dysfunction in many patients with the sick sinus syndrome.[88–90] Transient arrest of spontaneous sinus node activity follows cessation of overdrive atrial pacing as an apparent physiologic event. In general, patients with sinus node dysfunction demonstrate longer periods of sinus arrest than do healthy subjects (Fig. 6–9). The mechanism(s) by which overdrive pacing suppresses pacemaker automaticity has been the subject of much speculation. Two general hypotheses have received serious consideration in the clinical and experimental laboratory: (1) suppression is mediated by the release of autonomic neurotransmitters, and (2) overdrive pacing directly disrupts intrinsic mechanisms of pacemaker automaticity.[86, 91, 92]

Atrial overdrive pacing does result in a release of autonomic neurotransmitters from storage sites within myocardial tissue and nerve endings.[6, 93] Assuming that there is a net release of a negative chronotropic neurotransmitter, presumably acetylcholine, suppression of sinus node automaticity may indeed be mediated by this neurohumoral agent. Vagal stimulation or acetylcholine administration does in fact prolong sinus node recovery. That catecholamine release also plays a role in post-overdrive electrophysiologic events is suggested by the observation that post-overdrive acceleration of the sinus rate can be abolished by reserpine or propranolol pretreatment.[82] Moreover, isoproterenol infusion results in a predictable shortening of the sinus node recovery time (SNRT).

Recent observations in the microelectrode laboratory on the relationship between rate of overdrive pacing and SNRT have significantly advanced our understanding of the mechanisms and determinants of sinus node recovery time[94, 95]:

1. Using small sinus node preparations and pacing at a closer proximity to the pacemaker cell (<5 mm) minimizes acetylcholine release and unmasks the direct effects of overdrive pacing on pacemaker automaticity. These effects on the sinus pacemaker action potential are directly proportional to the rate of penetration of paced beats and are not reversed by atropine.

2. The extent of sinus node pacemaker suppression is directly related to the number of paced beats actually penetrating it per unit of time. Paced beats that fail to penetrate the sinus node do not suppress pacemaker automaticity to the same extent as paced beats penetrating the sinus pacemaker.

3. Overdrive pacing directly hypopolarizes the sinus node pacemaker cell, thus eliminating activation of the electrogenic sodium pump as a mechanism of pacemaker suppression in the sinus node.

4. Sinus node recovery time cannot be interpreted only in terms of overdrive suppression of sinus node automaticity but is the result of a complex interaction between conduction and impulse formation in the sinoatrial region. The faster the rate of overdrive pacing, the slower the retrograde sinoatrial conduction, because of progressive impingement on the relative refractory period of the perinodal zone. The faster the rate of overdrive pacing, the slower the anterograde sinoatrial conduction, because of decreased amplitude of the sinus node pacemaker action potential.

5. The mechanism by which overdrive pacing reduces the amplitude of the pacemaker action potential may be prevention of completion of phase 3 when pacing rates are rapid.

To date, abnormalities of only one potential intrinsic mechanism of sinus node automaticity have been studied with the object of uncovering the mechanism of suppression by overdrive pacing. When isolated rabbit sinus node preparations are perfused with the slow-channel inhibitor verapamil, the corrected sinus node recovery time is prolonged.[96] This finding is reproducible even when the influence of released autonomic neurotransmitters is blocked by atropine and propranolol added to the perfusate.[97] It is therefore reasonable to assume that some patients with the sick sinus syndrome demonstrating abnormal prolongation of the sinus node recovery time may have intrinsic slow-channel abnormalities.

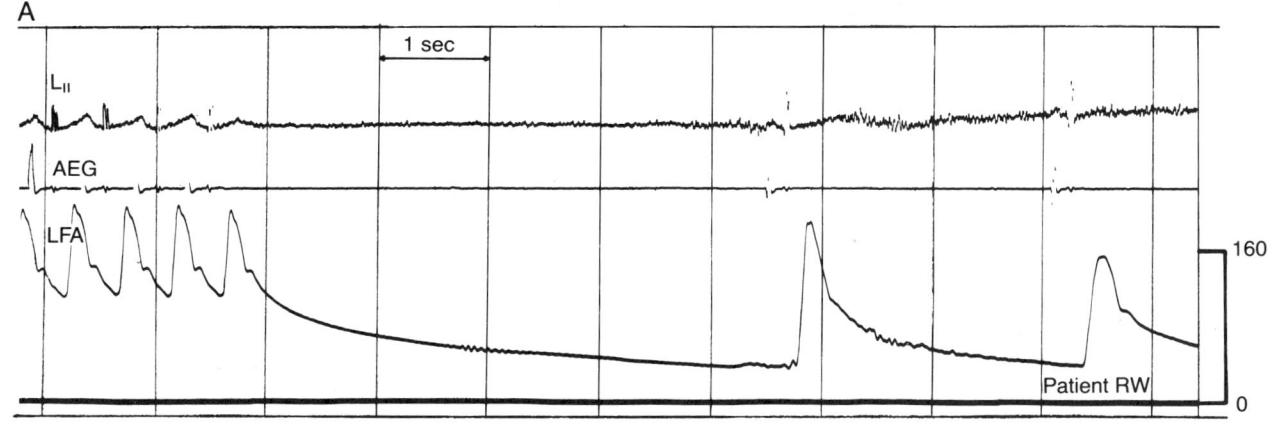

FIGURE 6–9
A typical example of marked suppression of sinus function following overdrive pacing. The tracings are, from above downward, lead II electrocardiogram, a high right atrial electrocardiogram, and left femoral artery blood pressure. Right atrial overdrive pacing at a rate of 130/min was abruptly turned off, resulting in a pause of approximately 5 seconds terminated by a sinus complex.

Another mechanism that has been considered as a possible etiology of overdrive suppression is the transient induction of ischemia of the sinus node by rapid atrial pacing. Against this hypothesis is the clinical finding that sinus node recovery time is not prolonged in patients with chronic or acute ischemia of the SA node.[98,99] The possibility that pH changes induced by rapid pacing may contribute to ionic current alterations and therefore to abnormal pacemaker suppression has not been specifically investigated. However, sinus node automaticity is certainly influenced by acid-base imbalance.[100]

Intracardiac pacing is performed in the cardiac catheterization laboratory with patients in the fasting state. All cardiac drugs known to interfere with sinus node or autonomic neural function should be withdrawn for at least 48 hours or 5 half-lives before the study; a quadripolar pacing catheter is positioned at the high right atrium. Multiple electrocardiographic leads as well as an intra-atrial electrogram are used for monitoring. Atrial pacing is performed at a milliamperage two times the diastolic threshold. An initial atrial pacing rate of approximately 20 bpm faster than the patient's resting heart rate is chosen, with increments of 20 bpm in succeeding pacing trials, up to a rate of 200 bpm. Pacing is continued for 30, 60, and 180 seconds at each pacing rate and abruptly terminated; 60 seconds is allowed to elapse between each pacing trial. The SNRT is measured in milliseconds as the time elapsing from the last paced P wave to the first spontaneous depolarization on the atrial electrogram. The shape of the P wave is noted to confirm that the complex ending the pause is indeed sinus in origin.

To control for differences in spontaneous sinus rate between patients and for the influence that it would have on the time it would take the sinus node to recover its automaticity, the sinus node recovery time may be corrected for the spontaneous sinus cycle length (SCL); thus the corrected sinus node recovery time (SNRTC) = SNRT − SCL. Benditt and associates[101] expressed SNRT as a ratio of SCL. Accordingly, SNRT/SCL ≤ 1.61 was used as the normal value for patients with sinus cycle lengths less than 800 ms. For patients with sinus cycle lengths greater than 800 ms, SNRT/SCL ≤ 1.83 was considered normal. Reported SNRT values for normal subjects include 1400 ms, 1040 ± 56 ms (M ± SEM), and 958 ± 149 ms.[87,102,103] Reported normal SNRTC values range from <450 ms to <525 ms.[89,104]

In humans and animals, SNRT increases slightly as the pacing rate increases. However, at rapid rates (>130 bpm) SNRT decreases somewhat.[87] In patients with the sick sinus syndrome, maximum SNRT often occurs at rates slower than the pacing rate at which $SNRT_{max}$ occurs in normal subjects.[105–107] It has been suggested that the pacing cycle length at which the longest postpacing pause occurs (peak paced cycle length, or PCL_p) be considered when interpreting the meaning of any particular SNRT value. Reiffel and colleagues[108] found that PCL_p was equal to or less than 600 ms in normal subjects and tended to be prolonged in patients with the sick sinus syndrome. The authors invoked the explanation that a prolonged PCL_p is a manifestation of disturbed atriosinus conduction during pacing and a prolonged perinodal refractory period.[109] Furthermore, they suggested that rate-dependent retrograde sinoatrial block during atrial pacing could result in spuriously short SNRT values in patients with the sick sinus syndrome because of failure of each paced beat to reach and depolarize sinus node pacemaker cells. Therefore, a patient with a normal SNRT but a long PCL_p may actually have a disorder of sinus node pacemaker function that escapes detection through overdrive atrial pacing if an abnormally prolonged PCL_p is not recognized. In microelectrode studies, Kerr and colleagues[110,111] have confirmed that the PCL_p is determined by the refractory period of the perinodal zone and the occurrence of retrograde sinoatrial block. In contrast, subsidiary pacemakers demonstrate significant proportional increases in recovery time with increasing pacing rates.[112] Of more importance clinically, subsidiary pacemakers have more sustained periods of suppression than the sinus node following overdrive.

Most normal subjects demonstrate little correlation between duration of pacing and SNRT.[112] The correlation in patients with the sick sinus syndrome is variable. Subsidiary pacemakers generally show a positive correlation between pacing duration and recovery time.[112] This finding may reflect different mechanisms mediating overdrive suppression in different pacemaker sites.

The proximity of the pacing catheter to the pacemaker being studied appears to be an important determinant of the magnitude of that pacemaker's overdrive suppression. Within the atrium, it has been demonstrated that a premature impulse results in a longer return cycle if delivered in the region of the coronary sinus or crista terminalis than in the intra-atrial septum.[113] In the clinical laboratory atrial pacing is performed in the high right atrium. Variations in pacing amperage cause no significant change in SNRT or SNRTC.[87] In normal subjects, the uncorrected SNRT is prolonged in a linear fashion with longer resting SCLs. However, at abnormally slow heart rates the recovery time generally becomes disproportionately prolonged.[87]

It has been shown that the sinus node recovery time in children and in elderly normal subjects is not significantly different from mean values found in the general population.[114, 115] The pacing rate at which there is a sudden decrease in SNRT seems to be slower in the elderly, suggesting that sinoatrial entrance block occurs at a slower rate.[105] This phenomenon may represent differential aging of the perinodal zone.

Generally, patients with the sick sinus syndrome with documented sinus arrest of marked duration (5 seconds or longer) and central nervous system symptoms have relatively longer SNRTC than asymptomatic patients with sinus arrest of lesser magnitude. However, exceptions to this rule demonstrate that there is probably no linear relationship between magnitude of sinus bradycardia or sinus arrest and the duration of SNRTC in patients with the sick sinus syndrome.

Patients with congestive heart failure, independent of etiology, have diminished sinus rate responses to variations in autonomic tone[69-72] as well as significantly slower intrinsic heart rates.[115] Jose suggested that in congestive heart failure the same biochemical abnormality exists in both myocardial and pacemaker cells.[115] However, the relationship between sinus node recovery time and the presence of heart failure has not been specifically investigated. Atherosclerotic disease of the sinus node artery is not associated with abnormalities of sinus node recovery time.[116] In addition, mild to moderate hypertension in the absence of cardiomegaly or heart failure does not influence sinus node response to overdrive pacing.[81]

Despite the theoretical potential for marked variations in autonomic tone, SNRT and SNRTC have been shown to be remarkably reproducible whether pacing is performed on consecutive days or at an interval of many months.[89, 105]

In some instances, sinoatrial conduction time (SACT) appears to be a clinically more sensitive indicator of electrophysiologic abnormalities of the sinoatrial region than SNRT (e.g., in the setting of atherosclerotic involvement of the sinus node artery). Even patients with gross manifestations of the sick sinus syndrome may have an abnormal SACT in association with a normal SNRT.[90, 117, 118] The comparative insensitivity of SNRT may be a consequence of sinoatrial entrance block in the diseased perinodal zone and inconsistent penetration of the sinus node.[109] The occasional finding of a paradoxical effect of atropine on SNRT (i.e., increased prolongation) may thus be accounted for on the basis of improved retrograde conduction of paced beats into the SA node.[119, 120]

That a disparity of sinus node recovery time and sinoatrial conduction time may be artifactual is suggested by observations in isolated tissue preparations in which the calcium current is abnormal. In these preparations, SNRT and SACT abnormalities invariably parallel one another.[97, 121] The relative magnitude of abnormalities of SNRT and SACT may depend on the mechanisms of sinoatrial dysfunction operative in any given patient with the sick sinus syndrome, the calcium current being equally important to both automaticity and sinoatrial conduction. Limited information suggests that sick sinus patients with abnormalities of AV nodal or intraventricular conduction may have a greater incidence of abnormal SNRT than patients without distal conduction abnormalities.[102]

Recently, the value of the sinus node recovery time as a diagnostic tool in the sick sinus syndrome has been questioned. Specifically, not all patients with the sick sinus syndrome demonstrate abnormal prolongation of the sinus node recovery time.[122] However, to expect the sinus node recovery time to be prolonged in all patients with the sick sinus syndrome presupposes that the technique of intra-atrial overdrive pacing tests an underlying pathophysiologic mechanism that is common to all cases. Based on knowledge of the large number of potential determinants of sinus node automaticity and overdrive suppression, it is unlikely that the sick sinus syndrome is a homogeneous entity in terms of pathophysiologic mechanisms and it is not surprising that all patients with the sick sinus syndrome do not demonstrate abnormal prolongation of the sinus node recovery time. In fact, Chadda and coworkers[123] have suggested that the finding of an abnormal corrected sinus node recovery time should be evaluated in terms of the role that autonomic tone plays in its value before concluding that sinus node dysfunction per se caused the abnormality.

Atropine shortens the sinus node recovery time in normal subjects. Many patients with the sick sinus syndrome have blunted sinus rate acceleration to the administration of atropine. Based on these observations, atropine has been employed to distinguish patients with the sick sinus syndrome with intrinsic sinus node disease from those with abnormally exaggerated parasympathetic influences. The effects of atropine on SNRT vary in patients with the sick sinus syndrome, shortening it in some, having no effect in others, and paradoxically prolonging it in a small number.[119, 120]

These different results may represent differences in residual parasympathetic tone.[124] Differences in resting sympathetic tone, now unopposed in the post-atropine state, also must be taken into account. All attempts to determine absolute normal values for SNRT in the post-atropine state may be thwarted because of the problems encountered in quantifying sympathetic and residual parasympathetic tone. The problems associated with determining normal values for post-propranolol SNRT are similar to those discussed for atropine. Standards for completeness of sympathetic blockade must be established, and differences in unopposed parasympathetic tone must be taken into account.

Most of the disadvantages of separate atropine and propranolol administration can be overcome by the simultaneous administration of these drugs and the determination of intrinsic heart rate at the time of atrial overdrive pacing. With the doses of atropine and propranolol employed with IHR_o determination (see above), sinus node recovery time can be automatically adjusted for the role that autonomic influences might play in its value. Alternatively, control sinus node recovery time can be adjusted mathematically for the role of autonomic influences.[81]

Adjusted SNRTC = SNRTC + SNRTC × (RHR/IHR − 1.00)

In our unit, observed intrinsic heart rates have been determined in 17 patients with symptomatic sinus bradycardia; 10 patients had normal IHR_o. Six of these patients had normal control SNRTC (<450 ms), and four had abnormal control SNRTC. Seven patients had abnormal IHR_o, and all seven patients had abnormal control SNRTC. When overdrive pacing was performed following autonomic blockade, all ten patients with normal IHR_o had normal adjusted SNRTC, whereas all seven patients with abnormal IRH_o continued to demonstrate abnormal corrected sinus node recovery times (Fig. 6–10). We concluded that: (1) the sick sinus syndrome is clearly not a homogeneous entity in terms of pathophysiologic mechanisms; (2) patients with sick sinus demonstrating normal sinus node recovery times corrected for the magnitude and direction of autonomic chronotropy consistently have normal intrinsic heart rates and, therefore, abnormalities of autonomic regulation of sinus node function; and (3) patients with sick sinus demonstrating abnormal adjusted sinus node recovery times consistently have abnormal intrinsic heart rates and, therefore, abnormalities of intrinsic sinus node function.

Subsequent investigators have demonstrated occasional exceptions to these results. However, most agree that the technique does improve the sensitivity and specificity of the sinus node recovery time as well as clarify mechanisms of sinus node dysfunction in patients with the sick sinus syndrome.

Mason[124] has reported results of overdrive atrial pacing in denervated transplanted human hearts. Sinus rate was significantly faster in denervated donor hearts than in remnant atrial and control subsets. No significant difference was found between donor SNRTC

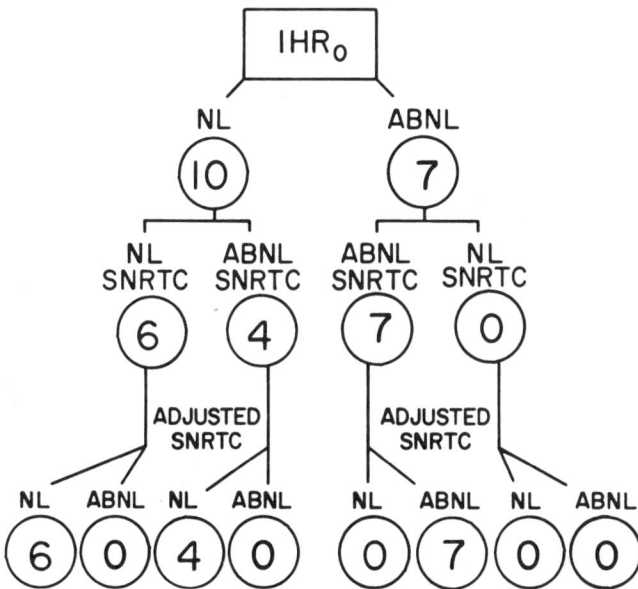

FIGURE 6–10
Use of the intrinsic heart rate to separate normal and abnormal sinus node recovery times based on intrinsic or extrinsic sinus node dysfunction. The flow diagram demonstrates that patients with normal intrinsic heart rates who have abnormal sinus node recovery times corrected for basic sinus cycle length will have corrected normal values if their SNRTC is adjusted from the degree of positive or negative chronotropic activity. The latter is based on differences between the observed intrinsic heart rate and the basal heart rate. (NL = normal; ABNL = abnormal; IHR_o = observed intrinsic heart rate; SNRTC = corrected sinus node recovery time)

(300 ± 117 ms) and recipient SNRTC (291 ± 171 ms) or control SNRTC (273 ± 171 ms). It is of clinical importance that these values compare favorably with SNRTC after pharmacologic blockade in patients with normal IHRs (287 ± 114 ms).[127] The most dramatic finding was that $SNRT_{max}$ resulted from shorter overdrive cycle lengths in donor hearts (359 ± 46 ms) than in recipient hearts (491 ± 111 ms) ($P<0.005$) or in control hearts (499 ± 82 ms) ($P<0.005$). This latter finding suggests that the sinoatrial junction is particularly sensitive to negative dromotropic effects of resting autonomic tone. Thus, elimination of resting autonomic tone resulted in shortening the retrograde sinoatrial refractory period, allowing more rapidly delivered paced beats to conduct into the sinus node.

There does not appear to be a correlation between the duration of overdrive pacing and the magnitude of SNRTC in patients with normal IHRs. However, preliminary observations suggest that patients with abnormal IHRs may show progressively longer recovery times with longer durations of pacing.[125] Recognizing this phenomenon as an abnormal response to overdrive pacing could potentially increase the sensitivity of the technique.

In the healthy subject, the sinus cycles following the first recovery sinus beat are either shorter (secondary acceleration) or initially longer than the basic sinus cycle with gradual but progressive return to the basic sinus cycle length. In some patients with the sick sinus syndrome the P-P interval immediately following cessation of pacing is neither the longest nor even abnormally prolonged, but is followed by longer P-P intervals (Fig. 6–11). This secondary suppression may persist for 10 to 20 beats or more. Instances of secondary suppression have been reported in patients with the sick sinus syndrome but less frequently in healthy subjects.

Desai and colleagues[126] reported that in the preautonomic blockade state, the incidence of secondary pauses was significantly higher in patients with abnormal IHRs than in those with normal IHRs (5 of 8 vs. 2 of 13) ($P<0.05$). Moreover, after autonomic blockade, secondary pauses in patients with abnormal IHRs persisted or increased, while secondary pauses in patients with normal IHRs tended to disappear. Similarly, Mason[124] reported that secondary pauses seen in 78% of recipient atria and in 45% of control atria were virtually absent in denervated donor hearts (6%). These observations suggest that careful examination of the phenomenon of secondary pauses, especially after autonomic block, increases the sensitivity and specificity of overdrive atrial pacing in the diagnosis of the sick sinus syndrome.

Sinoatrial Conduction Time—Atrial Premature Depolarizations

Analysis of sinus node responses to atrial premature depolarizations (APDs) has revealed important electrophysiologic features of normal and abnormal sinus node function and sinoatrial conduction.[117–130] Premature atrial stimuli are introduced in late diastole during spontaneous sinus rhythm after every eighth beat at progressively decreasing coupling intervals (in 10-ms increments). In this fashion, the sinus cycle length is scanned until atrial capture is lost.

Four types of sinus node responses to APDs have been identified, depending on the timing of the APDs in the sinus cycle (A_1–A_1) and whether the APDs retrogradely penetrate the sinus node: (1) *compensation* resulting from a late diastolic extra stimulus that fails to depolarize the sinus node because of collision with the normal sinus depolarization; (2) *reset*, produced by premature depolarization of the sinus node by the extra stimulus resulting in A_2–A_3 interval of shorter duration than a compensatory pause; (3) *interpolation*, produced by failure of the extra stimulus to enter the sinus node, but not barring conduction to the atrium of the next sinus impulse; and (4) *reentry* resulting from reflection of the premature complex, producing an early "sinus" depolarization (Fig. 6–12).

Identification of a perinodal zone of tissue in the right atrium of the rabbit by Strauss and Bigger[131] has contributed significantly to our understanding of the above events. The perinodal cells have electrophysiologic characteristics distinct from atrial muscle and sinus node cells and may represent a potential conduction barrier. The phenomenon of the compensatory pause may be attributed to the electrophysiologic properties of the perinodal zone because the APD does not penetrate or disturb the sinus node and the subsequent sinus beat occurs on time. If the perinodal zone is abnormal, the zone of compensation may be expected to occupy a greater percentage of the sinus cycle than in patients with normal perinodal tissue. Thus, even earlier APDs would encounter the exiting sinus beat in the perinodal zone. These events form the electrophysiologic basis of first-degree sinoatrial block, a manifestation of the sick sinus syndrome (Fig. 6–13).[132, 133]

During a portion of the zone of sinus node reset, the postextrasystolic pause (A_2–A_3) lengthens progressively as the premature beat is elicited earlier in the midportion of the atrial cycle. The proposed mechanisms of this lengthening include (1) a progressive slowing of the conduction velocity of the premature impulse, (2) a temporary depression of rhythmicity of sinus node pacemaker cells,[127, 129, 130, 134] and (3) intra-SA nodal pacemaker shifts. In patients with abnormalities of sinoatrial conduction, the zone of reset theoretically occupies less of the sinus cycle than in healthy subjects.[117]

Early APDs encounter a perinodal zone that remains effectively refractory in the wake of the preceding sinus impulse, are blocked from entering the sinus node, and fail to reset it. The next spontaneous impulse occurs on schedule, traverses a perinodal zone that has recovered from refractoriness, enters the atrium on schedule, and results in interpolation of the APD. Very early APDs may find a portion of the perinodal zone and sinus node recovered sufficiently from the previous spontaneous sinus beat to enter these tissues. However, retrograde conduction would be markedly slowed, allowing other portions of the sinus node and perinodal zone to recover excitability. Such an electrophysiologic circumstance would allow for reentry. Ab-

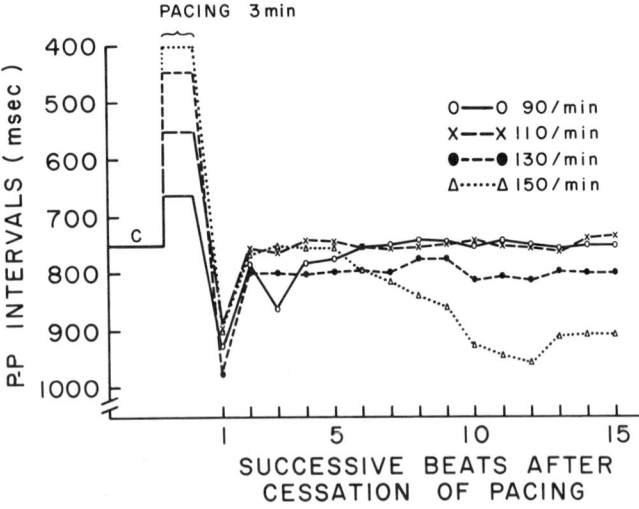

FIGURE 6–11
The influence of overdrive pacing at different rates on the sinus cycle length following termination of pacing. After overdrive pacing at rates of 90, 110, and 130 beats/min, sinus cycle length promptly returns to control values. However, following overdrive pacing at a rate of 150/min, initial overdrive suppression is followed, after approximately 10 beats, subsequent additional suppression (i.e., secondary suppression).

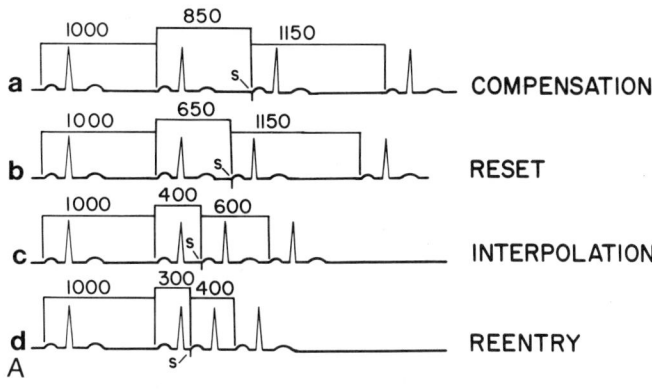

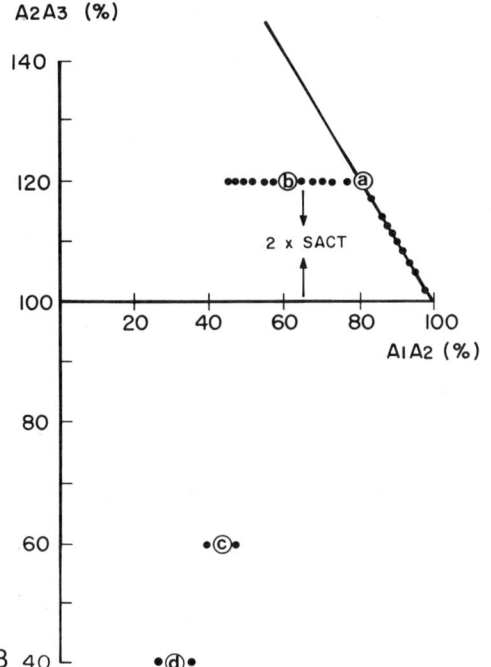

FIGURE 6–12
A, Diagrammatic representation of the various types of sinus node response to atrial extra stimuli (panels a to d)—compensation, reset, interpolation, and reentry. Compensation implies that the atrial premature depolarization did not depolarize the sinus node, leading to the development of a compensatory pause. Atrial premature complexes that occur earlier in the sinus cycle lead to the premature depolarization of the sinus node with subsequent reset (i.e., a less than compensatory pause). On rare occasions, an atrial premature depolarization can in fact be interpolated and not disturb the manifest sinus cycle length at all. On very rare occasions, an atrial premature depolarization that occurs early in the diastole can lead to delayed entrance into the sinus node region, followed by sinus node reentry. B, The horizontal axis identifies the test coupling interval (i.e., the A_1–A_2 interval expressed as a percentage of the basic sinus cycle, A_1–A_1 interval). The vertical axis identifies the return cycle length (i.e., the A_2–A_3 interval again expresses the percentage of basic sinus cycle length). Points a, b, c, and d in B refer to the similar points seen in A (i.e., compensation, reset, interpolation, and reentry). The oblique line at the upper right identifies the line of compensation.

normalities of the sinoatrial region should increase the probability of sinus node reentry and the occurrence of atrial arrhythmias.[50, 51, 135, 136] These events may be the underlying electrophysiologic basis for the observed increased frequency of occurrence of supraventricular tachyarrhythmias in patients with the sick sinus syndrome.

In summary, patients with the sick sinus syndrome with electrophysiologic abnormalities of the sinoatrial junction might be expected to demonstrate the following responses to premature atrial stimulation: (1) a prolonged zone of compensation, (2) a shortened zone of sinus node reset, (3) a prolonged zone of interpolation, and (4) a prolonged zone of sinus node reentry (see Fig. 6–13).

A fifth type of sinus node response to atrial premature depolarizations has been described: a second compensatory pause following very early APDs.[137] Collision between early APDs and the next sinus beat cannot be merely a consequence of fortuitous timing, as is the case with late APDs. The marked prematurity of early APDs should allow more than sufficient time for retrograde SA conduction before the next sinus discharge. Thus, conduction of these APDs must be significantly slowed in the sinoatrial junction. In short, early APDs followed by a compensatory sinus pause have encountered the relative refractory period of the sinoatrial junction, where decremental conduction becomes manifest.

In 1962, Langendorf and colleagues[138] deduced some of the functional characteristics of conduction between the sinoatrial node and the atrium from an analysis of the surface electrocardiogram in a patient with atrial parasystole. Based on their clinical observations and the experimental observations of Bonke and coworkers,[128] Strauss et al.[130] described how to assess sinoatrial conduction time using programmed atrial stimulation. The calculation of sinoatrial conduction time (SACT) assumes that the difference between the mean return cycle length (A_2–A_3) in the zone of sinus node reset and the spontaneous cycle length (A_1–A_1) is equal to the time required for the APD to conduct retrogradely through the perinodal zone plus the time required for the reset sinus impulse to traverse the perinodal zone anterogradely and enter the atrium (Fig. 6–14). An abnormally prolonged SACT is compatible with first-degree sinoatrial block, a characteristic of some patients with the sick sinus syndrome.[90, 131, 139–142]

However, this method requires certain assumptions: (1) all APDs resulting in a postextrasystolic pause that is less than compensatory must reset the sinus node; (2) APDs must not depress sinus node automaticity, an event that would cause an overestimation of SACT; (3) anterograde and retrograde conduction must be equally influenced by an APD; (4) SACT must be independent of variations in spontaneous sinus rate, a phenomenon common to many patients with sinus node dysfunction; and (5) the velocity of retrograde sinoatrial conduction must be independent of the site of atrial stimulation.

In isolated tissue, Miller and Strauss[143] demonstrated that the transition between compensatory postextrasystolic pauses included APDs that did not penetrate and reset the sinus node. Shortening of the sinus node return cycle in these cases was due to a shortening of the sinus node action potential by electrotonic inter-

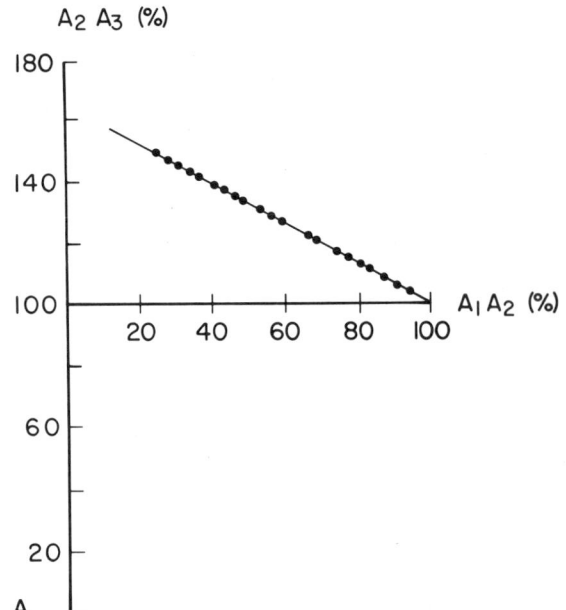 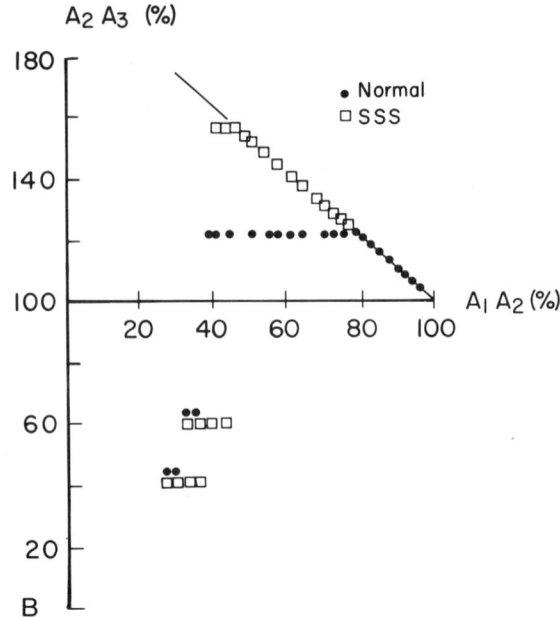

FIGURE 6–13
Diagrammatic representation of plots of the A_1-A_2/A_2-A_3 relationships that might be expected in normal patients (B, solid circles) and in patients with sinus node dysfunction (solid circles, A, and open squares, B). In A, all points fall on the line of identity, indicating inability of even early atrial premature depolarizations to enter the sinus node and reset it. This is an example of first degree SA block. In B, patients with sinus node dysfunction may be expected to have prolongation of the compensatory zone, a decrease in the reset zone, and an increase in the interpolation and reentry zone. (SSS = sick sinus syndrome.)

action between sinus node and adjacent cells during repolarization. This artifactual shortening of the return cycle resulted in underestimation of the actual SACT. Furthermore, APDs delivered in the middle of the

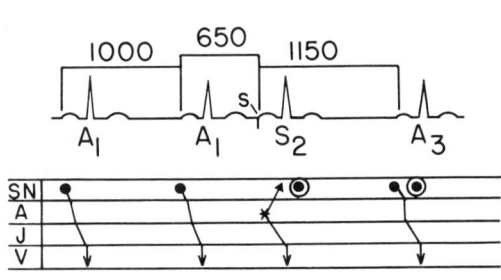

$$SACT = \frac{S_2A_3 - A_1A_1}{2}$$

FIGURE 6–14
Diagrammatic explanation of the method of calculating sinoatrial conduction time. The electrocardiographic strip identifies the events seen before and after an atrial premature complex. In the laddergram, the asterisk identifies the atrial premature depolarization that prematurely excites the sinus node (arrow); the double circles identify where the anticipated sinus node depolarization should normally have been; and the last solid circle identifies the reset sinus node discharge point. In the lowest portion of the diagram, SACT is calculated by subtracting the basal A_1-A_1 interval (1000 msec) from the observed recovery time S_2-A_3 interval (1150 msec). The total SACT (that is, the anterograde and retrograde conduction times) would be 150 msec; the unidirectional conduction time, as expressed in the formula, would be 75 msec. (SACT = sinoatrial conduction time.)

sinus cycle in animal hearts may depress sinus node automaticity and cause pacemaker shifts.[127] However, differences of opinion do exist concerning the magnitude of the influence of depressed pacemaker automaticity on estimated SACT in humans.[144] Miller and Strauss[143] noted that measured anterograde and retrograde conduction times are not equal, retrograde conduction usually being faster than anterograde conduction. In addition, SACT appears to vary as a function of the spontaneous sinus cycle length,[145, 146] at slower heart rates estimated SACT being shorter than at faster heart rates. Finally, Yamaguchi and Mandel[113] have demonstrated that the speed of retrograde conduction of an APD does depend on the site of atrial stimulation. This observation may relate to the existence of specialized functional pathways of conduction between the sinus node and the atrium.[147]

Despite these inherent problems, the method of Strauss and coworkers[130] has proved a valuable addition to the diagnostic modalities available for evaluating sinus node dysfunction. Differentiation between abnormalities of sinus node generator function and impulse conduction is now potentially possible.

Reported ranges of normal values for calculated sinoatrial conduction time in patients without apparent sinus node dysfunction include 56 ± 22 ms,[118] 70 ± 30 ms,[117] 84.5 ± 26 ms,[134] 92 ± 60 ms,[148] 82 ± 19.2 ms,[144] and 88 ± 7 ms.[105] However, many of these patients had evidence of organic heart disease, some with abnormalities of the distal conduction system, many with ischemic heart disease, and others with valvular abnormalities. Jordan and coworkers reported that patients with atherosclerotic involvement of the sinus node artery and no clinical or electrocardiographic evidence of sinus node dysfunction have significantly longer (although "normal") SACT values than do patients with coronary artery disease without such lesions.[116] Similar differences in SACT may eventually be found in patients without apparent sinus node dysfunction, dependent on other underlying pathologic processes. The important point is that sinoatrial disease progression to overt clinical and electrocardiographic manifestations may be a dynamic but gradual process.

As sinus node recovery time may be influenced by differences in autonomic tone, so may SACT be modified by changes in autonomic activity. Bonke et al.[127] and Klein and coworkers[129] could demonstrate no effect of atropine on sinoatrial conduction. Miller and Strauss[143] found that shortening of the sinus node action potential by APDs was not affected by atropine or propranolol. However, in 17 normal human subjects, Dhingra and colleagues[149] reported a significant shortening of calculated SACT following administration of 1 to 2 mg of atropine (from 103 ± 5.7 ms to 58 ± 3.9 ms) as well as a shortening of the zone of compensation. These authors did not find an overall shortening of the zone of compensation following atropine administration or a lengthening of the zone of sinus reset in patients with the sick sinus syndrome. Similarly, interpolation and echo responses were unaffected by atropine in these patients. Strauss and coworkers[150] found that propranolol, 1 mg/kg, significantly lengthened SACT in patients with the sick sinus syndrome. However, effects on sinus node automaticity may have contributed to this finding. In patients with the sick sinus syndrome, there appears to be no correlation between intrinsic heart rate and SACT.

Breithardt and coworkers[142] reported that 45% of 41 patients with various manifestations of sinus dysfunction had prolonged SACT when 120 ms was used as the upper limit of normal. Using a normal value of 215 ms for total anterograde plus retrograde conduction, Strauss et al.[90] reported that 38% of 16 patients with sinus node dysfunction demonstrated an abnormally long total SACT.

Breithardt and colleagues[142] attempted to correlate prolongation of SACT and sinus node recovery time (SNRT) with specific electrocardiographic abnormalities in patients with the sick sinus syndrome. Patients with asymptomatic sinus bradycardia did not have significantly longer SNRTC or SACT values than control subjects, whereas patients with symptoms did. Patients with the bradycardia-tachycardia syndrome or episodic sinoatrial block (or both) demonstrated significantly longer SNRT values than control subjects, although SACT in the bradycardia-tachycardia group did not differ from that of the control patients. SNRT was found to be a somewhat more sensitive measure than SACT, showing fewer false-negative results in patients with sinus node dysfunction (Fig. 6–15). Nonetheless, SACT determination proved to be a better method of distinguishing patients with sick sinus from healthy subjects than had previously been reported.[89]

Sinoatrial Conduction Time—Continuous Pacing Method

Limitations of the atrial premature stimulus technique for determining the sinoatrial conduction time have been reviewed. In order to circumvent sinus node suppression, pacemaker shift, and other variables, Narula described a new method for determining sinoatrial conduction time using overdrive atrial pacing.[151] The atrium is paced 10 beats per minute faster than the basic sinus rate for eight beats. The interval in milliseconds from the last paced beat to the first return sinus beat on the intra-atrial electrogram is taken as the total time of retrograde and anterograde sinoatrial conduction (Fig. 6–16). Clinically, at this pacing rate the sinus node pacemaker does not appear to be suppressed and there is no suggestion of pacemaker shift when post-return cycles (A_3-A_4, A_4-A_5, and so on) are examined. The measure appears to be reproducible. The advantages of the method are that it is reliable[152] and complex equipment (i.e., programmed stimulator) and laborious calculation are unnecessary.

Kang and colleagues[153] found that the two methods correlated very well ($r = 0.80$) during control and after autonomic blockade ($r = 0.85$). In addition, the directional changes in SACT after autonomic blockade were always similar. For each method, 8 of 12 patients with the sick sinus syndrome demonstrated shortening of SACT, and 4 of 12 demonstrated lengthening of SACT following autonomic blockade. The investigators suggested that prolongation of SACT after autonomic blockade is an abnormal response in patients in whom sinus node suppression cannot be demonstrated by examining postpacing or post–extra stimulus cycle lengths. They proposed that an increase in SACT may be related to intrinsic abnormalities of sinoatrial conduction previously masked by sympathetic activity. Breithardt and Seipel[154] reported a poor correlation between SACT by the constant atrial stimulation method and the premature atrial stimulation method ($r = 0.45$). The investigators suggested that poor correlation resulted from greater depression of sinus node automaticity by the premature atrial stimulus technique. However, Grant and associates[152] believe that the disparity was more likely related to failure of penetration and reset of the sinus node during pacing at slow pacing rates, an effect that disappeared when pacing rates were increased by as little as 3 beats per minute.

Sinus Nodal Refractoriness

Goldreyer and Damato[109] suggested that critically coupled atrial premature impulses that become interpolated are caused by sinus nodal refractoriness. Kerr et al.[110] verified this contention on isolated rabbit sinoatrial preparations with the microelectrode technique and concluded that the sudden transition between the zone of reset and the zone of incomplete interpolation was a good indication of the sinus node refractory period. These investigators extended these observa-

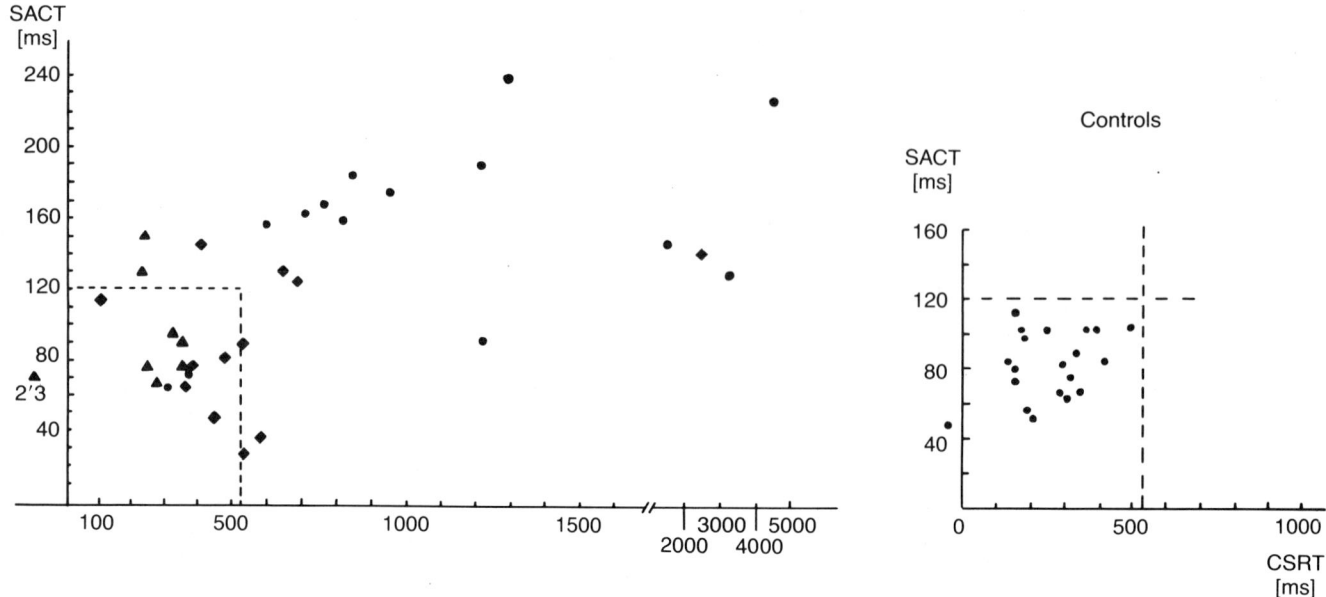

FIGURE 6-15
In this figure, the corrected sinus node recovery time is plotted on the horizontal axis and the sinoatrial conduction time is plotted on the vertical axis. In the right-hand graph, data on control patients without clinical evidence of sinus node dysfunction are plotted. Note that in all patients, corrected sinus node recovery times and sinoatrial conduction times fall within the normal zone. The left-hand graph shows data for patients with sinus bradycardia but no significant complaints (triangles) and sinus bradycardia with cardiovascular complaints (diamonds), as well as data for patients with bradycardia-tachycardia syndrome with SA block (circles). Note that the most abnormal data points for both sinoatrial conduction and sinus node recovery times occur with patients with bradycardia-tachycardia syndrome with SA block. The majority of patients with sinus bradycardia but no central nervous system symptomatology fall within the normal zone. (Reproduced by permission of the American Heart Association, Inc., from Breithardt G, Seipel L, Loogan F: Sinus node recovery time and calculated sinoatrial conduction time in normal subjects and patients with sinus node dysfunction. Circulation 56:43, 1977.)

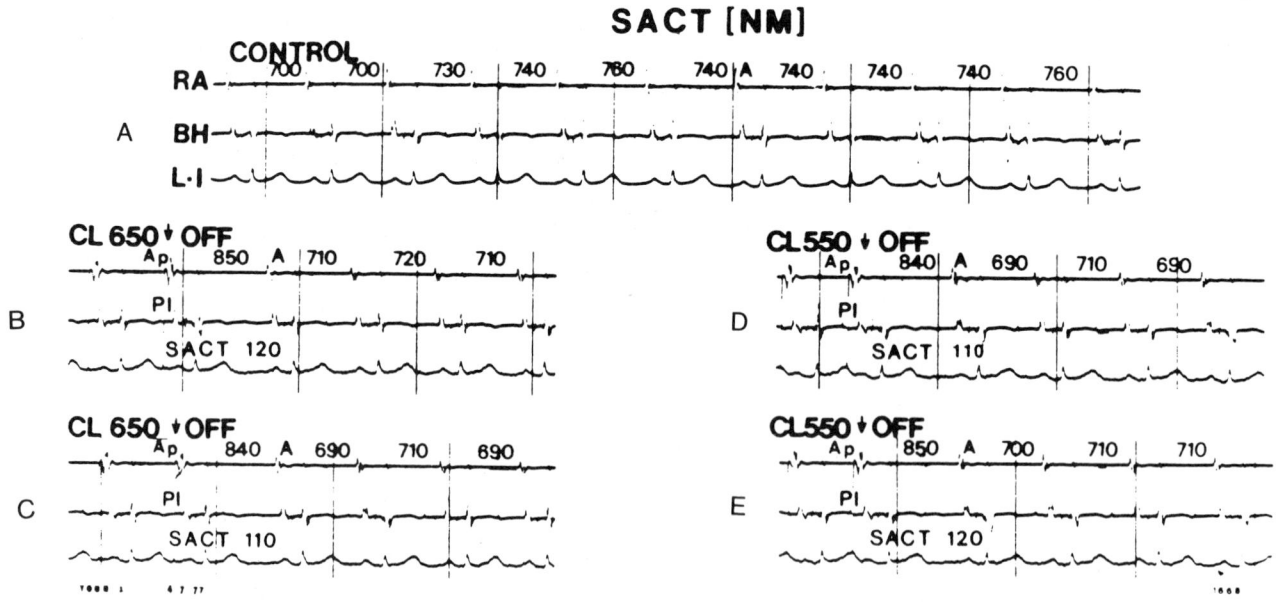

FIGURE 6-16
This figure shows the method used to calculate the sinoatrial condition time using the new method of Narula. In A to E, recordings are shown in the control state and following overdrive pacing at a cycle length of 650 and a cycle length of 550. Note the similarity of sinoatrial conduction times measured following the last paced beats to the onset of the next spontaneous sinus complex. (Reproduced by permission of the American Heart Association, Inc., from Narula OS, Narashimhan S, Vasquez M, et al.: A new method of measurement of sinoatrial conduction time. Circulation 58:706, 1978.)

tions to humans and demonstrated a clear difference between sinus nodal refractoriness in normal subjects (250–380 ms) and patients with sinus node dysfunction (500–550 ms).

Sinus Node Extracellular Potential Recordings

Developments in electrophysiologic techniques have permitted the recording of the sinus node action potential from the endocardial and epicardial surfaces of the intact heart.[155–158] With unipolar recordings through Ag–AgCl electrodes directly coupled to a preamplifier and positioned 0.2 to 0.5 mm above the sinus node, identification of pacemaker action potentials from the epicardial surface has been substantiated by simultaneous transmembrane recordings in isolated rabbit hearts.[155] A similar technique that obtains both unipolar and bipolar recordings has permitted extracellular action potentials to be recorded from the epicardial surface in humans during open-heart surgery (Fig. 6–17).[156] Hariman and colleagues[159, 162] found that sinoatrial conduction times were 32.4 ± 2.8 ms at sinus cycle lengths of 587.6 ± 35.6 ms for the bipolar method, and 38.2 ± 3.2 ms at sinus cycle lengths of 712.2 ± 50.7 ms for the unipolar method.

A transvenous catheter technique has been developed to record endocardial surface sinoatrial pacemaker potentials in the intact canine heart[157] and, more recently, in humans.[160,161] Gomes and coworkers[163] have reported that when the catheter was looped in the right atrium and advanced to the junction of the superior vena cava and right atrium so that the distal poles of the catheter were in direct contact with the right atrial endocardium underlying the area of the sinoatrial node, stable sinoatrial electrograms could be obtained in 18 of 21 (86%) patients. Their method was reported superior to the technique of Reiffel and colleagues,[161] in which only the catheter tip was in close proximity to the right atrial endocardium. The former technique minimized baseline drift of the sinoatrial electrograms. Patients with the sick sinus syndrome consistently had longer directly measured SACT (135 ± 30 ms) than did patients without the sick sinus syndrome (87 ± 12 ms), measurements in agreement with those found by Reiffel and coworkers. The discrepancy between SACT recorded from the endocardial surface and SACT recorded from the epicardial surface by Hariman and colleagues[159] was not explained. There was good correlation between direct and indirect SACT estimated by Narula's pacing method ($r = 0.843$, $N = 28$) and by the premature stimulation method ($r = 0.778$, $N = 18$). The direct method ($SACT_d$) appears superior to the indirect method ($SACT_i$) for measuring SACT in patients in whom no zone of reset can be obtained and in patients in whom frequent atrial premature complexes are present.

Reiffel and colleagues,[161] based on their findings that $SACT_i$ often overestimates $SACT_d$, have suggested that when $SACT_i$ is normal $SACT_d$ will be normal; however, if $SACT_i$ is prolonged, $SACT_d$ may be normal. On the other hand, and unexpectedly, Gomes and colleagues[163] found that $SACT_i$ often underestimates $SACT_d$. The discrepancy between these results is disturbing and requires explanation, although it may relate to differences in methodology.

Asseman and colleagues[164] studied eight patients with the sick sinus syndrome with SNRT greater than 1500 ms. In six patients, sinus node electrograms appearing at a rate similar to the basic sinus rate persisted during the postpacing pause. The authors concluded that the pause following cessation of atrial overdrive is often caused by overdrive-induced sinoatrial block rather than by sinus node pacemaker suppression. This conclusion is in direct conflict with findings in microelectrode studies that clearly demonstrate suppression of sinus node pacemaker activity by atrial overdrive pacing in both the normal sinus node[165] and in the sinus node made abnormal by the addition of verapamil to the preparation.[97] Moreover, microelectrode studies that do confirm alteration in sinoatrial conduction following overdrive pacing (as a consequence of decreased sinus pacemaker action potential amplitude) also show slowing of pacemaker rate.[166, 167] Curiously, Asseman and colleagues reported that overdrive pacing resulted in no sinus rate suppression, despite obvious changes in action potential characteristics.

More in keeping with microelectrode findings is the report of Gomes and coworkers.[168] Direct sinus node recordings in humans revealed that $SNRT_i$ reflects both sinus node automaticity and sinoatrial conduction. In all patients, overdrive atrial pacing appeared to result in marked prolongation of $SACT_d$ for the first postpacing beat, which was longer in patients with the sick sinus syndrome than in healthy subjects. Postpacing $SACT_d$ prolongation persisted for 3.6 ± 0.96 beats.

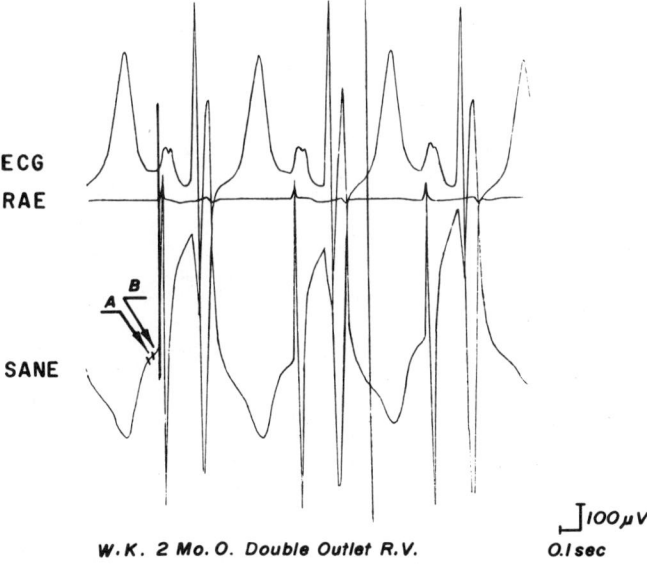

Figure 6–17
Extracellular recordings obtained from human sinus node at the time of open-heart surgery. From above downward; surface electrocardiogram (ECG), right atrial electrogram (RAE), and a sinoatrial node electrogram (SANE). Note the appearance of pre–P wave electrical activity in the SANE. (Courtesy of Robert Hariman, M.D.)

Sinus node suppression was seen in 56% of patients, sinus node acceleration was noted in 26%, and no appreciable change in sinus node automaticity was observed in 19%. Insensitive to the contribution of increased SACT to sinus node recovery after overdrive pacing, $SNRT_i$ consistently overestimated $SNRT_d$.

Direct sinoatrial electrogram recordings have exposed the importance of the role of alternations in sinoatrial conduction in other bradycardic situations previously ascribed to depression of sinus node automaticity alone. Using this recording technique, Gang and colleagues[169] have shown that sinoatrial block is an important component of the asystolic pause that occurs in patients with the cardioinhibitory form of the hypersensitive carotid sinus syndrome (Fig. 6-18).

Carotid sinus hypersensitivity may be manifested in two ways, apparently independent of each other.[170, 171] The cardioinhibitory type is expressed as an apparent slowing of the heart rate with mechanical stimulation of the carotid sinus and is inhibited by atropine. The less common vasodepressor type is accompanied by vasodilation and hypotension and is often inhibited by epinephrine. The cardioinhibitory type appears to be mediated by the parasympathetic nervous system and is most commonly found in elderly men with coronary atherosclerosis and hypertensive heart disease.[172-174] The precise mechanism of the cardioinhibitory type is not known, although four possibilities have been proposed: (1) a high level of resting vagal tone, (2) excessive release of acetylcholine, (3) inadequate cholinesterase activity, and (4) hyperresponsiveness to acetylcholine. If the latter mechanism is the predominant one, carotid hypersensitivity is properly part of the sick sinus syndrome. The majority of patients with carotid hypersensitivity have normal SNRT and SACT.[171, 175-177]

THE EFFECTS OF DRUGS ON NORMAL AND ABNORMAL SINUS NODE FUNCTION

Sinus node response to any particular pharmacologic agent can be extremely variable and may even appear to be almost idosyncratic. In any given person, a specific drug may have negligible, profound stimulatory, or marked inhibitory effects on sinus automaticity or sinoatrial conduction. Moreover, the electrophysiologic effects of any antiarrhythmic agents as observed in isolated tissue preparations often do not correspond to the clinical response witnessed in humans. Furthermore, the effect of a drug on sinus node function may

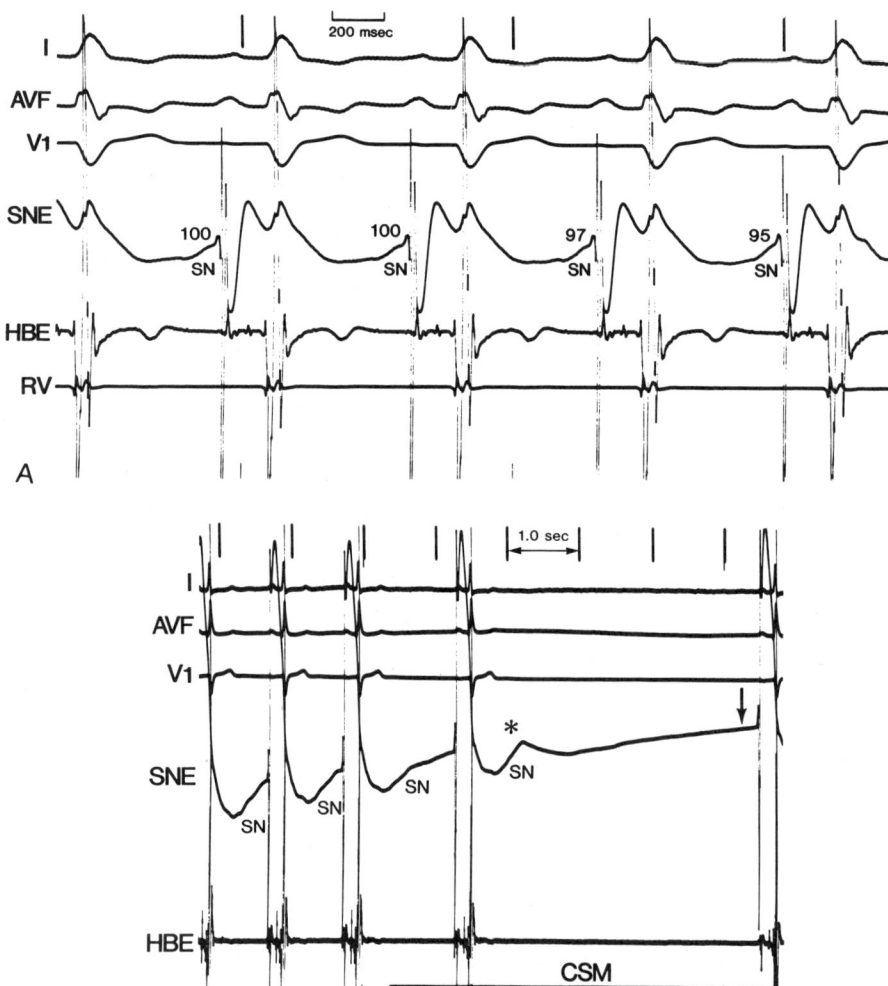

FIGURE 6-18
A, The sinus node electrogram. Surface electrocardiogram leads I, aVF and V_1 are displayed along with intracavitary electrocardiograms from the region of the sinus node, His bundle, and right ventricle. Sinus node potentials are the positive-going, low-frequency deflections preceding each atrial depolarization. The directly measured sinoatrial conduction times are labeled above each SN deflection. (SNE = sinus node; HBE = His bundle; RV = right ventricle; SN = sinus node potentials.) B, Carotid sinus massage in a patient with the hypersensitive carotid sinus syndrome. Surface and intracardiac electrocardiograms are labeled as in A. The onset of carotid sinus massage is followed by profound prolongation in the SN deflection, signifying probable prolongation in the sinoatrial conduction time. Sinoatrial block is then illustrated, since a sinus node impulse is shown to occur without subsequent atrial depolarization (asterisk). Sinus node quiescence is then recorded until the inscription of the next atrial impulse, which is not preceded by an SN potential (arrow). The absence of an SN potential suggests a shifting of the primary pacemaker focus out of the sinus node or to another region without the sinus node. (CSM = cardiac sinus massage.)

differ significantly when it is given as an acute single intravenous dose or a chronic oral administration. These apparent inconsistencies can be explained when several facts are considered:

1. The effects of a drug on sinus node function may be mediated by indirect (interaction with the autonomic and central nervous systems) as well as direct mechanisms of action.[178]

2. The sinus node response to a specific cardiac drug may differ in the setting of abnormal intrinsic sinoatrial function compared to when no intrinsic sinus node abnormalities are present. Patients with sinus node dysfunction are more sensitive to the depressant action of antiarrhythmic drugs and are more susceptible to manifest adverse side effects.[179]

3. In sinoatrial dysfunction, the clinical response to a pharmacologic agent may be determined by the specific electrophysiologic property that is abnormal as well as by the magnitude of the abnormality.

4. Drugs may have differential effects on properties of sinus node automaticity and sinoatrial conduction.

5. The electrophysiologic assumptions on which the technique of premature atrial stimulation is based may be invalid in the sinus node and sinoatrial junction made abnormal by cardioactive drugs.

Therefore, caution and constant monitoring are required when administration of cardioactive drugs is contemplated for patients with sinus node dysfunction. The mechanisms of this enhanced depressant action on sinus node function, causing symptoms, are uncertain at present and cannot be predicted with reasonable degree of accuracy in any given sick-sinus patient.[179]

Management of Patients with the Sick Sinus Syndrome

The indications for permanent pacing in patients with the sick sinus syndrome must be clearly defined.[180-185] The benefits to be realistically expected from pacemaker insertion must be understood by the clinician so that sound judgment may prevail. Thus the natural history, complications, morbidity, and mortality of the sick sinus syndrome must be elucidated. Furthermore, electrophysiologic and clinical predictors of the potential for complications must be developed to improve decisions concerning the timing of pacemaker insertion.

Not only is the sick sinus syndrome a heterogeneous entity in underlying pathophysiologic mechanisms, but it also occurs in a heterogeneous population having associated cardiovascular diseases. Patients with the sick sinus syndrome with ischemic heart disease, congestive heart failure, or primary cerebrovascular disease form a higher risk population for sudden death than patients without these associated risk factors.[185-188] Therefore, clinical data concerning the benefits of permanent pacing in terms of reduction in mortality and morbidity should be assessed independently in patients with and without other cardiovascular diseases. In addition, patients with the bradycardia-tachycardia syndrome present therapeutic challenges not encountered in patients with sinus bradycardia, sinus arrest, or sinoatrial block alone.

Provided that central nervous system symptoms have been shown to be unequivocally associated with episodes of sinus node dysfunction and failure of subsidiary pacemakers to escape, pacing has been consistently successful in eliminating cerebral symptoms.[180, 185-187] When an adequate cardiac output does not depend on atrial contribution, ventricular pacing has been as successful as atrial or dual-chamber pacing in eliminating dizziness or syncope. With severe heart failure, subtle symptoms of fatigue and failing mental acuity may be as much a consequence of diminished stroke volume as an inappropriately slow heart rate. Only prepacing and postpacing hemodynamic studies at a variety of rates will support an assumption that a faster heart rate will increase cerebral perfusion by increasing cardiac output. In patients with myocardial dysfunction, cardiac performance must be assessed in the basal state as well as with atrial, ventricular and dual-chamber pacing.

Improvements in symptoms of congestive heart failure, with and without the addition of digitalis, has been reported after pacemaker implantation in some patients with the sick sinus syndrome.[182, 185] An additional group of patients without overt congestive heart failure had improved exercise tolerance following pacemaker insertion.[186]

Since the sick sinus syndrome is probably a diffuse disease of the AV conduction system, His bundle recordings should be performed if atrial pacing is being considered. Frequently, abnormalities of AV nodal and distal pathways of conduction coexist with sinus node dysfunction. If atrial contribution to diastolic ventricular filling is necessary for adequate ventricular performance, dual-chamber pacing should be considered in these patients.

In general, pharmacologic approaches to the management of sinus bradycardia have been disappointing.[181, 189-191] However, notable exceptions have been reported, with symptom-free states lasting 5 years or longer. Atropine-like drugs and sublingual beta-adrenergic drugs have obvious disadvantages. These include short duration of action, intolerable side-effects, irregular and unreliable absorption, and the need for unfaltering patient compliance with a demanding dose schedule. Moreover, these drugs may worsen or precipitate atrial and ventricular tachyarrhythmias. Hydralazine may have some benefit and be better tolerated.

Bradyarrhythmias are less well tolerated by patients with significant cerebrovascular disease. In these patients, even short episodes of moderately slow heart rates can be catastrophic. Moreover, a stable sinus bradycardia may have variable central nervous system consequences depending on the relative distribution of blood flow during periods of stress or exercise; blood flow may be diverted to the periphery, "stealing" flow from the cerebral circulation in the absence of compensatory cardioacceleration. Thus, in patients with significant cerebrovascular disease, symptoms may occur even in the absence of gross changes in cardiac rhythm. In addition, cerebral atherosclerosis is a progressive disease, and some patients may have recurrences of central nervous system symptoms after a considerable period of being asymptomatic following artificial pacing. Failure of pacing to improve dizziness or syncopal episodes has been attributed to coexistent severe cerebrovascular disease in most series.[186]

The therapeutic approach to the patient with the bradycardia-tachycardia syndrome is complex and must be individualized. In the absence of central nervous system symptoms, the bradycardia may be observed very closely while antiarrhythmic agents alone are tried in progressive incremental doses. When the tachyarrhythmias are supraventricular, digitalis has been the mainstay of therapy. However, the effect of digitalis on sinus node function in these patients varies, and caution is warranted. Therapy is best started in the hospital while the patient is electrocardiographically monitored. Propranolol and verapamil, documented to be highly effective in treatment of supraventricular arrhythmias, probably carry a higher risk of suppressing sinus node function than do digitalis preparations, and the combination of the two drugs is contraindicated in patients with sinus node disease without permanent pacing.

Some investigators have suggested that artificial pacing not only may allow higher doses of antiarrhythmic drugs to be given, but also that many patients have better results with lower doses that failed to control the tachyarrhythmias before pacemaker application.[180, 182, 183] The potential for distal conduction system problems occurring secondary to the use of antiarrhythmic agents alone may be anticipated from the results of His bundle recordings.[185, 192, 193]

Considerable controversy exists regarding the efficacy of pacing alone for controlling the occurrence of supraventricular tachyarrhythmias in patients with the sick sinus syndrome. Rubenstein and others have been unable to limit the frequency of episodes or entirely suppress them without adding antiarrhythmic agents.[181, 190, 194] Others, however, have met with better success with atrial or coronary sinus pacing alone.[182, 195] Some investigators have reported successful prophylaxis with ventricular pacing when retrograde VA conduction is present.[196] At the other extreme, refractoriness to antiarrhythmic agents has continued in a few patients in spite of permanent pacing.[188]

Despite a potential electrophysiologic predisposition for ventricular arrhythmias to occur in the presence of slow heart rates, arrhythmias in patients with the sick sinus syndrome are more often supraventricular. When ventricular ectopy or malignant ventricular rhythms do occur, atrial or ventricular pacing may not abolish them without the assistance of antiarrhythmic drugs. However, pacing may facilitate pharmacologic management by shortening the Purkinje fiber refractory period, increasing the threshold for ventricular fibrillation, and minimizing asynchronous recovery of excitability in the ventricles.[197-200]

Prognosis in Patients with the Sick Sinus Syndrome

From the standpoint of mortality and morbidity, the sick sinus syndrome is a discouraging disease entity to treat. The 5-year mortality in these patients is high and does not appear to be significantly influenced by artificial pacing. Skagen and Hansen[187] followed 50 patients with sinoatrial block treated with permanent pacing for 1 to 14 years. They reported survival after 1, 2, 5, and 8 years to be 94%, 85%, 64%, and 48%, respectively. These figures indicate an excess yearly mortality in the first 5 years of 4 to 5% compared with a control population of the same age and sex. Mortality was significantly influenced by the coexistence of cardiovascular and valvular heart disease. (Fig. 6–19) Chokshi and coworkers[186] reported 1- and 4-year survival rates in 52 permanently paced patients with sick sinus of 85% and 47%, respectively. Krishnaswami and Geraci[188] followed 17 patients with sinus bradycardia or sinus arrest in a pacemaker clinic for a mean duration of 19.4 months and reported a 30% mortality over 16.3 months, half the deaths being secondary to massive cerebral infarction. In a follow-up study of 90 patients for a mean of 23 months after pacemaker implantation, Hartel and Talvensaari[185] reported an annual mortality of 11%. As a group, the patients who died did not differ significantly from the survivors with regard to type of sinus dysfunction, occurrence of tachyarrhythmias, or distal conduction abnormalities.

In all series, death in patients with this syndrome with permanent pacing most frequently resulted from complications of associated cardiovascular or cerebrovascular disease and not from complications of sinus node and subsidiary pacemaker dysfunction. However, a discouraging fact is that the incidence of embolic events involving the lungs, brain, and peripheral arterial tree remains distressingly high in patients with permanent pacing and the sick sinus syndrome. The frequency of embolic events suggests that the instances of alternating bradyarrhythmias and tachyarrhythmias are more common than appreciated from random electrophysiologic evaluation. Although more extensive use of Holter monitoring to detect cases of inadequate pharmacologic prophylaxis of tachyarrhythmias may reduce the incidence of embolization somewhat, the paroxysmal nature of these arrhythmias would allow many episodes to escape detection. Thus, it has been proposed that all patients exhibiting the bradycardia-tachycardia syndrome be fully anticoagulated. The benefit-risk argument of chronic anticoagulation has not been resolved, and the issue of anticoagulation in these patients is still controversial. Nevertheless, prevention of life-threatening embolization appears to be the only area in which the physcan can potentially favorably influence the high rate of mortality and morbidity in the permanently paced patient with the sick sinus syndrome. Thus, a strong case for chronic anticoagulation can be made. However, not all cerebrovascular accidents in these patients are secondary to embolic events. Elderly patients with atherosclerotic

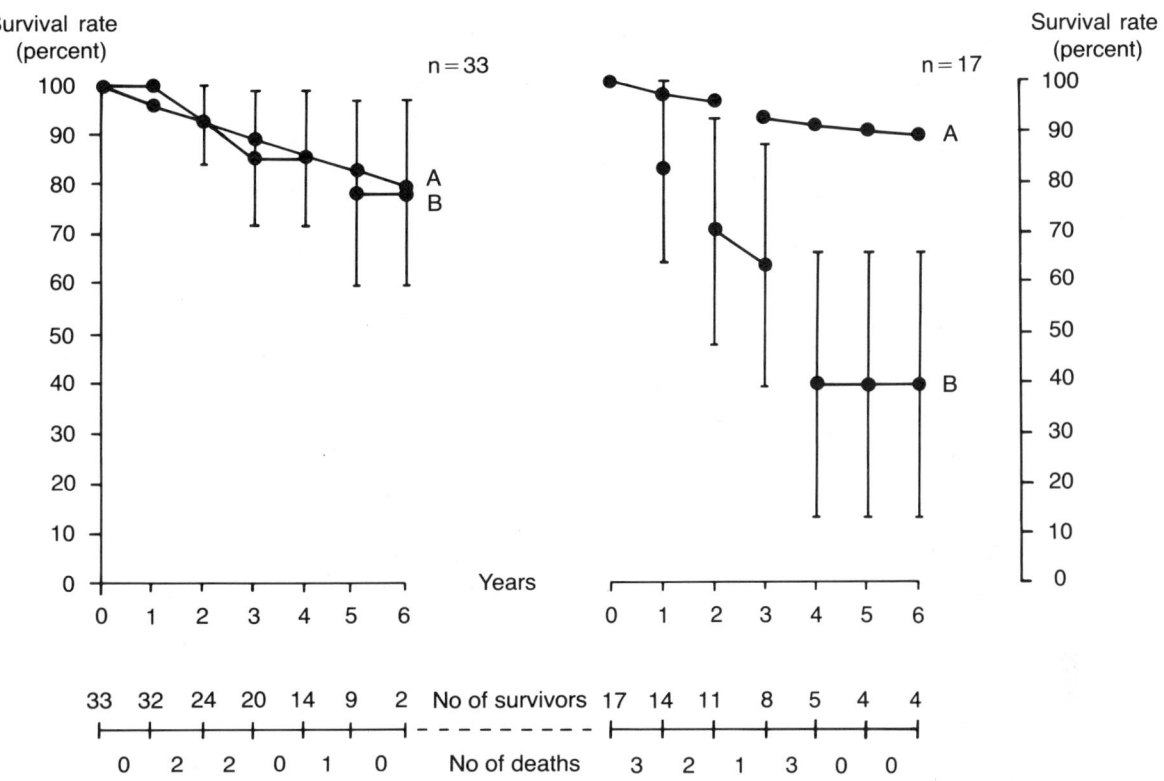

FIGURE 6–19
These graphs illustrate survival curves in two groups, one without significant cardiac disease (I) and one with significant cardiac disease (II). All of these patients had significant sinus node dysfunction and were treated with permanent cardiac pacing. In each graph, age-matched controls are illustrated by the line marked A, and the index patients are illustrated by the line marked B. Survival rates are shown for group I and group II patients. Note the significant deviation from the expected survival in group II patients without significant underlying disease. (Reproduced by permission from Skagen K, Hansen JF: The long-term prognosis for patients with sinoatrial block treated with permanent pacemaker. Acta Med Scand 199:13, 1975.)

cerebrovascular disease may have transient ischemic attacks or frank cerebral infarction if a tachyarrhythmia is associated with a fall in cardiac output. This group of patients will not benefit from anticoagulant therapy and must be distinguished from patients with cerebral embolization.

Finally, the issue of prophylactic permanent pacing in the asymptomatic patient with the sick sinus syndrome must be addressed. At present, the natural history of the disease is unknown; furthermore, clinical risk factors for the development of symptoms have not been defined, and no electrophysiologic measure of sinus node function has been demonstrated to have reliable predictive value. Therefore, common practice has been to withhold pacemaker therapy in the asymptomatic patient.

References

1. James TN: Anatomy of the human sinus node. Anat Rec 141:109, 1961.
2. Brown HF, Kimura J, Noble D, et al.: The ionic currents underlying pacemaker activity in rabbit sino-atrial node: experimental results and computer simulations. Proc R Soc London, 222:329, 1984.
3. Maylie J, Morad M: Ionic currents responsible for the generation of pacemaker current in rabbit sino-atrial node. J Physiol 355:215, 1984.
4. Jordan JL, Yamaguchi I, Mandel WJ: The effects of verapamil on sinoatrial conduction in isolated tissue. Clin Res 26:241, 1977.
5. Hutter OF, Trautwein W: Vagal and sympathetic effects on the pacemaker fibers in the sinus venous of the heart. J Gen Physiol 39:715, 1956.
6. Gaskell WH: The electrical changes in the quiescent cardiac muscle which accompany stimulation of the vagus nerve. J Physiol 7:451, 1886.
7. Lu HH, Lange G, Brooks C McC: Factors controlling pacemaker action in cells of the sinoatrial node. Circ Res 42:460, 1965.
8. Kassebaum DG: Membrane effects of epinephrine in the heart. In Krays O, Kovarikova A (eds.): Second International Pharmacologic meeting, vol. 5, Pharmacology of Cardiac Function, pp. 95–100. Oxford, Pergamon Press, 1964.
9. Mackary AJC, Hof TO, Bkeker WK, et al.: Interaction of adrenaline and acetylcholine on cardiac pacemaker function. Functional inhomogeneity of the rabbit sinus node. J Pharm Exp Therap 214:417, 1980.
10. Johnson PN, Freeberg AS, Marshall JM: Action of thyroid hormone on the transmembrane potentials from sinoatrial node cells and atrial muscle in isolated atria of rabbits. Cardiology 58:273, 1973.

11. James TN, Nadeau RA: Sinus bradycardia during injections directly into the sinus node artery. Am J Physiol 204:9, 1963.
12. James TN: Pulse and impulse formation in the sinus node. Henry Ford Hosp Med J 15:275, 1967.
13. Brooks C McC, Lange G, Lu HH: Effects of localized stretch of the sinoatrial node region of the dog heart. Am J Physiol 211:1197, 1966.
14. Lange G, Lu HH: Effect of stretch of the isolated cat sinoatrial node. Am J Physiol 211:1192, 1966.
15. Bouman LN, Van der Westen HM: Pacemaker shift in the sinoatrial node induced by a change of temperature. Pfluegers Arch 318:262, 1970.
16. Bouman LN, Mackaay AJC, Bleeker WK, et al.: Pacemaker shifts in the sinus node: effects of vagal stimulation, temperature and reduction of extracellular calcium. *In* Bonke FIM (ed.): The Sinus Node: Structure, Function and Clinical Relevance, p. 245. The Hague, Martinus Nijhoff, 1978.
17. Lown B: *In* Dreifus L, Likoff W, Moyer J (eds.): Fourteenth Hahnemann Symposium on Mechanisms and Therapy of Cardiac Arrhythmias, p. 185. New York, Grune & Stratton, 1966.
18. Ferrer MI: Sick sinus syndrome in atrial disease. JAMA 206:645, 1968.
19. Kulbertus HE, De Leval-Ruffen F, Demoulin JC: Sinoatrial disease: A report on 13 cases. J Electrocardiol 6:303, 1973.
20. Rasmussen K: Chronic sinoatrial heart block. Am Heart J 81:38, 1971.
21. Conde C, Leppo J, Lipski J: Effectiveness of pacemaker treatment in the bradycardia-tachycardia syndrome. Am J Cardiol 32:209, 1973.
22. Sigurd B, Jensen G, Meibom J: Adams-Stokes syndrome caused by sinoatrial block. Br Heart J 35:1002, 1973.
23. Rokseth R, Hatle L: Prospective study on the occurrence and management of chronic sinoatrial disease with follow-up. Br Heart J 36:582, 1974.
24. Radford DJ, Julian DG: Sick sinus syndrome: Experience of a cardiac pacemaker clinic. Br Med J 3:155, 1974.
25. Sowton E, Hendrix G, Roy P: Ten-year survey of treatment with implanted cardiac pacemaker. Br Med J 3:255, 1974.
26. Hartel G, Talvensaari T: Treatment of sinoatrial syndrome with permanent cardiac pacing in 90 patients. Acta Med Scand 198:341, 1975.
27. Rubenstein JJ, Schulman CL, Yurchok PM: Clinical spectrum of the sick sinus syndrome. Circulation 46:5, 1972.
28. Wan SH, Lee GS, Ton CS: The sick sinus syndrome. A study of 15 cases. Br Heart J 34:942, 1972.
29. Moss AJ, Davis RJ: Brady-tachy syndrome. Prog Cardiovasc Dis 16:439, 1974.
30. Fraser GR, Froggatt P, James TN: Congenital deafness associated with electrocardiographic abnormalities, fainting attacks and sudden death: A recessive syndrome. Q J Med 33:361, 1964.
31. Barks JB, Bosman CK, Cochrane JWC: Congenital cardiac arrhythmias. Lancet 2:531, 1964.
32. Metzger AL, Goldberg AN, Hunter RL: Sick sinus node syndrome as the presenting manifestation of reticulum cell sarcoma. Chest 60:602, 1971.
33. Kaplin BM, Langendorf FR, Lev M: Tachycardia-bradycardia syndrome (so-called "sick sinus syndrome"). Pathology, mechanisms and treatment. Am J Cardiol 31:497, 1973.
34. Jordan JL, Yamaguchi I, Mandel WJ: Characteristics of sinoatrial conduction in patients with coronary artery disease. Circulation 55:569, 1977.
35. Haden RF, Langsjoen PH, Rapoport MI, et al.: The significance of sinus bradycardia in acute myocardial infarction. Dis Chest 44:168, 1963.
36. Adgey AJJ, Geddes JS, Mulholland HE: Incidence, significance and management of early bradyarrhythmia complicating acute myocardial infarction. Lancet 2:1097, 1968.
37. Rokseth R, Hattle L: Sinus arrest in acute myocardial infarction. Br Heart J 33:639, 1971.
38. Thomas M, Goodgate D: Effect of atropine on bradycardia and hypotension in acute myocardial infarction. Br Heart J 28:409, 1966.
39. Brown AM: Excitation of afferent cardiac sympathetic nerve fibers during myocardial ischemia. J Physiol 190:35, 1967.
40. Botti C, et al.: Efectti imediati della legatura della "arteria del noda del seno" su la funzione ritmica sinusale ne cane. Rass Fisiof Cl Ten 29:149, 1957.
41. James TN, Reemtsma K: The response of sinus node function to ligation of the sinus node artery. Henry Ford Hosp Med Bull 8:129, 1960.
42. Billette J, Elharrar V, Porlier G: Sinus slowing produced by experimental ischemia of the sinus node in dogs. Am J Cardiol 31:331, 1973.
43. Meck WJ, Keenan M, Theisen HJ: Auricular blood supply in the dog. I. General auricular supply with special reference to sino-auricular node. Am Heart J 4:591, 1929.
44. Halpern MH: Arterial supply to the nodal tissue in the dog heart. Circulation 9:547, 1954.
45. Marriott HJL: Practical Electrocardiography, 5th ed., p. 128. Baltimore, Williams & Wilkins, 1972.
46. Freidman HH: Diagnostic Electrocardiography and Vectorcardiography, pp. 432. New York, McGraw-Hill, 1977.
47. Chung EK: Electrocardiography: Practical Applications with Vectorial Principles, p. 167. Hagerstown, MD, Harper & Row, 1974.
48. Han J, DeTraglia J, Millet D: Incidence of ectopic beats as a function of basic rate in the ventricle. Am Heart J 72:632, 1966.
49. Han J, Millet D, Chizzonezzi B: Temporal dispersion of recovery of excitability in atrium and ventricle as a function of heart rate. Am Heart J 71:481, 1966.
50. Han J, Malozzi AM, Moe GK: Sinoatrial reciprocation in the isolated rabbit heart. Circ Res 22:355, 1968.
51. Paulay KL, Varghese JP, Damato AN: Sinus node reentry. An in vivo demonstration in the dog. Circ Res 32:455, 1973b.
52. Narula OS: Sinus node reentry. A mechanism for supraventricular tachycardia. Circulation 50:1114, 1974.
53. Weisfogel GM, Bataford WP, Paulay KL: Sinus node reentrant tachycardia in man. Am Heart J 90:295, 1975.
54. Breithardt G, Seipel L: Sequence of atrial activation in patients with atrial echo beats. *In* Bonke FIM (ed.): The Sinus Node: Structure, Function and Clinical Relevance, pp. 389–408. The Hague, Martinus Nijhoff, 1978.
55. Allessie MA, Bonke FIM: Re-entry within the sino-atrial node as demonstrated by multiple microelectrode recordings in the isolated rabbit heart. *In* Bonke FIM (ed.): The Sinus Node: Structure, Function and Clinical Relevance, pp. 409–421. The Hague, Martinus Nijhoff, 1978.
56. Damato AN: Clinical evidence for sinus node reentry. *In* Bonke FIM (ed.): The Sinus Node: Structure, Function and Clinical Relevance, pp. 379–388. The Hague, Martinus Nijhoff, 1978.
57. Curry PVL, Callowhill E, Krikler DM: Paroxysmal re-entry sinus tachycardia. Br Heart J 38:311, 1976.
58. Curry PVL, Krikler DM: Paroxysmal reciprocating sinus tachycardia. *In* Kulbertus H (ed.): Re-entrant Arrhythmias, Mechanisms and Treatment, p. 39. Baltimore, University Park Press, 1977.
59. Karagueuzian HS, Jordan J, Sugi K, et al.: Appropriate diagnostic studies for sinus node dysfunction. PACE 8:242, 1985.
60. Balke B, Ware RW: An experimental study of physical fitness of Air Force personnel. U.S. Armed Forces Med J 10:675, 1959.
61. Goldberg AN, Moran JF, Resnekov L: Multistage electrocardiographic tests. Am J Cardiol 26:84, 1970.
62. Holden W, McAnulty JW, Rahimotoola SN: Characterization of heart rate response to exercise in the sick sinus syndrome. Br Heart J 40:923, 1978.
63. Ellestad MH: Stress Testing: Principles and Practice, p. 38. Philadelphia, F.A. Davis, 1975.
64. Agruss NS, Rosin EY, Adolph RJ, et al.: Significance of chronic sinus bradycardia in elderly people. Circulation 46:924, 1972.
65. Crook BRM, Cashman PM, Scott RD: Tape monitoring of the electrocardiogram in ambulant patients with sinoatrial disease. Br Heart J 35:1009, 1973.
66. Brasil A: Autonomic sinoatrial block. A new disturbance of the heart mechanism. Arg Bras Cardiol 8:159, 1955.
67. Dighton DH: Sinoatrial block: Autonomic influences and clinical assessment. Br Heart J 37:321, 1975.
68. Hamlin RL, Smith CR, Smeler DL: Sinus arrhythmia in the dog. Am J Physiol 210:321, 1966.

69. Covell JW, Chidsey CP, Braunwald E: Reduction of the cardiac responses to postganglionic sympathetic nerve stimulation in patients with cardiac decompensation. Circ Res 19:51, 1966.
70. Beiser GD, Epstein SE, Stampfer M: Impaired heart rate response to sympathetic nerve stimulation in patients with cardiac decompensation. Circulation 38:VI-40, 1968.
71. Eckberg DL, Drabinsky M, Braunwald E: Defective cardiac parasympathetic control in patients with heart disease. N Engl J Med 285:877, 1971.
72. Goldstein RE, Beiger GD, Stampfer M: Impairment of autonomically mediated heart rate control in patients with cardiac dysfunction. Circ Res 36:571, 1975.
73. Mandel WJ, Laks MM, Obayashi K: Sinus node function: Evaluation in patients with and without sinus node disease. Arch Intern Med 135:388, 1975.
74. Wang SC, Borison HL: An analysis of the carotid sinus cardiovascular reflex mechanism. Am J Physiol 150:712, 1947.
75. Glick G, Braunwald E: Relative roles of sympathetic and parasympathetic nervous systems in the reflex control of heart rate. Circ Res 16:363, 1963.
76. Robinson BF, Epstein SE, Beiger GD: Control of heart rate by the autonomic nervous system. Circ Res 19:400, 1966.
77. Deuleeschhouwer GC, Heymen E: In Kezdi P (ed.): Baroreceptors and Hypertension, pp. 187–190. New York, Pergamon Press, 1967.
78. Thomas MD, Kontos HA: Mechanisms of baroreceptor-induced changes in heart rate. Am J Physiol 218:251, 1970.
79. Dighton DH: Sinus bradycardia autonomic influences and clinical assessment. Br Heart J 36:791, 1974.
80. Jose AD, Collison D: The normal range and determinants of the intrinsic heart rate in man. Cardiovasc Res 4:160, 1970.
81. Jordan JL, Yamaguchi I, Mandel WJ: Studies on the mechanism of sinus node dysfunction in the sick sinus syndrome. Circulation 57:217, 1978.
82. Gaskell WH: On the innervation of the heart with especial reference to the heart of the tortoise. J Physiol 4:43, 1884.
83. Cohn AE, Lewis T: Auricular fibrillation and complete heart block: a description of a case of Adams-Stokes syndrome including the post-mortem examination. Heart 4:15, 1912.
84. Parkinson J, Papp C, Evans W: The electrocardiogram of the Stokes-Adams attack. Br Heart J 3:171, 1941.
85. Pick A, Langendorf R, Katz LN: Depression of cardiac pacemakers by premature impulses. Am Heart J 41:49, 1951.
86. Lange G: Action of driving stimuli from intrinsic and extrinsic sources on in situ cardiac pacemaker tissues. Circ Res 17:449, 1965.
87. Mandel WJ, Hayakawa H, Danzig R: Evaluation of sino-atrial node function in man by overdrive suppression. Circulation 44:59, 1971.
88. Mandel WJ, Hayakawa H, Allen HN: Assessment of sinus node function in patients with sick sinus syndrome. Circulation 43:761, 1972.
89. Narula OS, Samet P, Javier RP: Significance of the sinus node recovery time. Circulation 45:140, 1972.
90. Strauss HC, Bigger CMJT, et al.: Electrophysiologic evaluation of sinus node function in patients with sinus node dysfunction. Circulation 53:763, 1976.
91. Vincenzi FF, West TC: Release of autonomic mediators in cardiac tissue by direct subthreshold electrical stimulation. J Pharmacol Exp Ther 141:185, 1963.
92. Lu HH, Lange G, Brooks C McC: Factors controlling pacemaker action in cells of the sinoatrial node. Circ Res 17:461, 1965.
93. Furchgott RF, DeGubareff T, Grossman A: Release of autonomic mediators in cardiac tissue by subthreshold stimulation. Science 129:328, 1959.
94. Kodama I, Goto J, Anso S, et al.: Effects of rapid stimulation on the transmembrane action potentials of rabbit sinus node pacemaker cells. Circ Res 46:90, 1980.
95. Steinbeck G, Haberl R, Luderitz B: Effects of atrial pacing on atriosinus conduction and overdrive suppression in the isolated rabbit sinus node. Circ Res 46:859, 1981.
96. Konsai T: Electrophysiologic consideration of sick sinus syndrome. Jpn Circ J 40:194, 1976.
97. Jordan JL, Yamaguchi I, Mandel WJ: Studies on the mechanism of suppression of sinus node pacemaker automaticity by atrial overdrive pacing. Clin Res 26:241A, 1978.
98. Engel TR, Meister SG, Feitusa GS: Appraisal of sinus node artery disease. Circulation 52:285, 1975.
99. Singer D, Parameswaran R, Goldberg G: Sinus and AV nodal dysfunction following myocardial infarction. J Electrocardiol 8:281, 1975.
100. Mandel WJ, Yamaguchi I: The effects of changes in extracellular pH on sinoatrial conduction. Am J Cardiol 39:265, 1977.
101. Benditt DC, Strauss HC, Scheinman MM, et al.: Analysis of secondary pauses following termination of rapid atrial pacing in man. Circulation 54:436, 1976.
102. Rosen RM, Loeb HS, Sinno MZ: Cardiac conduction in patients with symptomatic sinus node disease. Circulation 43:836, 1971.
103. Engel TR, Schaal SF: Digitalis in the sick sinus syndrome: the effects of digitalis on sinoatrial automaticity and atrioventricular conduction. Circulation 48:1201, 1973.
104. Jordan JL, Yamaguchi I, Mandel WJ: The sick sinus syndrome: pathophysiology, significance and treatment. Cardiol Dig 12:11, 1977.
105. Kulbertus HE, De Leval-Ruffen F, Casters L: Sinus node recovery time in elderly. Br Heart J 37:420, 1975.
106. Strauss HC, Bigger JT Jr, Saroff AL, et al.: Electrophysiologic evaluation of sinus node function in patient with sinus node dysfunction. Circulation 53:763, 1976.
107. Scheinman MM, Strauss HC, Abbott JA: Electrophysiologic testing for patients with sinus node dysfunction. J Electrocardiol 12:211, 1979.
108. Reiffel JA, Gang E, Bigger JT Jr, et al.: Sinus node recovery time related to paced cycle length in normals and patients with sinoatrial dysfunction. Am Heart J 104:746, 1982.
109. Goldreyer BN, Damato AN: Sinoatrial node entrance block. Circulation 44:789, 1971.
110. Kerr CR, Prystowsky EN, Browning DJ, et al.: Characterization of refractoriness in the sinus node of the rabbit. Circ Res 47:742, 1980.
111. Kerr CR, Strauss HC: The measurement of sinus node refractoriness in man. Circulation 68:1231, 1983.
112. Jordan J, Yamaguchi I, Mandel WJ, et al.: Comparative effects of overdrive on sinus and subsidiary pacemaker function. Am Heart J 93:367, 1977.
113. Yamaguchi I, Mandel WJ: Alterations in measured and estimated sinus node conduction times: Effects of site stimulation and drug infusion. Arch Ven Cardiol 3:78, 1976.
114. Yabek SM, Jarmakani JM, Roberts NK: Sinus node function in children. Factors influencing its evaluation. Circulation 53:28, 1976.
115. Jose AD, Taylor RR: Autonomic blockade by propranolol and atropine to study myocardial function in man. J Clin Invest 48:2019, 1969.
116. Jordan JL, Yamaguchi E, Mandel WJ: Characteristics of sinoatrial conduction in patients with coronary artery disease. Circulation 55:569, 1977.
117. Massini G, Dianda R, Grazina A: Analysis of sino-atrial conduction in man using premature atrial stimulation. Cardiovasc Res 9:498, 1975.
118. Steinbeck G, Luderitz G: Comparative study of sino-atrial conduction time and sinus node recovery time. Br Heart J 37:956, 1975.
119. Bashour T, Hemb R, Wickramerekaran B: An unusual effect of atropine on overdrive suppression. Circulation 48:911, 1973.
120. Reiffel JP, Bigger JT Jr, Giardina EGV: "Paradoxical" prolongation of sinus nodal recovery time after atropine in the sick sinus syndrome. Am J Cardiol 36:98, 1975.
121. Jordan JL, Yamaguchi I, Mandel WJ: The effects of verapamil on sinoatrial conduction in isolated tissue. Clin Res 26:279A, 1978.
122. Gupta PK, Lichstein E, Chadda KD: Appraisal of sinus nodal recovery time in patients with sick sinus syndrome. Am J Cardiol 34:265, 1974.
123. Chadda KD, Banka VS, Bodenheimer MM: Corrected sinus node recovery: Experimental, physiological and pathologic determinants. Circulation 51:797, 1975.
124. Mason JW: Overdrive suppression in the transplanted heart: Effect of the autonomic nervous system on human sinus node recovery. Circulation 62:688, 1980.
125. Jordan JL, Mandel WJ: Comparative effects of duration of

atrial overdrive pacing in patients with and without intrinsic sinus node dysfunction. In preparation.
126. Desai JM, Scheinman MM, Strauss HC, et al.: Electrophysiologic effects of combined autonomic blockade in patients with sinus node disease. Circulation 63:953, 1981.
127. Bonke FIM, Bouman LN, VanRisn HE: Change of cardiac rhythm in the rabbit after an atrial premature beat. Circ Res 24:533, 1969.
128. Bonke FIM, Bouman LN, Schopman FJG: Effect of an early atrial premature beat on activity of the sinoatrial rhythm in the rabbit. Circ Res 24:704, 1971.
129. Klein HO, Singer DH, Hoffman BF: Effects of atrial premature systoles on sinus rhythm in the rabbit. Circ Res 32:480, 1973.
130. Strauss HC, Saroff AL, Bigger JT Jr, et al.: Premature atrial stimulation as a key to the understanding of sinoatrial conduction in man. Presentation of data and critical review of the literature. Circulation 47:86, 1973.
131. Strauss NC, Bigger JT Jr: Electrophysiological properties of rabbit sinoatrial perinodal fibers. Circ Res 31:490, 1972.
132. Rasmussen K: Chronic sinoatrial heart block. Am Heart J 81:38, 1971.
133. Scherf D: The mechanisms of sinoatrial block. Am J Cardiol 23:769, 1969.
134. Engel TR, Bond RC, Schaal SF: First degree sinoatrial heart block: Sinoatrial block in the sick sinus syndrome. Am Heart J 91:303, 1976.
135. Childers RW, et al.: Sinus node echoes. Am J Cardiol 31:220, 1973.
136. Paritsky Z, Obayashi K, Mandel WJ: Atrial tachycardia secondary to sinoatrial node reentry. Chest 66:526, 1974.
137. Tzivoni D, Jordan JL, Barrett P, et al.: Two zones of full compensation: An unexpected finding related to alterations in conduction at the sinoatrial junction. Clin Res 26:241, 1978.
138. Langendorf R, Lesser ME, Plotkin P: Atrial parasystole with interpolation: Observations on prolonged sinoatrial conduction. Am Heart J 63:649, 1962.
139. Scheinman MM, Runkel FW, Peters RW: Sinoatrial function and atrial refractoriness in patients with sick sinus syndrome. Circulation 48:IV-215, 1973.
140. Bigger JT: A simple, rapid method for the diagnosis of first-degree sinoatrial block in man. Am Heart J 87:731, 1974.
141. Dhingra RC, Amar-Y-Leon F, Wynham C: Clinical significance of prolonged sinoatrial conduction time. Circulation 55:8, 1977.
142. Breithardt G, Seipel L, Loogen F: Sinus node recovery time and calculated sinoatrial conduction time in normal subjects and patients with sinus node dysfunction. Circulation 56:43, 1977.
143. Miller HC, Strauss HC: Measurement of sinoatrial conduction time by premature atrial stimulation in the rabbit. Circ Res 35:935, 1974.
144. Breithardt G, Seipel L: The effect of premature atrial depolarization on sinus node automaticity in man. Circulation 53:920, 1976.
145. Denes P, Wu D, Dhingra R: The effects of cycle length on cardiac refractory periods in man. Circulation 49:32, 1974.
146. Reiffel JA, Bigger JT Jr, Konstam MA: The relationship between sinoatrial conduction time and sinus cycle length during spontaneous sinus arrhythmia in adults. Circulation 50:924, 1974.
147. Sanot T, Yamagishi S: Spread of excitation from the sinus node. Circ Res 16:423, 1965.
148. Dhingra RC, Wyndham C, Amar-Y-Leon F: Sinus nodal responses to atrial extrastimuli in patients without apparent sinus node disease. Am J Cardiol 36:445, 1975.
149. Dhingra RC, Amar-Y Leon F, Wyndham C: Electrophysiologic effects of atropine on sinus node and atrium in patients with sinus node dysfunction. Am J Cardiol 38:848, 1976.
150. Strauss HC, Gilbert M, Svenson R: Electrophysiologic effects of propranolol on sinus node function in patients with sinus node dysfunction. Circulation 54:452, 1976.
151. Narula OS, Narashimhan S, Vasquez M, et al.: A new method for measurement of sinoatrial conduction time. Circulation 58:706, 1978.
152. Grant AO, Kirkorian G, Benditt DG, et al.: The estimation of sinoatrial conduction time in rabbit heart by the constant atrial pacing technique. Circulation 60:597, 1979.
153. Kang PS, Gomes JAC, Keler G, et al.: Role of autonomic regulatory mechanisms in sinoatrial conduction and sinus node automaticity in sick sinus syndrome. Circulation 64:832, 1981.
154. Breithardt G, Seipel L: Comparative study of two methods of estimating sinoatrial conduction time in man. Am J Cardiol 42:965, 1978.
155. Cramer M, Siegal M, Bigger TJ, et al.: Characteristics of extracellular potentials recorded from the sinoatrial pacemaker of the rabbit. Circ Res 41L:292, 1977.
156. Hariman RJ, Krongrad E, Boxer RA: A new method for recording of extracellular sinoatrial electrograms during cardiac surgery in man. Am J Cardiol 41:375, 1978.
157. Cramer M, Hariman RJ, Boxer RA, et al.: Catheter recording of sinoatrial node potentials in the in situ canine heart. Am J Cardiol 41:374, 1978.
158. Cramer M, Seigal M, Hoffman BF: Electrogram of the canine sinus node. Circulation 54:II-156, 1976.
159. Hariman RJ, Krongrad E, Boxer RA, et al.: Methods for recording electrograms of the sinoatrial node during cardiac surgery in man. Circulation 61:1024, 1980.
160. Castillo-Fesnoy A, Thebaut JF, Achard F, et al.: Identification du potentiel sinusal chez l'homme. Arch Mol Coeur 72:948, 1977.
161. Reiffel JA, Gang E, Glicklich J, et al.: The human sinus node electrogram: A transvenous catheter technique and a comparison of directly measured and indirectly estimated sinoatrial conduction time in adults. Circulation 62:1324, 1980.
162. Hariman RJ, Krongrad E, Beyer RA, et al.: Method for recording electrical activity of the sinoatrial node and automatic atrial foci during cardiac catheterization in human subjects. Am J Cardiol 45:775, 1980.
163. Gomes JAC, Kang PS, El-Sherif N: The sinus node electrogram in patients with and without sick sinus syndrome. Techniques and correlation between directly measured and indirectly estimated sinoatrial conduction time. Circulation 66:864, 1982.
164. Asseman P, Berzun B, Desry DR, et al.: Persistent sinus nodal electrograms during abnormally prolonged post pacing atrial pauses in sick sinus syndrome in humans: Sinoatrial block vs. overdrive suppression. Circulation 68:33, 1983.
165. Koniski T: Electrophysiological consideration of sick sinus syndrome. Jpn Circ J 40:194, 1976.
166. Kodama I, Goto J, Ando S, et al.: Effects of rapid atrial stimulation on the transmembrane potentials of rabbit sinus node pacemaker cell. Circ Res 46:90, 1980.
167. Steinbeck G, Naberi R, Luderitz B: Effects of atrial pacing on atriosinus conduction and overdrive suppression in the isolated rabbit sinus node. Circ Res 46:859, 1980.
168. Gomes JA, Hariman BI, Chowdry IA: New application of direct sinus node recordings in man: Assessment of sinus node recovery time. Circulation 70:663, 1984.
169. Gang ES, Oseran DS, Mandel WJ, et al.: The sinus node electrogram in patients with the hypersensitive carotid sinus syndrome. J Am Cardiol 55:1525, 1985.
170. Weiss S, Baker JP: The carotid sinus reflex in health and disease: Its role in the causation of fainting and convulsions. Medicine 12:297, 1933.
171. Walter PF, Crawley IS, Derney ER: Carotid hypersensitivity and syncope. Am J Cardiol 42:396, 1978.
172. Thomas JE: Hyperactive carotid sinus reflex and carotid sinus syncope. Mayo Clin Prac 44:127, 1969.
173. Nathanson MH: Hyperactive cardioinhibitory carotid sinus reflex. Arch Intern Med 77:491, 1946.
174. Sigler LH: The cardioinhibitory carotid sinus reflex. Am J Cardiol 12:175, 1963.
175. Hartzler GO, Maloney JD: Cardioinhibitory carotid sinus hypersensitivity. Arch Intern Med 137:727, 1977.
176. Davis AB, Stephens MR, Davies AG: Carotid sinus hypersensitivity in patients presenting with syncope. Br Heart J 42:583, 1979.
177. Probst P, Muhlberger V, Lederbauer M, et al.: Electrophysiologic findings in carotid sinus massage. PACE 6:689, 1983.
178. Katoh T, Karagueuzian HS, Jordan JL, et al.: The cellular electrophysiologic mechanism of the dual actions of disopyramide on rabbit sinus node function. Circulation 66:1216, 1982.
179. Karagueuzian HS, Mandel WJ: The effects of drugs on sinus node function. *In* Masoni A, Alboni P (eds.): Cardiac Electrophysiology Today. New York, Academic Press, 1982.

180. Conde C, Leppo J, Lipski J, et al.: Effectiveness of pacemaker treatment in the bradycardia-tachycardia syndrome. Am J Cardiol 32:209, 1973.
181. Sigurd B, Jensen G, Melbom J, et al.: Adams-Stokes syndrome caused by sinoatrial block. Br Heart J 35:1002, 1973.
182. Rokseth R, Hatle L: Prospective study on the occurrence and management of chronic sinoatrial disease, with follow-up. Br Heart J 36:582, 1974.
183. Radford DJ, Julian DG: Sick sinus syndrome: Experience of a cardiac pacemaker clinic. Br Med J 3:504, 1974.
184. Sowton E, Hendrix G, Roy P: Ten-year survey of treatment with implanted cardiac pacemaker. Br Med J 3:155, 1974.
185. Hartel G, Talvensaari T: Treatment of sinoatrial syndrome with permanent cardiac pacing in 90 patients. Acta Med Scand 198:341, 1975.
186. Chokshi DS, Mascarenhas E, Sanet P, et al.: Treatment of sinoatrial rhythm disturbances with permanent cardiac pacing. Am J Cardiol 32:215, 1973.
187. Skagen K, Hansen JF: The long-term prognosis for patients with sinoatrial block treated with permanent pacemaker. Acta Med Scand 199:13, 1975.
188. Krishnaswami K, Geraci AR: Permanent pacing in disorders of sinus node function. Am Heart J 89:579, 1975.
189. Bayley TJ: Long-term ventricular pacing in treatment of sinoatrial block. Br Med J 3:456, 1971.
190. Rubenstein JJ, Schulman CL, Yurchak PM: Clinical spectrum of the sick sinus syndrome. Circulation 46:5, 1972.
191. Wan SH, Lee GS, Toh CCS: The sick sinus syndrome. A study of 15 cases. Br Heart J 34:942, 1972.
192. Rosen K, Loeb H, Sinno MZ: Cardiac conduction in patients with symptomatic sinus node disease. Circulation 43:836, 1971.
193. Narula O: Atrioventricular conduction defects in patients with sinus bradycardia. Analysis by His bundle recordings. Circulation 44:1096, 1971.
194. Easley RM, Goldstein S: Sinoatrial syncope. Am J Med 50:166, 1971.
195. Zipes DP, Wallace RG, Sealy WC, et al.: Artificial atrial and ventricular pacing in the treatment of arrhythmias. Ann Intern Med 70:885, 1969.
196. Chen TO: Transvenous ventricular pacing in the treatment of paroxysmal atrial tachyarrhythmias alternating with sinus bradycardia and standstill. Am J Cardiol 22:874, 1968.
197. Zoll PM, Linenthal DJ, Zarsky LRN: Ventricular fibrillation. Treatment and prevention by external cardiac currents. N Engl J Med 262:105, 1960.
198. Han J, Millet D, Chizzonitti B, et al.: Temporal dispersion of recovery of excitability in atrium and ventricle as a function of heart rate. Am Heart J 71:481, 1966.
199. Han J, De Traglia J, Miller D, et al.: Incidence of ectopic beats as a function of basic rate in the ventricle. Am Heart J 72:632, 1966.
200. Sandoe E, Flensted-Jensen E: Adams-Stokes seizures in patients with attacks of both tachy and bradycardia, a therapeutic challenge. Acta Med Scand 186:111, 1969.

7

Atrioventricular and Intraventricular Conduction Disorders: Clinical Aspects

Shantha Ursell
Moh'D. A. Habbab
Nabil El-Sherif

The earliest description of slow heart rate leading to symptoms of syncope was made by Adams[1] and Stokes[2] in the first half of the nineteenth century. In 1899, Wenckebach[3] described progressive atrioventricular (AV) block based on analysis of jugular venous pulse, and in 1924 Mobitz[4] described the criteria for the two types of second-degree AV block. Anatomic description of the different parts of the conduction system was made in the last few decades of the nineteenth century and early twentieth century.[5-7] Although the functional importance of some parts of the conduction system is still controversial, details of its structure, including electron microscopy studies of the specialized tissues, have been extensively described.[8,9]

The introduction of electrode catheter techniques for recording His bundle activity[10-12] has improved our understanding of AV conduction and helped to optimize the indications for cardiac pacing. Although the indications for pacing have increased over the years, AV block is still an important indication for pacemaker implantation.[13] For this reason, it is important to understand the electrophysiologic mechanisms, electrocardiographic characteristics, clinical presentations, and therapeutic options of the various types of AV and intraventricular conduction disorders.

Anatomy of the AV Conduction System

Tawara was the first to describe the connection between the atrium and the ventricle.[6] The "AV junction" encompasses the AV node with its atrial approaches, the penetrating His bundle and its bifurcation. The AV node tissue is epicardial during embryonic development and migrates inward as the dorsal endocardial cushion invaginates during formation of the AV valves. This position in contact with the posterior atrial wall is retained in the adult heart.[14] The AV node is an ovoid structure measuring $6 \times 3 \times 1$ mm^3 and situated just beneath the right atrial endocardium toward the apex of the triangle of Koch.[15,16] The latter is formed by the continuation of the eustachian valve (the tendon of Todaro[17]), the septal attachment of the tricuspid valve, and the orifice of the coronary sinus (Fig. 7-1). These landmarks are of considerable value as guidelines to the AV conduction tissue during surgery (see Chap. 24). The atrial approaches to the AV node extend toward the septal leaflet of the tricuspid valve, and the lower limb of the AV node extends into the mitral annulus. The anterior margin of the AV node is continuous with the His bundle. The AV node has an abundant blood supply, mostly from the AV nodal artery, which originates from the right coronary artery in 90% of the population and from the circumflex artery in the remaining 10%.[18] The AV nodal artery also supplies the proximal portion of the His bundle. The AV node is richly innervated by both sympathetic and parasympathetic fibers.[19]

Based on both functional and histologic differences, three regions are identified in the AV node[20,21]:

1. The atrial approaches to the AV node, which are also referred to as the transitional cell zone or AN region.
2. The midnodal or compact node (N region), which is made up of interconnecting fasciculi of small cells with extensions into the central fibrous body and the annulus of the mitral and tricuspid valves.

Supported by National Institutes of Health Grants HL 31341 and HL 36680 and Veterans Administration Medical Research Funds.

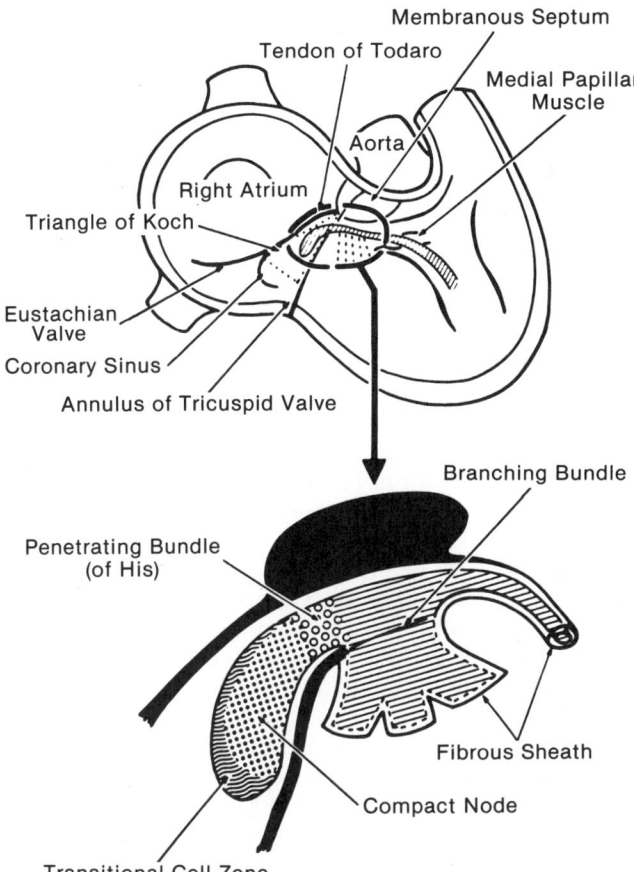

FIGURE 7–1
Diagrammatic illustration of the gross landmarks of the AV junctional area and its cellular components and zones. See text for details. (Reprinted with permission from Anderson RH, et al.: Br Heart J 45:67, 1981.)

3. The nodo-Hisian or penetrating bundle (NH region), which leads directly into the penetrating His bundle and its branching portion.

Microelectrode studies have shown that the AN zone has a high rate of spontaneous diastolic depolarizations, the NH zone has a lower rate, and the central compact node has no automaticity. This N zone appears to be the site for most of the delay in the AV node.[22,23]

The His bundle begins at an ill-defined point of the lower end of the AV node and penetrates the central fibrous body and descends through the membranous septum on the left side until the left bundle branch is given off. The His bundle then continues as the right bundle branch. The common bundle consists of cells larger than those in the AV node, and most of the cells resemble Purkinje fibers. These cells are arranged in longitudinal fascicles separated by a collagenous framework that is incompletely linked by some fibrous septa.[24] The bundle branches have in most cases a dual blood supply from both left and right coronary arteries. The proximal right bundle branch and the left bundle branch with its anterior fascicle receive their blood supply from the left anterior descending coronary artery and the AV node artery. The posterior fascicle of the left bundle branch receives its blood supply from the AV node artery and from branches of the posterior descending coronary artery and the circumflex artery.[25]

Normal AV Conduction

The AV conduction time is measured from the beginning of the P wave (atrial activation) to the onset of the QRS complex (ventricular activation). In the His bundle electrogram, the P-R interval can be divided into three subintervals (Fig. 7–2):

1. The P-A interval, which reflects the intra-atrial conduction time, is measured from the onset of the high right atrial electrogram to the onset of the low atrial electrogram in the His bundle area.
2. The A-H interval, which represents mostly AV nodal conduction time, is measured from the beginning of the low atrial electrogram to the beginning of the His bundle deflection.
3. The H-V interval represents the conduction time through the His bundle and the bundle branches until ventricular activation. It is measured from the beginning of the His bundle deflection to the beginning of earliest ventricular depolarization in either the intracardiac or surface electrograms.

The normal range and mean and standard deviations of these intervals are, respectively, P-A = 25 − 45 (37 ± 7) ms, A-H = 50 − 120 (77 ± 16) ms, and H-V = 35 − 45 (40 ± 3) ms. The duration of the His bundle is usually 15 to 20 ms.[26]

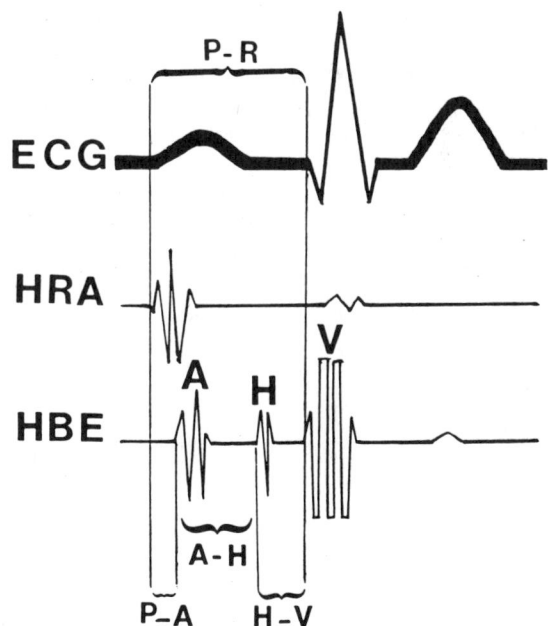

FIGURE 7–2
Schematic illustration of a single cardiac cycle showing the intervals measured during an electrophysiologic study. HRA = High right atrial electrogram; HBE = His bundle electrogram recording low right atrial activity (A), His bundle activity (H), and ventricular septal activity (V).

Abnormal AV Conduction

AV blocks have been classified into four types: first-degree, second-degree, high-degree, and third-degree (or complete) heart block.

FIRST-DEGREE AV BLOCK

First-degree AV block is characterized by prolongation of the P-R interval to more than 0.20 s on the surface electrocardiogram (ECG). It may result from prolongation of conduction in the atrium, AV node, bundle of His, bundle branches, or in a combination of more than one site.[26-28] In most cases, however, the AV node appears to be the site of delay. Conduction delays in the His-Purkinje system usually do not result in an abnormally prolonged P-R interval.

In the His bundle electrogram, first-degree AV nodal block is represented by a prolongation of the A-H interval (>120 ms), whereas the H-V interval is normal (Fig. 7-3). Occasionally, transient first-degree AV nodal block during sinus rhythm can be a manifestation of dual AV nodal pathways.[29] In this case, the prolonged P-R and A-H intervals are due to block in the fast AV nodal pathway and conduction in the slow pathway. Alternation between a short and long P-R interval can be seen with no perceptible change in the sinus rate (Figs. 7-4 and 7-5). In the majority of cases of first-degree AV block with narrow QRS, the AV node is the primary site of delay; however, in some patients intra-Hisian conduction delay may result in a split His potential and prolongation of the His potential duration, the H-V and the P-R intervals.[27] Intra-Hisian disease causing first-degree AV block can be diagnosed only from a His bundle electrogram.

The presence of first-degree AV block in association with a wide QRS complex raises the question of whether the delay is localized in the AV node or in the His-Purkinje system (Fig. 7-6) or is due to a combination of AV nodal and His-Purkinje delay (Fig. 7-7). In the presence of first-degree AV block, the pattern of intraventricular conduction disorder usually allows certain assumptions regarding the site of AV conduction delay. A right bundle branch block and normal frontal plane axis is often associated with AV nodal delay and normal His-Purkinje conduction.[30] On the other hand, a right bundle branch block and left axis deviation can be associated with AV nodal or His-Purkinje delay. A left right bundle branch block with right axis deviation is associated with His-Purkinje delay in more than 50% of cases.[31]

The prevalence of first-degree AV block in the young adult population ranges from 0.65 to 1.1%.[32, 33] A higher prevalence (1.3%) is found in subjects over 50 years of age; however, the longest P-R intervals tend to occur in the younger age groups.[32] In a study of highly trained athletes, first-degree AV block was detected in 8.7%.[34] During long-term ambulatory monitoring, subjects with first-degree AV nodal block not

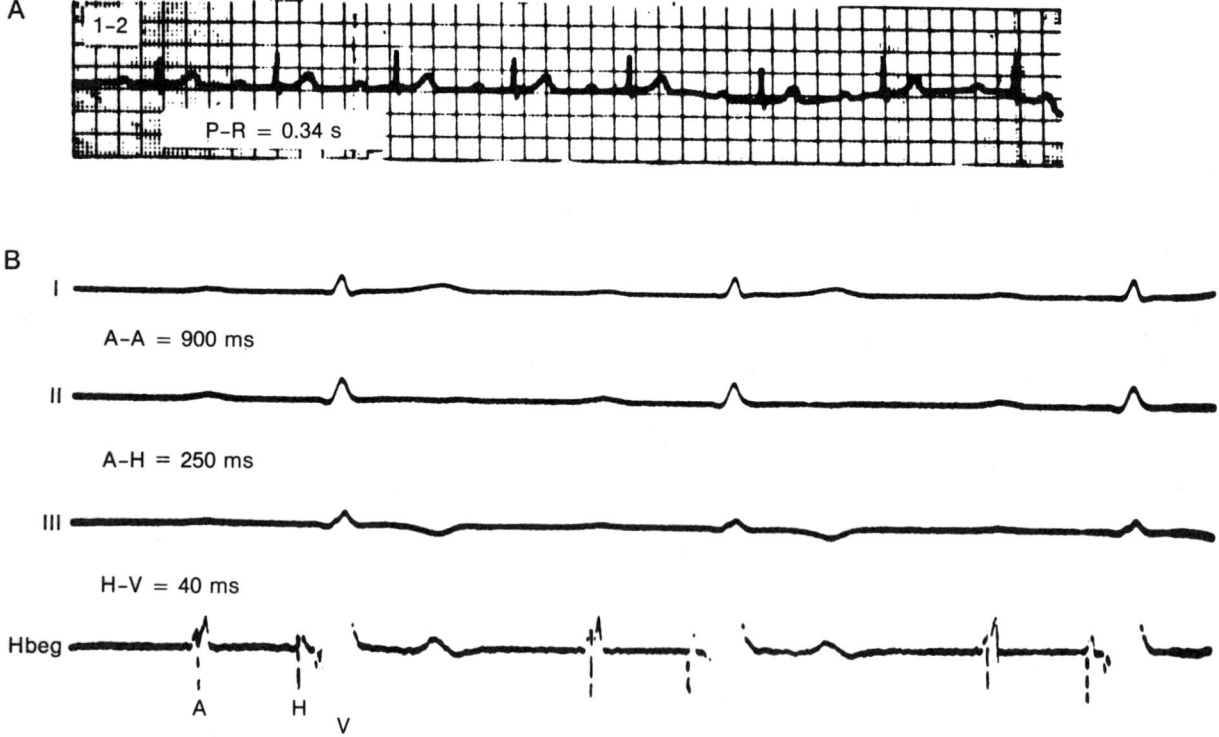

FIGURE 7-3
Recordings from a 76-year-old man with sclerodegenerative AV nodal disease showing first degree AV block (P-R interval = 0.34 seconds). The His bundle electrogram shows AV nodal conduction delay with a markedly prolonged A-H interval of 250 ms (normal, 60–120 ms). The H-V interval of 40 ms reflects normal His-Purkinje conduction. A, V, and H = atrial, ventricular, and His bundle deflections, respectively. Hbeg = His bundle electrogram.

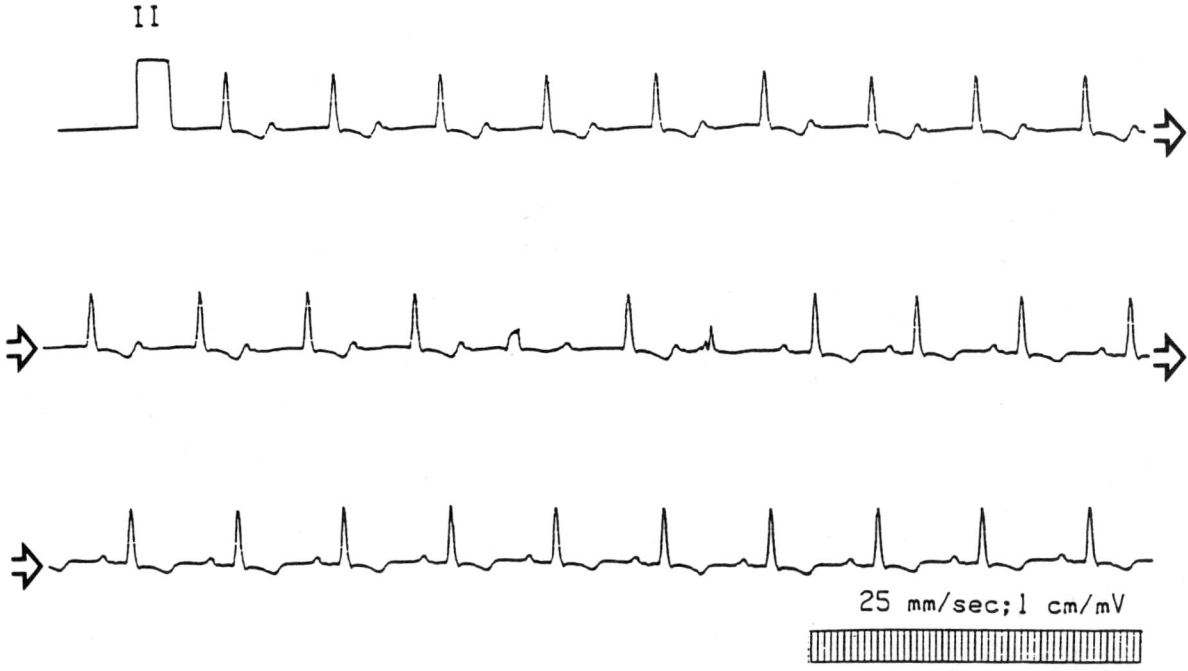

FIGURE 7-4
Continuous electrocardiographic recording showing sinus rhythm at a relatively constant rate of 95 beats per minute and two sets of P-R intervals (0.36 second in the top tracing and 0.16 second in the bottom tracing). The middle tracing shows the transition from a prolonged to a normal P-R interval following a ventricular ectopic beat but with no perceptible change of the sinus rate.

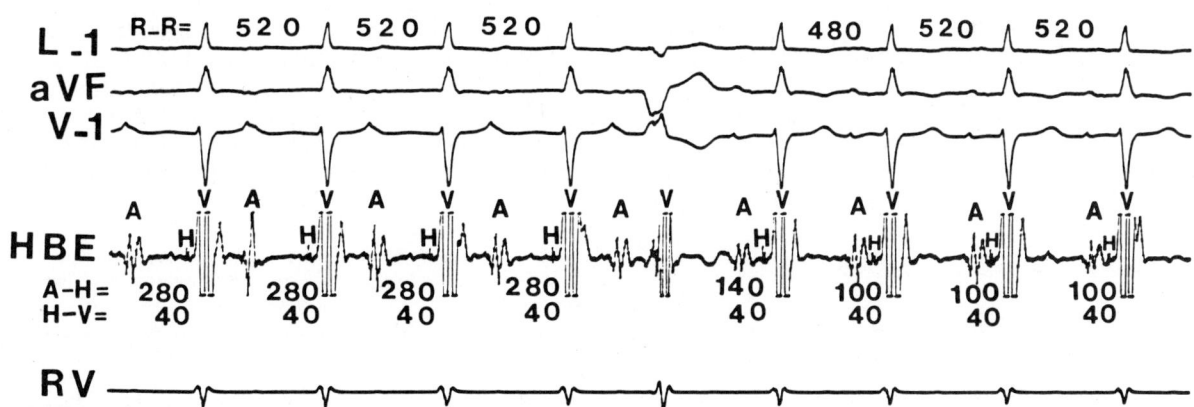

FIGURE 7-5
A His bundle recording (HBE) from the same case illustrated in Figure 7-4. Similar to Figure 7-4, the transition from a prolonged to a normal P-R interval followed a ventricular premature beat. The change in the P-R interval is due solely to shortening of the A-H interval from 280 ms to 100 ms at a constant sinus cycle of 520 ms. The long A-H interval is explained by block in an AV nodal fast pathway with conduction in a slow pathway. The transition from slow to fast pathway anterograde conduction following a ventricular premature beat may be due to retrograde concealed conduction in the slow pathway. RV = right ventricular electrogram.

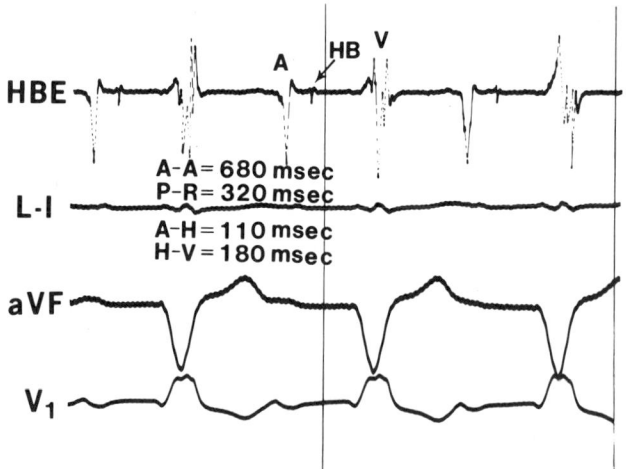

FIGURE 7–6
Recordings from a 58-year-old man with acute anterior wall myocardial infarction complicated by right bundle branch block, left anterior fascicular block, and first degree AV block (P-R interval = 0.32 second). The His bundle electrogram (HBE) shows normal AV nodal conduction (A-H interval = 110 ms) and markedly prolonged His-Purkinje conduction (H-V interval = 180 ms). A, V, and HB = atrial, ventricular, and His bundle deflections, respectively. Time lines are set at 1-s intervals.

uncommonly show instances of second-degree block of the Wenckebach type. Since the etiologies of both types of AV nodal block are usually similar, this is discussed under Wenckebach Block in the AV Node.

The prognosis and therapy of first-degree AV block depend mostly on the site of the delay. Intra-atrial delays rarely progress to second-degree block.[35] However, associated atrial arrhythmias due to diseased atria[36] may warrant therapy. First-degree AV block caused by AV nodal delay does not require any specific therapy. Drugs like digitalis and beta-adrenergic blocking agents are not contraindicated, although caution should be exercised because the degree of block may worsen. The prognostic significance of conduction delay in the His-Purkinje system (prolonged H-V interval) is discussed in detail later in the chapter.

SECOND-DEGREE AV BLOCK

Second-degree AV block has been classified into type I (Wenckebach or Mobitz I) and type II (Mobitz II) AV block.

Wenckebach AV Block

Wenckebach AV block is characterized on the surface ECG by progressive prolongation of the P-R interval until a P wave fails to conduct to the ventricle. In a typical Wenckebach arrangement, the degree of increment of the P-R interval is less in successive beats, with most of the increment occurring between the first and second beat in the cycle. This would result in progressive decrease of the R-R interval. Wenckebach AV block may result from conduction delay and block in the AV node, the bundle of His, or the bundle branch–Purkinje system.[27, 28, 37, 38]

WENCKEBACH BLOCK IN THE AV NODE

Wenckebach block in the AV node can be induced by rapid atrial pacing in a majority of subjects with normal AV conduction. Incremental atrial pacing progressively results in first-degree AV nodal delay, Wenckebach AV nodal block, and a 2:1 or higher degree AV nodal block (Fig. 7–8). The AV node is also the most frequent site for spontaneous Wenckebach type second-degree AV block, occurring in almost 75% of patients studied by His bundle recording.[27] In the His bundle electrogram, progressive prolongation of the A-H interval is seen until an atrial deflection is blocked within the AV node (i.e., is not followed by a His bundle deflection). In a typical Wenckebach periodicity, the increment in the A-H interval decreases progressively and the R-R interval becomes progressively shorter. However, typical features of Wenckebach periodicity are not common, and in fact the atypical forms are most commonly seen.[39] Both spontaneous and pacing-induced atypical Wenckebach periods increase as AV conduction ratios increase to 5:4 or greater.[40] Sometimes an atypical Wenckebach arrangement may resemble Mobitz II AV block.[41] This type, also called pseudo–Mobitz II is defined as a long

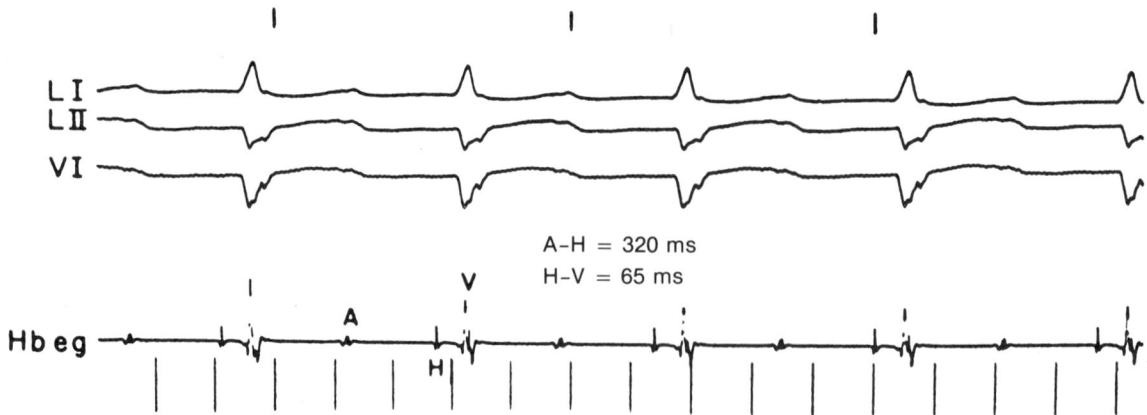

FIGURE 7–7
His bundle electrogram in a patient with first degree AV block and left bundle branch block. Note that the first degree AV block is due to conduction delay in the AV node (A-H interval = 320 msec) and His-Purkinje system (H-V interval = 65 ms). Time lines at top and bottom are set at 1-s and 200-ms intervals, respectively.

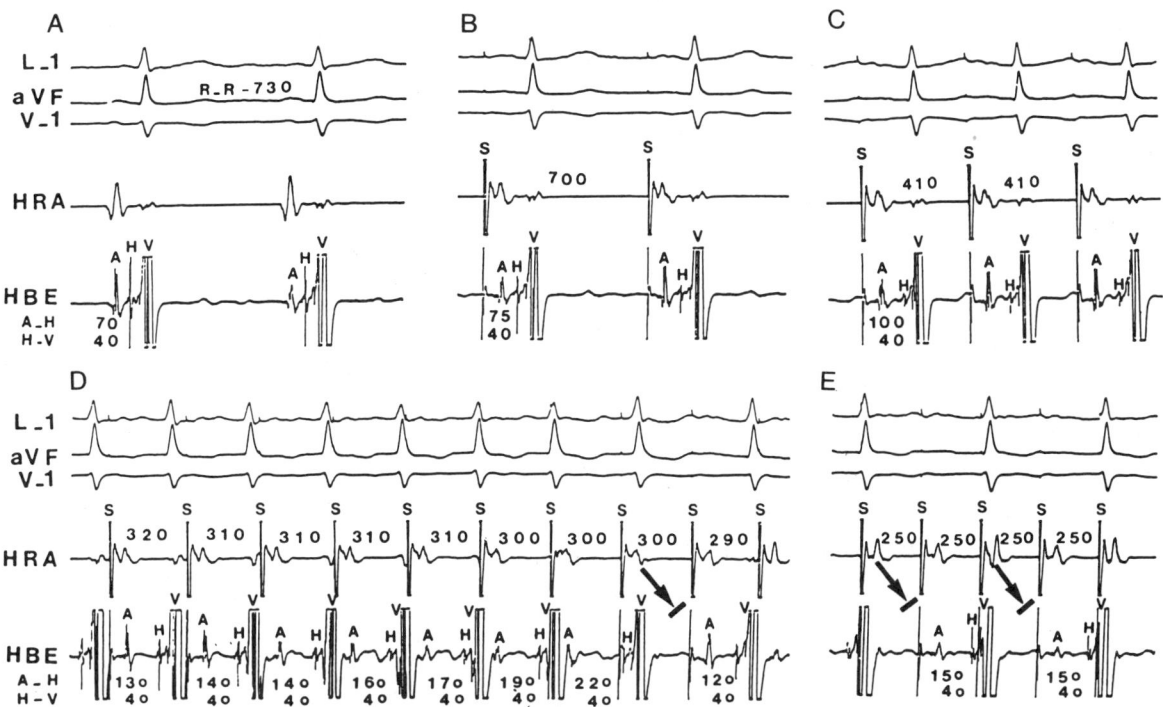

FIGURE 7–8
Effects of incremental atrial pacing on normal AV nodal conduction. A, Normal sinus rhythm. The A-H and H-V intervals are within normal limits (70 and 40 ms, respectively). Atrial pacing at cycle lengths of 700 ms (B) and 410 ms (C) resulted in a gradual increase in the A-H interval, but 1:1 AV conduction was maintained. D, Incremental atrial pacing from 370 to 290 ms resulted in gradual lengthening of the A-H interval before AV block occurred in the AV node (i.e., the atrial deflection was not followed by a His bundle potential). E, Atrial pacing at a cycle length of 250 ms resulted in a stable 2:1 AV nodal block. Note that the A-H interval during 2:1 block (150 ms) was longer than the A-H interval during 1:1 conduction in C (100 ms), even though the effective ventricular cycle length in E is longer compared with C (500 ms vs. 410 ms). This is explained by concealed conduction of the blocked atrial impulses during 2:1 AV block.

Wenckebach cycle in which, at least, the last three beats of the cycle show relatively constant P-R intervals (variations of no more than 0.02 seconds in the surface leads and no more than 10 ms in His bundle electrogram) and in which the P-R interval immediately following the blocked beat is shorter than the P-R interval before block by 0.04 second or more[41] (Figs. 7–9 and 7–10). In one study, the pseudo–Mobitz II block was seen in 19% of atypical AV nodal Wenckebach periods.[41] In contrast to Mobitz II block, a pseudo–Mobitz II block carries a very low risk for development of paroxysmal AV block.

Wenckebach AV block has been reported during routine ambulatory electrocardiographic monitoring in 6% of asymptomatic young medical students with no apparent heart disease[42] and was noted mostly during sleep. It has also been noted in young well-trained athletes and is thought to be due to conditioning and enhanced vagal tone.[34] These patients typically show significant improvement in AV nodal function during exercise or following atropine administration.[43, 44] However, in a small group of young children with Wenckebach AV block, progression to high-degree AV block was noted over the course of many years.[45] Hence, in children with or without heart disease, careful monitoring appears to be warranted when second-degree AV block is noted. Wenckebach AV nodal block can also be induced by a number of drugs that prolong AV nodal refractoriness, including digitalis, beta-adrenergic blocking agents, and the calcium channel blocking agents verapamil and diltiazem. Central and peripheral sympatholytic agents such as alpha-methyldopa and clonidine have also been implicated, as well as ophthalmologic preparations of beta-blockers such as timolol that may undergo systemic absorption.[46, 47]

AV nodal conduction disorders including Wenckebach block are not uncommon in acute inferior wall myocardial infarction. In this clinical setting, AV nodal blocks show a bimodal pattern.[48–50] During the first hour of myocardial infarction, AV nodal conduction disorders occur very frequently. Observations from mobile coronary care units have revealed that second- and third-degree AV blocks occur in approximately 11% of patients with inferior wall myocardial infarction seen within 1 hour after onset of symptoms.[48] In contrast, this incidence was extremely low in those seen during the second hour after onset of symptoms. The very short duration and its immediate response to atropine suggest that vasovagal mechanisms probably play a very important role in the genesis of these conduction disorders. More recently, the role of adenosine released during myocardial ischemia has been implicated.[51] AV nodal conduction disturbances in hospitalized patients occur in approximately 20% of

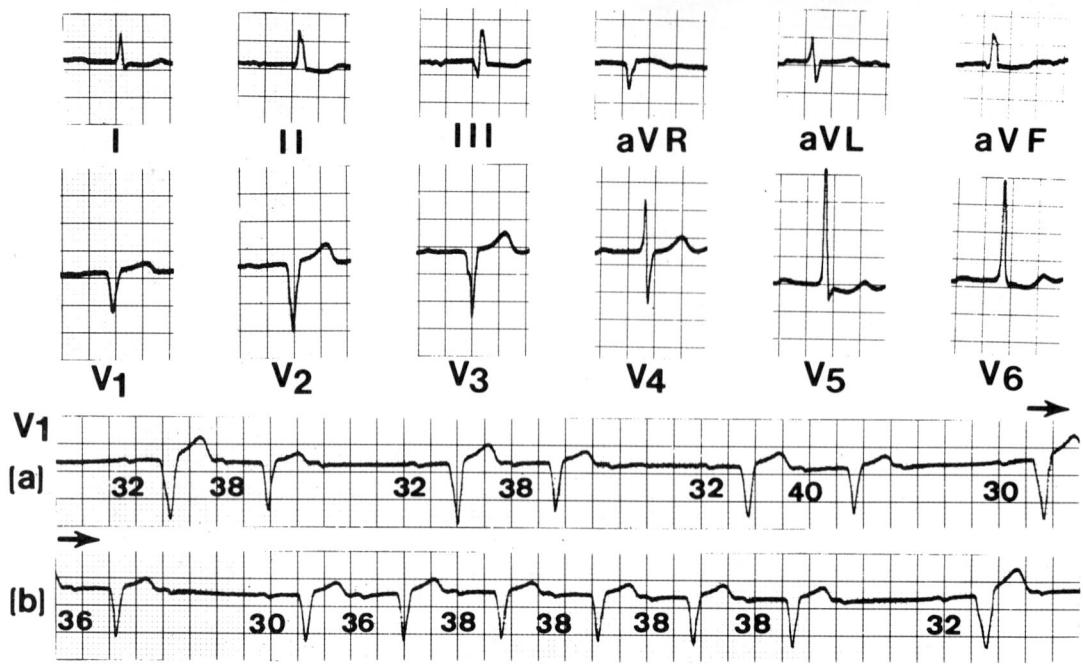

FIGURE 7–9
Pseudo–Mobitz II block in the AV node. Recordings were obtained from a 55-year-old man 2 days after the onset of an acute inferior wall myocardial infarction. The 12-lead electrocardiogram shows an old anteroseptal infarction and intraventricular conduction defect of the incomplete left bundle branch block pattern. Newly developed Q waves in leads II, III, and aVF were compatible with an acute inferior wall infarction. The continuous rhythm strip at the bottom (a–b) shows four successive 3:2 Wenckebach cycles followed by a long 7:6 cycle. P-R intervals are listed in hundredths of a second. During the long Wenckebach cycles, the main increment of AV conduction delay occurred between the first and second beats of the cycles. The P-R intervals remained almost constant (variation of 0.02 s or less) for five successive beats before the blocked P wave. This was followed by significant shortening of the P-R interval in the beat that immediately followed the blocked impulse. This represents a pseudo-Mobitz II arrangement. Also note the presence of varying degrees of bradycardia-dependent left bundle branch block pattern in the opening beats of the Wenckebach cycles that followed the longer pauses. (Reprinted with permission from El-Sherif N, et al.: Br Heart J 40:1376, 1978.)

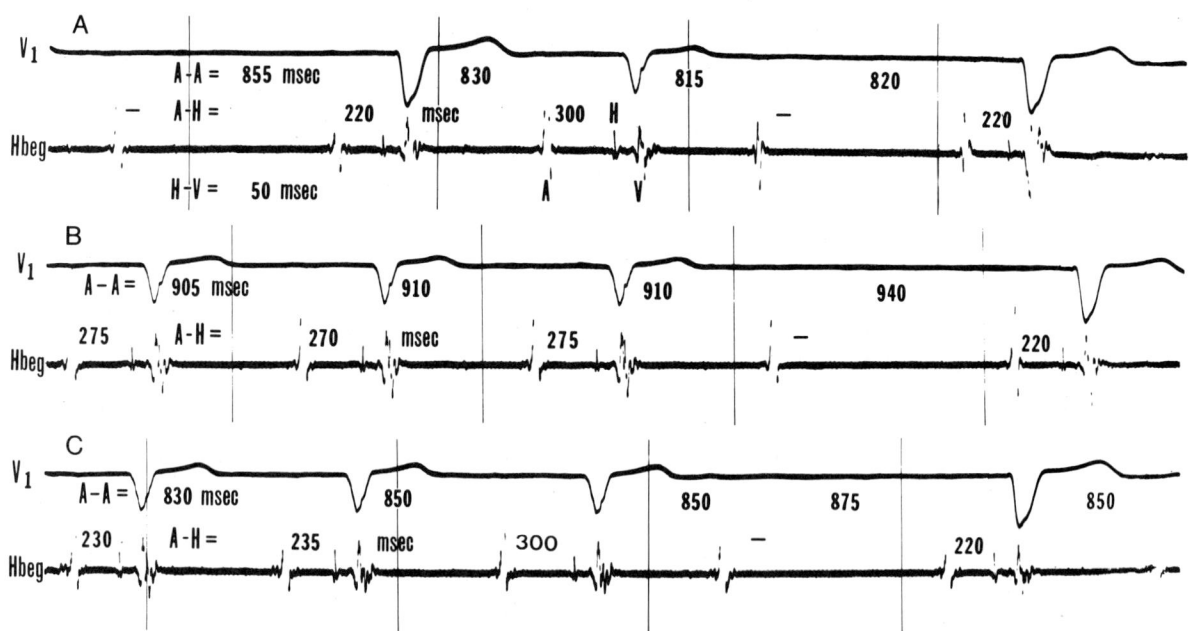

FIGURE 7–10
His bundle electrogram from the same patient as in Figure 7–9, obtained during the insertion of a temporary ventricular pacemaker. A, A 3:2 AV nodal Wenckebach cycle. Note that the P-R interval of the opening beat of the Wenckebach cycle that followed the long pause remained quite prolonged. This was accounted for by a long A-H interval. B illustrates the last three beats of a long 6:5 Wenckebach cycle and shows almost constant P-R and A-H intervals before the blocked P wave. After the blocked impulse, the A-H interval shortened. This represents a pseudo–Mobitz II pattern. C illustrates another variant of atypical Wenckebach periodicity in which the last increment is the largest. A, B, and C also show the bradycardia-dependent left bundle branch block. The change in intraventricular conduction was not accompanied by a change in H-V interval. A, V, and H = atrial, ventricular, and His bundle deflections, respectively; Hbeg = His bundle electrogram. Time lines are set at 1-s intervals. (Reprinted with permission from El-Sherif N, et al.: Br Heart J 40:1376, 1978.)

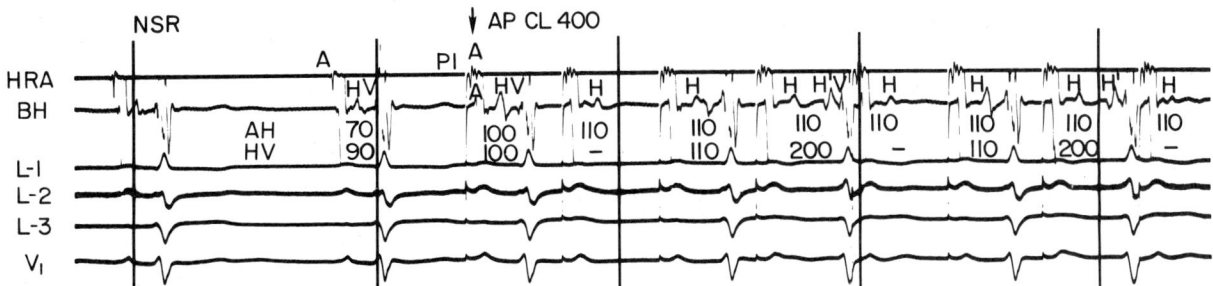

FIGURE 7–11
Second-degree Wenckebach AV block in the His bundle. During normal sinus rhythm (NSR) the His bundle potential was wide (50 ms) and the H-V interval was prolonged (90 ms). Atrial pacing at a cycle length of 400 ms induced 2:1 AV block followed by two 3:2 Wenckebach cycles. During the first conducted beat of the Wenckebach cycle, the His bundle potential was fractionated into two components. During the second conducted beat, the His potential became clearly split into H and H' deflections with marked lengthening of the H-V interval from 110 to 200 ms. During the last beat of the Wenckebach cycle, conduction block occurred distal to H and proximal to H' deflection. BH = His bundle electrogram; HRA = high right atrial electrogram; AP = atrial pacing; CL = cycle length; A, V, and H = atrial, ventricular, and His bundle deflections, respectively. Time lines are set at 1-s intervals.

patients with inferior wall myocardial infarction.[52] In-hospital AV nodal conduction disorders that occur in association with inferior wall myocardial infarction usually develop several hours after onset of symptoms. The majority of such patients exhibit the first appearance of block between 2 and 72 hours after onset of symptoms. The latest time of onset of AV conduction disorders was reported to be on the fifth day of infarction.[49]

WENCKEBACH BLOCK IN THE HIS BUNDLE SYSTEM

Wenckebach block in the His bundle is uncommon, occurring in approximately 9% of patients, and may be seen in the presence of narrow or wide QRS complex.[27] A His bundle recording is required to identify intra-Hisian Wenckebach block. The recording usually shows a split His bundle potential with progressive lengthening of the interval between the two deflections before failure of transmission in the distal His bundle (Fig. 7–11).

WENCKEBACH BLOCK DISTAL TO THE HIS BUNDLE

This type of block is manifested as either (1) progressive prolongation of the H-V interval until a sinus beat is blocked distal to the level of His bundle recording (Figs. 7–12 and 7–13) or (2) progressive change of the QRS configuration from normal to incomplete bundle branch block pattern and finally to complete bundle branch block with progressive increase in the H-V interval. As in the AV node, atypical Wenckebach periodicity is not uncommon in the His-Purkinje system. A Wenckebach arrangement similar to the pseudo-Mobitz II AV nodal block described earlier has been observed in 17% of Wenckebach cycles in the His-Purkinje system (see Figs. 7–12C and 7–13B).[41]

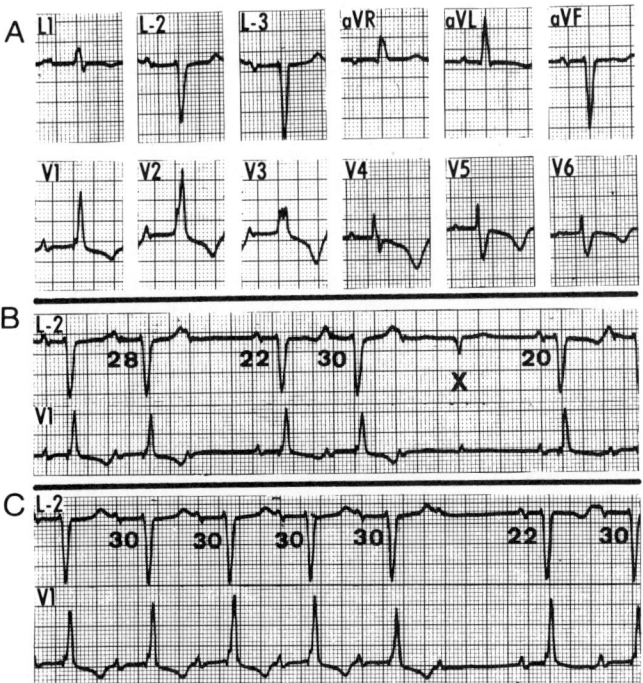

FIGURE 7–12
Pseudo–Mobitz II block in the His-Purkinje system. Recordings were obtained from a 69-year-old man with arteriosclerotic heart disease who was on digoxin for the last 3 years for congestive heart failure. Four months before admission, the patient noticed frequent episodes of dizzy spells. The 12-lead electrocardiogram showed right bundle branch block, left axis deviation, and inversion of T waves in precordial leads (A). A silent myocardial infarction was ruled out by the presence of normal levels of serum enzymes and the absence of serial changes in the QRS and ST-T complexes. The rhythm strip in B shows 3:2 Wenckebach cycles. C illustrates a pseudo–Mobitz II pattern. Note the presence of almost constant P-R intervals in the last four beats of a long Wenckebach cycle and significant shortening of the P-R interval after the blocked impulse. P-R intervals are listed in hundredths of a second. X = premature P wave.

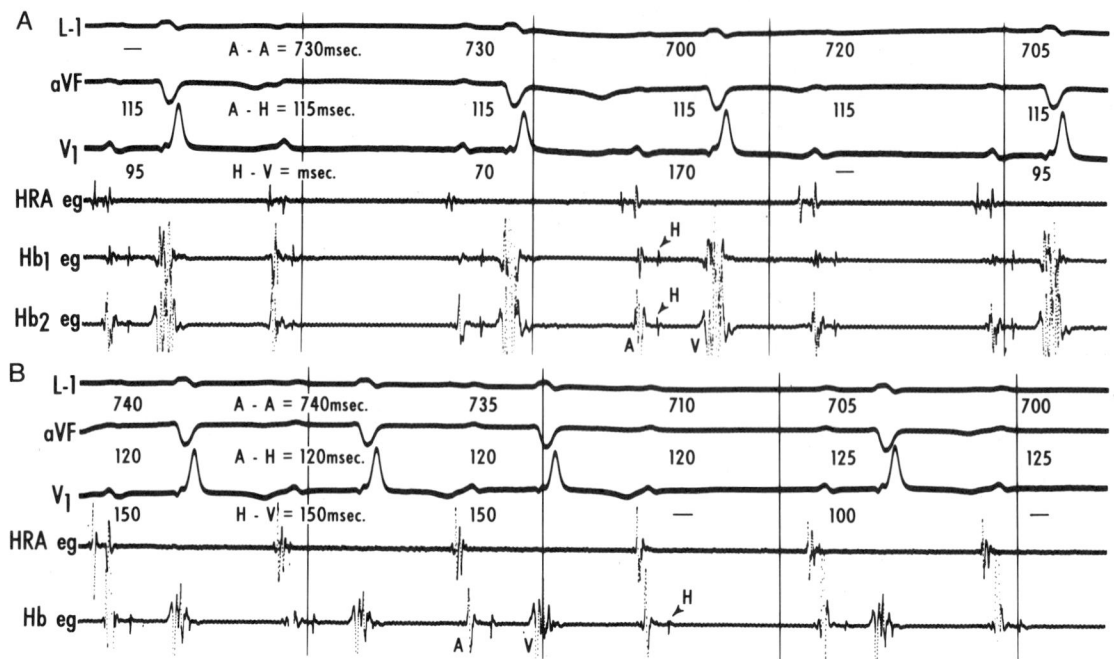

FIGURE 7–13
His bundle electrograms that correspond to the two rhythm strips (B and C) in Figure 7–12. A shows a 3:2 Wenckebach conduction in the His-Purkinje system distal to the site of the His bundle recording. B illustrates the last three beats of a long 7:6 Wenckebach cycle. Note the presence of markedly prolonged but constant H-V intervals before block distal to the His bundle deflection. The H-V interval shortened in the beat immediately after the blocked impulse. This represents a pseudo–Mobitz II pattern. A, V, and H = atrial, ventricular, and His bundle deflections, respectively; HRA eg = high right atrial electrogram; Hb_1 eg and Hb_2 eg = His bundle electrograms. Time lines are set at 1-s intervals.

Because Wenckebach block in the His bundle or the His-Purkinje system commonly progresses to high-degree block or to complete AV block, the implantation of a permanent pacemaker is usually justified in these patients.

Mobitz II AV Block

Mobitz II AV block is characterized by sudden failure of conduction of an atrial impulse without prior P-R interval prolongation. In contrast to Wenckebach AV block, the P-R interval of conducted beats remains constant before the block. Bundle branch block and bifascicular block patterns are commonly seen with Mobitz II AV block, and the block is either localized in the His bundle (35%) or in the bundle branch–Purkinje system (65%).[26–28, 38]

Relationship Between Mobitz II and Wenckebach AV Block (A Unified Hypothesis of Second-Degree AV Block)

The two types of second-degree AV block were originally described by Wenckebach[3, 53] and Hay[54] from analysis of the a-c interval of the jugular pulse. After the introduction of the ECG, these were classified by Mobitz[4] as types I and II. The clinical significance of the two types of second-degree AV block was first recognized by Mobitz,[4] who suggested that type II block may be the first step to Adams-Stokes attacks and complete, permanent AV dissociation.

With the introduction of intensive care and electrocardiographic monitoring for acute myocardial infarction, there was renewed interest in the distinction between type I and type II AV blocks. Several anatomic[55, 56] and clinical studies[57–59] have shown that the two types of second-degree AV block were associated with different anatomic localization of the infarction and have different electrophysiologic and clinical significance. Type I AV block is seen with diaphragmatic infarction, being associated with reversible ischemia of the AV node, and commonly runs a benign course. In contrast, type II AV block is observed in anterior infarction and is associated with necrosis of the bundle branches and a more grave prognosis.

Studies utilizing His bundle electrocardiographic techniques in patients with acute myocardial infarction have generally confirmed the specific localization of the two types of second-degree AV block.[60, 61] However, studies in experimental myocardial infarction have argued that types I and II AV conduction patterns may not represent two distinct electrophysiologic processes, but rather are manifestations of varying degrees of the same process.[62, 63] These studies have shown that under pathologic conditions, exemplified by acute myocardial ischemia, the normal His-Purkinje system may gradually lose the characteristics of the fast response and may begin to show properties of the slow response. At an early stage of departure from normal, the proximal His-Purkinje system may show second-degree A-V block with no perceptible to a few-ms increment

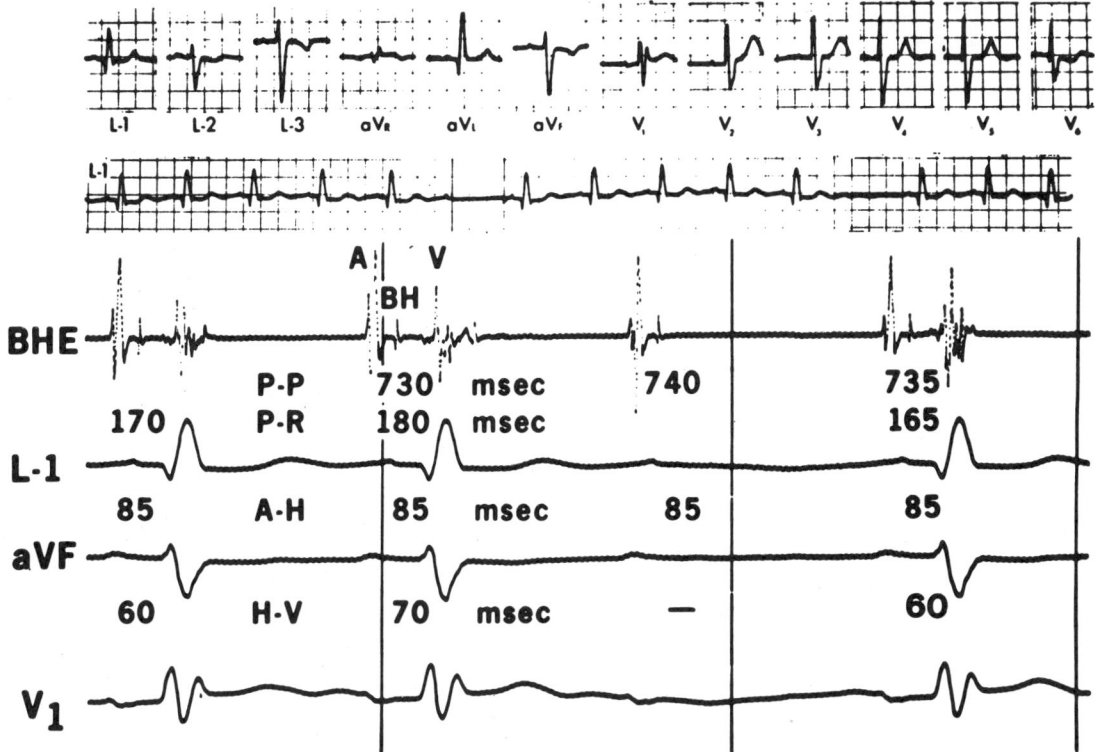

FIGURE 7–14
Electrocardiographic and His bundle recordings obtained from a 72-year-old man with old anteroseptal and recent lateroposterior infarctions. Previous 12-lead electrocardiogram showed right bundle branch block and left anterior fascicular block pattern. The 12-lead electrocardiogram obtained on admission is shown at top. The rhythm strip was obtained 18 hours after the onset of chest pain and showed a second-degree Mobitz II AV block. The His bundle electrogram (BHE) obtained during insertion of a temporary ventricular pacemaker showed second-degree AV block in the His-Purkinje system with 10-ms increment of H-V interval prior to blocked beat (i.e., the equivalent of Mobitz II block). A, V, and BH = atrial, ventricular, and bundle of His deflections, respectively. Time lines are set at 1-s intervals. (Reprinted with permission from El-Sherif N, et al.: Chest 71:615, 1977.)

of conduction delay (the equivalent of Mobitz type II block). On further departure from normal, the His-Purkinje system resembles the AV node in showing a significant increment of conduction delay prior to the blocked impulse (the equivalent of Wenckebach periodicity). Both in vivo and in vitro experimental observations demonstrated a clear propensity of the ischemic proximal His-Purkinje system to develop paroxysmal AV block during the stage of second-degree AV block when there is no perceptible to a few-ms increment of conduction delay.

At least one clinical study seemed to confirm the results of the experimental observations.[64] The evolution of ischemia-related second-degree AV block in the His-Purkinje system was studied utilizing continuous electrocardiographic monitoring and serial His bundle recordings in several patients. In some patients, second-degree AV block in the His-Purkinje system with minimal increment of conduction delay prior to block was seen within the first few hours of infarction. A few days later, second-degree AV block changed to a conduction pattern in which a significant increment of conduction delay preceded the block (Figs. 7–14, 7–15, and 7–16).

Pseudo–AV Block

In 1947, Langendorf and Mehlman,[65] utilizing deductive analysis of the ECG, suggested that concealed junctional premature systoles could simulate first- and second-degree AV block and nonconducted atrial premature beats. Langendorf and Pick[66] later proposed that concealed junctional premature systoles could also result in alternation of the P-R interval and pseudo-Wenckebach periods. However, it was not until 1970 that Rosen and associates,[67] through recording of the His bundle electrogram, provided the first documented example of concealed His bundle extra systoles producing intermittent first- and second-degree AV block. Concealed His bundle extrasystole was also shown to initiate reentrant rhythms (Fig. 7–17).[68]

Alternate Wenckebach Periodicity

Alternate Wenckebach periods are defined as episodes of 2:1 AV block associated with progressive prolongation of the conducted atrial impulses until two or three consecutive atrial impulses are blocked. Langendorf and Pick[66, 69] suggested that the block of two

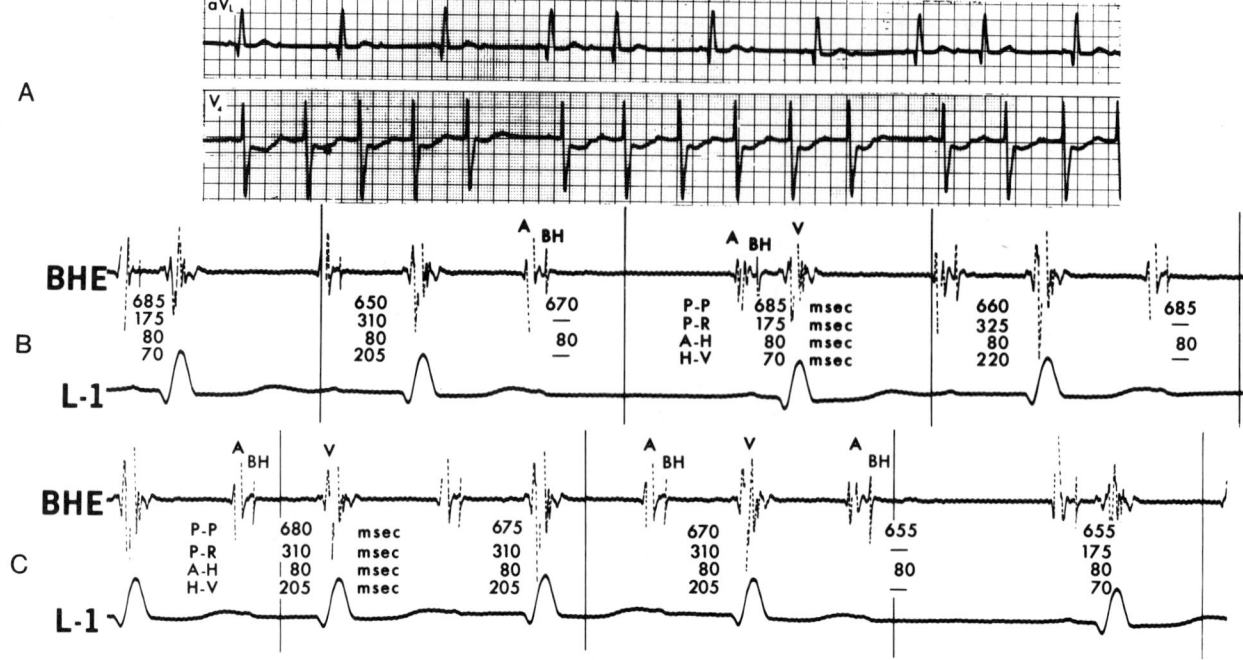

FIGURE 7–15

Recordings from the same patient shown in Figure 7–14 obtained 14 days after acute myocardial infarction. A, Upper rhythm strip shows 2:1 and 3:2 Wenckebach AV conduction, whereas lower rhythm strip illustrates long Wenckebach cycles with prolonged and almost constant P-R intervals prior to blocked beat and marked shortening of P-R interval following block. B and C, Bundle of His electrograms (BHE) corresponding to the two rhythm strips. B shows 3:2 Wenckebach conduction in the His-Purkinje system, with an increment of 135 to 150 ms in H-V intervals prior to block. C illustrates the last three beats of a long Wenckebach cycle, with constant H-V intervals prior to block. Note marked shortening of the H-V interval of the first conducted beat. This pattern represents one variant of atypical Wenckebach periodicity called pseudo–Mobitz II block. A, V, and BH = atrial, ventricular, and bundle of His deflections, respectively. Time lines are set at 1-s intervals. (Reprinted with permission from El-Sherif N, et al.: Chest 71:615, 1977.)

consecutive atrial impulses represented inhomogeneous penetration of the AV node with deeper penetration of the first impulse and more superficial penetration of the second. Electrophysiologic studies have confirmed these observations.[70] However, the areas of depressed conduction may not be limited to the AV node, and the bundle of His or the His-Purkinje system may be the site of distal block.[71] Alternate Wenckebach periodicity is commonly seen during atrial flutter with high-degree AV block (Fig. 7–18).[69] El-Sherif and

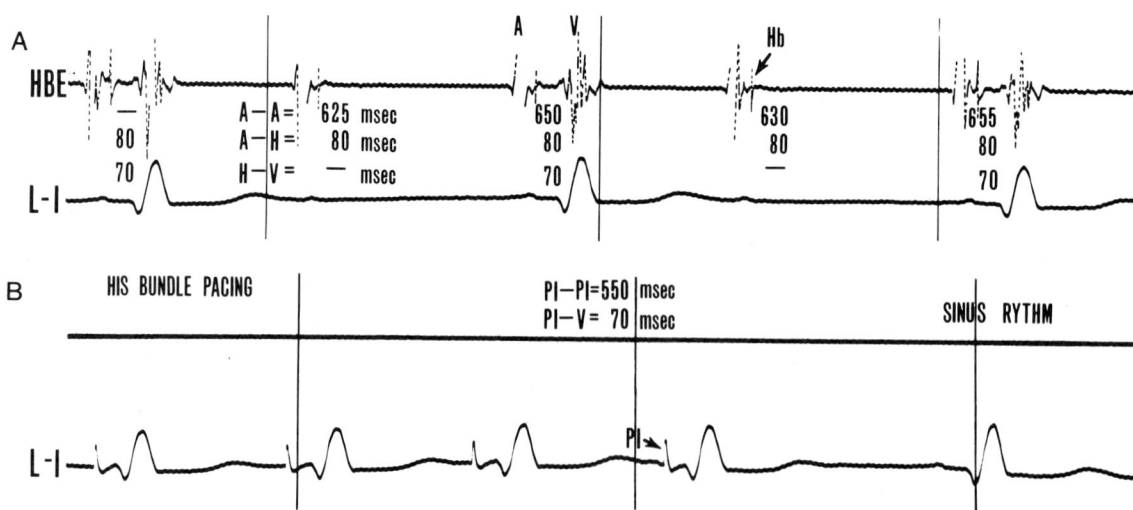

FIGURE 7–16

Recordings obtained during same study as those shown in Figure 7–15. A, Bundle of His electrogram (HBE) showing 2:1 block in the His-Purkinje system at a sinus rate of 92 to 95 beats per minute. B, 1:1 His bundle pacing at a faster rate of 109 beats per minute. This suggests that the block in conduction is localized in the His bundle. PI = Paced impulse. Time lines are set at 1-s intervals. (Reprinted with permission from El-Sherif N, et al.: Chest 71:615, 1977.)

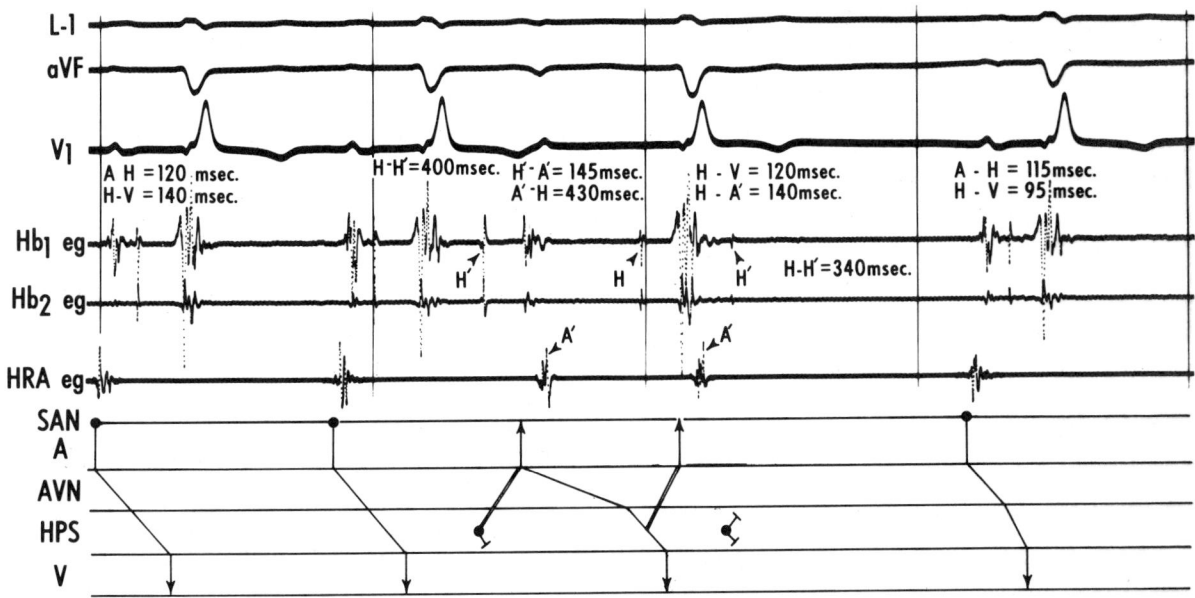

FIGURE 7-17
Reentry secondary to an ectopic His bundle systole. Diagrammatic analysis of the arrhythmia is shown below. A premature His bundle ectopic impulse (H′) conducted retrogradely to the atria but failed to conduct in antegrade direction. This beat is followed by a second His bundle deflection (H) that conducted in both antegrade and retrograde directions. The next H′ is blocked in both directions. The diagram suggests that the first H′ during its retrograde conduction to the atria entered a reentrant pathway and conducted antegradely to the ventricles. A second reentrant cycle conducted retrogradely to the atria before termination of reentry by block in the antegrade limb. Hb_1 eg and Hb_2 eg = His bundle electrograms; HRA eg = high right atrial electrogram; SAN = sinoatrial node; A = atria; AVN = atrioventricular node; HPS = His-Purkinje system; V = ventricles. Time lines are set at 1-s intervals. (Reprinted with permission of the American Heart Association, Inc., from El-Sherif et al.: Circulation 53:902, 1976.)

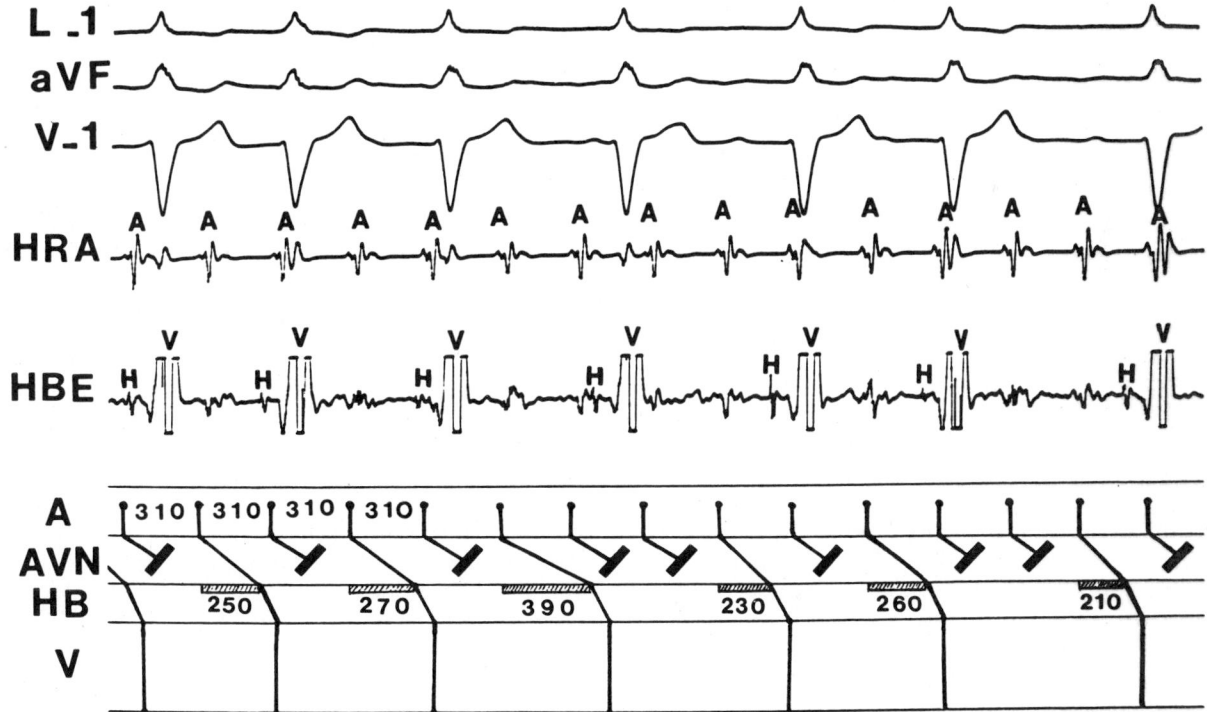

FIGURE 7-18
Recording obtained from a 71-year-old woman showing atrial flutter with alternate Wenckebach periodicity. Diagrammatic analysis of the arrhythmia is shown below. The arrhythmia is explained by two levels of block in the AV node: a 2:1 block at an upper level and a Wenckebach type conduction at a lower level. This results in gradual lengthening of the A-H interval of conducted atrial flutter impulses followed by AV block of two consecutive atrial flutter impulses. Following block the A-H interval shortened. Numbers refer to A-H intervals in mseconds. The A-H intervals are also marked by shaded bars. HRA = High right atrial electrogram; HBE = His bundle electrogram; A, H, and V = atrial, His bundle, and ventricular deflections, respectively.

colleagues[72] have shown that during experimental acute myocardial infarction, alternating Wenckebach periods in the His-Purkinje system may precede the development of paroxysmal AV block.

HIGH-DEGREE AV BLOCK

High-degree AV block refers to 2:1, 3:1, or higher AV ratios while AV synchrony is maintained. The block can be localized in the AV node, the bundle of His, or the bundle branch–Purkinje system. Sometimes high-degree AV block is due to conduction block at more than one level of the AV conduction system. The site of block can be precisely localized by recording a His bundle electrogram, although a careful examination of the surface ECG and clinical circumstances may lead to the correct diagnosis of the site of block.[73] Clinical and electrocardiographic features suggesting high-degree AV block caused by AV nodal block include the following:

1. Narrow QRS complexes in conducted beats, although rarely a narrow QRS complex is associated with intra-Hisian block.
2. Wenckebach periodicity prior to development of high-degree AV block.
3. Inferior wall myocardial infarction, digitalis intoxication, and therapy with beta-adrenergic or calcium channel blocking agents.
4. Reversion to 1:1 conduction following administration of atropine.

Clinical and electrocardiographic features suggesting high-degree AV block in the His-Purkinje system include the following:

1. Bundle branch block or bifascicular block in conducted beats.
2. Absence of a history of intake of digitalis or beta-adrenergic or calcium channel blocking agents.
3. Either no changes or an increase in conduction ratio with acceleration of the sinus rate after the administration of atropine.

A pacemaker is not indicated when 2:1 AV block is due to conduction block in the AV node if the patient is asymptomatic, the block is drug-related, or the ventricular response increases after the administration of atropine or isoproterenol or during exercise. However, a pacemaker *is* indicated if the patient is symptomatic or in congestive heart failure and if the ventricular response is less than 40 beats per minute without an appreciable increase in ventricular response after exercise or administration of atropine. Patients with high-degree AV block caused by block in or below the His bundle should have a permanent pacemaker, irrespective of the presence of symptoms.

COMPLETE AV BLOCK

In complete heart block, there is total absence of AV conduction with the ventricles beating independently of the atria, in response to a pacemaker in either the AV junction, the His bundle, or the bundle branch-Purkinje system. Some cases of 2:1 AV block in which an escape rhythm occurs at a cycle length slightly shorter than twice the atrial cycle may simulate complete AV block (Figs. 7–19 and 7–20). In complete AV block the ventricular rate varies depending on the site of the escape pacemaker. The site of block is localized distal to the His bundle in approximately 60% of patients; in the His bundle in 14 to 20%; and within the AV node in 16 to 25%.[26, 27] Complete AV block can be classified as congenital or acquired, and the latter can be either acute or chronic.

Congenital Complete AV Block

Congenital complete AV block can occur in an otherwise normal heart, but in 50% of cases it is seen in association with other congenital heart diseases.[74] Histologic studies indicate that congenital complete heart block may result from failure of a hypoplastic AV node to develop connections with the internodal pathway, failure of the developing His bundle to link with the AV node, or absence of a portion of the His bundle or bundle branches.[75, 76]

Congenital AV block is estimated to occur once every 25,000 live births.[77] In children with congenital heart disease, complete heart block occurs in 0.4 to 0.9%. An early age of discovery, additional structural heart defects, wide QRS escape rhythms, and a long QT interval were reported to be associated with increased risk.[78] Long-term follow-up of patients with isolated congenital complete heart block has shown that although a majority may remain asymptomatic, a sizable number may develop syncope and will require a permanent pacemaker, and a few patients may die suddenly.[79, 80] The response of the junctional pacemaker to atropine and the AV junctional recovery time[81] may be useful determinants of symptoms and prognosis.

Acute Acquired Complete AV Block

Acute acquired complete AV block can occur in the course of acute myocardial infarction or following the administration of some pharmacologic agents or can be post-traumatic during cardiac surgery, catheterization, or ablation.

Complete AV block during acute inferior wall myocardial infarction is usually localized in the AV node. The escape rhythm commonly arises from an AV junctional pacemaker and the QRS is narrow. In some cases, however, a bradycardia-dependent left bundle branch block of the AV junctional pacemaker is seen.[48] The pacemaker rate is usually 50 to 60 beats per minute (bpm) and can be accelerated by vagolytic drugs or by exercise. A temporary pacemaker may be indicated if the escape pacemaker has a right bundle branch block configuration, the ventricular rate is less than 40 bpm and is associated with hypotension or congestive heart failure, and for overdrive suppression of bradycardia-dependent ventricular arrhythmias.[82] In most instances

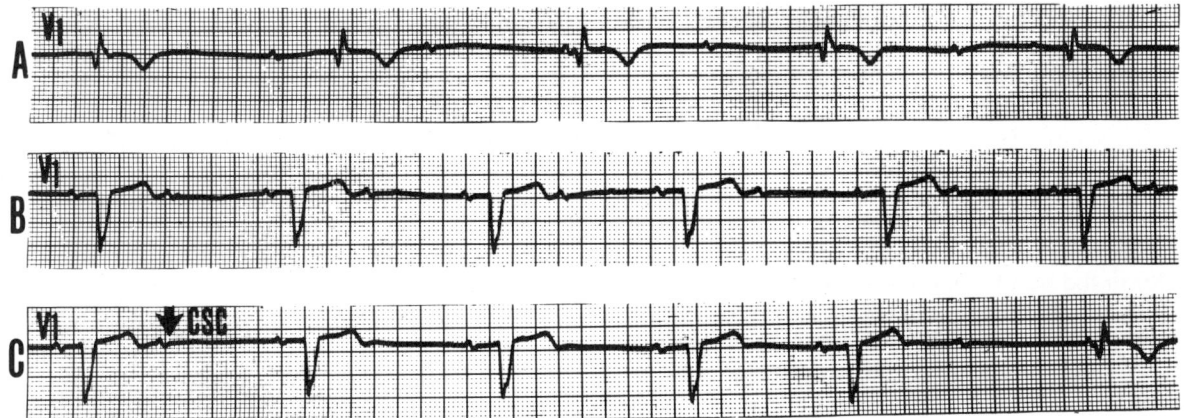

FIGURE 7–19
Recordings obtained from a 65-year-old man who had dizzy spells and was found to have complete AV dissociation with a slow idioventricular rhythm on the admission electrocardiogram. A, Rhythm strip on admission showing complete AV dissociation with a sinus cycle length of 1000 to 1200 ms and an idioventricular cycle length of 2120 ms. B, Rhythm strip recorded a few hours later showing a decrease of the sinus cycle length to 860 and 2:1 AV conduction and with conducted beats showing a left bundle branch block pattern. C, Rhythm strip recorded shortly after B; carotid sinus compression (CSC) resulted in marked lengthening of the sinus cycle length associated with 1:1 AV conduction. On release of carotid sinus compression, AV block recurred on critical shortening the sinus cycle to 1200 ms. Following the blocked P wave, an idioventricular escape beat occurred at a cycle length of 2320 ms and before the resumption of 2:1 AV block, as in B. The QRS configuration of the idioventricular escape beat is similar to that in A. This confirms that the apparent complete AV dissociation actually represented a slow idioventricular rhythm superimposed on tachycardia-dependent 2:1 AV block.

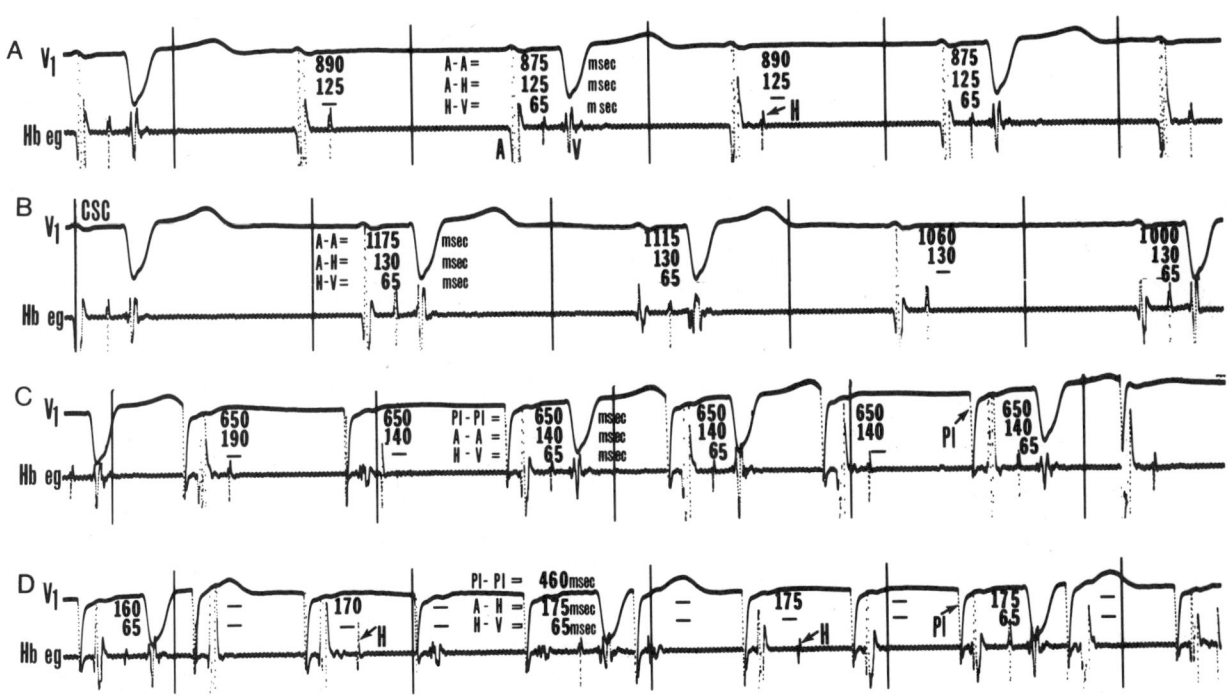

FIGURE 7–20
His bundle electrogram (Hb eg) recordings from the same patient shown in Figure 7–19. Recordings in A and B are equivalent to the cardiac rhythms shown in Figure 7–19 B and C respectively. A shows that the 2:1 AV block is due to conduction block distal to His bundle recording. The H-V interval of conducted beats is prolonged (65 ms). B, 1:1 AV conduction occurred on lengthening of the sinus cycle by carotid sinus compression (CSC). AV block occurred on critical shortening of the sinus cycle to 1060 ms. The AV block is of the Mobitz II type (i.e., associated with no perceptible increase of the P-R or H-V intervals). C and D, Atrial pacing at cycle lengths of 650 and 460 ms, respectively. In C, a 3:1 AV block distal to the His bundle was followed by 1:1 AV conduction. The 1:1 AV conduction occurred at a cycle length much shorter than the cycle length associated with the 2:1 AV block in A. This may be a manifestation of supernormal conduction. In D, a 4:1 AV block was due to superimposition of 2:1 AV nodal block on top of a 2:1 block distal to the His bundle. Time lines are set at 1-s intervals.

of inferior wall myocardial infarction, the heart block resolves within a few days and a permanent pacemaker is unnecessary. However, in about 10% of patients the block is localized in the His bundle. In these cases a permanent pacemaker is usually indicated because of the unstable nature of the escape rhythm.

Complete AV block during anterior wall myocardial infarction is usually associated with damage to the bundle branches.[56, 83] The ventricles are driven by a pacemaker in the bundle branch–Purkinje network that is characterized by a wide QRS complex and a rate of less than 40 bpm and is usually unstable. In these cases the damage may not be reversible, and a permanent pacemaker is indicated.

In patients with a diseased His-Purkinje system, some antiarrhythmic agents, particularly those that depress the fast sodium channel, such as lidocaine,[84] procainamide,[85] and disopyramide,[86] can induce second- and third-degree His-Purkinje block. A high incidence of complete heart block is also noted after surgical correction of aortic valve disease[87] and ventricular septal defect either with or without tetralogy of Fallot.[88] In these cases, usually the His bundle is the site of trauma, and prophylactic pacing is recommended if the escape pacemaker is slow or unstable.

Complete AV block can be induced inadvertently during catheter manipulation.[89, 90] In patients with a previous left bundle branch block, right heart catheterization can at times produce additional conduction block in the right bundle branch, hence resulting in complete AV block. In such patients, therefore, caution should be exercised during right heart catheterization, and temporary pacing should be available. Rarely, in some patients with a right bundle branch block pattern, catheter-induced conduction delay in the left bundle branch during left ventricular angiography has led to complete heart block. In most cases with catheter-induced trauma to the bundle branches, the damage is temporary and recovery is usual within a few hours.

Therapeutic AV block is now induced to treat intractable supraventricular tachyarrhythmias, utilizing a closed chest catheter ablation technique.[91, 92] High-energy impulses are usually delivered by catheter electrodes positioned close to the AV junction to induce AV block. However, other forms of ablative energy have also been utilized.[93]

Chronic Acquired Complete AV Block

Acquired complete AV block is usually seen with generalized myocardial scarring from various causes, especially atherosclerosis, dilated cardiomyopathy, and hypertension.[8] An entity known as idiopathic bilateral bundle branch fibrosis, or Lev's disease,[94] has been described and is characterized by slowly progressive replacement of specialized conduction tissue by fibrosis, resulting in progressive fascicular and bundle branch block. Lev has proposed that the damage to the proximal left bundle branch and adjacent main bundle, or to the main bundle alone at its junction between penetrating and bifurcating portions, is an aging process exaggerated by hypertension and arteriosclerosis of the blood vessels supplying the conduction system. Another variant of idiopathic conduction system disorder is Lenegre's disease,[95] which occurs in the younger population and is characterized by loss of conduction tissue predominantly in the peripheral parts of the bundle branches. Progression to AV block occurs over time.

Calcific degeneration involving the mitral or aortic annulus can produce AV block[96, 97] owing to proximity to the His bundle. Similarly, calcification from a stenotic bicuspid aortic valve can produce AV block.[98, 99] Chronic acquired complete AV block has also been described with infiltrative diseases like Chagas' disease[100], sarcoidosis,[101] rheumatoid arthritis,[102] and hemochromatosis,[103, 104] as well as with some hereditary neuromuscular disorders[105, 106] and with mesothelioma of the AV node.[107] In all these cases the block tends to be permanent, and prophylactic pacing is recommended.

Electrophysiologic Evaluation of Complete AV Block

In the His bundle electrogram, complete AV block localized in the AV node is characterized by atrial deflections that are not followed by a His bundle potential and by ventricular depolarizations that are preceded by a His bundle potential. The H-V interval can be either normal or prolonged if there is a preexisting bundle branch block pattern (Fig. 7–21A). When the block is localized in the His bundle, the His bundle potential is split with the atrial deflections followed by a proximal His bundle potential (h_1) and the ventricular deflections preceded by a distal His bundle potential (h_2) with a usually normal h_2-V interval (Fig. 7–21B). In the case of block distal to the His bundle, all atrial deflections are followed by a His bundle potential, whereas ventricular depolarizations are not preceded by a His bundle potential (Fig. 7–21C).

Once the site of block is established, it is important to evaluate the stability of the escape pacemaker rhythm. Intravenous atropine in a vagolytic dose can be administered to evaluate the potential of the escape pacemaker to accelerate.[81] Isoproterenol or exercise may also be used to evaluate the response of the pacemaker. Most escape rhythms in the AV node will increase in rate following administration of atropine or isoproterenol. Pacemakers in the His bundle accelerate modestly or not at all with the drugs, whereas distal pacemakers do not usually increase in rate with atropine but may do so with isoproterenol.

Junctional recovery time can be used as another index of stability of the escape pacemaker.[81] Ventricular pacing for 1-minute intervals is performed at rates faster than the rate of escape rhythm, and the interval between the last paced ventricular complex to the first beat of the escape rhythm is measured as the recovery time of the pacemaker (Figs. 7–22 and 7–23). When corrected for the underlying pacemaker interval (i.e.,

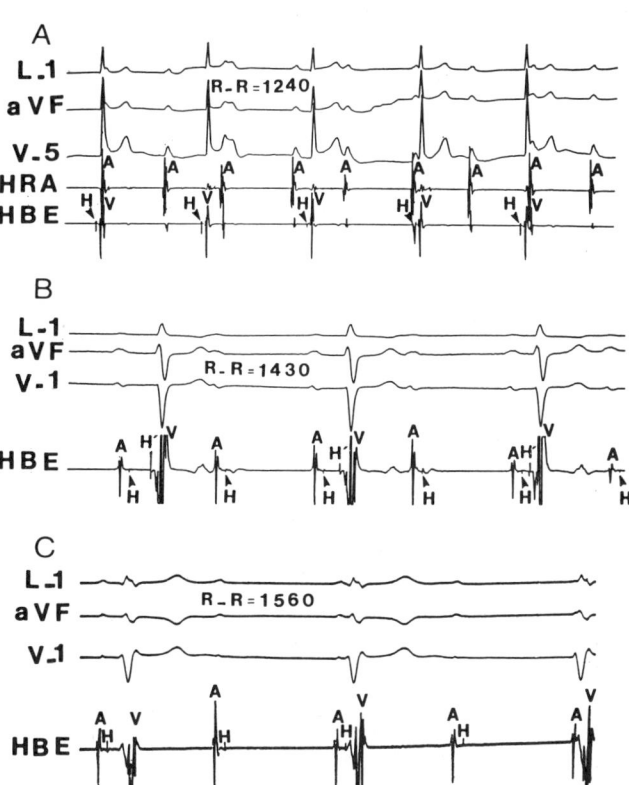

FIGURE 7-21
His bundle electrogram (HBE) recordings from three patients with complete AV block, showing different sites of block. A, AV nodal block; atrial deflections are not followed by His bundle potential, and the escape ventricular rhythm has a narrow QRS and is preceded by a His bundle potential with a normal H-V interval. B, Intra-Hisian block; atrial deflections are followed by a proximal His bundle potential (H), and the escape ventricular rhythm has a narrow QRS and is preceded by a distal His bundle potential (H′) with a normal H-V interval. C, Block distal to His; atrial deflections are followed by a His bundle potential, and the escape ventricular rhythm has a right bundle branch configuration and is not preceded by a His bundle potential. Note that the AV nodal escape rhythm in A is faster than the His bundle rhythm in B and the idioventricular rhythm in C.

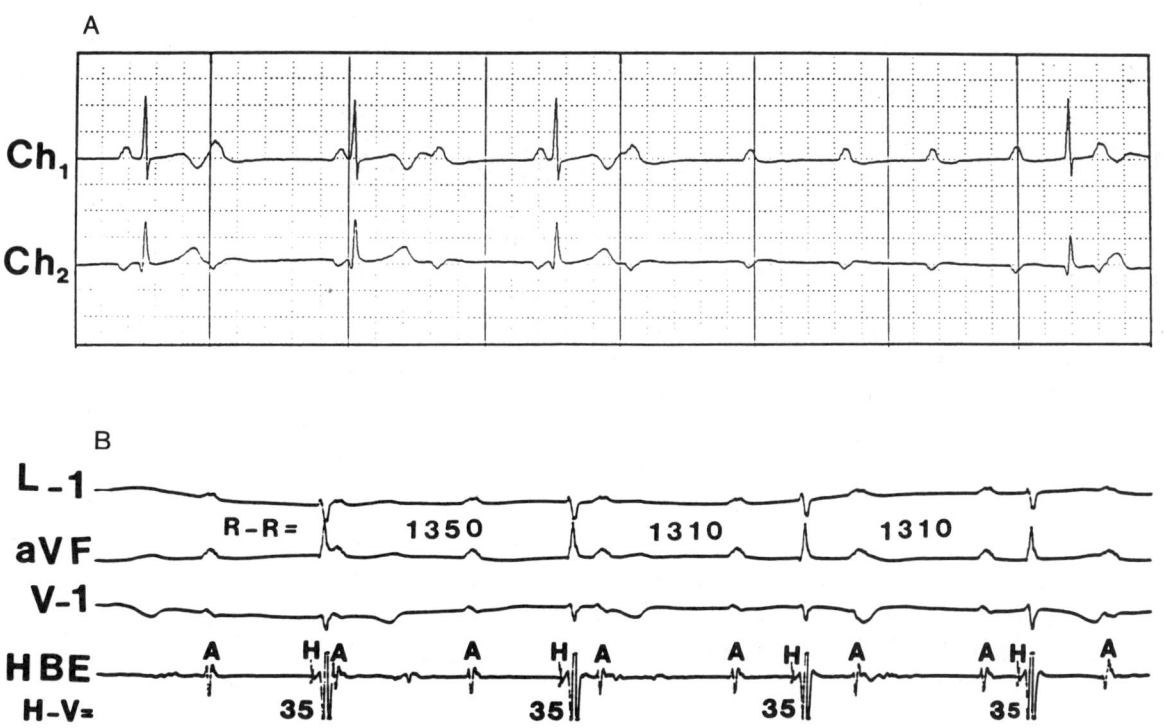

FIGURE 7-22
Congenital complete AV block. A, Representative recording of an ambulatory electrocardiogram from an 11-year-old girl with congenital heart block. The recording shows complete AV dissociation and a ventricular escape rhythm with narrow QRS at a rate of 45 beats per minute. The escape rhythm could increase up to 95 beats per minute during exercise. There were also frequent ventricular pauses of up to 4 seconds. B, His bundle electrogram showing an AV nodal site of block. A = atrial, H = His electrogram.

Atrioventricular and Intraventricular Conduction Disorders: Clinical Aspects

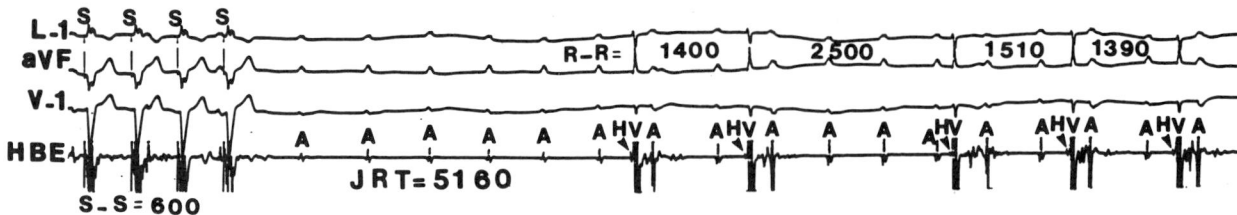

FIGURE 7–23
His bundle recording (HBE) from the same patient shown in Figure 7–22, illustrating a study of the recovery time of the AV junctional pacemaker. Following ventricular pacing at a cycle length of 600 ms for 1 minute, the AV junctional recovery time (JRT) was 5160 ms. The control cycle length of the AV junctional rhythm was approximately 1400 ms. Thus, the corrected AV junctional recovery time was 3760 ms, which was markedly prolonged. Note also the presence of a secondary pause of 2500 ms. A, H, V = atrial, His bundle, ventriculogram.

subtracting the control pacemaker interval from the recovery time interval), corrected junctional recovery time is obtained.[81] A corrected recovery time of less than 200 ms represents a stable AV junctional pacemaker, and in the absence of symptoms of dizziness or syncope prophylactic pacing may not be required.

Cardiac pacing is usually recommended for complete AV nodal block when (1) the ventricular rate is less than 40 bpm, (2) there is no significant increase in rate with atropine or exercise, and (3) symptoms suggestive of low cardiac output such as dizziness, syncope, or congestive heart failure are present. On the other hand, if complete AV block is localized in the His-Purkinje system, a permanent pacemaker is recommended even in the absence of symptoms.

PAROXYSMAL AV BLOCK

Paroxysmal AV block may be defined as the sudden occurrence of repetitive block of the atrial impulse during 1:1 AV conduction (or occasionally 2:1 AV block), resulting in a transient total interruption of AV conduction.[72] The onset of the arrhythmia is usually associated with a period of ventricular asystole before the return of conduction or the escape of a subsidiary pacemaker. This period of ventricular asystole, often exaggerated by delayed escape rhythms, frequently dramatizes the clinical picture of the arrhythmia. Since the early clinical observations by Mobitz,[4] type II second-degree AV block was associated with paroxysmal AV block and Adams-Stokes syndrome. An increase in atrial rate was postulated as a possible cause of intermittent complete AV block and Stokes-Adams attacks as early as 1905.[108] Wenckebach and Winterberg[109] and Gilchrist[110] have discussed the role of atrial rate in the change to higher-degree block in patients showing type II AV block. Repetitive concealed conduction has been suggested as the mechanism of prolonged ventricular asystole in cases of second-degree AV block.[111, 112] Experimental studies in the canine model of acute ischemia of the proximal His-Purkinje system have suggested that the His bundle is a critical site in the development of paroxysmal AV block.[72] This was the case even when a bundle branch block pattern was present in the ECG, which is usually considered to indicate the presence of bilateral bundle branch block in clinical records. In the experimental model a clear temporal association was observed between the occurrence of early stages of second-degree AV block with no perceptible or only a few-ms increment of conduction delay and the induction or spontaneous onset of paroxysmal AV block. Paroxysmal AV block occurring abruptly during sinus rhythm or that induced by rapid atrial pacing were both considered to be tachycardia-dependent, since slowing the heart rate in both instances allowed immediate resumption of 1:1 conduction.

Examples of tachycardia-dependent paroxysmal AV block in patients with acute myocardial infarction have been reported.[72] The increase in the atrial rate occurred either spontaneously (Fig. 7–24) or in response to pharmacologic agents (Fig. 7–25). In these patients paroxysmal AV block occurred in close association with Mobitz type II AV block, and the site of the block was most probably in the His-Purkinje system.

Cases of tachycardia-dependent paroxysmal AV block have been described in patients with Stokes-Adams syndrome not suffering from acute myocardial ischemia.[113, 114] In these patients there is also the close association of Mobitz type II block and paroxysmal AV block (Fig. 7–26).[115] Several patients showed what has been described as "labile" AV conduction, which, at least in some cases, represented a tachycardia-dependent 2:1 AV block.[116] However, many cases of paroxysmal AV block occur abruptly and without a perceptible increase in the atrial rate. In these cases, some variation in the degree of electrophysiologic disorder in the AV conduction system secondary to slight changes in coronary perfusion, autonomic tone, circulating catecholamines, and so forth could be involved.[72]

Most clinical examples with chronic "stable" lesions in the His-Purkinje system respond to rapid atrial pacing by AV nodal block of 2:1 or a higher degree of block in the His-Purkinje system, but not by paroxysmal AV block (Figs. 7–27 and 7–28). In those patients the propensity for repetitive concealed conduction in the His-Purkinje system may be absent. An alternative explanation would be that the critical short cycle necessary for repetitive block in the His-Purkinje system could not be achieved because of physiologic AV nodal refractoriness.[72]

In a few patients, tachycardia-dependent repetitive block seems to be localized in the AV node (Fig.

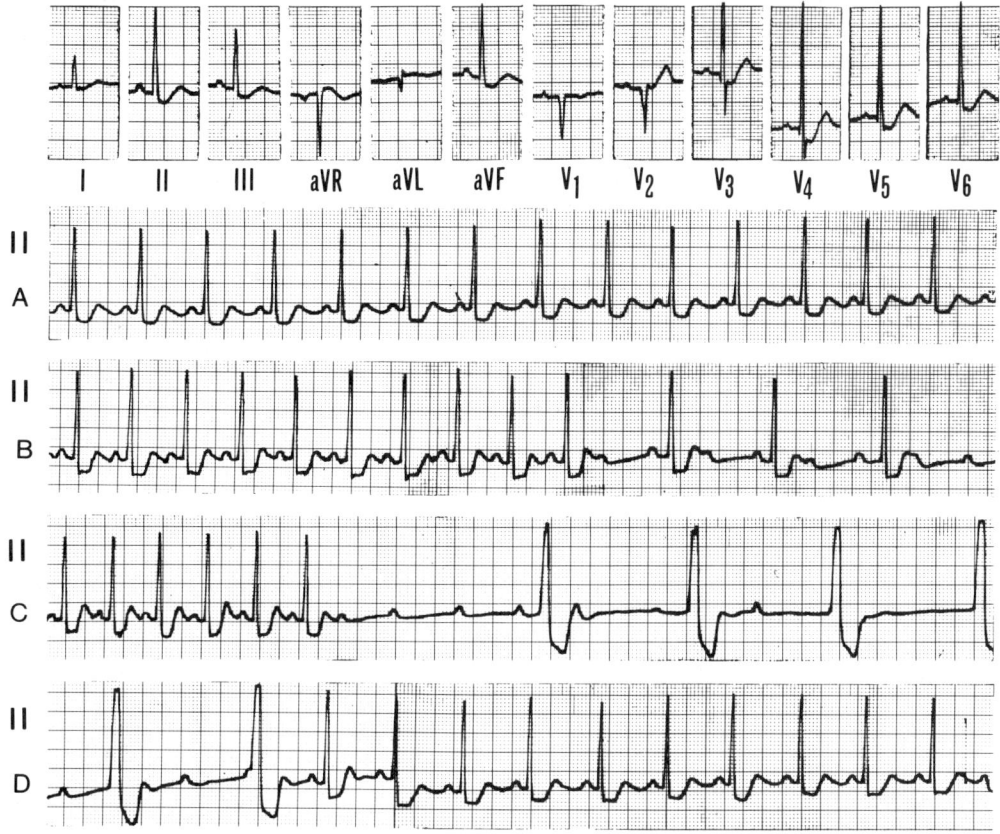

FIGURE 7–24
Representative electrocardiograms from a 71-year-old man with acute non–Q wave myocardial infarction showing paroxysmal AV block on acceleration of the sinus rate. The top recording illustrates the 12-lead electrocardiogram on admission, showing an old anteroseptal infarction and recent ST-T changes in inferolateral surface leads. A, 1:1 AV conduction at an average sinus rate of 87 beats per minute and a P-R interval of 0.18 s. B, A faster sinus rate of 102 to 108 beats per minute and sudden failure of AV conduction without an appreciable change in the sinus rate or the P-R interval (Mobitz type II block). C illustrates the onset of paroxysmal AV block, which was always preceded by an acceleration of the sinus rate to 115 to 120 beats per minute or higher. The recording shows a period of ventricular asystole of 2.5 seconds followed by the escape of an idioventricular rhythm at a rate of 40 beats per minute. Note that after the onset of ventricular asystole, spontaneous slowing of the sinus rate and shift of the sinus pacemaker occurred. D is a tracing recorded 45 seconds following the onset of paroxysmal AV block in C and illustrates the re-establishment of 1:1 AV conduction; 1:1 AV conduction usually resumed only when the sinus rate fell below 100 beats per minute. (Reprinted with permission of the American Heart Association, Inc., from El-Sherif N, et al.: Circulation 50:515, 1974.)

7–29).[117] In some of these cases an intra-Hisian block may be missed if the proximal His bundle deflection is not recorded. This may also explain the occasional reports of Mobitz II block in the AV node.[117] However, some experimental studies have demonstrated the occurrences of tachycardia-dependent paroxysmal AV block in the ischemic AV node.[118] Furthermore, this type of block was temporally related to the development of a characteristic type of second-degree AV block characterized by marked prolongation of AV nodal conduction time but with a minimal increment of conduction delay prior to the blocked beat, thus simulating Mobitz II block.

In some patients in whom tachycardia-dependent AV block in the His-Purkinje system could be demonstrated by incremental atrial pacing, rapid ventricular pacing may also induce a high-degree AV block (Fig. 7–30). Similar observations have been reported in the canine model of acute ischemia of the proximal His-Purkinje system, in which paroxysmal AV block could be induced by rapid atrial or ventricular pacing.[118] The AV block induced by ventricular pacing may represent a "fatigue" phenomenon caused by invasion and repetitive depolarization of Purkinje fibers at the critical site of AV block.

Although the majority of cases of paroxysmal AV block appear to be tachycardia-dependent, few example of bradycardia-dependent paroxysmal AV block have been described (Fig. 7–31).[119, 120] The phenomenon has been explained by spontaneous diastolic depolarization at the critical site of lesion in the His-Purkinje system. Some experimental studies, however, suggest that bradycardia-dependent conduction disorders may be associated with a positive shift of the threshold potential rather than an enhanced phase-4 depolarization.[118]

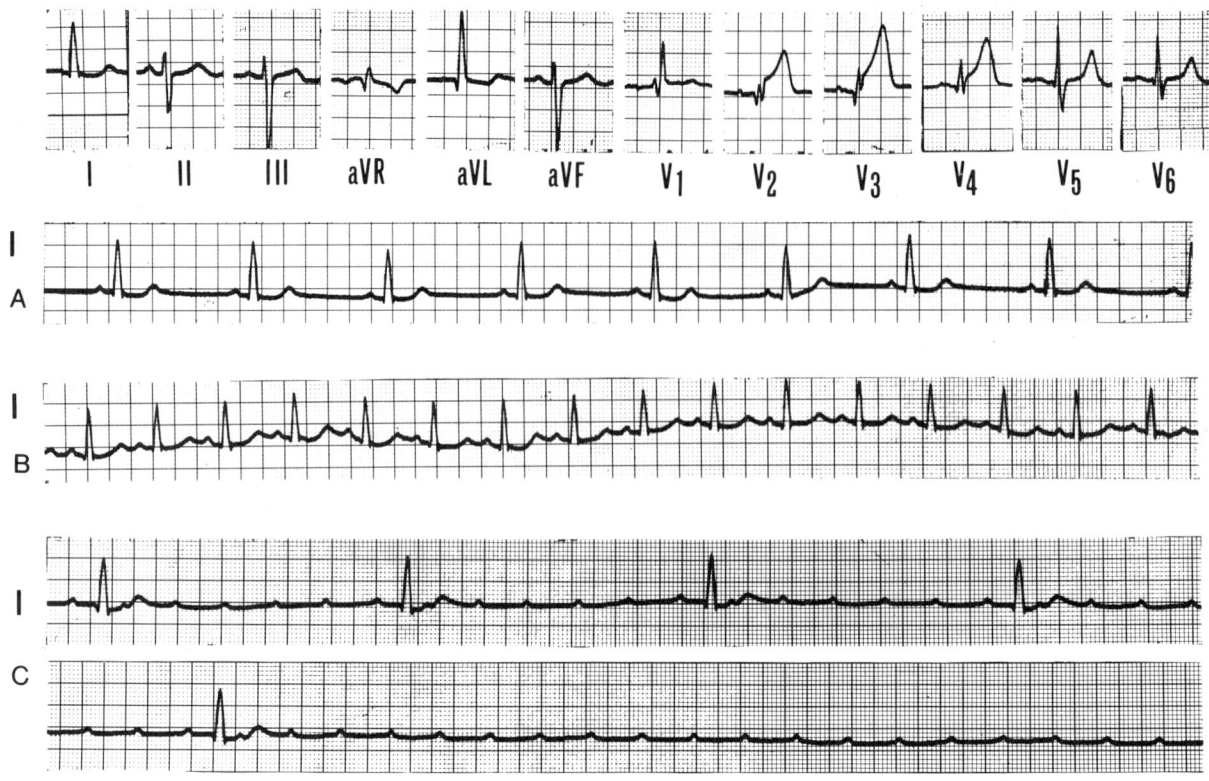

FIGURE 7–25
Representative electrocardiograms from a 75-year-old man with acute myocardial infarction, showing paroxysmal AV block that followed isoprenaline infusion with marked acceleration of the sinus rate. At top is a recording of the 12-lead electrocardiogram on admission, showing right bundle branch block, left axis deviation, and acute anteroseptal myocardial infarction. A shows the patient's cardiac rhythm on admission and reveals sinus bradycardia at a rate of 48 beats per minute. B, This rhythm strip was obtained shortly after the start of isoprenaline infusion and shows an increase of the sinus rate to 95 beats per minute with 1:1 AV conduction. C illustrates the development of sinus tachycardia (130 beats per minute) with a high-grade AV block that terminated in complete AV block and a prolonged ventricular asystole. Note the lengthening of the P-R interval of conducted beats in C (0.26 s) compared with a P-R interval of 0.16 s in B. This suggests concealed AV conduction in C. (Reprinted with permission of the American Heart Association, Inc., from El-Sherif N, et al.: Circulation 50:515, 1974.)

Intraventricular Conduction Disorders

According to the trifascicular concept,[121] the intraventricular conduction system is composed of three fascicles: the right bundle branch and the left anterior and posterior fascicles of the main left bundle branch. A possible third or septal fascicle was later described.[122] Some authors question the existence of discrete fascicles, since pathologic specimens of the conduction system reveal no discrete fascicles but rather a fan-shaped arrangement of the fibers of the left bundle branch.[123] However, the fascicular concept, whether anatomically proven or not, is useful in explaining functional abnormalities and electrocardiographic patterns associated with intraventricular conduction.

Bundle branch block occurs in about 0.6% of the population and in 1 to 2% of the population over 60 years of age. Up to 80% of these patients have organic heart disease, 50% of which is due to coronary artery disease.[124] Ventricular mapping studies have documented abnormal epicardial and endocardial activation in patients with fascicular and bundle branch blocks.[125, 126] On the other hand, pathologic studies have demonstrated widespread fibrotic lesions throughout the His-Purkinje system even when isolated fascicular patterns are observed on the ECG.[8, 95, 127]

ISOLATED BUNDLE BRANCH BLOCK AND FASCICULAR BLOCK

Left Bundle Branch Block

Complete left bundle branch block is uncommon in the absence of clinically evident heart disease[33, 128] and is rarely associated with AV block or syncope.[129, 130] Preexisting left bundle branch block in the absence of clinical evidence of disease carries a slightly higher mortality rate than normal (mortality risk ratio = 1.26–1.38),[131, 132] whereas newly acquired left bundle branch block carries a substantially higher mortality rate (mortality risk ratio = 10).[133] No adequate information is available on the prognosis of incomplete left bundle branch block.

Right Bundle Branch Block

Isolated complete right bundle branch block is about three times as common as isolated left bundle branch

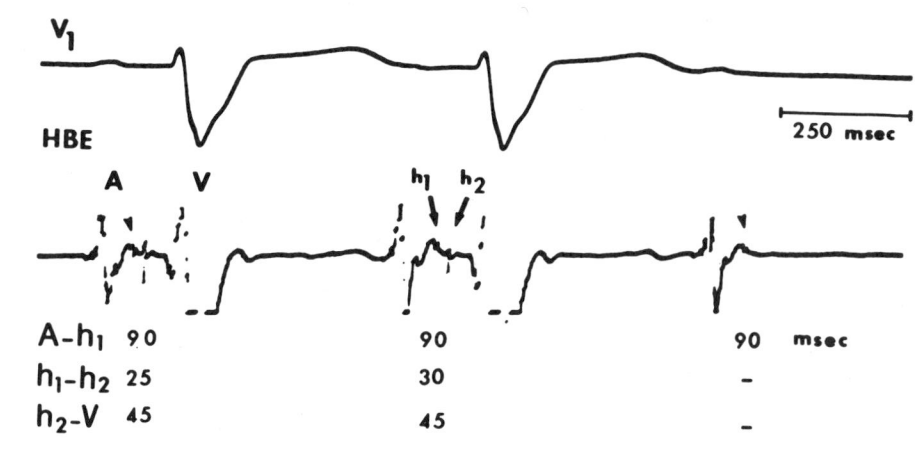
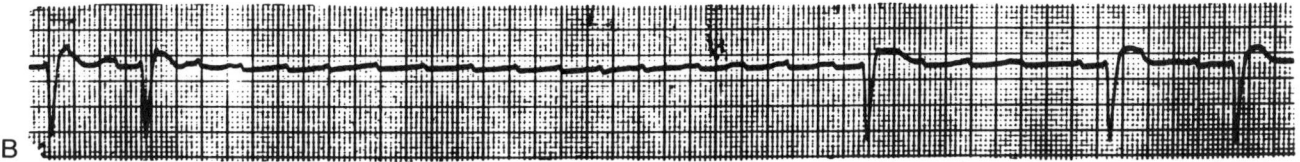

FIGURE 7–26
Recordings obtained from a 65-year-old woman with a history of dizzy spells. An echo-doppler study showed a calcified mitral annulus and mild mitral regurgitation. The electrocardiogram showed normal sinus rhythm, complete left bundle branch block pattern, and periods of Mobitz type II AV block. A, His bundle electrogram (HBE) showing a period of 3:2 AV block. The block is intra-Hisian with split His potential (h_1, h_2) and a 5-ms increment of the $h_1 h_2$ interval prior to block. The intra-Hisian block was not initially recognized because the h_1 deflection was overlooked. B, A rhythm strip obtained one day later showing the occurrence of an atrial tachycardia (rate 150–170 beats per minute) that resulted in a tachycardia-dependent paroxysmal AV block. AV conduction resumed at the end of the recording when the tachycardia slowed down and sinus rhythm resumed (last beat).

block in the general population,[33, 128] and it is rarely associated with AV block or syncope.[129, 130] Neither preexisting nor recently acquired (complete or incomplete) right bundle branch block appears to be associated with an increased mortality ratio or coronary risk ratio.[130, 134–136]

Left Anterior Fascicular Block

Isolated left anterior fascicular block is three to ten times more common than right bundle branch block,[33, 128] and it is not associated with an additional risk of sudden death or high-degree AV block.[128, 137] The risk of syncope in left anterior fascicular block is not documented.

Left Posterior Fascicular Block

Isolated left posterior fascicular block is less common than left bundle branch block and is substantially less common than right bundle branch block or left anterior fascicular block.[33, 128] There are no adequate data on isolated left posterior fascicular block and the risk of sudden death or of high-degree AV block.[138]

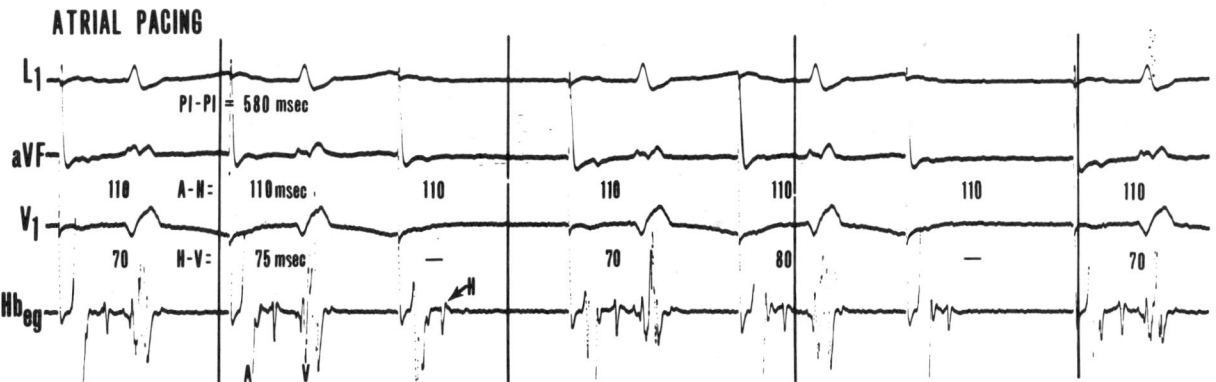

FIGURE 7–27
His bundle recording (Hb_{eg}) showing atrial pacing at a cycle length of 580 ms associated with 3:2 AV block distal to His bundle. Note 5 to 10 ms increment of H-V interval prior to block. Time lines are set at 1-s intervals.

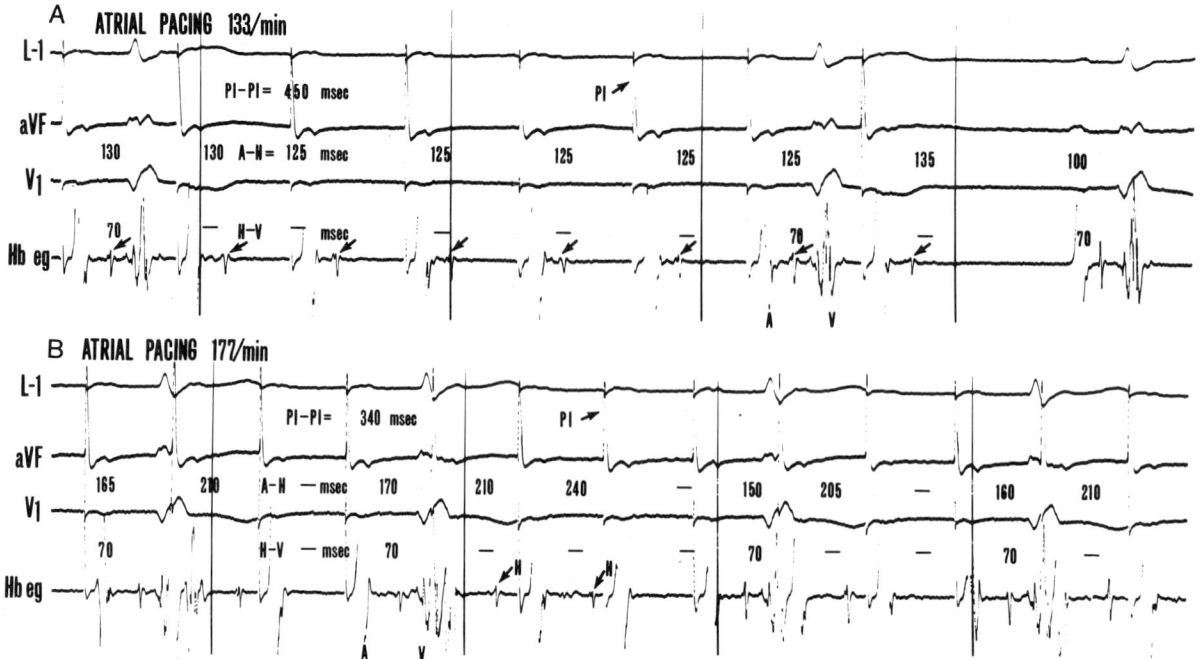

FIGURE 7–28
Tachycardia-dependent repetitive block in the His-Purkinje system. Recordings were obtained from the same patient shown in Figure 7–27. A, Atrial pacing at a shorter cycle length of 450 ms induced a 6:1 AV block distal to the His bundle. B, Further shortening of the atrial pacing cycle to 340 ms resulted in alternating 3:1 and 4:1 AV block due to interaction of AV nodal Wenckebach block and a block in the His-Purkinje system. Hb eg = His bundle electrogram. Time lines are set at 1-s intervals.

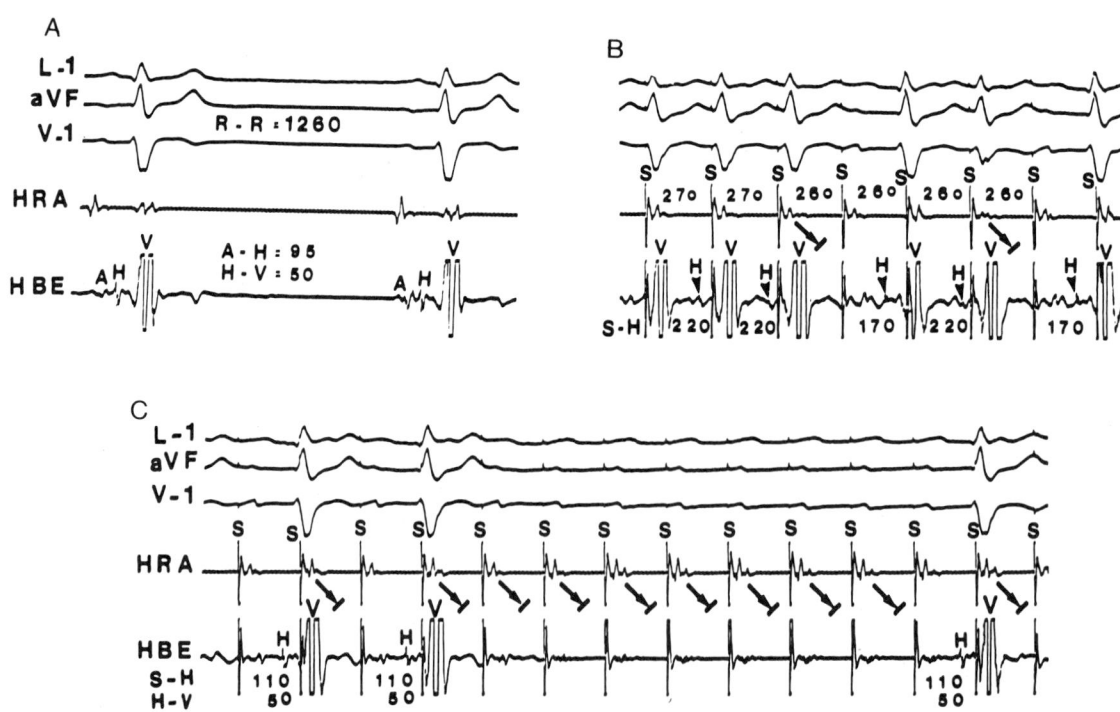

FIGURE 7–29
Tachycardia-dependent repetitive block in the AV node. A, His bundle electrogram (HBE) during sinus bradycardia, showing normal A-H and H-V intervals. B, Atrial pacing at a cycle length of 260 to 270 ms resulted in Wenckebach AV nodal block. C, Atrial pacing at a constant cycle length of 250 ms resulted in 2:1 AV block followed by 9:1 AV block in the AV node. Although the AV block occurred proximal to the recorded His bundle potential, the possibility that the block was localized in the proximal His bundle cannot be ruled out completely from this type of recording. HRA = High right atrial electrogram.

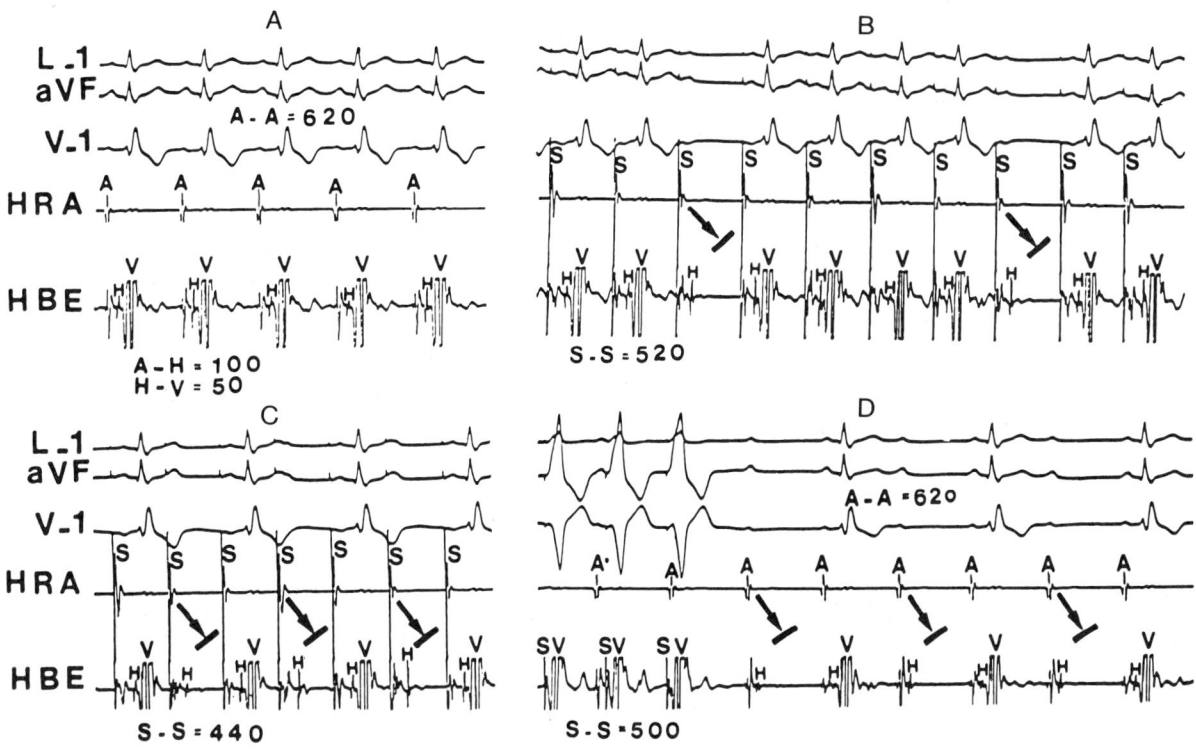

FIGURE 7–30
Effects of rapid ventricular pacing on His-Purkinje conduction. A, His bundle recording during sinus rhythm at a cycle of 620 ms, showing normal A-H and H-V intervals. The surface electrocardiogram showed a right bundle branch block pattern and normal frontal plane axis. B and C, Atrial pacing showing the development of tachycardia-dependent second-degree Mobitz II block distal to the His bundle at a cycle length of 520 ms in B and 2:1 AV block at a cycle length of 440 ms in C. D, Ventricular pacing at a cycle length of 500 ms for one minute was followed by 2:1 block distal to the His bundle during sinus rhythm at the same cycle length of 620 ms that was associated with 1:1 AV conduction in A. See text for explanation. S = pacing stimulus; A, H, V = atrial His bundle, and ventriculogram; SS = pacing interval.

INTERMITTENT AND RATE-RELATED BUNDLE BRANCH BLOCK

Transient bundle branch block is usually defined as an intraventricular conduction defect that subsequently returns, if only temporarily, to normal conduction, while intermittent bundle branch block is characterized in the same electrocardiographic recording of complexes showing bundle branch block pattern and normally conducted beats.[139] However, since some cases of bundle branch block are rate-dependent, and in many of these cases no attempt is usually taken to uncover probable instances of normal intraventricular conduction, it is difficult at times to make a clear-cut distinction not only between transient and intermittent bundle branch block but even between permanent and transient blocks. On the other hand, an electrocardiographic recording showing normal intraventricular conduction at "physiologic" heart rates does not exclude the presence of a latent degree of conduction delay in the bundle branch system.

The majority of cases of intermittent bundle branch block are rate-dependent, with the conduction disturbance usually associated with acceleration of the heart rate (tachycardia-dependent block) or slowing of the rate (bradycardia-dependent block).[140] Studies of the onset and course of transient bundle branch block in a canine experimental model of ischemia of the proximal His-Purkinje system revealed that the bundle branch block initially developed on increasing or slowing of

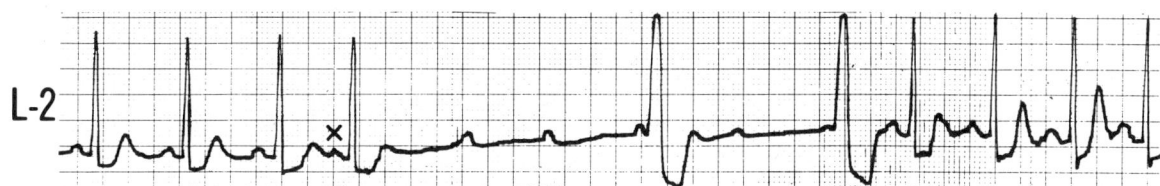

FIGURE 7–31
Bradycardia-dependent paroxysmal AV block. There is a brief period of complete AV block with the escape of an idioventricular rhythm initiated by a long atrial cycle that followed the atrial premature beat marked X. At the end of the recording, 1:1 AV conduction resumed on slight acceleration of the sinus rate.

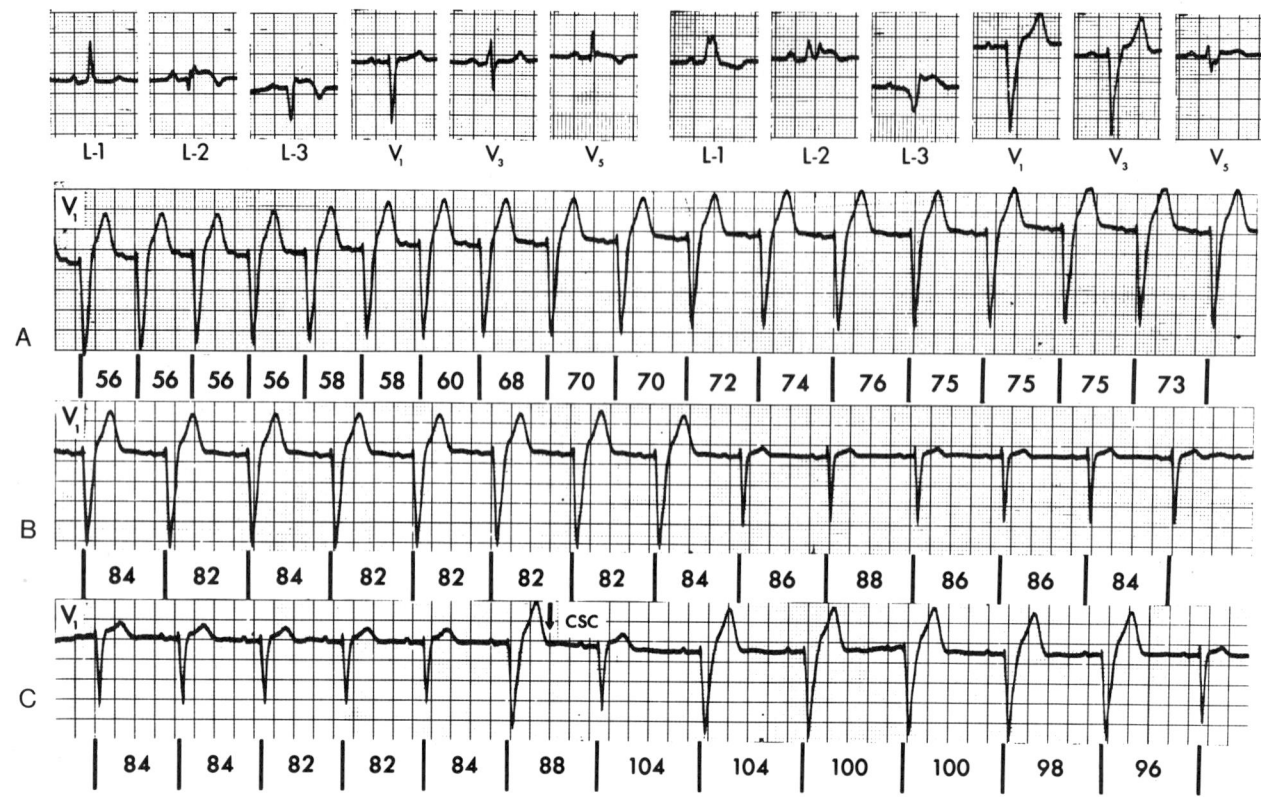

FIGURE 7–32
Tachycardia- and bradycardia-dependent left bundle branch block. Electrocardiographic recordings obtained from a 64-year-old woman with acute inferolateral wall myocardial infarction. Top, 12-lead electrocardiogram. A–C are consecutive recordings with only a few beats omitted. The first half of A shows sinus tachycardia at a cycle length of 560 ms and left bundle branch block during isoprenaline infusion. B, When the infusion was stopped, the heart rate slowed gradually and, at a critical cycle length of 840 ms, normal intraventricular conduction was observed, illustrating the presence of a tachycardia-dependent left bundle branch block. C, Further slowing of the heart rate by carotid sinus compression (CSC) revealed the presence of a bradycardia-dependent left bundle branch block that reverted to normal intraventricular conduction at critical shortening of R-R interval to 960 ms (the last beat in C). There is a narrow range of normal intraventricular conduction at cycle lengths of 840 to 960 ms. The numbers in A–C represent one hundredths of a second. (Reprinted with permission from El-Sherif N, et al.: Brit Heart J 36:291, 1974.)

the heart rate with a range of intermediate rates at which intraventricular conduction was normal.[141] At a later stage of ischemia, bundle branch block became constant at all heart rates before it was again replaced by normal intraventricular conduction at intermediate rates and finally consistent normal conduction. Similar observations have been reported during the course of transient bundle branch block in patients with acute myocardial infarction (Fig. 7–32)[142] as well as in other patients with intermittent bundle branch block not associated with acute infarction.[143]

A bradycardia-dependent conduction delay or block in the His-Purkinje system may explain clinical examples of unexpected improvement of intraventricular or AV conduction of beats terminating short cardiac cycles while impaired conduction is present at longer cycles. Some of these cases have been ascribed to supernormal conduction[144, 145] or to the Wedensky phenomenon.[146] The electrophysiologic mechanisms underlying both tachycardia-dependent and bradycardia-dependent conduction delays and block in the His-Purkinje system are discussed in detail in Part I of Chapter 18.

BUNDLE BRANCH BLOCK PATTERN DUE TO LONGITUDINAL DISSOCIATION IN THE HIS BUNDLE

Conventionally, fascicular and bundle branch block patterns in electrocardiographic leads are considered to represent conduction delay or block in the corresponding fascicle or bundle branch. The possibility that bundle branch block patterns in the ECG may be caused by more distal conduction delays in the Purkinje network, Purkinje-muscle junctions, and the working myocardium (so-called peripheral or parietal blocks) has been entertained for years.[147] Probably, for as many years, the alternative hypothesis that bundle branch block patterns can occur secondary to a more proximal lesion in the AV junction was suggested.[148] Several experimental studies[149–152] and a few clinical observations[153, 154] examined the concept that functional longitudinal dissociation in the AV node or the His bundle can result in significant alteration in the ventricular activation pattern. Some of these studies presented controversial evidence, especially in regard to the functional significance of the transverse interconnections of the His bundle that could militate against longitudinal dissociation of conduction under normal physiologic conditions. However, both experimental[155] and clinical studies[155, 156] have shown that under pathologic conditions, the His bundle may show asynchronous conduction delay and functional longitudinal dissociation, giving rise to altered intraventricular conduction and bundle branch block patterns. In those cases, normalization of intraventricular conduction by His bundle pacing at a site distal to the pathologic lesion has been used as evidence that the bundle branch block pattern is secondary to functional longitudinal dissociation in the pathologic His bundle (Fig. 7–33). Functional longitudinal dissociation in a pathologic His bundle can also explain the rare occurrence of alternating H-V intervals during a constant atrial rate (Fig. 7–34).

The prognostic significance of bundle branch block pattern secondary to longitudinal dissociation in the His bundle is primarily related to the His bundle lesion.[155] An example of a clinical situation in which a bundle branch block due to a His bundle lesion may carry a higher risk of complete AV block is postoperative left anterior hemiblock and right bundle branch block following repair of tetrology of Fallot. Two distinct groups of patients have been recognized: one group in which the electrocardiographic pattern is secondary to a His bundle lesion, and a second group in which the pattern is caused by lesions in the peripheral conduction system.[157] The first group of patients has a higher risk of complete AV block. Also, in these patients a prolonged H-V interval was suggested as a useful index to identify those at risk.[157]

BIFASCICULAR AND TRIFASCICULAR BLOCK

Bifascicular block includes the electrocardiographic patterns of right bundle branch block and left anterior fascicular block, right bundle branch block and left posterior fascicular block, and left bundle branch block. If conduction in the remaining fascicle is also impaired, an incomplete or complete trifascicular block will result. This usually is manifested as a prolonged H-V interval in the His bundle electrogram. However, in some of these cases the H-V interval prolongation may be due to an intra-His bundle delay rather than a conduction delay in the remaining fascicle. His bundle pacing could be used to discern the site responsible for prolonged H-V interval (see Fig. 7–16).

Right bundle branch block with left anterior fascicular block is the most common form of bifascicular block and is seen in approximately 1% of hospitalized patients. Left anterior fascicular block is diagnosed in the presence of left axis deviation greater than or equal to −30 degrees. It was reported that 59% of patients with AV block had right bundle branch block and left anterior fascicular block during periods of AV conduction.[158] However, progression to AV block in patients with right bundle branch block and left anterior fascicular block is estimated to be about 6% per year.

Right bundle branch block with left posterior fascicular block is much less frequent but potentially more dangerous. This is probably because these patients have a diffuse myocardial involvement. The diagnosis of left posterior fascicular block is made on the basis of abnormal right axis deviation of 120 degrees or more in the frontal plane in the absence of right ventricular hypertrophy, pulmonary disease, and extreme vertical position.

A combination of conduction delays in individual fascicles of the left bundle would be manifested as left bundle branch block. The incidence of complete AV block in patients with left bundle branch block is lower than in patients with right bundle branch block and left anterior fascicular block or left posterior fascicular block. Patients with left bundle branch block and left axis deviation had a greater incidence of myocardial dysfunction and long P-R, A-H, and H-V intervals when compared with those without left axis deviation.[159] Despite these findings, AV block developed in only 6% of patients with left bundle branch block and left axis deviation and in none of the patients with left bundle branch block and normal axis when prospectively followed for 30 to 2271 days.[159]

BUNDLE BRANCH AND BIFASCICULAR BLOCKS IN ACUTE MYOCARDIAL INFARCTION

Bundle branch and bifascicular blocks are seen in approximately 13% of patients with acute myocardial infarction.[160] These patients usually have extensive anteroseptal, anterior, or anterolateral infarction. The most commonly encountered bifascicular blocks are right bundle branch block and left anterior fascicular block and left bundle branch block. Right bundle branch block and left posterior fascicular block are much less frequent. The incidence of AV block in patients with acute myocardial infarction and bifascicular block varies from 8% to 47%.[161, 162] It is noteworthy that 33% of patients who develop complete AV block do so without prior first- or second-degree AV block.[163] Since the occurrence of bifascicular block in acute myocardial infarction can be the only warning of an impending complete AV block, these patients should have a temporary pacemaker. Permanent prophylactic pacing is usually indicated in patients who develop complete AV block in the His-Purkinje system, patients who demonstrate alternating bundle branch block, and perhaps those with a new right bundle branch block and left posterior fascicular block.[164]

Several reports have demonstrated that patients who developed bundle branch block during acute myocardial infarction had a higher in-hospital mortality than those who did not.[162, 163, 165–171] Those patients were older and had a larger infarct size and a higher incidence of anterior wall infarction, especially in cases of right bundle branch block, left ventricular failure, arrhythmias, and AV block. The long-term prognosis in patients with bundle branch block is also poor compared with patients without this conduction disor-

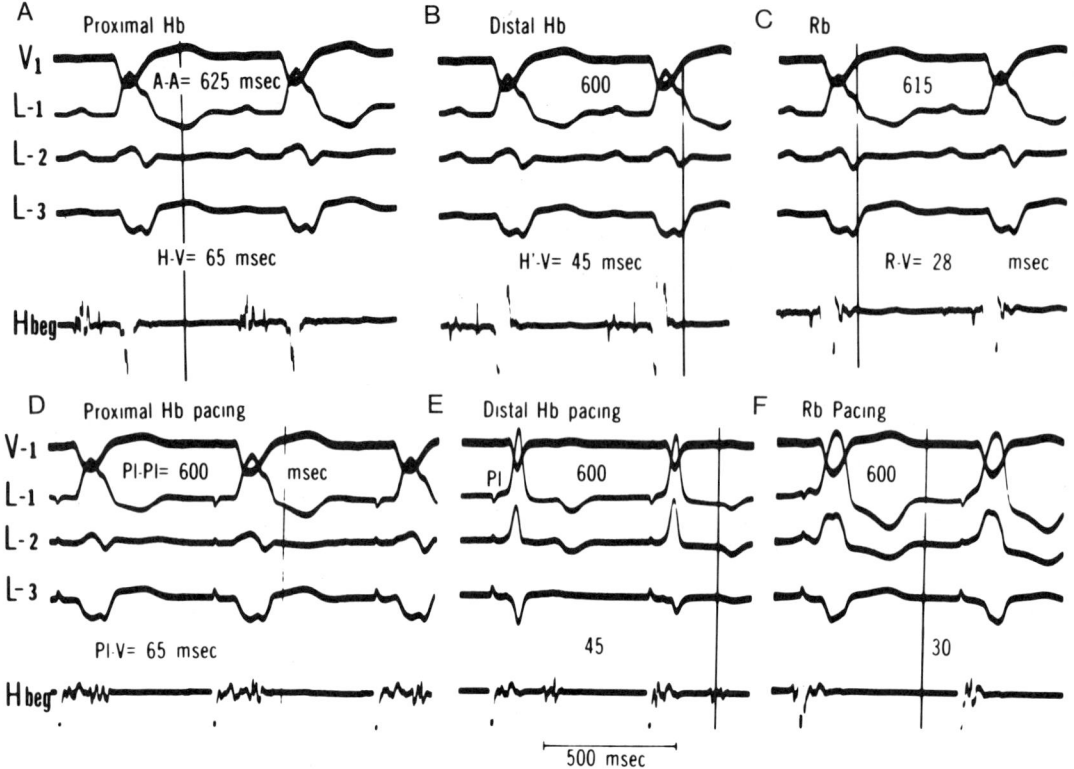

FIGURE 7–33
His bundle Hb recordings from a 60-year-old man with a chronic left bundle branch block (LBBB) pattern probably secondary to functional longitudinal dissociation in the His bundle. A, C, and E were obtained from different electrode catheter positions and illustrate, respectively, the proximal HB potential, the distal HB potential, and the right bundle spike (Rb). B, D, and F illustrate pacing from the three different sites utilizing the same stimulus strength and polarity. Proximal Hb pacing in B gave rise to a QRS configuration identical to conducted supraventricular beats and a PI-V interval similar to the H-V interval. On the other hand, distal Hb pacing in D resulted in disappearance of the LBBB pattern with decrease of the QRS duration from 0.14 to 0.08 sec. The frontal plane QRS axis also changed from −35 degrees during the LBBB pattern to +15 degrees during the normalized QRS pattern. The PI-V interval of 45 ms was identical to the H'-V interval. Right bundle pacing in F was obtained from an electrode positioned a few millimeters distal to that during distal Hb pacing. This resulted in paced beats with an LBBB pattern similar but not identical to conducted supraventricular beats. The difference was in the frontal plane QRS axis, which measured +15 degrees during right bundle pacing (compare lead 2 during both patterns). Hbeg = His bundle electrogram. (Reprinted with permission of the American Heart Association, Inc., from El-Sherif N, et al.: Circulation 57:473, 1978.)

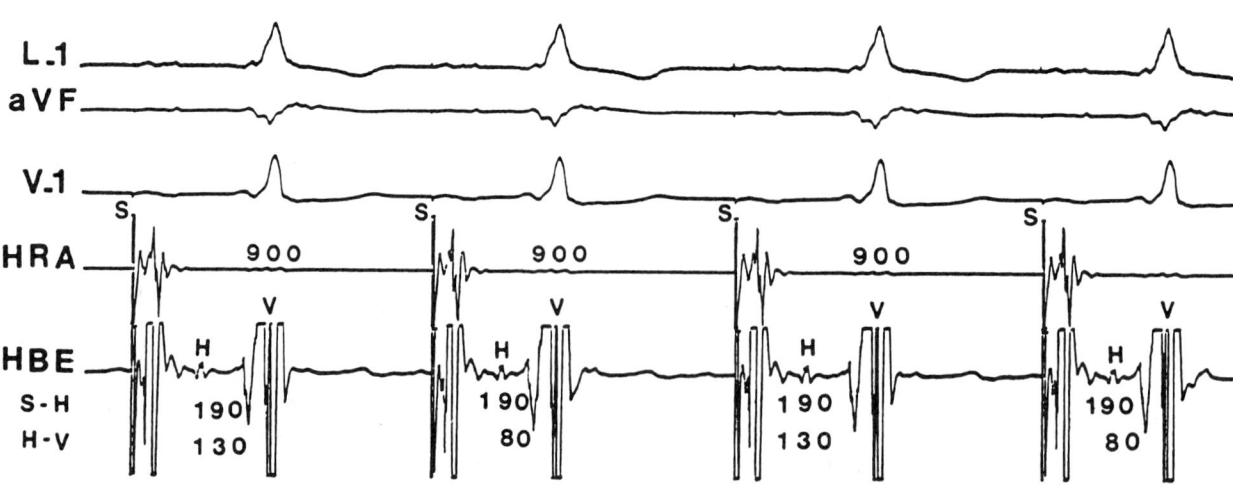

FIGURE 7–34
Atrial pacing at a cycle length of 900 ms showing alternation of the P-R interval due to alternation of the H-V interval. There was no associated change in QRS configuration, which shows right bundle branch block and left anterior fascicular block. Both sets of H-V intervals are prolonged compared with normal. The recording suggests longitudinal dissociation in a diseased His bundle. HRA = High right atrial electrogram; HBE = His bundle electrogram; S-H = stimulus to His interval.

der.[163, 167-170, 172] Some authors,[172] but not others,[163, 168] have found that right and left bundle branch block had the same deleterious long-term prognostic significance. Even if the bundle branch block was transient and absent at hospital discharge, the patient still had a poor long-term prognosis.[172, 173]

CHRONIC BIFASCICULAR BLOCK AND PROGNOSTIC SIGNIFICANCE OF PROLONGED H-V INTERVAL

Most patients with chronic bifascicular block have underlying heart disease, with a prevalence ranging from 74% to 88%.[174-176] The most common causes are coronary artery disease and hypertensive cardiovascular disease, which are frequently severe.[174-176]

Chronic bifascicular block is associated with substantial mortality.[177, 178] The bulk of this mortality is due to cardiovascular deaths, two thirds of which are sudden with a sudden death mortality rate of 12 to 27%.[174, 175, 179] However, this mortality generally reflects the presence and severity of underlying organic heart disease. Sudden cardiac death is frequently associated with ventricular tachyarrhythmias[175, 176, 180] and is only rarely due to paroxysmal AV block.[175, 176, 180, 181]

Although a prolonged H-V interval in patients with chronic bifascicular block may be associated with increased mortality,[174-176, 181] it is likely that this association merely reflects the relationship between the duration of the H-V interval and the extent of underlying heart disease.[182, 183] Thus, measurement of the H-V interval is considered to be, at best, only an indirect means of delineating prognosis in chronic bifascicular block.[182]

Although patients with bifascicular block and prolonged H-V interval are at increased risk of developing complete trifascicular block, the absolute risk remains very low (approximately 2% per year).[174-176] It is likely that this risk varies directly with the degree of H-V interval prolongation. However, it is not clear that even a grossly prolonged H-V interval (more than 100 ms) or atrial pacing-induced block distal to the His bundle indicate a likelihood of developing trifascicular block over a period of several years.[176, 184] Thus, at present there are no clinical indications for electrophysiologic studies in asymptomatic patients with chronic bifascicular block.

On the other hand, even syncope in patients with chronic bifascicular block is caused by transient AV block, albeit in a minority of cases.[176, 185, 186] If a thorough clinical evaluation including a neurologic workup and continuous electrocardiographic monitoring fails to reveal a probable cause for syncope, an electrophysiologic study would be recommended. If the H-V interval is markedly prolonged or if atrial pacing induces block distal to the His bundle, a prophylactic permanent pacemaker is usually indicated.[176, 187] The electrophysiologic study may also reveal other causes of syncope such as sinus node dysfunction and supraventricular or ventricular tachyarrhythmias. In some reports, 23 to 28% of patients with syncope and preexisting bundle branch block had inducible sustained ventricular tachyarrhythmias during electrophysiologic testing.[188, 189]

References

1. Adams R: Dublin Hospital Report 4:353, 1827.
2. Stokes W: Dublin Q J Med Sci 2:73, 1846.
3. Wenckebach KF: Zur Analyse des unregalmässigen Pulses. Z Klin Med 39:293, 1900.
4. Mobitz W: Uber die unvollstandige Storung der Erregungsuberleitung zwischen Vorhof und Kammer des menschlichen Herzens. Zschr Exper Med 41:180, 1924.
5. His W Jr: Die Tatigkeit des embryonalen Herzens und deren Bedentung fur die Lehre von Herzbewegung beim Erwach-Sener. Arkiv Medizinische Klinik Leipzig, 14, 1893.
6. Tawara S: Das Reitzleitungssystem des Saugetierherzens. Jena, Gustav Fischer, 1906.
7. Blair DM, Dairos F: Observations on the conducting system of the heart. J Anat 69:303, 1934–1935.
8. Davies MJ, Anderson RH and Becker AE: The Conduction System of the Heart, p 228. London, Butterworths, 1983.
9. James TN, Sherf L, Fine G, Morales AR: Comparative ultrastructure of the sinus node in man and dog. Circulation 34:139, 1966.
10. Scherlag BJ, Lau SH, Helfant RH, et al.: Catheter technique for recording His bundle activity in man. Circulation 39:13, 1969.
11. Damato AN, Lau SH: Clinical value of the electrogram of the conducting system. Prog Cardiovas Dis 13:119, 1970.
12. Narula OS, Cohen LS, Scherlag BJ, et al.: Localization of AV conduction defects in man by recording of the His bundle electrogram. Am J Cardiol 25:228, 1970.
13. Parsonnet V, Crawford C: United States survey on cardiac pacing. PACE 6:21A, 1983.
14. Patten BM: Development of the heart. In Development of the Sinoventricular Conduction System. University of Michigan Medical Bulletin 22.1, 1973.
15. Koch W: Weiter Mitteilungen uber den Sinnusknoter der Herzens. Verh Desch Pathol Ges. 13:85, 1909.
16. Koch W: Der Funktionelle Ban des Menschlichen Herzens, p. 92. Berlin, Urban V. Schwarzenburg, 1922.
17. Todaro F: Novelle richerche sopra la struttura muscolare delle Orechietta del Coure Umano e sopra la Valva d'Eustachio. Sperimentale 16:217, 1865.
18. James TN: Anatomy of the Coronary Arteries. New York, Hoeber Medical Division, Harper and Row, 1961.
19. James TN: Cardiac innervation: Anatomic and pharmacologic relations. Bull NY Acad Sci 43:1041, 1967.
20. Paes de Carvalho A, de Almeida DF: Speed of activity through the atrioventricular node. Circ Res 8:801, 1960.
21. Anderson RH, Janse MJ, Capelle FJ, et al.: A combined morphological and electrophysiological study of the atrioventricular node of the rabbit heart. Circ Res 35:909, 1974.
22. Scherlag BJ, Lazzara R, Helfant RH: Differentiation of "AV junctional rhythms." Circulation 48:304, 1973.
23. James TN, Isobe JH, Urthaler F: Correlative electrophysiological and anatomical studies concerning the site of origin of escape rhythm during complete atrioventricular block in the dog. Circ Res 45:108, 1979.
24. James TN, Scherf L: Fine structure of the His bundle. Circulation 44:9, 1971.
25. Frink RJ, James TN: Normal blood supply to the human His bundle and proximal bundle branches. Circulation 47:8, 1973.
26. Narula OS: Conduction disorders in the AV transmission system. In Dreifus LS, Likoff W (eds.): Cardiac Arrhythmias, p. 259. 25th Hahnemann Symposium. New York, Grune and Stratton, 1973.
27. Puech P, Grolleau R, Guimond C: Incidence of different types of AV block and their localization by His bundle recordings. In Wellens HJJ, Lie KI, Janse NJ (eds.): The Conduction System of the Heart: Structure, Function and Clinical Implications. Philadelphia, Lea & Febiger, 1976.

28. Gomes JAC, El-Sherif N: His Bundle recordings: Contributions to clinical electrophysiology. *In* Samet P, El-Sherif N (eds.): Cardiac Pacing, p. 375. New York, Grune and Stratton, 1980.
29. Rosen KM, Mehta A, Miller RA: Demonstration of dual atrioventricular pathways in man. Am J Cardiol 3:291, 1974.
30. Narula OS, Samet P: Right bundle branch block with normal, left or right axis deviation. Am J Med 51:432, 1971.
31. Haft JI, Levites R: Significance of first degree AV block (prolonged PR interval) in bifascicular block. Am J Cardiol 34:257, 1974.
32. Johnson RL, Averill KH, Lamb LE: Electrocardiographic findings in 67,375 asymptomatic subjects. VII. Atrioventricular block. Am J Cardiol 6:153, 1960.
33. Hiss RG, Lamb LE: Electrocardiographic findings in 122,043 individuals. Circulation 25:947, 1962.
34. Meyers I, Kaplinsky E, Yahini JH, Hanne-Paparo N, Neufeld HN: Wenckebach AV block: A frequent feature following heavy physical training. Am Heart J 90:426, 1975.
35. Narula OS, Runge M, Samet P: Second-degree Wenckebach type A-V block due to block within the atrium. Br Heart J 34:1127, 1972.
36. Leier DV, Meacham JA, Schall SF: Prolonged atrial conduction: A major predisposing factor for the development of atrial flutter. Circulation 57:213, 1978.
37. Narula DS, Samet P: Wenckebach and Mobitz II AV block due to lesions within the His bundle and bundle branches. Circulation 41:947, 1970.
38. Schuillenberg RM, Durrer D: Conduction disturbances located within the His bundle. Circulation 45:612, 1972.
39. Denes P, Levy L, Pica A, Rosen KM: The incidence of typical and atypical AV Wenckebach periodicity. Am Heart J 89:26, 1975.
40. Friedman HS, Gomes JAC, Haft JI: An analysis of Wenckebach periodicity. J Electrocardiol 8:307, 1975.
41. El-Sherif N, Aranda J, Befeler B, Lazzara R: Atypical Wenckebach periodicity stimulating Mobitz II AV block. Br Heart J 40:1376, 1978.
42. Brodsky M, Wu D, Denes P, et al.: Arrhythmias documented by 24-hour continuous electrocardiographic monitoring in 50 male medical students without apparent heart disease. Am J Cardiol 39:390, 1977.
43. Huston TP, Puffer JC, Rodney WM: The athletic heart syndrome. N Engl J Med 313:24, 1985.
44. DiMarco JP, Garan H, Harthorne JW, Ruskin JN: Intracardiac electrophysiologic techniques in recurrent syncope of unknown cause. Ann Intern Med 95:542, 1981.
45. Young D, Eisenberg R, Fisch B, Fisher JD: Wenckebach AV block (Mobitz I) in children and young adults. Am J Cardiol 40:393, 1977.
46. Kibler LE, Gazes PC: Effect of clonidine on atrioventricular conduction. JAMA 238:1930, 1977.
47. Gould L, Reddy R, Singh BK: Electrophysiologic properties of methyldopa in man. Chest 76:310, 1979.
48. Adgey AA, Pantridg JF: Acute phase of myocardial infarction. Lancet 2:501, 1971.
49. Lie KI, Duner D: Atrioventricular and intraventricular conduction disturbances in acute myocardial infarction: Clinical aspects. *In* Samet P, El-Sherif N (eds.): Cardiac Pacing, p. 439. New York, Grune and Stratton, 1980.
50. Sclarovsky S, Strasberg B, Hirshberg A, et al.: Advanced early and late atrioventricular block in acute inferior wall myocardial infarction. Am Heart J 108:19, 1984.
51. Clemo HP, Belardinelli L: Effect of adenosine on atrioventricular conduction. I: Site and characterization of adenosine action in the guinea pig atrioventricular node. Circ Res 59:427, 1986.
52. Meltzer LE, Cohen HE: The incidence of arrhythmias associated with acute myocardial infarction. *In* Meltzer LE, Dunning AJ (eds.): Textbook of Coronary Care, p. 197. Amsterdam, Experta Medica, 1972.
53. Wenckebach KF: Beitrage zur Kenntnis der menschlichen Herztatigkeit. Arch Anat Physiol 297–354, 1906.
54. Hay J: Bradycardia and cardiac arrhythmia produced by depression of certain of the functions of the heart. Lancet 1:139, 1906.
55. Blondeau M, Rizzon M, Lenegre J: Les troubles de la conduction auriculo-ventriculaire dans l'infarctus myocardique recent: 2. Étude anatomique. Arch Mal Coeur 54:1104, 1961.
56. Sutton R, Davies M: The conduction system in acute myocardial infarction complicated by heart block. Circulation 38:987, 1968.
57. Chamberlain D, Leinbach R: Electrical pacing in heart block complicating acute myocardial infarction. Br Heart J 32:2, 1970.
58. Rotman M, Wagner GS, Waugh RA: Significance of high-degree atrioventricular block in acute posterior myocardial infarction. Circulation 47:257, 1973.
59. Waugh RA, Wagner GS, Haney TL, et al.: Immediate and remote prognostic significance of fascicular block during acute myocardial infarction. Circulation 47:765, 1973.
60. Rosen KM, Loeb HS, Chuquimia R, et al.: Site of heart block in acute myocardial infarction. Circulation 42:925, 1970.
61. Touboul P, Clement C, Porte J, et al.: Étude électrophysiologique des troubles de conduction auriculoventriculaire dans l'infarctus myocardique récent. Arch Mal Coeur 65:1287, 1972.
62. El-Sherif N, Scherlag BJ, Lazzara R: Pathophysiology of second-degree atrioventricular block: A unified hypothesis. Am J Cardiol 35:421, 1975.
63. El-Sherif N, Scherlag BJ, Lazzara R: An appraisal of second-degree and paroxysmal atrioventricular block. Eur J Cardiol 4:117, 1976.
64. El-Sherif N, Scherlag BJ, Lazzara R: Second-degree atrioventricular block in the His-Purkinje system following acute myocardial infarction. Clinical observations on its evolution. Chest 71:615, 1977.
65. Langendorf R, Mehlman FS: Blocked (nonconducted) AV nodal premature systoles initiating first and second degree AV block. Am Heart J 34:500, 1947.
66. Langendorf R, Pick A: Concealed conduction in the A-V junction. *In* Dreifus LS, Likoff W, Meyer JH (eds.): Mechanisms and Therapy of Cardiac Arrhythmias, p. 395. New York, Grune and Stratton, 1966.
67. Rosen KM, Rahimtoola SH, Gunnar RM: Pseudo AV block secondary to premature non-propagated His bundle depolarizations. Documentation by His bundle electrocardiography. Circulation 42:367, 1970.
68. El-Sherif N, Befeler B, Aranda J, et al.: Re-entry due to manifest and concealed His bundle ectopic systoles. Circulation 53:402, 1976.
69. Besoain-Santander M, Pick A, Langendorf R: AV conduction in atrial flutter. Circulation 2:604, 1950.
70. Amat-Y-Leon F, Chuquimia R, Wu D et al.: Alternating Wenckebach periodicity: A common electrophysiologic response. Am J Cardiol 36:757, 1975.
71. Halpern MS, Nau GJ, Levi RJ, et al.: Wenckebach periods of alternate beats. Clinical and experimental observations. Circulation 48:41, 1973.
72. El-Sherif N, Scherlag BJ, Lazzara R, et al.: The pathophysiology of tachycardia-dependent paroxysmal atrioventricular block after myocardial ischemia. Experimental and clinical observations. Circulation 50:515, 1974.
73. Gomes JAC, El-Sherif N: Atrioventricular block. Mechanism, clinical presentation, and therapy. Med Clin North Am 68:955, 1984.
74. Nakamura FF, Nadas AS: Complete heart block in infants and children. New Engl J Med 270:1261, 1964.
75. Lev M: Pathogenesis of congenital AV block. Prog Cardiovasc Dis 15:145, 1972.
76. Carter JB, Blieden LC, Edwards JE: Congenital heart block. Anatomic correlations and review of literature. Arch Pathol 97:51, 1974.
77. McHenry MM, Cayler GG: Congenital complete heart block in newborns, infants, children and adults. Med Times 97:113, 1969.
78. Camm J, Bexton RS: Congenital complete heart block. Eur Heart J 5(Suppl A):115, 1984.
79. Esscher EF: Congenital complete heart block in adolescence and adult life. A follow-up study. Eur Heart J 2:281, 1981.
80. Karpawich PP, Gillette PC, Carson Jr A, et al.: Congenital

complete atrioventricular block: Clinical and electrophysiologic predictors of need for pacemaker insertion. Am J Cardiol 48:1098, 1981.
81. Narula OS, Narula JT: Junctional pacemaker in man. Response to overdrive suppression with and without parasympathetic blockade. Circulation 57:880, 1978.
82. Lie KI, Durrer D: Indications for temporary and permanent pacing in ischemic conduction disturbances. In Samet R, El-Sherif N (eds.): Cardiac Pacing, p. 459. New York, Grune and Stratton, 1980.
83. Hackel DB, Wagner G, Ratliff NB et al.: Anatomic studies of the cardiac conducting system in acute myocardial infarction. Am Heart J 83:77, 1972.
84. Kunkel R, Rowland M, Scheinman MM: The electrophysiologic effects of lidocaine in patients with intraventricular conduction defects. Circulation 49:894, 1974.
85. Scheinman MM, Weiss AN, Shafton E, et al.: Electrophysiologic effects of procainamide in patients with intraventricular conduction delay. Circulation 49:522, 1974.
86. Desai JM, Scheinman M, Peters RW, O'Young J: Electrophysiological effects of disopyramide in patients with bundle branch block. Circulation 59:215, 1979.
87. Sayed HM: Complete heart block following open heart surgery. J Cardiovasc Surg 6:426, 1965.
88. Sondheimer HM, Izukawa T, Olley DM, et al.: Conduction disturbances after total correction of tetralogy of Fallot. Am Heart J 92:278, 1976.
89. Gupta PK, Haft JI: Complete heart block complicating cardiac catheterization. Chest 61:185, 1972.
90. Abernathy WS: Complete heart block caused by the Swan-Ganz catheterization. Chest 65:349, 1974.
91. Scheinman MM, Morady F, Hess DS, Gonzales R: Catheter-induced ablation of the atrioventricular junction to control refractory supraventricular arrhythmias. JAMA 248:851, 1982.
92. Gallagher JJ, Svenson RH, Kassell JH, et al.: Catheter technique for closed chest ablation of the atrioventricular conduction system. N Engl J Med 306:194, 1982.
93. Schienman MM: Catheter Ablation of Cardiac Arrhythmias. Boston, Martinus Nijhoff, 1988.
94. Lev M: The pathology of complete AV block: Prog Cardiovasc Dis 6:317, 1964.
95. Lenegre J: Etiology and pathology of bilateral bundle branch fibrosis in relation to complete heart block. Prog Cardiovasc Dis 6:409, 1964.
96. Rytand DA, Lipsitch LS: Clinical aspects of calcification of mitral annulus. Arch Intern Med 78:544, 1946.
97. Narula OS, Samet P: Predilection of elderly females for intra-His bundle (BH) blocks. Circulation 50(Suppl):III-195, 1974.
98. Ablaza SG, Blanco G, Maranhao V, et al.: Calcific aortic valve disease associated with complete heart block. Dis Chest 54:457, 1968.
99. Harris A, Sleight P, Drew CE: The diagnosis and treatment of aortic stenosis complicated by AV block. Br Heart J 27:560, 1965.
100. Rosenbaum MB: Chagasic myocardiopathy. Prog Cardiovasc Dis 7:199, 1964.
101. Fawcett FJ, Goldberg MJ: Heart block resulting from myocardial sarcoidosis. Br Heart J 36:220, 1974.
102. Hoffman FG, Leight L: Complete AV block associated with rheumatoid disease. Am J Cardiol 16:585, 1965.
103. Aronow WS, Meister L, Kent JR: AV block in familial hemochromatosis treated by permanent synchronous pacemaker. Arch Intern Med 133:433, 1969.
104. Schellhammer PF, Engle M, Hagstrom JW: Histochemical studies of the myocardium and conduction system in acquired iron storage disease. Circulation 35:631, 1967.
105. Perloff JK: Cardiac involvement in heredofamilial neuromyopathic diseases. Cardiovasc Clin 4:33, 1972.
106. Prystowsky EN, Pritchett EL, Roses AD, Gallagher JJ: The natural history of conduction system disease in mytonic muscular dystrophy as determined by serial electrophysiologic studies. Circulation 60:1360, 1979.
107. Burucúa JE, Bellido CA, Vazquez ST, Casas JG, al.: Mesothelioma of AV node. N Engl J Med 289:753, 1973.
108. Erlanger J: On the physiology of heart block in mammals with special reference to causation of Stokes-Adams disease. J Exp Med 7:676, 1905.
109. Wenckebach KF, Winterberg H: Die unregelmaessige. Hertz-taetigkeit, pp. 305–310. Leipzig, Engellmann, 1927.
110. Gilchrist AR: Clinical aspects of high grade heart block. Scott Med J 3:53, 1958.
111. Langendorf R, Pick A: Concealed conduction. Further evaluation of a fundamental aspect of propagation of the cardiac impulse. Circulation 13:381, 1956.
112. Langendorf R, Pick A: Causes and mechanisms of ventricular asystole in advanced A-V block. In Schwarz B, Pellegrino B (eds.): Sudden Cardiac Death. New York, Grune and Stratton, 1964.
113. Stock RJ, Macken DL: Observations on heart block during continuous electrocardiographic monitoring in myocardial infarction. Circulation 38:993, 1968.
114. McHenry PL, Knoebel SB: Acceleration of the sinoatrial rate leading to complete heart block, an unusual mechanism for the Adams-Stokes syndrome. Am Heart J 72:681, 1966.
115. Donoso E, Adler N, Friedberg CK: Unusual forms of second-degree atrioventricular block, including Mobitz type II block associated with the Morgagni-Adams-Stokes syndrome. Am Heart J 67:150, 1964.
116. Schwartz SP, Schwartz LS: Adams-Stokes syndrome during normal sinus rhythm and transient heart block. III. The paradoxical effects of carotid sinus digital pressure and deep breathing on patients with Adams-Stokes seizures during normal sinus rhythm and transient heart block. Am J Cardiol 7:204, 1961.
117. Rosen KM, Loeb HS, Rahimtoola SH: Mobitz type II block with narrow QRS complex and Stokes-Adams attacks. Arch Intern Med 132:595, 1973.
118. El-Sherif N, Gann D, Samet P: Pathophysiology of atrioventricular and bundle branch block in acute myocardial infarction. In Samet P, El-Sherif N (eds.), Cardiac Pacing, p. 409. New York, Grune and Stratton, 1980.
119. Coumel P, Fabiato A, Waynberger M, et al.: Bradycardia-dependent atrio-ventricular block. Report of two cases of A-V block elicited by premature beats. J Electrocardiol 4:168, 1971.
120. Rosenbaum MB, Elizari MV, Levi RJ, Nau GJ: Paroxysmal atrioventricular block related to hypopolarization and spontaneous diastolic depolarization. Chest 63:678, 1973.
121. Rosenbaum MB, Elizari MV, and Lassari JO: Los Hemiblo-queos. Buenos Aires, Parados, 1968.
122. DeMoulin JC, Kulbertus HE: Left hemiblocks revisited from the histopathological viewpoint. Am Heart J 87:712, 1973.
123. Massing GK, James TN: Anatomical configuration of the His bundle and bundle branches in the human heart. Circulation 53:609, 1976.
124. McAnulty J, Rahimtoola S: Prognosis in bundle branch block. Ann Rev Med 32:499, 1981.
125. Wyndham CRC: Epicardial activation in bundle branch block. PACE 6:1201, 1983.
126. Vassallo JA, Cassidy DM, Marchlinski FE, et al.: Endocardial activation of left bundle branch block. Circulation 69:914, 1984.
127. DeMoulin JC, Simar LJ, Kulbertus HE: Quantitative study of left bundle branch fibrosis in left anterior hemiblock: A stereologic approach. Am J Cardiol 36:751, 1975.
128. Barrett PA, Peter T, Swan HJC, et al.: The frequency and prognostic significance of electrocardiographic abnormalities in clinically normal individuals. Prog Cardiovasc Dis 23:299, 1981.
129. Rotman M, Triebwasser JH: A clinical and follow-up study of right and left bundle branch block. Circulation 51:477, 1975.
130. Smith RF, Jackson DH, Hartborne JW, Sanders CA: Acquired bundle branch block in a healthy population. Am Heart J 80:746, 1970.
131. Singer RB: Mortality in 966 life insurance applicants with bundle branch block or wide QRS. Trans Assoc Life Ins Med Dir Am 52:94, 1969.
132. Brackenbridge RDC: Medical Selection of Life Risks. London, Undershaft Press, 1977.
133. Rabkin SW, Mathewson FAL, Tate RB: Natural history of left bundle branch block. Br Heart J 43:164, 1980.
134. Blackburn H, Taylor HL, Keys A: The electrocardiogram in prediction of 5-year coronary heart disease incidence among men aged 40 through 59. Circulation (Suppl)41:I-154, 1970.

135. Rodstein M, Gubner R, Mills JP, et al.: A mortality study in bundle branch. Arch Intern Med 87:663, 1951.
136. Massing GK, Lancaster MC: Clinical significance of acquired complete right bundle branch block in 59 patients without overt heart disease. Aerospace Med 40:967, 1969.
137. Rabkin SW, Mathewson FAL, Tate RB: Natural history of marked left axis deviation—left anterior hemiblock. Am J Cardiol 43:605, 1979.
138. Rowlands DJ: Left and right bundle branch block, left anterior and left posterior hemiblock. Eur Heart J 5:99, 1984.
139. Bauer GE: Transient bundle-branch block. Circulation 29:730, 1964.
140. El-Sherif N: Tachycardia-dependent versus bradycardia-dependent intermittent bundle branch block. Br Heart J 34:167, 1972.
141. El-Sherif N, Scherlag BJ, Lazzara R, Samet P: Pathophysiology of tachycardia- and bradycardia-dependent block in the canine proximal His-Purkinje system after myocardial infarction. Am J Cardiol 33:529, 1974.
142. El-Sherif N: Tachycardia and bradycardia-dependent bundle-branch block after acute myocardial ischemia. Br Heart J 36:291, 1974.
143. Rosenbaum MB, Lazzari JO, Elizari MV: The role of phase 3 and phase 4 block in clinical electrocardiography. In Wellens HJJ, Lie KI, Janse MJ (eds.): The Conduction System of the Heart: Structure, Function and Clinical Implications, pp 126–142. Philadelphia, Lea & Febiger, 1976.
144. Scherf D, Scharf MM: Supernormal phase of intraventricular conduction. Am Heart J 36:621, 1948.
145. Pick A, Langendorf R, Katz LN: The supernormal phase of atrioventricular conduction I. Fundamental mechanisms. Circulation 26:388, 1962.
146. Friedberg HD: Mechanism of Wedensky phenomena in the left bundle branch. Am J Cardiol 27:698, 1971.
147. Alboni P, Malacarne C, Masoni A: Physiopathological and diagnostic hypotheses in peripheral block. J Electrocardiol 10:87, 1977.
148. Kaufman R, Rothberger CJ: Beitrage zur enstehungsweise extrasystolischer allorhythmien (Zweite Mitteilung). Z Gesamte Exp Med 7:199, 1919.
149. Watt TB, Pruitt RD: Focal lesions in the canine bundle of His. Circ Res 31:531, 1972.
150. Lazzara R, Yeh BK, Samet P: Functional transverse interconnections within the His bundle and the bundle branches. Circ Res 32:509, 1973.
151. Bailey JC, Spear JF, Moore EN: Functional significance of transverse conducting pathways within the canine bundle of His. Am J Cardiol 34:790, 1974.
152. Fabregas RA, Tse WW, Han J: Conduction disturbances of the bundle branches produced by lesions in the nonbranching portion of the His bundle. Am Heart J 92:356, 1976.
153. Pick A: Aberrant ventricular conduction of escape beats: Preferential and accessory pathways in the A-V junction. Circulation 13:702, 1956.
154. Sherf L, James TN: New electrocardiographic concept: Synchronized sino-ventricular conduction. Dis Chest 55:127, 1969.
155. El-Sherif N, Amat-Y-Leon F, Schonfield C, et al.: Normalization of bundle branch block patterns by distal His bundle pacing. Clinical and experimental evidence of longitudinal dissociation in the pathologic His bundle. Circulation 57:473, 1978.
156. Narula OS: Longitudinal dissociation in the His bundle: Bundle branch block due to asynchronous conduction within the His Bundle in man. Circulation 56:996, 1977.
157. Steeg CN, Krongrad E, Davachi F, et al.: Postoperative left anterior hemiblock and right bundle branch block following repair of tetralogy of Fallot. Clinical and etiologic considerations. Circulation 51:1026, 1975.
158. Lasser RP, Haft JI, Friedberg CK: Relationship of right bundle branch block and marked left axis deviation (with left parietal or peri-infarction block) to complete heart block and syncope. Circulation 37:429, 1968.
159. Dhingra RC, Amat-Y-Leon F, Wyndham C, et al.: Significance of left axis deviation in patients with chronic left bundle branch block. Am J Cardiol 42:551, 1978.
160. Mullins CB, Atkins JN: Prognosis and management of ventricular conduction blocks in acute myocardial infarction. Mod Conc Cardiovasc Dis 45:129, 1976.
161. Goodman MJ, Lasser BW, Julian DG: Complete bundle branch block complicating acute myocardial infarction. N Engl J Med 282:237, 1970.
162. Scheinman M, Brennan B: Clinical and anatomic implications of intraventricular conduction block in acute myocardial infarction. Circulation 46:753, 1972.
163. Hindman MC, Wagner GS, Jaro M, et al.: The clinical significance of bundle branch block complicating acute myocardial infarction. 1. Clinical characteristics, hospital mortality and one-year follow-up. Circulation 58:679, 1978.
164. Rosenfeld LE: Bradyarrhythmias: Abnormalities of conduction, and indications for pacing in acute myocardial infarction. Cardiol Clin 6:49, 1988.
165. Col JJ, Weinberg SL: The incidence and mortality of intraventricular conduction defects in acute myocardial infarction. Am J Cardiol 29:344, 1972.
166. Basualdo CAE, Haraphongse M, Rossall RE: Intraventricular blocks in acute myocardial infarction. Chest 67:75, 1975.
167. Roos JC, Dunning AJ: Bundle branch block in acute myocardial infarction. Eur J Cardiol 6:403, 1978.
168. Norris RM, Woo HS: Bundle branch block after myocardial infarction. Short and long term effects. In Keely DT (ed.): Advances in the Management of Arrhythmias, p. 364. Sydney, Telectronics, 1978.
169. Ross DL: Approach to the patient with bundle branch block. In Wellens HJJ, Kulbertus HE (eds.): What's New in Electrocardiography, p. 1110. The Hague, Martinus Nijhoff, 1981.
170. Klein RC, Vera Z, Mason DT: Intraventricular conduction defects in acute myocardial infarction: Incidence, prognosis and therapy. Am Heart J 108:1007, 1984.
171. Opolski G, Kraska T, Ostrzycki A, et al.: The effect of infarct size on atrioventricular and intraventricular conduction disturbances in acute myocardial infarction. Int J Cardiol 10:111, 1986.
172. Dubois C, Pierard LA, Sweets J-P, et al.: Short- and long-term prognostic importance of complete bundle-branch block complicating acute myocardial infarction. Clin Cardiol 11:292, 1988.
173. Hauer RNW, Lie KI, Liem KL, Durrer D: Long-term prognosis in patients with bundle branch block complicating acute anteroseptal infarction. Am J Cardiol 49:1581, 1982.
174. Dhingra RC, Palileo E, Strasberg B, et al.: Significance of the H-V interval in 517 patients with chronic bifascicular block. Circulation 64:1265, 1981.
175. McAnulty JH, Rahimtoola SH, Murphy E, et al.: Natural history of "high-risk" bundle-branch block: Final report of a prospective study. N Engl J Med 307:137, 1982.
176. Scheinman MM, Peters RW, Sauve MJ, et al.: Value of the H-Q interval in patients with bundle branch block and the role of prophylactic permanent pacing. Am J Cardiol 50:1316, 1982.
177. Schneider JF, Thomas HE, Kreger BE, et al.: Newly acquired left bundle-branch block: The Framingham Study. Ann Intern Med 90:303, 1979.
178. Schneider JF, Thomas HE, Kreger BE, et al.: Newly acquired left bundle-branch block: The Framingham Study. Ann Intern Med 92:37, 1980.
179. Morady F, Higgins J, Peters RW, et al.: Electrophysiologic testing in bundle branch block and unexplained syncope. Am J Cardiol 54:587, 1984.
180. Denes P, Dhingra RC, Wu D, et al.: Sudden death in patients with chronic bifascicular block. Arch Intern Med 137:1005, 1977.
181. Narula OS, Gann D, Samet P: Prognostic value of H-V intervals. In Narula OS (ed.): His Bundle Electrocardiography and Clinical Electrophysiology, pp 129–134. Philadelphia, F.A. Davis, 1975.
182. Bauernfeind RA, Welch WJ, Brownstein SL: Distal atrioventricular conduction system function. Cardiol Clin 4:417, 1986.

183. Rosen KM, Palileo E, Westveer D, et al.: Sudden and nonsudden cardiovascular mortality in patients with chronic bifascicular block (Abstract). Am J Cardiol 49:1006, 1982.
184. Dhingra RC, Denes P, Wu D, et al.: Prospective observations in patients with chronic bundle branch block and marked H-V prolongation. Circulation 53:600, 1976.
185. Dhingra RC, Denes P, Wu D, et al.: Syncope in patients with chronic bifascicular block: Significance, causative mechanisms, and clinical implications. Ann Intern Med 81:302, 1974.
186. Peters RW, Scheinman MM, Modin G, et al.: Prophylactic permanent pacemakers for patients with chronic bundle branch block. Am J Med 66:978, 1979.
187. Dhingra RC, Wyndham C, Bauernfeind R, et al.: Significance of block distal to the His bundle induced by atrial pacing in patients with chronic bifascicular block. Circulation 60:1455, 1979.
188. Ezri M, Lerman BB, Marchlinski FE, et al.: Electrophysiologic evaluation of syncope in patients with bifascicular block. Am Heart J 106:693, 1983.
189. Morady F, Higgins J, Peters RW, et al.: Electrophysiologic testing in bundle branch block and unexplained syncope. Am J Cardiol 54:587, 1984.

8

Supraventricular Tachycardias: Clinical Characteristics, Diagnosis, and Management

Masood Akhtar
Patrick Tchou
Mohammad Jazayeri

The supraventricular tachycardias traditionally have been classified as atrioventricular (AV) junctional and atrial. This distinction is conceptually relevant because AV response during atrial arrhythmias is an incidental event, whereas intact conduction in both anterograde and retrograde direction is important for initiation and sustenance of most AV junctional tachycardias. The latter is related to the fact that an overwhelming majority of the AV junctional tachycardias are reentrant in nature, and the reentry circuits need intact bidirectional conduction to sustain the process. In this chapter SVT not directly utilizing the accessory pathways (APs) in the reentry loop will be discussed. Arrhythmias associated with AP are covered in detail in Chapter 10 in this book and will only be touched on where considered appropriate.

AV Junctional Tachycardias

AV NODAL REENTRY

In the absence of APs, the most frequent form of AV junctional tachycardia is due to AV nodal reentry.[1-4] The clinical presentation of this arrhythmia is that of paroxysms of SVT with long, asymptomatic intervening periods. This arrhythmia is commonly but incorrectly termed paroxysmal atrial tachycardia. Intracardiac electrophysiologic studies have now clearly identified that this type of arrhythmia can result from several possible underlying mechanisms, one being the reentry within the AV node, of which two forms have been described—the so-called common and uncommon types—with distinct electrocardiographic features.[4,5]

ELECTROPHYSIOLOGIC AND ELECTROCARDIOGRAPHIC FEATURES

The pattern of reentry depicted in Fig. 8–1D is usual for the common type of AV nodal reentry. This results in relatively slow anterograde conduction and relatively rapid retrograde conduction such that the AH interval during the tachycardia is significantly longer than the H-Ae interval (i.e., His bundle deflection to the atrial reciprocal beat) (Fig. 8–2A). On the surface electrocardiogram the appearance is that of simultaneous atrial and ventricular activation obscuring the P wave in most instances.[6,8,9] In some patients, however, the retrograde P wave may be detectable at the tail end of the QRS complex (Fig. 8–3). In a relatively small percentage of cases the conduction along the circuit of reentry may be reversed, and therefore the slow pathway is utilized in the retrograde direction, whereas the fast pathway is used in the anterograde direction (see Fig. 8–2B and Fig. 8–3).[4,5] Hence the P-R and R-P relationship is reversed, such that the R-P is much longer than the P-R interval. This pattern of AV nodal reentry is frequently referred to as the uncommon type and is seen in fewer than 10% of the patients with this type of arrhythmia.

The P-QRS relationship in these two forms of AV nodal reentry falls at the two extremes. An intermediate type of P-QRS relationship in which the P is obscured in the ST segment and the P-R approximates the R-P interval is more typical of reentry via accessory pathway of the Kent bundle type.[4,6,8,9] Since intact

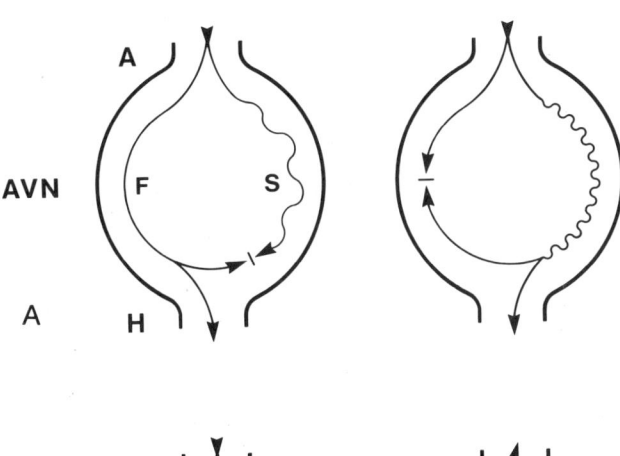

FIGURE 8–1
AV nodal reentry. The mechanism of AV nodal reentry is schematically depicted. See text for explanation. A = atrium; AVN = atrioventricular node; H = His bundle; S = slow pathway; F = fast pathway.

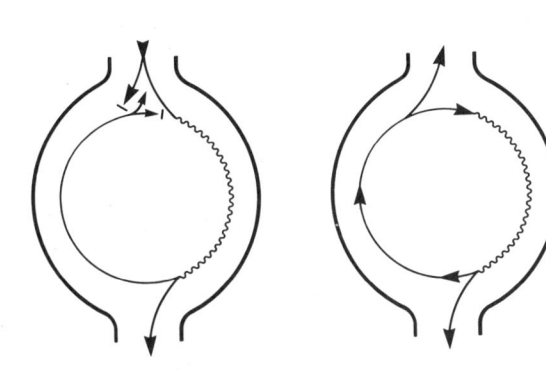

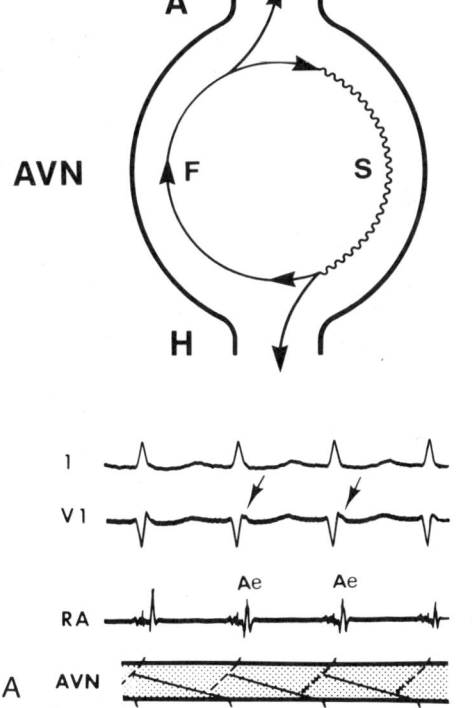
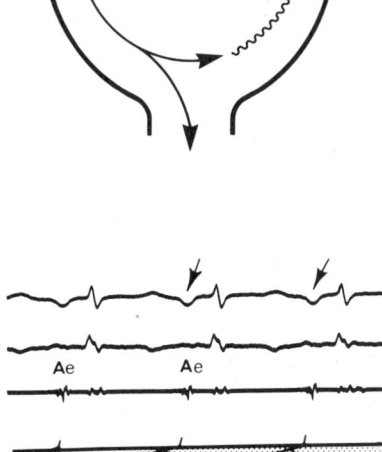

FIGURE 8–2
Common and uncommon types of AV nodal reentry. The two patterns, schematic representation and ladder diagrams, are depicted. A = atrium, AVN = atrioventricular node, H = His bundle; S = slow pathway; F = fast pathway; 1, 2, and V_1 = surface ECG leads; RA = right atrial electrogram; AE = atrial reciprocal or echo beat. The arrows on the surface electrocardiogram indicate the location of the retrograde P waves.

Supraventricular Tachycardias: Clinical Characteristics, Diagnosis, and Management

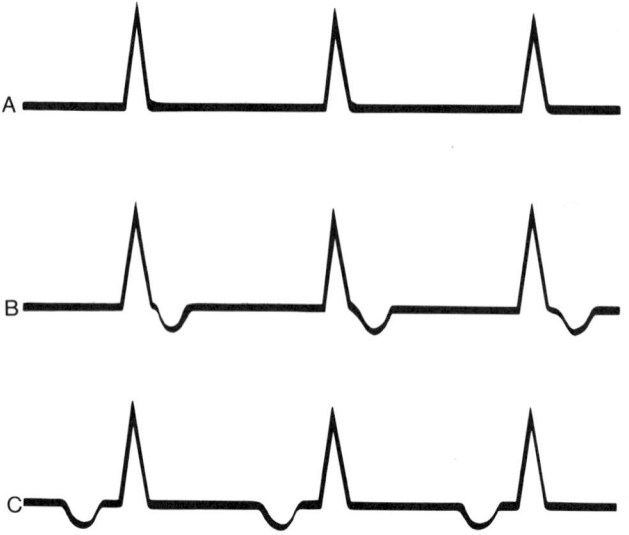

FIGURE 8–3
Surface electrocardiographic appearance of AV nodal reentry. A, In common AV nodal reentry the retrograde P wave is usually obscured by the QRS complex. B, Less frequently it may be seen at the tail end of the QRS. C, In the uncommon AV nodal reentry, the P-QRS relationship is characterized by a long R-P interval and shorter P-R interval such that the retrograde P wave precedes the next QRS complex.

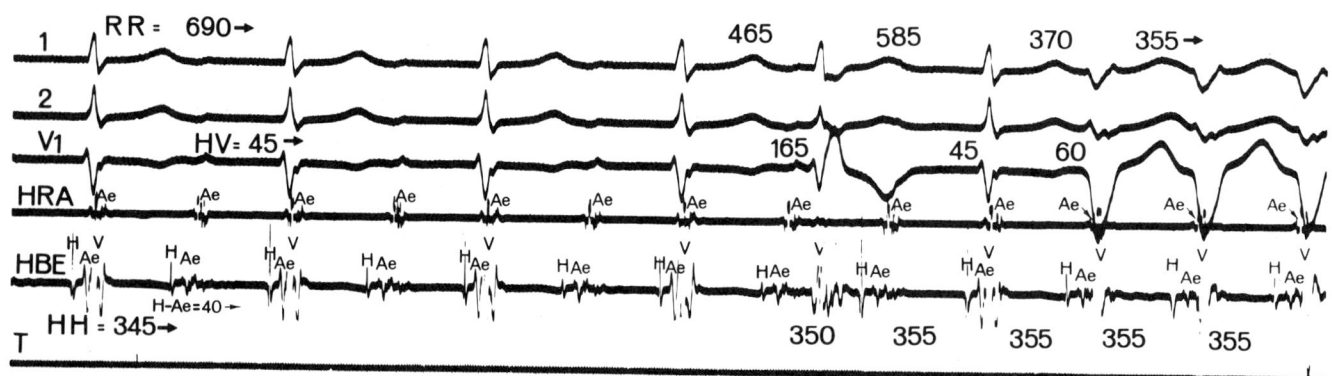

FIGURE 8–4
Block in the His-Purkinje system during common AV nodal reentry. The tracing shows a 2:1 block within the His-Purkinje system during tachycardia. The block shows a transition from 2:1 to 3:2 and then 1:1 conduction, with a left bundle branch block pattern. Note that the cycle length (CL) of SVT and H-Ae remain constant during bundle branch block, HV prolongation, and block in the HPS. Pertinent intervals are labeled. Aberrants 1, 2, V_1 surface ECG leads. Ae = Atrial reciprocal or echo beat; H-Ae = His bundle deflection to the Ae; HRA = high right atrial electrogram; HB = His bundle electrogram; T = time line. A similar format is used in subsequent tracings. (Reprinted by permission from Akhtar M: Supraventricular tachycardias; electrophysiologic mechanisms, diagnosis and pharmacologic therapy. In Josephson M, Wellens HJJ (eds.): Tachycardias: Mechanisms, Diagnosis and Treatment, p. 137. Philadelphia, Lea & Febiger, 1984.)

conduction in both anterograde and retrograde intranodal pathways is essential to sustain intranodal reentry, a 1:1 P-QRS relationship is the rule in both type of tachycardias. Spontaneous, vagal, or drug-induced intranodal block results in the termination of the tachycardia.[4] The spontaneous termination of the common type of AV nodal reentry can occur in either the anterograde or retrograde direction, whereas the uncommon type usually terminates in the retrograde direction.[4]

Since the entire circuit of reentry is intranodal, patients with second- or higher-degree AV nodal block during sinus rhythm are unlikely to manifest this type of arrhythmia. Continuation of supraventricular tachycardia with AV nodal block generally (but not always) excludes AV junctional tachycardias, and this finding strengthens the possibility of atrial origin.[4, 10] Abnormalities in the intraventricular conduction in the form of bundle branch block, fascicular block, or AV block in the His Purkinje system do not have any influence on the initiation or continuation of this type of arrhythmia (Fig. 8–4).[11, 12] Such findings constitute important clues for distinction between AV nodal reentry and those reentrant tachycardias associated with APs of the Kent bundle type.

Common AV Nodal Reentry

Although this arrhythmia can occur in the absence of any structural heart disease, a significant percentage of patients may have underlying organic heart disease. A high prevalence of AV nodal reentry in patients with any one specific form of structural heart disease has not been demonstrated.[6] The resting electrocardiogram in patients with AV nodal reentry is usually within normal limits but may reflect an underlying cardiac abnormality.

It has been suggested that patients with AV nodal reentry have at least two intranodal pathways with different conduction and refractory period properties (see Fig. 8–1).[7] These pathways are often labeled as having fast and slow conduction, respectively. During sinus rhythm and during atrial pacing at slow heart rates (when both pathways are capable of conduction) the atrial impulses preferentially reach the His bundle via the fast pathway (see Fig. 8–1A). At rapid pacing rates or with closely coupled atrial premature beats, the impulses could block in the fast pathway when it has longer refractory period (see Fig. 8–1B). Since the fast pathway beyond the area of block is not excited, it is engaged retrogradely by impulses crossing over from the distal common pathway. If the retrogradely conducting impulse does not find the area ahead recovered from prior excitation, the process will spontaneously terminate at this point. However, critically timed atrial premature beats can result in a more proximal block in the fast pathway and concomitantly in greater delay in the slow pathway (see Fig. 8–1C). This would allow recovery of excitability for the reentrant impulse, which can then negotiate the retrograde pathway, and this will result in reciprocal atrial response. Subsequent anterograde penetration of the reentrant impulse may initiate a sustained AV nodal reentrant tachycardia. Conceptually it has been implied that the entire process is localized to the AV node and that anterograde conduction in the direction of the His bundle and retrograde toward the atria is incidental to the reentrant process.

ELECTROPHYSIOLOGIC CHARACTERISTICS

During sinus rhythm the range of P-R intervals in patients with AV nodal reentry is similar to those without.[13, 14] There seems to be no direct relationship between the length of P-R interval and the occurrence of this type of arrhythmia. The initiation of AV nodal reentry is preceded by progressive prolongation of the P-R interval either during atrial pacing or with atrial

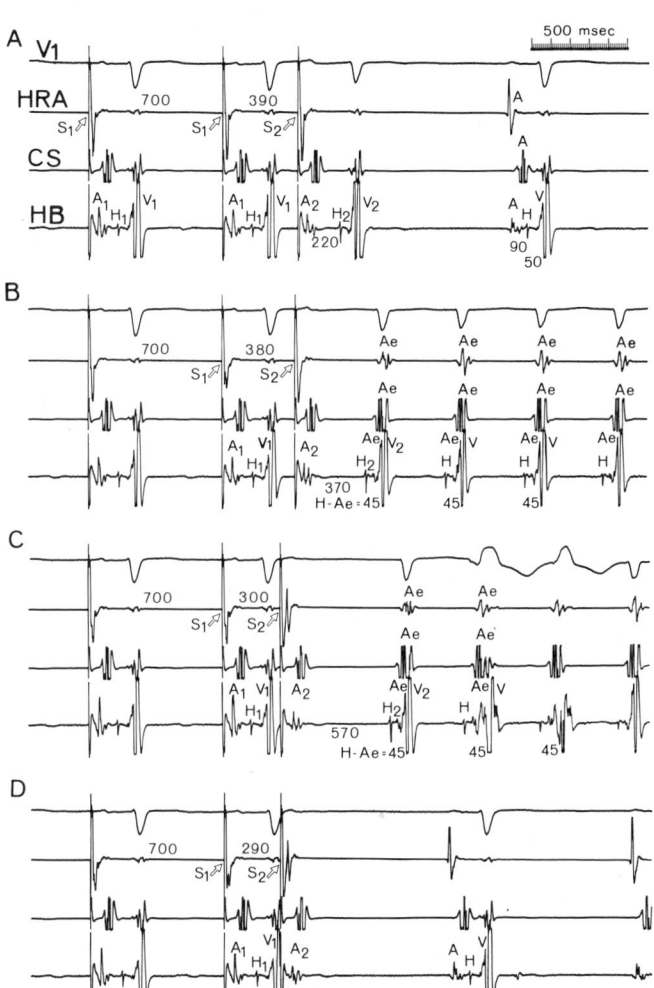

FIGURE 8–5
Initiation of common AV nodal reentry. A, At a basic cycle length of 700 ms, an atrial premature beat (A_2) conducts with an A_2H_2 interval of 210 ms. B, With a shorter A_1A_2 interval of 380 ms, a sudden jump in AV nodal conduction time (A_2H_2) coincides with the onset of tachycardia, during which the H-Ae interval measures 45 ms. C depicts the shortest A_1A_2 interval associated with onset of tachycardia. With a block in the AV node (D), the arrhythmia could not be induced, suggesting that propagation beyond the atria is important for induction. This finding also argues against intra-atrial reentry as the mechanism. See legend of Figure 8–4 for explanation of abbreviations. CS = coronary sinus electrogram.

premature stimulation (Figs. 8–5 and 8–6).[1-4] On the His bundle electrogram the main prolongation of conduction is seen within the AV node (i.e., the A-H interval). At critical A-H delays, this type of reentry starts.[1] Frequently the initiation of AV nodal reentry coincides with the jump in the A-H interval (see Fig. 8–6). This has been interpreted as manifestation of switch from a fast to a slow pathway with the encroachment of the effective refractory period of the fast pathway.[2, 3] In the retrograde direction these patients invariably show relatively rapid conduction from the His bundle to the atria.[4] This manifests in the form of rapid 1:1 ventriculoatrial (VA) conduction during ventricular pacing and a short H-A interval that can be directly documented during premature ventricular stimulation at various basic cycle lengths. During the process of ventricular premature stimulation with progressively shorter coupling intervals it can be usually demonstrated that progressive increase in the V_2-A_2 interval is primarily the result of V-H delays (Fig. 8–7).[4] The H_2-A_2 intervals generally remain constant during the process of scanning (see Fig. 8–7).[4]

DOCUMENTATION OF SITE OF REENTRY

Because of the difficulty in obtaining reliable recordings from the AV node it has not been possible to directly document that this reentry is localized to the AV node. Many criteria have been proposed that suggest but do not prove that this process may be localized to the AV node. These include (1) A predictable relationship between intranodal conduction delays and the occurrence of AV nodal reentry tachycardia in a given patient (see Figs. 8–5 and 8–6); (2) the demonstration of dual AV nodal refractory period curves coinciding with the onset of tachycardia when the effective refractory period of the fast pathway is reached (see Fig. 8–6); (3) an atrial activation sequence that is typical of impulse origin from the AV node; (4) continuation of reentry despite a concomitant block within the His-Purkinje system, indicating that the level of reentry is at or above the level of the His bundle recording site (see Fig. 8–4); and (5) the retrograde conduction time from the His to the atrium (i.e., H-A interval) with ventricular pacing exceeds the H-Ae interval, supporting the notion that the point of turnaround in the AV node is above the level of the His bundle recording site.[4, 15]

NATURE OF INTRANODAL PATHWAYS

Although many aspects of AV nodal reentry have been defined, several questions remain. Only the conduction characteristics of anterograde and retrograde pathways during established reentry are appreciated. Almost no information is available concerning the role of proximal and distal crossover connections. Similarly, in patients with common AV nodal reentry the characteristics of the slow pathway in the retrograde direction are essentially unknown. It is not even clear whether the so-called anterograde fast pathway is in fact the same as the retrograde fast pathway.

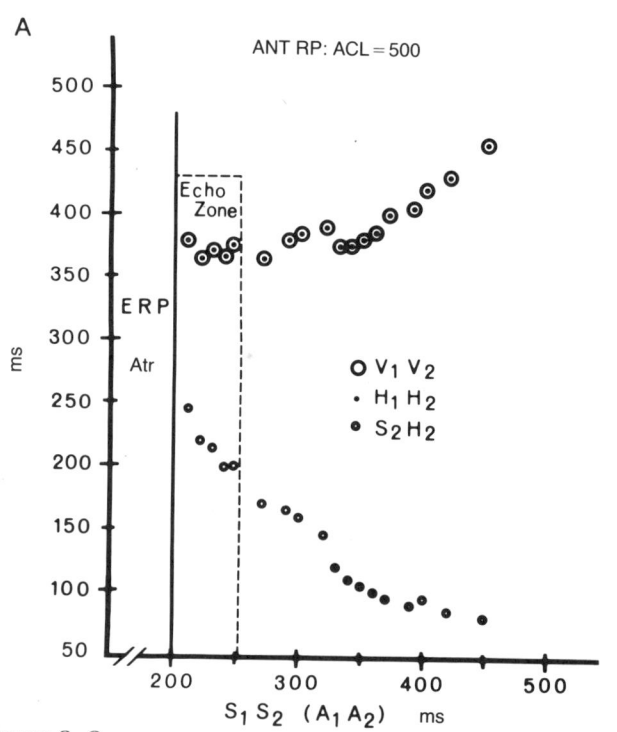 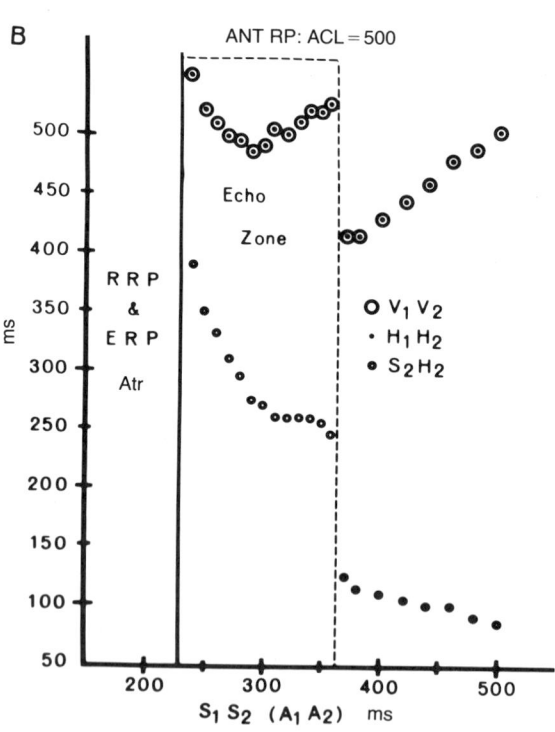

FIGURE 8–6
AV nodal refractory period curves in patients with AV nodal reentry. Atrial coupling intervals (A_1A_2) are plotted against A_2H_2, H_1H_2, and V_1V_2 intervals in two patients with AV nodal reentry. A shows no jump in AV nodal conduction (continuous refractory period curves), whereas a sudden break is noted in B. This discontinuous refractory period curve reflects onset of block in the fast pathway and coincides with initiation of AV nodal reentry. ERP = effective refractory period; RRP = relative refractory period; ANT RP = anterograde refractory period; Atr = atrium; echo zone = zone of A_1A_2 associated with onset of AV nodal reentry.

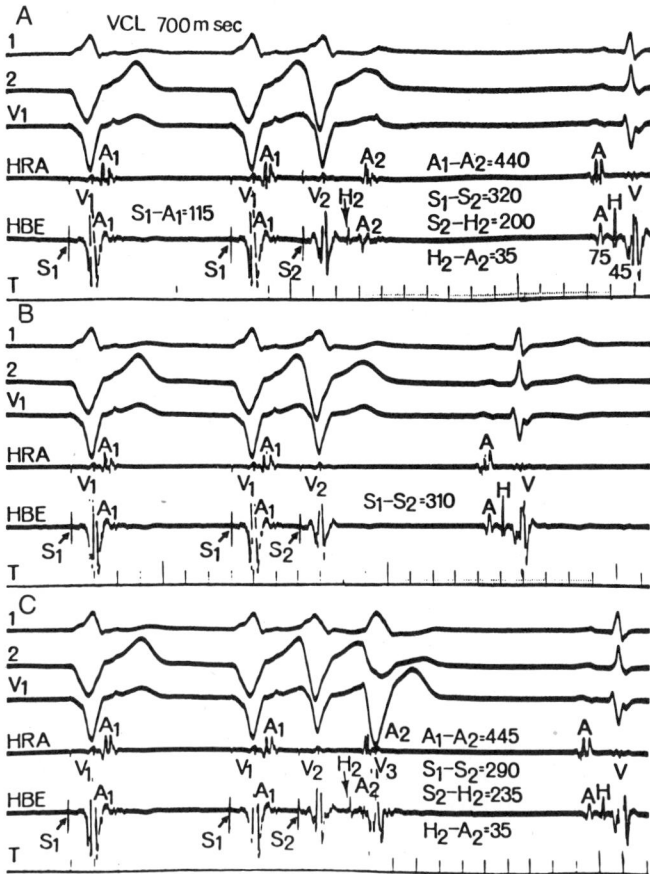

FIGURE 8–7
Retrograde conduction in patients with common AV nodal reentry. A, At a basic cycle length of 700 ms, the V_2 conducts to atria with a His Purkinje system delay (S_2H_2) of 200 ms and AV nodal conduction time (H_2A_2) of 35 ms. A ventriculoatrial block is seen in B in which the V_2 blocks below the His bundle recording site. A short H_2A_2 is typical of these cases, and when V_2 blocks, it is rarely above the His bundle. VCL = ventricular cycle length. See legend of Figure 8–4 for explanation of other abbreviations.

It seems that the anterograde conduction in these patients is typically AV-nodal, but the conduction behavior of the retrograde pathway is somewhat more puzzling. The retrograde pathway has rapid conduction and does not show the expected increase in conduction time with incremental ventricular pacing or premature stimulation; these characteristics can be interpreted as properties unlike that of the AV node and somewhat more suggestive of conduction via a bypass tract.[16] This issue has been further complicated by the observation that intravenous procainamide selectively blocks retrograde fast pathway conduction without much influence on the typical AV-nodal conduction of the anterograde limb.[17] The recent data suggesting surgical correction of AV nodal reentry without totally interrupting either anterograde or retrograde conduction has created some serious doubts about the intranodal location of these retrograde pathways.[18] However, the foregoing arguments are not necessarily indicative that these pathways are partial or complete AV nodal bypass tracts. These pathways will often respond to drugs like verapamil or beta blockers.[11] The exact anatomic boundaries of the AV node have not been clearly defined during surgical exploration or with subsequent dissection or ablation. The issue concerning intranodal versus extranodal location of reentrant pathways in the common type of AV nodal reentry, therefore, remains unresolved at the present time.

Uncommon AV Nodal Reentry

ELECTROPHYSIOLOGIC CHARACTERISTICS

This form of reentry tachycardia produces a pattern in which the H-Ae interval is longer than the Ae-H interval, consistent with anterograde conduction over a fast pathway and retrograde conduction over a slow pathway.[4, 5, 11] The corresponding electrocardiographic pattern is that of a longer R-P and a shorter P-R interval (see Figs. 8–2 and 8–3). This type of pattern is not specific for the uncommon type of AV nodal reentry and has also been seen in patients who have retrogradely conducting accessory pathways with relatively long conduction times.[19, 20] In fact, the available information on this type of supraventricular tachycardia suggests that in the majority of these people there indeed is an accessory pathway with relatively long conduction time. Therefore the documentation that the AV node is the site of reentry requires exclusion of an accessory pathway unrelated to the normal pathway. During ventricular stimulation, retrograde conduction is also relatively slow in these patients, due to prolonged H-A conduction. A progressive conduction delay can be shown with progressively earlier premature beats. The cycle length of tachycardia tends to be somewhat slower than the common type of AV nodal reentry, ranging from 350 to 600 ms. The spontaneous and vagally induced termination of this tachycardia occurs in the retrograde limb of the circuit (i.e., the H is not followed by a retrograde atrial echo response).

The role of the atrium or the His-Purkinje system in this type of reentry has seldom been documented. However, occasional examples show continuation of reentry despite a concomitant block in the His-Purkinje system.

NONPAROXYSMAL AV JUNCTIONAL TACHYCARDIA

A regular, narrow QRS complex tachycardia in which the atrial activity is dissociated from the ventricle is termed nonparoxysmal. This is not an uncommon rhythm and is frequently seen in association with acute events such as myocardial infarction, open heart surgery, and digitalis intoxication. The exact mechanism and origin of this type of arrhythmia has not been well defined. From a clinical standpoint, however, such arrhythmias generally do not pose a significant problem and therefore have seldom been extensively studied. Nonetheless, the treatment in this type of arrhythmia is often that of the underlying cardiovascular problem rather than of the arrhythmia per se.

AUTOMATIC JUNCTIONAL TACHYCARDIA

Automatic junctional tachycardia, a frequently misdiagnosed arrhythmia, is most often seen in infants and has recently been reported in young adults.[21,22] It is characterized by relatively rapid rates: 140 to 270 beats per minute (bpm). During the tachycardia there may be irregularity of the R-R intervals, and there is AV dissociation. Rate-related aberrant conduction is common and may therefore simulate episodes of polymorphic ventricular tachycardia. This tachycardia cannot be initiated or terminated with programmed stimulation; its lack of response to calcium channel blockers also suggests that delayed after-depolarizations are not involved. The weight of evidence suggests that it is probably abnormal automaticity localized to the AV junction, perhaps in the area above or within the His bundle.

Supraventricular Tachycardia Originating in the Atria

These tachyarrhythmias include those arising from above the level of the AV junction, including the sinus node.[23-29] Since the atrial arrhythmia is the primary event, the atrial rates are equal to or exceed ventricular rates. Unlike the reentrant AV junctional tachycardias, in which intact conduction in both directions is essential, presence of VA conduction is not relevant in these arrhythmias. The P-QRS relationship is therefore a function of AV conduction in response to the atrial rates. For lack of better classification, the origin of atrial arrhythmias can be broadly separated into two categories: (1) those arising in the region of the sinus node and (2) those outside the region of the sinus node. When the P wave morphology is suggestive of sinus origin (i.e., the P wave is upright in leads 2 and 3 and in aV_f and biphasic in V_1), the terminology of sinus is applied. All other P wave morphologies are considered to be of nonsinus origin.

SINUS TACHYCARDIA

The usual type of sinus tachycardia seen during exertion and congestive heart failure occurs as an appropriate response to increased demand. This arrhythmia is gradual in onset and termination and cannot be initiated or terminated by atrial premature beats or overdrive pacing. Overdrive suppression is generally noted following cessation of pacing. The underlying mechanism is enhanced automaticity produced by sympathetic stimulation or vagal withdrawal, and overall rates seldom exceed 160 bpm. Since the same triggering mechanisms also enhance AV nodal conduction, the P-R interval during this type of arrhythmia seldom exceeds the P-R interval during sinus rhythm.

SINUS NODE REENTRY

It has been demonstrated that an arrhythmia that arises within or around the environment of the sinus node can be initiated and terminated with appropriately timed atrial premature beats (Fig. 8-8).[23-25] Since no concomitant facilitation of AV nodal conduction is present, atrial impulses generally show delay or block in the AV node. The presence of upright P wave similar to sinus rhythm with first- or second-degree AV nodal block is often present. Longer P-R during supraventricular tachycardia, compared to the sinus beats, suggests this type of arrhythmia. Because it clinically presents as a paroxysmal tachycardia and can be initiated and terminated by programmed atrial stimulation, it is often classified as reentrant.

ATRIAL TACHYCARDIA

Atrial tachycardia[26,27,29] refers to tachyarrhythmias arising from the atrium, which have different P wave morphologies compared to sinus beats. When the P wave morphology is identical from beat to beat, the term unifocal is applied. Multifocal atrial tachycardia describes an arrhythmia in which the P wave morphology varies and at least three different P wave appearances can be identified. When such arrhythmias can be initiated and terminated with atrial premature stimulation or atrial pacing, the mechanism is considered to be reentry. When noninducible, it is assumed that the arrhythmia is non-reentrant in nature. It should be pointed out, however, that certain forms of atrial tachycardia may be due to triggered delayed after depolarizations. This may be particularly true of digitalis-induced atrial arrhythmias.[30]

In the clinical setting, however, limited data are available to characterize the various forms of atrial tachycardias that are commonly seen. As with all other arrhythmias, to establish reentry as the mechanism the ultimate proof lies in the demonstration of the reentry circuit. This has seldom been possible, because of the limited number of recordings that are generally available during the conduct of cardiac electrophysiologic studies. However, the occurrence of intra-atrial conduction delay or block in association with the initiation of tachyarrhythmias does provide support for a reentrant mechanism.[28]

ATRIAL FLUTTER

Atrial flutter[31] often presents as a regular tachycardia with the ventricular rates approaching 150 bpm as a result of 2:1 AV nodal block. In the so-called typical or common type of atrial flutter there is a saw tooth appearance with atrial rates approximately 300 beats per minute. Atrial flutter with flutter wave morphology different than described above and faster rates has also been described. A rapid atrial flutter with the rates exceeding 400 bpm is often difficult to distinguish from atrial fibrillation except that rates in atrial flutter are quite regular. Intracardiac electrocardiograms generally show a relatively regular atrial activity with a low to high atrial activation sequence during the common type of atrial flutter.

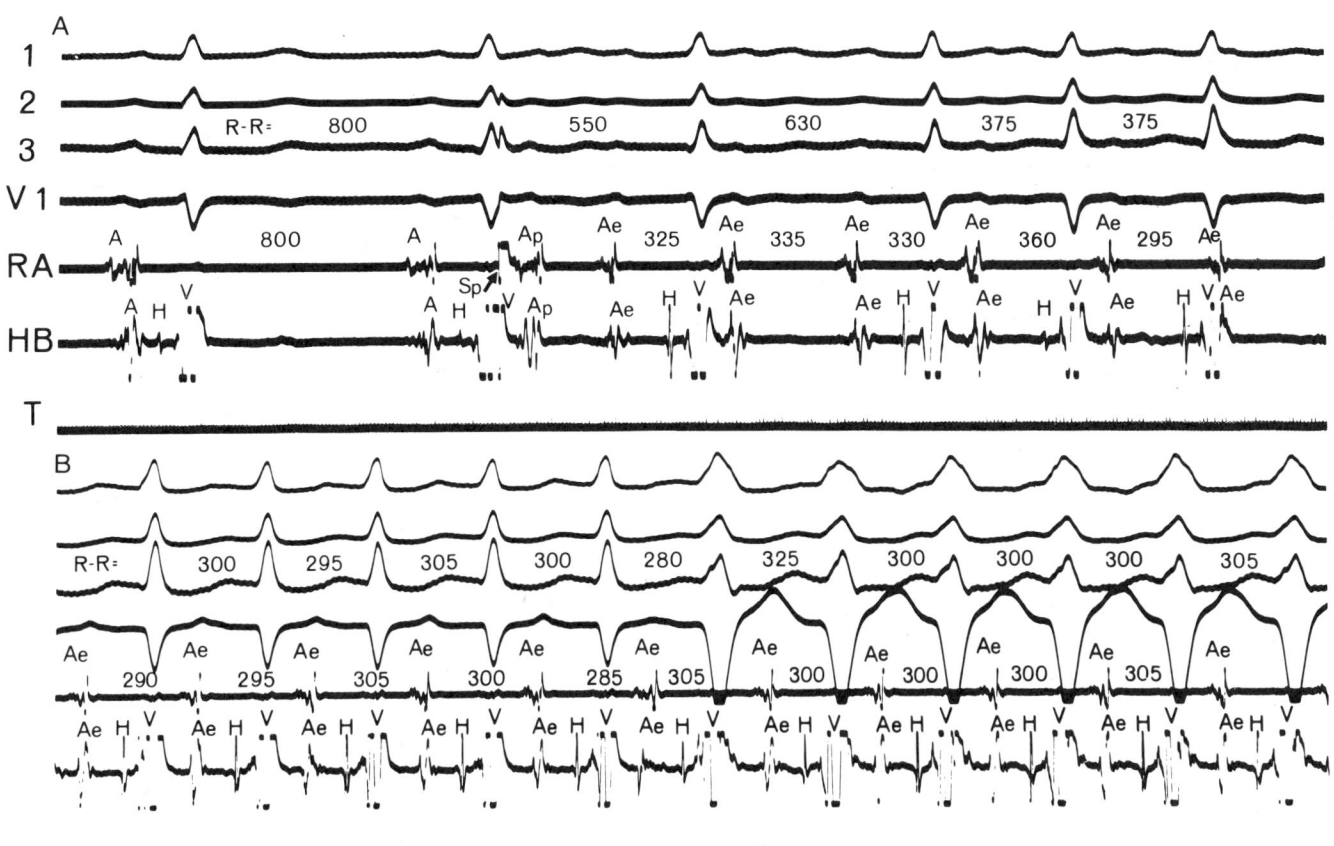

FIGURE 8-8
Sinus node reentry. The first two beats in A are of sinus origin, and the SVT is initiated with a single atrial premature beat. The concomitant AV nodal block (seen at the onset of SVT) suggests intra-atrial origin of the tachycardia. The atrial activation sequence and P wave (seen clearly during the block) suggest origin within or around the sinus node. B shows an acceleration of tachycardia rate and a 1:1 AV response that is associated with the onset of left bundle branch block. Note a relatively fast rate of SVT (cycle of approximately 300 ms). See legend of Figure 8-4 for explanation of abbreviations. (Reprinted by permission from Akhtar M: Supraventricular tachycardias; electrophysiologic mechanisms, diagnosis and pharmacologic therapy. In Josephson M, Wellens HJJ (eds.): Tachycardias: Mechanisms, Diagnosis and Treatment, pp. 137–140. Philadelphia, Lea & Febiger, 1984.)

ATRIAL FIBRILLATION

Atrial fibrillation[31] frequently starts as a transient, paroxysmal arrhythmia and becomes more persistent with the passage of time. Often the runs of atrial fibrillation will alternate with periods of bradycardia, and this is considered to be one manifestation of the sick sinus syndrome. Generally both atrial flutter and fibrillation are seen in patients who have underlying heart disease, often with dilated atria and chronic heart failure. Not uncommonly, however, atrial fibrillation can be seen in association with no clinically detectable structural heart disease.

During atrial fibrillation there is gross irregularity of the atrial activity wave forms, and the ventricular response is irregular. However, irregularity of R-R intervals can be less when the atrial fibrillation is associated with rapid ventricular response. The ventricular response via the normal pathway seldom exceeds 250 bpm during this arrhythmia. In patients with the Wolff-Parkinson-White syndrome, however, the ventricular response may be fairly rapid if the accessory pathway refractory period is short.[32] Atrial fibrillation associated with fast ventricular response over an accessory pathway is known to have been associated with the risk of lethal ventricular fibrillation. Intracardiac electrogram recordings during atrial fibrillation are characterized by beat-to-beat variability, thereby clearly distinguishing this rhythm from atrial flutter.

Therapy for Supraventricular Tachycardia

Although a variety of nonpharmacologic and pharmacologic methods have evolved for the management of supraventricular tachycardia, drug therapy remains the mainstay. In the treatment of atrial arrhythmia one can either target prevention of atrial tachycardia or control AV response.

DRUG THERAPY

Traditional drugs that are known to prevent the recurrence of atrial tachyarrhythmias such as atrial flutter-

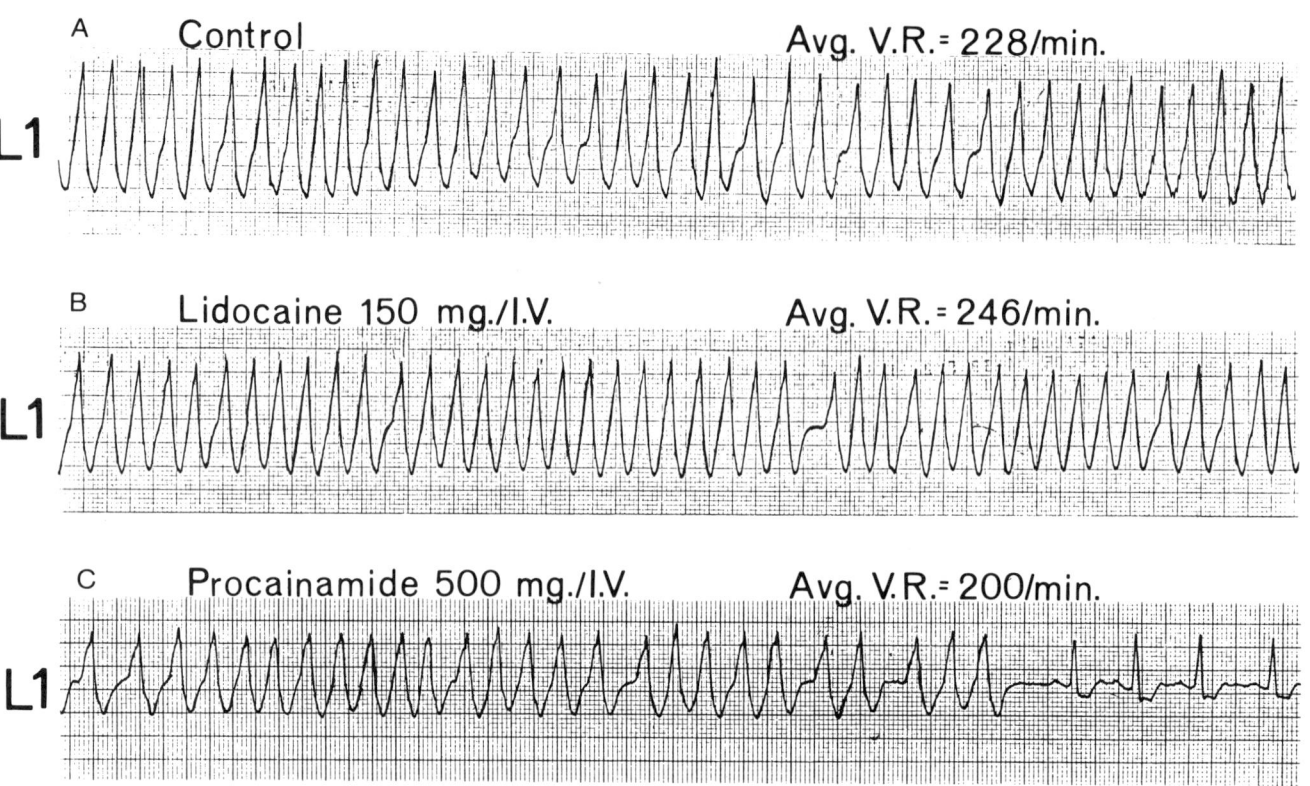

FIGURE 8–9
Atrial fibrillation and AV response over an accessory pathway of the Kent bundle type. A, A rapid ventricular response is seen in the unmedicated state in a patient with Wolff-Parkinson-White syndrome. Note acceleration of ventricular response after administration of lidocaine (B) and slowing and subsequent termination of atrial fibrillation following intravenous procainamide (C).

fibrillation include Class 1A agents (e.g., quinidine, procainamide, disopyramide).[31] Agents that belong to Class 1C (e.g., flecainide and encainide) are also promising. In difficult cases, amiodarone is often effective in prevention of atrial tachyarrhythmias. Agents such as digitalis, beta blockers, and calcium channel blockers including verapamil and diltiazem, although frequently employed during the management of atrial tachyarrhythmias, have never been shown conclusively to prevent atrial tachyarrhythmias. Pharmaceutic agents belonging to Class 1B, such as lidocaine, mexiletine, and tocainide, have no proven benefit for prevention of atrial tachycardias.

When atrial tachycardias cannot be completely prevented, AV response can be controlled via the AV node with digitalis, beta blockers, and calcium channel blockers (e.g., verapamil and diltiazem). These agents are titrated to achieve a ventricular rate acceptable for the individual patient. Frequently, however, the control achieved in this manner is unsatisfactory, since attempts to control ventricular response during activity may produce bradycardia during the resting state. Conversely, rate control during activity may not translate into acceptable ventricular response when the patient is more active physically. In patients who utilize accessory pathways such as the Kent bundle during atrial tachyarrhythmias, the AV response over the accessory pathway can be primarily controlled with Class 1A[33, 34] (Fig. 8–9) or Class 1C drugs. Amiodarone can also be used in difficult cases. In this context it is appropriate to point out that Class 1C agents (e.g., flecainide and encainide) seem to be especially promising agents.[35] Class IB drugs have no place in the management of ventricular response via the accessory pathway during atrial fibrillation. Digitalis is contraindicated and verapamil has no beneficial effect in this setting.[36, 37] The value of beta blockers in this situation remains uncertain. It is, however, quite possible that the beta blockers could prove useful, since endogenous catecholamine release can shorten the refractory period of the accessory pathway and this effect can be blocked with these agents.

In AV junctional tachycardias such as the common type of AV nodal reentry, the anterograde pathway frequently will respond to digitalis, beta blockers and calcium channel blockers (Fig. 8–10).[11, 38–40] The retrograde limb, however, is not drug selective; but often Class 1C and Class 1A agents are effective (see Fig. 8–10).[41] In some patients verapamil or beta blockers may block the conduction along the retrograde pathway, whereas Class 1A drugs fail (Fig. 8–11). Mexiletine, tocainide, and lidocaine usually have no beneficial or deleterious effect in this type of reentrant tachycardia. Amiodarone can be utilized both for block of anterograde as well as of retrograde conduction in the AV node.[42] Clinical experience comparing the efficacy of various antiarrhythmic agents in uncommon AV nodal reentry is limited; we have found that the agents

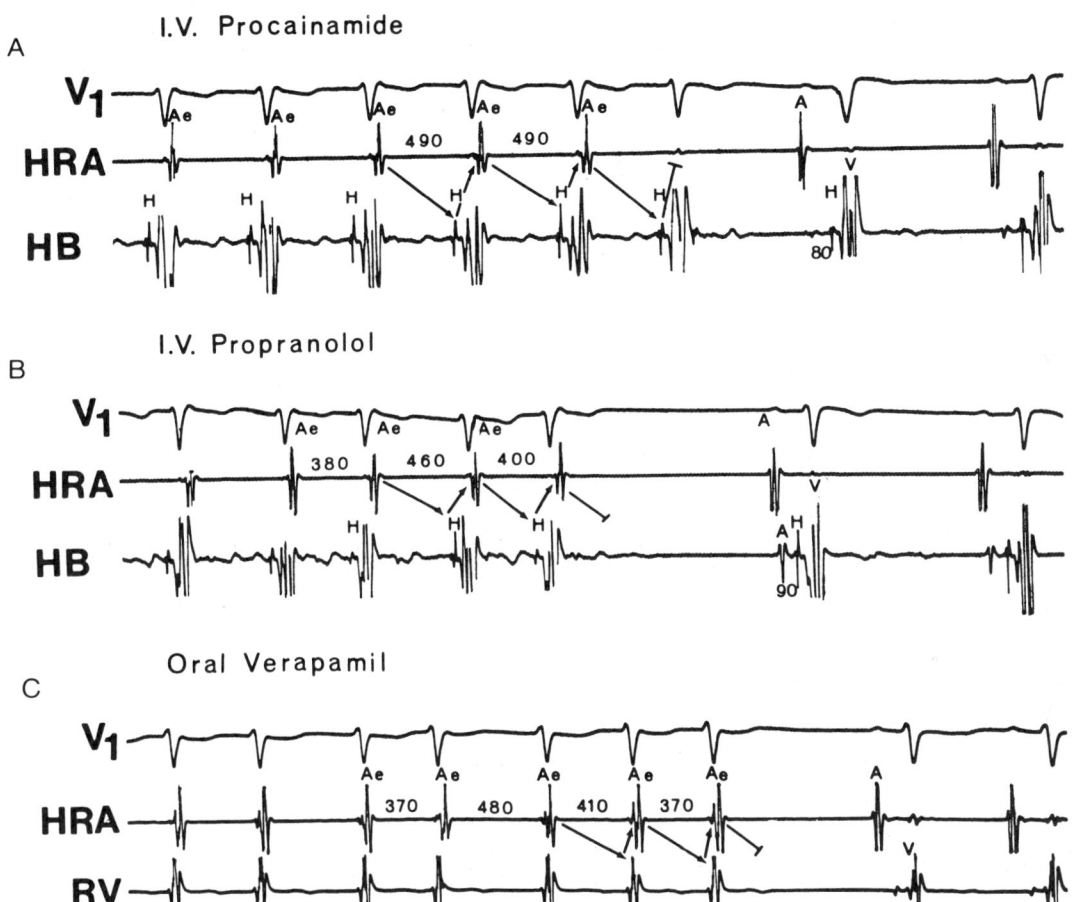

FIGURE 8–10
A, intravenous administration of procainamide terminates the PSVT with a retrograde block (i.e., H is not followed by an Ae). In the same patient, there is spontaneous termination of tachycardia in the anterograde direction (i.e., Ae is not followed by a His bundle deflection or a QRS complex) after intravenous administration of propranolol (B) and oral administration of verapamil (C). See legend of Figure 8–4 for explanation of abbreviations. (Reprinted by permission from Akhtar M: Supraventricular tachycardias; electrophysiologic mechanisms, diagnosis and pharmacologic therapy. In Josephson M, Wellens HJJ (eds.): Tachycardias: Mechanisms, Diagnosis and Treatment, pp. 137–140. Philadelphia, Lea & Febiger, 1984.)

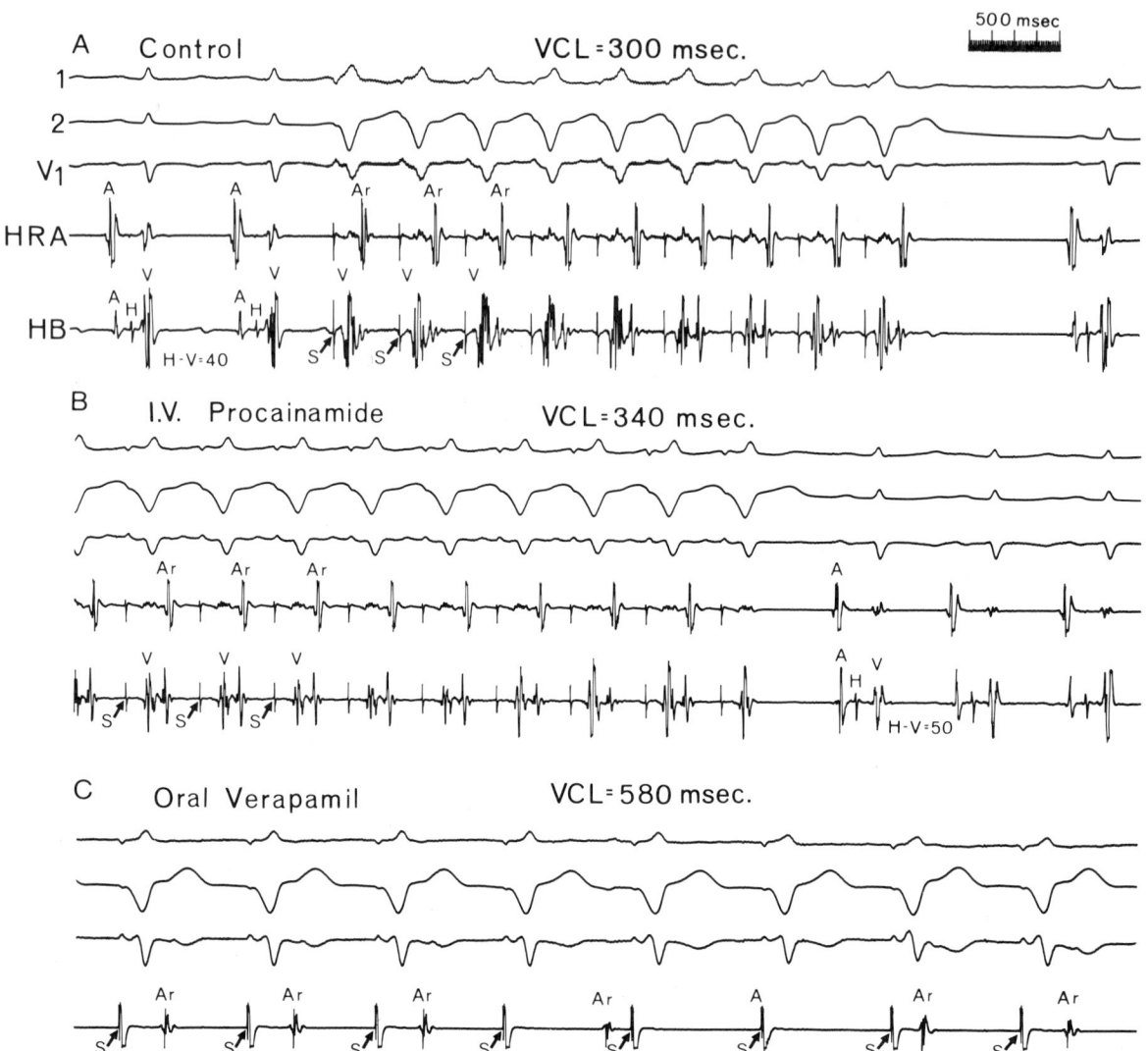

FIGURE 8-11
Effect of verapamil on retrograde pathway in common AV nodal reentry (same patient as in Figure 6-25). Control 1:1 ventriculoarterial (VA) response is seen in A at a paced ventricular cycle (VCL) of 300 ms. Intravenous administration of procainamide produces VA block at a paced VCL of 340 ms (B), a relatively modest effect. C, After 2 days of oral administration of verapamil, a marked depressant effect is noted on retrograde conduction, and the VA block occurs at a relatively long-paced VCL of 580 ms. HRA = high right atrial electrogram; HB = His bundle electrogram. (Reprinted by permission from Akhtar M: Supraventricular tachycardias; electrophysiologic mechanisms, diagnosis and pharmacologic therapy. In Josephson M, Wellens HJJ (eds.): Tachycardias; Mechanisms, Diagnosis and Treatment, pp. 137–140. Philadelphia, Lea & Febiger, 1984.)

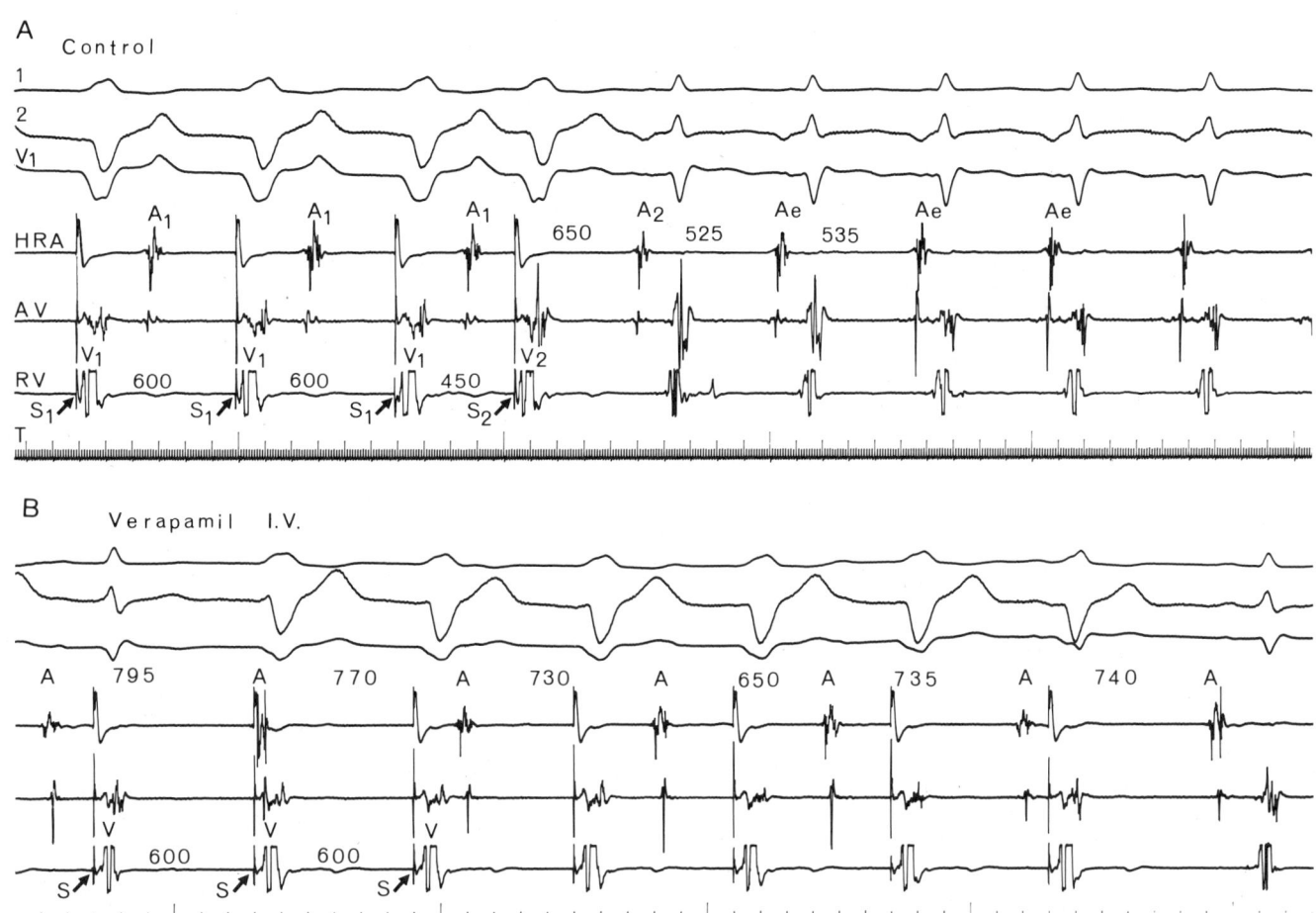

FIGURE 8–12
Effect of verapamil on uncommon AV nodal reentry. A shows initiation of an uncommon type of AV nodal reentry during ventricular premature stimulation. The pertinent A-A cycles are labeled. Note 1:1 ventriculoatrial (VA) conduction during paced basic cycle (CL) of 600 ms and long V_2-A_2 in response to ventricular premature beat. B shows complete VA block at the same paced CL as panel A after administration of 5 mg of IV verapamil. AV = electrogram from the region of the AV junction. See legend of Figure 8–4 for explanation of other abbreviations. (Reprinted by permission from Akhtar M: Supraventricular tachycardias; electrophysiologic mechanisms, diagnosis and pharmacologic therapy. In Josephson M, Wellens HJJ (eds.): Tachycardias: Mechanisms, Diagnosis and Treatment, pp. 137–140. Philadelphia, Lea & Febiger, 1984.)

used for control of common AV nodal reentry often are effective in this type of arrhythmia as well (Fig. 8–12).

CATHETER ABLATION

For all tachycardias that utilize anterograde conduction along the normal pathway, such as atrial flutter-fibrillation, as well as a variety of supraventricular tachycardias, catheter ablation has been applied to produce AV block.[43] A variety of energies are being tested at the present time; however, electrical energy via electrode catheters is currently used in clinical settings. Single or multiple shocks, with the current flowing between one of the electrodes of the catheter and an anode placed over the chest, result in production of AV block. The cumulative energy varies but has been as high as 500 joules.[44] Satisfactory AV block is achieved in approximately 75% of patients. Following production of AV block, permanent pacemaker placement is mandatory. Among the accessory pathways, posteroseptal location has been more amenable to catheter ablation via a catheter placed in the os of the coronary sinus.[45]

Surprisingly, catheter ablation techniques have not produced the kind of risk that one would anticipate with the use of high-energy delivered in the cardiac chambers; however, the procedure is not risk-free.[44] The majority of patients who have undergone catheter ablation of the His bundle were not responsive to treatment of atrial fibrillation with fast ventricular response. In this setting, it is imperative to document that the patient's symptoms are related to fast ventricular rates and not to loss of atrial kick, since the latter will not be restored with production of AV block.

SURGICAL THERAPY

A novel technique has been utilized for the control of AV nodal reentrant tachycardia by Ross and coworkers.[18] This form of surgery is relatively simple and can be curative without production of AV block. The isolation of the AV node and the His Bundle during right atriotomy is straightforward and can be accomplished with either recording techniques or constant monitoring of AV conduction during manipulation of the region of the AV node. Minor damage in the region with either cryoablation or incision or simple scratching may be sufficient to produce block in the retrograde direction, eliminate the AV nodal reentrant tachycardia, and still preserve AV conduction. This technique, which is in its early stages, has many of the advantages lacking in catheter ablation, such as the preservation of AV conduction. This is obviously important in young patients.

For atrial tachyarrhythmias, identification of an atrial focus in unifocal tachycardias can be accomplished at the time of surgery and the arrhythmia can also be controlled with catheter ablation of the focus.[46,47] In difficult patients with atrial fibrillation who are incapacitated by a rapid ventricular response, a unique surgical approach has been used by Guiraudon, termed a corridor operation, in which a tract of atrial tissue is isolated, connecting the sinus with the AV node and separating the rest of the atria.[48] Both of the two atria can continue in atrial fibrillation, whereas the ventricular response is controlled by sinus mechanism. Atrial mapping, excision, and isolation hold promise for control of an atrial flutter as well.

References

1. Goldreyer BN, Damato AN: The essential role of atrioventricular conduction delay in the initiation of paroxysmal supraventricular tachycardia. Circulation 43:679, 1971.
2. Denes P, Dhingra RC, Chuquimia R, et al.: Demonstration of dual A-V nodal pathways in patients with paroxysmal supraventricular tachycardia. Circulation 43:549, 1973.
3. Denes P, et al.: The determinants of atrioventricular re-entrance with premature atrial stimulation in patients with dual AV-nodal pathways. Circulation 56:253, 1977.
4. Akhtar M, et al.: Antegrade and retrograde conduction characteristics in three patterns of paroxysmal atrioventricular junctional reentrant tachycardia. Am Heart J 95:22, 1978.
5. Wu D, et al.: An unusual variety of atrioventricular nodal reentry due to retrograde dual atrioventricular nodal pathways. Circulation 56:50, 1977.
6. Wu D, et al.: Clinical electrocardiographic and electrophysiological observations in patients with paroxysmal supraventricular tachycardia. Am J Cardiol 41:1045, 1978.
7. Mendez C, Moe GK: Demonstration of a dual A-V nodal conduction system in the isolated rabbit heart. Circ Res 19:378, 1966.
8. Akhtar M, Damato AN: Determination of site of re-entry from antegrade and retrograde conduction ratios in paroxysmal atrioventricular junctional re-entrant tachycardia (Abstract). Clin Res, April, 1976.
9. Josephson ME: Paroxysmal supraventricular tachycardia. An electrophysiologic approach. Am J Cardiol 41:1123, 1976.
10. Hariman RJ, Chen C, Caracta AR, et al.: Evidence that A-V nodal reentrant tachycardia does not require participation of the entire A-V node. PACE 6:1252, 1983.
11. Akhtar M: Supraventricular tachycardias: electrophysiologic mechanisms, diagnosis and pharmacologic therapy. *In* Josephson M, Wellens HJJ, (eds.): Tachycardias: Mechanisms, Diagnosis and Treatment, pp. 137–169. Philadelphia, Lea & Febiger, 1984.
12. Akhtar M: Atrioventricular nodal reentry. Circulation 75(4):III:26, 1987.
13. Bauernfeind RA, et al.: Cycle length in atrioventricular nodal reentrant paroxysmal tachycardia with observations on the Lown-Ganong-Levine syndrome. Am J Cardiol 45:1148, 1980.
14. Akhtar M, et al.: A comparative analysis of antegrade and retrograde conduction patterns in man. Circulation 52:766, 1975.
15. Miller JM, Rosenthal ME, Vassallo JA, et al.: Atrioventricular nodal reentrant tachycardia: studies on upper and lower "common pathways." Circulation 75:930, 1987.
16. Gomes JAC, Dhatt MA, Damato AN, et al.: Incidence, determinants and significance of fixed retrograde conduction in the region of the atrioventricular node: evidence for retrograde atrioventricular nodal bypass tracts. Am J Cardiol 44:1089, 1979.
17. Wu B, et al.: Effect of procainamide on atrioventricular nodal re-entrant paroxysmal tachycardia. Circulation 57:1171, 1978.
18. Ross DL, Johnson DC, Denniss AR, et al.: Curative surgery for atrioventricular junctional ("A-V nodal") reentrant tachycardia. J Am Coll Cardiol 6:1383, 1985.
19. Coumel P, Attuel P, Leclercq JF: Permanent form of junctional reciprocating tachycardia: Mechanism, clinical and therapeutic implications. *In* Narula OS (ed.): Cardiac Arrhythmias: Electrophysiology, Diagnosis and Management, pp. 347–363. Baltimore, Williams & Wilkins, 1979.
20. Farre J, et al.: Reciprocal tachycardias using accessory pathways with long conduction times. Am J Cardiol 44:1099, 1979.
21. Garson A Jr, Gillette PC: Junctional ectopic tachycardia in children: electrocardiography, electrophysiology and pharmacologic response. Am J Cardiol 44:298, 1979.

22. Gillette PC, Garson A Jr, Porter CJ, et al.: Junctional automatic ectopic tachycardia: New proposed treatment by transcatheter His Bundle ablation. Am Heart J 106:619, 1983.
23. Paulay KL, Varghese PJ, Damato AN: Sinus node re-entry: An in vivo demonstration in the dog. Circ Res 32:455, 1973.
24. Narula OS: Sinus node re-entry. Circulation 50:1114, 1974.
25. Weisfogel GM, et al.: Sinus node re-entrant tachycardia in man. Am Heart J 90:295, 1975.
26. Goldreyer BN, Gallagher JJ, Damato AN: The electrophysiologic demonstration of atrial ectopic tachycardia in man. Am Heart J 85:205, 1973.
27. Wu D, et al.: Demonstration of sustained sinus and atrial reentry as a mechanism of paroxysmal supraventricular tachycardia. Circulation 51:234, 1975.
28. Akhtar M, et al.: Demonstration of intra-atrial conduction delay, block, gap and reentry. Circulation 58:947, 1978.
29. Scheinman MM, Basu D, Hollenberg M: Electrophysiologic studies in patients with persistent atrial tachycardia. Circulation 50:266, 1974.
30. Akhtar M, Tchou P, Jazayeri M: Mechanisms of clinical tachycardias. Am J Cardiol 61:9A, 1988.
31. Benditt DG, Benson DW Jr, Dunnigan A, et al.: Atrial flutter, atrial fibrillation, and other primary atrial tachycardias. The Med Clin North Am 68:895, 1984.
32. Wellens HJJ, Durrer D: Wolff-Parkinson-White syndrome and atrial fibrillation. Relation between refractory period of the accessory pathway and ventricular rate during atrial fibrillation. Am J Cardiol 34:777, 1974.
33. Bauernfeind RA, Swiryn SP, Strasberg B, et al.: Electrophysiologic drug testing in prophylaxis of paroxysmal atrial fibrillation: Technique, application, and efficacy in severely symptomatic preexcitation patients. Am Heart J 103:941, 1982.
34. Sellers TD Jr, Campbell RWF, Bashore TM, et al.: Effects of procainamide and quinidine sulfate in the Wolff-Parkinson-White syndrome. Circulation 55:15, 1977.
35. Prystowsky EN, Klein GH, Rinkenberger RL, et al.: Clinical efficacy and electrophysiologic effects of encainide in patients with the Wolff-Parkinson-White syndrome. Circulation 69:278, 1984.
36. Sellers TD, Bashore TM, Gallagher JJ: Digitalis in the preexcitation syndrome: Analysis during atrial fibrillation. Circulation 56:260, 1977.
37. Klein GJ, Gulamhusein S, Prystowsky EN, et al.: Comparison of the electrophysiologic effects of intravenous and oral verapamil in patients with paroxysmal supraventricular tachycardia. Am J Cardiol 49:117, 1982.
38. Wu D, et al.: The effects of ouabain on induction of atrioventricular nodal reentrant paroxysmal supraventricular tachycardia. Circulation 52:201, 1975.
39. Wu D, et al.: The effects of propranolol on induction of A-V nodal reentrant paroxysmal tachycardia. Circulation 50:665, 1974.
40. Krikler D, Rowland E: Management of supraventricular tachycardia with drugs and artificial pacing. *In* Narula OS (ed.): Cardiac Arrhythmias: Electrophysiology, Diagnosis and Management, pp. 382–396, Baltimore, Williams & Wilkins, 1979.
41. Kou HC, Hung JS, Lee YS, et al.: Effects of oral disopyramide phosphate on induction and sustenance of atrioventricular reentrant tachycardia incorporating retrograde accessory pathway conduction. Circulation 66:454, 1982.
42. Rosenbaum MB, et al.: Clinical efficacy of amiodarone as an antiarrhythmic agent. Am J Cardiol 38:934, 1976.
43. Scheinman MM, Morady F, Hess DS, et al.: Catheter-induced ablation of the atrioventricular junction to control refractory supraventricular arrhythmias. JAMA 248:851, 1982.
44. Evans G, Scheinman MM: The Percutaneous Cardiac Mapping and Ablation Registry: Summary of results. PACE 10:1395, 1987.
45. Morady F, Scheinman MM, Winston SA, et al.: Efficacy and safety of transcatheter ablation of posteroseptal accessory pathways. Circulation 72:170, 1985.
46. Silka MJ, Gillette PC, Garson A Jr, et al.: Transvenous catheter ablation of a right atrial automatic ectopic tachycardia. J Am Coll Cardiol 5:999, 1985.
47. Gillette PC, Wampler DG, Garson A Jr, et al.: Treatment of atrial automatic tachycardia by ablation procedures. J Am Coll Cardiol 6:405, 1985.
48. Guiraudon GM, Campbell CS, Jones DL, et al.: Combined sino-atrial node atrio-ventricular isolation: A surgical alternative to His bundle ablation in patients with atrial fibrillation. Circulation 72:220, 1985.

9

Atrial Flutter: Basic and Clinical Aspects

Albert L. Waldo
Mark D. Carlson
Richard W. Henthorn

Atrial flutter was first recognized almost eight decades ago and has been of interest to clinicians ever since. Until recently, there was much controversy concerning its mechanism, and little new about its treatment. In this chapter on atrial flutter, we will emphasize several practical aspects concerning its diagnosis and treatment. We will also discuss theoretic considerations, emphasizing mechanism.

Types of Atrial Flutter

It is now recognized that there are two types of atrial flutter in humans: type I (classical) and type II.[1] This classification is independent of the morphology or polarity of the atrial flutter waves in the ECG. When recording a bipolar atrial electrogram, each type has a remarkably constant beat-to-beat morphology, polarity, and amplitude (Fig. 9–1), although a beat-to-beat alternans of electrogram amplitude may be recorded. Also, both types have a strikingly constant beat-to-beat atrial cycle length, although on occasion the atrial electrogram of either type of atrial flutter may be associated with cycle length alternans.

Of course, there are distinct differences that separate the two types. Type I atrial flutter can always be interrupted by rapid atrial pacing, whereas type II atrial flutter cannot, at least from sites high in the right atrium (pacing of type II atrial flutter from other sites has not been reported).[1–3] It was this major difference that led to the identification of the two types of atrial flutter. Why type II atrial flutter cannot be interrupted

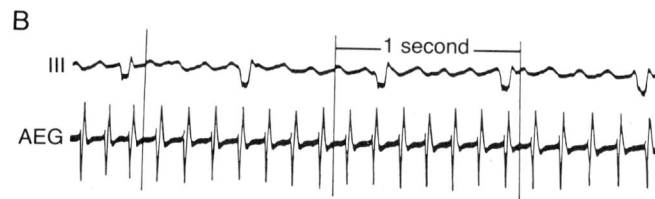

FIGURE 9–1
A and B demonstrate the simultaneous recording of ECG lead III and a bipolar atrial electrogram (AEG) during type I atrial flutter with an atrial rate of 296 beats per minute (bpm) (A) and type II atrial flutter at a rate of 420 bpm (B). Note that, in each instance, there is an irregular ventricular rate in response to the atrial flutter. However, the atrial electrograms have a constant polarity, morphology, and cycle length. Time lines are at 1-second intervals. (After Wells JL Jr, MacLean WAH, James TN, et al.: Circulation 60:665, 1979.)

with rapid atrial pacing from high right atrial sites is unknown. It may be that atrial refractoriness and prolonged atrial conduction time preclude the interruption of type II atrial flutter when pacing from this site (presumably because the site is too far from the flutter's reentrant circuit), or the mechanism of this type of atrial flutter may not be reentry with an excitable gap. In fact, it has been suggested that type II atrial flutter may be due to leading circle type reentry (i.e., a reentry circuit essentially without an excitable gap).[4]

The above observations permitted a further differ-

Supported in part by Grant # R01 HL38408 from the National Institutes of Health, National Heart, Lung, and Blood Institute, Bethesda, Md; and a Research Initiative Award from the American Heart Association, Northeast Ohio Affiliate, Cleveland, Oh.

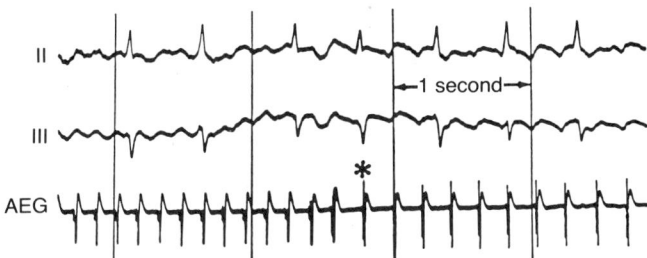

FIGURE 9–2
ECG leads II and III recorded simultaneously with a bipolar atrial electrogram (AEG) in a patient during the spontaneous conversion from type II atrial flutter to type I atrial flutter. The asterisk (*) marks the transition period. Paper recording speed is 50 mm/s. Time lines are at 1-second intervals.

entiation between the two types of atrial flutter based on rate. The ability of rapid high atrial pacing to interrupt atrial flutter permitted type I atrial flutter to be characterized by rates ranging from 240 to 340 beats per minute (bpm), and type II atrial flutter by rates ranging from 340 to 433 bpm. Some overlap probably exists between the upper range of rates for type I atrial flutter and the lower range of rates for type II, and type I may sometimes exist at rates less than 240 bpm.

If the only difference between type I and type II atrial flutter was the response to rapid atrial pacing from a high right atrial site, there might be skepticism regarding separation of atrial flutter into slower and faster types. Two additional observations have provided strong support for the presence of two types of atrial flutter.[1] First, type II atrial flutter has been observed to convert spontaneously to type I in a stepwise fashion (Fig. 9–2). Second, on occasion, when rapid atrial pacing from a high right atrial site is used to treat type I atrial flutter, type II may be present at the termination of the rapid pacing. Thus, it would appear that type I and type II atrial flutter are not really part of the same atrial flutter continuum; rather they are separate entities, although perhaps quite closely related.

Mechanism of Atrial Flutter

There has been much interest and controversy regarding the mechanism of atrial flutter. As summarized recently,[5] three theories for its mechanism have been proposed: (1) it is due to reentry with a large reentry circuit; (2) it is due to a reentry with a small, perhaps very small, reentry circuit; and (3) it is due to a single focus, presumably an abnormal automatic focus, firing rapidly. This controversy seems to have been resolved as a result of studies in both animal models and humans. Part of the problem was that until recently, in most of the animal models of atrial flutter, the flutter was created by placing substances on the heart or by creating lesions, making it unlikely that these models represented experimental counterparts of the clinical arrhythmia in humans.

The first experimental studies of atrial flutter were performed in the dog heart by Lewis and colleagues.[6] They employed neither destructive lesions nor application of substances to the atria. However, the atrial flutter they induced was rather brief, and the electrogram recording technology was quite limited, making the number of atrial recording sites that could be obtained for mapping purposes quite small. Therefore, much extrapolation had to be made regarding the sequence of atrial activation during atrial flutter in this model. Nevertheless, on the basis of these studies in experimental animals[6] and of studies of vector analysis of electrocardiograms in humans,[7] Lewis and colleagues concluded that atrial flutter was the result of circus movement in the atria.

Subsequently, primarily after the studies of Rosenbleuth and Garcia-Ramos,[8] in which a lesion was created between the vena cava, with the lesion occasionally extending into a portion of the free wall of the right atrium, it was demonstrated that atrial flutter could indeed be due to an intra-atrial reentrant mechanism. It had been assumed, and in some measure demonstrated, that the reentry circuit in this model was around the obstacle created by the atrial lesion. However, recently it has been shown by Frame et al.[9] that in the presence of a lesion similar to that created by Rosenbleuth and Garcia-Ramos (modified to create a Y incisional lesion in the right atrium), atrial flutter could be explained by circus movement around the tricuspid valve annulus.

Perhaps experimental atrial flutter that relies on a surgical incision or a crush lesion in the right atrium has a clinical counterpart in patients who have undergone a Mustard procedure for surgical correction of

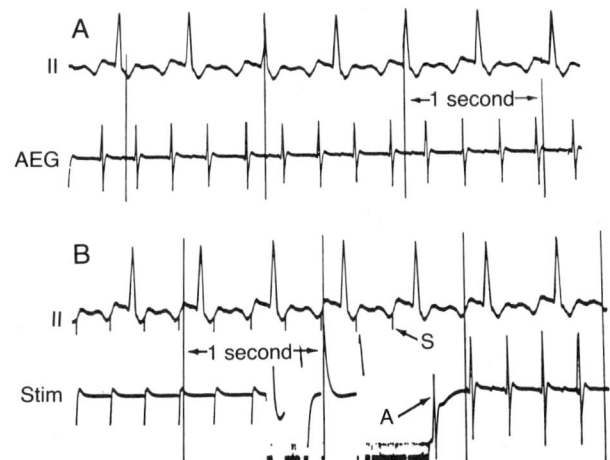

FIGURE 9–3
A, ECG lead II recorded simultaneously with a bipolar atrial electrogram (AEG) from a patient who developed type I (classical) atrial flutter following open heart surgery. The mean beat-to-beat atrial cycle length is 264 ms.

B, ECG lead II recorded simultaneously with a stimulus artifact (Stim) in the same patient at the end of 30 seconds of rapid atrial pacing from a high right atrial site with a cycle length of 254 ms. Note that during atrial pacing, although the atrial rate is increased to the pacing rate, the morphology of the atrial complexes in the ECG appears unchanged. S = stimulus artifact; A = atrial electrogram. Time lines are at 1-second intervals. (After Waldo AL, MacLean WAH, Karp RB, et al.: Circulation 56:737, 1977.)

transposition of the great vessels. These patients have a very high and seemingly unavoidable incidence of atrial flutter postoperatively, both short- and long-term. It seems reasonable to suggest that the large incisions made in the free-wall of the right atrium and in the interatrial septum required of this procedure essentially produce in humans the counterpart of the above experimental studies. This would explain why these patients have such a clinical problem with atrial flutter following this operation.

The recent studies of Allessie and colleagues[4] utilizing a Langendorff perfused canine atrial model have clearly shown that atrial flutter due to atrial reentry of the leading circle type can occur at numerous places in the atria and can occur in the absence of an anatomic obstacle (i.e., the reentrant wave front of the atrial flutter circulates around a functional obstacle). As indicated above, this group has suggested that this model may be the experimental counterpart of type II atrial flutter.

Three separate models of atrial flutter in the canine heart have been described (each of which legitimately could be considered an experimental counterpart of spontaneous atrial flutter in humans) that have demonstrated that reentry occurs in the free-wall of the right atrium. One model was a spontaneous example of atrial flutter in a single dog studied by Boineau and coworkers.[10] Another was Boyden's model of chronic right atrial enlargement caused by creating tricuspid regurgitation and banding of the pulmonary artery.[11] The third was the pericarditis model of atrial flutter

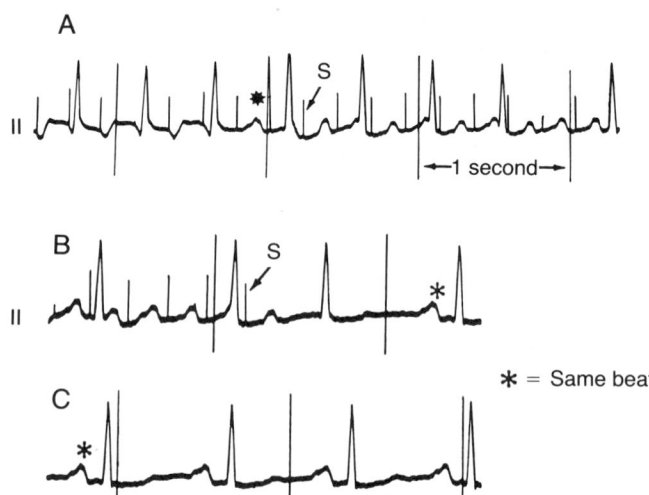

FIGURE 9–5
A, ECG lead II recorded in the same patient as the preceding two figures during high right atrial pacing at a cycle length of 224 ms. Note that with the seventh atrial beat in this tracing, and after 22 seconds of atrial pacing at a constant rate, the atrial complexes suddenly became positive (asterisk). B, ECG lead II recorded at the termination of atrial pacing in the same patient. Note that with abrupt termination of pacing, sinus rhythm recurs. C, The first beat in this panel (asterisk) is identical with the last beat in B (asterisk). S = stimulus artifact. Time lines are at 1-second intervals. (After Waldo AL, MacLean WAH, Karp RB, et al.: Circulation 56:737, 1977.)

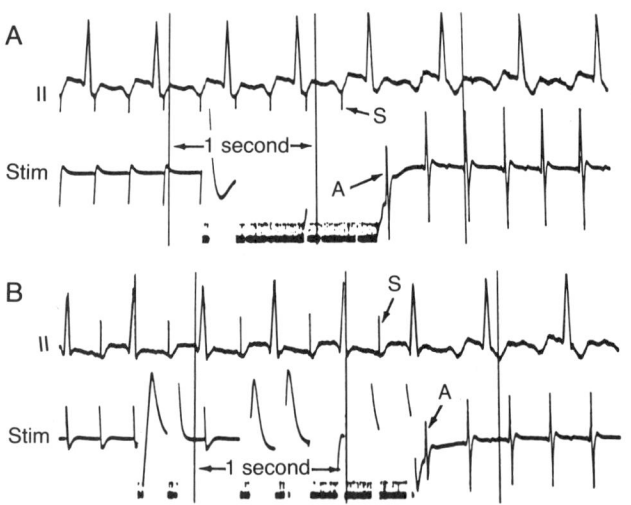

FIGURE 9–4
ECG lead II recorded simultaneously with the stimulus artifact (Stim) in the same patient as in Figure 9–3 recorded at the end of 30 seconds of high right atrial pacing at a cycle length of 242 ms (A) and at the end of 30 seconds of atrial pacing at a cycle length of 232 ms (B). Despite the fact that the atrial rate increased to the pacing rate in both A and B, note that the morphology of the atrial complexes during spontaneous atrial flutter is not very different from that during atrial pacing, although in B the atrial complexes during atrial pacing do appear to display fusion. S = stimulus artifact; A = atrial electrogram. Time lines are at 1-second intervals. (After Waldo AL, MacLean WAH, Karp RB, et al.: Circulation 56:737, 1977.)

described in our laboratory.[12] The location of the reentry circuit in these models is especially of interest in view of the catheter mapping studies (limited) performed in the 1950s and 1960s in humans, which used esophageal leads and selected intra-atrial leads, usually correlated with electrocardiographic recordings. As summarized by Rytand,[13] these data from humans support the notion that atrial flutter is an intra-atrial reentrant rhythm in which activation travels in a caudocranial direction in the left atrium and a craniocaudal direction in the right atrium. Based on their studies during cardiac catheterization, Puech and colleagues[14,15] suggested that the entire duration of the atrial flutter cycle length could be explained by activation of the right atrium alone and, in fact, that atrial flutter could be explained by circus movement in the right atrium. Most recently, mapping studies using cardiac catheterization techniques from our laboratory[16] and by Cosio and colleagues[17] and intraoperative mapping studies by Klein and coworkers[18] have provided additional support that type I, or classical, atrial flutter is due to reentry of the type initially described by Puech.

Unfortunately, the catheter electrode mapping techniques had intrinsic limitations which did not permit definitive conclusions about the mechanism of atrial flutter in humans. However, the demonstration of transient entrainment and interruption of atrial flutter in humans, using rapid atrial pacing techniques (Figs. 9–3, 9–4, and 9–5), provides additional strong evidence to support the notion that atrial flutter is due to reentry with an excitable gap.[2,3,19] Thus, although definitive, multiplex recording techniques to map atrial flutter in humans are not yet available, there is very strong evidence in experimental models, as well as clinical evidence in humans, that atrial flutter virtually always is due to reentry in the right atrium, with the reentry circuit being relatively large.

For completeness, it must be noted that experimental evidence exists to support the idea that atrial flutter can be produced by a single focus firing rapidly. This evidence comes primarily from studies that used the application to the heart of such substances as aconitine or delphinine[20-22] or that used atrial pacing from the coronary sinus at typical atrial flutter rates.[23] Also, data obtained during open heart surgery in humans by Prinzmetal et al.[24] and Wellens et al.[25] are consistent with atrial flutter emanating from a single focus. Nevertheless, it is now generally accepted that this mechanism is unlikely.

THE NATURE OF THE REENTRY CIRCUIT IN ATRIAL FLUTTER

Although it is now generally thought that atrial flutter in patients does indeed result from circus movement (i.e., reentry within the atria), many questions remain. Where is the precise location of the circus movement in patients? Does it involve circus movement in part or in full around an anatomic obstacle? Can the reentrant wave front be explained by circus movement in part or in full around a functional obstacle? The fact that, clinically, atrial flutter is so markedly similar from patient to patient and from circumstance to circumstance suggests that the site and characteristics of the reentry circuit are in some way anatomically determined. It has been suggested that the sinus node is critically involved in atrial flutter, because of either its location or an intrinsic abnormality.[26] It has also been suggested that functional or specialized intra-atrial or internodal pathways may be involved, although this has been largely speculative.[26, 27] The mechanism of the very rapid form of atrial flutter (type II) also is unknown, although, as indicated earlier, it has been suggested that it may be due to the leading circle type of reentry.[4]

In sum, particularly as a result of the recent entrainment and mapping data, it is generally accepted that classical (type I) atrial flutter in humans is due to reentry with an excitable gap. The nature and mechanism of type II atrial flutter remain speculative.

Practical Aspects of the Treatment of Atrial Flutter with Cardiac Pacing

As recently summarized,[28] many studies have used rapid atrial pacing techniques to treat atrial flutter. In most of those studies, atrial pacing was done not only unsystematically, but also at rates that often greatly exceeded the spontaneous atrial flutter rate, thereby

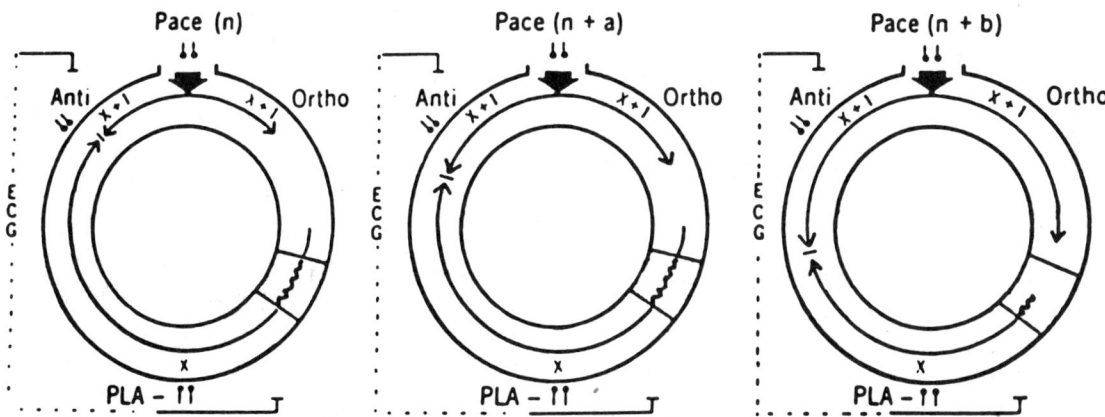

FIGURE 9–6
Reentry loops during overdrive pacing of atrial flutter at three different overdrive pacing rates (n, n + a, and n + b) diagrammatically showing progressive fusion (i.e., different degrees of fusion during transient entrainment at different overdrive pacing rates). The pacing cycle length of n is longer than the pacing cycle length of n + b. The arrowheads indicate the pacing impulse from the same high right atrial pacing site entering into the reentry loop. Note that, with pacing at each rate, the antidromic (Anti) wave front of each pacing impulse (x + 1) collides with the orthodromic (Ortho) wave front of the previous beat (x), and the orthodromic wave front of each pacing impulse (x + 1) resets and continues (i.e., entrains) the tachycardia. However, because the pacing cycle length of n + a is shorter than that of n, there is greater penetration of the wave fronts from the pacing impulse into the reentry loop both antidromically and orthodromically. This results in a different degree of atrial fusion during pacing at n + a than during pacing at n because the site of collision of the antidromic wave front (x + 1) with the orthodromic wave front of the previous beat (x) necessarily occurs at a different site. This also explains why a different degree of atrial fusion occurs during overdrive pacing at n + b than at n + a. PLA = posterior left anterior recording site. (Reprinted by permission from Waldo AL, Plumb VJ, Henthorn RW: Observations on the mechanism of atrial flutter. In Surawicz B, Reddy CP, Prystowsky EN (eds.): Tachycardias, pp. 213–229, Boston, Martinus Nijhoff Publishing, 1984.)

producing atrial fibrillation. The latter, in turn, quite often reverted spontaneously to sinus rhythm. There also have been several reports of failure to interrupt atrial flutter with rapid pacing. We now understand that such failure is virtually always due to a technical problem (e.g., failure to capture the atria because of inadequate stimulus strength, failure of the pacing electrode to make continuous contact with atrial tissue, or failure to pace at the proper rate for an appropriate period of time).[3, 27]

It is now clear that several important factors should always be considered when atrial pacing is used to interrupt atrial flutter.[3, 27] First, to interrupt type I atrial flutter, the atria have to be paced at a critical rate for a critical duration of time (see Figs. 9–3, 9–4, and 9–5). Pacing the atria at rates faster than the atrial flutter rate, but slower than a critical pacing rate, will only transiently entrain the atrial flutter (see Figs. 9–3 and 9–4). Thus, following termination of pacing at such rapid but inadequate rates will result in prompt return of the atrial flutter at its previous spontaneous rate.[2, 3, 14, 28] However, when the critically rapid pacing rate is achieved, atrial flutter can always be interrupted (see Fig. 9–5). In addition, our previous studies have shown that, even when pacing at the appropriate pacing rate, there is a critical duration of pacing (mean 11 s) at that rate before the atrial flutter is interrupted.[2] As a result, we usually recommend pacing for at least 15 seconds, with longer durations sometimes required, in order to interrupt atrial flutter. Finally, atrial pacing at rapid rates usually requires a relatively high stimulus strength, as the threshold for atrial capture increases at rapid rates.[3, 28, 29] Therefore, a pacemaker that is capable of delivering stimuli of at least 20 mA should be available for use.

Several other techniques should prove helpful when using rapid atrial pacing to interrupt atrial flutter. Pacing from the high right atrium is recommended because the interruption of atrial flutter is heralded by the appearance of positive atrial complexes in the inferior leads (II, III, aVF) of the ECG (see Fig. 9–5). During rapid atrial pacing from the high right atrium at rates that transiently entrain rather than interrupt the atrial flutter, the atrial complexes in the ECG will be fusion beats (Figs. 9–3, 9–4, and 9–6). Thus, they will not have the usual positive polarity in the inferior leads that normally occurs when overdrive pacing a sinus rhythm from this pacing site. When the atria are paced at the critically rapid rate so that the atrial flutter is interrupted, the atrial complexes in the ECG no longer are fusion beats; rather, they are the complexes one would expect to find when overdrive pacing a sinus rhythm. Thus, when atrial flutter is interrupted, the atrial complexes in leads II, III, and aVF will become positive (Figs. 9–5 and 9–7). In sum, the appearance of positive atrial complexes in leads II, III, and aVF is the hallmark that atrial flutter is no longer being transiently entrained, but rather has been interrupted. These principles of rapid atrial pacing in the treatment of atrial flutter are of value not only for use with temporary pacing techniques to interrupt atrial flutter but also in concert with the use of antitachycardia pacemakers permanently implanted to treat this arrhythmia.

Last, during rapid atrial pacing the simultaneous administration of a type IA antiarrhythmic agent increases the efficacy of conversion of atrial flutter to sinus rhythm.[30, 31] When a type 1A antiarrhythmic agent is not used, an important incidence of induction of atrial fibrillation results. While this rhythm often is transient, spontaneously reverting to sinus rhythm, many times the atrial fibrillation will revert to atrial flutter, or the atrial fibrillation will persist, so that DC cardioversion is required. Thus, we also recommend the administration of a type 1A antiarrhythmic agent whenever possible prior to initiating rapid pacing. It is

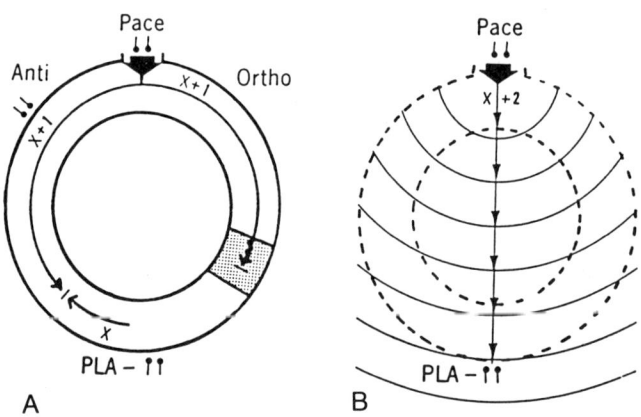

FIGURE 9–7
A, The arrowhead indicates the pacing impulse from an atrial site entering into the reentry loop, whereupon it is conducted orthodromically (Ortho) and antidromically (Anti). The antidromic wave front (x + 1) collides with the orthodromic wave front from the previous beat (x), resulting in atrial fusion. The orthodromic wave front (x + 1) also blocks, presumably in the area of slow conduction, so that the tachycardia is no longer reset. In fact, because the antidromic and orthodromic wave fronts of the same pacing impulse have blocked, the tachycardia has been interrupted. Note that block of both the antidromic and orthodromic wave fronts of the same pacing impulse is associated with absence of conduction of one pacing impulse to the posterior-inferior left atrial recording site (PLA).
B, The large arrow indicates the next pacing impulse (x + 2) from the same atrial pacing site as in the left diagram. The dashed circle shows the reentry loop present during both the previous period of spontaneous atrial flutter and that of transient entrainment of the atrial flutter. Because the atrial flutter has been interrupted by the previous pacing impulse (x + 1), the sequence of atrial activation of the next pacing impulse (x + 2) is the same as one would expect during overdrive pacing of a sinus rhythm. Therefore, the P wave in ECG lead II will be positive, and the PLA recording site will be activated from a different direction and with a shorter conduction time than during previous periods of transient entrainment from the same pacing site. The isochromes are drawn to indicate the general direction of spread of the impulse and are not meant to imply that the sequence of atrial activation from the pacing site to the PLA recording is radial. (Reprinted by permission from Waldo AL, Plumb VJ, Henthorn RW: Observations on the mechanism of atrial flutter. In Surawicz B, Reddy CP, Prystowsky EN [eds.]: Tachycardias, pp. 213–229, Boston, Martinus Nijhoff Publishing, 1984.)

of interest that type IA agents are not especially effective in interrupting atrial flutter when used alone, and their use to provide effective suppression of recurrent atrial flutter is unpredictable and often unsatisfactory. Recent studies suggest that the type IC agents may hold some hope in this regard.[32, 33]

Future Directions

While we have learned a great deal about atrial flutter over the years, there is still much to learn about it and its treatment. For instance, why does the reentry circuit occur in the right atrium, and what are the components of the reentry loop? Can atrial flutter be successfully prevented with surgical therapy or catheter ablation? Will the newer antiarrhythmic agents, particularly the type 1C agents, be more effective in suppressing recurrent atrial flutter? Amiodarone appears to be quite effective in suppressing recurrent atrial flutter, but because of the high incidence of adverse effects, its use to treat atrial flutter probably should be limited. Will a drug be found that will predictably interrupt atrial flutter acutely when given intravenously? These are only a few of the many remaining questions that will occupy investigators for many years to come.

References

1. Wells JL Jr, MacLean WAH, James TN, et al.: Characterization of atrial flutter. Studies in man after open heart surgery using fixed atrial electrodes. Circulation 60:655, 1979.
2. Waldo AL, MacLean WAH, Karp RB, et al.: Entrainment and interruption of atrial flutter with atrial pacing: Studies in man following open heart surgery. Circulation 56:737, 1977.
3. Waldo AL, MacLean WAH: Diagnosis and Treatment of Arrhythmias Following Open Heart Surgery—Emphasis on the Use of Epicardial Wire Electrodes. New York, Futura Publishing Co., 1980.
4. Allessie MA, Lammers WJEP, Bonke FIM, et al.: Intraatrial reentry as a mechanism for atrial flutter induced by acetylcholine in rapid pacing in the dog. Circulation 70:123, 1984.
5. Waldo AL: Mechanisms of atrial fibrillation, atrial flutter, and ectopic atrial tachycardia—a brief review. Circulation (Suppl 3) 75:III-37, 1987.
6. Lewis T, Feil HS, Stroud WD: Observations upon flutter and fibrillation. Part II. The nature of auricular flutter. Heart 7:191, 1920.
7. Lewis T, Drury AN, Iliescu CC: A demonstration of circus movement in clinical flutter of the auricles. Heart 8:341, 1921.
8. Rosenbleuth A, Garcia-Ramos J: Studies on flutter and fibrillation. II. The influence of artificial obstacles on experimental auricular flutter. Am Heart J 33:677, 1947.
9. Frame LH, Page RL, Hoffman BF: Atrial reentry around an anatomic barrier with a partially refractory excitable gap. A canine model of atrial flutter. Circ Res 58:495, 1986.
10. Boineau JP, Schuessler RB, Mooney CR, et al.: Natural and evoked atrial flutter due to circus movement in dogs. Am J Cardiol 45:1167, 1980.
11. Boyden PA: Activation sequence during atrial flutter in dogs with surgically induced right atrial enlargement. I. Observations during sustained rhythms. Circ Res 62:596, 1988.
12. Page PL, Plumb VJ, Okumura K, et al.: A new animal model of atrial flutter. Am J Coll Cardiol 8:872, 1986.
13. Rytand DA: The circus movement (entrapped circuit wave) hypothesis of atrial flutter. Arch Intern Med 65:125, 1966.
14. Puech P: L'Activité électrique Auriculaire Normale et pathologique. Paris, Masson & Cie, 1956, p. 214.
15. Puech P, Latour H, Grolleau R: Le flutter et ses limites. Arch Mal Coeur 63:116, 1970.
16. Olshansky B, Okumura K, Henthorn RW, et al.: Atrial mapping of human atrial flutter demonstrates reentry in the right atrium (Abstract). J Am Coll Cardiol 7:194A, 1986.
17. Cosio FG, Arribas F, Barbero JM, et al.: Validation of double spike electrograms as markers of conduction delayer block in atrial flutter. Am J Cardiol 61:775, 1988.
18. Klein GJ, Guiraudon GM, Sharma AD, et al.: Demonstration of macroreentry and feasibility of operative therapy in the common type of atrial flutter. Am J Cardiol 57:587, 1986.
19. Waldo AL, Plumb VJ, Henthorn RW: Observations on the mechanism of atrial flutter. In Surawicz B, Reddy CP, Prystowsky EN (eds.): Tachycardias, pp. 213–229. Boston, Martinus Nijhoff, 1984.
20. Scherf D: Studies on auricular tachycardia caused by aconitine administration. Proc Exp Biol Med 64:233, 1947.
21. Scherf D, Blumenfeld S, Taner D, et al.: Cardiac arrhythmias provoked by focal application of delphinine. Arch Kreisl Forsch 33:4, 1960.
22. Hayden WG, Hurley EJ, Rytand DA: The mechanism of canine atrial flutter. Circ Res 20:496, 1967.
23. Rosen K, Lau SH, Damato AN: Simulation of atrial flutter by rapid coronary sinus pacing. Am Heart J 78:635, 1969.
24. Prinzmetal M, Corday E, Oblath RW, et al.: Auricular flutter. Am J Med 11:410, 1951.
25. Wellens HJJ, Janse MJ, Van Dam RTH, et al.: Epicardial excitation of the atria in a patient with atrial flutter. Br Heart J 33:233, 1971.
26. James TN: The connecting pathways between the sinus node and the AV node and between the right and the left atrium in the human heart. Am Heart J 66:498, 1963.
27. Pastelin G, Mendez R, Moe GK: Participation of atrial specialized conduction pathways in atrial flutter. Circ Res 42:386, 1978.
28. Waldo AL: Some observations concerning atrial flutter in man. PACE 6:1181, 1983.
29. Plumb VJ, Karp RB, James TN, et al.: Atrial excitability and conduction during rapid atrial pacing. Circulation 63:1140, 1981.
30. Camm J, Ward D, Spurrell R: Response of atrial flutter to overdrive atrial pacing and intravenous dysopyramide phosphate singly and in combination. Br Heart J 44:240, 1980.
31. Olshansky B, Okumura K, Hess PG, et al.: Use of procainamide with atrial pacing for successful conversion of atrial flutter to sinus rhythm. J Am Coll Cardiol 11:359, 1988.
32. Anderson JL, Jolivette DM, Fredell PA: Summary of efficacy and safety of flecainide for supraventricular arrhythmias. Am J Cardiol 62:62D–66D, 1988.
33. Anderson JL, Gilbert EM, Alpert BL, et al.: Flecainide for prevention of symptomatic paroxysmal atrial fibrillation: a multicenter, double-blind, placebo-controlled, crossover study (abstr). J Am Coll Cardiol 11(2):77A, 1988.

10

The Pre-excitation Syndrome

Bruce D. Lindsay
Nancy A. Branyas
Michael E. Cain

The term pre-excitation was used originally by Ohnell to signify premature activation of the ventricles in patients with Wolff-Parkinson-White (WPW) syndrome.[109] Today, the term pre-excitation has been extended to include all disorders in which anterograde ventricular activation or retrograde atrial activation occurs in part or totally through anomalous pathways distinct from the normal cardiac conduction system. This chapter reviews the pathophysiology of these disorders, the noninvasive and invasive procedures used for diagnosis, and management strategies for patients with the pre-excitation syndrome.

Historical Perspective

The description of atrioventricular (AV) conduction by His[72] and the pioneering studies of the AV node by Tawara[142] were critical to the early understanding of normal AV synchrony during sinus rhythm. Kent first described muscular tissue that bridged the annulus fibrosus and proposed that it accounted for the transmission of electrical impulses from the atria to the ventricles.[77] The functional significance of these muscular AV bands aroused controversy and was dismissed by many of Kent's colleagues, including such leading authorities as Sir Thomas Lewis.[91] As early as 1914, Mines[102] speculated that episodes of paroxysmal tachycardia might be attributable to anterograde conduction through the normal AV conduction system with retrograde conduction through an anomalous AV muscle bundle described by Kent. Wilson[154] and Cohn and Fraser[33] recorded examples of ventricular pre-excitation from patients with paroxysmal tachycardia and demonstrated the dynamic relationship between vagal tone and intermittent QRS aberrancy, which they attributed to a variant of bundle branch block.

Collaborative efforts by Wolff, Parkinson, and White in 1930 drew attention to the clinical syndrome characterized by a short P-R interval, an abnormal QRS morphology, and paroxysmal tachycardia.[156] Two years later, Holtzmann and Scherf[73] proposed that the anomalous QRS complex was due to either bypass of the AV node or activation of an abnormal ventricular focus by the contraction of the atrium. Wolfarth and Wood[155] arrived at a similar conclusion and speculated that in such patients the QRS morphology depended on the location of the accessory pathway. They later demonstrated muscular AV bridges from a patient with pre-excitation who died during an arrhythmia.[157] Growing acceptance of this hypothesis was reflected in the electrocardiographic classification by Rosenbaum et al.[122] of pre-excitation into types A and B, based on the presumed order of ventricular activation.

Debate over the cause of ventricular pre-excitation persisted until 1967, when Durrer and Roos[51] recorded early ventricular activation over the right free-wall from a patient with the WPW syndrome, which they attributed to an anomalous pathway connecting the right atrium and adjoining ventricle. Results of pioneering studies by Durrer et al.[52] of patients with the WPW syndrome demonstrated that the atria, the normal AV conduction system, the ventricles, and an accessory pathway could be components of a macro-reentrant circuit. These observations confirmed the electrophysiologic basis of the WPW syndrome and provided a physiologic and anatomic basis for the development of new treatment strategies.

Traditionally, treatment had been limited to the administration of antiarrhythmic drugs. The observations of Durrer and coworkers suggested that surgical division of the AV node or the accessory pathway would interrupt the reentrant loop, precluding the occurrence of the tachycardia. During closure of an atrial septal defect in a patient with the WPW syndrome, Burchell used a unipolar electrode to identify an area of early epicardial activation that was presumed

---

Supported in part by NIH Grant HL17646, SCOR in Ischemic Heart Disease.

to be the site of an accessory pathway. Direct pressure or injection of procainamide at this site resulted in the transient loss of pre-excitation; however, an attempt to divide the accessory pathway by a transverse subendocardial incision was unsuccessful.[25] Dreifus and colleagues[50] described a patient with refractory tachycardia in whom surgical ligation of the AV node resulted in persistent pre-excitation without a recurrence of the tachycardia. In 1968 Cobb and coworkers[32] reported a patient with a right free-wall accessory pathway who had intractable episodes of tachycardia. The approximate location of the anomalous pathway was determined from body surface potential distribution maps and localized further by epicardial mapping at the time of surgery. Permanent ablation of ventricular pre-excitation was achieved by surgical dissection of the region identified by electrophysiologic mapping. Over the ensuing 20 years, investigators from many laboratories have further defined the pathophysiology of pre-excitation syndromes. Particular recognition should be extended to the groups at Duke University and the University of Limburg for their contributions to our understanding of these disorders and their treatment.

Anatomic and Developmental Aspects

During early fetal development, the atrial and ventricular myocardium are in continuity. The subsequent invagination of the atrial and ventricular septa and formation of the annulus fibrosus occur concomitantly with regression of muscle bands. Defects in the continuity of the annulus fibrosus have been observed in infants,[7, 120] but most often resolve during the first six months of life and do not necessarily have functional significance.[75, 146] Such defects, however, may account for the subendocardial location of many right-sided accessory pathways, particularly those associated with abnormalities in the development of the AV ring, and may explain the high incidence of the pre-excitation syndrome in patients with Ebstein's anomaly.[14] Left free-wall pathways are not usually associated with discontinuities of the annulus fibrosus and represent residual, subepicardial AV bridges of myocardium that failed to regress during fetal development.[8, 9]

Morphologically, accessory pathways are strands of normal myocardium that bridge the AV groove at any point around the annulus fibrosus on either side of the heart, except that portion of the mitral valve annulus between the right and left fibrous trigones.[38] For purposes of surgical or percutaneous ablation, the locations of accessory pathways are regionalized to left free-wall (58%), posterior-septal (24%), right free-wall (13%), and anterior-septal (5%) sites.[26] Accessory pathways at posterior-septal and anterior-septal sites have complex anatomic relationships with the coronary circulation and normal AV conduction system. Posterior-septal pathways are located within the pyramidal space, bound anteriorly by the insertion of the atrial extension of the membranous septum into the right fibrous trigone and posteriorly by the epicardium overlying the crux of the heart. The lateral boundaries are formed by divergent walls of the left and right atria. Within this space is the AV nodal artery, the tendon of Todaro, epicardial fat, and the proximal portion of the coronary sinus. The AV node and its proximal penetrating bundle lie within the triangle of Koch, immediately adjacent to the pyramidal space. Anterior-septal pathways, which are typically located just anterior to the AV node, pass through the fat pad between the right and left fibrous trigones and the insertion of the right coronary artery into the AV groove. This path lies anterior to the membranous portion of the interatrial septum and is bounded by the pericardial reflection of the ascending aorta and medial wall of the right atrium.

Mahaim fibers are composed of specialized tissue that connects components of the normal conduction system to the ventricular septum. They are often observed in histologic studies[59] but are functionally significant only when relatively abundant.[88] Nodoventricular fibers have their origin in the AV node, originating from the transitional or compact nodal zones of the AV junction.[6] They generally insert on the right side of the septum,[61] but left septal insertions have been described.[1, 87] Fasciculoventricular fibers arise from the His bundle or bundle branches and have variable septal insertions.[59]

Pre-excitation Syndromes

WOLFF-PARKINSON-WHITE SYNDROME

Figure 10–1 is a schematic representation of the critical anatomic components of the WPW syndrome. During sinus rhythm, AV conduction occurs through both the normal conduction system and the accessory pathway.

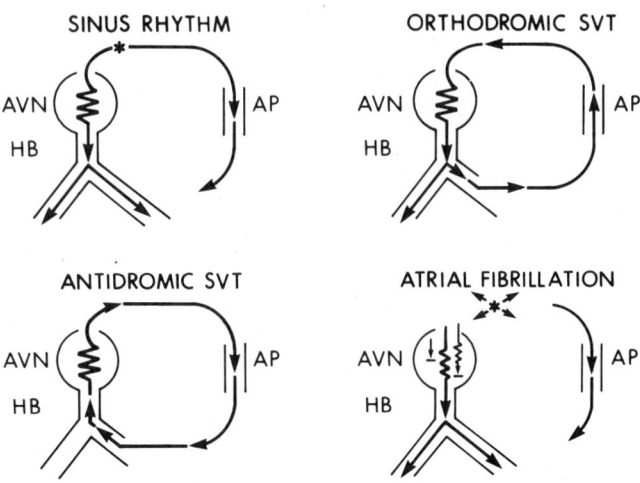

FIGURE 10–1
Schematic representation of the patterns of conduction through an accessory pathway (AP) and the normal conduction system (AVN-HB) during sinus rhythm, orthodromic supraventricular tachycardia (SVT), antidromic SVT, and atrial fibrillation.

Because accessory pathways do not usually exhibit the conduction delay characteristic of the AV node, activation of ventricular myocardium adjacent to the accessory pathway occurs before propagation through the normal AV conduction system is complete. In contrast to the sharp onset and relatively short QRS characteristic of ventricular activation through the normal AV conduction system, slow conduction from the insertion site of the accessory pathway through ventricular myocardium slurs the QRS upstroke and prolongs its duration. The eccentric and premature activation of the ventricle are responsible for the altered QRS morphology and short P-R interval that are the electrocardiographic hallmarks of the WPW syndrome. The QRS pattern and the P-R interval depend on the relative contribution of conduction through the accessory pathway to ventricular activation and may show considerable temporal variation. Perturbations that delay conduction through the AV node including premature atrial depolarizations and an increase of vagal tone result in preferential conduction over the accessory pathway, enhancing the degree of pre-excitation evident on the electrocardiogram.

Patients with accessory pathways are prone to AV reentrant supraventricular tachycardia (SVT) because the normal conduction system and the accessory pathway join proximally (atrium) and distally (ventricle) to form a closed circuit of conduction. Unidirectional block in one pathway and slow conduction through the unblocked pathway may allow the blocked pathway time to recover excitability and initiate reentry. Orthodromic SVT is most common and accounts for 90 to 95% of the arrhythmias observed clinically and inducible in the laboratory.[12] During orthodromic SVT (see Fig. 10–1) anterograde conduction to the ventricles is through the AV node/His-Purkinje system, and retrograde conduction to the atrium is through the accessory pathway. Because the ventricles are activated exclusively by the His-Purkinje system, the QRS morphology is normal unless aberration due to bundle branch block occurs. Orthodromic SVT depends on the participation of both the atria and the ventricles and is terminated by the development of AV or ventriculoatrial (VA) conduction block.

Antidromic SVT occurs spontaneously in 5% of and is inducible in 10% of patients with the WPW syndrome.[12] The anterograde limb (see Fig. 10–1) is the accessory pathway and the retrograde limb is either the normal conduction system or a second accessory pathway. Because the ventricles are activated exclusively through the accessory pathway, the QRS is maximally pre-excited and may be mistaken for ventricular tachycardia. Antidromic SVT also incorporates both the atria and the ventricles and is terminated whenever AV or VA conduction block occurs.

Atrial fibrillation is detectable in approximately 30% of patients with the WPW syndrome.[27] It may develop de novo or as a consequence of orthodromic or antidromic SVT.[13, 27, 35] During atrial fibrillation (see Fig. 10–1), the ventricles may be activated through the AV node/His-Purkinje system, the accessory pathway, or both, depending on the intrinsic electrophysiologic properties of each. Accordingly, the QRS morphology during atrial fibrillation varies with the contribution of conduction through the normal and anomalous AV pathways to ventricular activation. In patients with accessory pathways having short refractory periods, ventricular activation occurs predominantly through the accessory pathway, the QRS is maximally pre-excited, and ventricular rates exceeding 250 beats per minute (bpm) may be observed. The resultant short diastolic filling times reduce cardiac output and may result in profound hypotension and impaired coronary perfusion. It is likely that these conditions promote myocardial ischemia and that repetitive ventricular depolarizations at short coupling intervals precipitate ventricular fibrillation.

CONCEALED ACCESSORY PATHWAYS

Concealed accessory pathways conduct only retrogradely. The QRS morphology during sinus rhythm is normal. During atrial fibrillation, anterograde activation occurs exclusively through the AV node/His-Purkinje system. The ventricular rate and QRS morphology are similar to that from patients without accessory pathways. Concealed pathways compose the retrograde limb of the reentrant circuit during orthodromic SVT or the retrograde limb during antidromic SVT in patients with multiple pathways.[36, 133, 140, 162]

ACCESSORY PATHWAYS WITH DECREMENTAL PROPERTIES

The normal response of the AV node to incremental pacing or programmed atrial extrastimuli is a gradual prolongation of conduction. Similarly, retrograde conduction within the AV node is gradually prolonged by incremental ventricular pacing or programmed ventricular extrastimuli. This feature is often relied on clinically to distinguish conduction through the AV node/His-Purkinje system from that through an accessory pathway in which AV and VA conduction during programmed stimulation characteristically remains constant. An incessant form of AV reentry associated with an accessory pathway having decremental conduction properties was first described by Coumel et al.,[37] who coined the phrase "permanent junctional reciprocating tachycardia." The electrocardiographic features are a long R-P interval and an abnormal P wave axis. The P wave morphology is typically negative in leads II, III, and aVF. The onset of tachycardia is not generally preceded by a prolongation of the P-R interval; however, once established, the R-P interval may lengthen.

The observation that early retrograde atrial activation was recorded in the posterior-septal region initially raised speculation that conduction occurred through accessory AV nodal tissue.[60] Several studies, however, have confirmed that accessory pathways may exhibit features of decremental conduction retrogradely and may participate in AV reentry.[24, 53, 54, 60, 83] Moreover, patients have been identified recently with concealed pathways at left-sided sites that exhibit properties of decremental conduction,[110] further supporting the contention that these pathways are not composed of accessory AV nodal tissue. Most accessory pathways having features of decremental conduction are concealed. However, patients have been reported in whom ventricular pre-excitation became manifest following ablation of the AV node for the purpose of permanently interrupting incessant tachycardia. The antegrade refractory properties of these pathways were relatively long.[62, 127] A postmortem examination of the heart from one patient identified a tortuous accessory pathway composed of myocardial tissue with interstitial fibrosis, that was most pronounced at the site of the ventricular insertion.[40] Whether such structural features are typical and account for the unusual electrophysiologic properties of these accessory pathways requires further study.

Patients with incessant AV reentry frequently have left ventricular enlargement and impaired ventricular function. Myocardial biopsy has demonstrated myocytic hypertrophy and interstitial fibrosis without evidence of an acute inflammatory response. In some patients, ventricular function has improved dramatically following control of the arrhythmia, suggesting that the observed changes in ventricular function are the consequence of the tachycardia.[112]

MAHAIM FIBERS

Mahaim fibers are generally classified according to their origin from components of the normal conduction system (Fig. 10–2).[6] Nodoventricular fibers arise from the AV node and connect with the ventricular septum. The P-R interval is usually normal in the electrocardiograms from these patients but may be short if the nodoventricular fiber originates at the proximal portion of the AV node. The ventricular insertion is typically at the base of the interventricular septum, resulting in a posterobasal, right-to-left septal activation pattern. The QRS morphology resembles left bundle branch block.[61] Some patients have been identified in whom nodoventricular fibers insert into the left ventricle. The electrocardiographic pattern of pre-excitation from these patients resembles right bundle branch block.[1, 87] In most patients with nodoventricular fibers, pre-excitation is not evident at rest but becomes manifest only after a critical delay of propagation occurs in the normal AV conduction system. Premature atrial depolarizations, rapid atrial pacing, or atrial fibrillation may be required before the anomalous QRS morphology becomes evident. Participation of nodoventricular fibers in clinical arrhythmias may be active or passive. During tachycardias in which the nodoventricular fiber is a necessary component of the reentrant circuit (see Fig. 10–2), anterograde conduction occurs through the nodoventricular fiber activating the ventricles eccentrically and results in aberrant QRS complexes having a left bundle branch block morphology. Retrograde conduction through the His-Purkinje system to the AV node completes the reentrant loop.[61, 141, 145, 150] AV dissociation may be observed because the atria are not critical components of the reentrant circuit. A nodoventricular fiber may act as an innocent bystander during AV nodal reentry or other atrial arrhythmias.[106, 148] In such cases, ventricular pre-excitation is observed but the nodoventricular fiber is not essential to arrhythmogenesis.

Fasciculoventricular fibers, which are the type described by Mahaim,[96–98] arise from the His bundle or fascicles and insert on either side of the interventricular septum. Modest pre-excitation is generally evident on electrocardiograms recorded during sinus rhythm but remains constant despite lengthening of the P-R interval during incremental atrial pacing.[61] Fasciculoventricular fibers have not been demonstrated to participate actively in clinical arrhythmias.

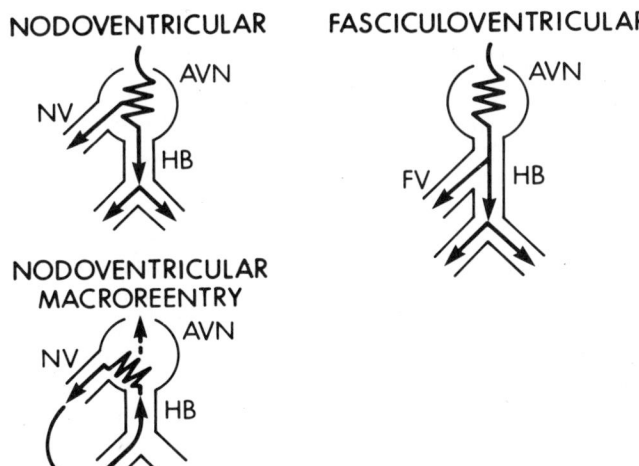

Figure 10–2
Schematic representation of the patterns of conduction through nodoventricular and fasciculoventricular fibers during sinus rhythm and during a macroreentrant circuit. During macroreentry, anterograde conduction occurs through the nodoventricular fiber and retrograde conduction occurs through the normal conduction system.

Incidence and Natural History of Pre-excitation Syndromes

The reported prevalence of ventricular pre-excitation based on analysis of electrocardiograms is 1 to 3 per 1000 persons.[30] The true prevalence of accessory pathways cannot be determined accurately, because some are concealed and only symptomatic patients are evaluated. While first-degree relatives of most patients do not have a higher prevalence of pre-excitation, a subset of patients with the WPW syndrome has been described in whom there is an autosomal dominant pattern of inheritance.[147] Individuals with pre-excitation and a positive family history often have multiple pathways. In the nonfamilial form, patients with a history of ventricular fibrillation have a greater prevalence of multiple accessory pathways compared to those without ventricular fibrillation.[80] It has not yet been determined whether the familial form is associated with an increased risk of sudden death.

Several congenital abnormalities are associated with pre-excitation syndrome. Foremost is Ebstein's anomaly, in which the incidence of the WPW syndrome has been reported to be as high as 25%.[64, 128, 135] Although accessory pathways can occur at any position around the annulus fibrosus, those at right free-wall and posterior-septal locations predominate in patients with Ebstein's anomaly, whereas multiple accessory pathways have been detected in up to 50% of patients.[34] In addition, Mahaim fibers have been described alone or in combination with an accessory pathway in patients with Epstein's anomaly. Ventricular pre-excitation is also found commonly in patients with coarctation of the aorta, hypertrophic cardiomyopathy, ventricular septal defects, and D-transposition of the great arteries.[114]

Most patients with the pre-excitation syndrome first experience arrhythmias early in life. Infants may experience heart rates up to 300 bpm. Congestive heart failure may complicate recurrent or prolonged episodes of tachycardia, whereas tachycardias that are incessant may lead to left ventricular dysfunction. The incidence of sudden death in infants with the pre-excitation syndrome has been reported to be 1%.[84] It is likely, however, that the true incidence of life-threatening arrhythmias has been underestimated because of the difficulty in documenting specific arrhythmias in this age group. Natural history studies have encompassed relatively small numbers of patients, but results suggest a variable course as children mature and enter adolescence. In one study of 40 patients who presented in infancy with paroxysmal tachycardia, only 50% continued to experience arrhythmias during the third decade of life.[95] In a similar study of 50 patients with pre-excitation syndrome followed for a period of 21 years, one patient died suddenly and 49% continued to experience symptomatic arrhythmias each year.[111]

Most arrhythmias experienced by patients with the pre-excitation syndrome are troublesome but not life-threatening. A small percentage of patients develop ventricular fibrillation and are at risk of sudden death. Although the incidence is low, ventricular fibrillation may be the presenting manifestation of the pre-excitation syndrome. Presently, there is no consensus regarding the need or method for determining risk in patients who are asymptomatic. Patients with the pre-excitation syndrome who have experienced ventricular fibrillation have a greater prevalence of both atrial fibrillation and reciprocating tachycardia than those without a history of ventricular fibrillation.[80] Ventricular fibrillation most commonly develops as a consequence of atrial fibrillation with a rapid ventricular rate.[80, 149] This fact poses a difficult problem, because the incidence of atrial fibrillation in patients with the pre-excitation syndrome increases during adolescence; however, neither the age of onset of symptoms nor the presence of associated congenital abnormalities helps to identify those who will develop ventricular fibrillation.

The prevalence of symptoms in patients with the pre-excitation syndrome varies considerably and ranges from 4 to 90%, depending on the population selected.[59] Based on results of one study, asymptomatic adults with ventricular pre-excitation are at low risk for sudden death.[18] In this study of 128 individuals (aged 25 years or older at time of entry) followed for 5 to 25 years, 17 (13%) had a documented tachycardia. Of these, 15 had clinical evidence or histories indicative of paroxysmal tachycardias at the time of the initial electrocardiogram. No deaths were attributable to arrhythmias or associated cardiovascular disease during the study.

Noninvasive Evaluation

Appropriate use of noninvasive techniques provides valuable information in the evaluation of patients with pre-excitation syndromes. Electrocardiographic patterns of pre-excitation recorded during sinus rhythm confirm the presence of a manifest accessory pathway and can be used to estimate its location.[92, 144] Although exercise testing is not a reliable method for inducing arrhythmias in patients with pre-excitation syndromes,[137] the presence or absence of pre-excitation during peak exercise has been used to stratify risk for the propensity to sustain a rapid ventricular rate during episodes of atrial fibrillation.[22, 41, 89, 131] Analysis of ventricular wall motion using radionuclide ventriculography and echocardiography has been used to estimate the location of accessory pathways.[20, 46] Each technique is limited by image resolution and the degree of pre-excitation present at the time of evaluation, and neither offers a distinct advantage over analysis of the 12-lead electrocardiogram. The echocardiogram is helpful in the detection of congenital abnormalities that may be associated with pre-excitation syndromes.

ELECTROCARDIOGRAPHIC FEATURES OF PRE-EXCITATION SYNDROMES

The electrocardiographic features of the WPW syndrome include (1) a short P-R interval (<120 ms) during sinus rhythm, (2) an initial slurring of the QRS complex (delta wave), (3) an abnormally wide QRS complex ($\geq$120 ms), and (4) secondary ST and T wave changes.[153] These features have been used to gain insight into the location of an accessory pathway. Rosenbaum et al.[122] classified electrocardiograms from patients manifesting pre-excitation into type A and B patterns. The type A pattern has positive delta waves and upright QRS complexes in all precordial leads and is attributed to early activation of the left ventricle. The type B pattern, associated with premature right ventricular activation, is characterized by negative delta waves in leads V_1–V_2 with positive delta waves and upright complexes in leads V_3–V_6. This classification scheme is based on deductive reasoning and does not take into consideration patterns of pre-excitation that are characteristic of accessory pathways located in the septum. Boineau et al.[19] and Tonkin and colleagues[144] detected a spectrum of electrocardiographic patterns in patients with the WPW syndrome and demonstrated the association of certain patterns with the anatomic location of the accessory pathway identified during intraoperative mapping. Composite delta wave patterns observed during maximal ventricular pre-excitation have been proposed, based on data derived from these studies.

We recently determined the concordance between electrocardiographic patterns recorded during sinus rhythm when pre-excitation was not maximal and the location of accessory pathways determined using catheter and intraoperative computer-assisted mapping.[92] Representative 12-lead electrocardiograms obtained from patients with accessory pathways at left-lateral (Fig. 10–3), left-posterior (Fig. 10–4), posterior-septal (Fig. 10–5), right free-wall (Fig. 10–6), and anterior-septal (Fig. 10–7) locations are shown. Propagation of the wavefront of excitation away from the accessory pathway results in negative delta waves in the electrocardiographic leads subtending this region of the heart. Moreover, the eccentric pattern of ventricular activation results in abnormalities of the mean frontal-plane QRS axis and the point of R wave transition in the horizontal plane. The combination of these three electrocardiographic features enables accurate identification of the region of an anatomic accessory pathway during sinus rhythm, provided that a sufficient degree of ventricular pre-excitation is present (Table 10–1). These characteristic patterns were detectable in 91% of electrocardiograms from patients with left-lateral pathways demonstrating pre-excitation during sinus rhythm, 88% of electrocardiograms in those with left-posterior pathways, and 100% of electrocardiograms in those with posterior-septal, right free-wall, or anterior-septal pathways.

There are obvious limitations to relying exclusively on electrocardiographic criteria for regionalizing accessory pathway locations. Temporal variation in the degree of pre-excitation results in variable QRS morphologies. QRS patterns are influenced by body habitus, orientation of the heart within the chest cavity, and the presence or absence of structural heart disease. Moreover, the proposed electrocardiographic criteria may not be applicable to patients with multiple accessory pathways, which are detectable in approximately 13% of patients with the pre-excitation syndrome.[34] However, as shown in Figure 10–8, electrocardiographic patterns that shift from region to region or have features characteristic of more than one region suggest the presence of multiple accessory pathways. Although definitive localization of an accessory pathway and exclusion of multiple pathways require an invasive electrophysiologic study, one may anticipate that results of catheter mapping will corroborate interpretation of the electrocardiogram. Moreover, in some patients the coronary sinus cannot be cannulated or right atrial endocardial mapping cannot be performed adequately. In such instances, the standard 12-lead electrocardiogram can be used to estimate reliably the location of the accessory pathway.

The electrocardiographic features of patients with nodoventricular fibers are variable and frequently masked due to accessory pathways that often occur concomitantly. Many patients with nodoventricular fibers do not have evidence of ventricular pre-excitation in electrocardiograms obtained during sinus rhythm.[10] The absence of apparent pre-excitation during sinus rhythm is attributable to the refractory properties of the AV node and nodoventricular fiber. In some, an increase in vagal tone or an acceleration of sinus rate may delay activation of the His-Purkinje system sufficiently and promote ventricular activation through the nodoventricular fibers. The QRS pattern during pre-excitation typically resembles left bundle branch block in those patients in whom nodoventricular fibers insert at the right ventricular septum.

ELECTROCARDIOGRAPHIC FEATURES OF RECIPROCATING TACHYCARDIAS

Standard 12-lead electrocardiograms obtained during orthodromic SVT demonstrate a normal QRS morphology in the absence of aberration in the His-Purkinje system. Electrical alternans is detectable in 38% of recordings and is most often observed in leads II, III, and V_1 to V_4.[65, 76] This pattern has also been observed in up to 23% of electrocardiograms recorded during AV nodal reentry and may be more sensitive to the rate of the tachycardia than to the underlying mechanism.[76] The relationship of the P wave to the QRS complex provides a more reliable criteria for distinguishing orthodromic SVT from AV nodal reentry. During orthodromic SVT, atrial activation begins 70 to 100 ms after the onset of the QRS and requires 50 to 60 ms for completion. Consequently, in 90% of patients, the P wave occurs after the QRS complex and distorts the ST segment in the first half of the R-R interval. Rarely, the P wave is detectable in the second half of the R-R interval (5%) or distorts the terminal QRS complex (5%). In contrast, during AV nodal reentry, the P wave is coincident with the QRS complex (40%) or evident during the first half of the R-R interval (55%). Rarely, the P wave is detectable during the second half of the R-R interval (5%).[76] AV dissociation excludes orthodromic SVT as the mechanism of a tachycardia because of the mandatory 1:1 relationship of the atria and ventricles.

Standard 12-lead electrocardiograms recorded during antidromic SVT show maximal pre-excitation with a pattern that is characteristic of the accessory pathway location. Retrograde P waves may be evident during the first half of the R-R interval but often are difficult to detect because of the marked repolarization abnor-

TABLE 10–1
Characteristic Electrocardiographic Patterns of Accessory Pathways in Specific Regions

Region	Negative Delta Waves	QRS Axis in Frontal Plane	Transition R > S
Left-lateral	I and/or aVL	Normal	V_1–V_3
Left-posterior	III and aVF	−75 to +75	V_1
Posterior-septum	III and aVF	0 to −90	V_2–V_4
Right free-wall	aVR	Normal	V_3–V_5
Anterior-septum	V_1 and V_2	Normal	V_3–V_5

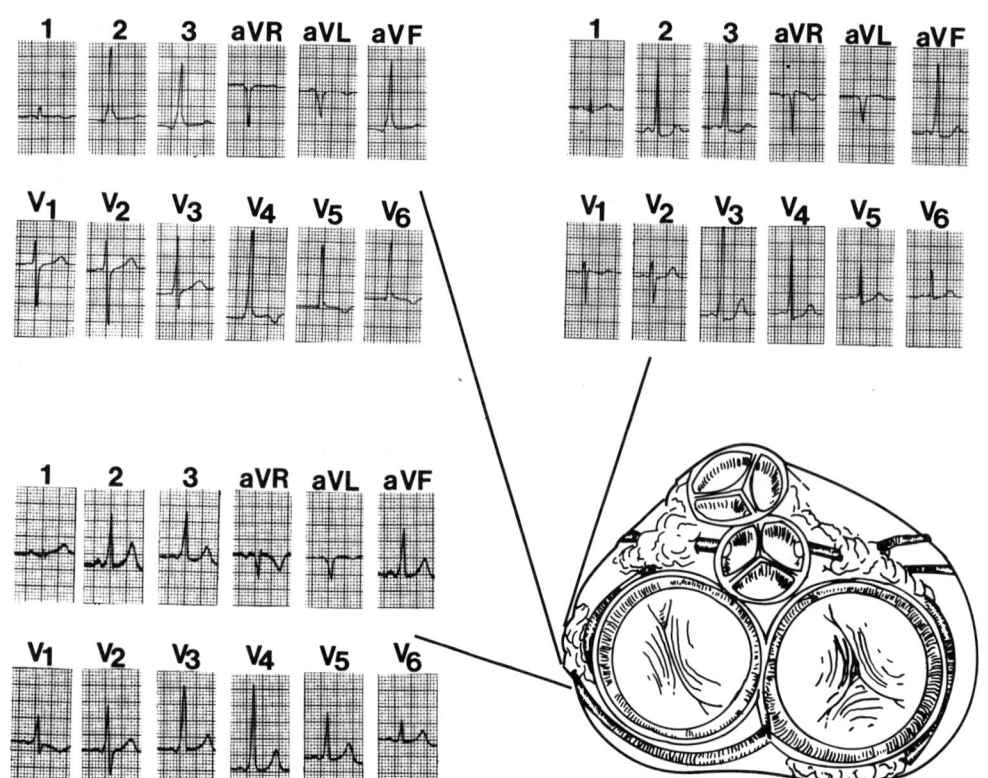

FIGURE 10–3
Representative electrocardiograms recorded during sinus rhythm from three patients with left-lateral accessory pathways. Characteristic features include negative delta waves in aVL and frequently in lead I, a normal QRS axis in the frontal plane, and early precordial R-wave transition. (Reprinted with permission from Lindsay BD, Crossen KJ, Cain ME. Am J Cardiol 59:1093, 1987.)

mality associated with pre-excited complexes. When evident, P waves have a 1:1 relationship with ventricular activation, since AV or VA block would terminate the tachycardia. The presence of AV dissociation suggests ventricular tachycardia, during which the QRS morphology may resemble pre-excitation.

Electrocardiograms (Fig. 10–9) from patients with tachycardia in which a nodoventricular fiber mediates the anterograde limb of the reentrant circuit typically exhibit a left bundle branch block configuration, a QRS duration of 0.12 to 0.15 seconds, a QRS axis from 0 to −75 degrees, and a precordial R wave

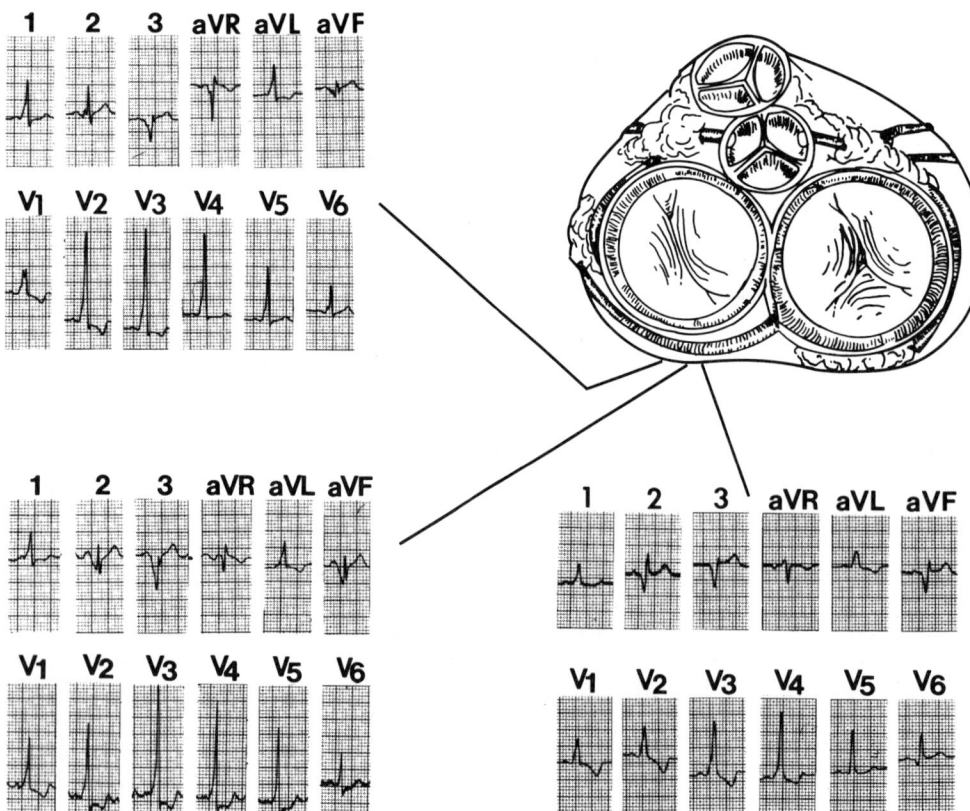

FIGURE 10–4
Representative electrocardiograms recorded during normal sinus rhythm from three patients with left-posterior accessory pathways. Characteristic features include negative delta waves in the inferior leads and a prominent R wave in V_1 (R/S ratio >1). (Reprinted with permission from Lindsay BD, Crossen KJ, Cain ME. Am J Cardiol 59:1093, 1987.)

FIGURE 10–5
Representative electrocardiograms recorded during sinus rhythm from three patients with posterior-septal accessory pathways. Characteristic features include negative delta waves in the inferior leads, left superior QRS axis, and an R/S ratio >1 in V_1. (Reprinted with permission from Lindsay BD, Crossen KJ, Cain ME. Am J Cardiol 59:1093, 1987.)

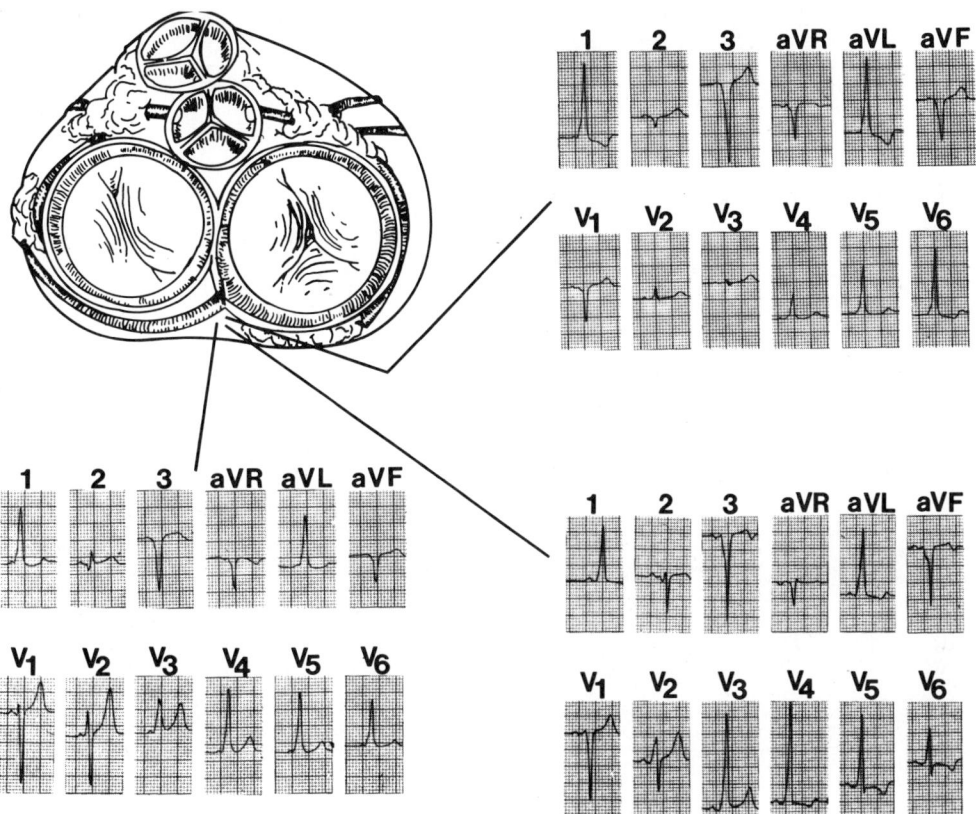

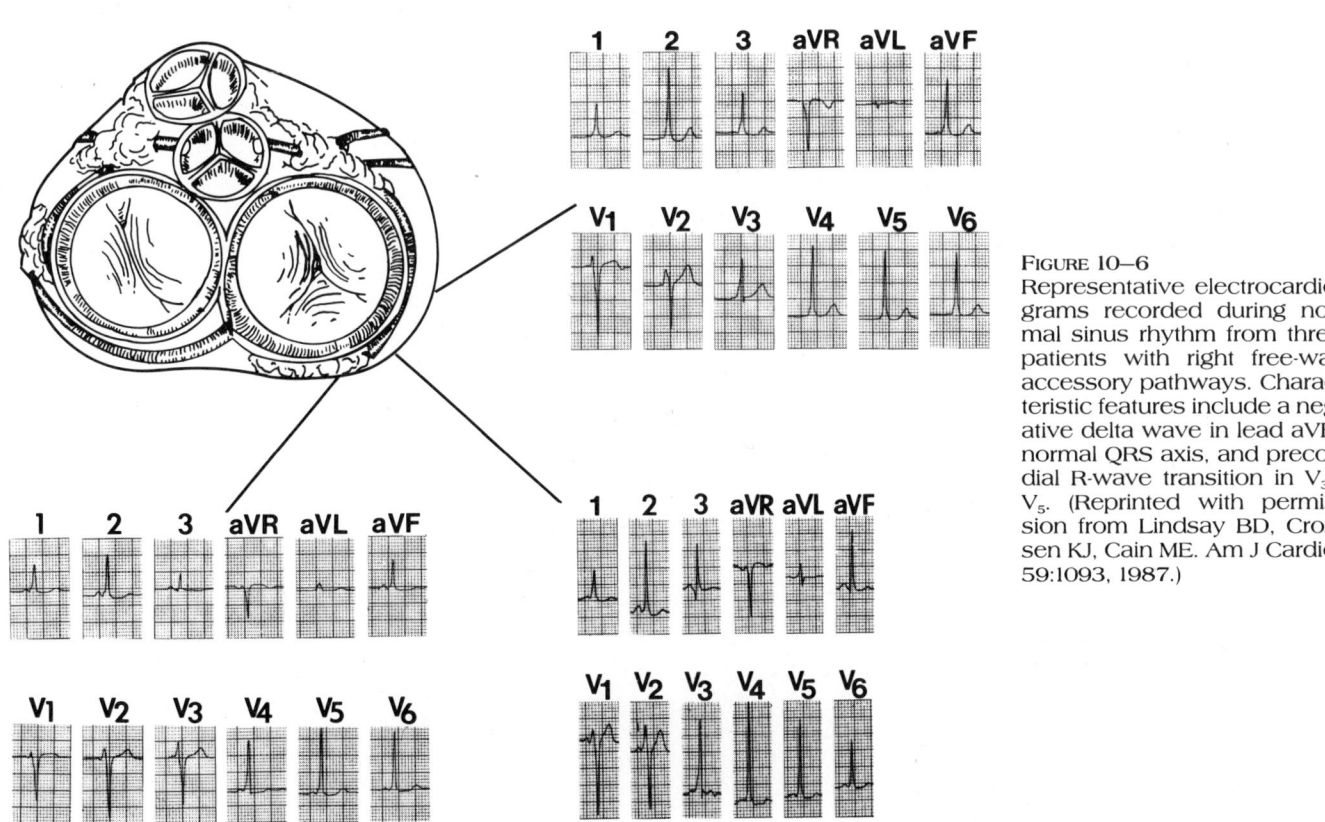

FIGURE 10–6
Representative electrocardiograms recorded during normal sinus rhythm from three patients with right free-wall accessory pathways. Characteristic features include a negative delta wave in lead aVR, normal QRS axis, and precordial R-wave transition in V_3–V_5. (Reprinted with permission from Lindsay BD, Crossen KJ, Cain ME. Am J Cardiol 59:1093, 1987.)

The Pre-excitation Syndrome

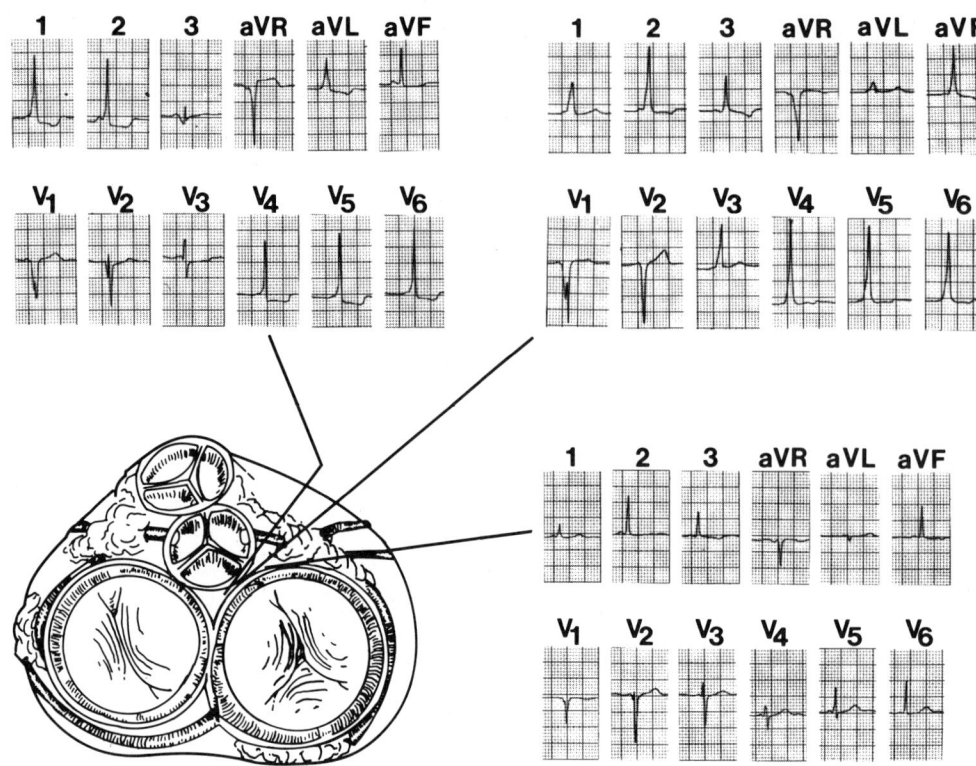

FIGURE 10–7
Representative electrocardiograms recorded during sinus rhythm from three patients with anterior-septal accessory pathways. Characteristic features include negative delta waves in V_1 and V_2, normal QRS axis, and precordial R-wave transition in V_3–V_5. (Reprinted with permission from Lindsay BD, Crossen KJ, Cain ME. Am J Cardiol 59:1093, 1987.)

transition in leads V_4 to V_6. Moreover, a small initial R wave is often observed in V_1. These criteria help differentiate a tachycardia mediated through a nodoventricular fiber from ventricular tachycardia or other tachycardias associated with a wide QRS complex.[10]

EXERCISE TESTING

The provocation of arrhythmias during exercise has been examined as a potential noninvasive technique for assessing drug efficacy. Unfortunately, arrhythmias are inducible by exercise in only 7% of patients with the pre-excitation syndrome.[22, 89, 137] Moreover, their induction is not sufficiently reproducible to enable accurate determination of drug efficacy.

The loss of pre-excitation during exercise has been advocated as a measure of low risk for the development of life-threatening ventricular rates during atrial fibrillation. Acceleration of the heart rate is associated with loss of pre-excitation in approximately 50% of pa-

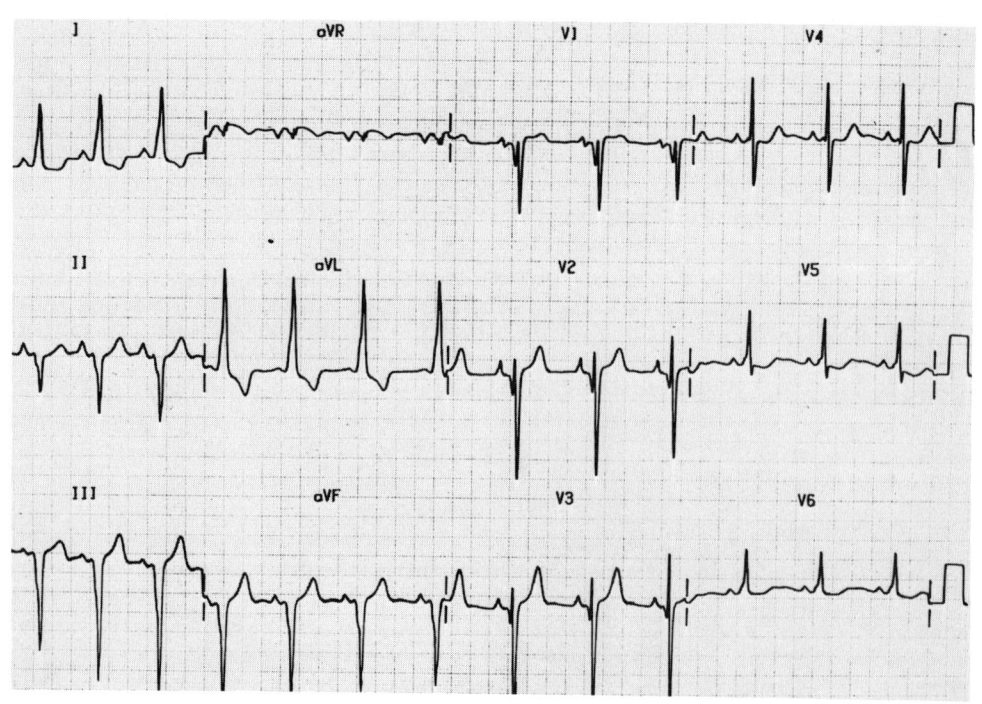

FIGURE 10–8
Standard electrocardiogram recorded during sinus rhythm from a patient with posterior-septal and anterior-septal accessory pathways. The negative delta waves inferiorly and anteriorly reflect features of pre-excitation that are characteristic of both regions.

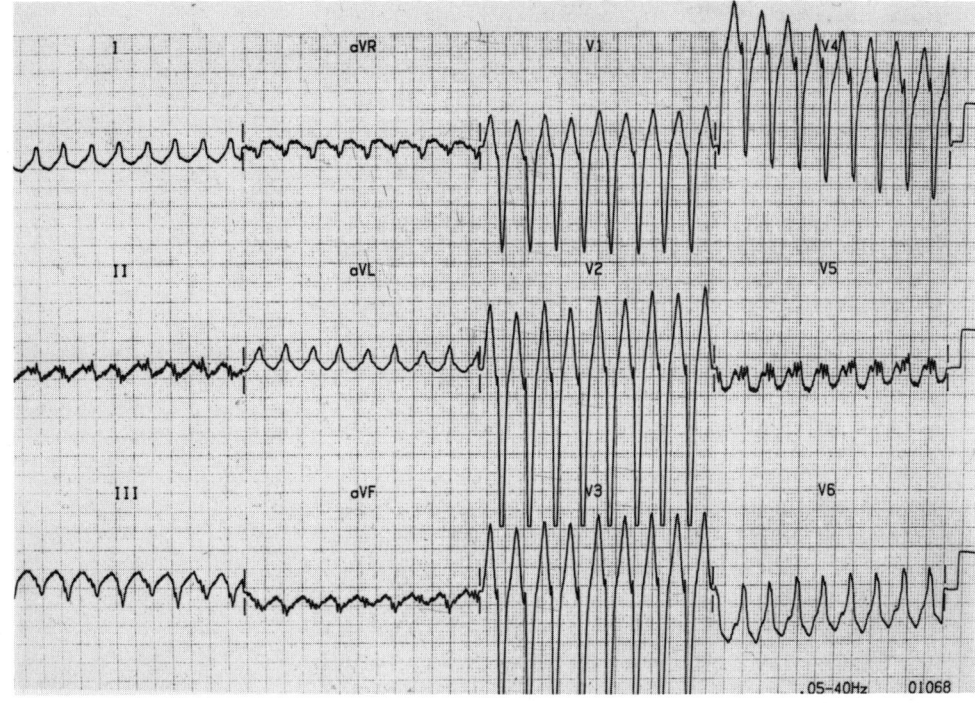

FIGURE 10–9
Representative electrocardiogram recorded during a reciprocating tachycardia in a patient with a nodoventricular fiber. Characteristic features include left bundle branch block morphology, leftward axis, R wave in lead I, rS in V_1, and precordial R-wave transition in V_5.

tients.[23, 137] Gradual loss of pre-excitation may occur because the loss of vagal tone enhances conduction through the AV node, or it may reflect the cessation of anterograde conduction over an accessory pathway. Sudden normalization of the QRS complex is more specific for anterograde block in the accessory pathway.

In one study of 56 patients with the pre-excitation syndrome, 6 of whom had a history of aborted sudden death,[131] the electrocardiograms of 34 (61%) showed continuous pre-excitation throughout exercise; 9 (16%) demonstrated gradual loss of pre-excitation; and 13 (23%) showed evidence of abrupt loss of pre-excitation. The mean shortest R-R interval during atrial fibrillation for each group was 236 ±64 ms, 242 ±37 ms, and 410 ±148 ms, respectively. While these results demonstrate a good concordance between the refractory properties of the accessory pathway measured indirectly and the presence or absence of pre-excitation during exercise, one of the 6 patients with a history of ventricular fibrillation had sudden loss of pre-excitation on the electrocardiogram during exercise, and gradual normalization of the QRS complex was observed in another patient. Analysis of the exercise test as a predictor of sudden death demonstrated a sensitivity of 80%, a specificity of 29%, and a predictive accuracy of 12%. In another study of 13 patients with a history of a rapid ventricular rate during atrial fibrillation (shortest R-R interval <250 ms) the electrocardiograms from 12 patients continued to demonstrate pre-excitation during maximal exercise.[41]

Thus, exercise testing has been shown to be of value in the differentiation of groups of patients at high or low risk for a life-threatening ventricular rate during atrial fibrillation. However, the proposed criteria must be interpreted cautiously when they are applied to individuals.

Invasive Electrophysiology Studies

INDICATIONS

Electrophysiology studies are used to (1) delineate the mechanism of arrhythmias, (2) measure the refractory periods of the accessory pathway as an indicator of the risk of sudden death in symptomatic patients, (3) assess the efficacy of antiarrhythmic agents, and (4) localize the accessory pathway in preparation for surgery. Concerns about the risk of sudden death as the presenting manifestation of pre-excitation syndromes have raised the issue of whether asymptomatic patients with pre-excitation should undergo invasive electrophysiology studies. Judging from results to date, there is no compelling evidence to support this approach.

TECHNICAL ASPECTS

During the initial electrophysiology study of patients with the pre-excitation syndrome, multi-electrode catheters are positioned in the high right atrium, coronary sinus, the AV junction, and the right ventricular apex. A No. 6 French decapolar catheter (USCI) facilitates recording close bipolar (interpole distance 5 mm) electrograms from multiple sites simultaneously in the coronary sinus. The distance between electrode pairs is 1 cm. Alternatively, a No. 7F catheter (Mansfield) with an orthogonal electrode array may be used to enhance direct recordings of accessory pathway potentials. In studies performed at Barnes Hospital, surface leads I, aVF, and V_1 are recorded simultaneously with intracardiac electrograms. Data are stored on magnetic tape (Honeywell 5600C) and electrograms are printed on a 16-channel Inkjet recorder (Siemens Mingograph) at paper speeds of 100 to 250 mm/s. Programmed stimulation is performed with a programmable stimulator and optically isolated constant source (Bloom Assoc.). Electrical stimuli are rectangular pulses 1 ms in duration delivered at twice diastolic threshold (<1 mA).

Anterograde ventricular activation is evaluated during incremental atrial pacing from the high right atrium and distal coronary sinus, programmed atrial extrastimuli from the high right atrium and distal coronary sinus, induced arrhythmias, and spontaneous junctional beats. The retrograde atrial activation pattern is evaluated during incremental ventricular pacing, the introduction of programmed ventricular extrastimuli, and induced arrhythmias. During atrial and ventricular pacing, the cycle length is decreased by 50-ms steps to a cycle length of 300 ms and then by 10-ms steps to a cycle length of 250 ms or until orthodromic or antidromic SVT is initiated. Pacing at each cycle length is continued until stable patterns of AV or VA conduction are obtained. The anterograde refractory periods of the accessory pathway are determined by the introduction of single atrial extrastimuli at paced cycle lengths of 600 and 400 ms. Coupling intervals are decreased by 10-ms steps to determine the presence or absence of dual AV nodal pathways. The retrograde refractory properties of the accessory pathway are determined by the introduction of single ventricular extrastimuli during paced cycle lengths of 600 and 400 ms.

DIAGNOSTIC CRITERIA FOR ATRIOVENTRICULAR REENTRY

Orthodromic SVT is the most common arrhythmia in patients with accessory pathways and is inducible by programmed stimulation in 90 to 95% of patients who have experienced this arrhythmia clinically. Figure 10–10 shows representative intracardiac recordings from a patient during orthodromic SVT. The criteria for diagnosis include (1) anterograde conduction through the AV node and His bundle, (2) eccentric retrograde atrial activation through the accessory pathway (may not be evident with septal pathways), (3) pre-excitation of the atria during SVT without a change in the activation sequence by premature ventricular extrastimuli introduced at a time when the His bundle is refractory, and (4) increase in the VA interval with bundle branch block ipsilateral to the accessory pathway (not observed with septal pathways).

Antidromic SVT occurs less commonly than orthodromic SVT but requires careful evaluation to exclude other wide-complex tachycardias. Multiple accessory pathways have been reported in up to 48% of patients with antidromic SVT.[12] The initiation of antidromic SVT in patients with single accessory pathways appears dependent on a critical distance (≥4 cm) between the location of the accessory pathway and the AV node/His bundle. In contrast, most patients with antidromic SVT in which a posterior-septal pathway functions as the anterograde limb utilize a second accessory path-

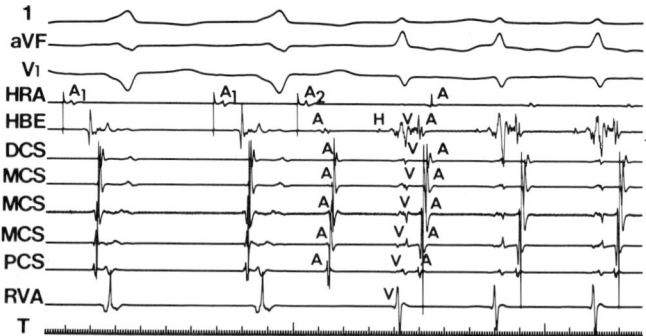

FIGURE 10–10
Induction of orthodromic supraventricular tachycardia (SVT) in a patient with a posterior-septal accessory pathway by a programmed atrial extrastimulus. The figure is organized from top to bottom with electrocardiographic leads I, aVF, and V_1, intracardiac recordings from the high right atrium (HRA); His-bundle region (HBE); distal (DCS), mid (MCS), and proximal coronary sinus (PCS); right ventricular apex (RVA); and time lines (T). Atrial pacing was performed at a cycle length of 600 ms (A_1–A_1). The accessory pathway was refractory when an atrial extrastimulus (A_2) was introduced at a coupling interval of 330 ms. Following the atrial extrastimulus the ventricle was activated exclusively by the normal conduction system, resulting in a normal QRS complex. The accessory pathway recovered and conducted retrogradely to initiate orthodromic SVT. Earliest retrograde atrial activation was recorded in the proximal coronary sinus (PCS).

way or a nodoventricular fiber as the retrograde component of the reentrant circuit. Figure 10–11 demonstrates representative intracardiac recordings from a patient during antidromic SVT. The criteria for diagnosis include (1) eccentric ventricular activation with a QRS morphology identical to that obtained during atrial pacing at a cycle length that produces maximal pre-excitation, (2) a 1:1 relationship between the atria and ventricles, (3) demonstration that the ventricle is an essential component of the reentrant circuit by

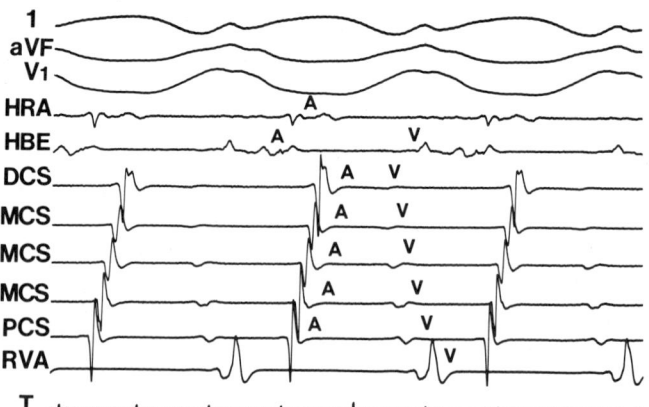

FIGURE 10–11
Intracardiac recordings during antidromic supraventricular tachycardia (SVT) from a patient with a left lateral accessory pathway. The figure is arranged using a format similar to that used in Figure 10–10. Anterograde activation of the ventricle occurs exclusively through the accessory pathway and is earliest in the distal coronary sinus (DCS), corresponding to a left-lateral site. Retrograde atrial activation occurs via the normal conduction system.

terminating the tachycardia with a premature ventricular depolarization without depolarizing the His bundle or the atria, and (4) demonstration that the sequence of retrograde atrial activation during ventricular pacing is identical to that during the tachycardia. Ventricular tachycardia virtually can be excluded if a premature atrial depolarization advances the next ventricular cycle without changing the QRS morphology or the earliest site recording ventricular activation.

METHODS FOR INDUCTION OF ATRIOVENTRICULAR REENTRY

Programmed stimulation facilitates induction of orthodromic and antidromic SVT because of differences in the refractory properties of components of the normal AV conduction system and the accessory pathway. In most patients in whom orthodromic SVT occurs spontaneously, the anterograde refractory period of the accessory pathway exceeds that of the AV node, thereby providing the substrate for unidirectional block required for initiation and maintenance of reentry.[45] Figure 10–10 illustrates induction of orthodromic SVT by a critically timed atrial extrastimulus that blocked in the accessory pathway but conducted through the normal AV conduction system to excite the ventricle, with sufficient delay to enable the accessory pathway time to recover and conduct retrogradely to initiate the tachycardia. Inducibility is enhanced by increasing the disparity between the anterograde refractory properties of the two pathways. The coupling interval of an extrastimulus that induces reentry has been shown to vary according to the paced cycle length[143] and the distance of the stimulus from the accessory pathway.[115] The activation wavefront of an extrastimulus from the right atrium must traverse the left atrium to depolarize a left-lateral pathway, which delays the effective prematurity of the excitation wavefront at the site of the accessory pathway. Stimulation in close proximity of the accessory pathway obviates this delay due to atrial conduction. Thus, in many patients with left free-wall pathways, the coupling interval of an atrial extrastimulus from the left atrium required to initiate orthodromic SVT is approximately 50 ms longer than that required for induction by right atrial stimulation. In patients in whom antidromic SVT is inducible by programmed atrial stimulation, the anterograde refractory periods of the accessory pathway are shorter than those of the AV node. The activation wavefront of a critically timed atrial extrastimulus encounters block anterogradely in the AV node, conducts exclusively through the accessory pathway to excite the ventricles, and re-excites the atria by conducting retrogradely through the normal conduction system or other accessory pathway tissue.

Induction of orthodromic or antidromic SVT by programmed ventricular stimulation is dependent on the retrograde refractory properties of the components of the normal conduction system and the accessory pathway.[138] In patients in whom orthodromic SVT is inducible by programmed ventricular stimulation, the retrograde refractory period of the normal AV conduction system exceeds that of the accessory pathway. A critically timed ventricular extrastimulus blocks in the AV node/His bundle, conducts retrogradely through the accessory pathway to the atria, and activates the AV node/His bundle anterogradely to complete the circuit. During initiation of antidromic SVT by programmed ventricular stimulation, retrograde block occurs first in the accessory pathway, whereas conduction retrogradely to the atria is through the normal AV conduction system or through another anomalous connection in those patients with multiple accessory pathways.

CATHETER MAPPING

Comprehensive catheter mapping provides accurate, detailed information pertinent to the number and location of accessory pathways. Initially, catheters are positioned in the coronary sinus, high lateral right atrium, low right atrial septum (His bundle), and right ventricular apex. The majority of mapping is performed using the coronary sinus and right atrial catheters.

Spatial location of electrode positions is determined using multiplane fluoroscopy. During mapping of the coronary sinus a 45-degree left-anterior oblique view is used to partition the coronary sinus into anterior-lateral, lateral, posterior-lateral, posterior, paraseptal, and septal segments. The decapolar mapping catheter is first advanced distally to record from anterior-lateral to posterior segments of the coronary sinus. The catheter is then withdrawn until the proximal electrode is at the os of the coronary sinus. With the catheter in this position, electrograms are recorded from posterior to septal segments of the coronary sinus. An abrupt decrease in the amplitude of electrograms measured from the proximal pair of electrodes occurs when cavity potentials are recorded and suggests that the catheter has been withdrawn too far. During right atrial mapping, the quadripolar catheter positioned initially at a high lateral right atrial site is used to map around the tricuspid annulus. A 45-degree right-anterior oblique view is used to distinguish anterior from posterior electrode sites and a 45-degree left-anterior oblique view is used to differentiate lateral from septal sites.

ANALYSIS OF VENTRICULAR ACTIVATION PATTERNS

Ventricular activation at each site is determined by measuring the interval between the onset of the delta wave on the surface electrocardiogram and the first major deflection of each local ventricular electrogram. The site at which the shortest delta-to-V interval is measured defines the region of the ventricular insertion of the accessory pathway. Incremental atrial pacing can be expected to increase the degree of ventricular pre-excitation and to accentuate early ventricular activation in the proximity of the accessory pathway. Pacing from the distal coronary sinus accentuates ventricular pre-excitation in patients with left-sided pathways, minimizing the effects of intra-atrial conduction delay and the relative contribution of conduction through the AV node/His-Purkinje system to ventricular activation. Figure 10–12 illustrates patterns of eccentric ventricular activation in patients with left-lateral, posterior-septal, and right free-wall accessory pathways. During atrial pacing, the degree of pre-excitation may vary depending on the paced cycle length; however, the delta-to-V interval remains relatively constant in the proximity of the accessory pathway. Pacing at shorter cycle lengths delays conduction through the AV node and accentuates patterns of pre-excitation. Changes in delta wave morphology or detection of a second site with a short delta-to-V interval suggest the presence of additional accessory pathways.

ANALYSIS OF RETROGRADE ATRIAL ACTIVATION PATTERNS

Retrograde atrial activation patterns are expressed as VA intervals measured from the onset of the QRS during orthodromic SVT or from the pacing stimulus during ventricular pacing to the first major deflection of each local atrial electrogram. In the absence of an accessory pathway, earliest retrograde atrial activation is recorded at the low right atrial septum from the His bundle catheter. In some individuals, atrial activation recorded from the os of the coronary sinus may occur simultaneously with that recorded from the low right atrial septum or may follow it closely. The atrial insertion of an accessory pathway is identified as the site demonstrating the shortest VA interval during orthodromic SVT. Figure 10–13 illustrates three representative patterns of retrograde atrial activation during orthodromic SVT from patients with accessory pathways at left-lateral, left-posterior, and posterior-septal sites.

Retrograde atrial activation during orthodromic SVT is typically detectable 70 to 100 ms after the onset of the surface QRS. As described by Coumel and Attuel[36] and illustrated in Figure 10–14, bundle branch block ipsilateral to a left- or right-sided accessory pathway lengthens the reentrant circuit, typically prolonging the VA interval by 25 to 70 ms. The standard electrocardiogram demonstrates a bundle branch block–dependent decrease in the rate of the tachycardia. If neither right nor left bundle branch block alters the VA

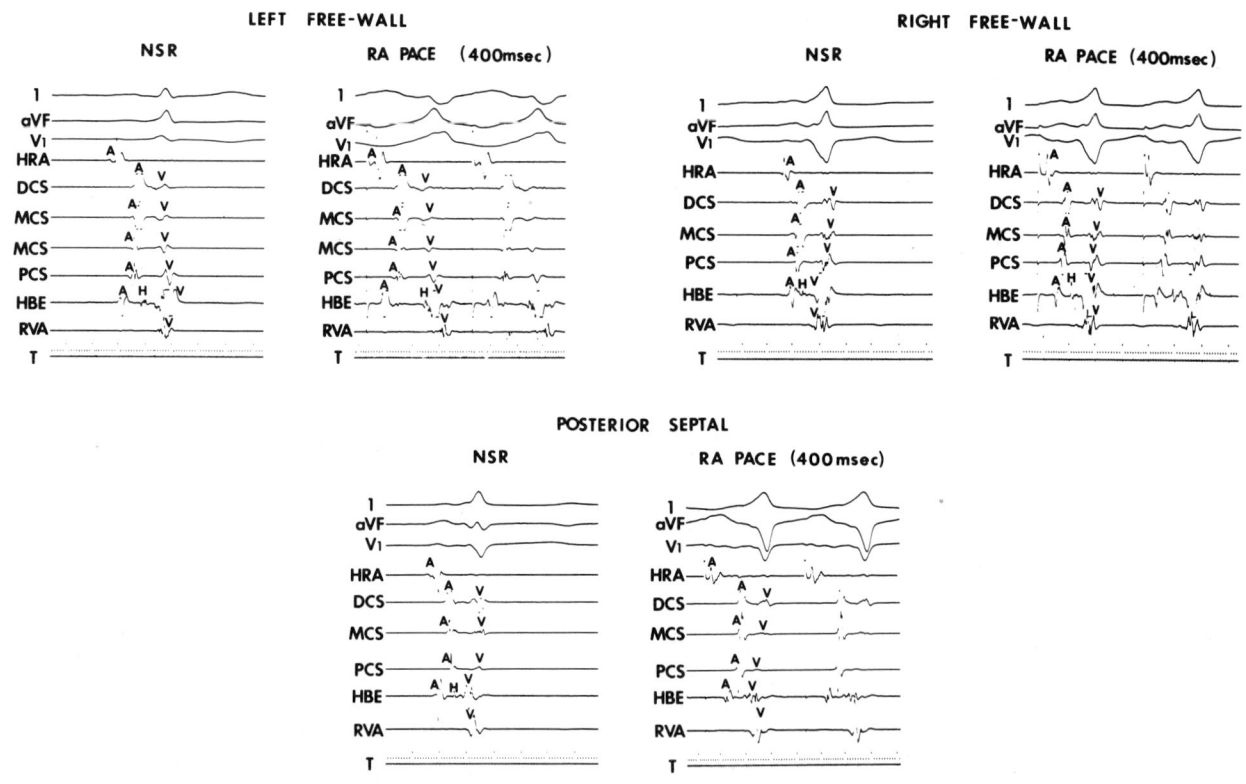

FIGURE 10–12
Representative patterns of anterograde ventricular activation during sinus rhythm and high right atrial pacing from three different patients with left free-wall, posterior-septal, and right free-wall accessory pathways, respectively. In the patient with a left free-wall pathway, earliest ventricular activation is recorded from the distal coronary sinus (DCS) electrode and corresponds to a left-posterior site. During sinus rhythm and atrial pacing at a cycle length of 400 ms in the patient with a posterior-septal accessory pathway, earliest ventricular activation is recorded from the HBE catheter. During atrial pacing, ventricular activation at the proximal coronary sinus (PCS) recording site is earlier than that during sinus rhythm. The PCS recording site corresponds to a left paraseptal location. The shortest delta-to-V interval was measured when the PCS electrodes were positioned at the os of the coronary sinus. In the patient with a right free-wall accessory pathway, earliest ventricular activation is recorded from the HBE and RVA catheters. Left ventricular activation as measured from the CS catheter recording sites occurs later. (Reproduced by permission From Cain ME, Cox JL: Surgical treatment of supraventricular tachyarrhythmias. In Platia EV (ed.): Management of Cardiac Arrhythmias—The Nonpharmacologic Approach, p. 311, 399. Philadelphia, J. B. Lippincott, 1987.)

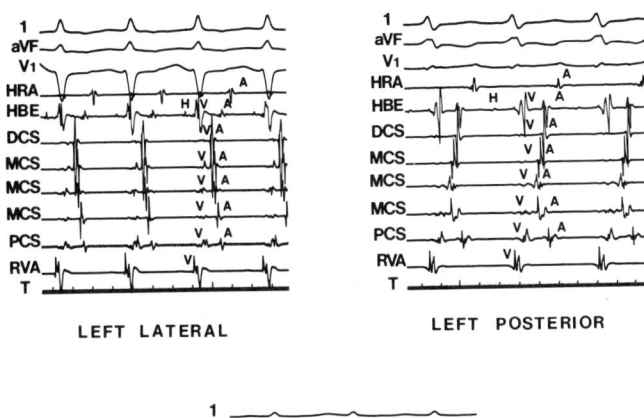
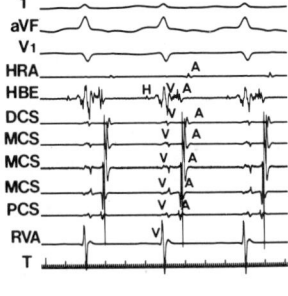

FIGURE 10–13
Representative patterns of retrograde atrial activation during orthodromic supraventricular tachycardia (SVT) from three different patients with left-lateral, left-posterior, and posterior-septal accessory pathways. Earliest atrial activation is recorded from the distal coronary sinus (DCS) electrode from the patient with a left-lateral accessory pathway and at the mid-coronary sinus (MCS) from the patient with a left-posterior pathway. Earliest atrial activation is recorded in the proximal coronary sinus (PCS) from the patient with a posterior-septal accessory pathway.

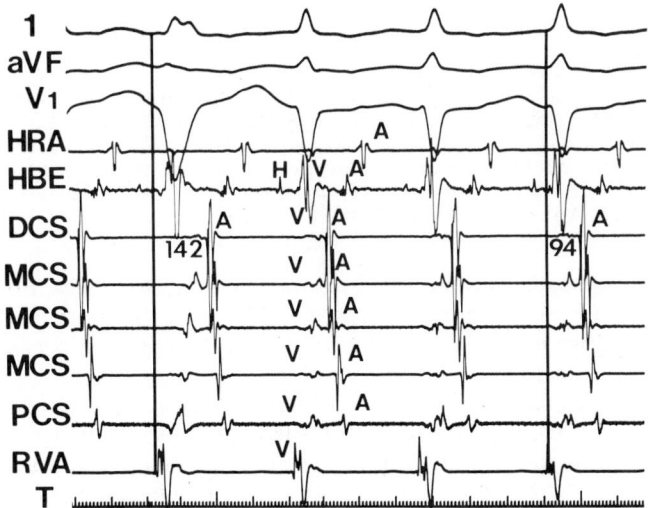

FIGURE 10–14
Effect of left bundle branch block on ventriculoatrial conduction during orthodromic supraventricular tachycardia (SVT) from a patient with a left-lateral accessory pathway. Because left bundle branch block (first beat) lengthened the reentrant circuit, earliest atrial activation in the distal coronary sinus (DCS) changed from 94 to 142 ms, an increment of 48 ms. The cycle length of the tachycardia was also prolonged.

interval, a septal pathway most likely is present. In patients with septal pathways, the pattern of retrograde atrial activation may be difficult to distinguish from that observed during retrograde propagation through the normal conduction system. Differentiation of orthodromic SVT from AV nodal reentry is best accomplished by analysis of the minimum VA conduction time and the response to programmed ventricular extrastimuli. During AV nodal reentry, activation of the atria and ventricles often is simultaneous. The interval from the onset of the QRS to the earliest atrial recording is generally less than 60 ms. In contrast, this interval during orthodromic SVT is rarely, if ever, less than 70 ms. A premature ventricular extrastimulus, introduced during orthodromic SVT when the His bundle is refractory, that prematurely depolarizes the atrium with the same retrograde sequence confirms that the retrograde limb of the circuit is composed of an accessory pathway.

Whenever possible, localization of the atrial insertion of the accessory pathway should be based on analysis of atrial activation during orthodromic SVT. In patients in whom the accessory pathway is concealed, localization is dependent solely on identification of the atrial insertion. There are practical limitations to this approach: for example, in some patients orthodromic SVT is not inducible by programmed stimulation or is associated with such deleterious hemodynamic effects that extensive mapping is precluded. In such instances, analysis of retrograde atrial activation during ventricular pacing is an alternative method to localize the atrial insertion of the accessory pathway. However, variability in retrograde conduction through the normal conduction system or multiple accessory pathways during ventricular pacing may result in atrial fusion that may obscure the location of the accessory pathway if one relies only on qualitative patterns of retrograde atrial activation.

During orthodromic SVT, when retrograde atrial activation occurs exclusively through the accessory pathway, the interval of time (ΔA-SVT) between the atrial electrogram recorded at the site of the accessory pathway and the atrial electrogram subtending the AV node (recorded from the His bundle catheter) reflects the distance of the accessory pathway from the AV node and can be used as an index of the eccentricity of the accessory pathway.[42] Characteristic values for the ΔA-SVT interval have been defined for left-lateral (66 $\pm$ 17 ms), left-posterior (50 $\pm$ 8 ms), posterior-septal (33 $\pm$ 7 ms), right free-wall (22 $\pm$ 15 ms), and anterior-septal (0 $\pm$ 0 ms) accessory pathway sites.

During ventricular pacing, the interval between the earliest atrial electrogram and the atrial electrogram recorded from the His bundle (ΔA-VP) can also be used as a measure of eccentricity and to identify the paced cycle length at which retrograde conduction occurs exclusively through the accessory pathway. The anatomic position of the electrode pair demonstrating the earliest atrial electrogram during ventricular pacing can thus be used to accurately identify the accessory pathway location if the ΔA-VP interval is comparable with the ΔA-SVT value characteristic of that accessory pathway location. Using this approach, we have found that values for the ΔA-VP interval are concordant with those for the ΔA-SVT (Fig. 10–15). Figure 10–16 illustrates representative recordings from a patient with a left free-wall accessory pathway in whom eccentric retrograde atrial activation during ventricular pacing became evident only during a paced cycle length of 280 ms. Thus, for patients in whom orthodromic SVT cannot be induced, the location of the accessory pathway can be determined accurately by the pattern of retrograde atrial activation during ventricular pacing.

EVALUATION OF PATIENTS WITH INCESSANT ATRIOVENTRICULAR REENTRY

Following the original description by Coumel et al.,[37] the incessant form of reentry has been widely recognized. Most commonly, the reentrant circuit is composed of anterograde conduction through the AV node/His bundle with retrograde propagation through a posterior-septal pathway exhibiting properties of decremental conduction;[67] one patient, however, has been described in whom the anterograde limb was a second accessory pathway located at a left-lateral site.[66] The A-H and H-V intervals recorded during the tachycardia are typically normal. Earliest retrograde atrial activation is usually recorded near the os of the coronary sinus. Premature activation of the atria by programmed ventricular extrastimuli introduced during the tachycardia when the His-Purkinje system is refractory confirms that the retrograde limb of the tachycardia is

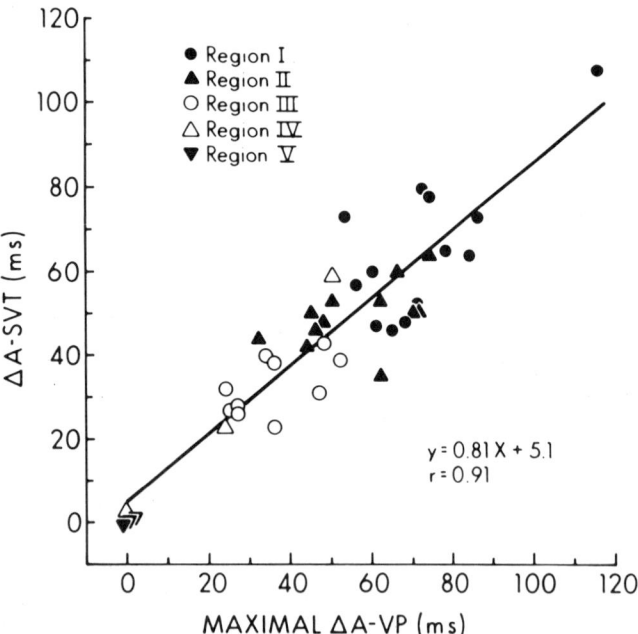

FIGURE 10–15
Comparison between values for the ΔA-SVT interval and maximum values for the ΔA-VP interval. Regions I through V correspond to left lateral, left-posterior, posterior-septal, right free-wall and anterior-septal sites, respectively. (Reprinted by permission of the American College of Cardiology from Crossen KJ, Lindsay BD, Cain ME: J Am Coll Cardiol 9:1279, 1987.)

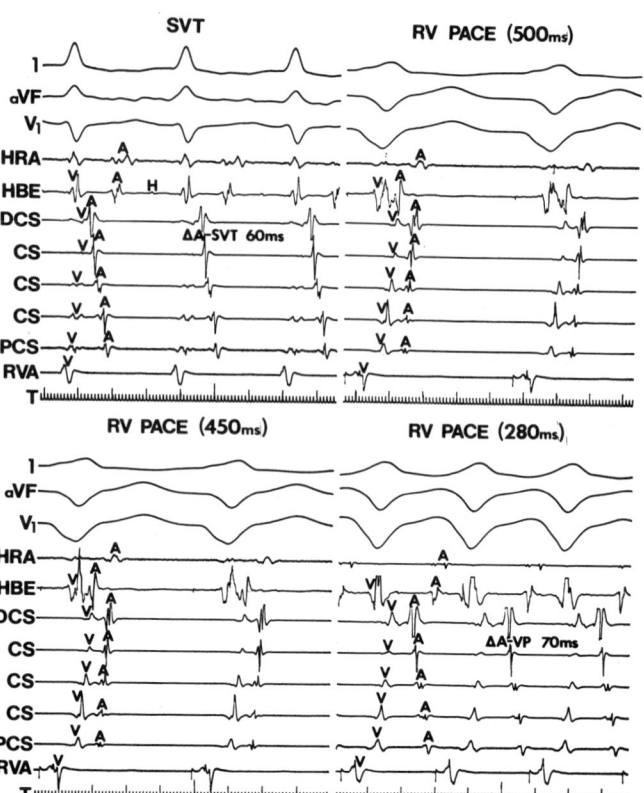

FIGURE 10–16
Retrograde atrial activation patterns from a patient with a left-lateral accessory pathway during orthodromic SVT and during right ventricular (RV) pacing at 500, 400, and 280 ms. During orthodromic supraventricular tachycardia (SVT), retrograde atrial activation is present with the earliest atrial electrogram recorded from the distal coronary sinus (DCS) electrodes. The value for the ΔA-SVT interval is 60 ms. During right ventricular pacing at 500 and 400 ms, eccentric atrial activation is not evident. The His-bundle atrial electrogram is earliest because of retrograde conduction occurring predominantly through the normal AV conduction system. Detection and localization of an accessory pathway are not possible during right ventricular pacing at these rates. During right ventricular pacing at 280 ms, however, eccentric atrial activation is present and a ΔA-VP interval comparable to that observed during SVT confirms the presence of an accessory pathway and allows accurate localization to a left-lateral site. (Reprinted by permission of the American College of Cardiology from Crossen KJ, Lindsay BD, Cain ME: J Am Coll Cardiol 9:1279, 1987.)

composed of an accessory pathway; paradoxically, delay in retrograde atrial activation may be observed because of decremental conduction through the accessory pathway.

Although retrograde conduction over a nodoventricular fiber provides an alternative explanation for these findings, the pattern of retrograde atrial activation has been most consistent with a posterior-septal accessory pathway. The atypical properties of these pathways may be attributable to structural and geometric considerations. In one postmortem study the accessory pathway exhibited a tortuous oblique course across the AV annulus. Histologic sections revealed interstitial fibrosis within the pathway and at the level of the ventricular insertion.[40]

Recently, we and others have identified patients in

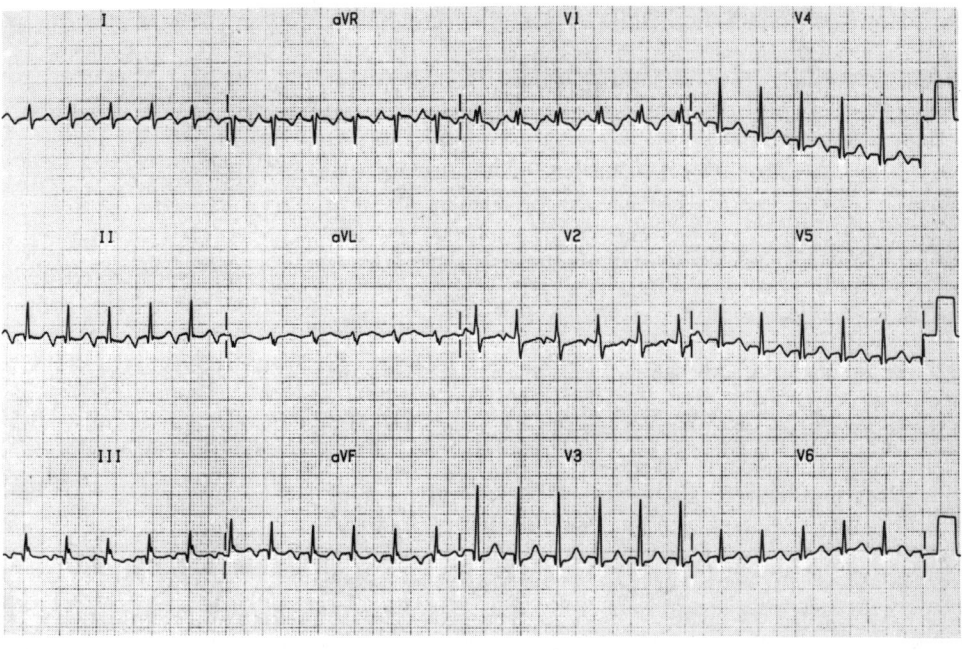

FIGURE 10–17
Standard electrocardiogram recorded from a patient with incessant AV reentry attributable to a left-lateral pathway with features of decremental conduction. The RP interval is prolonged. Negative P waves are apparent in the lateral leads. Right bundle branch block is evident during the tachycardia.

whom incessant AV reentry was attributable to a left-lateral accessory pathway.[110] Figure 10–17 shows a representative electrocardiogram recorded during an incessant tachycardia that utilizes a concealed left-lateral accessory pathway for the retrograde limb of the reentrant circuit. The R-P interval is prolonged and, as expected with retrograde conduction through a left lateral pathway, negative P waves were observed in leads I, II, III, aVF, and V_4–V_6. Figure 10–18 demonstrates the intracardiac recordings. The QRS complex is normal, and ventricular activation in the proximity of the accessory pathway is not delayed. The long R-P interval is attributable to prolonged conduction through the accessory pathway. Termination of the tachycardia occurred during block in either the anterograde or retrograde limb of the circuit. Epicardial mapping at the time of surgery confirmed the left-lateral location of the accessory pathway, which was divided successfully.

Irrespective of the location of the accessory pathway, the incessant form of AV reentry is often refractory to medical therapy. Antiarrhythimc medications that prolong AV nodal conduction or refractoriness of the accessory pathway may slow the rate of the tachycardia without terminating it.

EVALUATION OF PATIENTS WITH MULTIPLE ACCESSORY PATHWAYS

Evolving techniques of catheter and intraoperative mapping have led to improved recognition of patients with multiple accessory pathways. Clinical features that have been found to be associated with multiple pathways are Ebstein's anomaly and a history of antidromic SVT.[34] The prevalence of coexistent right-sided pathways may be increased in patients with posterior-septal pathways.[105] Preferential conduction through one accessory pathway may mask the detection of others, necessitating careful analysis of anterograde and retrograde activation sequences. Evidence supporting the presence of multiple pathways includes (1) multiple patterns of eccentric retrograde atrial activation during orthodromic SVT, (2) antidromic SVT with eccentric retrograde atrial activation, (3) multiple patterns of ventricular pre-excitation during programmed atrial stimulation or atrial fibrillation, and (4) early eccentric retrograde atrial activation at multiple sites during programmed ventricular stimulation.

To enhance detection of more than one pattern of anterograde ventricular activation, incremental atrial pacing and programmed atrial stimulation should be performed from both the right and left atria. Right atrial stimulation may facilitate conduction through a right free-wall or septal pathway without revealing a

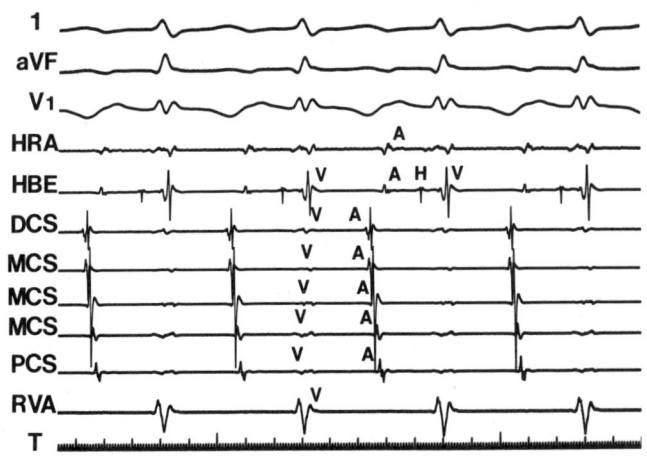

FIGURE 10–18
Intracardiac recording during incessant AV reentry in a patient with a left-lateral accessory pathway that exhibited properties of decremental conduction. Earliest atrial activation is recorded in the distal coronary sinus (DCS), corresponding to a left lateral site. VA conduction is delayed, resulting in a long RP interval detectable on the surface electrocardiogram.

coexistent left-sided pathway. Conversely, left atrial stimulation enhances preferential conduction through a left free-wall pathway. Multiple accessory pathways may also be exposed by introducing atrial extrastimuli at more than one paced cycle length to enhance differences in the refractory properties of the pathways. Figure 10–19 shows intracardiac recordings from a patient with posterior-septal and left-lateral accessory pathways in whom distinctive changes in QRS morphology and ventricular activation were observed when anterograde conduction alternated between the two pathways. In patients with antidromic SVT in whom retrograde atrial activation is through the normal conduction system, the earliest atrial activation is in the His bundle electrogram.

In some patients, a retrograde His deflection may not be evident during the tachycardia, and atrial activation may be recorded almost simultaneously at the region of the AV node and at the os of the coronary sinus. Exclusion of a concealed posterior-septal pathway as the retrograde limb is achieved best by careful mapping of the atrial septum between the os of the coronary sinus and AV nodal region. In addition, introduction of ventricular extrastimuli during the tachycardia should demonstrate decremental retrograde conduction if the normal conduction system composes the retrograde limb. A posterior-septal pathway with decremental conduction may be difficult to exclude if atrial activation in the His bundle atrial electrogram is not distinctly earlier than that recorded at the os of the coronary sinus.

The surgical approach to divide accessory pathways is dependent on the location of the accessory pathway. Incorrect identification of the location and failure to recognize the presence of additional pathways are among the most frequent causes of surgical failure. In addition, we have occasionally noted broad regions of early eccentric atrial activation during orthodromic SVT that appear to represent a relatively wide band of accessory pathway tissue. When these bands occur at the junction of the posterior-septal and left-paraseptal sites, it may be necessary to dissect both regions.

EVALUATION OF PATIENTS WITH MAHAIM FIBERS

Because nodoventricular fibers arise from the AV node rather than the atria, their electrophysiologic features differ from those of accessory pathways that bridge the annulus fibrosus. Depending on the level of the AV node from which a nodoventricular fiber arises, the P-R interval may be normal or short during sinus rhythm. Electrocardiographic evidence of ventricular pre-excitation is usually absent. Intracardiac recordings obtained during sinus rhythm typically demonstrate normal A-H and H-V intervals. However, with the introduction of premature atrial extrastimuli the A-H interval lengthens, the H-V interval shortens, and the QRS complex shows evidence of anomalous conduction despite a normal P-R interval. Changes in the QRS complex may occur gradually as the coupling interval of the extrastimuli become progressively shorter, or a critical increase in the AH interval may be associated with the sudden manifestation of pre-excitation, particularly in patients who also have dual AV nodal pathways. Most nodoventricular fibers insert at the right side of the ventricular septum, resulting in a QRS complex resembling left bundle branch block; however, left-sided insertions have been reported and are associated with variable QRS morphologies depending on the site of ventricular insertion.[1, 87] During programmed ventricular stimulation, retrograde atrial activation is recorded earliest from the His bundle catheter. Demonstration of a His deflection between the ventricular and atrial electrograms provides evidence of retrograde conduction through the normal His-Purkinje system.

Nodoventricular fibers may participate in a macro-reentrant circuit (Fig. 10–20) which is composed of the nodoventricular fiber, the ventricle, the His-Purkinje system, and the AV node.[61, 141, 145] The nodoventricular fiber is the anterograde limb of the circuit and the His-Purkinje system is the retrograde limb. Reversal of this circuit is rare but has been reported.[58] Because the atria are not part of the circuit, AV dissociation may be evident during the tachycardia. The site of earliest

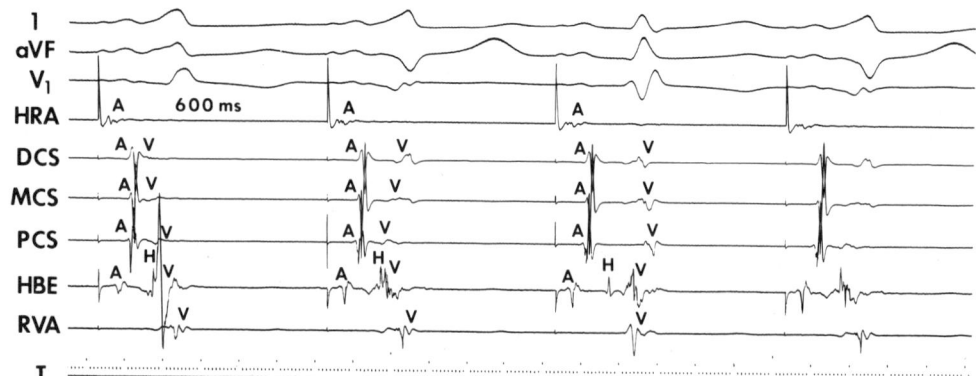

FIGURE 10–19
Two accessory pathways demonstrated during right atrial pacing. During the first beat, earliest ventricular activation is recorded from the distal coronary sinus (DCS) and corresponds to a left-posterior site. During the second paced beat, changes in QRS morphology and ventricular activation are evident with earliest ventricular activation recorded from the proximal coronary sinus (PCS). The PCS electrodes were positioned at the os of the coronary sinus, indicating the presence of a posterior-septal accessory pathway. In the third paced beat, anterograde block occurs in both pathways. Ventricular activation occurs through the normal AV conduction system and exhibits modest aberrancy. (Reprinted by permission from Cain ME, Cox JL: Surgical treatment of supraventricular tachyarrhythmias. In Platia EV (ed.): Management of Cardiac Arrhythmias—The Nonpharmacologic Approach, pp. 304–330. Philadelphia, J. B. Lippincott, 1987.)

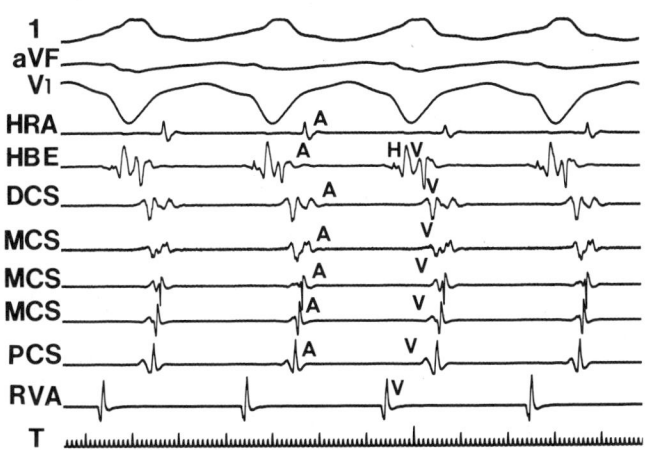

FIGURE 10–20
Reciprocating tachycardia in a patient with a nodoventricular fiber. Ventricular activation occurs via the nodoventricular fiber and is recorded in the right ventricular apex electrogram before the His-bundle deflection. Left bundle branch block morphology with left axis deviation is present. Retrograde atrial activation occurred by the normal conduction system.

ventricular activation always precedes the His deflection. If VA conduction is present, earliest retrograde atrial activation should be recorded by the His bundle catheter. Eccentric retrograde atrial activation indicates the presence of an additional accessory pathway. In addition, ventricular activation through the nodoventricular fiber may occur passively during other supraventricular arrhythmias, especially AV nodal reentry.[106, 148]

IDENTIFICATION OF PATIENTS AT RISK OF SUDDEN DEATH

An accurate method is not available for prospectively identifying patients with the WPW syndrome at high risk for sudden death. While results of some studies have shown an important association between the refractory period of an accessory pathway and the ventricular rate during atrial fibrillation,[28, 149] others have found great variability in this relationship.[80] Several factors may account for this discrepancy. In some patients, atrial refractoriness limits accurate assessment of the anterograde refractory periods of the accessory pathway. Moreover, refractoriness may increase or decrease substantially as the paced cycle length shortens.[143] In addition, the refractory properties of the accessory pathway are dependent on autonomic tone. The anterograde refractory period of an accessory pathway has been shown to decrease by 30 to 180 ms and the ventricular rate during atrial fibrillation to increase under conditions of exercise or the infusion of isoproterenol.[39, 63, 90] Accordingly, values measured at rest may not be representative of those encountered during the stress induced by a tachycardia or exercise. These dynamic characteristics of accessory pathways preclude accurate identification of patients at risk for sudden death based on a single electrophysiologic determinant.

Present strategies for defining risk for sudden death are based on retrospective analysis of patients with the WPW syndrome who have survived an episode of ventricular fibrillation. Klein and colleagues[80] compared the clinical and electrophysiologic characteristics from 31 patients with the WPW syndrome and a history of ventricular fibrillation with those from 73 patients with the WPW syndrome without ventricular fibrillation. The shortest R-R interval during atrial fibrillation best differentiated patients with a prior history of ventricular fibrillation from those without (180 ± 29 ms vs. 240 ± 63 ms) and did not exceed 250 ms in any patient with a history of ventricular fibrillation. Differences between groups were less striking when values of the anterograde refractory period of the accessory pathway or the mean R-R interval during atrial fibrillation were compared. Despite significant differences between groups in the values of the shortest R-R interval during atrial fibrillation, a significant overlap was evident. Among patients without ventricular fibrillation, 60% had an R-R interval during atrial fibrillation less than 250 ms. Studies by others reported R-R intervals during atrial fibrillation of less than 250 ms in up to 75% of patients with a history of atrial fibrillation but not ventricular fibrillation, 41% of patients with a history of atrioventricular reentry, 50% of patients with undocumented palpitations,[119] 50% of patients with syncope,[160] and 17% of asymptomatic patients.[101]

Thus, several clinical and electrophysiologic features are common to patients both with and without ventricular fibrillation. None can be used to accurately predict those patients who will develop ventricular fibrillation. Results of these studies do not support the routine electrophysiologic evaluation or treatment of asymptomatic patients with a pre-excitation syndrome.

EVALUATION OF DRUG THERAPY

Antiarrhythmic drugs are administered to patients with pre-excitation syndrome to prevent or reduce the occurrence of arrhythmias and decrease the ventricular rate during atrial fibrillation. Medical therapy that effectively prevents or decreases the occurrence of reentry is often difficult to achieve. The goal of medical therapy is to selectively block or impair conduction in one limb of the reentrant circuit. Unfortunately, changes in conduction and refractoriness induced by drugs are variable and are often dependent on the intrinsic electrophysiologic properties of the involved tissues.

Table 10–2 summarizes the disparate effects on inducibility observed from four patients. In the first patient, procainamide effectively prevented the initiation of orthodromic SVT through its effect on lengthening retrograde refractoriness in the accessory pathway. Changes in anterograde refractory properties of the AV node and accessory pathway were modest. In the second patient, refractoriness of the accessory pathway was prolonged to a greater extent anterogradely than retrogradely. As a result, the difference in refractory periods of the AV node and accessory

TABLE 10–2
Refractory Properties of AV Node and Accessory Pathway, Illustrating Variable Response to Antiarrhythmic Therapy

No. of Patients		A-ERP (ms):AVN	A-ERP (ms):AP	R-ERP (ms):AP	Cycle Length AVR (ms)
1	Control	260	280	320	350
	Procainamide	290	300	>600	NI
2	Control	250	360	260	290
	Procainamide	260	420	300	340
3	Control	240	270	220	290
	Procainamide	250	290	230	310
4	Control	260	—	230	300
	Flecainide	340	—	430	500

A-ERP = anterograde effective refractory period; AVN = atrioventricular node; AP = accessory pathway; R-ERP = retrograde effective refractory period; AVR = atrioventricular reentry; NI = not inducible.

pathway was exaggerated further and induction of orthodromic SVT was facilitated. Procainamide had little effect on either limb of the circuit in the third patient, and the tachycardia remained easily induced. The fourth patient had a concealed accessory pathway. During treatment with flecainide, the refractory properties of both the AV node and the accessory pathway were prolonged in parallel. As a result, orthodromic SVT remained readily inducible, but the rate of the tachycardia slowed moderately. These examples illustrate the variable response of antiarrhythmic drugs on inducibility.

Medications that prolong anterograde refractoriness but not retrograde refractoriness often facilitate induction of orthodromic SVT. Alternatively, when refractoriness is prolonged to a similar extent in both limbs of the circuit, episodes of SVT may be slower but more frequent. This effect may be observed during treatment with drugs that exert potent changes in the electrophysiologic properties of both the AV node and accessory pathway or during therapy with combinations of drugs that each affect a separate component of the reentrant circuit.

Despite the widespread use of electrophysiology studies, only limited information is available regarding the concordance of the response to programmed stimulation and long-term drug efficacy. Results of available studies suggest that antiarrhythmic agents that render arrhythmias noninducible also prevent or markedly reduce spontaneous episodes in 85 to 95% of patients when these drugs are administered long-term.[29, 79, 81, 93, 94, 100, 103, 124, 125, 158, 159] However, the clinical course of patients receiving treatment with drugs that fail to prevent induction of SVT has not been rigorously defined. It is possible that drugs that fail to prevent induction of SVT may still be beneficial if effective in suppressing spontaneous atrial or ventricular premature depolarizations that trigger the tachycardia. Moreover, changes in autonomic tone or other factors that modify the response to triggering events may not be replicated in the electrophysiology laboratory. Accordingly, a clinical trial of medical therapy may still be warranted for some patients in whom orthodromic or antidromic SVT remains inducible.

In patients with atrial fibrillation, the anterograde refractory period of an accessory pathway measured in the absence of antiarrhythmic drugs has been found by some to be predictive of the change in the refractory properties during treatment with antiarrhythmic agents.[151] When the anterograde refractory period exceeds 270 ms, treatment with procainamide, quinidine, ajmaline, or amiodarone markedly prolonged the anterograde refractory properties of the accessory pathway. A more modest change was observed on the retrograde refractory properties of the accessory pathway. When the anterograde refractory period was less than 270 ms, only amiodarone significantly prolonged the anterograde effective refractory period. In patients with accessory pathways that had short refractory properties, the change in retrograde refractoriness induced by drug therapy was variable. Thus, patients at highest risk for development of a life-threatening ventricular rate during atrial fibrillation are least likely to benefit from therapy with currently available antiarrhythmic drugs. Presently, the best measure of the effectiveness of antiarrhythmic drugs is the response to programmed stimulation and the ventricular rate measured directly during atrial fibrillation.

Management of Patients with Pre-excitation Syndromes

Decisions regarding the extent to which patients with pre-excitation syndromes should be evaluated are based on the severity of symptoms and on knowledge of the value of information to be gained from diagnostic studies. Most patients have a benign course. For those with recurrent or life-threatening arrhythmias, effective treatments are available.

INITIAL EVALUATION

Initial goals include (1) determination of the presence or absence of symptoms; (2) characterization of symptoms, including their frequency and severity; (3) elucidation of previous treatment regimens and effectiveness; (4) determination of the specific arrhythmia present during symptoms; and (5) determination of the presence or absence of concomitant heart disease. These data provide a foundation for treatment strategies.

Arrhythmias should be documented before contemplating therapy, a change of medication, or an invasive electrophysiology study. Patients with frequent arrhythmias that are associated with severe symptoms may require observation on a telemetry unit. In most patients, arrhythmias occur infrequently and are not severe enough to warrant admission to the hospital. Because they occur capriciously they are unlikely to be detected by 24-hour ambulatory monitoring. Transtelephonic monitoring devices provide a practical means of documenting the spontaneous heart rhythm during symptoms.

There is considerable variability in the degree of pre-excitation apparent on random electrocardiograms recorded from patients with the WPW syndrome. Concealed accessory pathways are not evident on electrocardiograms obtained during sinus rhythm. Abnormalities of the QRS complex during sinus rhythm are rarely detectable from patients with nodoventricular fibers. In patients with the WPW syndrome, intermittent loss of the delta wave may be observed when serial electrocardiograms are compared during 24-hour ambulatory recordings. Intermittent pre-excitation may be associated with accessory pathways having relatively long refractory periods. However, in one study, the shortest R-R interval recorded during atrial fibrillation was less than 250 ms in 4 of the 26 patients (15%) with intermittent pre-excitation. Moreover, the prevalence of symptoms in patients with intermittent pre-excitation was comparable to those from patients in whom pre-excitation was constant.[82] Thus, while patterns of pre-excitation provide information about the accessory pathway location, the electrocardiogram should not be used to predict whether an asymptomatic patient will develop arrhythmias or to identify those patients at high risk for development of a life-threatening ventricular rate during atrial fibrillation.

The merits and limitations of exercise testing and invasive electrophysiology studies for the identification of patients with pre-excitation syndrome at risk of ventricular fibrillation have been described in other sections of this chapter. At present, there is no objective evidence that results of these tests have a beneficial influence on the management of asymptomatic patients. It is our practice, however, to recommend evaluation for asymptomatic patients with pre-excitation syndrome whose occupation (e.g., pilot, professional athlete) places them or others at considerable risk of injury if an arrhythmia supervenes. In such patients an exercise test is performed first. Abrupt loss of pre-excitation during exercise implies a low risk of ventricular fibrillation. Patients with persistent pre-excitation throughout exercise are advised to undergo an invasive electrophysiology study. For asymptomatic patients, the decision to advise pharmacologic or nonpharmacologic therapy based on results of exercise testing or electrophysiology studies should be balanced by recognition that greater risk may attend the treatment than the underlying disorder.

ACUTE MANAGEMENT OF ARRHYTHMIAS ASSOCIATED WITH PRE-EXCITATION SYNDROME

In most patients, orthodromic SVT is not accompanied by life-threatening symptoms. Table 10-3 summarizes methods of terminating episodes of SVT. The arrhythmia may be terminated by prolonging refractoriness of the AV node or the accessory pathway. Increasing vagal tone by the valsalva maneuver or carotid sinus massage may terminate the tachycardia by altering the refractory properties of the AV node. When these measures are unsuccessful, 5 to 10 mg (0.075–0.15 mg/kg) of verapamil administered intravenously over 2 to 3 minutes is effective in terminating orthodromic SVT in up to 85% of patients.[69, 81, 113, 118, 139] Peak effects are achieved 3 to 5 minutes after administration as an intravenous bolus. It is eliminated biexpotentially with a rapid early distribution phase (half-life 4 minutes) and a slower terminal elimination phase (half-life 2–5 hours). A decrease in mean arterial pressure of 5 to 10 mm Hg in young patients and 10 to 20 mm Hg in elderly patients is observed commonly because of peripheral vasodilation.[3] The direct effects of verapamil on the refractory properties of accessory pathways are modest.[118, 136] In some patients, the reflex increase in symptomatic tone that occurs in response to peripheral vasodilation may be responsible for shortening of the anterograde effective refractory period of the accessory pathway. Occasionally, orthodromic SVT converts spontaneously to atrial fibrillation, which is a potential problem if verapamil has already been administered. If verapamil does not terminate the tachycardia and the patient subsequently develops atrial fibrillation, the effect of verapamil may enhance conduction through the accessory pathway and precipitate ventricular fibrillation.[68, 70, 118] For this reason a cardioverter/defibrillator should be available whenever verapamil is used intravenously.

Adenosine is an endogenously occurring nucleotide that is under investigation for the treatment of SVT. Its known electrophysiologic effects in humans include depression of sinus node automaticity and of AV conduction.[48, 134] These actions appear to be mediated by direct effects of adenosine on potassium and calcium conduction and by antagonism of the electrophysiologic actions of intracellular cyclic adenosine monophosphate.[15–17, 117, 121] After injection, adenosine is cleared rapidly from the circulation by cellular uptake and metabolism by vascular endothelium and formed ele-

TABLE 10-3
Acute Management of Arrhythmias in the Pre-excitation Syndrome

---

Orthodromic Atrioventricular Reentry
1. Valsalva maneuver/carotid sinus massage
2. IV Adenosine
3. IV Verapamil
4. IV Procainamide (1.0 g/100 ml D$_5$W over 30 min))
5. Cardioversion

Antidromic Atrioventricular Reentry
1. IV Procainamide
2. IV Flecainide encainide, propafenone
3. Cardioversion

Atrial Fibrillation
1. IV Procainamide
2. IV Flecainide, encainide, propafenone
3. Cardioversion

IV = intravenous.

ments of the blood, with an elimination half-life of less than 10 seconds.[71] Published studies have demonstrated uniform termination of orthodromic SVT within 30 seconds by an intravenously administered dose of 88 to 140 µg/kg.[31, 47, 48, 108] Adverse effects, which are minor and of short duration, include dyspnea or flushing in 15 to 20% of patients. Sinus arrest lasting 2 to 5 seconds has been observed in patients with sinus node dysfunction. Available evidence indicates that adenosine does not affect the refractory properties of accessory pathways.

Intravenous administration of procainamide (1.0 g in 100 ml D_5W over 30 minutes) prolongs refractoriness in the accessory pathway and provides an alternative treatment of orthodromic SVT for patients in whom verapamil is contraindicated.[99, 130, 158] The major disadvantage of procainamide is that it must be given slowly to avoid hypotension and may not be tolerated by patients who present with a systolic pressure less than 90 mm Hg.

Orthodromic SVT can be easily terminated in the majority of patients by the modes of therapy described above; however, cardioversion (25–100 J) may be required in an occasional patient. For patients in whom SVT promptly supervenes following cardioversion and cannot be easily controlled with medications, insertion of a temporary pacing electrode provides a means to terminate the tachycardia painlessly by rapid atrial or ventricular pacing until an effective medical regimen is identified.

Antidromic SVT is a regular reentrant tachycardia exhibiting ventricular pre-excitation in which retrograde conduction may occur via the normal conduction system or often by a second accessory pathway.[12] Treatment should be based on the recognition that retrograde conduction frequently occurs by a second accessory pathway and will not be terminated by agents that predominantly affect the AV node. Moreover, patients with antidromic SVT appear to be especially prone to the spontaneous transition to atrial fibrillation, in which case prior treatment with drugs that primarily prolong conduction in the AV node increases the risk of inducing ventricular fibrillation. In view of these considerations, it is advisable to treat patients who present with antidromic SVT with an intravenous infusion of procainamide or to proceed directly with cardioversion in patients who are compromised hemodynamically.

Patients with pre-excitation syndromes who develop atrial fibrillation may present with hypotension and rapid ventricular rate (300–400 bpm). This arrhythmia represents a medical emergency and should be treated promptly by DC cardioversion. Patients who have a more moderate ventricular rate and stable blood pressure may be treated less urgently by an infusion of procainamide, which may convert atrial fibrillation to sinus rhythm or prolong refractoriness of the accessory pathway and slow the ventricular rate. Lidocaine generally has little effect or may accelerate the ventricular rate during atrial fibrillation.[4]

Digoxin and verapamil have also been implicated as agents that accelerate the ventricular rate during atrial fibrillation.[43, 44, 49, 68, 129, 136] Digoxin shortens the anterograde refractoriness of the accessory pathway in some patients. The direct effects of verapamil on the refractory properties of accessory pathways are minimal; however, verapamil may accelerate the ventricular rate during atrial fibrillation by two indirect mechanisms: (1) conduction through the accessory pathway may be favored by slowing conduction through the AV node, which may decrease retrograde penetration into the accessory pathway; and (2) a reflex increase in adrenergic tone in response to vasodilation may shorten the refractory properties of the accessory pathway. The risk of this response may not be as great when verapamil is administered orally; however, until objective data demonstrate its safety, verapamil should not be used for the treatment of patients with anterograde pre-excitation who are at risk for atrial fibrillation. Propranolol has no direct effects on conduction or refractoriness in accessory pathways,[44] but an increase in the ventricular rate during atrial fibrillation has been reported.[104]

LONG-TERM MANAGEMENT OF PATIENTS WITH PRE-EXCITATION SYNDROME

Decisions regarding the management of symptomatic patients with pre-excitation are predicated on the necessity for treatment, the potential morbidity and mortality of the disorder, and the efficacy of therapy. Table 10–4 summarizes the approach to long-term management of patients with pre-excitation syndromes. Patients who experience infrequent, brief, self-terminating episodes of SVT without debilitating symptoms may not require treatment. Those with more prolonged episodes may prefer to take medications only at the time of their attacks. In our experience, most patients with symptomatic tachycardias prefer to take antiar-

TABLE 10–4
Long-Term Management of the Pre-excitation Syndrome

I. Candidates for empiric therapy
   A. Arrhythmias frequent
   B. Arrhythmias hemodynamically stable
II. Indications for electrophysiology study
   A. Determine mechanism of tachycardia
   B. Identify effective antiarrhythmic regimen
   C. Assess risk of a malignant ventricular rate during atrial fibrillation
   D. Determine the number of accessory pathways and their locations preoperatively
III. Pharmacologic management
   A. Concealed accessory pathway
     1. Digoxin/verapamil/beta-adrenergic antagonist
     2. Encainide/flecainide/propafenone
     3. Disopyramide/quinidine/procainamide
     4. Sotalol
   B. Manifest accessory pathway
     1. Encainide/flecainide/propafenone
     2. Disopyramide/quinidine/procainamide
     3. Sotalol
IV. Indications for surgery
   A. Medical therapy not effective
   B. Arrhythmias hemodynamically unstable
   C. Patient intolerant of medications
   D. Alternative to life-long therapy in young patients

rhythmic medications regularly to avert attacks. The majority can be treated effectively with antiarrhythmic medications, but nonpharmacologic therapy should be considered for selected patients.

Identification of an effective medical regime for the prevention of arrhythmias often proves difficult. Empiric therapy can be justified for patients who tolerate their arrhythmias without difficulty; however, the inadvertent selection of an agent that shortens the refractory properties of the accessory pathway may prove hazardous in patients who develop atrial fibrillation. In other cases, the agent selected may promote more frequent episodes of tachycardia, which can be debilitating. Moreover, it may take weeks or months to identify an effective regimen. For these reasons, we prefer to evaluate the effects of medical therapy in the electrophysiology laboratory to identify a regimen before the patient is discharged that prevents inducibility of SVT or a rapid ventricular rate during atrial fibrillation. If a regimen can be identified that achieves these goals, recurrences are infrequent.

The choice of antiarrhythmic medications includes those that interrupt episodes of tachycardia by their effects on refractoriness of the AV node, those that act primarily on the accessory pathway, and those that affect both the normal conduction system and the accessory pathway. Figure 10–21 illustrates the sites of action of antiarrhythmic agents that have been evaluated for the long-term treatment of SVT. To facilitate patient compliance it is advisable to identify a regimen that uses the least number of medications at the lowest effective dose.

Figure 10–22 summarizes the long-term efficacy of several antiarrhythmic agents for the prevention of orthodromic SVT.[2, 5, 21, 55, 74, 78, 79, 85, 86, 93, 94, 103, 113, 116, 123, 126, 152] Digoxin, beta-adrenergic antagonists, and verapamil affect electrophysiologic properties of the AV node. As shown, digoxin is generally not effective for treatment of AV reentry, and it has been implicated as a medication that accelerates the ventricular rate during atrial fibrillation. Although treatment with beta-adrenergic antagonists entails less risk in patients with atrial fibrillation, these agents have limited efficacy in the long-term management of patients with pre-excitation syndromes. Verapamil is relatively effective for the prevention of SVT but concerns persist about its safety in patients with atrial fibrillation.

Procainamide, quinidine, and disopyramide are class IA antiarrhythmic agents that may prolong anterograde and retrograde refractoriness of the accessory pathway and have comparable efficacy in the prevention of orthodromic SVT. Because of the incidence of a lupus

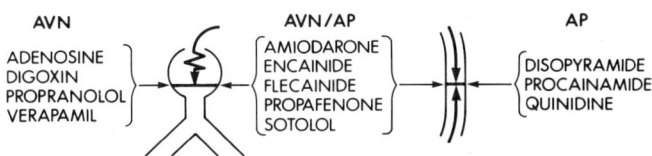

FIGURE 10–21
Schematic representation of sites of action of antiarrhythmic medications.

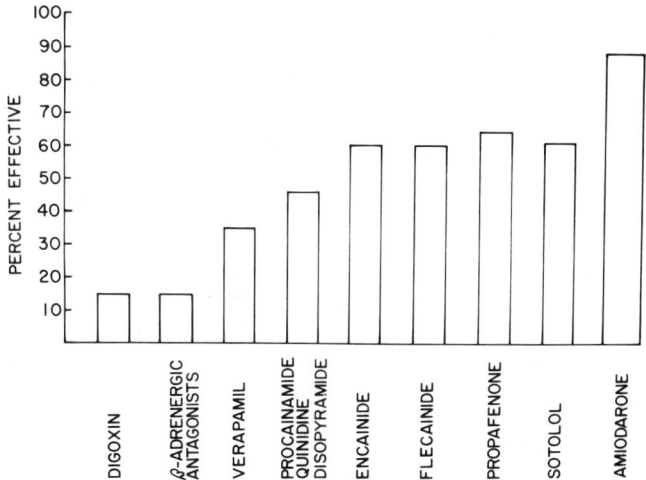

FIGURE 10–22
Efficacy of antiarrhythmic medications for the prevention of orthodromic SVT.

syndrome associated with long-term procainamide therapy, it is preferable to use quinidine or disopyramide. Sustained-release preparations facilitate patient compliance with these agents.

Flecainide, encainide, and propafenone are class IC agents that predominantly affect the electrophysiologic properties of the accessory pathway but also prolong refractoriness and delay conduction in the AV node. Treatment with these agents is usually well tolerated, and they prevent episodes of orthodromic SVT in up to 60% of patients during long-term therapy. Like class IA agents, these agents may reduce premature atrial or ventricular depolarizations that trigger arrhythmias, maintain sinus rhythm in patients with paroxysmal atrial fibrillation, and slow the ventricular rate during atrial fibrillation.

Amiodarone and sotalol are class III agents that affect the electrophysiologic properties of both the AV node and the accessory pathway. Although therapy with amiodarone has demonstrated exceptional long-term efficacy for prevention of AV reentry and atrial fibrillation, the toxicity associated with this drug renders it a poor choice for young patients. Sotalol is also effective for the prevention of AV reentry and reduces the ventricular rate during atrial fibrillation. Whether sotalol prevents recurrent episodes of atrial fibrillation requires further study.

To avoid repetitive visits to the emergency room, which are inconvenient and impractical, long-term daily administration of medication is necessary for patients with frequent arrhythmias. A recent study of 15 patients with pre-excitation syndromes demonstrated the feasibility of intermittent therapy with the single administration of combined doses of propranolol and diltiazem for acute attacks that are infrequent and associated with only mild symptoms.[161] The mean time to conversion of SVT in 14 of the patients was 27 ± 15 minutes. Results of this study demonstrate the safety and efficacy of this regimen in patients who do not experience severe symptoms during episodes of SVT. Although there is evidence that oral diltiazem does not accelerate the ventricular rate during atrial fibrillation,[132] a complete electrophysiologic evaluation of single-dose combination therapy with propranolol and diltiazem is advised to ensure its safety.

Refinements in surgical technique and improved understanding of the electrophysiologic mechanisms of the pre-excitation syndrome have provided alternative approaches to medical therapy. At experienced centers successful division of accessory pathways can be achieved in over 99% of patients. Surgical mortality is less than 1% for patients without associated anomalies undergoing elective operation.[38] Surgical techniques used to divide accessory pathways are described in Chapter 24. Although most patients can be treated effectively with antiarrhythmic medications, surgery should be considered for those who (1) have recurrent tachycardia that is refractory to medical management, (2) are unable to tolerate conventional medications, or (3) have life-threatening arrhythmias that may not be reliably prevented by treatment with antiarrhythmic drugs. In addition, younger patients may choose surgery as an alternative to the inconvenience of life-long medical therapy.

Nonpharmacologic alternatives to surgery include percutaneous catheter ablation and antitachycardia devices. Antitachycardia pacemakers can be programmed to detect SVT and are often effective in their termination.[57] However, they have several limitations, including (1) inability to prevent SVT, (2) complications and long-term follow-up similar to those with conventional pacemakers, and (3) the risk that pacing algorithms may induce atrial fibrillation.

Percutaneous catheter ablation of accessory pathways is under investigation for the treatment of patients with pre-excitation syndromes. Attempted ablation of left free-wall pathways using catheters positioned in the coronary sinus has been largely unsuccessful and is associated with an unacceptable risk of tamponade.[56] Results obtained in patients with posterior-septal accessory pathways have been more promising; however, the risk of tamponade remains a concern.[11, 107] The feasibility of this approach has been demonstrated; however, technical developments that provide for more controlled delivery of energy are needed to improve the efficacy of this technique and reduce the risk of tamponade, before percutaneous catheter ablative techniques can be widely applied in clinical practice.

Future Directions in the Treatment of the Pre-excitation Syndrome

Over the past two decades, results of electrophysiology studies have further defined the pathophysiology of the pre-excitation syndrome and its variants and have provided the foundation for the development of innovative therapeutic alternatives. Several new antiarrhythmic medications have demonstrated efficacy and are generally well tolerated. Surgery can be relied on to offer a cure for patients in whom antiarrhythmic medications are ineffective or cause intolerable effects. Percutaneous catheter ablation of accessory pathways, although still investigational, offers promise for a nonsurgical cure of the pre-excitation syndrome, but further technical developments are needed to enhance the safety and effectiveness of this approach.

As definitive therapy has become more available, the unresolved issue of patient management is changing from how to treat patients to whom to treat. As a group, asymptomatic patients and those with mild to moderate symptoms are at low risk for sudden death, yet the dilemma remains that some individuals will experience ventricular fibrillation.

The indications for electrophysiology studies and the prognostic value of information derived from these and noninvasive tests require clarification. To date, the standard index of risk for the development of ventricular fibrillation in patients with pre-excitation syndromes is the shortest R-R interval observed during atrial fibrillation, which has a positive predictive accuracy of approximately 35%. Before full advantage can be taken of the therapeutic advances that have been made or the modalities that will become available, a more accurate means must be identified to detect patients at risk of sudden death who will benefit from aggressive therapeutic interventions.

References

1. Abbott JA, Scheinman MM, Morady F, et al.: Coexistent Maheim and Kent accessory connections: diagnostic and therapeutic implications. J Am Coll Cardiol 10:364, 1987.
2. Abdollah H, Brugada P, Green M, et al.: Clinical efficacy and electrophysiologic effects of intravenous and oral encainide in patients with accessory atrioventricular pathways and supraventricular arrhythmias. Am J Cardiol 54:544, 1984.
3. Abernathy DR, Schumitz JB, Todd EL, et al.: Verapamil pharmacodynamics and disposition in young and elderly hypertensive patients. Altered electrocardiographic and hypotensive responses. Ann Intern Med 105:329, 1986.
4. Akhtar M, Gilbert CJ, Shenasa M: Effect of lidocaine on atrioventricular response via the accessory pathway in patients with Wolff-Parkinson-White syndrome. Circulation 63:435, 1981.
5. Alboni P, Narasimhan S, Pirani R, et al.: Effects of amiodarone on supraventricular tachycardia involving by-pass tracts. Am J Cardiol 53:93, 1984.
6. Anderson RH, Becker AE, Brechenmacher C, et al.: Ventricular preexcitation: a proposed nomenclature for its substrates. Eur J Cardiol 3:27, 1975.
7. Anderson RH, Becker AE, Wenink ACG, et al.: The development of the cardiac specialized tissue. In Wellens HJJ, Lie KI, Janse MJ (eds.): The Conduction System of the Heart: Structure, Function, and Clinical Implications, pp 3–28. Philadelphia, Lea and Febiger, 1976.
8. Anderson RH, Davies MJ, Becker AE: Atrioventricular ring specialized tissue in the normal heart. Eur J Cardiol 2:219, 1979.
9. Anderson RH, Ho SY, Smith A, et al.: Study of the cardiac conduction tissues in the pediatric age group. Diagn Histopathol 4:3, 1981.
10. Bardy GH, Fedor JM, German LD, et al.: Surface electrocardiographic clues suggesting presence of a nodofascicular Mahaim fiber. J Am Coll Cardiol 5:1161, 1984.
11. Bardy GH, Ivey TD, Coltorti F, et al.: Developments, complications, and limitations of catheter-mediated electrical abla-

tion of posterior accessory atrioventricular pathways. Am J Cardiol 61:309, 1988.
12. Bardy GH, Packer DL, German LD, et al.: Preexcited reciprocating tachycardia in patients with Wolff-Parkinson-White syndrome: incidence and mechanisms. Circulation 70:377, 1984.
13. Bauernfeind RA, Wyndham CR, Swiryn SP, et al.: Paroxysmal atrial fibrillation in the Wolff-Parkinson-White syndrome. Am J Cardiol 47:562, 1981.
14. Becker AE, Anderson RH, Durrer D, et al.: The anatomical substrates of Wolff-Parkinson-White syndrome: A clinicopathologic correlation in seven patients. Circulation 57:870, 1978.
15. Belhassen B, Pellig A: Electrophysiologic effects of adenosine triphosphate on the mammalian heart: clinical and experimental aspects. J Am Coll Cardiol 4:414, 1984.
16. Bellardinelli L, Isenberg G: Actions of adenosine and isoproterenol on isolated mammalian ventricular myocytes. Circ Res 53:287, 1983.
17. Bellardinelli L, Isenberg G: Isolated atrial myocytes: adenosine and acetylcholine increase potassium conductance. Am J Physiol 234:H734, 1983.
18. Berkman NL, Lamb LE: The Wolff-Parkinson-White electrocardiograms: A follow-up study of five to twenty-eight years. N Engl J Med 278:492, 1968.
19. Boineau JP, Moore EN, Spear JF, et al.: Basis of static and dynamic electrocardiographic variations in Wolff-Parkinson-White syndrome. Anatomic and electrophysiologic observations in right and left ventricular pre-excitation. Am J Cardiol 32:32, 1973.
20. Botvinick E, Frais M, O'Connell W, et al.: Phase image evaluation of patients with ventricular preexcitation syndromes. J Am Coll Cardiol 3:799, 1984.
21. Breithardt G, Borggrefe M, Wiebringhaus E, et al.: Effect of propafenone in the Wolff-Parkinson-White syndrome: electrophysiologic findings and long-term follow-up. Am J Cardiol 54:29D, 1984.
22. Bricker JT, Porter CJ, Garson A, et al.: Exercise testing in children with Wolff-Parkinson-White syndrome. Am J Cardiol 55:1001, 1985.
23. Broustet JP, Levy S, Viscoulon B, et al.: Syndrome de Wolff-Parkinson-White. Comportment au cours de l'épreuve d'effort limitée par les symptômes. Arch Mal Coeur 72:625, 1979.
24. Brugada P, Vanagt EJ, Bar FW, et al.: Incessant reciprocating atrioventricular tachycardia. Factors playing a role in the mechanism of the arrhythmias. PACE 3:670, 1980.
25. Burchell HB, Frye RL, Anderson MW, et al.: Atrioventricular and ventriculoatrial excitation in Wolff-Parkinson-White syndrome (type B): temporary ablation at surgery. Circulation 36:663, 1967.
26. Cain ME, Cox JL: Surgical treatment of supraventricular arrhythmias. In Platia EV (ed.): Management of Cardiac Arrhythmias: the Nonpharmacologic Approach, pp. 304–339, Philadelphia, J. B. Lippincott Co., 1987.
27. Campbell RWF, Smith RA, Gallagher JJ, et al.: Atrial fibrillation in the pre-excitation syndrome. Am J Cardiol 40:514, 1977.
28. Castellanos A, Myerburg RJ, Craparo K, et al.: Factors regulating ventricular rates during atrial flutter and fibrillation in pre-excitation (Wolff-Parkinson-White) syndrome. Br Heart J 35:811, 1973.
29. Chang M, Sung RJ, Tai T, et al.: Nadolol and supraventricular tachycardia: an electrophysiologic study. J Am Coll Cardiol 2:894, 1983.
30. Chung KY, Walsh TJ, Massie E: Wolff-Parkinson-White syndrome. Am Heart J 691:116, 1965.
31. Clarke B, Rowland E, Barnes PJ, et al.: Rapid and safe termination of supraventricular tachycardia in children by adenosine. Lancet 1:299, 1987.
32. Cobb FR, Blumenschein SD, Sealy WC, et al.: Successful surgical interruption of the bundle of Kent in a patient with Wolff-Parkinson-White syndrome. Circulation 38:1018, 1968.
33. Cohn AE, Fraser FR: Paroxysmal tachycardia and the effect of stimulation of the vagus nerves by pressure. Heart 5:93, 1913–1914.
34. Colavita PG, Packer KL, Pressley JC, et al.: Frequency, diagnosis, and clinical characteristics of patients with multiple accessory atrioventricular pathways. Am J Cardiol 59:601, 1987.
35. Cosio FG, Benson DW, Anderson RW, et al.: Onset of atrial fibrillation during antidromic tachycardia: Association with sudden cardiac arrest and ventricular fibrillation in a patient with Wolff-Parkinson-White syndrome. Am J Cardiol 50:353, 1982.
36. Coumel P, Attuel P: Reciprocating tachycardia in overt and latent preexcitation. Influence of functional bundle branch block on the rate of tachycardia. Eur J Cardiol 1:423, 1974.
37. Coumel P, Cabrol C, Fabiato A, et al.: Tachycardia permanente par rhythme réciproque. Arch Mal Coeur 60:1830, 1967.
38. Cox JL, Gallagher JJ, Cain ME: Experience with 118 consecutive patients undergoing operation for the Wolff-Parkinson-White syndrome. J Thor Cardiov Surg 90:490, 1985.
39. Crick JCP, Davies DW, Holt P, et al.: Effect of exercise on ventricular response to atrial fibrillation in Wolff-Parkinson-White syndrome. Br Heart J 54:80, 1985.
40. Critelli G, Gallagher JJ, Monda V, et al.: Anatomic and electrophysiologic substrate of the permanent form of junctional reciprocating tachycardia. J Am Coll Cardiol 4:601, 1984.
41. Critelli G, Gallagher JJ, Perticone F, et al.: Evaluation of noninvasive tests for identifying patients with preexcitation syndrome at risk of rapid ventricular response. Am Heart J 108:905, 1984.
42. Crossen KJ, Lindsay BD, Cain ME: Reliability of retrograde atrial activation patterns during ventricular pacing for localizing accessory pathways. J Am Coll Cardiol 9:1279, 1987.
43. Deal BJ, Keane JF, Gillette PC, et al.: Wolff-Parkinson-White syndrome and supraventricular tachycardia during infancy: management and follow-up. J Am Coll Cardiol 5:130, 1985.
44. Denes P, Cummings JM, Simpson R, et al.: Effects of propranolol on anomalous pathway refractoriness and circus movement tachycardias in patients with pre-excitation. Am J Cardiol 411:1061, 1978.
45. Denes P, Wu D, Amat-y-Leon F, et al.: Determinants of atrioventricular reentrant paroxysmal tachycardia in patients with Wolff-Parkinson-White syndrome. Circulation 58:415, 1978.
46. DiMaria AN, Vera Z, Newman A, et al.: Alternations in ventricular-contraction patterns in the Wolff-Parkinson-White syndrome. Circulation 53:249, 1976.
47. DiMarco JP, Sellers DT, Lerman BB, et al.: Diagnostic and therapeutic use of adenosine in patients with supraventricular tachyarrhythmias. J Am Coll Cardiol 6:417, 1985.
48. DiMarco JP, Sellers TD, Berne RM, et al.: Adenosine: electrophysiologic effects and therapeutic use for terminating paroxysmal supraventricular tachycardia. Circulation 68:1254, 1983.
49. Dreifus LS, Harat R, Watanabe Y, et al.: Ventricular fibrillation. A possible mechanism of sudden death in patients with Wolff-Parkinson-White syndrome. Circulation 43:520, 1971.
50. Dreifus LS, Nichols H, Morse D, et al.: Control of recurrent tachycardia of Wolff-Parkinson-White syndrome by surgical ligature of the A-V bundle. Circulation 38:1030, 1968.
51. Durrer D, Roos JP: Epicardial excitation of the ventricles in a patient with Wolff-Parkinson-White syndrome (type B). Circulation 35:15, 1967.
52. Durrer D, Schoo L, Schuilenburg RM, et al.: The role of premature beats in the initiation and the termination of supraventricular tachycardia in the Wolff-Parkinson-White syndrome. Circulation 36:644, 1967.
53. Epstein ML, Stone FM, Benditt DG: Incessant atrial tachycardia in childhood: association with rate-dependent conduction in accessory atrioventricular pathway. Am J Cardiol 44:498, 1979.
54. Farre J, Ross D, Wiener I, et al.: Reciprocal tachycardias using accessory pathways with long conduction times. Am J Cardiol 44:1099, 1979.
55. Feld GK, Nademanee K, Weiss J, et al.: Electrophysiologic basis for the suppression by amiodarone of orthodromic supraventricular tachycardias complicating pre-excitation syndromes. J Am Coll Cardiol 3:1298, 1984.
56. Fisher JD, Brodman R, Kim SG, et al.: Attempted nonsurgical electrical ablation of accessory pathways via the coronary sinus in the Wolff-Parkinson-White syndrome. J Am Coll Cardiol 4:685, 1984.

57. Fisher JD, Johnston DR, Kim SG, et al.: Implantable pacers for tachycardia termination: stimulation techniques and long-term efficacy. PACE 9:1325, 1986.
58. Gallagher JJ: Variants of preexcitation. In Zipes DP, Jalife J (eds.): Cardiac Electrophysiology and Arrhythmias, pp. 419–433. Orlando, Grune and Stratton, Inc., 1985.
59. Gallagher JJ, Pritchett ELC, Sealy WC, et al.: The preexcitation syndromes. Progr Cardiov Dis 20:285, 1978.
60. Gallagher JJ, Sealy WC: The permanent form of junctional reciprocating tachycardia. Further elucidation of the underlying mechanism. Eur J Cardiol 8:413, 1978.
61. Gallagher JJ, Smith WM, Kasell JH, et al.: Role of Maheim fibers in cardiac arrhythmias in man. Circulation 64:176, 1981.
62. Gallagher JJ, Svenson RH, Kasell J, et al.: Catheter technique for closed-chest ablation of the atrioventricular conduction system: a therapeutic alternative for the treatment of refractory supraventricular arrhythmias. N Engl J Med 306:194, 1982.
63. German LD, Gallagher JJ, Broughton A, et al.: Effects of exercise and isoproterenol during atrial fibrillation in patients with Wolff-Parkinson-White syndrome. Am J Cardiol 51:1203, 1983.
64. Giulani ER, Fuster V, Brandenburg RO, et al.: Ebstein's anomaly: the clinical features and natural history of Ebstein's anomaly of the tricuspid valve. Mayo Clin Proc 54:163, 1979.
65. Green M, Heddle B, Dassen W, et al.: Value of QRS alternation in determining the site of origin of narrow QRS supraventricular tachycardia. Circulation 68:368, 1983.
66. Guarneri T, Sealy WC, German LD, et al.: Utilization of an accessory pathway as the anterograde limb during the permanent form of junctional reciprocating tachycardia. Am J Cardiol 53:365, 1984.
67. Guarneri T, Sealy WC, Kasell JH, et al.: The nonpharmacologic management of the permanent form of junctional reciprocating tachycardia. Circulation 69:269, 1984.
68. Gulamhusein S, Ko P, Carruthers SG, et al.: Acceleration of the ventricular response during atrial fibrillation in the Wolff-Parkinson-White syndrome after verapamil. Circulation 65:348, 1982.
69. Hamer A, Peter T, Mandel WJ: Effects of verapamil on supraventricular tachycardia in patients with overt and concealed Wolff-Parkinson-White syndrome. Am Heart J 101:600, 1981.
70. Harper RW, Whiteford A, Middlebrook K, et al.: Effects of verapamil on the electrophysiologic properties of the accessory pathway in patients with Wolff-Parkinson-White syndrome. Am J Cardiol 50:1323, 1982.
71. Hirshborn R: Genetic deficiencies of adenosine deaminase and purine nucleoside phosphorylase. Overview, genetic heterogeneity and therapy. Birth Defects 3:73, 1983.
72. His W (trans. Bast TH, Gardner WD): The activity of the embryonic human heart and its significance for the understanding of the heart movement in the adult. J Hist Allied Sci 4:289, 1949.
73. Holtzmann M, Scherf D: Über elektrokardiogramme mit verkurzter vorhofkammer-distanz und positiven P-zacken. Z Klin Med 121:404, 1932.
74. Jackman WM, Zipes DP, Naccarelli GV, et al.: Electrophysiology of oral encainide. Am J Cardiol 419:1270, 1982.
75. Janse MJ, Anderson RH, van Capelle FJL, et al.: A combined electrophysiological and anatomical study of the human fetal heart. Am Heart J 91:556, 1976.
76. Kay GN, Pressley JC, Packer DL, et al.: Value of the 12-lead electrocardiogram in discriminating atrioventricular nodal reciprocating tachycardia from circus movement atrioventricular tachycardia utilizing a retrograde accessory pathway. Am J Cardiol 59:296, 1987.
77. Kent AFS: Researches on the structure and function of the mammalian heart. J Physiol 14:233, 1893.
78. Kerr CR, Prystowsky EN, Smith WM, et al.: Electrophysiologic effects of disopyramide phosphate in patients with Wolff-Parkinson-White syndrome. Circulation 65:869, 1982.
79. Kim SS, Lal R, Ruffy R: Treatment of paroxysmal reentrant supraventricular tachycardia with flecainide acetate. Am J Cardiol 58:80, 1986.
80. Klein GJ, Bashore TM, Selbers TD, et al.: Ventricular fibrillation in the Wolff-Parkinson-White syndrome. N Eng J Med 301:1080, 1979.
81. Klein GJ, Gulamhusein S, Prystowsky EN, et al.: Comparison of the electrophysiologic effects of intravenous and oral verapamil in patients with paroxysmal supraventricular tachycardia. Am J Cardiol 49:117, 1982.
82. Klein GJ, Gulamhusein SS: Intermittent pre-excitation in the Wolff-Parkinson-White syndrome. Am J Cardiol 52:292, 1983.
83. Klein GJ, Prystowsky EN, Prichett ELC, et al.: Atypical patterns of retrograde conduction over accessory atrioventricular pathways. Circulation 60:1477, 1979.
84. Kugler JD: Evaluation of pediatric patients with preexcitation syndromes. In Benditt DG, Benson DW (eds.): Cardiac Preexcitation Syndromes, p. 363. Boston, Martinus Nijhoff, 1986.
85. Kunze KP, Kuck KH, Schluter M, et al.: Electrophysiologic and clinical effects of intravenous and oral encainide in accessory atrioventricular pathway. Am J Cardiol 54:323, 1984.
86. Kunze KP, Schluter M, Kuck KH: Sotalol in patients with Wolff-Parkinson-White syndrome. Circulation 75:1050, 1987.
87. Lev M, Fox SM, Bharati S, et al.: Maheim and James fibers as a basis for a unique variety of pre-excitation. Am J Cardiol 36:880, 1975.
88. Lev M, Leffler WB, Langendorf R, et al.: Anatomic findings in a case of ventricular pre-excitation (WPW) terminating in complete atrioventricular block. Circulation 34:718, 1966.
89. Lévy PS, Broustet JP, Clémenty J, et al.: Syndrome de Wolff-Parkinson-White. Corrélations entre l'exploration électrophysiologique et l'effet de l'épreuve d'effort sur l'aspect électrocardiographique de préexcitation. Arch Mal Coeur 72:634, 1979.
90. Lévy S, Broustet JP, Metze M, et al.: Response of accessory AV pathways to exercise and catecholamines. In Benditt DG, Benson DW (eds.): Cardiac Preexcitation Syndromes, p. 154. Boston, Martinus Nijhoff, 1986.
91. Lewis T: The Mechanism and Graphic Registration of the Heart Beat. London, Shaw and Sons, Ltd., 1925.
92. Lindsay BD, Crossen KJ, Cain ME: Concordance of distinguishing electrocardiographic features during sinus rhythm with the location of accessory pathways in the Wolff-Parkinson-White syndrome. Am J Cardiol 59:1093, 1987.
93. Lindsay BD, Saksena S, Rothbart ST, et al.: Long-term efficacy and safety of beta-adrenergic receptor antagonists for supraventricular tachycardia. Am J Cardiol 60:63D, 1987.
94. Ludmer PL, McGowan NE, Autman EM, et al.: Efficacy of propafenone in Wolff-Parkinson-White syndrome: electrophysiologic findings and long-term follow-up. J Am Coll Cardiol 9:1357, 1987.
95. Lundberg A: Paroxysmal atrial tachycardia in infancy: long-term follow-up study of 49 subjects. Pediatrics 70:638, 1982.
96. Mahaim I, Winston WR: Recherches d'anatomic comparée et de pathologic expérimentale sur les connexions hautes de faisceau de His-Tawara. Cardiologia 45:189, 1941.
97. Maheim I: Kent's fibers and the AV paraspecific conduction through upper connections of the bundle of His-Tawara. Am Heart J 33:651, 1947.
98. Maheim I, Benott A: Nouvelles recherches sur les connexions supérieures de la branche gauche du faisceau de His-Tawara avec cloison interventriculaire. Cardiologia 1:61, 1938.
99. Mandel WJ, Kaks MM, Obayshi K, et al.: The Wolff-Parkinson-White syndrome: pharmacologic effects of procainamide. Am Heart J 90:744, 1975.
100. Markel ML, Prystowsky EN, Heger JJ, et al.: Encainide for treatment of supraventricular tachycardias associated with Wolff-Parkinson-White syndrome. Am J Cardiol 58:41C, 1986.
101. Milstein S, Sharma AD, Klein GJ: Electrophysiologic profile of asymptomatic Wolff-Parkinson-White pattern. Am J Cardiol 57:1097, 1986.
102. Mines GR: On circulating excitations in heart muscles and their possible relation to tachycardia and fibrillation. Trans R Soc Can (Ser. III, Sec. IV)8:43, 1914.
103. Mitchell BL, Wyse DG, Duff HJ: Electropharmacology of sotolol in patients with Wolff-Parkinson-White syndrome. Circulation 76:810, 1987.
104. Morady F, DiCarolo L, Berman JM, et al.: Effect of propranolol on ventricular rate during atrial fibrillation in the Wolff-Parkinson-White syndrome. PACE 10:492, 1987.
105. Morady F, Scheinman MM, DiCarlo LA, et al.: Coexistent posteroseptal and right-sided atrioventricular bypass tracts. J Am Coll Cardiol 5:640, 1985.

106. Morady F, Scheinman MM, Gonzalez R, et al.: His-ventricular dissociation in a patient with reciprocating tachycardia and a nodoventricular bypass tract. Circulation 64:839, 1981.
107. Morady F, Scheinman MM, Winston SA, et al.: Efficacy and safety of transcatheter ablation of posteroseptal accessory pathways. Circulation 72:170, 1985.
108. Munoz A, Leenhardt A, Sassine A, et al.: Therapeutic use of adenosine for terminating spontaneous paroxysmal supraventricular tachycardia. Eur Heart J 5:735, 1984.
109. Ohnell RF: Pre-excitation. A cardiac abnormality. Acta Med Scand (Suppl)152:9, 1944.
110. Okumura K, Henthorn R, Epstein A, et al.: "Incessant" atrioventricular (AV) reciprocating tachycardia utilizing left lateral AV bypass pathway with a long retrograde conduction time. PACE 9:332, 1986.
111. Orinius E: Pre-excitation: studies on criteria, prognosis, and heredity. Acta Med Scand (Suppl)465:1, 1966.
112. Packer D, Bardy GH, Worley SJ, et al.: Tachycardia induced cardiomyopathy: A reversible form of left ventricular dysfunction. Am J Cardiol 57:563, 1986.
113. Porter CJ, Gillette PC, Garson A, et al.: Effects of verapamil on supraventricular tachycardia in children. Am J Cardiol 48:487, 1981.
114. Porter CJ, Holmes DR: Preexcitation syndromes associated with congenital heart disease. In Benditt DG, Benson DW (eds.): Cardiac Preexcitation Syndromes, pp. 289–301. Boston, Martinus Nijkoff, 1986.
115. Pritchett ELC, Benditt DG, Smith WM, et al.: Effect of catheter position on the initiation of atrial echoes with atrial pacing and premature stimulation in patients with accessory pathways. Am J Cardiol 42:738, 1978.
116. Prystowsky EN, Klein GJ, Rinkenberger RL, et al.: Clinical efficacy and electrophysiologic effects of encainide in patients with Wolff-Parkinson-White syndrome. Circulation 69:278, 1984.
117. Rardon DP, Bailey JC: Adenosine attenuation of the electrophysiologic effects of isoproterenol on canine cardiac Purkinje fibers. J Pharmacol Exp Ther 228:792, 1984.
118. Rinkenberger RL, Prystowsky EN, Heger JJ, et al.: Effects of intravenous and chronic oral verapamil administration in patients with supraventricular tachyarrhythmias. Circulation 62:996, 1980.
119. Rinne C, Klein GJ, Sharma AD, et al.: Relation between clinical presentation and induced arrhythmias in the Wolff-Parkinson-White syndrome. Am J Cardiol 60:576, 1987.
120. Robb JS, Kaylor CT, Turman WG: A study of specialized heart tissue at various stages of development of the human fetal heart. Am J Med 5:324, 1948.
121. Rosen MR, Danilo P, Weiss RM: Actions of adenosine on normal and abnormal impulse initiation in canine ventricle. Am J Physiol H715, 1983.
122. Rosenbaum FF, Hecht HH, Wilson FN, et al.: The potential variations of the thorax and the esophagus in anomalous atrioventricular excitation (Wolff-Parkinson-White syndrome). Am Heart J 29:281, 1945.
123. Rosenbaum MB, Chiale PA, Ryba D, et al.: Control of tachyarrhythmias associated with Wolff-Parkinson-White syndrome by amiodarone hydrochloride. Am J Cardiol 34:215, 1974.
124. Saksena C, Calvo RA, Boccadamo R, et al.: Electrophysiologic effects, clinical efficacy, and safety of intravenous and oral nadolol in refractory supraventricular tachyarrhythmias: a multicenter study. Am J Cardiol 59:307, 1987.
125. Saksena S, Jacobs J, Rothbart ST: Role of electrophysiologic studies with acute drug testing in refractory supraventricular tachycardia. In Steinkopff D (ed.): Cardiac Pacing, pp. 711–718. Vienna, Verlag, 1983.
126. Sapire DW, O'Riordan AC, Black IFS: Safety and efficacy of short- and long-term verapamil therapy in children with tachycardia. Am J Cardiol 48:1091, 1981.
127. Scheinman M, Morady F, Hess D, et al.: Catheter induced ablation of the atrioventricular junction to control refractory supraventricular arrhythmias. JAMA 243:851, 1982.
128. Schiebler GL, Adams P, Anderson RC, et al.: Clinical study of twenty-three cases of Ebstein's anomaly of the tricuspid valve. Circulation 19:165, 1959.
129. Sellers TD, Bashore TM, Gallagher JJ: Digitalis in the preexcitation syndrome. Analysis during atrial fibrillation. Circulation 56:260, 1977.
130. Sellers TD, Campbell RWF, Bashore TM, et al.: Effects of procainamide and quinidine in Wolff-Parkinson-White syndrome. Circulation 55:15, 1977.
131. Sharma AD, Yee R, Guiradon G, et al.: Sensitivity and specificity of invasive and noninvasive testing for risk of sudden death in Wolff-Parkinson-White syndrome. J Am Coll Cardiol 10:373, 1987.
132. Shenasa M, Fromer M, Fangeri G, et al.: Efficacy and safety of intravenous and oral diltiazem for Wolff-Parkinson-White syndrome. Am J Cardiol 59:301, 1987.
133. Slama R, Coumel P, Bouvrain Y: Les syndromes de Wolff-Parkinson-White de type A inapparents ou latents en rhythme sinusal. Arch Mal Coeur 66:639, 1973.
134. Sollevi A, Lagerkranser M, Instedt L, et al.: Controlled hypotension with adenosine in aneurysm surgery. Anesthesiology 61:400, 1984.
135. Soulié P, Heulin A, Pauly-Laubry C, et al.: Maladie d'Ebstein étude clinique et évolution (à propos de 40 observations dont 9 chirurgicales). Arch Mal Coeur 63:615, 1970.
136. Spurrell RAJ, Krikler DM, Sowton E: Effects of verapamil on electro-physiological properties of anomalous atrioventricular connection in Wolff-Parkinson-White syndrome. Br Heart J 36:256, 1974.
137. Strasberg B, Ashley WW, Wyndham CRC, et al.: Treadmill exercise testing in Wolff-Parkinson-White syndrome. Am J Cardiol 45:742, 1980.
138. Sung RJ, Castellanos A, Mallon SM, et al.: Mode of initiation of reciprocating tachycardia during programmed ventricular stimulation in the Wolff-Parkinson-White syndrome. Am J Cardiol 40:24, 1977.
139. Sung RJ, Elser B, McAllister RG: Intravenous verapamil for termination of re-entrant supraventricular tachycardias. Ann Int Med 93:682, 1980.
140. Sung RJ, Geband H, Castellanos A, et al.: Clinical and electrophysiological observations in patients with concealed accessory bypass tracts. Am J Cardiol 40:839, 1977.
141. Sung RJ, Styperek JL: Electrophysiologic identification of dual atrioventricular nodal pathway conduction in patients with reciprocating tachycardia using anomalous bypass tracts. Circulation 60:1464, 1979.
142. Tawara S: Des Reizleitung des Sangetierherzens. Eine anatomisch-histologische studie uber das atrioventrikularbundel und die purkinjeschen faden. Jena, Verlag von Gustav Fischer, 1906.
143. Tonkin AM, Miller HC, Svenson RH, et al.: Refractory periods of the accessory pathway in Wolff-Parkinson-White syndrome. Circulation 52:563, 1975.
144. Tonkin AM, Wagner GS, Gallagher JJ, et al.: Initial forces of ventricular depolarization in the Wolff-Parkinson-White syndrome. Analysis based upon localization of the accessory pathway by epicardial mapping. Circulation 52:1030, 1975.
145. Touboul P, Vexler RM, Chatelain MT: Reentry via Maheim fibers as a possible basis for tachycardia. Br Heart J 40:806, 1978.
146. Truex RC, Bishof JK, Hoffman EL: Accessory atrioventricular muscle bundles of the developing human heart. Anat Rec 131:45, 1958.
147. Vaidailbet JH, Pressley JC, Henke E, et al.: Familial occurrence of accessory atrioventricular pathways (pre-excitation syndrome). N Engl J Med 317:65, 1987.
148. Ward DE, Camm AJ, Spurrell RAJ: Ventricular pre-excitation due to anomalous nodoventricular pathway. Report of 3 patients. Eur J Cardiol 9:111, 1979.
149. Wellens HJ, Durrer D: Wolff-Parkinson-White syndrome and atrial fibrillation: relation between refractory period of accessory pathway and ventricular rate during atrial fibrillation. Am J Cardiol 34:777, 1974.
150. Wellens HJJ: Electrical stimulation of the heart in the study and treatment of tachycardias, pp. 97–109. Baltimore, MD; University Park Press, 1971.
151. Wellens HJJ, Bar FW, Dassen WRM, et al.: Effect of drugs in the Wolff-Parkinson-White syndrome. Importance of initial length of effective refractory period of the accessory pathway. Am J Cardiol 46:665, 1980.

152. Wellens HJJ, Lie KI, Bar FW, et al.: Effect of amiodarone in the Wolff-Parkinson-White syndrome. Am J Cardiol 38:189, 1976.
153. Willems JL, et al.: World Health Organization/International Society and Federation for Cardiology Task Force Ad Hoc. Criteria for intraventricular conduction disturbances and pre-excitation. J Am Coll Cardiol 5:1261, 1985.
154. Wilson FN: A case in which the vagus influenced the form of the ventricular complex of the electrocardiogram. Arch Int Med 16:1008, 1915.
155. Wolfarth CC, Wood FC: The mechanism of production of short P-R intervals and prolonged QRS complexes in patients with presumably undamaged heart: hypothesis of an accessory pathway of auriculoventricular conduction (bundle of Kent). Am Heart J 8:297, 1933.
156. Wolff L, Parkinson J, White PD: Bundle-branch block with short P-R interval in healthy young people prone to paroxysmal tachycardia. Am Heart J 5:685, 1930.
157. Wood FC, Wolfarth CC, Geckeler GD: Histologic demonstration of accessory muscular connections between auricle and ventricle in a case of short P-R interval and prolonged QRS complex. Am Heart J 25:454, 1943.
158. Wu D, Amat-y-Leon F, Simpson RJ, et al.: Electrophysiology studies with multiple drugs in patients with atrioventricular reentrant tachycardia using an extranodal pathway. Circulation 56:727, 1977.
159. Yee R, Gulamhusein SS, Klein GJ: Combined verapamil and propranolol for supraventricular tachycardia. Am J Cardiol 53:757, 1984.
160. Yee R, Klein GJ: Syncope in the Wolff-Parkinson-White syndrome: incidence and electrophysiologic correlates. PACE 7:381, 1984.
161. Yeh SJ, Lin FC, Chow YY, et al.: Termination of paroxysmal supraventricular tachycardia with a single dose of diltiazem and propranolol. Circulation 71:104, 1985.
162. Zipes DP, DeJoseph RL, Rothbaum DA: Unusual properties of accessory pathways. Circulation 49:1200, 1974.

11

Complex Ventricular Arrhythmias and Nonsustained Ventricular Tachycardia: Risk Stratification and Management

Gioia Turitto
Nabil El-Sherif

Sudden cardiac death is currently the major contributor to overall cardiovascular mortality in the modern world. It accounts for approximately 60% of all coronary heart disease fatalities occurring annually.[1] The need for a systematic approach that can identify the high-risk patient, aid in initiating appropriate therapy, and prevent the occurrence of sudden cardiac death is paramount. It has been amply documented that patients with sustained ventricular tachyarrhythmias, including those resuscitated from cardiac arrest, have a high incidence of sudden cardiac death.[2-6] Those patients, however, represent only a small proportion of the total population with complex ventricular arrhythmias. The relationship of complex ventricular arrhythmias, short of sustained ventricular tachycardia (VT)/ventricular fibrillation (VF), to sudden cardiac "arrhythmic" death, however, remains controversial. A number of recent studies suggest that complex ventricular arrhythmias in the post-infarction patient are independent markers for risk of sudden cardiac arrest,[7-9] but there is a general agreement that their sensitivity and specificity are relatively low.[10]

In the last several years many studies have investigated the role of programmed electrical stimulation (PES) as a means of classifying patients with complex ventricular arrhythmias into low- and high-risk groups for sudden cardiac death.[11-37] This chapter reviews the role of PES and the recently introduced noninvasive technique of signal-averaged electrocardiography in risk stratification and management of patients with complex ventricular arrhythmias. Although complex ventricular arrhythmias are usually defined as frequent, multiform, and repetitive ventricular premature complexes (VPCs), the role of nonsustained VT (defined as three or more consecutive VPCs that are less than 30 seconds in duration at a rate of > 100/min) is particularly emphasized. Nonsustained VT is thought to represent a strong marker for sudden cardiac death.[10, 38-40]

Complex Ventricular Arrhythmias and Sudden Death in the Presence of a Normal Heart or Organic Heart Disease with or without Impaired Ventricular Function

Complex ventricular arrhythmias are uncommon in the absence of organic heart disease, and their presence does not increase the risk of either cardiac death or sudden death.[41] A long-term follow-up (average 6.5 years) of 73 asymptomatic subjects who had frequent and complex ventricular arrhythmias including nonsustained VT showed no increased risk of death compared with that of the healthy U.S. population.[42]

Supported by National Institutes of Health Grant HL31341 and Veterans Administration Medical Research Funds.

The incidence of complex ventricular arrhythmias increases in the presence of heart disease. However, in the absence of impaired ventricular function, the arrhythmia does not seem to be associated with an increased incidence of sudden death. Of 92 patients with normal left ventricular ejection fraction studied after coronary artery bypass surgery, 57% had complex ventricular arrhythmias, including 21.5% who had nonsustained VT. The incidence of complications in patients with complex ventricular arrhythmias was not higher than that in those with no arrhythmias, and there were no cardiac or sudden deaths during an average follow-up period of 16 months.[43] In another series of 130 patients with chronic stable angina pectoris, complex ventricular arrhythmias were not associated with an increased risk of sudden cardiac death.[44]

In the presence of impaired left ventricular function, complex ventricular arrhythmias may be an independent risk for sudden cardiac death. This view is not without controversy.[41] In the first quantitative study of the relationship between impaired left ventricular function and complex ventricular arrhythmias after myocardial infarction, cardiac death was strongly associated with a low left ventricular ejection fraction, and the independent role of the arrhythmia could not be established.[45] The interrelationship between impaired ventricular function, complex ventricular arrhythmias, and sudden cardiac death was systematically analyzed later in two groups of patients: (1) patients with congestive heart failure, commonly the result of ischemic or idiopathic dilated cardiomyopathy; and (2) patients who survived the early phase of myocardial infarction. Packer summarized the results of seven studies comprising 891 patients with congestive heart failure.[46] The incidence of nonsustained VT ranged from 39% to 60%. The total mortality rate averaged 37.4%, and the rate of sudden cardiac death was 14.3% per year. Surawicz reviewed eight additional studies comprising 398 patients with congestive heart failure.[41] The incidence of nonsustained VT ranged from 49% to 100% and averaged 65%, whereas the rates of total mortality and sudden cardiac death averaged 42.4% and 21.4%, respectively, during a follow-up period of 18.5 months (range of 11 to 34 months). In the majority of the above studies, sudden cardiac death was unrelated to nonsustained VT. In one study, nonsustained VT was present in 26 of 35 patients. Of these patients, 80% died within 2 years and only one of the deaths was attributed to arrhythmias.[47] Few studies found that complex ventricular arrhythmias were an independent risk factor for sudden cardiac death,[48-50] although the correlation was not strong.[41]

In survivors of myocardial infarction, three studies of a large series of patients addressed the interrelationship between impaired ventricular function, complex ventricular arrhythmias, and sudden cardiac death.[7-9] All three studies suggested that complex ventricular arrhythmias are an independent risk factor for sudden cardiac death. The multicenter post-infarction research group was a nine-hospital natural history study of patients under age 70 who had a proven myocardial infarction.[7] In 766 patients, 86 deaths occurred during a 3-year follow-up period. When multivariate survivorship techniques were used to evaluate the independent contribution of ventricular arrhythmias and impaired left ventricular function to post-infarction mortality, VPC frequency, VPC runs, and left ventricular ejection fraction were each independently associated with both total mortality and arrhythmia-specific mortality. The Multicenter Investigation of the Limitation of Infarct Size (MILIS) study was a five-hospital intervention study of the effect of hyaluronidase, propranolol, or both in patients under age 76 who had acute myocardial infarction.[8] In this study, 533 patients who survived 10 days after infarction were followed for a mean of 18 months. Frequent VPCs (>10/hour) and left ventricular ejection fraction of less than 40% were independently significant markers of risk for subsequent sudden death that was believed to be the result of primary ventricular arrhythmia. The incidence of sudden death was 18% in patients with both left ventricular dysfunction and frequent VPCs, which is an 11-fold increase compared with patients in whom neither risk factor was present; 79% of all sudden deaths occurred within 7 months after the index infarction. Maisel et al.[9] studied 191 survivors of non–Q wave myocardial infarction and 586 survivors of Q wave infarction. Complex ventricular arrhythmia at the time of hospital discharge was an important predictor of mortality only in patients with non–Q wave infarction. The 10% incidence of sudden cardiac death in this group was much higher than that in patients with Q wave infarction and the incidence of sudden death reported in most other studies. This was explained by the presence of an unstable ischemic state in these patients.

Although recent multicenter studies have shown that complex ventricular arrhythmias are an independent risk for sudden cardiac death, especially in survivors of myocardial infarction, the corollary observation that suppression of those arrhythmias will reduce the incidence of sudden death has not yet been demonstrated. Of seven trials of antiarrhythmic agents conducted so far (summarized by Furberg and May[51]), both the drug and the placebo produced the same result in one study; in two, the drug improved the outcome; in the remaining four, the drug worsened the outcome. These studies suffered from the small numbers of enrolled patients and the exclusion of patients with severe ventricular arrhythmias.

A large multicenter study, sponsored by The National Institutes of Health, that addresses some of the limitations of previous studies is currently under way. The goal of the Cardiac Arrhythmia Suppression Trial (CAST)[52] is to determine whether suppression of asymptomatic ventricular arrhythmias will reduce the incidence of sudden death in patients at moderate risk. This trial is being carried out at 27 sites in the United States, Canada, and Sweden; 4400 patients with previous myocardial infarction, asymptomatic ventricular arrhythmias, and reduced left ventricular function will be enrolled over a 3-year period. Patients whose arrhythmias are suppressed by antiarrhythmic drugs will be randomly assigned to receive either placebo or effective suppressive therapy during 2 to 5 years of follow-up, and the incidence of sudden death in the two groups will be compared.

An advantage of this study is that the hypothesis is being tested using three different, randomly assigned drugs, each of which can effectively suppress VPCs. Therefore, it is anticipated that the results of this study can be extrapolated to any safe drug that suppresses VPCs. Woosley[52] has argued that if the CAST study is successful, antiarrhythmic agents will join the beta-receptor antagonist as medications indicated for prevention of sudden death. If not, two possibilities should be considered: (1) the concept that ventricular arrhythmias in this population progress to cause sudden death is invalid, or (2) these agents prevent sudden death in some patients and cause sudden death in others, cancelling any overall benefit. In a preliminary report from CAST, patients treated with encainide or flecainide were found to have a higher rate of death from arrhythmia than the patients assigned to placebo during an average of 10 months of follow-up.[52a] Because of these results, the part of the trial involving encainide and flecainide, but not moricizine, has been discontinued.

Even if the CAST study eventually shows that suppression of complex ventricular arrhythmias decreases the incidence of sudden cardiac death in survivors of myocardial infarction, a risk stratification strategy other than the mere presence of complex ventricular arrhythmias on ambulatory monitoring would probably be required. This is because of the low sensitivity and specificity of Holter monitoring alone as a marker of sudden cardiac death in these patients. Because of the low sensitivity, a number of patients with no complex ventricular arrhythmias but who still may be at risk for sudden cardiac death could be deprived of appropriate therapy. Furthermore, the low specificity of this marker could lead to unnecessary chronic therapy in a large percentage of patients. This would be of relatively less concern if antiarrhythmic drugs (and other forms of antiarrhythmic therapy) are consistently effective, affordable, and without serious side effects. None of these premises are currently in sight. Because of this and similar arguments, the role of PES, and more recently of the signal-averaged electrocardiogram (ECG), in risk stratification and management of patients with complex ventricular arrhythmias has received considerable interest.

Programmed Electrical Stimulation in Patients with Complex Ventricular Arrhythmias

Several studies have investigated the role of PES in identifying subsets of patients with complex ventricular arrhythmias at low and high risk for sudden cardiac death.[11-37] Patients in whom PES fails to induce sustained VT may have a low risk of sudden cardiac death. In those patients, antiarrhythmic therapy may not be warranted. On the other hand, patients with inducible sustained VT may be at increased risk of sudden cardiac death. It is possible that antiarrhythmic therapy guided by the results of PES may decrease the risk of sudden death in this group.

STIMULATION PROTOCOLS

The incidence and type of ventricular arrhythmias induced by PES depend on the stimulation protocol. Table 11–1 lists studies of PES in patients with non-sustained VT in which details of the stimulation protocol were reported. The stimulation protocol varied with regard to the following factors:

1. The nature of the basic drive (sinus or ventricular paced rhythm)
2. The cycle length of the basic paced drive
3. The current strength of the stimulus
4. The nature of the stimulating train (basic drive followed by one or more extrastimuli, burst pacing, and alternation of short and long cycle)
5. The site of stimulation
6. The use of drugs such as isoproterenol to facilitate induction of VT
7. What constitutes a specific end point for the stimulation protocol

The introduction of a single ventricular extrastimulus during sinus rhythm rarely resulted in the induction of VT, which most often required two or more extrastimuli in patients with spontaneous nonsustained VT. In the studies of Estes and colleagues[53] and Prystowsky and coworkers,[54] approximately 20% of all episodes of VT (sustained or nonsustained) were induced by one to three extrastimuli delivered during sinus rhythm. Spielman et al.[19] reported that only 13% of all induced sustained VT was induced by triple extrastimuli during sinus rhythm. Extrastimuli applied during ventricular pacing were consistently more effective in inducing ventricular tachyarrhythmias. However, the optimal duration and cycle length of the pacing drive are not clearly established.[55] Based on results obtained both in patients with spontaneous sustained ventricular tachyarrhythmias[56, 57] and in those with nonsustained VT,[19] it seems advisable to use more than one pacing drive, with cycle lengths between 600 and 400 ms. In these studies, the yield of inducing sustained VT with up to three extrastimuli increased by approximately 20% with the use of a second pacing drive, and by an additional 20% when a third drive was included in the protocol. In a study by Breithardt and colleagues,[58] shortening the cycle length of the basic drive allowed induction of sustained VT by extrastimuli with longer coupling intervals. However, this finding was not reproduced by other groups.[59]

The incidence of inducible ventricular tachyarrhythmias varied directly with the number of extrastimuli applied during basic ventricular pacing both in patients with spontaneous sustained and nonsustained VT. In patients with spontaneous sustained VT, the probability of inducing sustained monomorphic VT ranged from 22% to 33% (mean, 27%) with one extrastimulus, from 47% to 73% (mean, 66%) with two extrastimuli,

TABLE 11–1
Techniques and End Points for Programmed Stimulation Studies in Patients with Spontaneous Nonsustained Ventricular Tachycardia*

Author	Basic Drive(s)	No. of Extrastimuli	Burst Pacing	Site(s) of Stimulation		Drugs (isop)	End Points
				RV	LV		
Vandepol (1980)[60]	SR, VP at ≥ 1 CL	2	yes	≥ 1	≥ 1	no	reproducible VT (≥3 RVR)
Naccarelli (1982)[11]	SR, VP at CL = 600, 500, 400 ms	2	yes	2 (apex, OT)	in some cases	no	VT
Livelli (1982)[69]	AP, VP at CL = 600, 400 ms	2	yes	2 (apex, OT)	no	no	reproducible sustained VT (requiring intervention for termination)
Buxton (1983)[13]	SR, VP at CL = 600–400 ms	2; 3 in some cases	yes	2 (apex, OT)	≥ 1 in some cases	yes	reproducible VT resembling clinical VT
Gomes (1984)[15]	SR, VP at CL = 600, 500 ms	2	yes	2 (apex, OT)	no	no	reproducible VT (≥5 RVR)
Veltri (1985)[18]	VP at CL = 600, 500, 450 ms	2	yes	2 (apex, OT)	2, in some cases	no	sustained VT (≥30 s)
Spielman (1985)[19]	SR, VP at CL = 600, 450 ms	3	no	2 (apex, OT)	no	no	sustained VT (≥15 s); VF
Schoenfeld (1985)[65]	SR, AP, VP at >1 CL	2; 3 in some cases	yes	1 (apex)	no	no	reproducible sustained VT (>100 complexes) or symptomatic nonsustained VT
Zheutlin (1986)[21]	SR, VP at CL = 600, 500, 400 ms	2	yes	≥1 (apex, OT in some cases)	no	no	reproducible VT (>6 RVR)
Breithardt (1986)[22]	SR, VP at CL = 500, 430, 370, 330 ms	2 or 3	no	1 or 2 (apex, OT)	no	yes, in some cases	VT
Poll (1986)[24]	VP at CL = 600, 400 ms	3	yes	2 (apex, OT)	no	no	sustained VT (>30 sec)
Estes (1986)[53]	SR, VP at ≥ 1 CL = 700–400 ms	2; 3 in some cases	yes	≥1 (apex, OT in some cases)	no	no	VT (≥5 RVR); VF
Prystowsky (1986)[54]	SR, VP at CL = 600, 500, 400 ms	2; 3 in some cases	yes	2 (apex, OT)	in some cases	no	VT (≥3 RVR) resembling clinical VT
Buxton (1987)[29]	VP at CL = 600, 400 ms	3	yes	2 (apex, OT)	no	no	reproducible sustained VT (> 30 s) resembling clinical VT
Sulpizi (1987)[30]	VP at CL = 600, 400 ms	2; 3 in some cases	no	1 (apex); >2 in some cases	in some cases	no	reproducible sustained VT (>15 complexes)
Zehender (1987)[63]	SR, VP at CL = 600, 500, 430 ms	3	no	1 (apex)	no	no	sustained monomorphic VT (≥30 s); VF
Turitto (1988)[33]	SR, VP at CL = 600, 500, 400 ms	3	no	2 (apex, OT)	no	no	sustained monomorphic VT (≥30 s); VF
Kharsa (1988)[35]	VP at CL = 600, 500, 400 ms	3	no	2 (apex, OT)	no	no	sustained monomorphic VT (≥30 s); VF

*The table lists, in chronological order, only those full reports in which patients with nonsustained VT represented all, or a significant fraction of, the study population.

RV = right ventricle; LV = left ventricle; isop = isoproterenol; SR = sinus rhythm; VP = ventricular pacing; CL = cycle length; VT = ventricular tachycardia; RVR = repetitive ventricular responses; OT = outflow tract; AP = atrial pacing; VF = ventricular fibrillation.

and from 72% to 94% (mean, 88%) with three extrastimuli.[56, 57, 60–63] Thus, the introduction of a second and a third extrastimulus increased the sensitivity of the stimulation protocol for sustained monomorphic VT by an average of 45% and 23%, respectively. The same phenomenon was reported in patients with spontaneous nonsustained VT. Four studies[19, 29, 33, 63] that utilized a similar stimulation protocol (three extrastimuli, one or two right ventricular pacing sites, and multiple basic drives) and similar end points (induction of sustained ventricular tachyarrhythmias) reported their data according to the number of extrastimuli required for induction. The fraction of patients who had sustained monomorphic VT induced by one extrastimulus was low (0–3%), rose substantially with two extrastimuli (9–24%), and showed further increase with three extrastimuli (21–39%). A similar trend was described for the induction of VF, which increased from 0% with one extrastimulus to 2% to 7% with two extrastimuli and to 10% to 14% with three extrastimuli.[19, 33, 63]

Burst pacing was used by several authors to induce ventricular tachyarrhythmias in patients with spontaneous nonsustained VT. The additional yield of this mode of stimulation above the use of two extrastimuli ranged from 3%[53, 54] to 11%.[60] Similar results were reported in patients with spontaneous sustained VT.[53, 60, 64, 65] However, burst pacing may have no advantage over the use of three extrastimuli.[54] Furthermore, animal studies[66] have shown that the technique of burst pacing is highly dependent on the number of beats in the paced train and the cycle length of stimulation in a fashion that makes it very difficult to standardize or to reproduce in the clinical setting. A protocol employing an abrupt short–long sequence of the basic drive before the introduction of one or more extrastimuli was reported to initiate sustained VT in patients not otherwise inducible with conventional protocols.[67] However, when the efficacy of such a technique was compared with the use of triple extrastimuli, no significant difference was found.[68]

Programmed stimulation is usually limited to right ventricular sites. In patients with spontaneous nonsustained VT, there was little advantage in stimulating a second right ventricular site (usually the outflow tract or the septum) after three extrastimuli applied at the right ventricular apex had failed to induce VT. In the studies by Turitto and coworkers[33] and Kharsa and colleagues,[35] VT initiated at the outflow tract represented 0% to 4% of all induced sustained VT. Similarly, Zheutlin et al.,[21] using up to two extrastimuli and VT lasting six or more complexes as the end point, found that only 3% of inductions occurred during stimulation at the outflow tract. However, Spielman and coworkers[19] reported that stimulation at the outflow tract was effective in 14% of patients and accounted for 53% of induced sustained VT.

SPECIFICITY OF INDUCED TACHYARRHYTHMIAS

In patients with recurrent sustained monomorphic VT, the sensitivity of the technique of programmed stimulation is defined as the ability to reproduce the clinical arrhythmia. Such a definition is not applicable in patients with spontaneous nonsustained VT. In these patients, programmed stimulation can induce nonsustained VT, sustained monomorphic or polymorphic VT, or VF. There is some evidence that the induction of sustained monomorphic VT, rather than that of nonsustained VT or VE, should be considered as the specific end point of PES in patients with spontaneous nonsustained VT. Nonsustained VT was as commonly induced in patients with as in those without heart disease (34% and 21%, respectively).[69–72] Induced nonsustained VT was polymorphic in 80% of the cases.[56, 68, 69, 71] Polymorphic nonsustained VT induced in patients without organic heart disease did not differ in its cycle length and mode of initiation from that elicited in post-infarction patients with spontaneous sustained ventricular tachyarrhythmias.[72] These data strongly suggest that the specificity of induced nonsustained VT is low. Although some authors tried to improve the specificity of induced nonsustained VT by comparing its QRS configuration[13] and/or cycle length[18, 54] to the spontaneous arrhythmia, this approach is fraught with difficulties. Careful comparison of the QRS configuration of spontaneous and induced rhythms may be difficult to accomplish because of limitations on the number of simultaneously recorded ECG leads. It is almost impossible to adequately compare the QRS configuration of polymorphic nonsustained VT. Furthermore, there is usually little correlation between the cycle lengths of spontaneous and induced VT.[19, 74, 75]

The induction of VF may be a nonspecific response to programmed stimulation in patients with nonsustained VT. Ventricular fibrillation was induced with comparable frequency in patients with spontaneous sustained ventricular tachyarrhythmias (3–13%),[63, 70, 73, 76, 77] survivors of myocardial infarction without documented sustained VT/VF (1–14%),[63, 78, 79] and patients with spontaneous nonsustained VT (0–15%) (see Table 11–2). The frequency of induced VF was related to the aggressiveness of the stimulation protocol.[19, 3, 70, 71]

On the other hand, sustained monomorphic VT could not be induced by PES in patients without organic heart disease; thus its specificity is close to 100%.[69, 70–72] The arrhythmia was considered a marker for an electrophysiologic substrate of reentry[80] and may not be induced in the absence of such a substrate. However, sustained monomorphic VT could be induced in patients with heart disease, regardless of the presence of spontaneous sustained VT. Its prevalence was less than 3% in studies of a miscellaneous population,[56, 60, 69–71, 73] but it was much higher in patients with spontaneous nonsustained VT (see Table 11–2) and in survivors of myocardial infarction. In the latter setting, sustained monomorphic VT was inducible in 28% to 51% of patients with spontaneous nonsustained VT,[33, 63, 81] as well as in 11% to 45% of those without documented arrhythmias.[63, 78, 79, 82]

In summary, the induction of sustained monomorphic VT in patients with spontaneous nonsustained runs may be interpreted as a demonstration of the ability of programmed stimulation to expose a fixed electrophsyiologic abnormality. Such an abnormality may be implicated in the high risk of sudden cardiac death in these patients.

RESULTS OF PROGRAMMED STIMULATION

Table 11–2 summarizes the results of PES in patients with complex ventricular arrhythmias and nonsustained VT in 25 studies published between 1980 and 1988. The table includes an early study from our laboratory by Gomes and coworkers[15] and a more recent series by Turitto and colleagues.[33]

PES initiated sustained monomorphic VT in 20% of patients (range, 0–50%), VF in 5% (range, 0–15%), and nonsustained VT in 38% (range, 10–64%); 43%

TABLE 11-2
Ventricular Tachyarrhythmias Induced by Programmed Electrical Stimulation in Patients with Spontaneous Nonsustained Ventricular Tachycardia and/or Complex Ventricular Ectopy*

Author	No. of Patients	S-VT	VF	ns-VT	NI	VT/VF
Vandepol (1980)[60]	29	0	0	62%	38%	
Naccarelli (1982)[11]	44	0	0	34%	66%	
Livelli (1982)[69]	18	11%	—	44%	44%	
Swerdlow† (1982)[12]	41	22%	7%	32%	39%	
Buxton‡ (1983)[13]	83	8% mono 10% poly	0	24% mono 24% poly	49%	
Gomes (1984)[15]	73	11%	7%	10%	73%	
Miles† (1984)[17]	139	16%	—	46%	38%	
Reddy† (1984)[16]	52	—	—	—	73%	27% (S-VT/VF)
Veltri (1985)[18]	33	21%	—	21%	58%	
Spielman (1985)[19]	58	26% mono	14%	3% mono 21% poly	36%	
Schoenfeld (1985)[65]	66	15%	2%	30% mono 14% poly	39%	
Zheutlin (1986)[21]	88	—	—	—	63%	38%
Breithardt (1986)[22]	106	12%	2%	44%	42%	
Poll (1986)[24]	20	10% mono 10% poly	10%	20% mono 25% poly	25%	
Estes (1986)[53]	110	—	—	—	38%	62%
Prystowsky (1986)[54]	104	15%	—	49%	36%	
Miles† (1986)[26]	53	25% (mono S-VT and VF by ≤2 extrastimuli)	15%	36%	25%	
Batsford† (1986)[28]	81	21%	—	44%	35%	
Klein† (1986)[27]	22	50% mono	0	—	50%	
Buxton (1987)[29]	62	39% mono 7%	0	24%	31%	
Buxton (1987)[81]	43	49% mono 2% poly	0	21% mono 5% poly	23%	
Sulpizi (1987)[30]	61	15% mono	0	28% mono 18% poly	39%	
Zehender‡ (1987)[63]	50	32% mono 16%	10%	20% mono 44% poly	18%	
Turitto (1988)[33]	105	21% mono	13%	8% mono 16% poly	43%	
Kharsa (1988)[35]	40	20% mono	5%	10% mono 20% poly	45%	

*The table lists first author only with year of report and reference source. Refer to Table 11–1 for details of the stimulation protocols used in the reported studies.
†Abstract report.
‡Study in which more than one induced arrhythmia was reported for some patients (total 100%).
S-VT = sustained ventricular tachycardia; VF = ventricular fibrillation; ns-VT = nonsustained ventricular tachycardia; NI = no induced arrhythmia; — = not reported; mono = monomorphic; poly = polymorphic.

of patients (range, 18–73%) did not have any inducible arrhythmias. Induced nonsustained VT was monomorphic in 46% of cases and polymorphic in the remaining 54%. The difference in the results of the reported studies may be related, in part, to the use of different stimulation protocols and end points (see Table 11–1). The proportion of patients with induced sustained monomorphic VT was lower (11%) when a maximum of two extrastimuli and burst pacing were delivered and higher (29%) when three extrastimuli were used. The use of three extrastimuli was associated with a proportional increase in the induction of VF. In studies by Turitto and associates[33] and Spielman and coworkers,[19] VF accounted for 31% and 44%, respectively, of sustained tachyarrhythmias induced by two extrastimuli, compared with 45% and 29%, respectively, of those induced by three extrastimuli, with no statistically significant differences.

The cycle length of induced sustained monomorphic VT was relatively short, ranging between 190 and 280 ms in most studies.[18, 19, 22, 26, 30, 33, 63, 81] These cycle lengths were shorter than those induced in patients with spontaneous sustained VT (285–370 ms).[56, 58, 59, 61, 63, 73, 75, 76] This may be due, at least in part, to the fact that the induction of sustained monomorphic VT usually required more extrastimuli in patients without than in those with spontaneous sustained VT.[63] The cycle length of induced VT tended to shorten as the number of extrastimuli necessary for induction increased. This was demonstrated in patients with spontaneous nonsustained VT[20, 21] as well as in those with sustained VT.[56]

NONINVASIVE PREDICTORS OF THE RESULTS OF PROGRAMMED STIMULATION

Because only a fraction of patients with spontaneous nonsustained VT had inducible sustained monomorphic VT on PES, several noninvasive determinants of VT inducibility have been investigated as means to screen patients for the invasive electrophysiologic procedure (Table 11–3). The presence and type of heart disease, other clinical variables, ECG characteristics of the spontaneous arrhythmia, and left ventricular function indices have been investigated separately or in combination. More recently, the value of the signal-averaged ECG was also assessed.

Clinical Variables

Induction of VT was more common in patients with than in those without heart disease.[11, 13, 15, 18, 30, 33, 35, 54] In a majority of studies, all patients with induced sustained VT[18, 30, 35] or induced nonsustained/sustained VT[15, 18] had structural heart disease. In a few reports, the incidence of induced nonsustained/sustained VT in patients with apparently normal hearts ranged from 12%[54] to 17%[13] to 40%.[11] Observed differences reach statistical significance when data from several reports are pooled together, even though this approach may not be entirely satisfactory because of the different design of individual studies. Eight investigative groups subjected to PES a total of 483 patients with heart disease and 112 subjects with apparently normal hearts.[11, 13, 15, 18, 30, 33, 35, 54] When inducible nonsustained VT and inducible sustained VT were considered together, these were significantly more frequent in patients with than in those without heart disease (48% versus 30%, respectively; p < 0.05). When inducible sustained monomorphic VT was considered alone, the difference between its incidence in patients with or without organic heart disease (20% versus 2%, respectively) became more statistically significant (p < 0.01). Organic heart disease was present in 86% of patients with induced nonsustained/sustained VT[11, 13, 15, 18, 54] and 98% of those with induced sustained VT.[13, 30, 33, 35]

The relationship between the type of heart disease and inducibility can be demonstrated by combining data from seven studies of a total of 315 patients with coronary artery disease and 152 patients with other types of organic heart disease, including 88 patients with idiopathic dilated cardiomyopathy.[13, 15, 18, 21, 33, 35, 54] Only induction of nonsustained/sustained VT was more frequent in the group with coronary artery disease compared with other groups (56% versus 29%; p <0.0001), whereas the induction of sustained VT occurred with similar frequency in the two groups (28% versus 16%). When patients with coronary artery disease were compared with those with idiopathic cardiomyopathy, the frequency of induced nonsustained/sustained VT was still higher in the group with coronary artery disease (56% versus 39%; p <0.05), whereas the frequency of induced sustained VT was not statistically different in the two groups (28% versus 16%).

A previous myocardial infarction was documented more often in patients with than in those without induced nonsustained/sustained VT in studies by Kharsa and associates[35] (88% versus 44%; p <0.05) and Gomes and coworkers[15] (85% versus 43%; p <0.001), whereas the difference was not statistically significant in the report from Zheutlin and colleagues[21] (73% versus 53%). In a study by Sulpizi et al.,[30] all

TABLE 11–3
Determinants of Ventricular Tachyarrhythmia Inducibility by Programmed Stimulation in Patients with Nonsustained Ventricular Tachycardia and/or Complex Ventricular Ectopy*

Variables	Predicted Arrhythmia (Author/Ref.)									
	VT (Buxton[13, 14])	S-VT/VF (Spielman[19])	VT (Veltri[18])	S-VT, m (Sulpizi[30])†	S-VT, m (Turitto[33])†	VT/VF (Gomes[15])	VT (Zheutlin[21])	VT (Gradman[84])	VT/VF (Schoenfeld[65])†	S-VT, m (Nalos[83])†
Age	–	no	–	–	no	–	no	–	no	yes
Sex	–	no	–	–	no	–	no	–	yes	no
Presence of HD	yes	–	yes	no	no	–	–	–	–	–
Ischemic HD	yes	no	–	no	no	yes	no	–	no	–
Prior MI	–	–	–	no	no	yes	no	–	yes	yes
Syncope	no	no	–	no	yes	–	–	–	yes	yes
VPCs/hour	–	no	–	–	no	–	–	yes	–	–
Couplets/24 hours	–	–	–	–	no	–	–	yes	–	–
Repetition index	–	–	–	–	no	–	–	yes	–	–
VT runs/24 hours	no	no	no	–	no	–	–	–	–	–
VT duration	no	no	no	–	no	–	–	–	–	–
VT rate	–	no	–	–	no	–	–	–	–	–
VT morphology	–	–	–	–	no	–	–	–	–	–
Ejection fraction	yes	no	no	yes	yes	yes	no	–	no	yes
LV dyskinesia	yes	yes	–	–	no	–	–	–	no	yes
Signal-averaged ECG	–	–	–	–	yes	–	–	–	–	yes

*The table lists the first author only with reference source and the induced arrhythmia that was predicted by the variables in the left-hand column that were analyzed in each study. The study population included (1) patients with spontaneous nonsustained VT and/or complex ventricular ectopy in the reports by Buxton, Sulpizi, and Turitto et al.; (2) patients with nonsustained VT and/or complex ventricular ectopy in the reports by Gomes and Zheutlin et al.; and (3) patients with various clinical presentations (e.g., sustained VT, cardiac arrest, non-sustained VT, syncope) in the reports by Gradman, Shoenfeld, and Nalos et al.

†Multivariate methods were used to predict inducibility of the index arrhythmia. (Univariate methods were utilized in the remaining studies.)

VT = ventricular tachycardia; VF = ventricular fibrillation; S-VT = sustained ventricular tachycardia; m = monomorphic; HD = heart disease; MI = myocardial infarction; VPCs = ventricular premature complexes; ECG = electrocardiogram. Yes = significant variable; no = variable not significantly related to inducibility; – = variable not studied.

patients with recent myocardial infarction (within 3 months of programmed stimulation) had inducible sustained or nonsustained VT, yielding a higher inducibility rate than in the remaining population (100% versus 54%; p <0.007). However, this variable was not considered to be independently related to VT inducibility by multivariate analysis. On the other hand, old myocardial infarction was a significant variable in multivariate models published by Schoenfeld et al.[65] (p <0.001) and Nalos and coworkers[83] (p <0.0002). The influence of the site of prior myocardial infarction on induction of sustained monomorphic VT was studied by Zehender and colleagues[63] in 106 postinfarction patients. In the group with spontaneous nonsustained VT or no documented VT, inducibility was 34% for inferior infarction, compared with 65% for anterior infarction (p <0.05).

Symptoms were significantly related to VT induction only in the series by Turitto and coworkers.[33] A history of syncope/presyncope was present in 50% of patients with and in 22% of those without induced sustained monomorphic VT (p <0.05). Other investigators did not find any significant difference in the frequency of syncope between patients with or without inducible VT.[13, 19, 30]

Electrocardiographic Variables

In a study by Gradman and associates,[84] three quantitative variables derived from 24-hour ambulatory ECG were found to be significantly related to the induction of VT by PES: a mean VPC frequency of 100 or more/1000 normal beats, a mean couplet frequency of 1 or more/1000 normal beats, and a repetition index value of 15 or more/1000 VPCs. The repetition index was defined as the ratio of the number of couplets to the total number of VPCs. These data are at variance with those of other studies, in which ECG characteristics of the spontaneous arrhythmia did not predict VT inducibility.[13, 18, 19, 33]

Left Ventricular Function Indices

Several studies found that patients with an ejection fraction <0.40 had a greater frequency of induced VT compared with those with an ejection fraction ≥0.40. This difference was significant in studies by Buxton et al.[14] (60% versus 22%; p <0.03), Gomes and colleagues[15] (85% versus 38%; p <0.0006), and Turitto and associates[33] (39% versus 5%; p <0.0001). Ejection fraction was a significant predictor of inducibility in multivariate analysis models reported by Turitto and coworkers[33] and Nalos and colleagues.[83] In a study by Sulpizi et al.,[30] impairment of left ventricular function, defined as an ejection fraction less than 0.35 or functional class III to IV with cardiomegaly on chest X-ray, was identified as the only variable independently related to the induction of sustained VT. On the other hand, the degree of left ventricular dysfunction was similar in patients with or without induced VT in reports from Zheutlin et al.,[21] Veltri and associates,[18] and Spielman and coworkers.[19]

Besides left ventricular ejection fraction, the relationship of wall motion abnormalities to inducibility was considered in a number of studies. Spielman and coworkers[19] found that induced sustained VT/VF was more frequent in patients with at least one akinetic or dyskinetic left ventricular segment, as shown by radionuclide angiography, compared with those without such abnormalities (69% versus 29%; p <0.01). Buxton and colleagues[13] reported that, among patients with coronary artery disease, sustained VT was induced more often in the presence of left ventricular aneurysm than in its absence (69% versus 20%; p <0.01). However, this finding was not corroborated by subsequent studies by the same authors[29] or by other groups.[33]

The Signal-Averaged ECG

The signal-averaged ECG is recorded by amplifying, averaging, and filtering the signal recorded on the body surface by orthognal leads.[85] The recording detects low-amplitude cardiac electrical signals in the late QRS/ST segment that may represent delayed activation of abnormal myocardial tissue.[86] These signals are usually called *late potentials*. The signal-averaged ECG was initially found to accurately predict the results of PES in patients with spontaneous sustained VT.[87-89] The predictive value of the signal-averaged ECG for the induction of sustained VT was confirmed in a study by Nalos and associates[83] in patients with miscellaneous presenting arrhythmias and by Buxton and coworkers[81] in patients with spontaneous nonsustained VT after healing of myocardial infarction.

The first prospective study of the value of the signal-averaged ECG as a predictor of the results of programmed stimulation in patients with nonsustained VT, using stepwise discriminant function analysis, was published from our laboratory by Turitto and colleagues.[33] The study found that the signal-averaged ECG is the single most accurate screening test to predict the inducibility of sustained VT in patients with spontaneous nonsustained VT. A consecutive series of 105 patients with spontaneous nonsustained VT on 24-hour ambulatory electrocardiography was studied. The study population consisted of 60 patients with coronary artery disease, 26 with idiopathic dilated cardiomyopathy, and 19 with no identifiable heart disease. Patients were divided into three groups according to the results of programmed stimulation (three extrastimuli, two right ventricular sites): group 1 included 22 patients with induced sustained monomorphic VT (Fig. 11–1); group 2, 14 patients with induced VF; and group 3, 69 patients without induced sustained ventricular tachyarrhythmias (Fig. 11–2).

Table 11–4 shows the characteristics of patients in the three groups. Group 1 patients showed a significantly higher frequency of syncope/presyncope, left ventricular ejection fraction <0.40, and late potentials on the signal-averaged ECG compared with group 3. Late potentials were defined as low-amplitude signals in the terminal part of the QRS with duration ≥38 ms and root mean square voltage ≤25 μV. The etiology of underlying heart disease, the ECG characteristics of

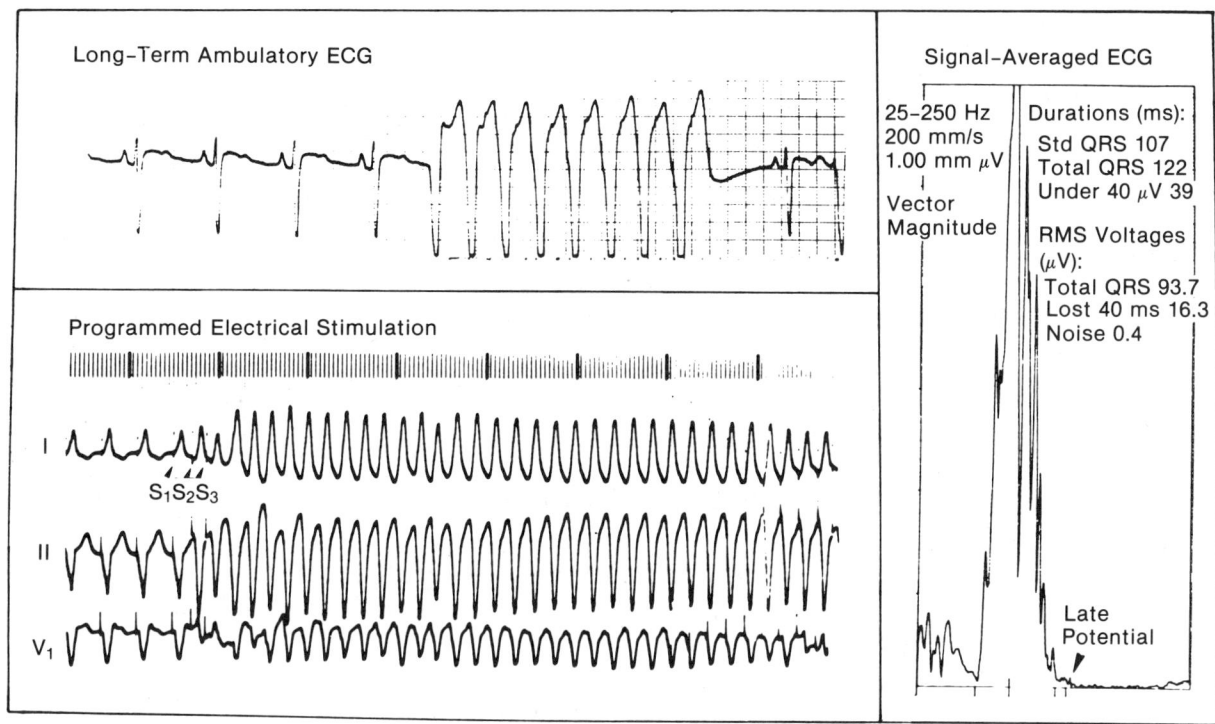

FIGURE 11—1
Recordings of ambulatory electrocardiogram (ECG), programmed electrical stimulation, and a signal-averaged ECG from a 56-year-old man with coronary artery disease. A 24-hour ambulatory ECG showed frequent ventricular premature complexes and runs of nonsustained ventricular tachycardia. The signal-averaged ECG showed late potentials: the root mean square (RMS) voltage of the last 40 ms of the filtered QRS = 16.3 μV and the duration of the low-amplitude signal under 40 μV = 39 ms. Programmed electrical stimulation utilizing an $S_1S_2S_3$ protocol from the right ventricular apex induced a sustained monomorphic tachycardia.

the spontaneous arrhythmia (number, duration, and cycle length of nonsustained VT runs), and the prevalence of left ventricular wall motion abnormalities were not significantly different in groups 1 and 3. On the other hand, when patients with induced VF (group 2) were compared with patients without induced sustained VT/VF (group 3), none of the variables showed significant differences. In further analysis of group 3 patients, clinical and ECG variables, left ventricular function indices, and the signal-averaged ECGs were not significantly different in patients in whom monomorphic nonsustained VT, polymorphic nonsustained VT, or no VT were induced.

Late potentials were recorded in 23 patients (23%): 14 in group 1, three in group 2, and six in group 3. The sensitivity, specificity, and positive, negative, and total predictive accuracy of late potentials for the induction of sustained monomorphic VT were 64%, 89%, 61%, 90%, and 84%, respectively. In other words, the probability of inducing sustained monomorphic VT was 61% in patients with late potentials and declined to 10% in those without late potentials. The frequency of late potentials was similar in patients with coronary artery disease (25%) and in those with idiopathic dilated cardiomyopathy (23%). Their predictive accuracy was also comparable in the two groups: 85% in coronary artery disease and 81% in cardiomyopathy patients. Among the 43 patients with prior myocardial infarction, late potentials showed high predictive accuracy both in anterior infarction (73%) and in inferior infarction (88%). Using stepwise discriminant function analysis, late potentials proved to be the variable most strongly correlated ($p < 0.00001$) with the induction of sustained monomorphic VT, with an overall predictive accuracy of 84%.

No combination of late potentials and other significant variables (ejection fraction and symptoms) provided an improvement in predicting sustained VT inducibility, in comparison with late potentials alone. When late potentials were removed from the analysis, the combination of other variables provided a predictive accuracy of 71%. Late potentials could still enter the model with a probability of improving it <0.05. Thus, the signal-averaged ECG offered predictive information above that found in clinical variables and other noninvasive tests. On the other hand, no single variable or combination of variables predicted the induction of VF.

In our series of 105 patients, concordance between the results of PES and those of the signal-averaged ECG was observed in 84% of cases. The largest subgroup consisted of patients who had no late potentials and no induced sustained monomorphic VT (70%). In these patients, it is reasonable to speculate that the spontaneous arrhythmia may be due to mechanisms other than reentry (e.g., abnormal automaticity[90] or triggered activity[91]). Patients with both late potentials and induced sustained monomorphic VT accounted for 14% of cases. The results of the two tests were discordant in the remaining 16%

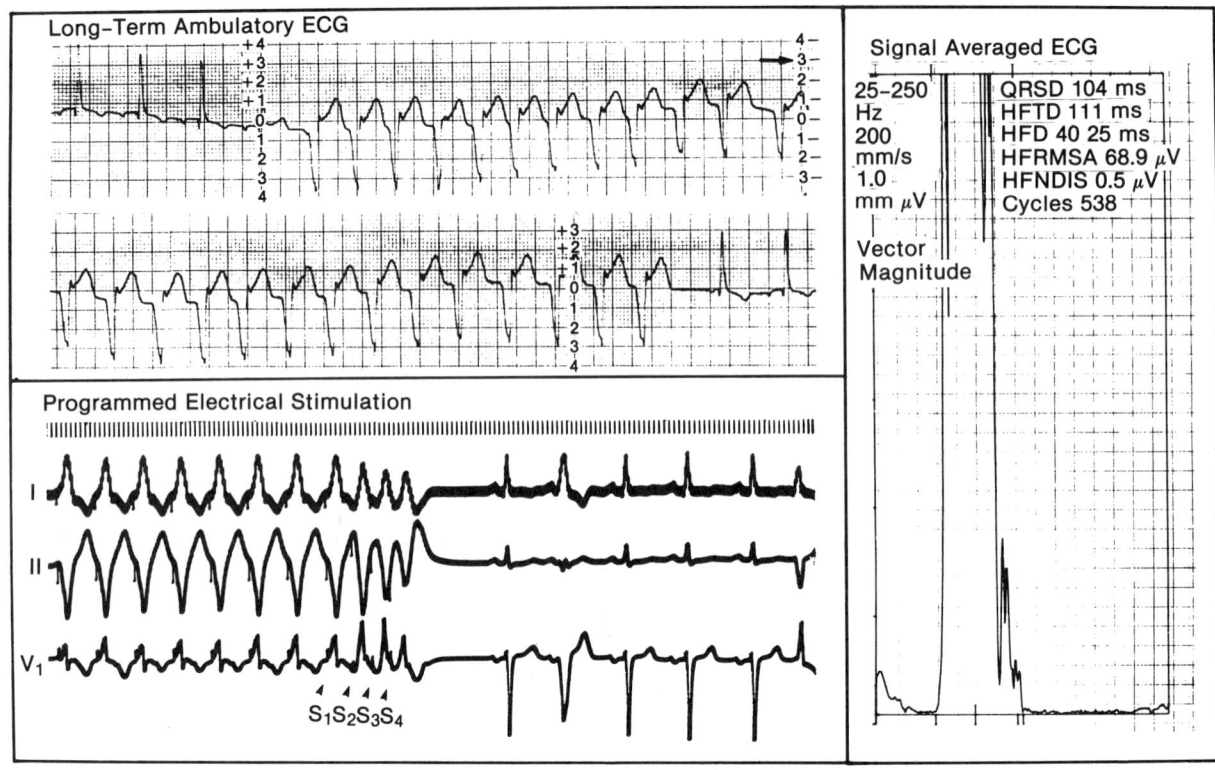

FIGURE 11—2
Recordings of ambulatory electrocardiograms (ECGs), programmed electrical stimulation, and a signal-averaged ECG from a 41 year old man with idiopathic dilated cardiomyopathy. The patient had no history of syncope/presyncope. The ejection fraction by radionuclide ventriculography was 16%. A 24-hour ambulatory ECG showed frequent ventricular premature complexes (average 240/hour) and 6 runs of nonsustained monomorphic ventricular tachycardia. The longest one is shown in the figure. It comprised 26 beats and had an averaged cycle length of 452 ms. The signal-averaged ECG was normal. There was no inducible arrhythmia on programmed electrical stimulation. (Reprinted by permission from: Turitto G, et al.: Am J Cardiol 61:1272, 1988.)

of cases. Nine patients had late potentials but failed to develop sustained monomorphic VT at PES. This may be explained by the electrophysiologic limitations of both PES[55] and signal-averaging techniques.[86] The relationship between myocardial zones with delayed conduction during sinus rhythm and the occurrence of reentrant arrhythmias is complex. Zones showing conduction delay (i.e., late potentials) during basic rhythm may completely block during premature stimulation and not participate in a reentrant pathway.[86] In eight patients, a sustained VT was induced in the absence of late potentials. Again, limitations of the signal-averaged ECG (e.g., inability to detect delayed activation potentials with a dynamic Wenckebach sequence) may have been a factor, as well as the possibility that some induced VT may have represented a nonspecific response to PES. In this regard, four of the eight patients in this group had a cycle length of induced sustained monomorphic VT of 190 to 195 ms.

Our observation that patients with induced VF could

TABLE 11—4
Characteristics of 105 Patients with Spontaneous Nonsustained Ventricular Tachycardia with or without Induced Ventricular Tachyarrhythmias*

	Group 1 (n = 22)	Group 2 (n = 14)	Group 3 (n = 69)	Probability	
				1 vs. 3	2 vs. 3
Heart disease	16 (73)	7 (50)	37 (54)	NS	NS
Ischemic (%)	12 (55)	5 (36)	26 (38)		
With prior MI (%)	5 (23)	3 (21)	18 (26)	NS	NS
Dilated CMP (%)	1 (5)	4 (29)	14 (20)	NS	NS
None (%)					
Syncope/presyncope (%)	11 (50)	7 (50)	15 (22)	<0.05	NS
LV ejection fraction <0.40 (%)	19 (86)	5 (36)	25 (36)	<0.0001	NS
LV segmental a/dyskinesia (%)	11 (50)	3 (21)	16 (23)	NS	NS
Late potentials on the signal-averaged ECG (%)	14 (64)	3 (21)	6 (9)	<0.00001	NS

*Group 1 = induced sustained monomorphic ventricular tachycardia; Group 2 = induced ventricular fibrillation; Group 3 = no induced sustained ventricular tachyarrhythmias.
NS = not significant; MI = myocardial infarction; CMP = cardiomyopathy; LV = left ventricle; ECG = electrocardiogram.

not be distinguished from patients with no induced VT/VF by the signal-averaged ECG or any other variable suggests that the induction of VF may represent a nonclinical response to PES in this group of patients. Furthermore, the fact that the induction of sustained monomorphic VT, rather than that of VF or nonsustained VT, was correlated with the presence or absence of late potentials on the signal-averaged ECG provides evidence for the hypothesis that late potentials represent abnormal myocardial zones with delayed activation potentials capable of providing the electrophysiologic substrate for reentrant rhythms.[86] It also emphasizes the specificity of induced sustained monomorphic VT, rather than of induced nonsustained VT or VF, as the end point of PES in patients with spontaneous nonsustained VT.

THE USE OF PES FOR RISK STRATIFICATION

In patients with no documented sustained ventricular tachyarrhythmias, the induction of sustained monomorphic VT by PES may either represent a mere laboratory finding or indicate patients at high risk for future serious arrhythmic events. The latter hypothesis was tested by a number of investigators. However, published reports on the prognostic significance of ventricular tachyarrhythmias induced by PES in patients with complex ventricular arrhythmias and nonsustained VT can be criticized for (1) small sample size,[12, 14–16, 18, 21, 26–30, 35] (2) retrospective data collection,[18, 29, 30] (3) study population not representative of the overall population with nonsustained VT (selection was based on the absence of symptoms in two studies),[18, 21] and (4) lack of uniform therapeutic approach. The indication for antiarrhythmic therapy varied in different studies. Patients with induced sustained VT[33, 35] were subjected to treatment, as well as those with induced nonsustained VT[13, 15, 18, 21] and induced VF.[15] In some studies, therapy was defined by means of repeat PES,[15, 21, 33, 35] whereas in other studies this was not always the case.[18, 29] On the other hand, guidelines for the management of patients without induced VT were disparate; in some instances, these patients did not receive any antiarrhythmic treatment,[21, 32, 33, 35] but in other studies subgroups were followed on or off antiarrhythmic drugs.[14, 15, 18, 29] In none of the published reports was treatment randomized.

Most studies reported a low risk of sudden cardiac death in patients with nonsustained VT who had no induced VT (Table 11–5).[14–16, 21, 28, 30, 32, 35–37] The risk of sudden death was equally low in patients with induced nonsustained VT in studies by Turitto and coworkers,[32, 33] Reddy and colleagues,[16] Miles and associates,[26] Buxton et al.,[29] and Kharsa et al.[35] Zheutlin and coworkers[21] followed 52 patients with asymptomatic spontaneous nonsustained VT who had no inducible VT on PES for 22 months off antiarrhythmic therapy; these authors found no instance of sudden cardiac death. Similarly, Kharsa and associates[35] reported no cases of sudden death among 32 patients without induced sustained VT followed for 17 months off antiarrhythmic drugs. In our recent series,[37] the 3-year sudden death rate was 9% in patients with no induced sustained VT/VF followed off antiarrhythmic drugs. The 3-year sudden death rate was the same (7%) in patients with ejection fractions ≥ 0.40 or < 0.40. On the other hand, the 3-year total cardiac mortality was significantly higher (27%) in those patients with ejection fraction < 0.40 compared with those with ejection fraction ≥ 0.40 (7%). It is interesting to note that the risk of serious arrhythmic events in the noninducible group of patients was low both in the presence[14, 15] and in the absence[15, 32, 35] of antiarrhythmic therapy. In an earlier study from our laboratory, Gomes et al.[15] followed 53 patients without induced VT/VF for 30 ± 15 months: among them, 27 did not receive any antiarrhythmic drugs, whereas 26 were randomly assigned to long-term oral antiarrhythmic therapy. No significant differences in the occurrence of sudden death were found between treated and untreated patients. Thus, it may be concluded that subjects with spontaneous nonsustained VT and no induced sustained VT can be managed safely without the use of antiarrhythmic drug therapy.[15, 21, 32, 33, 35]

There are few follow-up studies of patients with induced VF. In our series,[36, 37] all patients with spontaneous nonsustained VT who had induced VF remained alive off antiarrhythmic therapy during a follow-up of 30 ± 10 months. These findings are consistent with the findings of DiCarlo and colleagues[92] and Mahmud and coworkers.[93] These authors reported no major arrhythmic events in a total of 27 patients without documented spontaneous sustained VT/VF and with induced VF, who were followed for over 2 years. The arrhythmia was considered a nonclinical response to PES in patients without clinical sustained ventricular tachyarrhythmias.

On the other hand, VT inducibility seems to carry an increased risk of sudden death in patients with spontaneous nonsustained VT. The induced arrhythmia that portended a poor prognosis was identified as sustained VT by Buxton and associates,[14] Klein and coworkers,[27] Reddy et al.,[16] Miles and colleagues,[26] and Turitto et al.,[36, 37] and as both sustained and nonsustained VT by Gomes and associates,[15] Zheutlin and colleagues,[21] and Batsford and coworkers.[28] In the study by Buxton et al.,[14] sudden death occurred in four out of 15 patients (27%) with induced sustained VT, two out of 37 (5%) with induced nonsustained VT, and four out of 31 (13%) without induced VT, during a follow-up period of 33 months. Sudden death occurred only in patients with ejection fraction < 0.40. Using multivariate analysis, patients with one poor prognostic marker (induced sustained VT or low ejection fraction) were characterized by a threefold increased risk of sudden death, whereas patients with both markers had a sevenfold increased risk. Gomes et al.[15] reported major arrhythmic events in two out of eight patients (25%) with induced sustained VT, two out of five (40%) with induced VF, two out of seven (29%) with induced nonsustained VT, and one out of 53 (2%) without induced arrhythmias, during a follow-

TABLE 11-5
Outcome of Patients with Spontaneous Nonsustained Ventricular Tachycardia and/or Complex Ventricular Ectopy Studied with Programmed Stimulation*

Author	No. of Patients Induced/Not Induced	Follow-Up (Months)	Sudden Death or Major Arrhythmic Events (%) Induced/Not Induced	Relation of Induced Arrhythmias to Sudden Death	Role of Therapy	Significant Risk Factors for Sudden Death
Swerdlow† (1982)[12]	25/16	?	12/12	NS	Guided by PS; not predictive of outcome	None identified
Gomes (1984)[15]	20/53	30 ± 15	32/2	<0.001	Guided by PS; not effective in preventing SD	Induced VT/VF and ejection fraction <0.40
Reddy† (1984)[16]	14/38	23 ± 16	27/5	<0.001	Guided by PS; not effective in preventing SD	Induced sustained VT/VF
Buxton (1984)[14]	15/68	33	27/9	<0.00001	Similar mortality in patients treated empirically or by PS	Induced sustained VT and ejection fraction <0.40
Veltri (1985)[18]	14/19	23 ± 16	21/21	NS	Uncertain	Low ejection fraction
Zheutlin (1986)[21]	33/55	22	12/0	<0.02	Only to induced patients, guided by PS; not effective in preventing SD	Induced VT
Klein† (1986)[27]	11/11	2–32	45/9	<0.05	Uncertain	Induced sustained VT
Miles† (1986)[26]	13/40	8.6 ± 5.3	23/5	=0.08	Only to induced patients; when PS guided, effective in preventing SD	Induced sustained VT and VF by ≤2 extrastimuli
Batsford† (1986)[28]	53/28	17	17/0	<0.02	Uncertain	Induced VT sustained or nonsustained
Buxton (1987)[29]	28/34	28	25/12	Among induced patients, higher mortality in those treated empirically versus those receiving PS-guided therapy (<0.001)	PS-guided therapy effective in preventing SD	Induced sustained VT not treated with PS-guided therapy
Sulpizi (1987)[30]	9/52	26	11/6	NS	Uncertain	Low ejection fraction
Kharsa (1988)[35]	8/32	16.2	0/0	Low risk of SD both in untreated patients without induced sustained VT and induced patients on PS-guided therapy	Guided by PS, only for induced patients	
Turitto (1988)[36]	23/87	14 ± 7	4/3	Low risk of SD both in untreated patients without induced sustained VT and induced patients on PS-guided therapy	Guided by PS, only for induced patients	

*Table lists first author only with year of report and reference source.
†Abstract report.
NS = not significant; PS = programmed stimulation; SD = sudden death; VT = ventricular tachycardia; VF = ventricular fibrillation.

up period of 30 ± 15 months. Actuarial survival curves revealed that, at 1 year, 75% of patients with induced VT/VF and 100% of those without induced VT/VF were alive, whereas at 2 years the probability of survival declined, to 65% and 97%, respectively (p <0.0001). In the study by Batsford and coworkers,[28] the incidence of serious arrhythmic events was 57% (4/7) in patients with induced sustained VT, 14% (5/36) in those with induced nonsustained VT, and 0% (0/28) in those without induced VT. Differences in survival between patients with and without induced VT were statistically significant (p <0.02). The relationship between outcome and different types of induced arrhythmias was not specified by Zheutlin and colleagues.[21]

Few studies failed to find a correlation between the inducibility of VT and high risk for sudden cardiac death in patients with spontaneous nonsustained VT. Two of these studies were retrospective,[18, 30] and one was a preliminary report.[12] In the study by Sulpizi and associates,[30] the overall probability of sudden death was low (7% during a follow-up period of 26 months) and was not influenced by VT inducibility. On the other hand, poor left ventricular function was an important predictor of mortality. Similar findings were reported by Veltri and coworkers.[18] In their study, a 21% incidence of serious arrhythmic events was documented over a follow-up period of approximately 2 years. Ejection fraction was significantly lower in the group with than in the group without arrhythmic events (0.49 ± 0.18 versus 0.31 ± 0.17; p <0.04), and the ability to induce VT was not correlated to outcome.

The available literature concerning the effects of empirical antiarrhythmic therapy or therapy guided by PES on survival of patients with spontaneous nonsustained VT and induced VT is controversial. Most of the reported studies failed to demonstrate that PES-guided therapy improved survival of patients with induced VT or was superior to empirical therapy.[11, 12, 14, 17, 18, 27] Patients with induced VT treated with drug regimens selected by PES maintained an excess mortality, compared with those without induced VT, in studies by Gomes et al.[15] and Zheutlin and colleagues.[21] However, a study by Buxton and associates[29] that utilized only historical controls suggested that therapy guided by PES in this group was associated with a lower rate of sudden cardiac death, compared with empiric therapy. On the other hand, the significance of the finding that PES-guided therapy in patients with induced sustained VT was associated with a low risk of sudden death in the study by Kharsa et al.[35] and in our own series[36, 37] is limited by the lack of a controlled group followed off antiarrhythmic therapy.

The hypothesis that the induction of sustained VT in patients with complex ventricular arrhythmias and nonsustained VT identifies a subset of patients with increased risk of sudden cardiac death will remain unsubstantiated in the absence of a randomized study that compares the incidence of sudden death on and off antiarrhythmic therapy. The antiarrhythmic protocol probably should be based on the prevention of induction of sustained VT.

Recommended Protocol for Risk Stratification and Management of Patients with Nonsustained VT

A recent study from our laboratory[37] strongly suggests that an optimal protocol for risk stratification and management of patients with organic heart disease and spontaneous nonsustained VT should be based on the results of the signal-averaged ECG, left ventricular ejection fraction, and PES as follows (Fig. 11–3):

1. Patients with no late potentials in the signal-averaged ECG and with an ejection fraction ≥0.40 do not require testing by PES nor long-term antiarrhythmic therapy, since the incidence of inducible sustained monomorphic VT and the risk of sudden death are very low in this group of patients. There was no instance of induced sustained VT in 33 consecutive patients in this group.

2. Patients with no late potentials but with ejection fraction <0.40 and patients with late potentials should be recommended for electrophysiologic evaluation. The incidence of inducible sustained monomorphic VT was 21% in the former group and 65% in the latter group. In patients with late potentials, the high incidence of inducible VT was independent of the etiology of heart disease and the degree of ejection fraction (50% with ejection fraction ≥0.40 versus 68% with ejection fraction <0.40).

Based on the results of PES, patients with no inducible tachyarrhythmia as well as those with inducible

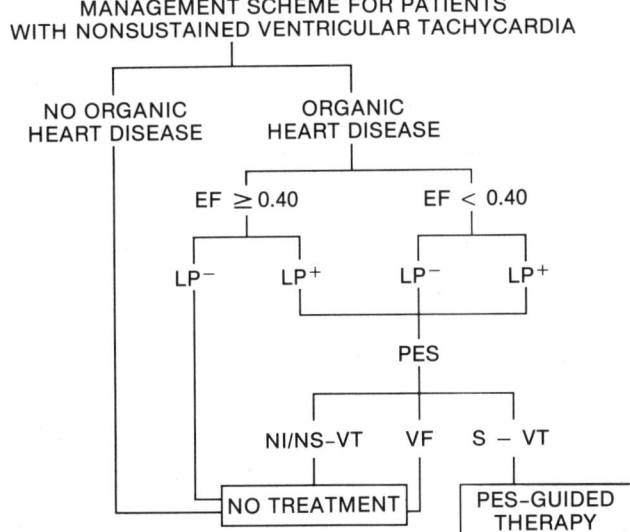

FIGURE 11–3
A suggested management protocol for patients with organic heart disease and spontaneous nonsustained ventricular tachycardia. See text for details. EF = left ventricular ejection fraction; LP– = no late potentials in the signal-averaged electrocardiogram; LP+ = late potentials in the signal-averaged electrocardiogram; PES = programmed electrical stimulation; NI = not inducible; NS-VT = inducible nonsustained ventricular tachycardia; VF = inducible ventricular fibrillation; S-VT = inducible sustained monomorphic ventricular tachycardia.

nonsustained VT or VF could be followed off antiarrhythmic therapy with a low risk of sudden death. However, if sustained monomorphic VT is induced, these patients should receive antiarrhythmic therapy guided by PES, with the understanding that the value of antiarrhythmic therapy in this group has not been definitely established. This can be achieved only through randomization of therapy in a large multicenter study. Considering the magnitude of the problem, such a study is long overdue.

References

1. Lown B: Sudden cardiac death—1978. Circulation 60:1593, 1979.
2. Mason J, Winkle R: Electrode-catheter arrhythmia induction in the selection and assessment of antiarrhythmic drug therapy for recurrent ventricular tachycardia. Circulation 58:971, 1978.
3. Horowitz L, Josephson M, Farshidi A, et al.: Recurrent sustained ventricular tachycardia. 3. Role of the electrophysiologic study in selection of antiarrhythmic regimens. Circulation 58:986, 1978.
4. Swerdlow CD, Winkle RA, Mason JW: Determinants of survival in patients with ventricular tachyarrhythmias. N Eng J Med 308:1436, 1983.
5. Myerburg RJ, Kessler KM, Estes D, et al.: Long-term survival after prehospital cardiac arrest: analysis of outcome during an 8-year study. Circulation 70:538, 1984.
6. Goldstein S, Landis JR, Leighton R, et al.: Predictive survival models for resuscitated victims of out-of-hospital cardiac arrest with coronary heart disease. Circulation 5:873, 1985.
7. Bigger JT Jr, Fleiss JL, Kleiger R, et al., and the Multicenter Post-Infarction Research Group. The relationships among ventricular arrhythmias, left ventricular dysfunction, and mortality in the 2 years after myocardial infarction. Circulation 69:250, 1984.
8. Mukharji J, Rude RE, Poole WK, et al., and the MILIS Group: Risk factors for sudden death after acute myocardial infarction: two-year follow-up. Am J Cardiol 54:31, 1984.
9. Maisel AS, Scott N, Gilpin E, et al.: Complex ventricular arrhythmias in patients with Q wave versus non–Q wave myocardial infarction. Circulation 72:963, 1985.
10. Josephson ME: Treatment of ventricular arrhythmias after myocardial infarction. Circulation 74:653, 1986.
11. Naccarelli GV, Prystowsky EN, Jackman WM, et al.: Role of electrophysiologic testing in managing patients who have ventricular tachycardia unrelated to coronary artery disease. Am J Cardiol 50:165, 1982.
12. Swerdlow CD, Echt DS, Soderholm-Difatte V, et al.: Limited value of programmed stimulation in patients with unsustained VT (Abstract). Circulation 66(Suppl II):II-145, 1982.
13. Buxton AE, Waxman HL, Marchlinski FE, et al.: Electrophysiologic studies in nonsustained ventricular tachycardia: relation to underlying heart disease. Am J Cardiol 52:985, 1983.
14. Buxton AE, Marchlinski FE, Waxman HL, et al.: Prognostic factors in nonsustained ventricular tachycardia. Am J Cardiol 53:1275, 1984.
15. Gomes JAC, Hariman RI, Kang PS, et al.: Programmed electrical stimulation in patients with high-grade ventricular ectopy: Electrophysiologic findings and prognosis for survival. Circulation 70:43, 1984.
16. Reddy CP, Jivrajka VB: Is programmed cardiac stimulation useful in risk stratification of patients with high-grade ventricular ectopy (Abstract)? Circulation 70(Suppl II):II-400, 1984.
17. Miles WM, Skale BT, Windle JR, et al.: Electrophysiologic characteristics and follow-up of 139 patients with nonsustained ventricular tachycardia (Abstract). Circulation 70(Suppl II):II-400, 1984.
18. Veltri EP, Platia EV, Griffith LSC, Reid PR: Programmed electrical stimulation and long-term follow-up in asymptomatic, nonsustained ventricular tachycardia. Am J Cardiol 56:309,1985.
19. Spielman SR, Greenspan AM, Kay HR, et al.: Electrophysiologic testing in patients at high risk for sudden cardiac death. 1. Nonsustained ventricular tachycardia and abnormal ventricular function. J Am Coll Cardiol 6:31, 1985.
20. Meinertz T, Treese N, Kasper W, et al.: Determinants of prognosis in idiopathic dilated cardiomyopathy as determined by programmed electrical stimulation. Am J Cardiol 56:337, 1985.
21. Zheutlin TA, Roth H, Chua W, et al.: Programmed electrical stimulation to determine the need for antiarrhythmic therapy in patients with complex ventricular ectopic activity. Am Heart J 111:860, 1986.
22. Breithardt G, Borggrefe M, Podczeck A: Electrophysiology and pharmacology of asymptomatic nonsustained ventricular tachycardia. Clin Progr Electrophysiol Pacing 4:81, 1986.
23. Das SK, Morady F, DiCarlo L Jr, et al.: Prognostic usefulness of programmed ventricular stimulation in idiopathic dilated cardiomyopathy without symptomatic ventricular arrhythmias. Am J Cardiol 58:998, 1986.
24. Poll DS, Marchlinski FE, Buxton AE, et al.: Usefulness of programmed stimulation in idiopathic cardiomyopathy. Am J Cardiol 58:992, 1986.
25. Friedman L, Yusuf S: Does therapy directed by programmed electrical stimulation provide a satisfactory clinical response? Circulation 73(Suppl II):II-59, 1986.
26. Miles WM, Heger JJ, Zipes DP, et al.: Management of patients with asymptomatic nonsustained ventricular tachycardia directed by electrophysiologic study (Abstract). Clin Res 34:326A, 1986.
27. Klein RC, Machell C: Electrophysiologic studies in patients with nonsustained ventricular tachycardia and coronary disease: relation of ventricular aneurysm to inducible tachycardia and prognosis (Abstract). J Am Coll Cardiol 7:71A, 1986.
28. Batsford WP, Sudbrink L, Stark SI, et al.: Outcome in nonsustained ventricular tachycardia: relation to clinical factors, spontaneous and induced ventricular arrhythmias (Abstract). J Am Coll Cardiol 7:71A, 1986.
29. Buxton AE, Marchlinski FE, Waxman HL, et al.: Nonsustained ventricular tachycardia in patients with coronary artery disease: Role of electrophysiologic study. Circulation 75:1178, 1987.
30. Sulpizi AM, Friehling TD, Kowey PR: Value of electrophysiologic testing in patients with nonsustained ventricular tachycardia. Am J Cardiol 59:841, 1987.
31. Fontaine JM, Turitto G, El-Sherif N: Prognostic significance of ambulatory electrocardiographic recording, programmed electrical stimulation and signal-averaged electrocardiogram in patients with complex ventricular arrhythmias. J Electrophysiol 1:204, 1987.
32. Turitto G, Fontaine J, Caref E, et al.: Low risk of sudden cardiac death in patients with non-sustained ventricular tachycardia and normal signal averaged electrocardiogram (Abstract). Circulation 76(Suppl IV):IV-32, 1987.
33. Turitto G, Fontaine JM, Ursell SN, et al.: Value of the signal-averaged electrocardiogram as a predictor of the results of programmed stimulation in nonsustained ventricular tachycardia. Am J Cardiol 61:1272, 1988.
34. El-Sherif N, Turitto G, Fontaine JM: Risk stratification of patients with complex ventricular arrhythmias. Herz 13:204, 1988.
35. Kharsa MH, Gold RL, Moore H, et al.: Long-term outcome following programmed electrical stimulation in patients with high-grade ventricular ectopy. PACE 11:603, 1988.
36. Turitto G, El-Sherif N: Role of the signal-averaged electrocardiogram and electrophysiologic study in the management of patients with non-sustained ventricular tachycardia. New Trends Arrhythm 5:431, 1988.
37. Turitto G, Fontaine JM, Ursell S, et al.: Risk stratification and management of patients with organic heart disease and non-sustained ventricular tachycardia. Role of programmed stimulation, left ventricular ejection fraction and the signal averaged electrocardiogram. Am J Med 88:1-35N, 1990.
38. Anderson KP, DeCamilla J, Moss AJ: Clinical significance of ventricular tachycardia (3 beats or longer) detected during ambulatory monitoring after myocardial infarction. Circulation 57:890, 1978.
39. Bigger JT, Weld FM, Rolinzky LM: Prevalence, characteristics and significance of ventricular tachycardia (three or more complexes) detected with ambulatory electrocardiographic recording in the late hospital phase of acute myocardial infarction. Am J Cardiol 48:815, 1981.

40. Kleiger RE, Miller JP, Thanavaro S, et al.: Relationship between clinical features of acute myocardial infarction and ventricular runs 2 weeks to 1 year after infarction. Circulation 63:64, 1981.
41. Surawicz B: Prognosis of ventricular arrhythmias in relation to sudden cardiac death: Therapeutic implications. J Amer Coll Cardiol 10:435, 1987.
42. Kennedy HL, Whitlock JA, Sprague MK, et al.: Long-term follow-up of asymptomatic healthy subjects with frequent and complex ventricular ectopy. N Engl J Med 312:193, 1985.
43. Rubin DA, Nieminski KE, Monteferrante JC, et al.: Ventricular arrhythmias after coronary artery bypass graft surgery: incidence, risk factors and long-term prognosis. J Am Coll Cardiol 6:307, 1985.
44. DeSoyza N, Murphy ML, Bissett JK, et al.: Ventricular arrhythmia in chronic stable angina pectoris with surgical or medical treatment. Ann Intern Med 89:10, 1978.
45. Schultze RA Jr, Strauss HW, Pitt B: Sudden death in the year following myocardial infarction. Relationship to ventricular premature contractions in the late hospital phase and left ventricular ejection fraction. Am J Med 62:192, 1977.
46. Packer M: Sudden unexpected death in patients with congestive heart failure: a second frontier. Circulation 72:681, 1985.
47. Maskin CS, Siskind SJ, LeJemtel TH: High prevalence of nonsustained ventricular tachycardia in severe congestive heart failure. Am Heart J 107:896, 1984.
48. Meinertz T, Hoffman T, Kasper W, et al.: Significance of ventricular arrhythmias in idiopathic dilated cardiomyopathy. Am J Cardiol 53:902, 1984.
49. Holmes J, Kubo SH, Cody RJ, et al.: Arrhythmias in ischemic and non-ischemic dilated cardiomyopathy: Prediction of mortality by ambulatory electrocardiography. Am J Cardiol 55:146, 1985.
50. Unverferth DV, Magorien RD, Moeschberger ML, et al.: Factors influencing the one-year mortality of dilated cardiomyopathy. Am J Cardiol 54:147, 1984.
51. Furberg CD, May GS: Effect of long-term prophylactic treatment on survival after myocardial infarction. Am J Med 76:76, 1984.
52. Woosley RL: Indications for antiarrhythmic therapy: A wealth of controversy, a dearth of data. Ann Intern Med 108:450, 1988.
52a. The Cardiac Arrhythmia Suppression Trial (CAST) Investigators: Preliminary report: Effect of encainide and flecainide on mortality in a randomized trial of arrhythmia suppression after myocardial infarction. N Engl J Med 321:406,1989.
53. Estes NAM III, Garan H, McGovern B, et al.: Influence of drive cycle length during programmed stimulation on induction of ventricular arrhythmias: Analysis of 403 patients. Am J Cardiol 57:108, 1986.
54. Prystowsky EN, Miles WM, Evans JJ, et al.: Induction of ventricular tachycardia during programmed electrical stimulation: Analysis of pacing methods. Circulation 73(Suppl II):II-32, 1986.
55. Mason JW, Anderson KP, Freedman RA: Techniques and criteria in electrophysiologic study of ventricular tachycardia. Circulation 75(Suppl III):III-125, 1987.
56. Buxton AE, Waxman HL, Marchlinski FE, et al.: Role of triple extrastimuli during electrophysiologic study of patients with documented sustained ventricular tachyarrhythmias. Circulation 69:532, 1984.
57. Brugada P, Wellens HJJ: Comparison in the same patient of two programmed stimulation protocols to induce ventricular tachycardia. Am J Cardiol 55:380, 1985.
58. Breithardt G, Borggrefe M, Podczeck A, et al.: Influence of the cycle length of basic drive on induction of sustained ventricular tachycardia associated with coronary artery disease. Am J Cardiol 60:1306, 1987.
59. Morady F, DiCarlo LA Jr, Baerman JM, et al.: Comparison of coupling intervals that induce clinical and nonclinical forms of ventricular tachycardia during programmed stimulation. Am J Cardiol 57:1269, 1986.
60. Vandepol CJ, Farshidi A, Spielman SR, et al.: Incidence and clinical significance of induced ventricular tachycardia. Am J Cardiol 45:725, 1980.
61. Morady F, DiCarlo L, Winston S, et al.: A prospective comparison of the role of triple extrastimuli and left ventricular stimulation in studies of ventricular tachycardia induction. Circulation 70:52, 1984.
62. Gottlieb C, Josephson ME: The preference of programmed stimulation guided therapy for sustained ventricular arrhythmias. In Brugada P, Wellens HJJ (eds.): Cardiac Arrhythmias: Where to Go from Here? (pp. 421–434) Mount Kisco, NY, Futura Publishing, 1987.
63. Zehender M, Brugada P, Geibel A, et al.: Programmed electrical stimulation in healed myocardial infarction using a standardized ventricular stimulation protocol. Am J Cardiol 59:578, 1987.
64. Platia EV, Greene HL, Vlay SC, et al.: Sensitivity of various extrastimulus techniques in patients with serious ventricular arrhythmias. Am Heart J 106:698, 1983.
65. Schoenfeld MH, McGovern B, Garan H, et al.: Determinants of the outcome of electrophysiologic study in patients with ventricular tachyarrhythmias. J Am Coll Cardiol 6:298, 1985.
66. El-Sherif N, Mehra R, Gough WB, et al: Reentrant ventricular arrhythmias in the late myocardial infarction period. II. Burst pacing versus multiple premature stimulation in the induction of reentry. J Am Coll Cardiol 4:295, 1984.
67. Denker S, Lehmann M, Mahmud R, et al.: Facilitation of ventricular tachycardia induction with abrupt changes in ventricular cycle length. Am J Cardiol 53:508, 1984.
68. Rosenfeld LE, McPherson CA, Kennedy EE, et al.: Ventricular tachycardia induction: Comparison of triple extrastimuli with an abrupt change in ventricular drive cycle length. Am Heart J 111:868, 1986.
69. Livelli FD Jr, Bigger JT Jr, Reiffel JA, et al.: Response to programmed ventricular stimulation: sensitivity, specificity and relationship to heart disease. Am J Cardiol 50:452, 1982.
70. Brugada P, Green M, Abdollah H, et al.: Significance of ventricular arrhythmias initiated by programmed ventricular stimulation: the importance of the type of ventricular arrhythmia induced and the number of premature extrastimuli required. Circulation 69:87, 1984.
71. Morady F, Shapiro W, Shen E, et al.: Programmed ventricular stimulation in patients without spontaneous ventricular tachycardia. Am Heart J 107:875, 1984.
72. Stevenson WG, Brugada P, Waldecker B, et al.: Can potentially significant polymorphic ventricular arrhythmias initiated by programmed stimulation be distinguished from those that are nonspecific? Am Heart J 111:1073, 1986.
73. Mann DE, Luck JC, Griffin JC, et al.: Induction of clinical ventricular tachycardia using programmed stimulation: Value of third and fourth extrastimuli. Am J Cardiol 52:501, 1983.
74. Kim SG, Mercando AD, Fisher JD: Comparison of characteristics of nonsustained ventricular tachycardia on Holter monitoring and sustained ventricular tachycardia observed spontaneously or induced by programmed stimulation. Am J Cardiol 60:288, 1987.
75. Kammerling JM, Miles WM, Zipes DP, et al.: Characteristics of spontaneous nonsustained ventricular tachycardia poorly predict rate of sustained ventricular tachycardia (Abstract). Clin Res 34:312A, 1986.
76. Doherty JU, Kienzle MG, Waxman HL, et al.: Programmed ventricular stimulation at a second right ventricular site: An analysis of 100 patients, with special reference to sensitivity, specificity and characteristics of patients with induced ventricular tachycardia. Am J Cardiol 52:1184, 1983.
77. Lin H-T, Mann DE, Luck JC, et al.: Prospective comparison of right and left ventricular stimulation for induction of sustained ventricular tachycardia. Am J Cardiol 59:559, 1987.
78. Denniss RA, Richards DA, Cody DV, et al.: Prognostic significance of ventricular tachycardia and fibrillation induced at programmed stimulation and delayed potentials detected on the signal-averaged electrocardiograms of survivors of acute myocardial infarction. Circulation 74:731, 1986.
79. Roy D, Arenal A, Godin D, et al.: The Canadian experience on the identification of candidates for sudden cardiac death after myocardial infarction. In Brugada P, Wellens HJJ (eds.): Cardiac Arrhythmias: Where to Go from Here? (pp. 343–351). Mount Kisco, NY, Futura Publishing, 1987.
80. Wellens HJJ, Brugada P, Stevenson WG: Programmed stimulation of the heart in life-threatening ventricular arrhythmias: What is the significance of induced arrhythmias and what is the correct stimulation protocol? Circulation 72:1, 1985.

81. Buxton, AE, Simson MS, Falcone RA, et al.: Results of signal-averaged electrocardiography and electrophysiologic study in patients with nonsustained ventricular tachycardia after healing of acute myocardial infarction. Am J Cardiol 60:80, 1987.
82. Marchlinski FE, Buxton AE, Waxman HL, et al.: Identifying patients at risk of sudden death after myocardial infarction: Value of the response to programmed stimulation, degree of ventricular ectopic activity and severity of left ventricular dysfunction. Am J Cardiol 52:1190, 1983.
83. Nalos PC, Gang ES, Mandel WJ, et al.: The signal-averaged electrocardiogram as a screening test for inducibility of sustained ventricular tachycardia in high-risk patients: A prospective study. J Am Coll Cardiol 9:539, 1987.
84. Gradman AH, Batsford WP, Rieur EC, et al.: Ambulatory electrocardiographic correlates of ventricular inducibility during programmed electrical stimulation. J Am Coll Cardiol 5:1087, 1985.
85. Simson MB: Use of signals in the terminal QRS complex to identify patients with ventricular tachycardia after myocardial infarction. Circulation 64:235, 1981.
86. El-Sherif N, Gomes JAC, Restivo M, et al.: Late potentials and arrhythmogenesis. PACE 8:440, 1985.
87. Denes P, Uretz E, Santarelli P: Determinants of arrhythmogenic ventricular activity detected on the body surface QRS in patients with coronary artery disease. Am J Cardiol 53:1519, 1984.
88. Freedman RA, Gillis AM, Keren A, et al.: Signal-averaged electrocardiographic late potentials in patients with ventricular fibrillation or ventricular tachycardia: Correlation with clinical arrhythmia and electrophysiologic study. Am J Cardiol 55:1350, 1985.
89. Lindsay BD, Ambos HD, Schechtman KB, et al.: Improved selection of patients for programmed ventricular stimulation by frequency analysis of signal-averaged electrocardiograms. Circulation 73:675, 1986.
90. Hoffman BF, Rosen MR: Cellular mechanisms for cardiac arrhythmias. Circ Res 49:1, 1981.
91. El-Sherif N, Gough WB, Zeiler RH, et al.: Triggered ventricular rhythms in 1-day-old myocardial infarction in the dog. Circ Res 52:566, 1983.
92. DiCarlo LA Jr, Morady F, Schwartz AB, et al.: Clinical significance of ventricular fibrillation-flutter induced by ventricular programmed stimulation. Am Heart J 109:959, 1985.
93. Mahmud R, Denker S, Lehmann MH, et al.: Incidence and clinical significance of ventricular fibrillation induced with single and double ventricular extrastimuli. Am J Cardiol 58:75, 1986.

12

Repetitive Monomorphic Ventricular Tachycardia

Philippe Coumel

History and Definition

Repetitive monomorphic ventricular tachycardia (RMVT) was first described by Gallavardin in 1922 as "extrasystolie ventriculaire à paroxysmes tachycardiques prolongés."[18] This curious arrhythmia, characterized by single and double premature ventricular complexes and bursts of ventricular tachycardia (VT), has also been called repetitive paroxysmal VT,[35] and a number of other terms have also been proposed: type II paroxysmal VT,[16] benign paroxysmal VT,[15] chronic recurrent right VT,[14] and tachycardie ventriculaire en salves.[6] The terms repetitive monomorphic benign VT or, more simply, repetitive monomorphic VT[38] tend to be preferred because they reflect the ECG pattern that is this arrhythmia's most important characteristic.

The definition of RMVT includes the absence of any patent heart disease, a condition that was easier to define when only clinical signs, x-ray studies, and standard surface ECG were available than presently, even if the criteria refer only to noninvasive investigations. In particular, 2-D echocardiography progressively reveals an increasing incidence of minor forms of arrhythmogenic right ventricular dysplasia,[30] while at the same time the limits of this disease become more difficult to define. For the clinician, the major points that make RMVT easy to recognize remain the absence of easily discernible cardiopathy and of myocardial dysfunction, good clinical tolerance that does not exclude symptoms (palpitations, light-headedness, and rarely pre-syncope or even syncope) but does include a good long-term prognosis, and a distinct ECG pattern. This last characteristic is most important and is discussed in detail in the following section.

Electrocardiographic Pattern

THE 12-LEAD ECG

The ECG pattern most frequently seen in RMVT is presented in Figure 12–1. The QRS complexes of sinus origin are normal, and those of ventricular origin have a right-axis deviation and a left bundle branch block pattern. This suggests the base of the right ventricle as the origin of the arrhythmia,[39] a location confirmed by endocavitary mapping and pace-mapping studies.[19, 21, 34, 36] In the systematic study that we carried out with 70 patients,[8] an inferiorly directed QRS axis in the peripheral leads was found in 75% of patients, and a left bundle branch block pattern in 58%. When a right bundle branch block pattern was present in V_1 (42%), it coexisted with an exclusive R wave in the left precordial leads in 50% of patients and an rS or RS pattern in the other 50%. Only in the last category (RS or rS pattern), which represents about 20% of cases, is the QRS axis outside the normal limits (0 and +120 degrees), suggesting that the arrhythmia origin may not be exclusively related to the right ventricle or the interventricular septum.

The QRS amplitude in the frontal plane is also significant. The sum of QRS in leads I, II, and III was 4.3 ± 1.3 mV (mean ± SD) in our 70 patients, and 3.8 ± 1.1 mV in the unipolar leads V_R, V_L, and V_F. In our experience,[11] these values are significantly higher than in any other form of VT: referring to the unipolar limb leads, the corresponding values are 3 ± 1.2 mV in paroxysmal idiopathic VT (n = 38), 2.5 ± 1 mV in arrhythmogenic right ventricular dysplasia VT (n = 33), 2.6 ± 0.8 mV in myocardial infarction VT (n = 100), and 2 ± 0.8 mV in cardiomyopathy VT (n = 43). There is an inverse relationship between the QRS amplitude and the QRS width in this spectrum of arrhythmias, the values for the QRS width being 135 ± 11 ms in RMVT, and 147 ± 16, 151 ± 19, 171 ± 32, and 214 ± 19 ms, respectively, in the other types. In conclusion, not only the basic ECG pattern but also easily measurable quantitative parameters aid in the differentiation of RMVT from other forms.

HOLTER MONITORING DATA

From a purely descriptive point of view, the main ECG characteristic of RMVT is to include all intermediate

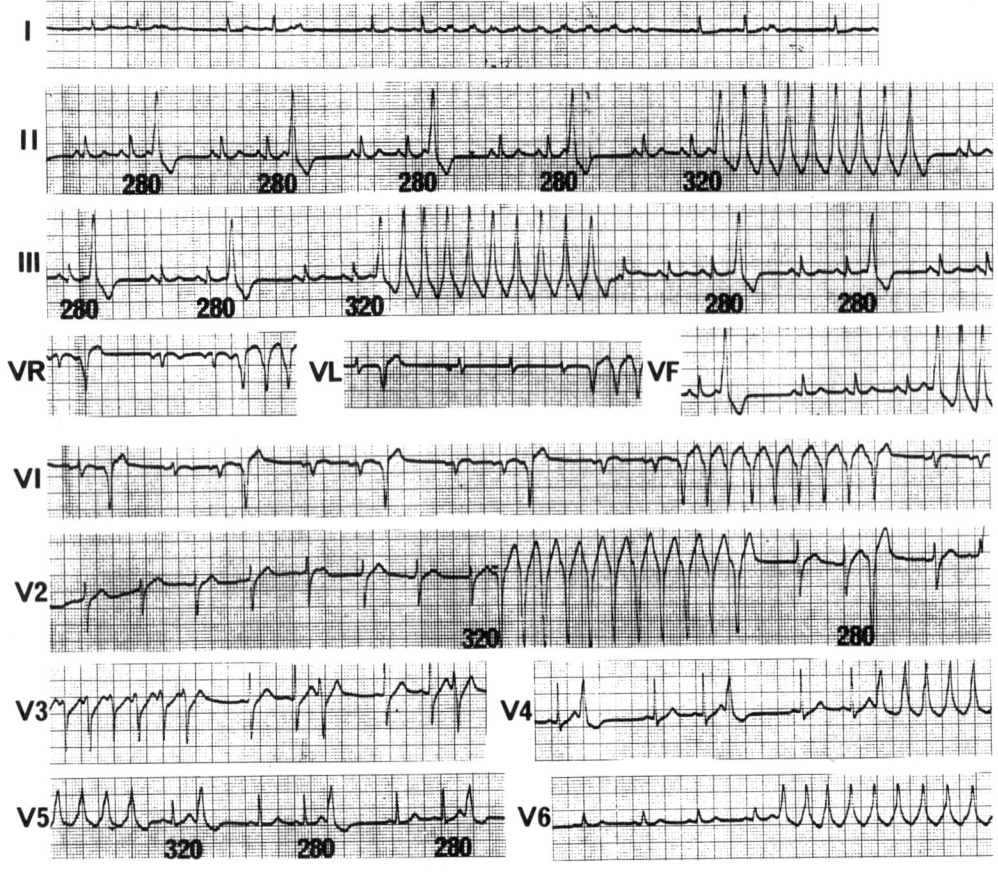

FIGURE 12–1
In the typical ECG pattern of RMVT, frequent isolated extrasystoles and runs of VT coexist. The QRS complexes of sinus origin are normal. The ventricular complexes have a vertical axis and a right bundle branch block pattern. Note that the coupling interval of the salvos is consistently longer than that of the isolated extrasystoles.

forms between isolated ventricular premature beats and sustained VT (of more than 3-minute duration): strictly speaking, this extends from a single couplet to a nonsustained VT in a 24-hour period. In practice, all patients with RMVT do have, at least during a period of their history, the typical pattern of frequent bursts of repetitive ventricular activity, which tend to occur in clusters. It should be emphasized, however, that in the long term it is usual to observe large variations in the activity of RMVT. Not only may the number and the duration of the bursts vary from day to day, but over long periods one may observe in the same patient only isolated premature beats or, conversely, their absence and the occasional occurrence of paroxysmal sustained VT. This is an important factor in the understanding of this arrhythmia. Although RMVT is a well-defined syndrome, there is no definite, clear-cut distinction from some forms of paroxysmal idiopathic VT. In fact, this characteristic was a part of the initial description, to the point that Gallavardin first suggested that the arrhythmia had two different components: the extrasystoles and the tachycardia—a hypothesis that we are tempted to endorse based on electrophysiologic evidence.

Electrophysiologic Studies

Ambulatory monitoring is probably the best tool for understanding RMVT, and we shall refer to it often in this discussion of the electrophysiologic characteristics and mechanism of RMVT. To approach apparently complex and contradictory aspects of the RMVT through various modes of exploration, we shall consider separately the isolated and/or initial extrasystoles, and the repetitive activity (even limited to one beat in a couplet). Their different behavior is probably the expression of different mechanisms, as suggested in Figure 12–2. Even though this hypothesis is not definitely established, it is clear that the presence and the

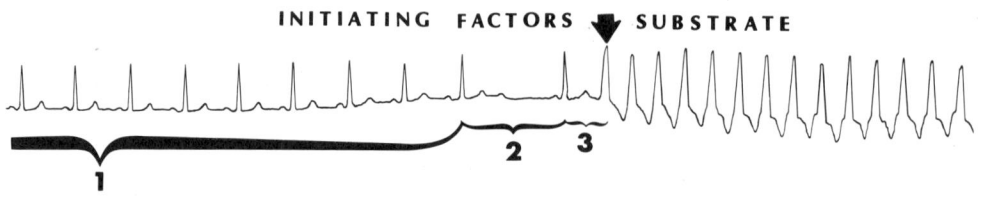

FIGURE 12–2
Components and determinants of RMVT. The substrate for the repetitive activity should be distinguished from the trigger that is formed by the initial extrasystole. The determinants of the two components are the coupling interval, the cycle that precedes the first extrasystole, and the mean heart rate that reflects the level of the adrenergic tone.

characteristics of the two components of RMVT depend on different factors or on the same factors to different extents; the preceding heart rate reflecting the level of the sympathetic drive, the immediately preceding cycle length reflecting the rate dependence, and the coupling interval. The fact that the origin of the two components is usually (but not necessarily) the same suggests that the causal mechanisms occur in the same area, which by no means implies that they are identical.

The response to exercise is variable: some authors[3, 4, 34] insist on the frequency of exercise-provokable right VT, while others[1] have reported a dramatic decrease in or the total suppression of VT, a behavior that confirms our experience and was nicely documented recently.[26] In many studies, isoprenaline infusion was used alone or in combination with programmed stimulation to reproduce arrhythmia, with variable effects. The general consensus was that between one quarter and one third of cases can be more or less easily induced, in a rather inconsistent way and with important inter- and intra-individual variations.[5, 31, 34, 38] It would be tedious to detail the results obtained, and the general conclusion was that invasive electrophysiology is certainly not the most rewarding mode for exploration of VT. We experienced similar difficulties in inducing arrhythmia, and determining whether it can be terminated is always uncertain in nonsustained arrhythmias: in the rare cases in which the duration of the runs was sufficiently stable, it appeared that the same premature stimulation may not or may stop the VT according to its delivery with respect to the expected spontaneous termination.[9]

ISOLATED OR INITIAL EXTRASYSTOLES

Extrasystoles and the Heart Rate: Adrenergic and Rate Dependence

The daily experience of disappearance of arrhythmias at rest or during exercise suggests that the electrophysiologic mechanism depends on the heart rate, a phenomenon first described as the rule of bigeminy.[25] The existence of an upper threshold for extrasystolic activity can be determined artificially using the exercise test or an isoprenaline infusion. It is occasionally possible, as shown in Figure 12–3, to determine also the existence of a lower threshold. However, because these artificial maneuvers cannot be repeated frequently, it is more convenient to follow these thresholds on ambulatory recordings. In a precise analysis that we performed in 30 patients, arrhythmia appeared in 43% only when the prevailing sinus rate increased and reached a certain value.[46] This lower threshold was most conveniently explored during the sleeping period and its value was 71 ± 13 beats per minute (bpm). In 67% of patients the arrhythmia disappeared at fast heart rates, and the maximal value of the sinus rate above which all arrhythmias disappeared was defined as the upper threshold, with a mean value of 113 ± 19 bpm. These lower and upper thresholds existed both for isolated extrasystoles and for extrasystoles initiating a run of VT.

In order to follow spontaneous changes of threshold values, ideally atrial pacing should be used, but this is by no means feasible in long-term studies. For this reason we designed the type of analysis displayed in Figure 12–4,[17] in which the sinus cycles are only considered during a certain period of time in the ambulatory recording, and the histograms are displayed in solid or open areas according to the presence or the absence of an extrasystole following the last sinus beat. In the example presented, the population of sinus cycles followed by extrasystoles had particularly sharp, narrow upper and lower limits (820 and 940 ms, respectively). The statistical significance of these limits can be evaluated if a sufficient number of cycles followed or not followed by extrasystoles can be collected during a single period of time. In our study including 10 patients with idiopathic isolated extrasystoles, these limits were determined on an hour-by-hour basis and were significant in all patients although not at any particular time during the 24-hour period: upper limits were seen more often during the day, whereas lower limits were evident more often at night for the obvious reason that the spontaneous variations of the sinus rate condition the feasibility of the determination.

The mean value of the lower limit in these 10 patients was 859 ± 136 ms, which corresponds to 70 bpm (extremes 101 and 54), a frequency that is quite consistent with the value of the lower threshold defined in our previous study dealing with 30 RMVT patients.[46] In contrast, the mean value of the upper limit was 693 ± 145 ms, which corresponds to 87 bpm (extremes 117 and 61) in patients with isolated extrasystoles, whereas in the 30 RMVT patients it was significantly higher (113 ± 19 bpm). As the occurrence of a repetitive activity precisely necessitates some degree of sympathetic stimulation (see below), the difference between these two groups most probably accounts for the existence of a repetitive activity following the initial premature beat only in cases where the upper threshold is high enough to allow its presence. The values of the limits are well correlated with the mean sinus cycle length. In spite of rather large interindividual variations, the pooled hourly data of the 10 recordings had a correlation coefficient of 0.98, and the calculated common slope was 0.93 for the upper limit. The correlation coefficient for the lower limit was 0.84, with a common slope of 0.81. These values apply to hourly determinations, although in fact they are changing very rapidly, within minutes, according to the patient's activity; for instance, when the patient stands up[26] or exercises moderately. Figure 12–5 shows diagrammatically the correspondence between these dynamic changes and the static image that we are only able to obtain.

In summary, the rate dependence of the extrasystoles is a reality that can be rather easily documented. However, this rate dependence is not fixed, and it does change according to the variations of the sympathetic drive. In any case, the presence of the extrasystole is

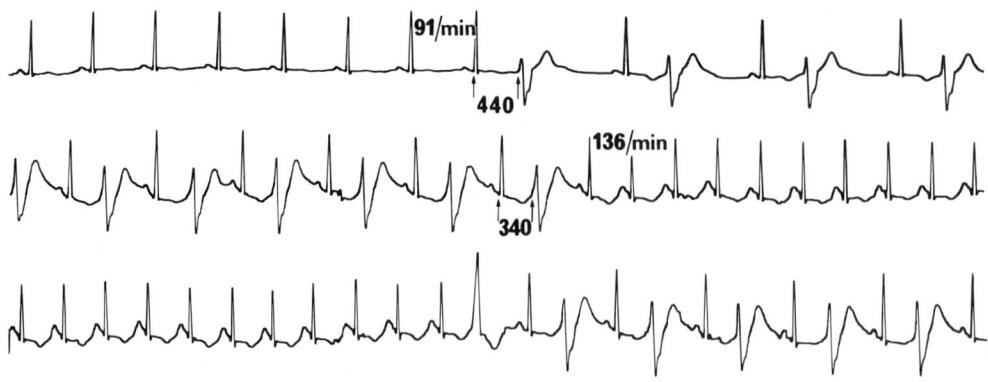

FIGURE 12–3
The effect of adrenergic stimulation on the presence of extrasystoles and their coupling interval. As the sinus rate is progressively accelerated by the infusion of isoprenaline, the lower threshold of the extrasystoles is attained at 91 bpm (top tracing). The extrasystolic phenomenon then persists up to the rate of 136 bpm (upper threshold) and the coupling interval is dramatically shortened (middle tracing). As the infusion is discontinued, the decreasing heart rate again allows the observation of the upper threshold (bottom tracing).

a necessary condition for repetitive activity to be observed; this is why the latter by definition disappears when the former is lacking. Exercise or isuprel may well favor repetitive activity, but on the condition that they do not increase the heart rate in such a way that the upper threshold is attained, thus explaining how the data provided by these modes of exploration can be totally inconsistent.

Distribution of Extrasystoles and Their Possible Mechanisms

The extrasystoles are usually abundant when present, and a frequent pattern is that of bi-, tri-, quadrigeminy, etc. It is a fascinating and difficult problem to understand this sort of distribution, which can be manipulated easily by atrial pacing (see Fig. 12–9), and the usually proposed explanation is reentry. It is indeed a convenient hypothesis: reentry has become such a flexible mode of reasoning that its rules can be adapted to practically any situation.[33] An important limitation is that in principle this mechanism can be accepted only when the reentrant circuit is defined anatomically, a condition that has not yet been filled. On the other hand, now that it has been experimentally demonstrated that coupled extrasystoles are indeed compatible with mechanisms of modulated parasystole, or reflection,[20, 32] it becomes necessary to check whether all the phenomena are really compatible with reentry.

In general, the number of extrasystoles diminishes as the rate accelerates, and the coupling interval does

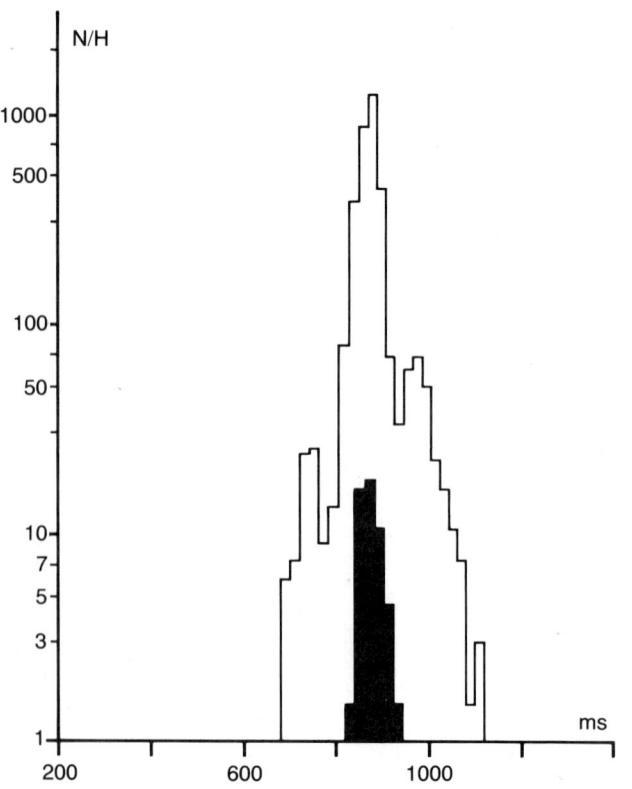

FIGURE 12–4
Rate dependence of extrasystoles. Determination of the limits of extrasystolic phenomena. The sinus cycles followed (solid area) or not followed (open area) by an extrasystole are from an ambulatory ECG during a stable 1-hour period. It is clear that the extrasystoles are consistently observed after sinus cycles composed between 820 and 940 ms, and that their occurrence is not compatible with higher or lower values.

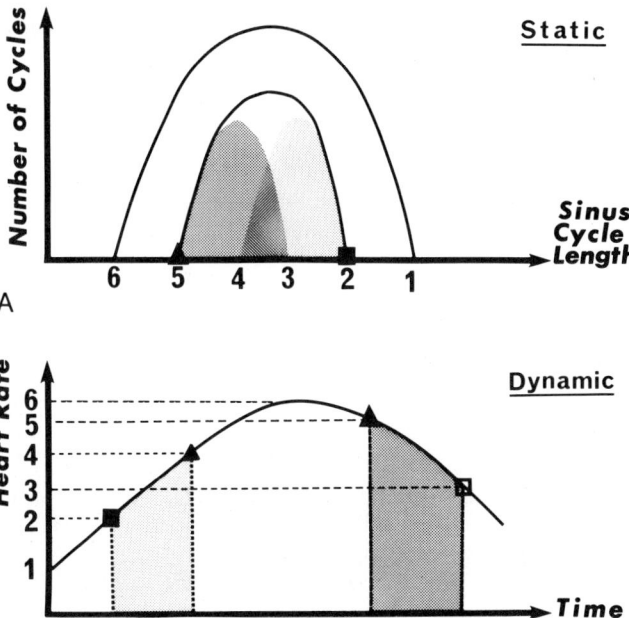

FIGURE 12–5
Variations of the rate dependence of extrasystolic phenomena. If the limits of the rate dependence of the extrasystoles are traced for a sufficient period of time (i.e., during various conditions of sympathetic stimulation reflected by the sinus frequency), the changing thresholds tend to widen the range of the limits if they are considered in a "static" (A) rather than in a "dynamic" (B) way. In fact, the entire population of sinus cycles followed by extrasystoles studied over a long period of time is formed by smaller groups with narrower limits corresponding to shorter periods.

vary, although the classical definition of a "fixed coupling interval" admits a variation of 100 to 120 ms[41] that is arbitrary. If in some instances the coupling interval increases with the appealing pattern of a Wenckebach phenomenon, more often its rate-related variations in either direction are not consistent with the reentry hypothesis. The coupling interval varies in fact according to the level of the sympathetic drive, as demonstrated by isoprenaline infusion (see Fig. 12–3) or by the comparison of circadian values that are shorter at daytime than at night. However, this is not the only determinant; the coupling interval also varies according to the distribution of extrasystoles into bi-, tri-, quadrigeminy, etc., thus demonstrating that it is also directly rate-dependent: the longer the preceding cycle, the shorter the coupling interval, a pattern suggesting a parasystole.

The mathematical rules defined for modulated parasystole are also flexible enough to fit with such patterns.[29] This model hypothesizes the adjustment between frequencies of the prevailing rate and the rate of the partially protected parasystolic focus. The complexity of the analysis of the clinical tracings results not only from the interplay of the sinus period, ectopic period, exit block, and ventricular refractoriness but also from the powerful synchronization of the two rhythms.[44] Reflection, which is part of a continuous electrophysiologic spectrum including triggered activity[22] and modulated parasystole, might fit better with the precise rate dependence of the distribution of

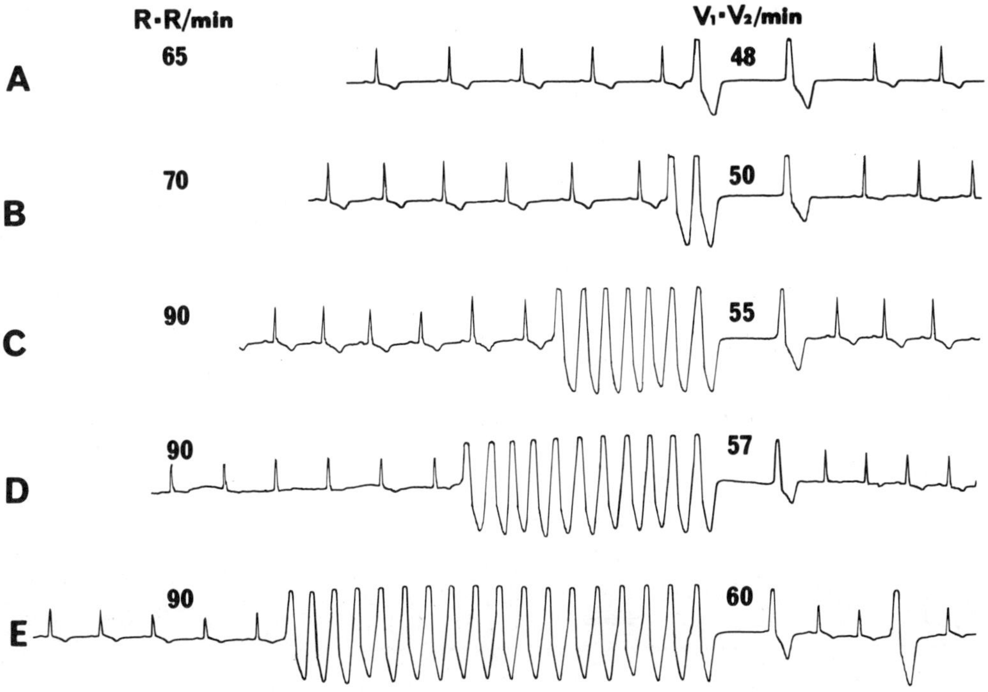

FIGURE 12–6
Parasystole and repetitive activity. A parasystole with its proper rate is occasionally visible in this patient after the appearance of an isolated extrasystole as well as couplets or runs of ventricular tachycardia. As the sinus rate increases (R-R/min), the parasystolic rate (V_1-V_2/min) also accelerates to a lesser extent. The duration of the repetitive activity increases as the level of sympathetic drive becomes higher and higher from A to E.

the extrasystoles. On the other hand, it is not unusual to find evidence of parasystole in ambulatory recordings, and in the example of Figure 12–6 the parasystolic cycle was patent after either isolated premature beats or shorter or longer runs of VT, with an intrinsic rate ranging from 48 to 60 bpm.

During the 24-hour period, we studied the number and characteristics of different types of events in 30 patients.[46] The mean total number of isolated extrasystoles per patient was $10{,}187 \pm 9933$ and 2933 ± 4087 for couplets, and 2356 ± 4241 for runs of three or more premature beats. The mean coupling interval of isolated extrasystoles (R-V_1) was 427 ± 76 ms. The mean R-V_1/R-R ratio was 0.62 ± 0.09 ms, and the coupling interval was variable (>120 ms) in 24 patients, with fusion beats in 10. The R-V_1 interval was longer for extrasystoles initiating a run of VT than for single extrasystoles (448 ± 63 ms). However, the difference was not statistically significant for the entire group because of the variability of the coupling interval. This is usually the case when the comparison includes a number of different parameters such as distribution into various form of bigeminy, day and night variations, and duration of the last sinus cycle. When considering individual groups that are homogeneous with regard to these variables, coupling intervals are indeed longer for initial than for isolated extrasystoles (see Fig. 12–1), a phenomenon signaled on different occasions in diseased as well as undiseased hearts.[2, 23, 37, 42, 43]

REPETITIVE ACTIVITY

As a rule, runs of VT occur exclusively or predominantly during patients' activity. In our 30 patients more than 90% of the total number of runs were observed during the day in 83% of patients, with peaks during the morning, the end of the afternoon, and on waking. The VT rate ranged from 110 to 250 bpm (158 ± 33). The first cycle of VT (V_1-V_2) was shorter than the initial coupling interval in 77% of cases and was the shortest of all tachycardia cycles in 47%. An inverse linear correlation was observed between the V_1-V_2 value and the length of the runs; that is, the shorter the V_1-V_2 interval, the longer the runs ($r = -0.97$, $p < 0.01$). Moreover, the V_1-V_2 value shortened linearly with increasing heart rate ($r = -0.89$, $p < 0.05$), in a proportion that usually does not parallel that of the coupling interval R-V_1 and further suggests that the V_1-V_2 interval forms a sort of junction between two different phenomena. A progressive shortening of the VT cycle length (warm-up), with R-$V_1 > V_1$-$V_2 > V_2$-V_3, was present in 33% of cases but was consistently limited to the first three tachycardia cycles. Termination of VT runs was characterized by a slowly progressive but significant increase in cycle length (cool-off) in all cases exhibiting runs of more than 10 complexes ($n = 8$).

Three determinants are responsible for the presence or absence of the repetitive response, and for its duration: (1) the level of the sympathetic drive, (2) the immediately preceding cycle length, and (3) the coupling interval (Fig. 12–2). Because they tend to interfere with each other, it is frequently difficult to obtain a pure analysis of each determinant independently from the others.

The Repetitive Response and the Heart Rate: Adrenergic Dependence

A computerized analysis permits selection of all the events of ventricular origin not preceded by any other extrasystole during a certain number of R-R intervals, e.g., 10 in the example shown in Figure 12–7. To avoid any interference with the role of the coupling interval, another technical precaution is to restrict the analysis to a homogeneous period of time that may cover from tens of minutes to several hours, thus considering stable conditions, such as day and night periods. Comparison of isolated extrasystoles with any type of repetitive response constantly shows that the former always occur in the setting of a lower heart rate. As the analysis usually involves hundreds of events, the differences are highly statistically significant because the value of the standard deviations are of the order of 100 ms for differences in the mean values that are of the same order. In a systematic study of this phenomenon,[46] we pooled the values obtained in 30 patients, and we extended the analysis to the mean heart rate during the 3 minutes preceding each of the events. This made it possible to obtain the correlation displayed in Figure 12–8. The high value of the correlation coefficient (0.98) applies to the duration of the repetitive activity: the higher the mean heart rate, the longer the duration of the salvos. Similar correlations were observed when the heart rate was calculated for the 14 cycles, or even when 4 cycles preceding the events were considered: this excludes the possibility of any bias in the evaluation of the mean heart rate in the 3-minute period, due for instance to the presence of numerous long salvos of VT. Of course, the favorable effect of adrenergic stimulation can also be demonstrated by isoprenaline infusion (Fig. 12–9); however, frequently it is difficult to consistently obtain the same effect in the same patient.

The Long Preceding R-R Interval and Rate Dependence

When highly active extrasystolic periods are not excluded from the analysis, the proper role of the duration of the last cycle preceding the isolated extrasystole (or the initial extrasystole followed by a repetitive response) can be explored. For instance, in Figure 12–9 (A and B) the occurrence of a single extrasystole or of a couplet relates to the duration of the last R-R interval shorter or longer than 800 ms. In our cohort of 30 patients, a long preceding R-R interval just before the VT runs was observed in 77% of cases, and in this subset of patients there was a positive linear correlation between the length of the runs and the mean value of this long preceding cycle ($r = 0.90$, $p < 0.05$); that is, the longer the preceding cycle, the longer the runs, independently of the role of the mean heart rate. In this subgroup of patients, an oscillatory pattern of

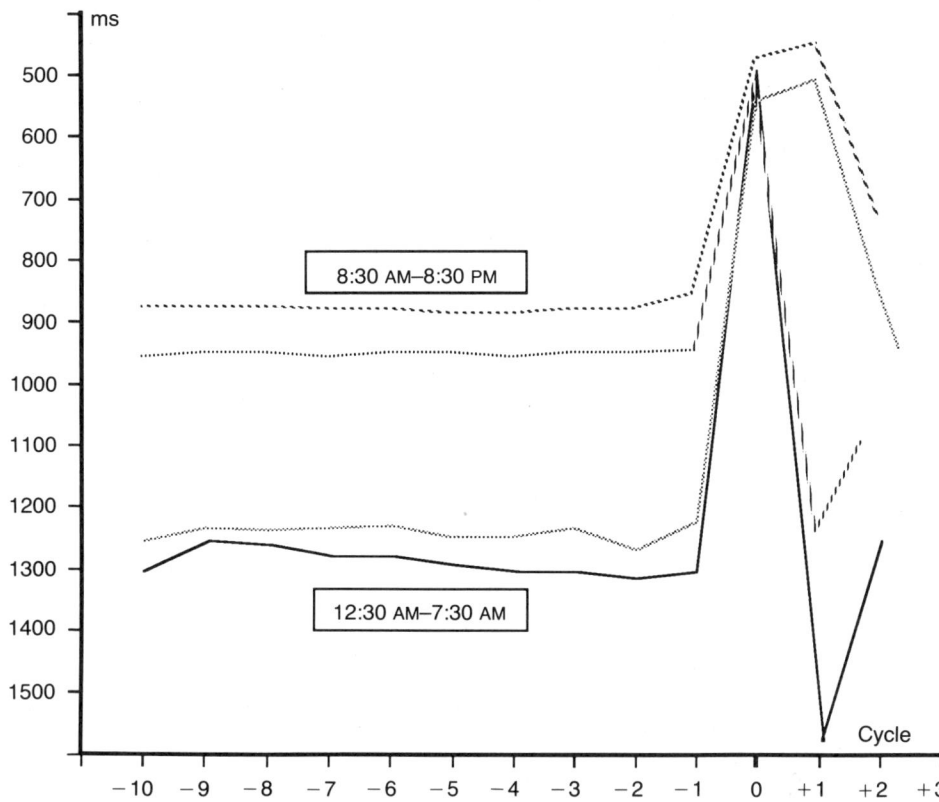

FIGURE 12–7
Mean heart rate relationships of isolated extrasystoles, repetitive phenomena, and coupling intervals. The 10 sinus cycles preceding several hundredths of isolated extrasystoles and couplets or runs of ventricular complexes were collected during the day (from 8:30 AM to 8:30 PM) and at night (from 12:30 AM to 7:30 AM). In both situations the sinus rate preceding isolated extrasystoles is significantly lower (p<0.01) than before couplets and runs. The coupling interval of isolated extrasystoles does not differ during the day and at night. However, extrasystoles followed by a repetitive activity have a significantly shorter coupling interval during the day and a longer coupling interval at night.

preceding R-R intervals due to bigeminy or trigeminy (Fig. 12–10) was observed in 14 cases, whereas in the other 9 cases the long preceding interval was due to the compensatory pause of an occasional extrasystole or the abrupt slowing of the sinus rate occurring in the penultimate cycle.

Comparison of the pooled data, including or excluding an oscillation phenomenon, allows evaluation of the relative role of the pause on the one hand, and the mean heart rate on the other (see Fig. 12–8). It then becomes clear that the heart rate level necessary for the occurrence of the repetitive phenomenon is lower when the oscillations exist than when they are absent, thus proving that the necessary amount of sympathetic stimulation to provoke the repetitive response is lower in the presence of a long preceding cycle: this differentiates once again adrenergic dependence and rate dependence of the repetitive phenomenon.

The Coupling Interval of the Initial Beat

In our study, the R-V_1 interval was longer for extrasystoles initiating a run of VT than for single extrasystoles in 18 patients, and in this subset of patients a positive linear correlation was observed between the value of the initial coupling interval and the length of

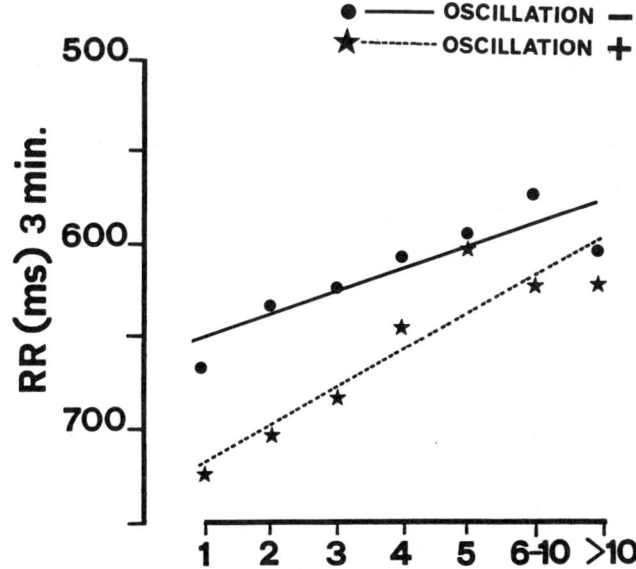

FIGURE 12–8
Pooled data from 30 patients with RMVT have been arranged in two populations according to the absence (circles; "–" oscillations) or the presence (stars; "+" oscillations) of oscillations of the cycle length related to bigeminy or trigeminy. Then the various types of events from isolated extrasystoles (1) to couplets (2), triplets (3), and runs of 4, 5, 6–10, and more than 10 QRSs have been correlated with the mean cycle length during the 3 minutes preceding each of the events. It is clear from the 2 regression lines that a correlation between the heart rate and the type of event observed exists in both situations. However, the sinus rate is always higher when the oscillations are lacking. The amount of adrenergic stimulation that is necessary to induce the repetitive phenomena is more important when there are no favoring oscillatory phenomena. (See text and the following figures for discussion.)

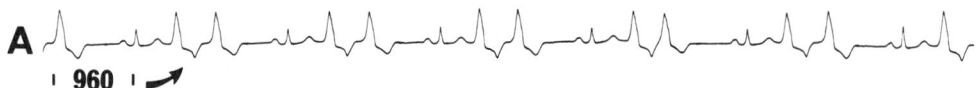

FIGURE 12–9
Rate dependence and adrenergic dependence of arrhythmias. *A* and *B*, The occurrence of a couplet rather than an isolated extrasystole clearly depends on the duration of the preceding cycle. Couplets are observed only after post-extrasystolic pauses longer than 900 ms. *C–E*, Atrial pacing conditions the presence or the absence of isolated extrasystoles distributed into bigeminy or trigeminy. *F*, Isoprenaline infusion induces prolonged runs of tachycardia that can be inconsistently stopped by premature ventricular stimulations.

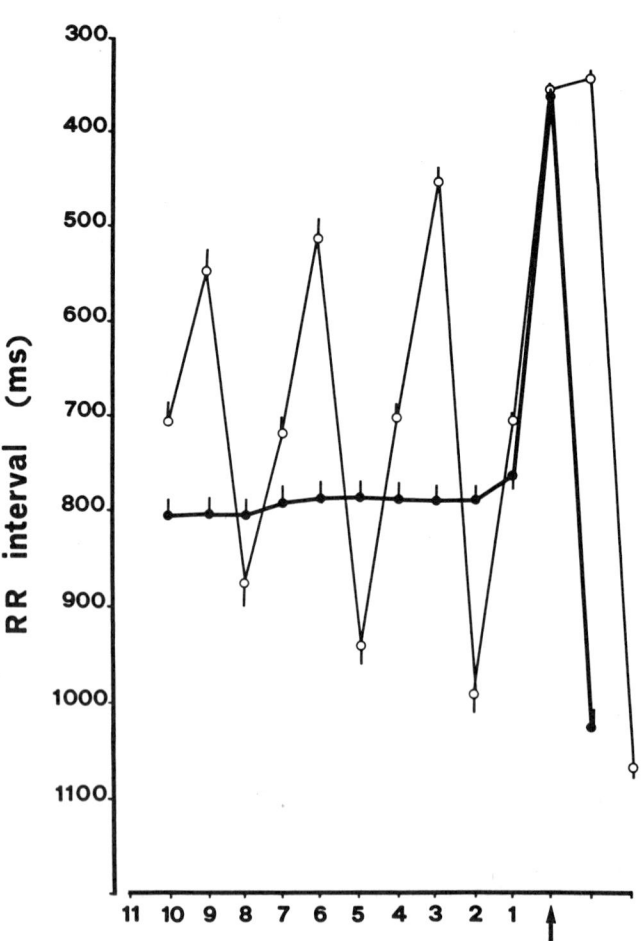

FIGURE 12–10
Cycle length oscillations and repetitive activity. Isolated premature beats and couplets have been recorded in a patient with occasional episodes of trigeminy over a 10-hour period of time. The 11 cycles preceding the initial extrasystole are represented, and it clearly appears that the oscillatory phenomenon favors the occurrence of couplets independently of the coupling interval (identical) and the heart rate level. Open and solid circles represent the mean values (±SEM) of the cardiac cycles for sequences terminated (open circles) or not (solid circles) by a repetitive activity.

the runs (r = 0.98, p <0.001). In the other 12 patients there were no variations of the coupling interval, which apparently played no role in the occurrence of repetitive phenomena.

Even in patients in whom there is no apparent relationship between the coupling interval and the occurrence of repetitive activity, further analysis may demonstrate that the phenomenon is operating consistently under various conditions, although this may not be apparent at first glance. In the example of Figure 12–7, the coupling interval for isolated premature beats does not change during the two periods considered. However, it is longer for the repetitive phenomena that occur at night and shorter for those occurring at daytime, simply because the coupling interval follows the general rule of becoming shorter as the sympathetic drive increases.

Figure 12–11 exemplifies the interplay between the coupling interval cycle 0 and the value of the immediately preceding sinus cycle length (cycle −1) in a patient having repetitive activity ranging from couplets to salvos of 5 beats. There is a complex balance between these two determinants: both cycles −1 and 0 depend on the sympathetic drive and tend to shorten when it increases; on the other hand, there is an inverse relationship between the value of cycle −1 and that of cycle 0. The net result of these two opposite trends appears in the lower diagram: if the value of these cycles in the case of isolated extrasystoles is taken as the reference point, the differences in the sinus cycles (negative) and in the coupling intervals (positive) according to the type of events are interchangeable: the probability of a repetitive activity becomes greater as the cycle −1 decreases or the cycle 0 increases.

Interaction of the Various Determinants of Repetitive Activity

We have tried to demonstrate the complexity of the action of the various determinants of repetitive phenomena in the diagram of Figure 12–12. No one factor is independent of the others, and they may even act on the repetitive response in opposite ways, according to their direct or indirect influence. We have seen that the lengthening of cycle 0 (coupling interval) has a positive effect on the repetitive response; this is true also of the lengthening of cycle −1 and of the sympathetic drive. At the same time, however, the sympathetic drive tends to shorten both the coupling interval and the −1 sinus cycle, thus having an indirect negative effect on the repetitive response. On the other hand, to a lesser extent the balance between the −1 and the 0 cycle contributes to the transformation of this negative, indirect influence to a positive, even more indirect, effect. These complex interactions explain why any global analysis of these different behaviors has not thus far resulted in the isolation of each of the determinants that are all interactive. As a matter of fact, every time they are looked for over periods including changes in the predominant role of one of them, the compensation between them tends to obscure the particular mode of action of each of them taken separately. A sophisticated, computerized analysis of spontaneous ambulatory tracings is the most effective method for isolation of the various determinants of the two components of RMVT, that is, the initial extrasystole and the repetitive activity.[10]

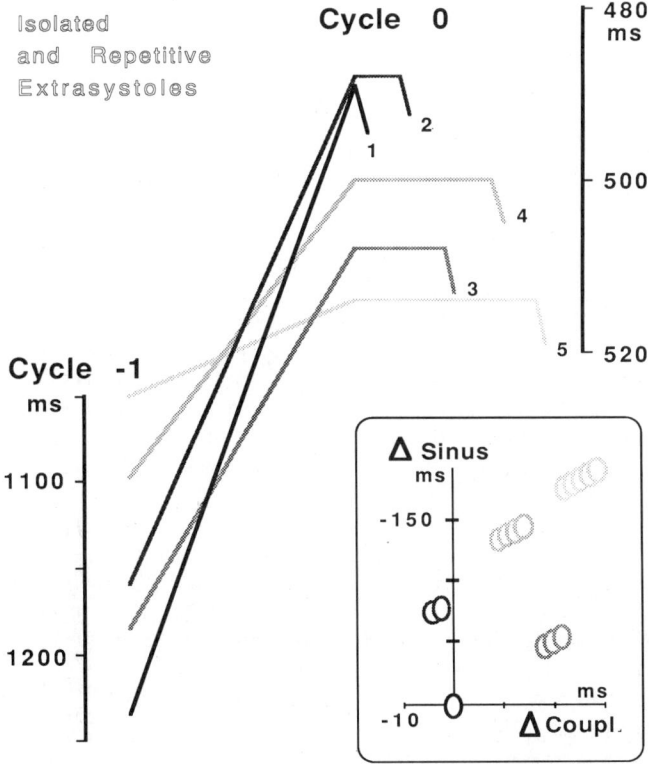

FIGURE 12–11
Relationships between the last sinus cycle length, the coupling interval, and repetitive activity. A number of events of different types (1 = isolated extrasystole, 2 = couplet, 3 = triplets, etc.) were collected during a stable 4-hour period of recording. The sinus cycle "−1" and the cycle "0" (coupling interval) are represented by different scales (in ms). There is obviously a balance between the duration of cycles 0 and −1, the combination of which is responsible for the type of the repetitive response. Taking cycles −1 and 0 of isolated extrasystoles as the reference point, the relative impact of their variations (Δ sinus and Δ coupling) on the type of event (2 to 5 ovals) observed is shown in the inset.

Possible Mechanisms of Repetitive Activity

Electrophysiologic studies suggest that triggered activity, rather than reentry, may be responsible for repetitive activity.[12] In animal experiments it has been shown that the presence and the amplitude of afterdepolarizations are favored not only by rapid pacing but by a preceding pause[13] and by the addition of catecholamines. A warm-up phenomenon is also frequently observed in a series of afterdepolarizations, as well as the lengthening of the cycles of the tachycardia before its spontaneous termination.[28, 45] Many of these phenomena are observed in RMVT, and the monomorphism of the initial extrasystole and the repetitive activity is not incompatible with the hypothesis that two different electrophysiologic mechanisms occur in the same area.[27] Reentry within the parasystolic focus has been

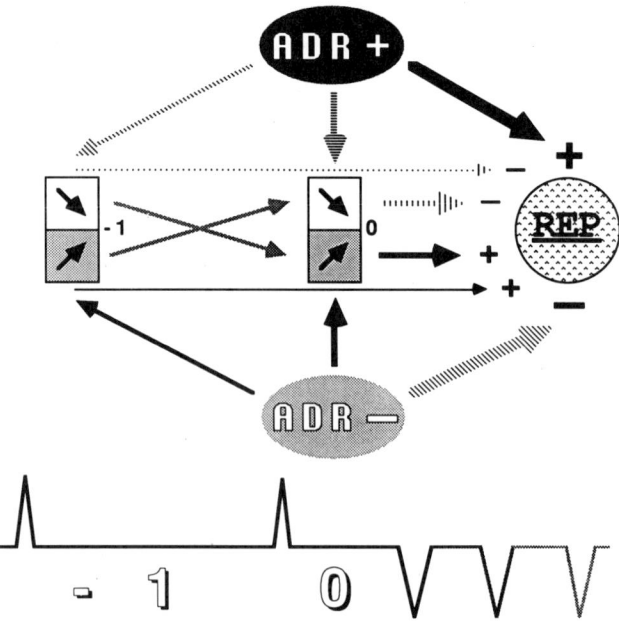

FIGURE 12–12
Complex direct and indirect interactions of the determinants of repetitive activity (REP) are diagrammed, including the positive (+) and negative (−) effects of its various determinants: adrenergic stimulation (ADR+) or depression (ADR−), shorter or longer cycle "0" (coupling interval), and shorter or longer sinus cycle "−1." An increased sympathetic drive, a shorter coupling interval, and a longer preceding sinus cycle have a direct positive effect on REP. However, indirect actions of the sympathetic drive or the sinus cycle on the coupling interval tend to have a negative effect on repetitive activity, so that their net effect may be difficult to analyze, especially when the action of a drug is to be evaluated. The bottom panel is a schematic representation of two sinus beats limits of the cycle −1, and three premature beats starting after cycle 0, as in the coupling interval.

proposed as a mechanism of repetitive activity,[24] but the difficulty in manipulating RMVT by programmed stimulation makes this hypothesis less attractive. Finally, the occurrence of afterdepolarization is related to the intracellular concentration of calcium; in this regard, the efficacy of calcium channel blockers observed in our laboratory[12] and by others[14, 38, 40] contrasts with studies of reentrant ventricular arrhythmias.

THE EFFECT OF DRUGS

Although not always explicitly specified in the literature, this model of ventricular arrhythmia is often used for testing the effects of antiarrhythmic drugs, because of its convenience for quantifying the events. The particular behavior of the two components of RMVT deserves to be considered because certain aspects may provide further information about the mechanisms of this arrhythmia.

TYPE I DRUGS

Extrasystoles usually are sensitive to all categories of type I drugs. Their effect on isolated premature beats may be dissociated from their effect on repetitive responses, particularly when a drug is used at low dosages. These cases, as shown in Figure 12–13, provide the opportunity to detect the dissociation in the effect on extrasystoles and on repetitive activity: although both components are clearly influenced by quinidine, the extrasystoles are almost suppressed, whereas during the periods that still include them, the salvos of tachycardia are still capable of occurring in long runs. Of course, the repetitive activity totally disappears when all the extrasystoles are suppressed.

BETA BLOCKERS

The primary effect of beta blockers is to diminish the heart rate, a fact that usually is not taken into account when their antiarrhythmic efficacy is evaluated. As we have just seen, because extrasystolic phenomena are so rate-dependent, it can be expected that the effect of beta blockers on the prevailing rate may be responsible for the increase as well as the decrease of arrhythmic activity; in fact, beta blockers are generally considered active in 50% of cases. They may favor the presence of extrasystoles simply by maintaining the heart rate at a value between the upper and the lower limits (that is, in front of the window of frequency); the drug is then defined as arrhythmogenic. In other cases, an opposite situation may occur, and then the drug is qualified as antiarrhythmic. Most probably in both situations the terms are not adequate; the main effect of the beta blocker is to unmask or mask the extrasystoles rather than actually to suppress or induce them.

The effect of beta blockers can be even more complex, because they may act on the thresholds themselves, as shown in Figure 12–14, in which the same amount of propranolol is administered on two different days to the same patient. Comparing the arrhythmia behavior as the sinus rate spontaneously decreases or when the heart rate is artificially maintained by atrial pacing demonstrates that the rate dependence of the extrasystoles is still present, but the values of the thresholds have changed.

The effect of beta blockers is more consistent on the salvos of tachycardia. Figure 12–13 demonstrates that the repetitive activity is completely abolished, whereas the isolated premature beats persist, a phenomenon that clearly confirms that the repetitive activity depends on the adrenegic drive. Conversely, when a beta-blocker with intrinsic sympathetic activity is used, frequently the number and duration of the salvos are dramatically augmented (Fig. 12–15).

CALCIUM ANTAGONISTS

The action of calcium antagonists, particularly of verapamil, is not simple. One can say that this drug, as well as bepridil, is approximately 50% effective in this type of arrhythmia (Fig. 12–16); this is equivalent to the efficacy of beta blockers, although the mechanism differs.

We studied 32 patients, divided into 3 subsets according to the presence or the absence of repetitive

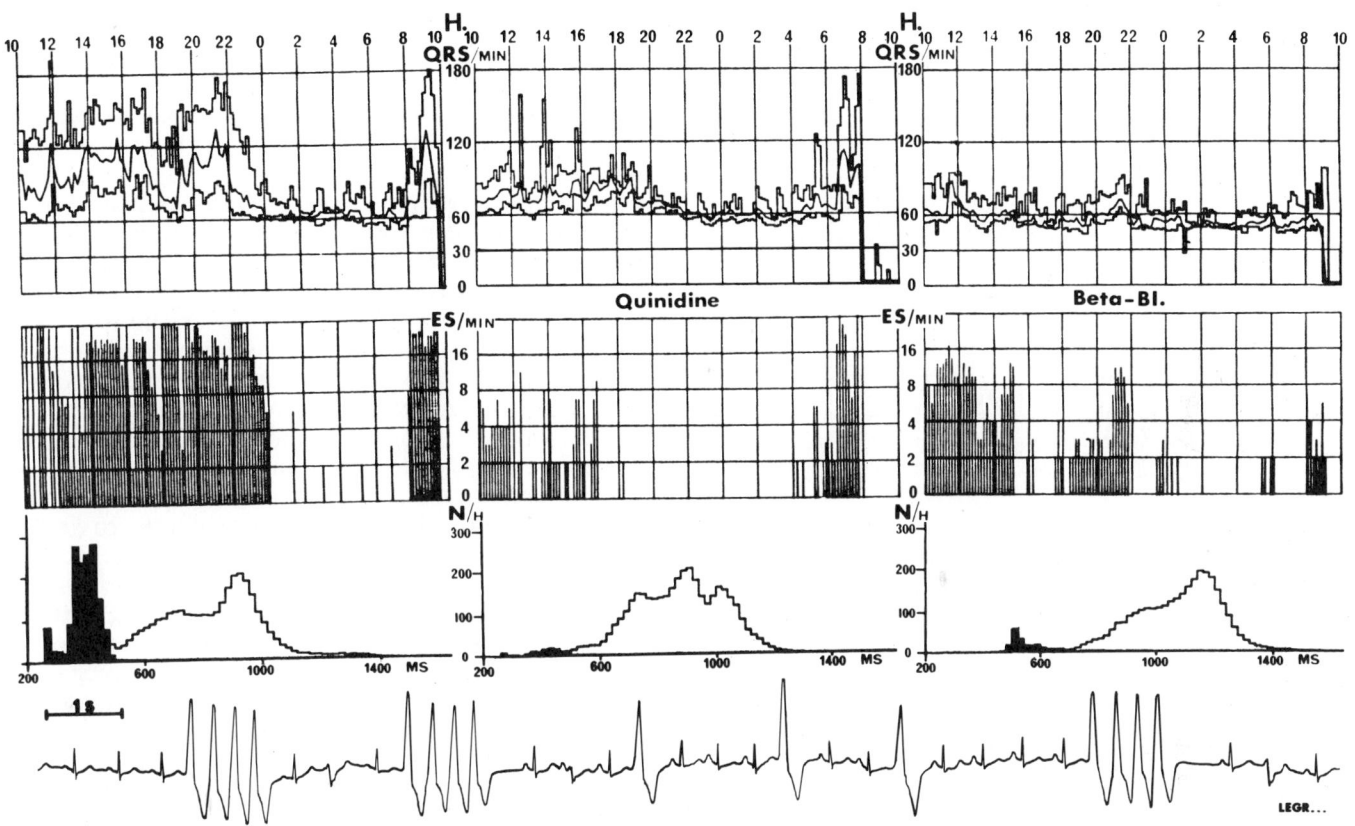

FIGURE 12-13
In a patient with numerous extrasystoles and runs of tachycardia occurring predominantly during the day (left panel), the effect of quinidine (middle panel) and a beta blocker (right panel) are successively analyzed. The diagrams display (from top to bottom) the heart (QRS/min) rate (mean, maximal, and minimal), the extrasystolic (ES/min) rate per minute, and the histograms of the populations of sinus beats (open area) and complexes of ventricular origin (solid area). Quinidine dramatically decreases the extrasystoles, but runs of ventricular tachycardia are still observed during the day. Therapy with beta blockers (Beta-bl.) is less effective on the isolated extrasystoles, but the salvos of tachycardia are totally suppressed. N/H = number of beats per hour; H = hour.

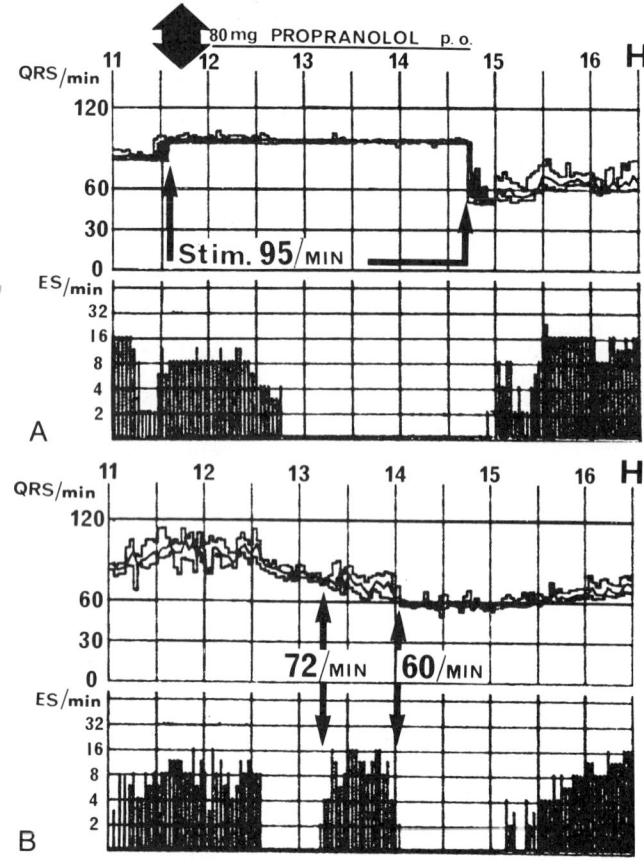

FIGURE 12–14
The complex effect of propranolol on ventricular extrasystoles. Propranolol (80 mg) was given orally to a patient with a chronic extrasystolic arrhythmia. *A*, When the heart rate was artificially maintained at 95/bpm by atrial pacing, the extrasystoles (ES) totally disappeared. In *B*, however, the drug-induced decrease of the sinus rhythm was responsible for a complex behavior: the extrasystoles first disappeared (1), then reappeared (2) when the rate was between 60 and 72/bpm, and then finally disappeared again (3) before reappearing (4) as the drug effect progressively vanished. This sequence can be explained by the successive occurrence of a prevailing heart rate below the lower threshold for extrasystoles (1), a dramatic change in the "window" rate so that the upper threshold can be seen (2) as well as the lower threshold (3), and the progressive return to the control situation (4).

activity and the temporal distribution of arrhythmia throughout a 24-hour period.[7] Group A consisted of 14 patients with isolated extrasystoles: their mean number was 792 ± 500 per hour, and there was no difference between daytime and nighttime periods. Group B consisted of 8 patients with not only isolated extrasystoles (492 ± 285/h) but also doublets (35 ± 25/h) and salvos (13 ± 10/h) concentrated in the daytime period so that if the total number of premature beats for the 24-hour period was 540 ± 270, the difference in daytime and nighttime occurrences was significant ($p < 0.05$). Finally, group C was composed of 10 patients differing from group B not only in the more numerous isolated extrasystoles (1237 ± 541/h) but overall in the greater number of doublets (240 ± 397/h) and salvos (140 ± 160/h) and in the more uniform distribution in the 24-hour period, so that no difference between the daytime and nighttime periods could be observed.

The effect of verapamil cannot be schematized in a simple way. Applying the usual but noncomprehensive statistical criteria to the total of the 32 patients, no significant antiarrhythmic effect of the drug could be demonstrated. However, this by no means signified that the drug was not active in some of the subsets. In group A (isolated extrasystoles), verapamil was not found effective for the entire group (-22%, $p > 0.9$), but this was only a balance between half responders and half nonresponders. In group B the total number of premature beats was reduced by 49% ($p < 0.05$), and the doublets and salvos totally disappeared. In group C the doublets and the salvos were only influenced at night (-44%, $p < 0.03$), thus giving to this treated group C a pattern that was no longer different from that of the untreated B group.

The interpretation of such results is as complex as the effect of the drug itself if one keeps in mind the different determinants of the two components, and their interactions. The most consistent effects of calcium antagonists are (1) to decrease the heart rate, (2) to prolong the coupling interval, and (3) to depress the repetitive activity. Each of these effects may contribute either directly or indirectly to the decrease or increase of isolated extrasystoles and to the decrease or increase

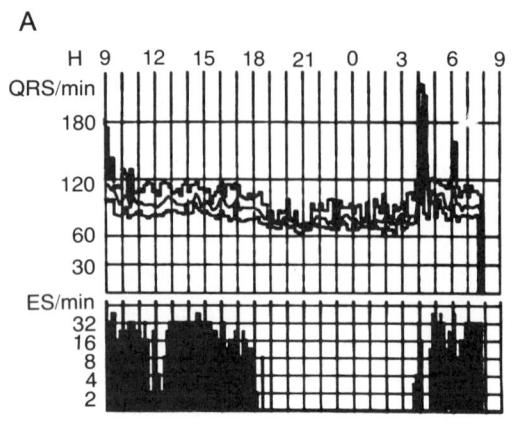
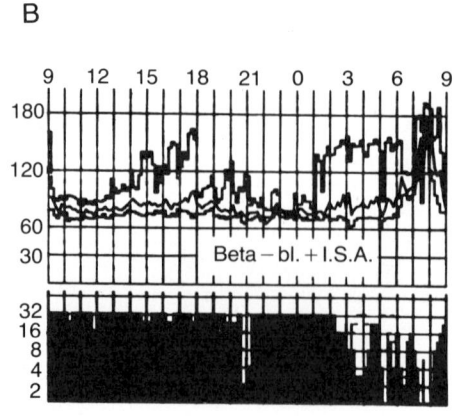

FIGURE 12–15
Arrhythmogenic effect of the intrinsic sympathetic activity of a beta blocker.

In a patient with isolated extrasystoles occurring exclusively during the day, with occasional salvos (*A*), the intrinsic sympathetic activity (I.S.A.) of a beta blocker (Beta-bl.) is responsible for the extension of the arrhythmia at night and for the occurrence of numerous salvos that are visible on the maximal heart rate (H) curve (*B*).

of the tendency of extrasystoles to be followed by repetitive activity (particularly by prolonging the coupling interval); all these effects are modulated by the vago-sympathetic balance.

The main clinical problem is to decide whether patients with RMVT should be treated, and the fact that the arrhythmia is fundamentally benign must be taken into account. It is necessary to weigh the inconvenience and dangers of available drugs and the satisfaction of the cardiologist when a clean Holter recording is obtained. For the asymptomatic patient, the choice is clear and no drug should be prescribed. When the patient has palpitations or dizziness related to rapid salvos, the cardiologist still has the choice of cleaning the Holter or relieving the symptoms by shortening the salvos and prolonging the coupling interval by either drug adapted to every case as a function of the response. However, the use of potent drugs such as amiodarone, although it is indeed effective on both components, should be discouraged in these usually young patients with a chronic arrhythmia because of the possible long-term side effects of the drug.

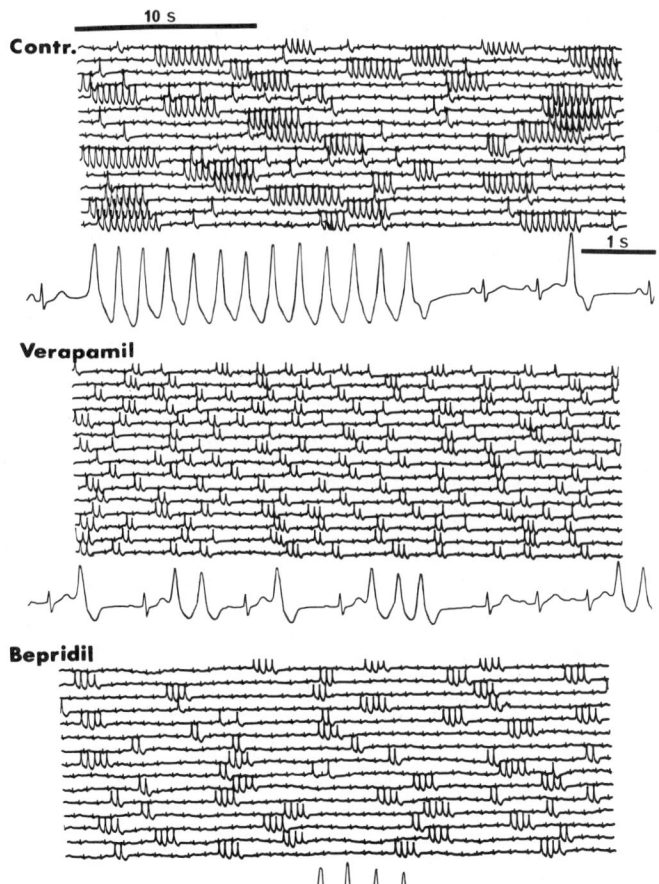

FIGURE 12–16
Usual effect of calcium antagonists. A dramatic shortening of the salvos of tachycardia is the most constantly observed effect of verapamil, which otherwise does not significantly influence the number of isolated or initial premature beats. Bepridil, a calcium antagonist with type I properties, has the same effect with an additional decrease of the extrasystolic activity. Contr. = control.

Conclusion

RMVT constitutes a clinical syndrome that summarizes all the complexity of ventricular arrhythmias. It is intermediate between "simple" (isolated extrasystoles) and "complex" (sustained ventricular tachycardias). The ECG pattern is appropriate for patients without evidence of heart disease if it suggests a right ventricular origin. The same type of arrhythmia may be observed in patients with diseased hearts, but the pattern of the QRS complexes of ventricular origin is usually different, suggesting a left-sided location. In both cases this type of arrhythmia constitutes an unique model for the study of the behavior of the two components and their determinants, which cannot be approached easily when simple and complex arrhythmias do not coexist in the same individuals.

Our experience with these determinants, particularly adrenergic dependence and rate dependence, is that they are also active in the arrhythmias observed in patients with heart disease, but their impact is quantitatively, but not qualitatively, different.[26, 47] In short, a continuous spectrum extends from the isolated extrasystole to sustained VT, as well as from normal to diseased hearts. The modes of exploration, the prognostic significance, and the treatment of RMVT may well be different according to the clinical situation and to the ECG pattern. From the electrophysiologic point of view, however, this arrhythmia should be considered a single entity.

References

1. Aliot E, Brembilla-Perrot B, Khalife K, et al.: Ventricular tachycardias in individuals with apparently normal hearts. *In* Aliot E, Lazzara R (eds.): Ventricular Tachycardias, pp. 95–112. Boston, Martinus Nijhoff, 1987.
2. Bigger JT, Weld FM, Rolnitzky LM: Prevalence, characteristics and significance of ventricular tachycardia (three or more complexes) detected with ambulatory electrocardiographic recordings in the late hospital phase of acute myocardial infarction. Am J Cardiol 48:815, 1981.
3. Buxton AE, Waxman HL, Marchlinski FE, et al.: Electrophysiologic studies in nonsustained ventricular tachycardia: Relation to underlying heart disease. Am J Cardiol 52:985, 1983.
4. Buxton AE, Waxman HL, Marchlinski FE, et al.: Right ventricular tachycardia: Clinical and electrophysiologic characteristics. Circulation 68:917, 1983.
5. Buxton AE, Marchlinski FE, Doherty JV, et al.: Repetitive monomorphic ventricular tachycardia: Clinical and electrophysiologic characteristics in patients with and without organic heart disease. Am J Cardiol 54:997, 1985.
6. Coumel P, Leclercq JF, Attuel P, et al.: Tachycardies ventriculaires en salves. Etude électrophysiologique et thérapeutique. Arch Mal Coeur 73:153, 1980.
7. Coumel P, Attuel P: Which arrhythmias are specifically susceptible to calcium antagonists? *In* Rosenbaum MB, Elizari MV (eds.): Frontiers of Cardiac Electrophysiology, pp. 341–348. Boston, Martinus Nijhoff, 1983.
8. Coumel P, Leclercq JF, Attuel P, et al.: The QRS morphology in post myocardial infarction ventricular tachycardia. A study of 100 tracings compared with 70 cases of idiopathic ventricular tachycardia. Eur J Cardiol 5:792, 1984.
9. Coumel P, Leclercq JF, Slama R: Repetitive monomorphic idiopathic ventricular tachycardia. *In* Zipes DP, Jalife J (eds.): Cardiac Electrophysiology and Arrhythmias, pp. 457–468. Orlando, Grune & Stratton, 1985.

10. Coumel P, Leclercq JF, Maisonblanche P, et al.: Computerized analysis of dynamic electrocardiograms: A tool for comprehensive electrophysiology. A description of the ATREC II system. Clin Progress 3:181, 1985.
11. Coumel P: Diagnostic significance of the QRS wave form in patients with ventricular tachycardia. *In* Barold S (ed.): Cardiol Clin 5:527–540,1987.
12. Cranefield PF: Action potentials, afterpotentials, and arrhythmias. Circ Res 41:415, 1977.
13. Dangman KH, Hoffman BF: In vivo and in vitro antiarrhythmic and arrhythmogenic effects of N-acetylprocainamide. J Pharmacol Exp Ther 217:851, 1981.
14. Denes P, Wu D, Dhingra RC, et al.: Electrophysiological studies in patients with chronic recurrent ventricular tachycardia. Circulation 54:229, 1976.
15. Dimond EG, Hayes WL: Benign paroxysmal ventricular tachycardia: Report of a case. Ann Intern Med 53:1255, 1960.
16. Froment R, Gallavardin L, Cahen P: Paroxysmal ventricular tachycardia: A clinical classification. Br Heart J 15:172, 1953.
17. Funck-Brentano C, Coumel P, Lorente P, et al.: Rate-dependence of ventricular extrasystoles. Computer identification and quantitative analysis. Cardiovasc Res, 22:101,1988.
18. Gallavardin L: Extrasystolie ventriculaire à paroxysmes tachycardiques prolongés. Arch Mal Coeur 15:298, 1922.
19. Holt PM, Smallpiece C, Deverall PB, et al.: Ventricular arrhythmias. A guide to their localisation. Br Heart J 53:417, 1985.
20. Jalife J, Antzelevitch C, Moe GK: Models of parasystole and reflection. *In* Rosenbaum MB, Elizari MV (eds.): Frontiers of cardiac electrophysiology, pp. 217–238. Boston, Martinus Nijhoff, 1983.
21. Josephson ME, Horowitz LN, Farshidi A, et al.: Recurrent sustained ventricular tachycardia. 2. Endocardial mapping. Circulation 57:440, 1978.
22. Kieval RS, Johnson NJ, Rosen MR: Triggered activity as a cause of bigeminy. J Am Coll Cardiol 8:644, 1986.
23. Kinoshita S, Fujita K, Kanda K, et al.: A cause of paired ventricular extrasystoles. Circulation 60:1395, 1979.
24. Kuo CS, Surawicz B: Coexistence of ventricular parasystole and ventricular couplets: Mechanism and clinical significance. Am J Cardiol 44:435, 1979.
25. Langendorf R, Pick A, Winternitz MI: Appearance of ectopic beats dependent upon length of the ventricular cycle, the "rule of bigeminy." Circulation 11:422, 1955.
26. Lombardi F, Malfatto G, Belloni A, et al.: Effects of sympathetic activation on ventricular ectopic beats in subjects with and without evidence of organic heart disease. Eur Heart J 8:1065, 1987.
27. Mendez C, Delmar M: Triggered activity: Its possible importance in cardiac arrhythmias. *In* Zipes DP, Jalife J (eds.): Cardiac electrophysiology and arrhythmias, pp. 457–468. Orlando, Grune & Stratton, 1985.
28. Moak JP, Rosen MR: Induction and termination of triggered activity by pacing in isolated canine Purkinje fibers. Circulation 69:149, 1984.
29. Moe GK, Jalife J, Mueller WJ, et al.: A mathematical model of parasystole and its application to clinical arrhythmias. Circulation 56:968, 1977.
30. Morgera T, Salvi A, Alberti E, et al.: Morphological findings in apparently idiopathic ventricular tachycardia. An echocardiographic haemodynamic and histologic study. Eur Heart J 6:323, 1985.
31. Nacarelli GV, Prystowsky EN, Jackman WM, et al.: Role of electrophysiologic testing in managing patients who have ventricular tachycardia unrelated to coronary artery disease. Am J Cardiol 50:165, 1982.
32. Nau GJ, Aldariz AE, Acunzo RS, et al.: Modulation of parasystolic activity by nonparasystolic beats. Circulation 66:402, 1982.
33. Nau GJ, Aldariz AE, Acunzo RS, et al.: Clinical studies on the mechanism of ventricular arrhythmias. *In* Rosenbaum MB, Elizari MV (eds.): Frontiers of cardiac electrophysiology, pp. 239–273. Boston, Martinus Nijhoff, 1983.
34. Palileo EV, Ashley WW, Swyrin S, et al.: Exercise provocable right ventricular outflow tract tachycardia. Am Heart J 104:185, 1982.
35. Parkinson J, Papp C: Repetitive paroxysmal tachycardia. Br Heart J 9:241, 1947.
36. Pietras RJ, Lam W, Bauernfeind R, et al.: Chronic recurrent right ventricular tachycardia in patients without ischemic heart disease: Clinical, hemodynamic, and angiographic findings. Am Heart J 105:357, 1983.
37. Qi WH, Fineberg NS, Surawicz B: The timing of ventricular premature complexes initiating chronic ventricular tachycardia. J Electrocardiol 17:377, 1984.
38. Rahilly GT, Prystowsky EN, Zipes DP, et al.: Clinical and electrocardiographic findings in patients with repetitive monomorphic ventricular tachycardia and otherwise normal electrocardiogram. Am J Cardiol 50:459, 1982.
39. Rosenbaum MB: Classification of ventricular extrasystoles according to form. J Electrocardiol 2:289, 1969.
40. Sung RJ, Shapiro WA, Shen EN, et al.: Effects of verapamil on ventricular tachycardias possibly caused by reentry, automaticity, and triggered activity. J Clin Invest 72:350, 1983.
41. Surawicz B, MacDonald MG: Ventricular ectopic beats with fixed and variable coupling: Incidence, clinical significance and factors influencing the coupling interval. Am J Cardiol 13:198, 1964.
42. Swerdlow B, Axelrod P, Kolman B, et al.: Ambulatory ventricular tachycardia: Characteristics of the initiating beat. Am Heart J 106:1326, 1983.
43. Thanavaro S, Kleiger RE, Miller JP, et al.: Coupling interval and types of ventricular ectopic activity associated with ventricular runs. Am Heart J 106:484, 1983.
44. Vellani CW, Murray A: Mechanisms of fixed coupled ventricular ectopic complexes. Cardiovasc Res 17:390, 1983.
45. Wit AL, Cranefield P, Gadsby DC: Electrogenic sodium extrusion can stop triggered activity in the canine coronary sinus. Circ Res 49:1029, 1981.
46. Zimmermann M, Maison-Blanche P, Cauchemez B, et al.: Determinants of the spontaneous ectopic activity in repetitive monomorphic idiopathic ventricular tachycardia. J Am Coll Cardiol 7:1219, 1986.
47. Zimmermann M, Maison-Blanche P, Cauchemez B, et al.: Déterminants de l'activité répétitive dans les tachycardies ventriculaires en salves. Arch Mal Coeur 79:1420, 1986a.

13

Sustained Ventricular Tachycardia: Clinical Aspects

Roger A. Freedman
Jay W. Mason

Ventricular tachycardia (VT) is a rhythm originating from the right or left ventricle with rate exceeding 100 beats per minute (bpm). The distinction between nonsustained and sustained VT is arbitrary; generally a duration of at least 15 to 30 seconds is required for the diagnosis of sustained VT.

History

Thomas Lewis[1] is credited with publishing the first electrocardiogram of VT in 1909, but the subject of that report had nonsustained VT, of no more than 11 beats. Sustained VT was documented electrocardiographically in a 1912 publication by T. S. Hart from Presbyterian Hospital in New York.[2] The patient was a 49-year-old man with a history of heavy alcohol use and paroxysmal palpitations lasting up to 3 minutes, during which sustained VT was documented. Similar descriptive reports followed from the U.S. and France.[3-11] These early reports stressed the causative roles of digitalis toxicity and acute myocardial ischemia, the criteria for bedside and electrocardiographic diagnosis, and the poor prognosis if there was accompanying structural heart disease.

A patient in whom quinidine was effective in terminating and preventing episodes of VT was described by Scott in 1921.[12] By 1930, Strauss[6] in reviewing the literature found 16 patients in whom quinidine therapy had been used, all successfully. However, the potential of quinidine to cause VT or ventricular fibrillation, especially in patients being treated for atrial fibrillation, was also recognized by this time,[6] and later reports describe treatment failures with quinidine.[7, 9, 10]

Although there was sporadic success in treating VT with quinine, morphine, magnesium sulfate, and potassium salts, quinidine remained the mainstay of therapy for nearly 30 years. Procainamide was not introduced until 1950,[13] and lidocaine was not widely used until the 1960s. The 1975 edition of Goodman and Gilman's *The Pharmacologic Basis of Therapeutics* mentions six approved antiarrhythmic drugs.[14] That number has more than doubled in the ensuing years. Overdrive suppression of VT with atrial or ventricular pacing was employed in patients with complete heart block in 1960[15] and in patients without heart block in 1964.[16] Aneurysmectomy was used to treat VT in 1959.[17] However, the variable response to all therapies was appreciated even as the therapies were initially introduced.

Initiation and termination of sustained VT by ventricular pacing was described by Wellens et al. in 1972.[18] This discovery facilitated the study of VT and has led to further progress in therapy for VT during the last two decades.

Pathophysiology

Sustained VT may occur in patients with any form of structural heart disease, as well as in patients with no discernible structural heart disease. Table 13–1 lists conditions commonly associated with sustained VT. Among patients with structural heart disease, the prevalence of all ventricular arrhythmias, including sustained VT, increases with worsening ventricular function.

The most common disease associated with VT is coronary artery disease. Sustained VT occurs in approximately 5% of patients hospitalized with acute myocardial infarction and is the initiating rhythm in about 20% of patients with primary ventricular fibrillation complicating the hospital phase of infarction.[19] Since the majority of episodes of ventricular fibrillation occur in the pre-hospital phase of infarction,[20] it is likely that many patients have early, undocumented

TABLE 13-1
Conditions Associated with Sustained Ventricular Tachycardia

Coronary artery disease
   Acute myocardial infarction
   Myocardial ischemia
   Recent or remote myocardial infarction
Idiopathic dilated cardiomyopathy
Hypertrophic cardiomyopathy
Valvular heart disease
Alcoholic cardiomyopathy
Acute myocarditis
Sarcoidosis
Mitral valve prolapse
Right ventricular dysplasia
Chronic Chagasic myocarditis
Idiopathic or acquired long QT syndrome
Antiarrhythmic and psychotropic medications

sustained VT, and that the actual incidence of sustained VT in acute infarction is substantially greater than 5%.

Among patients with sustained VT not associated with acute myocardial infarction, approximately 70% have had prior infarction.[21-23] A sustained ventricular tachyarrhythmia occurs in approximately 5% of patients in the first year after acute infarction.[24] Curiously, in many patients VT does not occur until years after an infarction, despite apparent stability of their cardiac disease. The cause for this latency is not known; it may be a result of remodeling of infarct architecture, progressive subclinical infarction or ischemia, or deterioration of left ventricular function. The age and gender distributions of patients with sustained VT and prior myocardial infarction parallel those of the general coronary disease population: about 80% are men and most are in their sixth or seventh decade.

Infarcts in patients with sustained VT are larger than those in patients without VT,[25] and most are associated with left ventricular aneurysm.[21, 22] The area of spared subendocardium underlying healed infarcts in patients with sustained VT is more extensive than in patients without VT.[25] These areas of subendocardium frequently contain bundles of apparently viable myocardial fibers embedded in fibrous tissue;[26] this anatomy may predispose to slow conduction and reentrant arrhythmias.

Idiopathic dilated cardiomyopathy is present in about 10% of patients with sustained VT; it is the second most common type of structural heart disease in patients with sustained VT.[22-23] Less frequent forms of structural disorders are valvular disease (usually associated with ventricular hypertrophy or dilatation), alcoholic cardiomyopathy, acute myocarditis, hypertrophic cardiomyopathy, and sarcoidosis. VT may also complicate mitral valve prolapse, right ventricular dysplasia, and other forms of congenital heart disease (before and after surgical correction). In Central and South America, chronic Chagasic myocarditis is an important cause of sustained VT.[27]

No structural heart disease is apparent in approximately 10% of patients with sustained VT.[21-23] VT in patients without structural heart disease is often precipitated by exercise, emotional stress, caffeine, and smoking.[10, 28-30] Patients with sustained VT in the absence of structural heart disease are younger and more likely to be female than patients with sustained VT and coronary artery disease.

A distinct category of patients with sustained VT have congenital or acquired long-QT syndrome and the torsade de pointes form of polymorphic VT. This syndrome is discussed elsewhere in this volume (see Chapter 15).

Virtually every antiarrhythmic drug may precipitate or increase the frequency of sustained VT.[31] This adverse drug effect may be seen with serum drug levels above, within, or below levels generally thought to be therapeutic. Drugs that prolong the QT interval are prone to cause the torsade de pointes form of polymorphic VT,[32] although this arrhythmia may also be precipitated by drugs such as lidocaine,[33] which do not prolong the QT interval. Flecainide and encainide may cause sustained monomorphic VT that is resistant to cardioversion;[34, 35] frequently the VT caused by these drugs is triggered by exercise.[36] VT is one of many arrhythmias that may be caused by digitalis in excessive doses; digitalis has been implicated as a frequent cause of bidirectional tachycardia, a wide-QRS tachycardia with alternation of QRS polarity, which is usually of ventricular origin.[37] Excessive doses of tricyclic antidepressant medications and phenothiazines may cause sustained VT, usually in the setting of a massive overdose[38, 39] but also with therapeutic dosage.[40]

Hypokalcmia, usually caused by therapy with diuretic medications, is well known to cause premature ventricular depolarizations.[41, 42] In some patients with recurrent sustained VT, the frequency of VT may be increased by hypokalemia. The risk of sustained VT resulting from hypokalemia in a patient not previously known to have VT is unknown. An excess of sudden death associated with diuretic therapy in a large trial of coronary risk factor interventions suggests that hypokalemia may result in malignant ventricular arrhythmias in patients without known predisposing disease.[43] A high incidence (41%) of hypokalemia is reported in the first 30 to 60 minutes following resuscitation from cardiac arrest; however, it is uncertain whether the hypokalemia is a cause or a result of the cardiac arrest.[44]

Clinical Electrophysiology

ELECTROPHYSIOLOGIC MECHANISMS

There is evidence for three mechanisms of sustained VT: (1) abnormal automaticity, (2) triggered automaticity, and (3) reentry. It is likely that other mechanisms exist.

Abnormal Automaticity

Abnormal automaticity has been suggested as the mechanism of recurrent, sustained VT in a limited subset of patients.[29, 30, 45] Features suggesting an automatic mechanism are precipitation of VT with catecholamine stimulation and inability to initiate or terminate VT by ventricular pacing. These patients are usually less than 40 years old and often have no identifiable structural cardiac abnormality; the presentation is often that of exercise-provoked VT.

Triggered Automaticity

Triggered automaticity also may be a mechanism of recurrent, sustained VT in a small number of patients.[45-50] The clinical presentation in these patients is similar to those in whom automaticity is a proposed mechanism, in that they are frequently young, often have no identifiable structural cardiac abnormality, and may have exercise-provoked VT. The principal feature suggesting triggered automaticity is initiation of VT with a premature beat, with the coupling interval of the first return cycle of VT proportional to the coupling interval of the premature beat.[45-47]

Efficacy of verapamil in terminating or preventing ventricular tachycardia has also been suggested as evidence favoring a triggered mechanism,[45,49] but other evidence suggests that response of VT to verapamil does not rule out a reentrant mechanism.[50,52] Recently, adenosine has been shown to terminate exercise-induced sustained VT in selected patients, and inhibition by adenosine of cyclic AMP–mediated triggered activity has been proposed as the mechanism.[53]

Experimental data indicate that abnormal automaticity or triggered automaticity are likely to be the cause of arrhythmias associated with digitalis toxicity.[54,55]

Reentry

Reentry is probably the most common cause of recurrent, sustained VT, especially in patients in whom VT is associated with healed myocardial infarction. In most patients who have VT inducible by pacing, the coupling interval of the first tachycardia beat is inversely related to the coupling interval of the initiating stimulus, a pattern suggestive of reentry.[56] Fractionated electrograms recorded directly from the myocardium and late potentials detected by signal-averaged ECG are usually present in patients with recurrent, sustained VT and suggest the presence of slowly conducting areas of myocardium that may participate in reentry.[57,58] Further evidence for reentry has been obtained by mapping the spread of activation during tachycardia at the time of surgery. In some patients, activation proceeds circumferentially around the border of the infarct or around an area of functional conduction block (macro-reentry).[59,60] In others, however, tachycardia appears to have a focal origin, which is consistent with either automaticity or a small reentrant circuit (micro-reentry).[59,60] Proximal His-Purkinje participation in reentry is thought to be unusual[61] but may occur.[62]

Few data are available in man concerning the mechanism of VT in the first hours or days of myocardial infarction. Sustained VT in humans within the first 24 hours of infarction can only rarely be terminated or initiated by pacing;[63] this suggests a non-reentrant mechanism. However, no data exist regarding inducibility of VT in humans during the first few hours of infarction. Data from experimental canine infarction suggest that reentry is the mechanism of "early" ventricular arrhythmias, occurring in the first 30 minutes of coronary occlusion.[64] Reentry early after coronary occlusion may be facilitated by the reduction in conduction velocity that results from elevation of extracellular potassium concentration and partial diastolic depolarization of myocytes in the area of ischemia.[65] In contrast, animal data suggest that arrhythmias 24 hours after infarction (corresponding to the "delayed" arrhythmias of Harris[66]) are either automatic or triggered.[67-69]

ELECTROPHYSIOLOGIC STUDIES

Recording and pacing with intracardiac electrodes is performed widely in patients with spontaneous sustained VT for research, diagnostic, and therapeutic purposes. Electrode catheters generally are introduced percutaneously into a vein or artery and advanced into one or more cardiac chambers, most commonly the right atrium, right ventricle, and the area of the His bundle.

The cornerstone of electrophysiologic studies of VT is the ability to induce sustained VT with pacing in the majority of patients with spontaneous, sustained VT (Table 13-2). Induction of VT not only has important diagnostic and therapeutic implications (see below) but also permits study of what is otherwise an unpredictable, transient, and unstable condition. Nonsustained VT, sustained polymorphic VT, and ventricular fibrillation may also be induced by pacing in patients with spontaneous, sustained VT, and in some patients these are the only inducible ventricular tachyarrhythmias. However, these rhythms also are frequently induced in patients without known spontaneous ventricular arrhythmias, which reduces their utility for evaluation of antiarrhythmic therapy of sustained VT. Therefore, for both diagnostic and therapeutic purposes, the appropriate end point of tachycardia induction is sustained, monomorphic VT.

A number of pacing techniques can be used to initiate sustained VT.[70] The most commonly used technique is the introduction of one or more closely coupled right ventricular extrastimuli during sinus rhythm or following a short period of ventricular drive pacing. A number of parameters can be varied within this technique, including stimulus strength, the rate of the drive, the number of extrastimuli, and the coupling interval of the extrastimuli. Each parameter can be varied from a less "aggressive" value to a more aggressive value. More aggressive stimulation modes (e.g., those that utilize higher stimulus strengths, faster drives, more extrastimuli, and shorter coupling intervals) are more likely to reproduce spontaneous arrhythmias, but are also more likely to result in ventricular tachyarrhythmias that have not occurred spontaneously.[71-75] Therefore, it is prudent to start with less aggressive stimulation methods and gradually increase the aggressiveness of the stimulation until the desired end point is reached.

The number of extrastimuli is the parameter that

TABLE 13–2
Ventricular Arrhythmias Induced during Electrophysiologic Study in Patients Presenting with Sustained VT

Study (Ref. #)	No. of Patients	Sustained VT (%)	Nonsustained VT (%)	Polymorphic VT or VF (%)	None (%)
Mason et al.[84]	226	78	8	6	7
Schoenfeld et al.[79]	91	67	22	0	11
Morady et al.[72]	101	89	4	6	1
Buxton et al.[77]	113	96	2	0	2

VT = ventricular tachycardia; VF = ventricular fibrillation.

has the greatest effect on induction of both clinical and nonclinical arrhythmias.[71, 72, 76–78] One or two extrastimuli will suffice to reproduce VT in most patients with spontaneous sustained VT; however, the addition of a third extrastimulus will induce arrhythmias in an additional 5 to 24% of patients.[71, 72, 77–79] More extrastimuli, rapid burst pacing, pacing from a second right ventricular site or the left ventricle, or infusion of isoproterenol occasionally will induce arrhythmias when other techniques fail.[73, 80–82]

Most episodes of sustained VT induced during electrophysiologic studies can be terminated with ventricular pacing. One or more ventricular extrastimuli, burst pacing, burst pacing followed by extrastimuli, and autodecremental burst pacing may be effective.[83] Like the methods used to induce VT, the methods most often successful in terminating VT (e.g., burst pacing) are also more likely to result in acceleration of VT.[83] If at any time the patient loses consciousness from VT or ventricular fibrillation, prompt cardioversion or defibrillation is necessary. Cardioversion or defibrillation is required in approximately 50% of patients undergoing ventricular arrhythmia induction studies[84, 85] and represents the major source of morbidity of these studies.

A single ventricular premature extrastimulus delivered during sustained VT frequently resets the timing of VT (i.e., the pause preceding the next VT beat is less than compensatory).[18, 86] As early as 1972 it was appreciated that such resetting suggested capture by the extrastimulus of an excitable portion of a reentrant circuit.[18] More recently, trains of ventricular extrastimuli have been shown capable of transiently accelerating and perturbing the morphology of VT in a pattern suggestive of fusion (Fig. 13–1).[87–89] This phenomenon, termed *entrainment*, is among the strongest evidence for reentry as a mechanism of VT.

In patients with recurrent sustained VT, bipolar electrograms recorded from the ventricular endocardium—both during VT and during sinus rhythm—may show abnormally long duration and decreased amplitude.[55, 90] Such fractionated electrograms most commonly are seen in the left ventricle in the vicinity of a healed infarct. During sinus rhythm, a fractionated electrogram may extend beyond the termination of the QRS complex. During VT, a fractionated electrogram may start before the onset of the QRS complex, persist beyond the termination of the QRS complex, or occasionally span the cardiac cycle (continuous electrical activity).[90] Detection of continuous electrical activity has been interpreted as evidence for localized reentry sustaining the VT.[90] However, more recent evidence indicates that most cases of continuous electrical activity can be interrupted without termination of VT and brings into question any causal relationship of continuous electrical activity with the reentrant mechanism.[91]

Ventricular arrhythmia induction should be performed only in experienced centers. As ventricular fibrillation and other malignant arrhythmias frequently are induced, personnel and equipment should be present to defibrillate and resuscitate patients. Generally, two experienced physicians, two experienced nurses, two defibrillators, and a full complement of medications and equipment useful in cardiopulmonary resuscitation should be present. With these precautions, the mortality and morbidity of ventricular arrhythmia induction has been low.[85, 92]

Clinical Presentation

Sustained VT occasionally is an isolated occurrence. A reversible cause, such as acute myocardial infarction or drug toxicity, may be identified. In most patients with sustained VT, the attacks recur. The frequency of the recurrences varies widely from patient to patient, ranging from multiple episodes daily to only a few episodes per annum. Furthermore, in a given patient the frequency of the episodes can vary over time just as widely, without obvious explanation.

Sustained VT is equally unpredictable in its duration, QRS morphology, and rate. Tachycardia duration ranges from seconds to days, and it is not unusual for a patient to exhibit a wide range of VT duration in consecutive paroxysms. Multiple QRS morphologies are frequently seen in a given patient; the likelihood of documenting more than a single QRS morphology during spontaneous VT increases with worsening left ventricular function, the number of episodes of VT recorded, and whether antiarrhythmic drug therapy varied between episodes of recorded VT.[93] Although patients often show a propensity toward either slow or fast rates during VT, the rate of tachycardia may vary considerably in a given patient, even within a single paroxysm. Most antiarrhythmic drugs slow the rate of VT, but acceleration of rate by an antiarrhythmic drug may occur unpredictably.

Symptoms associated with sustained VT include palpitations, dyspnea, chest pain, presyncope, syncope, and cardiac arrest. Rarely, a patient with VT will be asymptomatic. The severity of symptoms depends on the rate of VT, its duration, and the type and severity of associated cardiac disease. Among a series of patients who survived sustained VT and were seen at a

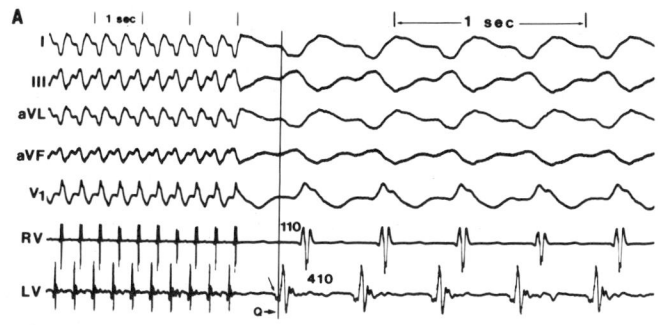
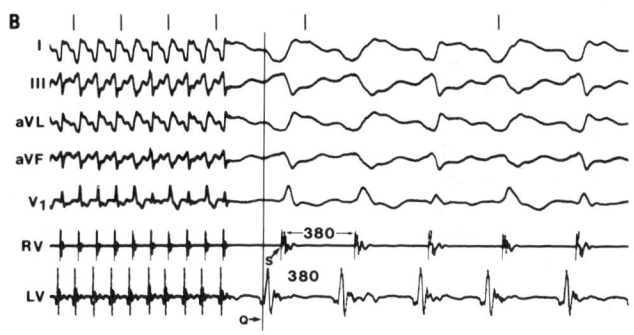
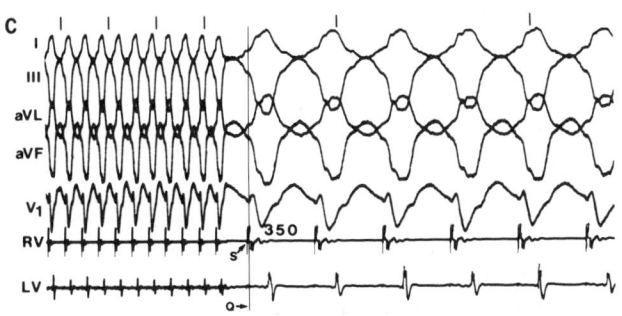

FIGURE 13–1

Entrainment of sustained ventricular tachycardia with right ventricular pacing. Each panel shows standard ECG leads I, III, aV$_L$, aV$_F$, V$_1$; a right ventricular (RV) electrogram; and a left ventricular (LV) electrogram. Q = onset of QRS complex; S = stimulus artifact. (Courtesy of Kelley P. Anderson, M.D. and reprinted by permission from Anderson KP, Swerdlow CD, Mason JW Am J Cardiol 5:781, 1985.)

A, Induced ventricular tachycardia has cycle length of 410 ms and right bundle branch block morphology. The LV electrogram precedes the onset of the surface ECG by 20 ms (arrow).

B, Pacing the right ventricle at cycle length of 380 ms results in acceleration of the ventricular tachycardia and perturbation of its morphology. Each paced impulse is conducted to the reentrant circuit and advances the next tachycardia beat. The entrained QRS morphology is intermediate between that of unperturbed ventricular tachycardia (A) and right ventricular pacing during sinus rhythm (C). The LV electrogram is unchanged compared to A with respect to its morphology and temporal relation to subsequent QRS complex.

C, Right ventricular pacing at cycle length of 350 ms during sinus rhythm results in QRS complexes with left bundle branch block morphology. The LV electrogram is changed in morphology and occurs later with respect to the QRS compared to A and B.

referral center, the most common initial symptom was palpitations (48%), followed by cardiac arrest (19%), syncope (13%), presyncope (4%), and pulmonary edema (1%).[21] However, such a sample of patients is probably overrepresented by patients with well-tolerated VT, and the percentage of patients with sustained VT in whom the initial symptom is cardiac arrest is likely to be higher.

VT is diagnosed in approximately 10% of patients evaluated for syncope.[94] Usually the diagnosis is apparent from ECG monitoring,[94] but when the cause of recurrent syncope is elusive, electrophysiologic studies may be required. Sustained VT is inducible during electrophysiologic studies in up to 28% of patients undergoing investigation of syncope of unknown cause.[95–99] The likelihood of inducing sustained VT in a patient with syncope increases when evidence of structural heart disease, such as an abnormal ECG or depressed ejection fraction, is present.[99,100]

Sustained VT is probably the initiating arrhythmia in most cases of sudden cardiac death. Although ventricular fibrillation often is the only arrhythmia documented at the time, sustained VT usually has been apparent as the initiating arrhythmia in patients fortuitously undergoing ambulatory electrocardiographic monitoring at the time of arrest.[101–103] Furthermore, among survivors of cardiac arrest, many of whom have not had documentation of spontaneous sustained VT, about half have sustained VT induced during electrophysiologic studies.[23,104–107] Thus sustained VT probably precedes ventricular fibrillation in the majority of instances of sudden cardiac death.

Diagnosis

THE ELECTROCARDIOGRAM

History, physical examination, and catheter electrophysiologic studies each have a role in the diagnosis of sustained VT, but in most patients the cornerstone of diagnosis is ECG recordings made during the tachycardia. Therefore, in a patient in whom sustained VT is suspected, every effort should be made to obtain as complete an ECG as possible, preferably all 12 standard leads, during tachycardia.

Obtaining the ECG

When confronted with a patient with a wide QRS complex tachycardia, there is often an urge to terminate the tachycardia before obtaining a 12-lead ECG. Immediate intervention without complete ECG documentation may be unavoidable in some patients with extremely poorly tolerated tachycardia. However, in the majority of patients presenting with VT without loss of consciousness, it is possible to delay tachycardia termination long enough to obtain an ECG, and the information gained almost always offsets the small risk and additional discomfort caused by the delay. Many portable defibrillators can record all 12 standard leads serially.

Electrocardiographic documentation of VT is more difficult when it is of only several minutes' duration and terminates before the patient is able to reach a hospital. Continuous, 24-hour tape recorders (Holter monitors) worn by ambulatory patients record one to three ECG leads simultaneously; they are most useful in patients with arrhythmias that recur at least daily; however, if worn on several consecutive days, they can be useful in patients with less frequently recurring arrhythmias. Hand-held, patient-activated ECG event recorders are useful in documenting infrequent arrhythmias; their capabilities include storage of 30 seconds of ECG in up to two leads and transtelephonic transmission of both stored and real-time ECGs. Some event recorders continuously record the ECG, with the last 30 to 60 seconds of data kept in memory; the patient may freeze the recording at the time of symptoms.

Diagnostic Electrocardiographic Features

RATE AND REGULARITY

By definition, the rate of sustained VT exceeds 100 bpm. Although paroxysmal ventricular rhythms with rates of 60 to 100 bpm may occur, these are more properly termed *accelerated idioventricular rhythms*.

The rate of VT in humans rarely exceeds 300 bpm. An episode of VT whose rate approaches 300 bpm often shows a sinusoidal morphology and may be termed *ventricular flutter*. Above 300 bpm, a ventricular tachyarrhythmia usually shows indistinct QRS complexes and therefore would be termed *ventricular fibrillation*.

The R-R interval during monomorphic sustained VT is regular or nearly so, with beat-to-beat variation usually less than 20 ms.[108] However, the tachycardia rate may change gradually over a period of minutes; for instance, following induction of sustained VT during electrophysiologic studies, the tachycardia rate typically slows over the first 1 to 2 minutes (Kelley P. Anderson, M. D., unpublished observation) (Fig. 13-2). In contrast to monomorphic VT, polymorphic VT usually has wide variation in R-R intervals.

QRS DURATION AND MORPHOLOGY

Because electrical activation during VT arises from the ventricular myocardium and the His-Purkinje system is not engaged early, the QRS complex is wide ($\geq$ 0.12 s). In about two thirds of cases, the QRS duration is >0.14 s.[108] Most antiarrhythmic drugs will further prolong QRS duration during VT.

About two thirds of cases of sustained, monomorphic VT show a QRS morphology simulating that of right bundle branch block (rsR', Rsr', qR, Rs, or monophasic R in lead V_1).[108] About one third of cases show a QRS morphology simulating that of left bundle branch block (predominantly negative QRS in V_1; rsR', Rsr', qR, Rs, or monophasic R in lead V_6).[108] Occasionally the QRS morphology during VT will resemble neither right nor left bundle branch block; for instance, the QRS will be predominantly positive in all precordial leads, or it will be predominantly negative in all precordial leads.

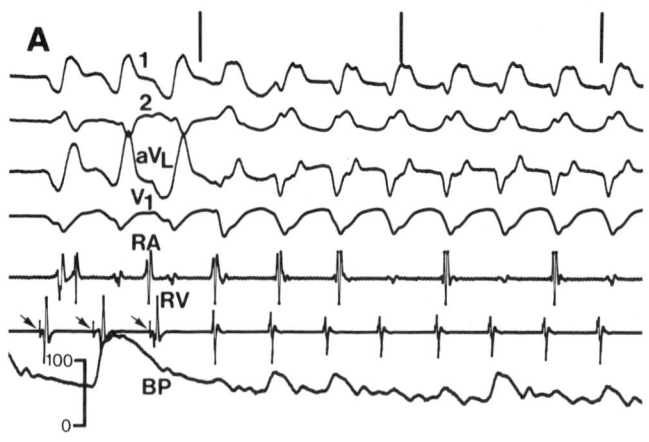

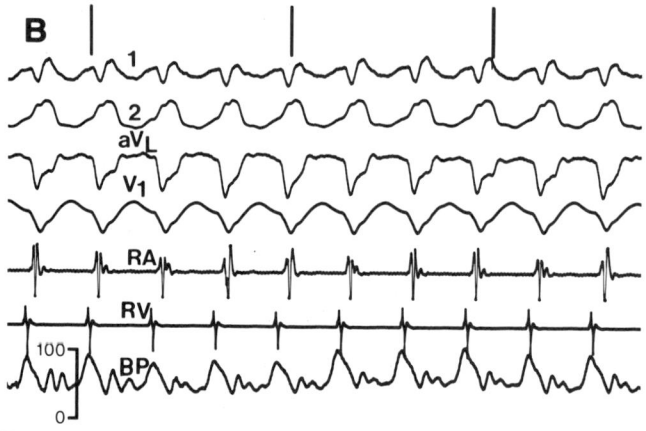

FIGURE 13-2

A, Sustained ventricular tachycardia induced with right ventricular pacing (arrows) in a 63-year-old man with a remote history of myocardial infarction. Shown are standard leads 1, 2, and aV_L; intracardiac recordings from the right atrium (RA) and right ventricle (RV); and blood pressure (BP). The initial cycle length of the tachycardia is 280 ms (rate 214 bpm). Initially, there is 2:1 ventriculoatrial conduction. P waves are difficult to see on the surface leads and are most evident in aV_L as an alternating deformation of the ST segment.

B, Three minutes after initiation of tachycardia, spontaneous prolongation of the cycle length to 315 ms (rate 190 bpm) and slight change of QRS morphology have occurred. Slowing of the tachycardia is accompanied by the development of 1:1 ventriculoatrial conduction and a rise in blood pressure.

Left axis deviation (mean frontal plane QRS axis between -30 and -90 degrees) is present in about two thirds of cases of monomorphic VT.[108] Of the remainder of cases, about half show right axis deviation (between $+90$ and $+270$ degrees) and half show a normal QRS axis.

ATRIAL-VENTRICULAR RELATIONSHIP

The atrial rhythm during VT depends on the pattern with which ventricular impulses are conducted retrogradely to the atria via the His bundle and atrioventricular node. P waves frequently are not discernible on the ECG during VT. Electrophysiologic studies have been helpful in defining the spectrum of atrial rhythms during VT.[108]

In about one third of cases, each ventricular depolarization is conducted retrogradely, resulting in a one-to-one atrioventricular relation (Figs. 13–2*B* and 13–3*B*). The retrograde P waves usually are negative in lead II, consistent with caudocranial atrial activation. Comparison of activation times of the low septal right atrium and high right atrium confirms retrograde atrial activation in such cases (Fig. 13–3*B*).

In about one half of cases, retrograde conduction is absent and the atrial rhythm will be completely dissociated from the ventricular rhythm (Fig. 13–4*B*). Faster VT is more often accompanied by complete ventriculoatrial block than is slower VT. This indicates that concealed conduction from the ventricle into the His bundle or atrioventricular node may contribute to high levels of ventriculoatrial block during VT. (Unfortunately, although faster tachycardias are more likely to result in dissociation, faster tachycardias are also more likely to obscure P waves, hindering the determination that dissociation is present.)

In the remainder of cases, some but not all ventricular depolarizations are retrogradely conducted to the atria (i.e., second-degree ventriculoatrial block is present); typical patterns are two-to-one block (see Fig. 13–2*A*), Wenckebach block (especially three-to-two), or only occasional retrograde capture.

More than a single pattern of retrograde conduction may be seen during an episode of VT (see Fig. 13–2). Carotid sinus massage may cause or increase the degree of ventriculoatrial block during VT.

CAPTURE BEATS AND FUSION (DRESSLER) BEATS

In episodes of VT with atrioventricular dissociation, there may be intermittent antegrade conduction of P waves to the ventricles that results in a normal QRS complex (capture beat) or fusion between normal ventricular activation and the idioventricular impulse (fusion beat) (see Fig. 13–4). Capture or fusion beats are seen in only approximately 5% of episodes of VT, and they are generally seen at slower rates of tachycardia (less than 180 bpm). The infrequency of capture or fusion beats suggests that there is concealed retrograde penetration of the atrioventricular conduction system during most episodes of VT with atrioventricular dissociation.

ONSET AND TERMINATION

The onset of VT is abrupt. The first beat of VT is usually premature; its morphology may be similar to that of the ensuing VT beats or it may have a different morphology. In the latter case, the first beat may appear to be a premature ventricular beat that "initiates" the ensuing VT. Occasionally, VT may be precipitated by a supraventricular tachycardia. In a patient with a bradyarrhythmia, VT may arise as an escape rhythm.

Without therapy, sustained VT either spontaneously terminates (i.e., converts to sinus or other supraventricular rhythm) or degenerates to ventricular fibrillation. Before spontaneous termination, the rate and morphology of VT often change for several beats or several seconds. Degeneration to ventricular fibrillation is usually preceded by gradual acceleration of the rate of tachycardia.

THE PHYSICAL EXAMINATION

The general appearance of the patient during sustained VT depends on the hemodynamic consequences of the tachycardia; the patient's appearance can range from normal to comatose. Most patients are in some distress during VT. The pulse may be easily palpable in the extremities; if not, it may be palpable only over central (carotid or femoral) arteries, or not at all. The amplitude of the pulse may vary from beat to beat, even in a regular tachycardia. Occasionally, a pulse deficit or pulsus alternans is present (see Fig. 13–3*B*). The blood pressure is usually decreased or unobtainable during tachycardia. Other physical findings of heart failure, shock, or both may be present.

Two physical findings are of special value, as they are suggestive of atrioventricular dissociation during tachycardia. First, the intensity of the first heart sound may vary perceptibly from beat to beat. This results from variation in the position of the atrioventricular valve leaflets just prior to their closure, which in turn depends on the relative timing of atrial and ventricular systole. Second, cannon A waves may be visible in the jugular veins. These result from atrial systoles coinciding with ventricular systole.

INVASIVE CARDIAC ELECTRICAL RECORDINGS AND PACING

Esophageal Electrocardiography

Esophageal electrocardiography is a minimally invasive technique for recording atrial activity, which may be useful when P waves are not clearly visible on the ECG. A miniature bipolar electrode within a gelatin capsule is well tolerated and, when coupled to a preamplifier and frequency filter, yields excellent atrial electrograms.[109]

Catheter Electrophysiologic Studies

RECORDINGS DURING TACHYCARDIA

Atrioventricular dissociation, if present, can be demonstrated by atrial electrograms recorded during tachycardia. If atrioventricular dissociation is not present, then atrial overdrive pacing is a useful maneuver. The diagnosis of VT is strongly supported if (1) the tachycardia is unaffected by atrial overdrive pacing or (2) the tachycardia accelerates to the atrial pacing rate and the QRS complex normalizes (see Fig. 13–3). On the other hand, if atrial overdrive pacing accelerates the tachycardia without change in the QRS complex, then a supraventricular tachycardia is more likely than VT.

Although the vast majority of wide QRS complex tachycardias that show atrioventricular dissociation are VT, there are rare instances of supraventricular tachycardias that arise from the atrioventricular junction and display atrioventricular dissociation. The only means of distinguishing these tachycardias from VT is by recording His bundle electrograms during tachycardia. A supraventricular rhythm will show a His bundle electrogram before each QRS, with an H-V interval equal to or longer than the H-V interval recorded

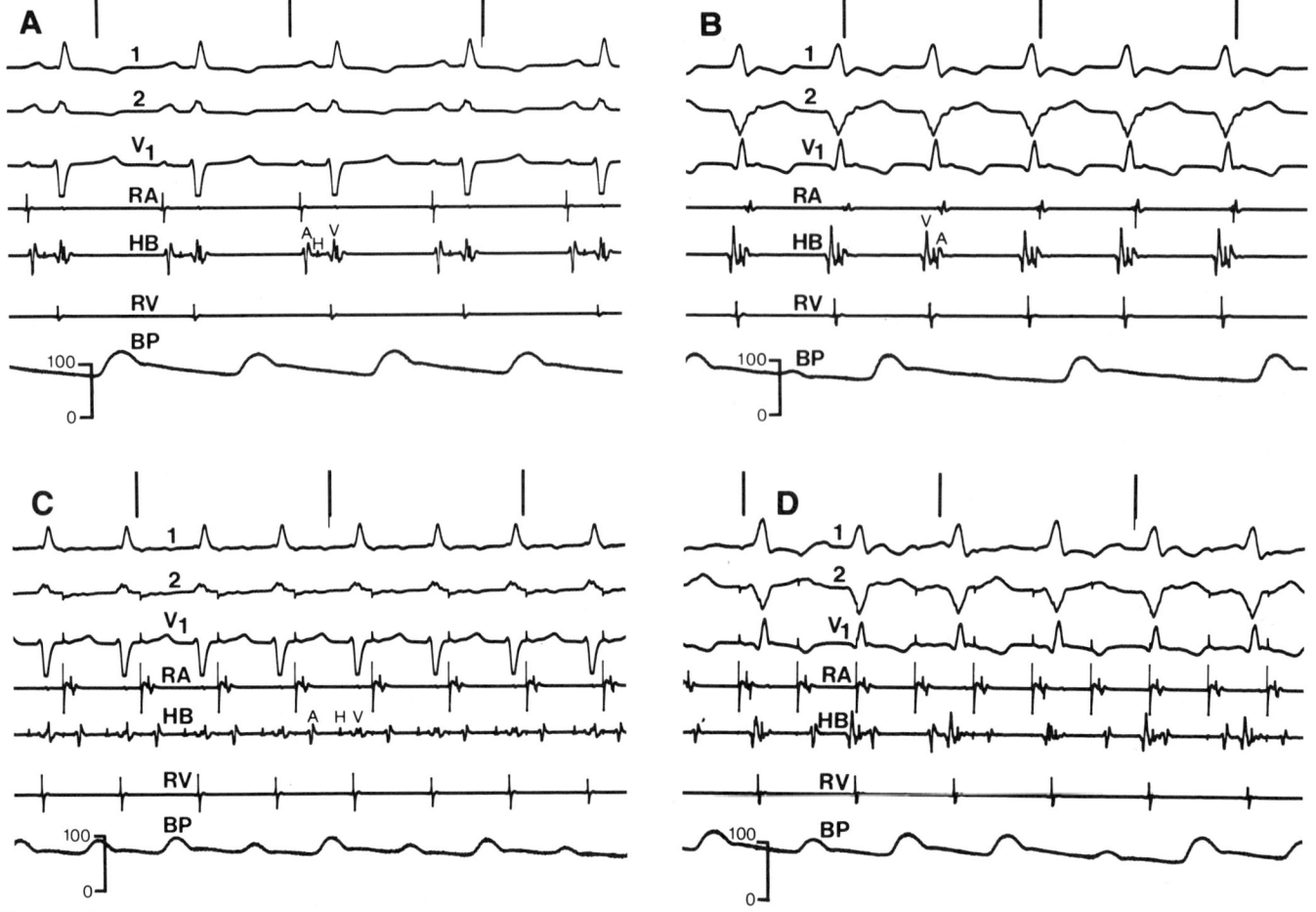

FIGURE 13–3

A, Sinus rhythm in a 56-year-old man with idiopathic dilated cardiomyopathy and recurrent, sustained ventricular tachycardia. Shown are standard leads 1, 2, and V_1; intracardiac recordings from the high right atrium (RA), area of the bundle of His (HB), and right ventricle (RV); and blood pressure (BP). In the HB recording, depolarization of the low septal right atrium (A), bundle of His (H), and right ventricle (V) are labeled.

B, Ventricular tachycardia, cycle length of 500 ms, recorded minutes after the recordings in A and without adjustment of catheter position. Note the 1:1 ventriculoatrial conduction. Despite a clear His bundle depolarization during sinus rhythm, none is clearly discernible during ventricular tachycardia, and it is presumed to be obscured by the ventricular electrogram. Note that depolarization of the low septal right atrium, recorded in HB, precedes depolarization of the high right atrium, consistent with retrograde, caudocranial atrial activation. Note also the pulsus alternans, despite the regularity of rate, during ventricular tachycardia.

C, During ventricular tachycardia, atrial pacing at cycle length of 400 ms results in normalization of the QRS complex, without termination of the tachycardia. (Ventricular tachycardia resumed when atrial pacing was discontinued.) Such a response to atrial pacing virtually excludes the possibility that the tachycardia in B is supraventricular with aberrant conduction.

D, Atrial pacing at cycle length 300 ms results in AV dissociation without perturbation of the tachycardia. This response is typical of ventricular tachycardia but very unusual for supraventricular tachycardia.

during supraventricular rhythm. By contrast, during most episodes of VT, no His bundle electrogram is recordable (see Figs. 13–3 and 13–4). Occasionally, a His bundle electrogram is visible after, within, or just preceding (with an H-V interval less than that during supraventricular rhythm) the QRS complex during VT.

Before concluding that a rhythm is VT on the basis of an absent His bundle electrogram, it is vital to validate the position of the His bundle catheter by demonstrating His bundle electrograms during sinus rhythm. Conversely, before concluding that a rhythm is supraventricular on the basis of a recordable His bundle electrogram, it is important to compare the HV interval during tachycardia with that during supraventricular rhythm and to be certain that the recorded electrogram is not arising from the right bundle branch.

An unusual class of supraventricular arrhythmias in which QRS complexes are not preceded by typical His bundle deflections occurs in some patients with accessory atrioventricular or nodoventricular pathways. Accordingly, His bundle recordings should be interpreted with caution in a patient with a known accessory pathway and wide QRS complex tachycardia.

ARRHYTHMIA INDUCTION WITH PACING

It is often impractical or impossible to obtain catheter recordings during spontaneous tachycardia. Therefore, the greatest diagnostic advantage of catheter electrophysiologic studies lies in the ability to reproduce

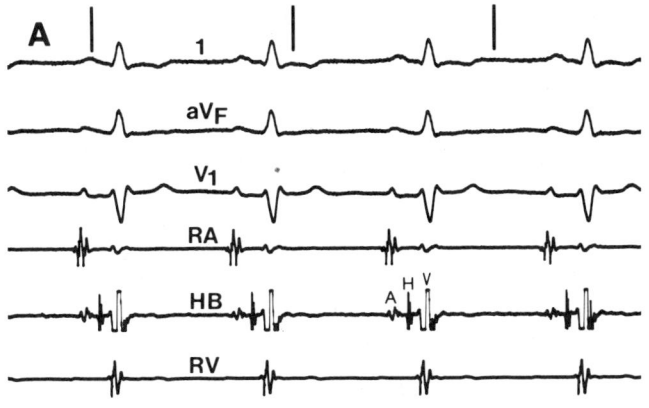

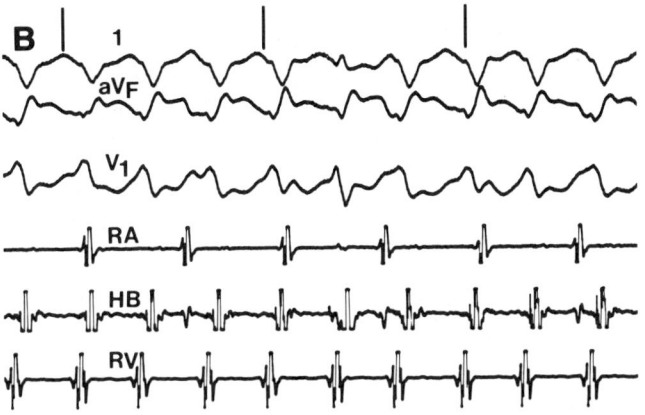

FIGURE 13–4

A, Sinus rhythm in a 41-year-old woman with idiopathic dilated cardiomyopathy and recurrent sustained ventricular tachycardia. Shown are standard leads 1, aV$_F$, V$_1$; and intracardiac recordings from the right atrium (RA), the area of the bundle of His (HB), and right ventricle (RV). The components of the HB recording are labeled as in Figure 13–3.

B, During ventricular tachycardia, atrioventricular dissociation is present. The sixth QRS complex results from fusion of ventricular activation between normal supraventricular activation (from the preceding P wave) and activation from ventricular tachycardia. Note that the sixth QRS complex is more narrow than the others and, in the HB lead, is preceded by a His bundle deflection.

clinical tachycardias at a later date by pacing. As sustained VT is rarely induced in patients without a history suggestive of spontaneous ventricular arrhythmias,[71] the ability to induce sustained VT in a patient with known or suspected ventricular arrhythmias is strongly suggestive that sustained VT has occurred spontaneously. When the QRS morphology of an induced VT is similar in all 12 leads to that of a spontaneous tachycardia, VT is nearly always the correct clinical diagnosis.

SIGNAL-AVERAGED ELECTROCARDIOGRAPHY

Signal-averaged ECG is a recently introduced technique that allows detection of low-amplitude components of the QRS complex by aligning and averaging several hundred complexes, thereby enhancing the signal-to-noise ratio. In most patients with a history of sustained VT, signal-averaged ECG performed during sinus rhythm reveals high-frequency (25–100 Hz), low amplitude signals at the terminus of the QRS complex.[56, 110] These signals, usually termed *late potentials*, are rarely present in normal subjects, but occasionally they are present in patients with heart disease without known or suspected VT.[111–113] Thus the finding of late potentials in a patient with suspected arrhythmias is suggestive, but not diagnostic, of sustained VT.

DIFFERENTIATION OF VT FROM SUPRAVENTRICULAR TACHYCARDIA (SVT) WITH ABERRANT CONDUCTION

Determining whether a wide QRS tachycardia is VT or SVT with aberrant conduction is a common clinical problem. Up to 40% of presenting episodes of sustained VT are misdiagnosed as SVT with aberrant conduction, and the clinical outcome in the misdiagnosed patients is often poor.[114] In many cases of wide QRS tachycardia, careful assessment of the history, physical examination, and 12-lead ECG will suggest the correct diagnosis. Often, however, invasive recordings are required for definitive diagnosis.

The single most useful finding to differentiate VT from aberrantly conducted SVT is atrioventricular dissociation. As noted above, second- or third-degree ventriculoatrial block is present in about two thirds of cases of VT, whereas such a pattern is rare in SVT. The ECG, physical examination, esophageal recordings, and electrophysiologic study may be used to determine the atrial-ventricular relationship.

When there is a one-to-one atrial-ventricular relationship, or when P waves are not discernible, the tachycardia may be either supraventricular or ventricular in origin. In such cases, Wellens et al.[108] have developed criteria to distinguish VT from SVT with aberrancy, based on features of the QRS during tachycardia (Fig. 13–5). A QRS duration >0.14 s is strongly suggestive of VT, whereas a QRS duration ≤0.14 s favors SVT (by about 3 to 1). Left axis deviation (less than −30 degrees) strongly favors VT (by about 10 to 1), whereas a normal QRS axis (between −30 and +90 degrees) favors SVT (by about 4 to 1). Findings of right axis deviation or an indeterminate axis were not helpful discriminators.

In ECGs showing a right bundle branch block QRS morphology, certain features of the QRS complexes in leads V$_1$ and V$_6$ were also found helpful by Wellens et al.[108] A monophasic (R) or biphasic (qR, QR, RS) complex in V$_1$ strongly favors VT. When a triphasic complex (RSR′) was present in V$_1$, an R′ > R strongly favors SVT, but an R > R′ favors VT (see Fig. 13–5). A triphasic QRS complex in V$_6$ strongly favors SVT, but a predominantly negative monophasic or biphasic complex favors VT.

In ECGs showing a left bundle branch block QRS morphology, features suggestive of VT are an R in V$_1$ with duration greater than 30 to 40 ms and a Q in V$_6$.[115, 116]

An important limitation of the Wellens criteria is

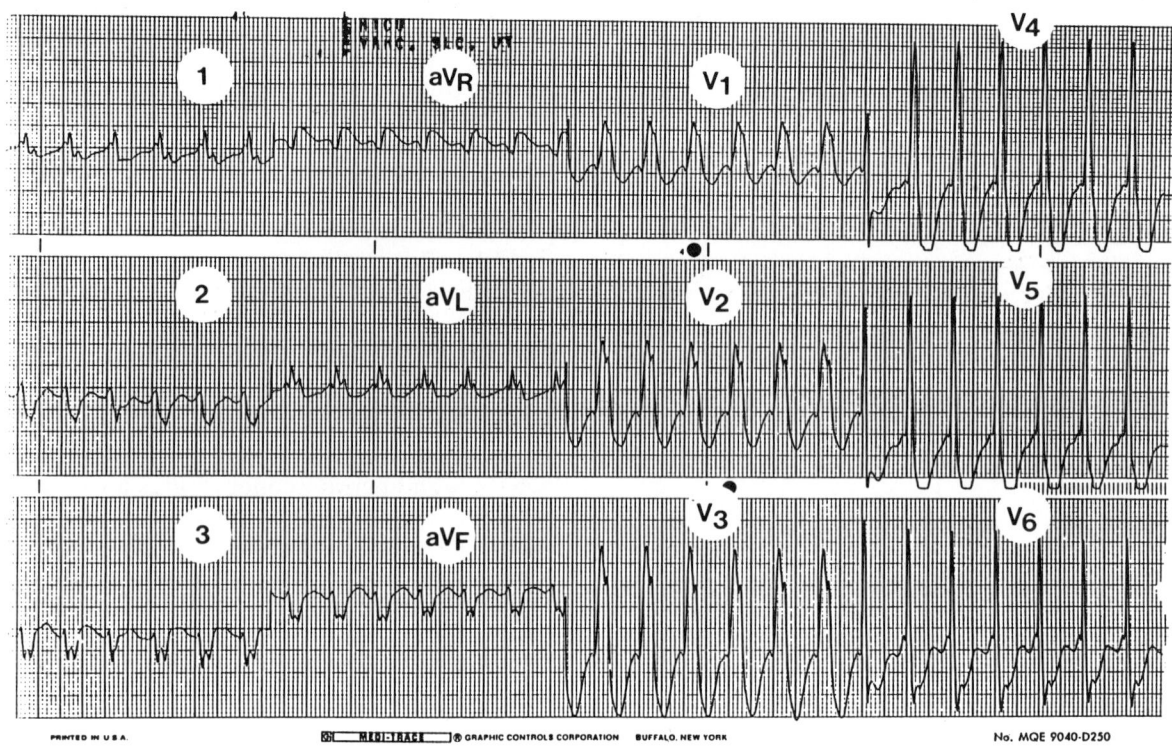

FIGURE 13–5
Standard 12-lead electrocardiogram showing a wide QRS tachycardia in a 60-year-old man with prior myocardial infarction but a normal QRS duration during sinus rhythm. Several features of the QRS morphology are suggestive that the rhythm is ventricular rather than supraventricular in origin: QRS duration greater than 140 ms, left axis deviation, and right bundle branch block morphology with the amplitude of R greater than the amplitude of R' in V_1. The diagnosis of ventricular tachycardia was subsequently confirmed by electrophysiologic studies. Note also the third QRS complex in lead 1 which, unlike the other QRS complexes, appears not to be followed by a P wave. This is also very suggestive of a ventricular origin of the tachycardia.

that they are not applicable to patients with prolonged QRS duration during sinus rhythm; therefore, caution is advised in applying these criteria in a patient presenting de novo with tachycardia, without an available ECG during sinus rhythm.

The clinical context often suggests the mechanism of a wide QRS complex tachycardia.[117] For instance, such a rhythm in a middle-aged man with a history of prior myocardial infarction and known left ventricular aneurysm is likely to be VT. Conversely, a wide QRS tachycardia in a younger patient without known structural heart disease, which terminates after Valsalva maneuvers, is more likely to be SVT with aberrant conduction. Often, however, the clinical context will be misleading, and it should never be used as the basis for a definitive diagnosis. A widespread misconception is that a wide QRS tachycardia that is hemodynamically well tolerated is likely to be supraventricular in origin.

The response of a tachycardia to medication is not a reliable means of differentiating VT from SVT. Furthermore, selecting the wrong medication may have hazardous consequences. For example, the use of intravenous verapamil in the setting of a well-tolerated wide QRS tachycardia of unknown mechanism often results in hypotension and the need for emergent cardioversion.[114, 118]

It is commonly stated that when a patient with a wide QRS tachycardia also displays isolated premature ventricular beats of similar morphology, the tachycardia is likely to be ventricular in origin.[119, 120] However, little documentation other than anecdote exists to support this statement, and a recent study suggests that VT and premature ventricular beats occurring in the same patient usually have different QRS morphologies.[121] It is possible that the coexistence of premature ventricular beats, regardless of their morphology, may favor the diagnosis of VT.

Therapy

TERMINATION OF SUSTAINED VT

The approach to the patient with sustained VT varies depending on the patient's toleration of the arrhythmia.

If at any time the patient loses consciousness, immediate institution of cardiopulmonary resuscitation and prompt electrical cardioversion are indicated. An initial synchronized shock of 100 to 200 joules is recommended; a shock of this energy will be effective in most patients, and shocks with energy less than 100 joules may be more likely to result in acceleration rather than in termination of the VT. If the initial shock is not effective, then repeat cardioversion using the maximum energy deliverable is indicated. Metabolic or electrolyte disorders and proarrhythmic drug toxicity should be suspected and corrected in patients with VT that repeatedly resists attempted cardioversion.

It is not infrequent for a patient to be in considerable physical distress from sustained VT and yet not to have lost consciousness. Prompt administration of a short-acting, general anesthetic (such as an intravenous benzodiazepine or a short-acting barbiturate) and then electrical cardioversion is indicated in such a patient. Electrical cardioversion of a conscious patient should be avoided.

Patients in whom sustained VT is well tolerated may be treated with medications or interventional pacing rather than electrical cardioversion. Usually, intravenously administered medications are used because of their more rapid onset of action. The antiarrhythmic medications appropriate for use in patients with sustained VT are lidocaine, procainamide, quinidine, and propranolol (and other beta-adrenergic antagonists). Loading doses of these medications should be used, followed by maintenance infusions if necessary. Magnesium sulfate is highly effective in terminating the torsade de pointes form of VT,[122] and occasionally it may also be effective in terminating monomorphic VT. Intravenously administered amiodarone, available only on an investigational basis, is effective in terminating VT in some patients. Bretylium and verapamil should only be administered with extreme caution to patients with well-tolerated VT, because their potent vasodilatory effects often result in profound hypotension.

Sustained VT often can be terminated with ventricular pacing. Generally, a temporary transvenous pacemaker is used with an external stimulator, but certain implantable pacing generators may be used to terminate VT. The same stimulation sequences that are utilized to terminate induced VT during electrophysiologic studies (such as one or more extrastimuli or burst pacing) may be used to terminate spontaneous VT. Portable stimulators capable of delivering critically timed extrastimuli and rapid bursts are available for bedside use. Also available are temporary pacing generators that can deliver burst pacing at rates up to 800 bpm. Conventional temporary pacing generators are limited to rates below 180 bpm and therefore are not suitable for termination of VT in most patients. The possibility of accelerating VT should be anticipated before pacing is performed, and a defibrillator should be immediately available in case an accelerated rhythm results in hemodynamic collapse. Pace termination of VT is sometimes facilitated by antiarrhythmic drugs and if not previously successful pacing may be tried after the addition of a drug.

LONG-TERM THERAPY FOR SUSTAINED VT

In most patients presenting with a first episode of sustained VT, it will be a recurring event, and long-term therapy will be required. However, in a minority of patients a reversible precipitating cause of the VT can be identified and corrected. Such precipitants include myocardial ischemia, infarction, hypokalemia, hypoxemia, acidosis, alkalosis, and drug toxicity (especially antiarrhythmic drugs).

Antiarrhythmic Drugs

Medications currently available for prevention of sustained VT are listed in Table 13-3. None is effective in all patients or even a majority of patients. Data on the efficacy rates of antiarrhythmic drugs for treatment of sustained VT are reported primarily in patients referred to tertiary centers (see below). This population is heavily weighted with drug-refractory patients, and therefore these data probably underestimate the efficacy of antiarrhythmic drugs in the general population of patients with sustained VT. Nevertheless, most patients need to be tested using more than one drug before an effective one is found. Despite considerable information on the electrophysiologic effects of these drugs, this information is not useful in determining which drug is likely to be effective in a given patient. The choice of drug to test in a given patient depends on (1) the patient's previous experience with the drug, (2) the pharmacokinetics of the drug and any abnormality of drug metabolism in the patient, and (3) the patient's predisposition to any potential side effect of the drug.

THE PATIENT WITH FREQUENTLY RECURRING VT

Patients with multiple daily recurrences of VT are managed in a coronary care or telemetry unit. Usually, drugs that can be administered intravenously are selected first, but drugs available only orally also may be used. Spontaneous VT may recur multiple times before an effective drug is identified; if the VT can be pace-terminated, then placement of a temporary pacing catheter may obviate the need for frequent cardioversions.

Generally, VT recurrence while the patient is re-

TABLE 13-3
Medications for Termination and Prevention of Sustained VT

Drug	Route of Administration
Lidocaine	Intravenous
Magnesium sulfate	Intravenous
Procainamide	Intravenous and oral
Quinidine	Intravenous and oral
Disopyramide	Oral
Tocainide	Oral
Mexiletine	Oral
Propranolol (and other beta-adrenergic antagonists)	Intravenous and oral
Verapamil	Oral*
Phenytoin	Intravenous and oral
Flecainide	Oral
Encainide	Oral
Imipramine	Oral
Amiodarone	Oral†

*An intravenous preparation is available, but it is not approved for therapy of sustained VT, and it should be used only with caution.
†An intravenous preparation is available for investigational use.

ceiving a maximally tolerated dose of a drug indicates drug inefficacy. Therapy with different drugs is tried until one is found that appears to have eliminated the VT. However, in many patients there is sufficient spontaneous variability in the frequency of episodes of VT that drug efficacy may be falsely suggested. Therefore, when practical it is prudent to discontinue an apparently effective drug under observation at least once to document return of the VT. If VT does not recur shortly after discontinuation of the drug, then one can be less certain of the drug's efficacy, and further evidence of drug efficacy should be sought (see below).

THE PATIENT WITH INFREQUENTLY RECURRING VT
The patient with infrequently recurring VT is a difficult management problem. VT may recur at intervals of weeks or longer, so that direct demonstration of a drug's efficacy in preventing recurrences will take at least as long. To hospitalize patients for this duration is impractical, but to discharge patients before confirming the efficacy of a drug subjects them to the risk of a catastrophic recurrence of VT. Even patients who have not had syncope or cardiac arrest from VT in the past are at risk of catastrophic consequences from subsequent episodes of VT, particularly if they are newly receiving a medication. Because of the difficulty in directly assessing medications in these patients, two indirect methods have been used.

The first method predicts the likelihood of efficacy by observation of the medication's effect on ventricular arrhythmias induced during electrophysiologic studies. Patients considered eligible for this method are those with reproducibly induced VT or ventricular fibrillation at an initial study when they were not receiving antiarrhythmic medications. Patients treated with drugs that render ventricular tachyarrhythmias noninducible during a subsequent electrophysiologic study have a much lower incidence of arrhythmia recurrence or sudden death (1-year actuarial incidence of 3–9%) than patients in whom no such drug can be identified (1-year actuarial incidence of 27–30%).[123, 124] There are several methodologic uncertainties and problems regarding this electrophysiologic method to assess drug efficacy. Obviously, patients with no inducible ventricular arrhythmias are not candidates for the electrophysiologic method. It is uncertain whether patients with inducible ventricular fibrillation or nonsustained VT should be assessed by serial electrophysiologic studies.[23, 125, 126] Among patients tested, there is often a disappointingly low fraction (30–38%) in whom any drug is predicted effective.[21, 22, 124] The precise number of nonstimulated beats induced that predict drug inefficacy is controversial.[127, 128] Finally, a drug may render an arrhythmia more difficult to induce or better tolerated, and there is uncertainty as to the prognostic significance of these.[129–132]

The second indirect method for predicting antiarrhythmic drug efficacy for therapy of sustained VT measures the extent of suppression of spontaneous and exercise-induced ventricular ectopy.[133] Candidates for this method are those in whom medication can be discontinued long enough to perform baseline 24-hour ambulatory monitoring. Data indicate that patients treated with medications that suppress frequent and complex ventricular ectopy are less likely to experience subsequent sudden cardiac death (1-year actuarial incidence of 5%) than patients in whom no such drug is used (1-year actuarial incidence of 42%).[133] As with the electrophysiologic method, however, there are methodologic uncertainties with ambulatory monitoring. Patients without frequent ectopy and those who cannot exercise are not candidates for this technique. Among patients with ectopy, there is a large degree of spontaneous variability in its frequency and complexity that may obscure or resemble drug effect; this has not been taken into consideration by some investigators.[133] Finally, criteria defining the desired end point of arrhythmia suppression during drug testing vary among investigators, with some requiring reduction of all forms of ventricular ectopy and others requiring elimination of only repetitive or closely coupled premature beats.[133–135]

Which method of drug assessment—electrophysiologic studies or ambulatory monitoring—is preferable? Patients who meet baseline criteria (e.g., inducible arrhythmias or sufficiently frequent ventricular ectopy) for only one method should be assessed using that method. Available data suggest that approximately 80% of patients with sustained ventricular arrhythmias completing 48 hours of ambulatory monitoring demonstrate at least 10 premature ventricular beats per hour.[136, 137] Similarly, about 80% of patients with sustained VT will have inducible sustained ventricular arrhythmias (see Table 13–2). Thus most patients will be eligible for either method. The only randomized study directly comparing the two methods in patients who qualify for both[135] suffers from small sample size.[138] A larger prospective, randomized, multicenter trial is under way in the United States.[139]

Surgery

Despite initial enthusiasm, coronary artery bypass graft surgery has not been demonstrated to be effective therapy for recurrent, sustained VT, except in the occasional patient in whom there is a clear causal relation between acute myocardial ischemia and sustained ventricular arrhythmias.[140, 141] Other surgical techniques with limited applicability and uncertain efficacy for prevention of sustained ventricular arrhythmias include cervicothoracic sympathectomy in patients with idiopathic long QT syndrome,[142] aortic valve replacement in patients with aortic stenosis,[143] mitral valve replacement in patients with mitral valve prolapse or obstructive hypertrophic cardiomyopathy,[144] and septal myotomy-myectomy in patients with obstructive hypertrophic cardiomyopathy.[145]

The most promising surgical techniques for recurrent VT are those that resect, devitalize, or isolate ventricular myocardium participating in the initiation or perpetuation of the VT. Historically, the first such surgical technique was left ventricular aneurysmectomy.[17] The success of simple aneurysmectomy depends on whether tissue necessary for perpetuation of the tachycardia is fortuitously removed. Without guidance by intraoperative recording of cardiac activation, aneurysmectomy is effective in only about 20 to 30% of patients.[146, 147] A second surgical technique, which also does not require intraoperative electrical recordings, is the encircling endocardial ventriculotomy.[148] The efficacy of this procedure appears comparable to that of more recently introduced techniques directed by intraoperative cardiac activation recordings,[149] but the extensive ventriculotomy frequently results in significant depression of left ventricular systolic function.[150, 151] A third surgical technique, also not requiring intraoperative electrical recordings, is resection of visually identified subendocardial scar; only limited data are available on the results of this technique.[152–154]

Most recently introduced surgical techniques for ablation of VT are directed by intraoperative recordings of cardiac activation. Generally, local activation time during VT is determined at a number of ventricular sites, a mechanism of the VT is surmized, and on that basis a limited resection (i.e., ventriculotomy, cryoablation, laser ablation, DC shock, or a combination of these) is performed.[57, 155–158]

In up to one third of patients, tachycardia cannot be reproducibly induced intraoperatively or its mechanism cannot be surmized.[57] In these patients, the operation can be guided by localization of abnormal electrograms during sinus rhythm[157] or by pace-mapping.[159] However, the ventricular sites implicated by these techniques frequently do not correlate with those implicated by the activation sequence during VT, and experience with these approaches is limited.[160]

Epicardial mapping is generally performed first, as it may suggest the mechanism of tachycardia, and the tachycardia may not be inducible following ventriculotomy.[57, 161] However, subendocardial tissue is more likely to be implicated in the tachycardia mechanism than subepicardial tissue, and endocardial mapping is desirable.[162] Multisite mapping systems with computer-assisted determinations of local activation time and activation sequence have recently been introduced.[163, 164] Novel endocardial mapping systems may obviate the need for ventriculotomy prior to endocardial mapping.[158, 165]

Operative mortality for activation sequence–guided VT surgery is 9 to 17%,[155, 161, 166] the most common causes being cardiogenic shock and arrhythmia recurrence. Surgical success, defined as prevention of induced and spontaneous VT by surgery alone, is reported in 60 to 70% of patients at mean follow-up of about 2 years.[155, 161, 166] In an additional 6 to 11% of patients, a drug ineffective at preventing VT induction preoperatively will be found to be so postoperatively.[161, 166]

Implantable Devices

Atrial or ventricular pacing at moderate rates (70–110 bpm) may prevent episodes of VT in selected patients, and in these patients implanted pacemakers may provide effective long-term prophylaxis of VT.[167–169] Most, but not all, of these are patients with VT arising as an escape rhythm following a bradyarrhythmia or with idiopathic long-QT syndrome complicated by torsade de pointes. Asynchronous ventricular underdrive pacing, initiated by magnet application to a conventional ventricular demand pacemaker, will terminate VT in occasional patients.

Several implantable pacemakers are capable of delivering bursts of rapid stimuli or critically timed extrastimuli, and these pacemakers can be used to terminate VT in selected patients.[169] In 1985, an implantable automatic cardioverter-defibrillator was approved for use in the United States.[170–171] (Antitachycardia pacemakers and the implantable automatic cardioverter-defibrillator are discussed in detail elsewhere in this volume.) Future implantable devices will be capable of both antitachycardia pacing and cardioversion-defibrillation. Until they are available, the combination of an automatic antitachycardia pacemaker and an automatic cardioverter-defibrillator may be used in some patients (Fig. 13–6).

When Not to Treat VT

Patients with structurally normal hearts and recurrent, slow, sustained VT may have a good prognosis. Therefore, if these patients have no symptoms or minimal symptoms from VT, then therapy, especially that which has major morbidity or side effects, may not be indicated.

The Economics of VT

Patients with sustained VT often require repeated, lengthy hospitalizations. The mean length of stay for serial antiarrhythmic drug testing and initiation of therapy at referral hospitals has been reported to be 20 to 33 days, with a mean hospital cost ranging from $7,000 to $14,000.[172, 173] These are much greater than the estimated average length of stay and reimbursement rate of the currently applicable Medicare diagnosis-related groups (DRGs), which are 3 to 10 days and $2,626 to $4,672, respectively.[174] Despite the fact that electrophysiologically guided therapy appears to result in fewer subsequent hospital days and charges than empirical therapy,[173] there is no DRG category for electrophysiologic studies that recognizes the expense and efficacy of the technique. The Health Care Financing Administration is currently considering separate DRG categories for electrophysiologic studies.

Perspectives

As recently as 1950, sustained VT was described as a rare condition.[10] The increased frequency of VT since then is a result of an epidemic of coronary heart disease and possibly the increased proportion of patients surviving acute myocardial infarction. Ultimately, VT will be most effectively controlled by prevention of coronary artery disease, cardiomyopathy, and other cardiac diseases that predispose to VT.

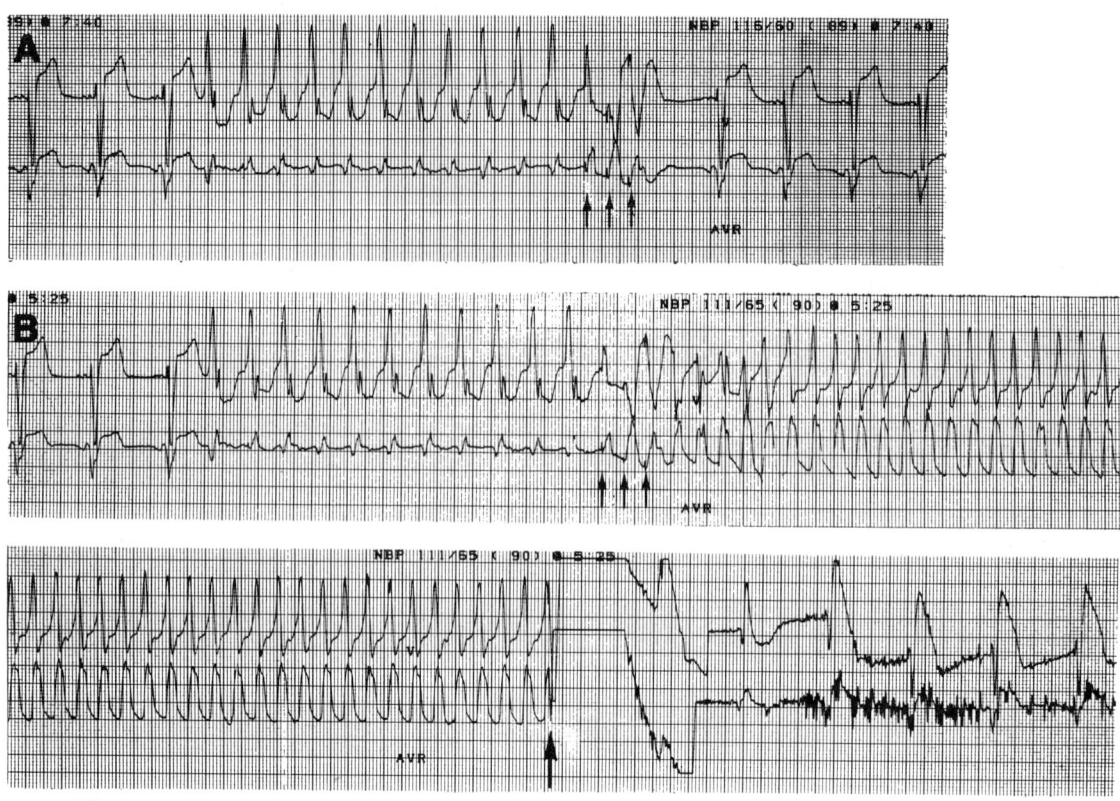

FIGURE 13–6
Tracings from a 64-year-old man with frequent sustained ventricular tachycardia, who received an implanted automatic antitachycardia ventricular pacemaker and an implanted automatic cardioverter-defibrillator. The pacemaker is programmed to detect tachycardia faster than 140 bpm, and the cardioverter-defibrillator is designed to detect tachycardia faster than 175 bpm.
A, Spontaneous ventricular tachycardia (rate 157 bpm) is terminated with three premature paced ventricular beats (arrows) automatically delivered by the antitachycardia pacemaker. Approximately 200 such terminations were documented during a 1-week period.
B, Identical spontaneous ventricular tachycardia accelerated to 240 bpm by three premature paced ventricular beats (arrows) from the antitachycardia pacemaker. The coupling intervals of these paced beats is identical to those that terminated tachycardia in *A*. The faster tachycardia is automatically sensed and terminated by a discharge (large arrow) from the cardioverter-defibrillator.

Some recent advances in therapy, such as surgical ablation, have paralleled advances in our understanding of the mechanism of VT. However, major deficiencies remain in our understanding of the mechanism of VT. The possible roles of anisotropy of conduction velocity, dispersion of refractoriness, the Purkinje-ventricular junction, and mechanically mediated changes in cellular electrophysiology require further investigation. Furthermore, despite our increased knowledge of the cellular effects of the various antiarrhythmic drugs, initial selection of an antiarrhythmic drug for a given patient is largely arbitrary. In the future, the particular combination of local conduction slowing and refractoriness that permits reentry may be defined in each patient, and a drug that modifies these so as to prevent reentry may be rationally selected.

Other improvements in therapy, such as implantable devices, have been made possible by technologic advances. The success of other emerging therapies—transcatheter endocardial ablation, subselective intracoronary infusion of ablative substances, and continuous ambulatory drug infusion, to name a few—may also depend on technologic innovations.

Apart from therapy, a major challenge remains to identify the patient at high risk for a first episode of sustained VT. Electrophysiologic studies, signal-averaged ECG, and ambulatory ECG monitoring have all shown promise in identifying patients at risk for VT after acute myocardial infarction.[175, 176] Other diagnostic tools, such as those involving body-surface ECG mapping techniques, show promise.[177] Much work remains in identifying high-risk subsets among other patients, such as those with idiopathic cardiomyopathy, heart failure, left ventricular hypertrophy, and mitral valve prolapse.

Acknowledgment

The expert secretarial assistance of Ms Karen Allen is appreciated.

References

1. Lewis T: Single and successive extrasystoles. Lancet 1:382, 1909.

2. Hart TS: Paroxysmal tachycardia. Heart 4:128, 1912.
3. Willins FA: Paroxysmal tachycardia of ventricular origin. Boston Med Surg J 178:40, 1918.
4. Gallavardin L: Tachycardie ventriculaire terminale. Arch Mol Cover 13:153, 1920.
5. Gallavardin L: Extra-systolie ventriculaire. Arch Mol Cover 15:298, 1922.
6. Strauss MB: Paroxysmal ventricular tachycardia. Am J Med Sci 179:337, 1930.
7. Cooke WT, White PD: Paroxysmal ventricular tachycardia. Br Heart J 5:33, 1943.
8. Williams C, Ellis LB: Ventricular tachycardia. Arch Intern Med 71:137, 1943.
9. Herrmann GR, Hejtmancik MR: A clinical and electrocardiographic study of paroxysmal ventricular tachycardia and its management. Ann Intern Med 28:989, 1947.
10. Armbrust CA, Levine SA: Paroxysmal ventricular tachycardia: A study of one hundred and seven cases. Circulation 1:28, 1950.
11. Herrmann GR, Park HM, Hejtmancik MR: Paroxysmal ventricular tachycardia: A clinical electrocardiographic study. Am Heart J 57:166, 1958.
12. Scott RW: Observations on a case of ventricular tachycardia with retrograde conduction. Heart 9:297, 1921.
13. Mark LC, Berlin I, Kayden HJ: The action of procaine amide (N^1-[2-diethylaminoethyl]-p-aminobenzamide) on ventricular arrhythmias. J Pharm Exper Therap 98:21, 1950.
14. Moe GK, Abildskov JA: Antiarrhythmic drugs. In Goodman LS, Gilman A (eds.): The Pharmacological Basis of Therapeutics (ed 5), pp. 683–704. New York, Macmillan Publishing Co., Inc., 1975.
15. Zoll PM, Linenthal AJ, Zarsky LRN: Ventricular fibrillation: Treatment and prevention by external electric currents. N Engl J Med 262:105, 1960.
16. Sowton E, Leatham A, Carson P: The suppression of arrhythmias by artificial pacemaking. Lancet 1098, 1964.
17. Couch OA: Cardiac aneurysm with ventricular tachycardia and subsequent excision of aneurysm. Circulation 20:251, 1959.
18. Wellens HJ, Schuilenburg RM: Electrical stimulation of the heart in patients with ventricular tachycardia. Circulation 46:216, 1972.
19. Lie KI, Wellens HJJ, Downar E, et al.: Observations on patients with primary ventricular fibrillation complicating acute myocardial infarction. Circulation 52:755, 1975.
20. Adgey AAJ, Allen JD, Geddes JS, et al.: Acute phase of myocardial infarction. Lancet 501, 1971.
21. Spielman SR, Schwartz JS, McCarthy DM, et al.: Predictors of the success or failure of medical therapy in patients with chronic recurrent sustained ventricular tachycardia: A discriminant analysis. J Am Coll Cardiol 1:401, 1983.
22. Swerdlow CD, Gong G, Echt DS, et al.: Clinical factors predicting successful electrophysiologic-pharmacologic study in patients with ventricular tachycardia. J Am Coll Cardiol 1:409, 1983.
23. Freedman RA, Swerdlow CD, Soderholm-Difatte V, et al.: Prognostic significance of arrhythmia inducibility or noninducibility at initial electrophysiologic study in survivors of cardiac arrest. Am J Cardiol 61:578, 1988.
24. Kiat H, Richards D, Ross D, et al.: Prediction of late sustained ventricular tachyarrhythmias after myocardial infarction. J Am Coll Cardiol 7:67A, 1986.
25. Bolick DR, Hackel DB, Reimer KA, et al.: Quantitative analysis of myocardial infarct structure in patients with ventricular tachycardia. Circulation 74:1266, 1986.
26. Fenoglio JJ, Pham TD, Harken AH, et al.: Recurrent sustained ventricular tachycardia: Structure and ultrastructure of subendocardial regions in which tachycardia originates. Circulation 68:518, 1983.
27. Mendoza I, Camardo J, Moleiro F, et al.: Sustained ventricular tachycardia in chronic chagasic myocarditis: Electrophysiologic and pharmacologic characteristics. Am J Cardiol 57:423, 1986.
28. Wu D, Kou HC, Hung JS: Exercise-triggered paroxysmal ventricular tachycardia. Ann Intern Med 95:410, 1981.
29. Palileo EV, Ashley WW, Swiryn S, et al.: Exercise provocable right ventricular outflow tract tachycardia. Am Heart J 104:185, 1982.
30. Sung RJ, Shen EN, Morady F, et al.: Electrophysiologic mechanism of exercise-induced sustained ventricular tachycardia. Am J Cardiol 51:525, 1983.
31. Velebit V, Podrid P, Lown B, et al.: Aggravation and provocation of ventricular arrhythmias by antiarrhythmic drugs. Circulation 65:886, 1982.
32. Keren A, Tzivoni D, Gavish D, et al.: Etiology, warning signs and therapy of torsade de pointes. Circulation 64:1167, 1981.
33. Burket MW, Fraker TD, Temesy-Armos PN: Polymorphous ventricular tachycardia provoked by lidocaine. Am J Cardiol 55:592, 1985.
34. Winkle RA, Mason JW, Griffin JC, et al.: Malignant ventricular tachyarrhythmias associated with the use of encainide. Am Heart J 102:857, 1981.
35. Morganroth J, Anderson JL, Gentzkow GD: Classification by type of ventricular arrhythmia predicts frequency of adverse cardiac events from flecainide. J Am Coll Cardiol 8:607, 1986.
36. Anastasiou-Nana MI, Anderson JL, Stewert JR, et al.: Exercise-induced ventricular tachycardia as a proarrhythmic effect of flecainide. Circulation 72:III, 1985.
37. Morris SN, Zipes DP: His bundle electrocardiography during bidirectional tachycardia. Circulation 46:32, 1973.
38. Marshall JB, Forker AD: Cardiovascular effects of tricyclic antidepressant drugs: Therapeutic usage, overdose, and management of complications. Am Heart J 103:401, 1982.
39. Crane GE: Cardiac toxicity and psychotropic drugs. Diseases Nervous System 31:534, 1970.
40. Fowler NO, McCall D, Chon TC, et al.: Electrocardiographic changes and cardiac arrhythmias in patients receiving psychotropic drugs. Am J Cardiol 37:223, 1976.
41. Whelton PK, Watson AJ: Diuretic-induced hypokalemia and cardiac arrhythmias. Am J Cardiol 58:5A, 1986.
42. Steiness E, Olesen KH: Cardiac arrhythmias induced by hypokalaemia and potassium loss during maintenance digoxin therapy. Br Heart J 38:167, 1976.
43. Multiple Risk Factor Intervention Trial Research Group: Baseline rest electrocardiographic abnormalities, antihypertensive treatment, and mortality in the multiple risk factor intervention trial. Am J Cardiol 55:1, 1985.
44. Salerno DM, Asinger RW, Elsperger J: Frequency of hypokalemia after successfully resuscitating out-of-hospital cardiac arrest compared with that in transmural acute myocardial infarction. Am J Cardiol 59:84, 1987.
45. Sung RJ, Shapiro WA, Shen EN, et al.: Effects of verapamil on ventricular tachycardias possibly caused by reentry, automaticity, and triggered activity. J Clin Invest 72:350, 1983.
46. Zipes DP, Foster PR, Troup PJ, et al.: Atrial induction of ventricular tachycardia: Reentry versus triggered automaticity. Am J Cardiol 44:1, 1979.
47. Wellens HJJ, Brugada P, Vanagt EJDM, et al.: New studies with triggered automaticity. In Harrison DC (ed.): Cardiac Arrhythmias: a decade of progress, pp. 601–610. Boston, G. K. Hall Medical Publishers, 1981.
48. Belhassen B, Rotmensch HH, Laniado S: Response of recurrent sustained ventricular tachycardia to verapamil. Br Heart J 46:679, 1981.
49. Wu D, Kou H, Hung J: Exercise-triggered paroxysmal ventricular tachycardia. Ann Intern Med 95:410, 1981.
50. Woelfel A, Foster JR, McAllister RG, et al.: Efficacy of verapamil in exercise-induced ventricular tachycardia. Am J Cardiol 56:292, 1985.
51. Lin FC, Finley D, Rahimtoola SH, et al.: Idiopathic paroxysmal ventricular tachycardia with a QRS pattern of right bundle branch block and left axis deviation: A unique clinical entity with specific properties. Am J Cardiol 52:95, 1983.
52. Ohe T, Shimomura K, Aihara N, et al.: Idiopathic sustained left ventricular tachycardia: Clinical and electrophysiologic characteristics. Circulation 77:560, 1988.
53. Lerman BB, Belardinelli L, West GA, et al.: Adenosine-sensitive ventricular tachycardia: Evidence suggesting cyclic AMP-mediated triggered activity. Circulation 74:270, 1986.
54. Rosen MR, Wit AL, Hoffman BF: Electrophysiology and pharmacology of cardiac arrhythmias. IV. Cardiac antiarrhythmic and toxic effects of digitalis. Am Heart J 89:391, 1975.
55. Cranefield PF: Action potentials, afterpotentials, and arrhythmias. Circ Res 41:415, 1977.

56. Wellens HJJ, Duren DR, Lie KI: Observations on mechanisms of ventricular tachycardia in man. Circulation 54:237, 1976.
57. Cassidy DM, Vassallo JA, Miller JM, et al.: Endocardial catheter mapping in patients in sinus rhythm: Relationship to underlying heart disease and ventricular arrhythmias. Circulation 73:645, 1986.
58. Freedman RA, Gillis AM, Keren A, et al.: Signal-averaged electrocardiographic late potentials in patients with ventricular fibrillation or ventricular tachycardia: Correlation with clinical arrhythmia and electrophysiologic study. Am J Cardiol 55:1350, 1985.
59. Mason JW, Stinson EB, Oyer PE, et al.: The mechanisms of ventricular tachycardia in humans determined by intraoperative recording of the electrical activation sequence. Int J Cardiol 8:163, 1985.
60. Downar E, Harris L, Mickleborough LL, et al.: Endocardial mapping of ventricular tachycardia in the intact human ventricle: Evidence for reentrant mechanisms. J Am Coll Cardiol 11:783, 1988.
61. Josephson ME, Horowitz LN, Farshidi A, et al.: Sustained ventricular tachycardia: Evidence for protected localized reentry. Am J Cardiol 42:416, 1978.
62. Wellens HJJ, Farre J, Brugada P, et al.: The method of programmed stimulation in the study of ventricular tachycardia. In Josephson ME (ed.): Ventricular Tachycardia Mechanisms and Management, pp. 237–283. New York, Futura Publishing Co., 1982.
63. Wellens HJJ, Lie KI, Durrer D: Further observations on ventricular tachycardia as studied by electrical stimulation of the heart. Circulation 49:647, 1974.
64. Janse MJ, van Capelle FJL, Morsink H, et al.: Flow of "injury current" and patterns of excitation during early ventricular arrhythmias in acute regional myocardial ischemia in isolated porcine and canine hearts: Evidence for 2 different arrhythmogenic mechanisms. Circ Res 47:151, 1980.
65. Gettes LS, Hill JL, Saito T, et al.: Factors related to vulnerability to arrhythmias in acute myocardial infarction. Am Heart J 103:667, 1982.
66. Harris AS: Delayed development of ventricular ectopic rhythms following experimental coronary occlusion. Circulation 1:1318, 1950.
67. Lazzara R, El-Sherif N, Scherlag BJ: Electrophysiologic properties of canine purkinje cells in one-day-old myocardial infarction. Circ Res 33:722, 1973.
68. El-Sherif N, Gough WB, Zeiler RH, et al.: Triggered ventricular rhythms in 1-day-old myocardial infarction in the dog. Circ Res 52:566, 1983.
69. Marec HL, Dangman KH, Danilo P, et al.: An evaluation of automaticity and triggered activity in the canine heart one to four days after myocardial infarction. Circulation 71:1224, 1985.
70. Mason JW, Anderson KP, Freedman RA: Techniques and criteria in electrophysiologic study of ventricular tachycardia. Circulation 75:III125, 1987.
71. Brugada P, Green M, Abdollah H, et al.: Significance of ventricular arrhythmias initiated by programmed ventricular stimulation: The importance of the type of ventricular arrhythmia induced and the number of premature stimuli required. Circulation 69:87, 1984.
72. Morady F, DiCarlo L, Winston S, et al.: A prospective comparison of triple extrastimuli and left ventricular stimulation in studies of ventricular tachycardia induction. Circulation 70:52, 1984.
73. Herre JM, Mann DE, Luck JC, et al.: Effect of increased current, multiple pacing sites and number of extrastimuli on induction of ventricular tachycardia. Am J Cardiol 57:102, 1986.
74. Kennedy EE, Rosenfeld LE, McPherson CA, et al.: Mechanisms and relevance of arrhythmias induced by high-current programmed ventricular stimulation. Am J Cardiol 57:598, 1986.
75. Morady F, DiCarlo LA, Baerman JM, et al.: Comparison of coupling intervals that induce clinical and nonclinical forms of ventricular tachycardia during programmed stimulation. Am J Cardiol 57:1269, 1986.
76. Echt D, Swerdlow C, Anderson K, et al.: Value of adding extrastimuli vs shortening drive cycle length in ventricular induction. PACE 6:A141, 1983.
77. Buxton AE, Waxman HL, Marchlinski FE, et al.: Role of triple extrastimuli during electrophysiologic study of patients with documented sustained ventricular tachyarrhythmias. Circulation 69:532, 1984.
78. Brugada P, Wellens HJJ: Comparison in the same patient of two programmed ventricular stimulation protocols to induce ventricular tachycardia. Am J Cardiol 55:380, 1985.
79. Schoenfeld MH, McGovern B, Garan H, et al.: Determinants of the outcome of electrophysiologic study in patients with ventricular tachyarrhythmias. J Am Coll Cardiol 6:298, 1985.
80. Doherty JU, Kienzle MG, Waxman HL, et al.: Programmed ventricular stimulation at a second right ventricular site: An analysis of 100 patients, with special reference to sensitivity, specificity and characteristics of patients with induced ventricular tachycardia. Am J Cardiol 52:1184, 1983.
81. Robertson JF, Cain ME, Horowitz LN, et al.: Anatomic and electrophysiologic correlates of ventricular tachycardia requiring left ventricular stimulation. Am J Cardiol 48:263, 1981.
82. Freedman RA, Swerdlow CD, Echt DS, et al.: Facilitation of ventricular tachyarrhythmia induction by isoproterenol. Am J Cardiol 54:765, 1984.
83. Charos GS, Haffajee CI, Gold RL, et al.: A theoretically and practically more effective method for interruption of ventricular tachycardia: Self-adapting autodecremental overdrive pacing. Circulation 73:309, 1986.
84. Mason JW, Swerdlow CD, Winkle RA, et al.: Ventricular tachyarrhythmia induction for drug selection: Experience with 311 patients. In Lucchesi BR, Dingell JV, Schwarz RP (eds.): Clinical Pharmacology of Antiarrhythmic Therapy, pp. 229–239. New York, Raven Press, 1984.
85. Horowitz LN, Kay HR, Kutalek SP, et al.: Risks and complications of clinical cardiac electrophysiologic studies: A prospective analysis of 1,000 consecutive patients. J Am Coll Cardiol 9:1261, 1987.
86. Almendral JM, Stamato NJ, Rosenthal ME, et al.: Resetting response patterns during sustained ventricular tachycardia: Relationship to the excitable gap. Circulation 74:722, 1986.
87. MacLean WAH, Plumb VJ, Waldo AL: Transient entrainment and interruption of ventricular tachycardia. PACE 4:358, 1981.
88. Anderson KP, Swerdlow CD, Mason JW: Entrainment of ventricular tachycardia. Am J Cardiol 53:335, 1984.
89. Mann DE, Lawrie GM, Luck JC, et al.: Importance of pacing site in entrainment of ventricular tachycardia. J Am Coll Cardiol 5:781, 1985.
90. Josephson ME, Horowitz LN, Farshidi A: Continuous local electrical activity. Circulation 57:659, 1978.
91. Brugada P, Abdollah H, Wellens HJJ: Continuous electrical activity during sustained monomorphic ventricular tachycardia. Am J Cardiol 55:402, 1985.
92. Dimarco JP, Garan H, Ruskin JN: Complications in patients undergoing cardiac electrophysiologic procedures. Ann Intern Med 97:490, 1982.
93. Wilber DJ, Davis MJ, Rosenbaum M, et al.: Incidence and determinants of multiple morphologically distinct sustained ventricular tachycardias. J Am Coll Cardiol 10:583, 1987.
94. Kapoor WN, Karpf M, Wieand S, et al.: A prospective evaluation and follow-up of patients with syncope. N Engl J Med 309:197, 1983.
95. DiMarco JP, Garan H, Harthorne JW, et al.: Intracardiac electrophysiologic techniques in recurrent syncope of unknown cause. Ann Intern Med 95:542, 1981.
96. Hess DS, Morady F, Scheinman MM: Electrophysiologic testing in the evaluation of patients with syncope of undetermined origin. Am J Cardiol 50:1309, 1982.
97. Morady F, Shen E, Schwartz A, et al.: Long-term follow-up of patients with recurrent unexplained syncope evaluated by electrophysiologic testing. J Am Coll Cardiol 2:1053, 1983.
98. Doherty JU, Pembrook-Rogers D, Grogan EW, et al.: Electrophysiologic evaluation of patients with recurrent unexplained syncope and presyncope. Am J Cardiol 55:703, 1985.
99. Krol RB, Morady F, Flaker GC, et al.: Electrophysiologic testing in patients with unexplained syncope: Clinical and noninvasive predictors of outcome. J Am Coll Cardiol 10:358, 1987.
100. Prystowsky EN, Klein GJ, Naccarelli GV, et al.: Electrophysiologic study in patients with syncope and normal resting electrocardiograms. Clin Res 29:697A, 1981.

101. Nikolic G, Bishop RL, Singh JB: Sudden death recorded during holter monitoring. Circulation 66:218, 1982.
102. Pratt CM, Francis MJ, Luck JC, et al.: Analysis of ambulatory electrocardiograms in 15 patients during spontaneous ventricular fibrillation with special reference to preceding arrhythmic events. J Am Coll Cardiol 2:789, 1983.
103. Panidis JP, Morganroth J: Sudden death in hospitalized patients: Cardiac rhythm disturbances detected by ambulatory electrocardiographic monitoring. J Am Coll Cardiol 2:798, 1983.
104. Roy D, Waxman HL, Kienzle MG, et al.: Clinical characteristics and long-term follow-up in 119 survivors of cardiac arrest: Relation to inducibility at electrophysiologic testing. Am J Cardiol 52:969, 1983.
105. Morady F, Scheinman MM, Hess DS, et al.: Electrophysiologic testing in the management of survivors of out-of-hospital cardiac arrest. Am J Cardiol 51:85, 1983.
106. Swerdlow CD, Bardy GH, McAnulty J, et al.: Determinants of induced sustained arrhythmias in survivors of out-of-hospital ventricular fibrillation. Circulation 76:1053, 1987.
107. Eldar M, Sauve MJ, Scheinman MM: Electrophysiologic testing and follow-up of patients with aborted sudden death. J Am Coll Cardiol 10:291, 1987.
108. Wellens HJJ, Bar FWHM, Lie KI: The value of the electrocardiogram in the differential diagnosis of tachycardia with a widened QRS complex. Am J Med 64:27, 1978.
109. Schnittger I, Rodriguez IM, Winkle RA: Esophageal electrocardiography: A new technology revives an old technique. Am J Cardiol 57:604, 1986.
110. Simson MB: Use of signals in the terminal QRS complex to identify patients with ventricular tachycardia after myocardial infarction. Circulation 64:235, 1981.
111. Breithardt G, Borggrefe M, Quantius B, et al.: Ventricular vulnerability assessed by programmed ventricular stimulation in patients with and without late potentials. Circulation 68:275, 1983.
112. Buckingham TA, Ghosh S, Homan SM, et al.: Independent value of signal-averaged electrocardiography and left ventricular function in identifying patients with sustained ventricular tachycardia with coronary artery disease. Am J Cardiol 59:568, 1987.
113. Gomes JA, Winters SL, Stewart D, et al.: Optimal bandpass filters for time-domain analysis of the signal-averaged electrocardiogram. Am J Cardiol 60:1290, 1987.
114. Stewart RB, Bardy GH, Greene HL: Wide complex tachycardia: Misdiagnosis and outcome after emergent therapy. Ann Intern Med 104:766, 1986.
115. Wellens HJJ, Bar FW, Vanagt EJ, et al.: The differentiation between ventricular tachycardia and supraventricular tachycardia with aberrant conduction: The value of the 12-lead electrocardiogram. In Wellens HJ, Kulbertus HE (eds.): What's New in Electrocardiography, pp. 184–199. Boston, Martinus Nijhoff, 1981.
116. Kindwall KE, Brown J, Josephson ME: Electrocardiographic criteria for ventricular tachycardia in wide complex left bundle branch block morphology tachycardias. Am J Cardiol 61:1279, 1988.
117. Tchou P, Young P, Mahmud R, et al.: Useful clinical criteria for the diagnosis of ventricular tachycardia. Am J Med 84:53, 1988.
118. Buxton EB, Marchlinski FE, Doherty JU, et al.: Hazards of intravenous verapamil for sustained ventricular tachycardia. Am J Cardiol 59:1107, 1987.
119. Marriott HJL: Practical Electrocardiography (ed. 6), p. 183. Baltimore, Williams & Wilkins Co., 1972.
120. Chou TC: Electrocardiography in Clinical Practice (ed. 2), p. 454. Orlando, Grune & Stratton, Inc., 1986.
121. Anderson KP, Lux RL, Nussbaum JA, et al.: Dissimilarity in morphology of premature ventricular complexes and ventricular tachycardia. Circulation 74:II, 1986.
122. Tzivoni D, Banai S, Schuger C, et al.: Treatment of torsade de pointes with magnesium sulfate. Circulation 77:392, 1988.
123. Swerdlow CD, Winkle RA, Mason JW: Determinants of survival in patients with ventricular tachyarrhythmias. N Engl J Med 308:1436, 1983.
124. Rae AP, Greenspan AM, Spielman SR, et al.: Antiarrhythmic drug efficacy for ventricular tachyarrhythmias associated with coronary artery disease as assessed by electrophysiologic studies. Am J Cardiol 55:1494, 1985.
125. Wellens HJJ, Brugada P, Stevenson WG: Programmed electrical stimulation of the heart in patients with life-threatening ventricular arrhythmias: What is the significance of induced arrhythmias and what is the correct stimulation protocol? Circulation 72:1, 1985.
126. Podrid PJ, Schoeneberger A, Lown B, et al.: Use of nonsustained ventricular tachycardia as a guide to antiarrhythmic drug therapy in patients with malignant ventricular arrhythmia. Am Heart J 105:181, 1983.
127. Swerdlow CD, Winkle RA, Mason JW: Prognostic significance of the number of induced ventricular complexes during assessment of therapy for ventricular tachyarrhythmias. Circulation 68:400, 1983.
128. Platia EV, Reid PR: Nonsustained ventricular tachycardia during programmed ventricular stimulation: Criteria for a positive test. Am J Cardiol 56:79, 1985.
129. Swerdlow CD, Blum J, Winkle RA, et al.: Decreased incidence of antiarrhythmic drug efficacy at electrophysiologic study associated with the use of a third extrastimulus. Am Heart J 104:1004, 1982.
130. Waller TJ, Kay HR, Spielman SR, et al.: Reduction in sudden death and total mortality by antiarrhythmic therapy evaluated by electrophysiologic drug testing: Criteria of efficacy in patients with sustained ventricular tachyarrhythmia. J Am Coll Cardiol 10:83, 1987.
131. Kadish AH, Buxton AE, Waxman HL, et al.: Usefulness of electrophysiologic study to determine the clinical tolerance of arrhythmia recurrences during amiodarone therapy. J Am Coll Cardiol 10:90, 1987.
132. Zhu J, Haines DE, Lerman BB, et al.: Predictors of efficacy of amiodarone and characteristics of arrhythmia patients with sustained ventricular tachycardia and coronary artery disease. Circulation 76:802, 1987.
133. Graboys TB, Lown B, Podrid PJ, et al.: Long-term survival of patients with malignant ventricular arrhythmia treated with antiarrhythmic drugs. Am J Cardiol 50:437, 1982.
134. Kim SG, Seiden SW, Felder DS, et al.: Is programmed stimulation of value in predicting the long-term success of antiarrhythmic therapy for ventricular tachycardia? N Engl J Med 315:356, 1986.
135. Mitchell LB, Duff HJ, Manyari DE, et al.: A randomized clinical trial of the noninvasive and invasive approaches to drug therapy of ventricular tachycardia. N Engl J Med 317:1681, 1987.
136. Swerdlow CD, Peterson J: Prospective comparison of Holter monitoring and electrophysiologic study in patients with coronary artery disease and sustained ventricular tachyarrhythmias. Am J Cardiol 56:577, 1985.
137. Kim SG, Katz G, Mercando AD, et al.: Qualification rates of various Holter monitoring criteria in patients with ventricular tachycardias. J Am Coll Cardiol 9:97A, 1987.
138. Mason JW: Treatment of ventricular tachycardia (letter to the editor). N Engl J Med 318:1693, 1988.
139. The ESVEM Investigators: The ESVEM Trial: Electrophysiologic study versus electrocardiographic monitoring for selection of antiarrhythmic therapy of ventricular tachyarrhythmias. Circulation 79:1354, 1989.
140. Bryson AL, Parisi AF, Schechter E, et al.: Life-threatening ventricular arrhythmia induced by exercise. Am J Cardiol 32:995, 1973.
141. Nordstom LA, Lillehei JP, Adicoff A, et al.: Coronary artery surgery for recurrent ventricular arrhythmias in patients with variant angina. Am Heart J 89:236, 1975.
142. Bhandari AK, Scheinman MM, Morady F, et al.: Efficacy of left cardiac sympathectomy in the treatment of patients with the long QT syndrome. Circulation 70:1018, 1984.
143. Schwarz F, Baumann P, Manthey J, et al.: The effect of aortic valve replacement on survival. Circulation 66:1105, 1982.
144. Ross A, DeWeese JA, Yu PN: Refractory ventricular arrhythmias in a patient with mitral valve prolapse. Successful control with mitral valve replacement. J Electrocardiol 11:289, 1978.
145. Beahrs MM, Tajik AJ, Sweard JB, et al.: Hypertrophic obstructive cardiomyopathy: Ten- to 21-year follow-up after partial septal myectomy. Am J Cardiol 51:1160, 1983.

146. Harken AH, Horowitz LN, Josephson ME, et al.: Comparison of standard aneurysmectomy and aneurysmectomy with direct endocardial resection for the treatment of recurrent sustained ventricular tachycardia. J Thorac Cardiovasc Surg 80:527, 1980.
147. Mason JW, Stinson EB, Winkle RA, et al.: Surgery for ventricular tachycardia: Efficacy of left ventricular aneurysm resection compared with operation guided by electrical activation mapping. Circulation 65:1148, 1982.
148. Guiraudon G, Fontaine G, Frank R, et al.: Encircling endocardial ventriculotomy: A new surgical treatment for life-threatening ventricular tachycardias resistant to medical treatment following myocardial infarction. Ann Thorac Surg 26:438, 1978.
149. Anderson KP, Mason JW: Surgical management of ventricular tachyarrhythmias. Clin Cardiol 6:415, 1983.
150. Waldo AL, Arciniegas JG, Klein H: Surgical treatment of life-threatening ventricular arrhythmias: The role of intraoperative mapping and consideration of the presently available surgical techniques. Prog Cardiovasc Dis 23:247, 1981.
151. Cox JL, Gallagher JJ, Ungerleider RM: Encircling endocardial ventriculotomy for refractory ischemic ventricular tachycardia. J Thorac Cardiovasc Surg 83:865, 1982.
152. Kehoe R, Zheutlin T, Finkelmeier B, et al.: Visually directed endocardial resection for ventricular arrhythmia: long term outcome and functional status. J Am Coll Cardiol 5:497, 1985.
153. Ruffy R, Connors JP, Sandza JG, et al.: Successful treatment of high-risk patients with non-guided surgery, supported by electrophysiologic testing and drug therapy. Circulation 72:III-220, 1985.
154. Gardner MJ, Landymore RW, Johnstone DE, et al.: Visually-directed endocardial resection for recurrent ventricular tachycardia: Long-term results and effect on LV function. Circulation 72:III-221, 1985.
155. Miller JM, Kienzle MG, Harken AH, et al.: Subendocardial resection for ventricular tachycardia: predictors of surgical success. Circulation 70:624, 1984.
156. Camm J, Ward DE, Spurrell RAJ, et al.: Cryothermal mapping and cryoablation in the treatment of refractory cardiac arrhythmias. Circulation 62:67, 1980.
157. Svenson RH, Gallagher JJ, Selle JG, et al.: Neodymium: YAG laser photocoagulation: A successful new map-guided technique for the intraoperative ablation of ventricular tachycardia. Circulation 76:1319, 1987.
158. Downar E, Mickleborough L, Harris L, et al.: Intraoperative electrical ablation of ventricular arrhythmias: A "closed heart" procedure. J Am Coll Cardiol 10:1048, 1987.
159. Josephson ME, Waxman HL, Cain ME, et al.: Ventricular activation during ventricular endocardial pacing. II. Role of pace-mapping to localize origin of ventricular tachycardia. Am J Cardiol 50:11, 1982.
160. Kienzle MG, Miller J, Falcone RA, et al.: Intraoperative endocardial mapping during sinus rhythm: Relationship to site of origin of ventricular tachycardia. Circulation 70:957, 1984.
161. Garan H, Nguyen K, McGovern B, et al.: Perioperative and long-term results after electrophysiologically directed ventricular surgery for recurrent ventricular tachycardia. J Am Coll Cardiol 8:201, 1986.
162. Horowitz LN, Harken AH, Kastor JA, et al.: Ventricular resection guided by epicardial and endocardial mapping for treatment of recurrent ventricular tachycardia. N Engl J Med 302:589, 1980.
163. Ideker RE, Smith WM, Wallace AG, et al.: A computerized method for the rapid display of ventricular activation during the intraoperative study of arrhythmias. Circulation 59:449, 1979.
164. Downar E, Parson ID, Mickleborough LL, et al.: On-line epicardial mapping of intraoperative ventricular arrhythmias: Initial clinical experience. J Am Coll Cardiol 4:703, 1984.
165. Taccardi B, Arisi G, Macchi E, et al.: A new intracavitary probe for detecting the site of origin of ectopic ventricular beats during one cardiac cycle. Circulation 75:272, 1987.
166. Swerdlow CD, Mason JW, Stinson EB, et al.: Results of operations for ventricular tachycardia in 105 patients. J Thorac Cardiovasc Surg 92:105, 1986.
167. Fisher JD, Kim SG, Furman S, et al.: Role of implantable pacemakers in control of recurrent ventricular tachycardia. Am J Cardiol 49:194, 1982.
168. Eldar M, Griffin JC, Abbott JA, et al.: Permanent cardiac pacing in patients with the long QT syndrome. J Am Coll Cardiol 10:100, 1987.
169. Fisher JD, Johnston DR, Furman S, et al.: Long-term efficacy of antitachycardia pacing for supraventricular and ventricular tachycardias. Am J Cardiol 60:1311, 1987.
170. Mirowski M, Reid PR, Mower MM, et al.: Termination of malignant ventricular arrhythmias with an implanted automatic defibrillator in human beings. N Engl J Med 303:322, 1980.
171. Echt DS, Armstrong K, Schmidt P, et al.: Clinical experience, complications, and survival in 70 patients with the automatic implantable cardioverter/defibrillator. Circulation 71:289, 1985.
172. Ferguson D, Saksena S, Greenberg E, et al.: Management of recurrent ventricular tachycardia: Economic impact of therapeutic alternatives. Am J Cardiol 53:531, 1984.
173. Mitchell LB, Wyse DG, Eliasoph HP, et al.: A randomized cost comparison of the invasive and noninvasive approaches to drug selection for ventricular tachyarrhythmias. Circulation 76:IV-509, 1987.
174. Saksena S, Greenberg E, Ferguson D: Prospective reimbursement for state-of-the-art medical practice: The case for invasive electrophysiologic evaluation. Am J Cardiol 55:963, 1985.
175. Denniss AR, Richards DA, Cody DV, et al.: Prognostic significance of ventricular tachycardia and fibrillation induced at programmed stimulation and delayed potentials detected on the signal-averaged electrocardiograms of survivors of acute myocardial infarction. Circulation 74:731, 1986.
176. The Multicenter Postinfarction Research Group: Risk stratification and survival after myocardial infarction. N Engl J Med 309:331, 1983.
177. Abildskov JA, Green LS, Lux RL: The present status of body surface potential mapping. J Am Coll Cardiol 2:394, 1983.

14

The Long QT Syndrome and Torsades de Pointes: Basic and Clinical Aspects

Dan M. Roden

The notion that abnormal cardiac repolarization might contribute to the genesis of cardiac arrhythmias evolved during the late 1950s and early 1960s. In 1957, Jervell and Lange-Nielsen[1] described a kindred in which congenital deafness was associated with abnormal QT prolongation and a high incidence of sudden death; they speculated that death was due to asystole. The following year, Ward[2] and Romano[3] independently described the syndrome of abnormal QT prolongation and sudden death without congenital deafness, which now bears their names. In 1966, Dessertenne[4] described an elderly patient with AV block who had intermittent syncope. When her rhythm was monitored, it was found that syncope was associated not with excessively slow heart rates but, in fact, with a morphologically distinctive ventricular tachycardia. Dessertenne noted that the electrical axis of the QRS appeared to shift slowly over time, giving the entire arrhythmia the appearance of a military braid ("torsade"); hence, he coined the term torsades de pointes (literally, twisting of the pointes) to describe this arrhythmia. Since the early description of the congenital cases and Dessertenne's index case, it has become clear that the most common etiology of this syndrome of polymorphic ventricular tachycardia in association with a prolonged QT interval is therapy with action potential–prolonging antiarrhythmic drugs.

The observation that a polymorphic ventricular tachycardia superficially resembling torsades de pointes can occur in patients with absolutely normal repolarization has given rise to some ambiguity with respect to the term *torsades de pointes*. In this review, as we and others have advocated,[5–8] the term torsades de pointes will be used exclusively to describe a ventricular tachycardia occurring in the setting of markedly delayed repolarization (Fig. 14–1). The two—abnormal QT-U intervals and torsades de pointes—are intimately linked clinically. Moreover, studies of underlying mechanisms have reinforced the link between abnormal repolarization and arrhythmias. Polymorphic ventricular tachycardia occurring in the absence of QT interval prolongation appears to be a separate syndrome, with its own electrocardiographic features, associated clinical entities, appropriate treatment modalities, and prognosis. Thus it seems reasonable to suggest that what we call "true" torsades de pointes may well be mechanistically different from polymorphic ventricular tachycardia in the absence of QT abnormalities.

Clinical Features

Torsades de pointes has been observed in all age groups from fetuses[9] and neonates[10] to the elderly; in adults, acquired cases are much more common than congenital ones, although the latter may present in adulthood.

ELECTROCARDIOGRAPHIC FEATURES OF THE LONG QT SYNDROME

Several distinctive electrocardiographic features of the congenital and acquired long QT–torsades de pointes syndromes deserve emphasis:

1. The QT interval is not always dramatically prolonged. This is particularly true in certain congenital cases in which recurrent syncope may occur in the face of a normal QT interval.[11–13] Some reports indicate that the QT interval may be normal except at slow rates.[14] If the index of suspicion is high, treadmill exercise or catecholamine challenge may reveal failure of the QT interval to shorten.[15] Modest QT prolongation has been associated with an exaggerated incidence of arrhythmia

---

Supported in part by a grant from the United States Public Health Service (HL-32694).

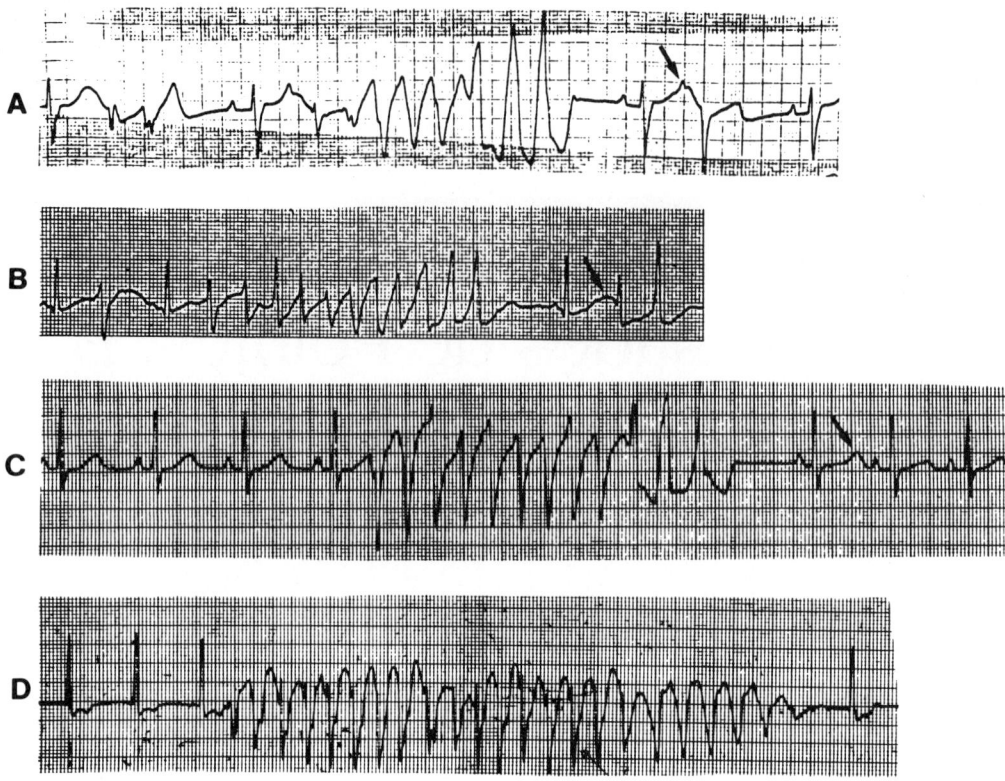

FIGURE 14–1
Four episodes of polymorphic ventricular tachycardia. A was recorded from a 65-year-old woman with a malfunctioning VVI pacemaker and recent initiation of quinidine therapy for ventricular ectopic beats. B was recorded from a 12-year-old boy with marked hypokalemia and an otherwise normal heart. C was recorded from a 32-year-old woman with a normal heart and recurrent ventricular tachycardia in whom sotalol therapy was being initiated. D was recorded from a 67-year-old man with an extensive anterior myocardial infarction and acute pulmonary edema whose serum electrolytes were normal and who was not receiving therapy with any QT-prolonging drugs. In A–C, the tachycardia develops after a pause or with bradycardia (C), and the post-tachycardia QT interval (arrows) is markedly prolonged. In D, on the other hand, no antecedent rate changes were evident, no post-tachycardia QT prolongation was noted, and clinical features of "typical" torsades de pointes were absent. A–C represent torsades de pointes, whereas D represents polymorphic ventricular tachycardia that is not typical torsades de pointes.

aggravation by antiarrhythmic drugs, raising the possibility that a forme fruste of the syndrome may exist.[16]

2. A very prominent U wave is often observed. Alternans in QT duration and T and U wave amplitude is also frequently reported.[17–19] As discussed further below, the mechanism responsible for the genesis of these changes is not completely established, although prolonged Purkinje repolarization appears to play a role.

3. QRS prolongation (a marker of slowed impulse propagation) is not a feature of either the congenital or the acquired syndromes.

4. The tachycardia itself may be monomorphic for at least three reasons: (a) Some patients with long QT syndromes appear to be prone to monomorphic, and not polymorphic, ventricular tachycardia (Fig. 14–2).[20] (b) The tachycardia may appear monomorphic if recorded for only brief periods in one lead; longer periods of recording and multiple leads will usually indicate the true polymorphic character of the tachycardia.[4] (c) In a number of patients, typical polymorphic torsades de pointes itself appears to elicit the typical sustained monomorphic ventricular tachycardia seen so commonly in patients with advanced coronary artery disease, remote myocardial infarction, and so forth;[21] in effect, the spontaneous development of torsades de pointes serves as a "autoprogrammed ventricular stimulation study" to induce monomorphic ventricular tachycardia. Indeed, the induction of typical ventricular fibrillation by typical torsades de pointes (Fig. 14–3) is one likely cause of deaths observed in the long QT syndrome, especially since torsades de pointes itself is frequently self-terminating.

Polymorphic ventricular tachycardia or coarse ventricular fibrillation associated with no QT abnormality (see Fig. 14–1D) may be distinguished from torsades de pointes by a number of clinical features (Table 14–1).[5, 6, 22] Also, the electrocardiogram recorded just prior to an episode of arrhythmia may be helpful. Marked QT-U prolongation is virtually always present in the last few supraventricular beats prior to the paroxysm and the first one(s) following it (see Fig. 14–1). In congenital cases, an increase in heart rate, often without commensurate shortening of the QT interval may be observed (Fig. 14–4). In many of the acquired or drug-associated cases, a stereotypical series of cycle length changes prior to the initiation of an episode of torsades de pointes has been described.[23–25] An extra-

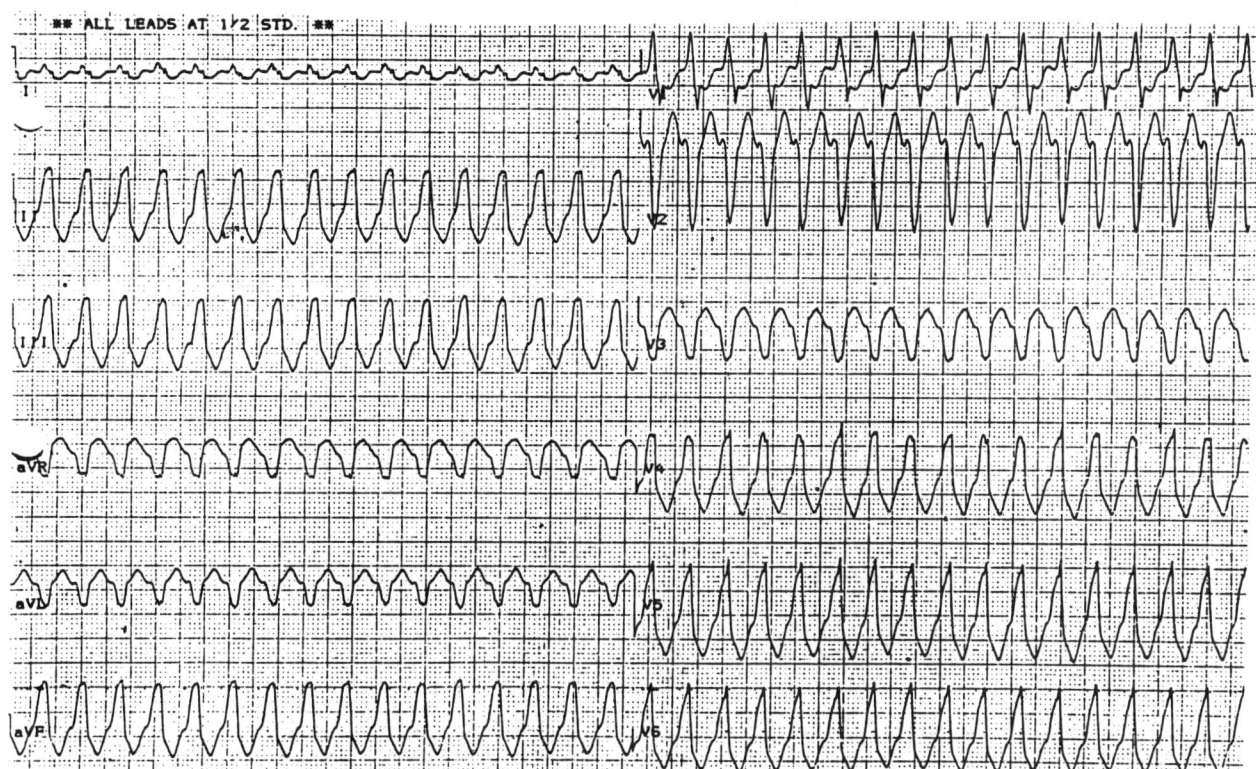

FIGURE 14–2
Monomorphic ventricular tachycardia in a 12-year-old boy with a normal heart and a rate-corrected QT interval during sinus rhythm of 480 ms. This may represent a variant of the long QT syndrome.

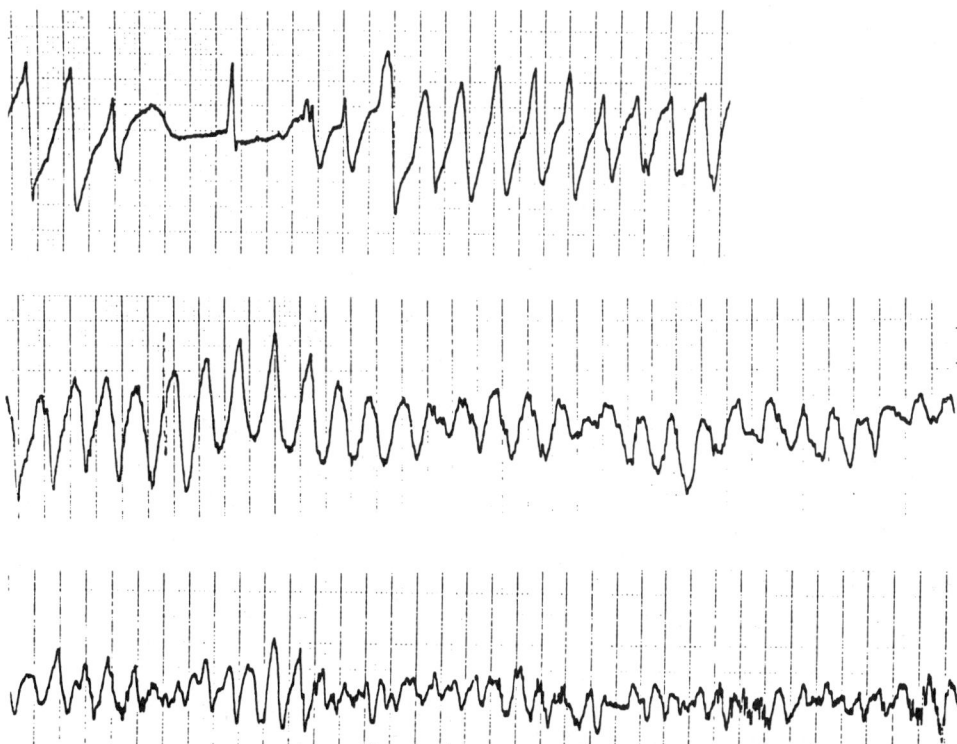

FIGURE 14–3
An episode of quinidine-associated torsades de pointes that degenerated into ventricular fibrillation (continuous strips).

The Long QT Syndrome and Torsades de Pointes: Basic and Clinical Aspects

TABLE 14–1
Long QT-Associated vs. Non–Long QT-Associated Polymorphic Ventricular Tachycardia

	Long QT-Associated	Non–Long QT-Associated
Initiation	Short-long-short cycles	Very short coupling without antecedent cycle length changes
Termination	Prominent post-tachycardia ↑ QT	No post-tachycardia ↑ QT
Type of Underlying Heart Disease	Left ventricular function often normal; atrial arrhythmias being treated with quinidine-like drugs	Often severe ischemic heart disease
Associated Clinical Features	At least one (often more) associated finding*: quinidine, hypokalemia, unrecognized congenital long QT syndrome, etc.	No associated findings*—often occurs in unstable ischemic syndromes
Treatment	*Acute:* Withdrawal of offending factor(s) K$^+$, Mg^{++}, catecholamines, pacing *Chronic (persistent ↑↑QT):* Beta-blockers QT-shortening drugs (lidocaine, etc.) (L) stellate ganglionectomy Permanent pacing Automatic implantable cardioverter/defibrillator	"Usual" antiarrhythmics, including quinidine, lidocaine, bretylium, aminodarone, etc. Anti-ischemic interventions
Prognosis	Excellent when associated with reversible causes* Variable when persistent or congenital	Depends on underlying heart disease; often very poor

*See Table 14–2.

systole or a brief episode of tachycardia is followed by an appropriate postextrasystolic pause. The next supraventricular beat has a markedly prolonged QT-U interval. The tachycardia itself starts after the peak of the T wave, i.e., during terminal repolarization (Fig. 14–5). A number of reports, in fact, suggest that the arrhythmia episodes are not so much characterized by marked QT prolongation as by a prominent "late diastolic" (or U) wave (Fig. 14–6).[26-27]

The "short-long-short" series of cycle length changes preceding a prolonged paroxysm is typical of drug-induced torsades de pointes but may not be present in congenital cases (see Fig. 14–4). Moreover, a number of records have been reported of patients with acquired torsades de pointes in whom these cycle length changes were absent (see Fig. 14–1C). It is unclear whether these cycle length changes indicate certain fundamental differences in etiology among the clinical syndromes. Moreover, the extrasystole preceding the long cycle presumably arises from a mechanism similar to the long paroxysm that follows the long cycle. The "short-long-short" series may thus merely represent the fact that long episodes are preceding by particularly long (postectopic) cycles. This would be consistent with the

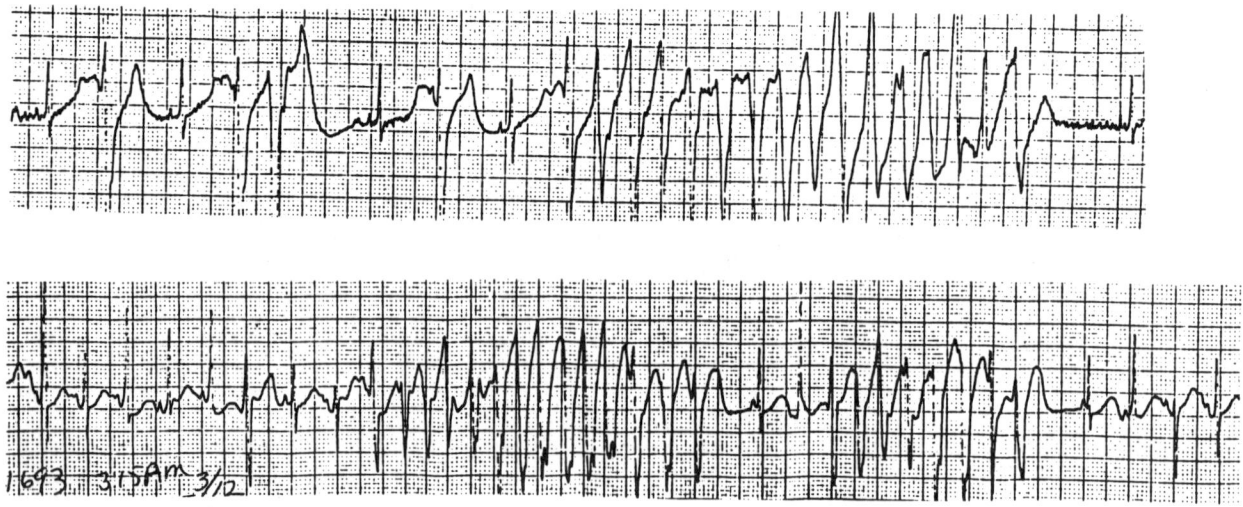

FIGURE 14–4
Two episodes of torsades de pointes 10 minutes apart in a 6-year-old girl with Romano-Ward syndrome. The episode in the top panel, like those shown in Figure 14–1A–C and Figure 15–5, is associated with relative bradycardia and marked QT prolongation. The episode in the bottom panel, however, appears to be triggered by an increase in heart rate.

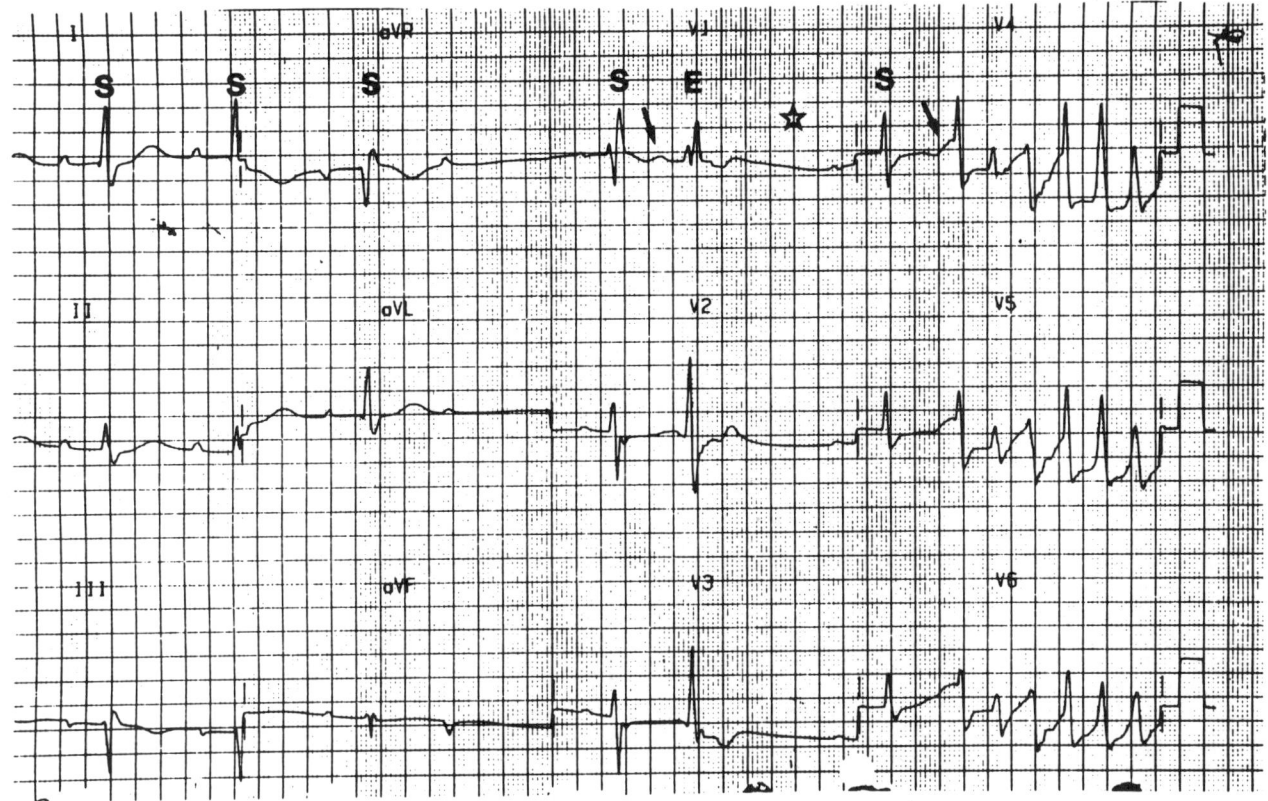

FIGURE 14–5
Onset of quinidine-induced torsades de pointes recorded during routine 12-lead electrocardiography. The patient was a 78-year-old man with recurrent, non-sustained ventricular tachycardia. Quinidine therapy had been started the day before this ECG was made. The underlying rhythm is sinus with right bundle branch block. The first three P waves are conducted (S: sinus) with a 320-ms PR, whereas the fourth is blocked, resulting in a long pause. The next conducted sinus beat has a particularly long QT interval (arrow) whose terminal portion is interrupted by an ectopic beat (E). These two beats are followed by another long pause (star), a sinus beat with a markedly prolonged QT-U interval (arrow), and torsades de pointes.

clinical observation (dating to the original case reports) that bradycardia is a precipitator of torsades de pointes.[4,18,25,28,29] Indeed, sinus bradycardia is common among patients with the congenital syndromes (Fig. 14–7) and has been attributed to an associated defect in autonomic control of heart rate.[30]

Left stellate ganglion stimulation prolongs the QT interval, particularly in patients with the congenital syndrome.[31] Acute beta-blockade generally shortens the QT interval and chronic beta-blockade appears to prolong it;[32–38] the latter is particularly intriguing in view of the efficacy of beta-blockade in the chronic management of the syndrome. QT-prolonging antiarrhythmic drugs increase the QT interval at all heart rates; thus the longest QT intervals in drug-treated patients are seen at slow rates.[39]

ETIOLOGIES AND ASSOCIATED CLINICAL FINDINGS

The congenital long QT syndromes are inherited in a typical autosomal recessive fashion. This, of course, suggests that an abnormal protein product is ultimately responsible for the expression of the clinical syndrome, although, as described below, the molecular mechanism has not yet been elucidated. Patients with the

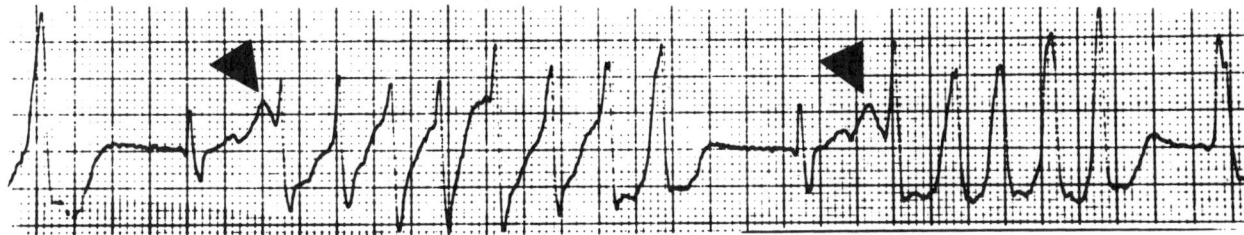

FIGURE 14–6
Typical torsades de pointes (in a patient who recently started quinidine therapy) initiated not by a long QT interval but, as indicated, by a prominent U wave.

The Long QT Syndrome and Torsades de Pointes: Basic and Clinical Aspects

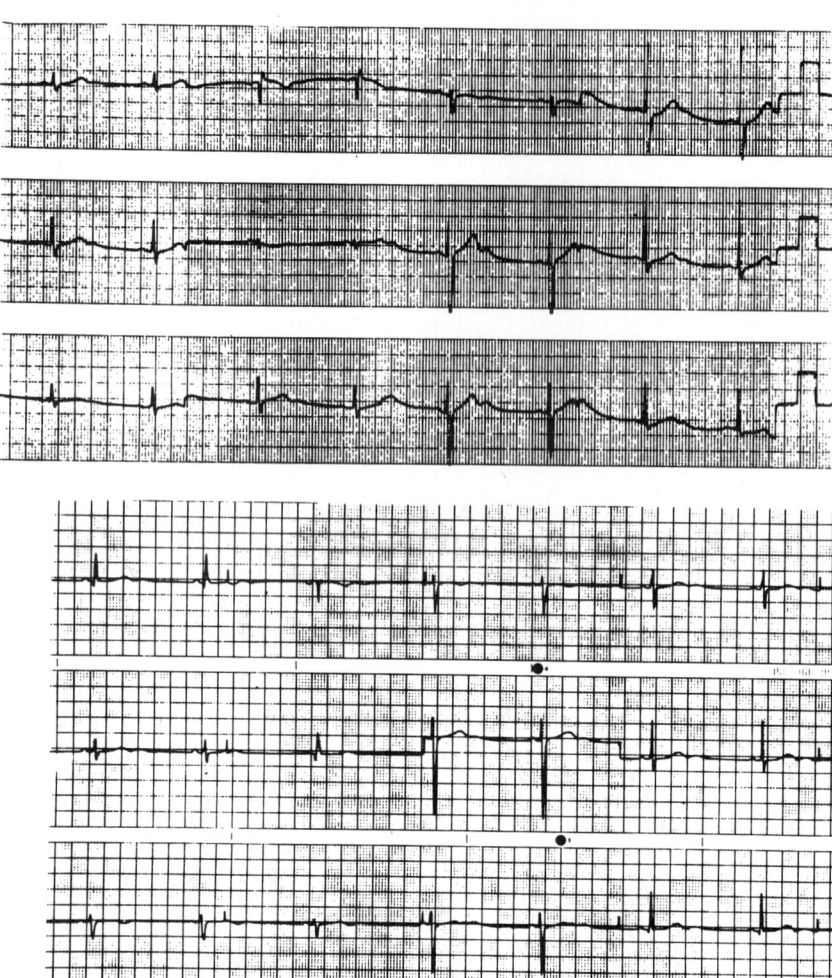

FIGURE 14–7
12-lead ECGs in a brother and sister with the Romano-Ward syndrome. Note sinus bradycardia, QT prolongation and prominent U waves. The family came to medical attention when the brother (top tracing) complained of palpitations, was given quinidine, and developed recurrent syncope due to torsades de pointes. Initial ECG screening of his sister demonstrated a normal ECG; the lower tracing was taken 3 years later. Aside from the quinidine-associated event in the propositus, neither patient has experienced syncope. Both are now treated with permanent pacing at rates of 70–80/min and beta-blockers.

congenital long QT syndromes typically develop episodes of arrhythmia during periods of sympathetic activation, such as treadmill exercise or sudden awakening. Sudden death in the absence of any premonitory symptom appears to be unusual; on the other hand, syncope or seizures[40] in a patient with the congenital (or acquired) long QT syndrome is a red flag that intervention is urgently required. The mortality rate for untreated symptomatic patients with the congenital syndrome has been cited as high as 71%, and this can probably be reduced by interventions described below.[11]

The most common etiology of the acquired long QT–torsades de pointes syndrome is treatment with action potential–prolonging antiarrhythmic drugs.[23-25, 41-44] Most patients develop symptoms (syncope) within several days of starting therapy. Multiple other etiologies have been described (Table 14–2) and it is not unusual for several inciting features to be present in a particular patient. For example, the administration of quinidine to a hypokalemic patient or a patient with unrecognized congenital long QT syndrome can precipitate an episode of torsades de pointes. Similarly, hypokalemia, hypomagnesemia, or slow heart rates due to sinus bradycardia or AV block are themselves associated with torsades de pointes and can precipitate torsades de pointes during long-term antiarrhythmic therapy.[41-51] The association between perturbations of the sympathetic nervous system, either in the brain itself or in the neck, and marked repolarization abnormalities (Fig. 14–8) and torsades de pointes is particularly intriguing in view of the suggested role of the autonomic nervous system.[52-54] Recently an association has been described between the administration of a variety of antibiotics, including ampicillin,[55] erythromycin,[56,57] trimethoprim-sulfa,[58] and pentamidine,[59] and the subsequent development of torsades de pointes. Other drugs, such as chloral hydrate,[60] the serotonin antagonist ketanserin,[61] the lipid-lowering agent probucol,[62] the anorexiant prenylamine,[63] the anthracycline doxorubicin,[64] alpha-blocking agents,[65] and even a Chinese herbal remedy,[66] have been shown to prolong QT and may cause torsades de pointes, although the association is far from conclusive. Sudden death in some patients receiving psychotropic drugs has been related to the development of torsades de pointes;[67] clearly, thioridazine (Mellaril)[68] can cause marked QT prolongation and torsades de pointes, however the association, although reported (e.g., for maprotiline),[69] is less certain for other drugs of this type. It is also possible that depression itself may alter autonomic tone, baseline QT, and/or QT response to drugs.[70] Intoxication with organophosphorus insecti-

TABLE 14–2
Associated Clinical Findings in Long QT-Related Polymorphic Ventricular Tachycardia (Torsades de Pointes)

Common Associations
Therapy with QT prolonging drugs
  Quinidine
  Procainamide (especially with NAPA accumulation, e.g., in patients with renal failure)
  Disopyramide
  Sotalol
  NAPA
  Thioridazine
Electrolyte abnormalities
  Hypokalemia
  Hypomagnesemia
Bradyarrhythmias
Unrecognized congenital long QT syndrome

Less Common (but Clear) Associations
Other QT prolonging drugs
  Amiodarone
  Bepridil
  Lidoflazine
  Aprindine
  Neuroleptics
  Prenylamine
Other disease
  Hypothyroidism
  Liquid protein and other diets
  Central nervous system abnormalities, especially those affecting sympathetic outflow (subarachnoid hemorrhage, lesions of brainstem, cervical cord, etc.)
Intoxication with organophosphorus insecticides

Other Associations, Not (Yet) Well-established
Antibiotics
  Ampicillin anaphylaxis
  Erythromycin
  Trimethoprim-sulfa
  Pentamidine
Other drugs
  Ketanserin
  Probucol
  Chloral hydrate
  Anthracyclines
  Encainide
Mitral valve prolapse and other structural heart disease

cides[71] and use of the liquid protein[72,73] and other low-calorie diets[74–77] have also been associated with torsades de pointes. QT changes and torsades de pointes–like arrhythmias may develop during coronary injection of ionic contrast media.[78–80] Similar arrhythmias have been provoked by (usually malfunctioning) pacemakers (see Fig. 14–1A), with long diastolic intervals preceding a paced beat with a long QT.[81,82] In general, with the exception of antiarrhythmic drugs, these are clinical associations, and studies of basic mechanisms such as those outlined below have not been conducted. Although a role for intrinsic myocardial disease (myocarditis, ischemic heart disease) has been proposed, the association is not strong.[83–88] Some case reports suggest a role for an inflammatory process in the cardiac sympathetic ganglia in both congenital and acquired non–drug-related cases.[73,89] The observation that torsades de pointes can occur in completely normal hearts (e.g., from sotalol overdose[90]) reinforces the notion that underlying myocardial disease is not a prerequisite for the development of this arrhythmia.

Another major question that remains unanswered is the arrhythmogenic potential of a prolonged QT interval per se. QT intervals > 600 ms or QT-U intervals > 600 ms with prominent U waves in patients receiving quinidine or in those with the congenital long QT syndromes appear to carry with them a substantial risk of syncope due to torsades de pointes.[25,41] Rate correction is a convenient method to normalize QT and for comparisons among populations;[91,92] however, it appears to be absolute QT duration (and not its rate-corrected value) which is associated with torsades de pointes.[23,25,41,42] The hallmark of treatment with amiodarone is QT prolongation but torsades de pointes appears to be quite unusual, although not unheard of.[46,93–95] In fact, isolated case reports suggest a role for amiodarone in the management of patients with congenital long QT syndromes.[96] Similarly, hypothyroidism usually slows heart rate and prolongs QT but, as with amiodarone therapy, torsades de pointes is unusual.[97–99] Hypocalcemia prolongs QT, but generally it is the ST segment and not the T wave which is abnormal; torsades de pointes is again quite unusual.

In most series,[20–25] quinidine is the most commonly implicated antiarrhythmic drug.[100–104] In fact, the association among quinidine therapy, marked QT prolongation, and generally self-terminating polymorphic ventricular tachycardia was recognized as the cause of quinidine syncope[100] prior to Dessertenne's report. Several series[25,26,105,106] have estimated the incidence between 0.5 and 8% within the first several days of treatment. Disopyramide is another leading cause and, in some series,[41] is more common than quinidine, presumably reflecting local prescribing habits. Other antiarrhythmic agents implicated include procainamide[110] and its active metabolite N-acetyl procainamide (NAPA),[111–114] sotalol,[47,90,115–117] amiodarone,[46,93–95] aprindine,[118] bepridil,[119–121] and lidoflazine.[122] Most of these agents not only prolong repolarization but also produce other electrophysiologic changes, which as described below may modulate the

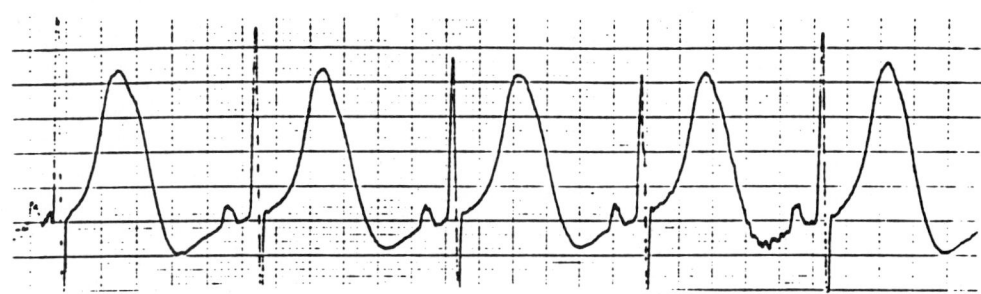

FIGURE 14–8
Monster U waves recorded from an otherwise healthy 80-year-old man who suffered a posterior fossa cerebrovascular accident.

development of torsades de pointes. These include beta-blockade and heart rate slowing (sotalol, amiodarone), calcium channel block (bepridil, lidoflazine), and sodium channel block (quinidine, disopyramide, procainamide, amiodarone). Other sodium channel blockers such as mexiletine and lidocaine do not cause true torsades de pointes and, in fact, sodium channel block can successfully reverse clinical and experimental torsades de pointes (see below). Encainide has rarely been associated with torsades de pointes; accumulation of 3-methoxy-O-desmethyl encainide, an active metabolite that appears to prolong repolarization, may be responsible.[123]

The short-long-short series of cycle length changes are typically seen in quinidine-associated cases, and electrolyte abnormalities, particularly hypokalemia, are common.[23–25] In our series, about half the patients developing torsades de pointes during quinidine therapy were receiving the drug for nonsustained ventricular arrhythmias; the remainder were being treated for atrial fibrillation or flutter.[25] In those patients being treated for atrial fibrillation, torsades de pointes almost inevitably develops following conversion to sinus rhythm and not during atrial fibrillation itself (Fig. 14–9).[25, 124] Whether this reflects differences in ventricular rate (and therefore in QT interval) or some fundamental electrophysiologic difference between sinus rhythm and atrial fibrillation is unclear. As outlined above, rules regarding the point beyond which QT interval prolongation during quinidine therapy becomes unacceptable have not been formulated. A QT interval greater than 550 ms, particularly following a postectopic pause, should at least alert the clinician to the possibility of impending torsades de pointes and prompt measurement of serum electrolytes and a reevaluation of the indication for therapy.[21, 25] Since the risk of developing torsades de pointes during the initiation of quinidine therapy may as high as 8%,[26, 106] brief hospitalization with monitoring of cardiac rhythm has been advocated. It is unclear whether patients who develop torsades de pointes during quinidine therapy probably can receive subsequent treatment with quinidine or other action potential–prolonging antiarrhythmics,[21, 23, 125] even if another factor such as hypokalemia is present. Our own philosophy is to avoid such treatment, since such patients have declared that they are "at risk," particularly should another inciting factor such as hypokalemia or bradycardia redevelop. Successful treatment with amiodarone may, however, be possible in these patients, although the data are conflicting.

One of the most striking features of quinidine-associated torsades de pointes is the failure of plasma concentration monitoring to predict this form of drug toxicity.[25, 100–104] In fact, in most series, plasma quinidine concentrations are at or below the lower limit of the

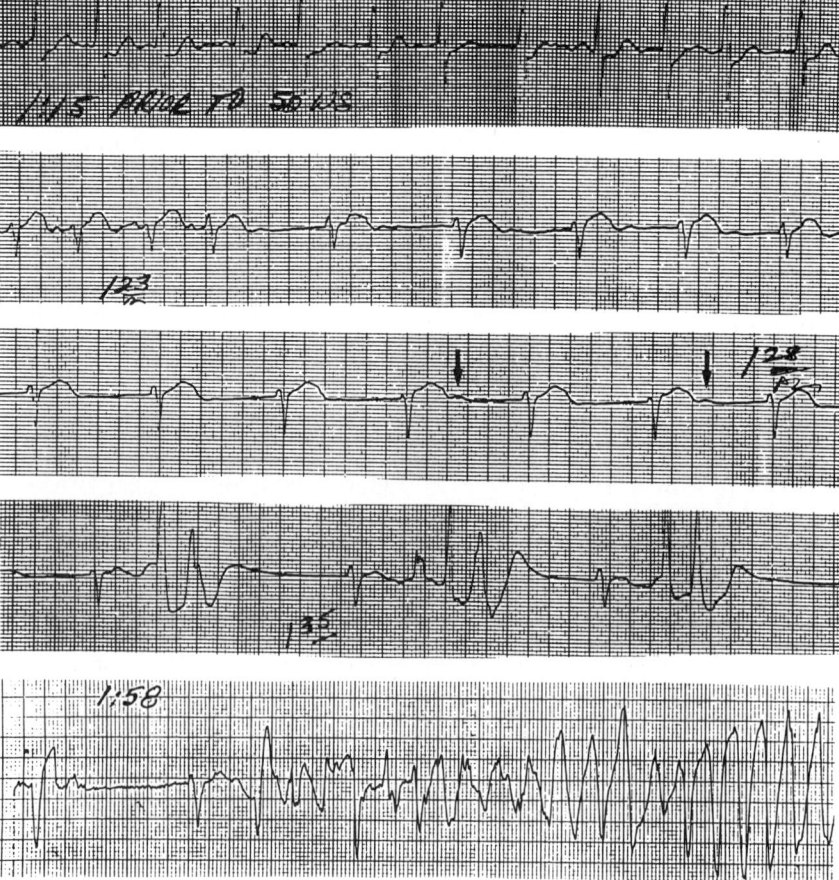

FIGURE 14–9
Serial rhythm strips over less than 45 minutes in a 77-year-old woman being treated with quinidine and digitalis for atrial fibrillation who underwent cardioversion shortly after the top panel was recorded. The second panel shows sinus rhythm followed by a junctional bradycardia. U wave alternans is evident in the third strip (arrows), brief episodes of polymorphic ventricular tachycardia preceded by short-long-short cycles in the fourth, and typical torsades de pointes in the fifth.

usual therapeutic range in many patients, and the arrhythmia may occur after only one or two doses of drug. It is possible that active metabolites[126, 127] whose concentrations are not routinely measured may contribute in part to the development of torsades de pointes. However, we have shown that unusual accumulation of such active metabolites does not explain the development of torsades de pointes at low plasma quinidine concentrations.[128] Interestingly, in contrast to quinidine therapy, currently available data suggest that QT prolongation during sotalol therapy is concentration-dependent[129, 130] and torsades de pointes occurs at a threshold dose and plasma concentration in a given individual;[131] successful treatment with lower doses of sotalol is frequently effective and well tolerated. As a corollary, torsades de pointes is a very frequent manifestation of sotalol overdose.[90] As with quinidine, hypokalemia usually due to thiazide diuretics appears to be a potent inciter of torsades de pointes in patients who are receiving sotalol.[47] Similarly, accumulation of NAPA during procainamide therapy[112–114] has been associated with torsades de pointes. When NAPA has itself been used as an antiarrhythmic, torsades de pointes has been described, again at high plasma concentrations.[111] Interestingly, NAPA appears to be just as potent as procainamide in prolonging repolarization, both in vitro[132] and in the intact canine[133] or human heart,[134] whereas it is considerably less potent as a sodium channel blocking agent.[132, 133] Thus the relationship between drug dose, plasma concentration, and development of torsades de pointes appears inconsistent; for example, the arrhythmia occurs even at very low doses and plasma concentrations of quinidine, whereas the arrhythmia seems more dose- and concentration-related for other drugs such as sotalol or NAPA. The role of inciters such as bradycardia or hypokalemia is clear, but even when these are taken into account, the reasons that only some patients develop torsades de pointes are not fully explained.

Attempts to elicit torsades de pointes by classic programmed ventricular stimulation techniques have met with conflicting results. Early reports indicated that polymorphic ventricular tachycardia with modest QT prolongation was a fairly regular feature of programmed ventricular stimulation in patients receiving procainamide or quinidine.[135] However, more recent reports indicate that these techniques do not usually result in reproduction of the syndrome in patients with marked QT prolongation.[136] The latter outcome appears more consistent with the notion that the arrhythmia is frequently exacerbated by slow heart rates and ameliorated by rapid pacing. Clinical electrophysiologic studies have indicated marked prolongation of right ventricular effective refractory period in patients with congenital long QT syndromes,[136–138] and a role for monophasic action potential recordings, described further below, has been advocated both in the diagnosis of the syndromes and in studies of underlying mechanisms.[19, 139, 140] Similarly, body surface mapping has been reported to provide further evidence of localized abnormal repolarization.[141]

Management

In the vast majority of acquired cases, the most important therapeutic maneuvers are recognition of the clinical syndrome, withdrawal of any offending agents, and correction of serum electrolyte deficits.[23–25, 41–44] In many patients these treatments will suffice. In others, paroxysms of torsades de pointes will persist for several days, and maneuvers to increase heart rate are then most important. Infusion of isoproterenol to raise the heart rate to 100–120 bpm is often effective, but if therapy for more than several hours is contemplated or if catecholamine infusion is contraindicated (as in the case of underlying myocardial ischemia), temporary pacing is indicated.[142] If there is any question about the adequacy of AV nodal transmission or the stability of an atrial pacing site, the ventricle should be paced. DC cardioversion is effective for prolonged episodes, but the paroxysms are frequently self-terminating. The use of antiarrhythmic drugs has met with variable success, perhaps because arrhythmia recurrence is unpredictable in an individual patient. Hence, an intervention such as lidocaine may be judged "successful" when torsades de pointes does not recur, even if it would not have recurred without intervention.[25] QT-prolonging agents should be avoided; lidocaine and other sodium channel blockers that do not increase QT (mexiletine, tocainide, phenytoin)[143, 144] may be effective. The anecdotal efficacy of bretylium[51] has been attributed to reduction in heterogeneity of repolarization. Potassium and magnesium supplementation may be helpful. Magnesium in particular has been reported effective in some[145, 146] (but not all[147]) series, even in non-hypomagnesemic patients. Non–QT prolonging calcium channel blockers and beta-blockers have not been systematically evaluated although, as described below, there is some rationale for their use.

The management of patients with congenital long QT syndromes is much more controversial. A very high mortality rate has been cited, particularly after an initial episode of syncope.[11] Treatment with beta-blockers has been effective in non-randomized clinical trials.[11, 148] If symptoms persist despite beta-blocker therapy, left stellate ganglionectomy has been advocated both to reduce sympathetic input into the heart as well as to correct a theorized imbalance between right and left stellate inputs.[148, 149] This approach has not proven to be uniformly successful[150] and other therapies, including permanent pacing[151, 152] and the use of an automatic implantable cardioverter/defibrillator,[153] have been employed. Drugs such as phenytoin, primidone, mexiletine, and tocainide may also have a useful ancillary role, particularly if suppression of arrhythmias with a non–QT prolonging agent is required.[143, 144, 154] Interestingly, management with beta-blockers generally does not always result in QT shortening,[36, 38] although syncope is frequently alleviated. An unresolved issue is whether asymptomatic patients with a congenital long QT syndrome require treatment. A registry of patients with this illness has been established by Moss and colleagues,[11] and it may be that the natural history of the asymptomatic case will result from such studies.[149, 155] Meanwhile, one approach is to withhold therapy until an episode of syncope occurs; exceptions may be those who are judged to be at particular risk, possibly those with the Jervell and Lange-Nielsen syndrome or those who have had an affected sibling die.[11]

Basic Mechanisms

HYPOTHESES

Two competing but not necessarily mutually exclusive mechanisms have been proposed for the association between abnormal repolarization and torsades de pointes.[148, 156, 157] The first is the notion that regional variations in cardiac repolarization result in heterogeneity of refractoriness and boundary currents, with the resultant development of arrhythmias. This point of view has been most forcefully expressed by Schwartz,[148] whose animal studies clearly indicate that regional alterations in sympathetic inflow due to imbalance between right and left stellate ganglia can result in arrhythmias in a wide range of circumstances. Moreover, as discussed above, left stellate ganglionectomy has been apparently effective in some beta-blocker resistant cases, although a controlled randomized trial has not been conducted.

The alternate hypothesis for the underlying mechanism of torsades de pointes is that early afterdepolarizations (EADs) are responsible (Fig. 14-10). EADs (i.e., prominent delays in late phase-3 repolarization that result in triggered activity[158]) develop in canine cardiac Purkinje fibers driven at slow rates and superfused with high concentrations of sotalol[159] or of NAPA.[132] When we examined the relationship among quinidine treatment, extracellular potassium (K_o), and cycle length in canine cardiac Purkinje fibers, we found that EADs, like torsades de pointes, were much more common at low K_o and at long drive-cycle lengths, even in the presence of only a low concentration of quinidine (1 μM = 0.3 μg/ml).[160] Moreover, EADs, like torsades de pointes, interrupt terminal repolarization and were reversed by shortening cycle length or raising K_o. Therefore, we and others have hypothesized that under appropriate conditions EADs may develop in the Purkinje system and propagate into ventricular muscle (or develop in ventricular muscle) to cause torsades de pointes. Clearly, the "dispersion" hypothesis and "EAD" hypothesis are not mutually exclusive, since one can envision the situation in which, for example, abnormal sympathetic innervation contributed to heterogeneity of repolarization, which facilitated EAD propagation.

MECHANISM OF ACTION POTENTIAL PROLONGATION

The development of drugs such as amiodarone, N-acetyl procainamide, sotalol, clofilium, and meobentine, whose primary mode of action is prolongation of

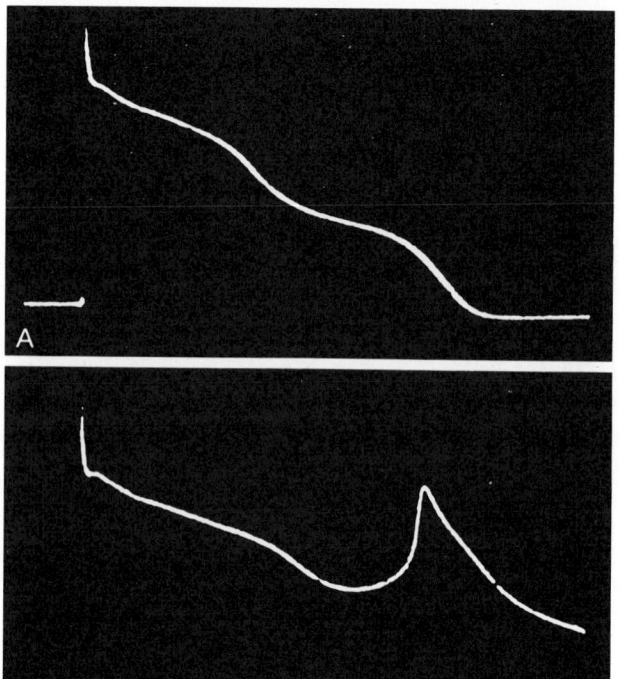

FIGURE 14–10
Transmembrane action potentials from canine cardiac Purkinje fibers being superfused with quinidine and low K_o and driven at a slow rate (cycle length 4 s). A shows a prominent interruption in terminal repolarization (an early afterdepolarization[158]). In B, triggered activity develops from the early afterdepolarization. Hence this triggered activity, like torsades de pointes, occurs in low K_o and quinidine at slow rates and interrupts terminal repolarization.

repolarization[162-165] rather than depression of the fast inward sodium current, has created an intense interest in the determinants of cardiac repolarization itself. Not only are such agents at least as effective as sodium channel blockers in patients with sustained atrial or ventricular tachyarrhythmias, but they also appear to render ventricular fibrillation more difficult to induce[166] and ventricular defibrillation easier to accomplish.[167] Interest in this mechanism of antiarrhythmic drug action is compounded by the fact that agents with this particular pharmacologic property would be viewed with considerably more enthusiasm were it not for the occasional development of torsades de pointes.[7, 168] Repolarization in ventricular muscle and in the Purkinje network reflects a predominance of outward (repolarizing) over inward (depolarizing) currents. Since membrane conductance is high during the plateau of the action potential, changes in repolarization may reflect even small perturbations in the balance between inward and outward currents. The major outward (repolarizing) currents in heart include:

1. I_{K1}:[169] A virtually time-independent potassium current that conducts a large inward current at potentials more negative than the resting potential and a small outward current at more positive potentials. This property is known as inward rectification.
2. I_K (or I_x):[170-173] A time-dependent potassium cur-

rent that activates slowly (over several hundred milliseconds) at potentials more positive than −40 mV. This current is known as the delayed rectifier; obviously its time course and voltage dependence suggest a major role in repolarization.

3. Other potassium currents including (at least) the rapidly (time constant approximately 50 ms) inactivating (probably) calcium-dependent transient outward current I_{to};[174] a recently described time-independent plateau current (I_{Kp});[175] a sodium-dependent potassium current;[176] a time-independent potassium current activated by ATP deficiency;[177–178] and a muscarinic potassium current most prominent in atria.[179]

4. Na-K pump: The pump normally extrudes 3 Na^+ ions for each 2 K^+ ions drawn in from the outside. Therefore, the act of pumping produces a current (i.e., this is an electrogenic pump). The pump is most active when intracellular sodium rises (e.g., at fast rates).

The major inward currents during the plateau include a small maintained current through the sodium channel; a maintained current through the calcium channel, and electrogenic Na-Ca exchange. In theory, although multiple underlying mechanisms can underlie action potential prolongation, only two major classes of drug action need to be considered: drugs can increase action potential duration only by augmenting inward current(s) or by decreasing outward current(s). This action may then produce EADs that can then be associated with a depolarizing upstroke (triggered activity); thus, the ionic mechanisms of action potential prolongation and EAD generation may be quite distinct from those of the triggered activity that results. In fact, Purkinje fibers appear to have two possible "resting" potentials:[180] a "normal" level of about −85 mV and a "depolarized" (EAD) level of around −60 mV, which may become manifest under appropriate conditions (slow rates, decreased outward current, etc.). Action potentials can be prolonged, EADs generated, and torsades de pointes–like arrhythmias elicited in the intact heart by drugs that delay sodium channel inactivation, such as batrachotoxin,[181] aconitine, veratridine,[182] and the sea anemone toxin anthopleurin-A (APA).[183, 184] Similarly, induction of a maintained inward calcium current by the calcium channel "agonist" Bay K8644 can result in EADs and triggered activity.[185]

Most useful antiarrhythmic drugs either have no effect on or actually decrease inward currents, so alternate mechanisms of action potential prolongation should be sought. (Interestingly an agent whose predominant electrophysiologic action appears to be the prolongation of inward sodium current [DPI-201] is now under development).[186] Cesium blocks potassium currents,[187] and prolongs cardiac action potentials, presumably by decreasing both I_K and I_{K1}; EADs and triggering are seen.[188] Block of potassium currents, particularly I_K and at higher concentrations I_{K1}, has also been described as a mechanism for action potential prolongation by quinidine (Fig. 14–11),[189–194] sotalol and its non–beta-blocking d-isomer,[195] amiodarone,[196, 197] and clofilium.[198, 199] Acidosis can clearly cause EADs and triggering; the mechanism is uncertain, but may

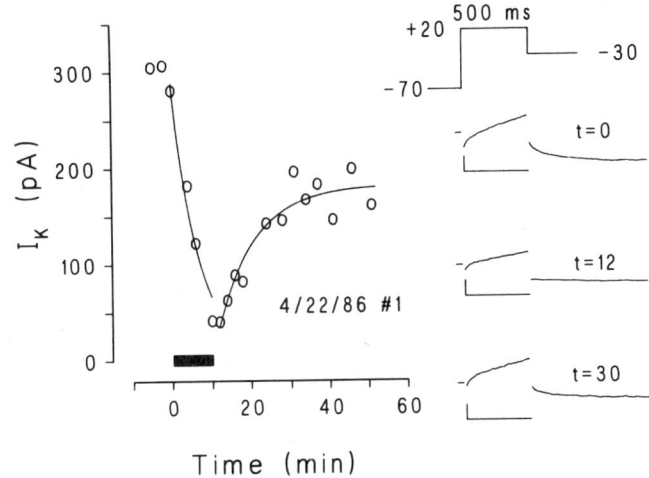

FIGURE 14–11
Block of the delayed outward rectifier I_K by quinidine in single heart cells. The magnitude of the time-dependent "tail" at −30 mV is shown as a function of time, where the black bar indicates a 10-minute exposure to 10 μM of quinidine. As the graph and the raw traces at right indicate, quinidine reversibly depressed this repolarizing potassium current. (Reprinted by permission of the authors and the American Heart Association, Inc., from Roden DM, Bennett PB, Synders DJ, et al: Circ Res 62:1055, 1988.)

reflect decreased outward I_{K1}.[200] The Na-H exchange inhibitor amiloride also prolongs action potential duration and causes EADs and triggered activity[201] in isolated Purkinje fibers, but the mechanism of this effect is not clear; Na-H inhibition (with intracellular acidosis?), Na-Ca exchange inhibition, or potassium channel block is possible. Interestingly, amiloride has recently been reported to be an effective agent in the management of some patients with inducible sustained ventricular tachycardia.[202] Thus, as interest in this mechanism of antiarrhythmic drug action increases, studies of the basic mechanism whereby antiarrhythmic drugs prolong action potential and whereby they enable abnormal depolarizing currents under conditions of prolonged action potential will allow better delineation of drug actions that may or may not be important to incorporate into subsequent drug entities.

MODULATION OF TRIGGERED ACTIVITY IN VITRO

An inward current obviously causes the depolarizing upstroke of triggered activity. This may be a depressed fast inward sodium current, the slow inward (calcium) current, Na-Ca exchange, or the transient inward current most often associated with digitalis intoxication. Interpretation of any data obtained in preparations with multiple currents is confounded by the dependence of repolarization on the delicate balance among multiple inward and outward currents. Hence, for example, studies that demonstrate abolition of EADs and/or triggering by any one of a number of sodium channel blockers (tetrodotoxin,[160] lidocaine,[160] mexiletine,[203] tocainide[204]) cannot be interpreted as showing that sodium current is responsible. Rather, sodium current block merely serves to shift the balance of repolarizing currents to the outward direction. Similarly, while low extracellular magnesium (Mg_o) promotes EADs[205] and high Mg_o abolishes them,[206] the mechanism(s) are unclear; high Mg_o may block the slow inward current or reverse the effects of high K_o.[207] Augmentation of outward potassium current(s), as has been reported with a number of potassium channel "activators" such as pinacidil[208] or BRL 34915, may also reverse action potential prolongation, EADs, and triggering induced by drugs such as quinidine.[209]

In most studies, the take-off potential for triggered activity is −60 mV or more positive, making a fast inward sodium current an unattractive mechanism to explain triggering. However, in some of the reported data with cesium, EADs can arise at potentials as low as −80 mV.[188, 210] More data are available to support the idea that the slow inward current may produce the depolarizing upstroke. Aliot et al.[211] reported that D600, a calcium channel antagonist, blocked triggering induced by cesium in Purkinje fibers without shortening action potential duration; as well, arrhythmias induced by cesium in the intact dog were reversed. We found that the action potential–prolonging calcium channel blockers bepridil and lidoflazine frequently produced either very prominent EADs or stable depolarized (−60 mV) membrane potentials when Purkinje fibers were driven at slow stimulation frequencies in low K_o.[212] Interestingly, triggered activity was distinctly uncommon until the preparations were superfused with epinephrine. Similarly, Quantz and Nattel[213] reported that nifedipine blocked quinidine-induced EADs and that subsequent treatment with isoproterenol was sufficient to re-elicit EADs. These data suggest that enhancement of an inward current, most likely the calcium current, by catecholamines can elicit triggered activity when action potentials are prolonged. Moreover, they may provide a link between abnormal repolarization and arrhythmias seen with adrenergic activation in the congenital long QT syndromes: as in the experiments with bepridil, lidoflazine, and quinidine plus nifedipine, patients with congenital long QT syndromes display abnormal repolarization and frequently develop their arrhythmia upon exposure to catecholamines. Higher concentrations of catecholamines in these in vitro studies lead to increased automaticity and shortening of rate-corrected repolarization (possibly due to increased I_K[214]). These latter actions no doubt underlie the efficacy of isoproterenol treatment in torsades de pointes. January et al. elicited EADs and triggered activity using the calcium channel agonist Bay K8644 in sheep Purkinje fibers.[185, 215] In parallel voltage clamp experiments, inward movement of calcium through calcium channels was found to be the most likely explanation. Marban and coworkers[216] compared the pharmacologic behavior of delayed afterdepolarizations elicited by ouabain and early afterdepolarizations and triggering elicited by cesium in ferret papillary muscle. (Interestingly, this is one of the few examples of EAD and triggered activity elicited in ventricular muscle; Sicouri and colleagues[217] recently reported EADs in ventricular muscle following prolonged superfusion with quinidine although triggered activity was absent.) Ryanodine inhibited ouabain-related arrhythmias, whereas verapamil but not ryanodine inhibited cesium-related arrhythmias. These data provide evidence that the cesium-related arrhythmias were not due to calcium-activated calcium release but rather to calcium entry through trans-sarcolemmal channels.

A competing hypothesis for the apparent calcium dependence of triggering is the notion that calcium loading by sodium-calcium exchange, particularly in the presence of prolonged repolarization (e.g., by cesium), can also elicit EADs and triggering.[218] No data are available to definitely exclude either possibility as the source of a transmembrane calcium transient, and both mechanisms may be operative, depending on the experimental situation. Calcium loading may also be involved in changes in monophasic action potential signals seen after valvuloplasty;[219] it has also been reported that such patients occasionally die suddenly. Another interesting possible clinical implication of these studies is the observation by Mason et al.[220] that amiodarone is a potent blocker of both sodium current and calcium current–dependent depolarization-induced automaticity.[221] Hence, the rarity of amiodarone-related torsades de pointes may reflect the drug's ability to block depolarization-induced automaticity arising from EADs. Alternatively, an effect on propagation of EADs from Purkinje to ventricular muscle sites may be important. In summary, although it is apparent that Purkinje fibers whose plateau phase is prolonged develop EADs and triggered activity, the mechanism underlying the triggered activity is not yet clear.

MODELS OF TORSADES DE POINTES IN THE INTACT HEART

Although it is fairly simple to elicit EADs and triggered activity in vitro, the corresponding convincing animal models have been more difficult to develop. When Dessertenne described the arrhythmia, he proposed that its distinctive morphology was related to the presence of multiple pacemakers with similar, but not completely identical, frequencies. Experimental studies have subsequently shown that pacing the heart from two different sites at slightly different frequencies does, indeed, give rise to a morphology similar to torsades de pointes.[222] Similarly, application of aconitine to multiple sites in the quinidine-treated dog heart results in a polymorphic ventricular tachycardia.[223] On the other hand, a number of investigators have described models in which coronary occlusion, intravenous infusion of large doses of quinidine, and rapid ventricular pacing with premature ventricular stimuli elicit modest QT prolongation and polymorphic ventricular tachycardia.[224-226] Although such models may well represent polymorphic ventricular tachycardia based on regional heterogeneity of repolarization, they are probably not sufficiently faithful to the clinical characteristics to the syndrome to allow any inferences on basic mechanisms in patients.

Quinidine does elicit a bradycardia-dependent arrhythmia in the isolated rabbit heart, but only at very slow pacing rates and with low K_o and low Mg_o.[227] Thus, other modulators may play a role if quinidine-associated EADs and triggering are involved as a cause of arrhythmias in vivo. We have noted that EADs and triggering develop much more frequently in isolated false tendons treated with quinidine, as opposed to false tendons whose attachment to papillary muscle has been left intact,[228] suggesting an important Purkinje-muscle interaction in preventing torsades de pointes. On the other hand, several groups have shown that EADs and triggered activity in Purkinje fibers can propagate to ventricular muscle when the two tissue types (Purkinje, muscle) are superfused with different media.[229, 230] These findings, therefore, further suggest that perturbed cell-to-cell coupling may an important modulator of the genesis and propagation of EADs and triggering in vivo.

Arrhythmias possibly related to EADs and triggering have been elicited in the intact dog. Dangman and Hoffman[132] showed that the administration of a large intravenous dose of NAPA to dogs with slow heart rates due to chronic AV block frequently caused arrhythmias, but these tended to be monomorphic. Brachmann et al.[188] showed that intravenous boluses of cesium readily elicited bradycardia-dependent arrhythmias in the intact dog; as with NAPA, the arrhythmias were usually monomorphic, although "typical" torsades de pointes with QT prolongation and antecedent cycle length changes was also reported. The sea anemone toxin APA also appeared to cause early afterdepolarizations in the intact dog.[183] Moreover, both Levine coworkers (using cesium),[231] and El-Sherif and colleagues (using APA),[183] demonstrated EAD-like activity more prominent in endocardial than in epicardial monophasic action potential recordings that was coincident with the development of experimental torsades de pointes, further strengthening the argument that EADs and triggering in an endocardial site (Purkinje) propagated to the remainder of the heart to cause torsades de pointes (Figs. 14–12 and 14–13). The studies with APA also provided evidence that ST/U alternans was attributable to alternans in the endocardial monophasic action potential signal (see Fig. 14–13). These findings provide direct in vivo confirmatory evidence for the hypothesis that the U wave represents Purkinje repolarization that follows ventricular muscle repolarization.[232] Giant inverted T waves may, on the other hand, represent a reversed epicardial-endocardial repolarization gradient.[233] Prominent U waves thus would indicate Purkinje EADs and a risk for associated triggered torsades de pointes. Other reports, using endocardial monophasic action potential signals[19, 139, 140] or filtered bipolar electrograms,[234] have also generated evidence for afterdepolarization-mediated arrhythmias in patients.

Torsades de Pointes: Unanswered Questions

The intense interest at both the clinical and basic levels in mechanisms of action potential control and associ-

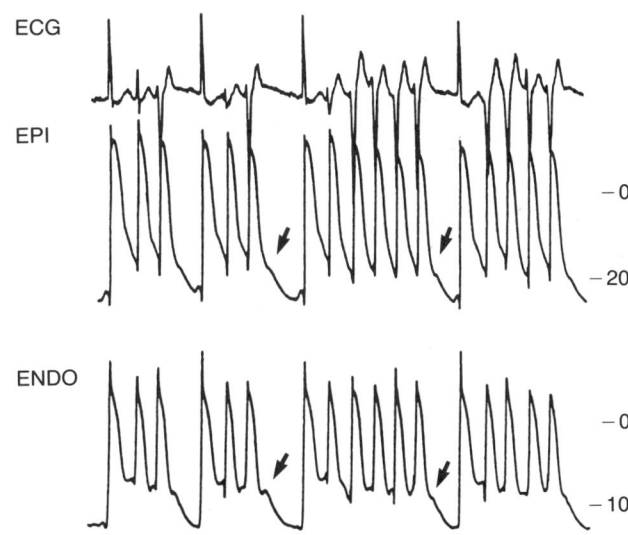

FIGURE 14–12
Endocardial (ENDO) and epicardial (EPI) monophasic action potential recordings from a dog given an intravenous bolus of cesium, an agent that blocks cardiac potassium channels (see text for explanation). The spontaneous ectopic activity that cesium elicits is associated with abnormalities of terminal repolarization (arrows), particularly on the endocardial record, providing evidence for an endocardial origin of "focal" automatic behavior due to cesium. (Reprinted by permission of the authors and the American Heart Association, Inc., from Levine JH, Spear JF, Guarnieri T, et al.: Circulation 72:1092, 1985.)

ated arrhythmias has, as described above, resulted in a range of new and potentially important information. Torsades de pointes is a clinical entity whose mechanism is likely distinct from the usual sustained ventricular tachycardia seen in patients with advanced coronary disease. Research into a number of major unanswered related questions, including those discussed below, may yield fundamental new information which will be important in managing patients with heart disease. These research areas include:

IS THERE A ROLE FOR ABNORMAL REPOLARIZATION IN SUDDEN CARDIAC DEATH FOLLOWING MYOCARDIAL INFARCTION? ■ A number of studies have indicated that even modest prolongation of the QT interval in patients following myocardial infarction identifies those at subsequent risk for sudden death.[235–237] A modestly prolonged QT interval may merely indicate heterogeneity of repolarization, antiarrhythmic drug use, more extensive myocardial damage, and so forth. On the other hand, it is intriguing to speculate that early afterdepolarizations and triggering related to abnormal repolarization may play a role in some ischemic sudden cardiac death. Rhythm strips obtained serendipitously in patients who died suddenly while wearing a Holter monitor frequently show modest QT increases and a short-long-short series of cycle length changes preceding rapid polymorphic ventricular tachycardia (Fig. 14–14); in some series, in fact, the recent initiation of quinidine therapy has been clearly implicated.[238–245] Moreover, recent reports have indicated that canine tissue previously damaged by a coronary occlusion is more susceptible to clofilium-

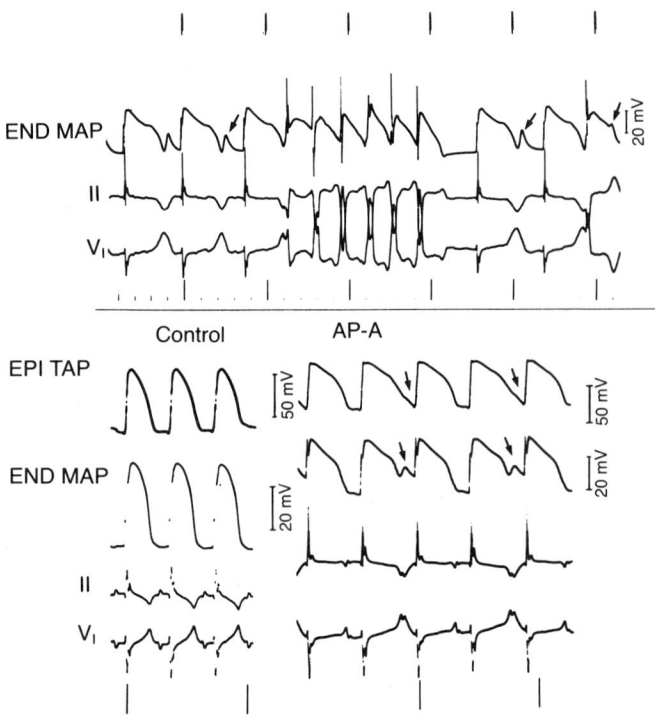

FIGURE 14–13
Endocardial (END) and epicardial (EPI) monophasic action potential recordings from a dog given an intravenous bolus of the sea anemone toxin anthopleurin-A, an agent that interferes with sodium channel inactivation. The top tracings show that, as with the cesium-induced ectopic activity shown in Figure 14–12, APA-induced arrhythmias are preceded by marked abnormalities of endocardial repolarization (arrows). The bottom series of tracings show that when these occur in alternate beats, T-wave alternans, a clinical feature of long QT-related arrhythmias, is recorded. (Reprinted by permission of the authors and the American Heart Association, Inc., from El-Sherif N, Zeiler RH, Craelius W, et al.: Circ Res 63:286, 1988.)

induced EADs and triggering than is normal tissue; triggered activity does propagate from abnormal to normal tissue in this experimental situation.[246] The possibility that even completely "atypical" torsades de pointes (see Fig. 14–1D) or other arrhythmias (e.g., monomorphic ventricular tachycardia in the normal heart[140]) might arise as a result of early afterdepolarizations is one that requires further study.

DOES PERTURBED REPOLARIZATION PLAY A ROLE IN THE SUDDEN INFANT DEATH SYNDROME (SIDS)? ■ Initial reports produced diametrically opposed conclusions as to the potential role for abnormal repolarization in infants with SIDS. Maron et al.[247] found abnormal QT intervals in parents and siblings of infants with SIDS and an abnormal QT interval in one infant with "near miss" SIDS. On the other hand, Kelly and colleagues[248] reported that post-resuscitation electrocardiograms of 21 infants with aborted SIDS were no different from those of control infants. Schwartz and coworkers,[249] in a prospective registry, found that the QT intervals of three infants with SIDS exceeded by 2 to 9 standard deviations those of the control infants. Guntheroth[250] disputed the notion that abnormal control of repolarization could be associated with SIDS, stating that "there is no possibility that the long QT, developmental or genetic, or even arrhythmias, can be a major cause of SIDS." The issue, however, appears unresolved,[251] especially since recent analysis of QT-RR relationships in infants with SIDS strongly suggests intermittently abnormal control of repolarization in some of these infants.[252] Whether this is merely reflective of an underlying defect in autonomic control or whether some SIDS cases might, in fact, be due to arrhythmias, remains uncertain.

WHAT IS THE UNDERLYING MOLECULAR DEFECT IN PATIENTS WITH THE CONGENITAL LONG QT SYNDROMES? ■ Although the genetic locus for the Romano-Ward syndrome has been tentatively localized to chromosome 6,[253] the abnormal protein product that is ultimately responsible for the clinical expression of this disease is unknown. Based on the concepts outlined above, a defect in sodium or calcium channel inactivation or a defect in potassium channel function appear to be the most likely causes. Identification of the abnormal protein product would be of more than passing interest, since screening large kindreds with electrocardiograms or even body surface maps may be insensitive because QT intervals are sometimes normal in afflicted individuals.

WHAT ARE THE ROLES OF THE AUTONOMIC NERVOUS SYSTEM AND OF CELL-TO-CELL COUPLING IN THE GENESIS OF THIS SYNDROME? ■ A considerable body of experimental and clinical data suggests that the autonomic nervous system plays at least a facilitatory

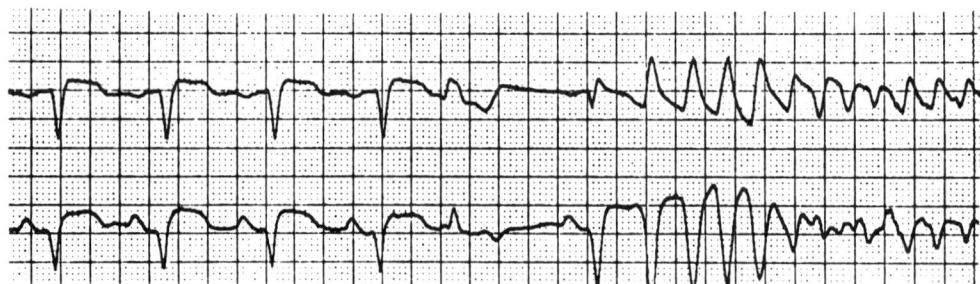

FIGURE 14–14
Routine Holter monitor recording in an ambulatory post-myocardial infarction out-patient who had no cardiac symptoms and was receiving no drugs. A single ventricular ectopic beat is followed by a pause, a sinus beat, and rapid ventricular tachycardia that resulted in the patient's death. This pattern is reminiscent of that seen with "typical" torsades de pointes, although marked QT prolongation is absent. Dispersion of repolarization is, in theory, also maximized by this series of alternating cycles.

role in the genesis of this syndrome. However, the underlying basic mechanisms whereby autonomic perturbations lead to changes in action potential duration and configuration and associated arrhythmias remain unclear. Similarly, if coupling between cells and between cell types is tightly preserved, arrhythmias related to heterogeneity of repolarization should, in theory, be unlikely, whereas if coupling is completely disrupted abnormal rhythms should develop but not propagate. The modulating role of cell-to-cell coupling and the factors that can perturb it, such as digitalis, extracellular calcium, or acidosis,[254] requires further study.

Summary

Studies of the long QT syndrome and its related arrhythmia provide a superb example of a fruitful interplay between basic and clinical electrophysiology. Recognition of the critical clinical features has prompted basic laboratory investigations at a number of levels that will not only be important for the delineation of mechanisms in this syndrome but also may ultimately lead to improved antiarrhythmic therapy.

References

1. Jervell A, Lange-Nielsen F: Congenital deaf-mutism, functional heart disease with prolongation of the Q-T interval and sudden death. Am Heart J 54:59, 1957.
2. Ward OC: A new familial cardiac syndrome in children. J Ir Med Assoc 54:103, 1964.
3. Romano C, Genrme G, Pongiglione R: Aritmie cardiache rare dell'eta pediatrica. Clin Pediatr 45:656, 1963.
4. Dessertenne F: La tachycardie ventriculaire à deux foyers opposés variables. Arch Mal Coeur 59:263, 1966.
5. Tzivoni D, Keren A, Stern S: Torsades de pointes versus polymorphous ventricular tachycardia. Am J Cardiol 52:639, 1983.
6. Soffer J, Dreifus LS, Michelson EL: Polymorphous ventricular tachycardia associated with normal and long Q-T intervals. Am J Cardiol 49:2021, 1982.
7. Roden DM, Thompson KA, Hoffman BF, et al.: Clinical features and basic mechanisms of quinidine-induced arrhythmias. The Proceedings of the 4th Annual Joint US-USSR Symposium on Sudden Cardiac Death. J Am Coll Cardiol 8:73A, 1986.
8. Motte G: True and false Torsade de pointes. Am Heart J 6:1404, 1985.
9. Morvill P, Mauran P, Motte J, et al.: Torsades de pointe foetales et syndrome du QT long. Arch Mal Coeur 78:781, 1985.
10. Southall DP, Arrowsmith WA, Oakley JR, et al.: Prolonged QT interval and cardiac arrhythmias in two neonates: Sudden infant death syndrome in one case. Arch Dis Child 54:776, 1979.
11. Moss AJ, Schwartz PJ, Crampton RS, et al.: The long QT syndrome: A prospective international study. Circulation 71:17, 1985.
12. Motte G, Coumel P, Abitbol G, et al.: Le syndrome QT long et syncopes par "torsades de pointe." Arch Mal Coeur 63:831, 1970.
13. Schwartz PJ: Idiopathic long QT syndrome: Progress and questions. Am Heart J 399, 1985.
14. Vincent JM, Timothy K, Jaiswal D: Disproportionate QT interval lengthening at long cycle lengths in Romano-Ward long QT patients. Circulation 76:SIV-414, 1987.
15. Santinelli V, Chiariello M: Heart rate acceleration without changes in the QT interval and severe ventricular tachyarrhythmias: A variant of the long QT syndrome? Int J Cardiol 4:69, 1983.
16. Levine JH, Luke R, Veltri EP, et al.: Proarrhythmia: A manifestation of latent long QT syndrome? Circulation 76:SIV-415, 1987.
17. Schwartz PJ, Malliani A: Electrical alternation of the T-wave: Clinical and experimental evidence of its relationship with the sympathetic nervous system and with the long QT syndrome. Am Heart J 89:45, 1975.
18. Sharma S, Nair KG, Gadekar HA: Romano-Ward prolonged QT syndrome and intermittent T wave alternans and atrioventricular block. Am Heart J 100:500, 1981.
19. Bonatti V, Finardi A, Botti G: Enregistrement des potentiels d'action monophasiques du ventricule droit dans un cas de QT long et alternance isolée de l'onde U. Arch Mal Coeur 72:1180, 1979.
20. Webb CL, Dick M, Rocchini AP, et al.: Quinidine syncope in children. J Am Coll Cardiol 9:1031, 1987.
21. Jackman WM, Clark M, Friday KJ, et al.: Ventricular tachyarrhythmias in the long QT syndrome. Med Clin North Am 68:1079, 1984.
22. Nguyen PT, Scheinman MM, Seger J: Polymorphous ventricular tachycardia: Clinical characterization, therapy, and QT interval. Circulation 74:340, 1986.
23. Kay GN, Plumb VJ, Arciniegas JG, et al.: Torsades de pointes: The long-short initiating sequence and other clinical features: Observations in 32 patients. J Am Coll Cardiol 2:806, 1983.
24. Bauman JL, Bauernfeind RA, Hoff JV, et al.: Torsades de pointes due to quinidine: Observations in 31 patients. Am Heart J 107:425, 1984.
25. Roden DM, Woosley RL, Primm RK: Incidence and clinical features of the quinidine-associated long QT syndrome: Implications for patient care. Am Heart J 111:1088, 1986.
26. Ejvinsson G, Orinius E: Prodromal ventricular premature beats preceded by a diastolic wave. Acta Med Scand 208:445, 1980.
27. Sarmiento JJ, Shea PM, Goldberger AL: Unusual ventricular depolarizations associated with torsade de pointes. Am Heart J 109:377, 1985.
28. Fontaine G, Frank R, Lascault G, et al.: Torsades de pointes favorisées par stimulations ventriculaires à rythme lent. Arch Mal Coeur 8:918, 1983.
29. Steinbrecher UP, Fitchett DH: Torsades de pointes: A cause of syncope with atrioventricular block. Arch Intern Med 140:1223, 1980.
30. Vincent GM: The heart rate of Romano-Ward syndrome patients. Am Heart J 112:61, 1986.
31. Crampton R: Preeminence of the left stellate ganglion on the long QT syndrome. Circulation 59:769, 1979.
32. Duff HJ, Roden DM, Reele SB, et al.: The electrophysiologic actions of high dose propranolol in man. J Am Coll Cardiol 2:1134, 1983.
33. Browne KF, Zipes DP, Heger JJ, et al.: Influence of the autonomic nervous system on the Q-T interval in man. Am J Cardiol 50:1099, 1982.
34. Milne JR, Ward DE, Spurrell AJ, et al.: The long QT syndrome: Effects of drugs and left stellate ganglion block. Am Heart J 104:194, 1982.
35. Mitsutake A, Takeshita A, Kuroiwa A, et al.: Usefulness of the valsalva maneuver in management of the long QT syndrome. Circulation 63:1029, 1981.
36. Vaughan Williams EM, Hassan MO, Floras JS, et al.: Adaptation of hypertensives to treatment with cardioselective and non-selective beta-blockers: Absence of correlation between bradycardia and blood pressure control, and reduction in slope of the QT/RR relation. Br Heart J 44:473, 1980.
37. Ahnve S, Vallin H: Influence of heart rate and inhibition of autonomic tone on the QT interval. Circulation 65:435, 1982.
38. Edvardsson N, Olsson SB: Induction of delayed repolarization during chronic beta-receptor blockade. Eur Heart J 6(Suppl D):163, 1985.
39. Echt DS, Kopelman HA, Lee JT, et al.: Control mechanisms for QT interval in man. Circulation 74:SII-401, 1986.
40. Sundaram MBM, McMeekin JD, Gulamhusein S: Cardiac tachyarrhythmias in hereditary long QT syndromes presenting as a seizure disorder. Can J Neurol Sci 13:262, 1986.

41. Keren A, Tzivoni D, Gavish D, et al.: Etiology, warning signs and therapy of torsade de pointes. Circulation 64:1167, 1981.
42. Khan MM, Logan KR, McComb JM, et al.: Management of recurrent ventricular tachyarrhythmias associated with Q-T prolongation. Am J Cardiol 47:1301, 1981.
43. Sclarovsky S, Strasberg B, Lewin RF, et al.: Polymorphous ventricular tachycardia: Clinical features and treatment. Am J Cardiol 44:339, 1979.
44. Smith WM, Gallagher JJ: "Les Torsades de Pointes": An unusual ventricular arrhythmia. Ann Intern Med 93:578, 1980.
45. Curry P, Stubbs W, Fitchett D, et al.: Ventricular arrhythmias and hypokalemia. Lancet 1:231, 1976.
46. Forfar JC, Gribbin B: Torsade de pointes after amiodarone withdrawal; effects of mild hypokalaemia on repolarization. Eur Heart J 5:510, 1984.
47. McKibbin JK, Pocock WA, Barlow JB, et al.: Sotalol, hypokalaemia, syncope, and torsade de pointes. Br Heart J 51:157, 1984.
48. Moro C, Romero J, Peiretti MAC: Amiodarone and hypolemia. A dangerous combination. Int J Cardiol 13:365, 1986.
49. Prandota J, Iwanczak F: Long Q-T syndrome precipitated by atropine and hypokalemia. Dev Pharmacol Ther 6:356, 1983.
50. Ramee SR, White CJ, Svinarich JT, et al.: Torsade de pointes and magnesium deficiency. Am Heart J 109:164, 1985.
51. Redleaf PD, Lerner IJ: Thiazide-induced hypokalemia with associated major ventricular arrhythmias: Report of a case and comment on therapeutic use of bretylium. JAMA 608:1302, 1968.
52. Hust MH, Nitsche K, Hohnloser S, et al.: Q-T prolongation and torsades de pointes in a patient with subarachnoid hemorrhage. Clin Cardiol 7:44, 1984.
53. Otteni JC, Pottecher T, Bronner G, et al.: Prolongation of the Q-T interval and sudden cardiac arrest following right radical neck dissection. Anesthesiology 59:358, 1983.
54. Rudehill A, Sundqvist K, Sylven C: QT and QT-peak interval measurements. A methodological study in patients with subarachnoid haemorrhage compared to a reference group. Clin Physiol 6:23, 1986.
55. Mehta D, Warwick GL, Goldberg MJ: QT prolongation after ampicillin anaphylaxis. Br Heart J 55:308, 1986.
56. McComb JM, Campbell NPS, Cleland J: Recurrent ventricular tachycardia associated with QT prolongation after mitral valve replacement and its association with intravenous administration of erythromycin. Am J Cardiol 54:922, 1984.
57. Freedman RA, Anderson KP, Green LS, et al.: Effect of erythromycin on ventricular arrhythmias and ventricular repolarization in idiopathic long QT syndrome. Am J Cardiol 59:168, 1987.
58. Lopez JA, Harold JG, Rosenthal MC, et al.: QT prolongation and torsades de pointes after administration of trimethoprim-sulfamethoxazole. Am J Cardiol 59:376, 1987.
59. Wharton JM, Demopulos PA, Goldschlager N: Torsade de pointes during administration of pentamidine isethionate. Am J Med 83:571, 1987.
60. Young JB, Vandermolen LA, Pratt CM: Torsade de pointes: An unusual manifestation of chloral hydrate poisoning. Am Heart J 112:181, 1986.
61. Aldariz AE, Romero H, Baroni M, et al.: QT prolongation and torsade de pointes ventricular tachycardia produced by ketanserin. PACE 9:836, 1986.
62. Probucol and the QT interval (Letter). Lancet 1:1179, 1982.
63. Abinader EG, Shahar J: Possible female preponderance in prenylamine-induced "torsade de pointes" tachycardia. Cardiology 70:37, 1983.
64. Bender KS, Shematek JP, Leventhal BG, et al.: QT interval prolongation associated with anthracycline cardiotoxicity. J Ped 105:442, 1984.
65. James MA, Culling W, Jones JV: Polymorphous ventricular tachycardia due to α-blockade. Int J Cardiol 14:225, 1987.
66. Bryer-Ash M, Zehnder J, Angelchik P, et al.: Torsades de pointes precipitated by a Chinese herbal remedy. Am J Cardiol 60:1186, 1987.
67. Liberatore MA, Robinson DS: Torsade de pointes: A mechanism for sudden death associated with neuroleptic drug therapy? J Clin Psychopharmacol 4:143, 1984.
68. Kemper AJ, Dunlap R, Pietro DA: Thioridazine-induced torsades de pointes: Successful therapy with isoproterenol. JAMA 249:2931, 1983.
69. Herrmann HC, Kaplan LM, Bierer BE: Q-T prolongation and torsades de pointes ventricular tachycardia produced by the tetracyclic antidepressant agent maprotiline. Am J Cardiol 51:904, 1983.
70. Rainey Jr JM, Pohl RB, Bilolikar SG: The QT interval in drug-free depressed patients. J Clin Psychiatry 43:39, 1982.
71. Ludomirsky A, Klein HO, Sarelli P, et al.: Q-T prolongation and polymorphous ("torsades de pointes") ventricular arrhythmias associated with organophosphorus insecticide poisoning. Am J Cardiol 49:1654, 1982.
72. Isner JM, Sours HE, Paris AL, et al.: Sudden, unexpected death in avid dieters using the liquid-protein-modified-fast diet. Circulation 60:1401, 1979.
73. Siegel RJ, Cabeen WR, Jr. Roberts, WC: Prolonged QT interval-ventricular tachycardia syndrome from massive rapid weight loss utilizing the liquid-protein-modified-fast diet: Sudden death with sinus node ganglionitis and neuritis. Am Heart J 102:121, 1981.
74. Frank S, Colliver JA, Frank A: Low-energy diets and prolonged QT intervals. JAMA 257:1601, 1987.
75. Isner JM, Roberts WC, Heymsfield SB, et al.: Anorexia nervosa and sudden death. Ann Intern Med 102:49, 1985.
76. Moss AJ: Caution: Very low-calorie diets can be deadly. Ann Intern Med 102:121, 1985.
77. Schmidinger H, Weber H, Zwiauer K, et al.: Potential life-threatening cardiac arrhythmias associated with a conventional hypocaloric diet. Int J Cardiol 14:55, 1987.
78. Smith RF, Harthorne JW, Sanders CA: Vectorcardiographic changes during intracoronary injections. Circulation 36:63, 1967.
79. Lehmann MH, Case RB: Reduced human ventricular fibrillation threshold associated with contrast-induced Q-T prolongation. J Electrocardiol 16:105, 1983.
80. Zukerman LS, Friehling TD, Wolf NM, et al.: Effect of calcium-binding additives on ventricular fibrillation and repolarization changes during coronary angiography. J Am Coll Cardiol 10:1249, 1987.
81. Evans TR, Curry PVL, Fitchett DH, et al.: "Torsade de pointes" initiated by electrical ventricular stimulation. J Electrocardiol 9:255, 1976.
82. Chung EK: Principles of Cardiac Arrhythmias, 3rd ed. p. 744. Baltimore, Williams & Wilkins, 1983.
83. Bissett JK, Watson JW, Scovil JA, et al.: Sudden death in cardiomyopathy: Role of bradycardia-dependent repolarization changes. Am Heart J 99:625, 1980.
84. Fung AY, Kerr CR, Maybee TK: QT prolongation and torsades de pointes: The sole manifestation of coronary artery disease. Int J Cardiol 7:63, 1985.
85. Griffin J, Most AS: Torsades de pointes complicating acute myocardial infarction. Am Heart J 107:169, 1984.
86. Mallion J-M, Avezou F, Denis B, et al.: Syndrome de QT long avec torsades de pointe, syncopes et insuffisance coronarienne. Arch Mal Coeur 65:1209, 1971.
87. Forssell G, Orinius E: QT prolongation and ventricular fibrillation in acute myocardial infarction. Acta Med Scand 210:309, 1981.
88. Grenadier E, Alpan G, Maor N, et al.: Polymorphous ventricular tachycardia in acute myocardial infarction. Am J Cardiol 53:1280, 1984.
89. James TN, Froggatt P, Atkinson WJ, et al.: Observations on the pathophysiology of the long QT syndromes with special reference to the neuropathology of the heart. Circulation 57:1221, 1978.
90. Neuvonen PJ, Elonen E, Vuorenmaa T, et al.: Prolonged Q-T interval and severe tachyarrhythmias, common features of sotalol intoxication. Eur J Clin Pharmacol 20:85, 1981.
91. Bazett HC: An analysis of the time relationship of the electrocardiogram. Am Heart J 7:353, 1920.
92. Ahnve S: Correction of the QT interval for heart rate: Review of different formulas and the use of Bazett's formula in myocardial infarction. Am Heart J 109:568, 1985.
93. Brown MA, Smith WM, Lubbe WF, et al.: Amiodarone-induced torsades de pointes. Eur Heart J 7:234, 1986.
94. Leroy G, Haiat R, Barthelemy M, et al.: Torsades de pointes during loading with amiodarone. Eur Heart J 8:541, 1987.

95. Sclarovsky S, Lewin RF, Kracoff O, et al.: Amiodarone-induced polymorphous ventricular tachycardia. Am Heart J 105:6, 1983.
96. Bashour T, Jokhadar M, Cheng TO: Effective management of the long Q-T syndrome with amiodarone. Chest 79:704, 1981.
97. Fredlund BO, Olsson SB: Long QT interval and ventricular tachycardia of "torsades de pointe" type in hypothyroidism. Acta Med Scand 213:231, 1983.
98. Hanslik R, Kaspar L, Kroiss A, et al.: Myxodem als ursache eines QT-syndroms und rezidivierender kammertachykardien. Kardiol 76:58, 1987.
99. Pechter RA, Osborn LA: Polymorphic ventricular tachycardia secondary to hypothyroidism. Am J Cardiol 57:882, 1986.
100. Selzer A, Wray HW: Quinidine syncope: Paroxysmal ventricular fibrillation occurring during treatment of chronic atrial arrhythmias. Circulation 30:17, 1964.
101. Jenzer HR, Hagemeijer F: Quinidine syncope: torsades de pointes with low quinidine plasma concentrations. Eur J Cardiol 4:447, 1976.
102. Koenig W, Schinz AM: Spontaneous ventricular flutter and fibrillation during quinidine medication. Am Heart J 105:863, 1983.
103. Seaton A: Quinidine-induced paroxysmal ventricular fibrillation treated with propranolol. Brit Med J 1:1522, 1966.
104. Koster RW, Wellens HJJ: Quinidine-induced ventricular flutter and fibrillation without digitalis therapy. Am J Cardiol 38:519, 1976.
105. Lown B, Wolf M: Approaches to sudden death from coronary heart disease. Circulation 44:130, 1971.
106. Radford MD, Evans DW: Long-term results of DC reversion of atrial fibrillation. Br Heart J 30:91, 1968.
107. Nicholson WJ, Martin CE, Gracey JG, et al.: Disopyramide-induced ventricular fibrillation. Am J Cardiol 43:1053, 1979.
108. Riccioni N, Castiglioni M, Bartolomei C: Disopyramide-induced QT prolongation and ventricular tachyarrhythmias. Am Heart J 105:870, 1983.
109. Wald RW, Waxman MB, Colman JM: Torsade de pointes ventricular tachycardia: a complication of disopyramide shared with quinidine. J Electrocardiol 14:301, 1981.
110. Strasberg B, Sclarovsky S, Erdberg A, et al.: Procainamide-induced polymorphous ventricular tachycardia. Am J Cardiol 47:1309, 1981.
111. Chow MJ, Piergies AA, Bowsher DJ, et al.: Torsade de pointes induced by N-acetylprocainamide. J Am Coll Cardiol 4:621, 1984.
112. Herre JM, Thompson JA: Polymorphic ventricular tachycardia and ventricular fibrillation due to N-acetyl procainamide. Am J Cardiol 55:227, 1985.
113. Olshansky B, Martins J, Hunt S: N-acetyl procainamide causing torsades de pointes. Am J Cardiol 50:1439, 1982.
114. Stratmann HG, Walter KE, Kennedy HL: Torsade de pointes associated with elevated N-acetylprocainamide levels. Am Heart J 109:375, 1985.
115. Kontopoulos A, Manoudis F, Filindris A, et al.: Sotalol-induced torsade de pointes. Postgrad Med J 57:321, 1981.
116. Kuck KH, Kunze KP, Roewer N, et al.: Sotalol-induced torsade de pointes. Am Heart J Jan:179, 1986.
117. Laakso M, Pentikainen PJ, Rehnberg S: Sotalol-induced prolongation of the Q-T interval and attacks of unconsciousness. Int J Clin Pharmacol Ther Toxicol 22:487, 1984.
118. Scagliotti D, Strasberg B, Hai HA, et al.: Aprindine-induced polymorphous ventricular tachycardia. Am J Cardiol 49:1297, 1982.
119. Chabanier A, Delforge J, Blanc P, et al.: Torsade de pointe du bepridil. Therapie 38:701, 1983.
120. LeClercq JF, Kural S, Valere PE: Bepridil et torsades de pointes. Arch Mal Coeur 76:341, 1983.
121. Manouvrier J, Sagot M, Caron C, et al.: Nine cases of torsade de pointes with bepridil administration. Am Heart J 111:1005, 1986.
122. Kennelly BM: Comparison of lidoflazine and quinidine in prophylactic treatment of arrhythmias. Br Heart J 39:540, 1977.
123. Barbey JT, Thompson KA, Echt DS, et al.: Antiarrhythmic activity, electrocardiographic effects and pharmacokinetics of the encainide metabolites O-desmethyl encainide and 3-methoxy-O-desmethyl encainide in man. Circulation 77:380, 1988.
124. Maisuls E, Lorber A: Quinidine-induced torsade de pointes suppressed by paroxysmal atrial fibrillation. Int J Cardiol 16:315, 1987.
125. Clark M, Friday K, Anderson J, et al.: Drug induced torsades de pointes: High concordance rate among type IA antiarrhythmic drugs and amiodarone. J Am Coll Cardiol 5:450, 1985.
126. Juliard JM, Heckle J, Jaillon P, et al.: Comparison of the cardiac electrophysiologic effects of quinidine, 3-hydroxyquinidine and 3-hydroxyhydroquinidine in the anesthesized dog. Study of plasma dose response relations. Arch Mal Coeur 76:670, 1983.
127. Thompson KA, Blair IA, Woosley RL, et al.: Comparative electrophysiologic effects of quinidine, its major metabolites and dihydroquinidine in canine cardiac Purkinje fibers. J Pharm Exp Ther 241:84, 1987.
128. Thompson KA, Murray JJ, Blair IA, et al.: Plasma concentrations of quinidine its major active metabolites, and dihydroquinidine in patients with torsades de pointes. Clin Pharmacol Ther 43:636, 1988.
129. Neuvonen PJ, Elonen E, Tanskanen A, et al.: Sotalol prolongation of the QTc interval in hypertensive patients. Clin Pharmacol Ther 32:25, 1982.
130. Wang T, Bergstrand RH, Siddoway LA, et al.: Concentration dependent pharmacologic properties of sotalol. Am J Cardiol 57:1160, 1985.
131. Friday KJ, Jackman WM, Lee IK, et al.: Torsades de pointes on sotalol: incidence and unique clinical features. Circulation 76:SIV-368, 1987.
132. Dangman KH, Hoffman BF: In vivo and in vitro antiarrhythmic and arrhythmogenic effects of N-acetyl procainamide. J Pharmacol Exp Ther 217:851, 1981.
133. Jaillon P, Winkle RA: Electrophysiologic comparative study of procainamide and N-acetylprocainamide in anesthetized dogs: concentration-response relationships. Circulation 60:1385, 1979.
134. Jaillon P, Rubenson D, Peters F, et al.: Electrophysiologic effects of N-acetylprocainamine in human beings. Am J Cardiol 47:1134, 1981.
135. Horowitz LN, Greenspan AM, Spielman SR, et al.: Torsades de pointes: electrophysiologic studies in patients without transient pharmacologic or metabolic abnormalities. Circulation 63:1120, 1981.
136. Bhandari AK, Shapiro WA, Morady F, et al.: Electrophysiologic testing in patients with the long QT syndrome. Circulation 71:63, 1985.
137. Hartzler GO, Osborn MJ: Invasive electrophysiological study in the Jervell and Lange-Nielsen syndrome. Br Heart J 45:225, 1981.
138. Hiejima K, Suzuki F, Satake S, et al.: Electrophysiologic studies of Jervell, Lange-Nielsen syndrome. Chest 79:446, 1981.
139. Gavrilescu S, Luca C: Right ventricular monophasic action potentials in patients with long QT syndrome. Br Heart J 40:1014, 1978.
140. Levine JH, Merillat JC, Singer I, et al.: Ventricular tachycardia in patients without underlying structural heart disease: evidence for triggered activity in humans. J Am Coll Cardiol 11:113a, 1988.
141. De Ambroggi L, Bertoni T, Locati E, et al.: Mapping of body surface potentials in patients with the idiopathic long QT syndrome. Circulation 74:1334, 1986.
142. DiSegni E, Klein HO, David D, et al.: Overdrive pacing in quinidine syncope and other long QT-interval syndromes. Arch Intern Med 140:1036, 1980.
143. Bansal AM, Kugler JD, Pinsky WW, et al.: Torsade de pointes: Successful acute control by lidocaine and chronic control by tocainide in two patients—one each with acquired long QT and the congenital long QT syndrome. Am Heart J 112:618, 1986.
144. Shah A, Schwartz H: Mexiletine for treatment of torsade de pointes. Am Heart J 107:589, 1984.
145. Perticone F, Adinolfi L, Bonaduce D: Efficacy of magnesium sulphate in the treatment of torsade de pointes. Am Heart J 112:847, 1986.
146. Tzivoni D, Banai S, Schugar C, et al.: Treatment of torsade de pointes with magnesium sulfate. Circulation 77:392, 1988.
147. Toivonen LK, Leinonen H: Limited effect of magnesium

sulphate on torsades de pointes ventricular tachycardia. Int J Cardiol 12:260, 1986.
148. Schwartz PJ, Locati E: The idiopathic long QT syndrome: Pathogenetic mechanisms and therapy. Eur Heart J 6:103, 1985.
149. Moss AJ, McDonald J: Unilateral cervicothoracic sympathetic ganglionectomy for the treatment of long QT interval syndrome. N Engl J Med 285:903, 1971.
150. Bhandari AK, Scheinman MM, Morady F, et al.: Efficacy of left cardiac sympathectomy in the treatment of patients with the long QT syndrome. Circulation 70:1018, 1984.
151. Eldar M, Griffin JC, Abbott JA, et al.: Permanent cardiac pacing in patients with the long QT syndrome. J Am Coll Cardiol 10:600, 1987.
152. DiSegni E, David D, Katzenstein M, et al.: Permant overdrive pacing for the suppression of recurrent ventricular tachycardia in a newborn with long QT syndrome. J Electrocardiol 13:189, 1980.
153. Echt DS, Armstrong K, Schmidt P, et al.: Clinical experience, complications, and survival in 70 patients with the automatic implantable cardioverter/defibrillator. Circulation 71:289, 1985.
154. DeSilvey DL, Moss AJ: Primidone in the treatment of the long QT syndrome: QT shortening and ventricular arrhythmia suppression. Ann Intern Med 93:53, 1980.
155. Schwartz PJ: The idiopathic long Q-T syndrome. Ann Intern Med 99:561, 1983.
156. Coumel P, Leclercq J-F, Lucet V: Possible mechanisms of the arrhythmias in the long QT syndrome. Eur Heart J 6:115, 1985.
157. Kuo CS, Reddy CP, Munakata K, et al.: Mechanism of ventricular arrhythmias caused by increased dispersion of repolarization. Eur Heart J 6:63, 1985.
158. Cranefield PF: Action potentials, afterpotentials, and arrhythmias. Circ Res 41:415, 1977.
159. Strauss HC, Bigger JT, Hoffman BF: Electrophysiological and beta-receptor blocking effects of MJ 1999 on dog and rabbit cardiac tissue. Circ Res 26:661, 1970.
160. Roden DM, Hoffman BF: Action potential prolongation and induction of abnormal automaticity by low quinidine concentrations in canine Purkinje fibers: Relationship to potassium and cycle length. Circ Res 56:857, 1985.
161. Damiano BP, Rosen MR: Effects of pacing on triggered activity induced by early afterdepolarizations. Circulation 69:1013, 1984.
162. Singh BN, Vaughan Williams EM: A third class of antiarrhythmic action. Effects on atrial and ventricular intracellular potentials, and other pharmacological actions on cardiac muscle, of MJ 1999 and AH 3747. Br J Pharmacol 39:675, 1970.
163. Williams EMV: QT and action potential duration. Br Heart J 47:513, 1982.
164. Williams EMV: Delayed ventricular repolarization as an antiarrhythmic principle. Eur Heart J 6:145, 1985.
165. Roden DM, Woosley RL: Antiarrhythmic effects of QT prolongation. Am Heart J 109:411, 1985.
166. Bacaner MB, Clay JR, Shrier A, et al.: Potassium channel blockade: a mechanism for suppressing ventricular fibrillation. Proc Natl Acad Sci USA 83:2223, 1985.
167. Echt DS, Black JN, Barbey JT, Coxe DR, Cato E: Evaluation of antiarrhythmic drugs on defibrillation energy requirements in dogs: Sodium channel block and action potential prolongation. Circulation 79:1106, 1989.
168. Surawicz B, Knoebel SB: Long QT: Good, bad or indifferent? J Am Coll Cardiol 4:398, 1984.
169. Sakmann B, Trube G: Conductance properties of single inwardly rectifying potassium channels in ventricular cells from guinea-pig heart. J Physiol 347:641, 1984.
170. Noble D, Tsien RW: Outward membrane currents activated in the plateau range of potentials in cardiac Purkinje fibres. J Physiol (Lond) 200:205, 1969.
171. McDonald TF, Trautwein W: The potassium current underlying delayed rectification in cat ventricular muscle. J Physiol 274:217, 1978.
172. Bennett PB, McKinney LC, Kass RS, et al.: Delayed rectification in the calf cardiac Purkinje fiber: Evidence for multiple state kinetics. Biophys J 48:553, 1985.
173. Gintant GA, Datyner NB, Cohen IS: Gating of delayed rectification in acutely isolated canine cardiac Purkinje myocytes: Evidence for a single voltage-gated conductance. Biophys J 48:1059, 1985.
174. Litovsky SH, Antzelevitch C: Transient outward current prominent in canine ventricular epicardium but not endocardium. Circ Res 62:116, 1988.
175. Yue DT, Marban E: A novel cardiac potassium channel that is active and conductive at depolarized potentials. Biophys J 53:641a, 1988.
176. Kameyama M, Kakei M, Sato R, et al.: Intracellular Na^+ activates a K^+ channel in mammalian cardiac cells. Nature 309:354, 1984.
177. Noma A: ATP-regulated K^+ channels in cardiac muscle. Nature 305:147, 1983.
178. Isenberg G, Vereecke J, van der Heyden G, et al.: The shortening of the action potential by DNP in guinea-pig ventricular myocytes is mediated by an increase of a time-independent K conductance. Pflugers Arch 397:251, 1983.
179. Sakmann B, Noma A, Trautwein W: Acetylcholine activation of single muscarinic K^+ channels in isolated pacemaker cells of the mammalian heart. Nature 303:250, 1983.
180. Gadsby DV, Cranefield PF: Two levels of resting potential in cardiac Purkinje fibers. J Gen Physiol 70:725, 1977.
181. Brown B: Early afterdepolarizations induced by batrachotoxin: Possible involvement of a sodium current. Fed Proc 42, 1983.
182. Swain HH, McCarthy DA: Veratrine, protoveratrine and andromedotroxin arrhythmias in the isolated dog heart. J Pharmacol Exp Ther 121:379, 1957.
183. El-Sherif N, Zeiler RH, Craelius W, et al.: QTU prolongation and polymorphic ventricular tachyarrhythmias due to bradycardia-dependent early afterdepolarizations. Circ Res 63:286, 1988.
184. Craelius W, Chen VKH, El-Sherif N: Sodium current modifications by anthropleurin-A and their role in early afterdepolarizations. J Am Coll Cardiol 11:253a, 1988.
185. January CT, Riddle JM, Salata JJ: A model for early afterdepolarizations: induction with the Ca^{2+} channel agonist Bay K 8644. Circ Res 62:563, 1988.
186. Scholtysik G, Williams FM: Antiarrhythmic effects of DPI 201–106. Br J Pharmacol 89:287, 1986.
187. Isenberg G: Cardiac Purkinje fibers: Cesium as a tool to block inward rectifying potassium currents. Pfluegers Arch 365:99, 1976.
188. Brachmann J, Scherlag BJ, Rosenshtraukh LV, et al.: Bradycardia-dependent triggered activity: relevance to drug-induced multiform ventricular tachycardia. Circulation 68:846, 1983.
189. Colatsky TJ: Mechanisms of action of lidocaine and quinidine on action potential duration in rabbit cardiac Purkinje fibers. Circ Res 50:17, 1982.
190. Hiraoka M, Sawada K, Kawano S: Effects of quinidine on plateau currents of guinea-pig ventricular myocytes. J Mol Cell Cardiol 18:1097, 1986.
191. Salata JJ, Wasserstrom JA: Effects of quinidine on action potentials and ionic currents in isolated canine ventricular myocytes. Circ Res 62:324, 1988.
192. Roden DM, Bennett PB, Snyders DJ, et al.: Quinidine delays I_K activation in guinea pig myocytes. Circ Res 62:1055, 1988.
193. Imaizumi Y, Giles WR: Quinidine-induced inhibition of transient outward current in cardiac muscle. Am J Physiol 253:H704, 1987.
194. Sato R, Hisatome I, Wasserstrom JA, et al.: Quinidine blocks the inward-rectifier K^+ channel (IK_1) from the inside of the membrane in guinea pig ventricular myocytes. Biophys J 53:642a, 1988.
195. Carmeliet E: Electrophysiologic and voltage clamp analysis of the effects of sotalol on isolated cardiac muscle and Purkinje fibers. J Pharmacol Exp Ther 232:817, 1985.
196. Balser JR, Hondeghem LM, Roden DM: Amiodarone reduces time dependent I_K activation. Circulation 76:SIV-150, 1987.
197. Sato R, Hisatome I, Singer DH: Amiodarone blocks the inward-rectifier K^+ channel in guinea pig ventricular myocytes. Circulation 76:SIV-150, 1987.
198. Snyders DJ, Katzung BG: Clofilium reduces the plateau potassium current in isolated cardiac myocytes. Circulation 72:SIII-233, 1985.
199. Arena JP, Kass RS: Pharmacological dissection of two heart K

channels: the inward rectifier and the delayed rectifier. Biophys J 51:367a, 1987.
200. Coraboeuf E, Deroubaix E, Coulombe A: Acidosis-induced abnormal repolarization and repetitive activity in isolated dog Purkinje fibers. J Physiol (Paris) 76:97, 1980.
201. Marchese AC, Hill JA, Xie P, et al.: Electrophysiologic effects of amiloride in canine Purkinje fibers: Evidence for a delayed effect on repolarization. J Pharmacol Exp Ther 232:485, 1985.
202. Duff HJ, Mitchell LB, Kavanaugh KM, et al.: Amiloride: Electropharmacologic actions in patients with sustained ventricular tachycardia. Circulation 76:SIV-174, 1987.
203. Roden DM, Iansmith DHS, Woosley RL: Frequency-dependent interactions of mexiletine and quinidine in canine cardiac Purkinje fibers. J Pharm Exp Ther 243:1218, 1987.
204. Valois M, Sasyniuk BI: Modification of the frequency- and voltage-dependent effects of quinidine when administered in combination with tocainide in canine Purkinje fibers. Circulation 76:427, 1987.
205. Roden DM, Iansmith DHS: Effects of low potassium or magnesium concentrations on isolated cardiac tissue. Am J Med 82:18, 1987.
206. Kaseda S, Gilmour RF Jr, Zipes DP: Magnesium abolishes early afterdepolarizations induced by cesium, 4-aminopyridine or quinidine in canine Purkinje fibers. J Am Coll Cardiol 11:254a, 1988.
207. Kraft LF, Katholi RE, Woods WT, et al.: Attenuation by magnesium of the electrophysiologic effects of hyperkalemia on human and canine heart cells. Am J Cardiol 45:1189, 1980.
208. Arena JP, Kass RS: Pinacidil, a putative K-channel agonist, enhances K-sensitive current in isolated guinea pig ventricular cells. Biophys J 53:461a, 1988.
209. Fish FA, Roden DM: *In vitro* and *in vivo* antiarrhythmic effects of K$^+$ channel activators in altered repolarization. Submitted, 62nd annual Scientific Sessions, American Heart Association, 1989.
210. Szabo B, Sweidan RR, Scherlag BJ, et al.: Cesium-induced late-coupled, triggered action potentials in Purkinje fibers. J Am Coll Cardiol 7:52A, 1986.
211. Aliot E, Szabo B, Sweiden R, et al.: Prevention of torsades de pointes with calcium channel blockade in an animal model. J Am Coll Cardiol 5:492, 1985.
212. Campbell RM, Woosley RL, Roden DM: Lack of early afterdepolarizations despite phase 3 repolarization abnormalities due to bepridil and lidoflazine. Circulation 72:SIII-381, 1985.
213. Quantz MA, Nattel S: The ionic mechanism for quinidine-induced early afterdepolarizations. Circulation 74:SII-420, 1986.
214. Bennett PB, McKinney LC, Begenisich T, et al.: Adrenergic modulation of the delayed rectifier potassium channel in calf cardiac Purkinje fibers. Biophys J 49:839, 1986.
215. January CT, Riddle JM: Early afterdepolarizations and Ca^{++}. Circulation 76:SIV-473, 1987.
216. Marban E, Robinson SW, Weir WG: Mechanisms of arrhythmogenic delayed and early afterdepolarizations and triggered activity in vivo. J Clin Invest 78:1185, 1986.
217. Sicouri S, Sitovsky S, Krishnan S, et al.: Quinidine-induced early afterdepolarizations (EAD) in canine ventricular muscle. Circulation 76:SIV-150, 1988.
218. Szabo B, Patterson E, Scherlag B, et al.: Early afterdepolarizations induced by Ca$^+$ are dependent on intra- and extracellular [Ca^{2+}] and [Na$^+$]. Circulation 76:SIV-115, 1987.
219. Martin GR, Stanger P: Transient prolongation of the QTc interval after balloon valvuloplasty and angioplasty in children. Am J Cardiol 58:1233, 1986.
220. Mason JW, Hondeghem LM, Katzung BG: Block of inactivated sodium channels and of depolarization-induced automaticity in guinea pig papillary muscle by amiodarone. Circ Res 55, 1984.
221. Grant AO, Katzung BG: The effects of quinidine and verapamil on electrically induced automaticity in the ventricular myocardium of guinea pig. J Pharmacol Exp Ther 196:407, 1976.
222. D'Alnoncourt CN, Zierhut W, Luderitz B: "Torsades de pointes" tachycardia: Re-entry or focal activity? Br Heart J 48:213, 1982.
223. Leichter DA, Danilo P, Rosen T, et al.: Torsades de pointes induced by aconitine and quinidine in the canine heart. Circulation 74:SII-349, 1986.
224. Bardy GH, Ungerleider RM, Smith WM, et al.: A mechanism of torsades de pointes in a canine model. Circulation 64:52, 1983.
225. Inoue H, Murakawa Y, Toda I, et al.: Epicardial activation patterns of torsades de pointes in canine hearts with quinidine-induced long QT interval but without myocardial infarction. Am Heart J 111:1080, 1986.
226. Inoue H, Matsuo H, Mashima S, et al.: Effects of atrial pacing, isoprenaline and lignocaine on experimental polymorphous ventricular tachycardia. Cardiovasc Res 18:538, 1984.
227. Roden DM, Arthur M, Woosley RL: Bradycardia-dependent triggered activity in the intact heart. J Am Coll Cardiol 5:390, 1985.
228. Balser JR, Roden DM: Inhibitory effect of ventricular muscle on induction of early afterdepolarizations in canine false tendons. Clin Res, 35:260A, 1987.
229. Mendez C, Delmar M: Triggered activity: Its possible role in cardiac arrhythmias. *In* Zipes D, Jalife J, eds: Cardiac Electrophysiology and Arrhythmias, pp. 311–313. New York, Grune & Stratton, 1985.
230. Kupersmith J, Hoff P: Occurrence and transmission of localized repolarization abnormalities in vitro. J Am Coll Cardiol 6:152, 1985.
231. Levine JH, Spear JF, Guarnieri T, et al.: Cesium chloride–induced long QT syndrome: Demonstration of afterdepolarizations and triggered activity in vivo. Circulation 72:1092, 1985.
232. Watanabe Y: Purkinje repolarization as a possible cause of the U wave in the electrocardiogram. Circulation 51:1030, 1975.
233. Higuchi T, Nakaya Y: T wave polarity related to the repolarization process of epicardial and endocardial ventricular surfaces. Am J Cardiol 108:290, 1984.
234. Schechter E, Freeman CC, Lazzara R: Afterdepolarizations as a mechanism for the long QT syndrome: Electrophysiologic studies of a case. J Am Coll Cardiol 3:1556, 1984.
235. Schwartz PJ, Wolf S: QT interval prolongation as a predictor of sudden death in patients with myocardial infarction. Circulation 56:1074, 1978.
236. Ahnve S, Gilpin E, Madsen EB, et al.: Prognostic importance of QT$_c$ interval at discharge after acute myocardial infarction: a multicenter study of 865 patients. Am Heart J 108:395, 1984.
237. Wheelan K, Murharji J, Rude RE, et al.: Sudden death and its relation to QT-interval prolongation after acute myocardial infarction: Two-year follow-up. Am J Cardiol 57:745, 1986.
238. Denes P, Gabster A, Huang SK: Clinical, electrocardiographic and follow-up observations in patients having ventricular fibrillation during Holter monitoring. Am J Cardiol 48:9, 1981.
239. Kempf FC Jr, Josephson ME: Cardiac arrest recorded on ambulatory electrocardiograms. Am J Cardiol 53:1577, 1984.
240. Lewis BH, Antman EM, Graboys TB: Detailed analysis of 24 hour ambulatory electrocardiographic recordings during ventricular fibrillation or torsades de pointes. J Am Coll Cardiol 2:426, 1983.
241. Nikolic G, Bishop RL, Singh JB: Sudden death recorded during Holter monitoring. Circulation 66:218, 1982.
242. Panidis IP, Morganroth J: Sudden death in hospitalized patients: Cardiac rhythm disturbances detected by ambulatory electrocardiographic monitoring. J Am Coll Cardiol 2:798, 1983.
243. Pool J, Kunst K, Van Wermeskerken JL: Two monitored cases of sudden death outside hospital. Br Heart J 40:627, 1978.
244. Savage HR, Kissane JQ, Becher EL, et al.: Analysis of ambulatory electrocardiograms in 14 patients who experienced sudden cardiac death during monitoring. Clin Cardiol 10:621, 1987.
245. Brembilla-Perrott B, Taggeddine R, Rebmann JP, et al.: Morts subites au cours d'un enregistrement Holter. Presse Med 31:103, 1987.
246. Gough WB, Hu D, El-Sherif N: Effects of clofilium on ischemic subendocardial Purkinje fibers 1 day postinfarction. J Am Coll Cardiol 11:431, 1988.
247. Maron BJ, Clark CE, Goldstein RE, et al.: Potential role of QT interval prolongation in sudden infant death syndrome. Circulation 54:423, 1976.
248. Kelly DH, Shannon DC, Liberthson RR: The role of the QT interval in the sudden infant death syndrome. Circulation 55:633, 1977.

249. Schwartz PJ, Montemerlo M, Facchini M, et al.: The QT interval throughout the first 6 months of life: A prospective study. Circulation 66:496, 1982.
250. Guntheroth WG: Editorial: The QT interval and sudden infant death syndrome. Circulation 66:502, 1982.
251. Schwartz PJ: The quest for the mechanisms of the sudden infant death syndrome: Doubts and progress. Circulation 75:677, 1987.
252. Sadeh D, Shannon DC, Abboud S, et al.: Altered cardiac repolarization in some victims of sudden infant death syndrome. N Engl J Med 317:1501, 1987.
253. Itoh S, Munemura S, Satoh H: A study of the inheritance pattern of Romano-Ward syndrome. Clin Pediatr 21:20, 1982.
254. Spray DC, White RL, Mazet F, et al.: Regulation of gap junctional conductance. Am J Physiol 249:H753, 1985.

15

Tachycardia in Infants

Paul C. Gillette
Fred A. Crawford Jr
Bertrand A. Ross
Vicki Zeigler
David Buckles
Mark Harold

Tachycardias are the most frequent dysrhythmias occurring in infants and children. They are subdivided in the same manner as in adults (i.e., into supraventricular and ventricular),[1,2] and their mechanisms are the same (i.e., reentry and automaticity).[3] The presentation, natural history, diagnostic evaluation, and treatment are somewhat different for adults than for infants and children. In this chapter we stress the care of infants with tachydysrhythmias, based primarily on our own experience. We define infancy as the age of 1 month through 12 months. We include fetal and neonatal tachycardias because of their importance and because they often lead into infantile tachycardias, and shall differentiate between paroxysmal and incessant tachycardias.

Clinical Presentation

In infants tachycardias usually present nonspecifically. Poor feeding, tachypnea, cyanosis, and respiratory distress are the most frequent symptoms. Occasionally the tachycardia is detected by a physician performing a routine physical examination. Rarely, tachycardia in infants presents as a cardiac arrest or shock (Fig. 15–1). This should always be kept in mind, and all shock in infants should not be assumed to be "sepsis." By the time the patient is resuscitated, the tachycardia may have temporarily stopped. The patient may show ECG activity typical of the Wolff-Parkinson-White (WPW) syndrome or a short P-R interval with normal QRS on the sinus rhythm ECG (Fig. 15–2). Patients who had ventricular tachycardia may still show premature ventricular contractions (PVCs). Thus, in an infant who presents with shock or cardiac arrest, close observation of the ECG and long-term monitoring are indicated.[4]

Tachycardias are frequently detected during routine monitoring in fetuses and neonates. In the fetus, signs of congestive heart failure may also be detected echocardiographically as cardiomegaly, scalp edema, or ascites. Fetuses and neonates may show marked changes in intra-atrial shunting during tachycardia. Cyanosis may be the presenting sign in neonates and may in some ways mimic cyanotic congenital heart disease.[5] Tachyarrhythmias in infants may be precipitated or exacerbated by respiratory infections or by the medications used to treat them. Extra observation is warranted during these episodes.

The clinical presentation of infantile tachycardia may be that of near-miss sudden infant death syndrome (SIDS). We have reported one case of ventricular tachycardia presenting as near-miss SIDS.[6]

Mechanisms

Ventricular tachycardia (VT) may be either reentrant or automatic. We have found each mechanism in infants, and they are about equally distributed. Most VT in infants becomes incessant.

Supraventricular tachycardias (SVTs) have a larger variety of mechanisms. They also can be classified as reentrant or automatic. Automatic tachycardias may occur in the right or left atrium or His bundle. Atrial automatic tachycardias occur rarely in neonates and infants,[7] and their rates are often only moderately high (170–210 bpm). They often do not cause heart failure.

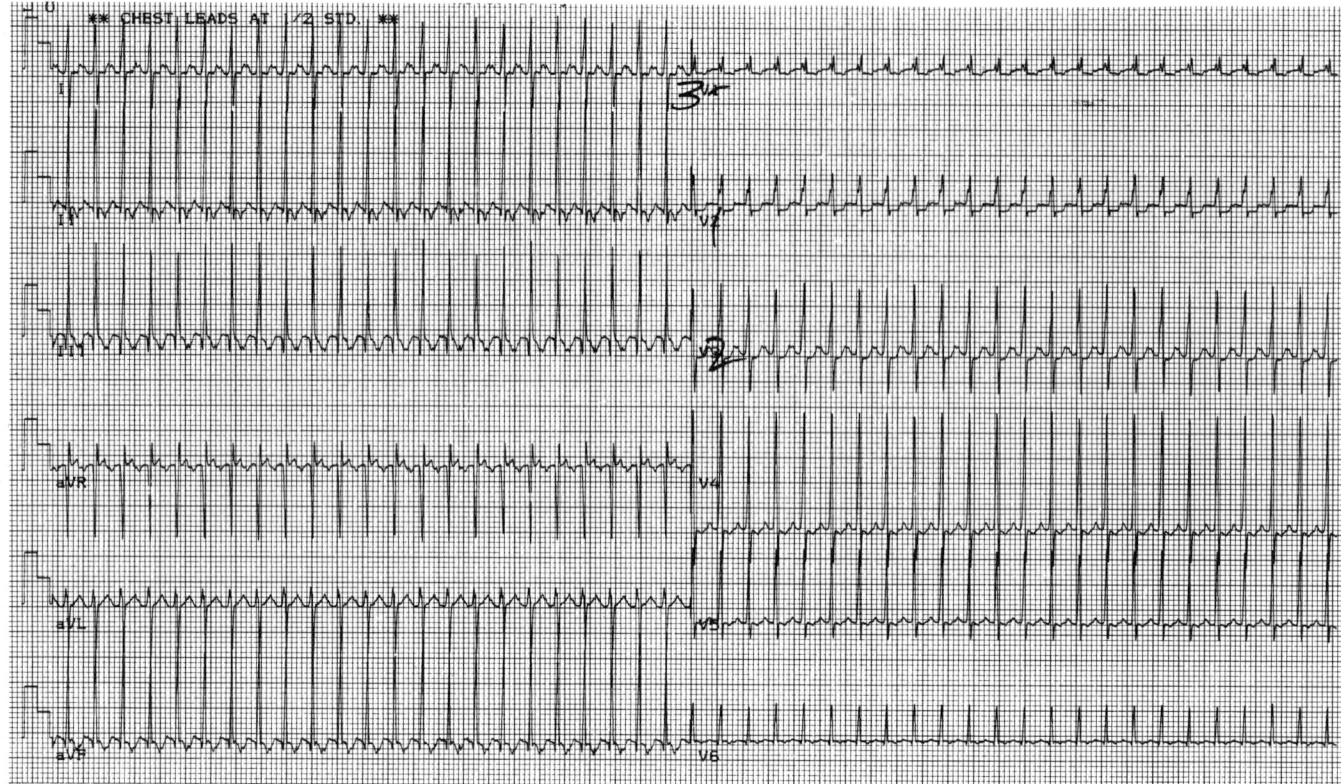

FIGURE 15–1
Twelve-lead surface ECG of an infant during supraventricular tachycardia. The rate is approximately 230 bpm. A clear negative P wave can be seen in lead 2, and it can be seen to begin negatively and then positively in lead 1. Because of the QRS-P relationship, it can be estimated with a high degree of probability that this tachycardia is due to accessory connection. Because of the P-wave morphology, it can be suspected that the accessory connection is posterior septal.

As opposed to atrial automatic tachycardias in teenagers, in whom automatic tachycardias rarely disappear spontaneously, infantile automatic tachycardias often stop within a number of months. Junctional automatic tachycardias often have very high rates with a high incidence of congestive heart failure and death.[8] Not only the rate but also the atrioventricular (AV) dissociation lead to myocardial dysfunction and death. Death may also result from sudden, complete AV block caused by an initially irritative lesion in the His bundle, which becomes destructive. Antiarrhythmic medications may suppress the escape focus.[9]

Reentrant SVTs in infants are most often due to accessory connections (Fig. 15–3).[10, 11] The accessory connection makes up the retrograde limb of the reentry circuit, and the AV node and His bundle make up the antegrade limb.[12] Since almost all accessory connections have rapid conduction, the function of the AV node is the variable most likely to influence the tachycardia rate. We have noted an association between the presence of a left free-wall accessory connection and enhanced AV node function.[13] Thus, patients with left-sided accessory connections whether manifest or concealed tend to have rapid tachycardias and to be more symptomatic. Approximately 50% of infants with SVT will be found to have manifest WPW syndrome activity on sinus rhythm surface ECG. Most of the remaining 50% probably have concealed accessory connections, based on both intracardiac and esophageal electrophysiologic studies. Patients with right-sided concealed accessory connections tend to have incessant tachycardias, whereas those with concealed left-sided pathways tend to have paroxysmal but very rapid tachycardias. Patients with slow-conducting posterior septal accessory pathways also tend to have incessant tachycardias. The sites of accessory connections in children are more evenly distributed than in adults. Right free-wall, left free-wall, and septal pathways each account for about one third of accessory connections. Multiple accessory connections make up less than 10% of accessory connections in pediatric patients. Multiple accessory connections often present as wide QRS tachycardia, due to the fact that the reentry circuit in these patients often involves antegrade conduction over one pathway and retrograde over the other. Atrial flutter or fibrillation associated with WPW syndrome may rarely lead to a wide QRS tachycardia in infants.

More than 90% of the time, a wide QRS tachycardia in an infant will be due to ventricular tachycardia.[1] Aberration due to bundle branch block rarely occurs persistently in infants (Fig. 15–4) and children, although it often occurs transiently at the onset of tachycardia. If a patient is being treated with a type I drug, particularly a type IC drug such as flecainide, bundle branch block aberrations will occur frequently.

Atrial muscle reentry tachycardia (atrial flutter) is a frequent mechanism of SVT in infancy[14] and may occur in infants with either normal or abnormal hearts. It is

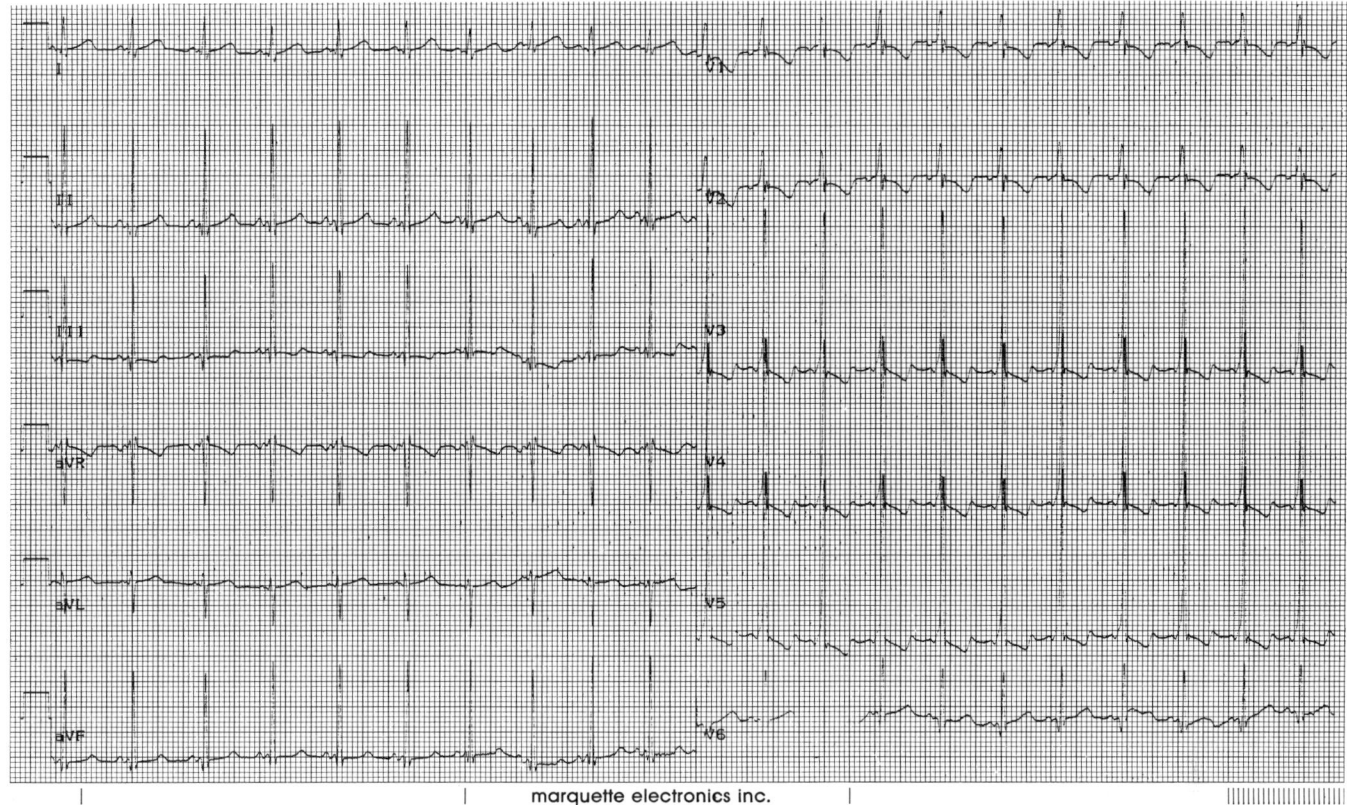

FIGURE 15-2
Twelve-lead ECG of an infant with Wolff-Parkinson-White syndrome. The delta waves are most prominent in leads V_3, V_4, and V_5 but are also prominent in V_1. The delta waves are subtle in the limb leads but can be seen well in the surface lead 2.

particularly frequent in patients after atrial surgery for transposition of the great arteries and less frequent in patients following surgery for atrial septal defect or anomalous venous return.[15] Infants with normal hearts often have a transient atrial flutter that may degenerate into chaotic atrial rhythm. These rhythms are thought to represent atrial reentry. Chaotic atrial rhythm bridges the gap between atrial flutter and atrial fibrillation.

Evaluation

The evaluation of an infant with a tachycardia should be comprehensive. Congenital heart disease or either primary or secondary cardiomyopathy are found more often in infants with tachycardia than in the general population. Complete cardiac history and physical examination should be performed. Extracardiac causes of tachycardia, including hyperthyroidism and medications, should be considered. An electrocardiogram both during tachycardia and during sinus rhythm should be obtained. In general, it is not acceptable to treat a tachycardia without performing an ECG during the tachycardia. Although SVTs make up the majority of pediatric tachycardias, VTs are not rare. The two can only be differentiated by electrocardiography. If a patient's tachycardia is transient, ambulatory monitoring and/or transtelephonic monitoring should be used before treatment is initiated.

Echocardiography should be performed during the initial evaluation of all infant with tachycardia. This will detect both occult congenital heart defects and abnormalities of myocardial function. A chest x-ray is usually part of the initial evaluation. Intracardiac elec-

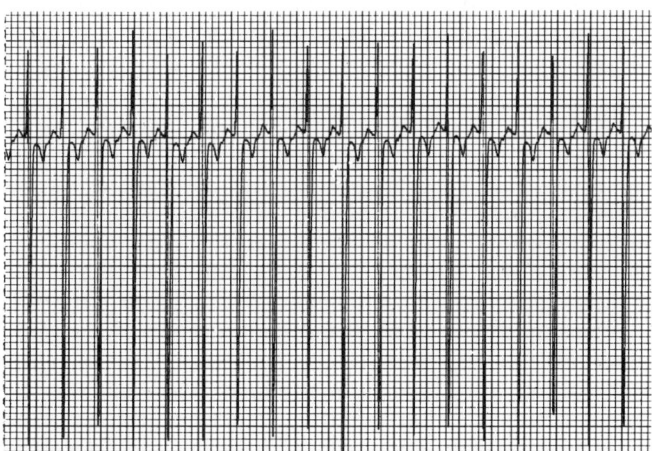

FIGURE 15-3
Surface ECG lead 2 of an infant with supraventricular tachycardia. The rate is approximately 270 bpm. Negative P waves can be seen following the QRS complex in a location suggestive of an accessory connection. The positive sharp spikes are probably T waves. A mild ST-segment depression is present.

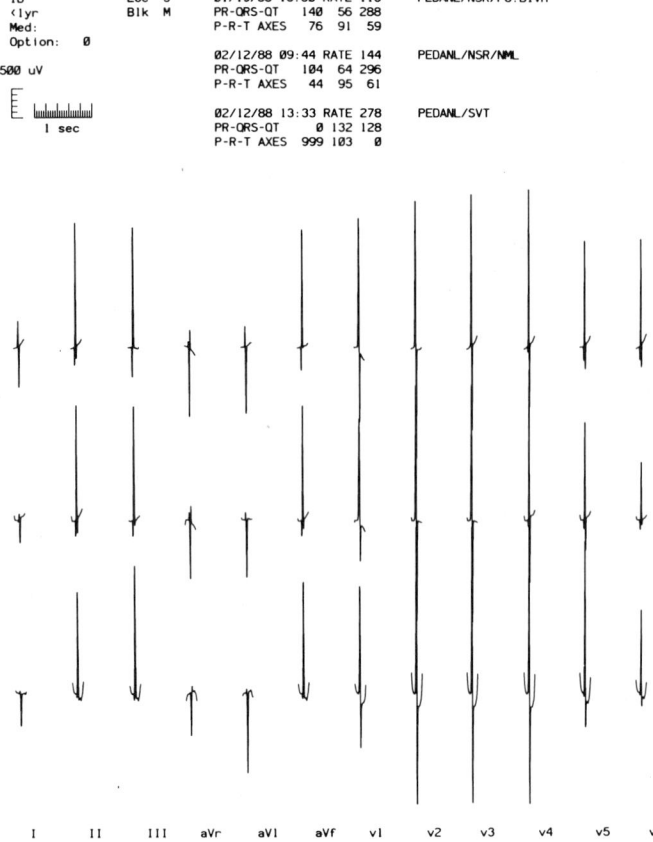

FIGURE 15–4
Three surface ECGs showing patient QRS complexes only during sinus rhythm in the top two tracings and supraventricular tachycardia in the bottom tracing. This demonstrates the nearly identical QRS complexes during sinus rhythm and during supraventricular tachycardia. Note also the marked ST-segment depression during tachycardia at a rate of 278 bpm.

trophysiologic testing is not part of a routine initial evaluation. In infants, it can be expected that if treatment is effective, a substantial percentage of patients may outgrow their tachycardia.

TACHYCARDIAS AND CARDIOMYOPATHIES

In recent years we have found that both SVT and VT may lead to chronic cardiomyopathies.[16] It takes days to years to develop a cardiomyopathy. The degree of cardiomyopathy depends on several factors, including the rate and duration of tachycardia, the presence or absence of a normal P-R interval during tachycardia, and the presence and degree of associated heart disease.

Thus VT with ventriculoatrial dissociation or an inappropriately long P-R interval due to rapid retrograde conduction and a rate of 300 beats per minute (bpm) could result in the development of a large dilated heart within several hours. A patient with an atrial tachycardia rate of 150 bpm with a normal P-R interval will take years to develop a detectable cardiomyopathy. The rapidity of recovery seems to be related to the severity of the cardiomyopathy and the duration of tachycardia. A tachycardia-related cardiomyopathy that develops within hours to days will often return to normal just as quickly if sinus rhythm resumes. On the other hand, a cardiomyopathy that develops over a period of years may take as long as a year to recover. The biochemical mechanism of tachycardia-related cardiomyopathy is unknown. We have yet to see a patient in whom the tachycardia was cured whose myocardium has not returned to normal. Both surgical and medical treatment of the tachycardia have been effective in returning myocardial function to normal.

Certain mechanisms of tachycardias are most likely to result in cardiomyopathy. The chronicity of tachycardia is the most important. Incessant VT and junctional ectopic, automatic tachycardias are the most frequent causes of tachycardia-related cardiomyopathy in infants. Atrial automatic tachycardias and those due to concealed accessory pathways also tend to cause cardiomyopathy. The cause of tachycardia-related cardiomyopathy is unknown. Chronic myocardial ischemia as is often seen on the surface ECG may be partly responsible (Fig. 15–4).

Treatment

The treatment of tachycardias in infants may be divided into medical and surgical. Each requires an understanding of the physiology and mechanisms of tachycardias.

INITIAL TREATMENT

The initial treatment of a tachycardia in an infant requires differentiation of SVT from VT. In an infant with SVT, the QRS complex is absolutely normal. Often retrograde P waves may be seen. VT is characterized by an abnormal but often not very wide QRS complex (Fig. 15–5).[17] There may be retrograde P waves or AV dissociation. The most common mistake made is the misdiagnosis of VT as SVT.

Ventricular Tachycardia (VT)

An algorithm outlining therapy for VT is shown in Figure 15–6. If VT is diagnosed and the patient is very stable, 1 mg/kg of xylocaine intravenously may be used. Procainamide, 15 mg/kg intravenously over 1 hour, may also be used. If procainamide is given too rapidly, hypotension will result. If an infant with VT is even slightly unstable, then synchronized DC cardioversion is the treatment of choice. This is also the case if the above medical treatment fails. The best way to cardiovert is to use adhesive pads in the anterior posterior position. Pediatric-size paddles are appropriate. The proper initial dose of electricity is 0.25 W·S/kg. If cardioversion converts the tachycardia for 1 or 2 beats and it resumes, then further cardioversion will also likely prove futile. Medication should then be given as above, and the cardioversion should be repeated. Intravenous phenytoin, 15 mg/kg over 1 hour,

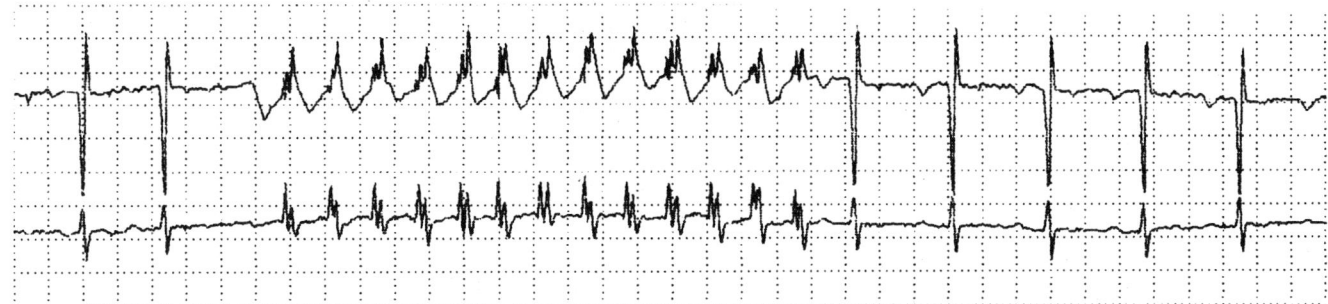

FIGURE 15–5
The patient is an infant with ventricular tachycardia. Shown are two simultaneously recorded surface ECGs from an ambulatory monitor showing a paroxysm of nonsustained ventricular tachycardia at a rate of 265 bpm. In this instance, the degree of abnormality of the surface ECG makes it easy to distinguish this ventricular tachycardia from supraventricular tachycardia.

is occasionally useful but has the same or greater hypotensive effects as procainamide. Intravenous propranolol, 0.1 mg/kg over 10 to 15 minutes, may be given, but temporary pacing (either transvenous or transcutaneous) must be available. Bretylium, 5 mg/kg intravenously, may rarely be effective but may worsen the arrhythmia or cause hypotension.

Volume expansion with saline or plasmanate is the best initial treatment for hypotension secondary to antiarrhythmic drug therapy. Dopamine may be used short-term but may increase the tachycardia rate.

Digitalis-induced VT or fibrillation is a special case. Digitalis antibody fragments (Digibind) are a specific treatment. Phenytoin and propranolol are also relatively specific for digitalis-induced arrhythmias. In this situation, as with other ventricular arrhythmias, maintenance of a normal serum potassium level is very important. Although cardioversion is more likely to cause secondary arrhythmias in digitalis-toxic patients, it is sometimes necessary.

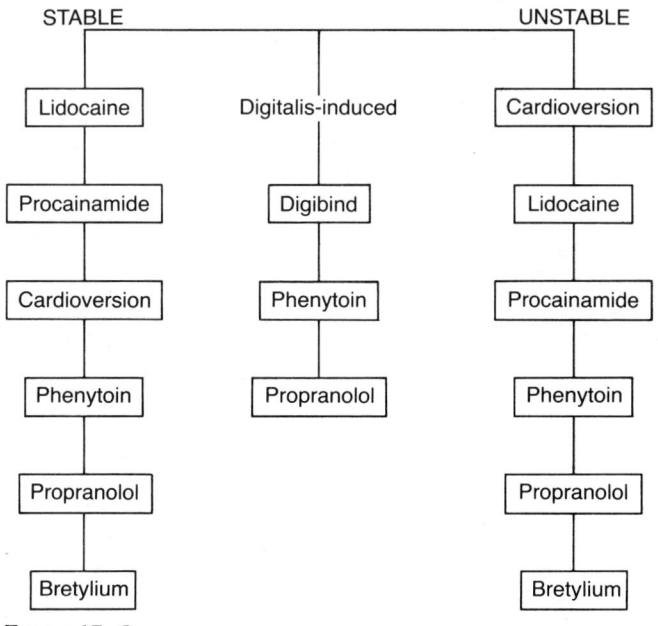

FIGURE 15–6
Algorithm for management of ventricular tachycardia in infants.

Supraventricular Tachycardia (SVT)

Figure 15–7 outlines general strategy for management of infants with SVT. Infants with a completely normal QRS complex during tachycardia may be treated as having SVT. If there is any question, it is better to treat for VT.

In very stable infants with SVT, the diving reflex may be used. This involves an ice bag application to the facial area. This therapy is not recommended for unstable infants who may decompensate due to the increased afterload this causes. Intravenous verapamil should never be given to infants, because the infantile myocardium is very sensitive to the negative inotropic effects of this drug, and cardiovascular collapse occurs all too often when verapamil is given to infants.[18] It has been proposed that pretreatment with calcium will prevent this problem, but the conditions under which this was tested were different than those when verapamil was given without calcium.

When the diving reflex fails, we use synchronized DC cardioversion as our primary treatment. The dose of electricity is 0.25 W·S/kg, best applied through adhesive pads. Resuscitation equipment must be available. Overdrive pacing through an esophageal electrode is an acceptable alternative. It is imperative that this procedure be carried out in the same setting and with the same resuscitation equipment as cardioversion.

We do not use intravenous digoxin or propranolol as first-line drugs in treating SVT. Digoxin is effective in greater than 50% of cases but it may take hours to be effective, and the patient may deteriorate during that period. Also, if digoxin fails, cardioversion may carry a greater danger of ventricular fibrillation. If the patient has WPW syndrome, and the SVT degenerates into atrial flutter or fibrillation, a rapid ventricular response may occur. Furthermore, digoxin may lower the ventricular fibrillation threshold. Intravenous beta-blockers may also be dangerous in patients in compensated congestive heart failure. The compensation is partially due to increased adrenergic agonists, and blocking their effect may lead to congestive heart failure and cardiovascular collapse.

If cardioversion fails, or if it is successful and tachycardia rapidly resumes, then procainamide or digoxin

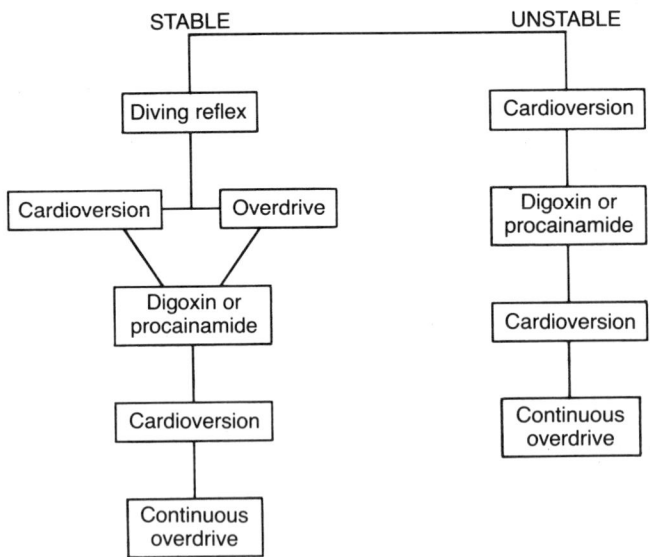

FIGURE 15–7
Algorithm for management of supraventricular tachycardia in infants.

may be given. We make this choice based on the patient's clinical status and ventricular function. If signs and symptoms of congestive heart failure are present, digoxin is used; if the patient is well compensated, procainamide is used.

In extremely critical situations when cardioversion and initial drugs fail, continuous overdrive pacing from the esophagus or right atrium may be used. If the patient has SVT with a rate of 250 bpm, and overdrive pacing is carried out at 300 bpm with 2:1 AV block, the ventricular rate will be 150 bpm. Although this restores blood pressure and cardiac output, it will lead to atrial dilatation. Paired pacing or rapid ventricular pacing may also temporarily control SVT symptoms.[19, 20]

CHRONIC TREATMENT

Supraventricular Tachycardia (SVT)

Once SVT has been converted, the question to be answered is whether WPW syndrome is present. This usually will not be known while the patient is in SVT, since the QRS is usually normal in SVT. If WPW syndrome is seen on a 12-lead ECG in sinus rhythm, digoxin should be avoided, since it may lead to sudden death in 2 to 4% of infants.[21] The speculated mechanism is described in the preceding section. Since most pediatric cardiologists may never see 50 infants with WPW syndrome, it has not been well recognized that digoxin can be dangerous.

Propranolol is a useful and effective alternative to digoxin for patients with WPW syndrome.[22] The fact that it has to be given four times a day is not a major problem because infants must be fed more often. Infants taking propranolol should be watched carefully for myocardial decompensation. For patients without manifest WPW syndrome (including those with concealed WPW syndrome) digoxin is a very effective treatment. For electrophysiologic effects, larger doses and higher serum concentration are required than those believed to be necessary for hemodynamic effect. Serum digoxin levels of 1.5 to 2 ng/ml are usual, and digoxin therapy should not be discontinued until these levels are achieved.

Verapamil given orally is safe and effective. The oral form does not lead to cardiovascular collapse, as does the intravenous form. We often try verapamil, 3 to 5 mg/kg/day in three divided doses, if digoxin and propranolol fail. We decrease the dose of digoxin and add verapamil to replace propranolol.

If digoxin, propranolol, and verapamil fail, we use a type IC drug such as flecainide or encainide. Flecainide has the advantage of twice-a-day dosing. These drugs have proved very effective in treating infants with SVT and VT. Flecainide is less effective against atrial flutter, but encainide may be effective.

Type IA drugs such as quinidine and procainamide are finding less favor for treatment of SVT because of their cardiac and noncardiac side effects. Serious ventricular arrhythmias and sudden death have been reported. Quinidine has frequent gastrointestinal side effects, and procainamide may cause lupus erythematosus. Amiodarone, a powerful but potentially toxic antiarrhythmic drug, is very effective in infants.

NONPHARMACOLOGIC THERAPY

Although implanted pacemakers may be used to treat infants with SVT, their size makes this difficult. Infants

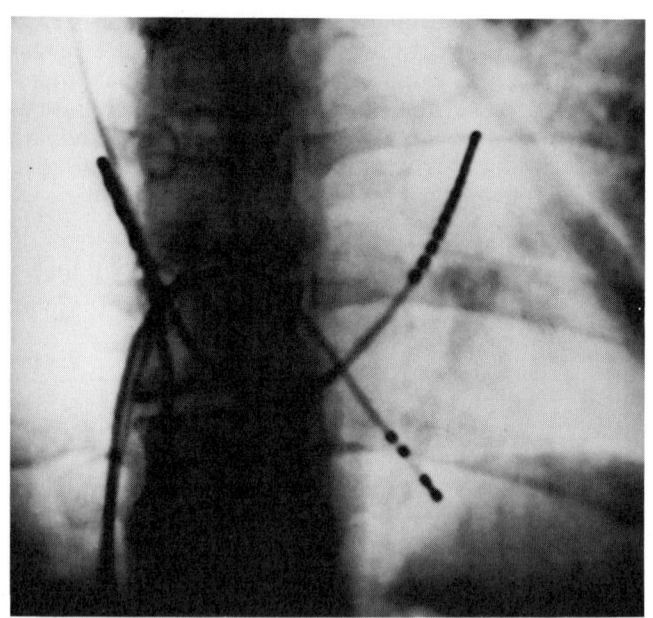

FIGURE 15–8
Demonstration of catheter position for pediatric supraventricular tachycardia study. Four catheters are positioned in the heart (one from the left arm into the coronary sinus with 1-mm electrode spacing), in this instance, mapping the distal coronary sinus including the lateral wall, the left atrium, and the posterior lateral wall left of the atrium. The remaining three catheters are positioned from the right femoral vein, with one quadripolar catheter in the right ventricular apex, the second quadripolar catheter in the right atrial appendage, and a tripolar catheter across the tricuspid valve for recording the low septal right atrium and His bundle potentials.

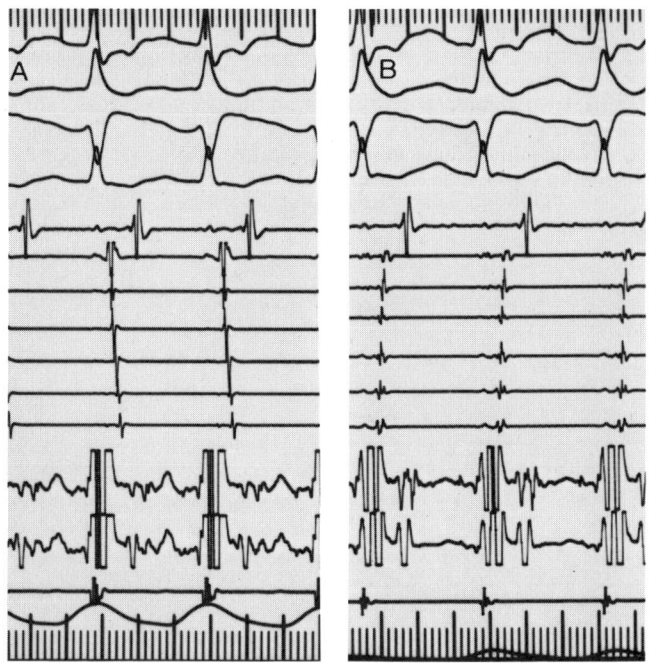

FIGURE 15–9
Two electrophysiology tracings from a patient with supraventricular tachycardia due to a left-sided accessory connection. Shown are simultaneously recorded surface ECG leads 1, AVF, V_1, and V_6; high right atrium; 6 bipolar coronary sinuses, 2 His bundles, and 1 right ventricular apex recording; and femoral artery blood pressure. A, This tracing was taken with the catheter position in the proximal coronary sinus; thus the distal (top) pair of coronary sinus electrodes was recording the earliest depolarization retrograde during supraventricular tachycardia. The tracing shown in B was taken with the catheter position more distally in the coronary sinus, with the proximal pair of electrodes in the catheter recording the earliest retrograde activation during supraventricular tachycardia.

with a postoperative bradycardia-tachycardia syndrome are the best candidates for atrial antitachycardia pacing.

Direct surgical treatment of supraventricular and ventricular tachycardias has been carried out successfully in infants and children. Before direct surgical therapy is considered, the exact mechanism of tachycardia must be defined. This is accomplished by intracardiac electrophysiologic studies (Figs. 15–8 and 15–9). Although SVT in most infants can be controlled medically, a few cases cannot. Some infants tolerate SVT poorly, and these are surgical candidates. In 1987 we successfully divided right and left free-wall and septal accessory connections using temporary cardiopulmonary bypass in infants as young as 3 months of age. The youngest child we have operated on for AV node reentry was 4 years of age. The technique of surgically treating AV node reentry would be difficult but not impossible in an infant.

Many cases of infantile VT are caused by small myocardial tumors. These tumors are usually invisible by all common techniques, but direct mapping and inspection will detect the tumors. They may be multiple and often are in areas which are inappropriate for excision. We currently use cryoablation for tumor removal in all but the best candidates for resection.

Incessant VT may present as near-miss SIDS. It is also frequently misdiagnosed as SVT, with disastrous results. With proper diagnosis and treatment, most children with incessant VT should be able to lead normal lives.

Summary

In summary, infants with tachycardia deserve specific diagnosis and rapid specific treatment. In general, efforts should be made to abolish all episodes of tachycardia during the first hospitalization. Infants sent home with small recurrences often return quickly with major recurrences. All infants with a tachycardia should eventually lead a normal life, either because of outgrowing the substate of the tachycardia or because of an easy non-toxic drug regimen or surgical treatment.

References

1. Garson A, Gillette PC, McNamara DG: Supraventricular tachycardia in children: Clinical features, response to treatment and long-term follow-up in 217 patients. J Pediatr 98:857, 1981.
2. Garson A, Gillette PC: Electrophysiologic studies of supraventricular tachycardia in children. II. Prediction of specific mechanism by noninvasive features. Am Heart J 102:383, 1981.
3. Gillette PC: The mechanisms of supraventricular tachycardia in children. Circulation 54:133, 1976.
4. Gillette PC, Garson A Jr, Porter CJ, et al.: Arrhythmias. In Anderson RH, Macartney FJ, Shinebourne EA, Tynan M (eds.): Pediatric Cardiology, Vol. 2, pp. 1273–1292. London, Churchill Livingstone, 1987.
5. Hesslein PS, Gillette PC: Tachycardia and cyanosis in a newborn. Pediatr Cardiol 1:163, 1980.
6. Buchanan D, Gillette PC, Zinner A, et al.: Ventricular tachydysrhythmias in an infant with near-miss SIDS. Am Heart J 111:398, 1986.
7. Gillette PC, Garson A Jr: Electrophysiologic and pharmacologic characteristics of automatic ectopic atrial tachycardia. Circulation 56:571, 1977.
8. Garson A Jr, Gillette PC: Junctional ectopic tachycardia in children: Electrocardiography, electrophysiology, and pharmacologic response. Am J Cardiol 44:298, 1979.
9. Gillette PC, Garson A Jr, Porter CJ, et al.: Junctional automatic ectopic tachycardia: New proposed treatment by transcatheter His bundle ablation. Am Heart J 106(4):619, 1983.
10. Gillette PC, Garson A Jr, Kugler JD: Wolff-Parkinson-White syndrome in children: Electrophysiologic and pharmacologic characteristics. Circulation 60:1487, 1979.
11. Gillette PC, Gallagher JJ, Sealy W: Concealed anomalous cardiac conduction pathway: An operable cause of supraventricular tachycardia. J Pediatr 90:427, 1977.
12. Orzan F, Gillette PC: Reciprocating tachycardia due to a right-sided unidirectional retrograde anomalous pathway. PACE 1:306, 1978.
13. Henglein D, Gillette PC, Garson A Jr, et al.: Antegrade conduction and A-V node function in patients with unidirectional retrograde accessory pathways. Am Heart J 107(3):411, 1984.
14. Dunnigan A, Benson W Jr, Benditt DG: Atrial flutter in infancy: Diagnosis, clinical features, and treatment. Pediatrics 75(4):725, 1985.
15. Gillette PC, Kugler JD, Garson A Jr, et al.: The mechanisms of cardiac dysrhythmias after the Mustard operation for transposition of the great arteries. Am J Cardiol 45:1225, 1980.
16. Gillette PC, Goh TH, Garson A Jr, et al.: Chronic supraventricular tachycardia: A curable cause of congestive cardiomyopathy. JAMA 253:391, 1985.
17. Garson A Jr, Gillette PC, Titus JL, et al.: Surgical treatment

of ventricular tachycardia in infants: Infant ventricular tachycardia surgery. N Engl J Med 310:1443, 1984.
18. Gibson R, Driscoll DJ, Hartley CJ, et al.: The comparative electrophysiologic and hemodynamic effects of verapamil in puppies and adult dogs. Dev Pharmacol Ther 2:104, 1981.
19. Waldo AL, Krongrad E, Kupersmith J, et al.: Ventricular paired pacing to control rapid ventricular heart rate following open heart surgery. Observations on ectopic automaticity. Report of a case in a four-month-old patient. Circulation 53(1):176, 1976.
20. Ward DE, Rigby M, Dawson P, et al.: Rapid ventricular pacing to control resistant neonatal atrioventricular reentrant tachycardias. Pediatr Cardiol 5(1):843, 1980.
21. Deal BJ, Keane JF, Gillette PC, et al.: Wolff-Parkinson-White syndrome and supraventricular tachycardia during infancy: Management and follow-up. J Am Coll Cardiol 5:130, 1985.
22. Gillette PC, Garson A Jr, Eterovic E, et al.: Oral propranolol treatment in infants and children. J Pediatr 92:141, 1978.
23. Porter CJ, Gillette PC, Garson A, et al.: The effects of verapamil on supraventricular tachycardia in children. Am J Cardiol 48:487, 1981.

16

Electrophysiologic Evaluation of Syncope of Unexplained Origin

Joseph Borbola
Pablo Denes

"People who have frequent and severe fainting fits for no definable reason die suddenly."
Hippocrates (Aphorisms)

Syncope is defined as a sudden and transient loss of consciousness, with absence of postural tone, followed by spontaneous recovery. It is a common medical problem affecting all age groups. Syncopal episodes account for about 3% of emergency room visits and 1% of a general hospital's medical admissions.[8, 34] Many patients who experience syncopal attacks describe premonitory symptoms or a prodrome that is characterized by generalized weakness and a feeling of impending loss of consciousness. This prodrome is called presyncope or near-syncope, which may or may not progress to a complete loss of consciousness. Syncopal attacks can be single or multiple (recurrent), frequent or infrequent, associated with or without injuries. Management of patients with syncope is often difficult because of the wide variety of cardiac and noncardiac etiologies. Syncope may be a harbinger of sudden death, especially in the presence of cardiovascular disease.

A recent prospective study of patients presenting with syncopal events showed that in approximately 50% of cases the etiology remains undetermined, despite a thorough noninvasive clinical assessment.[18] The term *syncope of unexplained origin* (SUO) applies to this important subset of patients who, after a complete clinical and noninvasive assessment including ambulatory ECG monitoring and neurologic workup, remain without a definitive or strongly suggestive diagnosis.[12, 35] Today, syncope of unexplained origin still represents a diagnostic challenge and a therapeutic dilemma.

The purpose of this article is to review the currently available scientific data on the diagnostic, therapeutic and prognostic role of clinical electrophysiologic testing in patients with unexplained syncope. The use of electrophysiologic studies (EPS) in the assessement of patients with SUO has been the subject of several recent reviews.[7, 12, 21, 26, 30, 32, 34] These reviews detail the concepts and the rationale underlying the use of this invasive technique. At the time of this report at least 17 major series had been published,[2–5, 8, 10, 12, 13, 15, 16, 22, 24, 27–29, 31, 35] including more than 1000 patients.

Importance of Initial Noninvasive Clinical Evaluation

A likely cause of syncope in many patients can be identified on the basis of a carefully taken history, physical examination, 12-lead standard electrocardiogram (ECG), and noninvasive laboratory assessment (echocardiogram, dynamic electrocardiographic recording, treadmill test). Exercise electrocardiography may uncover occult arrhythmias and is particularly useful in patients with exercise-induced syncopal attacks.[30] On the basis of these evaluations, patients can also be separated into prognostic subgroups.[9, 18] Eagle et al.[9] reported that over 70% of patients with syncope can be placed into either a very-high or a very-low risk group. Patients with presumed cardiovascular mechanism of syncope have a strikingly higher one year mortality rate (30%) than patients with noncardiovascular cause (12%) or patients with syncope of unknown origin (6%).[18]

Prolonged ambulatory (Holter) or extended in-hospital ECG monitoring have been considered to have an important role as a screening test in the evaluation of patients with an episode of syncope. Unfortunately, the diagnostic yield of Holter monitoring is relatively low and plagued with unresolved issues regarding sensitivity and specificity of the findings and other limitations.[3, 4, 8, 20, 21, 30-32] The limitations include: the unpredictable and sporadic nature of syncopal attacks and the fact that symptoms rarely occur during monitoring; the poor correlation between reported symptoms and the presence of brady and tachyarrhythmias; the difficulty in differentiating meaningful arrhythmias from ambient rhythm disturbances which are common in the elderly asymptomatic population. Neither the optimal duration of ambulatory monitoring nor its impact on patient management has been clearly established.[21] According to one review, 24 hours is the minimum acceptable duration of monitoring, but because of the variability in frequency of arrhythmias, at least 48 hours is advisable.[35] The current clinical practice of performing ambulatory ECG monitoring first, and electrophysiologic study thereafter in patients with SUO appears justified when the results of ambulatory ECG monitoring are nondiagnostic.[35]

New noninvasive screening tests (signal-averaged ECG, head-up tilt testing) have emerged and may increase the yield of the clinical assessment.[1, 14, 23, 25, 36] Signal-averaging of the surface QRS complex can identify patients with inducible ventricular arrhythmias who subsequently should undergo programmed ventricular stimulation. In those patients with syncope but without late potentials, the incidence of inducible ventricular tachyarrhythmias is low.[14, 25, 36] Head-up tilt testing is a safe and valuable provocative tool for detecting patients with autonomic dysfunction presenting with syncopal episodes.[1, 23]

In the last decade, a growing body of information has accumulated suggesting that clinical intracardiac EPS is a useful provocative tool to uncover the otherwise occult pathology responsible for unexplained syncope.[2-5, 7, 8, 10, 13, 15, 16, 21, 22, 24, 26-32, 35] Moreover, EPS can play an active role in guiding therapy of patients who have recurrent episodes of syncope.

Indications for Intracardiac Electrophysiologic Study (EPS)

The goal of the EPS is to uncover the probable arrhythmic cause(s) of syncope, to guide rational therapeutic interventions, and to assess the prognosis.[7] EPS is particularly well suited for the diagnostic and therapeutic evaluation of patients with unexplained syncope, since sporadic arrhythmic events of paroxysmal nature can be reproduced by cardiac stimulation techniques.[5]

The use of clinical presentation as a guide for indication for EPS is highly controversial. A recent review[26] dealing with selection of patients with syncope for EPS emphasized that EPS should be reserved for those with recurrent syncope of unknown origin (i.e., only if the syncope recurred after an initial negative noninvasive assessment). In contrast, another study[35] with the largest patient population and longest follow-up showed that a significant number of patients could benefit from EPS even when only a single event had occurred. Akhtar et al.[2] suggested that EPS may uncover arrhythmic causes of syncope more frequently in patients with recurrent syncope as opposed to those with single events. In 1985, Doherty and coworkers[8] reported on the finding that multiple events had proved to be a useless clinical predictor of a positive EPS response. In 1987, Krol and colleagues[24] found that all patients who have had more than six syncopal episodes or had lost consciousness for >5 minutes have had a negative EPS test. In contrast, history of injury occurring as a result of syncope proved to be predictive of positive EPS findings.[24] The Framingham study has shown that isolated syncopal episodes (i.e., transient loss of consciousness in the absence of neurologic or cardiovascular disease stigmata) was reported by 2.4% of the men and 3.1% of the women during 26 years of surveillance. Isolated syncope was not associated with any excess of all causes of cardiovascular mortality, including sudden death.[33]

Reports from the literature indicate that EPS is not equally helpful in all sub-groups of patients presenting with SUO.[7, 21, 27] Therefore, selection of the appropriate subjects for EPS will enhance the yield of this invasive test. The diagnostic yield of EPS for detecting a cause presumed to be related to patients' syncope varies from 18 to 96%.[2-5, 7, 8, 13, 16, 24, 27, 35] This wide range is due mostly to the highly selected patient populations that form the basis of these studies. Patients with recurrent syncopal episodes who are likely to benefit from EPS are described below.[7, 10, 12, 20-22, 24, 26-30, 32, 34]

PATIENTS WITH EVIDENCE OF ORGANIC HEART DISEASE.[2, 4, 5, 8, 16, 21, 24, 27, 30, 32, 34] ■ Based on the results of reported series, the yield of EPS appears to be determined by the presence or absence of underlying cardiac disease. In patients with no evident heart disease, the sensitivity of EPS for diagnosing the cause of syncope is low and varies between 12 and 64%.[4, 5, 13, 32, 35] In 1982, Gulamhusein et al.[13] reported on the results of EPS in 34 patients with unexplained syncope and no organic heart disease. The EPS results were abnormal in 6 patients (18%). Of these, the findings were considered to be diagnostic, leading to appropriate therapy in 4 patients (12%). In contrast, in the presence of underlying organic heart disease, EPS findings are positive in the majority (45 to 96%) of patients assessed.[2-5, 16, 27, 30] In reported series between 35 and 72% of patients have evidence of organic heart disease.[2, 4, 5, 8, 16, 24, 27, 29, 35]

PATIENTS WITH ECG EVIDENCE OF BIFASCICULAR BLOCK.[10, 21, 22, 28, 30] ■ It is well known that patients with bifascicular block have an increased incidence of syncope and sudden cardiac death due to either episodic high-degree atrioventricular (AV) block or ventricular tachyarrhythmias. The incidence of syncope in these patients is reported to vary between 10 and 15% over a 3-year follow-up.[10, 28] The increased risk for the development of episodic third-degree AV block is 17 to 36%.[22] Reports have shown that approximately 50 to 60% of patients with bundle branch block and unexplained syncope have significant electrophysiologic abnormalities: H-V interval of 70 ms or more, infranodal block during atrial pacing, and inducible ventricular tachycardia (VT). Some patients have more than one abnormality.[10, 22, 28] Patients with negative EPS have a benign prognosis.[28]

PATIENTS WITH DOCUMENTED VENTRICULAR TACHYARRHYTHMIAS.[20, 21, 24] ■ Complex ventricular arrhythmias are defined as the presence of frequent, multiform and repetitive ventricular premature complexes (VPCs) and nonsustained ventricular tachycardia (three or more consecutive VPCs and <30 s in duration at a rate of >100/min). Patients with SUO and ventricular arrhythmias require EPS to define whether VT can be initiated by programmed ventricular stimulation. The induced VT in these patients is considered a probable cause of syncopal episodes. This is particularly true when only single or double extrastimulus techniques are required for induction.[4, 5, 7, 8, 13, 16, 24, 26, 27, 29] In 1987, Kapoor et al.[20] reported on the results and prognostic importance of prolonged electrocardiographic monitoring in 235 patients with unexplained syncope. At 2 years of follow-up, patients with frequent or repetitive ventricular ectopy, compared with patients with rare VPCs, had a significantly higher incidence of sudden death and overall mortality. Therefore, they suggested that patients with syncope and frequent or repetitive ventricular ectopy constitute a high-risk subgroup and may be candidates for more extensive diagnostic evaluation. Programmed ventricular stimulation appears to be useful in stratifying patients with complex ventricular arrhythmias into low- and high-risk groups for sudden death.[15] Recent studies suggest that signal-averaging of the surface QRS complex is a useful noninvasive tool for identifying the presence of late potentials and thus for selecting patients with syncope of unknown origin who should undergo programmed ventricular stimulation.[14, 25, 36]

RECURRENT SYNCOPAL EPISODES IN PATIENTS WITH WOLFF-PARKINSON-WHITE SYNDROME WITHOUT DOCUMENTED CARDIAC TACHYARRHYTHMIAS.[30] ■ There is a high probability that in patients with the Wolff-Parkinson-White (WPW) syndrome the cause of syncope is related to cardiac arrhythmias. However, the empirical treatment of undocumented arrhythmias is frequently inefficacious. There are multiple arrhythmic causes for syncopal events in patients with WPW syndrome. These arrhythmic causes include (1) orthodromic and antidromic AV reentrant tachycardias, (2) atrial fibrillation with rapid ventricular response, and (3) ventricular tachycardia or fibrillation.[11] The EPS in these patients is especially helpful in defining the arrhythmic cause(s) and as a guide to therapy.

Electrophysiologic Technique and Study Protocol

EPS is performed in the nonsedated, postabsorptive state. All antiarrhythmic drugs are discontinued for at least 48 to 72 hours prior to the study. Patients may be rechallenged with drugs if there is a strong suspicion that the syncopal episode was related to the proarrhythmic effects of antiarrhythmic drugs, particularly after a negative baseline study. In 1987, Krol and colleagues[24] reported that almost 50% of patients with SUO were being treated with type I antiarrhythmic drugs at the time of syncope.

Using local anesthesia, usually three electrode catheters (two quadripolar and one tripolar) are inserted percutaneously and advanced to the heart by using established catheterization procedures and fluoroscopic guidance.[6] Electrode catheters are positioned in the right atrium, in the right ventricular apex or outflow tract, and across the septal leaflet of the tricuspid valve for His bundle recording. In selected patients, an additional catheter is placed in the left ventricular apex or in the coronary sinus to record and/or stimulate from the left ventricle and left atrium, respectively. Surface electrocardiographic leads I, II, aV_F, V_1 and intracardiac electrograms filtered at 30 and 500 Hz are recorded at a paper speed of 100 mm/s. Programmed electrical stimulation (PES) is carried out using a programmable stimulator with isolated current source. The electrical stimuli are rectangular impulses, 1 to 2 ms in duration, delivered at twice diastolic threshold.

Evaluation of syncope of unknown origin includes assessment of sinoatrial node function, determination of AV node and His-Purkinje system conduction and refractoriness, and characterization of spontaneous or induced arrhythmias. The method of initiation and termination, the possible mechanism of induced tachyarrhythmias, the location of the site of origin, and the response to antiarrhythmic drugs and/or to antitachycardia pacing are evaluated.

A standard protocol of complete evaluation for all patients should be employed. A complete and meticulous protocol is of paramount importance, because patients with SUO may have more than one arrhythmic etiology[11] or abnormal EPS finding.[22, 28, 35] An arrhythmia and/or conduction disturbance leading to syncope in the laboratory during the study makes the diagnosis highly probable. Otherwise, positive EPS findings represent only a presumed, undocumented cause of previous syncope.[7] To elucidate the role of supraventricular tachycardia induced by stimulation techniques as a potential cause of the unexplained syncope, the measurement of the hemodynamic response during supine and upright positions is recommended. Specific stimulation protocols are used for evaluating patients with the WPW syndrome and unexplained syncope.[6, 12, 15]

The following baseline electrophysiologic parameters need to be determined in order to evaluate EPS results:[2–8, 10–13, 16, 21, 24, 26–28, 29–32, 34, 35]

1. *Sinus node function evaluation:* Sinus node and corrected sinus node recovery times (SNRT, CSNRT), the presence of secondary pauses following overdrive suppression of the sinus node by pacing in the high right atrium at incremental rates for a period of 30 seconds; measurement of sinoatrial conduction time (SACT) with direct recording or programmed atrial stimulation during sinus rhythm.

2. *Atrial conduction and electrical instability:* Right atrial conduction time (PA interval); atrial programmed stimulation during sinus rhythm and at one or more additional paced cycle lengths with one or more extrastimuli, to attempt induction of supraventricular tachyarrhythmias.

3. *AV node function:* AV nodal conduction time (A-H interval); incremental atrial pacing to determine the cycle length of AV nodal Wenckebach periodicity; atrial programmed stimulation to determine refractoriness and AV conduction patterns.

4. *His-Purkinje system function:* Intra-His conduction time (His bundle potential duration, split or multiphasic His); infra-His conduction time (H-V interval) during sinus rhythm and incremental atrial pacing; refractoriness of the His bundle and the bundle branches during atrial programmed stimulation.

5. *Ventricular electrical instability:* Inducibility of nonsustained or sustained ventricular tachyarrhythmias by electrical stimulation techniques; right ventricular PES during sinus rhythm and two or more paced cycle lengths from one or more ventricular sites (apex and/or outflow tract); incremental right ventricular pacing to a cycle length of at least 300 m to evaluate ventriculoatrial conduction and in an effort to induce ventricular tachyarrhythmias. In some studies, more aggressive ventricular pacing protocols were utilized, including the use of three extrastimuli, left ventricular stimulation, and/or isoproterenol infusion.[8, 16, 27, 29, 35] The use of a third extrastimulus increases sensitivity, but at the same time it also considerably decreases specificity of the pacing protocol.[4] The most appropriate ventricular stimulation techniques to be used in evaluating patients with unexplained syncope remain to be determined (Table 16–1).[34]

6. *Carotid sinus hypersensitivity:* In the absence of carotid bruits or history of cerebrovascular accidents, ECG and intracardiac recordings are taken during carotid sinus massage of left, then right carotid arteries to detect carotid sinus hypersensitivity (>3 s asystole).[4] Carotid sinus massage is usually repeated during pacing with measurement of arterial blood pressure to detect a significant drop (>50 mm Hg) in systolic blood pressure.

7. *Pharmacologic stresses:* In some centers, specific pharmacologic agents are used to uncover abnormalities when borderline values are found in conduction parameters or in an attempt to modify the autonomic tone. Drugs chosen for this use will depend on the suspected abnormality of the individual patient. The following drugs may be used: edrophonium (10–20 mg IV) to increase vagal tone; verapamil (0.10 mg/kg IV) to depress AV nodal conduction; procainamide (10 mg/kg IV) or ajmaline (1 mg/kg IV) (especially in Europe) to depress His-Purkinje conduction;[22] isoproterenol (2–4 μg/min IV) to increase sympathetic tone; and atropine (1–2 mg IV) to decrease parasympathetic influence. The interpretation of the results of pharmacologic stresses remains controversial.[21]

8. *Serial antiarrhythmic drug testing:* Patients with inducible, sustained supraventricular or ventricular tachycardia can undergo serial drug testing protocols to define an effective antiarrhythmic drug regimen. Most of the studies utilizing this approach to evaluate drug efficacy have shown an improved prognosis for patients compared to empirical management.[2, 4, 5, 12, 16, 18, 27]

Diagnostic Criteria of Positive Electrophysiologic Findings

The interpretation of the findings of EPS in patients with recurrent unexplained syncope is plagued with problems.[7, 21, 26, 34, 35] There is no consensus on how to interpret specific EPS findings and what to consider a positive EPS response.

Some prior EPS reports on patients with SUO considered all electrophysiologic abnormalities as a positive result. However, some EPS findings may be abnormal but nonspecific (pleomorphic VT or ventricular fibrillation [VF]) or of uncertain clinical significance (nonsustained VT). The difference between abnormal and positive (diagnostic) findings based on available studies[2, 4, 5, 13, 24, 27, 35] is presented in Table 16–2. The percentage of abnormal EPS has proved to be higher than the percentage of positive EPS in all but one study.[27] Sinus node dysfunction, conduction blocks, brady- or tachyarrhythmias induced during the EPS should be considered positive when they reproduce the

TABLE 16–1
Comparison of Ventricular Stimulation Protocols of Ten Major Studies in Patients with Unexplained Syncope

Authors/Ref./Year	RVA	RVOT	Multiple Rates	S_3	S_4	Burst	LV	Isoproterenol
DiMarco et al.[5] (1981)	+	+	+	+	–	+	–	–
Gulamhusein et al.[13] (1982)	+	+	+	+	–	+	–	–
Hess et al.[16] (1982)	+	+	+	+	+	+	+	+
Akhtar et al.[2] (1983)	+	+	+	+	–	+	–	–
Morady et al.[27] (1983)	+	+	+	+	+	+	+	+
Denes and Ezri[4] (1985)	+	+	+	+	–	+	–	–
Doherty et al.[8] (1985)	+	+	+	+	+	–	–	–
Teichman et al.[35] (1985)	+	+	+	+	+	+	+	+
Olshansky et al.[29] (1985)	+	+	+	+	+	+	+	+
Krol et al.[24] (1987)	+	+	+	+	+	–	–	–

LV = left ventricular; RVA = right ventricular apex; RVOT = right ventricular outflow tract; S_3 = two extrastimuli; S_4 = three extrastimuli; + = done; – = not done.

TABLE 16–2
Abnormal and Positive EPS Findings in Patients with Unexplained Syncope

Authors/Ref.	Abnormal (%)	Positive (%)
DiMarco et al.[5]	76	68
Gulamhusein et al.[13]	18	12
Morady et al.[27]	56	56
Akhtar et al.[2]	66	53
Denes and Ezri[4]	74	46
Teichman et al.[35]	75	36
Krol et al.[24]	—	30

individual patient's symptoms during the study. Otherwise, as stated by DiMarco,[7] findings represent the presumed but undocumented cause of previous syncope. If symptoms recur despite a negative EPS response, cardiac arrhythmias still have to be considered, and further evaluation, such as long-term ambulatory ECG monitoring, is needed to provide the clue for the diagnosis.[7, 26, 34] In 1981, DiMarco et al.[5] reported on a case history with recurrent unexplained syncope and negative initial EPS. After 30 days of consecutive ambulatory ECG monitoring, a syncopal episode occurred and was found to be associated with a rapid, nonsustained VT that was followed by a prolonged period of asystole.

Attempts have been made to differentiate between abnormal and positive EPS response, or between borderline and definitely positive EPS in patients with SUO.[24, 31, 35] In 1985, Reiffel and coworkers[31] reported on the results of EPS in 59 patients with one or more unexplained syncopal episodes; 29 of these patients (49%) had organic heart disease. Results of EPS were graded according to the type and severity of the abnormality, using the following four-class grading system:

Grade I: Normal or minor abnormalities.

Grade II: Corrected sinoatrial node recovery time 525–1000 ms; sinoatrial conduction time 120–220 ms; AV nodal block during incremental atrial pacing at cycle lengths >600 ms; supraventricular tachycardia >180 bpm; A-H interval 240–400 ms; H-V interval 55–75 ms.

Grade III: WPW syndrome with inducible atrial fibrillation, with ventricular rate >200 bpm and/or shortest R-R interval <220 ms; H-V interval 75–100 ms; nonsustained VT.

Grade IV: Corrected sinoatrial recovery time >1000 ms; sinoatrial conduction time >210 ms; A-H interval >400 ms; H-V interval >100 ms; induced intra- or infra-His block; sustained VT.

In 1985, Teichman et al.[35] reported on the results of EPS in 150 cases with unexplained syncope or near-syncope; 75 patients (50%) had concomitant heart disease. Abnormal electrophysiologic findings were categorized as either borderline (diagnostic yield: 75%), or clearly abnormal (diagnostic yield: 36%). Both categories were thought to be potential causes of syncope. The definitions for borderline and clearly abnormal EPS findings are summarized in Table 16–3. Most recently, a positive EPS was defined by Krol and colleagues[24] as the presence of sinus node recovery time > 3 s; H-V interval >100 ms; infranodal block during atrial pacing; monomorphic VT; and supraventricular tachycardia (SVT) associated with a fall in systolic blood pressure to 80 mm Hg supine. In contrast, a negative EPS was characterized by the following findings: an entirely normal EPS; supraventricular tachycardia without hypotension; H-V interval 55–99 ms; and polymorphic VT or VF.

The most frequent disagreements regarding the definition of a positive EPS response include (1) the definition of the degree of sinus node dysfunction; (2) the extent of the prolongation of HV interval; (3) the type, rate, and duration of the induced SVT; and (4) the morphology, duration, and rate of induced VT (Table 16–4).

Electrophysiologic Study Findings

As shown in Table 16–2, the overall incidence of abnormal EPS findings considered by the authors to be related positively to the cause of syncope ranges from 12 to 68%. The type of abnormalities that are identified vary among the different reports, depending on the presence or absence of organic heart disease, the criteria for choosing patients for EPS, the protocol of evaluation, the definition of an abnormal electrophysiologic finding.[4, 7, 26] For example, in some studies[2, 4, 8, 35] carotid sinus massage was used as a part of the EPS protocol; in others[13, 16, 24] it was used as a bedside maneuver before EPS. Denes and Ezri[4] reported that a previously negative test might become positive when performed in the electrophysiologic laboratory with the safeguards of pacing back-up. Some of the reported studies were also selective; one study included only patients without organic heart disease,[13] and others specifically excluded patients with bifascicular block with first-degree AV block,[5] sinus node dysfunction (sinus bradycardia, sinus arrest, sinus exit block),[2, 16, 27] transient second- or third-degree AV block,[2, 16, 24, 27] or frequent PVCs.[16, 27] Other studies[4, 24, 35] included unselected, consecutive patient populations. Also, the number and characteristics of syncopal episodes were varied; in some reports the number of syncopal events was one or more,[4, 8, 13, 16, 24, 31, 35] whereas other studies included patients with two or more syncopal episodes.[2, 5, 27] Patients with pre- or near-syncopal episodes also were included in some studies.[8, 13, 35]

In 1978, Boudoulas et al.[3] reported on the findings of EPS in 65 patients with underlying heart disease in whom no obvious cause of syncope could be detected. These patients were compared to a control group without syncopal episodes. In contrast to 96% in the group with syncopal events, 29% of the control group had abnormal EPS findings. The prevalence of syncope was 93% in patients with three or more electrophysiologic abnormalities.

Later, between 1981 and 1987, various reports[2, 4, 5, 8, 13, 16, 24, 27, 29, 31, 35] described the EPS findings in patients with SUO. On the basis of these studies in 702 patients,

TABLE 16–3
Definitions of Borderline and Clearly Abnormal EPS Findings in Patients with Unexplained Syncope[35]

EPS Finding	Borderline	Clearly Abnormal
Sinus node dysfunction	SNRT > 1600 ms SACT > 145 ms or PSB < 40 bpm	SNRT > 3000 ms or PSB < 30 bpm
AV node dysfunction	AH > 150 ms W < 100 bpm DAVNP, EAVNC or ERP, FRP ↑ 2 S.D.	W < 80 bpm
Induced SVT	asympt SVT > 130 bpm or unsust SVT ≥ 10 beats	sympt SVT or SVT + BP of <90 mm Hg
His-Purkinje system dysfunction	HV ≥ 60 ms pHV ≥ 70 ms multiphasic H	HV ≥ 70 ms H > 40 ms or split H
Induced VT	sust VT or VF with S_2–S_4 coupling interval <200 ms unsust VT > 7 beats	sust. VT or VF with S_2–S_4 coupling interval ≥ 200 ms unsust. VT ≥ 10 beats 200 bpm
Carotid sinus hypersensitivity	CSM >2.0 sec or CSM→AV block	CSM ≥ 3.0 s

AH = A-H interval; asympt = asymptomatic; AV = atrioventricular; W = Wenckebach rate; CSM = carotid sinus massage; DAVNP = dual atrioventricular nodal pathways; EAV = enhanced atrioventricular node conduction; ERP/FRP = effective/functional refractory period; HV = H-V interval; pHV = paced H-V interval; PSB = paradoxic sinus bradycardia after atropine; SACT = sinoatrial conduction time; SNRT = sinus node recovery time; SVT = supraventricular tachycardia; sust = sustained; S = extrastimulus; VT = ventricular tachycardia; VF = ventricular fibrillation; unsust = unsustained; BP = systolic blood pressure; 2 S.D. = two standard deviations of published norms.
Data from Teichman SL, Felder SD, Matos JA, et al.: Am Heart J 110:469, 1985.

the diagnostic yield was approximately 57%. The most common abnormality found during EPS was the induction of ventricular tachyarrhythmias, with a prevalence of 27% (range, 8–53%). Inducible supraventricular tachycardia was found in 11% (range, 9–20%) of patients, sinus node dysfunction in 8% (range, 2–30%), His-Purkinje system dysfunction in 8% (range, 6–34%), hypertensitive carotid sinus in 6% (range, 2–24%), and AV node dysfunction in 4% (range, 1–14%) (Table 16–5).

Inducible ventricular tachyarrhythmia was the abnormality detected most frequently in patients with syncope of undetermined origin who had undergone EPS.[2, 5, 8, 16, 24, 27, 29] The comparison of ventricular stimulation protocol of ten major studies in patients with unexplained syncope is shown in Table 16–1. A higher yield for VT induction was found in those studies with a more aggressive stimulation protocol (three extrastimuli, left ventricular stimulation, and isoproterenol infusion).[8, 16, 24, 27, 29, 35] The comparison of induced ventricular tachyarrhythmias in ten major studies with patients of unexplained syncope is summarized in Table 16–6. In 179 patients with induced VT/VF, 53% had sustained VT, 44% had nonsustained VT, and only 3% had inducible ventricular fibrillation. Only limited data are available to compare monomorphic versus polymorphic, and nonsustained versus sustained VTs. However, all studies included some patients with inducible nonsustained VT.

Patients with bundle branch block have an increased incidence of syncope and sudden cardiac death.[7, 10, 22, 26, 28] Prospective studies indicate that approximately 10

TABLE 16–4
Diagnostic Criteria for An Abnormal/Positive EPS in Patients with Unexplained Syncope

Authors/Ref.	SVT	HPS	VT
DiMarco et al.[5]	—	HV > 55 ms	≥4 beats
Gulamhusein et al.[13]	—	HV > 55 ms	—
Hess et al.[16]	—	HQ > 70 ms	≥6 beats
Morady et al.[27]	—	HV > 70 ms	≥6 beats
Akhtar et al.[2]	—	HV > 55 ms	≥3 beats
Denes and Ezri[4]	—	HV > 55 ms	≥3 beats
Olsansky et al.[29]	≥5 beats	HV > 60 ms	≥5 beats
Doherty et al.[8]	>1 min	HV > 100 ms	>4 beats
Reiffel et al.[31]	>180 bpm	HV > 55 ms	>3–9 beats
Teichman et al.[35]	SVT + 90 mm Hg	HV > 70 ms HH ≥ 40 ms	>10 beats >200 bpm
Krol et al.[24]	SVT + 80 mm Hg	HV > 100 ms	>6 beats

HPS = His-Purkinje system dysfunction; HV = H-V interval; HH = intra-His conduction time; SVT = induced supraventricular tachycardia; VT = induced ventricular tachycardia.

TABLE 16–5
Comparison of EPS Findings of Ten Major Studies in Patients with Unexplained Syncope

Authors/Ref.	SND	AVN	HPS	SVT	VT/VF	HSCS	Normal
DiMarco et al.[5]	1(4%)	3(12%)	3(12%)	3(12%)	9(36%)	—	6(24%)
Gulamhusein et al.[13]	3(9%)	—	—	3(9%)	—	—	28(82%)
Hess et al.[16]	5(6%)	—	11(34%)	—	11(34%)	—	14(44%)
Akhtar et al.[2]	4(13%)	—	2(6%)	5(17%)	11(36%)	—	10(34%)
Morady et al.[27]	2(4%)	—	—	—	28(53%)	—	23(43%)
Denes and Ezri[4]	15(30%)	7(14%)	7(14%)	6(12%)	4(8%)	12(24%)	13(26%)
Doherty et al.[8]	4(3%)	5(4%)	*	23(19%)	31(26%)	7(6%)	41(34%)
Teichman et al.[35]	14(17%)	12(14%)	27(33%)	17(20%)	36(43%)	13(16%)	17(21%)
Olshansky et al.[29]	8(8%)	1(1%)	13(12%)	13(12%)	28(27%)	2(2%)	58(55%)
Krol et al.[24]	2(2%)	—	4(6%)	2(2%)	22(21%)	—	73(70%)

AVN = atrioventricular node dysfunction; HPS = His-Purkinje system dysfunction; HSCG = hypersensitive carotid syndrome; SVT = induced supraventricular tachycardia; VT/VF = induced ventricular tachycardia/ventricular fibrillation; SND = sinus node dysfunction; * = a single result; 5(4%) was reported for AVN + HPS.

to 15% of these patients develop syncope during a 3-year follow-up.[10, 22, 28] EPS findings in patients with bifascicular block and syncope have been variable. In 1983, Ezri et al.[10] reported on the findings of EPS in 13 patients (mean age, 62 years) with bifascicular block and syncope; 79% of these patients were male and 69% had organic heart disease. Nine patients (69%) had abnormal electrophysiologic findings. EPS demonstrated inducible sustained VT in 4 patients (31%), and His-Purkinje system dysfunction in 5 (38%). These workers concluded, that VT may be a significant cause of syncope in patients with bifascicular block. In 1984, Morady and colleagues[28] reported on EPS findings in 32 patients (mean age, 62 years) with bifascicular block and syncope; 78% of the patients were male, and 87% had structural heart disease. Abnormal electrophysiologic findings were detected by EPS in 47% of patients. His-Purkinje system dysfunction was found in 14 patients (44%), and monomorphic VT was induced in 9 (28%). They concluded that approximately 50% of patients with bundle branch block and syncope who undergo EPS are found to have significant abnormalities. Most recently, Kaul and coworkers,[22] reported on the evaluation of patients (mean age, 47 years) with bundle branch block and syncope; 79% were male, and 57% had organic heart disease. The study was based on EPS testing and ajmaline stress. Kaul et al. found that approximately 60% of patients had clinically significant electrophysiologic abnormalities (His-Purkinje system dysfunction and/or inducible VT). They suggested that the ajmaline stress test is a useful adjunct to unmask infra-His block.

On the basis of the results of these studies,[10, 22, 28, 47] 47 to 69% of patients with bundle branch block and syncope had an electrophysiologic abnormality—mainly His-Purkinje system dysfunction (prolonged H-V interval and/or intra- and infra-His block with atrial pacing) or inducible VT. Some patients had more than one electrophysiologic abnormality. Long-term management guided by EPS proved to be successful in preventing recurrent syncopal episodes in most patients. The ultimate prognosis of this patient population appears to be related to the severity of the underlying organic heart disease.

Clinical and Noninvasive Predictors of EPS Outcome

Selection of patients with a high probability of positive electrophysiologic response would allow more rational and cost-effective use of EPS in clinical practice. Gulamhusein et al.[13] reported that the diagnostic yield of EPS is low in patients without ECG abnormality or clinical evidence of underlying organic heart disease. Morady and coworkers[27] demonstrated that female gender and lack of structural heart disease were inde-

TABLE 16–6
Comparison of Induced Ventricular Tachyarrhythmias in Patients with Unexplained Syncope

| Authors/Ref. | No. of Patients | Nonsustained VT | | | Sustained VT | | | VF |
		All	Mono	Poly	All	Mono	Poly	
DiMarco et al.[5]	9	7	—	—	2	—	—	0
Gulamhusein et al.[13]	0	0	—	—	0	—	—	0
Hess et al.[16]	11	4	—	—	7	—	—	0
Morady et al.[27]	27	15	4	11	9	8	1	3
Akhtar et al.[2]	11	5	—	—	4	—	—	2
Denes and Ezri[4]	4	1	—	—	2	—	—	1
Doherty et al.[8]	31	7	—	—	24	—	—	0
Teichman et al.[35]	36	16	—	—	20	—	—	0
Olshansky et al.[29]	28	22	14	8	6	4	2	0
Krol et al.[24]	22	1	—	—	21	—	—	0
Total	179	78(44%)			95(53%)			6(3%)

Mono = monomorphic; Poly = polymorphic; VT = ventricular tachycardia; VF = ventricular fibrillation.

pendently associated with negative EPS response. In 1985 Doherty et al.[8] examined the clinical and electrocardiographic predictors of a positive EPS response in 119 patients with unexplained syncope and presyncope. The only predictors of a positive EPS response were the presence of structural heart disease and previous myocardial infarction. Recently Krol and colleagues[24] examined the clinical and noninvasive predictors of EPS outcome in 104 patients with unexplained syncope. They also classified the EPS response as positive or negative. Left ventricular dysfunction (ejection fraction < 0.40) was the most powerful predictor of a positive EPS response, followed by the presence of bundle branch block, coronary artery disease, remote myocardial infarction, use of type I antiarrhythmic drugs at the time of syncope, injury related to loss of consciousness, and male gender. A negative EPS response was associated with normal left ventricular ejection fraction, lack of structural heart disease, normal ECG and long-term ambulatory ECG monitoring, and increased number (>5) and duration of syncopal episodes. The authors concluded that on the basis of clinical and noninvasive variables, a majority of patients with unexplained syncope can be categorized into subgroups with low and high probability of having a positive EPS response.

In conclusion, in patients with unexplained syncope, EPS findings can be predicted from clinical and noninvasive laboratory data. The presently available clinical and noninvasive predictors of EPS outcome in patients with unexplained syncope are summarized in Table 16–7. These results may help to better select patients with recurrent syncopal episodes for EPS and provide prognostic information regarding recurrence and survival.

Therapy and Prognosis

Therapeutic options can be selected on the basis of a negative or a positive response to EPS. In our practice patients with inducible sustained SVT or VT undergo serial drug testing guided by EPS. Others receive antiarrhythmic treatment guided by noninvasive methods (ambulatory ECG monitoring and treadmill testing). Patients with sinus node, AV node, and/or His-Purkinje system dysfunction are generally treated with pacemaker insertion. Patients with multiple abnormalities may receive both drug and pacemaker therapy. Finally, patients with negative EPS response usually receive no specific therapy.

The effectiveness of EPS-guided therapy for unexplained syncope in ten major studies is shown in Table 16–8. A total of 346 patients had positive EPS findings, and 285 patients (82%) became asymptomatic when treated with EPS-guided therapy during a mean follow-up of 21 months.[2, 4, 5, 8, 13, 16, 27, 29, 35] In contrast, the majority of reports have indicated a higher incidence of recurrence in patients in whom treatment was not directed by abnormal EPS findings.[2, 5, 13, 27, 35] In the combined series of 200 patients with normal EPS findings and SUO, there were 70 recurrences (35%)[2, 4, 5, 8, 13, 16, 27, 29, 35] and seven deaths (4%) (Table 16–9). In one study[8] no significant difference in recurrence was reported between patients with positive and with negative EPS findings. In another study[4] the incidence of recurrence was somewhat higher in patients with positive EPS findings. A summary of reports on the different therapy in patients with unexplained syncope and EPS is presented in Table 16–10. In the published reports, a total of 448 cases have been studied.[2, 4, 5, 8, 13, 16, 27, 29] Of these, 40% received antiarrhythmic drugs, 16% received pacemaker implantation, and 44% were given no specific therapy. Recurrence of syncope during the follow-up period has generally been used as an end point to evaluate effectiveness of a specific therapy.[21] In the combined series of 448 patients with a mean follow-up of 22 months, the recurrence rate of syncope was 22%, and the overall mortality was 5% (2–12%), (see Table 16–10). All but 2 patients who died had underlying organic heart disease. Thus, there were 18 deaths in 226 patients (8%) with underlying organic heart disease. In contrast, in the prospective study of Kapoor et al.,[18] in which EPS was not used in the majority of patients, the mortality was 30% for those with cardiovascular diagnosis of syncope. In the study of Doherty and colleagues,[8] the total cardiovascular mortality was 13% in the positive EPS group and 4% in the negative EPS group during a mean follow-up of 27 months. There was a high spontaneous remission rate in the untreated EPS-negative group. The presence of a negative EPS response was helpful in defining a patient subset with a high rate of remission of syncope and a low risk of sudden cardiac death.[8] Denes and Ezri[4] reviewed the recurrence/death rates and noted that it varied with the type of treatment, being 16% in patients treated by antiarrhythmic drugs, 39% in those receiving pacemaker implantation, and 44% in those with no specific therapy. On the other hand, spontaneous remission of syncope was found in about 50% (44–70%) of patients with negative EPS response and without any specific therapy.[7, 13, 16, 18, 26] No clinical variables predict remission of syncope in the absence of therapy.[8] The presence of multiple abnormal electrophysiologic findings does not increase the subsequent incidence of recurrence or death.[35]

In conclusion, it appears from the results of the reported studies that the incidence of recurrence is generally higher, whereas the overall mortality rate is lower, in patients with negative EPS and unexplained

TABLE 16–7
Clinical and Noninvasive Predictors of EPS Outcome in Patients with Unexplained Syncope

Negative EPS Response	Positive EPS Response
No organic heart disease[24,27]	Organic heart disease[8]
LVEF >40%	LVEF ≤40%
Normal ECG[24]	Bundle branch block[24]
Normal Holter[24]	Coronary artery disease[24]
Female gender[27]	Remote MI[8,24]
>5 syncope[24]	Injury with syncope[24]
	Use of type I AAD[24]
	Male gender[24]

AAD = antiarrhythmic drugs; LVEF = left ventricular ejection fracture; MI = myocardial infarction.

TABLE 16-8
Effectiveness of EPS-Guided Therapy for Unexplained Syncope in Ten Major Studies

Authors/Ref.	No. of Patients with Abnormal EPS	No. of Patients Who Became Asymptomatic	Follow-up (Months)
DiMarco et al.[5]	17	15(88%)	18
Fischer[12]	54	38(89%)	14
Gulamhusein et al.[13]	4	4(100%)	15
Hess et al.[16]	18	16(83%)	21
Morady et al.[27]	19	16(86%)	19
Akhtar et al.[2]	16	14(88%)	17
Denes and Ezri[4]	35	28(80%)	23
Doherty et al.[8]	57	46(81%)	25
Teichman et al.[35]	103	88(85%)	31
Olshansky et al.[29]	23	20(87%)	25
Total	346	285(82%)	21

syncope. EPS-guided therapy in patients with a positive EPS finding is associated with a good outcome with a low rate of recurrence and mortality. Patients with normal EPS response have a low risk of sudden cardiac death and a high rate of remission of symptoms without any specific therapy.[8]

RISK AND COMPLICATIONS OF ELECTROPHYSIOLOGIC STUDIES

Recent reports confirm the safety of EPS even in patients with advanced heart disease.[6, 15, 17] The reported complication rates are less than 0.7%. The most common complications were local hematoma, deep venous thrombosis, pulmonary embolism, and infections. However, the potential risk of complications should not be underestimated; study-related deaths have been reported.[15, 17]

Limitations

The following limitations must be considered when evaluating patients with unexplained syncope by EPS:

- The sensitivity and specificity of EPS varies with the study population, the protocol for evaluation and the criteria for a positive finding.
- A positive EPS finding represents only the presumed but undocumented cause of a previous syncope.[5, 7]
- A normal EPS does not exclude with certainty the diagnosis of cardiac arrhythmias;[7, 13] false negative results do occasionally occur.
- Abnormal EPS findings may be unrelated to the cause of syncope.
- There are controversies on how to interpret the findings of EPS and what to consider a positive or negative response.
- There is a lack of agreement on the clinical and prognostic significance of certain EPS findings, such as nonsustained VT, polymorphic sustained VT/VF, pharmacologic stress tests, and abnormal refractoriness of the conduction system.
- In some patients treated with antiarrhythmic drugs at the time of a syncopal episode, loss of consciousness may be related to the proarrhythmic effect of antiarrhythmic drugs; baseline EPS in such cases may be negative.
- Long-term follow-up studies are needed to evaluate the efficacy of specific therapeutic interventions and to elucidate the spontaneous remission rate of syncope.[34]

The challenge for the 1990s will be the continued refinement of present electrophysiologic study protocol, standardization of the evaluation of the results, and an improved identification of patients who are at high risk for recurrence or sudden cardiac death. A prospective randomized trial is required to define the

TABLE 16-9
Results of Follow-up in Patients with Normal EPS and Unexplained Syncope

Authors/Ref.	No. of Patients with Normal EPS	Follow-up (Months)	Recurrence	Death
DiMarco et al.[5]	8	26	4(50%)	0
Gulamhusein et al.[13]	28	15	13(46%)	N/A
Hess et al.[16]	14	23	4(29%)	0
Akhtar et al.[2]	14	15	11(79%)	N/A
Morady et al.[27]	23	31	10(43%)	1(4%)
Denes and Ezri[4]	13	25	0 —	1(7%)
Doherty et al.[8]	28	32	4(14%)	1(4%)
Teichman et al.[35]	22	26	12(54%)	3(14%)
Olshansky et al.[29]	50	26	12(18%)	1(2%)
Total	200	24	70(35%)	7(4%)

N/A = not applicable.

TABLE 16–10
Therapy and Follow-up in Patients with Syncope of Unknown Origin

Authors/Ref.	No. of Patients	Follow-up (Months)	AAD	PM	No Therapy	Recurrence	Death
DiMarco et al.[5]	25	21	14(56%)	7(28%)	4(16%)	7(28%)	1(4%)
Gulamhusein et al.[13]	34	15	4(12%)	—	30(88%)	14(41%)	N/A
Hess et al.[16]	32	19	11(34%)	12(38%)	9(28%)	6(19%)	2(6%)
Morady et al.[27]	53	24	36(68%)	5(9%)	12(23%)	18(34%)	1(2%)
Akhtar et al.[2]	30	16	11(36%)	5(17%)	14(47%)	13(43%)	N/A
Denes and Ezri[4]	50	23	17(34%)	20(40%)	13(26%)	2(4%)	6(12%)
Olshansky et al.[29]	105	26	40(38%)	7(7%)	58(55%)	22(21%)	3(3%)
Doherty et al.[8]	119	28	47(39%)	14(12%)	58(49%)	15(18%)	7(8%)
Total	448	22	180(40%)	70(16%)	198(44%)	97(22%)	20(5%)

AAD = antiarrhythmic drugs; PM = pacemaker.

exact role of EPS, comparing the outcome of patients with SUO who are treated with an EPS approach with the outcome of patients whose diagnosis and therapy are guided by noninvasive methods.

Acknowledgment

We wish to thank Ms. Lillian Linares for her invaluable secretarial help.

References

1. Abi-Samra FM, Maloney JD, Fouad FM, et al.: Head-up tilt testing: an important tool in the work-up of recurrent syncope of unknown etiology. J Am Coll Cardiol 7:126A, 1986.
2. Akhtar M, Shenasa M, Denker S, et al.: Role of cardiac electrophysiologic studies in patients with recurrent unexplained syncope. PACE 6:192, 1983.
3. Boudoulas H, Schaal S, Lewis RP: Electrophysiologic risk factors of syncope. J Electrocardiol 11:339, 1978.
4. Denes P, Ezri MD: The role of electrophysiologic studies in the management of patients with unexplained syncope. PACE 8:424, 1985.
5. DiMarco JP, Garan H, Harthorne JW, et al.: Intracardiac electrophysiologic techniques in recurrent syncope of unknown cause. Ann Intern Med 95:542, 1981.
6. DiMarco JP: Intracardiac electrophysiology. In Grossman W (ed.): Cardiac Catheterization and Angiography, ed 3, pp. 339–355. Philadelphia, Lea & Febiger, 1986.
7. DiMarco JP: Electrophysiologic studies in patients with unexplained syncope. Circulation 75:III-140, 1987.
8. Doherty JU, Pembrook-Rogers D, Grogan E, et al.: Electrophysiologic evaluation and follow-up characteristics of patients with recurrent unexplained syncope and presyncope. Am J Cardiol 55:703, 1985.
9. Eagle KA, Black HR, Cook EF, et al.: Evaluation of prognostic classifications for patients with syncope. Am J Med 79:455, 1985.
10. Ezri M, Lerman BB, Marchlinski FE, et al.: Electrophysiologic evaluation of syncope in patients with bifascicular block. Am Heart J 106:693, 1983.
11. Ezri MD, Jacobs LG, Denes P: Unexpected coexistence of supraventricular and ventricular tachycardia in patients with syncope. PACE 8:329, 1985.
12. Fischer JD: Role of electrophysiologic testing in the diagnosis and treatment of patients with known and suspected bradycardias and tachycardias. Progr Cardiovasc Dis 24:25, 1981.
13. Gulamhusein S, Naccarelli GV, Ko PT, et al.: Value and limitations of clinical electrophysiologic study in assessment of patients with unexplained syncope. Am J Med 73:700, 1982.
14. Gang ES, Peter T, Rosenthal ME: Detection of late potentials in the surface electrocardiogram in unexplained syncope. Am J Cardiol 58:1014, 1986.
15. Hammill SC, Sugrue DD, Gersh BJ, et al.: Clinical intracardiac electrophysiologic testing: Technique, diagnostic indications and therapeutic uses. Mayo Clin Proc 61:478, 1986.
16. Hess DS, Morady F, Scheinman MM: Electrophysiologic testing in the evaluation of patients with syncope of undetermined origin. Am J Cardiol 50:1309, 1982.
17. Horowitz, LN, Kay HR, Kutalek SP, et al.: Risks and complications of clinical cardiac electrophysiologic studies: A prospective analysis of 1000 consecutive patients. J Am Coll Cardiol 9:1261, 1987.
18. Kapoor WN, Karpf M, Wieand S: A prospective evaluation and follow-up of patients with syncope. N Engl J Med 309:197, 1983.
19. Kapoor WN, Snustad D, Peterson J, et al.: Syncope in the elderly. Am J Med 80:419, 1986.
20. Kapoor WN, Cha R, Peterson JR, et al.: Prolonged electrocardiographic monitoring in patients with syncope: Importance of frequent and repetitive ventricular ectopy. Am J Med 82:20, 1987.
21. Kapoor WN: The use of electrophysiologic studies in unexplained syncope. Practical Cardiol 13:53, 1987.
22. Kaul U, Dev V, Narula J, et al.: Evaluation of patients with bundle branch block and unexplained syncope: A study based on comprehensive electrophysiologic testing and ajmaline stress. PACE 11:289, 1988.
23. Kenny RA, Ingram A, Bayliss J, et al.: Head-up tilt: A useful test for investigating unexplained syncope. Lancet 1:982, 1986.
24. Krol RB, Morady F, Flaker GC, et al.: Electrophysiologic testing in patients with unexplained syncope: Clinical and non-invasive predictors of outcome. J Am Coll Cardiol 10:358, 1987.
25. Kuchar DL, Thorburn CW, Sammel NL: Signal-averaged electrocardiogram for evaluation of recurrent syncope. Am J Cardiol 58:949, 1986.
26. McAnulty JH: Syncope of unknown origin: The role of electrophysiologic studies. Circulation 75:III-144, 1987.
27. Morady F, Shen E, Schwartz A, et al.: Long-term follow-up of patients with recurrent unexplained syncope evaluated by electrophysiologic testing. J Am Coll Cardiol 2:1053, 1983.
28. Morady F, Higgins J, Peters RW, et al.: Electrophysiologic testing in bundle branch block and unexplained syncope. Am J Cardiol 54:587, 1984.
29. Olshansky B, Mazuz M, Martins JB: Significance of inducible tachycardia in patients with syncope of unknown origin: A long-term follow-up. J Am Coll Cardiol 5:216, 1985.
30. Radack KL: Syncope. Cost-effective patient workup. Postgrad Med 80:169, 1986.
31. Reiffel JA, Wang P, Bower R, et al.: Electrophysiologic testing in patients with recurrent syncope: Are results predicted by prior ambulatory monitoring? Am Heart J 110:1146, 1985.
32. Reiffel JA: Electrophysiologic testing for recurrent syncope. Cardiol Board Rev 3:65, 1986.
33. Savage DD, Corwin L, McGee DL, et al.: Epidemiologic features of isolated syncope: the Framingham Study. Stroke 16:626, 1985.
34. Sharma AD, Klein GJ, Milstein S: Diagnostic assessment of recurrent syncope. PACE 7:749, 1984.
35. Teichman SL, Felder SD, Matos JA, et al.: The value of electrophysiologic studies in syncope of undetermined origin: Report of 150 cases. Am Heart J 110:469, 1985.
36. Winters SL, Stewart D, Gomes JA: Signal averaging of the surface QRS complex predicts inducibility of ventricular tachycardia in patients with syncope of unknown origin: A prospective study. J Am Coll Cardiol 10:775, 1987.

17

Risk Stratification for Arrhythmic Death After Myocardial Infarction

A. An Overview

J. Thomas Bigger, Jr.
Jonathan S. Steinberg

The identification of patients with risk of increased mortality and morbidity after myocardial infarction provides a rationale and cost-effective basis for individualizing diagnostic and therapeutic strategies. Risk stratification can provide valuable insight into risk mechanisms, thereby advancing our understanding of disease processes and providing a rationale for large-scale intervention trials and for decisions about conventional diagnostic or therapeutic procedures. This chapter will review information related to identifying those patients after myocardial infarction who are at high risk for sudden or arrhythmic death. We will review primarily the evaluation of (1) left ventricular function, (2) spontaneous ventricular arrhythmias, (3) ability of the scar to support sustained ventricular arrhythmias, and (4) the autonomic nervous system. We have selected these topics based on the concept that spontaneous ventricular arrhythmias act as "triggers" than can provoke a vulnerable myocardium into sustained ventricular tachycardia (VT) or ventricular fibrillation (VF). The myocardium may be vulnerable to VT or VF due to permanent factors, such as the scarring of previous myocardial infarction, or due to transient factors, such as drugs, electrolyte abnormalities, or changes in autonomic nervous system activity. We recognize that transient factors may be difficult to assess because they may be absent when assessed by routine screening. Also, we will discuss problems with using sudden or arrhythmic deaths in controlled trials that are evaluating arrhythmic treatment.

Left Ventricular Dysfunction

INFARCT SIZE

Infarct size has an important role to play in the development of left ventricular dysfunction, or cardiac arrhythmias. Also, it is a prime determinant of sudden or arrhythmic death as well as total mortality early and late after myocardial infarction. The major cause of hospital death in acute myocardial infarction is mechanical pump failure, which is primarily related to the fraction of left ventricle that is infarcted.[1] Recent animal and patient studies indicate that the evolution of myocardial infarction is a dynamic and time-dependent process. Infarct size is dependent on the amount of myocardium supplied by the occluded or stenotic coronary artery; the extent and timing, if any, of spontaneous or therapeutic thrombolysis, the extent and effectiveness of coronary collaterals, and the mag-

---

Supported in part by NIH grants HL-22982 and HL-70204 from the National Heart, Lung, and Blood Institute; by grant RR-00645 from the Research Resources Administration, Bethesda, MD; and by the Winthrop and Chernow Foundations, New York, NY.

nitude of the myocardial oxygen demand. In 1971, quantitative estimates of infarction size became possible through the analysis of serial changes in serum creatine kinase (CK) activity.[2] Refined methods that measure the myocardial band CK (CK-MB) provide more precise quantitation.[3, 4]

Determining infarct size requires serial CK-MB enzyme samples at least every 4 hours for 3 days, to determine the time-activity curve for enzyme release. The algorithm for calculating infarct size accounts for the rate of CK-MB release into the blood, the elimination rate, and body weight.[5] The infarct size index determined from CK-MB curves is expressed in units of g-Eq/m^2.

Studies using these methods showed that infarction size was a major determinant of outcome during all phases of myocardial infarction.[4-7] Geltman et al.[4] studied 173 patients younger than 66 years of age who survived their first acute myocardial infarction for at least 24 hours. The mean infarct size index of those who died averaged 46.5 ± 5.8 (SEM) units, compared with 21.1 ± 1.4 units for survivors (p <0.001). Overall survival was significantly better after small (infarct size index <15 units) or moderate-size infarcts (15 to 30 units) than with large infarcts (>30 units). Regardless of the infarct location, patients with small infarcts had a better prognosis than those with larger infarcts. Patients with anterior infarcts had higher mortality than those with interior infarcts, but this difference in survival was accounted for by infarct size (i.e., anterior infarcts were larger than inferior infarcts). Multivariate analysis indicated the importance of infarct size as an independent predictor of outcome in patients experiencing their first infarct. Ventricular premature depolarizations (VPDs) in the CCU phase of myocardial infarction were more frequent among patients with infarct size >15 units than those with smaller infarcts, regardless of infarct location.[4]

Marmor and colleagues[6] explored the relationship between the infarct size in Q wave and non–Q wave infarcts and the significance of a second enzyme peak several days after the onset of myocardial infarction. These authors studied a sample of 200 patients and found that non–Q wave infarctions were associated with less myocardial damage than Q wave infarctions (i.e., 11 versus 25 CK-MB units). Furthermore, 43% of the non–Q wave and 8% of the Q wave infarctions exhibited early recurrence or an extension of the initial infarct, manifest by a second rise in CK-MB activity beginning ≥48 hours after the onset of the primary infarct. The hospital mortality in patients with non–Q wave infarcts that extended was 16%, compared to 7% for those that did not. Also, in patients with infarct extension, left ventricular ejection fraction decreased from $56 \pm 11\%$ to $34 \pm 10\%$ 10 days later (p <0.01). Roberts[7] concluded that the second episode of necrosis was attributable to occlusion of the same vessel that caused the initial episode of infarction. Furthermore, extension of the necrosis in patients with non–Q wave infarctions was associated with an increased 1-year mortality compared to patients without extension. Thus, a secondary increase in infarct size evidenced by a secondary rise in CK-MB activity occurs predominantly in patients with non–Q wave infarctions, is associated with a reduction in the left ventricular ejection fraction, and is associated with increased hospital and post-hospital mortality rates. Recognition of the pathophysiology and identification of patients at high risk for early infarct extension provides a rationale for attempts to prevent infarct extension.

The pattern of CK-MB release after myocardial infarction is quite variable, and slow and rapid release patterns have been noted. Rapid release patterns have been observed in animal models and in patients undergoing therapeutic intra-coronary thrombolysis,[8, 9] and it is presumed that these patterns result from washout with reperfusion. This enzyme washout has been used as an indicator of successful recanalization. Ong et al.[10] studied the time to peak CK-MB in a sample of 52 patients with myocardial infarction. Patients were divided into two groups, according to whether the time from baseline to peak CK-MB enzyme activity was rapid or slow. Patients with slow release (n=28, time to peak 19 ± 4.9 hours) had no significant change in global or regional ejection fraction pattern from the time of admission to discharge. In contrast, patients with rapid release (n=24, time to peak 9 ± 2.5 hours), showed an increase in global ejection fraction from $38 \pm 9\%$ to $48 \pm 8\%$ (p <0.001) and regional ejection fraction showed similar improvement. The early reperfusion may be due to spontaneous thrombolysis, relaxation of coronary spasm, or enhanced collateral flow. This study provided a rationale for trials to limit infarct size and preserve ventricular function by early administration of fibrinolytic therapy.

Several other techniques are available for the direct measurement of infarct size, but they have not gained wide clinical acceptance. Myocardial scintigrams with ^{99m}Tc stannous pyrophosphate imaging provides useful qualitative data about the extent and anatomic location of the infarction.[11] Nuclear magnetic resonance[12] and proton emission tomography[13] have potential, but high cost and lack of availability limit their use. Among the new imaging techniques, positron emission tomography has the best potential to provide new insights into the metabolic evolution of myocardial infarction and thereby lead to therapeutic advances. Positron emission tomography uses labeled compounds, (e.g., ^{11}C-palmitate) for the study of myocardial metabolism.[14] During radioactive decay, the ^{11}C atom emits a positron that collides with an electron and creates a photon. Photons are sensed by detectors positioned in a circle around the subject to make cross-sectional images of the myocardial uptake of ^{11}C-palmitate. Palmitate uptake is markedly slowed in the presence of ischemia, and there is no uptake in the presence of infarction. These characteristics of palmitate metabolism permit positron emission tomography to quantify the fraction of myocardium that is infarcted, ischemic, and normal. Also, the time course of changes in myocardial metabolism during ischemia can be elucidated, and the metabolic effects of treatment can be assessed.

INVASIVE HEMODYNAMIC EVALUATION OF LEFT VENTRICULAR FUNCTION DURING THE CORONARY CARE UNIT (CCU) PHASE OF ACUTE MYOCARDIAL INFARCTION

Since the introduction of the Swan-Ganz catheter in the early 1970s, numerous groups have documented the therapeutic and prognostic value of hemodynamic monitoring for patients with myocardial infarction.[15-18] The combined use of serial cardiac index, pulmonary capillary wedge pressure, and arterial pressure measurements is useful for assessing prognosis and guiding treatment in critically ill patients. Patients with a depressed cardiac index (<2.2 L/min/m^2), an elevated wedge pressure (≥ 18 mm Hg), or reduced blood pressure (<100 mm Hg systolic) have a poor prognosis. Forrester et al.[17] reported a hospital mortality of 5% in 95 patients with a cardiac index >2.2 L/min/m^2 compared to a mortality of 45% in 105 patients with a cardiac index <2.2 L/min/m^2. Shell and coworkers[19] observed a 10% 30-day mortality in patients with pulmonary capillary wedge pressures <18 mm Hg, compared to 33% in patients with higher filling pressures. Similar findings were reported by Cohn et al.[20] Classification of patients in the coronary care unit (CCU) phase of myocardial infarction using hemodynamic measurements permits an estimate of mortality risk. The hemodynamic classification scheme and the associated in-hospital mortality rates developed by Forrester et al.[17] are presented in Table 17-1. The ordinal increase in mortality with progressive hemodynamic embarrassment is clearly evident. A cardiac index <2.2 L/min/m^2 carries greater risk than a wedge pressure elevation >18 mm Hg. When these two hemodynamic abnormalities coexist, the risk of dying in hospital is about 50%. When both variables are normal, the in-hospital mortality is less than 5%. Left ventricular dysfunction during the early phase of infarction also has serious long-term prognostic implications. Patients with this problem should be evaluated intensively before discharge.

CLINICAL VARIABLES DURING THE CCU PHASE OF ACUTE MYOCARDIAL INFARCTION THAT PREDICT SHORT- AND LONG-TERM RISK

Many clinical variables that can be assessed during the CCU phase of acute myocardial infarction have value in risk stratification. Most of these reflect marked left ventricular dysfunction (e.g., shock, low blood pressure, rales, increased heart rate, increased respiratory rate, and pulmonary venous congestion or cardiomegaly on chest x-ray). Prognostic indices derived from these data, such as the Norris[21] and Peel[22] indices, can predict short- and long-term outcome, and these findings indicate that extensive myocardial damage at the time of infarction is a permanent liability. ST segment mapping has been used to evaluate infarct size in anterior myocardial infarction.[23] The accuracy of this method has been challenged,[24] and the cumbersome methodology and analysis involved have limited the application of this method.

NONINVASIVE EVALUATION OF LEFT VENTRICULAR FUNCTION

Radionuclide ventriculograms and echocardiography are two commonly used noninvasive laboratory techniques for evaluation of ventricular function after myocardial infarction. Radionuclide methods for measuring global ventricular function have been used more commonly in clinical trials and clinical practice, but newer echocardiographic methods are gaining wider acceptance.[25]

Radionuclide Methods

Ejection fraction can be measured early after myocardial infarction and periodically during convalescence to determine whether ventricular function is improving or deteriorating. In 1975, Schultz et al.[26] studied 81 post-infarction patients and found an association between left ventricular ejection fraction $<40\%$ and mortality events during a six-month follow-up. The Multicenter Post-Infarction Program (MPIP) obtained a radionuclide ejection fraction on 811 of their 867 patients during hospitalization for acute myocardial infarction.[27] One-year cardiac mortality increased progressively as the ejection fraction decreased below 40% (Fig. 17-1). Cox survival analyses identified an ejection fraction $<40\%$ and rales heard in the upper two thirds of the lung fields while the patient was in the CCU as the two most significant independent risk factors. Patients with both of these indicators of left ventricular dysfunction had an eightfold mortality risk compared to patients without these factors. In a comparison report of the same study population, Greenberg and colleagues[28] concluded that rales in the CCU provide information about acute phase ventricular dysfunction, possibly ischemic-related reduction in ventricular com-

TABLE 17-1
Prognostic Significance of Hemodynamic Findings Early After Myocardial Infarction

Cardiac Index <2.2 L/min/m^2	Pulmonary Wedge Pressure >18 mm Hg	No. of Patients	Mortality Rate	Relative Risk
No	No	62	3.2%	
	Yes	33	9.1%	2.8
Yes	No	35	22.9%	
	Yes	70	51.4%	2.2
	Total	200	24.5%	

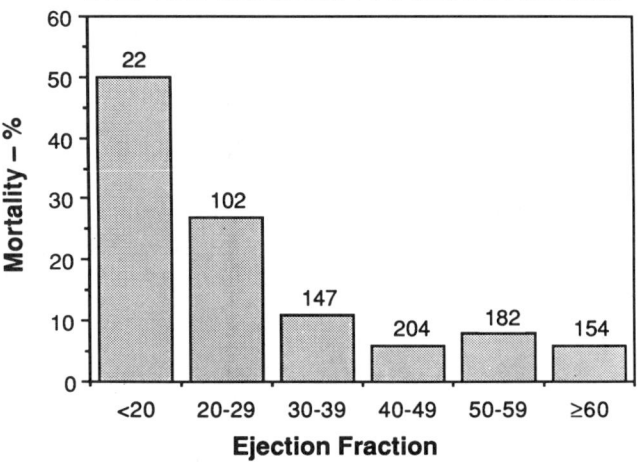

FIGURE 17–1
Two-year mortality rate as a function of left ventricular ejection fraction (LVEF) in the Multicenter Post-Infarction Program. Radionuclide ventriculograms were done about 10 days after infarction. The numbers above the columns indicate the number of patients in each group. With a left ventricular ejection fraction greater than 40%, 2-year mortality is about 6%. With a left ventricular ejection fraction less than 30%, 2-year mortality rises sharply.

pliance, whereas the radionuclide ejection fraction obtained a week or so later provides information about residual ventricular performance after the infarct has stabilized. The rales and low ejection fraction findings provide different hemodynamic information at different chronological periods during the acute infarctive process. These interpretations are further substantiated by the observations of Warnowicz et al.,[29] who noted a marked disparity between acute phase ventricular dysfunction (pulmonary edema) and recovery phase ventricular performance (normal ejection fraction) in selected patients with acute myocardial infarction. Additional studies by our research group highlighted the usefulness of radionuclide studies for identifying patients at risk for certain morbidity events after hospital discharge. Dwyer and coworkers[30] found that an ejection fraction <40% was as significant independent predictor of nonfatal cardiac rehospitalization events (angina, heart failure, arrhythmia, and coronary artery surgery), but not of reinfarction in the first year after the index infarction.

The resting radionuclide ejection fraction clearly has prognostic value, and high-risk patients with ejection fractions <40% can be easily identified. A significant percentage of patients with ejection fractions >40% still experience mortality and morbidity events, and it is in this subgroup that exercise radionuclide ejection fraction studies may have their greatest value. Corbett et al.[31] studied 67 post-infarction patients with submaximal exercise ejection fractions before hospital discharge. The mean ejection fraction in this population was 55%, the patients with major cardiac events the during 6-month follow-up had a significant reduction in peak exercise ejection fraction (44% rest to 37% exercise), compared to minimal charge in patients with minor cardiac events and an increase in patients with no cardiac events (66% rest to 76% exercise). These findings are in contrast to those of Borer and colleagues,[32] who did not find the exercise ejection fraction a prognostically useful test in post-infarction patients. Borer's population generally had a low resting ejection fraction, and this finding alone carries such adverse prognostic information that exercise studies provide minimal additional information. It is likely that, in patients with normal resting ejection fraction, a reduction in the exercise ejection fraction suggests multivessel coronary disease,[33] and this may explain the unfavorable outcome in this group of patients.

Echocardiographic Methods

The echocardiogram has proved useful in evaluating ventricular function and in risk stratification after infarction. The rationale for use of the echocardiogram is that postmortem studies in patients dying within 30 days after acute myocardial infarction have shown that 72% of the hearts have some thinning and dilation of the infarcted area of the myocardium within one week of the acute infarction.[34] Furthermore, approximately one third of hearts with transmural infarction had significant expansion of the infarct zone with obvious cardiac dilation. It is likely that infarct expansion is deleterious to the heart as a result of the increased demands associated with increased wall tension. Two-dimensional echocardiography echocardiography can detect acute alterations in cardiac topography, including regional myocardial dilation and wall thinning. Eaton et al.[35] assessed these changes by serial echocardiography in 28 patients during the first 2 weeks after acute transmural myocardial infarction. Regional end-diastolic segment lengths and wall thickness for anterior and posterior left ventricular walls were calculated. Eight patients showed infarct expansion with disproportionate dilation and transmural thinning in the infarcted zone that was significantly different ($p <0.005$) from changes in noninfarcted regions. This regional expansion led to an overall left ventricular dilation in these eight patients of 25%, compared to 5% in the 20 patients without infarct expansion. The eight patients with regional expansion had similar peak CK levels and Killip classification to those without this finding; however, their 8-week mortality was significantly higher.

Several echocardiographic studies have been reported in which the extent of left ventricular dysfunction complicating an acute myocardial infarction has been determined from a "wall motion index."[36–38] The wall motion index is derived from visualized alterations in segmental left and right ventricular free wall movement and thickening. Each of 11 segments is assigned a numerical value based on the normality or abnormality of wall motion in terms of hypokinesis, akinesis, and dyskinesis. Adding all the values for the segments analyzed and dividing by the number of segments gives an average wall motion index. Gibson et al.[37] used this approach to evaluate ventricular function in 75 consecutive patients with acute myocardial infarction. Akinesia or dyskinesia was detected in at least one of the

11 segments in all patients. Severe wall motion abnormalities remote from the infarct zone were observed in 47% of patients and correlated with greater prevalence of death (p <0.05), shock (p <0.01), progression to a worse Killip class (p <0.001), reinfarction (p <0.01), and angina (p <0.10). In 66 patients initially assigned to Killip class I or II, the wall motion index was highly predictive of later hemodynamic deterioration. This study corroborated the earlier work of Heger[36] by demonstrating the value of early echocardiography for predicting later hemodynamic deterioration.

The relationship between coronary anatomy and left ventricular wall motion abnormalities detected by two-dimensional echocardiography during the acute phase myocardial infarction has been correlated with coronary angiography. Stamm and coworkers[39] identified ventricular asynergy (lack of systolic thickening) during an acute myocardial infarction in three locations (infarct zone, adjacent to infarct zone, and remote region) by echocardiography and compared segmental wall motion abnormalities with predischarge coronary angiograms in 30 patients. Myocardial infarction in the distribution of a single coronary vessel produces a distinctive, recognizable pattern of asynergy. The stress of infarction was associated with remote compensatory hyperkinesis in 50% of patients with single-vessel disease. In 75% of patients with multivessel coronary disease, the infarction stress exceeded the perfusion capacity of the additionally stenosed vessels and resulted in remote asynergy; this was rarely seen in patients with single-vessel disease. The authors also found that the extent of asynergy during acute myocardial infarction overestimated the extent of wall motion abnormality present after recovery from the infarct. Thus, the pathophysiology is in keeping with that proposed by Greenberg et al.[28] One third of patients with single-vessel disease and more than two thirds of patients with multivessel disease had improvement in the extent of asynergy during follow-up echocardiography 1 to 2 weeks later. The authors concluded that remote asynergy identifies a subset of patients with significant residual myocardium at risk (i.e., jeopardized myocardium). Remote asynergy is associated with early reinfarction,[35] further myocardial events, and a poor prognosis when compared to patients with normal contractility in adjacent and remote areas of the acute infarction.

It would seem reasonable to perform coronary angiography in patients with remote asynergy detected by echocardiography. Patients with critical coronary lesions in non–infarct vessels should be considered for revascularization, especially when left ventricular ejection fraction is <40%.

Ventricular Arrhythmias

HOLTER STUDIES

Asymptomatic spontaneous ventricular arrhythmia after myocardial infarction have been the object of a great deal of study over the past 20 years. The significance of these arrhythmias, their variability and secular trends, and their relationship to left ventricular dysfunction have been clarified. However, the pathophysiologic link between spontaneous asymptomatic ventricular arrhythmias after myocardial infarction and sustained ventricular arrhythmias that cause arrhythmic death has not been clarified.

Three large studies have analyzed 24-hour ECG recordings made about 10 days after myocardial infarction, using accurate computerized arrhythmia detectors.[27,40–42] The prevalence of ventricular premature depolarizations (VPDs) is not high at this time. Only 15 to 20% have ≥10 VPDs per hour (Table 17–2). The S-shaped curve relating VPD frequency to mortality is shown in Figure 17–2. Two weeks after myocardial infarction, 50 to 60% of patients have an average VPD frequency below 1 per hour, and they have a 2-year mortality of about 8%. The curve rises steeply between 1 and 10 VPDs per hour to reach mortality rates between 20 and 30% depending on the study.[27,40,41] As VPD frequency rises from 10 per hour to 1000 per hour, mortality rates increase very little. Mortality rates are 2.5 to 4 times as great for patients with ≥10 VPDs per hour in a 24-hour ECG recording as for patients with lower VPD frequencies (see Table 17–2). Also, the shape of the VPD mortality curve suggests that studies done to determine whether suppression of VPDs after myocardial infarction will reduce mortality should use a VPD frequency of 3 to 10 per hour as the eligibility criterion.

Previous studies suggest that "complex" VPD features are at least as important as frequency (i.e., have as strong an association with death during follow-up). Early studies proposing this concept used short ECG recordings and various definitions of complex ventricular arrhythmias.[43,44] We have looked carefully at the relationship between individual complex VPD features and mortality in two separate large samples of post-infarction patients using 24-hour recordings and have concluded that repetitive (i.e., pairs or runs of VPDs) are very important predictors of subsequent mortality.[40,41,45] Figure 17–3 shows survivorship over three years as a function of repetitive VPD. An increasing degree of repetitiveness of VPD is associated with decreasing survivorship. Unsustained ventricular tachycardia occurring in a predischarge 24-hour ECG recording has a very strong relationship with subsequent mortality (odds ratio = 4.2) but occurs relatively infrequently (i.e., in about 12% of the patients at 10 days after myocardial infarction).[40,41,46] Using multivariate statistical techniques, two studies found that repetitive VPDs are associated with death independent of VPD frequency.[40,41]

THE RELATIONSHIP BETWEEN LEFT VENTRICULAR DYSFUNCTION AND VENTRICULAR ARRHYTHMIAS AFTER MYOCARDIAL INFARCTION

The first quantitative study of the relationship between left ventricular dysfunction and ventricular arrhythmias

TABLE 17–2
Frequency and Characteristics of Ventricular Arrhythmias Two Weeks After Acute Myocardial Infarction*

Institution/Program	Duration of Recording (hours)	No. of Patients	Frequency of VPDs (%)			VPD Characteristics (%)			
			0	≥1/hour	≥10/hour	Multiform	Pairs	VT	R-on-T
Stanford University	10	95	24	76	30	43	16	17	—
University of Rochester	6	500	47	—	5	10	3	1	10†
University of Ghent	6–8	150	41	58	23	24	24	15	2‡
Washington University	10	238	26	43	17	45	15	2	18†
Columbia University	24	616	16	50	25	54	31	12	27†
MPIP	24	819	14	41	20	64	17	11	24†
MILIS	24	533	16	—	15	66	26	11	10†

MILIS = Multicenter investigation of the Limitation of Infarct Size; MPIP = Multicenter Post-Infarction Program; VPD = ventricular premature depolarization.
*Reproduced by permission from Bigger JT Jr, Rolnitzky LM, Merab JP: In: Fozzard HM, Haber E, Jennings RB, Katz AM, Morgan HE (eds.): Handbook of Experimental Cardiology, pp. 1405–1449. New York, Raven Press, 1986.
†R-V/QT <1.00.
‡R-V/QT <0.85.

after myocardial infarction was done by Schulze et al.,[26, 47] who measured left ventricular ejection fraction using gated blood pool radionuclide ventriculograms and quantified ventricular arrhythmias in 24-hour ECG recordings in 81 patients.[26, 47] Eight deaths occurred during about 18 months of follow-up, all in the subgroup with left ventricular ejection fraction <40% and "high grade" arrhythmias, making it impossible to evaluate the relative importance of these two risk predictors. This ambiguity permitted two conflicting views on the relationships among the two risk predictors and mortality: (1) ventricular arrhythmias are strongly associated with left ventricular dysfunction and are not independently associated with mortality,

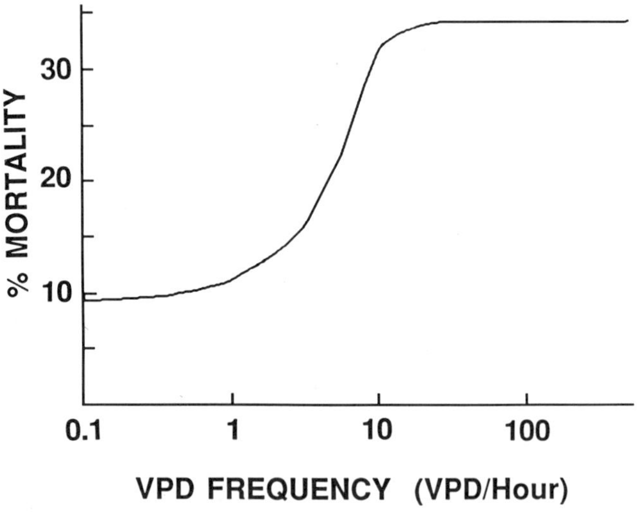

FIGURE 17–2
Two-year mortality rate as a function of 24-hour average ventricular polar depolarization (VPD) frequency in Multicenter Post-Infarction Program. Twenty-four–hour ECG recordings were obtained 11±3 days after myocardial infarction in 820 patients, who were then followed for 2 to 4 years. Patients with <1 VPD per hour have a low mortality rate. As VPD frequency increases from 1 to 10 per hour, mortality increases sharply. At VPD frequency >10 per hour, mortality increases only slightly as VPD frequency increases. (Reprinted by permission from Multicenter Post-Infarction Research Group: Progr Cardiovasc Dis 29:389, 1987.)

and (2) the presence of ventricular arrhythmias is a risk indicator for subsequent mortality independent of their association with left ventricular dysfunction. The distinction is important because the rationale for treating certain post-infarction ventricular arrhythmias and for performing studies to determine the effect of antiarrhythmic drugs on mortality in patients with potentially malignant ventricular arrhythmias depends on the validity of the second hypothesis.

Recently, two multicenter studies have evaluated the relationships among left ventricular dysfunction, ventricular arrhythmias, and mortality after myocardial infarction.[41, 42, 48] The Multicenter Post-Infarction Program (MPIP) was a nine-hospital natural history study of patients under age 70 who had a proven myocardial infarction. The Multicenter Investigation of the Limitation of Infarct Size (MILIS) study was a five-hospital intervention study of the effect of hyaluronidase, propranolol, or both in patients under age 76 who had acute myocardial infarction. In both studies a 24-hour ECG recording and a radionuclide ventriculogram were performed about 2 weeks after infarction. Both studies used accurate computer programs to analyze the 24-hour ECG recordings[49-51] and standardized procedures for analyzing the radionuclide left ventricular function studies. In both the MILIS and MPIP, repetitive VPDs were strongly related to mortality after adjusting for left ventricular dysfunction with left ventricular ejection fraction <40% (Table 17–3). Since the risk of dying in the 2 years after myocardial infarction is independently increased by left ventricular dysfunction and ventricular arrhythmias, the multivariate hazard ratios of these two risk indicators are multiplied to give the risk of dying during follow-up when both factors are present. In the MPIP, the risk of dying in patients with low left ventricular ejection fraction, high VPD frequency, and repetitive VPDs is increased about 12-fold. In the MILIS, the risk was increased about 16-fold when both repetitive VPDs and low left ventricular ejection fraction were present. In the MPIP, low values of left ventricular ejection fraction predicted early deaths better than late deaths, whereas the converse was true of ventricular arrhythmias (Fig. 17–4). The group with low left ventricular

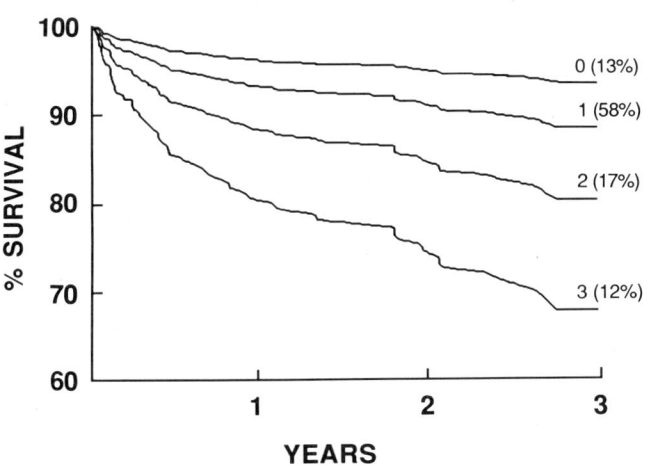

FIGURE 17-3
Survival over 3 years of 820 patients in the Multicenter Post-Infarction Program as a function of repetitive ventricular polar depolarization (VPD). 0-no VPD; 1-single (isolated) VPD; 2-paired VPD (couples); 3-runs of three or more consecutive VPD. The numbers in parentheses indicate the frequency of occurrence (e.g., 13% had no VPD at all in the 24-hour recording made 11 ± 3 days after myocardial infarction). (Reprinted by permission from Multicenter Post-infarction Research Group: Progr Cardiovasc Dis 29:389, 1987.)

ejection fraction and ventricular arrhythmias had high mortality rates early and late after infarction (see Fig. 17-4).

NON–Q WAVE MYOCARDIAL INFARCTION, COMPLEX VENTRICULAR ARRHYTHMIAS, AND MORTALITY

Maisel et al.[52] suggested that the presence of complex VPD during the recovery phase of acute myocardial infarction indicate high risk only in patients with non–Q wave infarction. This group studied a group of 1783 patients from San Diego and Vancouver, 777 of whom had a 24-hour ECG continuous recording prior to discharge from hospital. Complex ventricular arrhythmias were defined as multiform VPDs, paired VPDs, or VT (three or more consecutive VPDs at a heart rate >100/min). Of the 777 subjects, 566 had left ventricular ejection fraction measured with radionuclide methods or during cardiac catheterization. Non–Q wave infarction was present in 25% of the patients, and Q wave infarction was present in 75%

(41% inferior, 34% anterior). There was no difference between patients with non–Q and Q wave infarction in the prevalence of complex VPDs (41% vs. 36%) or in average left ventricular ejection fraction (48% vs. 49%). The patients were cross-classified by type of infarct (Q vs. non-Q) and presence or absence of complex VPDs, and the 1-year cardiac mortality was compared between the two groups. The mortality rate was 10% or less for all subgroups except the group with non–Q wave infarction and complex VPDs, which had a 1-year mortality rate of 27%. Interestingly, there was a significant association between the presence of complex VPDs and left ventricular ejection fraction ≤45% in the patients with Q wave infarction (odds ratio = 2.30) but not in the group with non–Q wave infarction (odds ratio = 0.86).

There are a number of problems with this study. First, the particular subgroup analysis addressed in this paper was not prespecified at the beginning of the study, which makes the study hypothesis generating rather than definitive. Second, the 24-hour ECG was not part of the protocol, so that it was the primary physician's decision that determined whether or not a patient would have a recording; similarly, left ventricular ejection fraction was obtained at the discretion of the primary physician. The selection of patients to have tests in this manner is likely to introduce bias. Third, the presence of complex ventricular arrhythmias is strongly dependent on multiform VPDs, which are common even in patients with low VPD frequency. Fourth, the prevalence of multiform VPDs, paired VPDs, and VT were all about half those usually found in 24-hour ECG recordings when they were analyzed using sensitive and specific computer algorithms. Finally, the high prevalence of digitalis and diuretic use in the non–Q wave infarction group is hard to explain. Nevertheless, the finding that the association of complex ventricular arrhythmias with mortality is restricted to patients with non–Q wave infarction is interesting and has provoked stimulating speculation on mechanism by the authors. Two hypotheses were (1) the ventricular arrhythmias may be responsible for the unexpectedly high mortality rate in patients with non–Q wave infarction by increasing the chance of nonischemic sustained ventricular arrhythmias; and (2) unsustained ventricular arrhythmias may provoke sustained ventricular arrhythmias during the ischemic episodes that are so common in patients with non–Q

TABLE 17-3
Left Ventricular Dysfunction, Ventricular Arrhythmias, and Mortality After Myocardial Infarction

LVEF <40%	VPDs >10/hour	No. of Patients		Mortality Rate		Relative Risk	
		MPIP*	MILIS†	MPIP	MILIS	MPIP	MILIS
No	No	433	314	10%	5%		
	Yes	78	38	15%	18%	1.5	3.6
Yes	No	184	141	27%	19%		
	Yes	72	40	47%	40%	1.7	2.1
	Total	767	533	17%	12%		

LVEF = left ventricular ejection fraction; MPIP = Multicenter Post-Infarction Program; MILIS = Multicenter Investigation of the Limitation of Infarct Size; VPD = ventricular premature depolarization.
*Average follow-up for MPIP was 33 months.
†Average follow-up for MILIS was 18 months.

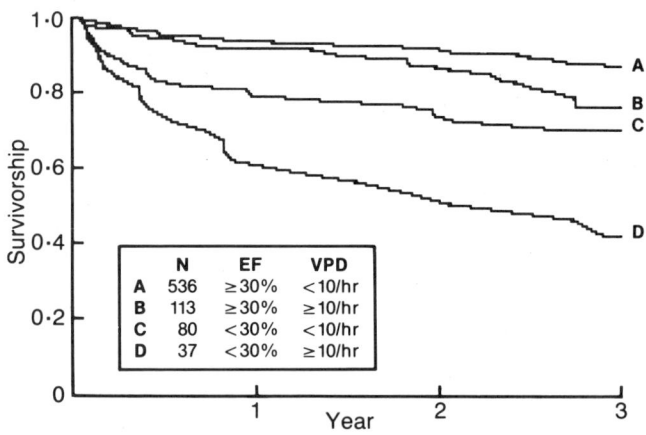

FIGURE 17–4
Survivorship as a function of left ventricular dysfunction and ventricular arrhythmias in 766 patients in the Multicenter Post-Infarction Program who had both a 24-hour continuous ECG recording and a radionuclide ventriculogram. N = number of patients in the group; EF = left ventricular ejection fraction; VPD = ventricular premature depolarizations. The survival curves were calculated by the method of Kaplan and Meier. Mortality tended to occur late in patients who had VPD ≥ 10 per hour and an EF ≥30% (B) and early in patients who had an EF <30% and VPD <10 per hour (C). The group that had both (D) had a high early and late mortality rate.

wave infarction. Certainly the findings of this study are worthy of further study to confirm or deny the special importance of complex VPD in patients with non–Q wave infarction.

INCREASE IN SPONTANEOUS VENTRICULAR ARRHYTHMIAS AFTER MYOCARDIAL INFARCTION

Kleiger et al.[53] made monthly ambulatory ECG recordings in a group of patients for a year after myocardial infarction and showed that the frequency of ventricular arrhythmias rises substantially from 2 weeks to 3 months after discharge and then remains approximately constant. The Beta Blocker Heart Attack Trial attempted to obtain a 24-hour ECG recording in all patients at baseline and in a 25% random sample at 6 weeks after myocardial infarction.[54] Table 17–4 shows that there was a three- to fourfold increase in the prevalence of ventricular arrhythmias between 2 and 6 weeks after discharge. The increase was substantially less in the group of patients treated with propranolol (180 to 240 mg per day).

EXERCISE VENTRICULAR ARRHYTHMIA AFTER MYOCARDIAL INFARCTION

Unsustained ventricular arrhythmias occurring during exercise testing after myocardial infarction have not been as extensively studied as those recorded by Holter techniques. Although exercise testing is commonly done between 7 days and 6 months after myocardial infarction, very few studies have made continuous recordings and analyzed them quantitatively for ventricular arrhythmias. The arrhythmias recorded during exercise may assess a variety of arrhythmic mechanisms: (1) increased heart rate, (2) ischemia, (3) decreased parasympathetic nervous system tone, (4) increased sympathetic nervous system tone, (5) increased ventricular wall tension due to augmented venous return, and (6) increased blood pressure. The extent to which each of these pathophysiologies is assessed by exercise is not known.

In 1977, Granath et al.[55] reported a study of the prevalence and prognostic significance of ventricular arrhythmias during treadmill exercise 3 weeks after myocardial infarction. These authors studied 183 men and 22 women with a mean age of 59 ± 9 years. The treadmill test started with a load of 16 or 33 watts and was advanced every 4 to 6 minutes by 16 watts. Exercise was discontinued because of (1) angina pectoris or dyspnea, (2) frequent VPDs, or (3) heart rate >140 per minute; 75% of the patients stopped exercise at ≤50 watts of effort. During exercise, ventricular arrhythmias occurred in 34 patients (17%). During an average follow-up of over 2 years, 47% of the 34 patients with exercise-induced ventricular arrhythmias died, compared to 24% of the 171 patients without exercise-induced ventricular arrhythmias (p <0.05). The odds of dying were 2.8 times greater for those who had exercise-induced ventricular arrhythmias than for those who did not. The exercise test was repeated 9 weeks after myocardial infarction in 174 of the patients, and 40 (23%) had ventricular arrhythmias. During follow-up, 40% of the 40 patients with ventricular arrhythmias died, compared to 19% of the 134 patients without ventricular arrhythmias (p <0.05). The odds of dying for patients with exercise ventricular arrhythmias was 2.9 times greater than for those who did not.

Weld and coworkers[56] evaluated exercise-induced ventricular arrhythmias in 236 patients who performed a low-level exercise test just before hospital discharge. They studied 190 men and 46 women (mean age 57 ± 9 years). The exercise test was done an average of 16 ± 4

TABLE 17–4
Effect of Propranolol on Unsustained Ventricular Arrhythmias After Myocardial Infarction in The Beta-Blocker Heart Attack Trial*

	Placebo		Propranolol		
	N	% with VA	N	% with VA	Propranolol/Placebo
Baseline	1635	7.2	1644	8.1	1.13
Six weeks	407	25.6	419	14.6	0.57
Six weeks/baseline		3.56		1.80	0.51

VA = ventricular arrhythmias (i.e., ≥10 VPDs per hour and repetitive VPDs).
*Based on data from Lichstein E, Morganroth J, Harris K, et al.: Circulation 67:I-5, 1983

days after infarction. Patients with complicated myocardial infarction were enrolled if they were able to walk 100 feet. Patients were excluded because of unstable angina pectoris, systolic blood pressure less than 90 mm Hg, or unsteady gait. The 9-minute exercise protocol was performed 1 or 2 days before anticipated hospital discharge. The final 3-minute stage was identical to stage I of the standard Bruce exercise protocol (approximately 4 METS). To evaluate ventricular arrhythmias, the ECG was recorded continuously for 9 minutes prior to exercise, during exercise, and for 10 minutes after exercise was completed. Average VPD frequency was calculated by dividing the number of VPDs by the duration of the recording interval. Of the 236 participants, 102 (43%) had one or more VPDs during the exercise session, and 56 patients (24%) had 10 or more VPDs per hour. Fifty patients (22%) had one of the following complex forms: multiform VPDs, R-on-T VPDs, paired VPDs, or VT. Weld et al.[56] examined the association of VPD and other risk indicators, especially left ventricular dysfunction. There was no significant association between VPD during the exercise test and left ventricular failure in the CCU, left ventricular failure at the time of exercise, cardiomegaly or pulmonary congestion in the discharge chest x-ray, or exercise duration of less than 9 minutes. VPDs were associated significantly with digoxin treatment at the time of the exercise test. Exercise VPDs showed a strong univariate association with cardiovascular death within a year of the infarct. Multiple logistic regression analysis indicated that exercise ventricular arrhythmias were significantly and independently associated with mortality after adjusting for age, previous myocardial infarction, cardiomegaly on chest x-ray, pulmonary vascular congestion on chest x-ray, exercise ST depression, and exercise duration. In the study by these authors, ventricular arrhythmias were relatively common after myocardial infarction, had a weak association with left ventricular dysfunction, and contributed dependently to the prediction of 1-year cardiovascular mortality when adjusting for several important clinical variables and other exercise variables that indicate left ventricular dysfunction and myocardial ischemia.

Krone and colleagues[57] reported the exercise results from MPIP. This study used the same predischarge treadmill exercise test protocol as described by Weld and coworkers[53] to study 530 men and 137 women 15 ± 6 days after infarction. The exercise test consisted of three 3-minute stages and stopped before completion because of decrease in systolic blood pressure, ST depression ≥4 mm, or heart rate >150 per minute. The presence of any VPD (43%) or paired VPDs (7%) before, during, or after the exercise test was associated significantly with increased cardiac mortality in the first year. In a stepwise logistic regression model, paired VPDs were used as the ventricular arrhythmia variable and were significantly associated with mortality after adjusting for other clinical and exercise variables (e.g., pulmonary congestion on chest x-ray, heart rate ≥90 per minute, and exercise systolic blood pressure >110 mm Hg). Thus, in this study also, Krone et al. confirmed the prevalence of exercise-induced ventricular arrhythmias and their significant independent value in predicting cardiac mortality after myocardial infarction.[57]

To evaluate the possible confounding effect of treatment on the relationship between ventricular arrhythmias during or after an exercise test and on cardiac mortality, Krone and coworkers[57] analyzed separately the subgroups who took or did not take beta-blockers or digitalis.[57] A total of 187 patients (28%) were taking digoxin, and 207 patients (31%) were taking a beta-blocker at the time of the exercise test. The policy of the study was not to take patients off either of these drugs for the test. An interaction was found for beta-blocker treatment: VPDs predicted cardiac mortality in patients not treated with beta-blockers, but not in those treated with beta-blockers. The opposite kind of interaction was found for digitalis. Only patients who were taking digitalis showed a significant association between exercise VPD and mortality during follow-up. These results suggest significant interactions between exercise-induced ventricular arrhythmias and treatment with either digitalis or beta-blocking drugs (i.e., suggest harm from digitalis and benefit from beta-blocking drugs). However, the results should be interpreted with caution because patients were not randomly selected for treatment with beta-blockers or digitalis, and thus many other important variables aside from treatment are likely to be different between patients taking drugs and those not taking drugs. Patients on beta-blockers had much less left ventricular dysfunction than those taking digitalis.

All studies that have recorded the ECG continuously and evaluated the association between ventricular arrhythmias and death have found a significant association that is stronger than the association of ST segment depression and death. However, there have been no trials that have selected patients for antiarrhythmic treatment on the basis of exercise ventricular arrhythmias.

ELECTROPHYSIOLOGIC STUDIES AFTER MYOCARDIAL INFARCTION

Electrophysiologic studies are used to evaluate nearly all patients who have sustained ventricular arrhythmias. These studies characterize the type and severity of ventricular arrhythmias and can be used to predict the efficacy and safety of antiarrhythmic drug treatment. Programmed ventricular stimulation has excellent sensitivity, specificity, and reproducibility in patients with chronic coronary heart disease and sustained VT.[58] Also, the response of inducible ventricular arrhythmias to drug therapy or surgery has excellent predictive accuracy for subsequent death and symptomatic arrhythmias.[59-63] The utility of electrophysiologic studies to assess risk early after acute myocardial infarction has been controversial. Patients with complicated or uncomplicated myocardial infarction have been studied, using programmed ventricular stimulation,[64-70] but most of the studies were small, were done on biased samples, and were difficult to interpret. Four studies that include more than 100 patients[64, 69-71] provide the best estimate of the prevalence and significance of inducible ventricular arrhythmias after myocardial infarction (see Table 17-5).

Prevalence of Inducible Ventricular Tachycardia

The prevalence of inducible, unsustained or sustained VT after acute myocardial infarction varies with the selection of patients, time after infarction, arrhythmia definitions, and stimulation protocol. Haerten et al.[65] studied 64 patients an average of 25 days after myocardial infarction. Four basic ventricular pacing rates (120, 140, 160, and 180 per minute) were used, and one or two premature stimuli were delivered to the right ventricular apex. This protocol provoked unsustained VT in 30% of the patients and sustained VT or VF in 20%. Hamer et al.[66] studied 70 patients, all of whom had arrhythmias or left ventricular failure in the CCU phase of myocardial infarction. Each patient had an electrophysiologic study while off antiarrhythmic medications. Two ventricular pacing rates (120 and 150 per minute) were used and single premature stimuli were delivered to the right ventricular apex in all 70 patients. High current (20 mA) and two premature stimuli were used in 33 patients. A second right ventricular site was stimulated in 50 patients. Of the 37 patients who underwent the entire protocol, eight had sustained ventricular tachycardia (22%) and four had unsustained ventricular tachycardia (11%) (i.e., more than five consecutive VPDs). Richards et al.[68] studied 165 patients 6 to 28 days after uncomplicated myocardial infarction. All electrophysiologic studies were done with the patients off antiarrhythmic drugs. Ventricular pacing at a rate of 100 per minute with one or two premature stimuli was applied to the right ventricular apex and outflow tract at both low (twice threshold) and high (20 mA) current amplitudes. In 38 patients (23%), sustained VT (>10 seconds) or VF was induced. In 1986, Denniss and coworkers[71] reported on a study of 403 patients done an average of 12 days after myocardial infarction. One and two premature stimuli were delivered at the right ventricular apex and outflow tract; stimulation amplitude was twice threshold and 20 mA. Stimulation was stopped if VT lasting ≥10 seconds occurred. Sustained VF was induced in 20%, and ventricular fibrillation in 14%. The prevalence of VT or VF was about twice as great for stimulation with 20 mA pulses as for stimulation at twice diastolic threshold. Patients with left ventricular ejection fraction <40% were 11.5 times more likely (52% versus 5%) to have sustained ventricular tachycardia induced by programmed ventricular stimulation.[71] Ventricular arrhythmias by Holter recording and late potentials in the signal-averaged ECG increased the likelihood of inducing sustained VT by programmed ventricular stimulation; exercise-induced ST depression did not.

Time Course of Inducible Ventricular Tachycardia

Klein and colleagues[72] studied 70 patients 3 to 4 weeks after myocardial infarction and found that 16% had inducible, sustained VT or VF. Subsequent studies done at 6 months in 40 patients and at 12 months in 35 patients showed no significant difference in the proportion with inducible ventricular arrhythmias. Costard et al.[73] studied 18 patients 6 and 24 days after infarction with up to three premature stimuli. They found that arrhythmias were inducible in two patients (11%) on day 6, and in nine (50%) on day 24. Denniss and coworkers[71] studied 29 patients a second time for an average of about 8 months after acute myocardial infarction. Seven patients who had inducible, sustained VT at baseline were studied after they developed spontaneous VT or VF during follow-up, and 6 (86%) were inducible. Nine patients who were not inducible at baseline were studied again after they developed spontaneous VT or VF during follow-up, and 67% were inducible. Thirteen patients who had sustained VT induced at baseline but remained free of sustained ventricular arrhythmias for 1 year after myocardial infarction were studied, and only 46% were inducible. Thus, some patients become inducible more than 1 month after myocardial infarction, and this indicates an increased risk for developing spontaneous sustained ventricular arrhythmias. Some patients who were inducible less than 1 month after myocardial infarction became uninducible later during the year after myocardial infarction.[71]

Infarct Size and Prevalence of Inducible Ventricular Tachycardia Early After Acute Myocardial Infarction

In dogs with experimental myocardial infarction, the probability of having sustained VT as a response to programmed ventricular stimulation is strongly related to infarct size (Fig. 17-5).[74, 75] In studies involving more than 100 dogs, infarct size expressed as percentage of left ventricular mass was related to the probability of inducing sustained VT as follows: infarct size <10%, 5% inducible; infarct size 10-19%, 20-25% inducible; and infarct size >20%, 70% inducible.[74, 75] Wilber et al.[76] showed that dogs with large myocardial infarcts were not only more likely to have inducible VT but also they were more likely to have spontaneous VF during a period of myocardial ischemia. Richards et al.[68] studied 165 survivors of myocardial infarction and found that inducible patients had lower left ventricular ejection fractions, (47±3%) than uninducible patients, (58±2%) (p <0.01). These findings suggest that inducible VT is more likely in patients who have large infarcts. Denniss et al.[71] found a strong relationship between left ventricular ejection fraction and the probability of inducing sustained VT. The overall probability of inducing sustained VT was 20%. The probability of inducing sustained VT in patients with left ventricular ejection fraction <40% was 52% versus 5% in patients with left ventricular ejection fraction ≥40%.

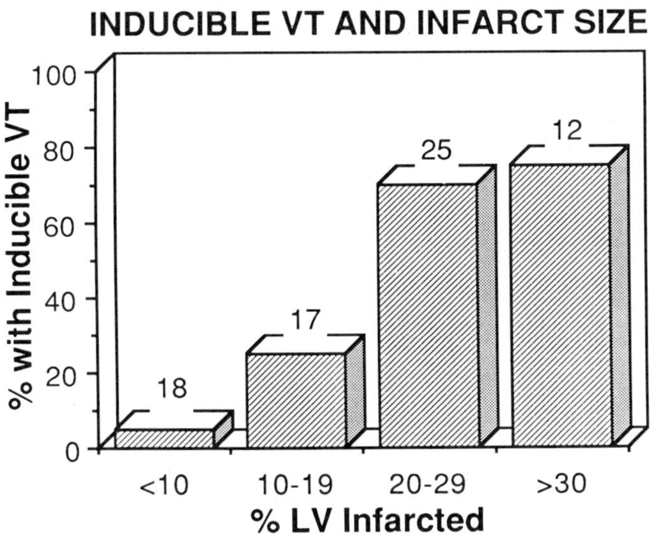

INDUCIBLE VT AND INFARCT SIZE

FIGURE 17–5
The relationship between the size of experimental myocardial infarcts in dogs and inducible ventricular tachycardia (VT).

Patients with chronic coronary heart disease and large scars, particularly those with ventricular aneurysms, are more likely to have sustained VT induced during electrophysiologic studies. Spielman[77,78] studied 58 patients with previous myocardial infarction, who had at least 10 VPDs per hour and left ventricular ejection fraction less than 50%.[77,78] In this group, 50% had inducible, sustained VT, a much higher rate than those found in studies of unselected patients. Although the human data are still meager, they suggest that large infarcts are strongly associated with inducible, sustained VT in humans just as in dogs.

Prediction of Mortality by Programmed Ventricular Stimulation

Data from four studies of programmed ventricular stimulation early after myocardial infarction, which enrolled more than 100 patients, are summarized in Table 17–5. In the 1983 Westmead Hospital report,[68] patients with ≥10 seconds of VT or VF had a 1-year mortality rate of 26%, contrasted with 6% for patients who did not have one of these arrhythmias induced (p <0.01). In inducible patients, 80% of the deaths were instantaneous, and ventricular tachyarrhythmias were documented in 63%; none of the noninducible patients died instantaneously. In 1986; the same group[71] reported another study in which 22% of those with inducible sustained ventricular tachycardia early after myocardial infarction developed spontaneous sustained ventricular tachycardia, ventricular fibrillation, or instantaneous death by 2 years of follow-up compared to 5% in those without inducible sustained ventricular tachycardia (p <0.01) (Fig. 17–6).[71] Ventricular fibrillation induced by programmed stimulation did not predict spontaneous sustained VT, VF, or death during follow-up (see Fig. 17–6). In the study by Roy and coworkers,[69] the incidence of spontaneous sustained VT and sudden cardiac death did not differ between the groups with and without inducible ventricular tachyarrhythmias, although the overall spontaneous event rate was low (two sudden cardiac deaths and two sustained VTs in 10 months of follow-up) and limited the power to detect a difference between the two groups. Much of the controversy about postinfarction electrophysiologic studies may be attributable to the lack of association of inducible VF with subsequent death. Nearly all of the smaller studies that did not find an association between inducible ventricular arrhythmias and death used VT and VF as a combined end point. In patients who had inducible, sustained VT less than 1 month after myocardial infarction, the factors that predicted death were anterior myocardial infarction, left ventricular ejection fraction <30%, presence of ventricular aneurysm, increased QRS duration in the signal-averaged ECG, and slower induced VT rates.[68] Studies are not available to show whether inducible sustained ventricular tachycardia predicts death or spontaneous sustained ventricular arrhythmias independent of left ventricular ejection fraction. Such studies are badly needed.

The findings early after myocardial infarction (see above) are similar to those in chronic coronary heart

TABLE 17–5
Significance of Programmed Ventricular Stimulation Early After Myocardial Infarction

	Richards et al.[65]	Breithardt et al.[61]	Roy et al.[69]	Denniss et al.[68]
Year of study	1983	1985	1985	1985
Number of patients	165	132	150	306
Days between infarction and electrophysiologic study	10	22	12	12
Stimulus amplitude (mA)	<2, 20	<2	<1.5	<2, 20
Follow-up (months)	8 ± 4	15 ± 11	10 ± 5	12 ± 6
Prevalence of inducible VT-s	23% *	21%	11%	20%
Number of deaths	17	8	5	22
Mortality rate				
With inducible VT-s	35% *	3%	3%	22%
Without inducible VT-s	9%	8%	4%	5%
Occurrences of spontaneous VT-s	6*	9	2	6
Spontaneous VT-s during follow-up				
With inducible VT-s	11% *	25%	3%	8%
Without inducible VT-s	1.6% *	2%	1%	0.4%

VT-s = sustained ventricular tachycardia.
*Sustained ventricular tachycardia or ventricular fibrillation.

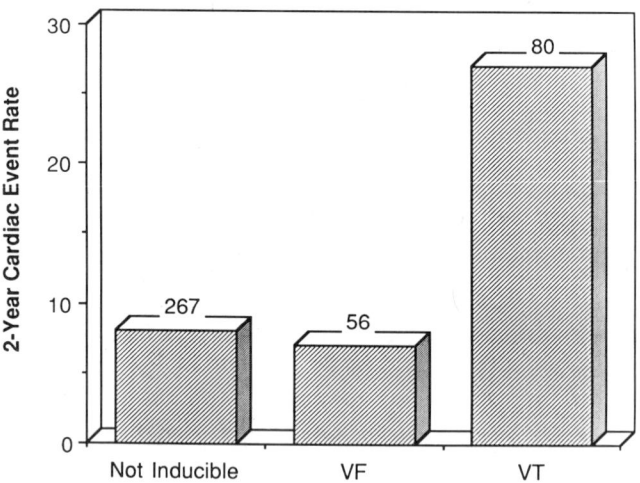

FIGURE 17–6
The relationship between ventricular arrhythmias induced by programmed ventricular stimulation and 2-year cardiac event rate in the Westmeade Hospital study. Patients who had ventricular fibrillation (VF) induced or who were not inducible had a low cardiac event rate, whereas the group with inducible ventricular tachycardia (VT) were at high risk. (After Denniss AR, Richards DA, Cody DV, et al.: Circulation 74:731, 1986.)

disease, in which about 50% of the patients who have left ventricular dysfunction and ventricular arrhythmias have inducible sustained ventricular tachycardia.[77, 78] In chronic coronary heart disease after the occurrence of at least one episode of sustained ventricular tachyarrhythmia, inducible VT predicts mortality. Studies so far suggest that programmed ventricular stimulation early after myocardial infarction predicts mortality as well.

Programmed ventricular stimulation to search for VT is minimally invasive, involving only percutaneous venipuncture and catheterization of the right side of the heart. Also, it is a relatively brief (1–2 hours) and safe procedure. It has a morbidity similar to that of Swan-Ganz catheterization. Patients with left ventricular dysfunction (left ventricular ejection fraction <40%) have about a 50% chance of having sustained VT induced by programmed ventricular stimulation when studied between 1 week and 1 month after myocardial infarction. Most investigators have found that inducible, sustained VT predicts arrhythmic death, sustained VT, and nonfatal VF (resuscitated) during follow-up. These facts indicate that the diagnostic use of clinical electrophysiologic studies may help stratify risk in patients with low left ventricular ejection fraction after myocardial infarction. Furthermore, we now have treatments that are effective in reducing the arrhythmic death rate in patients who have survived VT or VF. For example, the automatic implantable cardioverter defibrillator can reduce arrhythmic mortality in patients with malignant ventricular arrhythmias from 20% per year to about 2% per year.[79] Given these facts, it is reasonable to perform programmed ventricular stimulation in all patients with a left ventricular ejection fraction <40%, with the intention of enrolling patients who are inducible into controlled clinical trials to test the overall benefit of treatments. Because of the risks attributable to recurrent ischemia or heart failure, it will require trials to establish overall benefit.

THE SIGNAL-AVERAGED ELECTROCARDIOGRAM

The signal-averaged ECG is obtained by signal averaging, amplifying, and filtering orthogonal ECG leads to detect low amplitude cardiac electrical activity in the ST segment of the ECG, which is presumed to represent delayed conduction in abnormal tissue. Late, low-amplitude potentials in the signal-averaged ECG are associated with sustained ventricular arrhythmias. Thus, the signal-averaged ECG provides insight into cardiac electrical events that previously were detectable only by recording directly from the heart.

Table 17–6 summarizes the results of the published trials that have collected prospective data on the use of signal-averaged ECGs after myocardial infarction. Breithardt and his colleagues in West Germany[80–85] have the largest experience with the signal-averaging technique following myocardial infarction. This group recorded the signal-averaged ECG from four bipolar leads and averaged 150 to 300 beats according to the background noise level. A single pole analog filter with a bandwidth of 100 to 300 Hz was applied to the averaged QRS, which was then amplified. A late potential was identified visually as "low-amplitude activity" ≥ 10 ms duration at the end of the QRS. The study comprised 132 patients with a mean age of 56 ± 8 years studied a median of 22 days after myocardial infarction.[83] The site of infarct was evenly divided between anterior (n = 64) and inferior (n = 68). Of the 132 patients, 45% had late potentials of the following duration: 10 to 19 ms, 10%; 20 to 39 ms, 19%; and ≥ 40 msec, 16%. The prevalence of late potentials was 54% for inferior infarcts and 35% for anterior infarcts. In 15 ± 11 months of follow-up, eight deaths occurred; four were sudden. Sustained VT occurred in nine patients. Three of the four patients with sudden death and seven of the nine patients with sustained VT had late potentials in their signal-averaged ECG. The sensitivity of the signal-averaged ECG was 77% and the specificity was 59%. The odds of having sudden death or a sustained ventricular arrhythmia during follow-up was 4.3 times greater in patients with late potentials than in those without late potentials. The risk was greatest in the subset with the longest late potentials (i.e., ≥ 40 ms), of whom 25% went on to have sustained VT. Similar proportions of patients with and without late potentials received antiarrhythmic drugs and beta-adrenergic blockers during follow-up. Breithardt et al.[84] have continued to accumulate data and at last count had a cohort of 628 patients with coronary artery disease, 469 of whom had a prior myocardial infarction and 258 of whom were studied within 4 weeks of infarction. Of the 628 patients, 40% had late potentials; in 9%, late potentials

TABLE 17-6
Prognostic Value of Signal-Averaged Electrocardiogram Post-Myocardial Infarction

Authors/Ref.	No. of Patients	SAECG Day No.	No. of Positive Late Potential	Duration of Follow-up (months)	Arrhythmic Events		Prognostic Value of Late Potential				
					SCD	VT-s	Sensitivity	Specificity	+ Predictive Value	− Predictive Value	Odds Ratio (Corrected)
Breithardt et al.[83]	132	22 (median)	59 (45%)	15 ± 11	4 (3%)	9 (7%)	77%	59%	17%	96%	4.3
Gomes et al.[86]	102	10 ± 6	45 (44%)*	12 ± 6	5 (5%)	10 (10%)	87%	63%	29%	97%	9.2
Kuchar et al.[87]	210	11 ± 6	78 (39%)	14 (median)	8 (4%)	7 (3%)	93%	65%	17%	99%	18.1
Denniss et al.[71]	306	11 (mean)	80 (26%)	12 (mean)	10 (3%)	13 (4%)	65%	77%	19%	96%	6.1
Hopp et al.[90]	50	7, 14, 28	30 (60%)	24 ± 5	5 (10%)	—	100%	44%	17%	100%	8.8†

SAECG = signal-averaged ECG; SCD = sudden cardiac death; VT-s = sustained ventricular tachycardia.
*Presence of abnormal signal-averaged ECG.
†Values for sudden cardiac death only.

were ≥40 ms in duration. During 39±15 months of follow-up, there were 38 cardiac deaths (6%), 21 (3%) sudden deaths, and 14 (2%) patients who had episodes of sustained VT. Arrhythmic events were more likely to occur if a late potential was present, particularly if it was ≥40 ms. Less than 1% of patients without late potentials had sustained VT, and 1.6% had sudden cardiac death. When the late potential was present but was <40 ms, 1.6% had VT, and 5.2% died suddenly. If the late potential duration was ≥40 ms, the VT incidence jumped to 13.8%, and the sudden death incidence to 8.6%. The results were most impressive for patients with anterior myocardial infarction. In this subset, the incidence of VT increased from 1.5% if the late potential was absent, and to 25% if it was present and ≥40 ms.

Denniss et al.[71] tested the prognostic utility of the duration of the unfiltered averaged QRS or ventricular activation time (which was termed "delayed" if it exceeded 140 ms) in a cohort of 306 patients followed for a mean of 12 months. The mean ventricular activation time was 133±2 ms, and 80 patients (26%) had a delayed potential. Cardiac death (5.5% overall) was more likely to occur in the presence of delayed potential (10% vs. 2%, p <0.01), as were sudden cardiac death and nonfatal VT/VF events (15% vs. 2%, p <0.001). The risk of the occurrence of arrhythmic events was increased to a similar degree if delayed potential was present or if VT was induced by programmed stimulation, and the sensitivity for these end points was high if either delayed potential or induced VT was present. The presence of delayed potential was associated with a higher CK value, indicative of a larger myocardial infarction, but left ventricular ejection fraction was not measured in many patients. Multiple logistic regression analysis indicated that the signal-averaged ECG results were not independent predictors of fatal or nonfatal events. Of the 13 variables tested, only anterior site of infarct and pulmonary congestion on chest x-ray were independent predictors of clinical events. The presence of delayed potential did predict the inducibility of VT (sensitivity = 53%, specificity = 81%).

The studies of Gomes and colleagues[86] and Kuchar and coworkers[87] have provided important findings regarding the independent predictive ability of the signal-averaged ECG. Gomes et al.[83] performed signal-averaged ECG, 24-hour ECG recording, and radionuclide ventriculography in 102 patients about 2 weeks after acute myocardial infarction. All three studies were performed in more than three fourths of the patients. Three orthogonal ECG leads were averaged for 200 beats and then filtered with a bidirectional filter at a bandpass of 40 to 250 Hz with an Arrhythmia Research Technology-101 System. An abnormal signal-averaged ECG was defined by either root mean square voltage of ≤20 μV in the terminal 40 ms, a low amplitude signal duration under 40 μV >38 ms, or signal-averaged QRS duration >114 ms. The correlation coefficient between signal-averaged ECG results with either left ventricular ejection fraction or 24-hour ECG results was low. During a follow-up of 12±6 months, 15 arrhythmic events (VT, VF, or sudden cardiac death) occurred. The presence of an abnormal signal-averaged ECG, left ventricular ejection fraction <40%, or frequent or complex ventricular ectopy (defined as ≥10 VPDs per hour or presence of couplets or nonsustained VT) on 24-hour ECG recordings, were all associated with increased risk of an arrhythmic event. Of 28 clinical and noninvasive parameters tested, the duration of the filtered QRS on the signal-averaged ECG was the most significant predictor of arrhythmic events by the Cox proportional hazards regression model.[88] Together, an abnormal signal-averaged ECG and low left ventricular ejection fraction yielded a greatly increased (about 30 times) risk of an arrhythmic event. Regression analysis found left ventricular ejection fraction, several signal-averaged ECG variables, and unsustained VT in the 24-hour ECG independently related to the occurrence of an arrhythmic event. Gomes et al.[86] concluded that this "new noninvasive index for selecting a high risk subset of patients after infarction" could be used to select patients "for future studies of other interventions."

In the study by Kuchar and coworkers,[87] 210 patients were followed for a median of 14 months after myocardial infarction. The signal-averaged ECG technique and parameters are similar to those described above for Gomes et al.[86] and were performed 11±6 days after infarction. Only 5% of patients were receiving antiarrhythmic drugs at the time the signal-averaged ECG was recorded. Antiarrhythmic drugs can alter the results of signal averaging.[89] In this study, 98% of patients had a 24-hour ECG recording and 100% had left ventriculography (radionuclide or contrast), as well as a signal-averaged ECG recording. The 78 patients (39%) with an abnormal signal-averaged ECG tracing had a greater peak CK, a greater prevalence of inferior infarcts, and a lower prevalence of treatment with beta-blockers and surgical revascularization than the group with a normal signal-averaged ECG. In the group with an abnormal signal-averaged ECG, 17% had an arrhythmic event during follow-up, whereas only 1% of the group with a normal signal-averaged ECG had an arrhythmic event. Thus, the sensitivity was 93%, and the odds ratio was 18:1. The signal-averaged ECG, the left ventricular ejection fraction, and the complexity of ventricular ectopy on 24-hour ECG recording each contributed independently to the prediction of arrhythmic events. The combination of an abnormal signal-averaged ECG and a left ventricular ejection fraction <40% provided a sensitivity of 80% and a specificity of 89%.

Fifty patients who had suffered their first myocardial infarction were studied by Hopp et al.[90] A 6-lead signal-averaged high gain amplified ECG was recorded in all patients. Ventricular late potentials were defined as signals that outlasted the amplified QRS by ≥10 ms in ≥3 leads. The signal-averaged ECG was performed several times following infarction. The prevalence of late potentials increased from 34 to 40% from week 1 to week 2, and to 55% by week 4. With a mean follow-up of 2 years, the incidence of sudden cardiac death was 17% in the 30 patients who manifested a late potential on any study performed up to 4 weeks after infarction, and 0% in the group of 20 patients who never demonstrated a late potential.

Von Leitner et al.[91] reported in an abstract that the signal-averaged ECG identified a high-risk group for sudden cardiac death and cardiac mortality in a population of 518 patients who were seen during cardiac rehabilitation after myocardial infarction. In patients with an abnormal signal-averaged ECG, the sudden death rate was 3.6%, compared to a rate of 0.9% in patients whose signal-averaged ECG was normal.

The signal-averaged ECG is a noninvasive method that evaluates ventricular activation patterns associated with ventricular tachyarrhythmias. The accumulated evidence suggests that the signal-averaged ECG can predict the risk of sudden cardiac death or sustained ventricular arrhythmias after myocardial infarction. Further studies are needed to define its association with other post-infarction risk indicators and how the test should be used to select patients for treatment with drugs and implantable defibrillators or antitachycardia devices. Also, the methodology needs to be standardized and the best time to make recordings after infarction should be clarified.

HEART RATE VARIABILITY

Until recently, we have not had a noninvasive tool for assessment of autonomic nervous system activity in intact humans. Recently, evaluation of heart rate or heart period variability has filled this void and is under active investigation. Having such a tool should increase our knowledge of the pathophysiologic role of the autonomic nervous system in cardiac arrhythmias occurring after myocardial infarction.

A wealth of experimental evidence links abnormalities of the autonomic nervous system to ventricular arrhythmias during myocardial ischemia or infarction. Under these circumstances, increased activity in the sympathetic nervous system is engendered as a reflex response to myocardial ischemia or to decreased cardiac output. The release of norepinephrine from sympathetic nerve terminals can cause ventricular arrhythmias by a variety of mechanisms.[92] Factors that increase sympathetic nervous system activity increase the likelihood of ventricular arrhythmias, and those that decrease sympathetic nervous system decrease the likelihood of ventricular arrhythmias.[92, 93] Conversely, an increase in parasympathetic nervous system (vagal) activity tends to prevent ventricular arrhythmias, and a decrease in parasympathetic nervous system activity tends to promote ventricular arrhythmias.[92, 93] Schwartz has shown that experimental myocardial infarction in the dog causes a decrease in the baroreceptor reflex slope measured as the increase in R-R interval as a function of an increase in blood pressure engendered by phenylephrine injection. Dogs with the greatest decrease in baroreceptor reflex slope were most susceptible to VF caused by a combination of exercise and myocardial ischemia. Exercise training of dogs after myocardial infarction increased the baroreceptor reflex slope and decreased susceptibility to VF. La Rovere and colleagues[95] showed that baroreceptor reflex slope was reduced in some of their 78 patients with recent myocardial infarction. They found that, after myocardial infarction, the baroreceptor reflex slope was inversely correlated with age and, surprisingly, not related to left ventricular ejection fraction or exercise capacity. The baroreceptor reflex slope was significantly lower for the six patients who died during follow-up than for the 72 survivors. These authors concluded that, as in the dog model, many patients develop reduced parasympathetic activity, tipping the autonomic balance in favor of the sympathetic nervous system. Sympathetic predominance during the year after myocardial infarction may be related to a higher death rate.[95]

Lombardi and coworkers[96] compared sympathovagal interactions in 70 patients studied 2 weeks after myocardial infarction with 26 age-matched controls, by analyzing spectral components of heart rate. These authors found that, after myocardial infarction, patients had smaller high-frequency (HF) peaks (vagal activity) and larger low-frequency (LF) peaks (sympathetic activity), compared to the control group. This finding was interpreted as a shift in autonomic balance toward sympathetic predominance at 2 weeks after infarction. About 30 patients were studied at 6 months and 1 year after myocardial infarction. These late studies suggested that autonomic balance returned to normal by 6 months (i.e., the LF/HF ratio was lower). Since paired observations were not reported, it is possible that the patients who were studied late had more normal autonomic balance to begin with. The increase in the amplitude of the LF peak to passive tilt to 90° was markedly blunted at 2 weeks after myocardial infarction in the 24 subjects tested. The interpretation of this finding is uncertain; the increased sympathetic tone at rest may have down-regulated myocardial beta receptors. This interesting finding needs further investigation.

Kleiger et al.[97] used the 24-hour standard deviation of normal R-R intervals (HP-24) as a measure of heart rate variability in the 808 MPIP patients, who had a 24-hour ECG recording 11 ± 3 days after myocardial infarction that was suitable for analyzing heart rate variability. HP-24 is a broad band measure responding to ultralow frequency variability as well as low and high frequency variability.[98] HP-24 was related to mortality during an average follow-up of 31 months (Fig. 17-7). Patients with HP-24 <50 ms represented 16% of the sample and had a relative risk of dying 5.3 times higher than those with an HP-24 >100 ms (upper 25% of the sample). These authors looked for correlations of HP-24 and other risk predictors. HP-24 had its strongest correlations with average R-R interval (r = 0.52), left ventricular ejection fraction (r = 0.24), rales in the CCU (r = −0.25), and age (r = −0.19). Its correlations with VPD frequency (r = 0.07) and VPD runs (r = −0.02) were very weak. Cox proportional hazards models were fitted using the best MPIP predictors of mortality (i.e., rales in the CCU, left ventricular ejection fraction <30%, VPD frequency ≥ 10/hour, New York Heart Association functional Class

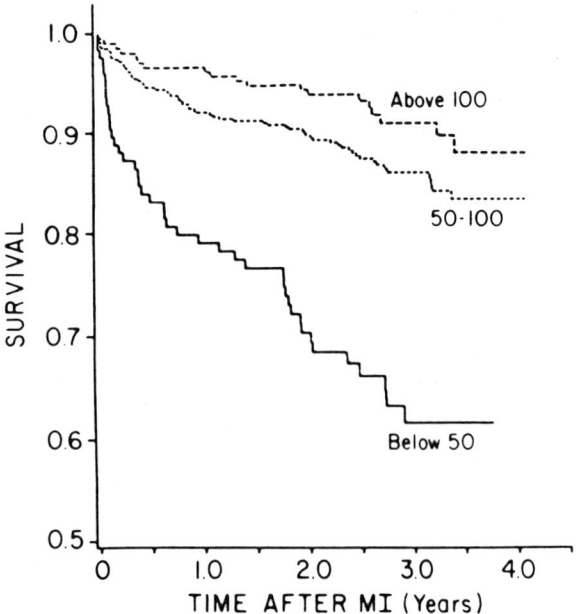

FIGURE 17–7
Survivorship as a function of heart period variability in 808 patients in Multicenter Post-Infarction Program. The standard deviation of the normal R-R intervals computed over a 24-hour period (HP-24) was related to survival over the subsequent 2 to 4 years. The survival curves were calculated by the method of Kaplan and Meier for three groups: HP-24 > 100 ms (n = 211, HP-24 50–100 ms (n = 472), and HP 24 <50 ms (n = 125). The groups with HP-24 <50 ms had a significantly worse survival rate than the other two groups. MI = myocardial infarction. (Reprinted by permission from Kleiger RE, Miller JP, Bigger JT, et al.: Am J Cardiol 59:256, 1987.)

III or IV), and HP-24 was then added to the model. Simultaneously adjusted for these other risk predictors and for heart rate, HP-24 was significantly associated with mortality. Kleiger and colleagues suggested that the low values of HP-24 that were associated with mortality independent of other important risk indicators were due to increased sympathetic tone, decreased parasympathetic tone, or both.[97] In a follow-up study to dissect the sources of variability that contribute to HP-24, Bigger and colleagues[99] found that various sources of heart period variability were reduced in patients with low HP-24. A time domain measure of parasympathetic nervous system activity, the proportion of successive differences between adjacent normal R-R intervals >50 ms (pNN-50), was markedly reduced in patients who had low HP-24, compared to those with high values of HP-24 (Fig. 17–8), indicating that atients with low heart period variability after myocardial infarction have reduced vagal (parasympathetic) activity.

In summary, three studies using very different measures have concluded that vagal activity was reduced in some patients after myocardial infarction. This finding seems established. The evidence for increased sympathetic nervous system activity 2 to 4 weeks after myocardial infarction is only suggestive. The relationship between reduced vagal activity early after myocardial infarction and subsequent mortality is also only suggestive at this time. It does seem that noninvasive methods are now available to study the autonomic nervous system in intact humans and to define better its role in the pathophysiology of arrhythmias, ischemia, and ventricular function.

Sudden Cardiac Death as an End Point for Observational Studies and Clinical Trials

A serious issue in risk stratification of patients after myocardial infarction is that of assessing mechanisms of death. If the mechanisms of death could be determined accurately, then the type of death and proportion of patients dying of each mechanism (e.g., arrhythmic or myocardial failure deaths) would suggest which treatments might have the greatest impact and how to allocate limited resources. An important issue for clinical trials is the end point(s) by which the treatment will be judged. If sudden cardiac death could be equated with an arrhythmic mechanism of death, then this would be the most appropriate end point to assess for benefit of treatment aimed at reducing death due to ventricular arrhythmias. Using sudden death instead of total mortality or total cardiac mortality would reduce the sample size required to determine whether an antiarrhythmic treatment has a significant effect in terms of survival, because it would remove from consideration those deaths (e.g., myocardial failure deaths) that the treatment has little chance of influencing. Unfortunately, neither sudden cardiac

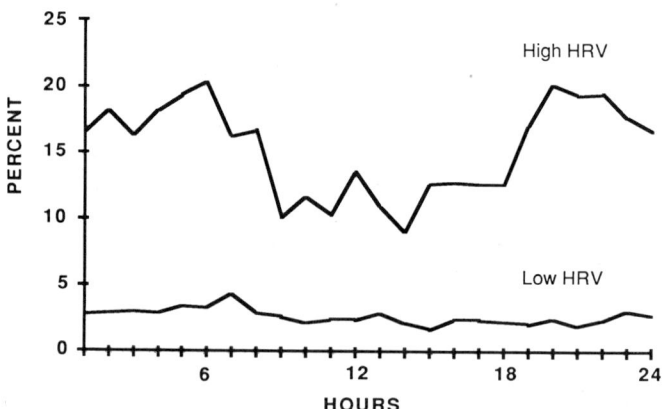

FIGURE 17–8
Vagal activity in a group of 10 patients with high (i.e., HP-24) heart period variability (HRV), compared to a group of 10 patients with low heart period variability. The mean hourly percentages of successive N-N intervals differing by >50 ms (pNN-50) was used as a measure of vagal activity. The percentages for the patients with low and high variability were averaged for each hour starting at midnight (00:00). The difference between the two groups was four- to sixfold. The lower number of differences between successive N-N intervals of >50 ms for the patients with low values of HP-24 indicates a lower level of parasympathetic nervous (vagal) activity in this group. (Reprinted by permission from Bigger JT, Kleiger RE, Fleiss JL, et al.: Am J Cardiol 61:208, 1988.)

death nor the arrhythmic death category in the Hinkle-Thaler classification has been validated. Classification of deaths as due to myocardial failure has not been validated either.

The Multicenter Post-Infarction Program (MPIP) investigators classified deaths as sudden or non-sudden, and also by mechanism.[100] The MPIP was based on a longitudinal natural history that sampled both university and community hospital populations.[27] During an average of 31 months of follow-up after myocardial infarction, 143 deaths occurred. Carefully designed mortality forms were used to collect information on the location of death, whether it was sudden, and whether symptoms suggesting ischemia were present during the terminal event.[100] Data on the forms were supplemented by a narrative summary of the terminal event prepared by the research nurse and principal investigator in each enrolling center. Mortality information was reviewed and classified at regular meetings of a four-man Mortality Review Committee.

To assign a mechanism to each death, the classification by Hinkle and Thaler[101] was used (Table 17–7). The major categories in this classification are arrhythmic death, death due to circulatory failure, and noncardiac death. Arrhythmic death is defined by Hinkle and Thaler as "abrupt loss of consciousness and disappearance of pulse without prior collapse of the circulation." Arrhythmic deaths also are subclassified with respect to heart failure: (1) not preceded by congestive heart failure; (2) preceded by chronic congestive heart failure that was not disabling; and (3) preceded by chronic, disabling congestive heart failure. Circulatory failure is defined as collapse of circulation before disappearance of the pulse and is subdivided into two subclasses: (1) failure of peripheral circulation and (2) myocardial failure. Category III (i.e., noncardiac deaths) includes death due to cancer, cerebral emboli, accidents, suicide, and complications of procedures.

Of the 143 deaths in the MPIP, 53% occurred outside-hospital, 42% in-hospital, and 5% in emergency rooms.[100] Death was witnessed in 70% of the cases. Almost 25% of the deaths were not cardiac. Of the 104 cardiac deaths with known onset of symptoms, 43% were sudden (<1 hour). By the Hinkle-Thaler classification, 56% of the deaths were arrhythmic, 20% were due to myocardial failure, and 24% were not cardiac. The subgroups of arrhythmic deaths are shown in Table 17–7. About two-thirds of the arrhythmic deaths were not preceded by disabling heart failure. Even deaths that were preceded by disabling heart failure were abrupt and occurred without prior evidence of circulatory collapse. By the Hinkle-Thaler classification, 98% of the sudden deaths, were classified as arrhythmic and 54% of the non-sudden cardiac deaths were arrhythmic.

THE VALIDITY OF SUDDEN DEATH

A common method for validating a mechanistic classification of death is by relating the mechanism of death to functional risk indicators found at baseline. Sudden or arrhythmic death is expected to have a stronger association with arrhythmias detected at baseline than with other risk indicators. Similarly, deaths classified as myocardial failure could be validated by finding that reduced left ventricular ejection fraction at baseline was more strongly associated with failure deaths than with other mechanisms. In the MPIP, patients were characterized for functional risk indicators using the following tests: 24-hour continuous ECG recording (arrhythmias), radionuclide ventriculogram (left ventricular dysfunction), and treadmill exercise (ischemia). Patients were then followed 2 to 4 years. An intensive effort was made to determine the mechanisms of death in terms of arrhythmias, left ventricular dysfunction, and ischemia. The classification of sudden cardiac death was not validated. Patients with spontaneous ventricular arrhythmias at baseline were not much more likely to die from sudden or arrhythmic mechanisms than from other mechanisms. The classification of myocardial failure death was not validated either. Patients with low ejection fractions at baseline were more likely to die from arrhythmias than from myocardial failure. This lack of validity for classification of the mechanism of death, could be due to inability of the baseline tests to characterize important functional abnormalities, changes in functional risk due to interim events, or to confounding by competing risks.

Multiple and Competing Risks After Myocardial Infarction

The MPIP investigators found that patients with coronary heart disease usually have multiple functional deficits as they approach death. Many have both arrhythmias and heart failure, and about half have either angina pectoris or recurrent myocardial infarction in the last few weeks of life. How the three important mechanisms interact pathophysiologically to lead to death is almost impossible to determine. A single functional mechanism of death is difficult to identify, even when a patient dies in an intensive care unit

TABLE 17–7
Hinkle-Thaler Classification of Deaths After Myocardial Infarction*

Classification	Number of Deaths
I. Arrhythmic Deaths	
1. not preceded by heart failure	26
2. preceded by heart failure, not disabling	26
3. preceded by heart failure, disabling	28
Subtotal	80
II. Circulatory Failure Deaths	
1. peripheral circulatory failure	0
2. myocardial failure	28
Subtotal	28
III. Not Classifiable	35
Total	143

*Data from Marcus FI, Cobb LA, Edwards JE, et al.: Am J Cardiol 61:8, 1988.

under continuous electrocardiographic and hemodynamic observation.

Because several pathophysiologic factors often contribute to death in coronary heart disease, it is difficult to link baseline indicators (i.e., arrhythmias, left ventricular dysfunction, or ischemia) to the mechanism of death. Competing risks can confound functional classifications of death. A post-infarction patient who has frequent and repetitive ventricular arrhythmias in a baseline 24-hour ECG recording may experience a second myocardial infarct and die a few days later of myocardial failure. If the death is classified as primarily due to heart failure or ischemia, this case represents a lack of validity (i.e., arrhythmic risk was detected on baseline examination, but the death was not arrhythmic). Had the fatal infarct not occurred, the patient may have died an arrhythmic death at some later point in time, but we can never know. The competing risk concept makes it clear why it is difficult to validate mechanistic classifications of death.

The difficulty in validating sudden death will cloud the interpretation of studies that attempt to show treatment effects on sudden or arrhythmic death. However, collateral information can strengthen the inference that a reduction in sudden death indicates an effect on lethal arrhythmias. For example, the inference would be strengthened if the treatment reduces arrhythmias and known arrhythmogenic factors as well as sudden death.

References

1. Miller RR, Olson HG, Vismara LA, et al.: Pump dysfunction after myocardial infarction: Importance of location, extent and pattern of abnormal left ventricular segmental contraction. Am J Cardiol 37:340, 1976.
2. Shell WE, Kjekshus JK, Sobel BE: Quantitative assessment of the extent of myocardial infarction in the conscious dog by means of analysis of serial changes in serum creatine phosphokinase activity. J Clin Invest 50:2614, 1971.
3. Roberts R, Sobel BE, Parker CW: Radioimmunoassay for creatine kinase isoenzymes. Science 194:855, 1976.
4. Geltman EM, Ehsani AA, Campbell MK, et al.: The influence of location and extent of myocardial infarction on long-term ventricular dysrhythmia and mortality. Circulation 60:805, 1979.
5. Roberts R, Henry PD, Sobel BE: An improved basis for enzymatic estimation of infarct size. Circulation 52:743, 1975.
6. Marmor A, Sobel BE, Roberts R: Factors presaging early recurrent myocardial infarction ("extension"). Am J Cardiol 48:603, 1981.
7. Roberts R: Non-transmural myocardial infarction. Council Clin Cardiol Newslet 11:1, 1985.
8. Vatner SF, Baig H, Manders WT, et al.: Effects of coronary artery reperfusion on myocardial infarct size calculated from creatine kinase. J Clin Invest 61:1048, 1978.
9. Ganz W, Buchbinder N, Marcus H, et al.: Intracoronary thrombolysis in evolving myocardial infarction. Am Heart J 101:4, 1981.
10. Ong L, Reiser P, Coromilas J, et al.: Left ventricular function and rapid release of creatine kinase MB in acute myocardial infarction: Evidence for spontaneous reperfusion. N Engl J Med 309:1, 1983.
11. Holman BL, Chisholm RJ, Braunwald E: The prognostic implications of acute myocardial infarct scintigraphy with ^{99m}Tc pyrophosphate. Circulation 57:320, 1978.
12. Weshey G, Higging CB, Lanzer P, et al.: Imaging and characterization of acute myocardial infarction in vivo by gated nuclear magnetic resonance. Circulation 69:125, 1984.
13. Holman BL, Goldhaber SZ, Kirsch CM, et al.: Measurement of infarct size using single photon emission computed tomography and technetium-^{99m}pyrophosphate: A description of the method and comparison with patient prognosis. Am J Cardiol 50:503, 1982.
14. Schelbert HR, Henze E, Schron HR, et al.: C-11 palmitate for the noninvasive evaluation of regional myocardial fatty acid metabolism with positron computed tomography. III. In vivo demonstration of the effects of substrate availability of myocardial metabolism. Am Heart J 105:492, 1983.
15. Rutherford BD, McCann WD, O'Donnovan TPB: The value of monitoring pulmonary artery pressure for early detection of left ventricular failure following myocardial infarction. Circulation 43:655, 1971.
16. Ratshin RA, Rackley CE, Russell RO: Hemodynamic evaluation of left ventricular function in shock complicating myocardial infarction. Circulation 45:127, 1972.
17. Forrester JS, Diamond GA, Swan HJC: Correlative classification of clinical and hemodynamic function after myocardial infarction. Am J Cardiol 39:137, 1977.
18. Weber KT, Janicki JJ, Russell RO, et al.: Identification of high risk subsets of acute myocardial infarction. Am J Cardiol 41:197, 1978.
19. Shell W, Peter T, Mickle D, et al.: Prognostic implications of reduction of left ventricular filling pressure in early transmural acute myocardial infarction. Am Heart J 102:334, 1981.
20. Cohn JA, Franciosa JA, Francis GA, et al.: Effects of short term infusion of sodium nitroprusside on mortality rate in acute myocardial infarction complicated by left ventricular failure. N Engl J Med 306:1129, 1982.
21. Norris RM, Brandt PWT, Caughey DE, et al.: A new coronary prognostic index. Lancet 1:274, 1969.
22. Peel AAF, Semple T, Wang I, et al.: A coronary prognostic index for grading the severity of infarction. Br Heart J 24:745, 1962.
23. Maroko PR, Libby P, Covell JW, et al.: Precordial S-T segment elevation mapping: An atraumatic method for assessing alterations in the extent of myocardial ischemic injury. Am J Cardiol 29:223, 1972.
24. Heng Mk, Singh BN, Norris RM, et al.: Relationship between ST-segment elevation and myocardial ischemic damage after experimental coronary artery occlusion in dogs. J Clin Invest 58:1317, 1976.
25. Schelbert H, Verba J, Johnson A, et al.: Nontraumatic determination of left ventricular ejection fraction by radionuclide angiocardiography. Circulation 51:902, 1975.
26. Schulze RA Jr, Rouleau J, Rigo P, et al.: Ventricular arrhythmias in the late hospital phase of acute myocardial infarction: Relation to left ventricular function detected by gated cardiac blood pool scanning. Circulation 52:1006, 1975.
27. Multicenter Post-infarction Research Group: Risk stratification after myocardial infarction. N Engl J Med 309:331, 1983.
28. Greenberg H, McMaster P, Dwyer EM Jr, et al.: Left ventricular dysfunction after acute myocardial infarct: Results of a prospective multicenter study. J Am Coll Cardiol 4:867, 1984.
29. Warnowitz MA, Parker H, Cheitlin MD: Prognosis of patients with acute pulmonary edema and normal ejection fraction after myocardial infarction. Circulation 67:330, 1983.
30. Dwyer EM Jr, McMaster P, Greenberg H, et al.: Non-fatal cardiac events and recurrent infarction in the year following acute myocardial infarction. J Am Coll Cardiol 4:695, 1984.
31. Corbett JR, Dehmer GJ, Lewis SE, et al.: The prognostic value of submaximal exercise testing with radionuclide ventriculography before hospital discharge in patients with recent myocardial infarction. Circulation 65:535, 1981.
32. Borer JS, Roding DR, Miller RH, et al.: Natural history of left ventricular function during 1 year after acute myocardial infarction: Comparison with clinical, electrocardiographic and biochemical determinations. Am J Cardiol 46:1, 1980.
33. Wasserman AG, Katz RJ, Cleary P, et al.: Noninvasive detection of multivessel disease after myocardial infarction by exercise radionuclide ventriculography. Am J Cardiol 50:1242, 1982.
34. Hutchins GM, Bukley BH: Infarct expansion versus extension:

Two different complications of acute myocardial infarction. Am J Cardiol 41:1127, 1978.
35. Eaton LW, Weiss JL, Bukley BH, et al.: Regional cardiac dilatation after acute myocardial infarction. N Engl J Med 300:57, 1979.
36. Heger JJ, Weyman AE, Wann LS, et al.: Cross-sectional echocardiographic analysis of the extent of left ventricular asynergy in acute myocardial infarction. Circulation 61:113, 1980.
37. Gibson RS, Bishop HL, Stamm RB, et al.: Value of early two-dimensional echocardiography in patients with acute myocardial infarction. Am J Cardiol 49:1110, 1982.
38. Nixon JV, Narahara A, Smitherman TC: Estimation of myocardial involvement in patients with acute myocardial infarction by two-dimensional echocardiography. Circulation 62:1248, 1980.
39. Stamm RB, Gibson RS, Bishop HL, et al.: Echocardiographic detection of infarct-localized asynergy and remote asynergy during acute myocardial infarction: Correlation with extent of angiographic coronary disease. Circulation 67:233, 1983.
40. Bigger JT Jr, Weld FM, Coromilas J, et al.: Prevalence and significance of arrhythmias in 24-hour ECG recordings made within one month of acute myocardial infarction. In Kulbertus H, Wellens HJJ (eds.): The First Year after a Myocardial Infarction, pp. 161–175. Boston, Martinus Nijhoff, 1983.
41. Bigger JT Jr, Fleiss JL, Kleiger R, et al.: The relationships among ventricular arrhythmias, left ventricular dysfunction, and mortality in the 2 years after myocardial infarction. Circulation 69:250, 1984.
42. Mukharji J, Rude RE, Poole WK, et al.: Risk factors for sudden death after acute myocardial infarction: Two-year follow-up. Am J Cardiol 54:31, 1984.
43. Bigger JT Jr, Rolnitzky LM, Merab JP: Epidemiology of ventricular arrhythmias and clinical trials with antiarrhythmic drugs. In Fozzard HM, Haber E, Jennings RB, et al. (eds.): The Heart and Cardiovascular System: Scientific Foundations, pp. 1405–1449. Boston, Martinus Nijhoff, 1986.
44. Moss AJ, Davis HT, DeCamilla J, et al.: Ventricular ectopic beats and their relation to sudden and nonsudden cardiac death after myocardial infarction. Circulation 60:998, 1978.
45. Bigger JT Jr, Weld FM: Analysis of prognostic significance of ventricular arrhythmias after myocardial infarction. Shortcomings of Lown grading system. Br Heart J 45:717, 1981.
46. Bigger JT Jr, Weld FM, Rolnitzky LM: The prevalence and significance of ventricular tachycardia detected by ambulatory ECG recording in the late hospital phase of acute myocardial infarction. Am J Cardiol 48:815, 1981.
47. Schulze RA Jr, Strauss HW, Pitt B: Sudden death in the year following myocardial infarction. Relation to ventricular premature contractions in the late hospital phase and left ventricular ejection fraction. Am J Med 62:192, 1977.
48. Mukharji J, Rude RE, Poole K, et al.: Late sudden death following acute myocardial infarction, importance of combined presence of repetitive ventricular ectopy and left ventricular dysfunction. Clin Res 30:108A, 1982.
49. Clark KW, Hitchens RE, Ritter JA, et al.: Argus/2H: a dual-channel Holter-tape analysis system. In Computers in Cardiology (IEEE Computer Society), pp. 191–196, 1977.
50. Birman KP, Rolnitzky LM, Bigger JT: A shape oriented system for automated Holter ECG analysis. In Computers in Cardiology (IEEE Computer Society), pp. 217–220, 1978.
51. Clark KW, Rolnitzky LM, Miller JP, et al.: Ambulatory ECG analysis shared by two independent computer labs in a multicenter post-infarction program (MPIP). In Computers in Cardiology (IEEE Computer Society), pp. 271–275, 1981.
52. Maisel AS, Scott N, Gilpin E, et al.: Complex ventricular arrhythmias in patients with Q wave versus non–Q wave myocardial infarction. Circulation 72:963, 1985.
53. Kleiger RE, Miller JP, Thanavaro S, et al.: Relationship between clinical features of acute myocardial infarction and ventricular runs two weeks to one year following infarction. Circulation 63:64, 1981.
54. Lichstein E, Morganroth J, Harrist R, et al.: Effect of propranolol on ventricular arrhythmia. The beta-blocker heart attack trial experience. Circulation 67:I-5, 1983.
55. Granath A, Sodermark T, Winge T, et al.: Early work load tests for evaluation of long-term prognosis of myocardial infarction. Br Heart J 39:758, 1977.
56. Weld FM, Chu K-L, Bigger JT Jr, et al.: Risk stratification with low-level exercise testing 2 weeks after acute myocardial infarction. Circulation 64:306, 1981.
57. Krone RJ, Gillespie JA, Weld FM, et al.: Low-level exercise testing after myocardial infarction: Usefulness in enhancing clinical risk stratification. Circulation 71:80, 1985.
58. Bigger JT Jr, Reiffel JA, Livelli FD Jr, et al.: Sensitivity, specificity, and reproducibility of programmed ventricular stimulation. Circulation 73(Suppl 2):II-73, 1986.
59. Horowitz L, Josephson M, Farshidi A, et al.: Recurrent sustained ventricular tachycardia. 3. Role of the electrophysiologic study in selection of antiarrhythmic regimens. Circulation 58:986, 1978.
60. Mason JW, Winkle RA: Electrode-catheter arrhythmia induction in the selection and assessment of antiarrhythmic drug therapy for recurrent ventricular tachycardia. Circulation 58:971, 1978.
61. Podrid PJ, Schoeneberger A, Lown B, et al.: Use of nonsustained ventricular tachycardia as a guide to antiarrhythmic drug therapy in patients with malignant ventricular arrhythmia. Am Heart J 105:181, 1983.
62. Swerdlow CD, Winkle RA, Mason JW: Prognostic significance of the number of induced ventricular complexes during assessment of therapy for ventricular tachyarrhythmias. Circulation 68:400, 1983.
63. Zipes DP, Prystowsky EN, Heger JJ: Electrophysiologic testing of antiarrhythmic agents. Am Heart J 103:610, 1982.
64. Breithardt G, Borggrefe M, Haerten K: Role of programmed ventricular stimulation and noninvasive recording of ventricular late potentials for the identification of patients at risk of ventricular tachyarrhythmias after acute myocardial infarction. In Zipes DP, Jalife J (eds.): Cardiac Electrophysiology and Arrhythmias, pp. 553–561. New York, Grune & Stratton, Inc., 1985.
65. Haerten K, Abendroth RR, Breithardt G: Programmierte stimulation zur prufung der vulnerabilitat der kammern in der postinfarktphase. Z Kardiol 70:325, 1981.
66. Hamer A, Vohra J, Hunt D, et al.: Prediction of sudden death by electrophysiologic studies in high risk patients surviving acute myocardial infarction. Am J Cardiol 50:223, 1982.
67. Marchlinski FE, Buxton AE, Waxman HL, et al.: Identifying patients at risk of sudden death after myocardial infarction: Value of the response to programmed stimulation, degree of ventricular ectopic activity and severity of left ventricular dysfunction. Am J Cardiol 52:1190, 1983.
68. Richards DA, Cody DV, Denniss AR, et al.: Ventricular electrical instability: A predictor of death after myocardial infarction. Am J Cardiol 51:75, 1983.
69. Roy D, Marchand E, Theroux P, et al.: Programmed ventricular stimulation in survivors of an acute myocardial infarction. Circulation 72:487, 1985.
70. Santarelli P, Bellocci F, Loperfido F, et al.: Ventricular electrical instability in acute myocardial infarction: Clinical, angiographic and electrophysiologic correlations. Circulation 68(Suppl 3):108, 1983.
71. Denniss AR, Richards DA, Cody DV, et al.: Prognostic significance of ventricular tachycardia and fibrillation induced at programmed stimulation and delayed potentials detected on the signal-averaged electrocardiograms of survivors of acute myocardial infarction. Circulation 74:731, 1986.
72. Klein H, Trappe HJ, Hartwig CA, et al.: Repeated programmed stimulation within the first year after myocardial infarction. Circulation 72:III-359, 1985.
73. Costard A, Schluter M, Geiger M: Inducibility of ventricular arrhythmias after myocardial infarction. Influence of time on stimulation results and prognostic significance. Circulation 72:III-477, 1985.
74. Gang ES, Bigger JT Jr, Livelli FD Jr: A model of chronic ischemic arrhythmias: The relationships among electrically inducible ventricular tachycardia, ventricular fibrillation threshold and myocardial infarct size. Am J Cardiol 50:469, 1982.
75. Coromilas J, Bigger JT Jr, Gang ES, et al.: Relationship between infarct size and ventricular arrhythmias. In Zipes DP, Jalife J (eds.): Cardiac Electrophysiology and Arrhythmias, pp. 523–530. New York, Grune & Stratton, 1985.

76. Wilber DJ, Lynch JJ, Montgomery D, et al.: Postinfarction sudden death: Significance of inducible ventricular tachycardia and infarct size in a conscious canine model. Am Heart J 109:8, 1985.
77. Spielman SR, Yacone LA, Greenspan AM, et al.: Electrophysiologic testing in high-risk patients with nonsustained ventricular tachycardia and abnormal ventricular function. Circulation 68(Suppl 3):III-56, 1983.
78. Spielman SR, Greenspan AM, Kay HR, et al.: Electrophysiologic testing in patients at high risk to sudden death. Nonsustained ventricular tachycardia and abnormal ventricular function. J Am Coll Cardiol 6:31, 1985.
79. Winkle RA, Thomas A: The automatic implantable cardioverter defibrillator: The U.S. experience. *In* Brugada P, Wellens HJJ (eds.): Cardiac Arrhythmias: Where do we go from here? pp. 663–680. Mt. Kisco, New York, Futura Publishing Co., 1987.
80. Breithardt G, Schwarzmaier J, Borggrefe M, et al.: Prognostic significance of late ventricular potentials after acute myocardial infarction. Eur Heart J 4:487, 1983.
81. Breithardt G, Borggrefe M, Haerten K: Ventricular late potentials and inducible ventricular tachyarrhythmias as a marker for ventricular tachycardia after myocardial infarction. Eur Heart J 7:127, 1986.
82. Breithardt G, Borggrefe M: Pathophysiological mechanisms and clinical significance of ventricular late potentials. Eur Heart J 7:364, 1986.
83. Breithardt G, Borggrefe M, Haerten K: Role of programmed ventricular stimulation and noninvasive recording of ventricular late potentials for the identification of patients at risk of ventricular tachyarrhythmias after acute myocardial infarction. *In* Zipes D, Jalife J (eds.): Cardiac Electrophysiology and Arrhythmias, pp. 553–561. Orlando, Fla., Grune and Stratton, 1984.
84. Breithardt G, Borggrefe M: Recent advances in the identification of patients at risk of ventricular tachyarrhythmias: Role of ventricular late potentials. Circulation 75:1091, 1987.
85. Breithardt G, Borggrefe M, Podczek A, et al.: Prognostic significance of late potentials in patients with coronary heart disease (Abstract). Circulation 76(Suppl 4):IV-344, 1987.
86. Gomes JA, Winters SL, Stewart D, et al.: A new noninvasive index to predict ventricular tachycardia and sudden death in the first year after myocardial infarction: Based on signal averaged electrocardiogram, radionuclide ejection fraction and Holter monitoring. J Am Coll Cardiol 10:349, 1987.
87. Kuchar DL, Thorburn CW, Sammel NL: Prediction of serious arrhythmic events after myocardial infarction: Signal-averaged electrocardiogram, Holter monitoring and radionuclide ventriculography. J Am Coll Cardiol 9:531, 1987.
88. Gomes JA, Winters SW, Stewart DW, et al.: The duration of the signal averaged QRS complex is the best non-invasive parameter to predict malignant arrhythmic events post-myocardial infarction: A prospective study (Abstract). Circulation 76(Suppl 4):IV-344, 1987.
89. Steinberg JS, Freedman RA, for the ESVEM investigators: The signal averaged ECG does not predict drug efficacy in sustained ventricular arrhythmias (Abstract). Circulation 76(Suppl 4):IV-344, 1987.
90. Hopp HW, Hombach V, Osterpey A, et al.: Clinical and prognostic significance of ventricular arrhythmias and ventricular late potentials in patients with coronary heart disease. *In* Hombach V, Hilger HH (eds.): Holter Monitoring Technique: Technical Aspects and Clinical Applications, pp. 297–307. Stuttgart, Schattauer, 1985.
91. Von Leitner E, Oeff M, Loock D, et al.: Value of noninvasively detected delayed ventricular depolarizations to predict prognosis in postmyocardial infarction patients (Abstract). Circulation 68(Suppl 3):III-83, 1983.
92. Sharma AD, Corr PB: Adrenergic factors in arrhythmogenesis in the ischemic and reperfused myocardium. Eur Heart J 4(Suppl D):79, 1983.
93. Lown B, Verrier RL: Neural activity and ventricular fibrillation. N Engl J Med 294:1165, 1976.
94. Schwartz PJ: Manipulation of the autonomic nervous system in the prevention of sudden cardiac death. *In* Brugada P, Wellens HJJ (eds.): Cardiac Arrhythmias: Where Do We Go from Here? pp. 741–765. Mt. Kisco, Futura Publishing Co., 1987.
95. La Rovere MT, Specchia G, Mazzoleni C, et al.: Baroreflex sensitivity in post-myocardial infarction patients. Correlation with physical training and prognosis. Circulation 74(Suppl IV):514, 1986.
96. Lombardi F, Sandrone G, Pernpruner S, et al.: Heart rate variability as an index of sympathovagal interaction in patients after myocardial infarction. Am J Cardiol 60:1239, 1988.
97. Kleiger RE, Miller JP, Bigger JT Jr, et al.: Decreased heart rate variability and its association with increased mortality after acute myocardial infarction. Am J Cardiol 59:256, 1987.
98. Myers GA, Martin GJ, Magid NM, et al.: Power spectral analysis of heart rate variability in sudden cardiac death: Comparison to other methods. IEEE Trans Biomed Eng BME-33:1149, 1986.
99. Bigger JT Jr, Kleiger RE, Fleiss JL, et al.: Components of heart rate variability measured during healing of acute myocardial infarction. Am J Cardiol 61:208, 1988.
100. Marcus FI, Cobb LA, Edwards JE, et al.: Mechanism of death and prevalence of myocardial ischemic symptoms in the terminal event after acute myocardial infarction. Am J Cardiol 61:8, 1988.
101. Hinkle LE, Thaler JT: Clinical classification of cardiac deaths. Circulation 65:457, 1982.

B. Role of Programmed Stimulation and the Signal-Averaged Electrocardiogram

A. Robert Denniss
David A. Richards
David L. Ross
John B. Uther

Contribution of Ventricular Tachyarrhythmias to Mortality after Myocardial Infarction

Approximately 50% of deaths in the year following myocardial infarction occur unexpectedly, with little or no warning.[2, 3, 11, 42, 45, 64, 68] These deaths are usually referred to as "sudden" deaths, although there is no uniform definition as to what constitutes sudden or unexpected death.[37] The majority of sudden deaths are due to ventricular tachycardia (VT) or ventricular fibrillation (VF).[8, 23, 40] When the onset of cardiac arrest has been documented by ambulatory electrocardiographic monitoring, VF was almost invariably initiated by VT.[48, 49]

Patients who die suddenly or who are resuscitated from VT or VF fit into two main groups. Many patients (the majority in most reported series) die virtually instantaneously following the onset of spontaneous VT or VF and have neither clinical evidence of fresh ischemia or infarction nor postmortem evidence of acute coronary thrombosis or recent infarction. The other large group of patients, who usually have prodromal symptoms, die rapidly in VT or VF associated with acute ischemia with or without reinfarction.[8, 11, 26, 40, 58] In the former group of patients, the scarred myocardium appears to provide the substrate for reentrant ventricular tachyarrhythmias and sudden death, in the absence of further acute myocardial ischemia.[10, 67]

Anatomic and Electrophysiologic Substrate for Reentrant Ventricular Tachyarrhythmias

The presence of patchy scar tissue after myocardial infarction permits intraventricular reentry. Reentry may be promoted by slowing conduction or shortening refractory periods or both,[31, 71] but a key prerequisite for reentry is that activation through one part of the potential circuit must persist beyond the refractory period of the excitable adjacent myocardium.[4] The reentrant pathways may be relatively constant for VT but may change their size and location with time in VF.[31, 71]

There are probably several causes for the slowed conduction and block required for reentrant excitation. It has been proposed that reduced resting membrane potentials and reduced amplitude and maximum upstroke velocity of action potentials may be contributing factors,[28, 63, 71] as may the anisotropic structure of cardiac muscle, which can promote asymmetry of activation due to the relationship of fiber orientation and the direction of propagation of excitatory wavefronts.[62] In some cases, intraventricular reentry may result from functional unidirectional block in the absence of a well-defined anatomic pathway.[1, 25, 50, 71]

However, the major contributors to the milieu of anatomic and electrophysiologic heterogeneity that predisposes to the initiation of reentrant ventricular tachyarrhythmias are the physical changes in intercellular coupling resulting from cell necrosis and scarring. The usual anatomic basis for conduction delay in sinus rhythm is the presence of patchy areas of scar tissue interdigitating with viable bundles of myocardium that have distorted orientation and tortuous interconnections.[16, 27, 50] Action potentials recorded from the surviving myocardial cells are almost always normal,[27, 65] but within a relatively small area of tissue there is heterogeneity of conduction, reflected in asynchrony of action potentials as adjacent regions are activated. The different components of the fractionated and delayed electrograms coincide with the asynchronous but normal action potentials.[65]

The anatomy of the infarct edge appears to be a determinant of the degree of localized conduction delay present in sinus rhythm. In a canine model of chronic myocardial infarction, the viable muscle bundles interdigitating with scar tissue were much larger and the edge of the infarct was much more irregular at sites

---

Grants were received from the National Health and Medical Research Council of Australia and the National Heart Foundation of Australia.

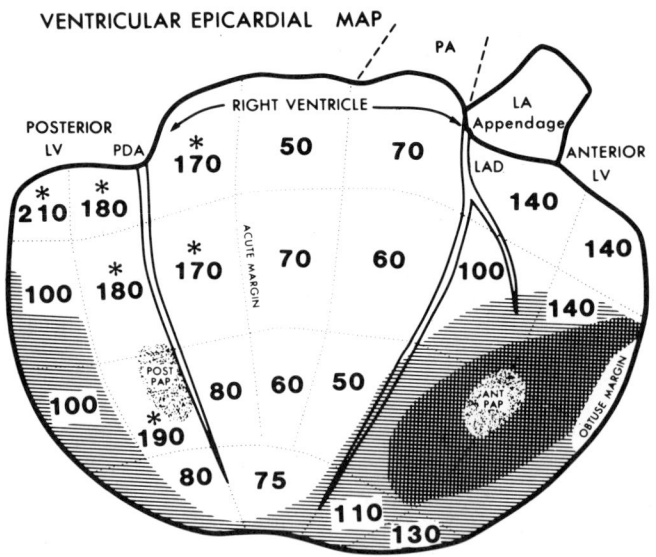

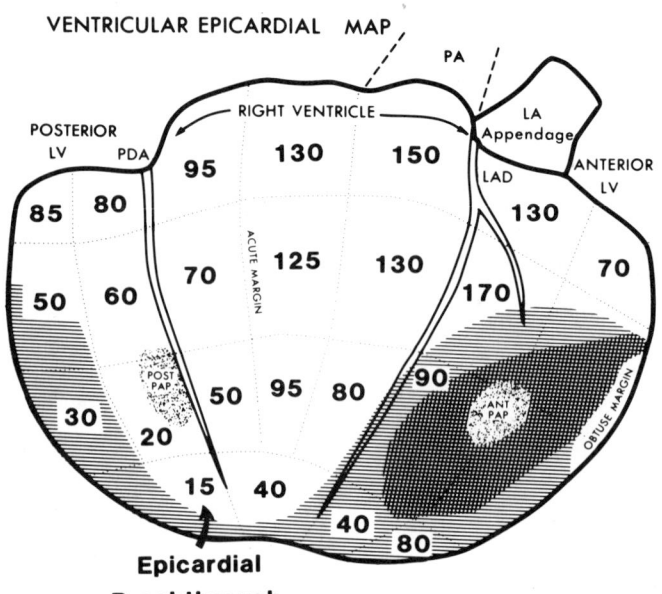

FIGURE 17–9
Ventricular epicardial map in sinus rhythm. Ventricular activation times (ms), measured from QRS onset to the end of local electrograms, are shown for epicardial sites from which electrograms were recorded intraoperatively in a patient with ventricular tachycardia.

The free wall of the left ventricle (LV) has been incised and laid open. The landmarks are the left anterior descending (LAD) and posterior descending (PDA) coronary arteries. The hatched areas depict macroscopic scar tissue, with the dark cross-hatching in the anterior left ventricle representing electrically inert scar. The sites with particularly marked conduction delay in sinus rhythm are highlighted by asterisks. LA = left atrium; PA = pulmonary artery; ANT PAP and POST PAP = anterior and posterior papillary muscles, respectively.

FIGURE 17–11
Ventricular epicardial map in ventricular tachycardia. Epicardial activation times during ventricular tachycardia are shown for the same patient as in Figures 17–9 and 17–10. Activation times (ms) are measured from QRS onset.

Earliest epicardial activation in ventricular tachycardia occurred 15 ms after QRS onset at the left ventricular apex posteriorly at the edge of the infarct and adjacent to an epicardial site with delayed activation in sinus rhythm (see legend of Figure 17–9 for explanation of abbreviations and hatched areas).

with conduction delay than at sites with no conduction delay.[16]

Conduction delay through small areas of myocardium, manifested as fractionated or delayed electrograms, has been detected consistently at epicardial and endocardial mapping in patients with VT associated with chronic myocardial infarction.[12, 32, 34] Conduction delay in sinus rhythm therefore appears to be a marker for the substrate for reentrant ventricular tachyarrhythmias, and earliest epicardial or endocardial activation in VT usually occurs at or near sites with delayed conduction (Figs. 17–9 through 17–12). However, not all sites with conduction delay in sinus rhythm appear to be intimately associated with reentrant circuits for

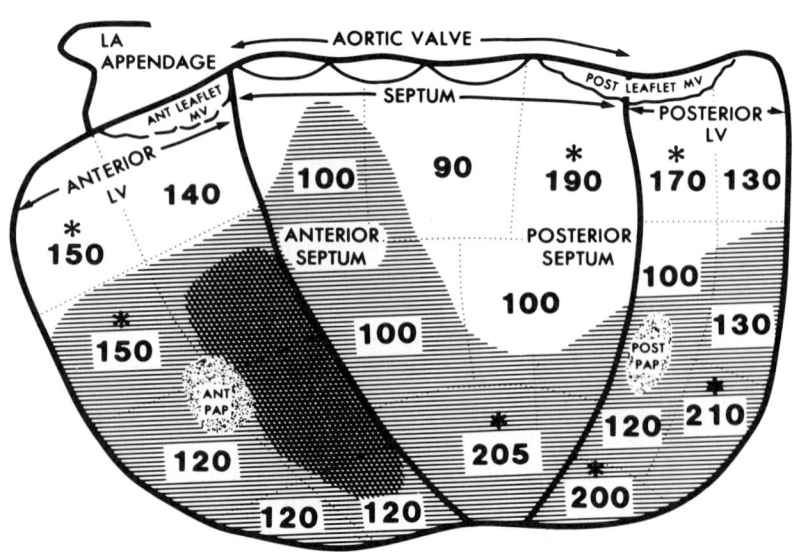

FIGURE 17–10
Ventricular endocardial map in sinus rhythm. Ventricular activation times (ms) are shown for left ventricular endocardial sites mapped intraoperatively in the same patient whose epicardial map is shown in Figure 17–9. The free wall of the left ventricle has been incised and laid open. The sites with particularly marked conduction delay in sinus rhythm are highlighted by asterisks. Abbreviations and hatching are same as for Figure 17–9. MV = mitral valve.

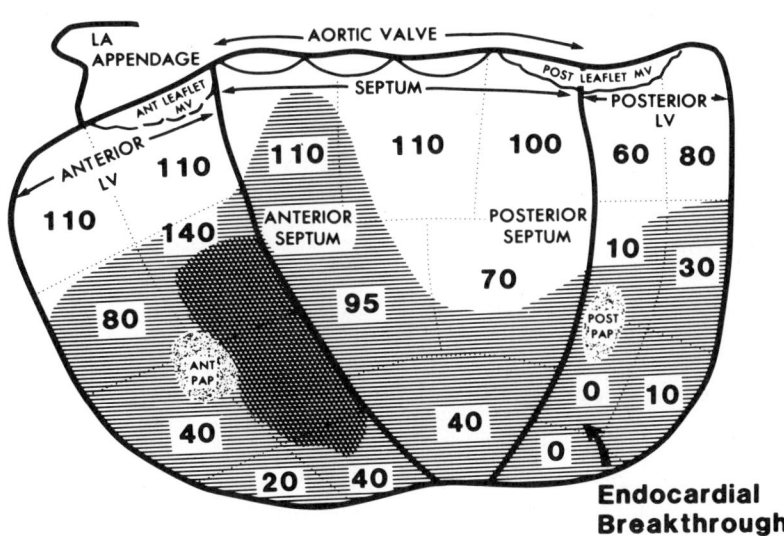

FIGURE 17–12
Ventricular endocardial map in ventricular tachycardia. Left ventricular activation times during ventricular tachycardia are shown for the same patient as in Figures 17–10 and 17–11. Activation times (ms) are measured from QRS onset.

Earliest endocardial activation occurred coincident with QRS onset at the posterior left ventricle near the apex. This was adjacent to sites with delayed ventricular activation in sinus rhythm (see Fig. 17–10) and was deep to the site at which earliest epicardial breakthrough occurred 15 ms later (see Fig. 17–11). See legend of Figure 17–9 for explanation of abbreviations and hatched areas.

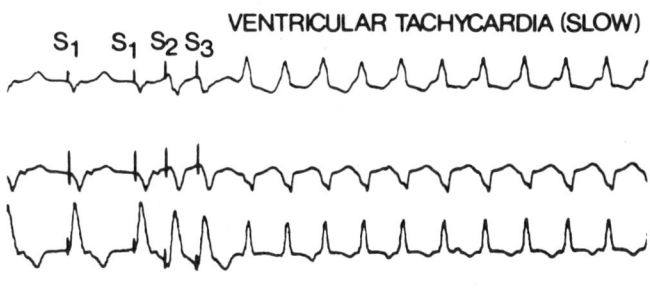

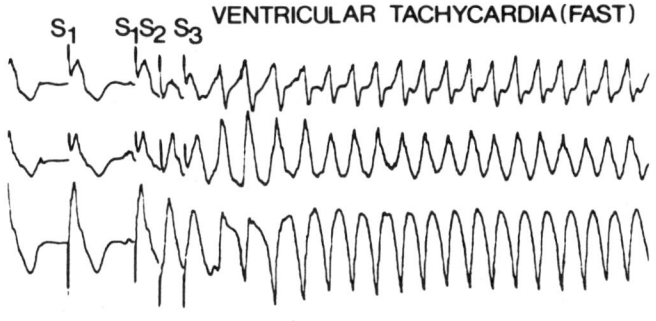

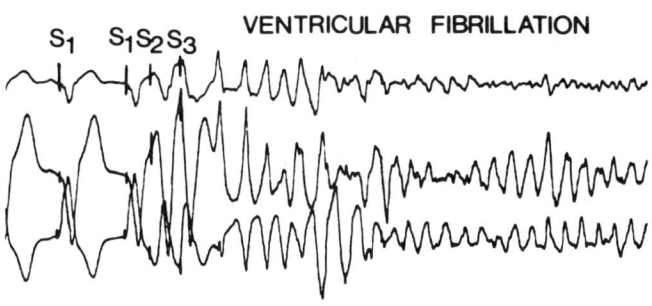

FIGURE 17–13
Induction of ventricular tachycardia (slow and fast) and ventricular fibrillation at programmed stimulation. The stimulation protocol used a drive train of 8 paced beats (S_1-S_1 = 600 ms) followed by 2 extrastimuli (S_2 and S_3).

VT (see Figs. 17–9 through 17–12), and there may be other factors such as the timing and location of ventricular premature complexes that determine whether an arrhythmia will be initiated and which sites with delayed conduction will be involved in the reentrant circuit.[4]

Role of Programmed Stimulation in Assessing Prognosis

Premature ventricular extrastimuli can be applied at programmed stimulation to induce reentrant ventricular tachyarrhythmias as part of electrophysiologic evaluation of patients who have been resuscitated from spontaneous VT and VF (Fig. 17–13). While multiple extrastimuli and sites of stimulation may have to be applied to induce arrhythmias, it is clear that programmed stimulation can be used in patients with spontaneous arrhythmias to identify the substrate for malignant reentrant arrhythmias.[18, 33, 41, 44, 52]

There has been much interest in the last decade in assessing the clinical implications of inducing ventricular tachyarrhythmias at programmed stimulation in survivors of acute myocardial infarction who have not exhibited such arrhythmias spontaneously. At least seven groups[6, 13, 30, 43, 51, 53, 55, 57, 70] have published studies examining the prognostic implications of inducible ventricular tachyarrhythmias in patient groups with either complicated or uncomplicated myocardial infarction. Besides large differences in patient selection, the studies have differed with respect to stimulation protocols and end points of stimulation. Only three centers have reported studies that have included more than 100 patients.[6, 13, 51, 53, 55]

The pattern that emerges from these investigations is that those studies with greater numbers of end points during follow-up[6, 13, 30, 51, 53, 70] showed that programmed stimulation was a significant predictor of sudden death or subsequent ventricular tachyarrhythmias. Those studies examined either patients who were considered to have complicated myocardial infarctions or else recruited large numbers of patients (up to 628).[6] In general, those studies with few end points during follow-up[43, 55, 57] did not find programmed stimulation to be useful prognostically; however, such studies examined only small numbers of patients (46–150 in each study) who were not typical of uncomplicated survivors of infarction, since they were clearly at unusually low risk of developing events.

The largest experience in the use of programmed stimulation as a predictive test in non-selected populations of clinically well survivors of infarction comes from the three Westmead Hospital studies, which investigated a total of 768 patients between 1980 and 1986.[13, 51, 53] The three Westmead studies will be considered in greater detail because they illustrate the progressive realization that not only the morphology of the inducible arrhythmia is important prognostically but also the cycle length.

WESTMEAD STUDIES

Patient Selection

Patients with acute myocardial infarction who fulfilled the following criteria were recruited: age less than 76 years; no spontaneous VT or VF beyond 48 hours after infarction; no persistent angina at rest; no cardiac failure, or else cardiac failure controlled with digitalis and diuretics; no significant comorbidity; and written informed consent.

Programmed Stimulation Protocols

Each patient underwent right ventricular programmed stimulation 6 to 28 days following infarction. All cardioactive medications other than digitalis and diuretics were suspended for at least 5 days prior to programmed stimulation.

The protocol applied to all 768 patients has been described in detail in the report by Richards.[52] A basic cycle length as close as possible to 600 ms was used; single and then double extrastimuli were introduced in diastole from 300 ms in 10-ms decrements to ventricular refractoriness. Pacing was performed at two right ventricular sites (apex and outflow tract), first at twice diastolic threshold current intensity and then at 20 mA. Stimuli were rectangular pulses 2 ms in duration, and there was a 3-s delay between each stimulus train.

In the third study (last 200 patients) a second protocol[53] was employed in addition to the first protocol described above. Each of the 200 patients was studied using the two protocols, applied in random order, with a break of 5 to 10 minutes between the completion of one protocol and the commencement of the other. The second protocol differed from the first in that only the right ventricular apex was stimulated, and all stimuli were at twice diastolic threshold. Each extrastimulus (from 300 ms in 10-ms decrements) was applied three times at each coupling interval before proceeding to the next coupling interval. Up to five extrastimuli were applied. The end points for stimulation using either protocol were completion of the protocol or induction of VT or VF lasting at least 10 seconds.[52]

Study End Points

The study end points were death or documented spontaneous sustained VT or VF. Ventricular tachyarrhythmias were presumed to be the cause of death if VT or VF was documented and had not been associated with antecedent chest pain or ischemic ECG changes, or if the death was instantaneous and not associated with prodrome or postmortem evidence of another cause of death.

Incidence of Inducible Arrhythmias

As shown in Table 17–8, the combined incidence of inducible VT and inducible VF in the first month after infarction was 23 to 34% using protocol 1 (two sites, two current intensities).[13, 51, 53] In the largest of the three studies,[13] the incidence of inducible arrhythmias 1 to 4 weeks after infarction was 20% for VT and 11% for VF. Of the patients with inducible VT, 30% had inducible slow VT (with a cycle length at least 230 ms). The patients with slow VT thus made up 6% of the study population. In that study,[13] the incidence of inducible arrhythmias declined with time after infarction, as only one half of the patients with inducible VT who remained well at 12 months after infarction still had inducible VT when retested using the identical protocol of programmed stimulation at 12 months.

Use of protocol 2, involving stimulation of 2 mA at the right ventricular apex and a variable number of extrastimuli,[53] resulted in a 16% incidence of inducible arrhythmias (VT + VF) with two extrastimuli. The incidence of inducible arrhythmias increased to 49% with three extrastimuli (see Table 17–8), to 73% with four extrastimuli and to 85% with five extrastimuli. The incidence of inducible slow VT was 3.5% for two extrastimuli, 7.5% for three extrastimuli, 8% for four extrastimuli, and 9% for five extrastimuli.

TABLE 17–8
Westmead Hospital Studies of Programmed Stimulation After Myocardial Infarction

	Author/Ref. No.		
	Richards[51]	Denniss[13]	Richards[53]
n	165	403	200
Inducible arrhythmias			
Protocol 1			
VT + VF	23%	34%	33%
Slow VT		6%	5.5%
Protocol 2 (3 ES)			
VT + VF			49%
Slow VT			7.5%

ES = extrastimuli; slow VT = VT with cycle length of at least 230 ms; Protocol 1 = 2 sites, 2 stimulus intensities, 1–2 ES[52]; Protocol 2 = 1 site, 1 stimulus intensity, 1–5 ES.[53]

Characteristics of Patients with Inducible Arrhythmias

Patients with inducible arrhythmias (VT + VF) have long been known to have worse left ventricular function than patients with no inducible arrhythmias.[51] More recently, it has been appreciated that patients with inducible arrhythmias do not constitute a homogeneous group and that there are differences between patients with inducible VT and patients with inducible VF.[13] When compared with inducible VF, inducible VT was associated with evidence of more extensive infarction (higher Norris coronary prognostic index,[46] lower left ventricular ejection fraction) and more marked conduction delay in sinus rhythm (longer ventricular activation time on signal-averaged ECG). As shown in Table 17–9, extrastimulus coupling intervals were shorter for induction of VF than for induction of VT. There was no correlation between ability to induce VT and the presence of complex ventricular ectopy, ST segment change at exercise testing, or angiographically defined coronary artery disease.[13]

Prognostic Implications of Inducible Arrhythmias

The first Richards study[51] showed that the presence of inducible arrhythmias (VT + VF) carried adverse implications, both for mortality and for occurrence of electrical events (instantaneous death + nonfatal VT or VF) in the first year after myocardial infarction. These findings were subsequently confirmed in the Denniss study.[13]

However, it was not until the Denniss study[13] that it was appreciated that only inducible VT had adverse prognostic implications. Patients with inducible VF were a low-risk group, comparable to the group with no inducible arrhythmias. Patients with nonsustained ventricular beating lasting less than 10 seconds were found to be at low risk of spontaneous arrhythmias. Besides the importance prognostically of the morphology of the inducible arrhythmia, the cycle length of the inducible arrhythmia was also found to be important. The majority of patients with events during follow-up had inducible slow VT,[13] an observation also made by Breithardt.[6] The adverse prognostic implications of inducible slow VT were subsequently confirmed by the second Richards study.[53]

For prediction of mortality or electrical events, the finding of inducible VT using protocol 1 had a positive predictive accuracy that was less than 25%.[53] Sensitivity was low (45–55%), but specificity exceeded 80% and negative predictive accuracy exceeded 90%.[13] Richards[53] set out to refine the protocol of programmed stimulation in order to improve the positive predictive accuracy of programmed stimulation. Using induction of slow VT as the predictor, Richards demonstrated that varying the number of extrastimuli rather than the site of stimulation and current intensity resulted not only in a simpler protocol but also in a more aggressive protocol in which positive predictive accuracy could be enhanced. It appeared that use of three extrastimuli in protocol 2 gave better positive predictive accuracy and sensitivity than did protocol 1 for prediction of electrical events, without loss of specificity or negative predictive accuracy.

In patients with a history of spontaneous VT associated with chronic myocardial infarction, the possibility of death or recurrence in untreated patients is only about 35%.[9] Therefore, the maximum positive predictive accuracy possible for any test after myocardial infarction would be about 35%.[53]

The optimum time at which to perform programmed stimulation for assessment of prognosis after recent myocardial infarction has yet to be determined. However, since a high proportion of patients who developed cardiac events did so within one month of infarction,[13] it would seem best to perform programmed stimulation within the first month.

Role of Signal-Averaged Electrocardiogram in Assessing Prognosis

The use of signal averaging and spatial averaging techniques to optimize the information content available from the surface electrocardiogram has enabled noninvasive detection of the conduction delay demonstrable at direct cardiac mapping in patients with VT.[5, 15, 24, 56, 59, 66] The conduction delay present in sinus rhythm can be recorded from the body surface as delayed (or late) potentials (Fig. 17–14) using averaging techniques, provided that the delayed conduction outlasts normal ventricular activation.[20, 61]

The prognostic implication of finding delayed potentials in patients in the convalescent phase of myocardial infarction (1 week–2 months) has been investigated in several large studies of at least 200 patients.[6, 13, 36, 53, 69] Despite the use of different averaging techniques, which were not strictly comparable with each other,[15, 47] all studies found that the presence of delayed potentials in the convalescent phase of infarction was correlated with subsequent cardiac mortality and/or occurrence of spontaneous sustained ventricular tachyarrhythmias.

In addition, there is evidence that delayed potentials detected in the first 10 days after infarction carry adverse prognostic implications.[29, 39] However, the optimal time after infarction at which to record the signal averaged ECG has yet to be established.

The incidence of delayed potentials in the convalescent phase after infarction varied from 20 to 40% in several studies.[6, 13, 36, 69] Two groups,[21, 35] restudied patients later after myocardial infarction and noted that the incidence of delayed potentials declined in the

TABLE 17–9
Extrastimulus Coupling Intervals for Arrhythmia Induction*

	Ventricular Tachycardia	Ventricular Fibrillation	p
S_1-S_2	228 ± 3	219 ± 3	<0.02
S_2-S_3	214 ± 4	198 ± 5	<0.01

*Values are means ± SEM (ms).

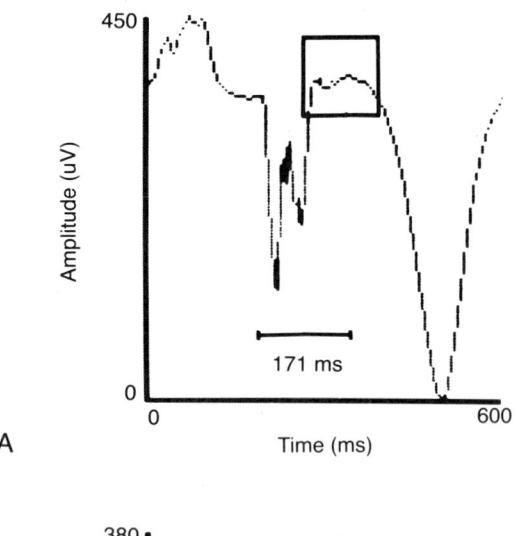

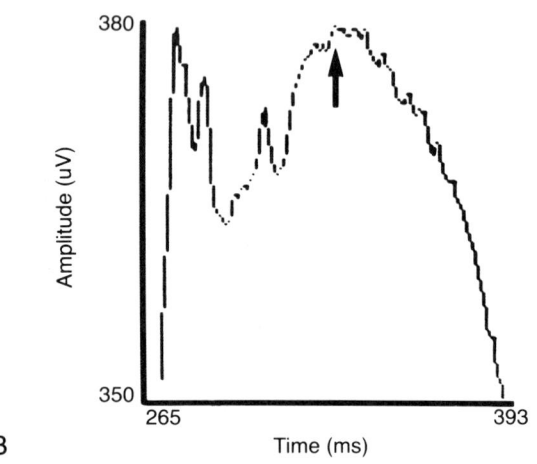

FIGURE 17-14
Signal-averaged Y trace from a patient who developed ventricular tachycardia late after myocardial infarction. *A*, Averaged Y trace at low amplification. Ventricular activation time in this lead was 171 ms; the determinations of QRS onset and offset (boxed area) were made at high amplification. *B*, QRS offset shown at high amplification. QRS offset (arrow) occurred at the end of low-amplitude signals extending into the ST segment. These signals were well above the noise level of 0.5 μV (not shown).

first 6 months after infarction but then remained relatively stable after 6 months. This was due to loss of delayed potentials in 30 to 45% of patients who had delayed potentials within the first month after myocardial infarction. Patients with no delayed potentials 1 to 6 weeks after infarction rarely developed delayed potentials in the next 12 months in the absence of further ischemia or reinfarction.

The findings of the two Westmead studies,[13, 54] which investigated a total of 506 patients between 1981 and 1986, will be considered in detail.

WESTMEAD STUDIES

Patient Selection

Patient selection was the same as that described earlier for the studies of programmed stimulation, except that patients were not studied by signal-averaged electrocardiography if they had bundle branch block or were on digitalis therapy.

Protocol for Signal Averaging

Each patient underwent signal averaging of the ECG 6 to 28 days following infarction (on the same day as programmed stimulation). All cardioactive medications other than diuretics were suspended at least 5 days prior to study. The signal-averaging technique has been described in detail in the report by Denniss.[15] X, Y, and Z leads of the Frank vectorcardiogram were recorded for 5 minutes, filtered (0.05–500 Hz), and digitized simultaneously, at 1000 samples/s. Signal averaging was performed after an iterative cross-correlation procedure was used to optimize QRS alignment.

QRS onset and offset in the averaged recordings were determined by displaying segments of each trace at high amplification. For a particular patient, ventricular activation time was measured as the total time from earliest QRS onset in any lead to latest QRS offset in any lead. QRS offset was measured to the end of any low-amplitude, high-frequency components extending into the ST segment, provided they had an amplitude more than twice that of the simultaneously displayed noise level (0.5–1.0 μV). Low amplitude signals extending into the ST segment were defined as delayed (late) potentials. Determination of ventricular activation time by this method has been shown to be free from significant interobserver variability, and day-to-day reproducibility of delayed potential detection exceeds 90%.[64]

Study End Points

The study end points were death or documented spontaneous sustained VT or VF.

Characteristics of Patients with Delayed Potentials

Patients with and without delayed potentials were not significantly different with respect to clinical profiles, although mean maximum creatine kinase levels and Norris coronary prognostic index were higher in the group with delayed potentials.[13] Left ventricular ejection fraction, number of diseased coronary arteries, and incidence of ST segment change of at least 2 mm at exercise testing were all similar in patient groups with and without delayed potentials (Table 17–10).

However, patients with delayed potentials had a higher incidence of inducible VT than did patients without delayed potentials (Table 17–10). Although there was a significant correlation between the presence or absence of delayed potentials and the presence or absence of inducible VT, overlap was not complete.

Prognostic Implications of Delayed Potentials

The Westmead studies[13, 54] showed that delayed potentials could predict either mortality or electrical events

TABLE 17–10
Characteristics of Patients with Delayed Potentials

	Delayed Potentials	No Delayed Potentials	p
Left ventricular ejection fraction*	0.34 ± 0.01	0.36 ± 0.01	NS
Diseased coronary vessels*	1.7 ± 0.1	1.8 ± 0.1	NS
Inducible ventricular tachycardia	41%	13%	<0.001
ST segment change ≥ 2 mm at exercise testing	21%	23%	NS

*Values are means ± SEM (ms). NS = not significant.

after myocardial infarction. Sensitivity for prediction of cardiac events and positive predictive accuracy were less than 25% and 70%, respectively. Specificity and negative predictive accuracy exceeded 70% and 90%, respectively.[13]

Events during follow-up were more likely the longer the ventricular activation time and the lower the ejection fraction.[13] As shown in Figure 17–15, patients with both delayed potentials and low ejection fraction fared much worse than did patients with delayed potentials who had relatively well-preserved left ventricular function.[13]

Multiple logistic regression analysis showed that delayed potentials and inducible VT did not provide independent prognostic information.[13] However, patients with both delayed potentials and inducible VT were at higher risk of having cardiac events in follow-up than patients with only delayed potentials or only inducible VT. The additive prognostic value of signal-averaged ECG and programmed stimulation has also been appreciated by Breithardt,[6] although Richards[54] suggested that delayed potentials did not give added predictive information if a patient was already known to have inducible VT of long cycle length. Delayed potentials have been shown, however, to give prognostic information independent of the presence of complex ventricular ectopy and independent of the degree of left ventricular dysfunction assessed at the time of hospital discharge.[36] Data from the study of Denniss[13] also shows that delayed potentials have superior predictive value compared with ST segment change of at least 2 mm (Table 17–11).

Patients at particularly low risk of any events during follow-up are those with the combination of no delayed potentials, no inducible VT, and well-preserved left ventricular function (Fig. 17–16).

Comparison of Programmed Stimulation and Signal-Averaged Electrocardiogram in Assessing Prognosis

Since there is a strong correlation between the results of programmed stimulation and the results of signal averaging,[13, 14] it is not surprising that inducible VT and delayed potentials have been found to be comparable in predicting mortality and electrical events after myocardial infarction. However, there is recent evidence that inducible *slow* VT is a better predictor of electrical events after myocardial infarction than is the presence of delayed potentials.[54] Multiple logistic regression analysis has shown that, after allowing for inducible slow VT, the presence of delayed potentials or complex ventricular ectopy or low ejection fraction or a positive exercise test did not provide additional predictive information. It would appear, therefore, that inducible slow VT is the most significant end point of programmed stimulation protocols.

Programmed stimulation and signal-averaged ECG appear to be able to identify, albeit with incomplete overlap, patients with the substrate for reentrant arrhythmias after myocardial infarction. Many of these patients appear to lose this substrate with time as the infarct heals, as judged by the decreased incidence of either inducible VT or delayed potentials 6 to 12 months after infarction. These patients appear to do well in follow-up. Whether programmed stimulation or the signal-averaged ECG will prove superior in serial monitoring of a patient's ongoing risk of developing VT and VF later after infarction has yet to be determined.

Clinical Implications

Inducible VT at programmed stimulation or delayed potentials at signal averaging can each identify patients at increased risk of cardiac death or of spontaneous VT or VF after myocardial infarction. Patients with either or both of these findings constitute 27% of the clinically well survivors of recent myocardial infarction.[13] The majority of patients have neither of these findings and are at very low risk for cardiac events and therefore do not require antiarrhythmic medication.

Not only do inducible slow VT and delayed potentials identify higher-risk patients, they also indicate a pathogenetic mechanism for adverse outcome—namely, propensity to reentrant ventricular tachyarrhythmias. Although predictive accuracy is no better for inducible VT and delayed potentials than for other indicators of high risk,[38] the finding of either of those

TABLE 17–11
Predictive Value of Delayed Potentials and ST Segment Change at Exercise Testing in 250 Survivors of Recent Myocardial Infarction*

	Death + Non-fatal Ventricular Tachyarrhythmias		
DP	16/50	32%	} p < 0.001; OR = 7.4
No DP	12/200	6%	
ST change	8/55	15%	} p = NS; OR = 1.5
No ST change	20/195	10%	

*Follow-up of 2 years.
DP = delayed potentials; ST change = ST segment change ≥ 2 mm; NS = not significant; OR = odds ratio.

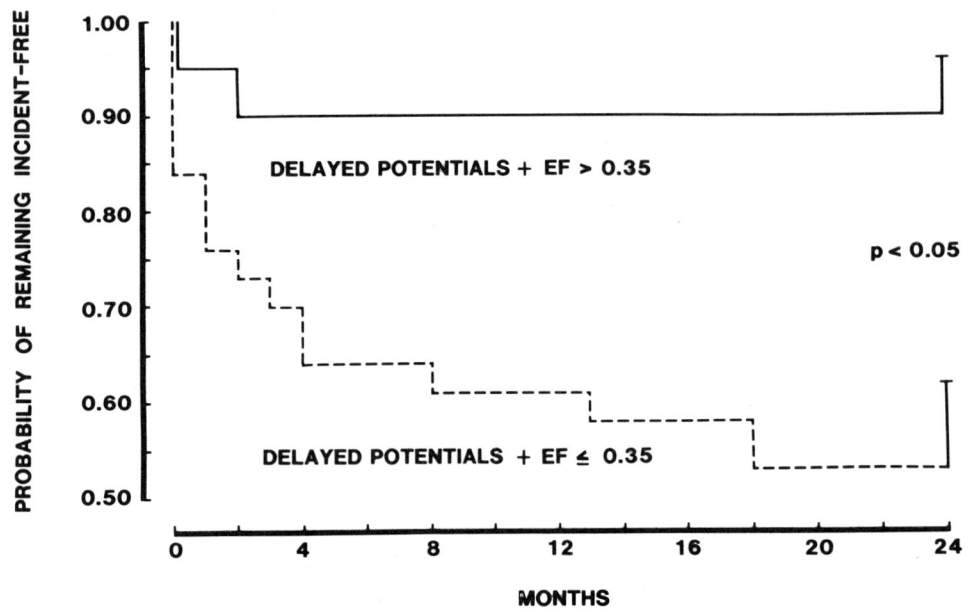

FIGURE 17–15
Prediction of death and non-fatal ventricular tachycardia or fibrillation (VT/VF) in patients with delayed potentials subdivided according to left ventricular ejection fraction (EF).

abnormalities does have potential usefulness by indicating that treatment should be directed at preventing arrhythmias. Other indices showing reduced ventricular function (e.g., left ventricular ejection fraction) are deficient in this respect, as there is no therapeutic maneuver available that can improve ventricular function and prolong life.

The predictive accuracy of inducible VT and delayed potentials may be increased by using both programmed stimulation and signal-averaged ECG to assess prognosis. Other investigations, looking at factors other than arrhythmogenic substrate (e.g., ventricular ectopy, extent of myocardial damage or ongoing ischemia) may also be added to define a very high risk group of patients with greater predictive accuracy than is possible when any of these investigations is used alone.

While inducible slow VT appears to be the single best predictor of electrical events after myocardial infarction,[54] it has the disadvantage that patients must be assessed by programmed stimulation, an invasive study. However, programmed stimulation is superior to the signal-averaged ECG in assessing antiarrhythmic drug therapies.[10] Even if patients are screened with the signal-averaged ECG, the high-risk patients with delayed potentials may still need to undergo programmed

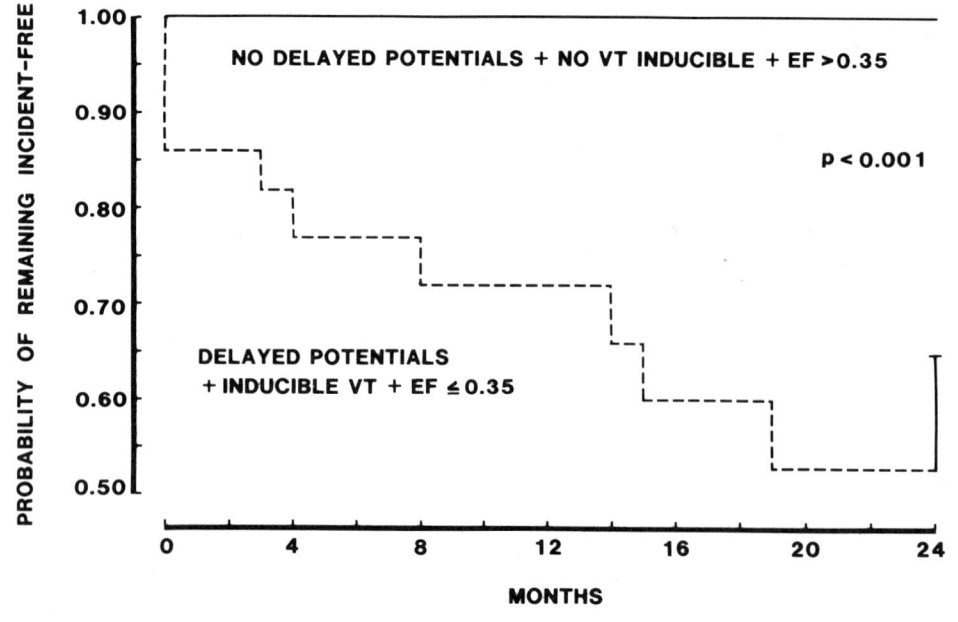

FIGURE 17–16
Prediction of death and non-fatal ventricular tachycardia or fibrillation (VT/VF) in a patient group with delayed potentials plus inducible VT plus low left ventricular ejection fraction (EF), compared with another patient group with no delayed potentials, no inducible VT, and high EF.

stimulation if antiarrhythmic drug therapies are under consideration, because the currently available antiarrhythmic drugs of classes I, II, and III only rarely abolish delayed potentials and have no therapeutically useful effects on ventricular activation time.[7, 19, 60]

Although no drug therapies have as yet been documented to improve the outcome of patients with inducible VT after recent myocardial infarction,[17] programmed stimulation does have an educational role for those patients with inducible VT. Such patients learn to recognize VT and are counseled that palpitations, presyncope, and syncope should not be ignored after hospital discharge.[53] Extra effort should be made to teach cardiopulmonary resuscitation techniques to the families of these patients. The best method of treatment of these high-risk patients has yet to be determined.

Acknowledgment

The typographical assistance of Sharon Galea is gratefully acknowledged.

References

1. Allessie MA, Bonke FI, Schopman FJ: Circus movement in rabbit atrial muscle as a mechanism of tachycardia. III. The "leading circle" concept: A new model of circus movement in cardiac tissue without the involvement of an anatomical obstacle. Circ Res 41:9, 1977.
2. Beta-blocker Heart Attack Trial Research Group: A randomized trial of propranolol in patients with acute myocardial infarction. 1. Mortality results. JAMA 247:1707, 1982.
3. Bigger JT, Heller CA, Wenger TL, et al.: Risk stratification after acute myocardial infarction. Am J Cardiol 42:202, 1978.
4. Boineau JP, Cox JL: Rationale for a direct surgical approach to control ventricular arrhythmias. Relation of specific intraoperative techniques to mechanism and location of arrhythmic circuit. Am J Cardiol 49:381, 1982.
5. Breithardt G, Becker R, Seipel L, et al.: Noninvasive detection of late potentials in man—a new marker for ventricular tachycardia. Eur Heart J 2:1, 1981.
6. Breithardt G, Borggrefe M, Haerten K: Role of programmed ventricular stimulation and non-invasive recording of ventricular late potentials for the identification of patients at risk of ventricular tachyarrhythmias after acute myocardial infarction. In Zipes DP, Jalife J (eds.): Cardiac Electrophysiology and Arrhythmias, pp. 53–61. New York, Grune and Stratton, 1985.
7. Breithardt G, Borggrefe M, Karbenn U, et al.: Effects of pharmacological and non-pharmacological interventions on ventricular late potentials. Eur Heart J 8(Suppl A):97, 1987.
8. Cobb LA, Baum RS, Alvarez HA, et al.: Resuscitation from out-of-hospital ventricular fibrillation: Four years follow-up. Circulation 52(Suppl. 3):223, 1975.
9. Cooper MJ, Hunt LJ, Palmer KJ, et al.: Prediction of proarrhythmic drug effects at electrophysiologic study for ventricular tachycardia. Circulation 74(Suppl. 2):482, 1986.
10. Cooper MJ, Hunt LJ, Richards DA, et al.: Antiarrhythmic drugs retard rather than suppress induction of ventricular tachycardia. Circulation 76(Suppl. 4):510, 1987.
11. Denniss AR, Baaijens H, Cody DV, et al.: Value of programmed stimulation and exercise testing in predicting one-year mortality after acute myocardial infarction. Am J Cardiol 56:213, 1985.
12. Denniss AR, Johnson DC, Richards DA, et al.: Effect of excision of ventricular myocardium on delayed potentials detected by the signal-averaged electrocardiogram in patients with ventricular tachycardia. Am J Cardiol 59:591, 1987.
13. Denniss AR, Richards DA, Cody DV, et al.: Prognostic significance of ventricular tachycardia and fibrillation induced at programmed stimulation and delayed potentials detected on the signal-averaged electrocardiograms of survivors of acute myocardial infarction. Circulation 74:731, 1986.
14. Denniss AR, Richards DA, Cody DV, et al.: Correlation between signal-averaged electrocardiogram and programmed stimulation in patients with and without spontaneous ventricular tachyarrhythmias. Am J Cardiol 59:586, 1987.
15. Denniss AR, Richards DA, Farrow RH, et al.: Technique for maximising the frequency response of the signal averaged Frank vectorcardiogram. J Biomed Eng 8:207, 1986.
16. Denniss AR, Richards DA, Waywood JA, et al.: Electrophysiological and anatomic differences between canine hearts with inducible ventricular tachycardia and fibrillation associated with chronic myocardial infarction. Circ Res 64:155, 1989.
17. Denniss AR, Ross DL, Cody DV, et al.: Randomized controlled trial of antiarrhythmic drugs in patients with inducible ventricular tachyarrhythmias after recent myocardial infarction. Eur Heart J 9:746, 1988.
18. Denniss AR, Ross DL, Johnson DC, et al.: Abnormalities on signal-averaged electrocardiogram and electrophysiologic study in patients with ventricular tachyarrhythmias not associated with ischemic heart disease. J Appl Cardiol 2:251, 1987.
19. Denniss AR, Ross DL, Richards DA, et al.: Effect of antiarrhythmic therapy on delayed potentials detected by the signal-averaged electrocardiogram in patients with ventricular tachycardia after acute myocardial infarction. Am J Cardiol 58:261, 1986.
20. Denniss AR, Ross DL, Richards DA, et al.: Differences between patients with ventricular tachycardia and ventricular fibrillation as assessed by signal-averaged electrocardiogram, radionuclide ventriculography and cardiac mapping. J Am Coll Cardiol 11:276, 1988.
21. Denniss AR, Ross DL, Richards DA, et al.: Changes in ventricular activation time on signal-averaged electrocardiogram in the first year after acute myocardial infarction. Am J Cardiol 60:580, 1987.
22. Denniss AR, Ross DL, Uther JB: Reproducibility of measurements of ventricular activation time using the signal-averaged Frank vectorcardiogram. Am J Cardiol 57:156, 1986.
23. Doyle JT: Profile of risk of sudden death in apparently healthy people. Circulation 52(Suppl. 3):176, 1975.
24. El-Sherif N, Mehra R, Gomes JAC, et al.: Appraisal of a low noise electrocardiogram. J Am Coll Cardiol 1:456, 1983.
25. El-Sherif N, Smith RA, Evans K: Canine ventricular arrhythmias in the late myocardial infarction period. 8. Epicardial mapping of re-entrant circuits. Circ Res 49:255, 1981.
26. Friedman M, Manwaring JH, Rosenman RH, et al.: Instantaneous and sudden deaths. Clinical and pathological differentiation in coronary artery disease. JAMA 225:1319, 1973.
27. Gardner PI, Ursell PC, Fenoglio JJ, et al.: Electrophysiologic and anatomic basis for fractionated electrograms recorded from healed myocardial infarcts. Circulation 72:596, 1985.
28. Gilmour RF, Heger JJ, Prystowsky EN, et al.: Cellular electrophysiologic abnormalities of diseased human ventricular myocardium. Am J Cardiol 51:137, 1983.
29. Gomes JA, Mehra R, Barreca P, et al.: Quantitative analysis of the high frequency components of the signal-averaged QRS complex in patients with acute myocardial infarction: A prospective study. Circulation 72:105, 1985.
30. Hamer A, Vohra J, Hunt D, et al.: Prediction of sudden death by electrophysiologic studies in high risk patients surviving acute myocardial infarction. Am J Cardiol 50:223, 1982.
31. Holley LK, Uther JB: A computer model of ventricular electrical activity and its application to ventricular arrhythmias. Australas Phys Eng Sci Med 8:88, 1985.
32. Horowitz LN, Josephson ME, Harken AH: Epicardial and endocardial activation during sustained ventricular tachycardia in man. Circulation 61:1227, 1980.
33. Kastor JA, Horowitz LN, Harken AH, et al.: Clinical electrophysiology of ventricular tachycardia. N Engl J Med 304:1004, 1981.
34. Klein H, Karp RB, Kouchoukos NT, et al.: Intraoperative electrophysiologic mapping of the ventricles during sinus rhythm in patients with a previous myocardial infarction. Identification of the electrophysiologic substrate of ventricular arrhythmias. Circulation 66:847, 1982.

35. Kuchar DL, Thorburn CW, Sammel NL: Late potentials detected after myocardial infarction: Natural history and prognostic significance. Circulation 74:1280, 1986.
36. Kuchar DL, Thorburn CW, Sammel NL: Prediction of serious arrhythmic events after myocardial infarction: Signal-averaged electrocardiogram, Holter monitoring and radionuclide ventriculography. J Am Coll Cardiol 9:531, 1987.
37. Kuller LH: Sudden death—definition and epidemiologic considerations. Progr Cardiovasc Dis 23:1, 1980.
38. Lesch M, Kehoe RF: Predictability of sudden cardiac death. A partly fulfilled promise. N Engl J Med 310:255, 1984.
39. Lewis SJ, Lauder PT, Taylor PA, et al.: The natural history of ventricular late potential activity in acute myocardial infarction. J Am Coll Cardiol 9:151A, 1987.
40. Liberthson RR, Nagel EL, Hirschman JC, et al.: Pathophysiologic observations in prehospital ventricular fibrillation and sudden cardiac death. Circulation 49:790, 1974.
41. Livelli FD, Bigger JT, Reiffel JA, et al.: Response to programmed ventricular stimulation: Sensitivity, specificity and relation to heart disease. Am J Cardiol 50:452, 1981.
42. Lown B: Sudden cardiac death: The major challenge confronting contemporary cardiology. Am J Cardiol 43:313, 1979.
43. Marchlinski FE, Buxton AE, Waxman HL, et al.: Identifying patients at risk of sudden death after myocardial infarction: Value of the response to programmed stimulation, degree of ventricular ectopic activity, and severity of left ventricular dysfunction. Am J Cardiol 52:1190, 1983.
44. Mason JW, Winkle RA: Accuracy of ventricular tachycardia-induction study for predicting long-term efficacy and inefficacy of antiarrhythmic drugs. N Engl J Med 303:1073, 1980.
45. Moss AJ, De Camilla J, Davis H: Cardiac death in the first 6 months after myocardial infarction: Potential for mortality reduction in the early posthospital period. Am J Cardiol 39:816, 1977.
46. Norris RM, Caughey DE, Mercer CJ, et al.: Coronary prognostic index for predicting survival after recovery from acute myocardial infarction. Lancet 2:485, 1970.
47. Oeff M, von Leitner ER, Sthapit R, et al.: Methods for non-invasive detection of ventricular late potentials—a comparative multicentre study. Eur Heart J 7:25, 1986.
48. Panidis I, Morganroth J: Sudden death in hospitalized patients: Cardiac rhythm disturbances detected by ambulatory electrocardiographic monitoring. J Am Coll Cardiol 2:798, 1983.
49. Pratt CM, Francis MJ, Luck JC, et al.: Analysis of ambulatory electrocardiograms in 15 patients during spontaneous ventricular fibrillation with special reference to preceding arrhythmic events. J Am Coll Cardiol 2:789, 1983.
50. Richards DA, Blake GJ, Spear JF, et al.: Electrophysiologic substrate for ventricular tachycardia: Correlation of properties in vivo and in vitro. Circulation 69:369, 1984.
51. Richards DA, Cody DV, Denniss AR, et al.: Ventricular electrical instability: A predictor of death after myocardial infarction. Am J Cardiol 51:75, 1983.
52. Richards DA, Cody DV, Denniss AR, et al.: A new protocol of programmed stimulation for assessment of predisposition to spontaneous ventricular arrhythmias. Eur Heart J 4:376, 1983.
53. Richards DA, Taylor A, Fahey P, et al.: Identification of patients at risk of sudden death after myocardial infarction: The continued Australian experience. *In* Brugada P, Wellens HJJ (eds.): Cardiac Arrhythmias. Where to Go From Here?, pp. 329–341. Mount Kisco, Futura Publishing Co., 1987.
54. Richards DA, Taylor A, Wallace E, et al.: What is the best predictor of sudden death after myocardial infarction? Aust NZ J Med 17:579, 1987.
55. Roy D, Marchand E, Theroux P, et al.: Programmed ventricular stimulation in survivors of an acute myocardial infarction. Circulation 72:487, 1985.
56. Rozanski JJ, Mortara D, Myerberg RJ, et al.: Body surface detection of delayed depolarizations in patients with recurrent ventricular tachycardia and left ventricular aneurysm. Circulation 63:1172, 1981.
57. Santarelli P, Bellocci F, Loperfido F, et al.: Ventricular arrhythmia induced by programmed ventricular stimulation after acute myocardial infarction. Am J Cardiol 55:391, 1985.
58. Schwartz CJ, Gerrity RG: Anatomical pathology of sudden unexpected cardiac death. Circulation 52(Suppl. 3):18, 1975.
59. Simson MB: Use of signals in the terminal QRS complex to identify patients with ventricular tachycardia after myocardial infarction. Circulation 64:235, 1981.
60. Simson MB, Falcone RA, Kindwall E: The signal-averaged electrocardiogram does not predict antiarrhythmic drug success. Circulation 72(Suppl. 3):7, 1985.
61. Simson MB, Untereker WJ, Spielman SR, et al.: Relation between late potentials on the body surface and directly recorded fragmented electrograms in patients with ventricular tachycardia. Am J Cardiol 51:105, 1983.
62. Spach MS, Kootsey JM: The nature of electrical propagation in cardiac muscle. Am J Physiol 244:H3, 1983.
63. Spear JF, Horowitz LN, Hodess AM, et al.: Cellular electrophysiology of human myocardial infarction. 1. Abnormalities of cellular activation. Circulation 59:247, 1979.
64. The Norwegian Multicenter Study Group: Timolol-induced reduction in mortality and reinfarction in patients surviving acute myocardial infarction. N Engl J Med 304:801, 1981.
65. Ursell PC, Gardner PI, Albala A, et al.: Structural and electrophysiological changes in the epicardial border zone of canine myocardial infarcts during infarct healing. Circ Res 56:436, 1985.
66. Uther JB, Dennett CJ, Tan A: The detection of delayed activation potentials of low amplitude in the vectorcardiogram of patients with recurrent ventricular tachycardia by signal averaging. *In* Sandoe E, Julian DG, Bell JW (eds.): Management of ventricular tachycardia—role of mexiletine, pp. 80–82. Amsterdam, Excerpta Medica, 1978.
67. Uther JB, Richards DA, Denniss AR, et al.: The prognostic significance of programmed ventricular stimulation after myocardial infarction: A review. Circulation 75(Suppl 3):161, 1987.
68. Vismara LA, Amsterdam EA, Mason DT: Relation of ventricular arrhythmias in the late hospital phase of acute myocardial infarction to sudden death after hospital discharge. Am J Med 59:6, 1975.
69. Von Leitner ER, Oeff M, Loock D, et al.: Value of noninvasively detected delayed ventricular depolarizations to predict prognosis in post myocardial infarction patients. Circulation 68(Suppl 3):83, 1983.
70. Waspe LE, Seinfeld D, Ferrick A, et al.: Prediction of sudden death and spontaneous ventricular tachycardia in survivors of complicated myocardial infarction: Value of the response to programmed stimulation using a maximum of three ventricular stimuli. J Am Coll Cardiol 5:1292, 1985.
71. Wit AL, Rosen M: Pathophysiologic mechanisms of cardiac arrhythmias. Am Heart J 106:798, 1983.

18

Management of the Patient with Sudden Cardiac Arrest

Eric Berger
Hasan Garan
Jeremy N. Ruskin

Despite recent advances in our understanding of cardiac pathology and the proliferation of increasingly sophisticated diagnostic techniques and treatment modalities, over 400,000 people die of sudden cardiac arrest each year in the United States alone.[1-3] Unfortunately, easily accessible and cost-effective means of identifying such cases before the index event are not yet available. While several important risk factors have been identified for cardiac arrest, individuals and physicians are often unaware of their presence, the arrest being the first clinical (and often fatal)[4] event for these individuals. However, when identified prospectively, modification of these risk factors may lead to a reduced risk of cardiac arrest.

For those people who do survive an episode of sudden cardiac arrest there is clearly a significant risk of recurrence in the first 1 to 2 years if no therapy or only empiric therapy is offered.[4-7] Advances in antiarrhythmic therapy,[8] especially when guided by electrophysiologic studies,[9] have reduced the subsequent mortality of these patients from 30 to 40% in the first year with empiric treatment to approximately 10% and 15% at 1 and 2 years, respectively. It is well established that the evaluation and therapy of patients surviving cardiac arrest must be aggressive and usually invasive to best establish a proper treatment regimen for each individual.

In this chapter, the current diagnostic and therapeutic approaches to such patients will be reviewed. It should be noted that considerable debate persists among many cardiologists with regard to the particular tests used to identify high-risk patients; the proper use, timing, and interpretation of these tests; and the relative efficacy and merits of various therapeutic options. These areas were discussed in detail in Chapter 17. A brief review of the pathophysiology and risk factors associated with sudden cardiac arrest is first presented.

Pathophysiology and Risk Factors

Early studies of patients who experienced cardiac arrest revealed the presence of significant arteriosclerotic heart disease (ASHD) in a majority of cases.[1, 10-21] The Tecumseh study prospectively identified coronary artery disease, hypertensive heart disease, and diabetes mellitus as significant risk factors present in 62% of people who subsequently sustained an episode of sudden cardiac arrest.[10] These findings were extended by Kuller et al.[1] in 1972. It is notable that the postmortem examination of sudden cardiac arrest patients in this study revealed extensive ASHD, usually involving three or four coronary arteries. Later studies similarly demonstrated multivessel coronary artery disease in a majority of these patients.[11-16, 20] An angiographic study of 64 patients resuscitated from cardiac arrest revealed advanced atherosclerosis in 94%, with 33% having triple vessel coronary artery disease. Thirty per cent had total occlusion of one or more coronary vessels. Importantly, ventricular fibrillation (VF) was the first manifestation of coronary artery disease in almost 30% of these patients.[20] Oberman and colleagues[18] similarly observed angiographically proven multivessel coronary artery disease in their evaluation of over 900 patients.

In addition to advanced atherosclerotic disease, the possible role of acute coronary thrombosis as a cause of cardiac arrest has been postulated. A study of over 200 patients who succumbed to cardiac arrest revealed thrombosis in 30% of cases, generally in the presence of advanced hemorrhagic atherosclerotic plaques.[14] Schwartz and Gerrity[17] noted this finding as well but cited the relatively small numbers of patients with sudden cardiac arrest and associated thrombi as opposed to the high frequency of thrombosis seen in patients with acute myocardial infarction (90%).[17] Reichenbach and colleagues[12,19] similarly found coronary thrombosis to be present only rarely in cardiac arrest patients. However, Reichenbach also observed that 8% of patients had no significant vascular disease and that the severity of coronary stenoses did not distinguish between those patients who survived an episode of sudden cardiac arrest and those who did not. These data imply that factors other than the severity of atherosclerosis alone play a role in the etiology of cardiac arrest. Platelet microemboli and alterations of the cardiac conduction system have been evaluated in this regard, although no specific lesions of the conduction system have been observed in patients succumbing to cardiac arrest.[16]

Several studies have sought to identify important clinical parameters that would serve to identify individuals at higher risk for sudden cardiac death. Weaver and coworkers[20] followed patients who survived an episode of out-of-hospital VF for a mean period of 20 months. Patients who experienced a second episode of VF tended to have a greater likelihood of triple vessel coronary artery disease, lower ejection fractions, and more extensive and severe left ventricular (LV) wall motion abnormalities, compared to patients who remained free of a secondary event. In an evaluation of over 150 survivors of out-of-hospital cardiac arrest, Ritchie et al.[22] found radionuclide ejection fraction to be the best predictor of recurrent arrest. The presence of a previous myocardial infarction was associated with an increased risk of cardiac arrest in a previous study.[21]

Oberman and colleagues[18] described five variables predictive of sudden death, including number of coronary vessels with $\geq$ 70% stenosis, the need for inotropic and diuretic therapy, presence of premature ventricular contractions (PVCs) and intraventricular conduction defects.[18] A review by Moss[25] employing univariate analysis of patients with coronary artery disease listed extent of atherosclerotic disease, as well as frequency of PVCs as risk factors for mortality. Finally, univariate and multivariate analyses by Hammermeister and coworkers[24] of over 700 patients with known coronary artery disease revealed LV ejection fraction as being most predictive of survival, and that age, number of diseased coronary vessels, and presence of ventricular ectopic activity on resting ECG were significant risk factors for medically treated patients.

Indeed, beyond the severity of ASHD and reduced LV function[17,20,23,76,77] as major risk factors for cardiac mortality and sudden cardiac arrest, the frequency and complexity of ventricular ectopic activity (VEA) was found to have prognostic import as well. An early study by Ruberman et al.[26] in which men with coronary artery disease underwent electrocardiographic monitoring for 1 hour revealed a higher mortality rate after 10 months of follow-up among those individuals with PVCs, compared to patients free of ventricular ectopy.[26] Moss et al.[27] employed 6-hour monitoring periods in 193 post–myocardial infarction patients and noted that patients with $\geq$ 20 PVCs per hour had a higher complication rate after discharge. Kotler and colleagues[28] employed 12-hour recordings to stratify patients according to the level of VEA (Lown criteria). In this study only patients with good LV function (N.Y. Heart Association classes I and II) were evaluated. PVCs and complex VEA (multiform PVCs and ventricular tachycardia [VT]) were found to have independent prognostic significance. PVCs were also found to have independent significance in a later study, especially in the presence of LV dysfunction.[29]

Observing patients with both acute and chronic coronary artery disease, Vismara et al.[30] found that VEA in the coronary care unit was not predictive of late mortality. However, complex VEA detected by Holter monitoring before discharge was significantly and independently correlated with later cardiac arrest. Of importance, these studies established the independent prognostic significance of VEA in patients with coronary artery disease. Earlier studies had suggested that complex VEA was a non-independent risk factor associated secondarily with more extensive atherosclerotic disease.[31]

From the preceding data it is apparent that the majority of sudden cardiac arrests are associated with atherosclerotic disease, which is often extensive. Unfortunately, a significant number of these cases will have a vague or absent prodromal symptom complex complicating the physician's ability to prospectively identify such patients. While patients with significant coronary artery disease, LV dysfunction, and complex VEA are at greater risk for cardiac arrest than other patients, defining the precise risk and optimal course of therapy in individual patients remains a significant challenge. The following sections describe the diagnostic and therapeutic options that may be employed by physicians in the evaluation and management of the patient who has survived cardiac arrest.

Management: Diagnosis and Therapy

Patients with coronary artery disease and impaired LV function have an increased risk of sudden cardiac arrest and cardiac mortality[20,24] as do patients with coronary artery disease and VEA.[28,31] The evaluation of a patient's risk for spontaneous VT or VF may be assessed invasively by programmed stimulation, or noninvasively by Holter monitoring.

NONINVASIVE EVALUATION

Ambulatory Electrocardiographic (Holter) Monitoring

Most episodes of sudden cardiac death are thought to be due to an episode of VF; however, little direct evidence to support this was available until several reports described Holter tracings that were recorded at the time of cardiac arrest. One case report documented ventricular flutter that degenerated to VF as the terminal event in a patient with evidence of ischemic ECG changes on the Holter tracing prior to his arrhythmia. Also of interest was the frequent and increasingly complex VEA recorded before the event, accompanied by an increase in resting heart rate.[32] Similar findings were documented for six cases of sudden cardiac arrest in a later report. Five of the six cases revealed VF as the underlying arrhythmia, with complex VEA present beforehand.[33] A subsequent report of 15 patients who sustained a cardiac arrest while being monitored similarly revealed increasing frequency of PVCs and VT, particularly in the 2 hours preceding the event. The runs of VT were noted to be relatively long (mean of 560 beats) and rapid (241 beats per minute [bpm]).[34] Kempf and Josephson[35] analyzed the Holter recordings of 27 patients who had sudden cardiac arrest and confirmed the presence of VT degenerating to VF as the mechanism in the majority of cases. In seven cases a bradyarrhythmia was the underlying cause. As noted previously, 11 of 20 patients succumbing to VT/VF had a ≥20% increase in resting heart rate prior to the event, often associated with complex VEA. Although the genesis of the increase in heart rate remained unclear, the authors speculated that such a rate increase might be associated with conduction delays in areas of myocardial ischemia, predisposing the patient to VT and VF.

A more recent study by Martin et al.[36] analyzed heart rate variability by Holter recordings in patients who experienced an episode of cardiac arrest while being monitored. In contrast to control patients, a significant reduction in heart rate variability was observed, defined as the standard deviation of R-R intervals during successive 5-minute periods during a 24-hour recording. The authors hypothesized that altered autonomic tone, specifically a relative reduction in parasympathetic input, may have contributed to this phenomenon. A preponderance of sympathetic tone, known to increase susceptibility to VF in animal models,[37] may have played a role in the occurrence of VT/VF in these cases. The potential use of heart rate variability analysis by Holter monitoring as a noninvasive aid to assess risk for cardiac arrest requires further evaluation, although the sensitivity and specificity of this finding are likely to be quite low.

Having established the presence of VT degenerating to VF as the cause of cardiac arrest in a majority of cases, the Holter monitor may also be employed as a means to identify patients with cardiac disease who are at a higher risk for this event. Unfortunately, spontaneous variability and the lack of sensitivity and specificity of VEA detected by ambulatory monitoring limits the usefulness of this test to define such risk in individual patients.

In a study by Schulze et al.,[38] post–myocardial infarction patients were evaluated with 24-hour ambulatory monitoring and radionuclide ventriculograms 2 weeks after admission to the hospital. The use of complex VEA on these recordings (≥ Lown III) as well as an ejection fraction <40% allowed for risk stratification of these patients. All patients who died suddenly during follow-up had significant VEA as well as depressed LV function. While low ejection fraction alone increased the risk of subsequent mortality, the presence of complex VEA appeared to further increase this risk. However, since all deaths occurred in the subgroup with both risk factors, the independent contribution of VEA could not be assessed.[38]

In 144 patients previously resuscitated from an episode of VF, Weaver and coworkers[41] performed 24-hour ambulatory monitoring approximately 5 months after the event; 90% of these patients had single PVCs and 66% had complex VEA, usually associated with a history of congestive heart failure or remote myocardial infarction. These clinical histories were more common in patients who died during the follow-up period. Uniform PVCs, even when frequent, did not predict mortality; complex VEA (defined in this study as bigeminy, trigeminy, multiform beats, and repetitive forms) was, however, significantly associated with subsequent cardiac arrest. For complex VEA as recorded on the Holter monitor, sensitivity was 80%; specificity, however, was only 40%.

A later report evaluated the risk of cardiac arrest in 533 patients with a history of myocardial infarction.[39] After a mean follow-up period of 18 months, analysis revealed that PVCs ≥10 per hour on Holter monitoring and an ejection fraction ≤40% were independent and significant risk factors. Cardiac arrest occurred in 18% of patients with both findings, an 11-fold increase compared to patients in whom neither risk factor was present. Almost 80% of cardiac arrests occurred within 7 months of the date of infarction.

Bigger et al.[40] examined over 700 patients after myocardial infarction by performing pre-discharge 24-hour Holter recordings and radionuclide ventriculography. By their analyses, an LV ejection fraction <30% strongly predicted subsequent mortality, especially within 6 months of the infarction, whereas the frequency of PVCs and repetitive forms was independently related to mortality, especially when occurring later than 6 months after infarction. Interestingly, a PVC rate of only 3 per hour was associated with a significantly greater risk of sudden death.[40]

From the foregoing observations, it is clear that ambulatory monitoring can be useful in detecting VEA in patients who may be at increased risk of cardiac arrest. The significance of VEA detected by Holter monitoring in predicting risk for sudden death in patients with recent myocardial infarction has been established. Furthermore, the risk associated with the presence of frequent and complex VEA is independent of and additive to the increased risk for sudden death associated with the presence of LV dysfunction.

However, significant problems exist that limit the use of Holter monitoring alone for clinical guidance in the management of individual patients; these problems are due, in part, to the test's relatively low specificity and sensitivity. In a study comparing Holter monitoring and electrophysiologic testing in patients with coronary artery disease and a history of sustained ventricular tachyarrhythmias, Holter monitoring detected arrhythmias suitable for guiding only 50% of patients. This was significantly less than programmed stimulation, during which sustained, monomorphic VT was induced in 87%.[42]

In addition, with respect to prophylactic antiarrhythmic drug therapy, it is important to note that treatment of "high-risk" patients, as defined by significant VEA and LV dysfunction after myocardial infarction, would lead to the unnecessary use of potentially toxic agents on a long-term basis in a large number of patients. For example, in the previously cited study by Mukharji et al.,[39] in which a PVC rate >10 per hour and a LV ejection fraction < 40% were defined as significant predictors of cardiac arrest, 80% of patients who were so identified remained free of a major arrhythmic event during the follow-up period. In this study, 18% of such patients experienced a cardiac arrest. Hence, treatment of this entire group would have led to chronic therapy in 80% of patients who, in retrospect, would not have required it. The same holds true for the data presented by Bigger and coworkers.[40] This problem would be of minor consequence if antiarrhythmic drugs were inexpensive and free of toxic side effects. It is well established, however, that a wide spectrum of potentially serious side effects occur with these medications, including the possibility of drug-induced proarrhythmic events.[105] Hence, the widespread use of these agents for all potentially high-risk patients as defined by Holter monitoring and LV function is untenable. Indeed, some mortality must be expected from these medications, perhaps in patients who would have otherwise remained free of a major arrhythmic event without them. Furthermore, whether prophylactic treatment with antiarrhythmic agents in this group of patients would actually lead to a significant reduction in mortality remains unknown. At present, there is one large-scale, prospective randomized trial in progress that may provide an answer to this crucial question.

A recent editorial by Josephson[43] highlighted the potential problems encountered with drug therapy in patients with VEA detected by Holter monitoring after myocardial infarction. Citing several reports, he suggested that the relatively low sensitivity of asymptomatic complex VEA would leave undetected a considerable number of patients at risk for sudden death. Conversely, the low specificity of this marker would lead to unnecessary chronic therapy in an even larger percentage of patients, this being of considerable importance given the cost, unproven efficacy, and potential toxicity of these agents. The author concluded that prophylactic therapy for infarct patients with asymptomatic complex VEA was not justified, based on the data presently available.

This viewpoint was also taken in a recent review by Surawicz,[45] in which the relatively low risk of cardiac arrest in patients with complex VEA and well preserved LV function was cited as evidence against the use of prophylactic therapy in this patient group. For post–myocardial infarction patients, this author explained the difficulty in initiating drug therapy as follows. If one assumes approximately one million myocardial infarctions per year in the United States, with an average mortality rate of 8% in the first year, approximately 830,000 1-year survivors of myocardial infarction remain in this country. The estimated number of sudden cardiac arrests in this group of patients, based on previously cited data, is 36,000 to 45,000. If a drug is employed that causes a 25% reduction in the incidence of cardiac arrest, 9000 to 11,000 lives will be saved, at the expense of treating over 800,000 patients for an extended period.

It is also important, when studying antiarrhythmic therapy with Holter guidance, to recognize that spontaneous variability of VEA may hinder the ability to gauge drug efficacy. An investigation of this variability by Pratt et al.[47] employed two 24-hour Holter recordings (average 8 days apart) in post–myocardial infarction patients enrolled in the Cardiac Arrhythmia Pilot Study (CAPS).[46] CAPS was a multicenter, prospective, randomized double-blind trial evaluating post–myocardial infarction patients with ≥ 10 PVCs/hour detected on Holter recordings 6 to 60 days after their infarction. Patients with severe LV dysfunction were excluded. Patients were randomized to therapy with encainide, flecainide, imipramine, ethmozine, or placebo to evaluate drug efficacy (≥ 70% reduction of PVCs) as well as side effects and proarrhythmia in these patients. The results of this trial will soon be published.

Of note from the analysis by Pratt and colleagues,[47] spontaneous variability of VEA in the CAPS patients was such that a 95% reduction of PVCs was required to establish a significant drug effect if Holter recordings during 1 day of control and 1 day of treatment are compared. The variability of VEA was independent of LV function. Interestingly, those patients on beta-blocker therapy had even greater spontaneous variability than patients not receiving these medications.

In addition, work done by Morganroth et al.[44] has revealed the need to guide antiarrhythmic therapy with Holter monitoring only if frequent VEA is recorded during baseline. Using analysis of variance, these authors showed that a reduction of PVC frequency by >80% was required to distinguish spontaneous variation from drug effect. This effect, combined with the abolition of repetitive forms, is required by most electrophysiologists to accept a drug regimen as being efficacious. These criteria cannot be applied to patients with only infrequent complex VEA or rare PVCs on ambulatory ECG recordings. Such patients are more suitably evaluated by electrophysiologic studies, as will be discussed in a later section.

Treadmill Stress Testing

In addition to Holter monitoring, treadmill stress testing (exercise testing) has been used to identify patients at increased risk for sudden death. In one study, exercise testing and ambulatory monitoring were performed in 81 patients referred for coronary artery disease or arrhythmias. Comparison was made for each test's ability to detect VEA. In 66 patients without arrhythmia on a 3-minute EKG, 18 had VEA detected by Holter monitoring, and 26 had VEA during treadmill stress testing. The authors concluded that exercise testing was an effective means for detecting potentially significant arrhythmias.[48]

In a later review, Lown et al.[49] found Holter monitoring to be more sensitive than exercise testing for detecting VEA but noted that over 40% of patients with known coronary artery disease manifested VEA on the treadmill. Discussing the arrhythmogenic properties of exercise, the authors cited human and animal studies that documented an increase in the frequency of PVCs during myocardial ischemia. The acceleration of heart rate, increase in sympathetic activity, rise in blood pressure and ventricular preload, as well as the presence of hypoxia and acidosis during exercise likely contributed to the occurrence of myocardial ischemia and secondary ectopy. In line with this reasoning, the authors found more advanced VEA in patients with severe ASHD as they underwent treadmill testing. These results were extended by Sheps and coworkers,[50] who noted a significant decrease in the frequency of exercise-induced PVCs during the second of two treadmill tests performed within 5 minutes of each other. Because of the reduced myocardial oxygen demand during the second test (decreased rate-pressure product during recovery), the role of ischemia in the genesis of VEA was again suggested.

In terms of prognostic information, VEA during exercise testing was evaluated in over 1200 patients in a study by Califf et al.[52] Stress tests were performed within 6 weeks of cardiac catheterization. Patients with more extensive coronary artery disease and LV dysfunction had significantly more PVCs and complex ventricular arrhythmias during exercise. Moreover, patients without VEA had a lower 3-year mortality rate than patients with simple PVCs, whereas those with complex VEA had even lower survival rates. The presence of ventricular arrhythmias added independent prognostic information to the other exercise test variables analyzed, although not to the cardiac catheterization data. In patients without significant ASHD, the presence of ventricular arrhythmias was found to have no prognostic import.

For post–myocardial infarction patients, there is evidence that supports the use of low-level exercise testing to stratify patients into high- and low-risk groups.[51] In one study, 210 stable post–myocardial infarction patients underwent limited treadmill testing prior to discharge. During a follow-up period of 1 year, a mortality rate of 2% was observed in patients without ischemic EKG changes during their exercise test, as opposed to a 27% mortality rate for patients with ischemic changes. Cardiac arrest, in particular, occurred in 1 of 146 patients with normal EKG tracings and in 10 of 64 patients having ischemic changes. These differences were statistically significant. As these findings were corroborated in a number of follow-up studies, the use of low-level exercise testing in stable post–myocardial infarction patients has become widely employed.

An evaluation of the results of exercise testing, specifically in patients resuscitated from an episode of out-of-hospital VF, was reported by Weaver and coworkers[53] in a study involving 90 patients. Those patients who were known to have developed VF with physical exertion had significantly less complex VEA during stress testing than patients who experienced VF at low activity levels, although ST segment depression occurred with equal frequency in both groups. After a 24-month follow-up period, significant predictors of recurrent cardiac arrest included the presence of angina and hypotension during the exercise test. Exercise duration, heart rate, ST segment response, and exercise-induced VEA were not useful predictors.

In summary, exercise testing alone is of little use in stratifying patients who have survived an episode of cardiac arrest. The test's ability to indicate the presence of extensive coronary artery disease might lead to therapy that would subsequently reduce the risk of a cardiac arrest. However, the value of exercise testing in detecting ventricular arrhythmias as a means of identifying patients at high risk for sudden death is limited.

Signal Averaging

In recent years signal averaging, a relatively new noninvasive test, has been employed for the identification of high-risk patients with cardiac disease.[54-59] The basis of this test involves the recording of multiple QRS complexes with standard bipolar orthogonal (X,Y,Z) leads during sinus rhythm. The recorded signals are amplified, digitized, averaged, and passed through a bidirectional filter to eliminate artifact. The signals are then combined into a vector magnitude representing the high frequency content from the 3 leads. The resulting signal-averaged electrogram is then analyzed for the presence of late potentials and for QRS prolongation (>120 ms). Late potentials are generally defined as being high-frequency, low-voltage (<20 μV) signals present at the terminal portion of the QRS complex. It is hypothesized that late potentials reflect the slow fractionated conduction that takes place at the border zones of infarcted tissue. Conduction characteristics such as these are known to favor the development of reentrant ventricular arrhythmias.[60, 61]

Early work with this technique was done by Simpson,[54] who studied signal-averaged electrograms in groups of post–myocardial infarction patients with and without a history of VT. Patients in the former (VT) group were noted to have a high incidence of late potentials and prolonged QRS durations compared to patients without VT. A later study supported these results and also found a significantly greater prevalence of late potentials in patients with documented LV aneurysms, consistent with the theoretical basis for the presence of the signals described above. In an evaluation of 174 patients after myocardial infarction, Kanovsky et al.[56] found the presence of late potentials or prolonged QRS intervals, a PVC rate >100 per hour on Holter monitoring, and the presence of LV aneurysm to be significant independent predictors of risk for VT. Ninety per cent of the VT group, as opposed to 30% of patients without VT, had abnormal signal-averaged electrograms. This test had a sensitivity of 89% and a specificity of 69% for patients with VT. Patients with both positive signal-averaged electrograms and >100 PVCs per hour had a 91% probability of developing VT. When these parameters were combined with the presence of LV aneurysm, patients had a 99% probability of developing VT. Patients with only one parameter had a probability of approximately 30%.

Although having independent prognostic import, it should be noted that the specificity of an abnormal signal-averaged electrogram is relatively low. Hence, if one were to initiate drug therapy in all patients with a positive test, a significant number would be exposed to long-term therapy, who in fact do not require it. In an effort to ameliorate this problem, a prospective analysis of 210 post–myocardial infarction patients was undertaken by Kuchar and colleagues,[59] in which the results of signal-averaged electrograms, Holter recordings, and radionuclide ventriculography were evaluated independently and in combination as a means of predicting which patients were at high risk for a major arrhythmic event. Patients with an abnormal signal-averaged electrogram had a 17% incidence of VF or VT during follow-up, as opposed to 1% of patients with a normal test. Use both of late potentials and of prolonged QRS resulted in an overall sensitivity of 50%, a specificity of 90%, and a predictive value of 28%. For complex VEA detected on 24-hour Holter monitoring the incidence of an arrhythmic event was 13%, whereas an ejection fraction <40% was associated with a 20% incidence. Multivariate analysis revealed each of these factors to be significant independent predictors of subsequent major arrhythmic events. The combination of signal-averaged electrograms with either of the other tests resulted in a specificity of 89% and a sensitivity of 65 to 80%.[59] Thus, noninvasive testing of post–myocardial infarction patients appears to be useful in defining patients at high risk for subsequent VT or VF when the results of several tests are combined. Problems with an ideal balance between sensitivity and specificity remain. Whether antiarrhythmic therapy in these high-risk patients will lead to a significant reduction in mortality remains unclear.

INVASIVE EVALUATION

Cardiac Catheterization and Surgical Correction of Coronary Artery Disease

In the previous sections we have reviewed the use of noninvasive tests to identify patients who appear to have an increased risk for sudden cardiac arrest. The following sections will deal with evaluation and treatment options for patients who have survived an episode of out-of-hospital VF.

As has been previously emphasized, a high percentage of survivors of sudden cardiac arrest have extensive coronary artery disease.[10–21] Given this fact, and the potential contribution of myocardial ischemia to the development of life-threatening arrhythmias, it is strongly recommended that cardiac catheterization be performed in such patients. Indeed, at our institution, virtually all sudden death survivors undergo initial evaluation with cardiac catheterization not only to define the extent of ASHD but also to assess overall LV function and regional wall motion.

It has been established that some groups of patients who undergo successful surgical revascularization will have a significant improvement in their prognosis.[62–66] Confirmation of severe coronary artery disease, especially of the left main artery or advanced three-vessel disease, generally warrants therapy with bypass surgery. Lesser degrees of disease may be adequately addressed with drug therapy, possibly in conjunction with percutaneous transluminal coronary angioplasty (PTCA) in appropriately selected patients. Evaluation with exercise testing (with thallium imaging) assists in assessing the need for and efficacy of such therapy.

An improvement in myocardial oxygen supply by one of the therapeutic modalities described above may reduce the incidence of ventricular arrhythmias resulting from ischemia. By producing profound alterations in the electrophysiologic properties of affected myocardial cells and their connections, ischemia sets the stage for slow conduction and reentrant ventricular arrhythmias.[67] In addition, the threshold for VF is lowered significantly during both acute and chronic ischemic conditions. In a study of 28 patients, VT thresholds in patients with ≥ 75% stenoses of the left anterior descending artery were found to be significantly lower than VF thresholds measured in patients without coronary artery disease.[68] An earlier study similarly revealed a 60% decrease in the VF threshold when a 75% stenosis was produced in a coronary artery.[68]

In clinical terms, the effect of revascularization on an individual patient's propensity for ventricular arrhythmia is often difficult to predict. When programmed electrical stimulation of the heart is employed in patient evaluation, the continued presence of inducible ventricular arrhythmias after bypass surgery may be due to the presence of a fixed anatomic substrate, usually scar, which may serve as a focus for the generation of VT or of other myocardial abnormalities not corrected with bypass alone. To evaluate the effect of revascularization on inducible ventricular arrhythmias, 17 patients with significant ASHD involving proximal stenoses of at least two major vessels and ejection fractions >30% underwent electrophysiologic studies (EPS) at our institution. Thirteen of these patients were survivors of out-of-hospital cardiac arrest. Prior to surgery VT or VF were induced in 15 patients. Postoperative EPS performed an average of 19 days after revascularization surgery revealed no inducible VT or VF in 10 patients. These patients were on no antiarrhythmic agents at the time of study. Both these patients and those whose postoperative VT was suppressed with medical therapy remained free of major arrhythmic events after a mean follow-up period of 23 months.[70]

We have recently extended our observations on the effect of myocardial revascularization both in survivors of cardiac arrest and in patients who presented with sustained VT. Data from 50 patients who experienced cardiac arrest (not associated with acute infarction) and who underwent bypass grafting were reviewed. All patients underwent EPS before and/or after surgery. There were 4 arrhythmia recurrences in four patients over a mean follow-up period of 39 months, three of whom had no inducible arrhythmias postoperatively. Cox analysis revealed no clinical, angiographic, or electrophysiologic variable to be predictive of arrhythmia recurrence. However, the 1- and 5-year probabilities of arrhythmia-free survival were 96% and 88%, respectively. Hence, the long-term prognosis appears to be good for selected survivors of cardiac arrest with operable coronary disease.

We have also observed the greater suppression of preoperatively induced VF with coronary revascularization, compared to induced sustained VT. Nine of nine patients with preoperative VF were noninducible after surgery, whereas 19 of 24 patients with sustained VT continued to have inducible, sustained VT postoperatively. The LV ejection fraction was also predictive of arrhythmia suppression: mean 43% versus 33% for nonsuppressed patients (unpublished observations). Hence, in a select group of patients with well-preserved LV function and inducible VF during preoperative EPS, revascularization with bypass surgery may substantially reduce the incidence of inducible ventricular arrhythmias. Considering this, it is advised that survivors of cardiac arrest undergo EPS before and after coronary artery bypass grafting or PTCA to assess for the continued presence of inducible VT or VF. In patients whose spontaneous and inducible arrhythmia is monomorphic VT, the arrhythmia almost always occurs in association with a fixed anatomic substrate (i.e., a major scar). In such patients, revascularization alone is almost never sufficient to suppress either the spontaneous or inducible VT.

Some survivors of cardiac arrest have no inducible ventricular arrhythmias during programmed cardiac stimulation. A report of 19 such patients indicated that those patients with documented coronary artery disease, many of whom sustained their arrest during physical activity and were treated with bypass grafting or antianginal medications alone, had an excellent prognosis, with only one death occurring in this group after a mean follow-up of over 2 years. The authors speculated that ischemia was the most likely initiating factor for cardiac arrest in these patients. They suggested that aggressive anti-ischemic therapy in such patients may improve their prognosis without the concomitant use of antiarrhythmic agents.[71]

Electrophysiologic Studies (EPS)

The use of EPS for the evaluation and management of survivors of out-of-hospital cardiac arrest, especially those having significant underlying coronary artery disease, is now widely applied. Most patients (70–80%) are found to have inducible ventricular arrhythmias such as sustained monomorphic ventricular tachycardia, polymorphic VT, or VF, with the former induced in 36 to 51% of patients.[72–74, 76] A number of controversial issues remain regarding the performance and interpretation of EPS in this patient population. These will be discussed in the final section of this chapter.

The use of EPS in survivors of out-of-hospital cardiac arrest enhances the ability of the physician to (1) detect and characterize a clinically significant arrhythmia (i.e. the ease of inducibility and the morphology, rate, and hemodynamic consequences of the arrhythmia), and (2) use serial electrophysiologic testing to guide the selection of antiarrhythmic therapy or to evaluate a patient's suitability for antiarrhythmic surgery or implantation of an automatic implantable cardioverter/defibrillator (AICD).

Early work in this area was performed by Ruskin et al.,[9] in which programmed stimulation was performed in 31 survivors of cardiac arrest. Complete suppression of the inducible VT or VF seen at baseline EPS was achieved with antiarrhythmic therapy in 19 of 25 patients. Over a mean follow-up period of 15 months, none of these 19 patients had a recurrent major arrhythmic event or sudden death. However, 3 of 6 patients in whom inducible arrhythmias could not be suppressed suffered a recurrent cardiac arrest. This study indicated that EPS could be used to unmask clinically significant ventricular arrhythmias in cardiac arrest survivors and, more important, that EPS-guided drug therapy appeared to be efficacious in preventing recurrent episodes of cardiac arrest. Interestingly, patients without inducible, sustained VT or VF at baseline EPS also remained free of major arrhythmic events.

These observations were extended by Morady and colleagues,[73] who used a more aggressive stimulation protocol involving up to three extrastimuli (as opposed to two extrastimuli employed by Ruskin et al.[9]). Survivors of cardiac arrest were evaluated in a baseline study, in which 76% manifested inducible sustained or nonsustained VT. In agreement with Ruskin and coworkers, these investigators found that patients without inducible VT at baseline EPS rarely experienced recurrent episodes of sustained VT or VF during follow-up. For those patients with inducible arrhythmias, suppression with conventional antiarrhythmic agents could be achieved in only 9 of 34 patients; 6 of these 9 patients remained free of major arrhythmic events over a 20-month follow-up period. Twenty-three of 25 patients whose arrhythmias remained inducible on conventional antiarrhythmic agents were placed on amiodarone, and 91% remained free of recurrent VT or VF. Overall patient mortality was 9%—a significant reduction in mortality compared to untreated cardiac arrest survivors.[73]

Although the latter findings were supported in a study by Roy and colleagues,[74] a degree of controversy was established with regard to the prognosis of cardiac arrest survivors who had no inducible VT or VF at baseline study. These investigators, in contrast to the findings of Ruskin et al.[9] and Morady et al.,[73] observed a high rate of recurrent cardiac arrest (32%) during a follow-up period of 20 months. However, important differences in the studies cited could account for this discrepancy. Stimulation protocols varied, and patient numbers in the noninducible subgroups were small. In addition, no randomization of therapy was made for these patients, some of whom received empiric antiarrhythmic treatment. Determining the potentially beneficial or proarrhythmic effects of these agents in this setting is not possible. Finally, Roy et al.[74] chose not to treat patients with inducible nonsustained VT, in contrast to Ruskin et al. and Morady et al., who relied on stricter criteria for defining "noninducibility." This may account for the higher mortality rate noted in the Roy's study.

Finally, Zheutlin and coworkers[75] reported a more recent evaluation of cardiac arrest survivors without inducible VT or VF, in which they observed a high incidence of potentially significant causative factors (such as reversible myocardial ischemia). With interventions directed at the treatment of these factors, a low mortality rate (3%) was seen after 2 years of follow-up in the absence of antiarrhythmic medications.[75] However, because of conflicting data, different patient populations, and the small patient numbers involved in these four studies, the prognostic significance of noninducibility in the baseline state in survivors of cardiac arrest remains a controversial issue.

At our institution we have examined the role of EPS and EPS-guided therapy in 166 survivors of out-of-hospital cardiac arrest.[80] Ventricular arrhythmias were inducible in 79% (sustained VT, 37%; polymorphic VT/VF, 15%; reproducible nonsustained VT, 27%) of patients at baseline EPS. Treatment with antiarrhythmic medications and/or surgery resulted in suppression of these arrhythmias in 75% of patients. Suppression of sustained VT was defined as the induction of less than 10 complexes during the stimulation protocol, while suppression of nonsustained VT was defined as induction of less than 5 complexes. Patients without inducible arrhythmias at baseline were significantly less likely to have coronary artery disease, and they had significantly higher ejection fractions (mean 50% vs. 39%) than patients with inducible arrhythmias. Approximately 30% of patients without inducible arrhythmias were discharged on empiric antiarrhythmic therapy to suppress complex VEA. Ten patients underwent implantation of an AICD for persistently inducible arrhythmias. Patients were followed for a mean of 28 ± 22 months, and cardiac arrest recurred in 16%. Of note, patients discharged without inducible ventricular arrhythmias had significantly fewer episodes of recurrent cardiac arrest and total arrhythmia recurrences. No significant differences in outcome were found with regard to the specific type of arrhythmia induced at baseline. The persistence of inducible VT was a significant independent predictor of recurrent cardiac arrest, as was LV dysfunction. The cumulative incidence of recurrent cardiac arrest was 10% after follow-up of 1 year. After 5 years of follow-up, no patient discharged with inducible VT remained alive, whereas 60% of patients in whom VT was suppressed were still living.

The major findings of this study can be summarized as follows (Fig. 18–1).

1. Suppression of inducible VT/VF with antiarrhythmic medications and/or surgery is a powerful predictor of freedom from recurrent cardiac arrest and sudden death in survivors of cardiac arrest, independent of left ventricular function.

2. Persistent inducibility of ventricular arrhythmias and reduced ejection fraction not only are significant independent predictors of recurrent cardiac arrest, but also the relative risks associated with these factors are multiplicative; patients with ejection fraction <30% (relative risk 2.6) and persistent inducibility (relative risk 4.0) have an almost tenfold increase in the risk of recurrent arrest.

3. The absence of inducible ventricular arrhythmia during baseline EPS does not necessarily indicate a favorable outcome. However, consistent with studies discussed earlier, those patients with coronary artery disease and well-preserved LV function who received aggressive anti-ischemic therapy, including bypass surgery, were at low risk for recurrent arrest. Patients with poor ventricular function and no inducible arrhythmia at baseline EPS had a substantial risk of recurrent cardiac arrest (25% at 1-year follow-up).

This study and others[74–76, 80] have demonstrated the frequent inducibility of potentially lethal ventricular arrhythmias in survivors of cardiac arrest. The continued presence of inducible sustained VT or VF in these patients despite treatment with antiarrhythmic agents portends a poor prognosis. Unfortunately, complete suppression of inducible VT and VF with conventional agents appears to be achievable in only a minority of patients.[79] Not infrequently, however, antiarrhythmic agents will reduce the rate of induced VT to the degree that the patient experiences no symptoms or hemodynamic instability.

The prognostic significance of this response was addressed in a recent study by Waller et al.[81] Serial EP tests were performed in 258 patients who were divided into three groups, based on the response of their induced VT to medical therapy. Group 1 had suppression of their arrhythmia; group 2 had a "beneficial response," defined as an increase in VT cycle length greater than 100 ms and no associated symptoms; group 3 had no beneficial response to therapy. Patients in groups 1 and 2 had mortality and recurrent cardiac arrest rates of < 10% after 1 year of follow-up, compared to a mortality rate of approximately 20% in group 3 patients. This difference was statistically significant and was maintained throughout 4 years of follow-up. With respect to nonfatal arrhythmic events, however, group 2 patients experienced a significantly greater frequency of recurrence (32%) as did group 3 patients (35%), compared to patients whose arrhythmias were suppressed (4%) at 1 year of follow-up. No differences were noted between those patients treated with amiodarone and those who received conventional agents. Hence, continued inducibility after serial EPS appears to be associated with a significantly increased risk of arrhythmia recurrence, whereas the risk of a fatal event remains low if the induced VT is well

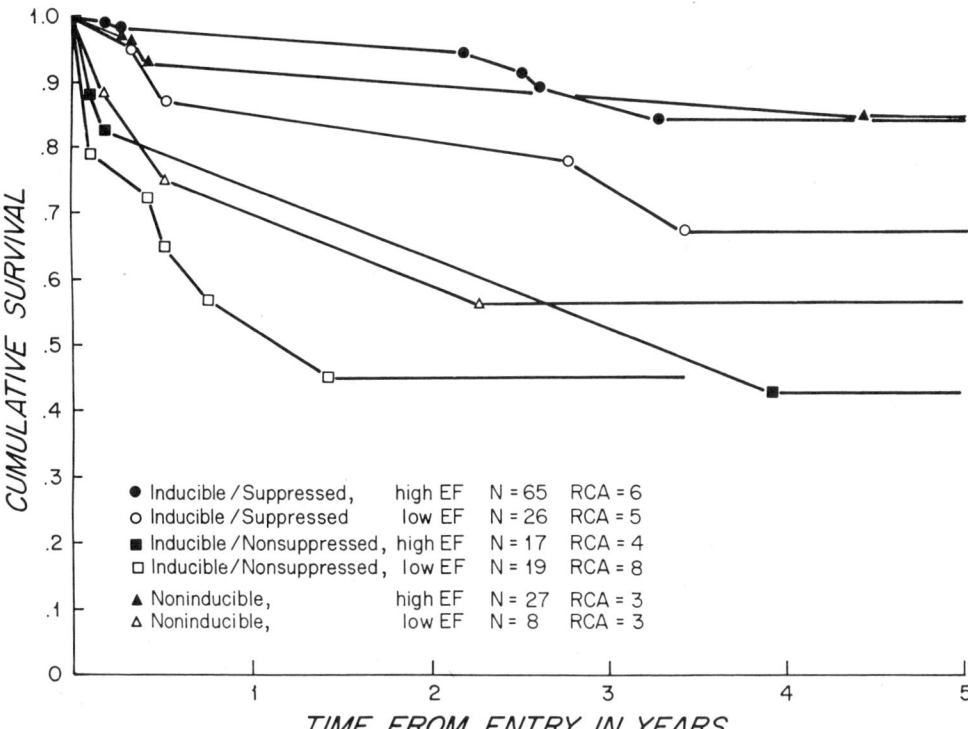

FIGURE 18–1
Cumulative survival without recurrent cardiac arrest stratified by the results of electrophysiologic studies and left ventricular ejection fraction (EF). The EF was classified as low (≤ 30%) or high (> 30%). (Reprinted by permission of The New England Journal of Medicine from Wilber JD, Garan H, Kelly E, et al. N Engl J Med 318:19, 1988.)

tolerated clinically. It should be noted that this was a retrospective analysis, and most patients were not survivors of out-of-hospital cardiac arrest. Prospective studies in appropriate patient populations will be required to further examine this hypothesis.

The use of programmed cardiac stimulation in patients with a previous episode of life-threatening VT or VF is well established. However, an important clinical scenario with which the physician must frequently deal involves patients with organic heart disease and nonsustained VT who are at increased risk for, but have not yet experienced, a life-threatening ventricular arrhythmia. The role of programmed stimulation in such patients is controversial at the present time. Nevertheless, a number of small clinical studies provide some provocative observations on this issue.

In 1984, Gomes et al.[82] prospectively evaluated 73 patients in whom high-grade VEA was documented. These patients had no prior history of sustained VT, sudden death, or syncope. All patients underwent electrophysiologic evaluation: 27% had inducible VT or VF, whereas 73% had less than four repetitive ventricular responses. The inducible group was significantly different with respect to the presence of atherosclerotic disease, previous infarct, and ejection fraction <40%. Most of these patients were treated with antiarrhythmic agents, guided by programmed stimulation, while noninducible patients were randomly assigned to therapy. After mean follow-up of 30 months, 31.5% of the inducible group and 2% of the noninducible group had an episode of sustained VT or VF. The probability of surviving 2 years (35% vs. 67%) was significantly lower for the inducible group. These results indicated that EPS might be useful for risk stratification of patients with spontaneous high-grade VEA.[82]

In 1985, Veltri and coworkers,[83] evaluated 33 patients with programmed stimulation who had asymptomatic nonsustained VT associated with coronary artery disease, dilated cardiomyopathy, and mitral valve prolapse. No patient had a prior major arrhythmic event. Programmed stimulation induced sustained VT in 21% of these patients, and nonsustained VT in 21% as well. Those patients without structural heart disease had no inducible VT. The ejection fraction was not significantly different in patients with and without inducible VT. After a mean follow-up period of 23 months, 85% of patients were alive, and 12% had died from cardiac causes, the latter group having a significantly lower E compared to survivors. Twenty-one per cent of the patients had arrhythmic events, with 9% being sudden cardiac deaths. These patients also had comparatively low ejection fractions compared to the arrhythmia-free group. The results of programmed stimulation, however, did not correlate well with such clinical events.[83]

Spielman and colleagues[84] performed EPS in 58 patients with a variety of underlying cardiac diseases, in whom nonsustained VT was detected on Holter monitoring and who had depressed LV function (ejection fraction < 50%). Using up to three extrastimuli, sustained VT was induced in 40% of patients. This response was found to correlate with the presence of LV akinesis or aneurysm but not with ejection fraction or the presence or absence of coronary artery disease. Data from Holter monitoring, including the frequency, rate, and duration of VT, did not predict which patients would subsequently have inducible sustained VT. The authors concluded that patients with spontaneous nonsustained VT and LV dysfunction were more likely to have sustained VT induced during programmed stimulation, and that this might allow for further risk stratification with regard to a future major arrhythmic event.

Buxton et al.[85] recently reported on 62 patients with documented ASHD and nonsustained VT, who underwent EPS. Sustained VT was induced in 45% of patients and was associated with a greater mortality during follow-up (7 of 11 patients who died suddenly had inducible sustained VT). Those patients in whom treatment of sustained VT led to ≤10 beats of inducible VT had an improved survival rate (three sudden deaths among 44 patients). Patients with asymptomatic nonsustained VT who were free of inducible sustained VT during programmed stimulation had a relatively low probability of cardiac arrest (one death in 19 patients).[85]

In summary, patients with nonsustained VT and significant LV dysfunction appear to be at high risk for cardiac arrest. Holter data, while identifying patients with nonsustained VT, appears to be of limited value in identifying which patients might benefit from antiarrhythmic therapy. Electrophysiologic testing may identify individuals (with induced sustained VT) who are at particularly high risk for spontaneous VT or sudden death. Those patients without inducible sustained VT appear to have a benign prognosis without antiarrhythmic therapy. It must be emphasized, however, that these issues remain controversial. In the studies cited here, as well as others, the patient numbers were small, therapy was not randomized, and the patients studied often had a variety of underlying cardiac diseases. Well-designed, large-scale prospective trials will be needed to resolve these issues.

The role of EPS in the management of survivors of cardiac arrest is of primary importance. The positive predictive value of the technique is reported to be between 70% and 90% over follow-up periods of 2 years.[86–88] Patients with inducible ventricular arrhythmias that are suppressed have a significantly lower mortality than patients with persistently inducible VT or those who receive empiric antiarrhythmic therapy. However, controversy exists with regard to a number of aspects of EPS. A standard stimulation protocol has not been agreed upon. The variety of pacing cycle lengths, number of extrastimuli (2–4), and the use of burst pacing by some investigators have made comparison of different studies difficult. Furthermore, investigators often employ different definitions of arrhythmia suppression[89–93] and, hence, use different end points to guide therapy. Obviously, comparison of survival and arrhythmic event data is complicated by this problem. Despite these shortcomings, there is consensus on the indication for programmed stimulation in survivors of cardiac arrest not associated with acute transmural myocardial infarction. Inducible sustained arrhythmias at baseline EPS should be treated aggressively to optimize a patient's prognosis. A review of the currently available treatment modalities is presented in the following section.

Therapy

ANTIARRHYTHMIC MEDICATIONS

The use of antiarrhythmic medications to suppress inducible VT/VF in cardiac arrest survivors has been discussed previously. Unfortunately, this end point is achieved in only a minority of patients when conventional agents alone are employed. Empiric long-term use of these drugs has also been shown to be without clinical efficacy, a fact reported before the advent of invasive evaluation.[94] When patients receiving chronic antiarrhythmic therapy are followed noninvasively, Holter monitoring should be employed to ensure the abolition of high-grade VEA.[95, 96] In addition, a report by Myerburg et al.[97] suggested the need for maintaining stable therapeutic plasma levels of antiarrhythmic agents to reduce the risk of recurrent arrest; however, most investigators believe this to be an unreliable standard by which to assess drug efficacy.

When a patient's arrhythmia cannot be suppressed by conventional medications, therapy with amiodarone should be considered. Early reports suggested that continued inducibility of VT in patients treated with this drug did not predict clinical outcome.[98–101] However, several studies have contested this notion. McGovern and colleagues[102] reported on 42 patients treated with amiodarone for recurrent VT or VF. Logistic regression revealed two independent predictors of recurrent arrhythmia: reduced ejection fraction and the persistence of inducible VT during therapy. The predictive accuracy of programmed stimulation in this setting was 67%, with a specificity of 91%. Using clinical variables, DiCarlo and coworkers[103] similarly identified reduced ejection fraction as well as the presence of VT on pre-discharge Holter recordings as predictors of subsequent major arrhythmic events in patients treated with amiodarone.[103] Finally, Horowitz and colleagues reported a prospective evaluation of 100 patients treated with this drug, in which patients were divided into noninducible and persistently inducible groups (as defined at EPS). Patients in the former group remained free of arrhythmia recurrence after a mean follow-up period of 18 months, whereas almost 50% of patients in the second group sustained a recurrent arrhythmic event. Of note, patients in whom the induced VT was hemodynamically well tolerated tended to have nonfatal events. No significant differences in the blood levels of amiodarone were seen in these two groups.

Therefore, it appears that programmed stimulation provides useful information with regard to the risk for recurrent major arrhythmic events and prognosis in patients treated with amiodarone. In survivors of cardiac arrest who receive this medication, we recommend the use of EPS to assess efficacy. Persistently inducible

VT or VF should prompt the physician to consider the addition of a second antiarrhythmic agent or to pursue nonpharmacologic therapeutic options.

As noted earlier, successful treatment of cardiac arrest survivors is associated with a 1-year mortality of 6 to 15%,[79, 80] in contrast to an almost threefold increase in mortality in patients treated empirically. It must be emphasized, however, that antiarrhythmic agents themselves may be responsible for the occurrence of arrhythmic events, including cardiac arrest in some patients. Ruskin et al.[105] evaluated six patients with out-of-hospital cardiac arrest who were on antiarrhythmic therapy at the time of their event and who manifested no inducible arrhythmia in the absence of antiarrhythmic drugs. However, when given the same antiarrhythmic agent that had been present at the time of cardiac arrest, four patients had inducible VT during repeat programmed stimulation. After a mean follow-up period of 32 months, only one noncardiac death occurred in the patients who had no inducible VT at baseline EPS and who received no subsequent antiarrhythmic medications. Clearly, the potential for these agents to cause a major arrhythmic event must be borne in mind when they are used in therapy. For a more complete review of the proarrhythmic effects of antiarrhythmic medications the reader is referred elsewhere.[106]

NONPHARMACOLOGIC THERAPY

Surgery

When antiarrhythmic agents fail to adequately suppress ventricular arrhythmias in survivors of cardiac arrest, other therapeutic options should be pursued. One consideration in patients with monomorphic VT should be map-guided endocardial resection. By excising the region of origin of VT, usually present at the border zone between normal myocardium and scar, ventricular arrhythmias can be ablated or rendered more easily manageable with antiarrhythmic medications.[107–114] Early work in this area was reported by Josephson et al.,[107] in which 12 patients with medically refractory VT underwent intraoperative mapping and excision of the region of earliest activation during VT (usually localized at the border zones of LV aneurysms). Before hospital discharge, programmed stimulation was performed in the absence of antiarrhythmic medications. Ventricular tachycardia could be induced in none of the patients. Ten surviving patients remained free of sustained VT during a follow-up period of up to 20 months.[107]

A later report from this laboratory[108] presented data on 119 patients who underwent map-guided subendocardial resection for refractory VT. All patients had previous infarctions. The authors defined two patient groups: those who underwent ablative surgery within 4 months of their infarct and those in whom surgery was performed at least 1 year after. Operative mortality (approximately 10%), late mortality (32%), and the frequency with which surgery, without adjunctive therapy, prevented postoperative VT (approximately 27%) were not significantly different for the two groups. The authors suggested that subendocardial resection, when indicated early after acute infarction, was associated with an acceptable risk of operative mortality.

More recently, Krafchek and colleagues[109] reported improved results when regional endocardial resection was performed with pre- and postoperative mapping. In their series, patients with recurrent sustained VT or VF underwent extensive mapping from 10 to 40 sites during induced VT. Having identified the site of origin of VT, 10 patients subsequently had localized endocardial resection with removal of only the earliest site of activation. In another 25 patients, surgical resection was extended to include all endocardial sites from which activation preceded the QRS during the mapping procedure. Operative mortality was 10%. During follow-up, a significantly greater proportion of patients in whom localized resection was performed experienced recurrent VT or VF (38%), in contrast to a 4% recurrence rate in the group of patients who underwent more extensive resection. Based on these results, the authors recommended surgical ablation of all sites showing presystolic activation during the mapping procedures, as a means to improve the surgical outcome.

Following ablative surgery, many patients are noted to have complex VEA; however, this does not appear to have prognostic significance. Evaluation of 36 patients who underwent study after endocardial resection revealed no significant change in the level of complex VEA recorded pre- and postoperatively by ambulatory monitoring. Furthermore, the level of VEA did not correlate with inducibility of VT by postoperative EPS. Finally, there was a suggestion that neither high-grade VEA nor inducible VT postoperatively precluded a good clinical outcome. However, patient numbers were too small to confirm this.[110]

Several factors, beside severe LV dysfunction, may aid in predicting the failure of endocardial resection to ablate VT. Disparate sites of VT separated by >5 cm and the presence of morphologically distinct VT also appear to be associated with surgical failure, as noted in a retrospective report of 100 patients.[111] An inferior site of VT and right bundle branch block morphology (free-wall site of origin) were similarly associated with failure of surgery to cure VT, mainly because of the greater technical difficulties involved in performing adequate resection in these areas. In agreement with this finding are the surgical results reported by Garan et al.,[113] in which the extent of resection was shown to affect late surgical outcome. Thirty-six patients underwent aneurysmectomy and map-guided endocardial resection for recurrent VT. In six cases resection was limited because of technical factors, such as proximity to a papillary muscle or the membranous septum. Postoperatively, VT recurred in five of the six patients. Only one of 27 patients in whom resection was not limited experienced VT recurrence during a mean follow-up of 25 months.

Most centers presently employ cryothermal ablation ($-60°C$ for 2–3 minutes) as well as endocardial resection for the surgical management of medically refractory VT. This technique appears to enhance the surgeon's ability to ablate sites on the septum or at the base of papillary muscles, where excision cannot be safely performed. A recent study evaluated the efficacy of cryothermal ablation in 15 patients with previous inferior infarction. Endocardial mapping localized the origin of VT to the septum, inferior wall, and/or posterior papillary muscle. Cryoablation alone was performed in these patients, with a postoperative VT suppression rate (defined by programmed stimulation) of 79%. In addition, no significant mitral regurgitation was detected in patients who underwent cryoablation on the posterior papillary muscle or near the mitral annulus. The LV ejection fraction was unchanged or improved postoperatively. Thus, cryotherapy may improve the success rate of ablative surgery, especially in cases in which endocardial resection is technically difficult, as discussed above.[114]

Although this procedure is clearly beneficial in selected patients with VT, problems remain with ablative surgery with respect to the accuracy of endocardial mapping, the difficulties of performing adequate resection in some areas of the heart, as well as the mortality (usually ≥10%) and morbidity associated with open heart surgery in this patient population. Survivors of cardiac arrest who have inducible sustained monomorphic VT refractory to medical therapy, and in whom residual LV function is not severely depressed, are reasonable candidates and may benefit from this form of therapy.

Automatic Implantable Cardioverter/Defibrillator (AICD)

A relatively new and highly effective means of prolonging survival in cardiac arrest patients involves the implantation of an automatic implantable cardioverter/defibrillator (AICD). This device, developed by Dr. Michel Mirowski, is capable of sensing and converting VT or VF to sinus rhythm by delivering one or more synchronized DC shocks. The AICD has produced a dramatic reduction of cardiac mortality in patients at high risk for sudden death.[115–119, 121, 122] As discussed previously, a number of patients continue to have inducible VT and recurrent arrhythmic events despite treatment with antiarrhythmic medications and, occasionally, surgical therapy. Such patients are ideal candidates for the implantation of an AICD. The device at present weighs approximately 300 grams and has a volume of 162 cc. Because of its size, which is rather large compared to a standard pacemaker, the device is implanted in a paraumbilical pocket, and leads from the heart are tunneled subcutaneously to the device.

The AICD is capable of sensing ventricular tachycardia or ventricular fibrillation and then delivering up to four sequential shocks (25–35 joules) to the heart for a single arrhythmic event. The sensing function always involves measurement of the heart rate, and in some units, the probability density function (PDF). The latter function examines the amount of time the cardiac electrogram spends at the isoelectric point. During sinus rhythm a relatively greater proportion of time is spent at the isoelectric line, compared to a wide QRS complex rhythm such as VT or VF. In "rate only" units any rhythm (including sinus tachycardia or supraventricular tachycardia) whose rate exceeds the preprogrammed rate cut-off of the device will lead to a discharge. In units employing PDF, both heart rate and PDF criteria must be fulfilled before a shock is delivered.

Several sensing and shocking lead configurations[120] have been employed and will not be extensively reviewed in this chapter. Rate sensing may be achieved either with two small epicardial electrodes that are anchored into the myocardium or with a bipolar endocardial lead placed in the RV apex, similar to a standard pacemaker electrode. Shocks are delivered between two titanium mesh patches placed intra- or extrapericardially or between an apical patch and a coiled spring electrode placed transvenously at the junction of the right atrium and superior vena cava. Operative mortality is approximately 2 to 3%. Approximately two thirds of patients are discharged on at least one antiarrhythmic agent in an attempt to minimize the number of spontaneous episodes of VT and VF.

Several investigators[119, 121, 122] have reported impressive survival data in patients in whom the AICD has been implanted. Sudden death mortality 1 year after implantation is approximately 2%, and approximately 5% after 3 years of follow-up. These figures are far below the best attainable survival statistics achieved with other forms of therapy. Present indications for implantation include survivors of one or more episodes of cardiac arrest in whom inducible VT or VF cannot be suppressed with aggressive medical, or in some cases, surgical therapy. Patients surviving an arrest in whom no arrhythmias are induced at baseline EPS may be candidates as well, especially when correctible causes such as extensive coronary artery disease are not present. Patients without prior cardiac arrest but with spontaneous hypotensive sustained VT refractory to medical therapy and who are not candidates for surgery are also candidates for an AICD.

Problems involving the AICD include the inability to adjust the rate cutoff and delivered energy, as well as the inability to interrogate the device about the rhythm present at the time of a spontaneous discharge. This complicates the detection of possible inappropriate shocks by the device. In addition, implantation presently requires extensive surgery, with exposure of the heart, usually via left thoracotomy or median sternotomy. Finally, while most patients tolerate the AICD well, a number experience considerable anxiety after implantation and require ongoing psychological support.

Many of these problems will be resolved or ameliorated as technological refinements are made on the device. It is anticipated that future AICDs will not only be smaller and widely programmable but will also incorporate bradycardia and antitachycardia pacing functions as well. Should pacing fail to convert or accelerate VT, back-up low-energy cardioversion and high-energy defibrillation functions will be activated.

It is anticipated that generator life, presently about 2 years or 100 discharges, will also be extended. Finally, devices employing subcutaneous or submuscular patches and endocardial leads (inserted transvenously) are being developed and may, in many patients, obviate the need for extensive surgery for implantation. With these improvements and the impressive survival statistics already obtained, it is likely that AICDs will assume a major role in the management of patients at high risk for sudden death.

Summary

Sudden cardiac arrest continues to be a major cause of mortality in the United States and other industrialized Western nations. Prospective identification of patients at high risk for cardiac arrest is difficult. The detection of impaired LV function, the presence of complex VEA, and the use of signal averaging in post–myocardial infarction patients may aid in the identification of one subset of high-risk patients who may warrant further evaluation and therapy. However, the majority of patients at risk will not be defined with acceptable specificity, using currently available screening techniques.

Once a patient has sustained and survived an episode of cardiac arrest, aggressive diagnostic and therapeutic measures must be taken in an attempt to reduce the otherwise considerable mortality associated with this problem. As most patients have significant coronary artery disease, cardiac catheterization should be performed. Anti-ischemic therapy with medications, percutaneous transluminal angioplasty, or bypass surgery should be implemented when appropriate. Evaluation of LV function is important for determining prognosis and is integral to many therapeutic decisions involving antiarrhythmic medications (some of which have significant negative inotropic properties) and to assessment of the risk of cardiac surgery. Finally, all patients should undergo baseline EPS with programmed stimulation. Those with inducible VT or VF should have their arrhythmias suppressed with medications or, in appropriate cases, surgical therapy. This approach leads to a significant reduction of late mortality. Patients whose arrhythmias remain persistently inducible despite medical therapy should be considered for implantation of an AICD.

Those survivors of cardiac arrest in whom no arrhythmias are induced with programmed stimulation may not have a benign prognosis. Correctible causes for their cardiac arrest, such as extensive atherosclerotic heart disease, should be sought and treated aggressively. Ischemia contributes to the risk of VT or VF, and treatment of severe coronary lesions with bypass surgery may reduce the risk of a recurrent event in selected patients. In general, however, the ultimate prognosis of patients without inducible arrhythmias remains unclear, and implantation of an AICD should be considered, particularly in patients without a definable and treatable cause for their arrest and in those with advanced LV dysfunction.

References

1. Kuller L, Cooper M, Perper J: Epidemiology of sudden death. Arch Intern Med 129:714, 1972.
2. Kuller L: Sudden death in arteriosclerotic heart disease: The case for preventive medicine. Am J Cardiol 24:617, 1969.
3. Adelson L, Hoffman W: Sudden death from coronary disease. JAMA 176:131, 1961.
4. Liberthson R, Nagel E, Hirschman J, et al.: Prehospital ventricular defibrillation. N Engl J Med 291:317, 1974.
5. Cobb L, Baum R, Alvarez H, et al.: Resuscitation from out-of-hospital ventricular fibrillation: Four years follow-up. Circulation 51&52(Suppl 3):223, 1975.
6. Schaffer W, Cobb L: Recurrent ventricular fibrillation and mode of death in survivors of out-of-hospital ventricular fibrillation. N Engl J Med 293:259, 1975.
7. Baum R, Alvarez H, Cobb L: Survival after resuscitation from out-of-hospital ventricular fibrillation. Circulation 50:1231, 1974.
8. Myerburg R, Kessler K, Estes D, et al.: Long-term survival after pre-hospital cardiac arrest: Analysis of outcome during an 8 year study. Circulation 70:538, 1984.
9. Ruskin J, DiMarco J, Garan H: Out-of-hospital cardiac arrest. N Engl J Med 303:607, 1980.
10. Chiang B, Perlman L, Fulton M, et al.: Predisposing factors in sudden cardiac death in Tecumseh, Michigan. Circulation 41:31, 1970.
11. Perper J, Kuller L, Cooper M: Arteriosclerosis of coronary arteries in sudden unexpected deaths. Circulation 51&52(Suppl 3):27, 1975.
12. Reichenbach D, Moss N, Meyer E: Pathology of the heart in sudden cardiac death. Am J Cardiol 39:865, 1977.
13. Bashe W, Baba N, Keller M, et al.: Pathology of atherosclerotic heart disease in sudden death. Circulation 51&52(Suppl 3):63, 1975.
14. Baba N, Bashe W, Keller M, et al.: Pathology of atherosclerotic heart disease in sudden death. Circulation 51&52(Suppl 3):53, 1975.
15. Doyle J, Kannel W, McNamara P, et al.: Factors related to suddenness of death from coronary disease: Combined Albany-Framingham studies. Am J Cardiol 37:1073, 1976.
16. Lie J, Titus J: Pathology of the myocardium and the conduction system in sudden coronary death. Circulation 51&52(Suppl 3):41, 1975.
17. Schwartz C, Gerrity R: Anatomical pathology of sudden unexpected cardiac death. Circulation 51&52(Suppl 3):18, 1975.
18. Oberman A, Ray M, Turner M, et al.: Sudden death in patients evaluated for ischemic heart disease. Circulation 51&52(Suppl 3):170, 1975.
19. Riechenbach D, Moss N: Myocardial cell necrosis and sudden death in humans. Circulation 51&52(Suppl 3):60, 1975.
20. Weaver W, Lorch G, Alvarez H, et al.: Angiographic findings and prognostic indicators in patients resuscitated from sudden cardiac death. Circulation 54:895, 1976.
21. Friedman G, Klatsky A, Siegelaub A: Predictors of sudden cardiac death. Circulation 51&52(Suppl 3):164, 1975.
22. Ritchie J, Hallstrom A, Troubaugh G, et al.: Out-of-hospital sudden coronary death: Rest and exercise radionuclide left ventricular function in survivors. Am J Cardiol 55:645, 1985.
23. Goldstein S, Landis J, Leighton R, et al.: Characteristics of the resuscitated out-of-hospital cardiac arrest victim with coronary heart disease. Circulation 64:977, 1981.
24. Hammermeister K, DeRouen T, Dodge H: Variables predictive of survival in patients with coronary disease. Circulation 59:425, 1979.
25. Moss A: Profile of high risk in people known to have coronary heart disease: A review. Circulation 51&52(Suppl 3):147, 1975.
26. Ruberman W, Weinblatt E, Frank C, et al.: Ventricular premature beats and mortality of men with coronary heart disease. Circulation 51&52(Suppl 3):199, 1975.
27. Moss A, DeCamilla J, Mietlowski W, et al.: Prognostic grading and significance of ventricular premature beats after recovery

from myocardial infarction. Circulation 51&52(Suppl 3):204, 1975.
28. Kotler M, Tabatznik B, Mower M, et al.: Prognostic significance of ventricular ectopic beats with respect to sudden death in the late post-infarction period. Circulation 47:959, 1973.
29. Davis H, DeCamilla J, Bayer L, et al.: Survivorship patterns in the post-hospital phase of myocardial infarction. Circulation 60:1252, 1979.
30. Vismara L, Vera Z, Foerster J, et al.: Identification of sudden death risk factors in acute and chronic coronary artery disease. Am J Cardiol 39:821, 1977.
31. Schulze R, Humphries J, Griffith L, et al.: Left ventricular and coronary angiographic anatomy. Circulation 55:839, 1976.
32. Gradman A, Bell P, DeBusk R: Sudden death during ambulatory monitoring. Circulation 55:210, 1977.
33. Nikolic G, Bishop R, Singh J: Sudden death recorded during Holter monitoring. Circulation 66:218, 1982.
34. Pratt C, Francis M, Luck J, et al.: Analysis of ambulatory electrograms in 15 patients during spontaneous ventricular fibrillation with special reference to preceding arrhythmic events. J Am Coll Cardiol 2:789, 1983.
35. Kempf F, Josephson M: Cardiac arrest recorded on ambulatory electrograms. Am J Cardiol 53:1577, 1984.
36. Martin G, Magrid N, Myers G, et al.: Heart rate variability and sudden death secondary to coronary artery disease during ambulatory electrocardiographic monitoring. Am J Cardiol 60:86, 1987.
37. Lown B, Verrier R: Neural activity and ventricular fibrillation. N Engl J Med 294:1165, 1976.
38. Schulze R, Strauss H, Pitt B: Sudden death in the year following myocardial infarction. Am J Med 62:192, 1977.
39. Mukharji J, Rude R, Poole W, et al.: Risk factors for sudden death after acute myocardial infarction: Two-year follow-up. Am J Cardiol 54:31, 1984.
40. Bigger J, Fleiss J, Kleiger R, et al.: The relationships among ventricular arrhythmias, left ventricular dysfunction and mortality in the two years after myocardial infarction. Circulation 69:250, 1984.
41. Weaver W, Cobb L, Hellstrom A: Ambulatory arrhythmias in resuscitated victims of cardiac arrest. Circulation 66:212, 1982.
42. Swerdlow C, Peterson J: Prospective comparison of Holter monitoring and electrophysiologic study in patients with coronary artery disease and sustained ventricular tachyarrhythmias. Am J Cardiol 56:577, 1985.
43. Josephson M: Treatment of ventricular arrhythmias after myocardial infarction. Circulation 74:653, 1986.
44. Morganroth J, Michelson E, Horowitz L: Limitations of routine long-term electrocardiographic monitoring to assess ventricular ectopic frequency. Circulation 58:408, 1978.
45. Surawicz B: Prognosis of ventricular arrhythmias in relation to sudden cardiac death: Therapeutic complications. J Am Coll Cardiol 10:435, 1987.
46. The CAPS Investigators: Cardiac Arrhythmia Pilot Study. Am J Cardiol 57:91, 1986.
47. Pratt C, Theroux P, Slymen D, et al.: Spontaneous variability of ventricular arrhythmias in patients at increased risk for sudden death after acute myocardial infarction. Am J Cardiol 59:278, 1987.
48. Kosowsky B, Lown B, Whiting R, et al.: Occurrence of ventricular arrhythmias with exercise as compared to monitoring. Circulation 44:826, 1971.
49. Lown B, Calvert A, Armington R, et al.: Monitoring for serious arrhythmias and high risk of sudden death. Circulation 51&52(Suppl 3):189, 1975.
50. Sheps D, Ernst J, Briese F, et al.: Decreased frequency of exercise-induced ventricular ectopic activity in the second of two consecutive treadmill tests. Circulation 55:892, 1977.
51. Theroux P, Waters D, Halphen C, et al.: Prognostic value of exercise testing soon after myocardial infarction. N Engl J Med 301:341, 1979.
52. Califf R, McKinnis R, NcNeer J et al.: Prognostic value of ventricular arrhythmias associated with treadmill exercise testing in patients studied with cardiac catheterization for suspected ischemic heart disease. J Am Coll Cardiol 2:1060, 1983.
53. Weaver W, Cobb L, Hallstrom A: Exercise and exercise testing in victims of out-of-hospital ventricular fibrillation (Abstract). Circulation 60(Suppl 3):269, 1979.
54. Simson M: Use of signals in the terminal QRS complex to identify patients with ventricular tachycardia after myocardial infarction. Circulation 64:235, 1981.
55. Breithardt G, Borggrefe M, Karbenn V, et al.: Prevalence of late potentials in patients with and without ventricular tachycardia: Correlation with angiographic findings. Am J Cardiol 49:1932, 1982.
56. Kanovsky M, Falcone R, Dresden C, et al.: Identification of patients with ventricular tachycardia after myocardial infarction: Signal-averaged electrocardiogram, Holter monitoring and cardiac catheterization. Circulation 70:264, 1984.
57. Gomes J, Mehra R, Barreca P, et al.: Quantitative analysis of the high-frequency components of the signal-averaged QRS complex in patients with acute myocardial infarction: A prospective study. Circulation 72:105, 1985.
58. Coto H, Maldonado C, Palakurthy P, et al.: Late potentials in normal subjects and in patients with ventricular tachycardia unrelated to myocardial infarction. Am J Cardiol 55:384, 1985.
59. Kuchar D, Thorburn C, Sammel N: Prediction of serious arrhythmic events after myocardial infarction: Signal-averaged electrocardiogram, Holter monitoring and radionuclide ventriculography. J Am Coll Cardiol 9:531, 1987.
60. Waldo A, Kaiser G: A study of ventricular arrhythmias associated with acute myocardial infarction in the canine heart. Circulation 47:1222, 1973.
61. El-Sherif N, Scherlag B, Lazzara R: Electrode catheter recordings during malignant ventricular arrhythmias following experimental acute myocardial ischemia. Circulation 51:1003, 1975.
62. Myerburg R, Ghahramani A, Mallon S, et al.: Coronary revascularization in patients surviving unexpected ventricular fibrillation. Circulation 51&52(Suppl 3):219, 1975.
63. Chaitman B, Fisher L, Bourassa M, et al.: Effect of coronary bypass surgery on survival patterns in subsets of patients with left main coronary artery disease. Am J Cardiol 48:765, 1981.
64. Veterans Administration Cooperative Group for the Study of Surgery for Coronary Arterial Disease: The VA Cooperative study of stable angina: current status. Circulation 65(Suppl II):II–60, 1982.
65. European Coronary Surgery Study Group: Prospective randomized study of coronary artery bypass surgery in stable angina pectoris. Lancet 11:491, 1980.
66. Takaro T, Hultgren H, Lipton M, et al.: The VA Cooperative randomized study of surgery for coronary arterial occlusive disease. Circulation 54(Suppl 3):107, 1976.
67. Krikler D, Perelman M, Rowland E: Ventricular tachycardia and ventricular fibrillation. In Mandel W (ed.): Cardiac Arrhythmias, Their Mechanisms, Diagnosis and Management. Philadelphia, J. B. Lippincott Co, 1987, p. 517.
68. Horowitz L, Spear J, Josephson M, et al.: The effects of coronary artery disease as the ventricular fibrillation threshold in man. Circulation 60:792, 1979.
69. Dixon M, Trank J, Dobell A: Ventricular fibrillation threshold: Variation with coronary flow and its value in assessing experimental myocardial revascularization. J Thorac Cardiovasc Surg 47:620, 1964.
70. Garan H, Ruskin J, DiMarco J, et al.: Electrophysiologic studies before and after myocardial revascularization in patients with life-threatening ventricular arrhythmias. Am J Cardiol 51:519, 1983.
71. Morady F, DiCarlo L, Winston S, et al.: Clinical features and prognosis of patients with out-of-hospital cardiac arrest and a normal electrophysiologic study. J Am Coll Cardiol 4:39, 1984.
72. Kehoe R, Moran J, Zheutlin T, et al.: Electrophysiologic study to direct therapy in survivors of pre-hospital ventricular fibrillation (Abstract). Am J Cardiol 49:928, 1982.
73. Morady F, Scheinman M, Hess David, et al.: Electrophysiologic testing in the management of survivors of out-of-hospital cardiac arrest. Am J Cardiol 51:85, 1983.
74. Roy D, Waxman H, Krienzle M, et al.: Clinical characteristics

and long-term follow-up in 119 survivors of cardiac arrest: Relation to inducibility at electrophysiologic testing. Am J Cardiol 52:969, 1983.
75. Zheutlin T, Steinman R, Summers C, et al.: Long-term outcome in survivors of cardiac arrest with non-inducible ventricular tachycardia during programmed stimulation. Circulation 70(Suppl 3):399, 1984.
76. Benditt D, Benson D, Klein G, et al.: Prevention of recurrent sudden cardiac arrest: Role of provocative electrophysiologic testing. J Am Coll Cardiol 2:418, 1983.
77. Myerburg R, Conde C, Sung R, et al.: Clinical electrophysiologic and hemodynamic profile of patients resuscitated from pre-hospital cardiac arrest. Am J Med 68:568, 1980.
78. Swerdlow C, Winkle R, Mason J: Determinants of survival in patients with ventricular tachyarrhythmias. N Engl J Med 308:1436, 1983.
79. Eldar M, Sauve M, Scheinman M: Electrophysiologic testing and follow-up of patients with aborted sudden death. J Am Coll Cardiol 10:291, 1987.
80. Wilber JD, Garan H, Kelly E, et al.: Out-of-hospital cardiac arrest: Role of electrophysiologic testing in the prediction of long-term outcome. N Engl J Med 318:19, 1988.
81. Waller T, Kay H, Spielman S, et al.: Reduction in sudden death and total mortality by antiarrhythmic therapy evaluated by electrophysiologic drug testing: criteria of efficacy in patients with sustained ventricular tachyarrhythmia. J Am Coll Cardiol 10:83, 1987.
82. Gomes J, Hariman R, Kang P, et al.: Programmed electrical stimulation patients with high-grade ventricular ectopy: Electrophysiologic findings and prognosis for survival. Circulation 70:43, 1984.
83. Veltri R, Platia E, Griffith L, et al.: Programmed electrical stimulation and long-term follow-up in asymptomatic, nonsustained ventricular tachycardia. Am J Cardiol 56:309, 1985.
84. Spielman S, Greenspan A, Kay H, et al.: Electrophysiologic testing in patients at high risk for sudden death. I. Nonsustained ventricular tachycardia and abnormal ventricular function. J Am Coll Cardiol 6:31, 1985.
85. Buxton A, Marchlinski F, Flores B, et al.: Nonsustained ventricular tachycardia in patients with coronary artery disease: role of electrophysiologic study. Circulation 75:1178, 1987.
86. Mason J, Winkle R: Electrode-catheter arrhythmia induction in the selection and assessment of antiarrhythmic drug therapy for recurrent ventricular tachycardia. Circulation 58:971, 1978.
87. Horowitz L, Josephson M, Farshidi A, et al.: Recurrent sustained ventricular tachycardia. 3. Role of the electrophysiologic study in selection of antiarrhythmic regimens. Circulation 58:986, 1978.
88. Horowitz L, Spielman S, Greenspan A, et al.: Role of programmed stimulation in assessing vulnerability to ventricular arrhythmias. Am Heart J 103:604, 1982.
89. Brugada P, Green M, Abdollah H, et al.: Significance of ventricular arrhythmias initiated by programmed ventricular stimulation: The importance of the type of ventricular arrhythmia induced and the number of premature stimuli required. Circulation 69:87, 1984.
90. Buxton A, Waxman H, Marchlinski F, et al.: Role of triple extrastimuli during electrophysiologic study of patients with documented sustained ventricular tachyarrhythmias. Circulation 69:532, 1984.
91. Bigger J, Reiffel J, Livelli F, et al.: Sensitivity and criteria in electrophysiologic study of ventricular tachycardia. Circulation 75(Suppl 3):125, 1987.
92. Mason J, Anderson K, Freedman R: Techniques and criteria in electrophysiologic study of ventricular tachycardia. Circulation 75(Suppl 3):125, 1987.
93. Wellens H, Brugada P, Stevenson W: Programmed electrical stimulation of the heart in patients with life-threatening ventricular arrhythmias: What is the significance of induced arrhythmias and what is the correct stimulation protocol? Circulation 72:1, 1985.
94. Lovell R: Arrhythmia prophylaxis: Long-term suppressive medication. Circulation 51&52(Suppl 3):236, 1975.
95. Graboys T, Lown B, Podrid P, et al.: Long-term survival of patients with malignant ventricular arrhythmia treated with antiarrhythmic drugs. Am J Cardiol 50:437, 1982.
96. Bigger J: Identification of patients at high risk for sudden cardiac death. Am J Cardiol 54:30, 1984.
97. Myerburg R, Conde C, Sheps D, et al.: Antiarrhythmic drug therapy in survivors of pre-hospital cardiac arrest: Comparison of effects on chronic ventricular arrhythmias and recurrent cardiac arrest. Circulation 59:855, 1979.
98. Heger J, Prystowsky E, Jackman W, et al.: Amiodarone: Clinical efficacy and electrophysiology during long-term therapy for recurrent ventricular tachycardia or ventricular fibrillation. N Engl J Med 305:539, 1981.
99. Kim S, Fisher J, Matos J: Poor predictive value of ventricular tachycardia induced by programmed stimulation in patients taking amiodarone (Abstract). PACE 5:305, 1982.
100. Hamer A, Finerman W, Peter T, et al.: Disparity between the clinical and electrophysiologic effects of amiodarone in the treatment of recurrent ventricular arrhythmias. Am Heart J 102:992, 1981.
101. Veltri E, Reid P, Platia E, et al.: Results of late programmed electrical stimulation and long-term electrophysiologic effects of amiodarone therapy in patients with refractory ventricular tachycardia. Am J Cardiol 55:375, 1985.
102. McGovern B, Garan H, Malacoff R, et al.: Long-term clinical outcome of ventricular tachycardia or fibrillation treated with amiodarone. Am J Cardiol 53:1558, 1984.
103. DiCarlo L, Morady F, Sauve J, et al.: Cardiac arrest and sudden death in patients treated with amiodarone for sustained ventricular tachycardia or ventricular fibrillation: Risk stratification based on clinical variables. Am J Cardiol 55:372, 1985.
104. Horowitz L, Greenspan A, Spielman S, et al.: Usefulness of electrophysiologic testing in evaluation of amiodarone therapy for sustained ventricular tachyarrhythmias associated with coronary heart disease. Am J Cardiol 55:367, 1985.
105. Ruskin J, McGovern B, Garan H, et al.: Antiarrhythmic drugs: A possible cause of out-of-hospital cardiac arrest. N Engl J Med 309:1302, 1983.
106. Horowitz L, Zipes D (eds.): A Symposium: Perspectives on Proarrhythmia. Am J Cardiol 59:2E, 1987.
107. Josephson M, Harken A, Horowitz L: Endocardial excision: A new surgical technique for the treatment of recurrent ventricular tachycardia. Circulation 60:1430, 1979.
108. Miller J, Marchlinski F, Harken A, et al.: Subendocardial resection for sustained ventricular tachycardia in the early period after acute myocardial infarction. Am J Cardiol 55:980, 1985.
109. Krafchek J, Laurie G, Roberts R, et al.: Surgical ablation of ventricular tachycardia: Improved results with a map-directed regional approach. Circulation 73:1239, 1986.
110. Kienzle M, Doherty J, Roy D, et al.: Subendocardial resection for refractory ventricular tachycardia: Effects on ambulatory electrocardiogram, programmed stimulation and ejection fraction and relation to outcome. J Am Coll Cardiol 2:853, 1983.
111. Miller J, Kienzle M, Harken A, et al.: Subendocardial resection for ventricular tachycardia: Predictors of surgical success. Circulation 70:624, 1984.
112. Waspe L, Brodman R, Kim S, et al.: Activation mapping in patients with coronary artery disease with multiple ventricular tachycardia configurations: Occurrence and therapeutic implications of widely separate apparent sites of origin. J Am Coll Cardiol 5:1075, 1985.
113. Garan H, Nguyen K, McGovern B, et al.: Perioperative and long-term results after electrophysiologically directed ventricular surgery for recurrent ventricular tachycardia. J Am Coll Cardiol 8:201, 1986.
114. Caceres J, Werner P, Jazayeri M, et al.: Efficacy of cryosurgery alone for refractory monomorphic sustained ventricular tachycardia due to inferior wall infarction. J Am Coll Cardiol 11:1254, 1988.
115. Mirowski M: The automatic implantable cardioverter-defibrillator: An overview. JACC 6:461, 1985.
116. Mirowski M, Reid P, Winkle R, et al.: Mortality in patients with implanted automatic defibrillators. Ann Intern Med 98:585, 1983.
117. Mirowski M: Management of malignant ventricular tachyarrhythmias with automatic implanted cardioverter-defibrillators. Mod Concepts Cardiovasc Dis 52:41, 1983.

118. Mirowski M, Reid P, Watkins L, et al.: Clinical treatment of life-threatening ventricular tachyarrhythmias with the automatic implantable defibrillator. Am Heart J 102:265, 1981.
119. Echt D, Armstrong K, Schmidt P, et al.: Clinical experience complications and survival in 70 patients with the automatic implantable cardioverter/defibrillator. Circulation 71:289, 1985.
120. Winkle R, Stinson E, Echt D, et al.: Practical aspects of automatic cardioverter/defibrillator implantation. Am Heart J 108:1335, 1984.
121. Gabry M, Grodman R, Johnston D, et al.: Automatic implantable cardioverter/defibrillator: Patient survival, battery longevity and shock delivery analysis. J Am Coll Cardiol 9:1349, 1987.
122. Kelly P, Cannom D, Garan H, et al.: The automatic implantable cardioverter/defibrillator: Efficacy, complications and survival in patients with malignant ventricular arrhythmias. J Am Coll Cardiol 11:1278, 1988.

19

The High-Resolution Electrocardiogram: Technical and Basic Aspects

Nabil El-Sherif
Mark Restivo
William Craelius
Rahul Mehra
Raphael Henkin
Edward B. Caref
George Kelen

Introduction

There are several low level electrocardiographic potentials whose manifestations on the body surface are too small to be detected by routine measurement techniques. These include the potentials produced by the His-Purkinje system and by slow conduction in depressed ventricular myocardium (usually called *late potentials*). These potentials are small because the activation front is slow and fractionated or the mass of tissue undergoing depolarization is small, or both. However, the measurement of the bioelectric potentials produced by these tissues is important for diagnostic purposes. Identification of the His-Purkinje potential can localize the site of atrioventricular conduction disorders, and the detection of late potentials may identify patients at high risk for malignant ventricular tachyarrhythmias. The problem in identifying these potentials is that the signal is smaller than the electrical noise produced by various sources. Two different techniques have been utilized to improve signal-to-noise (S/N) ratio:

1. *Ensemble or temporal averaging* (usually referred to as *signal averaging*). This technique is applicable only to repetitive electrocardiographic signals and cannot detect moment-by-moment dynamic changes in the signals.
2. *Spatial averaging.* This technique can record the His-Purkinje signal and late potentials on a beat-to-beat basis.

The signal-averaged technique has been utilized more often in the last few years, and the averaged signal can be analyzed in either time domain, frequency domain, or a combination of both time and frequency display in the form of spectro-temporal maps. The term high-resolution ECG should be considered to encompass any technique that results in improvement of ECG S/N ratio. This includes both temporal and spatial averaging techniques.

In this chapter we review system design and electrophysiologic instrumentation of the high-resolution ECG as well as the electrophysiologic substrate of late potentials. Clinical applications of both signal averaging and beat-to-beat recording techniques will be discussed in Chapters 20 and 21, respectively. Chapter 11 discusses the use of the signal-averaged (SA) ECG for risk stratification and management of patients with

---

Supported by National Institutes of Health Grants HL36680 and HL31341 and Veterans Administration Medical Research Funds.

complex ventricular arrhythmias and nonsustained ventricular tachycardia (VT).

Noise Sources in Electrophysiologic Signal Measurements

There are four primary noise sources in electrophysiologic signal measurements: (1) power frequency, (2) electrode–tissue interface, (3) amplifier, and (4) electromyographic potentials.

POWER FREQUENCY NOISE

A major source of artifact when one is recording physiologic signals is the electrical power system. Power lines are connected to other pieces of equipment in the typical hospital environment. Electrical field and magnetic field coupling can both give rise to power interference. A typical monitoring configuration uses two active electrodes as differential inputs to an amplifier and a third common electrode. This technique is used almost universally because differential amplifiers can be designed to give a high common mode rejection ratio and input impedance, both of which reduce interference. However, one has the choice of grounding the common or using different configurations of two-electrode recording systems. A theoretical analysis of the problem reveals that least interference would be expected with an ungrounded three-lead system. Lowering skin-electrode impedance and minimizing the difference between the two skin-electrode impedances is also important. Shielding the input cables and twisting them to reduce magnetic induction can further lower the interference. Power spectra of ECGs in a hospital environment show that sharp impulses occur not only at 60 Hz (50 Hz in Europe) but at many harmonics of the fundamental frequency. Although the higher harmonics are lower in magnitude, frequencies as high as 1500 Hz can sometimes be observed. One of the best ways to reduce interference is to enclose the patient and the recording system in a Faraday cage. Since this cage is grounded, most of the displacement currents are shunted. This technique, however, sacrifices the mobility of the measuring system. Low-noise electrophysiologic signal measurements such as evoked responses are frequently done in shielded rooms. A shielded room was also used by some investigators for their high-resolution ECG measurements.[1] Notch filters for 60 Hz and its harmonics can further reduce noise from the output signal.

ELECTRODE–TISSUE INTERFACE NOISE

The primary function of an electrode is to convert ionic conduction in tissue to electronic conduction in the measuring system. Silver–silver chloride electrodes are the least polarizable, and they result in a low impedance, low offset potential interface. The electrical stability of the electrode is considerably enhanced by mechanical stabilization of the electrode-tissue interface by interposing an electrolyte between the electrode and the tissue. Most commercial ECG electrodes are of this indirect-contact design. In addition to their nonpolarizable behavior, the silver–silver chloride electrode exhibits less electrical noise than other metal electrodes. It has also been observed that newly prepared electrodes are often noisy; however, with the passage of time the noise decreases. Electrodes with a peak-to-peak noise of about 1 μV (measured in 0.9% saline) at a bandwidth of 0.1 to 1000 Hz can be commercially purchased with a minimal amount of electrode "popping." Typical offset voltages range between 0 and 4 μV.[2] Sanding of the skin lightly with fine sandpaper (3M Type 220) and wiping with alcohol can significantly reduce electrode impedance, resulting in recordings with less interference.

AMPLIFIER NOISE

The noise associated with a differential amplifier stage is the result of Schottky, or shot noise; Johnson, or thermal noise and flicker; or low-frequency (l/f) noise.[3] Shot noise is due to the discrete particle nature of current carriers in semiconductors; the origin of the l/f noise is not well understood. Representation of all the noise sources by equivalent noise generators results in an equivalent input noise voltage and current with thermal noise of source resistance. All these noise sources are proportional to the square root of the bandwidth considered. Typically, with bipolar devices the input noise voltage is lower and the noise current higher than in field-effect transistor devices. In most applications, since the source resistances are low, the current noise figure does not add appreciably to the total noise as compared to the thermal noise of the source resistances. Most semiconductor devices have specified noise figures. As the technology changes, manufacturers continually introduce devices with lower input voltage and current noise specifications.

ELECTROMYOGRAPHIC POTENTIALS

Physiologic signals recorded via body surface electrodes reflect the asynchronous firing at motor units that are dispersed temporally and spatially with a superimposed ECG signal. Attempts have been made to separate the two by optimal bandpass filtering but significant overlap exists between the power spectra of the two signals. About 95% of the electromyographic power is between 25 and 250 Hz, with the remaining 5% above this frequency.[4] Most of the spectral power of the ECG lies below 40 Hz, although small amounts of power have been measured in some patients at frequencies up to 500 Hz.[5] A spectral analysis of the His bundle electrogram recorded from the body surface indicates that most of the power spectrum is below 100 Hz.[1] Due to this overlap of spectral components, it becomes difficult to measure the electrical activity of the heart independent of skeletal muscle activity. The latter can be reduced by relaxing the patient or by the use of muscle relaxants. Significant variations can exist between muscle tone of patients during relaxation. Cyclic variation in electromyography (EMG) can also be observed with respiration. Administration of succinylcholine chloride during anesthesia virtually eliminates skeletal muscle activity, and heart activity up to 300 to 400 Hz can be measured.[5] This technique is obviously not applicable to routine clinical measurements. EMG noise could be reduced in relation to the ECG signal by a number of techniques that are discussed in some detail under the section on "Beat-to-beat recording of the high-resolution electrocardiogram."

Temporal Signal Averaging

Temporal signal averaging is a process whereby fixed intervals of a noisy signal are aligned temporally with respect to a reference point and then summed. A signal-averaging system stores the information of a designated interval of the ECG and sums the information received from successive intervals. Division of the sum of stored information by the number of cycles yields an ensemble average. In this average, the components of the information arising from the noise sources diminish because they are random, and the desired repetitive signal is accentuated, thus resulting in an improved S/N ratio. In fact, the averaging process reduces to a simple summation, with the signal present in the summations building up linearly owing to the coherent timings with which the samples were taken. The noise, if it is random, adds up in a root-mean-square sense with the net result that after X signal repetitions have been combined, the S/N ratio has been improved by $\sqrt{X}$. There are, however certain assumptions inherent in the use of an averaging procedure for noise reduction. First, the characteristics of the signal must be uniform during the averaging period.[6, 7] Second, the noise must exhibit "stationarity"—that is, its probability distribution function must not change throughout the averaging period. The independence of "signal" and "noise" are important for improvement of S/N ratio. The noise produced by the amplifier and the electrode–tissue interface is primarily random and undergoes a $\sqrt{X}$ improvement in S/N ratio. However, the power line frequency and the EMG potentials related to respiration may be periodic. It has been shown that S/N ratio in such cases will be less than for random noise, even when the sampling of data is asynchronous with respect to the periodic noise. If periodic noise is present in the original signal, it is almost certain to produce a periodic component in the average, however small. Also, if an average contains components due to asynchronous periodic noise, repeated averages will show different configurations.

A basic averaging system consists of (1) an ECG amplifier having high resolution and gain, (2) high-fidelity bandpass filters, (3) a method for temporally aligning successive cardiac cycles, and (4) a digital computer system for the storage, averaging, and display of signals. Several such systems have been used, with designs ranging widely in complexity. Filter designs include analog bandpass circuits, linear digital filters,[8] and bidirectional digital filters.[9, 10] Temporal alignment schemes range in complexity from simple R wave amplitude triggers to QRS cross-correlation algorithms.[11, 12] Some alignment methods use the derivative of the QRS as the alignment signal[13, 14] whereas others use the wideband QRS.[10] Some QRS recognition algorithms, although not specifically designed for signal averaging, use an adaptive QRS threshold, whereby the waveforms from multiple beats specify threshold or contour limits, in order to optimize QRS detection.[15-18]

SIGNAL ALIGNMENT FOR TEMPORAL AVERAGING

The use of a precise fiducial or reference mark with a fixed temporal relationship to the signal of interest is essential for signal averaging. One obstacle to establishing standards for signal averaging has been the inability to directly measure the temporal misalignment. Because the wave shapes themselves are complex and vary from cycle to cycle, there are no a priori criteria by which to predict or quantify their alignment in time. Some attempts have been made to estimate alignment errors by modeling the QRS as a regular wave, such as sine, and calculating the effects of amplitude variations and added noise on a trigger system;[19, 20] however, they offer no direct measure of alignment errors. A common method used to estimate alignment error is to measure a quantity called "trigger jitter." This is done by observing the range in temporal displacements of successive triggered QRS complexes on an oscilloscope screen. Reported values of jitter have ranged between 0.5 and 2 ms. Since the QRS shapes change in complex ways from beat to beat within that time resolution, the measurement of trigger jitter suffers from considerable arbitrariness. A more systematic method will be preferable. Craelius and colleagues[21] have described a QRS detector system whereby temporal alignment accuracy and frequency response can be monitored during averaging and can be optimized for each patient. The system consists of two comparators, one based on amplitude and the other based on slope within a specified interval (Fig. 19–1). The ECG signal is high-pass filtered at a cutoff of 1 Hz to reduce baseline drift, and low-pass filtered at a cutoff of 500 Hz. The signal is fed into two circuits: (1) an amplitude level detector, consisting of a comparator, and (2) a differentiator. The level detector triggers a timing circuit that sends a variable width pulse after a delay to an analog switch. The switch gates a selected portion of the differentiated signal and transmits this to a second comparator. If the slope is above the specified threshold, the final trigger pulse is generated. This final pulse is known as the "window trigger," since it is based on a windowed portion of the QRS slope. It is used as the QRS alignment point for signal averaging, has a duration set just below the expected minimum ST interval of 300 ms, and is nonretriggerable. While alignment systems are subject

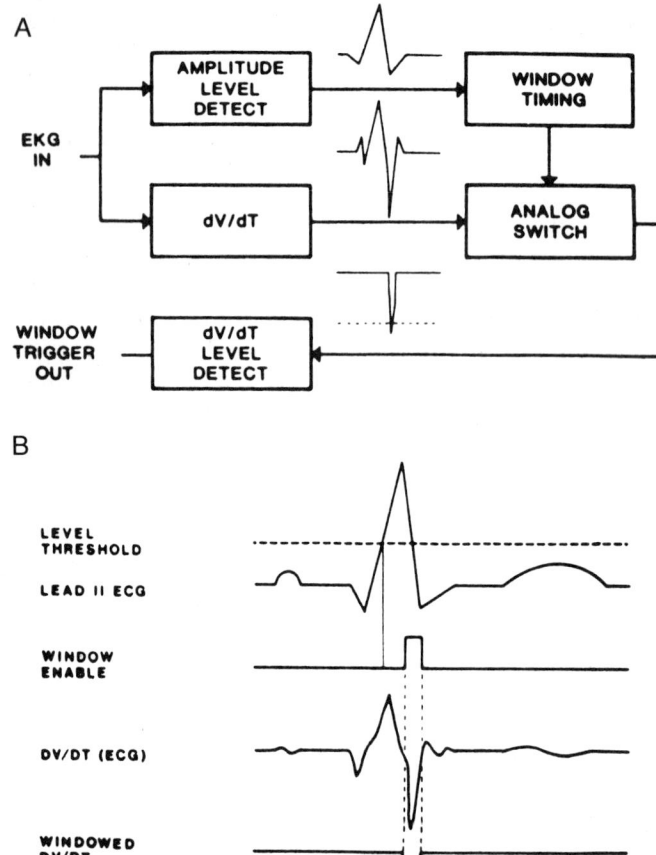

FIGURE 19–1
Design of QRS recognition system. A, Schematic diagram; B, timing diagram. (Reprinted with permission from Craelius W, et al.: IEEE Trans Biomed Eng 33:957, 1986.)

to some arbitrariness, one whose accuracy can be empirically measured and adjusted seems preferable. The window trigger system offers this advantage: it is not based on computed estimates and it can operate in real time. Moreover, the step response estimator of temporal misalignment can readily be incorporated into any alignment system, such as cross-correlation, in order to provide feedback on its accuracy.

LEAD SYSTEMS FOR TEMPORAL AVERAGING

Most investigators use an XYZ lead system formed by three orthogonal bipolar electrode combinations. The standard XYZ lead positions are as follows. The X lead electrodes are positioned at the right (−) and left (+) mid-axillary line at the V_5 level; the Y lead electrodes are positioned at the superior aspect of the manubrium (−) and at the inferior part of the sternum (+) and the Z lead electrodes at the fifth intercostal space at the left lateral sternal border (+) and at an identical position on the posterior chest (−). Other investigators have used different unipolar and bipolar leads.[22–24] The optimal lead system for recording the high-resolution ECG will probably depend on the electrical signal of interest (e.g., the His-Purkinje potential or ventricular late potentials). A few studies have compared different lead systems for recording of late potentials and found that left ventricular leads tend to have more abnormal measurements compared with the standard orthogonal lead system.[25] If late potentials represent a localized electrical source, they could be retrieved better by electrodes placed in proximity of the left ventricle. Faugere and associates[26] characterized the spatial distribution of late potentials by body surface mapping in patients with VT. They found that late potentials can be well detected with only three orthogonal leads because their distributions are bipolar. However, body surface maps could provide additional information about the location of late potentials that may be related to conduction delay sites and possibly site of origin of VT.

Other body surface potential mapping techniques have been used for morphologic analysis of the high-resolution ECG. Horan and coworkers[27] described a technique for the extraction of low-level His potentials from the larger atrial repolarization potentials. A spatial filter is first adapted to the morphology of atrial depolarization distribution and is then used to detect and cancel the atrial repolarization. A technique described by Horacek and coworkers[28] detects local extrema on the unfiltered body surface potential map and plots their trajectory over the torso during the entire heart beat.

ROLE OF BANDPASS FILTERS IN TEMPORAL AVERAGING

Most investigators have used bandpass digital filters[29] for time-domain analysis of the temporal averaged signal. Low-pass filters are utilized to remove high-frequency noise such as EMG noise. High-pass filters are used to eliminate the low-frequency components of the ST segment and T wave. However, the morphology of the signal is altered by the high-pass filtering, whatever the type and cutoff frequency of the filter. For example, a late potential signal composed of a series of positive peaks with no repolarization component will appear after filtering as a series of positive and negative peaks. Digital filters introduce two other types of distortion of the signal. One is "phase shift," whereby there is a change in timing of the signal after filtering, compared with the unfiltered signal. The second is "impulse ringing," which is oscillation occurring after an abrupt transient such as that occurring after the termination of a high-amplitude signal like the QRS. This artifact can thus simulate late potentials. Symmetric finite impulse response filters can prevent both phase shift and ringing, but their response will be affected by the proximity of the QRS. Simson[9] utilized a bidirectional infinite impulse response filter to prevent impulse ringing at the end of the QRS. The filter operates by processing the ECG

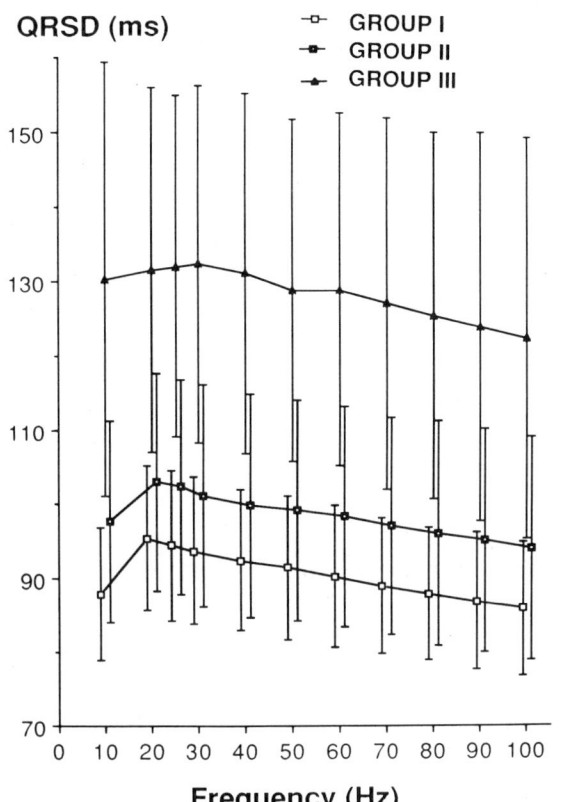

FIGURE 19–2
Mean ± standard deviation of filtered QRS duration (QRSD) at 11 high-pass filter settings in 100 normal subjects (group I), 52 patients with spontaneous nonsustained ventricular tachycardia (VT) and no inducible sustained monomorphic VT (group II), and 28 patients with spontaneous nonsustained VT and inducible sustained monomorphic VT (group III). The low-pass filter was fixed at 250 Hz. (Reprinted with permission from Caref EB, et al.: Am J Cardiol 64:16, 1989.)

forward in time until the middle of the QRS (40 ms from onset of the QRS). The ECG signal is processed retrograde, starting late in the ST segment, until the middle of the QRS is reached again. This filter, however, shifts the ringing to the middle of the QRS and still produces phase shifts.

Inappropriate high-pass filters can also attenuate or exclude signals of interest. Several investigators have evaluated the effects of high-pass filters on late potentials measurements.[30, 31] Caref et al.[31] analyzed the effects of 11 high-pass filters (10, 20, 25, 30, 40, 50, 60, 70, 80, 90, and 100 Hz) on the common scoring parameters of the signal-averaged ECG (SAECG). The low-pass cutoff frequency was fixed at 250 Hz. Three groups of patients were evaluated: group I, 100 normal subjects; group II, 52 patients with spontaneous nonsustained VT and no inducible monomorphic VT on programmed stimulation; and group III, 28 patients with spontaneous nonsustained VT and inducible sustained monomorphic VT on programmed stimulation. Four SAECG parameters were analyzed: (1) the duration of the filtered QRS (QRSD); (2) the duration of low-amplitude signals measured from the filtered QRS offset backward to when the signal reaches 40 μV (LAS40); (3) the root mean square voltage of the terminal 40 ms of the filtered QRS (RMS40); and (4) the root mean square voltage of the filtered QRS (RMSQRS).

The mean values of SAECG parameters were significantly influenced by the high-pass filter setting, both in normal subjects (group I) and in patients with spontaneous nonsustained VT (groups II and III). The QRSD increased between 10 and 20 Hz in groups I and II and between 10 and 30 Hz in group III before it gradually decreased at higher filter settings (Fig. 19–2). The LAS40 showed a gradual stepwise increase between 10 and 100 Hz in all three groups (Fig. 19–3), whereas the RMS40 (Fig. 19–4) and RMSQRS (Fig. 19–5) showed a nonlinear, gradual stepwise decrease. A typical effect of high-pass filters on the SAECG of a patient in group III is shown in Figure 19–6. The noise levels for all three groups showed a marked decline between 10 and 20 Hz, followed by a more gradual decrease between 20 and 50 Hz. From 50 to 100 Hz, the noise levels remained relatively stable. The algorithm for defining the filtered QRS offset was directly linked to the noise level, whereas RMS40 was more sensitive to the high-pass filter setting. Although RMS40 continued to decrease at higher high-pass filter settings, the reduction in noise level

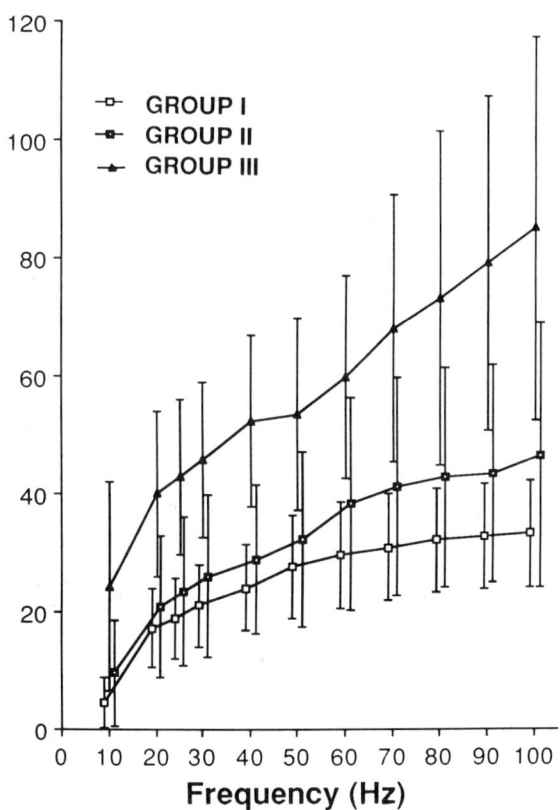

FIGURE 19–3
Mean ± standard deviation of low-amplitude signal < 40 μV (LAS40) at 11 high-pass filter settings in groups I, II, and III (described in Fig. 19–2). The low-pass filter was fixed at 250 Hz. (Reprinted with permission from Caref EB, et al.: Am J Cardiol 64:16, 1989.)

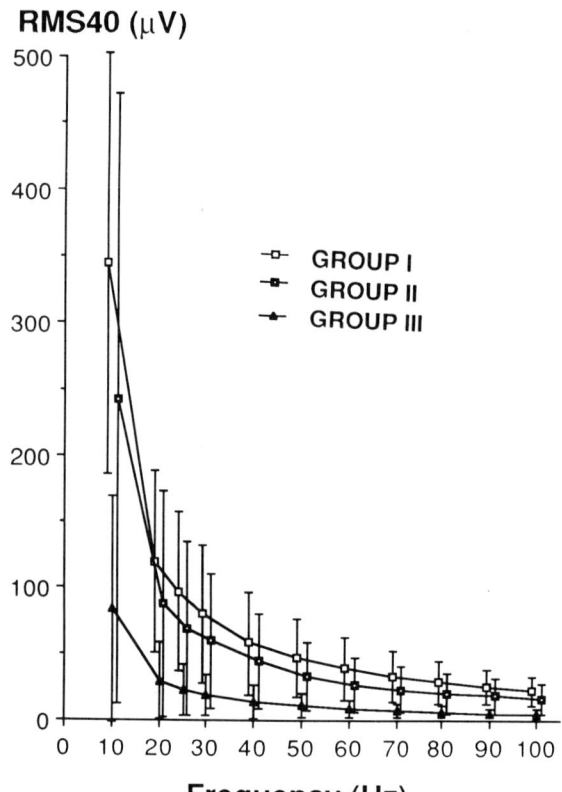

FIGURE 19–4
Mean ± standard deviation of root mean square voltage of the last 40 ms (RMS40) of the filtered QRS at 11 high-pass filter settings in groups I, II, and III (described in Fig. 19–2). The low-pass filter was fixed at 250 Hz. (Reprinted with permission from Caref EB, et al.: Am J Cardiol 64:16, 1989.)

had leveled off and remained fairly stable. The decrease in RMS40 without a corresponding decrease in noise could result in the inclusion of part of the low-amplitude signal at the end of the filtered QRS as baseline noise.

The loss of voltage, exemplified by RMSQRS, at high-pass filter settings ≥60 Hz prevented the analysis of LAS40 in 24 of 180 (13%) study subjects because no portion of the QRS signal reached 40 μV (see Fig. 19–6F). This phenomenon was observed three times at 60 Hz, five times at 70 Hz, 10 times at 80 Hz, 15 times at 90 Hz, and 24 times at 100 Hz. In some patients, a marked and abrupt attenuation of late potentials to below the baseline noise level occurred when the high-pass filter was increased from 20 to 40 Hz. In this case, late potentials seen at lower filter settings became invisible at higher filter settings (Fig. 19–7). This suggests that low-amplitude late potentials had a preponderance of relatively low-frequency signals in these patients.

The frequency characteristics of late potentials have not been adequately investigated. In a preliminary report by Craelius and colleagues,[32] direct endocardial mapping techniques in patients with VT showed that fragmented delayed depolarizations, which possibly contribute to late potentials on the body surface, had a peak frequency in the range of 25 to 110 Hz. Cain and associates,[33,34] using fast Fourier transform analysis (FFTA), found that frequencies greater than 50 Hz did not contribute significantly to the energy spectrum of the terminal QRS and ST segment in patients with VT. The distinguishing features between patients with or without VT was not due to the difference of frequency content of terminal QRS/early ST segment but rather to differences in amplitudes within a relatively narrow range of frequencies (20–50 Hz). In a study by Haberl and coworkers,[35] using a different FFTA technique, the frequency content of late potentials ranged from 40 to 240 Hz (mean 123±57), and all patients with VT had at least one spectral peak within the range of 60 to 120 Hz.

SIGNAL-AVERAGED ELECTROCARDIOGRAMS FROM HOLTER TAPE RECORDINGS

The high-frequency content of late potentials can be attenuated if signal averaging is performed on Holter tape recordings. Kelen and colleagues[36] compared SAECGs obtained from three-channel Holter record-

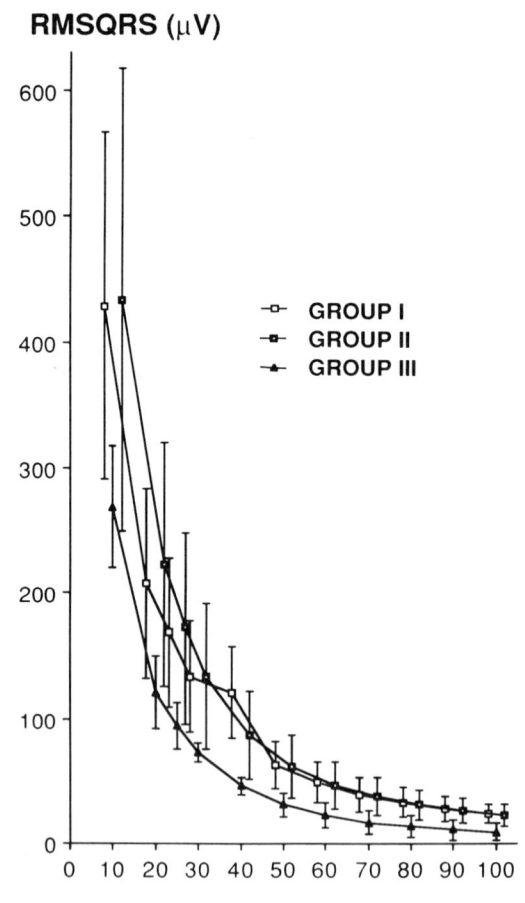

FIGURE 19–5
Mean ± standard deviation of root mean square voltage of the filtered QRS (RMSQRS) at 11 high-pass filter settings in groups I, II, and III (described in Fig. 19–2). The low-pass filter was fixed at 250 Hz. (Reprinted with permission from Caref EB, et al.: Am J Cardiol 64:16, 1989.)

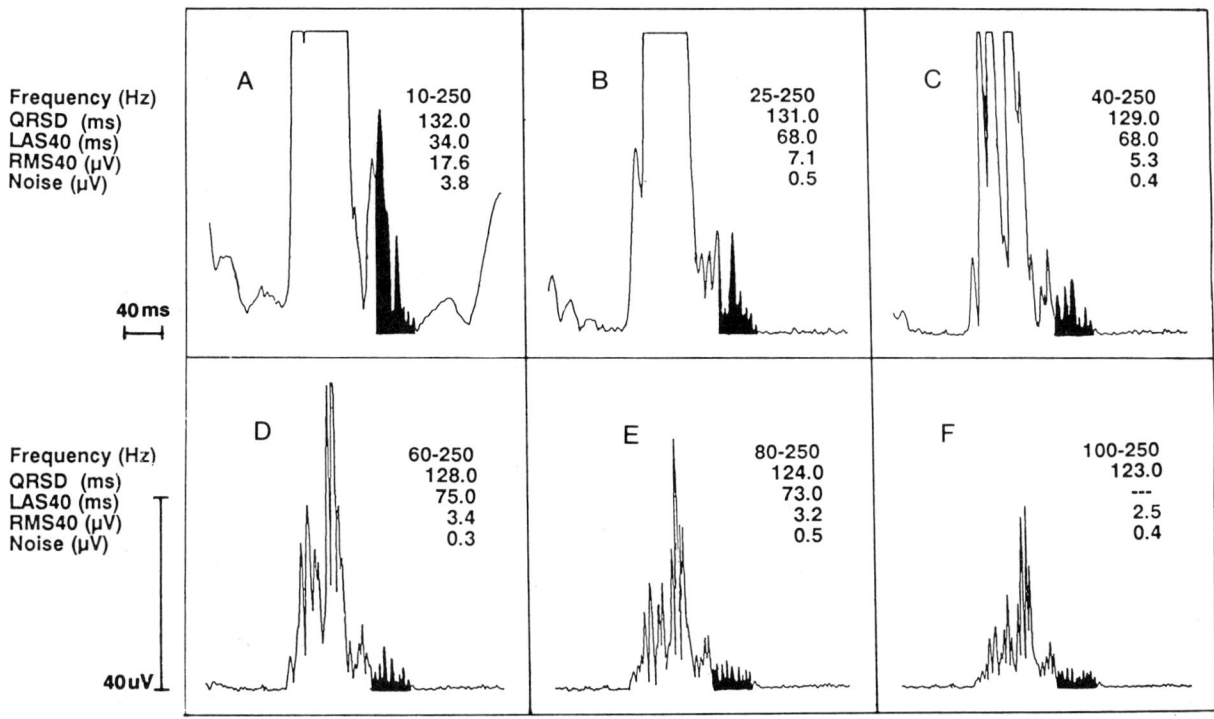

FIGURE 19–6
Typical effect of high-pass filters on signal-averaged electrocardiogram (SAECG) parameters in a patient with inducible sustained monomorphic ventricular tachycardia. The QRS duration shows a slight, gradual decrease at higher filter settings (A–F), whereas the RMS40 shows a significant, nonlinear decrease. The LAS40 shows a significant increase between 10 and 60 Hz (A–D) and then a slight decrease at 80 Hz (E). It could not be measured due to low amplitude of the filtered QRS at 100 Hz (F). The RMS40 is highlighted in each panel. Note the high noise level at 10 Hz (A), which significantly decreases and stabilizes at higher filter settings. QRSD = QRS duration; LAS40 = low-amplitude signal <40 μV; RMS40 = root mean square voltage of the last 40 ms. (Reprinted with permission from Caref EB, et al.: Am J Cardiol 64:16, 1989.)

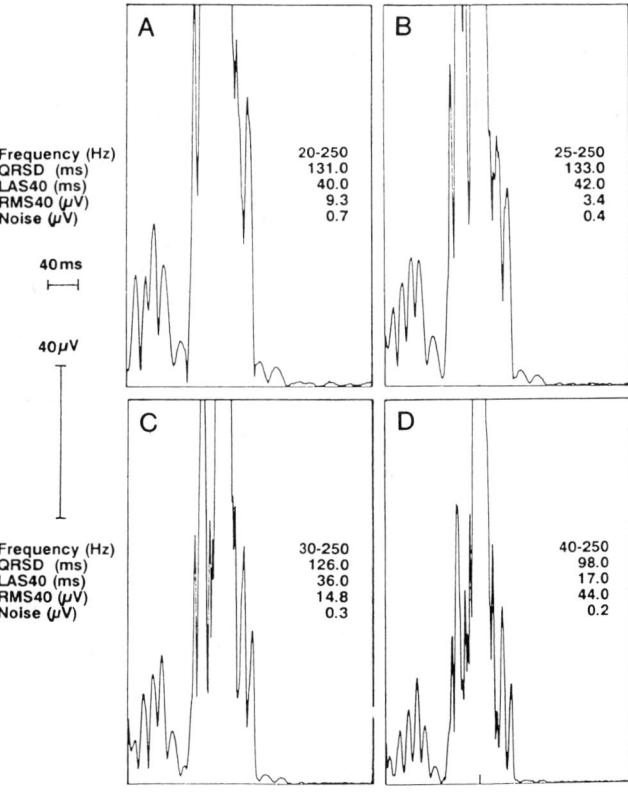

FIGURE 19–7
Signal-averaged electrocardiogram (SAECG) analyzed at four high-pass filter settings. Note marked attenuation of late potentials as the high-pass filter increases from 20 to 30 Hz (A–C). At 40 Hz (D), late potentials are no longer discernible. (See Fig. 19–6 for abbreviations.) (Reprinted with permission from Caref EB, et al.: Am J Cardiol 64:16, 1989.)

The High-Resolution Electrocardiogram: Technical and Basic Aspects   355

ings with signal-averaged real-time recordings. Both recordings were obtained from the same skin electrodes. The study was designed to determine whether the restricted frequency bandwidth (0.1–100 Hz ± 3dB), lower sampling rate (694 Hz), and additional background noise inherent in the recording/playback process of the Holter system result in significantly reduced reliability in the detection and quantification of clinically significant late potentials. The numerical late potential parameters and morphologic appearances correlated closely between the two methods (Fig. 19–8). However, high-frequency spikes were markedly attenuated on the Holter plot.

The attenuation of signals above 100 Hz inherent in the Holter recording and playback system would have the following predictable effects on the measured late potential parameters:

1. To the extent that they contain frequency components above 100 Hz, all ECG waveforms, including QRS proper and the late potentials "tail," will be of smaller amplitude; likewise, background "noise" is likely to be of smaller amplitude.

2. The RMS40 is likely to be smaller, leading to the possibility of false-positive diagnosis when the late potentials region contains many high-frequency spikes.

3. However, when the exclusion of high frequencies significantly alters the apparent time of QRS termination, the opposite may actually occur—that is, the LAS40 is likely to be longer, also leading to possible false-positive diagnosis, especially in the situation in which the sharp spike within the trailing edge of the QRS complex proper is attenuated to below 40 μV, thereby substantially changing the calculated value of LAS40.

Despite the differences in measured parameters, there was not a single example of a patient who had a convincing low-amplitude "tail" on real-time recording who did not also have an equally convincing "tail" on the Holter study. The study suggested that a minor modification to the RMS40 and LAS40 diagnostic criteria, appropriate to a signal bandwidth of 0.1 to 100 Hz, may result in even better diagnostic accuracy.

QUANTITATIVE ANALYSIS OF TIME-DOMAIN SIGNAL-AVERAGED ELECTROCARDIOGRAMS

Late potentials in the time-domain SAECG were initially identified visually. Later, computer algorithms have been used for quantitative analysis. In an attempt to standardize the measurement of late potentials, Simson[9] combined the signals from three orthogonal XYZ leads into a vector magnitude waveform. The latter was defined as

$$\sqrt{X^2 + Y^2 + Z^2}$$

This facilitated the measurement of some empirically defined parameters from the terminal QRS and late potential signals. However, Lander and associates[37] have pointed out some limitations of the vector magnitude formula that uses absolute values of the signal and noise in the three leads in the calculations, and not the relative values used to express the S/N ratio. There are two situations in which the presence of late potentials may not be recognized from the vector magnitude signal. The first is that of small signals present in one or more leads, but accompanied by a significant amount of residual noise in any lead. Late potentials will not be detected if the threshold value of the vector magnitude S/N ratio is not reached (Fig. 19–9). The second situation occurs when large signals accompanied by residual noise exceed the adopted threshold voltage value and hence may not be considered significant.

Computer algorithms for quantitative analysis of the time-domain SAECG depend on identification of the onset and offset of the QRS complex. The algorithm for the offset of the QRS complex depends on the S/N ratio. For example, in the algorithm described by Simson,[9] the mean noise level is found by averaging the values in 5-ms windows at the end of the signal-averaged window. Shifting the window backward in time, late potential activity is detected when the level of the waveform rises above the noise level by 3.5 standard deviations. This approach has the advantage

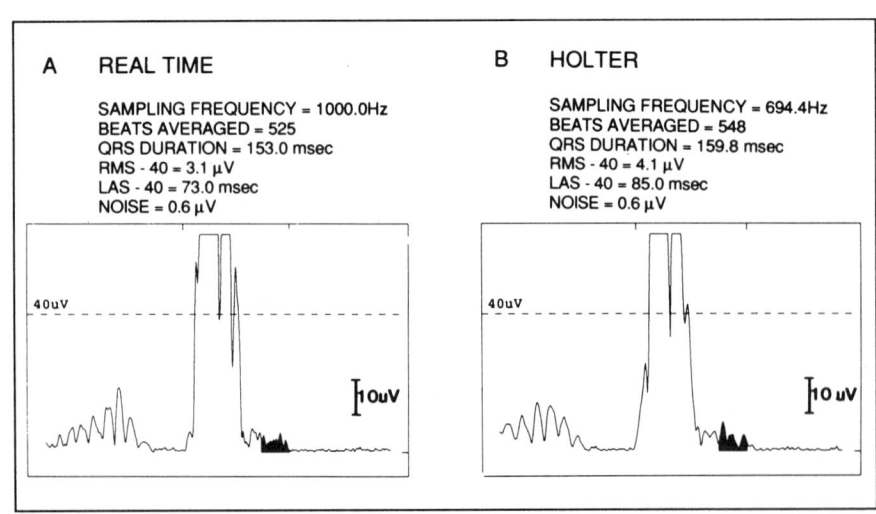

FIGURE 19–8
Vector sum plots of the signal-averaged electrocardiogram from real-time (A) and Holter (B) recordings from a subject with late potentials. The shaded areas are of 40-ms duration. Note close morphology and numerical correlation between the two plots. (See Fig. 19–6 for abbreviations.) (Reprinted with permission from Kelen G, et al.: Am J Cardiol 63:1321, 1989.)

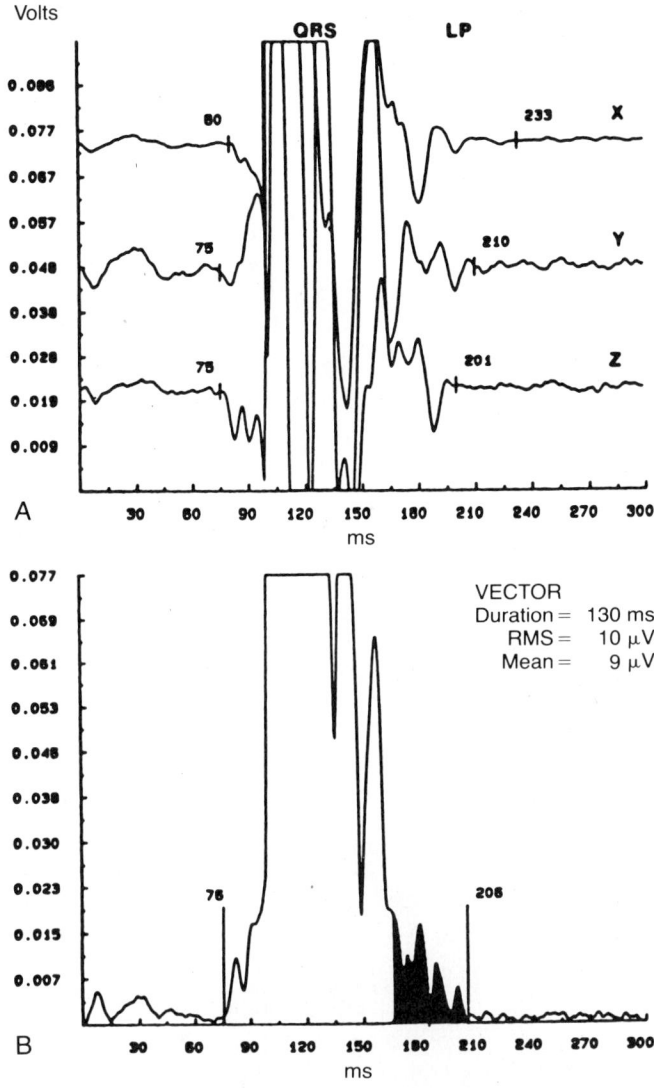

FIGURE 19–9
Signal-averaged and bandpass filtered XYZ leads *(A)* and the vector magnitude waveform *(B)* from a patient with late potentials. The duration of late potentials in the vector magnitude is underestimated, compared with lead X. The magnitude of late potentials is overestimated, due to the noise contributed by leads Y and Z. RMS = root mean square voltage. (Reprinted with permission from Lander P, et al.: IEEE Trans Biomed Eng 35:629, 1988.)

of applying the same set of quantitative parameters to the SAECG of all subjects. The disadvantage is that most of these parameters become exquisitely sensitive to the mean noise level achieved after signal averaging. Furthermore, the distribution of the S/N ratio on the body torso may not be uniform, and the quantitative parameters may vary with the lead system.[38]

Henkin and coworkers[39] used identical averaged data files to identify discordances due solely to differences in analysis algorithms used for QRS offset determination by three commercial devices. There was no significant difference between devices when QRSD and LAS40 measurements were compared, but RMS40 was significantly different. RMS40 discrepancies among the three devices amounted to 23% of the entire group and 46% of all discordancies. Although the difference between the morphologies of the vector magnitude was negligible, wide variation in the numerical values was evident. The RMS40 was the most sensitive of the numerical parameters to device idiosyncrasies (Fig. 19–10). At the sampling interval commonly used of 1000 Hz, each real data point is 1 ms from the next. A QRS offset defined by different noise algorithms may range over only a few milliseconds, yet translate into significantly different values for RMS40.

The commonly utilized quantitative parameters for scoring the time-domain SAECG, as defined previously, are the QRSD, LAS40, RMS40, and RMSQRS. Numerical values for normal SAECG parameters have usually been described based on comparative analysis of data derived from subjects with or without spontaneous or inducible VT. Recently, a study to establish normal values of SAECG parameters at different high-pass filter settings in 100 normal subjects was reported by Caref and coworkers.[31] QRSD and LAS40 were found to have normal distribution at all filter settings, and their normal values could be described at the 95% confidence limit. This was not the case for RMS40, which had a distribution significantly different from the expected normal values between 20 and 70 Hz. Normal values for RMS40 were obtained by first transforming the RMS40 data into its natural logarithm, which was found to be normally distributed. Cutoff values based on the mean −2 standard deviations were calculated and then exponentiated to allow for easier use in the clinical setting (Fig. 19–11). The lack of a normal distribution of RMS40 was most probably responsible for the need to resort to empirical selection of normal values both at 25 Hz by Simson[9] and at 40 Hz by Denes and coworkers.[40] In another study of a small group of normal subjects by Gomes and colleagues,[30] statistically valid techniques could not be applied to select normal values for RMS40. It is interesting that the normal value for RMS40 at 25 Hz of 25 μV was similar to that selected empirically by Simson.[9] This value had been commonly adopted by other investigators.

In the study by Caref and colleagues,[31] normal values were used in a systematic approach to optimize the accuracy of the SAECG to predict the results of programmed stimulation in patients with spontaneous nonsustained VT. Three SAECG parameters (QRSD, LAS40, and RMS40) at each high-pass filter were categorized as normal or abnormal and were evaluated singly or as a combination of two or three. The study found that in general SAECG parameters—whether analyzed singly or in combination—have higher specificity than sensitivity for the prediction of induced sustained monomorphic VT. The best total predictive accuracy of a single SAECG parameter was 85%, provided by RMS40 at 40 or 60 Hz. The predictive accuracy of the SAECG could be improved to 89% by the use of one of 32 different combinations. The top combinations were mostly in triplets and included RMS40 and LAS40, but not QRSD recorded at different high-pass filter settings. The only two paired com-

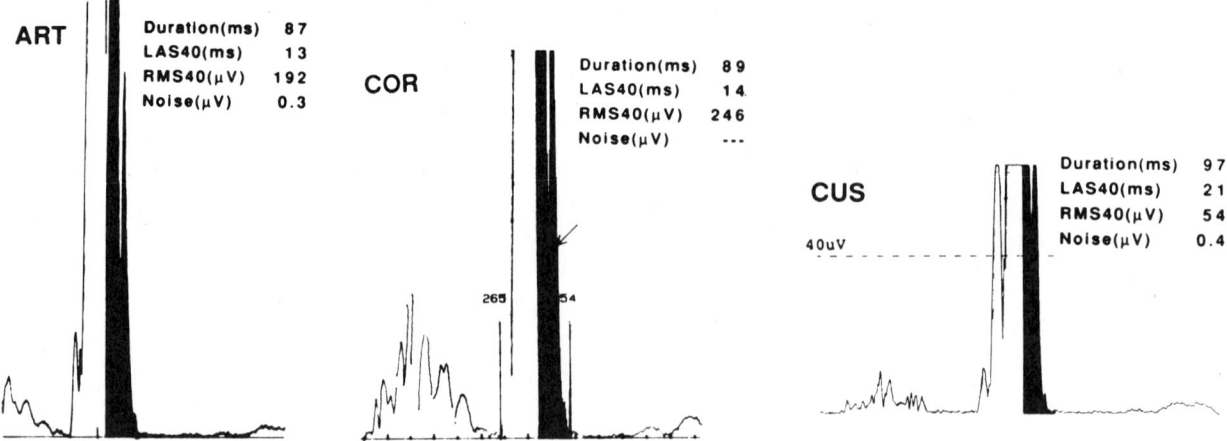

FIGURE 19–10
A composite of three vector magnitudes analyzed from an identical data file by the Arrhythmia Research Technology 1200 EPX (ART), the Corazonix Predictor (COR) and custom-designed, real-time version of the Del Mar Avionics Micropotential Analysis package for signal averaging directly from Holter tapes (CUS). Note the significant differences especially between the RMS40 values. This is due in part to the different algorithms used for the definition of QRS offset based on the calculation of baseline noise. (See Fig. 19–6 for abbreviations.) (Reprinted with permission from Henkin R, et al.: J Electrocardiol 22(Suppl 1):19, 1990.)

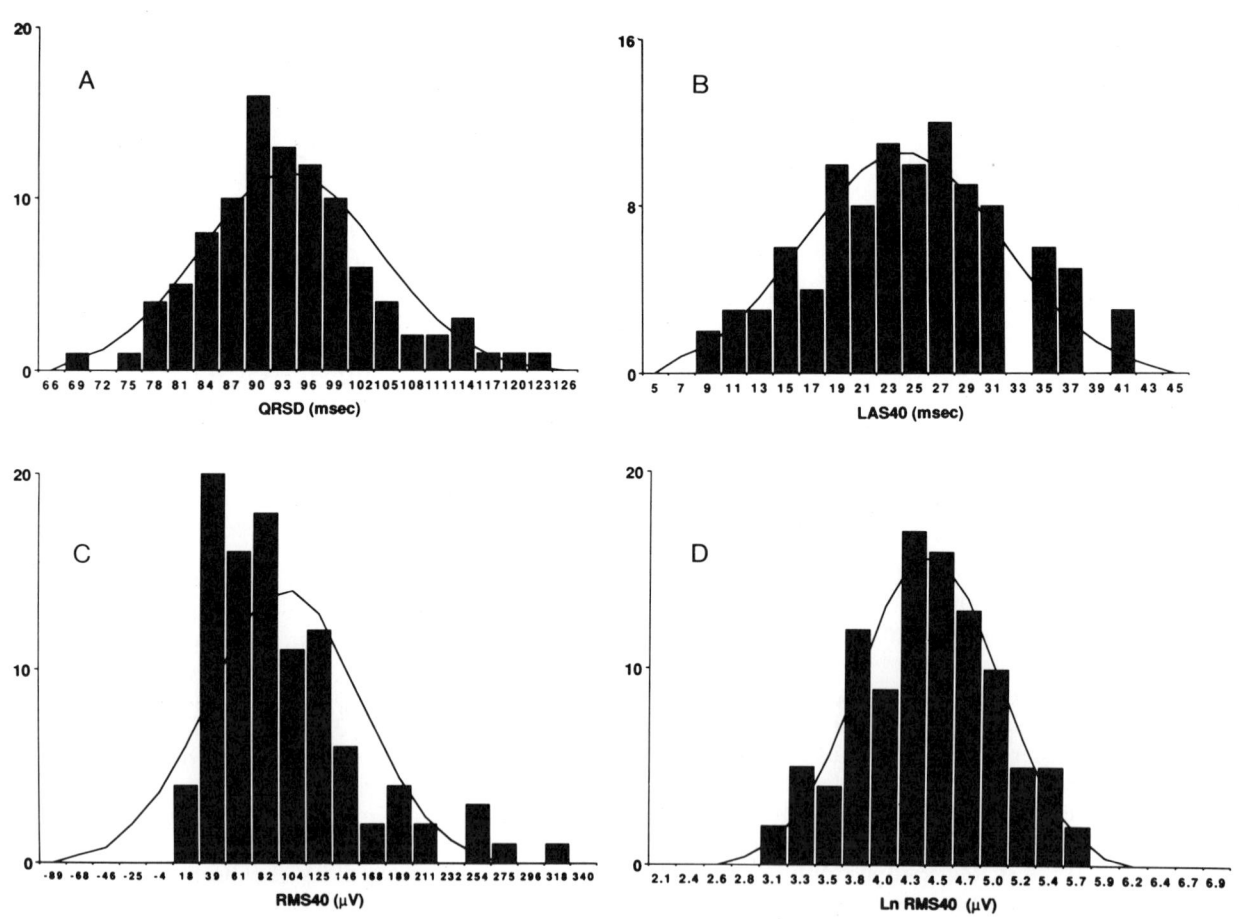

FIGURE 19–11
Histograms showing the distribution of signal-averaged electrocardiogram (SAECG) parameters from 100 normal subjects at 40 Hz, with overlaid, bell-shaped curves representing their expected normal distribution. A, Normal distribution for filtered QRS duration (QRSD). B, Similar results for duration of low amplitude signals < 40 μV (LAS40). C, The distribution of the root mean square voltage of the last 40 ms (RMS40) is significantly different from normal ($p < 0.002$). D, The transformation of each value of RMS40 into its natural logarithm (Ln RMS40) results in normal distribution. (Reprinted with permission from Caref EB, et al.: Am J Cardiol 64:16, 1989.)

binations with the best total predictive accuracy were RMS40 at 20 and 25 Hz paired with RMS40 at 40 Hz. The absence of QRS duration in any of the 32 top combinations was most probably related to the criteria for selection of patients into the study. Because the study excluded patients with a bundle branch block pattern, it may have unfairly restricted the representation of filtered QRS duration as a predictive criterion. The difference between a left bundle branch block pattern and an intraventricular conduction defect in a standard ECG can be subtle, and the decision to exclude some of these patients from the study based on a QRS duration greater than 120 ms in a standard ECG was empirical. The criteria for an abnormal SAECG in the presence of a left bundle branch block, intraventricular conduction defect, or both have not been definitely established[41,42] and continue to represent a limitation of time-domain analysis of the SAECG.

Besides enhancing the predictive accuracy of the SAECG, the study provided an insight into the most optimal high-pass filter settings. The frequencies at both ends of the analyzed high-pass filter settings (<20 Hz and >60 Hz) were not represented in the top predictive combinations. This argues for a narrower useful frequency range. High noise levels at high-pass filter settings greater than 20 Hz could be attributed to the failure of these filter settings to amply suppress skeletal muscle myopotentials, with the result that late potentials could be easily masked. On the other hand, it is possible that at higher bandpass frequencies, some late potentials could be filtered out and therefore may not be detected by the SAECG (see Fig. 19–8). The SAECG parameters analyzed at 40 Hz were represented more frequently in the top predictive combinations. This suggests that the SAECG may have the best total predictive accuracy at this filter setting and agrees with previous observations of Denes and coworkers.[40] Nevertheless, a combination of two or three SAECG parameters at more than one filter setting has a higher predictive accuracy than any single or combined parameter at 40 Hz.

Another interesting observation in the above study was the finding that the best total predictive accuracy of the SAECG for the results of programmed stimulation in patients with nonsustained VT was as high as 89%. Simson[43] recently analyzed various SAECG parameters at high-pass filter settings of 25 and 40 Hz in postinfarction patients with spontaneous monomorphic sustained VT who also were inducible at programmed stimulation; he found a best total predictive accuracy of 89%. These observations may argue that the fixed anatomic or electrophysiologic substrate responsible for an abnormal SAECG during sinus rhythm is similar in patients with inducible sustained monomorphic VT, whether they manifest with spontaneous nonsustained or sustained VT. However, the electrophysiologic factor(s) responsible for the expression of a reentrant substrate as spontaneous nonsustained or sustained VT is (or are) not definitely established at present.

Frequency-Domain Analysis of the Signal-Averaged Electrocardiogram

Cain and associates[33,34] introduced spectral analysis of the SAECG to take advantage of the possibility that late potentials may have different spectral characteristics (i.e., high-frequency components, compared with the QRS and ST segment waveforms. FFTA was used to quantitate late potential activity. This technique is a powerful computer-based mathematical algorithm that can determine the amplitudes and frequencies of the various harmonic components of a complex periodic signal such as the ECG. Frequency-domain analysis of the SAECG can avoid some of the inherent limitations of time-domain analysis, such as the need for exact localization of the signal and for bandpass filtering. The latter results in an unavoidable distortion of the signal. Cain and coworkers[33,34] and Lindsay and colleagues[44] advocated the use of the area ratio of the terminal QRS and ST segment to differentiate normal subjects or patients without a history of VT from those with a history of sustained VT. The area ratio was expressed as the area under the curve for frequencies between 20 Hz and 50 Hz divided by the area under the curve for frequencies between 0 and 20 Hz. An area ratio of less than 20 was considered normal. These results, however, could not be confirmed by other investigators.[45-47] One disadvantage of the technique is that the onset (terminal 40 ms of the QRS) and the offset (start of the T wave) of the analyzed signal were usually visually identified and marked with a computer graphic censor.[33,34] Kelen and coworkers[45] have shown that the technique is sensitive to slight changes in the duration and position of the analyzed segment (Figs. 19–12 and 19–13). In subjects with, as well as without, late potentials, area ratios increase as analyzed segment length decreases. A very small change in analyzed segment length of the order of 10 ms may change the area ratio by several hundred per cent, sufficient to cross any suggested boundary of normalcy[33,34,44] in either direction (Fig. 19–14).

Although referred to as a fast Fourier transform, the technique implemented on digitized sampled data is more correctly referred to as a discrete Fourier transform.[48] Albeit the mathematical algorithm used is the same as for a fast Fourier transform, the operation that is in fact performed is the calculation of the relative proportions of exact multiples (harmonics) of the fundamental frequency corresponding to the length of the analyzed sample that combine to make up the signal. This restriction to exact multiples of the fundamental frequency represented by the length of the sampled signal gives rise to the phenomenon of spectral leakage, wherein the spectra are distorted if the signal is not continuous at its boundaries.[49] That is, the technique assumes that the signal analyzed is repetitive and that the last data point would be immediately followed by another repetition of the same data sequence, which is

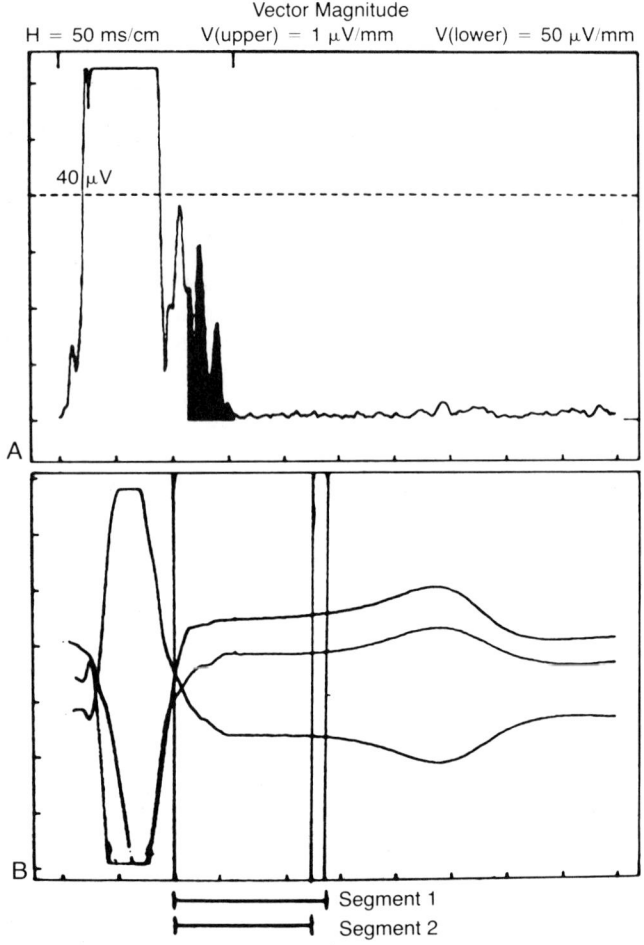

FIGURE 19–12
Signal-averaged electrocardiogram (SAECG) in the time domain from a 57-year-old man with anterior wall myocardial infarction and recurrent ventricular tachycardia. A, Vector magnitude; B, the X, Y, and Z leads. Note the presence of late potentials (the RMS40 is highlighted). (See Fig. 19–6 for abbreviations.) (Reprinted with permission from Kelen G, et al.: Am J Cardiol 60:1282, 1987.)

is precisely the case in the present application, in which the length of the hump representing the signal to be analyzed dominates the contribution to the overall frequency spectrum. Such an effect could in theory be overcome by performing an FFTA of the same (variable) number of data points to be analyzed, but it would be computationally much more difficult (FFTA is usually performed on powers of 2) and it would provide inadequate frequency resolution to be useful. Multiplication by the hump-shaped windows has a further highly undesirable effect in the case of late potentials. The latter, if present, occur predominantly in the very early part of the segment analyzed near the end of the QRS complex. This is precisely where the hump-shaped window attenuates (near its edges), tending thereby to mask the contribution of late potentials should they be present.

Spectro-Temporal Analysis of the Signal-Averaged Electrocardiogram

Because of limitations of traditional FFTA techniques, our group as well as a few other investigators[35, 50, 51] explored a novel technique to record a time-varying spectrum utilizing the running Fourier transform technique. The rationale for this technique is the observation that the QRS, late potentials, and ST segment waveforms in the SAECG have different spectral characteristics or, in other words, that the ECG signal has a time-varying spectrum. When analyzing late potentials, the duration of the analyzed segment should be optimally increased to get higher spectral resolution. However, this means including QRS and/or ST segment samples as well as the late potential waveform in the time period for spectral analysis. The attempt to measure this time-varying spectrum results in the power-density spectrum obtained being an average of all the spectra that exist within the analyzed segment. A spectro-temporal map is obtained by placing a short-time window of duration T, at the start of the signal, computing a power density spectrum, and plotting it on the time axis. The window is then shifted in time by a small amount (t), and another spectrum is computed and plotted. This procedure is repeated throughout the time period of interest. As the duration of T is increased, the resolution of changes in the temporal energy of the signal is decreased, but the spectral resolution of each spectral slice is increased. The choice of t affects only the temporal resolution of the spectro-temporal map.

Examples of time-domain SAECG and corresponding spectro-temporal maps, or spectrocardiograms, are shown in Figures 19–15 through 19–18. The durations of T and t were 24 and 2 ms, respectively. The spectrocardiogram is a three-dimensional frequency plot, since it represents the relative contributions of signals of differing frequencies to the ECG waveform throughout the cardiac cycle. For descriptive and orientation purposes, it is convenient to think of the

clearly not the case in this application. Kelen and colleagues[45] have shown that when FFTA is applied to a mathematically synthesized signal consisting of pure sine waves of different frequencies, the results are markedly influenced by both the duration and the phase of the analyzed segment.

To minimize the effect of discontinuity at the signal boundaries and spectral leakage, it is common practice in scientific applications to multiply the data by a "window" that smoothly attenuates the signal near the boundaries. However, to achieve the intended result of the performed FFTA, the sampled data and the length of the window should all be the same number of points; otherwise, the "hump-shaped" window itself represents a distortion of the analyzed signal.[48, 49] This

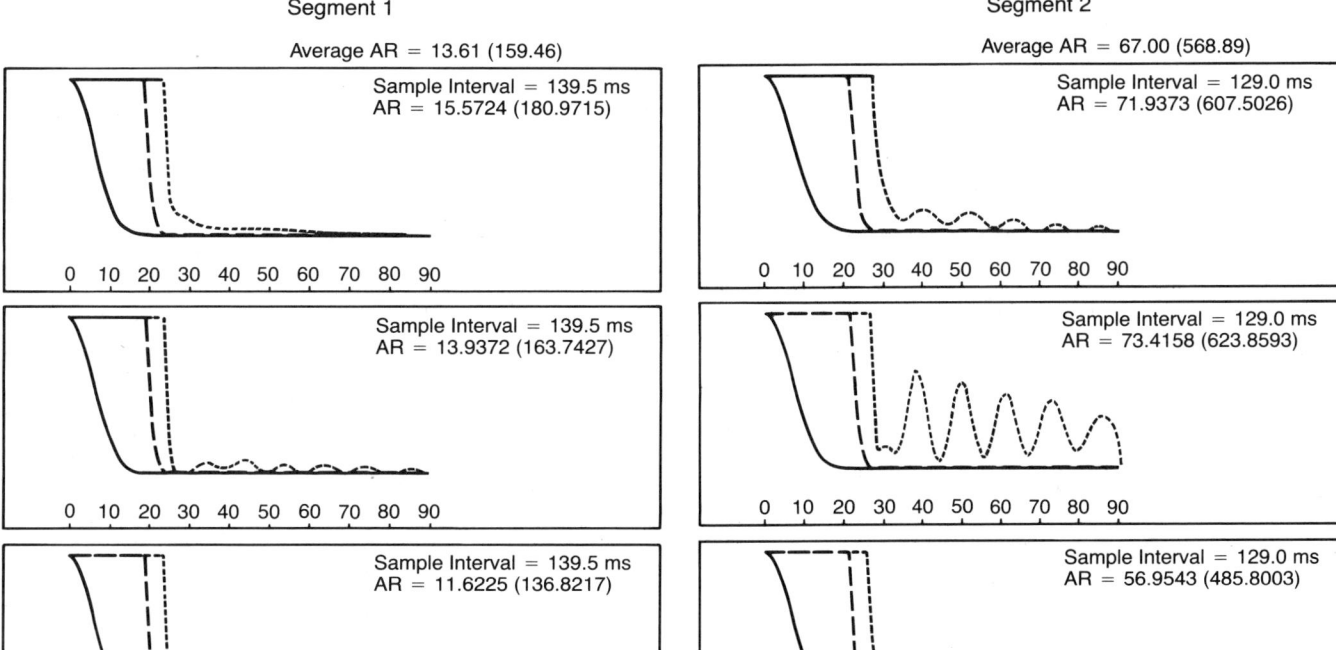

FIGURE 19–13
Fast Fourier transform (FFT) analysis from the same patient shown in Figure 19–12. The FFT plots of the two segments outlined in Figure 19–12 are shown. Segment 1 comprised the last 40 ms of the QRS and the ST segment up to what was visually considered to be the onset of the T wave. Segment 2 was 10.5 ms shorter in duration compared with segment 1 and was obtained by moving the rightward cursor to the left. Note that the ratio of the area under the spectral curve between 20 and 50 Hz divided by the area between 0 and 20 Hz is markedly different in the two segments. (Reprinted with permission from Kelen G, et al.: Am J Cardiol 60:1282, 1987.)

spectrocardiogram plots as views of a mountain range composed of stacked vertical slices, arising from a plain, with the observer looking obliquely downward from above. The spectrocardiogram can be displayed in different views. In Figure 19–16A, the mountain range (and the time axis) runs from top right to bottom left, with the P wave to the top right and the T wave to the bottom left. Frequency increases linearly from left to right, whereas the height of the range at each point represents the relative power at each frequency and each point in time during the QRS complex. This view is called the "oblique T view." In Figure 19–16B, the same data is viewed with the mountain range (i.e., time axis) running from left to right with the P wave to the left, the T wave to the right, and the lowest frequencies farthest from the highest frequencies closest to the observer. This view is referred to as the "horizontal view." Figure 19–16C shows the range running from top to bottom with the P wave farthest from and the T wave closest to the observer, whereas frequency increases from left to right. This presentation is referred to as the "solid vertical T view." In all views thus far, each slice is opaque and may hide features in slices behind (i.e., situated farther away) from the observer. In Figure 19–16D, which is called the "wire frame vertical T view" and is identical in orientation and data content to Figure 19–16C, the slices are transparent, so that features buried deep

FIGURE 19–14
Effects of the duration of the analyzed segment on the area ratio of spectral energy between 20 and 50 Hz and 0 and 20 Hz of the FFT plot of the signal-averaged electrocardiogram (SAECG) from 10 normal subjects and 10 patients with ventricular tachycardia (VT). The mean area ratio was calculated for 10 segments. The figure shows that area ratios increase as segment length decreases. (Reprinted with permission from Kelen G, et al.: Am J Cardiol 60:1282, 1987).

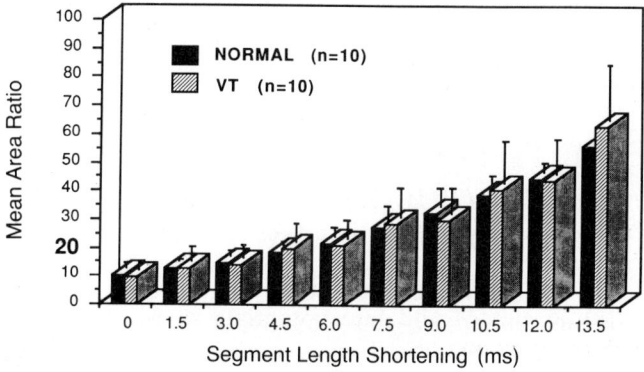

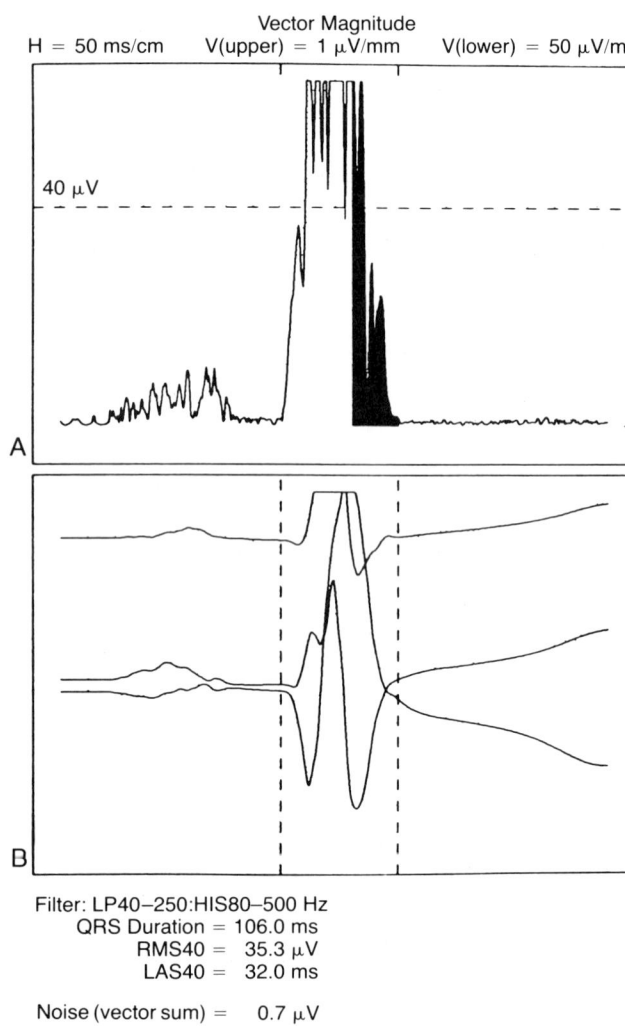

FIGURE 19–15
The time-domain signal-averaged electrocardiogram (SAECG) from a normal subject that shows no late potentials. A, Vector magnitude; B, the X, Y, and Z leads. (See Fig. 19–6 for abbreviations.)

within the mountain range or behind a larger feature are still visible. However, it may be impossible to identify a feature using a particular slice because of the complexity of intersecting lines.

The spectrocardiograms in Figure 19–16 were obtained from a normal subject whose time-domain SAECG (Fig. 19–15) showed no late potentials. The spectrocardiograms show no particular features in the late QRS/early ST periods. In contrast, the spectrocardiograms in Figure 19–18 were obtained from a post–myocardial infarction patient who had spontaneous inducible sustained VT. The time-domain SAECG showed late potentials (Fig. 19–17). The spectrocardiograms show significant spectro-temporal energy in the late QRS/early ST segment. The most optimal methods for quantitative analysis of the spectrocardiogram have yet to be defined.

Beat-To-Beat Recording of the High-Resolution Electrocardiography

There are two major limitations for recording the His-Purkinje signals and late potentials by the temporal averaging technique.[52, 53]

1. It will not be able to detect dynamic (beat-to-beat) changes in the signal during sinus rhythm.
2. The SAECG cannot be recorded during complex cardiac arrhythmias.

The clinical advantage of identifying the His-Purkinje signals on a beat-to-beat basis is obvious when there is a dynamic change of the temporal relation between the atrial and ventricular potentials. On the other hand, late potentials may vary from beat to beat. Electrophysiologic observations in the canine post-infarction model of reentry suggest that spontaneous reentrant arrhythmias may be associated with a Wenckebach-like conduction pattern in a potentially reentrant pathway.[54–58] Recording of late potentials on a beat-to-beat basis has the potential of directly identifying reentrant "malignant" versus focal "benign" ventricular rhythms.[52, 53] Several investigators have utilized different techniques to reduce the S/N ratio and to record His-Purkinje potentials or late potentials on a beat-to-beat basis.[52, 59–66]

To enhance the S/N ratio in a beat-to-beat recording, a spatial-averaging technique is frequently employed. In this technique, potentials recorded from multiple pairs of electrodes are averaged. The averaging reinforces the identical signals and attenuates the uncor-

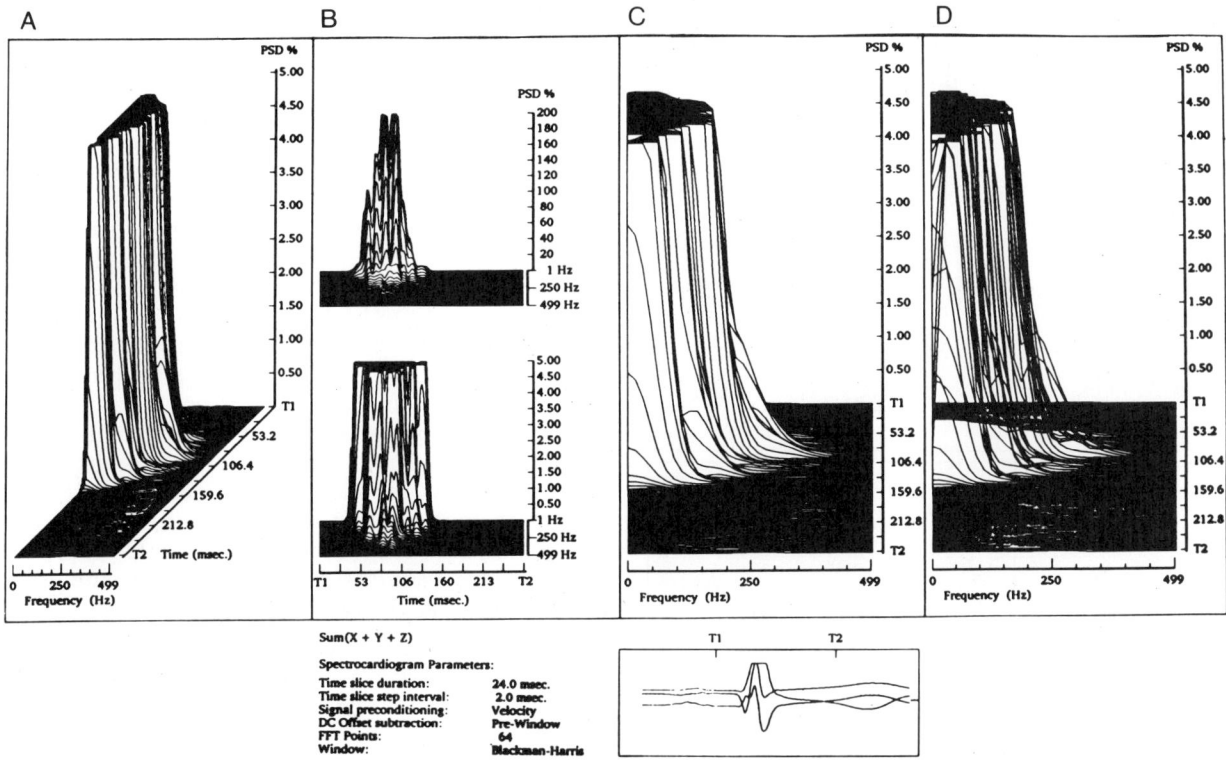

FIGURE 19–16
The spectro-temporal plots (spectrocardiograms) of the same subject shown in Figure 19–15. See text for details.

related potentials. If the distance between pairs of surface electrodes is small, the EMG noise as well as the ECG signal from each pair would be correlated and spatial averaging would not enhance the S/N ratio. However, since the EMG potential source consists of multiple muscle units distributed proximal to the skin surface, and because the ECG biogenerator is more distal to the recording electrodes, increasing the distance between the pairs of electrodes should improve the S/N ratio, as the EMG signal would be less correlated compared with the ECG potential.

Measurements of the coherence function of the EMG potentials during the ECG isoelectric interval from two pairs of surface leads has shown that the coherence function for the EMG potentials can be low and be almost unity for ECG signals.[5] The technique, therefore, has the potential to accentuate ECG and reduce EMG signals and was, in fact, first used to reduce noise in exercise electrocardiography.[67] However, the improvement in ECG signal/EMG noise depends primarily on the distance between electrode pairs and their position on the chest surface. In a study by Mehra et al.[68] it was found that significant improvement in the ratio of ECG signal to EMG noise can be obtained by spacing electrode pairs 6 inches apart.[3] A somewhat closer interelectrode distance (2–4 inches) may be more practical, given the constraints of the number of electrodes that could be spatially averaged and, at the same time, maintain similar vectorial orientation of each electrode in reference to the ECG signal.

The resolution of spatial averaging is limited by the size of the torso, the perimeters of the positive and negative fields on the chest, and the size of electrodes. Therefore, additional measures to improve the S/N ratio have been suggested. Shvartsman and associates[69] utilized a digital logic circuit that examines instantaneous polarity from each of the parallel input signals. The system would enhance signals with identical polarities and suppress those with nonidentical polarities. Although this technique can reduce electrode and amplifier noise, it will be less helpful in reducing synchronous EMG potentials from closely spaced electrodes.

Mehra and coworkers[68] have shown that an improvement in the ratio of ECG signal to EMG noise can be obtained by recording signals not from the precordial surface but a certain distance away from it with the help of a volume conductor electrode. When an electrode is placed directly on the chest surface, the potential recorded can be expressed by the solid angle model. It is directly proportional to the product of the potential difference of the activating biogenerator, the solid angle subtended by it, and a constant incorporating the conductivity of the medium. It is evident that if other variables do not change and if the electrodes are moved distal to the chest surface with a conducting medium in between, the reduction in the solid angle of the cardiac biogenerator will be less than for the EMG biogenerator. This is so because the ECG biogenerator is more distal to the skin surface than the EMG biogenerator. Hence, an improvement in the S/N ratio would occur even though both signals undergo attenuation. The concept of the volume con-

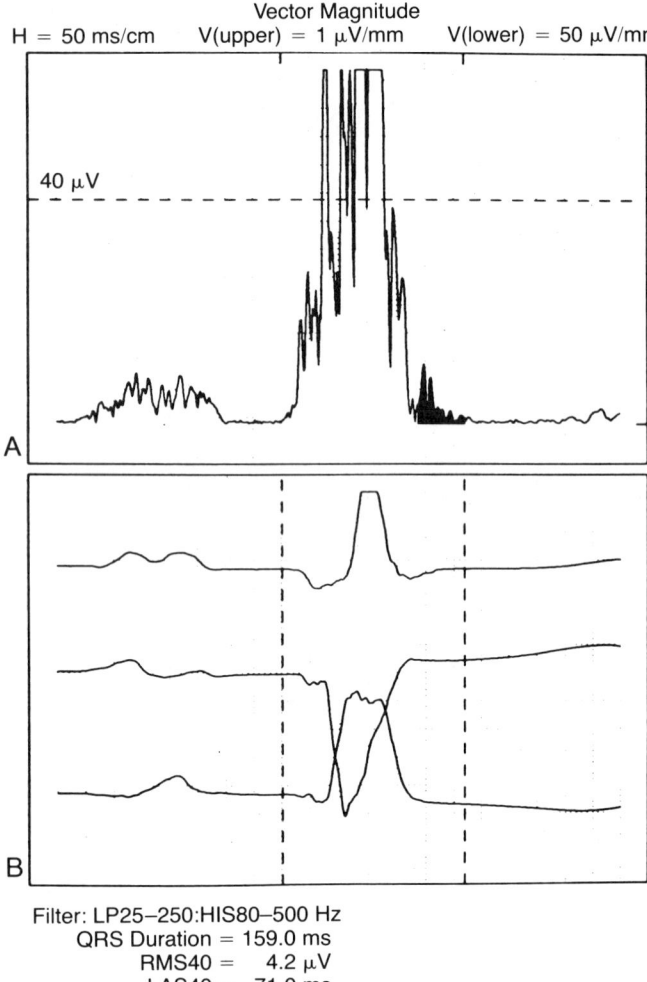

FIGURE 19–17
The time-domain signal-averaged electrocardiogram (SAECG) from a patient with sustained VT showing late potentials. *A*, Vector magnitude; *B*, the X, Y, and Z leads.

ductor electrode was tested experimentally and the electrode was shown to result in significant reduction of EMG noise as compared to the ECG signal[68] (Fig. 19–19). Figures 19–20 and 19–21 illustrate, respectively, beat-to-beat recording of the His-Purkinje potential and late potentials with use of a volume conductor electrode.

Electrophysiologic Substrate of Late Potentials

The origin of late potentials is believed to be myocardial zones with depressed electrophysiologic properties that may provide the substrate for reentrant excitation. Delayed activation potentials were initially described from the ischemic regions of the canine heart.[54–57, 70, 71] The relation between delayed ventricular activation in ischemic myocardial zones and ventricular arrhythmias based on a circus movement of excitation in the post-infarction heart has been extensively investigated.[58, 72–75] Several investigators have shown that late potentials appear to correspond to delayed and fragmented activation, which has been observed in epicardial and endocardial electrograms recorded in animals[76, 77] and in patients with ventricular tachyarrhythmias.[78]

None of these studies, however, correlated the presence of late potential recordings on the body surface with ventricular activation maps of reentrant circuits. This was investigated by Restivo and colleagues, utilizing the post-infarction canine model of reentrant excitation.[79] In this model, reentrant circuits commonly develop in the surviving ischemic epicardial layer overlying the infarction and analysis of epicardial activation usually reflects the entire reentrant circuit. Epicardial activation maps were constructed from 62 epicardial electrograms, using a computerized multiplexer system. To assess the relative contribution of electrically active regions to their detection on the body surface, a synthesized root mean square (RMS) composite electrogram was constructed by squaring the individual epicardial electrograms, adding them, and then taking the square root of the sum. This eliminates the possibility of electrogram cancellation. Body surface X, Y, and Z leads were signal-averaged, high-pass filtered, and vector summed to record an SAECG. Late potentials in the SAECG correlated in time with those in the 62 electrograms and with the synthesized composite electrogram. Although the synthesized composite electrogram showed late potentials that bridged the diastolic interval, in the SAECG 20 to 80 ms of the mid-diastolic interval sometimes failed to show late potentials. The late potential–free diastolic interval corresponded to very slow conduction of the reentrant wavefront and to electrograms greater than 0.1 mV.

Figure 19–22 illustrates the results of one of the experiments. In this experiment, a reentrant beat, V_1, was consistently induced by a single premature stimulus, S_2. A polar projection of epicardial activation of the reentrant circuit is shown on the right. Isochrones of activation are drawn at 20-ms intervals, and the arcs of functional conduction block are represented by the heavy solid lines. The XYZ vector sum of the SAECG is shown at the left in Figure 19–22. Diastolic activity is seen following the S_2 and preceding V_1. During a period of 70 ms in the mid-diastolic interval, activity was not present or was less than the noise level of the recording technique. The mid-diastolic interval corresponded in time to the slowly conducting common reentrant wavefront, as shown in the map at the right. On the other hand, continuous diastolic activity was evident in the epicardial electrograms and in the composite electrogram. The selected epicardial electrograms shown in Figure 19–22 corresponded to the interval from 160 to 230 ms, where surface activity was not detected. The electrograms in this interval were recorded from a thin (1–2 mm) surviving epicardial layer overlying the core of the infarct. Some electrograms in this area were of reasonable amplitude (>1 mV); other electrograms exhibited multiphasic electrotonic deflections and/or had low-amplitude slow deflections (<0.1 mV). These electrograms reflected very

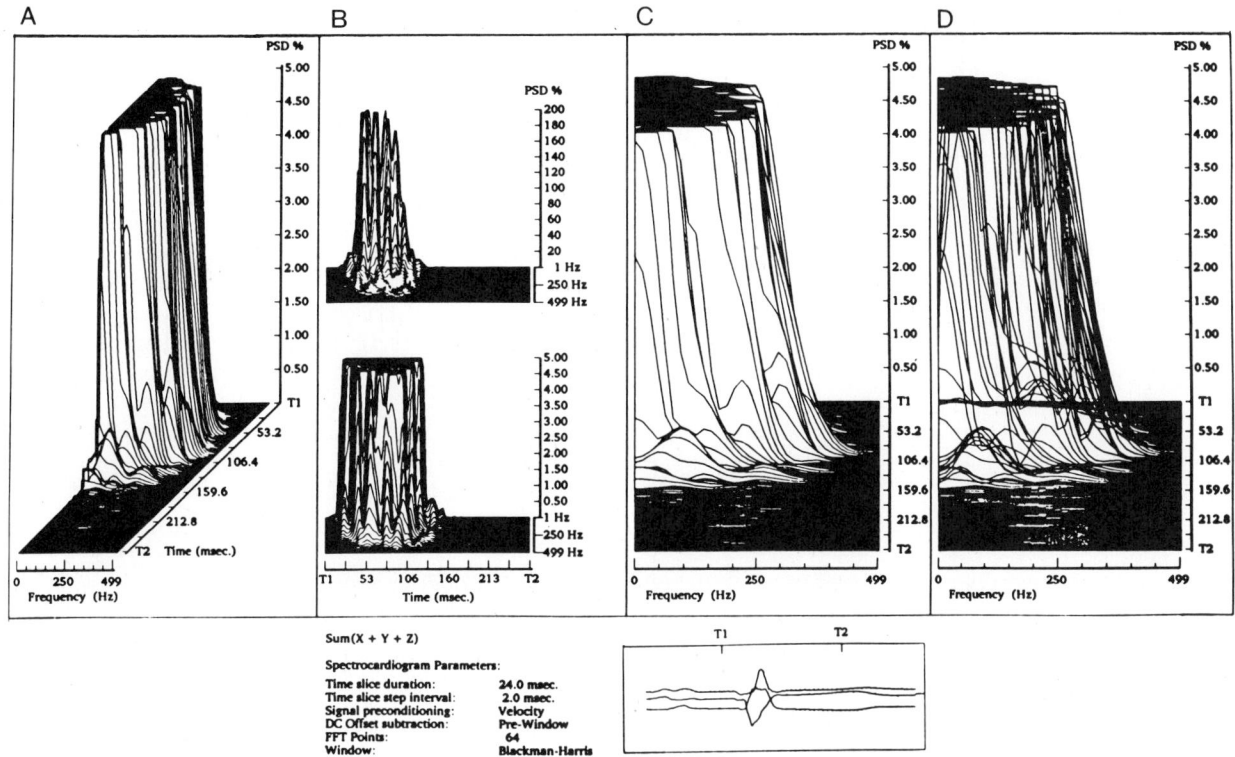

FIGURE 19–18
Spectro-temporal plots (spectrocardiograms) of the same subject shown in Figure 19–17. See text for details.

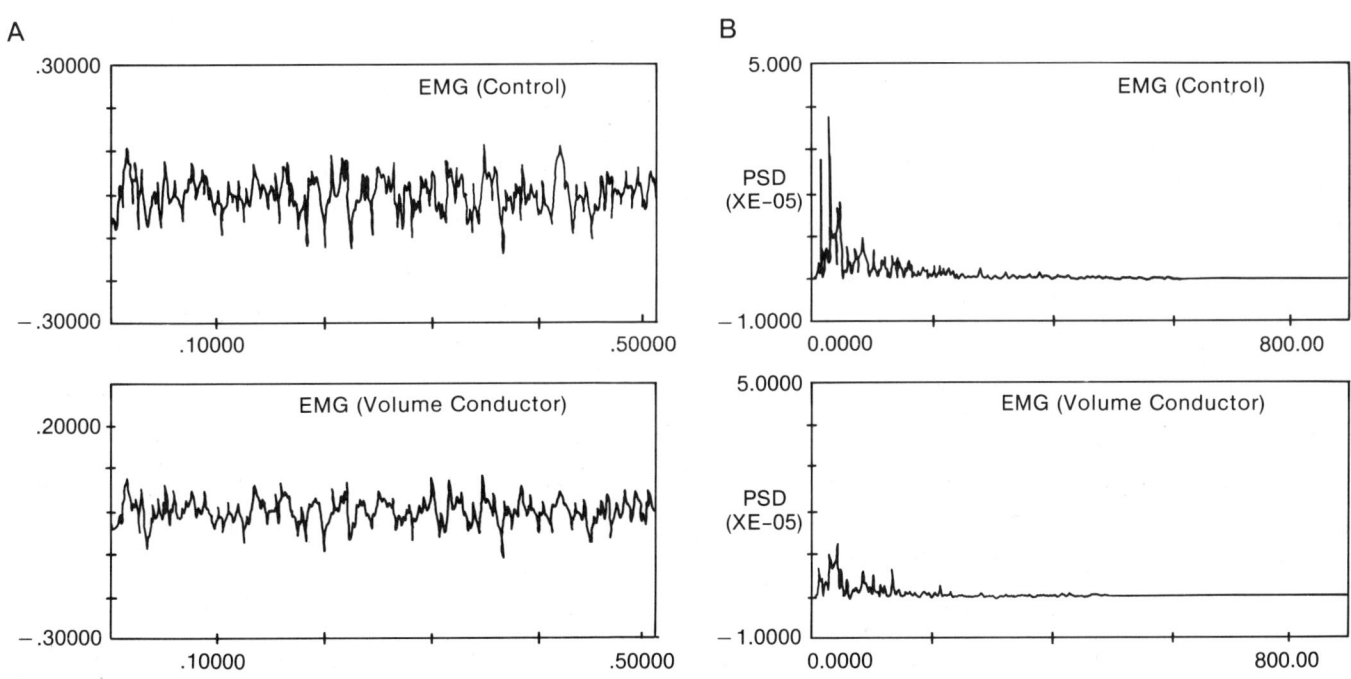

FIGURE 19–19
A, Simultaneous electromyographic potentials recorded from the skin surface with a standard ECG electrode (top) and with a "volume conductor" electrode (bottom). Note the significant reduction in electromyographic potentials with the "volume conductor" electrode. (Horizontal axis = seconds). B, The corresponding power spectral density function at frequencies up to 800 Hz (horizontal axis = hertz). (Reprinted with permission from Mehra R, et al.: Electromyographic noise reduction for high-resolution electrocardiography. In IEEE Frontiers of Engineering and Computing in Health Care, p. 298. IEEE Press, New York, 1983.)

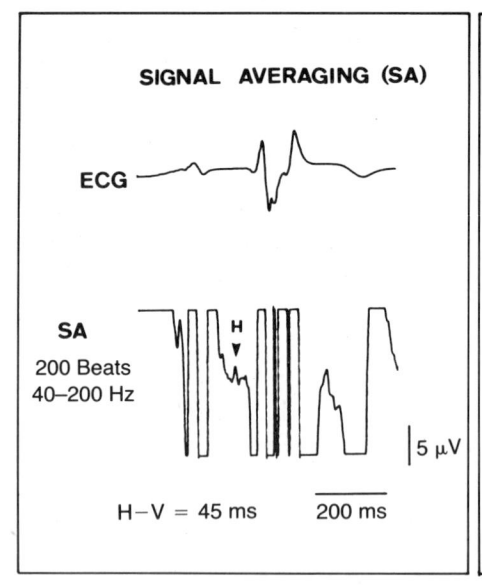
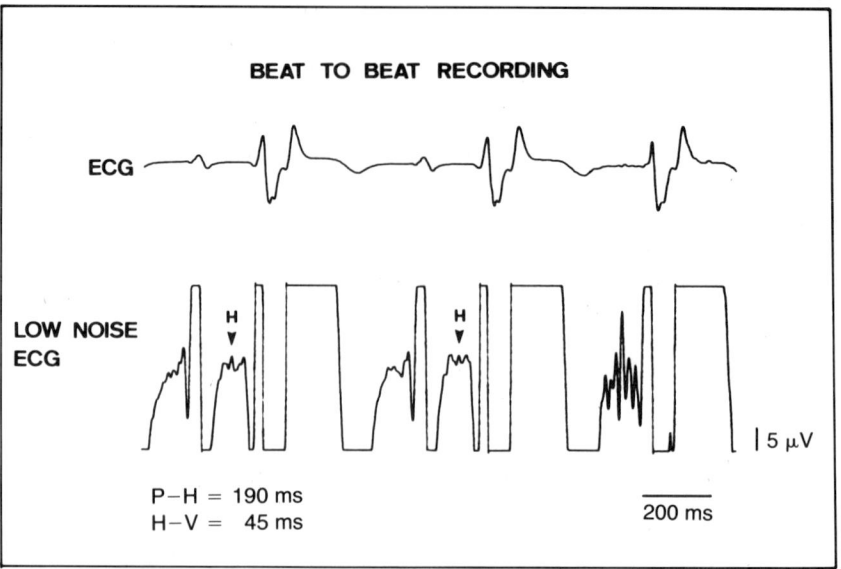

FIGURE 19–20
Beat-to-beat high-resolution electrocardiogram (ECG) using the volume conductor electrode in a 76-year-old man. The 12-lead ECG showed sinus rhythm with first-degree AV block and right bundle branch block. Signal averaging (SA) of 500 beats in the X lead (left panel) shows a discrete triphasic His bundle potential (H) with an H-V interval of 45 ms. The high-resolution ECG (right panel) reveals a remarkably similar H potential with an H-V interval of 45 ms. Of the three consecutive beat-to-beat recordings, the third is a supraventricular premature beat. The preventricular segment of this beat is obscured by potentials originating from an ectopic P wave with a short P-R interval. The possibility of electromyographic noise contributing to the preventricular potential cannot be excluded. (Reprinted with permission from El-Sherif N, et al.: J Am Coll Cardiol 1:456, 1983.)

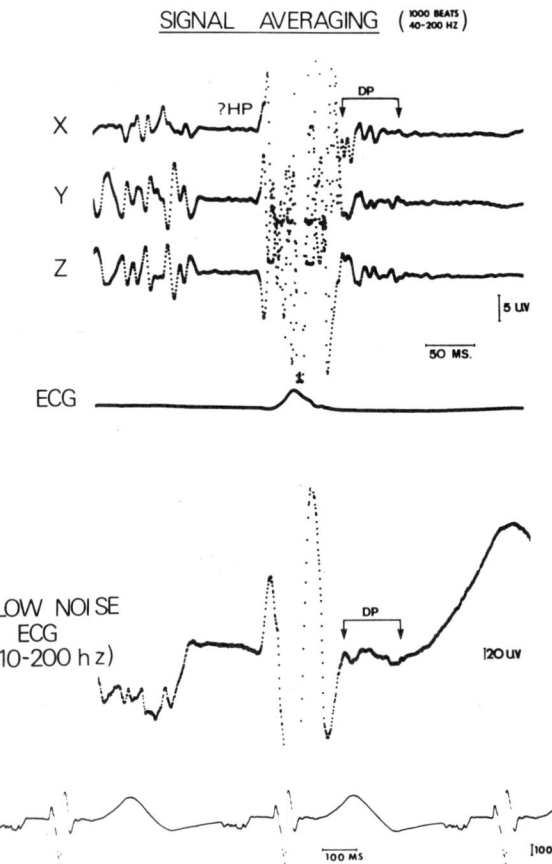

FIGURE 19–21
Beat-to-beat high-resolution electrocardiogram (ECG) in a 51-year-old man with 1-week-old inferior wall myocardial infarction. The patient had several runs of ventricular tachycardia during the first week after infarction. A, Signal averaging of sinus beats in the X, Y, and Z leads shows late diastolic potentials (DP) in the early part of the ST-T segment that extends for 150 ms from the onset of the QRS complex. B, The high-resolution beat-to-beat ECG with the same time scale as that of the signal-averaged leads shows the presence of diastolic potentials up to 25 μV in amplitude in the early part of the ST segment that correspond in duration to the diastolic potentials in the signal-averaged lead. C, A continuous recording of the high-resolution ECG is shown. The His-Purkinje potential (HP) seen in the signal-averaged recording is labeled ? because the amplitude of the signal is less than 2.5 times the average noise signal as measured from the late ST-T segment. (Reprinted with permission from El-Sherif N, et al.: J Am Coll Cardiol 1:456, 1983.)

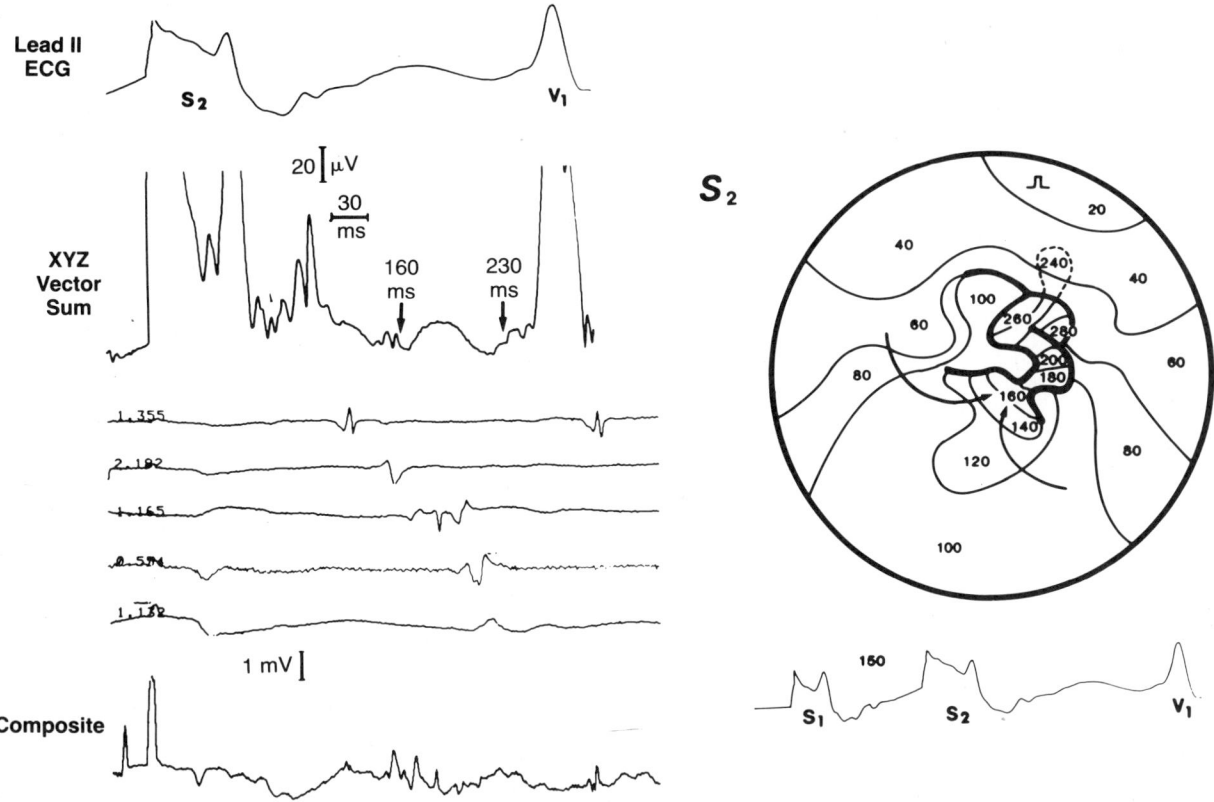

FIGURE 19-22
Recordings obtained from a 4-day-old canine post-infarction heart, showing that the electrical activity of the slowly conducting part of the reentrant circuit could not be detected as mid-diastolic potentials in the body surface signal-averaged electrocardiogram (SAECG). See text for details.

slow conduction through a narrow pathway surrounded by functionally blocked tissue. The small mass of active tissue that comprised the slowest part of the reentrant circuit was not reflected in the body surface recordings. Restivo and coworkers[79] concluded that, in this canine model, late potentials correlated with delayed epicardial activation in an area overlying the infarct. During reentrant activation, however, complete diastolic activity on the body surface may not be detected if the mass of electrically active cells is too small or if very slow conduction in part of the circuit generates low-amplitude extracellular potentials.

An important question in relation to the electrophysiologic significance of late potentials is whether regions of delayed activation during basic rhythms are the responsible arrhythmogenic substrate for reentry. The relationship between myocardial zones showing conduction delay during sinus rhythm and spontaneous or induced reentrant rhythms is complex. Reentry requires a critical balance between the length of the zone of unidirectional block and the degree of conduction delay of the circulating wavefront. The zones of unidirectional block are not represented in the SAECG, and the degree of conduction delay necessary for reentry may bear little relationship to the degree of conduction delay during sinus rhythm.

Restivo and coworkers[80] conducted a study in the canine post-infarction model of reentry to determine if regions of delayed activation during a basic rhythm (sinus rhythm or S_1-S_1 ventricular pacing) are the responsible arrhythmogenic substrate for reentry. Reentrant rhythms were induced by programmed electrical stimulation. The SAECG during basic rhythm at a cycle length of 400 to 500 ms detected late potentials, which corresponded temporally with the region of latest epicardial activation times. Subsequent signal averaging of reentrant circuits revealed that sites of late potentials during the basic rhythm were not always responsible for late potentials detected during reentrant activation. Examination of activation maps of these beats confirmed that the regions responsible for late potentials during a basic rhythm were not part of the final common reentrant pathway during reentrant activation.

Regions of marked delay, Wenckebach, or 2:1 conduction during the basic rhythm usually blocked during S_2 stimulation and did not participate in the reentrant process. This is illustrated in Figure 19-23, obtained from one of the experiments. Shown from top to bottom are the epicardial activation map, surface ECG, selected epicardial electrograms, and X, Y, and Z leads of the SAECG. Recordings on the left were obtained during basic right ventricular pacing at an S_1-S_1 cycle of 400 ms. Recordings on the right were obtained during premature stimulation (S_2) that initiated a reentrant beat (V_1). During S_1 stimulation, the most delayed epicardial activation sites were in the center of the ischemic zone, represented by epicardial

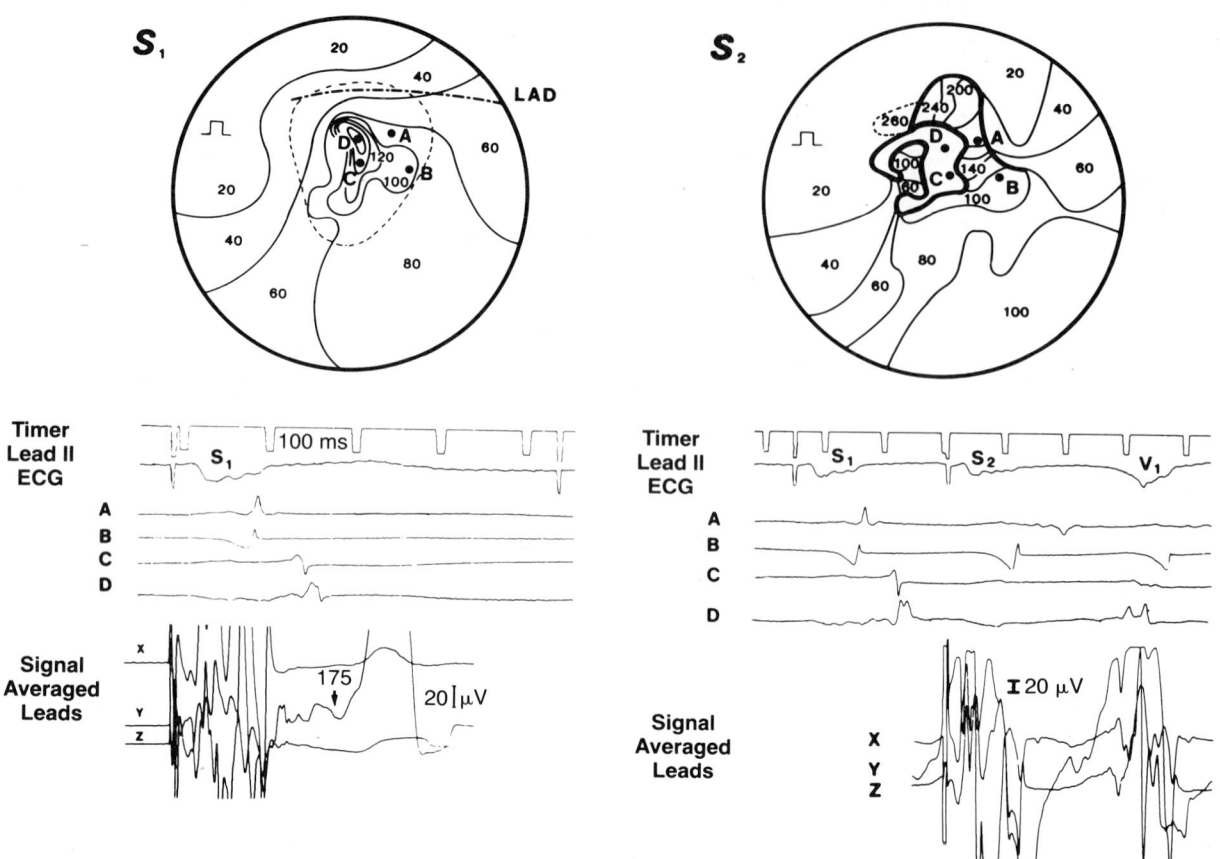

FIGURE 19–23
Recordings obtained from a 4-day-old canine post-infarction heart, showing that regions responsible for late potentials during the basic rhythm were not part of the slow common reentrant pathway during reentrant activation. See text for details.

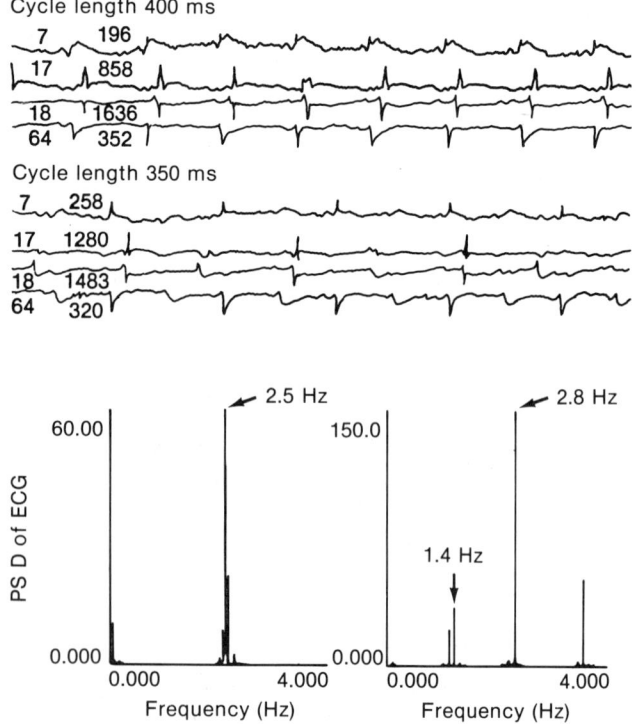

FIGURE 19–24
Time and spectral analyses of ECG signals from a 4-day-old post-infarction canine heart. A tachycardia-dependent 2:1 conduction block in some of the epicardial electrograms obtained from the ischemic epicardial zone was associated with the appearance of a subharmonic at 1.4 Hz in the spectral recording. See text for details. (Reprinted with permission from Craelius W, et al.: IEEE Trans Biomed Eng 33:1166, 1986.)

electrograms C and D. These sites were reflected by late potentials in the SAECG. However, during reentrant activation induced by S_2 stimulation, electrograms C and D showed conduction block and their sites did not participate in the reentrant circuit as shown in the activation map on the right. Mid-diastolic activity during reentry is represented by electrograms A and B. These sites contributed to the diastolic potentials during reentry but not to the late potentials during the basic rhythm.

Analysis of Periodicity of Late Potentials

Electrophysiologic observations of the post-infarction canine heart suggest that there is a close association between myocardial zones showing a Wenckebach-like conduction pattern and the development of spontaneous reentrant rhythms.[54-58] The presence of areas of 2:1 block also may prove to be a strong marker for spontaneous reentry. The rationale is as follows: Since conduction in ischemic myocardium is characteristically tachycardia-dependent,[55] it is expected that zones showing a 2:1 pattern usually will revert to a Wenckebach-like conduction pattern, and then to a 1:1 delayed conduction pattern on slowing of the heart rate. Thus, a body surface recording that is able to discern the presence of myocardial zones showing 2:1 or Wenckebach periodicity may prove to represent a better electrophysiologic marker for the propensity to develop reentrant arrhythmias, compared with a recording that primarily reflects areas of conduction delays in a 1:1 pattern. An SAECG will not be able to detect periodicity of late potentials, since the periodic absence of signals simply reduces the averaged signal. A low-noise ECG can potentially record dynamic beat-to-beat changes of late potentials. However, because of the very low amplitude of these potentials in relation to noise, a high degree of resolution of S/N ratio is required.

Craelius and coworkers[81] investigated a novel approach to detect periodicity of late potentials, using FFTA techniques. In the frequency domain, patterns that occur with any regularity, whether their period is the basic heart rate or some fraction of the heart rate, can be detected as subharmonics. An example of the Fourier analysis of the ECG is shown in Figure 19–24. The top record shows selected bipolar electrograms recorded from the epicardial surface of a 4-day-old post-infarction canine heart. The recording at a cardiac cycle length of 400 ms shows a 1:1 conduction pattern. When the cycle length was shortened to 350 ms, 2:1 conduction block developed in the ischemic epicardial zone, resulting in alternation of the electrogram configuration. The bottom of Figure 19–24 shows the power spectral densities of the surface ECG lead recorded from the post-infarction canine heart whose epicardial recordings are shown on top. The record on the left shows the spectrum of the ECG recorded during a 5-minute period at a constant cycle length of 400 ms. The spectrum has a single peak at a frequency of 2.5 Hz, as expected if a 1:1 activation pattern occurred every 400 ms. In the record on the right, the cardiac cycle length was decreased to 350 ms. A major peak occurred at 2.8 Hz, corresponding to the cardiac cycle length; however, a second peak became evident at 1.48 Hz, one half of the basic cycle length. This subharmonic is evidence of an event occurring with 2:1 periodicity induced by shortening the cardiac cycle length—most probably 2:1 conduction block in one or more ischemic epicardial zones. Further experimental and clinical studies will be required to investigate the feasibility of detecting periodicity of late potentials from spectral analysis of the ECG and its predictive value as a marker of reentrant ventricular arrhythmias.

Conclusions

In the last two decades, a number of techniques for obtaining a high-resolution ECG were investigated and were shown to be able to detect His-Purkinje and late potentials from body surface recordings. Although the retrieval rate is currently limited, the recording of the His-Purkinje potential, particularly on a beat-to-beat basis, can provide valuable clinical information. On the other hand, late potentials are proving to be a valuable marker for the propensity to develop malignant "reentrant" ventricular tachyarrhythmias, particularly in the post-infarction period. The high-resolution ECG owes a large part of its appeal to its being a relatively simple noninvasive test. However, there is an urgent need to establish standardized criteria for equipment design and methods of recording and analysis of the ECG signal in order to foster a better climate for the exchange of clinical data. Furthermore, more basic studies are needed to understand the electrophysiologic substrate of late potentials, and large-scale multicenter clinical studies are required to provide a definitive evaluation of their prognostic significance.

References

1. Berbari EJ, Scherlag BJ, Lazzara R: A computerized technique to record new components of the electrocardiogram. IEEE Trans Biomed Eng 65:799, 1977.
2. Patterson S: The electrical characteristics of some commercial ECG electrodes. J Electrocardiol 11 (1):23, 1978.
3. Tobey GE, Graeme G, Huelsman LP: Operational Amplifiers: Design and Applications, pp. 51–89. New York, NY, McGraw-Hill Book Co., 1971.
4. Schweitzer TW, Fitzgerald JW, Bowden JA, et al.: Spectral analysis of human inspiratory diaphragmatic electromyograms. J Appl Physiol 46(1):152, 1979.
5. Santipetro RF: The origin and characterization of the primary signal, noise and interference sources in the high frequency electrocardiogram. Proc IEEE 65:707, 1977.
6. Evanich MJ, Newberry O, Partridge LD: Some limitations of the removal of periodic noise by averaging. J Appl Physiol 33:536, 1972.
7. Schmitt OH: Averaging techniques employing several physiological variables. Ann NY Acad Sci 115:952, 1964.
8. Abboud S, Belhassen B, Laniado S, et al.: Non-invasive recording of late ventricular activity using an advanced method in

patients with a damaged mass of ventricular tissue. J Electrocardiol 16:245, 1983.
9. Simson MB: Use of signals in the terminal QRS complex to identify patients with ventricular tachycardia after myocardial infarction. Circulation 64:235, 1981.
10. Berbari EJ, Collins S, Salu Y, et al.: Orthogonal surface lead recordings of His-Purkinje activity: Comparison of actual and simulated waveforms. IEEE Trans Biomed Eng BME-30:160, 1983.
11. Abboud S, Sadeh D: The waveforms alignment procedure in the averaging process for external recording of the His bundle activity. Comput Biomed Res 15:212, 1982.
12. Wolf HK, MacInnis PJ, Stock S, et al.: Computer analysis of rest and exercise electrocardiograms. Comput Biomed Res 5:329, 1972.
13. Wajszczuk WJJ, Moskowitz MS, Bauld T, et al.: Non-inverse external recording of cardiac conduction system (His bundle) activity. Med Instrum 12:282, 1978.
14. Brandon CW, Brody DA: A hardware trigger for temporal indexing of the electrocardiographic signal. Comput Biomed Res 3:47, 1970.
15. Goovaerts HG, Ros HH, Van Der Akker TJ, et al.: A digital QRS detector based on the principle of contour limiting. IEEE Trans Biomed Eng BME-23:154, 1976.
16. Borjesson PO, Pahlm O, Sornmo L, et al.: Adaptive QRS detection based on maximum a posteriori estimation. IEEE Trans Biomed Eng BME-29:341, 1982.
17. Thakor NV, Webster JG, Tompkins WJ: Optimal QRS detector. Med Biol Eng Comput 21:343, 1983.
18. Tremblay G, LeBlanc AR: Near-optimal signal preprocessor for positive cardiac arrhythmia identification. IEEE Trans Biomed Eng BME-32:141, 1985.
19. Uijen GJH, deWeerd JPC, Vendrik AJH: Accuracy of QRS detection in relation to the analysis of high-frequency components in the electrocardiogram. Med Biol Eng Comput 17:492, 1979.
20. Fraden J, Neuman MR: QRS wave detection. Med Biol Eng Comput 18:125, 1980.
21. Craelius W, Restivo M, Assadi MA, et al.: Criteria for optimal averaging of cardiac signals. IEEE Trans Biomed Eng BME-33:957, 1986.
22. Breithardt G, Borggrefe M, Karbenn A, et al.: Prevalence of late potentials in patients with and without ventricular tachycardia. Correlation with angiographic findings. Am J Cardiol 49:1932, 1982.
23. Rozanski JJ, Mortara D, Myerburg RJ, et al.: Body surface detection of delayed depolarizations in patients with recurrent ventricular tachycardia and left ventricular aneurysm. Circulation 63:1172, 1981.
24. Hombach V, Braun V, Hopp HW, et al.: The application of signal-averaging technique in clinical cardiology. Clin Cardiol 5:107, 1982.
25. Atwood JE, Myers JJ, Forbes S, et al.: High-frequency electrocardiography: An evaluation of lead placement and measurements. Am Heart J 116:733, 1988.
26. Faugere G, Savard P, Nadeau RA, et al.: Characterization of the spatial distribution of late ventricular potentials by body surface mapping in patients with ventricular tachycardia. Circulation 74:1323, 1986.
27. Horan LG, Flowers NC, Sohi GS: A dynamic electrical record of the pathway of human His bundle activation from surface mapping. Circ Res 50:47, 1982.
28. Horacek BM, Montague TJ, Gardener MJ, Smith ER: Arrhythmogenic conditions. In Mirvis D (ed.): Electrocardiographic Body Surface Mapping. Boston, Martinus Nijhoff, 1988, pp. 214–236.
29. Oppenheim AV, Schaeffer RW: Digital Signal Processing. Englewood Cliffs, NJ, Prentice-Hall, 1975.
30. Gomes JAC, Winters SL, Stewart D, et al.: Optimal bandpass filters for time-domain analysis of the signal-averaged electrocardiogram. Am J Cardiol 68:1290, 1987.
31. Caref EB, Turitto G, Ibrahim BB, et al.: Role of bandpass filters in optimizing the value of the signal-averaged electrocardiogram as a predictor of the results of programmed stimulation. Am J Cardiol 64:16, 1989.
32. Craelius W, Hussain SM, Pantapoulos D, et al.: Intraoperative spectral analysis of ventricular potentials during sinus rhythm and ventricular tachycardia (Abstr). PACE 6:321, 1983.
33. Cain ME, Ambos HD, Witkowski FX, et al.: Fast Fourier transform analysis of signal-averaged ECGs for identification of patients prone to sustained ventricular tachycardia. Circulation 69:711, 1984.
34. Cain ME, Ambos HD, Markham J, et al.: Quantitation of differences in frequency content of signal-averaged ECGs in patients with compared to those without sustained ventricular tachycardia. Am J Cardiol 55:1500, 1985.
35. Haberl R, Jilge G, Pulter R, et al.: Comparison of frequency and time-domain analysis of the signal-averaged electrocardiogram in patients with ventricular tachycardia and coronary artery disease: Methodologic validation and clinical relevance. J Am Coll Cardiol 12:150, 1988.
36. Kelen G, Henkin R, Lannon M, et al.: Correlation between the signal-averaged electrocardiogram from Holter tapes and from real-time recordings. Am J Cardiol 63:1321, 1989.
37. Lander P, Deal RB, Berbari EJ: The analysis of ventricular late potentials using orthogonal leads. IEEE Trans Biomed Eng 33:629, 1988.
38. Berbari EJ, Friday K, Jackman WM, et al.: Precordial mapping of signal averaged late potentials compared to XYZ leads (Abstr). J Am Coll Cardiol 7:127, 1986.
39. Henkin R, Caref EB, Kelen G, et al.: The signal-averaged electrocardiogram and late potentials. A comparative analysis of commercial devices. J Electrocardiol 22(Suppl 1):19, 1990.
40. Denes P, Santarelli P, Hauser RG, et al.: Quantitative analysis of the high-frequency components of the terminal portion of the body surface QRS in normal subjects and in patients with ventricular tachycardia. Circulation 5:1129, 1983.
41. Fontaine JM, Henkin R, Howard M, et al.: Establishing criteria for the presence of late potentials in patients with left bundle branch block (Abstr). PACE 10:675, 1987.
42. Buckingham TA, Thessen CC, Stevens LL, et al.: Effect of conduction defects on the signal-averaged electrocardiographic determination of late potentials. Am J Cardiol 61:1265, 1988.
43. Simson MB: Optimal identification of late potentials. In Santini M, Pistolese M, Alliegro A (eds.): Progress in Clinical Pacing, pp. 225–238. Amsterdam, Excerpta Medica, 1988.
44. Lindsay BD, Ambos HD, Schechtman K, et al.: Improved selection of patients for programmed ventricular stimulation by frequency analysis of signal-averaged ECGs. Circulation 73:675, 1986.
45. Kelen GJ, Henkin R, Fontaine JM, et al.: Effects of analyzed signal duration and phase on the results of fast Fourier transform analysis of the surface electrocardiogram in subjects with and without late potentials. Am J Cardiol 60:1282, 1987.
46. Machac J, Weiss A, Winters SL, et al.: A comparative study of frequency domain analysis of signal-averaged ECGs in patients with ventricular tachycardia. J Am Coll Cardiol 11:284, 1988.
47. Worley SJ, Mark DB, Smith WM, et al.: Comparison of time domain and frequency domain variables from the signal-averaged electrocardiogram: A multivariable analysis. J Am Coll Cardiol 11:1041, 1988.
48. Kay SM, Marple SL Jr.: Spectrum analysis—a modern perspective. Proc IEEE 69:1380, 1981.
49. Harris FJ: On the use of windows for harmonic analysis with the discrete Fourier transform. Proc IEEE 66:51, 1978.
50. Haberl R, Jilge G, Pulter R, et al.: Spectral mapping of the electrocardiogram with Fourier transform for identification of patients with sustained ventricular tachycardia and coronary artery disease. Eur Heart J 10:316, 1989.
51. Lander P, Albert D, Berbari EJ: Principles of frequency domain analysis. In El-Sherif N, Hombach V (eds.): High Resolution Electrocardiography. New York, Futura Publishing Company, 1990. In press.
52. El-Sherif N, Mehra R, Gomes JAC, et al.: Appraisal of a low noise electrocardiogram. J Am Coll Cardiol 1:456, 1983.
53. El-Sherif N: The low noise (high resolution) electrocardiogram. Int J Cardiol 6:185, 1984.
54. El-Sherif N, Scherlag BJ, Lazzara R: Electrode catheter recordings during malignant ventricular arrhythmias following experimental acute myocardial ischemia. Circulation 51:1003, 1975.
55. El-Sherif N, Scherlag BJ, Lazzara R, et al.: Reentrant ventricular arrhythmias in the late myocardial infarction period. I.

Conduction characteristics in the infarction zone. Circulation 55:586, 1977.
56. El-Sherif N, Hope RR, Scherlag BJ, et al.: Reentrant ventricular arrhythmias in the late myocardial infarction period. 2. Patterns of initiation and termination of re-entry. Circulation 55:702, 1977.
57. El-Sherif N, Lazzara R, Hope RR, et al.: Reentrant arrhythmias in the late myocardial infarction period. 3. Manifest and concealed extrasystolic grouping. Circulation 56:225, 1977.
58. El-Sherif N, Gough WB, Zeiler RH, et al.: Reentrant ventricular arrhythmias in the late myocardial infarction period. 12. Spontaneous versus induced reentry and intramural versus epicardial circuits. J Am Coll Cardiol 6:124, 1985.
59. Flowers NC, Shvartsman V, Kennelly BM, et al.: Surface recordings of His-Purkinje activity on an every beat basis without digital averaging. Circulation 63:948, 1981.
60. Kepski R, Plucinski Z, Walczak F: Noninvasive recording of His-Purkinje system (HPS) activity in man on beat-to-beat basis. PACE 5:506, 1982.
61. Erne SN, Fenici RR, Hahlbohm HE, et al.: Beat-to-beat surface recording and averaging of His-Purkinje activity in man. J Electrocardiol 16:355, 1983.
62. Flowers NC, Schvartsman V, Horan LG, et al.: Analysis of the PR subinterval in normal subjects and early studies in patients with abnormalities of the conduction system using surface His bundle recordings. J Am Coll Cardiol 2:93, 1983.
63. Hombach V, Kebbel U, Hopp HW, et al.: Noninvasive beat by beat registration of ventricular late potentials using high resolution electrocardiography. Int J Cardiol 6:167, 1984.
64. El-Sherif N, Gomes JAC, Restivo M, et al.: Late potentials and arrhythmogenesis. PACE 8:440, 1985.
65. Hombach V, Hopp H-W, Kebbel U, et al.: Recovery of ventricular late potentials from body surface using the signal averaging and high resolution ECG techniques. Clin Cardiol 9:361, 1986.
66. Ishijima M, Kimata S, Kasanuki H, et al.: The feasibility of beat-to-beat detection of His-Purkinje activity by finite element method. PACE 10:1107, 1987.
67. Winter DA, Rautaharju PM, Wolf KH: Measurement and characteristics of over-all noise content in exercise electrocardiograms. Am Heart J 74:324, 1967.
68. Mehra R, Restivo M, El-Sherif N: Electromyographic noise reduction for high-resolution electrocardiography. In IEEE Frontiers of Engineering and Computing in Health Care, p. 298. IEEE Press, New York, 1983.
69. Shvartsman V, Barnes GR, Schvartsman L, et al.: Multi-channel signal processing based on logic averaging. IEEE Trans Biomed Eng 29:531, 1982.
70. Waldo AL, Kaiser GA: A study of ventricular arrhythmias associated with myocardial infarction in the canine heart. Circulation 47:1222, 1973.
71. Boineau JP, Cox JL: Slow ventricular activation in acute myocardial infarction in the canine heart. A source of reentrant premature ventricular contractions. Circulation 48:702, 1973.
72. Janse MJ, VanCapelle FJL, Morsink M, et al.: Flow of "injury" current and patterns of excitation during early ventricular arrhythmias in acute regional myocardial ischemia in isolated porcine and canine hearts. Circ Res 47:151, 1980.
73. El-Sherif N, Smith RA, Evans K: Ventricular arrhythmias in the late myocardial infarction period in the dog. 8: Epicardial mapping of reentrant circuits. Circ Res 49:225, 1981.
74. Mehra R, Zeiler RH, Gough WB, et al.: Reentrant ventricular arrhythmias in the late myocardial infarction period. 9. Electrophysiologic-anatomical correlation of reentrant circuits. Circulation 67:11, 1983.
75. El-Sherif N, Mehra R, Gough WB, et al.: Reentrant ventricular arrhythmias in the late myocardial infarction period. Interruption of reentrant circuits by cryothermal techniques. Circulation 68:644, 1983.
76. Berbari EJ, Scherlag BJ, Hope RR, et al.: Recording from the body surface of arrhythmogenic ventricular activity during the S-T segment. Am J Cardiol 41:697, 1978.
77. Simson MB, Euler D, Michelson EL, et al.: Detection of delayed ventricular activation on the body surface in dogs. Am J Physiol 24:H363, 1981.
78. Simson MB, Untereker WJ, Spielman SR, et al.: The relationship between late potentials in the body surface and directly recorded fragmented electrograms in patients with ventricular tachycardia. Am J Cardiol 51:105, 1983.
79. Restivo M, El-Sherif N, Kelen GJ, et al.: Correlation of late potentials in the body surface and ventricular activation maps of reentrant circuits in the post-infarction dog heart (Abstr). Circulation 72 (Suppl III):11, 1985.
80. Restivo M, Henkin R, Craelius W, et al.: Are regions of delayed activation during a basic rhythm the responsible arrhythmogenic substrate for reentry (abstr)? J Am Coll Cardiol 7:85A, 1986.
81. Craelius W, Chen VKH, Restivo M, et al.: Rhythm analysis of arterial blood pressure. IEEE Trans Biomed Eng BME-33:1166, 1986.

20

The High-Resolution Electrocardiogram: Clinical Aspects

Vinzenz Hombach

The conventional surface electrocardiogram (ECG) provides information on atrial and ventricular depolarization, atrioventricular conduction, and ventricular repolarization.[34] Abnormalities of sinus node function can only be derived from short- and long-term (Holter) ECGs, whereas the exact electrophysiologic mechanisms (e.g., sinoatrial block, sinus node standstill) remain undetected from the body surface, because the low-voltage sinus node depolarization (in the range of 10–30 μV) will be buried in the baseline noise of conventional ECG amplifiers. The same holds true for AV conduction blocks, the site of which (e.g., supra- and infra-His), cannot be exactly localized by the normal ECG. Prolongation of intraventricular conduction of larger myocardial areas due to bundle branch block can be recognized in the conventional ECG from the typical hemiblock or RBBB-LBBB patterns of the QRS complex. However, delayed activation of smaller areas of damaged myocardium in patients with acute or chronic myocardial infarction or with right ventricular dysplasia will be invisible on the surface ECG, due to the small amplitudes of the signals in the microvolt range.[21]

Some of these special electrophysiologic problems can be solved by direct intracardiac catheter recordings in the laboratory or by direct hand-held electrode mapping during open-heart surgery.[51] However, for routine detailed studies of the electrical behavior of the heart, noninvasive surface recordings would be highly desirable. The history of surface high-resolution electrocardiography began in 1973 with the attempt of three groups to record His bundle potentials, using the signal-averaging technique.[1, 24, 61] Since that time, different types of signal-averaging computers have been designed, and many investigators have reported on recordings of sinus node ECGs,[11, 42, 53, 72] His bundle potentials,[35, 43, 50, 68, 69] and ventricular late potentials.[1, 12, 25, 41, 46, 58]

In the following chapters, the spectrum of clinical application of the high-resolution ECG technique will be described, and the diagnostic and prognostic significance of the signals recorded with this technique will be described.

Pre-Atrial Activity (Sinus-Node Potentials)

From animal experiments it is well known that the depolarization of sinus node pacemaker cells resembles a slowly up- or down-sloping wave or ramp, both in transmembrane and in extracellular recordings, which precedes atrial depolarization by 30 to 40 ms.[10, 60, 62, 72] Such pre-atrial depolarizations have also been found in humans, using intracardiac catheter electrode recordings from the endocardial surface of the sinus node area.[28, 39, 40] In these studies, the time interval from the beginning of pre-atrial to atrial depolarization was found to be 40 to 80 ms in normal subjects, and more than 100 ms in patients with sinus node disease.

From these results it seems clear that such pre-atrial activity may represent sinus node depolarization and may be retrieved from the body surface by high-resolution electrocardiography if the following conditions are met:

1. No cut-off of lower frequencies; that is, DC 0.05 Hz high-pass filtering must be used.
2. The signals of interest should resemble slowly depolarizing ramp- or wavelike depolarizations, which are separated from or merging into the P wave.
3. The range of presumed sinoatrial conduction times should be 40 to 80 ms in normal individuals.

Using these criteria, several groups reported successful ECG recordings of pre-atrial activity in humans by means of the signal-averaging technique.[11, 42, 72] In the study by Wajsczuk et al.[72] of 40 consecutive patients, successful noise-free recordings were obtained in 36 individuals, and in 32, low-voltage deflections were seen before the onset of the P wave in the reference lead (highly filtered bipolar surface lead) and before the onset of the first large voltage deflection of atrial activity in the averaged leads. Using band-pass filtering of 30 to 300 Hz, these potentials preceded the onset of atrial activity by 24 to 40 ms, and their voltage varied from 4 to 15 μV. Ten patients from this study were additionally investigated with 0.1 Hz high-pass filtering, which revealed recordings with a long diastolic depolarization slope, followed by a steeper upstroke that made a transition into the P wave. Obviously, all these recordings were performed in patients with normal sinus rhythm, and none of them had evidence of overt sinus node disease.

Various precordial and transthoracic leads were tested for their efficacy in representing pre-atrial activity best with the longest intervals to the P wave. The transthoracic Z-lead appeared to detect the most and the earliest activity of the sinus node region. Our group studied a total of 37 patients by averaging 3 bipolar precordial leads; the one from the second right intercostal space (ICS) to the fourth left ICS was the most effective for retrieving clear and reproducible pre-atrial signals in 23 of 37 patients.

In principle, two types of pre-atrial signals can be observed: One type has a small base width, rapid upstroke, and higher frequency components that are still visible with 50-Hz high-pass filtering, and with intervals to the atrial deflection of 30 to 45 ms. The second type is characterized by a wider base width, a more wavelike structure (mono- or biphasic), with lower frequency components that are lost with 50-Hz high-pass filtering, and with intervals to the atrial depolarization of 50 to 165 ms. Drug testing with intravenous (IV) atropine decreased the interval of the pre-atrial i to atrial depolarization in two patients (Fig. 20–1), whereas this interval was prolonged after beta-blockade with pindolol. From this study it was concluded that only the second type of pre-atrial depolarizations met the characteristics of sinus node depolarization (as described above) and thus could represent true sinus node activity in the averaged low-noise ECG.

In a second study by our group, the efficacy of the beat-to-beat high-resolution ECG technique was tested for continuous recording of pre-atrial activity.[46] Pre-atrial potentials were not reproducibly found in any of eight normal subjects, whereas such signals were seen in 2 of 5 patients with coronary heart disease (Fig. 20–2). By comparison, pre-atrial activity was detected in 7 of 12 patients, using the signal-averaged surface ECG. Based on these preliminary reports, the high-resolution technique seems to be less efficient for noninvasive retrieval of sinus node depolarizations in humans. Moreover, no systematic studies have been conducted as yet in patients with normal and disturbed sinus node function, in whom the underlying pathophysiologic mechanisms of sinus node dysfunction could be documented with the low-noise ECG.

SUMMARY AND CONCLUSIONS

- Successful surface ECG recordings of pre-atrial activity are feasible by means of both the signal-averaging and the high-resolution beat-to-beat technique.
- The success rates for recording pre-atrial potentials seem to be higher with the signal averaging than with the beat-to-beat high-resolution technique.
- With the signal-averaging technique, pre-atrial potentials can be recorded only in patients with regular sinus rhythm, whereas dynamic changes of these potentials, which are lost by the signal-averaging process, may be recorded only by the beat-to-beat high-resolution technique.
- No systematic studies have been published directly validating externally recorded pre-atrial potentials as true sinus node depolarizations by simultaneous intracardiac catheter recordings from the SN area.
- Based on the presently available data, the clinical

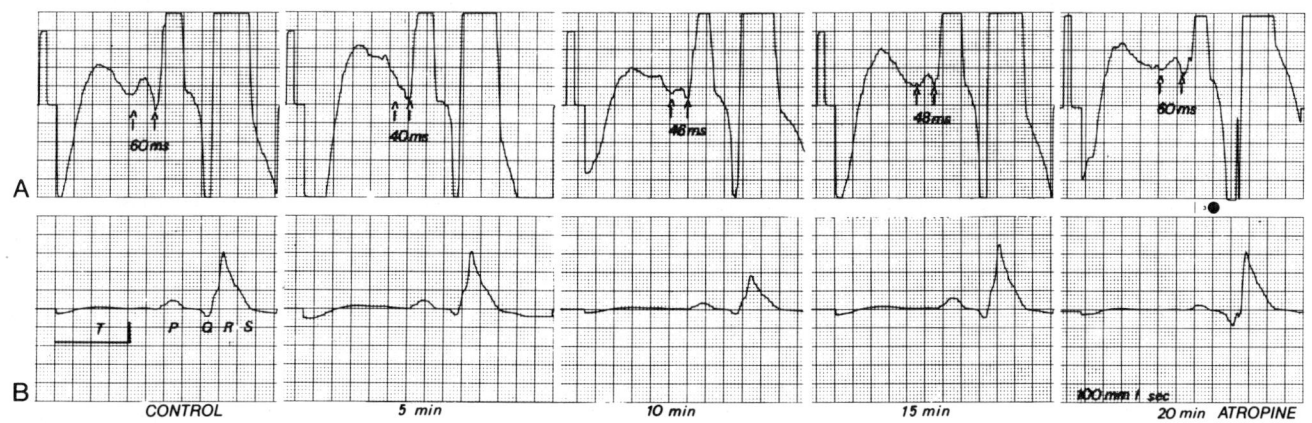

FIGURE 20–1
Pre-atrial potential recorded from body surface by the signal averaging technique before (Control) and up to 20 min. after administration of atropine. Note the wave-like shape of the pre-atrial signal, with an interval of 60 ms between the beginning of the pre-atrial potential to the beginning of atrial depolarization. This interval is shortened by atropine up to 15 min and returns to the control value after 20 min A, High-resolution ECG; B, conventional ECG.

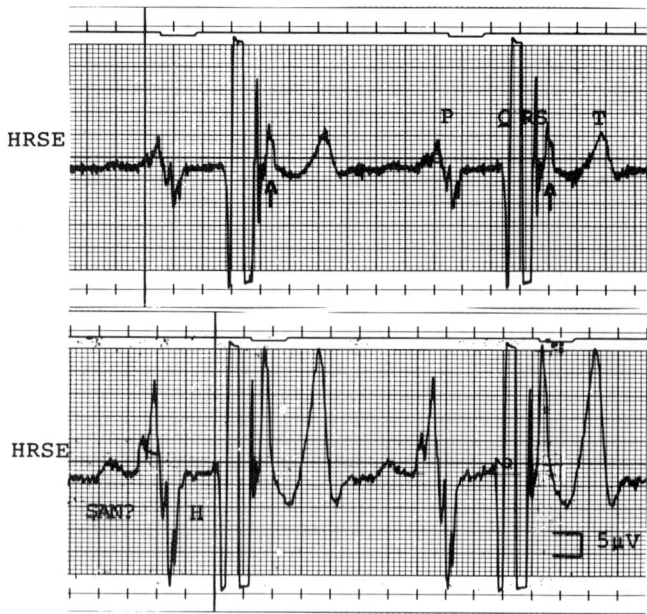

FIGURE 20–2
Pre-atrial potential (SAN?), recorded beat by beat with the high-resolution real-time technique in a patient with a left ventricular aneurysm. Note the wave-like pre-atrial signal that merges into the rapid upstroke of atrial depolarization. The interval from the beginning of the pre-atrial signal to the beginning of atrial depolarization is 60 ms. HRSE = High-resolution surface electrocardiogram; SAN? = possible sinus node potential; H = His bundle depolarization. Arrows denote ventricular late potential.

value of noninvasive recordings of pre-atrial activity is extremely limited. This holds particularly true for its contribution to clinical decision making (e.g., whether a patient should receive a cardiac pacemaker) and its prognostic significance for detecting high-risk patients prone to syncope or severe bradyarrhythmias.

Recordings of His Bundle Potentials

Surface recordings of His bundle activity represented the first clinical application of the signal-averaging technique.[1, 23, 61] Since these initial reports numerous studies have been published dealing with surface His bundle recordings, which have been performed with different kinds of signal-averaging computers.[27, 35, 43, 44, 50, 67–69, 71] In the earlier reports, successful His bundle recordings were made in 30 to 50% of cases, depending on the limited recording technology at that time and on problems with instability of the trigger mechanism. Reasons for failure to record His bundle activity included excessive trigger jitter and/or slight variations of the conduction velocity within the His-Purkinje-system, as shown by Tonkin and coworkers.[66] In more recent studies, the success rates for recording His bundle potentials were reported to be in the range of 50 to 75%, mostly due to better hardware and software technology. Some groups tried to confirm their surface His bundle electrograms by off-line intracardiac catheter recordings.[2, 44, 54, 56, 70]

In most of these studies, good to excellent correlations were found, with correlation coefficients well beyond 0.90 (Fig. 20–3). However, in none of these evaluation studies were direct on-line recordings performed, which may be a general limitation, since intraindividual variations of the AV conduction intervals are well known, depending on physical exercise or emotional stress during daily life.[66] His bundle spikes can be evaluated semidirectly in the signal-averaged ECG by IV administration of drugs that change the AV nodal conduction velocity such as, catecholamines, oxyfedrine or atropine for accelerating AV conduction (shortening of the P-H interval), and beta-blockers or verapamil for slowing AV conduction (prolongation of the P-H interval). In a pilot study performed by our group (unpublished data) in a series of 15 patients with bradyarrhythmias during sinus rhythm, the effect of oxyfedrine, (96 mg/day), on heart rate and cardiac conduction was evaluated, using the MAC-I averaging computer. In 11 of 15 patients a relatively stable and reproducible His bundle spike with an isoelectric interval to the preceding atrial complex was recorded, whereas in the remaining 4 patients the His bundle potential was obscure. In 8 of 15 patients the P-H interval decreased significantly (Fig. 20–4); it remained unchanged in 3 of 15 patients, and in the remaining 4 patients the P-H interval increased by the effect of oxyfedrine. In the whole group the P-H interval decreased from 131.5 ± 38.0 ms before to 123.3 ± 40.2 ms after administration of oxyfedrine (statistically insignificant), whereas the H-V interval remained virtually unchanged (41.3 ± 5.2 ms before and 42.0 ± 4.9 ms after oxyfedrine). The observations on apparent prolongations of the P-H interval in 4 patients of the latter group may be explained by the fact that in these individuals the His bundle spike could not be exactly separated from atrial depolarization and/or from background noise; thus the supposed negative dromotropic effect of oxyfedrine may be mimicked by the poor technical quality of the signal-averaged surface ECG. Nevertheless, these results show that with success rates of 60 to 80% of surface His bundle recordings, the influence of cardioactive drugs on AV and His-Purkinje system conduction may be tested noninvasively by the signal-averaged high-resolution ECG. This may be particularly helpful in screening the effect of new cardiovascular drugs in the preclinical phase of evaluation, as well as for monitoring possible side effects of clinically used drugs in patients on oral maintenance therapy. The latter may be particularly important in patients receiving antiarrhythmic drugs, and the side effects of these drugs can be documented when the patient is in regular sinus rhythm. Two severe limitations of surface His bundle electrocardiography with the averaging technique have to be mentioned:

1. Overlap of the His bundle potential by atrial activity
2. Failure to document second- or third-degree AV blocks beat-by-beat.

Atrial overlapping of His bundle spikes may be

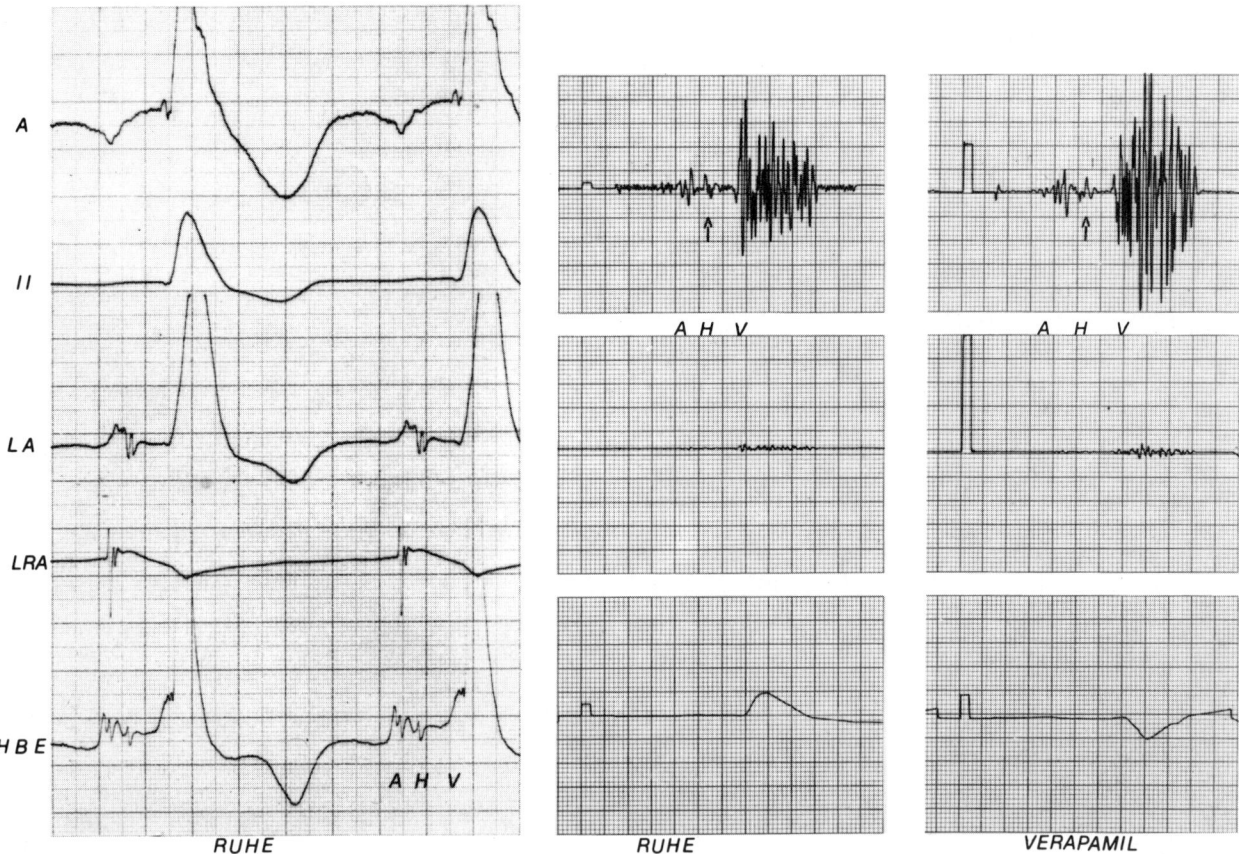

FIGURE 20–3
His bundle ECG obtained by intracardiac catheter recording (left panel) and by signal averaging of the high-gain amplified surface ECG at control (RUHE) and following IV administration of 10 mg of verapamil. Note the relatively short AH interval. The His bundle spike (arrows) is somewhat more separated from atrial depolarization after administration of verapamil. A = Surface ECG lead A according to Trethewie; II = Einthoven lead II; LA = left atrial ECG; LRA = low right atrial ECG; HBE = His bundle ECG.

observed in 20 to 40% of cases. In a study performed by McKenna et al,[54] of 70 individuals (5 normal subjects, 21 patients with arrhythmias, and 44 patients with surgically corrected tetralogy of Fallot), a clear His bundle potential was seen in 31 of the 70 subjects (44%). Atrial overlap was observed in 25 individuals; in 10 patients no His bundle spike was present, and in the remaining 4 patients electrical interference prevented successful His bundle recordings. IV administration of verapamil prolonged the P-H interval, and in 48 individuals (69%) a His bundle potential of good quality was recorded, mainly due to the fact that in 23 of 25 individuals with atrial overlap, verapamil separated the end of atrial depolarization from the beginning of His bundle activation. These results show that the problem of atrial overlap in surface His bundle recordings may be overcome by IV administration of verapamil or by beta-blocking drugs, and the success rates of His bundle recordings may be improved by 40 to 60%. This may be particularly helpful in patients with P-Q intervals of less than 160 ms (see Fig. 20-3) who have relatively short P-H intervals (i.e., faster AV nodal conduction, in which atrial overlap is very likely to occur).

The second problem, failure to document the site of AV block, may be overcome by selective triggering on blocked P and R waves, using the so-called automated discrimination circuit.[64, 65] By means of this technique, superimposed P and R wave segments can be excluded, and signal-averaging of the post–P intervals makes it possible to determine whether a His bundle potential exists (infra-His block) or not (supra-His block). In their recent study Takeda and colleagues[65] described the results in 10 patients with a complete AV block, 6 of whom had supra-His blocks, and 4 infra-His blocks. In the selectively triggered and signal-averaged electrograms, 5 patients had no His spike in the post–P interval but did have a His-bundle potential preceding the averaged pre-R interval. Four patients had no His bundle activity prior to the QRS complex but had consistent His spikes following the blocked P waves. Thus, in 9 of 10 patients, the site of complete AV block could be localized by an intelligent surface ECG signal-averaging method, the results of which corresponded perfectly to catheter recordings from the His bundle area. However, in one patient with block proximal to the His bundle, the correct diagnosis could not be achieved by the surface averaging method.

In this special study an esophageal atrial electrogram was taken for triggering the averager on the P wave, because its amplitude was much higher than that of

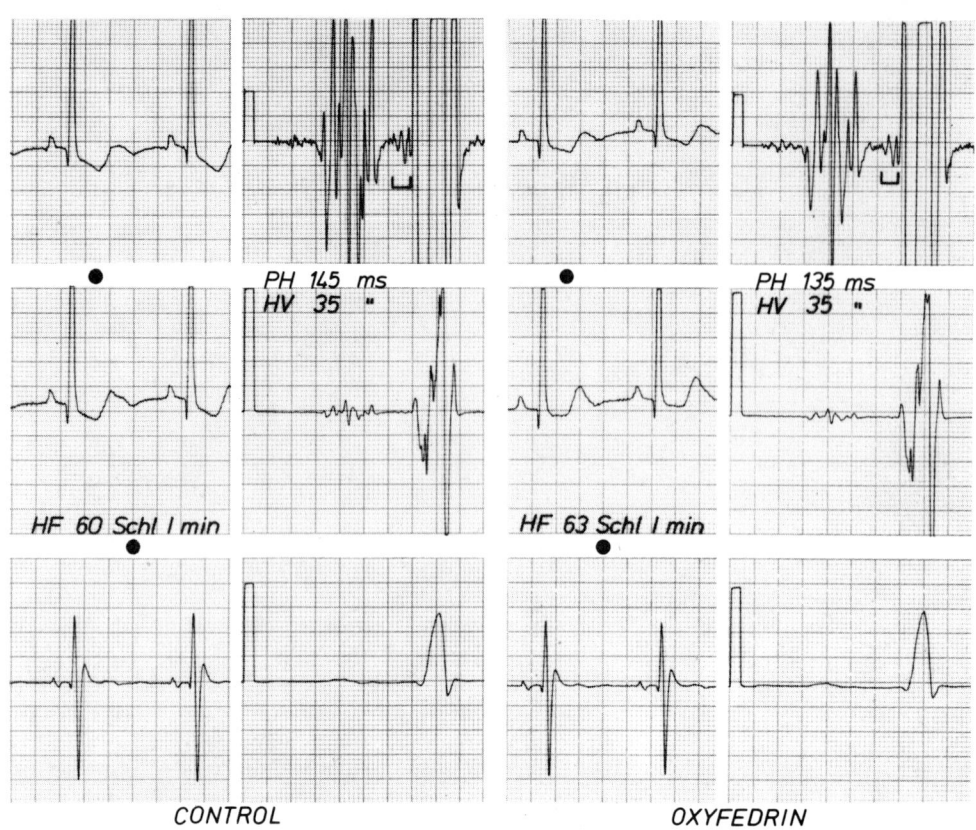

FIGURE 20-4
Signal-averaged surface His bundle ECG before (Control) and after administration of 96 mg of oxyfedrine. Note two cycles of the conventional ECG on the left and one cycle of the signal averaged high-gain amplified surface ECG on the right of each half of the figure. The heart rate (HF) increased slightly and the PH interval was shortened by the administration of oxyfedrine. HF = Heart rate (beats per minute); PH = PH interval; HV = HV interval.

the conventional bipolar surface ECG. This is a serious limitation of a "completely noninvasive" method, because many patients may feel much discomfort when swallowing a catheter electrode for recording the esophageal ECG. In addition, because the technical requirements are demanding, and the signal-averaging process is complicated, methodology may not receive widespread application. Ultimately the clinical information on the site of AV block seems to be rather limited, because, for example, patients with a complete AV block are absolute candidates for pacemaker implantation (with the exception of congenital complete heart block). In some patients with a second-degree AV block, the localization of the site of block might be helpful; for example, a Wenckebach supra-His block may be more benign than an infra-His block, which may also hold true for the Mobitz-type of second-degree AV block. However, the full dynamic behavior of AV conduction under various physiologic conditions can be documented more precisely by Holter long-term ECG monitoring, and the decision on pacemaker implantation will be made primarily by the patient's symptoms and the results of the Holter ECG, rather than by a short-term signal-averaged surface His bundle ECG.

One last peculiarity of surface His bundle electrocardiography with the signal-averaging technique should be mentioned. In about 20 to 50%, the His bundle potential may appear bi-, tri- or quadriphasic (see Fig. 20–4). It has been supposed that at least quadriphasic complexes might represent delayed intra-His activation (so-called split-His) or depolarization of both the His bundle and its branches. The clinical and prognostic significance of such findings remains unclear because corresponding correlative studies with intracardiac catheter recordings and follow-up of these patients have not yet been conducted.

Since the introduction of spatial averaging technology the low-noise ECG can be recorded from the body surface on a beat-to-beat basis, and the first applications of this technique were again recordings of His bundle potentials.[24, 63] In the study of Flowers et al,[24] 25 healthy individuals were investigated and their His bundle potentials were recorded. The mean P-H interval values were 115.0 ± 12.3 ms and the H-V intervals were 40.5 ± 3.5 ms. Owing to special computer algorithms and filtering procedures, relatively sharp spikelike His potentials were described. Occasional reports on continuous His bundle recordings from body surface have been published. El-Sherif and colleagues[19] reported recovery rates of His bundle potentials of 43% using high resolution beat-to-beat technique compared with a 71% recovery rate when using the signal-averaging technique. Our group reported successful His bundle recordings with the beat-to-beat technique in 9 of 14 subjects,[47] in whom His bundle potentials were found to be spikelike in 2 individuals (Fig. 20–5), and ramplike in 7 patients.

In all of these studies the surface beat-to-beat ECG recordings of His-Purkinje activity were not validated by intracardiac catheter studies. Moreover, although experiences with this new technique in patients with higher-degree AV blocks have not been published as yet, theoretically real-time electrocardiography repre-

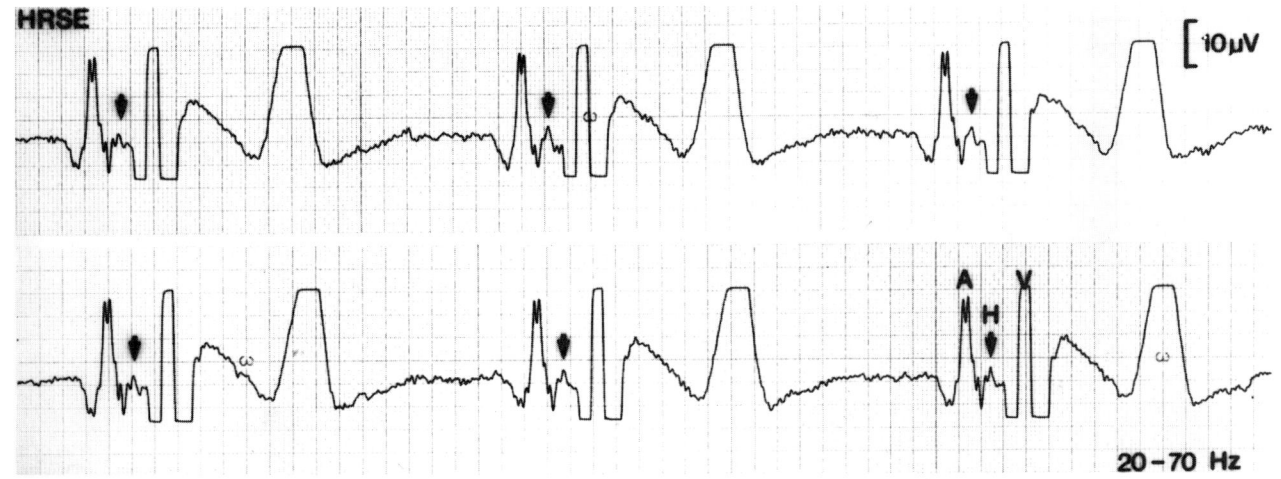

FIGURE 20–5
High-resolution real-time surface ECG (continuous strip) showing a spike-like His bundle potential (arrows). HRSE = High-resolution surface ECG; A = atrial depolarization; H = His bundle deflection; V = ventricular depolarization.

sents the most promising noninvasive technique for the detection of the site of AV block (e.g., second-degree block of Wenckebach-type or Mobitz-type and complete AV block). The presently available real-time ECG recording equipment apparently does not have enough noise-reduction capabilities to retrieve His-Purkinje activity from baseline noise in a high—and for clinical purposes, sufficient—percentage of cases. Thus, improvements in recording technology are necessary, before the high-resolution beat-to-beat technique will become a routine measure to study and screen larger patient populations with normal and disturbed AV conduction.

SUMMARY AND CONCLUSIONS

- His bundle potentials can be recorded from the body surface by both the signal-averaging and the high-resolution real-time technique.
- The recovery rates of His bundle potentials are presently higher with the signal-averaging (60 to 80%) than with the real-time technique (40 to 60%).
- The site of AV block (supra-His, infra-His) may be differentiated by a special averaging procedure (the application of the so-called automated discrimination circuit), but the beat-to-beat real-time technique is superior as an approach to this problem. However, the present experience with both techniques in larger patient groups with various types of AV blocks is greatly limited.
- In 20 to 40% of cases, the signal-averaged His bundle potential appears tri- or quadriphasic, which may possibly indicate intra-His conduction disturbances (so-called split-His) or may represent both His bundle and bundle branch depolarization.
- The knowledge of the A-V conduction subintervals (P-H and H-V intervals) through noninvasive electrocardiography seems to be limited, so far as decisions from these values for treatment (e.g., pacemaker implantations) are concerned. More important information will be derived from the patient's symptoms and from the results of 24-hour ambulatory ECG monitoring.
- His bundle electrocardiography with the signal-averaging and the high-resolution real-time technique may be useful for noninvasive screening of new cardiovascular drugs that influence AV conduction and for monitoring the effect of clinically established drugs during chronic maintenance therapy. The latter will be of particular importance for monitoring the effect of antiarrhythmic drugs that exert negative dromotropic effects mainly on intraventricular conduction (prolongation of the H-V interval).

Recordings of AV Nodal Potentials

Attempts to record AV nodal activity itself by the extracellular route date back to 1907.[22] Since that time several groups have described AV nodal potentials by direct needle or catheter recordings; however, much controversy existed about the true waveform and the validation of these so-called AV nodal potentials in dogs by means of the signal-averaging technique, the data of which was updated and reviewed in 1981 during the International Symposium on the Signal-Averaging Technique in Cologne.[6]

In 15 dogs, high-gain amplified electrograms from catheter recordings, obtained from the His bundle region, were analyzed by signal averaging during junctional rhythms. One or more low-frequency wavelike potentials, with a duration of 26 to 47 ms and amplitudes of 1 to 15 μV, were observed, which preceded the His bundle deflection. These potentials were characterized and discussed as AV nodal potentials, and the underlying rhythm was confirmed as a true AV nodal rhythm rather than a His bundle rhythm. Similar results were obtained by our group from 1979 to 1981 in patients by signal-averaging His bundle ECGs obtained by conventional catheter techniques. In 15 of

20 patients, reproducibly low-frequency wavelike potentials were recorded, which preceded the His bundle deflections by 20 to 106 ms. The amplitude of these potentials ranged from 1 to 12 μV, and their ratio to the amplitude of the His bundle potentials was 4:1 to 32:1. During sinus rhythm, 10 of 15 patients were studied with the MAC-I computer, and the following conduction times of the subintervals were recorded: A-H = 114 ± 30 ms; A-N = 85 ± 18 ms; and N-H = 29 ± 17 ms. During atrial pacing, AV nodal conduction was considerably prolonged, as indicated by the prolonged N-H intervals: A-H = 133 ± 38 ms; A-N = 85 ± 18 ms; and N-H = 45 ± 21 ms (Fig. 20–6). In two patients AV nodal tachycardias were initiated by programmed atrial pacing, and the antegrade AV conduction intervals were considerably prolonged: A-H = 240 ms and 260 ms; A-N = 95 ms and 80 ms; and N-H = 145 ms and 160 ms. From this study it was concluded that additional potentials can be retrieved between the end of atrial depolarization and the beginning of His bundle activation by averaging high-gain amplified His bundle ECGs from catheter recordings, and that these potentials may reveal functional characteristics of AV nodal cells (i.e., low-amplitude wavelike potentials and slowing of nodal conduction velocity during atrial pacing and during phases of AV nodal tachycardias).

Since the publication of these two reports, no further similar investigations have been conducted, although it might be of some clinical and theoretical interest to study the behavior of AV nodal conduction in humans under various physiologic and pathophysiologic conditions (e.g., exercise, drug administration).

SUMMARY AND CONCLUSIONS

- Extracellular recordings of AV nodal potentials in animals and in humans are feasible by signal-averaging high-gain amplified intracardiac catheter recordings from the region of His bundle.
- Validations of these potentials as being true AV nodal activity are crucial, at least in humans. This problem may be approached by testing the behavior of these "nodal" potentials during atrial pacing or following IV administration of drugs that are known to delay AV nodal conduction.
- AV nodal recordings in man may be of some theoretical and clinical interest in order to test the influence of various physiologic conditions and pharmacologic interventions on AV nodal conduction by means of a direct recording technology.
- The true practical value of this technique may be limited. Because an invasive approach is required it cannot be performed in larger groups of patients for screening purposes, and the results of AV nodal recordings cannot support in any way the clinical decision of what type of treatment should be applied in an individual patient.

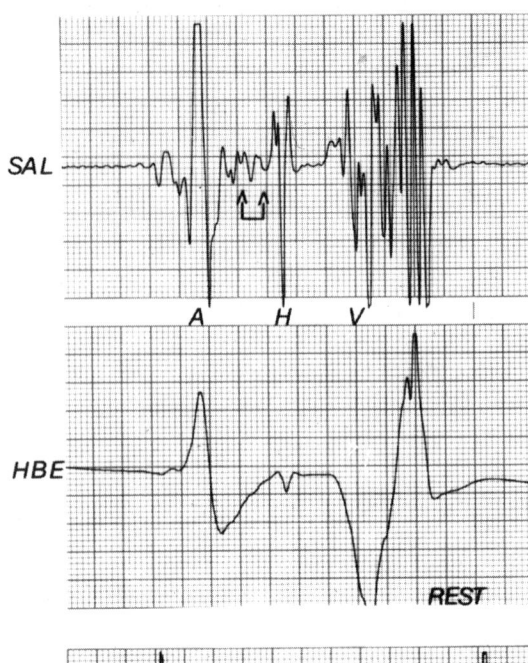

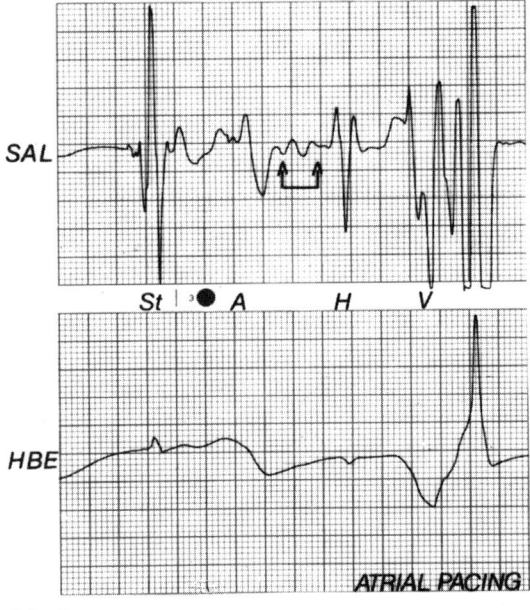

FIGURE 20–6
Signal-averaged high-gain amplified His bundle ECG. During sinus rhythm at resting conditions (REST) there are additional low amplitude signals between the end of atrial (A) and the beginning of His bundle (H) depolarizations, possibly indicating A-V nodal activity. During atrial pacing (bottom), the interval from the end of atrial (A) and the beginning of His bundle (H) depolarizations is considerably prolonged, possibly indicating a rate-dependent conduction delay within the AV node. SAL = Signal-averaged lead; HBE = Intracardiac catheter His bundle ECG; ST = stimulus artifact; A = atrial depolarization; H = His bundle deflection; V = ventricular depolarization.

Recordings of Ventricular Late Potentials

Experimental and clinical data has convincingly shown that reentry plays a major role in the genesis of ventricular tachyarrhythmias. Prerequisites of reentry are unidirectional block, slow conduction, and recovery of excitability of the tissue ahead of the excitation wavefront. As an expression of slow conduction, delayed and fractionated electrical activity during diastole has been documented both in experimental infarction and in the border zones of infarcted human myocardium.[3, 9, 17, 20, 25] Such late diastolic activity, commonly called "ventricular late potentials," may be recorded by direct intraoperative mapping during open-heart surgery, by intracardiac catheter mapping, and noninvasively from the body surface by high-resolution electrocardiography (signal-averaging technique and beat-to-beat high-resolution technique).[49, 58, 59]

Larger studies of the diagnostic and prognostic significance of ventricular late potentials have been performed almost exclusively with the signal-averaging technique. Several investigators have studied different patient groups according to the type of underlying heart disease and/or the prevailing type of ventricular arrhythmias. Our own group found that ventricular late potentials are an extremely rare finding in patients with congestive cardiomyopathy, aortic stenosis, and the so-called small vessel disease type of coronary heart disease, irrespective of whether the patients were suffering from potentially dangerous repetitive ventricular ectopic activity.[36, 37] Thus, ventricular late potentials seem to occur most frequently in patients with coronary heart disease, particularly in those with "regional" myocardial damage.

In a study of 50 patients with acute myocardial infarction, the spectrum of ventricular arrhythmias and the presence of ventricular late potentials was investigated, starting from the first day of illness, and the patients were followed for a mean of 30 ± 6 months.[36] Seven patients died within 3 to 6 days after myocardial infarction (MI), and six of these patients had ventricular late potentials. In the total group of MI patients, ventricular late potentials were relatively rare during the acute phase (17 of 50 = 34%), and this finding has been corroborated by subsequent studies.[29, 57] The predictive power of ventricular late potentials in the acute phase of MI was evaluated only in the study of Höpp and coworkers, and the predictive value of ventricular late potentials for in-hospital sudden cardiac death was 67%.[36] In contrast, ventricular late potentials recorded in the acute phase of illness were not helpful in predicting an increased risk in the posthospital period (predictive value for sudden cardiac death, 17%). The pre-discharge prevalence of ventricular late potentials post-MI is in the range of 21 to 55%; that is, within the healing and reparative phase of MI, delayed activation of circumscribed myocardial areas is more common than in the first hours of coronary artery occlusion.

Many prospective studies have been conducted to evaluate the long-term predictive power of ventricular late potentials post-MI.[8, 13, 14, 16, 21a, 30, 31, 38, 51a] The mean follow-up periods in these studies varied from 6 to 30 months. In two studies the occurrence of new attacks of ventricular tachycardias could be predicted by the presence of ventricular late potentials (predictive value of 24%). In two further studies,[30] the risk of sudden cardiac death and/or ventricular tachycardia could be prognosticated by ventricular late potentials, with a predictive value of 50%. In the study by our own group,[37] sudden cardiac death was predictable by ventricular late potentials in 30% of cases. By combining both variables (i.e., the presence of late potentials and the occurrence of repetitive forms of ventricular arrhythmias), the predictive value could be improved to 40%, but the sensitivity decreased from 88 to 50%.

Several reports have been published regarding the prevalence and prognostic significance of ventricular late potentials in patients with chronic coronary heart disease. In the study by Breithardt and Boggrefe,[12] 146 patients (20 without coronary heart disease, 126 with coronary heart disease, and 16 with dilatative cardiomyopathy) were prospectively followed; 49 patients had ventricular late potentials, with a mean duration of 31 ± 15.3 ms in patients without documented ventricular tachycardia, and of 51 ± 31.5 ms in those with documented ventricular tachycardia. The predictive value for sudden cardiac death was not reported in this study.

In another study, by our group 200 patients with chronic coronary heart disease were investigated prospectively.[37] In 108 patients (54%) ventricular late potentials were found at entry into the study. After a follow-up period of 32 ± 8 months, 25 patients died (18 from sudden cardiac death). The predictive value of ventricular late potentials for this event was 16%, and its sensitivity was 94%. The predictive value of spontaneous ventricular tachycardia (VT)–ventricular fibrillation (VF) attacks was 8%, and its sensitivity was 7%; the predictive value of left ventricular (LV) dysfunction (ejection fraction <40%) for sudden cardiac death was 21%, and its sensitivity was 72%. When combining the criteria of reduced LV function and the presence of ventricular late potentials, the sensitivity for predicting sudden cardiac death was 67%, and the predictive value was 21%. Thus the sensitivity of ventricular late potentials in the diagnosis of patients prone to sudden cardiac death was relatively high, whereas the predictive value was disappointingly low, due to the large number of false-positive late potential recordings.

Similar results were obtained by Zimmermann and coworkers,[73] who found ventricular late potentials in 32 of 92 (35%) patients with coronary heart disease. For predicting sudden cardiac death, the detection of ventricular late potentials revealed a high sensitivity (100%) and a predictive value of 19%. The corresponding values of ventricular late potentials for predicting the occurrence of VT/VF were sensitivity = 90%, predictive value = 31%.

Patients with spontaneous, documented VT/VF and those resuscitated from VF represent a special group of high-risk individuals. Ventricular late potentials were detected in 16 of 20 patients with coronary heart disease and documented VT/VF (Fig. 20–7). During the follow-up period of 26 ± 5 months, six patients died (five from sudden cardiac death). The sensitivity of ventricular late potentials for predicting sudden

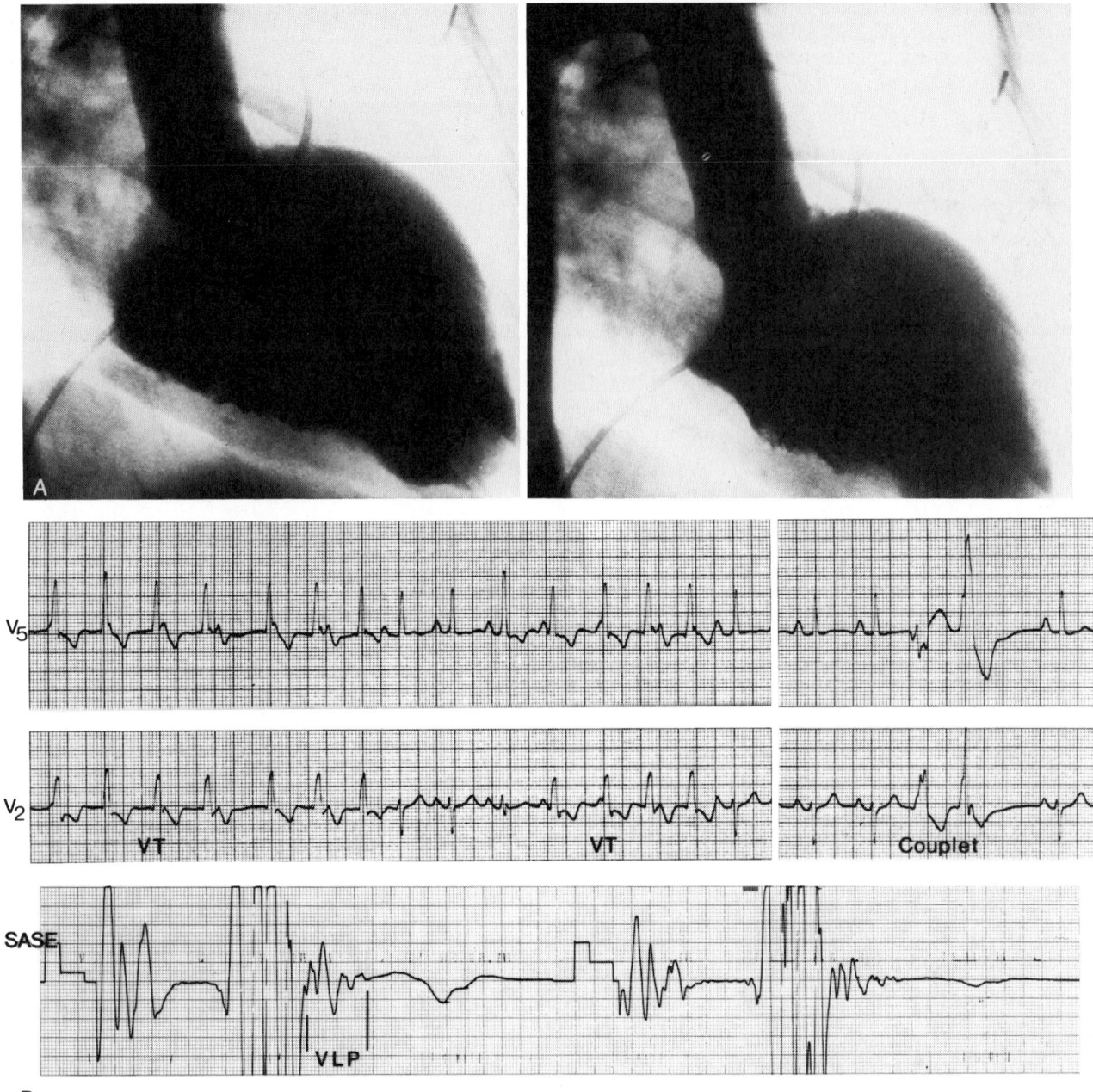

FIGURE 20–7

A, Left ventricular angiogram in a 46-year-old man with large anterior wall myocardial infarction, showing LV silhouette in diastole (top) and in systole (bottom). Note the large aneurysm of the whole anterior wall and of the left ventricular apex.

B, Holter ECG (top) and signal-averaged surface ECG (bottom) in the same patient as in A. Note short runs of ventricular tachycardias (top left), a ventricular couplet (top right) and a large ventricular late potential (VLP) at the end of the QRS complex (bottom). V 5 = thoracic bipolar lead V 5; V 2 = thoracic bipolar lead V 2; VT = ventricular tachycardia; SASE = signal-averaged surface ECG.

cardiac death was 100%, and the predictive value was 31%. Reduced LV ejection fraction (<40%) revealed a sensitivity of 80% and a predictive value of 44% for sudden cardiac death. A combination of three parameters (ventricular late potentials, plus VT/VF during Holter monitoring, plus reduced LV ejection fraction) showed the highest prognostic accuracy: sensitivity = 80%, predictive value = 67%.[37] In a further group of 22 patients with coronary heart disease, who were resuscitated from ventricular fibrillation, 15 (68%) had ventricular late potentials in the signal-averaged ECG. During a follow-up period of 29 ± 8 months, eight patients died (six from sudden cardiac death). The prognostic power of ventricular late potentials for predicting the recurrence of sudden cardiac death was sensitivity = 100%, predictive value = 40%. The corresponding values for a reduced LV ejection fraction (<40%) were sensitivity = 67%, predictive value = 50%. The highest diagnostic accuracy was found by a combination of the presence of ventricular late poten-

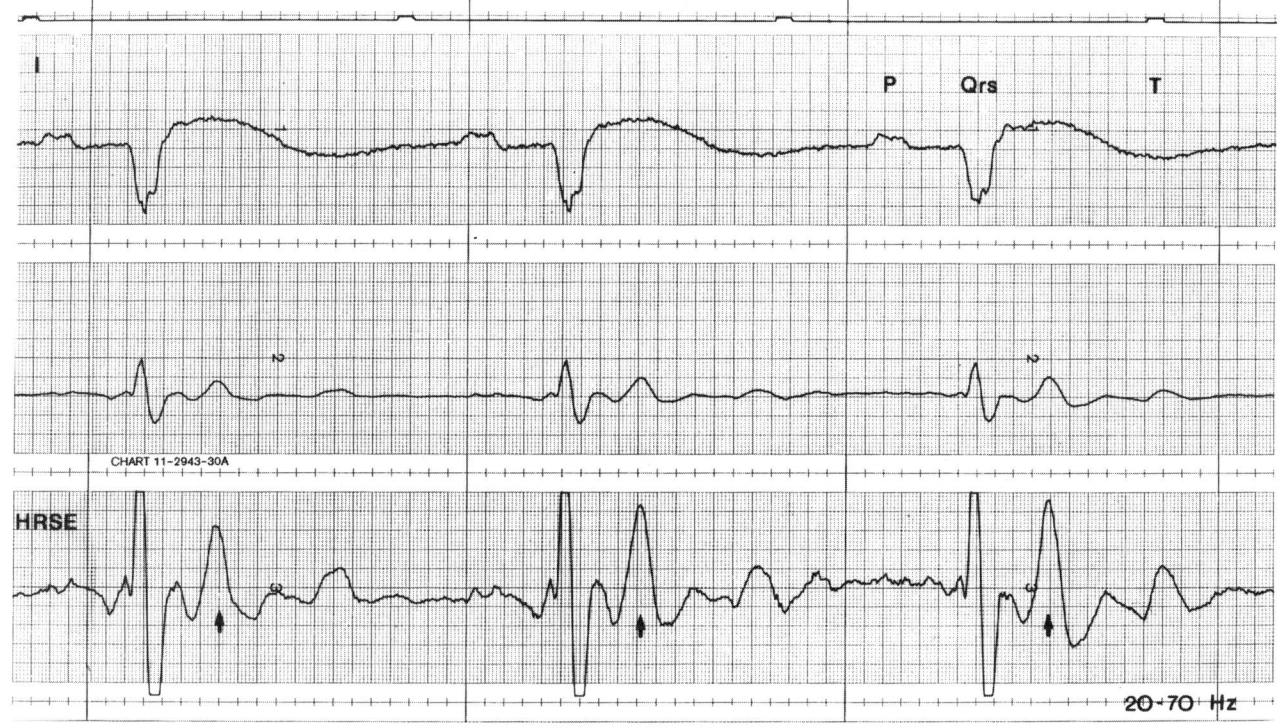

FIGURE 20-8
Continuous recording of the low-noise ECG in a patient with a large anterior wall aneurysm and repetitive attacks of sustained ventricular tachycardias. Note persistent ST segment elevations in Einthoven's lead I (top) as the electrocardiographic sign of aneurysm, and the large ventricular late potentials (arrows) extending to the entire ST segment of the low-noise real-time ECG (bottom). HRSE: High-resolution surface ECG.

tials, reduced LF ejection fraction and a repetitive ventricular response on programmed ventricular stimulation: sensitivity = 50%, predictive value = 100%.[37]

The disappointingly low predictive power of static ventricular late potentials obtained by the signal-averaging technique have stimulated several groups to develop high-resolution ECG equipment that permits continuous recording of ventricular late potentials and, thus, the study of the dynamic properties of ventricular late potentials. El-Sherif and colleagues[20] have pointed out that a Wenckebach conduction pattern in the peri-infarct zone may be the mechanism for initiating reentrant VT/VF. Such dynamic conduction implies a continuously increasing length of post–QRS activation (i.e., of ventricular late potentials that can only be detected by dynamic high-resolution surface ECG technology). Therefore, it is most important to investigate the transition of the last normal ventricular beat to the following single or repetitive ventricular ectopic beat, and to detect the functional role of ventricular late potentials between both. Using a special high-resolution ECG unit, El-Sherif and coworkers reported the following recovery rates of ventricular late potentials: In none of 18 healthy volunteers, in 2 of 20 patients with various cardiac disorders, and in 15 of 21 patients within the first 3 weeks following acute myocardial infarction. Twelve of 15 patients in the last group had episodes of VT/VF, either spontaneously or induced by programmed ventricular stimulation. Ventricular late potentials remained constant in successive sinus beats in 9 of 15 patients, indicating a 1:1 conduction pattern in the ischemic myocardium, and varied in configuration and timing in successive sinus beats in 6 of 15 patients, probably reflecting a Wenckebach conduction pattern.

In our initial study in 1984, we found ventricular late potentials in 12 of 30 patients with cardiac disease: using our own high-resolution ECG equipment (Fig. 20–8), and in 5 of 12 patients, ventricular late potentials occurred intermittently (Fig. 20–9).[47]

In a further expanded series of 44 patients, the incidence and dynamicity of ventricular late potentials was studied by our group.[49] Ventricular late potentials were found in 27 patients within the ST segment and in 21 patients following the T wave. Ventricular late potentials occurred intermittently in 11 of 27 patients within the ST segment, and in 5 of 21 individuals after the T wave. In 1 of 22 patients with single ventricular ectopic beats, a Wenckebach conduction pattern of ventricular late potentials was found (Fig. 20–10), whereas a "focal" type of late potential–ectopic beat interaction was seen in 13 of 22 patients (Fig. 20–11). During episodes of VT, slowly depolarizing diastolic potentials prior to each VT-QRS complex were seen in 3 of 4 patients, and "stressing" of ventricular late potentials by high ventricular rate or programmed pacing was achieved in 9 of 15 patients.

These studies show that ventricular late potentials may reveal dynamic properties during spontaneous sinus rhythm, during episodes of single or repetitive ventricular ectopic activity, and during programmed ventricular stimulation. However, up to now the prog-

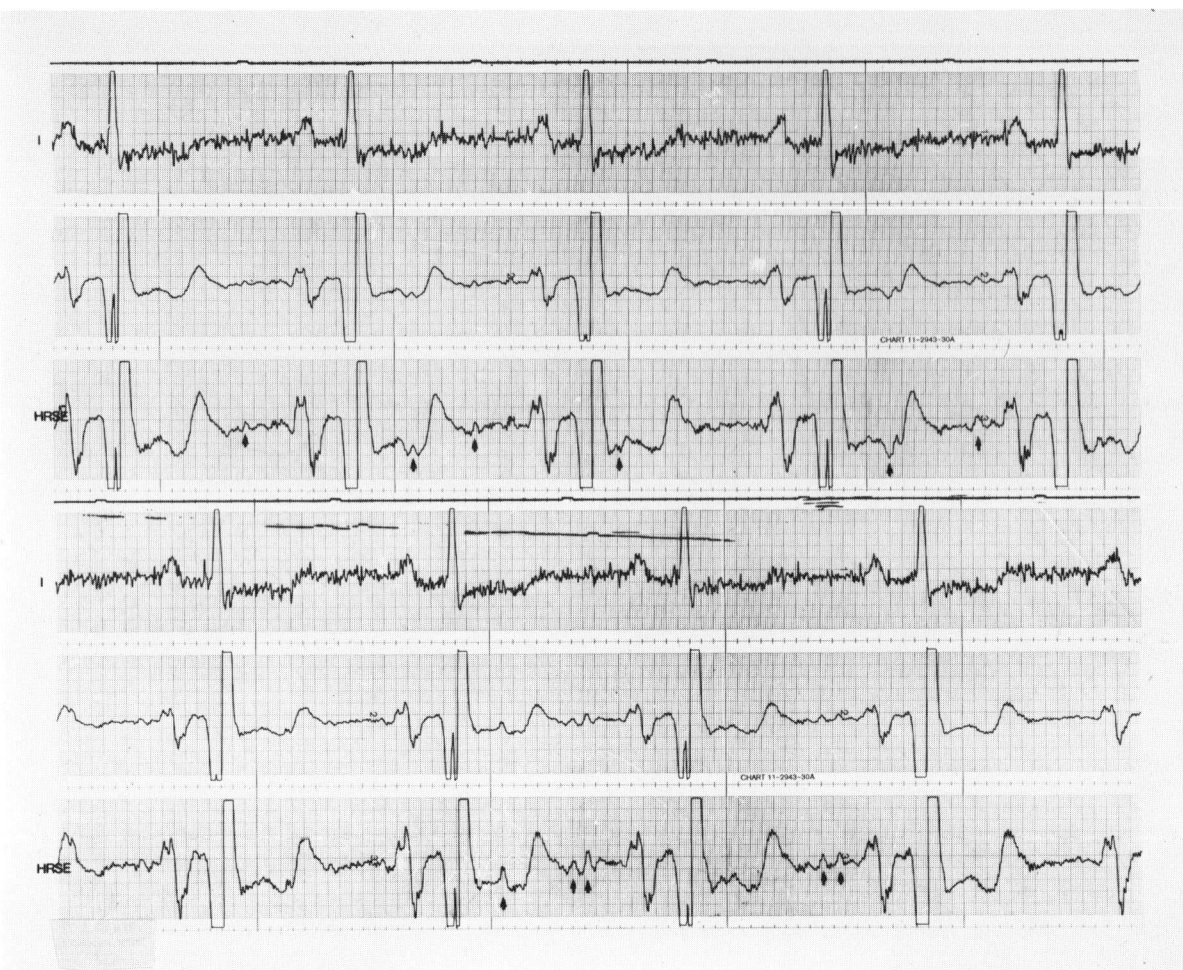

FIGURE 20–9
Einthoven's lead I and the low-noise electrocardiogram (HRSE) in a patient with left ventricular aneurysm and repetitive attacks of ventricular tachycardias. Note the intermittent occurrence of ventricular late potentials with varying timing to the preceding QRS complex and the T wave (arrows). For comparison the last ventricular depolarization (bottom right) does not show any abnormal depolarization within the ST and post-T segment. I = Einthoven lead I; HRSE = high-resolution surface ECG.

nostic significance of such findings has not been studied, although long-term recordings of the high-resolution ECG are now feasible which allow a more comprehensive documentation of the dynamic behavior of ventricular late potentials.[48]

It should be mentioned that, mostly due to dynamic properties of ventricular late potentials, the beat-to-beat technique provides higher detection rates of these potentials than does the signal-averaging technique.[21, 49] This holds particularly true for patients with the congenital long QT syndrome.

Eggeling and coworkers[18] found ventricular late potentials in six of seven patients with the congenital long QT syndrome by means of the high-resolution beat-to-beat technique, but in only three of seven patients with the signal-averaging technique. It is interesting that

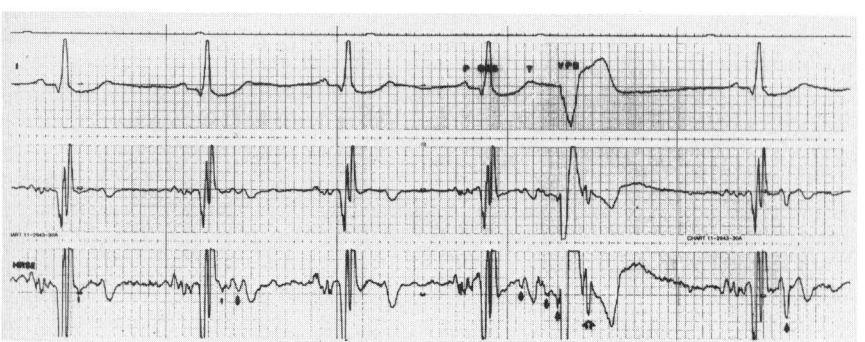

FIGURE 20–10
Low-noise ECG in real-time of a 66-year-old patient with coronary heart disease and single and repetitive ventricular ectopic activity. Note the intermittent, variable occurrence of ventricular late potential (arrows). Following the fourth normal ventricular complex, fractionated activity is seen within the ST and post-T segment, and this fractionation merges into the ventricular ectopic beat, indicating a Wenckebach-type of slowed ventricular conduction with one reentrant cycle. I = Einthoven lead I; HRSE = high-resolution surface ECG; VPB = ventricular premature beat.

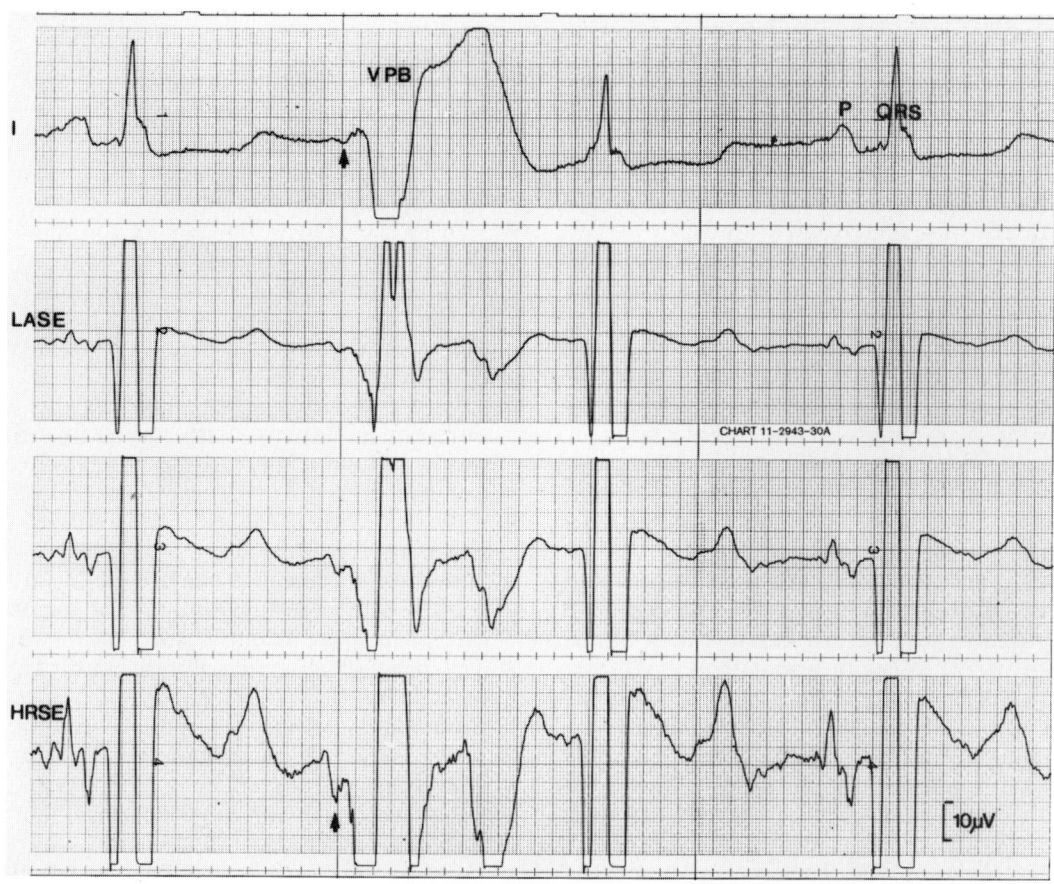

FIGURE 20-11
Low-noise ECG of a 28-year-old man with dilatative cardiomyopathy and repetitive attacks of sustained ventricular tachycardia. Note a single slowly depolarizing potential (arrow), that precedes and merges into the ventricular ectopic beat (VPB), indicating an ectopic type of ventricular premature depolarization. I = Einthoven lead I; LASE = low-amplified surface ECG; HRSE = high-resolution surface ECG.

patients with the long QT syndrome reveal ventricular late potentials not only within the ST segment but also following the T wave, and that these potentials are extremely variable with respect to timing to the QRS complex or to the T wave, amplitudes, and their appearance per se. These parameters may show hour-to hour, day-to-night, or day-to-day variability, depending on the level of sympathetic activity of the individual patient. Moreover, the amplitudes of the post–T wave late potentials in those patients can be enhanced by IV administration of catecholamines and can be diminished by IV beta-blockade (unpublished observations). In our experience, in patients with the long QT syndrome the detection of ventricular late potentials by high-resolution electrocardiography proved to be the most accurate indicator of increased ventricular vulnerability, compared to the spontaneous occurrence of VT during exercise or emotional stress, the spontaneous occurrence of VT during Holter ECG monitoring, and the response to programmed ventricular stimulation.

Ventricular late potentials may also be found in patients with right ventricular outflow tract obstructions, particularly in those with corrected Fallot's tetralogy. In a preliminary study by our group, ventricular late potentials were detected in 26 of 29 patients who were corrected for right ventricular outflow tract obstructions plus ventriculotomy, using the high-resolution surface ECG method. Twenty-three patients were studied both by endocardial right ventricular catheter mapping and by high-resolution electrocardiography; in 21 of these patients, catheter electrograms revealed clear to massive fractionated late potentials within the ST segment and after the T wave, whereas in 22 patients similar fractionated late potentials were seen within the ST segment and the post-T segment of the low-noise ECG. These late potentials correlated well with the spontaneous occurrence of VT in this special group of patients, in whom the prevalence of VT was known to be very high. Thus, ventricular late potentials seem to be a valuable noninvasive marker of right ventricular electrical instability in those patients with surgically corrected right ventricular outflow tract obstructions.

A separate technique has been devised to discover abnormal electrical activity within the ST segment, based on the analysis in the frequency domain by means of the fast Fourier transform analysis (FFTA). Ventricular late potentials within the ST segment represent electrical signals with higher-frequency components than are usually encountered in the normal ST segment. High-gain amplified signal-averaged or single-beat low-noise ECGs may be analyzed by FFTA, using special window functions (e.g., Blackman-Harris window).

Cain and coworkers[15] described a device, that performs FFTA of high-gain amplified signal-averaged X/Y/Z leads for noise reduction. For each ECG segment (e.g., QRS complex, terminal 40 ms of QRS/ST segment, T wave) spectral curves of the X/Y/Z leads are generated, and for quantitative comparison the energy spectra are calculated. Among three parameters of abnormal FFTA findings, the ratio of the area under the curve between 20 Hz and 50 Hz to the area under curve between 0 and 20 Hz was used for defining normal or abnormal frequency contents of the ST-segment. In a group of 20 patients with spontaneous VT, this criterion was compared with the results of programmed ventricular stimulation. A logistic regression, with inducibility of VT as the dependent variable, was used to help define area ratio values greater than 20 as abnormal. Sustained monomorphic VT was induced in 18 patients, each with an area ratio value greater than 20. Sustained VT was not induced in 2 patients, each with an area ratio value less than 20. In a group of 38 patients (12 with nonsustained VT and 26 with syncope), FFTA data were compared prospectively with the results of programmed ventricular stimulation. VT was not inducible in any of the 26 patients in this group with normal FFTA values. Sustained monomorphic VT was induced in 5 of 12 patients with abnormal FFTA values. Thus, the results of FFTA correctly predicted the results of programmed ventricular stimulation in 88% of patients studied and in 82% of patients with syncope or nonsustained VT.[52]

FFTA of single-beat-high resolution ECGs has been reported by Haberl and coworkers[32] and by Oeff and coworkers,[55] with results similar to those of Cain and colleagues.[15] A similar technique has been described by our own group,[49] using FFT analysis of the ST segment in single-beat low-noise ECGs. In a preliminary pilot study on 14 patients with coronary heart disease, 3 patients with sustained VT, 1 patient with ventricular fibrillation, and 4 healthy individuals, FFTA revealed higher-frequency components of the ST segment in the range of 0 to 100 Hz in the 3 VT patients, compared to the CHD patients without VT. Completely concordant results with the three methods (signal-averaged ECG, low-noise real-time ECG, and FFTA) were obtained in 11 of 14 patients (3 patients with VT and late potentials had abnormal FFT results, and 8 patients without VTs had negative results with all three methods). Thus, preliminary data on FFTA of the ST segment suggest that patients prone to VT may be identified by certain characteristics of the frequency components of the ST segment. The prognostic significance of these FFTA findings has not yet been investigated.

SUMMARY AND CONCLUSIONS

- Recordings of ventricular late potentials from body surface represent the most important and clinically relevant application of high-resolution electrocardiography.
- Animal experiments have shown that ventricular late potentials represent slowed conduction within an area of depressed myocardium (mostly following myocardial infarction), thus representing one determinant of a reentrant circuit at the level of ventricular myocardium.
- Ventricular late potentials as the electrical sign of slowed conduction may be detected in humans not only by intracardiac catheter mapping or direct intraoperative mapping but also noninvasively from the body surface by means of the high-resolution ECG technique.
- The prevalence of late potentials is considerably different in patients with various cardiac disorders (e.g., coronary heart disease, dilated cardiomyopathy, hypertrophic obstructive cardiomyopathy, aortic stenosis, long QT syndrome, surgically corrected Fallot's tetralogy).
- Based on numerous correlative clinical studies, ventricular late potentials may be considered a parameter of increased ventricular electrical instability.
- The prognostic power of ventricular late potentials, as detected by the signal-averaging technique, for predicting episodes of VT/VF or sudden cardiac death, seems to be limited.
- The prognostic significance of late potentials may be enhanced if a dynamic Wenckebach conduction pattern can be demonstrated.
- Dynamic properties of ventricular late potentials can be detected only by the low-noise real-time ECG technique. Mainly owing to the variability of timing and amplitudes of ventricular late potentials, the detection rates are higher with the beat-to-beat than with the signal-averaging technique.
- Dynamic changes of ventricular late potentials such as intermittent occurrence and variations in amplitude and timing to the QRS complex or to the T wave may occur during spontaneous sinus rhythm, during episodes of single or repetitive ventricular ectopic beats, and following programmed ventricular stimulation.
- Ventricular late potentials are extremely variable in patients with the congenital long QT syndrome. In these patients, late potentials seem to be the most sensitive parameter of ventricular vulnerability.
- The prognostic significance of the dynamic properties of late potentials, particularly the Wenckebach type of slowed conduction, is as yet unknown.
- Abnormal diastolic electrical activity may also be retrieved by FFT analysis, which detects higher-frequency components within the ST segment than are usually encountered in normal individuals.
- Abnormal results of the FFT analysis seem to correlate well with increased ventricular electrical instability, as documented by spontaneous or induced VT. However, the prognostic significance of abnormal FFT results in predicting sudden cardiac death is as yet unknown.

References

1. Berbari EJ, Lazzara R, Samet P, et al.: Noninvasive technique for detection of electrical activity during the P-R segment. Circulation 48:1005, 1973.
2. Berbari EJ, Scherlag BJ, Lazzara R: Recordings of A-V nodal potentials during junctional rhythms utilizing signal averaging. Am J Physiol 235:110, 1978.
3. Berbari EJ, Scherlag BJ, Hope R, et al.: Recordings from body surface of arrhythmogenic ventricular activity during the ST segment. Am J Cardiol 41:697, 1978.
4. Berbari EJ, Scherlag BJ, El-Sherif N, et al.: The His-Purkinje electrocardiogram in man. Circulation 54:219, 1976.
5. Berbari EJ, Brachmann J, Scherlag BJ, et al.: Recording late depolarization in dogs: Correlation with ventricular arrhythmias. In Hombach V, Hilher HH (eds.): Signal Averaging Technique in Clinical Cardiology, pp. 163–176. Stuttgart, Schattauer Publishers, 1981.
6. Berbari EJ, Scherlag BJ, Lazzara R: Recordings of A-V nodal potentials in dogs with junctional rhythms. In Hombach V, Hilger HH (eds.): Signal Averaging Technique in Clinical Cardiology, pp. 121–130. Stuttgart, Schattauer Publishers, 1981.
7. Berbari EJ: High resolution electrocardiography. Crit Rev Biomed Eng 16:67–103, 1988.
8. Billhardt RA, Mayerhofer KE, Uretz EF, et al.: Serial signal averaged ECGs in acute myocardial infarction patients. Circulation 72:III-213, 1985.
9. Boineaux JP, Cox JL: Slow ventricular activation in acute myocardial infarction. A source of reentrant premature ventricular contractions. Circulation 48:702, 1973.
10. Bonke FIM: Electrophysiology of the sinus node. In Hombach V, Hilger HH (eds.): Signal Averaging Technique in Clinical Cardiology, pp. 23–32. Stuttgart, Schattauer Publishers, 1981.
11. Braun V, Hombach V, Höpp HW, et al.: Preatrial activity recorded from intracardiac and surface leads by signal averaging. In Hombach V, Hilger HH (eds.): Signal Averaging Technique in Clinical Cardiology, pp. 81–94. Stuttgart, Schattauer-Publishers, 1981.
12. Breithardt G, Becker R, Seipel L, et al.: Noninvasive detection of late potentials in man—a new marker for ventricular tachycardias. Eur Heart J 2:1, 1981.
13. Breithardt G, Boggrefe M: Pathophysiological mechanisms and clinical significance of ventricular late potentials. Eur Heart J 7:364, 1986.
14. Breithardt G, Boggrefe M, Haerten K, et al.: Prognostische Bedeutung ventrikulärer Spätpotentiale bei Postinfarktpatienten und Patienten mit stabiler koronarer Herzkarnkheit. In Steinbeck G (ed.): Lebensbedrohliche Ventrikuläre Herzrhythmusstörungen, pp. 93–99. Darmstadt, Steinkopff Publishers, 1987.
15. Cain ME, Ambos HD, Witkowski FX, et al.: Fast-Fourier transform analysis of signal-averaged electrocardiograms for identification of patients prone to sustained ventricular tachycardia. Circulation 69:711, 1984.
16. Denniss A, Richards D, Cody D, et al.: Prognostic significance of ventricular tachycardia and fibrillation induced at programmed stimulation and delayed potentials detected on signal-averaged electrocardiograms of survivors of acute myocardial infarction. Circulation 74:731, 1986.
17. Durrer D, Van Lier A, Buller J: Epicardial and intramural excitation in chronic myocardial infarction. Am Heart J 68:765, 1964.
18. Eggeling T, Höpp HW, Schickendantz S, et al.: Diastolic microvolt potentials within the high resolution surface ECG in long QT syndrome. Z Kardiol 75:410, 1986.
19. El-Sherif N, Mehra R, Gomes JAC, et al.: Appraisal of a low noise electrocardiogram. J Am Coll Cardiol 1:456, 1983.
20. El-Sherif N, Gomes JAC, Restivo M, et al.: Late potentials and arrhythmogenesis. PACE 8:440, 1985.
21. El-Sherif N, Restivo M, Craelius W, et al.: High resolution electrocardiography—Basic and clinical aspects. In Hombach V, Hilger HH, Kennedy HL (eds.): Electrocardiography and Cardiac Drug Therapy, pp. 395–410. Dordrecht, Kluwer Academic Publishers, 1988.
21a. El-Sherif N, Ursell SN, Bekheit S, et al.: Prognostic significance of the signal-average ECG depends on the time of recording in the postinfarction period. Am Heart J 118:256, 1989.
22. Erlanger J, Blackman JR: A study of the relative rhythmicity and conductivity in various regions of the auricles of the mammalian heart. Am J Physiol 19:125, 1907.
23. Flowers NC, Horan LG: His bundle and bundle-branch recordings from the body surface. Circulation 48:IV-102, 1973.
24. Flowers NC, Shvartsman V, Sohi GS, et al.: Signal averaged versus beat-by-beat recording of surface His-Purkinje potentials. In Hombach V, Hilger HH (eds.): Signal Averaging Technique in Clinical Cardiology, pp. 329–349. Stuttgart, Schattauer Publishers, 1981.
25. Fontaine G, Guiraudon G, Frank R: Intramyocardial conduction defects in patients prone to ventricular tachycardia. III. The post-excitation syndrome in ventricular tachycardia. In Sandøe E, Julian DG, Bell JW (eds.): Management of ventricular tachycardia—Role of mexiletine, pp. 67–69. Amsterdam, Excerpta Medica, 1978.
26. Fontaine G, Pierefitte M, Tonet JL, et al.: Interpretation of afterpotentials registered from epicardium, endocardium and body surface in patients with chronic ventricular tachycardia. In Hombach V, Hilger HH (eds.): Signal Averaging Technique in Clinical Cardiology, pp. 175–203. Stuttgart, Schattauer Publishers, 1981.
27. Furness A, Sharratt GP, Carson P: The feasibility of detecting His bundle activity from the body surface. Cardiovasc Res 9:390, 1975.
28. Gebhardt-Seehausen U, Bethge C, Bonke FIM, et al.: Continuous recordings of sinus nodal potentials. In Hombach V, Hilger HH (eds.): Signal Averaging Technique in Clinical Cardiology, pp. 41–52. Stuttgart, Schattauer Publishers, 1981.
29. Goedel-Meinen L, Schmidt G, Jahns G, et al.: Spätpotentiale in den ersten 10 Tagen nach Myokardinfarkt. Z Kardiol 75:121, 1986.
30. Gomes J, Winters SL, Stewart D, et al.: A new noninvasive index to predict sustained ventricular tachycardia and sudden death in the first year after myocardial infarction based on signal-averaged electrocardiogram, radionuclide ejection fraction and Holter monitoring. J Am Coll Cardiol 2:349, 1987.
31. Grigg LE, Chan W, Hamer A, et al.: Correlation between electrophysiological studies, Holter recordings, and signal averaged ECGs in the post-infarction period. Circulation 76:IV-32, 1987.
32. Haberl R, Pulter R, Steinbeck G: Einzelschlaganalyse des Frequenzinhaltes von Spätpotentialen von der Körperoberfläche bei Patienten mit koronarer Herzkrankheit. Z Kardiol 75-4:98, 1986.
33. Haberl R, Steinbeck G: Frequenzanalyse von Einzelschlagelektrokardiogrammen zur Diagnostik von Kammertachykardien bei Patienten mit koronarer Herzkrankheit. In Steinbeck G (ed.): Lebensbedrohliche Ventrikuläre Herzrhythmusstörungen, pp. 123–127. Darmstadt, Steinkopff Publishers, 1987.
34. Heinecker R: Klinische Elektrokardiographie. Stuttgart, Thieme Publishers, 1986.
35. Hishimoto Y, Sawayama T: Non-invasive recording of His bundle potential in man—simplified method. Brit Heart J 37:635, 1975.
36. Höpp HW, Hombach V, Braun V, et al.: Ventricular delayed depolarisations in patients with chronic stable coronary heart disease and with acute myocardial infarction. In Hombach V, Hilger HH (eds.): Signal Averaging Technique in Clinical Cardiology, pp. 233–252. Stuttgart, Schattauer Publishers, 1981.
37. Höpp HW: Der Plötzliche Herztod—Pathophysiologie und Klinik bei koronarer Herzerkrankung. Stuttgart, Schattauer Publishers, 1987.
38. Höpp HW, Treis-Müller I, Osterspey A, et al.: Ventricular late potentials in acute myocardial infarction. Herz 13:169, 1988.
39. Hombach V, Zanker R, Behrenbeck DW, et al.: Recording of sinus node potentials in man. Z Kardiol 67:155, 1978.
40. Hombach V, Gil-Sanchez D, Zanker R, et al.: An approach to direct detection of sinus nodal activity in man. J Electrocardiol 12:343, 1979.
41. Hombach V, Höpp HW, Braun V, et al.: Significance of post-excitation potentials within the ST segment in the surface ECG of patients with coronary heart disease. Dtsch Med Wochenschr 105:1457, 1980.
42. Hombach V, Höpp HW, Braun V, et al.: Pre-P-potentials in the conventional body surface ECG. Dtsch Med Wochenschr 106:771, 1981.

43. Hombach V, Braun V, Höpp HW, et al.: Recordings of A-V nodal potentials in man using the signal averaging technique. *In* Hombach V, Hilger HH (eds.): Signal Averaging Technique in Clinical Cardiology, pp. 131–144. Stuttgart, Schattauer Publishers, 1981.
44. Hombach V, Braun V, Höpp HW, et al.: Noninvasive detection of potentials of the bundle of His from the body surface. Münch Med Wochenschr 123:173, 1981.
45. Hombach V, Braun V, Höpp HW, et al.: The applicability of the signal averaging technique in clinical cardiology. Clin Cardiol 5:107, 1982.
46. Hombach V, Kebbel U, Höpp HW, et al.: Continuous registration of micropotentials of the human heart: Preliminary results with a new high resolution ECG-amplifier system. Dtsch Med Wochenschr 107:1951, 1982.
47. Hombach V, Kebbel U, Höpp HW, et al.: Noninvasive beat-by-beat registration of ventricular late potentials using high resolution electrocardiography. Int J Cardiol 6:167, 1984.
48. Hombach V, Kebbel U, Höpp HW, et al.: Longterm recording of the low noise ECG from body surface—technical development and clinical significance. Herz 13:147, 1988.
49. Hombach V, Eggeling T, Höher M, et al.: Methods for detection of ventricular late potentials—high resolution ECG, signal averaging technique, frequency analysis, intracardiac mapping. Herz 13:147, 1988.
50. Honda N, Tanaka S, Kohno N, et al.: Clinical studies on noninvasive investigation of the His bundle electrogram. Proc VIth Int Symp Card Pac, pp. 19–25. Amsterdam, Excerpta Medica, 1977.
51. Josephson ME, Horowitz LN, Spielman SR, et al.: Role of catheter mapping in the preoperative evaluation of ventricular tachycardia. Am J Cardiol 49:207, 1982.
51a. Kuchar D, Thorburn C, Sammel N: Late potentials after myocardial infarction: Natural history and prognostic significance. Circulation 74:1280, 1986.
52. Lindsay BD, Ambos HD, Schechtman KB, et al.: Improved selection of patients for programmed ventricular stimulation by frequency analysis of signal-averaged electrocardiograms. Circulation 73:675, 1986.
53. Mackintosh AF, English MJ, Vincent R, et al.: Low-voltage electrical activity preceding right atrial depolarisation in man. Brit Heart J 42:117, 1979.
54. McKenna WJ, Rowland E, Mortara D, et al.: Non-invasive recording of the His bundle electrogram: Evaluation of the Marquette high resolution MAC unit. *In* Hombach V, Hilger HH (eds.): Signal Averaging Technique in Clinical Cardiology, pp. 301–310. Stuttgart, Schattauer Publishers, 1981.
55. Oeff M; Einzelschlagregistrierung verspäteter ventrikulärer Depolarisationen und ihre Frequenzanalyse mit der Fast-Fourier-Transformation-Methodische Aspekte. *In* Steinbeck G (ed.): Lebensbedrohliche Ventrikuläre Herzrhythmusstörungen, pp. 129–135. Darmstadt, Steinkopff Publishers, 1987.
56. Pernod J, Court L, Duret JC, et al.: Possibilité de détection des potentiels hisiens à partir d'electrodes thoraciques de surface. Nouv Presse Med 6:2963, 1977.
57. Potratz J, Djonlagic H, Mentzel H, et al.: Verlaufbeobachtung von Spätpotentialen bei akuten Infarktpatienten innerhalb der ersten drei Wochen. Herz/Kreisl 8:397, 1985.
58. Simson MB: Identification of patients with ventricular tachycardia after myocardial infarction from signals in the terminal QRS complex. Circulation 64:235, 1981.
59. Simson MB: Signalmittelung des Oberflächen-Elektrokardiogramms zur Erkennung von Spätpotentialen. *In* Steinbeck G (ed.): Lebensbedrohliche ventrikuläre Herzrhythmusstörungen, pp. 85–92. Darmstadt, Steinkopff Publishers, 1987.
60. Steinbeck G, Haberl R, Lüderitz B, et al.: Comparison of true and calculated sinoatrial conduction time by atrial pacing in the isolated rabbit heart. *In* Hombach V, Hilger HH (eds.): Signal Averaging Technique in Clinical Cardiology, pp. 33–39. Stuttgart, Schattauer Publishers, 1981.
61. Stopczyk MJ, Kopec J, Zochowski RJ, et al.: Surface recording of electrical heart activity during the P-R segment in man by a computer averaging technique. Int Res Com Syst 1973, 73–8, 11, 21–2.
62. Stopczyk MJ, Pieniak M, Wajszczuk W, et al.: Sinus node activity in man and animal studies recorded intraatrially by on-line pre-memorized averaging technique. Proc Vth Int Symp Card Pac, pp. 13–18. Amsterdam, Excerpta Medica, 1976.
63. Stopczyk MJ, Walczak F, Kepski R, et al.: The history of noninvasive His-bundle recording: From averaging to continuous record. *In* Hombach V, Hilger HH (eds.): Signal Averaging Technique in Clinical Cardiology, pp. 283–289. Stuttgart, Schattauer Publishers, 1981.
64. Takeda H, Kitamura K, Takamashi T, et al.: Non-invasive recording of His-purkinje activity in patients with complete atrioventricular block. Clinical application of an "automated discrimination circuit." Circulation 60:421, 1979.
65. Takeda H, Kitamura K, Tsujimura T, et al.: Non-invasive localization of A-V block by an "automated discrimination circuit." *In* Hombach V, Hilger HH (eds.): Signal Averaging Technique in Clinical Cardiology, pp. 311–327. Stuttgart, Schattauer Publishers, 1981.
66. Tonkin AM, Blood RJ, Riggs AR, et al.: Non-invasive recording of His-bundle potentials: Limitations of existing signal averaging techniques. *In* Hombach V, Hilger HH (eds.): Signal Averaging Technique in Clinical Cardlology, pp. 291–299, Stuttgart, Schattauer Publishers, 1981.
67. Tournoux B, Poindessault JP, Gargouil YM, et al.: Intérêt et limites de l'enregistrement des potentiels du fasceau de His par voie externe chez l'homme. Ann Cardiol Angeiol 29:327, 1980.
68. Van den Akker TJ, Goovaerts HG, Schneider H: Realtime method for noninvasive recording of His bundle activity of the electrocardiogram. Comp Biomed Res 9:559, 1976.
69. Vincent R, Stroud NP, Jenner R, et al.: Noninvasive recording of electrical activity in the PR segment in man. Brit Heart J 40:124, 1978.
70. Vincent R, English MJ, Woollons DJ, et al.: Surface His bundle potentials and other low amplitude cardiac signals by signal averaging. *In* Hombach V, Hilger HH (eds.): Signal Averaging Technique in Clinical Cardiology, pp. 351–362. Stuttgart, Schattauer Publishers, 1981.
71. Wajszczuk WJ, Stopczyk MJ, Moskowitz MS, et al.: Noninvasive recording of His-Purkinje activity in man by QRS-triggered signal averaging. Circulation 58:95, 1978.
72. Wajszczuk WJ, Palko T, Przybylski J, et al.: External recording of sinus node region activity in animals and in man. *In* Hombach V, Hilger HH (eds.): Signal Averaging Technique in Clinical Cardiology, pp. 65–79. Stuttgart, Schattauer Publishers, 1981.
73. Zimmermann M, Adamec R, Simonin P, et al.: Prognostic significance of ventricular late potentials in coronary artery disease. Am Heart J 109:725, 1985.

21

Ventricular Late Potentials: Clinical Aspects

Günter Breithardt
Martin Borggrefe
Antoni Martínez-Rubio

For many years, signal averaging has been used to detect low-amplitude signals from the body surface using high-gain amplification and subsequent signal averaging to reduce randomly occurring noise. Low-amplitude signals that appear at the end of and after the QRS complex within the ST segment have been called "ventricular late potentials" (LP) (Fig. 21-1). They originate from areas of previous myocardial infarction that may leave a zone of electrically abnormal ventricular myocardium as a potential site of origin for ventricular tachycardia (VT).[1-6] This tissue is normally located at the border zone of the previous infarction and is characterized by islands of relatively viable muscle alternating with areas of necrosis and later fibrosis. Such tissue may result in fragmentation of the propagating electromotive forces, owing to slow asynchronous conduction, with the consequent development of high-frequency components that can be recorded directly from these areas.[7-15] Regional slow conduction alone, obviously, is not sufficient to cause fragmented activity.[13, 14] Highly fractionated electrograms occurred only in preparations of chronic infarcts, with interstitial fibrosis forming insulating boundaries between muscle bundles. The individual components of fragmented electrograms, therefore, most probably represent asynchronous electrical activity in each of the separate bundles of surviving muscle under the electrode. The slow activation might result from conduction over circuitous pathways caused by the separation and distortion of the myocardial fiber bundles. The low amplitude of the electrograms from these regions probably results from the paucity of surviving muscle fibers under the electrode because of the large amount of connective tissue, and not from depression of the action potentials.[13, 14]

Prolonged, fractionated electrograms recorded in these regions reflect a slow, dissociated conduction that may cause an increase in the duration of the local electrogram, whereas the intrinsic activation time of the local electrogram may be normal, as the time required for an impulse to conduct through the remaining myocardium to that site may not be altered. The prolonged duration of the local electrogram depends on the impulse traversing the immediate field of view of a local recording electrode, and thus reflects more local conduction characteristics.[15] Local fractionated low-amplitude activity may extend beyond normal ventricular activation into the ST segment of the surface electrocardiogram (ECG). Fragmented electrograms possibly may be found wherever myocardial fibers are separated by connective tissue, even if reentry does not occur in this region.[16]

The areas from which ventricular late potentials can be recorded have been considered the "arrhythmogenic electrophysiologic substrate" for reentrant VT. The presence of an arrhythmogenic electrophysiologic substrate in the form of regional slow ventricular activation is, however, not sufficient to develop VT. Instead, some additional factor (such as ventricular ectopic beats) is necessary to initiate reentrant VT by triggering the arrhythmogenic substrate. Once initiated, reentrant VT may perpetuate itself within the reentrant circuit if the conditions are adequate.

A zone with arrhythmogenic properties may arise acutely (and be present only transiently) or it may exist chronically in the form of myocardium interspersed with fibrosis after a previous myocardial infarction. The classic example of an acutely developing arrhythmogenic tissue leading to ventricular tachyarrhythmias is acute myocardial infarction that is frequently accompanied by ventricular fibrillation (VF). The changes that occur in this situation are frequently transient in nature and may subside as soon as the tissue is completely necrotic. In contrast, strands of surviving myo-

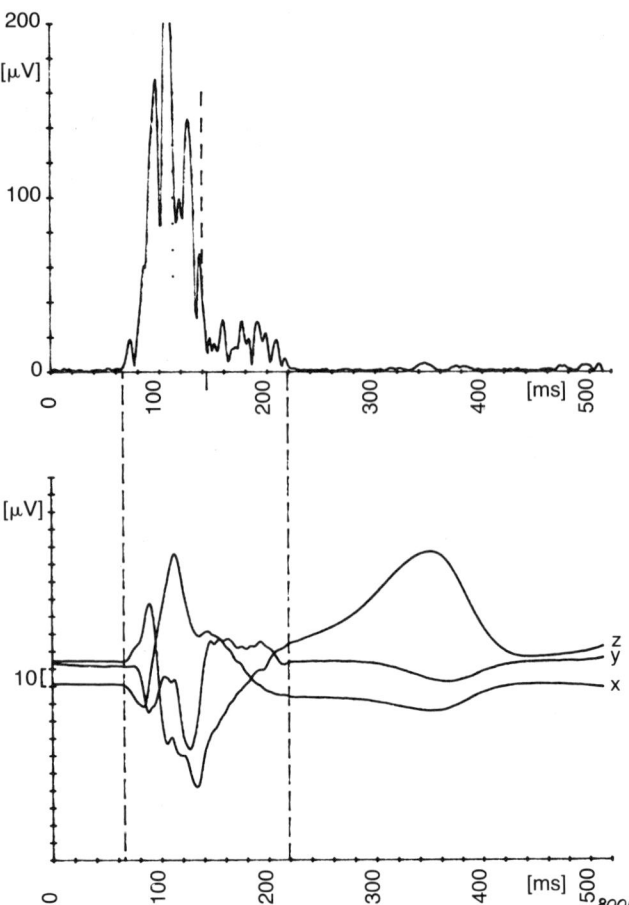

FIGURE 21–1
Signal-averaged and filtered recording of leads X, Y, and Z (vector magnitude) using the software of M. Simson in a patient with ventricular tachycardia. QRS duration in the highly amplified recording was 153 ms. The program automatically identified the end of the total QRS complex at 219 ms on the x-axis. The amplitude in the terminal 40 ms was low (V(40) = 16.69 µV), which was automatically measured by the program. Additionally, the onset of low-amplitude activity was automatically identified at 66 ms on the horizontal axis by the automatic recognition program. The latter program additionally measured the mean voltage of the late potential (V(LP) = 17.49 µV), the maximal voltage of the late potential (V_{max}(LP) = 29.76 µV), and the mean voltage of the true QRS complex (V(QRS) = 115.33 µV). (Modified from Simson MB. Circulation 64:235, 1981; and Karbenn U, Breithardt G, Borggrefe M, et al.: J Electrocardiol 18:123, 1985.)

mapping in patients with VT.[3,5] The amplitude of these potentials is in the low millivolt range even if direct recordings are used. With conventional methods of ECG recording, these signals therefore cannot be recovered from the body surface except in very rare cases.[18,19] However, they can be recorded from the body surface by the use of high-gain amplification, signal filtering and computer-averaging techniques, as was shown for the first time by Berbari et al.[20] in experimental animal studies, and by Fontaine et al.[1] in patients with idiopathic VT. Subsequently, Simson,[21] Rozanski et al.,[22] Breithardt et al.,[23] and Hombach et al.[24] presented their initial experience in patients with ventricular tachyarrhythmias. Since then a great number of clinical studies, mostly in patients with documented VT, have been published using the signal-averaging technique in the time domain[1,20–27] as well as in the frequency domain.[28–30]

The amplitude of ventricular late potentials on the body surface normally is smaller than the electrical noise produced by various sources.[31] Therefore, besides careful shielding of all cables and the use of preamplifiers with a very high signal-to-noise ratio, signal-averaging is used to eliminate the remaining random noise. This technique is applicable only to repetitive electrocardiographic signals and cannot detect moment-to-moment dynamic changes of the signal. (A more detailed review on the basic principles is presented in Chapter 19).

In principle, three different approaches have been used in patients for detection of ventricular late potentials (Fig. 21–2): (1) signal averaging in the time domain, (2) spatial averaging on a beat-to-beat basis, and (3) signal averaging in the frequency domain.

SIGNAL AVERAGING IN THE TIME DOMAIN ■ This approach[21–24,32–34] is based on high-gain amplification, band-pass filtering, and signal averaging of a given number of identical beats to eliminate random noise and to improve the signal-to-noise ratio (Fig. 21–3). One of the prerequisites for signal averaging is that the timing and morphology of late potentials is identical for beats of similar QRS morphology. Whether this is correct is still unsettled. Variation of the timing and configuration of ventricular late potentials may occur on a beat-to-beat basis and may thus cause progressive attenuation during the averaging process. Another

cardial fibers surrounded by fibrous tissue may develop during the healing phase of myocardial infarction and may persist chronically, even for many years.[15] A more detailed discussion of the pathophysiologic mechanisms of ventricular late potentials has previously been presented.[17]

Techniques to Detect Late Potentials

Delayed and fractionated potentials have been observed during intraoperative epicardial and endocardial mapping[1,2,4,6] as well as during endocardial catheter

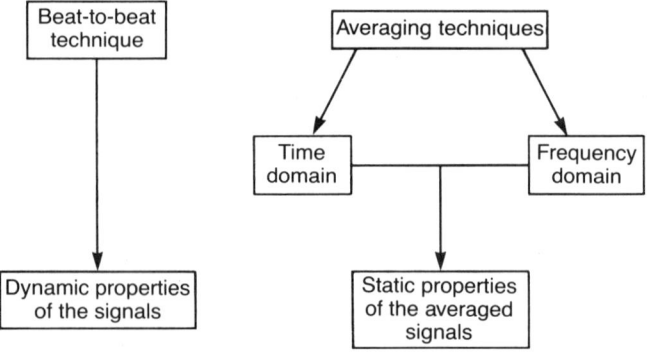

FIGURE 21–2
Noninvasive techniques for detecting low potentials.

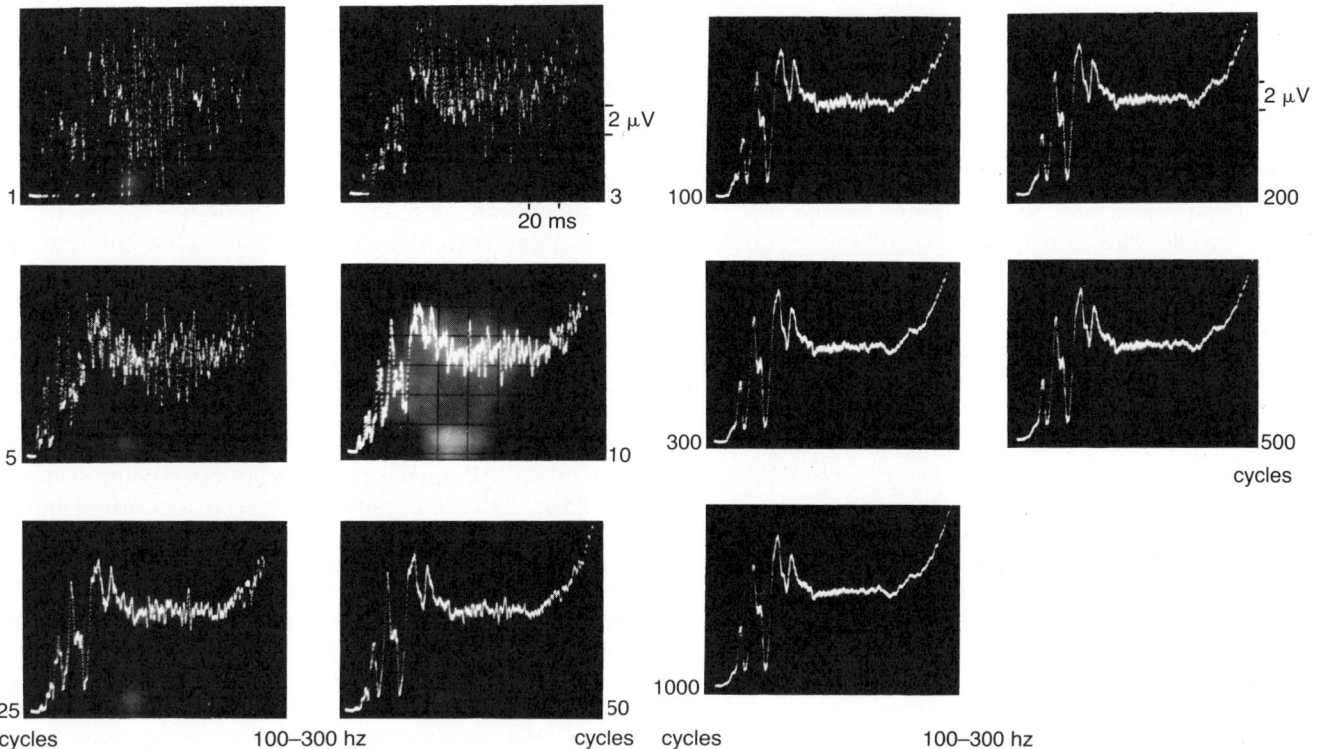

FIGURE 21–3
Improvement in the signal-to-noise ratio with evolution of the final signal during the averaging process with increasing number of cardiac cycles (from 1 to 1000 cycles) in a patient with a left ventricular aneurysm and a history of sustained ventricular tachycardia. A circumscribed high frequency activity represents a late potential shortly after the QRS complex.

problem is instability (jitter) of the trigger point for the QRS complex, which also may attenuate the signals and act as a low-pass filter. This is a limitation of signal averaging not only in the time domain but also in the frequency domain. In previous studies, values for the instability of the trigger point of QRS (jitter) between 0.5 to 2.0 ms have been reported.[20–23, 27, 28, 33, 35, 36]

For better identification of late potentials, elimination of low-frequency components of the signal is mandatory. This prevents the ST segment from saturating at extremely high amplifications and excludes respiratory movements. Depending on the characteristics of the filters, high-pass cut-off points between 25 and 100 Hz have been suggested.[21, 23, 33, 37, 38] Filter ringing after an abrupt transient in the voltage of the signal, especially if short high-pass filters are used,[39] represents a major problem with conventional filters. To prevent filter ringing, either filters with flat characteristics should be used or the signal should be analyzed retrogradely, as suggested by Simson.[21] In the latter approach, a bidirectional filter is used that first processes forward in time up to 40 ms into the QRS complex and then backward in time up to the same point within the QRS complex.

Reproducibility of signal averaging in the time domain depends on interobserver and day-to-day variability. The major factors responsible for this variability are the electrode position, noise level, stability of the triggering of QRS, stability of the cardiac status and medication, use of identical criteria to judge the onset and offset of QRS, and of the terminal low-voltage portion. Available evidence suggests that day-to-day reproducibility is high, with a high percentage of patients (>90%) still having late potentials detectable at a second recording, provided that no change in clinical status has occurred.[21, 23, 32, 33, 40]

SPATIAL AVERAGING ■ Spatial averaging has been used on a beat-to-beat basis to reduce the level of noise by electronic summation of potentials recorded from multiple pairs of electrodes.[32, 34, 41] This approach assumes that the signals developed between any pair of electrodes are almost identical, whereas the noise from electromyographic sources, electrode-tissue interface, and amplifiers are not completely correlated. Using a specially designed volume conductor electrode with 16 pairs of electrodes, noise could be reduced to 1.0 to 1.4 μV.[41] Others have used especially shielded rooms to reduce interference from external sources, mainly alternating current.[32, 37] (For a more detailed review of this technique, refer to Chapters 19 and 20.)

SIGNAL AVERAGING IN THE FREQUENCY DOMAIN ■
Besides signal averaging in the time domain,[21–24, 33, 34, 40] signal averaging in the frequency domain, using fast Fourier transform analysis (FFTA) has been suggested as an alternative approach by Cain et al.[28, 29] to circumvent the limitations of signal averaging in the time domain (such as filter ringing or attenuation of the signal by filtering). Signals are processed for their frequency content (frequency domain) by analyzing all signals for higher sinusoidal components (harmonics) in relation to the sinusoidal component with the lowest frequency. All harmonics have frequencies that are

integer multiples of the fundamental frequencies. FFTA for a discrete sample of a periodic waveform, such as the terminal portion of the QRS complex, is based on the assumption that the signal is a repetitive function and that the initial and final sample points are at a potential of zero. If this is not the case, a sharp-edged discontinuity would be introduced between the end of one cycle and the beginning of the next that would artifactually add both high and low frequencies to the original signal. To eliminate this source of harmonic error, time-domain samples are multiplied by a window function (e.g. the four-term Blackman-Harris window,[28]), which smoothes the initial and final sampling points to zero at the boundaries, allowing periodic extension of the finite signal.[42] This window function reduces spectral leakage owing to edge discontinuities associated with analysis of a discrete subset of the complex periodic waveform.

Haberl and colleagues[30] recently reported on the use of FFTA to perform a single-beat analysis of the total and terminal QRS and ST segment after high-gain low-noise amplification (0–300 Hz).

INCIDENCE OF LATE POTENTIALS IN PATIENTS WITH DOCUMENTED VENTRICULAR TACHYCARDIA

Ventricular late potentials have rarely been detected in subjects with normal left ventricular function.[21, 24, 36, 43–48] This is in contrast to patients with previously documented sustained VT and/or VF (outside the acute phase of myocardial infarction), in whom there is a high incidence of ventricular late potentials (see Fig. 21–1).[21–23, 36, 48–51] We previously reported that 54 of 63 patients (71%) with documented sustained VT/VF had ventricular late potentials of any duration. The proportion of patients with late potentials increased to 37 of 47 patients (79%) if only patients with coronary artery disease were considered.[36] Simson,[21] who was the first to use an algorithm for quantification of the terminal portion of the QRS complex, reported that patients with sustained VT had a low-amplitude signal in the last 40 ms of the filtered QRS complex that was not detectable in the filtered output from patients without VT. He found that the voltage in the last 40 ms of the filtered QRS complex was able to discriminate well between patients with and without VT. Patients with VT had 15 ± 14.4 μV of high-frequency signals in this segment; in contrast, patients without VT had 74 ± 77.7 μV (p< 0.0001). 25 μV was the best threshold to discriminate patients with and without VT.[21] Only three of 39 patients (8%) with VT exceeded 25 μV. The filtered QRS voltage tended to be lower in patients with VT than in those without (103 ± 30 vs. 127 ± 43 μV; non-significant). The QRS duration was longer in patients with VT than in those without VT (139 ± 26 vs. 95 ± 10 ms; p < 0.0001). Freedman et al.,[49] who used a similar methodology, found late potentials in 33 of 53 patients (62%) with ventricular tachycardia. Kanovsky and coworkers[51] studied 174 patients after myocardial infarction; 89 of these patients had recurrent sustained VT. By multivariate logistic regression analyses, the signal-averaged ECG, peak premature ventricular contractions >100 per hour, and the presence of a left ventricular aneurysm were found to be independently significant. Patients with nonsustained VT in whom sustained VT can be induced by programmed ventricular stimulation also have been shown to have a significantly higher incidence of late potentials (67%) than patients without inducible, sustained VT (25%).[52] The filtered QRS duration was also longer (127 vs. 100 ms).[52] Similar to patients with VT after myocardial infarction, patients with congestive cardiomyopathy with a history of sustained VT had a significantly greater incidence of late potentials and a longer QRS duration than those without VT.[53]

Using FFTA, it has been shown that patients with sustained VT have a higher-frequency content in their terminal QRS complex, compared to normal individuals.[28–30] Cain et al.[28] demonstrated an increase in the amplitude of high-frequency components in the terminal QRS in 88% of patients with sustained VT, in contrast to 15% in patients without VT. In a subsequent report, these authors[29] studied 87 patients (23 patients with and 53 patients without VT after myocardial infarction, as well as 11 normal subjects) in whom the terminal 40 ms of the QRS complex and the ST segment were analyzed as a single unit to enhance the frequency resolution. The terminal QRS and ST segment from patients with sustained VT contained 10- to 100-fold greater amplitudes of components in the 20- to 50-Hz range, compared to corresponding electrocardiographic segments in patients without sustained VT. There were no significant differences in the peak frequencies among the patient groups; however, the relative contribution of the magnitudes of these peak frequencies to the overall magnitude of the spectral plot differed significantly. No frequencies above 50 Hz contributed substantially to the energy spectra of the terminal QRS and ST segments in any group.

Similar results have been reported by Haberl et al.[54] using spectral analysis of single beats. The frequency content of the terminal QRS complex, expressed as area under the spectral plot, was significantly lower in patients with VT than in patients without any arrhythmias (p <0.01). Additionally, the frequency content of the ST segment in the range 10 to 40 Hz was higher in patients with VT than in patients without arrhythmias and in control subjects (p <0.01). Thus, spectral analysis of single-beat ECGs is promising for the noninvasive identification of patients prone to sustained VT owing to coronary artery disease.

Presently, it remains unclear whether FFTA is superior to signal averaging in the time domain. Both methods were assessed in 54 subjects comprising 26 patients with sustained VT, 18 control patients with organic heart disease but without sustained VT, and 11 normal volunteers.[55] Time domain analysis was performed with high-pass filtering of 25, 40, and 80 Hz and low-pass filtering of 250 Hz. Frequency-domain analysis was performed on the terminal 40 ms of the QRS complex, either alone or with 216 or 150 ms of the ST segment. Absolute summed energies of discrete frequency bands and band energy ratios were calculated. Frequency domain analysis was not considered as an improvement over time-domain analysis in differentiating patients with VT from those without. This is in contrast to the results by Haberl et al.,[56] who demonstrated superiority of frequency-domain analysis. These differences in results may be due to different methodology and require further evaluation. Table 21-1 presents criteria used in previous studies to define abnormal results of signal averaging.

Duration of Late Potentials

The duration of late potentials varies between 50 ms and 180 ms.[23, 36, 57] The median duration of late potentials in patients with one (40 ms) or more than one episode of VT (35 ms) was longer than in those with previous VF (16 ms). Kertes and colleagues[48] reported mean values for the duration of late potentials of 35 ms (range 15 to 70 ms) in 12 of 15 patients with VT.

The factors that govern the duration of late potentials have not yet been studied sufficiently. Data by Berbari et al.[58] suggest that an increase in atrial rates by pacing does not exert any influence on the duration of a late potential, whereas the high-frequency components of the signal do change. There was an inverse relationship between the duration of late potentials and the rate of sustained VT, which, however, was not significant due to a large scatter of data.[57]

The effect of spontaneous or pacing-induced changes in ventricular rate on ventricular late potentials also needs further evaluation. Studies by El-Sherif et al.[9, 11] showed that conduction in a reentrant pathway is markedly rate-dependent. Berbari and coworkers,[20] in preliminary experimental studies, reported that the duration of fractionated activity increased with increasing rates of atrial pacing. In contrast, Landreneao[59] reported a decrease in duration of late potentials in dogs with 2- to 10-day-old myocardial infarction during atrial pacing. This response was attributed to the creation of block in the region of slow conduction. This was in contrast to ventricular pacing, which caused a significant increase in the duration of late potentials compared to sinus rhythm.[59] Stimulation of the ventricles during the vulnerable period, using either single pulses or a train, showed marked fragmentation in electrograms recorded within 2 mm of the stimulation site. With stimulus intensities that evoked multiple ventricular extrasystoles or VF, the fragmented ventricular activity became continuous and bridged the diastolic interval between successive ectopic beats.[60]

The effects of atrial pacing on the ST segment and the terminal portion of the QRS in normal individuals and patients with VT were examined by Berbari et al.[58] Pacing up to the fastest conducted atrial rate showed no significant changes in the high-frequency components of the late potential in seven of eight patients with VT. There was no change in late potential duration. In two patients, VT was not inducible. One patient had late potentials without rate-induced changes, and the other had no late potentials or changes in terminal QRS with atrial pacing.

Reasons for Insufficient Sensitivity of Signal Averaging to Detect Late Potentials

Not all patients with documented VT/VF have late potentials detectable in body surface recordings. One explanation may be that their VT is not of the reentry type but instead may be due to some form of triggered automaticity. In the latter case, no regional slow conduction can be anticipated. How frequently this occurs has not yet been determined. However, several other reasons exist why late potentials may not be detectable on body surface electrograms.

1. The amount of tissue with regional slow conduction, and thus late activation, may be too small. In a recent study, we compared the results of signal averaging and of intraoperative endocardial mapping.[61] The extent of regional slow conduction during intraoperative mapping (i.e., the duration of local activation) did not correlate with the duration of late potentials on body surface recordings. However, the greater the number of sites with abnormal slow activation during endocardial mapping, the greater the chance of recording ventricular late potentials on the body surface. Thus, a given amount of abnormal slow activation probably was necessary to be detected from the body surface.
2. Fragmented activation of an area of the myocardium may occur so early that it takes place at the time of activation of the remaining normal myocardium. Therefore, its activity will be hidden within the QRS complex.[62] The finding that various left ventricular sites are activated at different times may also be of importance.[57] The inferoposterobasal areas of the left ventricle are activated later than the other areas; thus an electrogram of a given duration from an inferoposterobasal area may clearly extend beyond the QRS complex, because this area starts to be activated later than, for instance, the anterior wall of the left ventricle.
3. The signals may be too short and may occur immediately at the end of the QRS complex at a time when filter ringing occurs. This may be a problem

TABLE 21-1
Various Definitions of Ventricular Late Potentials Determined Noninvasively

Definitions
1. Presence of low-amplitude signals in the last 40 ms of the filtered and averaged QRS complex (<25 μV).[21]
2. Higher-frequency content in the terminal 40 ms of the QRS complex and ST segment (between 20-50) Hz,[28, 29] between 10-40 Hz[55])
3. Duration of late potentials ≥ 40 ms.[23, 36, 58, 59]
4. Long QRS duration in the absence of bundle branch block (>120 ms).[43, 53, 54]

if filters with steep characteristics are used. As a solution to this problem, Simson[21] suggested analyzing the QRS complex retrogradely, starting within the ST segment. To avoid filter ringing, we used single-pole filters with flat characteristics in our initial system, which showed a negligible degree of filter ringing.[23]

4. Unstable triggering of the QRS complex (jitter) may prevent the recording of late potentials that may be canceled by the always changing timing in relation to the trigger point. This seems to be of minor importance, as the jitter for triggering is relative small in available systems. However, there may be beat-to-beat variations in the configuration and timing of late potentials that may lead to cancellation during the averaging process. This, at least, may cause some attenuation in the high-frequency components, thus acting as a low-pass filter.

5. The level of base-line noise originating from muscular activity or from interference of alternating current, may hide ventricular late potentials, if it is too high.[63]

SPECIFICITY OF SIGNAL AVERAGING

The signal-averaged ECG proved to be very specific, as it did not detect late ventricular activity in patients in whom there was no delayed activity during intraoperative mapping.[64] However, as discussed above, it may miss delayed activity on the body surface in patients in whom it can be demonstrated by epicardial mapping. Studies have shown that the mean number of epicardial sites with a delayed activity was greater in patients with concordant results than in patients with discordant results.[64] Total ventricular activation time in the concordant groups with delayed activity was 199 ± 16 ms at mapping and 167 ± 17 ms on the signal-averaged ECG.

Although comparison of signal-averaged ECGs with intraoperative or catheter mapping has shown the specificity of the signal-averaging technique for the detection of late potentials, comparative studies of patients with and without a history of VT have shown that even those without a history of VT may exhibit late potentials.[36] The detection of late potentials in patients without a history of a sustained VT may be explained in two different ways. First, this may be a true false-positive finding due to some methodological inadequacy of the technique. Second, the presence of late potentials in a patient free of sustained VT may herald the propensity to VT, although it has not yet been manifested. To address this question, we prospectively studied 110 patients without a history of sustained VT, in whom programmed ventricular stimulation was performed.[65] There was a significant correlation between left ventricular function and the presence and duration of late potentials and between left ventricular function and the results of programmed ventricular stimulation. Thus, in these patients, late potentials indicated an increase in the propensity to VT in patients who had been free of symptomatic tachyarrhythmias up to the time of the study. Late potentials may therefore be considered an indicator of the presence of an arrhythmogenic substrate. Subsequent follow-up studies of larger groups of patients have shown that a significant proportion of these patients developed a spontaneous episode of VT or died suddenly (see below).

Late Potentials in Patients with Ventricular Tachycardia (VT) Versus Ventricular Fibrillation (VF)

The type of documented ventricular tachyarrhythmia has some influence on the incidence and duration of ventricular late potentials. Among patients with chronic recurrent VT, 46 of 62 patients (74%) had late potentials, which was similar to patients with only one documented episode of VT (21 of 26 patients; 80%). In contrast, in several studies of patients with a history of VF outside acute myocardial infarction, with no previous documentation of sustained VT, late potentials occurred in 8 of 15 patients (53%),[57] in 6 of 27 patients (22%),[49] and in 1 of 14 patients (7%).[48] Denniss et al.[66] detected late potentials in only 32% of patients with previous ventricular fibrillation, but in 58% of those with sustained ventricular tachycardia with rates greater than 270 beats per minute (bpm), and in 95% of those with rates of 270 bpm or less. Late potentials were significantly more frequent in those patients in whom the cycle length of induced ventricular tachycardia was greater than 250 ms (90%), compared to those with cycle lengths less than 250 ms (40%).[49] A similar relation was reported by Spielman et al.,[67] using left ventricular catheter mapping.

A short duration of a late potential may be due to a small area with slow fractionated conduction or to more rapid conduction in a larger area. However, as the wavefront of excitation probably travels along multiple pathways and in various directions, no calculations of conduction velocity or of wave length can be performed. In experimental studies, the amplitude and duration on electrograms in dogs with inducible VF were more normal than those recorded in animals with inducible VT.[12] There was an inverse relation between cycle length of VT and duration of late potentials.

This inverse relation between the rate of VT and the duration of late potentials points to one of the limitations of this technique. Especially in those patients at highest risk of sudden cardiac death (i.e., those with a propensity to very rapid rates), ventricular late potentials may be too short to be detected or to extend beyond the end of the QRS complex on the body surface. Therefore, techniques that exert a "stress," causing a prolongation and thus appearance of hidden late potentials, would be desirable.

Incidence of Late Potentials in Patients with Recurrent Syncope

Syncope may result from many conditions[68] and has a variable prognosis.[69] Analysis of the high-frequency components of the terminal QRS complex, using signal-averaged electrocardiography, may identify patients with a propensity to VT after myocardial infarction,[70] especially in the presence of a left ventricular aneurysm[70–72] or of arrhythmogenic right ventricular disease.[2] Therefore, signal averaging also may be useful for identifying those patients with recurrent syncope in whom VT may be the underlying mechanism.

Gang et al.[71] assessed the usefulness of signal averaging for detecting hitherto undocumented VT in 24 patients with unexplained syncope. Sustained ventricular tachycardia was documented in nine patients (eight with inducible VT and one with a spontaneous episode). The signal-averaged ECG contained a late potential and a filtered QRS complex longer than 120 ms in eight of these nine patients (sensitivity 89%). None of the remaining 15 patients had these electrocardiographic abnormalities.

We studied 40 patients (mean age 54 years) with syncope of unknown origin even after thorough medical and neurologic evaluation.[70] Twenty-two patients had late potentials (mean duration 34 ± 10.2 ms). In 18 of these 22 patients with late potentials, sustained VT or VF was inducible, whereas only 8 of 18 patients without late potentials had inducible sustained VT ($p < 0.05$).

A larger group of 150 consecutive patients presenting with syncope was studied by Kuchar et al.[72] Twenty-nine patients had late potentials, 107 patients had a normal signal-averaged ECG, and 14 patients had bundle branch block on the 12-lead ECG. The signal-averaged ECG identified late potentials in 16 of 22 patients with VT and was normal in 101 of 114 patients in whom syncope was attributed to causes other than VT or remained unexplained (sensitivity 73%, specificity 89%, predictive accuracy 54%). Absence of late potentials identified a group of patients with a very low incidence of VT. During a follow-up period of 1 to 20 months (mean 11 months), 15 patients (10%) died, 6 of whom died suddenly. There was no significant difference in survival or recurrence of syncope between patients with or without late potentials.

These results suggest that signal averaging of the surface ECG may be a useful noninvasive test for detecting a high-risk subset of patients prone to lethal tachyarrhythmias.

Effects of Antiarrhythmic Drugs on Late Potentials

Class I antiarrhythmic drugs characteristically slow conduction in normal and abnormal tissue.[73] Therefore, one might expect that this group of antiarrhythmic drugs would also affect the duration of ventricular late potentials. This might provide a means for controlling antiarrhythmic drug effects noninvasively in patients with documented VT, in whom ventricular late potentials are detectable on the body surface.

However, none of the presently available studies has shown any significant correlation between the effect of antiarrhythmic drugs on signal-averaged ventricular late potentials and parameters of drug efficacy. In all studies, drug efficacy has been assessed by use of programmed ventricular stimulation, whereas no sufficiently large group of patients has been studied in whom a possible correlation between the effects of antiarrhythmic drugs on late potentials and spontaneous recurrence rate of ventricular tachycardia was assessed.

In an early report, Rozanski and coworkers[22] suggested that lidocaine had little if any effect on late potentials. Similar results were reported by Simson et al.[74] in a study of 36 patients with a history of recurrent sustained ventricular tachycardia. In this study, late potentials were not abolished by antiarrhythmic agents, and successful pharmacologic control of the arrhythmia could be achieved despite the persistence of late potentials. We also were not able to show any significant correlation between changes in the duration of ventricular late potentials before and during therapy with various antiarrhythmic drugs and changes in the inducibility of ventricular tachycardia in 20 patients (unpublished).

Denniss and colleagues[75] studied whether the timing of ventricular late potentials was modified by antiarrhythmic agents, and whether any such changes correlated with suppression of clinical and inducible VT in 32 patients. There was no consistent effect of quinidine, mexiletine, and metoprolol on the timing of late potentials. Late potentials were abolished in five trials of antiarrhythmic agents (9.4%), whereas VT was not inducible after administration of antiarrhythmic agents in seven trials (13.4%). Both late potentials and inducibility of VT were abolished only in one trial. During long-term follow-up (mean 6 months), ventricular tachycardia recurred in four of nine patients in whom it was still inducible on these antiarrhythmic agents, and in one of seven patients in whom it was no longer inducible. The five patients with a recurrence of VT had persistent late potentials on antiarrhythmic agent therapy.

Höpp et al.[76] studied the effect of intravenous injections of lidocaine, propafenone, and ajmaline on ventricular late potentials in 10 patients. In all patients, there was no change in the pattern of ventricular late potentials after drug injection. These authors concluded that ventricular late potentials probably are not useful for assessment of antiarrhythmic drug efficacy.

Jauernig and coworkers[77] reported the effects of various class I and class II antiarrhythmic drugs on late potentials in 16 patients with documented sustained VT. During sinus rhythm, antiarrhythmic drugs produced no consistent change of late potential duration or amplitude. The prolongation of late potentials ranged from 2 to 26 ms. A shortening of late potentials occurred in 20% and ranged from 1 to 10 ms. During atrial pacing, the duration of late potentials was consistently prolonged from a mean of 42 ± 18 ms to 48 ± 20 ms (p <0.01) after administration of antiarrhythmic drug. Shortening of late potentials did not occur, and the amplitude of late potentials remained unchanged. Changes in duration of late potentials induced by antiarrhythmic drugs were not related to their antiarrhythmic efficacy, as assessed by programmed right ventricular stimulation.

Gessman et al.[78] described two patients with recurrent VT in whom the appearance or prolongation of late potentials recorded during sinus rhythm after administration of class I antiarrhythmic drugs coincided with the ability to induce VT by programmed stimulation. In the first case, endocardial and epicardial electrogram mapping during sinus rhythm was performed intraoperatively before aneurysmectomy. No late potentials were recorded, and VT could not be induced. After administration of 1 gram of procainamide, late potentials could be recorded at three of 22 sites that exceeded QRS duration by 10 ms. Thereafter, sustained VT was inducible. This tachycardia could be terminated by cryoablation at the site of recording of late potentials. In the second case, late potentials that exceeded the QRS duration by 55 ms were recorded in the highly amplified surface ECG. Nonsustained VT at a rate of 140 bpm could be induced. The duration of late potentials increased after administration of quinidine (1 g). During programmed stimulation, a morphologically identical but slower VT could be induced (rate 110 bpm).

Cain et al.[79] characterized the effects of antiarrhythmic drugs on ventricular late potentials by frequency analysis of signal-averaged ECGs. Squared FFTA data of signal-averaged orthogonal ECGs were compared in 14 patients with ventricular tachycardia before and during treatment with antiarrhythmic drugs. A total of 20 trials was performed. The ratio of the amplitudes of 20- to 50-Hz components to the total spectral amplitudes decreased substantially (81 ± 19%) in eight of ten successful trials, compared to control values, but in only one of ten unsuccessful trials (p <0.001). Thus, effective drugs were associated with a significant decrease in the proportion of relatively high-frequency components in the terminal QRS and ST segment. In contrast, Simson et al.[80] found no correlation between changes in the high-frequency content of the signal-averaged ECG and successful control by antiarrhythmic drug therapy in patients with VT. These authors studied 49 patients with sustained VT after myocardial infarction. For all trials, the drugs prolonged the filtered QRS complex by 7.4%, decreased the high-frequency content in the first 80 ms of the QRS complex by 7.8% and in the last 40 ms by 9.6%, and extended the time during which the high-frequency content stayed under 40 μV at the end of the QRS. No differences were found in the four measured parameters between 21 successful and 49 unsuccessful trials.

The reasons for the lack of predictive value of late potentials for antiarrhythmic drug efficacy are still obscure. The persistence of late potentials with therapy indicates that slow conduction in damaged tissue is still present, at least during sinus rhythm. There is no apparent, convincing explanation for the lack of correlation between the effect of antiarrhythmic drugs on noninvasively recorded late potentials and antiarrhythmic drug efficacy. However, with regard to the recent study by Gardner et al.,[15] it may be speculated that antiarrhythmic drugs do not affect that type of slow propagation that is produced by diminished intercellular connections, at least not during basic sinus rhythm.

Simson and coworkers[74] suggested several possible mechanisms by which antiarrhythmic agents could disrupt a reentrant rhythm without affecting slow conduction during sinus rhythm. First, the drugs could prolong the refractory period of normal myocardium and thereby isolate the slowly conducting tissue. Second, a prolongation of conduction time within infarcted tissue has been noted with premature beats. If the antiarrhythmic agents prevented very early ectopic beats from occurring, then a sufficient degree of conduction delay might not be achieved to allow the establishment of a reentrant arrhythmia. Third, the agents could promote block within the slowly conducting tissue with premature stimulation or at rapid heart rates. Fourth, the agents could cause excessive decrease of conduction slowing with premature beats, which can destabilize a reentrant circuit. Using signal-averting techniques as they are currently applied, these changes cannot be detected. However, beat-to-beat analysis may allow other insights into these pathophysiologic mechanisms.

Effect of Ablation Techniques on Ventricular Late Potentials

ANTITACHYCARDIA SURGERY

During recent years, map-guided cardiac surgery has proved to be an effective measure in the treatment of drug-resistant VT. The aim of this approach is to identify the site of origin of VT and to take appropriate measures of ablation such as partial or complete endomyocardial ventriculotomy, endomyocardial resection, and cryosurgery. Because, at the site of origin of VT, late fractionated electrical activity can often be found during sinus rhythm, one might expect that successful abolition of the propensity to VT would be accompanied by loss of ventricular late potentials (Fig. 21–4).

Early reports included only small numbers of patients. Uther and coworkers[27] reported that in two of three patients who had surgery for their ventricular tachycardia with excision of diseased myocardium, VT could no longer be induced and late potentials were no longer detectable. In the third patient, ventricular tachycardia could still be induced, and late potentials were still present. Rozanski et al.[22] reported data on four patients in whom ventricular late potentials were abolished by aneurysmectomy.

We were able to confirm these results in a series of

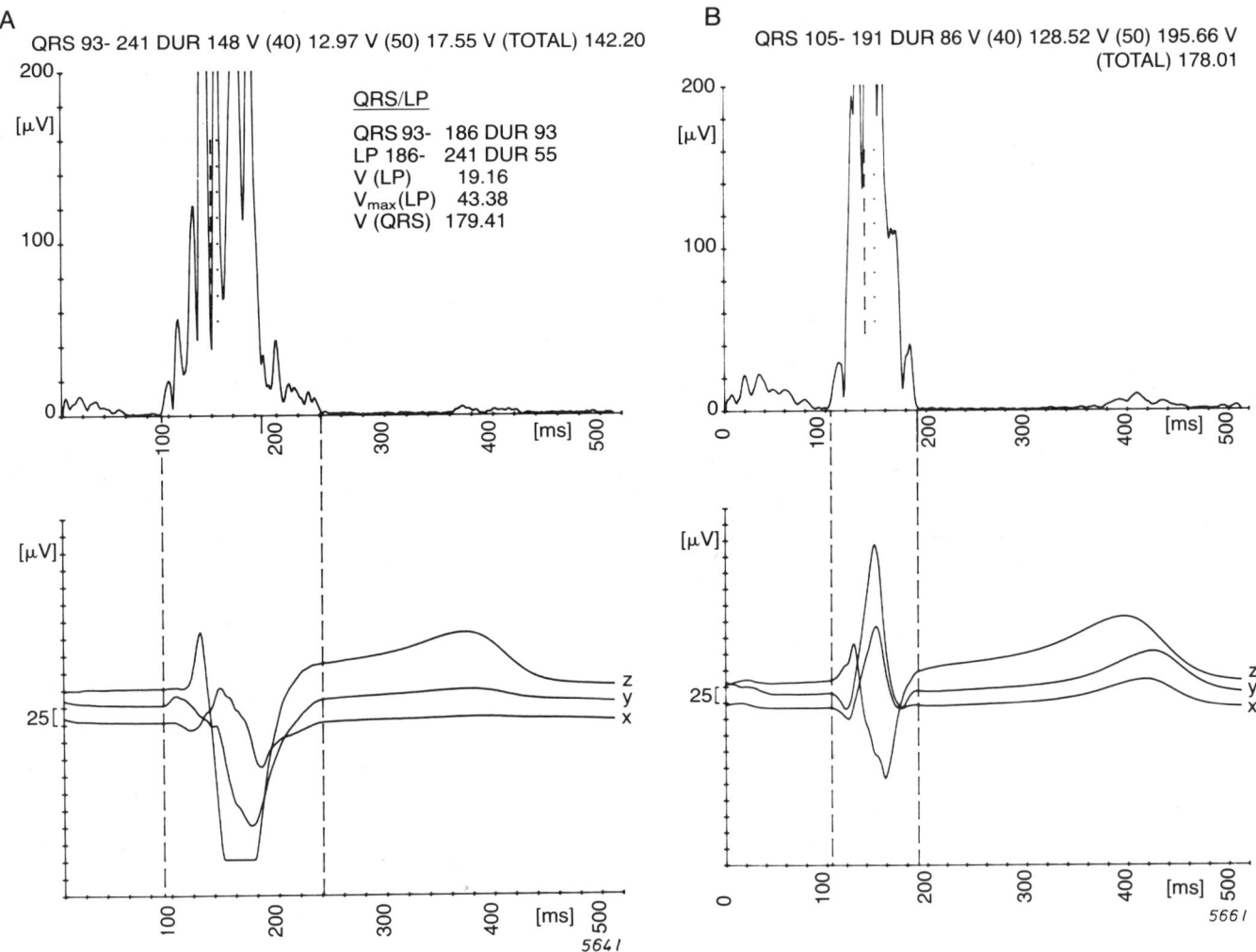

FIGURE 21-4
Pre- and postoperative signal-averaged recording in a patient with recurrent sustained ventricular tachycardia. Before surgery (A), the amplitude in the terminal 40 ms of the filtered (total) QRS complex was low (V[40] = 12.97 μV) and a late potential of 55 ms duration was automatically identified. After map-guided surgery (B), the amplitude in the terminal 40 ms of the QRS complex was normal (V[40] = 128.52 μV); there was no longer any low-amplitude tail at the end of QRS complex. Postoperatively, the patient was free of inducible and spontaneous ventricular tachycardia.

19 patients.[81] All patients were operated on for recurrent sustained VT, using a map-guided approach. During postoperative electrophysiologic studies, sustained VT was no longer inducible in 12 of 13 patients (92.3%) in whom late potentials disappeared after surgery, compared to 4 of 6 patients (66.7%) in whom late potentials were still present. Noninducibility of ventricular tachycardia and absence of late potentials after surgery correlated with a favorable long-term prognosis. Similar data were recently reported by Marcus et al.[82] in 37 patients in whom endocardial resection for VT has been performed. In 24 patients in whom VT became noninducible after surgery, QRS duration decreased and the voltage in the terminal 40 ms of the averaged and filtered QRS complex increased, indicating that low-amplitude electrical activity had been removed. The presence of late potentials decreased from 71 to 33%. In contrast, in 13 patients in whom ventricular tachycardia was still inducible, there was no significant change either in QRS duration or in the voltage of the last 40 ms. Late potentials were still present in 85% of these patients.

Recently, we[83] have reviewed our pre- and postoperative recordings of the signal-averaged ECG, using the same algorithm as reported by Simson et al.[21, 82] Our objectives were to gain some insight into whether the absence or presence of late potentials prior to surgery may predict outcome after surgical ablation of the site of origin of VT and to assess whether changes in these noninvasive recordings may predict surgical outcome. In our study, 86 patients underwent direct, map-guided antitachycardia surgery. Postoperatively, VT in 41 patients was rendered noninducible (48%); in 26 patients (30%), only nonsustained tachyarrhythmias were inducible. Sustained VT was still inducible in 19 patients (22%). In the majority of this last group of patients, VT was controlled by previously ineffective antiarrhythmic agents. Thus the overall surgical efficacy rate was 78%. Of the 86 patients, 40 (46%) did not have late potentials prior to surgery. Thus, in only

46 patients (54%) this noninvasive test could be used to assess surgical efficacy. The presence or absence of late potentials prior to surgery did not predict surgical outcome, as 34 of 67 patients (51%) who were treated successfully did not have late potentials prior to surgery, compared to 6 of 19 patients (31%) with VT still inducible up to surgery. These differences were not significantly different. Patients with noninducible VT after surgery showed a significant increase in the voltage in the last 40 ms of the signal-averaged QRS complex ($p < 0.03$), whereas this parameter remained unchanged in patients with inducible sustained and nonsustained VT postoperatively. Overall, the presence or absence of late potentials after antitachycardia surgery can be useful in noninvasive assessment of the efficacy of this procedure. The sensitivity was 36%, the specificity 69%, and the predictive accuracy 46%.

Based on these results, subgroups of patients can be identified after antitachycardia surgery, in whom the outcome can be predicted. For the individual patient, however, postoperative programmed stimulation is mandatory to assure postoperative noninducibility, as the sensitivity and specificity of noninvasive recording of late potentials are too low. Despite these limitations, the changes of the signal-averaged QRS complex after direct surgery have provided increasing insight into the pathophysiologic mechanisms underlying late potentials.

The mechanisms by which various techniques lead to a cure of VT have not been clearly established. In the encircling endocardial ventriculotomy approach, which has been mainly used by our group, the arrhythmogenic tissue is theoretically isolated from the pumping ventricular chamber. Thus, the reentrant circuit is prevented from engaging the normal portion of the ventricle. According to this concept, one might therefore expect that late potentials do persist postoperatively. However, this was not the case in many of the patients. One explanation might be that by the combined surgical procedure used (subendocardial encircling ventriculotomy and aneurysmectomy), the arrhythmogenic zone is not only isolated but also devitalized. Another explanation might be that in this zone, electrical activity still persists but is no longer synchronized to the normal heart beat by entrance and exit block and, thus, will go undetected during signal averaging. Conversely, the endocardial excision approach of controlling ventricular tachyarrhythmias theoretically either damages or completely excises the reentrant circuit; thus, in patients successfully treated, late potentials should not exist postoperatively. Even if late potentials still persist after surgery, VT has not been found to be inducible in all patients. This might be explained by the observation that low-amplitude fractionated activity during endocardial mapping can be found also in regions of the left ventricle that are at some distance from the site of origin of VT and that probably do not participate in the reentrant circuit. Removal of the arrhythmogenic tissue at the site of origin of VT, thus, cannot be expected to lead to a loss of ventricular late potentials on the body surface if abnormal electric activity at a distant site persists.

CATHETER ABLATION

Catheter ablation is a new, nonpharmacologic approach to control drug-refractory VT.[84] Its effects on the signal-averaged QRS complex are presently unknown. Because the overall clinical efficacy of this new approach is reported to range between 60 and 80%, one might expect that recording of late potentials would be useful in assessing acute and long-term outcome of patients after catheter ablation. We have recently analyzed 12 patients[85] who underwent catheter ablation and in whom signal averaging was performed prior to and after ablation. Overall, the QRS duration and the voltage in the last 40 ms of the filtered QRS did not reveal any significant changes after ablation. Furthermore, analysis of successful and ineffective ablation attempts did not show any differences in measured parameters of the filtered QRS complex. Although the number of patients studied was relatively small, the results indicate that recording of late potentials does not seem to be helpful in assessing acute and long-term outcome of patients undergoing catheter ablation. The underlying mechanisms are presently not understood. Probably the area of damage created by catheter ablation is too small to have any effects on low-amplitude fragmented endocardial activation. Previous studies have shown that many endocardial sites outside the area of origin of VT show low, fragmented endocardial activation. Thus, one cannot expect catheter ablation to eliminate these areas completely. However, probably the critical part of the reentrant circuit is sufficiently altered without an effect on areas of slowed myocardial activation. Further studies are needed to elucidate the underlying mechanisms.

Prognostic Significance of Late Potentials

During recent years, several studies have addressed the prognostic value of ventricular late potentials.[86, 87, 89–94] Our own experience is primarily based on two studies both using signal averaging in the time-domain. The first prospective trial, which was initiated at Düsseldorf University in 1980, used the methodology for signal averaging that had been developed in our department between 1978 and 1979. This system was based on a hard-wired signal averager,[23, 36, 65, 86, 87] which has subsequently also been used by other groups.[44, 77, 88] The second study, started in January, 1983, is the Post-Infarction Late Potential (PILP) study. It has recently been completed after inclusion of almost 800 patients. Data analysis has not yet been completed.

The results of the first prospective pilot study in 160 patients were reported in 1983.[86] Subsequently, another 788 patients without a history of sustained VT or VF outside the acute phase of myocardial infarction were studied. Mean duration of follow-up was 39 ± 15.0 months. A major arrhythmic event occurred in 35 patients, with 21 sudden deaths (3.3%) and 14 episodes of symptomatic, spontaneous sustained VT (2.2%).

The risk of major arrhythmic complications was 2.8 times greater in patients with late potentials <40 ms in duration than in those without any late potentials, and 9.3 times greater in those with late potentials with a duration of 40 ms or more. The chance of sudden cardiac death within 1 hour was 3.3 and 5.4 times greater, respectively, whereas the chance for symptomatic sustained ventricular tachycardia was 2.0 and 17.4 times greater, respectively, depending on the duration of late potentials (less than or greater than 40 ms). The chance of major arrhythmic complications such as sudden cardiac death or sustained symptomatic ventricular tachycardia was greatest in those patients who were studied within the first 4 to 8 weeks after their qualifying myocardial infarction and who had late potentials.

These data are supported by other studies also using signal averaging in the time-domain. Denniss et al.[89] studied 110 patients 7 to 28 days after acute myocardial infarction. Follow-up of these patients ranged from 2 to 12 months (mean, 5 months). There was a significant difference in the subsequent occurrence of symptomatic sustained VT during follow-up in patients without late potentials (1.1%) compared to those with late potentials (17.4%). The incidence of sudden cardiac death was not reported in this study.

In a more recent report, the same group presented the results of long-term observation in 403 clinically well survivors of transmural infarction who were 65 years old or younger.[90] Of these patients, 26% had late potentials. After 2 years, the probability of remaining free from cardiac death or nonfatal VT or VF was 0.73 for patients with late potentials and 0.95 for patients without. For patients with late potentials, the probability of remaining free from instantaneous death or nonfatal VT or VF was 0.85 at 1 year and 0.79 at 2 years, much lower than the corresponding figures of 0.98 ($p<0.001$) and 0.96 ($p<0.001$) for patients without late potentials.[90] Within the group of patients with late potentials, the patients who either died instantaneously or had nonfatal VT or VF, had a longer mean ventricular activation time, a lower mean left ventricular ejection fraction, and a higher incidence of left ventricular aneurysms than patients who were event-free.

Kacet and coworkers[91] studied a population of 104 patients who were followed for 8.5 ± 4 months. The incidence of subsequent, symptomatic sustained VT in patients without late potentials was 4.5%, compared to 28.9% in patients with late potentials. None of the patients without late potentials died suddenly, in contrast to 13% of patients with late potentials. In another study, Kuchar et al.[92] reported the results of follow-up (3 to 12 months) of 123 patients who were studied 10 days (mean) after acute myocardial infarction. The incidence of major arrhythmic complications such as sudden death or symptomatic sustained VT was only 1.4% in patients without late potentials, compared to 20.5% in patients with late potentials. In a study by Höpp et al.,[93] 50 patients were studied in the early post-infarction period. These patients were followed for 24 ± 5 months. Twelve of 30 patients who had late potentials (37%) died suddenly; on the contrary, none of the 20 patients without late potentials died suddenly. The same authors studied another group of 200 patients with chronic, stable coronary artery disease.[93] Mean follow-up was 20 ± 5 months, and 108 of 200 patients had ventricular late potentials. Fifteen of these patients (13.9%) died suddenly, compared to 4 of 92 patients (4.3%) without late potentials ($p<0.001$). Von Leitner and colleagues[94] followed 518 patients who took part in a rehabilitation program after myocardial infarction. These patients were studied between 6 and 8 weeks after onset of myocardial infarction. During a mean follow-up period of 10 months, cardiac mortality was 1.5% in patients without late potentials, compared to 7.3% in patients with late potentials. Sudden cardiac death occurred in 0.9% of patients without late potentials, compared to 3.6% in patients with late potentials. Symptomatic sustained VT was not reported in any of these patients.

In contrast to this extensive information on the prognostic significance of signal-averaging in the time-domain, there have been no prospective large-scale studies using signal averaging in the frequency-domain.

Significance of Late Potentials to Predict Rejection After Heart Transplantation

Recently, Haberl and coworkers[95, 96] have reported the use of frequency analysis of low-noise electrocardiographic recordings as a new noninvasive approach to detect early rejection after cardiac transplantation. Thirty-six acute rejection crises requiring treatment in heart-transplanted patients were diagnosed by cytoimmunologic monitoring and endomyocardial biopsy. In 33 of these cases, a significant increase in the frequency content of the QRS complex between 70 and 110 Hz was observed on the days of rejection. The frequency content of the ST segment in a 300-ms window was found to be decreased between 10 and 30 Hz. These changes in the frequency content were reversible within 1 to 2 weeks in most patients after successful treatment. These authors found only two false-positive results (two patients with acute mediastinitis). The mechanism of these changes and the potential use of this method for the evaluation of acute and chronic rejection after orthotopic heart transplantation seems a promising new approach that needs further evaluation.

Conclusions and Clinical Implications

Based on the presently available prospective studies, the presence of ventricular late potentials obviously heralds an increased risk for subsequent occurrence of sudden cardiac death or symptomatic sustained VT. This applies mainly to patients who are studied after recent myocardial infarction,[89, 91–93] whereas patients who are included later and/or who are considered to be eligible for a cardiac rehabilitation program[94] obviously have a much lower incidence of arrhythmic events. Thus the predictive value of the presence of ventricular late potentials largely depends on the clinical circumstances in which they can be detected. Patients who have survived for a long period after their myocardial infarction have a much lower risk of subsequent development of sudden cardiac death or symptomatic sustained VT. This is obviously based on a selection process, as patients at greater risk might have died meanwhile. In addition, our results show that the duration of late potentials may be of prognostic significance. The chance for development of an arrhythmic event, mainly symptomatic sustained VT, is proportional to the duration of the late potentials.

With regard to the complex mechanisms that may lead to sudden cardiac death, it cannot be expected that any single method will be able to predict the occurrence of sudden cardiac death with a sensitivity of 100%. Sudden cardiac death may be due to chronic electrophysiologic abnormalities as a consequence of regional slow conduction in the border zone of a previous myocardial infarction, which is conventionally considered to be the electrophysiologic substrate for ventricular late potentials.

The presence of regional slow conduction generally is not sufficient for the spontaneous occurrence of ventricular tachyarrhythmias. Rather, some trigger factor such as spontaneous ventricular ectopic beats are necessary to alter the electrophysiologic milieu in such a way that tachycardia originates. However, most spontaneous ventricular arrhythmias detected during long-term ECG recording are not harmful to the patient, as they obviously do not induce VT. Instead, some change in, for example, the coupling interval or the sequence of ectopic beats, including the occurrence of short runs, may alter the electrophysiologic milieu in such a way that the prerequisites for reentry are met. Such transient occurrence of complex ventricular arrhythmias acting as trigger factor may also be induced by short, regional episodes of ischemia due to embolization of platelet aggregates into the peripheral coronary system.[97]

Another mechanism that may lead to sudden cardiac death is the occurrence of more extensive ischemia due to re-infarction. There is no doubt that this may also lead to VF and, thus, to sudden cardiac death. Such a type of event, of course, cannot be predicted on the presence of preexisting indicators of regional slow conduction such as late potentials. However, it has been shown that preexisting myocardial damage increases the chance of VF if regional ischemia occurs at a site remote from that of preexisting cardiac damage.[98]

Thus, with regard to the complex mechanisms that may lead to sudden cardiac death, only a combination of various parameters, including late potentials, spontaneous ventricular arrhythmias during long-term ECG recording, results of programmed ventricular stimulation, extent of myocardial contractile disturbance (ejection fraction), and estimates of central nervous activity,[99,100] may allow further risk stratification in patients after recent myocardial infarction.

References

1. Fontaine G, Frank R, Gallais-Hamonno F, et al.: Electrocardiographie des potentiels tardifs du syndrome de post-excitation. Arch Mal Coeur 71:854, 1978.
2. Fontaine G, Guiraudon G, Frank R: Intramyocardial conduction defects in patients prone to ventricular tachycardia. III. The post-excitation syndrome in ventricular tachycardia. In Sandoe E, Julian DG, Bell JW (eds.): Management of ventricular tachycardia—Role of mexiletine, pp. 67–79. Amsterdam, Excerpta Medica, 1978.
3. Josephson ME, Horowitz LN, Farshidi A, et al.: Sustained ventricular tachycardia: Evidence for protected localized reentry. Am J Cardiol 42:416, 1978.
4. Ostermeyer J, Breithardt G, Kolvenbach R, et al. Intraoperative electrophysiologic mapping during cardiac surgery. Thorac Cardiovasc Surgeon 27:260, 1979.
5. Spielman SR, Untereker WJ, Horowitz LN, et al.: Fragmented electrical activity—relationship to ventricular tachycardia (Abstract). Am J Cardiol 47:448, 1981.
6. Klein H, Karp RB, Kouchoukos NT, et al.: Intraoperative electrophysiologic mapping of the ventricles during sinus rhythm in patients with previous myocardial infarction. Identification of the electrophysiologic substrate of ventricular arrhythmias. Circulation 66:847, 1982.
7. Durrer D, Formaijne P, Van Dam R, et al.: Electrogram in normal and some abnormal conditions. Am Heart J 61:303, 1961.
8. Flowers NC, Horan LG, Thomas JR, et al.: The anatomic basis for high frequency components in the electrocardiogram. Circulation 39:531, 1969.
9. El-Sherif N, Scherlag BJ, Lazzara R, et al.: Reentrant ventricular arrhythmias in the late myocardial infarction period. I. Conduction characteristics in the infarction zone. Circulation 55:686, 1977.
10. El-Sherif N, Scherlag BJ, Lazzara R, et al.: Reentrant ventricular arrhythmias in the late myocardial infarction period. II. Patterns of initiation and termination of reentry. Circulation 55:702, 1977.
11. El-Sherif N, Lazzara R, Hope RR, et al.: Reentrant arrhythmias in the late myocardial infarction period. III. Manifest and concealed extrasystolic grouping. Circulation 56:225, 1977.
12. Richards DA, Blake GJ, Spear JF, et al.: Electrophysiologic substrate for ventricular tachycardia: Correlation of properties in vivo and in vitro. Circulation 69:369, 1984.
13. Gardner PI, Ursell PC, Fenoglio JJ, et al.: Electrophysiologic and anatomic basis for fractionated electrograms recorded from healed myocardial infarcts. Circulation 72:596, 1985.
14. Gardner PI, Ursell PC, Pham TD, et al.: Experimental chronic ventricular tachycardia: Anatomic and electrophysiologic substrates. In Josephson ME, Wellens HJJ (eds.): Tachycardias: Mechanisms, Diagnosis, Treatment, pp. 29–60. Philadelphia, Lea & Febiger, 1984.
15. Hanich RF, de Langen CDJ, Kadish AH, et al.: Inducible sustained ventricular tachycardia 4 years after experimental canine myocardial infarction: Electrophysiologic and anatomic comparisons with early healed infarcts. Circulation 77:445, 1988.
16. Kienzle MG, Miller J, Falcone R, et al.: Intraoperative endocardial mapping during sinus rhythm: Relationship to site of origin of ventricular tachycardia. Circulation 70:957, 1984.
17. Breithardt G, Borggrefe M: Pathophysiological mechanisms and clinical significance of ventricular late potentials. Eur Heart J 7:364, 1986.
18. Zuckermann R: Postexzitation. Z Kreislauff 4:654, 1960.
19. Fontaine G, Guiraudon G, Frank R, et al.: Stimulation studies and epicardial mapping in ventricular tachycardia: Study of mechanisms and selection for surgery. In Kulbertus HE (ed.): Reentrant Arrhythmias, Mechanisms and Treatment, pp. 333–350. Lancaster, MTP Press, 1977.
20. Berbari EJ, Scherlag BJ, Hope RR, et al.: Recording from the body surface of arrhythmogenic ventricular activity during the ST-segment. Am J Cardiol 41:697, 1978.
21. Simson MB: Use of signals in the terminal QRS-complex to identify patients with ventricular tachycardia after myocardial infarction. Circulation 64:235, 1981.

22. Rozanski JJ, Mortara D, Myerburg RJ, et al.: Body surface detection of delayed depolarizations in patients with recurrent ventricular tachycardia and left ventricular aneurysm. Circulation 63:1172, 1981.
23. Breithardt G, Becker R, Seipel L, et al.: Non-invasive detection of late potentials in man—a new marker for ventricular tachycardia. Eur Heart J 2:1, 1981.
24. Hombach V, Höpp HW, Braun V, et al.: Die Bedeutung von Nachpotentialen innerhalb des ST-Segmentes im Oberflächen-EKG bei Patienten mit koronarer Herzkrankheit. Dtsch Med Wochenschr 105:1457, 1980.
25. Breithardt G, Becker R, Seipel L: Non-invasive recording of late ventricular activation in man. Circulation 62 (Suppl. III):320, 1980.
26. Simson M, Horowitz L, Josephson M, et al.: A marker for ventricular tachycardia after myocardial infarction (Abstract). Circulation 7(Suppl III):262, 1980.
27. Uther JB, Dennett CJ, Tan A: The detection of delayed activation signals of low amplitude in the vectorcardiogram of patients with recurrent ventricular tachycardia by signal averaging. In Sandoe E, Julian DG, Bell JW (eds.): Management of Ventricular Tachycardia—Role of Mexiletine, pp. 80–82. Amsterdam, Excerpta Medica, 1978.
28. Cain ME, Ambos D, Witkowski FX, et al.: Fast-Fourier transform analysis of signal-averaged electrocardiograms for identification of patients prone to sustained ventricular tachycardia. Circulation 69:711, 1984.
29. Cain ME, Ambos HD, Markham J, et al.: Quantification of differences in frequency content of signal-averaged electrocardiograms in patients with compared to those without sustained ventricular tachycardia. Am J Cardiol 55:1500, 1985.
30. Haberl R, Hengstenberg E, Pulter R, et al.: Frequenzanalyse des Einzelschlag-Elektrokardiogrammes zur Diagnostik von Kammertachykardien. Z Kardiol 75:659, 1986.
31. Santipetro RF: The origin and characterization of the primary signal, noise and interface sources in the high frequency electrocardiogram. IEEE Trans Biomed Eng 65:707, 1977.
32. Hombach V, Kebbel V, Höpp HW, et al.: Fortlaufende Registrierung von Mikropotentialen des menschlichen Herzens. Dtsch Med Wochenschr 107:1951, 1982.
33. Denes P, Santarelli P, Hauser RG, et al.: Quantitative analysis of the high frequency components of the terminal portion of the body surface QRS in normal subjects and in patients with ventricular tachycardia. Circulation 67:1129, 1983.
34. Hombach V, Kebbel V, Höpp HW, et al.: Noninvasive beat-by-beat registration of ventricular late potentials using high resolution electrocardiography. Int J Cardiol 6:167, 1984.
35. Simson MB, Euler D, Mickelson EL, et al.: Detection of delayed ventricular activation on the body surface in dogs. Am J Physiol 241 (Heart Circ Physiol 10):H363–H369, 1981.
36. Breithardt G, Borggrefe M, Karbenn U, et al.: Prevalence of late potentials in patients with and without ventricular tachycardia: Correlation to angiographic findings. Am J Cardiol 49:1932, 1982.
37. Oeff M, von Leitner ER, Erne SN, et al.: Failure of signal-averaging technique to record arrhythmogenic diastolic potentials: Advantage of non-invasive beat for beat recording. Circulation 68:III-218, 1983.
38. Karbenn U, Breithardt G, Borggrefe M, et al.: Automatic identification of late potentials. J Electrocardiol 18:123, 1985.
39. Graene JG, Tobey GE, Huelsman LE: Operational Amplifiers, p. 191. New York, McGraw-Hill, 1971.
40. Goedel-Meinen L, Hofmann M, Schmidt G, et al.: Reproducibility of data of the signal-averaged electrocardiogram (Abstract). Circulation 76(Suppl 4):124, 1987.
41. El-Sherif N, Mehru R, Gomes JAC, et al.: Appraisal of a low noise electrocardiogram. J Am Coll Cardiol 1:456, 1983.
42. Harris FJ: On the use of windows for harmonic analysis with the discrete Fourier transform. Proc. IEEE 66:51, 1978.
43. Oeff M, Leitner ER von, Brüggemann T, et al.: Methodische Probleme bei der Registrierung ventrikulärer Spätpotentiale (Abstract). Z Kardiol 71:204, 1982.
44. Flowers NC, Shvartsman V, Horan LG, et al.: Analysis of PR subintervals in normal subjects and early studies in patients with abnormalities of the conduction system using surface His bundle recordings. J Am Coll Cardiol 2:939, 1983.
45. Abboud S, Belhassen B, Laniado S, et al.: Non-invasive recording of late ventricular activity using an advanced method in patients with a damaged mass of ventricular tissue. J Electrocardiol 16:245, 1983.
46. Klempt HW, Wulschner W: Die Analyse des QRS-Komplexes sowie des ST-Abschnittes mit der Signalmittelungstechnik bei Herzgesunden. Z Kardiol 72:369, 1983.
47. Wilner J, Mindlich B: Fragmented endocardial electrical activity in patients with ventricular tachycardia: A guide to surgical therapy. Am J Cardiol 49:946, 1982.
48. Kertes PJ, Glaubus M, Murray A, et al.: Delayed ventricular depolarization—correlation with ventricular activation and relevance to ventricular fibrillation in acute myocardial infarction. Eur Heart J 5:974, 1984.
49. Freedman RA, Gillis AM, Keren A, et al.: Signal-averaged ECG late potentials correlate with clinical arrhythmia and electrophysiology study in patients with ventricular tachycardia or fibrillation. Circulation 70:II-252, 1984.
50. Höpp HW, Hombach V, Deutsch HJ, et al.: Assessment of ventricular vulnerability by Holter ECG, programmed ventricular stimulation and recording of ventricular late potentials. In Steinbach K, Glogar D, Laszkovics A, Scheibelhofer W, Weber H (eds): Cardiac Pacing, pp. 625–632. Darmstadt, Steinkopff Verlag, 1983.
51. Kanovsky MS, Falcone RA, Dresden CA, et al.: Identification of patients with ventricular tachycardia after myocardial infarction: Signal-averaged electrocardiogram, Holter monitoring, and cardiac catheterization. Circulation 70:264, 1984.
52. Buxton AE, Simson MB, Falcone R, et al.: Signal averaged ECG in patients with nonsustained ventricular tachycardia: Identification of patients with potential for sustained ventricular arrhythmias (Abstract). J Am Coll Cardiol 3:495, 1984.
53. Poll DS, Marchlinski FE, Falcone RA, et al.: Abnormal signal averaged ECG in nonischemic congestive cardiomyopathy: Relationship to sustained ventricular tachyarrhythmias. Circulation 70:II-253, 1984.
54. Haberl R, Weber M, Reichenspurner H, et al.: Frequency analysis of the surface electrocardiogram for recognition of acute rejection after orthotopic cardiac transplantation in man. Circulation 76(Suppl 1):101, 1987.
55. Machac J, Weiss A, Winters SL, et al.: A comparative study of frequency-domain and time-domain analysis of signal averaged electrocardiograms in patients with ventricular tachycardia. J Am Coll Cardiol 11:284, 1988.
56. Haberl R, Jilge G, Pulter R, et al.: Vergleich von Frequenzanalyse des EKG und Spätpotentialnachweis zur Erkennung von Patienten mit Kammertachykardien bei koronarer Herzkrankheit. Z Kardiol 76:8, 1987.
57. Borggrefe M, Karbenn U, Breithardt G: Spätpotentiale und elektrophysiologische Befunde bei ventrikulären Tachykardien (Abstract). Z Kardiol 71:627, 1982.
58. Berbari EJ, Friday KJ, Jackmann WM, et al.: Effects of atrial pacing on surface recorded late potentials in patients with ventricular tachycardia. Circulation 70(Suppl 2):II-373, 1984.
59. Landreneau JW, Arenburg JH, Hanley HG, et al.: Effect of atrial and ventricular pacing on the incidence and duration of signal averaged ECG late potentials in canine myocardial infarction. Circulation 72(Suppl 3):162, 1985.
60. Euler DE, Moore EN: Continuous fractionated electrical activity after stimulation of the ventricles during the vulnerable period: Evidence for local reentry. Am J Cardiol 46:783, 1980.
61. Schwarzmaier J, Karbenn U, Borggrefe M, et al.: Quantitative relation between intraoperative registration of late endocardial activation and late potentials in signal-averaged electrocardiogram (Abstract). Circulation 76(Suppl. 4):1363, 1987.
62. Simson MB, Untereker WJ, Spielman SR, et al.: Relation between late potentials on the body surface and directly recorded fragmented electrocardiograms in patients with ventricular tachycardia. Am J Cardiol 51:105, 1983.
63. Steinberg JS, Bigger T Jr, Bernstein F: Results of signal averaged ECG are dependent upon endpoint of noise reduction (Abstract). Circulation 76(Suppl 4):342, 1987.
64. Denniss AR, Ross DL, Johnson DC, et al.: Comparison of ventricular activation times obtained by signal averaged ECG and epicardial mapping (Abstract). J Am Coll Cardiol 3:623, 1984.

65. Breithardt G, Borggrefe M, Quantius B, et al.: Ventricular vulnerability assessed by programmed ventricular stimulation in patients with and without late potentials. Circulation 68:275, 1983.
66. Denniss AR, Holley LK, Cody DV, et al.: Ventricular tachycardia and fibrillation: Differences in ventricular activation times and ventricular function (Abstract). J Am Coll Cardiol 1:606, 1983.
67. Spielman SR, Horowitz LN, Greenspan AM, et al.: Activation mapping in sinus rhythm in patients with ventricular tachycardia—relationship to cycle length and site of origin (Abstract). Am J Cardiol 47:497, 1981.
68. Wright KE, McIntosch HD: Syncope: A review of pathophysiologic mechanisms. Progr. Cardiovasc. Dis 13:580, 1971.
69. Silverstein MB, Singer DE, Mulley AG, et al.: Patients with syncope admitted to medical intensive units. JAMA 248:1185, 1982.
70. Borggrefe M, Karbenn U, Breithardt G: Usefulness of Holter monitoring and non-invasive recording of late potentials in selection of patients for programmed ventricular stimulation (Abstract). Circulation 74(Suppl II):745, 1986.
71. Gang ES, Peter TH, Rosenthal ME, et al.: Detection of late potentials on the surface electrocardiogram in unexplained syncope. Am J Cardiol 58:1014, 1986.
72. Kuchar DL, Thorburn CW, Sammel NL: Signal-averaged electrocardiogram for evaluation of recurrent syncope. Am J Cardiol 58:949, 1986.
73. El-Sherif N, Scherlag BJ, Lazzara R, et al.: Reentrant ventricular arrhythmias in the late myocardial infarction period: 4. Mechanisms of action of lidocaine. Circulation 56:395, 1977.
74. Simson MB, Waxman HL, Falcone R, et al.: Effects of antiarrhythmic drugs on noninvasively recorded late potentials. In Breithardt G, Loogen F, (eds.): New Aspects in the Medical Treatment of Tachyarrhythmias, pp. 80–86. Munich, Urban & Schwarzenberg, 1987.
75. Denniss AR, Ross DL, Cody DV, et al.: Effect of antiarrhythmic therapy on delayed potentials in patients with ventricular tachycardia. J Am Coll Cardiol 3:495, 1984.
76. Höpp HW, Deutsch H, Hombach V, et al.: Medikamentöse Beeinflussbarkeit ventrikulärer Spätpotentials. Z Kardiol 71:206, 1982.
77. Jauernig RA, Senges J, Langfelder W, et al.: Effect of antiarrhythmic drugs on ventricular late potentials at sinus rhythm and at constant heart rate. In Steinbach D, Glogar D, Laszkovics A, et al. (eds.): Cardiac Pacing, pp. 767–772. Darmstadt, Steinkopff Verlag, 1983.
78. Gessman L, Gallagher J, Del Rossi A, et al.: Prolongation of late potentials by type I antiarrhythmic drugs coincident with inducibility of ventricular tachycardia. Circulation 68(Suppl 3):173, 1983.
79. Cain ME, Ambos HD, Fischer AE, et al.: Noninvasive prediction of antiarrhythmic drug efficacy in patients with sustained ventricular tachycardia from frequency analysis of signal average ECGs. Circulation 70(Suppl 2):252, 1984.
80. Simson MB, Falcone R, Kindwall E: The signal average electrocardiogram does not predict antiarrhythmic drug success. Circulation 72(Suppl 3):7, 1985.
81. Breithardt G, Seipel L, Ostermeyer J, et al.: Effects of antiarrhythmic surgery on late ventricular potentials recorded by precordial signal averaging in patients with ventricular tachycardia. Am Heart J 104:966, 1983.
82. Marcus NH, Falcone RA, Harken AH, et al.: Body surface late potentials: Effects of endocardial resection in patients with ventricular tachycardia. Circulation 70:632, 1984.
83. Borggrefe M, Schwarzmaier J, Karbenn U, et al.: Limitations of the signal-averaged ECG in predicting antiarrhythmic efficacy after antitachycardia surgery. In preparation.
84. Breithardt G, Borggrefe M, Zipes D: Non-pharmacological therapy of tachyarrhythmias. Mount Kisco, Futura, 1987.
85. Borggrefe M, Seifert D, Karbenn U, et al.: Effects of catheter ablation on late potentials. In preparation.
86. Breithardt G, Schwarzmaier J, Borggrefe M, et al.: Prognostic significance of ventricular late potentials after acute myocardial infarction. Eur Heart J 4:487, 1983.
87. Breithardt G, Borggrefe M, Haerten K: Role of programmed ventricular stimulation and noninvasive recording of ventricular late potentials for the identification of patients at risk of ventricular tachyarrhythmias after acute myocardial infarction. In Zipes DP, Jaliffe J (eds.): Cardiac Electrophysiology and Arrhythmias, pp. 553–561, New York, Grune and Stratton. 1985.
88. Oeff M, von Leitner ER, Sthapit R, et al.: Methods for noninvasive detection of ventricular late potentials—A comparative multicenter study. In Steinbach K, Glogar D, Laszkovics A, et al. (eds.): Cardiac Pacing, pp. 641–647. Darmstadt, Steinkopff Verlag, 1983.
89. Denniss AR, Cody DV, Fenton SM, et al.: Significance of delayed activation potentials in survivors of myocardial infarction (Abstract). J Am Coll Cardiol 1:582, 1983.
90. Denniss AR, Richards DA, Cody DV, et al.: Prognostic significance of ventricular tachycardia and fibrillation induced at programmed stimulation and delayed potentials detected on the signal-averaged electrocardiogram of survivors of acute myocardial infarction. Circulation 74:731, 1986.
91. Kacet S, Libersa C, Caron J, et al.: The prognostic value of signal-averaged late potentials in patients suffering from coronary artery disease (personal communication).
92. Kuchar D, Thorburn C, Sammel N: Natural history and clinical significance of late potentials after myocardial infarction. Circulation 72:III-477, 1985.
93. Höpp HW, Hombach V, Osterspey A, et al.: Clinical and prognostic significance of ventricular arrhythmias and ventricular late potentials in patients with coronary heart disease. In Hombach V, Hilger HH (eds.): Holter Monitoring Technique: Technical Aspects and Clinical Applications, pp. 297–307. Stuttgart, Schattauer Verlag, 1985.
94. von Leitner ER, Oeff M, Loock D, et al.: Value of non invasively detected delayed ventricular depolarizations to predict prognosis in post myocardial infarction patients. Circulation 68:III-83, 1983.
95. Haberl R, Weber M, Kemkes B, et al.: Frequency analysis of the QRS-complex and ST-segment for noninvasive detection of acute rejection after orthotopic heart transplantation (Abstract). Circulation 76(Suppl. 4):204, 1987.
96. Haberl R, Weber M, Reichenspurner H, et al.: Frequency analysis of the surface electrocardiogram for recognition of acute rejection after orthotopic cardiac transplantation. Circulation 76:101, 1987.
97. Davies MJ, Path FRC, Thomas AC, et al.: Intramyocardial platelet aggregation in patients with instable angina pectoris suffering sudden ischemic cardiac death. Circulation 73:418, 1986.
98. Patterson E, Holland K, Eller BT, et al.: Ventricular fibrillation resulting from ischemia at a site remote from previous myocardial infarction. A conscious canine model of sudden coronary death. Am J Cardiol 50:1414, 1982.
99. Malliani A, Schwartz PJ, Zanchetti A: Neural mechanisms in life-threatening arrhythmias. Am Heart J 100:705, 1980.
100. Tavazzi L, Zotti AM, Rondanelli R: The role of psychologic stress in the genesis of lethal arrhythmias in patients with coronary artery disease. Eur Heart J 7(Suppl. A):99, 1986.

22

Antiarrhythmic Drugs

Michael R. Rosen

Antiarrhythmic drugs exert their effects on cardiac rhythm by binding to specific loci on cardiac cell membranes. In some instances, these loci are integrally involved in the electrophysiologic function of the heart. Included here are drugs that interact with cardiac channels, such as the local anesthetic antiarrhythmics, drugs that modify phase-3 repolarization and drugs that are calcium channel blocking agents. In other instances, the loci are sites that modulate electrophysiologic function of the heart: representative drugs are beta-adrenergic blockers, which counteract the effects of sympathetic stimulation. Finally, there are drugs that, via a variety of means, modify (and chiefly enhance) vagal input to the heart: included here are drugs as diverse as digitalis (which increases acetylcholine release) and edrophonium (which inhibits acetylcholinesterase and thereby reduces the breakdown of acetylcholine). In this chapter, I shall concentrate on those drugs that act at specific loci on the cardiac cell membrane. Moreover, the purpose will be to emphasize the mechanisms whereby these drugs modify electrophysiologic function at the cellular level.

FUNCTION OF THE CELL MEMBRANE AND ION-SELECTIVE CHANNELS

The cardiac cell membrane is a lipid bilayer that serves as an electrical insulator between the highly conductive aqueous environments of the cytosol and the extracellular space (Fig. 22–1). The lipid bilayer is minimally permeable to ionic constituents of the intra- and extracellular spaces, thereby serving as a barrier to their passage between these two compartments. There are two primary means whereby ions can traverse the membrane, and such passage is essential both for the maintenance of the normal resting potential and for the occurrence of the action potential. The first such means is the ionic pump mechanism (see Fig. 22–1). An example is the enzyme Na-K ATPase, which moves Na^+ and K^+ across the membrane in an electrogenic fashion, such that a transmembrane potential is maintained.[26, 40] As a result, in the resting state the membrane interior is negatively charged. The pumping process requires energy, obtained from the breakdown of ATP. The need for energy is seen in the fact that pumping is not a passive event but must move ions against gradients that would otherwise not favor their passage. For example, the Na-K pump moves sodium out of the cell, where its concentration is low, to the extracellular space, where its concentration is already high. Similarly, potassium is moved from the relatively low concentration of the extracellular space to the high concentration of the intracellular space. Other exchange and/or pumping processes exist as well for ion pairs such as Na^+ and Ca^{2+} and for the pumping of Ca^{2+}.[31] Hence, pumping processes are responsible for the maintenance of ionic gradients and they function to establish concentration and charge disequilibria.

In contrast, channels function to permit the movement of ions passively *along* their concentration and electrical gradients, thereby tending to restore equilib-

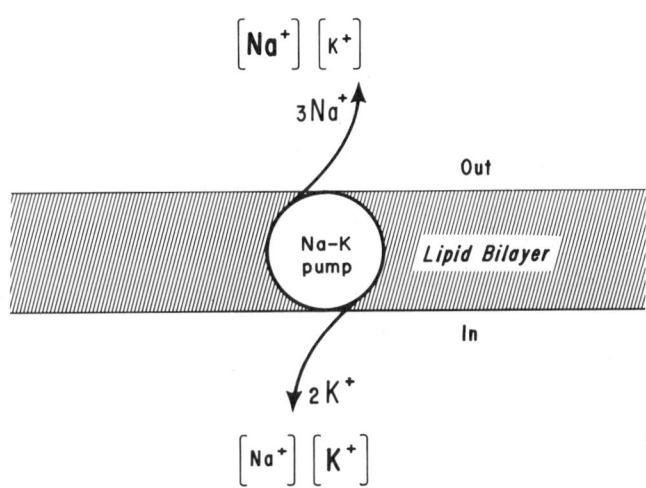

FIGURE 22–1
The cell membrane consists of a lipid bilayer, largely impermeable to the passage of ions. The Na-K pump exchanges Na for K in electrogenic fashion. (See text for explanation.)

Supported by USPHS-NHLBI grants HL-28958 and HL-28223

ria. This may best be understood by referring to Figure 22–2, in which a transmembrane action potential in the Purkinje system is depicted. During the resting state, in which the membrane potential is about -90 mV, this electronegative potential is maintained primarily by Na-K pumping. When the cell is stimulated, its permeability to Na^+ is increased (see below) as its sodium channels open, and the rapid entry of Na^+ ions along concentration and electrical gradients is responsible for phase-0 depolarization of the cell.[28] As Na^+ nears its equilibrium potential, the gradient for its entry decreases and the net charge carried in by sodium decreases as well. This is accompanied by a transient outward current carried by K^+ through a potassium channel, which removes positive charge from the cell (again, along a concentration gradient) and results in a negative-going notch, or phase 1.[34] During phase 0, calcium channels open, and the positive charge carried slowly inward by Ca^{2+} results in inscription of the action potential plateau, or phase 2.[3, 32] Also contributing to the plateau is a residual component of the inward sodium current, referred to as "window" current.[2] During phase 2, potassium channels commence to open and these carry K^+ out via concentration and electrical gradients (at the start of phase 2, the cell's interior is positive with respect to the extracellular space), ultimately returning the cell to its resting potential.[28] Hence, it can be seen that the movement of ions through channels is passive. It is this movement that is responsible for the generation of the cardiac impulse. Moreover, the above discussion ascribes certain characteristics to channels: they provide a pathway for ions to traverse the membrane; certain channels have specificity for the passage of certain ions; and there are specific factors that govern the opening and closing of channels.

We can begin to consider these factors by referring to Figure 22–3, in which I have depicted the lipid bilayer of the membrane, with a channel protein inserted into it. This protein contains a pore through which the aqueous solutions of the intra- and extracellular space can make contact. However, if these were all the components of a channel, ions would rapidly equilibrate through it and the cell could maintain neither an ionic gradient nor a charge. Hence, two additional structures are minimum requirements for its function.[21] The first is a selectivity filter, which resides near the outside of the pore and, via its diameter, configuration, and charge, favors the passage of certain ions along with their waters of hydration—to the relative exclusion of others. Hence the fast sodium channel most readily admits Na^+, but also admits H^+ (and other ions, with diminishing frequency). The slow calcium channel is most highly selective for Ca^+ but also admits Na^+, and so forth.

The second important structure is the channel gate.[21] This may be thought of as a protein at or near the inner side of the channel, which may be in an open or closed position. Consider, in Fig. 22–3, the situation with respect to a channel that is selective for some ion, X^+, which is in high concentration outside the cell and low concentration inside. The selectivity filter will readily permit the passage of X^+. Alternatively, another ion, Y^+, whose entry is not favored by dimension or by charge and concentration gradients can pass the filter to only a limited extent (or not at all). With respect to X^+, if the channel gate is open, it can enter the cell; if the gate is closed, it cannot. Hence, we can see that the filter and the gate act in a complementary fashion; the former establishes the species of ion that can enter the cell via a specific channel, and the latter determines when it can and cannot enter. I must stress that these considerations are not merely theoretical; they have been established experimentally. The ionic selectivity of Na^+, K^+, and Ca^{2+} channels has been documented,[21] and in neurophysiologic experiments, enzymes such as pronase have been used to digest off specific channel gates, thereby changing the functional state of the channel both predictably and reproducibly.[1]

To further explore the role of channel function, I shall consider the fast Na^+ channel as an example (Fig. 22–4). The fast channel has a selectivity filter, as described earlier, as well as two gates—an activation, or "m" gate, and an inactivation, or "h" gate. The functions of these gates were described experimentally in the giant axon of the squid and mathematically by Hodgkin and Huxley some years ago.[22-25] In the resting state, the m gate is closed and the h is open. At this time, recording of the transmembrane potential would reveal no electrical activity. When the cell is stimulated, by a pacemaker wire or a depolarizing impulse from an adjacent cell, the resultant change in voltage induces the opening of the m gate. In other words, the channel is voltage-dependent, and when a shift from resting to threshold potential occurs, the m gate responds to this by opening and permitting Na^+ to enter. As a result, phase 0 of the action potential is inscribed. The h gate, too, is voltage-dependent, and as voltage becomes more positive it commences to close. With

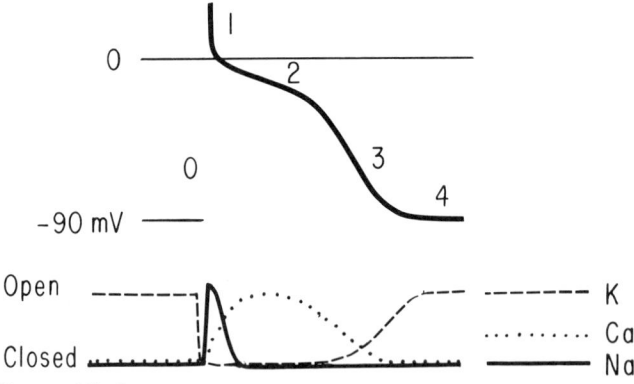

FIGURE 22–2
The transmembrane action potential of a Purkinje fiber showing rapid phase 0 depolarization and three phases of repolarization (1–3), followed by a return to the maximum diastolic potential (4). The legend on the bottom indicates sodium, calcium, and potassium channels, but ignores the fact that channel subtypes exist. Hence the early outward current carried by $[K^+]_o$ is not depicted, nor are the Ca^{2+} channel subtypes. The open and closed channel states are depicted. The indication that any channel (e.g., Na) is in the open or closed state does not mean that all channels of that type are open simultaneously, but rather that a preponderance is.

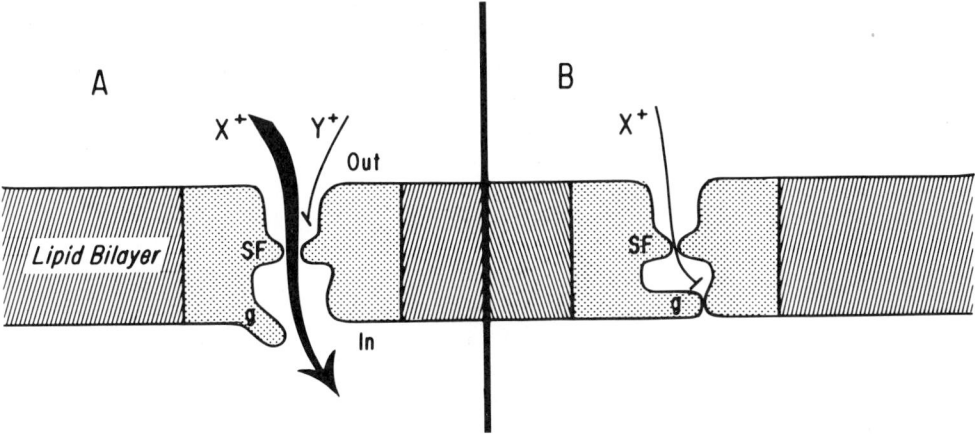

FIGURE 22–3
An idealized channel in the membrane, having a selectivity filter (SF) and gate (G), which may be open (A) or closed (B). Two ionic species X^+ and Y^+ are depicted. (See text for explanation.)

the h gate closed and the m gate open, no more sodium ion can enter, and Na^+ entry through that specific channel can no longer contribute to that action potential. Once the gates have attained their new positions, the channel is said to be in the inactivated state. The return of the gates to their initial states is both voltage and time dependent. When the process is complete, the cell is once again in the resting state and the process can be reinitiated.

It is important to stress that the above process is not entirely uniform. Recent studies of channels in membrane patches have revealed that in any state (resting, open, and inactivated), there is a high probability that all the channels in the membrane will share that particular state, but a subset will be in one of the other states.[21] In other words, there is a randomness to channel openings and closings that is not necessarily consonant with the state of the cell as a whole. Referring to the above processes and to Figure 22–4, one can appreciate the factors required for the cell to be excitable (i.e., the presence of a high resting membrane potential, a closed m gate, and an open h gate). One can also appreciate that once a cell has been excited and is in the inactivated state, it is refractory to additional electrical stimuli. That is, its m gate already is open, the h gate closed and both time and voltage dependent processes must occur before the channels can again open, en masse, to initiate an action potential. Nonetheless, in any state, some channels will be in a position to respond to a second stimulus, and channels *can* move from one state to another.[21]

Potassium channels and calcium channels differ from the fast sodium channel in terms of their ionic selectivity and their gating characteristics. There appears to be a family of potassium channels rather than a single channel subtype. Because the potassium equilibrium potential is negative, the function of open potassium channels will be to move membrane potential in the direction of the potassium equilibrium (i.e., in a repolarizing direction). Hence, potassium channels are concerned with various aspects of repolarization or hyperpolarization of the membrane. The various subtypes of potassium channels are reviewed in detail elsewhere.[9, 13, 35] Of particular importance, however, is that both the selectivity of K channels and their gating differ importantly from those of the sodium channel. The delayed rectifier K channel has received, perhaps, the greatest attention.[21, 35] Like most K channels it is

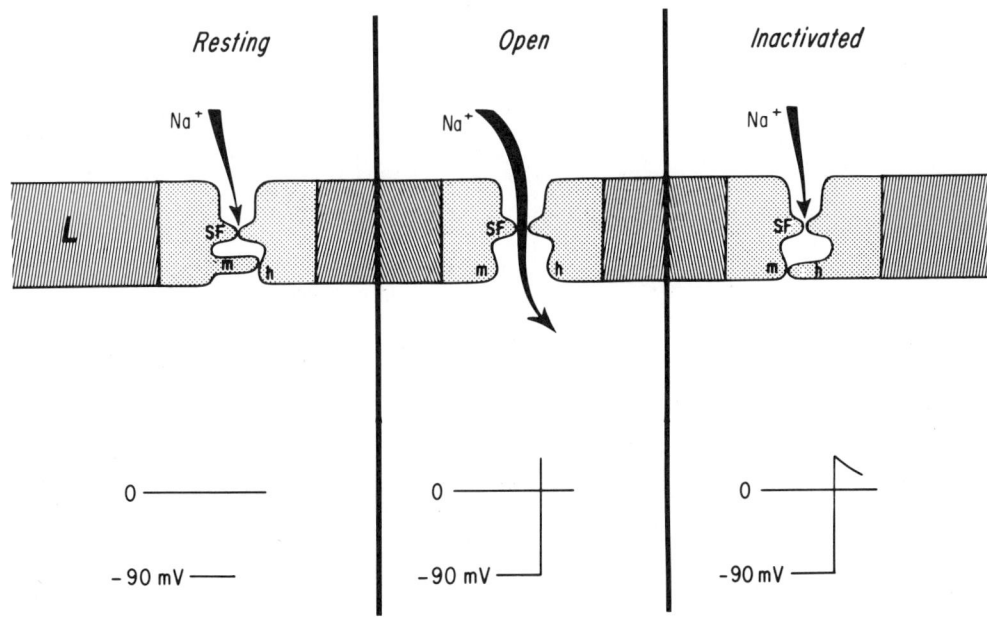

FIGURE 22–4
The resting, open, and inactivated states of the fast Na^+ channel. L = lipid bilayer; SF = selectivity filter; m and h = channel gates. The status of the transmembrane potential is depicted below each channel state. In the resting state (m gate closed) a resting membrane potential is recorded. In the open state (m and h open) the upstroke of the action potential is recorded, and in the inactivated state (h gate closed) the membrane is repolarizing. (See text for explanation.)

Antiarrhythmic Drugs 403

voltage sensitive. Its role is to modulate the duration of repolarization as well as pacemaker potentials. For this reason, drugs that modify the conductance of this channel will tend to modify the duration of the action potential, as well as pacemaker activity.

Calcium channels achieve their open state when the membrane is depolarized (e.g., during the upstroke of the action potential).[21] Although there appear to be a family of calcium channels in the heart, I will refer here to a channel that is voltage dependent for its activation and that contributes inward current to the plateau of the transmembrane action potential. The current density carried by the calcium channel is smaller than those of the sodium and potassium channels. Moreover, the slow inward current that occurs as the result of Ca^{2+} entry into the cell is slowly inactivating. As a result, the calcium-dependent action potentials referred to as "slow responses" have low amplitudes and rates of rise, and they propagate quite slowly.[11] This type of action potential occurs normally in the sinus and AV nodes and is thought to contribute to some reentrant rhythms in fibers of the atrial and ventricular conducting systems.

Local Anesthetic Antiarrhythmics

The primary effect of local anesthetic antiarrhythmic drugs is on the fast sodium channel. This does not mean they have no additional effects: for example, quinidine blocks K^+ and Ca^{2+} channels as well, and quinidine and disopyramide also are muscarinic blockers. However, the antiarrhythmic effect that is common to all local anesthetic drugs is attributable to their action on the fast channel.

Figure 22–5 depicts the interaction of a drug (D) with the fast sodium channel. The first important factor to consider is that the putative binding sites for local anesthetic drugs reside between the selectivity filter and the channel gates.[21, 33] In other words, drugs do not act to occlude the channel pore from the outside (in contrast to toxins like tetrodotoxin, which bind to the outside of the channel and have positively charged guanidinium groups that seem to be involved in occlusion of the channel).[6, 29] Furthermore, the drugs are too large and inappropriately configured to traverse the selectivity filter. Whether, in fact, all local anesthetics share the same specific binding site between the selectivity filter and the gates is still a matter that is unsettled. Moreover, whether this local anesthetic binding site has the same "lock and key" characteristics attributed to beta-adrenergic receptors and their agonists and antagonists is even less certain. These questions will be considered subsequently.

When drugs are in the extracellular space, they may be uncharged (D) or ionized (D^+). Both of these forms can equilibrate with the membrane, but in different fashions. D, which is not ionized, has a high lipid solubility; as a result, it can pass more readily through the lipid bilayer and attain its binding site, between the selectivity filter and the channel gates.

The ionized form of a local anesthetic moves slowly through the lipid bilayer but is freely soluble in the cytosol. To attain the local anesthetic binding site, it must pass an additional barrier. This is the channel gate(s). Hence, the ionized molecule can enter the channel only when the gates are open. This limitation of access to binding sites initially was noted in neuropharmacologic experiments in which permanently charged local anesthetics were iontophoresed into the cytosol.[15, 19, 20, 38] The requirement that channel gates must be in the open state to permit entry of drugs provides the basis for frequency or "use" dependence.[19, 20, 27, 33] Use dependence refers to the fact that the faster the heart or stimulus rate, the more a channel is "used." Increasing use means more frequent opening and closing. If a channel spends more time in the open state, there is increased opportunity for a local anesthetic to gain access to its binding site. Drugs that show use dependence (and this is a characteristic of most local anesthetic antiarrhythmics) will increasingly

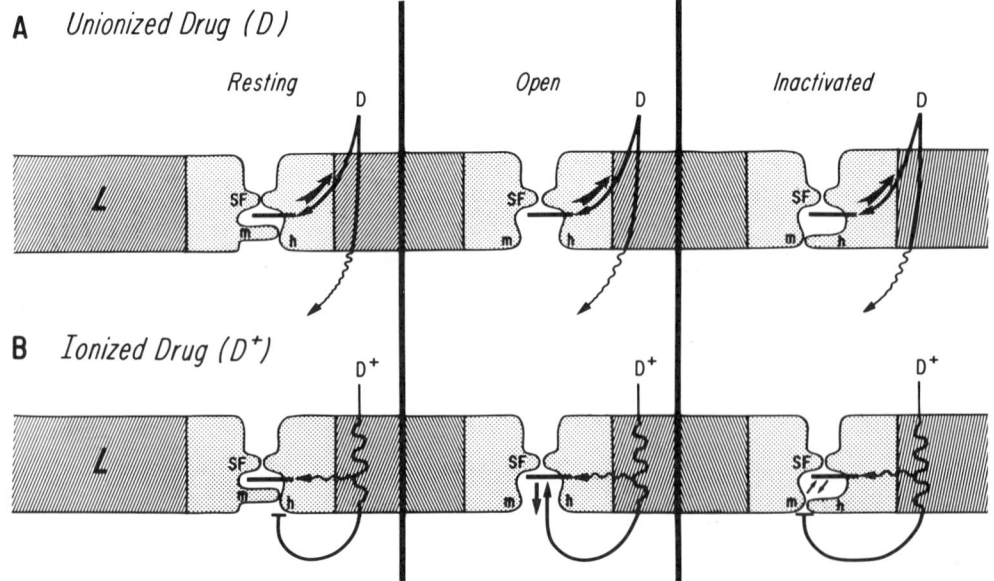

FIGURE 22–5

Interaction of an un-ionized (D, panel A) and an ionized (D^+ panel B) drug molecule with the fast Na^+ channel. The unionized molecule passes readily through the lipid bilayer and interacts with the channel in all three states, attaining its binding site (horizontal bar) and establishing an equilibrium. The ionized molecule passes slowly through the lipid bilayer. When it reaches the cytosol it passes readily through the aqueous environment but has access to the binding site only when the channel is open, again establishing an equilibrium. (See text for explanation.)

block the channel at faster stimulation rates or at faster heart rates.[19, 20, 27] In other words, in the presence of tachycardia there will be more channel block than during bradycardia. This use-dependent blocking characteristic is in contrast to the "tonic blocking" actions of uncharged drug molecules.[27] The latter can gain access to their binding sites regardless of channel state.

As for any drug-receptor interaction, the equilibrium between the local anesthetic molecule and its putative receptor site is characterized by specific rate constants. These rate constants differ from drug to drug but, for each drug, they describe the kinetics for binding to and unbinding from a channel site during any channel state (resting, open, and inactivated).[27, 41] In other words, the drug's affinity for the channel is modulated by the channel state. It must be understood as well that following drug binding, the state of the channel itself is affected. This behavior is described by the "modulated receptor hypothesis" presented in Figure 22–6.[19, 20, 27, 33] As shown here, the interactions among resting, open, and inactivated states of the membrane are described by Hodgkin and Huxley kinetics. Drugs can bind to and unbind from the receptor in any channel state—but with different kinetics. Implicit in this hypothesis is the idea that there is a specific local anesthetic receptor in the fast sodium channel, for which individual drugs and metabolites appear to have varying affinities. The demonstration of varying affinity is consistent with the presence of one binding site for which different molecules have different binding characteristics or with the presence of more than one type of binding site. There is experimental support for the hypothesis of a single, variable affinity binding site, but some studies have suggested that more than one local anesthetic receptor may exist in the channel.[30, 39]

More recently, an alternative hypothesis has been forwarded to explain the drug-receptor interaction. This is the guarded receptor hypothesis.[36, 37] Rather than assuming a specific local anesthetic receptor in the fast channel, this hypothesis assumes that drug binding in the channel may be a simpler process, perhaps requiring only a hydrogen bonding link between the drug and the channel wall. In this case, the entire channel between selectivity filter and gates may be thought of as the "receptor," with the gates themselves and the ability of a specific drug molecule to traverse the gates determining the drug-receptor interaction. In this way, the receptor may be thought of as being "guarded" by the gates, with its function determined by the kinetics for the drug's entry to, and its egress from, the channel.

Additional processes influence the drug-receptor interaction. For some drugs, such as lidocaine, there is a profound membrane potential dependence to channel binding.[7, 17] That is, as the membrane is depolarized, lidocaine binds more completely and readily to the channel, inducing greater channel block (Fig. 22–7). This explains in part the greater efficacy of lidocaine in depressing the phase-0 upstroke and conduction of action potentials in infarcted tissues having low membrane potentials than in normal tissues. It also provides a basis for understanding why an antiarrhythmic like lidocaine—which is effective in suppressing arrhythmias arising in diseased (and depolarized) tissues—exerts only minimal toxic effects on conduction in normal cardiac tissues.

A second factor influencing the drug-receptor interaction is pH.[18] Most local anesthetic antiarrhythmics exist in both ionized and unionized forms in the plasma.[16] For most of these drugs, acidosis will increase the proportion of ionized drug molecules present, thereby increasing their use-dependent actions (see above). Moreover, in settings where pH is changing, one can expect the actions of the drug to vary, based on the relationship of the pK_a of the drug to the pH.[18]

Another important variable is molecular weight (Fig. 22–8).[10, 41] As the molecular weight of a molecule increases, the rate at which it unbinds from the receptor tends to decrease. In other words, with other factors being equal, a drug of high molecular weight can be expected to bind more persistently to the channel than one of low molecular weight, thereby sustaining any channel blocking therapeutic or toxic effects it may be exerting. A final consideration is molecular structure. It has been shown for specific molecules, such as aprindine,[14] that minor modifications in the structure can bring important changes in the drug-receptor interaction. Hence, this factor must be taken into account, as well.

Given the above information, a fair amount of work has been done to characterize the binding to and unbinding from the fast channel of local anesthetic antiarrhythmics. These are summarized in Table 22–1. Although the information here is complex, it is no more complex than the many responses seen when

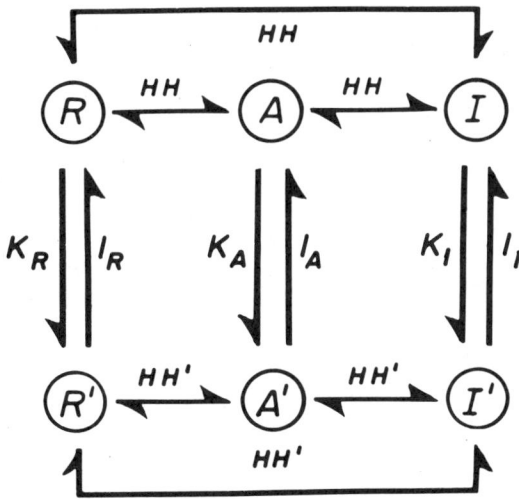

FIGURE 22–6
The modulated receptor hypothesis. Depicted are the three channel states: resting (R), activated or open (A), and inactivated (I). The interchange among channel states is described by Hodgkin-Huxley kinetics (H H). A drug can bind and unbind to its channel site in all three states (leading to the R', A', I' status). Here the interchange is described by modified Hodgkin-Huxley kinetics (H H'). The different on and off binding constants for a drug in each channel state (K) are indicated. (Reprinted by permission from Hondeghem LM, Katzung BG: Biochim Biophys Acta 472:373, 1977.)

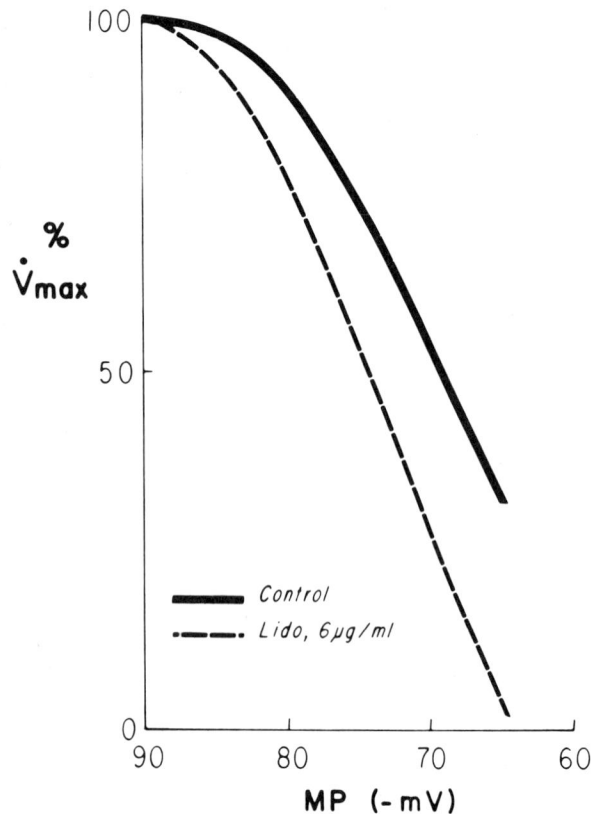

FIGURE 22-7
Effects of lidocaine (Lido; 6 μg/ml) on $\dot{V}_{max}$ of canine Purkinje fibers at different levels of membrane potential (MP). $\dot{V}_{max}$ is expressed as % of control. Note that as the membrane is depolarized there is an accentuated reduction of $\dot{V}_{max}$, demonstrating a voltage-dependent action of the drug. (Modified from Morikawa Y and Rosen M: Circ Res 55:637, 1984.)

local anesthetic antiarrhythmics are administered to patients with arrhythmias. Why two patients with apparently identical pathophysiologic processes and arrhythmias do not respond to the same drug, whereas two patients with apparently different processes do respond to the same drug has perplexed clinical and basic investigators alike. To be sure, some of these differences may be related to differences in drug absorption, binding, and metabolism among patients. However, it is clear that the differences do not stop with pharmacokinetics. Rather, different drugs in the same drug "category" (e.g., Vaughan Williams class IA, IB, or IC[41]) have quantitatively different interactions with the sodium channel. Moreover, depending on the cellular substrate in an individual patient, differences in membrane potential, extracellular [K^+] (which influences membrane potential), and pH will provide further cause for differences in the individual response to the same drug.

Drugs that Block Other Channels

There is not the same volume of information available for drugs that block potassium and calcium channels as for the Na^+ channel. Considering potassium first, there are relatively few drugs that affect a K^+ channel uniquely. A drug such as quinidine,[8] which prolongs phase-3 repolarization, has important depressant effects on the fast Na^+ channel which probably are equally if not more important in its overall antiarrhythmic effect. A prototypical drug that affects the K^+ channel is D-sotalol,[5] which reduces time-dependent K current activated during the action potential plateau, as well as background K current. The result is prolongation of action potential duration.

With respect to voltage-dependent calcium channels, verapamil is an example of drugs having important, blocking effects.[4] The major action of these drugs is on nodal tissues, which have calcium-dependent action potentials. Moreover, in pathologic settings in which cells are depolarized to the extent that the fast inward current is inactivated and slow channel–dependent "slow response" action potentials are occurring, these same drugs can have an important effect on action potential initiation and propagation.

Conclusions

Not long ago, it was believed that the actions of antiarrhythmic drugs might be readily explicable, based on their effects on the transmembrane action potential. This type of categorization of drug effects, although a useful stage in the evolution of our understanding of mechanisms of drug action, clearly has been superseded as our understanding of the complexity of cardiac channels and drug receptor interactions has increased. Although clinical antiarrhythmic therapy was and remains today largely an empirical phenome-

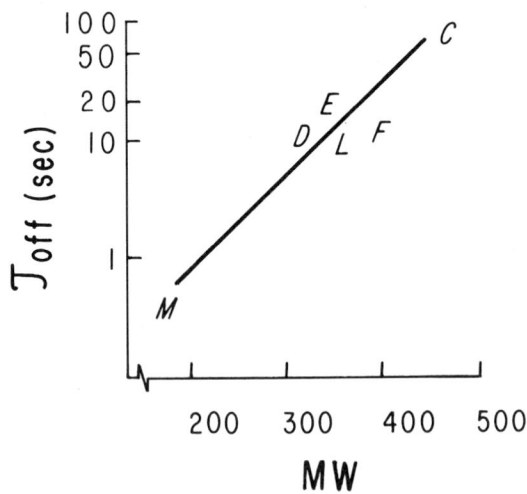

FIGURE 22-8
The time constant for unbinding of drugs (T_{off}) following use-dependent block, expressed as a function of molecular weight (MW). M = mexiletine; D = disopyramide; E = encainide; L = lidocaine; F = flecainide; C = CCI 22277. As molecular weight increases, the time constant for unbinding also increases. (Modified from Vaughan Williams EM: In Mechanisms and Treatment of Cardiac Arrhythmias: Relevance of Basic Studies to Clinical Management, pp 165–172. Baltimore, Urban & Swarzenberg, 1985.)

TABLE 22-1
Representative Rates of Onset and Offset of Use-Dependent Block.*

Drug	Fat Solubility (log P)	pK_a	Concentration (μM)	Block Onset Rate (AP^{-1})	Offset Rate (T_{off})	MW
Lidocaine	2.8	7.8	200	>.6		234
Mexiletine	1.3	9.3	20	>.6	.47	179
Tocainide	0.8	7.8	300	.277		190
Disopyramide	1.8	8.4	100	.113	12.2	339
Flecainide	1.2	9.3	5	.029	15.5	408
Encainide	0.9	10.2	3	.025	20.3	358

*These data obtained from Vaughan Williams, 1985.[41] They refer to ventricular muscle paced at a drive cycle length = 300 ms. The rate of onset of block was calculated at AP^{-1}.

non, we at last have the information available to understand why earlier attempts to predict and prescribe drug actions in a rational, mechanistic way have failed. Nonetheless, as we learn more about drugs and their receptors, it is likely that we are building the kind of information that will lead to more predictable and improved means for developing and administering antiarrhythmic drugs.

Acknowledgments

The author expresses his gratitude to Dr. Walter Spinelli for his thoughtful critique of the manuscript, and to Susan McMahon for her careful attention to its preparation.

References

1. Armstrong CM, Bezanilla F: Currents related to movement of the gating particles of the sodium channels. Nature (Lond.) 242:459, 1973.
2. Attwell D, Cohen I, Eisner D, et al.: The steady state TTX-sensitive ("window") sodium current in cardiac Purkinje fibers. Pflugers Arch 379:137, 1979.
3. Beeler GW Jr, Reuter H: Membrane calcium current in ventricular myocardial fibres. J Physiol (London) 207:191, 1970.
4. Boyden PA, Wit AL: Pharmacology of the antiarrhythmic drugs. In Rosen MR, Hoffman BF (eds.): Cardiac Therapy, pp. 171–234. Boston, Martinus Nijhoff, 1983.
5. Carmeliet E: Electrophysiologic and voltage clamp analysis of the effects of sotalol on isolated cardiac muscle and Purkinje fibers. J Pharmacol Exp Ther 232:817, 1985.
6. Catterall WA: Neurotoxins that act on voltage-sensitive sodium channels in excitable membranes. Ann Rev Pharmacol Toxicol 20:15, 1980.
7. Chen CM, Gettes LS: Combined effects of rate, membrane potential and drugs on maximum rate of rise (V_{max}) of action potential upstroke of guinea pig papillary muscle. Circ Res 38:464, 1976.
8. Colatsky TJ: Mechanisms of action of lidocaine and quinidine on action potential duration in rabbit cardiac Purkinje fibers. Circ Res 50:17, 1982.
9. Conti F, Hille B, and Nonner W: Nonstationary fluctuations of the potassium conductance at the node of Ranvier of the frog. J Physiol (Lond.) 353:199, 1984.
10. Courtney KR: Review: Quantitative structure/activity relations based on use-dependent block and repriming kinetics in myocardium. J Molec Cell Cardiol 19:319, 1987.
11. Cranefield PF: The Conduction of the Cardiac Impulse: The Slow Response and Cardiac Arrhythmias. Mt. Kisco, Futura Publishing Company, 1975.
12. Dubois JM: Evidence for the existence of three types of potassium channels in the frog Ranvier node membrane. J Physiol (Lond.) 318:297, 1981.
13. Dubois JM: Potassium currents in the frog node of Ranvier. Prog Biophys Molec Biol 42:1, 1983.
14. Ehring GR, Moyer JW, Hondeghem LM: Implications from electrophysiological differences resulting from small structural changes in antiarrhythmic drugs. Proc West Pharmacol Soc 25:65, 1982.
15. Frazier DT, Narahashi T, Yamada M: The site of action and active form of local anesthetics. Experiments with quaternary compounds. J Pharmacol Exp Ther 171:45, 1970.
16. Gintant GA, Hoffman BF, Naylor RE: The influence of molecular form of local anesthetic-type antiarrhythmic agents on reduction of the maximum upstroke velocity of canine cardiac Purkinje fibers. Circ Res 52:735, 1983.
17. Grant AO, Starmer CF, Strauss HC: Antiarrhythmic drug action: Blockade of the inward sodium current. Circ Res 55:427, 1984.
18. Grant AO, Strauss LJ, Wallace AG, et al.: The influence of pH on the electrophysiological effects of lidocaine in guinea pig ventricular myocardium. Circ Res 47:542, 1980.
19. Hille B: The pH-dependent rate of action of local anesthetics on the node of Ranvier. J Gen Physiol 69:475, 1977.
20. Hille B: Local anesthetics: Hydrophilic and hydrophobic pathways for the drug-receptor reaction. J Gen Physiol 69:497, 1977.
21. Hille B: Ionic Channels of Excitable Membranes. Sunderland, Mass., Sinauer Associates, 1984.
22. Hodgkin AL, Huxley AF: Currents carried by sodium and potassium ions through the membrane of the giant axon of Loligo. J Physiol (Lond.) 116:449, 1952.
23. Hodgkin AL, Huxley AF: The components of membrane conductance in the giant axon of Loligo. J Physiol 116:473, 1952.
24. Hodgkin AL, Huxley AF: The dual effect of membrane potential on sodium conductance in the giant axon of Loligo. J Physiol (Lond.) 116:497, 1952.
25. Hodgkin AL, Huxley AF: A quantitative description of membrane current and its application to conduction and excitation in nerve. J Physiol (Lond.) 117:500, 1952.
26. Hoffman BF, Cranefield PF: Electrophysiology of the Heart. New York, McGraw-Hill, 1960.
27. Hondeghem LM, Katzung BG: Time- and voltage-dependent interactions of antiarrhythmic drugs with cardiac sodium channels. Biochim Biophys Acta 472:373, 1977.
28. Jack JJB, Noble D, Tsien RW: Electric Current Flow in Excitable Cells. Oxford, Clarendon Press, 1975.
29. Kao CY, Walker SE: Active groups of saxitoxin and tetrodotoxin as deduced from actions of saxitoxin analogues on frog muscle and squid axon. J Physiol (Lond.) 323:619, 1982.
30. Mrose HE, Ritchie JM: Local anesthetics: Do benzocaine and lidocaine act at the same single site? J Gen Physiol 71:223, 1978.
31. Mullins LJ: Ion Transport in Heart. New York, Raven Press, 1981.
32. Reuter H: Divalent cations as charge carriers in excitable membranes. In Butler JAV, Noble D (eds.): Progress in Biophysics and Molecular Biology, pp. 3–43. New York, Pergamon Press, 1973.
33. Schwarz W, Palade PT, Hille B: Local anesthetics: Effect of pH on use-dependent block of sodium channels in frog muscle. Biophys J 20:343, 1977.
34. Siegelbaum SA, Tsien RW, Kass RS: Role of intracellular calcium in the transient outward current of calf Purkinje fibers. Nature 269:611, 1977.

35. Stanfield PR: Tetraethylammonium ions and the potassium permeability of excitable cells. Rev Physiol Biochem Pharmacol 97:1, 1983.
36. Starmer CF, Courtney KR: Modeling ion channel blockade at guarded binding sites: application to tertiary drugs. Am J Physiol 251:H848, 1986.
37. Starmer CF, Grant AO, Strauss HC: Mechanisms of use-dependent block of sodium channels in excitable membranes by local anesthetics. Biophys J 46:15, 1984.
38. Strichartz GR: The inhibition of sodium currents in myelinated nerve by quaternary derivatives of lidocaine. J Gen Physiol 62:37, 1973.
39. Ritchie JM: The action of local anesthetics on ion channels of excitable tissues. In Strichartz GR (ed): Local Anesthetics, Vol. 81 of The Handbook of Experimental Pharmacology, pp. 21–52. New York, Springer-Verlag, 1987.
40. Thomas RC: Electrogenic sodium pump in nerve and muscle cells. Physiol Rev 52:563, 1972.
41. Vaughan Williams EM: Subdivisions of Class I drugs. *In* Reiser HJ, Horowitz LN (eds.): Mechanisms and Treatment of Cardiac Arrhythmias: Relevance of Basic Studies to Clinical Management, pp. 165–172. Baltimore, Urban & Schwarzenberg, 1985.

23

Current Antiarrhythmic Agents: Clinical Pharmacology

Christian Funck-Brentano
Raymond L. Woosley

Ventricular and supraventricular arrhythmias can be associated with significant morbidity and mortality, with the prognosis for patients with ventricular arrhythmias depending mainly on the type of arrhythmia and the underlying heart disease.[1-11] The severity of symptoms varies among patients and is not necessarily correlated with the severity of the arrhythmia in terms of vital risk. Highly symptomatic arrhythmias may not be lethal; asymptomatic arrhythmias may degenerate into arrhythmias leading to sudden death. Among the numerous approaches to the treatment of arrhythmias, pharmacotherapy remains the cornerstone of treatment when therapy is indicated. Many antiarrhythmic agents are now available; all have a narrow therapeutic index in general,[12] and this is even more so in certain subsets of patients, such as those with depressed left ventricular function.[13] Although antiarrhythmic drugs have different potencies when groups of patients are considered[14] the antiarrhythmic response in a given patient cannot be predicted from such a classification. Most often, antiarrhythmic drug prescription remains empirical.[15]

For all these reasons, knowledge of the clinical pharmacology of antiarrhythmic drugs is essential to maximize response and limit the risks of administration. In this chapter, we will briefly review concepts of clinical pharmacology applicable to the administration of antiarrhythmic drugs and we will discuss the objectives of antiarrhythmic treatments. We will then review the clinical pharmacology of individual agents currently available and discuss their use in combination.

Concepts in Clinical Pharmacology

Administration of drugs, particularly those with a narrow therapeutic index, is guided by the knowledge of their fate in humans. Understanding the primary concepts of pharmacokinetics helps to better understand the variations within and among patients in response to the administration of drugs.

DRUG RELEASE

Patient compliance to treatment is better when infrequent dosing is possible. Recently, sustained release preparations of several cardioactive drugs have been marketed. In these preparations, the drug is in a form that is released slowly into the gut lumen.[16] While this is of potential benefit in terms of patient compliance with treatment, it may also lead to interindividual differences in completeness of absorption of drug. In cases of decreased bowel transit time or decreased intestinal surface for absorption, slow-release preparations may be carried past the absorptive sites before the drug has been completely absorbed or before complete tablet dissolution has occurred.[17]

ABSORPTION AND BIOAVAILABILITY

Bioavailability is the fraction of an orally administered drug that reaches the systemic circulation. It represents the sum of several processes that may lead to drug elimination prior to arrival in the systemic circulation: essentially, absorption and presystemic elimination. Absorption is the process by which a drug leaves the site where it is being released. The major determinants of the absorption of a drug are either properties of the drug itself (formulation, lipid solubility, pK, molecular size) or of the subject (gastrointestinal motility, absorptive area).

Presystemic elimination represents the sum of all processes that lead to drug elimination before the drug is made available to the systemic circulation to be distributed to its sites of action. For an orally administered drug, this may occur in the gut lumen, the gut wall, and in the liver.[18] Presystemic elimination does not always lead to inactivation of the parent drug and reduced pharmacodynamic activity. If a drug is extensively metabolized in the liver to form an active metabolite, bioavailability of the parent drug will be reduced without loss of overall pharmacodynamic activity.[19]

DISTRIBUTION

Once drugs reach the systemic circulation, they are distributed throughout the body. The rate of distribution depends on several factors, including the physicochemical properties of the drug considered, the type of tissue to which it is distributed, the extent of protein binding both in plasma and in tissues, and the rate of distribution to non-eliminating organs relative to the rate of distribution to eliminating organs. The volume of distribution is a calculated theoretical volume that has no strict anatomic counterpart. It is assumed that only unbound and non-ionized drug diffuses through membranes. For practical purposes, kinetics of distribution are often described using compartmental models, with drugs being characterized according to the rate at which they diffuse in and out of "mathematically determined" compartments. The initial volume into which a drug distributes (the central volume of distribution) includes blood volume and body tissues that are highly perfused. For most drugs, a slower distribution can be demonstrated to occur from the central compartment to a second "peripheral" compartment, which usually accumulates larger quantities of drug. The clinical significance of these compartments is evident in the relationship between drug plasma concentration and effect and in the dosing regimens designed to achieve a rapid effect (i.e., loading doses).

CLEARANCE

Drugs can be cleared from plasma at several sites, with the liver and kidneys being the most important for most drugs.[18] Clearance of drugs eliminated predominantly by the kidneys may be affected by alteration of any of the components of renal elimination, which include renal blood flow, glomerular filtration rate, tubular secretion, and tubular reabsorption.

Clearance of drugs eliminated predominantly by the liver may be affected by the rate of drug delivery to that organ (rate of absorption or liver blood flow) and the hepatic extraction ratio of the drug (which represents the extent to which liver enzymes are able to metabolize the drug). Each of these two factors can be altered in many clinical circumstances.

HALF-LIFE AND STEADY STATE

Half-life is the time required for a 50% change in any first-order process. A first-order process is one in which the rate of drug elimination is directly proportional to the serum concentration. The concept of half-life can be applied to both distribution and elimination. One half-life represents the time required for drug plasma concentration to decrease by 50%. After administration of a drug is discontinued, a time equal to 4 elimination half-lives is required to reduce drug concentration to less than 7% of its original level. Elimination of a drug from plasma does not necessarily correlate with an equivalent loss of pharmacologic activity, although this is often the case. The half-life is mathematically derived from the elimination rate constant (K_e):

$$t_{1/2} = 0.693/K_e$$

and may be thought of as the fractional rate of drug elimination from the body. If $K_e = 0.10$ h^{-1}, then 10% of the amount of drug in the body will be eliminated per hour at any given moment in time.

Steady state represents the condition in which drug uptake and elimination are equal, resulting in reproducible drug concentrations after each dose. Its time course is dependent on elimination rate. By analogy to drug elimination, it takes 4 or 5 half-lives from the time of initiation of therapy (or of change in dosage) to achieve a new steady state (Fig. 23–1). *In a first-order process, the time course of reaching steady state depends only on elimination half-life, whereas the magnitude of steady state concentration depends only on clearance and dose.*

PROTEIN BINDING

It is assumed that only that portion of drug not bound to plasma proteins diffuses through membranes and is pharmacologically active. Acidic drugs predominantly bind to albumin, whereas basic drugs, a class that includes most antiarrhythmic drugs, primarily bind to alpha$_1$-acid glycoprotein. Hence, factors causing changes in protein binding or protein content in plasma

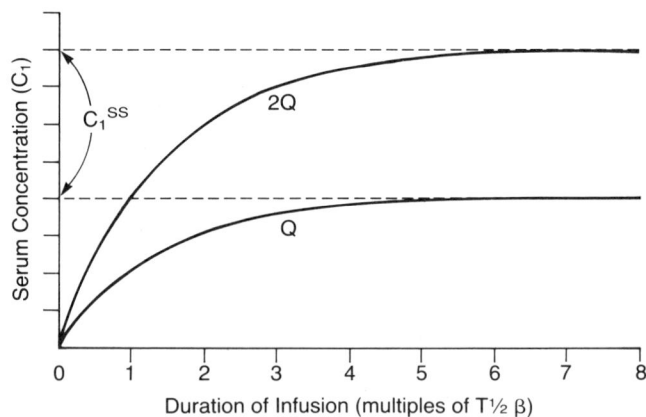

FIGURE 23–1
Concept of half-life and steady state in a first-order process. A constant-rate infusion of a given amount of drug is shown. Doubling the amount of drug infused (Q vs. 2Q) doubles the steady-state plasma concentration but does not alter the time needed to reach steady state. This time represents approximately 5 elimination half-lives of the drug. (Reprinted by permission from Woosley RL, Roden DM. Basic principles of clinical pharmacology. In Parmley WW, Chatterjee K (eds.): Cardiology, Chapter 15, p. 11. Philadelphia J. B. Lippincott Co. 1988.)

can cause an alteration in the actions of a drug at a given drug dosage.

Protein binding may also play a major role with respect to drug elimination in the liver and kidneys. In the kidney, only unbound drug is cleared by glomerular filtration; however, total drug is potentially available for active secretion in the proximal tubule, since this process may be sufficiently efficient to "strip" the bound drug from the protein.

In the liver, protein binding affects drug extraction to a variable extent, depending on the intrinsic ability of the liver to metabolize the drug.[20] When the extraction ratio, an index of metabolizing activity, is low (<25%) (i.e., when intrinsic clearance of the unbound drug is small compared to liver blood flow), protein binding is a limiting factor to clearance across the whole binding range. In contrast, if the liver is very efficient at drug removal, elimination is less affected by the extent of binding.[18]

FACTORS INFLUENCING DRUG DISPOSITION

Discussion of all possible factors that may alter pharmacokinetics is beyond the scope of this chapter. We will focus on those factors that are more relevant to administration of antiarrhythmic drugs and to patients with cardiovascular diseases.

Absorption and Presystemic Elimination

Absorption can be altered by concomitant administration of several drugs, as has been shown for propranolol and aluminum hydroxide gel.[21] Presystemic elimination can be altered in a major way by concomitant administration of drugs that enhance[22] or inhibit[23] hepatic enzymatic activity. Coadministration of drugs that compete for the same liver enzymes can also modify the bioavailability of those drugs having lower affinity for the enzymes. This type of interaction has been shown for propafenone and metoprolol.[24] Only drugs that are highly extracted by the liver (i.e., drugs with low or intermediate systemic bioavailability) are likely to demonstrate significant changes in bioavailability as a consequence of disease or drug-drug interaction.

Distribution and Protein Binding

The volume of the central compartment (i.e., the initial volume into which a drug distributes very rapidly) can be reduced, both in certain disease states and for certain drugs. For example, the volume of the central compartment for lidocaine is decreased in congestive heart failure.[25] Protein binding can be altered by changes in the amount of protein or by competition of several molecules for the same binding sites. For example, severe renal insufficiency is associated with decreased plasma levels of albumin, whereas myocardial infarction is associated with increased levels of alpha$_1$-acid glycoprotein.[26, 27] Competition between several molecules for the same binding sites is likely to cause significant alteration in pharmacologic response if the competing compounds are highly protein-bound (>90%), the volume of distribution is small, and the therapeutic index is narrow.[28] Protein binding can also be concentration-dependent, as is the case for disopyramide (Fig. 23–2), in which saturation of protein binding occurs in the range of usual plasma concentrations.[29]

Clearance

Drugs highly extracted by the liver are subject to potentially significant alterations of their clearance. In addition to factors discussed above for presystemic elimination, genetic influences in drug metabolism can play a major role in variations in hepatic elimination among patients.[30, 31] Elimination of drugs that are metabolized in the liver and that have a high hepatic extraction ratio depends mainly on liver blood flow. Change in clearance will be a function of change in liver blood flow. Liver blood flow can be affected by diseases such as congestive heart failure[32] or agents such as beta-adrenergic antagonists or calcium channel blockers.[33] Elimination of drugs metabolized in the liver that have a low extraction ratio depends on protein binding (see above) and the activity of hepatic enzymes responsible for their metabolism.

Alteration in elimination of drugs cleared by the kidney depends on alteration in renal blood flow, glomerular filtration rate, tubular secretion, and reabsorption. These factors can be affected by renal diseases,[34] age,[35] urinary pH,[36] and competition among drugs for tubular reabsorption or secretion.[37, 38]

DRUG ADMINISTRATION

The basic concepts discussed above help one to design rational regimens for drug administration. In nonurgent situations, drugs are administered as a maintenance dose. As previously described, it will take 4 to 5 half-lives before steady state in plasma is reached

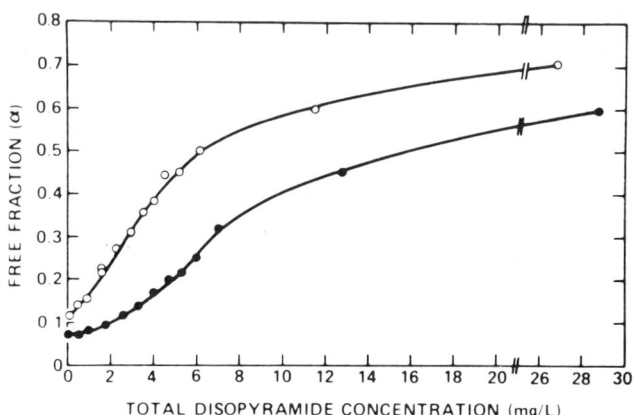

FIGURE 23–2
Saturable nature of disopyramide binding to plasma proteins. As the total disopyramide concentration increases, the free fraction (α) increases disproportionately. The two lines represent the extremes of values obtained from a population of 12 subjects. (Reprinted by permission from Meffin P, Robert EW, Winkle RA, et al.: J Pharmacokinet Biopharm 7:29, 1979.)

and a stable pharmacodynamic response can be expected to occur. However, in more urgent circumstances a loading dose may be administered. This loading dose does not reduce the time needed to reach steady state (which depends only on elimination half-life in a first-order process), but it will allow plasma concentrations, and concentrations in highly perfused tissues, to reach higher levels early after initiation of therapy. If the site of drug action can be reached early, loading doses can reduce the time before onset of a pharmacologic response. Depending on the pharmacokinetic characteristics of the drug administered and the therapeutic index, several loading regimens may be proposed. Simultaneous administration of loading and maintenance doses, of several consecutive loading doses, or of an exponentially decreasing infusion of drug following the loading infusion are examples of such regimens (Fig. 23–3).

PLASMA CONCENTRATIONS OF ANTIARRHYTHMIC DRUGS

It is generally recognized that the effects of antiarrhythmic drugs are manifested by their actions at unidentified active cellular sites and that the concentration at these sites is in equilibrium with that in plasma during steady state conditions. An optimal range of plasma concentrations may exist for which arrhythmia suppression might be reached without the occurrence of adverse effects.[39] This is called the "therapeutic range," and represents a statistical range of therapeutic plasma concentrations that provides rough but useful general guidelines for therapy. This can be misleading, however, for an individual patient. It must be remembered that most analytical methods for antiarrhythmic drugs do not assay unbound (free) drug concentration but only the total concentration of the drug. Many factors can modify protein binding of drugs (see above). For those drugs that are highly protein-bound, almost undetectable changes in total concentration may be associated with major changes in the unbound, presumably active, fraction of the drug. In addition, antiarrhythmic drugs can form active metabolites which contribute to, or are responsible for, substantial antiarrhythmic efficacy (Table 23–1).[19]

Plasma concentrations of antiarrhythmic drugs are not good predictors of their potential for arrhythmia aggravation.[40] Plasma concentrations of antiarrhythmic drugs associated with arrhythmia suppression may also differ depending on the arrhythmia being treated.[39] Only limited data indicate that maintaining plasma concentrations of antiarrhythmic drugs in the proposed therapeutic range can provide clinical benefit.[39] Despite all these limitations, plasma level measurements of antiarrhythmic drugs have a definite place in the management of arrhythmias. For example, they are helpful in documenting treatment failure due to inadequate dosage or in monitoring therapy in patients when disposition is difficult to predict, such as patients with cardiac, hepatic, or renal failure and patients receiving concomitant medications having the potential to interfere with antiarrhythmic therapy.

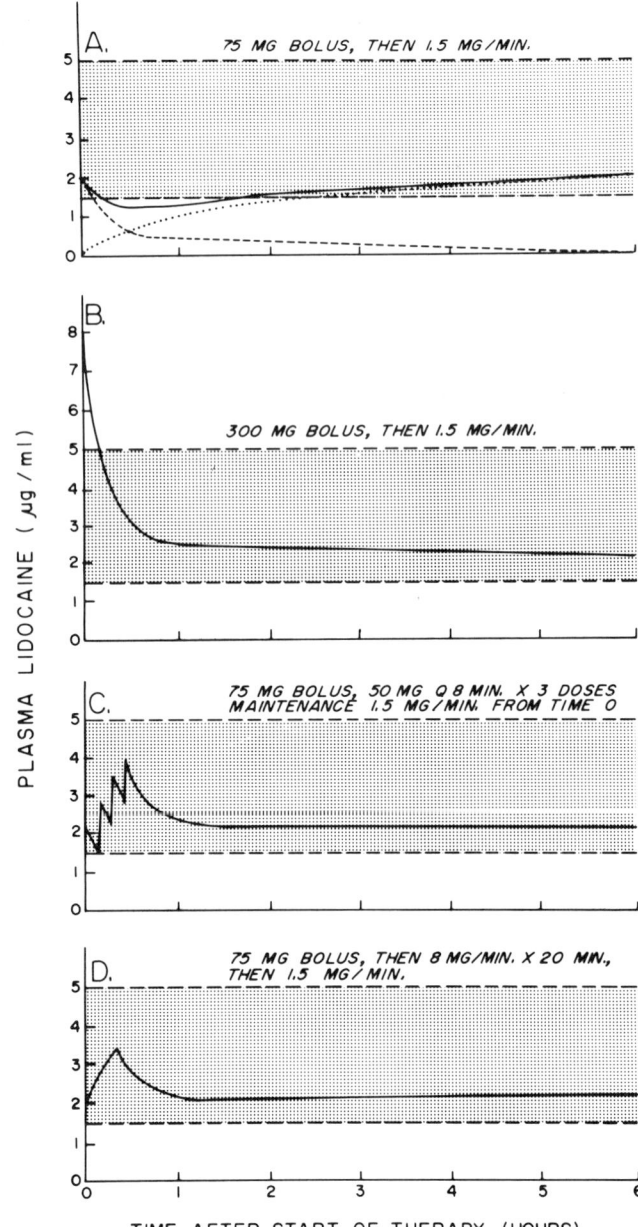

FIGURE 23–3
Examples of loading doses applied to the intravenous administration of lidocaine. In each panel, the loading regimen is indicated. In panel A, the dashed line represents the plasma concentration achieved following administration of a 75-mg bolus loading dose, and the dotted line represents the plasma concentration following the 1.5-mg/min maintenance dose. The sum of these two concentrations at any given time is the observed plasma concentration shown by the solid curve. (Adapted with permission from Woosley RL, Shand DG: Am J Cardiol 41:986–995, 1978.)

Classification of Antiarrhythmic Drug Action

The most widely used classification of antiarrhythmic drug action is that proposed by Vaughan Williams,[41] as modified by Harrison.[42] It is based on the electrophysiologic properties of drugs that might be antiar-

TABLE 23–1
Active Metabolites of Antiarrhythmic Drugs

Drug	Metabolite
Quinidine	3-Hydroxyquinidine
	2'-Oxoquinidinone
	O-desmethylquinidine
Procainamide	N-acetylprocainamide
Disopyramide	N-desisopropyldisopyramide
Lidocaine	Monoethylglycinexylidide
	Glycinexylidide
Encainide	O-desmethylencainide
	3-Methoxy-O-desmethylencainide
Propafenone	5-Hydroxypropafenone
Amiodarone	Desethylamiodarone

rhythmic. Although this classification has many limitations, it provides a useful framework for communication and consideration of antiarrhythmic action.[43]

CLASS I *Local anesthetics* ■ These drugs act primarily by blocking the rapid inward sodium current. Drugs with class I activity have been divided into three subclasses, Ia, Ib, and Ic, depending on their relative actions on repolarization and refractoriness. They increase intracardiac conduction times and widen the surface electrocardiogram QRS complex, with the order of potency being Ic > Ia > Ib. Drugs with Ia activity may also prolong effective refractory periods in atrium and ventricle.

CLASS II *Beta-adrenergic receptor antagonists* ■ Drugs with this action slow sinus rate and atrioventricular conduction, and increase atrioventricular nodal refractory period by antagonizing the intrinsic beta adrenergic stimulation.

CLASS III *Increase refractoriness* ■ Drugs with this action cause an increase in atrial and ventricular monophasic action potential duration and effective refractory period.

CLASS IV *Slow calcium inward current inhibition* ■ Drugs with this action act predominantly by slowing atrioventricular nodal conduction and increasing atrioventricular nodal refractoriness.

Antiarrhythmic drugs often have multiple actions overlapping several of these classes. Therefore, response, or lack thereof, to one drug in a given class does not necessarily predict success or failure of another with the same class of action.

Objectives of Antiarrhythmic Drug Therapy

There are two objectives of antiarrhythmic drug therapy: (1) prevention of death due to ventricular tachycardia/fibrillation, and (2) improvement in the quality of life through suppression or prevention of symptomatic arrhythmias. Attempts at prevention of sudden death due to arrhythmia assume that the physician can both identify patients at risk for sudden death and effectively prevent the responsible arrhythmias. This is currently feasible in some clinical conditions, but not in all. Patients who have been resuscitated from sudden cardiac death or who have had sustained ventricular tachycardia in the absence of acute myocardial infarction are at the highest known risk of sudden death. In these patients, drug therapy that has been found "effective" in suppressing ambient and exercise-induced arrhythmias or in preventing induction of arrhythmia by programmed ventricular stimulation has been shown to reduce the incidence of sudden death and recurrence of ventricular tachycardia.[44,45] However, many criticize these studies because they are not controlled; critics feel that "response" to therapy may simply identify a population at lower risk for sudden death or recurrence of arrhythmia. Ethical concerns make controlled studies in this population unlikely, unless the availability of the automatic implantable defibrillator/cardioverter will make such studies feasible.

The second indication for use of antiarrhythmic drugs, as stated above, is the suppression of symptomatic arrhythmias, either supraventricular or ventricular. When the association between the occurrence of symptoms and the arrhythmia has been firmly established, drug therapy can be very effective. However, many antiarrhythmic agents have severe side effects, and a consideration of the potential for overall improvement in quality of life and the risk/benefit ratio is essential before initiating drug therapy or even before increasing the dose of one of these agents.[46,47]

There is a known risk of sudden death in patients who have had a prior myocardial infarction and have asymptomatic ventricular arrhythmias. Many physicians have assumed that the suppression of these arrhythmias will reduce the incidence of sudden death and/or the development of symptomatic arrhythmias.[48] However, although many studies have been carried out, none have reported a reduction in sudden death, due to antiarrhythmic drug therapy, in patients with asymptomatic arrhythmias.[49,50] There were deficiencies in these studies, and more extensive investigations are now being performed with a better chance at answering this question. The Cardiac Arrhythmia Suppression Trial, CAST, is one such trial that is testing the hypothesis that suppression of asymptomatic ventricular ectopy in a post–mycocardial infarction population will reduce sudden arrhythmic death.[319] An early report of the outcome with two of the three drugs being evaluated in CAST has markedly changed the treatment of arrhythmias. Both encainide and flecainide were removed from the study because of a twofold increase in total mortality and a threefold increase in sudden arrhythmic death in the patients whose ectopy had been suppressed by these drugs compared with the experience in those who "responded" but were continued on placebo. The study is continuing to determine if suppression by the remaining drug in the study, moricizine, will be effective in reducing mortality.

Clinical Pharmacology of Individual Drugs

Basic pharmacokinetic and clinical information about the drugs discussed in this chapter is outlined in Tables 23–2 and 23–3.

TABLE 23–2
Pharmacokinetics of Antiarrhythmic Drugs

Drug	Main Activity in Vaughan Williams Classification	Inactivation or Route of Elimination[a]	Protein Binding (%)	Vd (L/kg)	Elimination Half-life (hours)	Oral Bioavailability (%)	Oral Clearance (ml/min)
Quinidine	Ia	Liver (60–80%) Kidney (10–30%)	80–90	2.5	4–17	70–80	200–400
Procainamide	Ia	Liver (40–70%) Kidney (30–60%)	15	2	3–6	80	400–700
Disopyramide	Ia	Liver (10–30%) Kidney (25–50%)	50–65	1.5	4–10	80–90	90
Lidocaine	Ib	Liver (90%)	40–70	2	1.5–4	35[c]	700–1000[c]
Mexiletine	Ib	Liver (90%)	70	6–12	12–24	85	400–700
Tocainide	Ib	Liver (50–60%) Kidney (40–50%)	50	2.8	12–15	98	150–200
Flecainide	Ic	Liver (70%)[b] Kidney (30%)	35–45	7–10	15–30[b]	90	200–800[b]
Encainide	Ic	Liver (90%)[b]	70	3.8–5.7	2[d]; 10[e]	25[d]; 90[e]	200[e]–12,000[d]
Propafenone	Ic	Liver (99%)[b]	90	3–4	2–24[b]	10–50[b]	800–5000[b]
Bretylium	III	Kidney (70–80%)	? (low)	3–4	4–16	20	1300
Amiodarone	III	Liver (99%)	95	20–200	13–103 days	20–80	6500–11,000

[a]Kidney refers to renal elimination of unchanged drugs.
[b]Dependent on metabolic phenotype (see text).
[c]Lidocaine should not be used orally.
[d]In poor metabolizers.
[e]In extensive metabolizers.

QUINIDINE

Quinidine has been widely used since 1918 for the treatment of ventricular and supraventricular arrhythmias.

Electrophysiologic Effects

Quinidine primary electrophysiologic effects are related to its class I activity. Inhibition of inward sodium current is rate-, pH-, and voltage-dependent and is most marked at increased heart rate or less negative potentials.[51–54] This effect results in slowed conduction, especially in the His-Purkinje system. Effective refractory periods and, to a lesser degree, action potential duration are increased by quinidine.[51–54] It has recently been shown that quinidine blocks the outward potassium current (I_k).[55]

Quinidine decreases automaticity by decreasing the slope of phase-4 depolarization and by raising the diastolic threshold for the action potential.[56] The direct electrophysiologic effects of quinidine in humans[57] are modified by its anticholinergic[58] and vasodilator actions.[59] On the surface ECG, quinidine causes dose-related increases in PR, QRS, and QTc intervals.[61]

Hemodynamic Effects

Quinidine has mild negative inotropic effects,[62] which are offset by its vasodilator properties during administration in humans.[59] Quinidine does not decrease the left ventricular ejection fraction when prescribed in patients with moderately depressed myocardial contractility.[60]

Clinical Pharmacokinetics

After oral administration, quinidine bioavailability is high (70-80%).[63, 64] Quinidine sulfate is absorbed more rapidly than quinidine gluconate.[63] Quinidine is 80 to 90% bound to plasma protein,[65] predominantly to alpha$_1$-acid glycoprotein.[66] Quinidine is 60 to 80% metabolized in the liver.[67, 68] Metabolites of quinidine observed in humans are 3-hydroxyquinidine, O-desmethylquinidine, 2′-oxoquinidinone and quinidine-N-oxide. There is considerable evidence that these metabolites might contribute to the overall pharmacodynamic response to quinidine,[69–71] probably less so for quinidine-N-oxide. Approximately 10 to 27% of quinidine is excreted unchanged in the urine.[64] Dihydroquinidine is an impurity constituting up to 20 to 30% of commercial preparations, which has electrophysiologic actions similar to quinidine.[70]

Dosage and Plasma Concentrations

Quinidine treatment should start at low doses, equivalent to 200 mg of quinidine sulfate every 6 hours, carefully titrated with changes in dosage after allowing at least 2 to 3 days for accumulation to steady state if clinically feasible. The usual range of dosages is 200 to 600 mg of quinidine sulfate every 4 to 8 hours. There is no firm evidence that dosage adjustments of quinidine are required in disease states. However, this is

TABLE 23–3
Dosages and Plasma Concentrations of Drugs Used in Treatment of Ventricular Arrhythmias*

Drug	Usual Initial Dosage†	Dosage Modification in Presence of Disease	Range of Dosages	Maximum Single Dose (mg)	Therapeutic Range‡ (μg/ml)
Quinidine (sulfate)	200 mg q 6 h	No	800–2400 mg/day	600	0.7–5
Procainamide (sustained-release)	500 mg q 6 h	↓ CHF, RI	2000–6000 mg/day	1500	4–8
Disopyramide	100 mg q 6 h	↓ CHF, HI, RI	300–1200 mg/day	300	2–5
Lidocaine	See text	↓ CHF, ↓ HI?	1–4 mg/min IV	—	1.5–5
Mexiletine	200 mg q 8 h	↓ CHF, ↓ HI	600–1200 mg/day	400	0.7–2
Tocainide	400 mg q 8 h	↓ HI, RI	1200–2400 mg/day	800	4–10
Flecainide	100 mg q 12 h	↓ CHF, RI, ↓ HI?	200–400 mg/day	200	0.2–1
Encainide	25 mg q 8 h	↓ RI	75–200 mg/day	75	—
Propafenone	150 mg q 8 h	See text	450–900 mg/day	300	0.5–3?
Bretylium	See text	↓ RI	1–4 mg/min IV	—	—
Amiodarone	600–1400 mg/day (load)	No	200–600 mg/day	600	1–2

*This table provides general guidelines. Dosage should be determined in light of clinical response and tolerance. CHF = congestive heart failure; HI = hepatic insufficiency; RI = renal insufficiency. See text for details.
†Dosage recommended in absence of significant cardiac, renal, or hepatic failure.
‡Therapeutic range of plasma concentrations represents a statistical range that should not be rigidly relied on when treating individual patients. See text for details.

probably due to a combination of assay variability, marked interindividual variability in disposition, and possibly the presence of active metabolites. Limited data in a small number of patients suggest that elderly patients may require a smaller dosage of quinidine than other patients because of reduced clearance and volume of distribution.[72] This should be confirmed in larger numbers of patients. With the newer, more specific assay methods, the therapeutic range for quinidine is 2 to 5 μg/ml.[73] Decreased protein binding in patients with liver failure[74] may lead to enhanced pharmacodynamic activity of quinidine at lower than usual total plasma concentrations. On the other hand, raised plasma concentrations of alpha$_1$-acid glycoprotein, such as can be observed after acute myocardial infarction, may decrease free plasma concentration of quinidine, and thus decrease efficacy, or lead to a normal pharmacodynamic response despite high total plasma concentrations of quinidine.[75] Free unbound quinidine plasma concentrations correlate better with changes in heart rate, QRS duration, and QTc interval than total quinidine concentration.[76]

Indications

Quinidine has been successfully used in the treatment or prevention of atrial fibrillation or flutter,[77] supraventricular tachycardia,[61, 78] ventricular extrasystoles,[79] ventricular tachycardia, and ventricular fibrillation.[80, 81] It is also useful in the treatment of Wolff-Parkinson-White syndrome, although there are reports of worsening arrhythmia, possibly due to quinidine's vagolytic actions. When treating atrial fibrillation or atrial flutter, quinidine should be used only after the ventricular response has been controlled by atrioventricular nodal slowing of conduction with a digitalis glycoside or a beta-blocker.

Drug Interactions

Several liver enzymes can be involved in metabolism of a given drug. The activity of some of them can be genetically determined. In the case of the antihypertensive drug debrisoquine, two phenotypes of metabolism have been identified: extensive metabolizers have a high enzymatic activity for debrisoquine hydroxylation, whereas poor metabolizers lack the hydroxylase activity (or enzyme) involved in this route of metabolism. Several drugs, including sparteine, bufuralol, encainide, propafenone, and metoprolol, are metabolized by the same enzymatic system, and their metabolism is therefore also genetically determined. Quinidine oxidation in the liver occurs independently of the enzymes responsible for oxidation of debrisoquine, sparteine, and bufuralol.[68, 82] However, quinidine is a potent inhibitor of these enzymes[83–85] and could therefore alter the disposition of drugs using them. Quinidine can also modify the results of tests used to phenotype patients for their ability to oxidize drugs dependent on the same enzymes as debrisoquine.[86] Smoking, which increases the activity of several oxidases in the liver, does not increase quinidine elimination.[87]

Quinidine increases plasma digoxin concentrations by mechanisms involving (1) displacement of digoxin from tissue binding sites[88] and (2) reduced renal[89, 90] and non-renal[91] elimination. This interaction may result in symptoms of overdosage of digoxin, although this is not always the case.[92] Digoxin dosage should be decreased by 50% in patients beginning quinidine therapy. Although quinidine also reduces the elimination of digitoxin,[93] there is currently no clear recommendation for adjustment of digitoxin dosage with quinidine. Quinidine oxidation to 3-hydroxyquinidine is reduced by verapamil.[94] Cimetidine decreases quinidine elimination.[92] When combined with organic nitrates, the additive vasodilator effects of these drugs and of quinidine may cause orthostatic hypotension. Quinidine worsens neuromuscular blockade in patients with myasthenia gravis[95] and may prolong the effects of succinylcholine.[96] Quinidine may decrease the liver synthesis of vitamin K–dependent clotting factors in certain patients and may produce additive anticoagulant effects when administered with warfarin-type anticoagulants.[97]

Adverse Effects

Over one half of patients starting quinidine therapy discontinue treatment within the first year because of side effects.[98] The most common side effects include diarrhea, nausea, and vomiting, which are more frequent at higher dosages. Hypersensitivity reactions such as fever, hepatitis, rashes, thrombocytopenia, and hemolytic anemia are less frequent.[99] The most severe side effects of quinidine are due to aggravation of arrhythmia.[40] Among these arrhythmias, torsades de pointes is of special interest.[100] This arrhythmia is a polymorphic ventricular tachycardia with progressive change of QRS axis occurring in the presence of marked QT prolongation and favored by hypokalemia and bradycardia; it typically occurs early in treatment and at a time when plasma quinidine concentrations are within or below therapeutic range.[101–104] Treatment of torsades de pointes includes discontinuation of quinidine, correction of hypokalemia, and maneuvers to increase heart rate and shorten QT intervals (e.g., pacing or isoproterenol). Patients who develop torsades de pointes with quinidine should not receive other drugs with the potential for prolonging the QTc interval. Quinidine can produce sinus arrest and sinoatrial block in patients with the sick sinus syndrome.[99] Quinidine generally does not cause heart failure.[60, 99] Parenteral administration of quinidine should not exceed a rate faster than 16 mg per minute to avoid excessive hypotension[60] or conduction slowing.

PROCAINAMIDE

Procainamide has been in clinical use for the treatment of arrhythmias for more than three decades. Its major metabolite, N-acetylprocainamide (NAPA), has antiarrhythmic properties with a different electrophysiologic and toxic profile.[105–107]

Electrophysiologic Effects

Like quinidine, the primary electrophysiologic effects of procainamide are related to its class I activity. It slows conduction velocity, prolongs refractoriness, decreases automaticity and excitability of atrial and ventricular myocardium and Purkinje fibers, and decreases conduction in bypass tracts.[61, 107–110] Procainamide causes less marked action potential duration and QTc prolongation than quinidine and has little vagolytic activity in humans.[61] Whereas procainamide prolongs QRS and QTc intervals on the surface ECG, N-acetylprocainamide has predominantly class III activity and prolongs action potential duration and refractoriness in atrial and ventricular myocardium with prolongation of the QT interval on the surface ECG.[106, 107, 111, 112] N-acetylprocainamide has little potency as a sodium channel blocker.

Hemodynamic Effects

In isolated muscle preparations, therapeutic levels of procainamide have little effect on or may slightly increase myocardial contractility.[113] Procainamide produces weak autonomic ganglia blockade that in high dosages can impair cardiovascular reflexes and cause hypotension.[114] Procainamide causes clinically apparent decreased myocardial contractility in patients with poor ventricular function or when given intravenously at a rapid rate.[115–117] N-acetylprocainamide has been found to increase contractility in isolated tissues and cardiac index in humans.

Clinical Pharmacokinetics

Procainamide is well absorbed after oral administration.[118] Binding to serum proteins is only about 15%; approximately 50 to 70% of procainamide is eliminated unchanged in the urine whereas 20 to 40% undergoes hepatic conversion to N-acetylprocainamide, which is eliminated unchanged in urine.[119–121] Acetylation of procainamide to N-acetylprocainamide is genetically determined,[120] with 45% of white and black populations and 10 to 20% of Orientals carrying the slow acetylator trait. Both procainamide and N-acetylprocainamide accumulate to high and potentially toxic concentrations in patients with renal failure.[121]

Dosage and Plasma Concentrations

Procainamide is available for parenteral and oral administration. The oral sustained-release form can be administered at intervals of 6 to 8 hours, thus overcoming the problem of 3- to 4-hour dosing intervals required with conventional tablets and capsules. In patients with normal renal and cardiac function, an initial oral maintenance dose of 15 mg per kg of body weight per day of the conventional form has been recommended.[122] Dosage should be lowered in patients with a low cardiac output or renal insufficiency.[121] When administered intravenously, procainamide can be given as a loading infusion of 275 µg per kg per minute over 25 minutes, or by a series of 100-mg doses delivered over 3 minutes every 5 minutes, up to a total dose of 1 g.[123, 124] If the loading infusion is well tolerated (no hypotension and less than 25% QRS or QT widening), a maintenance intravenous infusion of 20 to 60 µg per kg per minute can be given. A second loading infusion of 0.5 to 1 g has been given in some instances in which the initial loading infusion was well tolerated but ineffective. The range for procainamide therapeutic plasma concentrations is reported to range from 4 to 8 µg per ml.[121] However, the therapeutic range may be higher in patients with ventricular tachycardia.[125] The usual therapeutic range may be different during chronic therapy when N-acetylprocainamide is present; in this case, the range for procainamide plasma concentrations should not be rigidly considered, since the metabolite N-acetylprocainamide contributes in part to procainamide pharmacodynamic activity in some but not all patients.[126, 127] When NAPA was given alone, concentrations of 7 to 15 µg/ml were antiarrhythmic in 7 of 23 patients, and response did not correlate with response to procainamide.[127]

Indications

Procainamide has been successfully used for the same broad spectrum of arrhythmias as that responding to quinidine.[61, 108] N-acetylprocainamide (Acecainide) is currently an investigational drug with predominant class III activity. It has been shown to be effective in the treatment of ventricular arrhythmias, but its use is limited by a narrow therapeutic index.[106, 127, 128]

Drug Interactions

Cimetidine decreases procainamide clearance, predominantly by a reduction of its renal clearance.[38, 129] The mechanism of this interaction is thought to be a competition for the tubular secretion of both drugs. A similar interaction has been found between procainamide and its main metabolite, N-acetylprocainamide.[126] Ranitidine also interacts with procainamide pharmacokinetics by reducing its renal clearance and absorption.[130]

Adverse Effects

One of the most troublesome adverse effects encountered in patients receiving chronic procainamide treatment is the lupus syndrome, which is seen in approximately 20% of patients. Serologic and clinical signs of the lupus syndrome appear to be related to the cumulative dose of procainamide as well as to the duration of administration. Antinuclear antibodies can be found in more than 80% of patients taking procainamide for 1 year, but patients with positive antinuclear antibodies need not be withdrawn from therapy unless they become symptomatic.[131–133] Because N-acetylprocainamide very rarely causes positive antinuclear antibodies and has not been found to cause lupus, rapid acetylators of procainamide tend to develop the lupus syndrome later than slow acetylators.[133] The lupus syndrome is reversible upon discontinuation of procainamide, but antinuclear antibodies can persist in serum for years. Other side effects of procainamide include nausea, anorexia, diarrhea, and, more rarely, agranulocytosis, fever, and hepatitis.[134] Heart block and sinus node dysfunction can occur in patients with pre-existing conduction system abnormalities.[135] Like quinidine, procainamide and N-acetylprocainamide can cause torsades de pointes, although less frequently.[104, 136]

DISOPYRAMIDE

Disopyramide has been marketed in France since 1969 and in the United States since 1977. Its antiarrhythmic profile is similar to that of procainamide and quinidine.

Electrophysiologic Effects

Disopyramide's predominant electrophysiologic effects are due to its class I action. It has effects similar to those of quinidine and procainamide on automaticity, conduction, and refractoriness in atrial and ventricular tissue.[137–139] Disopyramide prolongs action potential duration of normal and ischemic cells and reduces dispersion of repolarization between ischemic and normal tissues.[140, 141] Its direct action on the sinus node tends to slow the heart rate.[142] However, the strong anticholinergic properties of disopyramide[138, 139, 142, 143] are such that heart rate is unchanged or tends to increase. The direct actions of disopyramide on the sinus node can lead to excessive bradycardia in patients with sinus nodal dysfunction.[144] The enantiomers and metabolites of disopyramide have different pharmacodynamic effects. Anticholinergic effects are predominantly due to R-(-) disopyramide and to R-(-) nordisopyramide.[145, 146] Prolongation of action potential duration is caused mainly by S-(+) disopyramide.[147, 148]

Hemodynamic Effects

One of the major limitations of disopyramide is its ability to decrease left ventricular function, causing new or worsening of congestive heart failure.[13, 149–151] This effect is due to direct negative inotropic action[13] and to vasoconstriction causing increased peripheral vascular resistance.[152] The S-(+) disopyramide enantiomer has a less negative inotropic effect, and it has been estimated that 70% of the negative inotropic action of disopyramide could be avoided by using the S-(+) enantiomer.[153]

Clinical Pharmacokinetics

Disopyramide is well absorbed after oral administration and has 80 to 90% systemic bioavailability.[154] The drug is eliminated primarily by the kidneys, with 50% excreted unchanged and 20% as mono-N-desalkyldisopyramide excreted in the urine.[155, 156] Protein binding of disopyramide is complex and variable because of inter-individual differences in affinity and the capacity of alpha$_1$-acid glycoprotein to bind the drug. This leads to nonlinear (concentration-dependent) plasma protein binding at plasma concentrations within the range attained with usual doses (see Fig. 23–2).[155, 157–161] Pharmacokinetics are further complicated by different plasma protein binding and elimination kinetics of the two enantiomers.[162]

Dosage and Plasma Concentrations

As with all antiarrhythmic drugs, but even more so because of its adverse reaction profile, the dosage of disopyramide should initially be low and carefully titrated upward. Usual dosages are 100 to 400 mg of the conventional release formulation every 6 to 8 hours. Disopyramide is also available as a controlled-release formulation that allows administration every 8 to 12 hours. The initial dosage of disopyramide should be reduced (50–100 mg every 12 hours) in patients with renal insufficiency[163] or decreased hepatic function[164] and, if disopyramide is absolutely necessary, in patients with a history of compensated congestive heart failure. Because previous studies have not always measured the free fraction of disopyramide in plasma, the generally accepted therapeutic range of 2 to 5 µg per milliliter for total concentration of disopyramide in plasma should not strictly be relied upon.[165] Monitoring of free concentrations of disopyramide has been recommended,[39] but the range of free concentrations associated with arrhythmia suppression has not been clearly delineated.

Indications

Disopyramide's antiarrhythmic efficacy is similar to that of quinidine. Disopyramide has been successfully used for the treatment of both supraventricular and ventricular arrhythmias, as well as in patients with the Wolff-Parkinson-White syndrome.[166, 167] Because of its negative inotropic actions, discussed above, disopyramide should be avoided in patients with clinical signs of congestive heart failure.

Drug Interactions

Plasma concentrations of disopyramide are decreased in patients treated with phenytoin[168] because of hepatic enzyme induction.[169] Disopyramide does not alter digoxin steady-state plasma concentrations[170] nor does it interact with warfarin.[171]

Adverse Effects

The two major side effects of disopyramide are its potential to aggravate congestive heart failure in susceptible patients[13, 149-151] and to cause symptoms related to its anticholinergic activity.[172] Impairment of left ventricular function is more likely to develop in patients with a previous history of congestive heart failure, and disopyramide administration should therefore be avoided in this population. However, as many as 5% of patients without a previous history of congestive heart failure develop symptoms of acquired heart failure on disopyramide therapy.[151]

The most frequent adverse effects of disopyramide are related to its anticholinergic activity. Side effects may occur in as many as 20 to 67% of patients receiving disopyramide; they include urinary retention, dry mouth or eyes, and constipation. Adverse effects related to the anticholinergic activity of disopyramide represent the major limitation to the clinical use of the drug. Disopyramide administration should therefore be avoided in patients with a previous history of urinary hesitancy, prostatism, glaucoma, or severe constipation. The combination of disopyramide with a cholinesterase inhibitor has been shown to reduce the severity of these symptoms without modifying antiarrhythmic activity.[173]

LIDOCAINE, MEXILETINE, AND TOCAINIDE

These three drugs will be discussed together because of their close chemical relationship (Fig. 23-4). Their main difference is that tocainide and mexiletine can be given orally because of the absence of significant presystemic elimination, whereas lidocaine is given only intravenously for this reason.

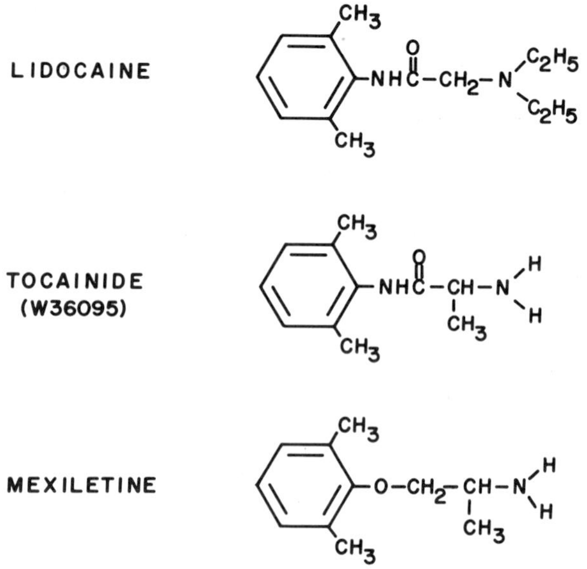

FIGURE 23-4
Chemical structure of lidocaine, tocainide, and mexiletine.

Electrophysiologic Effects

Lidocaine, mexiletine, and tocainide are drugs with predominantly class Ib activity. They depress the maximum upstroke velocity (V_{max}) of phase 0 of the action potential and slow impulse conduction velocity in Purkinje fibers in a frequency- and voltage-dependent manner.[174-176] Because of the frequency-dependence of their action on sodium channels, these drugs exert their maximum effect at rapid heart rates (>175 beats per minute). This may explain why they appear to have greater efficacy in "rapid" rather than "slow" ventricular tachycardia. Lidocaine decreases automaticity in Purkinje fibers,[174, 177] whereas this effect is less in ischemic tissues.[178] Lidocaine has little effect on atrial myocardium[179] and does not alter sinus function or His-Purkinje conduction in normal heart.[179, 180] However, it can decrease sinus automaticity[181] and His-Purkinje conduction[182] when they are abnormal. Lidocaine shortens action potential duration and to a lesser degree effective refractory periods in Purkinje fibers in ventricular myocardium.[183] Mexiletine and tocainide share most of these effects.[175, 184] On the surface ECG, PR and QRS intervals are unchanged, whereas QTc may shorten. Preliminary data in animals suggest that tocainide enantiomers may have different pharmacologic activity.[185]

Hemodynamic Effects

These drugs cause little hemodynamic change.[13, 184, 186] Intravenous tocainide has been shown to have mild negative inotropic action and to increase systemic vascular resistances.[13]

Clinical Pharmacokinetics

Lidocaine undergoes extensive first pass metabolism after oral administration and causes intolerable central nervous system side effects when administered orally.[187] For this reason, lidocaine is only used intravenously. Under normal conditions, clearance of lidocaine depends mainly on liver blood flow.[32, 188] Lidocaine binds predominantly to alpha$_1$-acid glycoprotein. Two metabolites of lidocaine, monoethylglycinexylidide and glycinexylidide, have been shown to have weak antiarrhythmic efficacy.[189] Mexiletine and tocainide are rapidly and very well absorbed after oral administration, with high systemic bioavailability.[175, 184] Their pharmacokinetic profile is similar, except for the fact that mexiletine is mainly cleared by the liver whereas tocainide is cleared by both renal and hepatic routes. Tocainide and its glucuronide conjugate are excreted in the urine.

Dosage and Plasma Concentrations

To rapidly achieve antiarrhythmic response, lidocaine must be infused as a loading dose. Several loading regimens have been shown to be useful (see Fig. 23–3). Because lidocaine distributes very rapidly into tissues, theoretically the ideal regimen would be an exponentially decreasing infusion (paralleling distribution) following a bolus loading infusion, an approach which has been successfully used.[190] One satisfactory regimen for patients without heart failure consists of the infusion of a 75-mg IV bolus over 2 minutes, followed by the administration of 150 mg over the next 18 minutes, with a subsequent maintenance infusion at a rate of 2 mg per minute.[191] Systemic clearance of lidocaine is markedly reduced in patients with liver cirrhosis.[25] Patients with congestive heart failure have a reduced clearance of lidocaine and reduced volume of distribution, the former possibly due to decreased liver blood flow.[32] Loading infusions should therefore be reduced by 50% in patients with heart failure, and the maintenance infusion should be reduced in patients with impaired clearance (i.e., liver disease) and in some patients with heart failure.

In patients with myocardial infarction, total plasma concentrations of lidocaine can rise without a corresponding increase in pharmacodynamic response. This is due to an increase in the level of alpha$_1$-acid glycoprotein, associated with myocardial infarction, leading to an increase in protein binding; the pharmacodynamic consequence of this action remains uncertain.[192] Renal insufficiency does not require dosage adjustment of lidocaine.[25] The usual therapeutic range of lidocaine is 1.5 to 5 µg per milliliter.

Mexiletine and tocainide should be started at low doses and increased at an interval of 3 days, if possible, to avoid side effects. The range of usually effective dosages is wide for both agents. No clear recommendation regarding dosage of mexiletine in patients with renal, cardiac, or hepatic insufficiency have been made. The pharmacokinetics of mexiletine suggest that dosages should be reduced in patients with severe liver insufficiency. Elimination of tocainide is reduced in patients with renal failure or severe hepatic disease, and reduced dosage is recommended in these populations.[184]

Indications

Lidocaine, mexiletine, and tocainide have been used in the treatment of ventricular arrhythmia. They have not been shown to be useful in the treatment of supraventricular arrhythmias. Lidocaine can increase the ventricular rate in patients with atrial fibrillation, atrial flutter, or supraventricular tachycardia associated with the Wolff-Parkinson-White syndrome. Lidocaine is most often used during the acute phase of myocardial infarction. Although its overall beneficial effect on mortality is uncertain,[50] its early use prior to hospitalization reduces the incidence of ventricular fibrillation.[193] Use of mexiletine following the acute phase of myocardial infarction has not been shown to reduce mortality.[194, 195] The antiarrhythmic potency of mexiletine and tocainide for the treatment of ventricular arrhythmia is within the range of that observed with quinidine.[184, 194] Long-term treatment with either of these two agents is limited mainly by troublesome side effects.

Drug Interactions

Hepatic enzyme induction increases the clearance of lidocaine and mexiletine.[175, 194] Because mexiletine metabolism in the liver involves mainly a conjugation reaction, cimetidine does not impair mexiletine elimination.[196] To date, no pharmacokinetic drug interaction has been reported with tocainide.[184]

Adverse Effects

The main limitation of treatment with lidocaine, mexiletine, and tocainide is the high frequency of dose-related side effects, which have been reported in as many as 50% of patients. Most of these side effects are related to the actions of these drugs on the central nervous system: tremor, visual blurring, dizziness, dysphoria, nausea, and paresthesia. Because the adverse effects of mexiletine and tocainide are dose-related, they can often be used at lower doses in combination with drugs with class Ia action (see below).

Thrombocytopenia has rarely been reported with mexiletine,[194] and interstitial pneumonitis has been reported with tocainide.[184] Agranulocytosis has been estimated to occur with tocainide therapy in 0.18% of patients.[184] As previously mentioned, excessive slowing of His-Purkinje conduction is possible with these drugs, when it is abnormal before therapy. Torsades de pointes is unlikely to be caused by these agents, and they have been proposed as therapy for this arrhythmia. Although lidocaine, mexiletine, and tocainide can worsen ventricular arrhythmias, the incidence of this side effect is probably lower than for other antiarrhythmic agents.[197]

FLECAINIDE

Flecainide is a new drug with potent antiarrhythmic properties. It has a narrow therapeutic index with significant cardiotoxicity. Although cardiac side effects are not predictable, patients at higher risk for these adverse reactions can be identified. Recent data indicating that flecainide and encainide increased mortality in patients with prior myocardial infarction and asymptomatic ventricular ectopy have led to restricted use of these two drugs.[319]

Electrophysiologic Effects

Flecainide is a sodium channel blocker with predominant class 1c activity. It markedly depresses V_{max} in Purkinje fibers and ventricular muscle.[198] As with other sodium channel blockers, this effect is frequency-dependent, with more block occurring at rapid stimulation rates. However, because flecainide dissociates from the sodium channel much more slowly than other agents with class I activity, the rate dependence of sodium channel block appears at lower heart rates in the case of flecainide. This may explain lengthening of the QRS interval on the surface ECG at physiologic heart rates.[199] Flecainide slows intraventricular conduction velocity more than it prolongs effective refractory periods.[200] It prolongs P-A, A-H, and H-V intervals and measurably increases P-R and QRS intervals on the surface ECG at therapeutic doses. QTc is slightly increased, primarily due to prolongation of QRS. Flecainide can depress sinus node activity in patients with pre-existing sinus node dysfunction.[201] Flecainide increases pacing thresholds by as much as 200% and should therefore be used with caution in patients dependent on pacemakers.[202]

Hemodynamic Effects

Flecainide has a significant potential for causing heart failure. Intravenously administered flecainide decreases cardiac output and increases pulmonary capillary wedge pressure, in patients with both normal and abnormal left ventricular function.[13] Generally, oral administration of flecainide is hemodynamically well tolerated in patients with good ventricular function and without a history of congestive heart failure. Patients with decreased (< 30%) ejection fraction have a high risk of flecainide-induced worsening or provocation of heart failure.[203] When possible, flecainide should be avoided in this population.

Clinical Pharmacokinetics

Flecainide is well absorbed after oral administration, and its systemic bioavailability is high[204]; 27% of flecainide is excreted unchanged in urine. Alkalinization of urine reduces flecainide renal elimination, probably by increasing tubular reabsorption of the non-ionized form of the drug.[36] Most of flecainide is metabolized in the liver to compounds unlikely to contribute to overall antiarrhythmic activity.[199] Elimination half-life is 15–30 hours in normal subjects and tends to be longer in patients with stable ventricular ectopy even in the absence of heart failure. Flecainide has a very large volume of distribution and high tissue uptake.[204]

Dosage and Plasma Concentrations

The relatively long elimination half-life of flecainide allows effective administration of the drug every 12 hours. For the same reason, dosage adjustment, if possible, should not be made before at least 4 days of oral administration have allowed accumulation to steady state. Patients with congestive heart failure have only a slight prolongation of elimination half-life,[199, 204] so that dosage intervals should remain at 12 hours. However, total clearance of flecainide is reduced in patients with congestive heart failure; thus if flecainide must be administered in such patients, the total dose should be reduced. Dosage should also be reduced in patients with renal failure. The usual dosage of flecainide is 100 to 150 mg every 12 hours in patients without cardiac or renal failure, and 50 to 100 mg every 12 hours in patients with cardiac or renal failure. A total daily dosage of more than 400 mg may be used but should be administered under close medical monitoring (see below). The therapeutic plasma concentration range of flecainide is often reported to be between 200 and 1000 ng per milliliter. However, the upper limit should not be rigidly considered since adverse effects may occur at lower concentrations,[205, 206] and many patients tolerate concentrations above this range. As with other antiarrhythmic agents, monitoring of the patient's clinical condition remains the cornerstone of evaluation. Prolongation of QRS and PR intervals on the surface ECG are common and do not necessarily indicate overdosage. However, prolongation of QRS or PR intervals of 40 ms or more, especially in the presence of a flecainide plasma concentration of more than 1000 ng per milliliter, may be useful indicators of possible cardiotoxicity.[206]

Indications

Flecainide is effective in both ventricular and supraventricular tachycardias.[199] Overall, the antiarrhythmic response to flecainide in patients with ventricular arrhythmias is higher than with agents having predominantly class Ia or Ib activity.[199, 207] However, the results of the CAST study—doubling of mortality in patients with asymptomatic ventricular arrhythmias—necessitate reserving this drug for patients with life-threatening arrhythmias. More information is needed to fully assess the risk/benefit ratio of flecainide in the treatment of supraventricular arrhythmias. Promising results have been obtained in patients with atrioventricular (AV) accessory pathways and AV nodal reentrant tachycardias.[208]

Drug Interactions

Cimetidine reduces flecainide clearance and prolongs flecainide elimination half-life.[209] In normal volunteers, plasma concentrations of digoxin and propranolol have been shown to rise when flecainide is co-administered.[210, 211] Propranolol and flecainide have been found to have additive negative inotropic effects.

Adverse Effects

The adverse effects resulting from the negative inotropic action and the electrophysiologic properties of flecainide (aggravation of pre-existing bundle branch block or sinus node dysfunction, worsening of congestive heart failure, and rise in pacing threshold), have been discussed above. In addition to worsening of congestive heart failure, provocation of serious ventricular arrhythmias by flecainide is a major concern. This proarrhythmic effect is more likely to occur in patients with severe arrhythmias and/or heart failure or when doses above 400 mg per day are administered.[199] It has been shown to occur in as many as 20% of patients with these three risk factors. The increased mortality seen with flecainide in CAST[319] is unlikely to be due to this type of proarrhythmia. The deaths were seen in patients whose arrhythmias had been suppressed and occurred evenly over 10 months of therapy.

Most side effects of flecainide appear to be concentration-related and can often be managed by a reduction in dose. They include transient symptoms involving the central nervous system, such as dizziness and difficulty in visual accommodation.[199, 206] In occasional cases of severe flecainide intoxication, acute sodium administration (sodium bicarbonate or lactate) and alkalinization has been shown to reverse the electrophysiologic and hemodynamic consequences of overdosage.[212]

ENCAINIDE

Encainide is an antiarrhythmic drug recently approved in the United States, with a potency profile similar to that of flecainide. Its clinical pharmacology is complicated by the formation of metabolites that may be responsible for a major part of its pharmacological activity. As with flecainide, there was an increase in mortality in patients receiving encainide in CAST.[319]

Electrophysiologic Effects

Encainide is a sodium channel blocker with predominantly class Ic activity. The characteristics of sodium channel blockade by encainide are similar to those of flecainide, and QRS prolongation on the surface ECG occurs at therapeutic doses. The electrophysiologic response to encainide is complicated by the presence of active metabolites found in 93% of patients (see below)—namely, O-desmethylencainide (ODE) and 3-methoxy-O-desmethylencainide (MODE)—which have different electrophysiologic potencies and properties. Encainide metabolism is genetically determined, with a bidomal distribution of metabolic phenotypes cosegregating with those of debrisoquine metabolism (see below). About 7% of the American population lack the ability to produce significant quantities of ODE and MODE. More prominent electrophysiologic effects of encainide are seen in these individuals.

Encainide itself slows conduction velocity in the His-Purkinje system and ventricle more than in the atrium or AV node.[213] It has little effect on the ventricular and AV nodal effective refractory periods but prolongs these parameters at short cycle lengths. ODE is more potent than encainide in its ability to slow conduction velocity throughout the heart and to prolong ventricular refractoriness.[214] MODE has potency similar to encainide but prolongs repolarization, whereas encainide and ODE do not.[215] The effects of encainide and its metabolites on sinus node automaticity have not been extensively studied.[216] In humans, encainide administration prolongs the QRS interval on the surface ECG, an effect mainly due to ODE and MODE in most patients.[217] The QTc interval is slightly prolonged, primarily due to prolongation of the QRS interval. The JTc interval (QTc − QRS) prolongation is minor and, when present, is possibly due to the formation of MODE.[215] Encainide and ODE raise the electrical threshold for defibrillation, whereas MODE does not.[218]

Hemodynamic Effects

One of the advantages of encainide is that it has very little negative inotropic effect (Fig. 23–5).[219] In vitro and in vivo studies have shown that encainide exerts only minimal negative inotropic effects at and above therapeutic levels.[216]

Clinical Pharmacokinetics

The pharmacokinetics of encainide are complex, owing to the variable rate with which it is transformed into

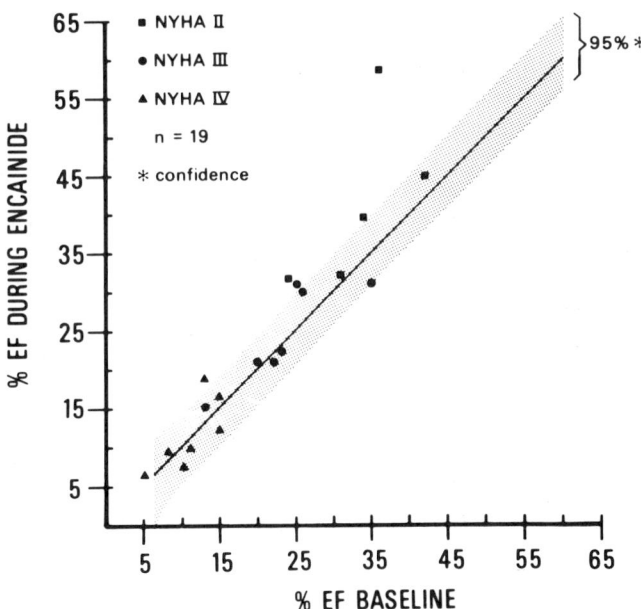

FIGURE 23–5
Absence of significant change in left ventricular ejection fraction (EF) after administration of encainide. (Reprinted by permission from Sami MH, Derbekyan VA, Lisbona R: Am J. Cardiol 52:507, 1983.)

its active metabolites ODE and MODE (Fig. 23-6). The biotransformation of encainide into ODE and that of ODE into MODE is genetically determined, with 93% of the American population being extensive metabolizers and 7% being slow metabolizers.[220] The liver enzymes involved in this metabolism are either the same as, or co-inherited with, those involved in the metabolism of the antihypertensive drug debrisoquine; because of this, the systemic bioavailability of encainide is highly variable. However, this variability does not necessarily lead to a great variability in antiarrhythmic response, because both encainide and its metabolites are active. In slow metabolizers, encainide accumulates in high concentrations and is the active drug in these individuals. In extensive metabolizers of encainide, antiarrhythmic actions are seen after transformation of encainide into ODE and MODE.

The elimination half-life of encainide is also highly variable depending on metabolism phenotype. Slow metabolizers of encainide have a much longer elimination half-life than rapid metabolizers, but the latter maintain prolonged efficacy because the apparent elimination half-lives of ODE and MODE are prolonged.[215] The recommended dosage interval and total daily dosage is therefore similar for both slow and rapid metabolizers.

Dosage and Plasma Concentrations

The starting dose of encainide is 25 mg 3 times a day. Doses may be titrated up to 35 or 50 mg 3 times a day. Preliminary data suggest that encainide may be administered effectively every 12 hours in some individuals.[221] Dosage adjustments should be made at not less than intervals of 4 or 5 days.[222] Occasionally, total daily doses of more than 150 mg and up to 300 mg can be administered, if they are initiated under carefully monitored conditions. Encainide disposition is altered in patients with renal[223] or hepatic[224] insufficiency. However, because of the accumulation of the parent molecule, the overall pharmacodynamics of encainide are not altered in liver cirrhosis, and dosage usually does not need to be decreased.[224] In renal insufficiency, encainide dosage should be reduced because of both a reduced encainide clearance and increased accumulation of active metabolites.[223] A correlation has been found between QRS prolongation and ventricular arrhythmia suppression in patients being treated with encainide.[217] This correlation is stronger in extensive metabolizers than in slow metabolizers. In the former, ventricular arrhythmia suppression is usually associated with a 20 to 35% increase of QRS from baseline. Because of the variable production of active metabolites, recommendations regarding the target plasma concentrations to be reached during encainide therapy are difficult to assess. When encainide and its metabolites are given separately it has been suggested that minimal effective plasma concentrations are approximately 250 ng/ml for encainide, 50 ng/ml for ODE, and 100 ng/ml for MODE.[215, 217]

Indications

Encainide is effective for the treatment of ventricular arrhythmias and supraventricular arrhythmias, including those associated with the Wolff-Parkinson-White syndrome.[219] When used in the treatment of ventricular arrhythmias, its efficacy is comparable to that of flecainide.[225] However, because of the increased mortality seen with encainide in CAST, it is now recommended only for patients with life-threatening arrhythmias. The metabolic phenotype does not appear to alter in a major way the response to encainide. As discussed above, slow metabolizers of encainide accumulate the drug to high concentrations, whereas in rapid metabolizers antiarrhythmic efficacy occurs after transformation of encainide into ODE and MODE.

Drug Interactions

Cimetidine has been shown to increase plasma concentrations of encainide and its metabolites.[226] Although unknown at this time, it is likely that this interaction may have clinical consequences such that the dosage of encainide should be reduced when cimetidine is co-administered. Drugs that inhibit or induce liver enzymes involved in the metabolism of encainide may alter the ratio of encainide and its metabolites. Because the overall response to encainide is similar in rapid and slow metabolizers of the drug, this interaction might not alter drug efficacy in patients.

Adverse Effects

Except for its relatively good tolerance in most patients with heart failure, encainide shares most of the side effects of flecainide therapy, including its adverse effects seen in CAST. Although the effects of encainide administration on sinus node automaticity are not well known, it is wise to avoid encainide administration in patients with the sick sinus syndrome unless a pacemaker is implanted. Encainide also should be used with caution in patients with pre-existing conduction defects. Pro-arrhythmia has been reported with encainide, with an occurrence similar to that with flecainide. The risk of arrhythmia exacerbation during encainide therapy is increased with dosages causing greater than 50% QRS prolongation, with rapid increases in dosage, with dosages greater than 200 mg per day, and in patients with a history of sustained ventricular tachycardia, this last finding being the most predictive.[227] Experimental data in animals suggest that sodium administration load can reverse the adverse electrophysiologic effects of encainide overdosage.[228] The most frequent noncardiac adverse reactions are dizziness, blurred vision, headache, taste disturbances, and tremor.

PROPAFENONE

Propafenone is a new antiarrhythmic drug with original pharmacokinetic and pharmacodynamic profiles due to the presence of a genetically determined active metab-

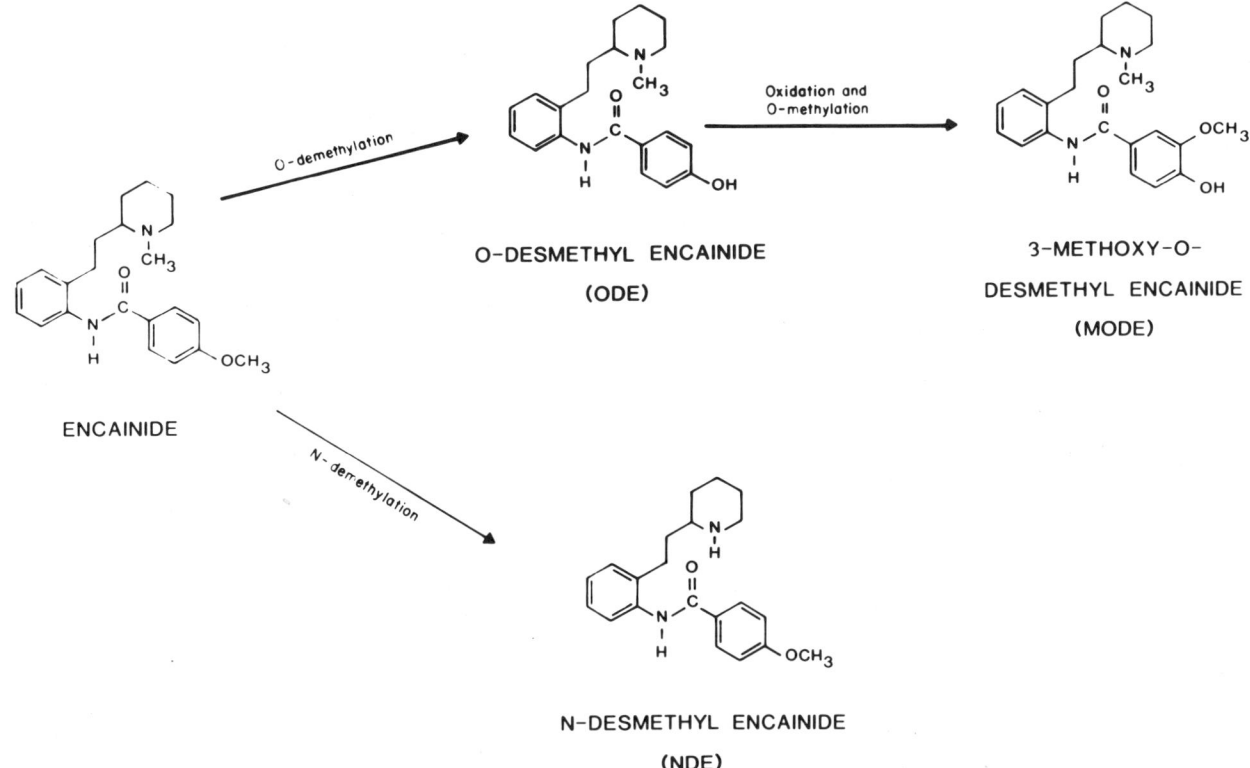

FIGURE 23–6
Metabolic pathways of encainide. In extensive metabolizers (EM) of encainide, metabolism proceeds via the pathway leading to the production of active metabolites ODE and MODE. In poor metabolizers (PM) of encainide, NDE is formed.

olite, and a potential for producing beta-adrenergic receptor antagonism.

Electrophysiologic Effects

Propafenone has mixed electrophysiologic properties consistent with class Ic, class II (beta-blocking), and class IV (calcium channel blocking) activities. It is presumed that its major antiarrhythmic effects are due to sodium channel blockade. Its active metabolite, 5-hydroxypropafenone, probably contributes to its actions. Propafenone slows conduction velocity in the atrium, AV node, and ventricle and prolongs the effective refractory periods in these tissues.[229] The blockade of sodium channel by propafenone is voltage- and rate-dependent. In vitro studies have shown that 5-hydroxypropafenone shares these electrophysiologic effects.[229, 230] In ventricular muscle fibers, action potential duration is not altered by propafenone or 5-hydroxypropafenone but both increase the ratio of effective refractory period to action potential duration.[230] Animal and in vitro studies have shown that propafenone decreases the slope of spontaneous diastolic depolarization in Purkinje fibers and decreases the rate of automatic impulse initiation without affecting automaticity of sinoatrial fibers.[231] However, high concentrations of propafenone depress sinus node automaticity, an effect that is counterbalanced in humans by propafenone's weak vagolytic properties.[231] Both propafenone and 5-hydroxypropafenone have weak calcium antagonist effects whereas 5-hydroxypropafenone's beta-receptor antagonist properties are half those of propafenone.[229] The clinical relevance of these class II and IV properties remains uncertain. During chronic oral administration of propafenone, QRS and PR intervals are prolonged on the surface ECG without significant change in the QTc interval.[232]

Hemodynamic Effects

Both propafenone and 5-hydroxypropafenone have significant negative inotropic action.[229, 233] Although it has been suggested that these negative inotropic actions are unlikely to become clinically significant at usual plasma concentrations required for antiarrhythmic efficacy,[229] this deserves further evaluation.

Clinical Pharmacokinetics

After oral administration, propafenone is very well absorbed but undergoes extensive (variable and saturable) presystemic elimination.[234] Propafenone is metabolized into 5-hydroxypropafenone in the liver; enzymes involved in this biotransformation are the same as those involved in debrisoquine (or encainide) metabolism.[235] As previously discussed for encainide, there is a genetic polymorphism of this metabolism, with approximately 93% of the American population being extensive metabolizers of the drug. The clinical pharmacokinetics of propafenone vary according to metabolic phenotype (Fig. 23–7). However, because propafenone and 5-hydroxypropafenone have similar

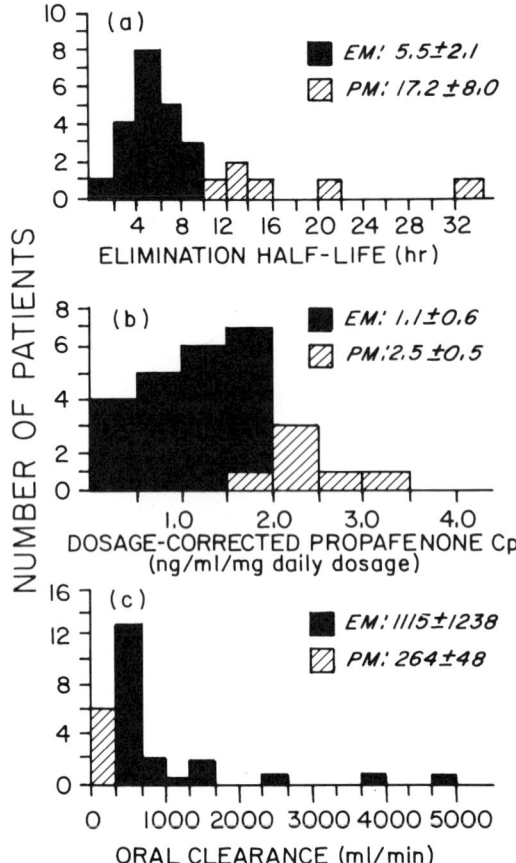

FIGURE 23-7
Pharmacokinetics of propafenone related to debrisoquine metabolic phenotype (extensive metabolizer, EM, or poor metabolizer, PM). (Reprinted by permission of the American Heart Association, Inc., from Siddoway LA, Thompson KA, McAllister CB, et al.: Circulation 75:785, 1987.)

pharmacologic profiles, the antiarrhythmic response to propafenone is not different between extensive and slow metabolizers.[235] One important fact is that the pharmacokinetics of propafenone show a nonlinear increase in plasma concentrations with increasing dosage.[232, 234, 235] This is probably due to saturability of hepatic metabolism, with consequent rise in plasma concentrations of propafenone in excess of those expected from the dosage increment. Because propafenone has greater beta-blocking potency than 5-hydroxypropafenone, it might be expected that slow metabolizers of propafenone (in whom high concentrations of propafenone can be found) will have more beta-blockade than extensive metabolizers.

Dosage and Plasma Concentrations

Usual dosages of propafenone are 450 to 900 mg per day administered in 3 divided doses. There is currently no recommendation concerning the need for dosage adjustments in patients with cardiac, renal, or hepatic insufficiency. Slow and extensive metabolizers appear to require the same range of dosages.[235] Because of the variable metabolism of propafenone, plasma concentrations associated with efficacy are not useful.

Indications

Propafenone is an effective drug for the treatment of ventricular and supraventricular arrhythmias.[232, 235-237] It also has been shown to be useful in the management of atrial fibrillation, atrial flutter, AV nodal reentrant tachycardia, and arrhythmias associated with the Wolff-Parkinson-White syndrome.[238, 239] However, its electrophysiologic similarity to encainide and flecainide have led many to reserve it for life-threatening arrhythmias.

Drug Interactions

Co-administration of propafenone and metoprolol leads to increased plasma concentrations of metoprolol and increased beta-blockade.[24] Because propafenone metabolism is saturable and involves a specific group of hepatic enzymes that can metabolize other xenobiotics, it is likely that other drug interactions will occur with propafenone. The pharmacodynamic consequences of such interactions will depend on the relative affinity of the two competing substrates for the hepatic enzymes. Food has already been shown to dramatically increase propafenone bioavailability in rapid but not in slow metabolizers of the drug.[240] Because extensive and poor metabolizers of propafenone have the same general pattern of clinical response,[235] such interactions might not modify antiarrhythmic efficacy of propafenone. However, since propafenone and its main metabolite (and probably their enantiomers) have different beta-blocking potencies,[229] differences in the two phenotypes might alter the incidence of side effects.

Adverse Effects

As with other antiarrhythmic agents, propafenone has the potential to worsen preexisting arrhythmias.[40] Although preliminary data indicates that this may be less of a problem with propafenone than with similar agents,[197] large prospective comparative studies are not available. The clinical relevance of the beta-blocking properties of propafenone with respect to its side effect profile has not been fully elucidated, although it has been suggested that propafenone does not exert a clinically significant beta-blocking effect in patients.[241] However, there is no doubt that beta-blockade can be clinically significant in certain patients such as those with asthma.[235, 242] Bundle branch block or AV nodal block has been reported occasionally with propafenone,[235, 241] and left ventricular function can be depressed by this drug.[233] The incidence and clinical consequences of these effects will remain uncertain until larger trials are performed. Neurologic side effects observed with flecainide and encainide have also been reported with propafenone. These include visual blurring, dizziness, paresthesia, and taste disturbance.[235, 236]

AMIODARONE

Amiodarone is an iodinated benzofuran that is structurally similar to thyroxine and procainamide. Originally developed as an antianginal agent, it was found to suppress effectively a wide variety of ventricular and supraventricular arrhythmias. This efficacy has been assumed to be due to prolongation of both refractoriness and action potential duration in myocardial tissue (Vaughan Williams class III activity). However, amiodarone has been found to have many diverse pharmacologic actions, and those responsible for its high degree of antiarrhythmic efficacy remain unidentified.

Electrophysiologic Effects

Intracellular recordings in cardiac tissues from rabbits chronically treated with amiodarone demonstrated prolongation of action potential duration and increased refractoriness of both atrial and ventricular myocardium, Purkinje fibers, and sinus and AV nodal tissues. Amiodarone decreases phase-0 depolarization of myocardial cells and blocks sodium channels that are in the inactivated state.[243,244] It also slows phase-4 depolarization of the sinus node as well as conduction through the AV node. Talajic et al.[245] have found that the electrophysiologic actions of the major metabolite of amiodarone, desethylamiodarone (DEA), are different from those of amiodarone, with the metabolite having greater effects on conduction, due to effects on sodium channels (and hence, on conduction).

The electrophysiologic changes seen in humans must be considered with respect to the route of drug administration and the duration of therapy. Following acute intravenous amiodarone administration, prolongation of the A-H interval and an increase in the refractory periods of the AV node and bypass tracts are seen; however, some of these changes may be due to the presence of the solubilizing agent polysorbate 80 (Tween 80) in the intravenous formulation. No changes are seen in sinus rate or atrial or ventricular refractoriness, whereas these are prolonged during chronic oral therapy. Chronic amiodarone therapy also prolongs the A-H and H-V and the P-R and QT intervals of the surface ECG. There are conflicting data on the time course of the development of these changes and how they might relate to the antiarrhythmic efficacy of amiodarone. The changes in action potential duration and refractoriness that are seen in hypothyroidism are similar to changes resulting from oral amiodarone therapy.[246] Since these changes can be prevented in animals by co-administration of thyroid hormone with amiodarone,[247] some have concluded that amiodarone's antiarrhythmic efficacy is due to production of "cardiac hypothyroidism." Amiodarone's major metabolite does cause noncompetitive inhibition of thyroid hormone binding to nuclear membrane receptors.[248] However, amiodarone also causes noncompetitive blockade of alpha- and beta-receptors,[249] muscarinic receptors,[250] and both calcium and sodium channel blockade—any combination of which may contribute to its antiarrhythmic efficacy.

Hemodynamic Effects

Intravenous administration of amiodarone at dosages greater than 5 mg/kg decreases contractility and peripheral vascular resistance, producing severe hypotension in some instances. It is possible that some of this effect, like the electrophysiologic effects described earlier, may be due to the effects of polysorbate 80 or benzyl alcohol present in this formulation. After oral administration at usual dosages, no change in myocardial contractility has been observed.

Clinical Pharmacokinetics

Amiodarone is a highly lipid-soluble compound having extremely variable and complex pharmacokinetics. It is slowly absorbed from the gastrointestinal tract, and bioavailability varies from 20 to 80%.[251] Amiodarone is extensively metabolized to DEA, and little if any is excreted unchanged in the urine. During chronic therapy, concentrations of DEA in plasma vary from 0.4 to 2.0 times that of amiodarone.[252] This metabolite has antiarrhythmic potency equal or greater to amiodarone when compared in in vitro and animal models.[253]

Amiodarone is rapidly concentrated in some tissues (including myocardium), but accumulates more slowly in others (e.g., adipose tissue). Significantly, it redistributes out of myocardial tissue while still accumulating in adipose and other tissues (Fig. 23–8).[252,254] Until all tissues are saturated, rapid redistribution out of the myocardium may be responsible for early recurrence of arrhythmias after discontinuation of therapy or rapid reduction of dosage. Because of drug accumulation in tissues, the volume of distribution for amiodarone is very large, (20–200 L/kg).[254] After intravenous administration, the measured half-life in plasma is from 4.8 to 68.2 hours[255] because tissue uptake is primarily responsible for the decline in plasma concentration. However, as tissues become saturated, the decline in plasma levels is slow, reflecting elimination and slow redistribution of drug out of adipose and muscle tissues. This leads to slow and extremely variable elimination from plasma; half-life ranges from 23 to 103 days.[254] It is also possible that amiodarone inhibits its own elimination after chronic therapy, contributing to the differences between half-life early in therapy to that after prolonged therapy.

Dosage and Plasma Concentration

Without a loading dose, amiodarone requires several days to weeks before producing its antiarrhythmic action. Large intravenous dosages or oral loading dosages can hasten the onset of therapeutic effects, but no prospective studies have determined the optimal method for administering loading dosages. Loading dosages reported in the literature have varied from 600 to 1800 mg per day for 2 to 21 days.[256] Because of relatively rapid redistribution out of myocardial tissue, the dosage should be tapered over a period of several weeks. The usual maintenance dose varies from 200 to 600 mg per day; because of the severe nature of adverse reactions, the lowest effective dosage should be prescribed. It is thought that patients with supraventricular arrhythmias will respond to lower dosages than those with ventricular arrhythmias, but there are many ex-

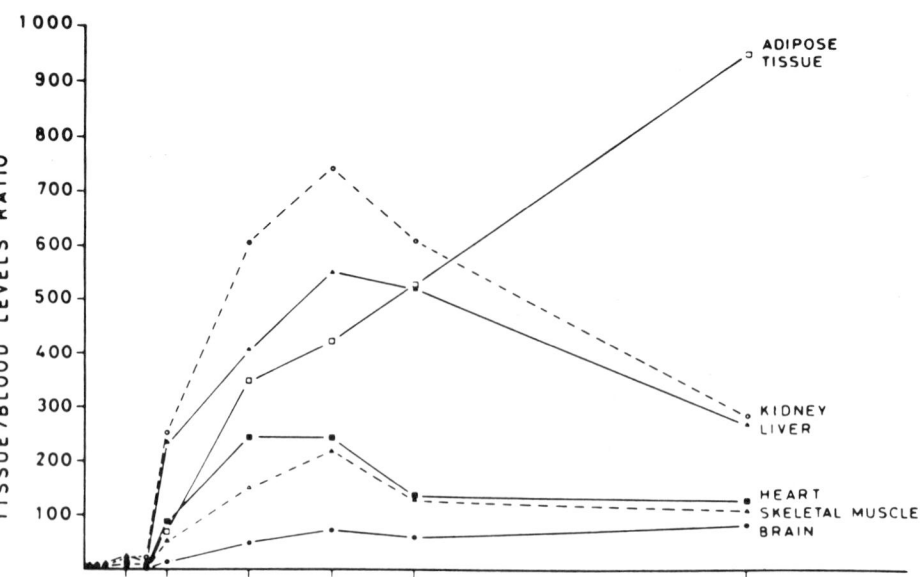

FIGURE 23-8
Tissue distribution of amiodarone after intraperitoneal administration in rats. (Reprinted by permission of the Raven Press Publishers, New York from Riva E, Gerna M, Neyroz P, et al.: J Cardiovasc Pharmacol 4-207, 1982.)

ceptions to this, and no comparative trials are available. Because of the variable pharmacokinetics and oral bioavailability, it is unlikely that generalizations such as this will be reliable.

Plasma concentrations of amiodarone are usually between 1 and 2 µg/ml during effective therapy.[257, 258] Similar concentrations of the desethyl metabolite (DEA) accumulate during therapy and are likely to contribute to antiarrhythmic efficacy. However, because of extensive overlap between the range of concentrations required for arrhythmia suppression and those associated with toxicity, monitoring of plasma concentrations is of limited value. Clearly, levels of amiodarone above 3 to 4 µg/ml for prolonged periods of time are associated with a higher incidence of adverse effects.[259]

Indications

Although amiodarone has been reported to have efficacy in a wide range of arrhythmias, the Food and Drug Administration in the United States has recommended it only as therapy for life-threatening ventricular arrhythmias refractory to all other available forms of therapy. Nevertheless, there are numerous reports in the literature documenting the efficacy of amiodarone in the conversion and slowing of atrial fibrillation, AV nodal reentrant tachycardia, and tachycardias associated with the Wolff-Parkinson-White syndrome.[260-262] The reasons for amiodarone's limited labeling are (1) the lack of controlled trials to support its use for other indications, (2) the documented potentially lethal complications of chronic amiodarone therapy, and (3) the difficulties associated with variable time for onset of action and drug interactions.

Drug Interactions

Amiodarone has been found to interfere with the clearance of many drugs. A partial explanation for these interactions may involve the formation of a metabolically inactive cytochrome P-450(II)–metabolite complex, which has been described in animals treated with amiodarone.[263] This may explain the unexpected accumulation of warfarin,[264] quinidine, procainamide, disopyramide, mexiletine, and propafenone[265] and the respective resultant bleeding, heart block, or torsades de pointes. However, it does not explain the interaction between amiodarone and drugs eliminated predominantly by the kidneys, such as digoxin.[266] It is likely that the elimination of many other drugs can be impaired by amiodarone, and the physician should titrate any concomitant therapy to the lowest effective dosage.

Adverse Reactions

The medical literature for amiodarone is replete with conflicting opinions regarding its safety. The early reports found it to be very well tolerated. Some studies continue to find that it is safe and effective, even in the treatment of arrhythmias in children.[267] The reason for these differences is not apparent, but clearly the experience with amiodarone in the United States, with a very high incidence of intolerable and sometimes lethal reactions, is different from that in Europe. The discrepancy may be due to differences in dosage, the patient population, drug interactions, or some unknown genetic or geographic factors. It is very difficult to determine the incidence of adverse reactions with amiodarone because most studies in the literature report the incidence in populations having highly variable durations of treatment. An actuarial analysis of the rate of occurrence would be much more helpful, and preliminary data from such an analysis by Mason et al.[268] indicate that the toxicity may be more frequent than previously appreciated.

The most serious reaction is the potentially lethal interstitial pneumonitis,[243, 269] which may be more common in patients with pre-existing lung disease. It is important that physicians monitor their patients carefully, because the pneumonitis is reversible if detected early. Serial pulmonary function tests are helpful for follow-up of patients, and most physicians familiar with the drug monitor their patients by having them obtain a chest x-ray every 3 months. Both hyper- and hypothyroidism are fairly common.[246] Accumulation of corneal microdeposits is almost uniform during therapy, and in many cases can progress to the point of interfering with vision.[270] Many caucasian patients notice a slate-gray or bluish discoloration of the sun-exposed areas of the skin.[271] Many also complain of photosensitivity, which can sometimes be alleviated by sun screens and protective clothing. More than 30% of patients have abnormally elevated hepatic enzyme levels in their serum, and progression to jaundice and cirrhosis has been reported.[272, 273] Serial laboratory tests to screen for amiodarone toxicity can be costly and generally are of little value. However, it is wise to obtain a reliable assessment of baseline tests (complete blood count, blood chemistry, tests of thyroid and pulmonary function, a slit-lamp examination, and measurement of blood levels of other drugs whenever possible). Careful instructions to patients and their family members are important in screening for toxicity.

BRETYLIUM TOSYLATE

Because of its sympatholytic activity, bretylium tosylate was first evaluated in the 1950s for the treatment of hypertension. However, a very high incidence of orthostatic hypotension and unreliable oral absorption led to its disfavor for chronic therapy. Bacaner[274] first discovered its antiarrhythmic activity in animals, and bretylium was eventually marketed in the Unites States as intravenous therapy for life-threatening ventricular arrhythmias. Because of its complex effects on the autonomic nervous system, it is usually reserved for those patients who have failed to respond to lidocaine.

Electrophysiologic Effects

In addition to the indirect electrophysiologic changes caused by the drug's action on postganglionic autonomic neurons, bretylium has a direct class III action that causes an increase in action potential duration and refractoriness in ventricular muscle and Purkinje fibers.[275] When clinically relevant concentrations of bretylium are studied in normal tissues, no changes are seen in $\dot{V}_{max}$, maximum velocity of phase 0 depolarization or conduction velocity. Studies by Cardinale and Sasyniuk[276] have found that bretylium reduces the degree of dispersion of repolarization across the boundary between normal and ischemic tissue. Transient increases in membrane potential and conduction velocity are seen early after bretylium administration and are presumed to be due to the local release of catecholamines. Bretylium has been found to elevate the threshold for electrically induced fibrillation in a variety of animal models.

When initially administered, bretylium causes the release of norepinephrine from postganglionic adrenergic neurons.[277] Bretylium is transported into the neuron by the norepinephrine pump (termed uptake 2), and extensive accumulation in the neuron is then associated with a blockade of further release or uptake of norepinephrine by the neuron. Blockade of uptake of circulating or infused catecholamines leads to supersensitivity functionally similar to a denervated state.

In assessing the effects of bretylium, it is essential that one distinguish between its direct effects and the indirect effects of bretylium on the autonomic nervous system. This may be difficult in clinical research, in which patients are studied under conditions very different from the usual clinical situation. Patients with ventricular tachycardia or experiencing recurrent ventricular fibrillation have striking adrenergic stimulation, and the effects of bretylium on myocardial tissue may be overwhelmed.

Anderson et al.[278] performed serial evaluations of the electrophysiologic actions of bretylium in patients given a 5 mg/kg loading dose and again after a 1-hour infusion at 1.5 mg/minute. They found changes compatible with catecholamine release during both periods (i.e., shortening of the refractory periods of the AV node, right atrium, and right ventricle).

Hemodynamic Effects

Studies in stable patients found that low and high dosages of bretylium cause a transient increase in heart rate, blood pressure, contractility, peripheral vascular resistance, and arrhythmia frequency. This was followed by a fall in standing blood pressure and peripheral vascular resistance.[279] Orthostatic hypotension is almost uniformly seen in patients receiving bretylium and sometimes lasts for days after discontinuation of therapy. Dosages that are well below those required for antiarrhythmic efficacy are capable of causing orthostatic hypotension. Therefore, when hypotension develops during bretylium therapy, it should be corrected with intravenous volume expansion, and adequate doses of bretylium should be given to suppress arrhythmias. After the initial phase of catecholamine release, bretylium has little effect on myocardial contractility at clinically achieved levels.

The postural hypotension induced by bretylium can be reversed by concomitant administration of tricyclic antidepressants, which compete for transport into the adrenergic neuron. This has been used experimentally in a few patients given chronic oral bretylium therapy without interfering with the antiarrhythmic actions of bretylium.[280] However, this may not be safe or feasible in patients for whom the anti-adrenergic actions of bretylium are essential for arrhythmia control.

Clinical Pharmacokinetics

Bretylium is poorly absorbed after oral administration, with a bioavailability of approximately 25%. It is eliminated almost entirely unchanged in the urine, and clearance correlates well with creatinine clearance.[281] It is probably actively secreted by the base transport system in the distal tubules. Clearance is reduced and half-life prolonged in patients with renal insufficiency.

Dosage and Plasma Concentrations

The usual intravenous dosage for bretylium is 5 mg/kg given at a rate dependent on the clinical setting.[282] During cardiac emergencies, it should be given by rapid injection into a central intravenous line. In less acute situations, a loading infusion of the same dose should be given over 10 to 20 minutes to reduce the incidence of nausea and vomiting. The loading dose should be repeated after 10 to 20 minutes if the arrhythmia is still present. A total loading dose of 20 mg/kg may be required, and dosages of up to 9 g in 24 hours have been given without serious adverse effects. Maintenance infusions of 1 to 4 mg/minute should be given, depending on body size and renal function. Heart rhythm and blood pressure should be monitored carefully, especially during the first few hours of bretylium therapy.

Studies in animals have found that the electrophysiologic effects of bretylium correlate better with myocardial concentrations than with plasma concentrations early after the first dose. Plasma concentrations of 1 to 2 µg/ml have been reported in a few patients with antiarrhythmic response to bretylium.[278] However, the wide therapeutic index and variable myocardial accumulation make plasma level monitoring of limited clinical utility.

Indications

Bretylium is effective for acute therapy of ventricular tachycardia and/or ventricular fibrillation. Because of its complex effects on the autonomic nervous system and orthostatic hypotension, it should be reserved for patients who have failed to respond to lidocaine.

Drug Interactions

No drug interactions have been reported. However, one would expect that there might be competition for renal tubular secretion with procainamide, NAPA, cimetidine, and other organic bases.

Adverse Effects

When bretylium is given by rapid intravenous injection, many patients experience nausea and vomiting. The release of norepinephrine has the potential to cause increased blood pressure, but severe hypertension has not been described. Increased frequency of ventricular arrhythmias is often seen at this time and can lead to the need for more frequent cardioversion. The reduction in peripheral vascular resistance can cause symptomatic hypotension in volume-depleted patients, but this can be readily corrected if recognized. Hypotension could prove dangerous in patients with fixed valvular obstruction. Bradycardia has been reported in some patients with abnormalities of the conduction system when given large intravenous dosages of bretylium.

Other Antiarrhythmic Agents

The beta-receptor antagonists are the only agents that have been shown to reduce mortality in the early period and 1 to 2 years following acute myocardial infarction.[283] It has been suggested that these results can in part be explained by an antiarrhythmic effect of adrenergic blockade.[283] Studies have shown that chronic ventricular arrhythmias can be suppressed by propranolol,[284] metoprolol,[285] timolol,[286] acebutolol,[287] pindolol,[288] nadolol,[289] and atenolol.[290] It has been consistently noted that beta-receptor antagonists suppress repetitive ventricular arrhythmias more than isolated ectopic beats. Some of the beta-adrenergic blocking agents have been shown to have antiarrhythmic properties independent of their anti-ischemic or beta-receptor blocking properties.[291–293] Sotalol is a beta-adrenergic antagonist with additional class III properties, which has been shown to be useful in the treatment of ventricular and supraventricular arrhythmias.[294] Beta-receptor antagonists can also be very useful for control of ventricular rate in atrial fibrillation or flutter, paroxysmal supraventricular tachycardia, and symptomatic sinus tachycardia and in the management of catecholamine-related ventricular arrhythmias and ischemia-related arrhythmias. The clinical pharmacokinetics of the beta-adrenergic antagonists has been reviewed recently.[295] These agents have proved to be very useful as an adjunct to therapy with agents with class I or class III antiarrhythmic actions.[44, 296]

Calcium channel blockers can also be used as antiarrhythmic agents.[297, 298] Verapamil and diltiazem are useful in the management of supraventricular tachycardia. They are administered to slow the ventricular rate in patients with atrial fibrillation or flutter and to treat and prevent AV nodal reentrant tachycardia. Although the intravenous administration of verapamil is dangerous in the acute treatment of ventricular tachycardia in patients with chronic or acute ischemic heart disease, verapamil has been shown to suppress a rare form of ventricular tachycardia with a right bundle branch block pattern and left axis deviation.[299] The electrophysiology[300] and pharmacokinetics[301] of calcium antagonists have been recently reviewed. Verapamil and diltiazem have been shown to decrease antipyrine clearance, often considered an index of oxidative metabolism in the liver.[33] Verapamil, but not diltiazem, increases liver blood flow as assessed by indocyanine green clearance.[33] Both drugs raise the plasma concentration of digoxin. Verapamil and diltiazem may sometimes increase the bioavailability and decrease the systemic elimination of drugs with low hepatic extraction ratios. Verapamil may also increase the systemic elimination of drugs with a high hepatic extraction ratio.

Other miscellaneous antiarrhythmic agents such as recainam,[302] moricizine,[303] and pirmenol[304] are currently being investigated and may prove to be useful in the future.

Combination of Antiarrhythmic Agents

When an antiarrhythmic agent fails to suppress an arrhythmia or when intolerable side effects appear, combining two antiarrhythmic agents has proved to be useful. For some combinations of antiarrhythmic drugs, enhanced pharmacologic response occurs and lower doses of each drug can be given, thus avoiding side effects present at full dosage. When combining antiarrhythmic drugs it should be kept in mind that pharmacokinetic interactions may occur. Some drugs can cause major alterations in the hepatic elimination of others. Amiodarone has been shown to inhibit hepatic mixed function oxidase in vitro[163] and in vivo.[305] Quinidine is a potent inhibitor of the cytochrome P450 responsible for the metabolism of debrisoquine.[83-86] Elimination of other drugs that use the same cytochrome P450, such as encainide or propafenone, may be altered by co-administration of quinidine. The effects of calcium channel blockers on hepatic mixed-function oxidase and on liver blood flow may also have clinical consequences (see above). Finally, most antiarrhythmic drugs are basic compounds. Some of them are actively secreted in the proximal tubule of the kidney, and competition for this route of elimination has been proposed as a mechanism for pharmacokinetic interactions.[126, 306] Combination of several antiarrhythmic drugs with predominant class Ia activity does not appear to be effective.[307, 308] Combination of mexiletine with quinidine,[309] tocainide with quinidine,[310] amiodarone with procainamide,[311, 312] mexiletine with disopyramide,[313] lidocaine with encainide,[314] and propafenone with quinidine[315] have been shown to be useful.

Conclusion

Several antiarrhythmic drugs are now available that can potentially suppress both ventricular and supraventricular arrhythmias. All these agents have significant toxicity, which can sometimes be lethal. Therefore, the decision to treat an arrhythmia should be based on the analysis of the risk/benefit ratio of the pharmacological therapy. If antiarrhythmic drugs are clearly indicated, their administration should start at low doses and titration should take into account the pharmacokinetics of the parent and any active metabolites. Since all these drugs have a low therapeutic index, the possibility of drug interaction should always be kept in mind.

As a general guideline, one should first administer one antiarrhythmic drug with predominant class Ia activity. If this fails, one can try combining an antiarrhythmic drug with predominant class Ia activity and one with predominant class Ib or class II activity. If the patient responds to the combination, evaluation of the second drug alone should also be considered, to reduce the possibility that the patient is being given unnecessary therapy. If this also fails, more potent antiarrhythmic agents such as flecainide, encainide, or propafenone can be tried alone. In patients where it is clearly indicated, amiodarone should be tried; however, because of its significant toxicity, this agent should be used only after all antiarrhythmic drugs or combinations of drugs have failed. Finally, combination of a beta-blocker with other antiarrhythmic drugs, if tolerated, can be very helpful in the management of arrhythmias.

References

1. Ruberman W, Weinblatt E, Goldberg JD, et al: Ventricular premature complexes and sudden death after myocardial infarction. Circulation 64:297, 1981.
2. Fuster V, Gersh BJ, Giuliani ER, et al.: The natural history of idiopathic dilated cardiomyopathy. Am J Cardiol 47:525, 1981.
3. Bjarnason I, Hardarson T, Jonsson S: Cardiac arrhythmias in hypertrophic cardiomyopathy. Br. Heart J 48:198, 1982.
4. McKenna WJ, Deanfield JE, Faruqui AM, et al.: Prognosis in hypertrophic cardiomyopathy: Role of age and clinical echocardiographic and hemodynamic features. Am J Cardiol 47:532, 1981.
5. Kligfield P, Levy D, Devereux RB, et al.: Arrhythmias and sudden death in mitral valve prolapse. Am Heart J 113:1298, 1987.
6. Olshausen KV, Schwarz F, Apfelbach J, et al.: Determinants of the incidence and severity of ventricular arrhythmias in aortic valve disease. Am J Cardiol 51:1103, 1983.
7. Kostis JB, Byington R, Friedman LM, et al: Prognostic significance of ventricular ectopic activity in survivors of acute myocardial infarction. J Am Coll Cardiol 10:231, 1987.
8. Bigger JT Jr, Fleiss JL, Kleiger R, et al.: The relationship among ventricular arrhythmias, left ventricular dysfunction, and mortality in the two years after myocardial infarction. Circulation 69:250, 1984.
9. Goldberg RJ, Gore JM, Haffajee CI, et al.: Outcome after cardiac arrest during acute myocardial infarction. Am J Cardiol 59:251, 1987.
10. Tofler GH, Stone PH, Muller JE, et al.: Prognosis after cardiac arrest due to ventricular tachycardia or ventricular fibrillation associated with acute myocardial infarction (the MILIS Study). Am J Cardiol 60:755, 1987.
11. Kennedy HL, Whitlock JA, Sprague MK, et al.: Long-term follow-up of asymptomatic healthy subjects with frequent and complex ventricular ectopy. N Engl J Med 312:193, 1985.
12. Nygaard TW, Sellers TD, Cook TS, et al.: Adverse reactions to antiarrhythmic drugs during therapy for ventricular arrhythmias. JAMA 256:55, 1986.
13. Wilson JR: Use of antiarrhythmic drugs in patients with heart failure: Clinical efficacy, hemodynamic results, and relation to survival. Circulation 75 (Suppl 4):IV-64, 1987.
14. Morganroth J: Comparative evaluation of antiarrhythmic agents. Drugs 29 (Suppl 4):14, 1985.
15. Zipes DL: A consideration of antiarrhythmic therapy. Circulation 72:949, 1985.
16. Goldman P: Rate-controlled drug delivery. N Engl J Med 307:286, 1982.
17. Flanagan AD: Pharmacokinetics of sustained release procainamide preparations. Angiology 33:71, 1982.
18. Wilkinson GR: Clearance approaches in pharmacology. Pharmacol Rev 39:1, 1987.
19. Woosley RL, Roden DM: Importance of metabolites in antiarrhythmic therapy. Am J Cardiol 52:3C, 1983.
20. Wilkinson GR, Shand DG: A physiological approach to hepatic drug clearance. Clin Pharmacol Ther 18:377, 1975.
21. Wood AJJ, Feely Jr: Pharmacokinetic drug interactions with propranolol. Clin Pharmacokinet 8:253, 1983.

22. Okey AB, Roberts EA, Harper PA, et al.: Induction of drug-metabolizing enzymes: Mechanisms and consequences. Clin Biochem 19:132, 1986.
23. Testa B, Jenner P: Inhibitors of cytochrome P450 and their mechanisms of action. Drug Metab Rev 12:1, 1981.
24. Wagner F, Kalusche D, Trenk D, et al.: Drug interaction between propafenone and metoprolol. Br J Clin Pharmacol 24:213, 1987.
25. Thompson PD, Melmon KL, Richardson JA, et al.: Lidocaine pharmacokinetics in advanced heart failure, liver disease and renal failure in humans. Ann Intern Med 78:499, 1973.
26. Odar-Cedarlof I, Borga O: Kinetics of diphenylhydantoin in uraemic patients: consequences of decreased plasma protein binding. Eur J Clin Pharmacol 7:31, 1974.
27. Barchowsy A, Shand DG, Stargel WW, et al.: On the role of alpha-1-acid glycoprotein in lignocaine accumulation following myocardial infarction. Br J Clin Pharmacol 13:411, 1982.
28. Jusko WM, Gretch M: Plasma and tissue protein binding of drugs in pharmacokinetics. Drug Metab Rev 5:43, 1976.
29. Lima JJ, Boudoulas H, Blanford M: Concentration-dependence of disopyramide binding to plasma protein and its influence on kinetics and dynamics. J Pharmacol Exp Ther 219:741, 1981.
30. Drayer DE, Reidenberg MM: Clinical consequence of polymorphic acetylation of basic drugs. Clin Pharmacol Ther 22:251, 1977.
31. Jacqz E, Hall SD, Branch RA: Genetically determined polymorphisms in drug oxidation. Hepatology 6:1020, 1986.
32. Stenson RE, Constantino RT, Harrison DC: Interrelationships of hepatic blood flow, cardiac output, and blood levels of lignocaine in man. Circulation 43:205, 1971.
33. Bauer LA, Stenwall M, Horn JR, et al.: Changes in antipyrine and indocyanine green kinetics during nifedipine, verapamil, and diltiazem therapy. Clin Pharmacol Ther 40:239, 1986.
34. Reidenberg MM, Drayer DE: Effects of renal disease upon drug disposition. Drug Metab Rev 8:293, 1977.
35. Ritschel WA: Pharmacokinetic changes in the elderly. Methods Find Exp Clin Pharmacol 9:161, 1987.
36. Johnston A, Warrington S, Turner P: Flecainide pharmacokinetics in healthy volunteers: The influence of urinary pH. Br J Clin Pharmacol 20:333, 1985.
37. Moller JV, Sheikh MI: Renal organic amine transport systems: Pharmacological, physiological, and biochemical aspects. Pharmacol Rev 34:315, 1983.
38. Somogyi A, McLean A, Heinzow B: Cimetidine-procainamide pharmacokinetic interaction in man: Evidence of competition for tubular secretion of basic drugs. Eur J Clin Pharmacol 25:339, 1983.
39. Edvardsson N, Olsson SB: Clinical value of plasma concentrations of antiarrhythmic drugs. Eur Heart J 8:83, 1987.
40. Podrid PJ, Lampert S, Graboys TB, et al.: Aggravation of arrhythmia by antiarrhythmic drugs. Incidence and predictors. Am J Cardiol 59:38E, 1987.
41. Vaughan Williams EM: A classification of antiarrhythmic actions reassessed after a decade of new drugs. J Clin Pharmacol 24:129, 1984.
42. Harrison DC: Introduction of the symposium on perspectives on the treatment of ventricular arrhythmias. Am J Cardiol 52:1C, 1983.
43. Cobbe SM: Clinical usefulness of the Vaughan Williams classification system. Eur Heart J 8 (Suppl A):65, 1987.
44. Graboys TB, Lown B, Podrid PJ, et al.: Long-term survival of patients with malignant ventricular arrhythmias treated with antiarrhythmic drugs. Am J Cardiol 50:437, 1982.
45. Hohnloser SH, Raeder EA, Podrid PJ, et al.: Predictors of antiarrhythmic drug efficacy in patients with malignant ventricular tachyarrhythmias. Am Heart J 114:1, 1987.
46. Woosley RL: Risk/benefit considerations in antiarrhythmic therapy. JAMA 256:82, 1986.
47. Bigger JT Jr: Antiarrhythmic treatment. An overview. Am J Cardiol 53:8B, 1984.
48. Vlay S: How the university cardiologist treats ventricular premature beats: A nationwide survey of 65 University Medical Centers. Am Heart J 110:904, 1985.
49. Gottlieb SH, Achuff SC, Mellits ED, et al.: Prophylactic antiarrhythmic therapy of high risk survivors of myocardial infarction: Lower mortality at 1 month but not at 1 year. Circulation 75:792, 1987.
50. Furberg CD: Effect of antiarrhythmic drugs on mortality after myocardial infarction. Am J Cardiol 52:32C, 1983.
51. Hondeghem LM, Katzung BG: Time- and voltage-dependent interactions of antiarrhythmic drugs with cardiac sodium channels. Biochim Biophys Acta 474:373, 1977.
52. Chen C-M, Gettes LS, Katzung BG: Effects of lidocaine and quinidine on steady-state characteristics and recovery kinetics (dV/dT)max in guinea pig ventricular myocardium. Circ Res 37:20, 1975.
53. Johnson EA, McKinnion MG: The differential effect on quinidine and pyrilamine on the myocardial action potential at different rates of stimulation. J Pharmacol Exp Ther 120:460, 1957.
54. Nattel S, Elharrar V, Zipes DP, et al.: pH-dependent electrophysiological effects of quinidine and lidocaine on canine cardiac Purkinje fibers. Circ Res 48:55, 1981.
55. Balser JR, Hondeghem LM, Roden DM: Quinidine block of Ik accumulates at negative potentials (Abstract). Circulation 76 (Suppl IV):IV-149, 1987.
56. Carmeliet E, Sairawa T: Shortening of the action potential and reduction of pacemaker activity by lidocaine, quinidine and procainamide in sheep cardiac Purkinje fibers: an effect on Na or K currents. Circ Res 50:257, 1982.
57. Mason JW, Winkle RA, Rider AK, et al.: The electrophysiologic effects of quinidine in the transplanted human heart. J Clin Invest 59:481, 1977.
58. Mirro MJ, Manalan AS, Bailey JC, et al.: Anticholinergic effects of disopyramide and quinidine on guinea-pig myocardium: Mediation by direct muscarinic receptor blockade. Circ Res 47:855, 1980.
59. Schmid PG, Nelson LD, Mark AL, et al.: Inhibition of adrenergic vasoconstriction by quinidine. J Pharmacol Exp Ther 188:124, 1974.
60. Mahmarian JJ, Verani MS, Hohmann T, et al.: The hemodynamic effects of sotalol and quinidine: Analysis by use of rest and exercise gated radionuclide angiography. Circulation 76:324, 1987.
61. Hoffman BF, Rosen MR, Wit AL: Electrophysiology and pharmacology of cardiac arrhythmias. VII. Cardiac effects of quinidine and procainamide. Am Heart J 90:117, 1975.
62. Parmley WW, Braunwald E: Comparative myocardial depressant and antiarrhythmic properties of D-propranolol, DL-propranolol, and quinidine. J Pharmacol Exp Ther 158:11, 1967.
63. Covinsky JO, Ruso J Jr, Kelly KL, et al.: Relative bioavailability of quinidine gluconate and quinidine sulfate in healthy volunteers. J Clin Pharmacol 19:261, 1979.
64. Ochs HR, Greenblatt DJ, Woo E, et al.: Single and multiple dose pharmacokinetics of oral quinidine sulfate and gluconate. Am J Cardiol 410:770, 1978.
65. Edwards DJ, Axelson JEE, Slaughter RL, et al.: Factors affecting quinidine protein binding in man. Clin Pharmacokinet 9:596, 1984.
66. Mihaly GW, Ching MS, Klejn MB, et al.: Differences in the binding of quinine and quinidine to plasma proteins. Br J Clin Pharmacol 24:769, 1987.
67. Palmer K, Martin B, Baggett B, et al.: The metabolic fate of orally administered quinidine gluconate in humans. Biochem Pharmacol 18:1845, 1969.
68. Guengerich FP, Muller-Enoch D, Blair IA: Oxidation of quinidine by human liver cytochrome P-450. Mol Pharmacol 30:287, 1986.
69. Vozeh S, Bindschedler M, Huy-Riem HA, et al.: Pharmacodynamics of 3-hydroxyquinidine alone and in combination with quinidine in healthy persons. Am J Cardiol 59:681, 1987.
70. Thompson KA, Blair A, Woosley RL, et al.: Comparative in vitro electrophysiology of quinidine, its major metabolites and dihydroxyquinidine. J Pharmacol Exp Ther 241:84, 1987.
71. Vozeh S, Oti-Amoako K, Uematsu T, et al.: Antiarrhythmic activity of two quinidine metabolites in experimental reperfusion arrhythmia: Relative potency and pharmacodynamic interaction with the parent drug. J Pharmacol Exp Ther 243:297, 1987.
72. Ochs HR, Greenblatt DJ, Woo E, et al.: Reduced quinidine clearance in elderly persons. Am J Cardiol 42:481, 1978.
73. Guentert TW, Upton RA, Holford NHG, et al.: Divergence in pharmacokinetic parameters of quinidine obtained by specific

and non-specific assay methods. J Pharmacokinet Biopharm 7:303, 1979.
74. Ochs HR, Greenblatt DJ, Woo E: Clinical pharmacokinetics of quinidine. Clin Pharmacokinet 5:150, 1980.
75. Garfinkel D, Mamelok RD, Blaschke TF: Altered therapeutic range for quinidine after myocardial infarction and cardiac surgery. Ann Intern Med 107:48, 1987.
76. Woo E, Greenblatt DJ: Pharmacokinetic and clinical implications of quinidine-protein binding. J Pharm Sci 68:466, 1979.
77. Levi GF, Proto C: Combined treatment of atrial fibrillation with quinidine and beta-blockers. Br Heart J 34:911, 1972.
78. Wu D, Hung J, Kuo C, et al.: Effects of quinidine on atrioventricular nodal reentrant paroxysmal tachycardia. Circulation 64:823, 1981.
79. Bloomfield SS, Romhilt DW, Chou T, et al.: Natural history of cardiac arrhythmias and their prevention with quinidine in patients with acute coronary insufficiency. Circulation 47:967, 1973.
80. Carliner NH, Crouthamel WG, Fisher ML, et al.: Quinidine therapy in hospitalized patients with ventricular arrhythmias. Am Heart J 98:708, 1979.
81. Belhassen B, Shapira I, Shoshani D, et al.: Idiopathic ventricular fibrillation: Inducibility and beneficial effects of class I antiarrhythmic agents. Circulation 75:809, 1987.
82. Mikus G, Ha HR, Vozeh S, et al. Pharmacokinetics and metabolism of quinidine in extensive and poor metabolizers of sparteine. Eur J Clin Pharmacol 31:69, 1986.
83. Brinn R, Brosen K, Gram LF, et al.: Sparteine oxidation is practically abolished in quinidine-treated patients. Br J Clin Pharmacol 22:194, 1986.
84. Inaba T, Tyndale RE, Mahon WA: Quinidine: Potent inhibition of sparteine and debrisoquine oxidation in vivo. Br J Clin Pharmacol 22:199, 1986.
85. Spiers CJ, Murray S, Boobis AR, et al.: Quinidine and the identification of drugs whose elimination is impaired in subjects classified as poor metabolizers of debrisoquine. Br J Clin Pharmacol 22:739, 1986.
86. Brosen K, Gram LF, Haghfelt T, et al.: Extensive metabolizers of debrisoquine become poor metabolizers during quinidine treatment. Pharmacol Toxicol 60:312, 1987.
87. Edwards DJ, Axelson JE, Visco JP, et al.: Lack of effect of smoking on the metabolism and pharmacokinetics of quinidine in patients. Br J Clin Pharmacol 23:351, 1987.
88. Doherty JE, Straub KD, Murphy ML, et al.: Digoxin-quinidine interaction. Changes in canine tissue concentration from steady state with quinidine. Am J Cardiol 45:1196, 1980.
89. Leahey EB, Reiffel JA, Drusin RE, et al.: Interactions between quinidine and digoxin. JAMA 240:533, 1978.
90. Hager WD, Fenster P, Mayersohn M, et al.: Digoxin-quinidine interaction: Pharmacokinetic evaluation. N Engl J Med 300:1238, 1979.
91. Angelin B, Arvidsson A, Dahlqvist R, et al.: Quinidine reduces biliary clearance of digoxin in man. Eur J Clin Invest 17:262, 1987.
92. Jaillon P: Antiarrhythmic drug interactions: Are they important? Eur Heart J 8 (Suppl A):127, 1987.
93. Kuhlman J: Effects of quinidine, verapamil and nifedipine on the pharmacokinetics and pharmacodynamics of digitoxin during steady state conditions. Arzneimittelforschung 37:545, 1987.
94. Edwards DJ, Lavoie R, Beckman H, et al.: The effect of coadministration of verapamil on the pharmacokinetics and metabolism of quinidine. Clin Pharmacol Ther 41:68, 1987.
95. Kornfield P, Horowitz SH, Genkins G, et al.: Myasthenia gravis unmasked by antiarrhythmic agents. Mt Sinai J Med 43:10, 1976.
96. Grogono AW: Anesthesia for atrial fibrillation: Effect of quinidine on muscle relaxation. Lancet 2:1039, 1963.
97. Udall JA: Drug interference with warfarin therapy. Clin Med 77:20, 1970.
98. Jelinek MV, Lehrbauer L, Lown B: Antiarrhythmic drug therapy for sporadic ventricular ectopic arrhythmias. Circulation 49:659, 1974.
99. Cohen IS, Jick H, Cohen SI: Adverse reactions to quinidine in hospitalized patients: Findings based on data from the Boston Collaborative Drug Surveillance Programs. Prog Cardiovasc Dis 20:151, 1977.
100. Roden DM, Woosley RL, Primm PK: Incidence and clinical features of the quinidine-associated long QT syndrome: Implications for patient care. Am Heart J 111:1088, 1986.
101. Jenzer HR, Hagemeijer F: Quinidine syncope: Torsade de pointes with low quinidine plasma concentration. Eur J Cardiol 4:447, 1976.
102. Tzivoni D, Keren A, Stern S: Torsades de pointes versus polymorphous ventricular tachycardia. Am J Cardiol 52:639, 1983.
103. Webb CL, Dick M, Rocchini AP, et al.: Quinidine syncope in children. J Am Coll Cardiol 9:1031, 1987.
104. Jackman WJ, Clark M, Friday KJ, et al.: Ventricular tachyarrhythmias in the long QT syndrome. Med Clin North Am 68:1079, 1984.
105. Elson J, Strong JM, Lee WK, et al.: Antiarrhythmic potency of N-acetylprocainamide. Clin Pharmacol Ther 17:134, 1975.
106. Jaillon P, Rubenson D, Peters F, et al.: Electrophysiologic effects of N-acetylprocainamide in human beings. Am J Cardiol 47:1134, 1981.
107. Jaillon P, Winkle RA: Electrophysiologic comparative study of procainamide and N-acetylprocainamide in anesthetized dogs: Concentration-response relationships. Circulation 60:1385, 1979.
108. Wellens HJJ, Durrer D: Effect of procainamide, quinidine and ajmaline in the Wolff-Parkinson-White syndrome. Circulation 50:114, 1974.
109. Rosen MR, Merker C, Gelband H, et al.: Effects of procaine amide on the electrophysiologic properties of the canine ventricular conduction system. J Pharmacol Exp Ther 185:438, 1973.
110. Arnsdorf MF, Bigger JT Jr.: The effect of procaine amide on components of excitability in long mammalian cardiac Purkinje fibers. Circ Res 38:115, 1976.
111. Lee WK, Strong JM, Kehoe RF, et al.: Antiarrhythmic efficacy of N-acetylprocainamide in patients with premature ventricular contractions. Clin Pharmacol Ther 19:508, 1976.
112. Winkle RA, Jaillon P, Kates RE, et al.: Clinical pharmacology and antiarrhythmic efficacy of N-acetylprocainamide. Am J Cardiol 47:123, 1981.
113. Williams JF Jr, Mathew B.: Effect of procainamide on myocardial contractile function and digoxin inotropy. J Am Coll Cardiol 4:1184, 1984.
114. Schmid PG, Nelson LD, Heistad DD, et al.: Vascular effects of procainamide in the dog: Predominance of the inhibitory effect on ganglionic transmission. Circ Res 35:948, 1974.
115. Miller RR, Hillard G, Lies JE, et al.: Hemodynamic effects of procainamide in patients with acute myocardial infarction and comparison with lidocaine. Am J Med 55:161, 1973.
116. McLendon RL, Hansen WR, Kinsman JM: Hemodynamic changes following procainamide administered intravenously. Am J Med Sci 222:375, 1951.
117. Jawad-Kanber G, Sherrod TR: Effect of loading dose of procaine amide on left ventricular performance in man. Chest 66:269, 1974.
118. Manion CV, Lalka D, Baer DT, et al.: Absorption kinetics of procainamide in humans. J Pharm Sci 66:981, 1977.
119. Giardina EGV, Dreyfuss J, Bigger JT Jr, et al.: Metabolism of procainamide in normal and cardiac subjects. Clin Pharmacol Ther 19:339, 1976.
120. Reidenberg MM, Drayer DE, Levy M, et al.: Polymorphic acetylation of procainamide in man. Clin Pharmacol Ther 17:722, 1975.
121. Karlsson E: Clinical pharmacokinetics of procainamide. Clin Pharmacokinet 3:97, 1978.
122. Koch-Weser J, Klein SW: Procainamide dosage schedules, plasma concentrations, and clinical effects. JAMA 215:1454, 1971.
123. Giardina EGV, Heissenbuttel RH, Bigger JT Jr.: Intermittent intravenous procainamide to treat ventricular arrhythmias. Correlation of plasma concentration with effect on arrhythmia, electrocardiogram and blood pressure. Ann Intern Med 78:183, 1973.
124. Lima JJ, Goldfarb AL, Conti DR, et al.: Safety and efficacy of procainamide infusions. Am J Cardiol 43:98, 1979.
125. Myerburg RJ, Kessler KM, Kiem I, et al.: Relationship between plasma levels of procainamide, suppression of premature

ventricular complexes and prevention of recurrent ventricular tachycardia. Circulation 64:280, 1981.
126. Funck-Brentano C, Jared LL, Roden DM, et al.: Interaction of procainamide and N-acetylprocainamide in man (Abstract). Circulation 76(Suppl 4):IV:520, 1987.
127. Roden DM, Reele SB, Higgins SB, et al.: Antiarrhythmic efficacy, pharmacokinetics and safety of N-acetylprocainamide in human subjects: Comparison with procainamide. Am J Cardiol 46:463, 1980.
128. Kluger J, Drayer D, Reidenberg M, et al.: The clinical pharmacology and antiarrhythmic efficacy of acetylprocainamide in patients with arrhythmias. Am J Cardiol 45:1250, 1980.
129. Christian CD Jr, Meredith CG, Speeg KV Jr.: Cimetidine inhibits renal procainamide clearance. Clin Pharmacol Ther 36:221, 1984.
130. Somogyi A, Bochner F: Dose and concentration dependent effect of ranitidine on procainamide disposition and renal clearance in man. Br J Clin Pharmacol 18:175, 1988.
131. Davies DM, Beedie MA, Rawlins MD: Antinuclear antibodies during procainamide treatment and drug acetylation. Br Med J 3:682, 1975.
132. Blomgren SE, Condemi JJ, Vaughan JH: Procainamide-induced lupus erythematosus—clinical and laboratory observations. Am J Med 52:338, 1972.
133. Woosley RL, Drayer DE, Reidenberg MM, et al.: Effect of acetylator phenotype on the rate at which procainamide induces antinuclear antibodies and the lupus syndrome. N Engl J Med 298:1157, 1978.
134. Berger BE, Hauser DJ: Agranulocytosis due to new sustained-release procainamide. Am Heart J 105:1035, 1983.
135. Wyse DG, McAnulty JH, Rahimtoola SH: Influence of plasma drug level and the presence of conduction disease on the electrophysiologic effects of procainamide. Am J Cardiol 43:619, 1979.
136. Olshansky B, Martins J, Hunt S: N-acetylprocainamide causing torsades de pointes. Am J Cardiol 50:1439, 1982.
137. Danilo P Jr, Hordof AJ, Rosen MR: Effects of disopyramide on electrophysiologic properties of canine cardiac Purkinje fibers. J Pharmacol Exp Ther 201:701, 1977.
138. Mirro MJ, Watanabe AM, Bailey JC: Electrophysiological effects of disopyramide and quinidine on guinea pig atria and canine Purkinje fibers. Circ Res 46:660, 1980.
139. Befeler B, Castellanos A, Wells DE, et al.: Electrophysiologic effects of the antiarrhythmic agent disopyramide phosphate. Am J Cardiol 35:282, 1975.
140. Kus T, Sasyniuk BI: Electrophysiological actions of disopyramide phosphate on canine ventricular muscle and Purkinje fibers. Circ Res 37:844, 1975.
141. Levites R, Anderson GJ: Electrophysiological effects of disopyramide phosphate during experimental myocardial ischemia. Am Heart J 98:339, 1979.
142. Birkhead JS, Vaughan Williams EM: Dual effects of disopyramide on atrial and atrioventricular conduction and refractory periods. Br Heart J 39:657, 1977.
143. Josephson ME, Caracta AR, Lau SH, et al.: Electrophysiological evaluation of disopyramide in man. Am Heart J 86:771, 1973.
144. LaBarre A, Strauss HC, Scheinman MM, et al.: Electrophysiologic effects of disopyramide phosphate on sinus node function in patients with sinus node dysfunction. Circulation 59:226, 1979.
145. Burke TR, Nelson WL, Mangion M, et al.: Resolution, absolute configuration and antiarrhythmic properties of enantiomers of disopyramide. J Med Chem 23:1044, 1980.
146. Giacomini KM, Cox BM, Blaschke TF: Comparative anticholinergic potencies of R- and S-disopyramide in longitudinal muscle strips from guinea pig ileum. Life Sci 27:1191, 1980.
147. Kidwell GA, Schaal SF, Muir WW III: Stereospecific effects of disopyramide enantiomers following pretreatment of canine cardiac Purkinje fibers with verapamil and nisoldipine. J Cardiovasc Pharmacol 9:276, 1987.
148. Dubray C, Boucher M, Paire M, et al.: Comparative effects of disopyramide and its mono-N-dealkylated metabolite in conscious dogs with chronic atrioventricular block: Plasma concentration-response relationships. J Cardiovasc Pharmacol 8:1229, 1986.
149. Silke B, Frais MA, Verma SP, et al.: Comparative hemodynamic effects of intravenous lignocaine, disopyramide, and flecainide in uncomplicated acute myocardial infarction. Br J Clin Pharmacol 22:707, 1986.
150. Ronnevik PK, Gundersen T, Abrahamsen AM: Tolerability and antiarrhythmic efficacy of disopyramide compared to lignocaine in selected patients with suspected acute myocardial infarction. Eur Heart J 8:19, 1987.
151. Podrid PJ, Schoenberger A, Lown B: Congestive heart failure caused by oral disopyramide. N Engl J Med 302:614, 1980.
152. Kotler V, Lindererer T, Schroder R: Effects of disopyramide on systemic and coronary hemodynamics and myocardial metabolism in patients with coronary artery disease: Comparison with lidocaine. Am Heart J 46:469, 1980.
153. Lima JJ, Boudoulas H: Stereoselective effects of disopyramide enantiomers in humans. J Cardiovasc Pharmacol 9:594, 1987.
154. Dubetz DK, Brown NN, Hooper WD, et al.: Disopyramide pharmacokinetics and bioavailability. Br J Clin Pharmacol 6:279, 1978.
155. Hinderling PH, Garrett ER: Pharmacokinetics of the antiarrhythmic disopyramide in healthy humans. J Pharmacokinet Biopharm 4:199, 1976.
156. Hinderling PH, Garrett ER: Pharmacodynamics of the antiarrhythmic disopyramide in healthy humans. J Pharmacokinet Biopharm 4:231, 1976.
157. Meffin P, Robert EW, Winkle RA, et al.: Role of concentration dependent plasma protein binding in disopyramide disposition. J Pharmacokinet Biopharm 7:29, 1979.
158. Lima JJ, Boudoulas H, Blanford MF: Concentration dependence of disopyramide binding to serum protein and its influence on kinetics and dynamics. J Pharmacol Exp Ther 219:741, 1981.
159. Haughey DB, Lima JJ: Influence of concentration dependent protein binding on serum concentrations and urinary excretion of disopyramide and its metabolite following oral administration. Biopharm Drug Dispos 4:103, 1983.
160. Bredeson JE, Kierulf P: Relationship between alpha 1-acid glycoprotein and distribution of disopyramide and mono-N-dealkyldisopyramide in whole blood. Br J Clin Pharmacol 22:281, 1986.
161. Upton RA, Williams RL: The impact of neglecting nonlinear plasma-protein binding on disopyramide bioavailability studies. J Pharmacokinet Biopharm 14:365, 1986.
162. Giacomini KM, Nelson WL, Pershe RA, et al.: In vivo interaction of the enantiomers of disopyramide in human subjects. J Pharmacokinet Biopharm 14:335, 1986.
163. Johnston A, Henry JA, Warrington SJ, et al.: Pharmacokinetics of oral disopyramide phosphate in patients with renal impairment. Br J Clin Pharmacol 10:245, 1980.
164. Bonde J, Gradual NA, Pedersen LE, et al.: Kinetics of disopyramide in decreased hepatic function. Eur J Clin Pharmacol 31:73, 1986.
165. Pedersen LE, Bonde J, Graudal NA: Quantitative and qualitative binding characteristics of disopyramide in serum from patients with decreased renal and hepatic function. Br J Clin Pharmacol 23:41, 1987.
166. Ribeiro C, Longo A: Procainamide and disopyramide. Eur Heart J 8(Suppl A):11, 1987.
167. Willis PW III: The clinical scope of disopyramide seven years after introduction—an overview. Angiology 38:165, 1987.
168. Kessler JM, Keys PW, Stattford RW: Disopyramide and phenytoin interaction. J Clin Pharmacol 1:263, 1982.
169. Aitio M, Mansury L, Tala E, et al.: The effect of enzyme-induction on the metabolism of disopyramide in man. Br J Clin Pharmacol 11:297, 1981.
170. Risler T, Burk M, Peters U, et al.: On the interaction between digoxin and disopyramide. Clin Pharmacol Ther 34:176, 1983.
171. Sylvan C, Anderson P: Evidence that disopyramide does not interact with warfarin. Br Med J 286:1181, 1983.
172. Morady F, Sacheinman MM, Desai J: Disopyramide. Ann Intern Med 96:339, 1982.
173. Teichman SL, Ferrick A, Kim SG, et al.: Disopyramide-pyridostigmine interaction: Selective reversal of anticholinergic symptoms with preservation of antiarrhythmic effect. J Am Coll Cardiol 10:633, 1987.
174. Hondeghem L, Katzung BG: Test of a model of antiarrhythmic drug action: effects of quinidine and lidocaine on myocardial conduction. Circulation 61:1217, 1980.

175. Woosley RL, Wang T, Stone W, et al.: Pharmacology, electrophysiology, and pharmacokinetics of mexiletine. Am Heart J 107:1058, 1984.
176. Campbell TJ: Kinetics of onset of rate-dependent effects of class I antiarrhythmic drugs are important in determining their effects on refractoriness in guinea-pig ventricle, and provide a theoretical basis for their subclassification. Cardiovasc Res 17:344, 1983.
177. Bigger JT Jr, Mandel WT: Effect of lidocaine on transmembrane potentials of ventricular muscle and Purkinje fibers. J Clin Invest 49:63, 1970.
178. Imanishi S, McAllister RG Jr, Surawicz B: The effects of verapamil and lidocaine on the automatic depolarization in guinea-pig ventricular myocardium. J Pharmacol Exp Ther 207:294, 1978.
179. Mandel WJ, Bigger JT Jr: Electrophysiologic effects of lidocaine on isolated canine and rabbit atrial tissues. J Pharmacol Exp Ther 178:81, 1971.
180. Rosen KM, Lau SH, Weiss MB, et al.: The effect of lidocaine on atrioventricular and intraventricular conduction in man. Am J Cardiol 25:1, 1970.
181. Lippestad CT, Forgang K: Production of sinus arrest by lignocaine. Br Med J 1:537, 1971.
182. Gupta PK, Lichstein E, Chadda KD: Lidocaine-induced heart block in patients with bundle branch block. Am J Cardiol 33:487, 1974.
183. Davis LD, Temte JV: Electrophysiological actions of lidocaine on canine ventricular muscle and Purkinje fibers. Circ Res 24:639, 1969.
184. Roden DM, Woosley RL: Tocainide. N Engl J Med 315:41, 1986.
185. Block AJ, Merrill D, Smith ER: Stereoselectivity of tocainide pharmacodynamics in vivo and in vitro. J Cardiovasc Pharmacol 11:216, 1988.
186. Shanks RG: Hemodynamic effects of mexiletine. Am Heart J 107:1065, 1984.
187. Boyes RN, Scott DB, Jebson PJ, et al.: Pharmacokinetics of lidocaine in man. Clin Pharmacol Ther 12:105, 1971.
188. Nies AS, Shand DG, Wilkinson GR: Altered hepatic blood flow and drug disposition. Clin Pharmacokinet 1:135, 1976.
189. Burney RG, DiFazio GA, Peach MJ, et al.: Antiarrhythmic effects of lidocaine metabolites. Am Heart J 88:765, 1974.
190. Riddell JG, Mc Allister CB, Wilkinson GR, et al.: A new method for constant plasma drug concentrations: Application to lidocaine. Ann Intern Med 100:25, 1984.
191. Stargel WW, Shand DG, Routledge PA, et al.: Clinical comparison of rapid infusion and multiple injection methods for lidocaine loading. Am Heart J 102:872, 1981.
192. Routledge PA, Stargel WW, Wagner GS, et al.: Increased alpha$_1$-acid glycoprotein and lidocaine disposition in myocardial infarction. Ann Intern Med 93:701, 1980.
193. Koster RW, Dunning AJ: Intramuscular lidocaine for prevention of lethal arrhythmias in the prehospitalization phase of acute myocardial infarction. N Engl J Med 313:1105, 1985.
194. Campbell RWF: Mexiletine. N Engl J Med 316:29, 1987.
195. Impact Research Group. International mexiletine and placebo antiarrhythmic coronary trial. I: Report on arrhythmia and other findings. J Am Coll Cardiol 4:1148, 1984.
196. Klein AL, Sami MH: Usefulness and safety of cimetidine in patients receiving mexiletine for ventricular arrhythmia. Am Heart J 109:1281, 1985.
197. Creamer JE, Nathan AW, Camm AJ: The proarrhythmic effects of antiarrhythmic drugs. Am Heart J 114:397, 1987.
198. Ikeda N, Singh BN, Davis LD, et al.: Effects of flecainide on the electrophysiologic properties of isolated canine and rabbit myocardial fibers. J Am Coll Cardiol 5:303, 1985.
199. Roden DM, Woosley RL: Flecainide. N Engl J Med 315:36, 1986.
200. Estes NAM III, Garan H, Ruskin JN: Electrophysiological properties of flecainide acetate. Am J Cardiol 53:26B, 1984.
201. Vik-Mo H, Ohm OJ, Lund-Johansen P: Electrophysiological effects of flecainide acetate in patients with sinus nodal dysfunction. Am J Cardiol 50:1090, 1982.
202. Hellestrand KJ, Nathan AW, Bexton RS, et al.: Electrophysiologic effects of flecainide acetate on sinus node function, anomalous atrioventricular connections and pacemaker thresholds. Am J Cardiol 53:30B, 1984.
203. De Paola AAV, Horowitz LN, Morganroth J, et al.: Influence of left ventricular dysfunction on flecainide therapy. J Am Coll Cardiol 9:163, 1987.
204. Conard GJ, Ober RE: Metabolism of flecainide. Am J Cardiol 53:41B, 1984.
205. Winkelman BR, Leinberger H: Life-threatening flecainide toxicity. Ann Intern Med 106:807, 1987.
206. Salerno DM, Granrud G, Sharkey P: Pharmacodynamics and side effects of flecainide acetate. Clin Pharmacol Ther 40:101, 1986.
207. Flecainide-Quinidine Research Group. Flecainide versus quinidine for treatment of ventricular arrhythmias: A multicenter clinical trial. Circulation 67:1117, 1983.
208. Hellestrand KJ, Nathan AW, Bexton RS, et al.: Cardiac electrophysiologic effects of flecainide acetate for paroxysmal reentrant junctional tachycardias. Am J Cardiol 51:770, 1983.
209. Tjandra Maga TB, van Hecken A, van Melle P, et al.: Altered pharmacokinetics of oral flecainide by cimetidine. Br J Clin Pharmacol 22:108, 1986.
210. Weeks CE, Conard GJ, Kvam DC, et al.: The effect of flecainide acetate, a new antiarrhythmic, on plasma digoxin levels. J Clin Pharmacol 26:27, 1986.
211. Lewis GP, Holtzman JL: Interaction of flecainide with digoxin and propranolol. Am J Cardiol 53:52B, 1984.
212. Chouty F, Funck-Brentano C, Landau JM, et al.: Efficacité de fortes doses de lactate molaire par voie veineuse lors des intoxications au flecainide. Presse Med 16:808, 1987.
213. Carmeliet E: Electrophysiologic effects of encainide in isolated cardiac muscle and Purkinje fibers and on the Langendorff perfused guinea pig heart. Eur J Pharmacol 61:247, 1980.
214. Davy J-M, Dorian P, Kantelip J-P, et al.: Qualitative and quantitative comparison of the cardiac effects of encainide and its three major metabolites in the dog. J Pharmacol Exp Ther 237:907, 1986.
215. Barbey JT, Thompson KA, Echt DS, et al.: Antiarrhythmic activity, electrocardiographic effects and pharmacokinetics of the encainide metabolites O-desmethyl encainide and 3-methoxy-O-desmethyl encainide in man. Circulation, 77:380, 1988.
216. Gomoll AW, Byrne JE, Antonaccio MJ: Electrophysiology, hemodynamic and arrhythmia efficacy model studies on encainide. Am J Cardiol 58:10C, 1986.
217. Carey EL, Duff HJ, Roden DM, et al.: Encainide and its metabolites. Comparative effects in man on ventricular arrhythmia and electrocardiographic intervals. J Clin Invest 73:539, 1984.
218. Fain ES, Dorian P, Davy J-M, et al.: Effects of encainide and its metabolites on energy requirements for defibrillation. Circulation 73:1334, 1986.
219. Somberg JC, Zanger D, Levine E, et al.: Encainide: A new and potent antiarrhythmic. Am Heart J 114:826, 1987.
220. Wang T, Roden DM, Wolfenden HT, et al.: Influence of genetic polymorphism on the metabolites and disposition of encainide in man. J Pharmacol Exp Ther 228:605, 1984.
221. Hohnloser SH, Meinertz T, Geibel A, et al.: BID versus TID administered encainide for complex ventricular arrhythmia (Abstract). Circulation 76(Suppl 4):IV-368, 1987.
222. Antonaccio MJ, Verjee S: Dosing recommendations for encainide. Am J Cardiol 58:114C, 1986.
223. Bergstrand RH, Wang T, Roden DM, et al.: Encainide disposition in patients with renal failure. Clin Pharmacol Ther 40:64, 1986.
224. Bergstrand RH, Wang T, Roden DM, et al.: Encainide disposition in patients with chronic cirrhosis. Clin Pharmacol Ther 40:148, 1986.
225. Morganroth J: Encainide for ventricular arrhythmias: Placebo-controlled and standard comparison trials. Am J Cardiol 58:74C, 1986.
226. Quart BD, Gallo DG, Sami MH, et al.: Drug interaction studies and encainide use in renal and hepatic impairment. Am J Cardiol 58:104C, 1986.
227. Tjordman T, Podrid PJ, Raeder E, et al.: Safety and efficacy of encainide for malignant ventricular arrhythmias. Am J Cardiol 58:87C, 1986.
228. Bajaj A, Woosley RL, Roden DM: Acute reversal of O-desmethyl encainide induced conduction slowing (Abstract). J Am Coll Cardiol 7(Suppl):82A, 1986.

229. von Philipsborn G, Gries J, Hofmann HP, et al.: Pharmacological studies on propafenone and its main metabolite 5-hydroxypropafenone. Arzneimittelforschung 34:1489, 1984.
230. Valenzuela C, Delgardo C, Tamargo J: Electrophysiological effects of 5-hydroxypropafenone on guinea pig ventricular muscle fibers. J Cardiovasc Pharmacol 10:523, 1987.
231. Katoh T, Karaguezian HS, Sugi K: Effects of propafenone on sinus nodal and ventricular automaticity: In vitro and in vivo correlation. Am Heart J 113:941, 1987.
232. Connolly SJ, Kates RE, Lebsack CS, et al.: Clinical pharmacology of propafenone. Circulation 68:589, 1983.
233. Baker BJ, Dinh HA, Kroskey D, et al.: Effect of propafenone on left ventricular ejection fraction. Am J Cardiol 54:20D, 1984.
234. Siddoway LA, Roden DM, Woosley RL: Clinical pharmacology of propafenone: Pharmacokinetics, metabolism and concentration-response relations. Am J Cardiol 54:9D, 1984.
235. Siddoway LA, Thompson KA, McAllister CB, et al.: Polymorphism of propafenone metabolism and disposition in man: Clinical and pharmacokinetic consequences. Circulation 75:785, 1987.
236. Harron DWG,, Brogden RN: Propafenone. A review of its pharmacodynamic and pharmacokinetic properties, and therapeutic use in treatment of arrhythmias. Drugs 34:617, 1988.
237. Chilson DA, Heger JJ, Zipes DP, et al.: Electrophysiologic effects and clinical efficacy of oral propafenone therapy in patients with ventricular tachycardia. J Am Coll Cardiol 5:1407, 1985.
238. Connolly SJ, Mulji AS, Hoffert DL, et al.: Randomized placebo-controlled trial of propafenone for treatment of atrial tachyarrhythmias after cardiac surgery. J Am Coll Cardiol 10:1145, 1987.
239. Breithardt G, Borggrefe M, Wiebringhaus E, et al.: Effect of propafenone in the Wolff-Parkinson-White syndrome: Electrophysiologic findings and long-term follow-up. Am J Cardiol 54:29D, 1984.
240. Axelson JE, Chan GLY, Kirsten EB, et al.: Food increases the bioavailability of propafenone. Br J Clin Pharmacol 23:735, 1987.
241. Cheriex EC, Krijne R, Brugada P, et al.: Lack of clinically significant beta-blocking effect of propafenone. Eur Heart J 8:54, 1987.
242. Hill MR, Gotz VP, Harman E, et al.: Evaluation of the asthmogenicity of propafenone, a new antiarrhythmic drug. Comparison of spirometry with metacholine challenge. Chest 90:698, 1986.
243. Mason JW. Amiodarone. N Engl J Med 316:455, 1987.
244. Mason JW, Hondeghem LM, Katzung BG: Amiodarone blocks inactivated cardiac sodium channels. Pflugers Arch 396:79, 1983.
245. Talajic M, DeRoode MR, Nattel S: Comparative electrophysiologic effects of intravenous amiodarone and desmethylamiodarone in dogs: Evidence for clinically relevant activity of the metabolite. Circulation 75:265, 1987.
246. Albert SG, Alves LE, Rose EP: Thyroid dysfunction during chronic amiodarone therapy. J Am Coll Cardiol 9:175, 1987.
247. Singh BN, Nademanee K: Amiodarone and thyroid function: Clinical implications during antiarrhythmic therapy. Am Heart J 106:857, 1983.
248. Latham KR, Sellitti DF, Goldstein RE: Interaction of amiodarone and desethylamiodarone with solubilized nuclear thyroid hormone receptors. J Am Coll Cardiol 9:872, 1987.
249. Charlier R, Deltour G, Baudine A, et al.: Pharmacology of amiodarone, an anti-anginal drug with a new biological profile. Arzneimittelforschung 18:1408, 1968.
250. Cohen-Armon M, Schreiber G, Sokolovsky M: Interaction of the antiarrhythmic drug amiodarone with the muscarinic receptor in rat heart and brain. J Cardiovasc Pharmacol 6:1148, 1984.
251. Pourbaix S, Berger Y, Desager J-P, et al.: Absolute bioavailability of amiodarone in normal subjects. Clin Pharmacol Ther 37:118, 1985.
252. Adams PC, Holt DW, Storey GC, et al.: Amiodarone and its desethyl metabolite: Tissue distribution and morphologic changes during long-term therapy. Circulation 72:1064, 1985.
253. Nattel S, Davies M, Quantz M: The antiarrhythmic efficacy of amiodarone and desethylamiodarone, alone and in combination, in dogs with acute myocardial infarction. Circulation 77:200, 1988.
254. Holt DW, Tucker GT, Jackson PR, McKenna WJ. Amiodarone pharmacokinetics. Br J Clin Pract (Symp Suppl)44:109, 1986.
255. Plomp TA, van Rossum JM, Robles de Medina EO, et al.: Pharmacokinetics and body distribution of amiodarone in man. Arzneimittelforschung 34:513, 1984.
256. Siddoway LA, McAllister CB, Wilkinson GR, et al.: Amiodarone dosing: a proposal based on its pharmacokinetics. Am Heart J 106:951, 1983.
257. Escoubet B, Coumel P, Poirier J-M, et al.: Suppression of arrhythmias within hours after a single oral dose of amiodarone and relation to plasma and myocardial concentrations. Am J Cardiol 55:696, 1985.
258. Mostow ND, Vrobel TR, Noon D, et al.: Rapid suppression of complex ventricular arrhythmias with high-dose oral amiodarone. Circulation 73:1231, 1986.
259. Greenberg ML, Lerman BB, Shipe JR, et al.: Relation between amiodarone and desethylamiodarone plasma concentrations and electrophysiological effects, efficacy and toxicity. J Am Coll Cardiol 9:1148, 1987.
260. Graboys TB, Podrid PJ, Lown B: Efficacy of amiodarone for refractory supraventricular tachyarrhythmias. Am Heart J 106:870, 1983.
261. Gold RL, Haffajee CI, Charos G, et al.: Amiodarone for refractory atrial fibrillation. Am J Cardiol 57:124, 1986.
262. Horowitz LN, Spielman SR, Greenspan AM, et al.: Use of amiodarone in the treatment of persistent and paroxysmal atrial fibrillation resistant to quinidine therapy. J Am Coll Cardiol 6:1402, 1985.
263. Larrey D, Tinel M, Letteron P, et al.: Formation of an inactive cytochrome P:450 Fe(II)-metabolite complex after administration of amiodarone in rats, mice and hamsters. Biochem Pharmacol 35:2213, 1986.
264. Almog S, Shafran N, Halkin H, et al.: Mechanism of warfarin potentiation by amiodarone: dose- and concentration-dependent inhibition of warfarin elimination. Eur J Clin Pharmacol 28:257, 1985.
265. Marcus FI: Drug interactions with amiodarone. Am Heart J 106:924, 1983.
266. Fenster PE, White NW Jr, Hanson CD: Pharmacokinetic evaluation of the digoxin-amiodarone interaction. J Am Coll Cardiol 5:108, 1985.
267. Coumel P, Fidelle J: Amiodarone in the treatment of cardiac arrhythmias in children: one hundred thirty-five cases. Am Heart J 100:1063, 1980.
268. Mason JW, The Amiodarone Toxicity Study Group. Toxicity of amiodarone (Abstract). Circulation 72(Suppl 3):III:272, 1985.
269. Veltri EP, Reid PR: Amiodarone pulmonary toxicity: Early changes in pulmonary function tests during amiodarone rechallenge. J Am Coll Cardiol 6:802, 1985.
270. Orlando RG, Dangel ME, Schaal SF: Clinical experience and grading of amiodarone keratopathy. Ophthalmology 91:1184, 1984.
271. Zachary CB, Slater DN, Holt DW, et al.: The pathogenesis of amiodarone-induced pigmentation and photosensitivity. Br J Dermatol 110:451, 1984.
272. Simon JB, Manley PN, Brien JF: Amiodarone hepatotoxicity simulating alcoholic liver disease. N Engl J Med 311:167, 1984.
273. Rigas B, Rosenfeld LE, Barwick KW, et al.: Amiodarone hepatotoxicity: A clinicopathologic study of five patients. Ann Intern Med 104:348, 1986.
274. Bacaner MB: Treatment of ventricular fibrillation and other acute arrhythmias with bretylium tosylate. Am J Cardiol 21:530, 1968.
275. Bigger JT Jr, Jaffee CC: The effect of bretylium tosylate on the electrophysiologic properties of ventricular muscle and Purkinje fibers. Am J Cardiol 27:82, 1971.
276. Cardinale R, Sasyniuk BI: Electrophysiological effects of bretylium tosylate on subendocardial Purkinje fibers from infarcted canine hearts. J Pharmacol Exp Ther 204:159, 1978.
277. Nishimura M, Watanabe Y: Membrane action and catecholamine release action of bretylium tosylate in normoxic and hypoxic canine Purkinje fibers. J Am Coll Cardiol 2:287, 1983.

278. Anderson JL, Brodine WN, Patterson E, et al.: Serial electrophysiologic effects of bretylium in man and their correlation with plasma concentration. J Cardiovasc Pharmacol 4:871, 1982.
279. Duff HJ, Roden DM, Yacobi A, et al.: Bretylium: Relations between plasma concentrations and pharmacologic actions in high-frequency ventricular arrhythmias. Am J Cardiol 55:395, 1985.
280. Woosley RL, Reele SB, Roden DM, et al.: Pharmacologic reversal of hypotensive effect complicating antiarrhythmic therapy with bretylium. Clin Pharmacol Ther 32:313, 1982.
281. Narang PK, Adir J, Josselson J, et al.: Pharmacokinetics of bretylium in man after intravenous administration. J Pharmacokinet Biopharm 8:363, 1980.
282. Chow MSS, Kluger J, DiPersio DM, et al.: Antifibrillatory effects of lidocaine and bretylium immediately postcardiopulmonary resuscitation. Am Heart J 110:938, 1985.
283. Yusef S, Peto R, Lewis J, et al.: Beta blockade during and after myocardial infarction: An overview of the randomized trials. Prog Cardiovasc Dis 27:335, 1985.
284. Duff HJ, Mitchell LB, Wyse DG: Antiarrhythmic efficacy of propranolol: Comparison of low and high serum concentrations. J Am Coll Cardiol 8:959, 1986.
285. Pratt CM, Yepson SC, Bloom MGK, et al.: Evaluation of metoprolol in suppressing complex ventricular arrhythmias. Am J Cardiol 52:73, 1983.
286. Von Der Lippe G, Lund-Johansen P, Kjekshus J: Effect of timolol on late ventricular arrhythmias after acute myocardial infarction. Acta Med Scand 651(Suppl):256, 1981.
287. deSoyza N, Shapiro W, Chandraratna PAN, et al.: Acebutolol therapy for ventricular arrhythmia. Circulation 65:1129, 1982.
288. Podrid PJ, Lown B: Pindolol for ventricular arrhythmia. Am Heart J 104:491, 1982.
289. Nademanee K, Schleman NM, Singh BN, et al.: Beta-adrenergic blockade by nadolol in control of ventricular tachyarrhythmias. Am Heart J 108:1109, 1984.
290. Fenster PE, Reynolds D, Horowitz LD, et al.: Atenolol for ventricular ectopy: A dose-response study. Clin Pharmacol Ther 41:118, 1987.
291. Coumel P, Leclercq JF, Escoubet B: Beta-blockers: Use for arrhythmias. Eur Heart J 8(Suppl A):41, 1987.
292. Thompson KA, Roden DM, Wood AJJ, et al.: Suppression of ventricular arrhythmias by dextro-propranolol in man independent of beta-adrenergic receptor blockade. Submitted.
293. Drayer DE: Pharmacodynamic and pharmacokinetic differences between drug enantiomers in humans: An overview. Clin Pharmacol Ther 40:125, 1986.
294. Singh BN: Sotalol: A beta-blocker with unique antiarrhythmic effects. Am Heart J 114:121, 1987.
295. Riddell JG, Harron DWG, Shanks RG: Clinical pharmacokinetics of beta-adrenoceptor antagonists: An update. Clin Pharmacokinet 12:305, 1987.
296. Tonet JL, Cazaux P, Chevalier B: Efficacy of low dose of beta-blocker agents combined with amiodarone in refractory ventricular tachycardia. Circulation 76(Suppl IV):IV-367, 1987.
297. Rowland E, Antiarrhythmic drugs—class IV. Eur Heart J 8(Suppl A):61, 1987.
298. Singh BN, Nademanee K, Baky S: Calcium antagonists. Clinical use in the treatment of arrhythmias. Drugs 25:125, 1983.
299. Ward DE, Nathan AW, Camm AJ: Fascicular tachycardia sensitive to calcium antagonists. Eur Heart J 5:896, 1984.
300. Sperelakis N: Electrophysiology of calcium antagonists. J Mol Cell Cardiol 19(Suppl 2):19, 1987.
301. Echizen H, Eichelbaum M: Clinical pharmacokinetics of verapamil, nifedipine and diltiazem. Clin Pharmacokinet 11:425, 1986.
302. Anderson JL, Anastasiou Nana MI, Heath BM, et al.: Efficacy of recainam, a new antiarrhythmic drug, for control of ventricular arrhythmias. Am J Cardiol 60:281, 1987.
303. Singh SN, DiBianco R, Gottdiener JS, et al.: Effect of moricizine-hydrochloride in reducing chronic high-frequency ventricular arrhythmia: Results of a prospective, controlled trial. Am J Cardiol 53:745, 1984.
304. Anderson JL, Lutz JR, Nappi JM: Pirmenol for control of ventricular arrhythmias: Oral dose-ranging and short-term maintenance study. Am J Cardiol 53:522, 1984.
305. Staigor C, Jauernig R, DeVris, et al.: Influence of amiodarone on antipyrine pharmacokinetics in three patients with ventricular tachycardia. Br J Clin Pharmacol 18:263, 1984.
306. Hughes B, Dyer JE, Schwartz AB: Increased procainamide plasma concentrations caused by quinidine: A new drug interaction. Am Heart J 114:908, 1987.
307. Ross DL, Sze DY, Keefe DL, et al.: Antiarrhythmic drug combinations in the treatment of ventricular tachycardia. Circulation 66:1205, 1982.
308. Duffy CE, Swiryn S, Bauernfeind RA, et al.: Inducible sustained ventricular tachycardia refractory to individual class I drugs: Effects of adding a second class I drug. Am Heart J 106:450, 1983.
309. Duff HJ, Roden D, Primm RK, et al.: Mexiletine in the treatment of resistant ventricular arrhythmias: Enhancement of efficacy and reduction of dose-related side effects by combination with quinidine. Circulation 67:1124, 1983.
310. Kim SG, Mercando AD, Fisher JD: Combination of tocainide and quinidine for better tolerance and additive effects in patients with coronary artery disease. J Am Coll Cardiol 9:1369, 1987.
311. Marchlinski FE, Buxton AE, Miller JM, et al.: Amiodarone versus amiodarone and a type IA agent for treatment of patients with rapid ventricular tachycardia. Circulation 74:1037, 1986.
312. Windle J, Prystowsky EN, Miles WM, et al.: Pharmacokinetic and electrophysiologic interactions of amiodarone and procainamide. Clin Pharmacol Ther 41:603, 1987.
313. Kim SG, Mercando AD, Fisher JD: Combination of disopyramide and mexiletine for additive efficacy for ventricular arrhythmias without additive side effects (Abstract). Circulation 76(Suppl IV):IV-512, 1987.
314. Lineberry MD, Davies RF, Chaffin PL, et al.: Safety and efficacy of combining encainide and lidocaine (Abstract). Circulation 76(Suppl 4):IV-511, 1987.
315. Klein RC, Huang SK, Marcus FI, et al.: Enhanced antiarrhythmic efficacy of propafenone when used in combination with procainamide or quinidine. Am Heart J 114:551, 1987.
316. Woosley RL, Roden DM: Basic principles of clinical pharmacology. In Parmley WW, Chatterjee K (eds.): Cardiology. Philadelphia, J.B. Lippincott, 1988, Chapter 15, pp. 1–19.
317. Sami MH, Derbekyan VA, Lisbona R: Hemodynamic effects of encainide in patients with ventricular arrhythmia and poor ventricular function. Am J Cardiol 52:507, 1983.
318. Riva E, Gerna M, Neyroz P, et al.: Pharmacokinetics of amiodarone in rats. J Cardiovasc Pharmacol 4:270, 1982.
319. The CAST investigators, Preliminary report: Effect of encainide and flecainide on mortality in a randomized trial of arrhythmia suppression and myocardial infarction. N Engl J Med 321:406–412, 1989.

24

Surgical Management of Cardiac Arrhythmias

James L. Cox

Recently, surgical techniques have been devised for the treatment of most types of supraventricular tachyarrhythmias and for both nonischemic and ischemic ventricular tachyarrhythmias. The development of these surgical techniques has paralleled the evolution of our understanding of cardiac arrhythmias and the availability of more sophisticated methods for their electrophysiologic evaluation. In some cases, these arrhythmias can be treated by electrical devices such as antitachycardia pacemakers, internal cardioverters, and automatic internal defibrillators. The implantation of these devices represents a surgical procedure designed to *terminate* the arrhythmias once they have developed rather than to *ablate* arrhythmogenic substrates responsible for the arrhythmias. This chapter will not address the role of these electrical devices in the management of cardiac arrhythmias but rather will be confined to a discussion of direct surgical techniques employed to either ablate or isolate arrhythmogenic myocardium in the atria and ventricles.

Supraventricular Tachyarrhythmias

WOLFF-PARKINSON-WHITE (WPW) SYNDROME

Indications for Surgery

The major indication for surgical intervention in the WPW syndrome is medical refractoriness. Other common surgical indications include patient intolerance to drug therapy, detrimental side effects of antiarrhythmic agents, and poor patient compliance. Major additions to these surgical indications include (1) recurrent supraventricular tachycardia in young, otherwise healthy patients and (2) spontaneous atrial fibrillation that conducts rapidly enough antegrade to allow the induction of ventricular fibrillation from the atrium.

Preoperative Electrophysiologic Evaluation

All patients who are to be subjected to surgery for the WPW syndrome should first undergo an endocardial catheter electrophysiologic study. The purposes of the preoperative electrophysiological study are (1) to document that the arrhythmia is supraventricular in origin, (2) to evaluate the response of the supraventricular tachycardia to programmed electrical stimulation (PES) to determine if it is reentrant or automatic in nature, (3) to establish the conduction properties of the normal specialized conduction tissue, (4) to document that the etiology of the arrhythmia is on the basis of the WPW syndrome rather than other types of supraventricular tachyarrhythmias, and (5) to define the location of the accessory atrioventricular connection responsible for the WPW syndrome.

Intraoperative Electrophysiologic Mapping

The intraoperative mapping system currently used in our operating theater was developed and reported by Witkowski and Corr in 1984.[1] The system is presently capable of recording 160 bipolar electrograms simultaneously, analyzing the data, and displaying it in various forms within 2 minutes after data acquisition. Analog data recorded from the heart enter the front-end system located in the operating theater, where each electrogram is individually filtered and digitized. The digitized data are then transferred across a fiber-optic cable to a remote computer facility located approximately 1500 meters away. The personnel in the operating theater and those in the computer facility are connected by both an audio system (headphones) and a video camera and display system for constant communication during the mapping procedure. Only 16 channels of the mapping system are used for patients undergoing surgery for the WPW syndrome; however, all 160 channels are used to map atrial flutter, atrial fibrillation, ectopic atrial tachycardia, and ventricular tachyarrhythmias.

Surgical Technique

The surgical procedure for interruption of accessory pathways responsible for the WPW syndrome consists of two steps: (1) localization of the accessory pathway by intraoperative electrical mapping techniques and (2) division of the accessory pathway.

The computerized mapping system has obviated the need to use cardiopulmonary bypass for intraoperative mapping of patients with the WPW syndrome. After performing a median sternotomy, fixed epicardial electrodes are sutured to the appropriate atrium and ventricle for purposes of pacing and recording. Generally, the electrodes are positioned as close as possible to the suspected site of the accessory pathway. In our institution, a "band electrode" is then placed around the ventricular side of the A-V groove (Fig. 24–1) and atrial pacing is commenced to effect maximal ventricular preexcitation across the accessory pathway.[2] Individual epicardial electrograms are recorded from 16 bipolar pairs located along the length of the band electrode around the base of the heart. A specially designed computer program then constructs an activation sequence map that is displayed on a color graphics terminal in the operating room and accurately localizes the site of insertion of the ventricular end of the accessory atrioventricular connection.

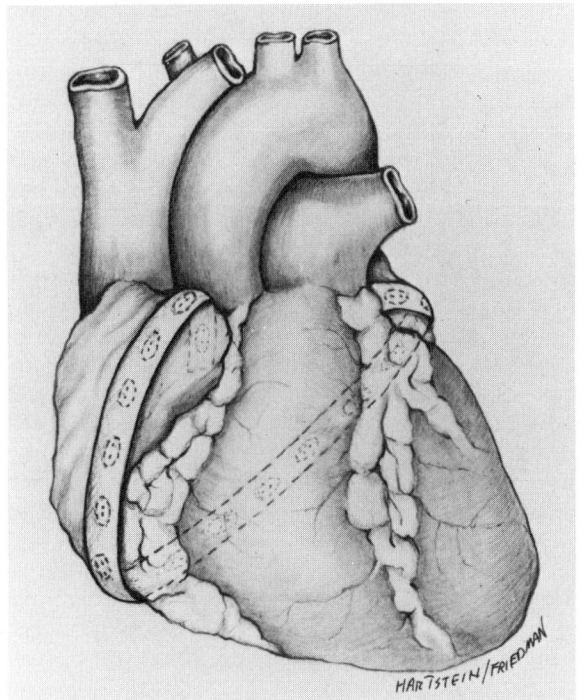

FIGURE 24–2
The band electrode with 16 bipolar electrodes is placed around the atrial side of the AV groove. The electrograms are recorded simultaneously from the bipolar electrodes to document the earliest site of atrial activation during retrograde conduction across the accessory atrioventricular connection. Retrograde conduction across the accessory pathway is accomplished either by ventricular pacing or by induction of reciprocating tachycardia. (Reprinted by permission of Futura Publishing Co., from Cox JL: In Brugada P, Wellens HJJ (eds.) Cardiac Arrhythmias: Where to Go From Here? pp. 613–637.)

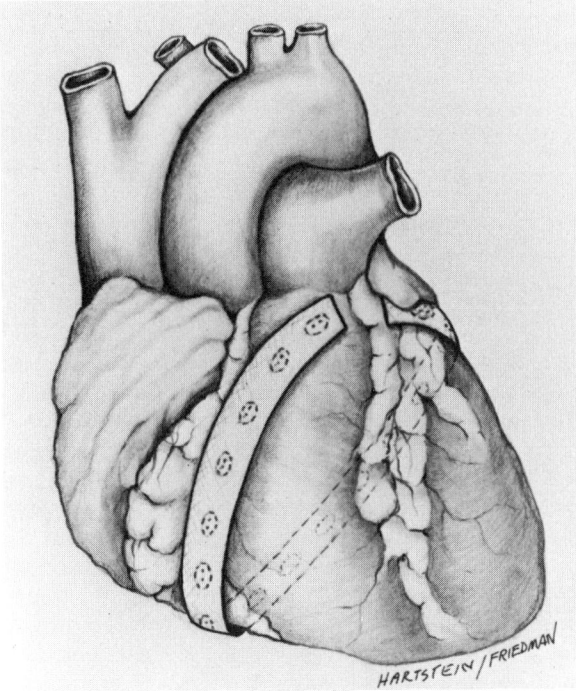

FIGURE 24–1
A flexible band containing 16 bipolar epicardial electrodes is placed around the ventricular side of the AV groove. Electrograms are recorded simultaneously from each of the 16 bipolar electrodes to document the earliest site of ventricular activation during antegrade conduction across the accessory atrioventricular connection. (Reprinted by permission of Futura Publishing Co., from Cox JL: In Brugada P, Wellens HJJ (eds.) Cardiac Arrhythmias: Where to Go From Here? pp. 613–637.)

The band electrode is then moved to the atrial side of the AV groove (Fig. 24–2), and reciprocating tachycardia is induced by programmed electrical stimulation. Atrial electrograms are recorded from the 16 bipolar pairs along the band electrode and, within 2 minutes, a retrograde atrial map delineating the site of insertion of the atrial end of the accessory pathway is displayed in the operating room. In this manner, the precise location of all accessory pathways, whether manifest or concealed, can be determined within approximately 5 minutes and without instituting cardiopulmonary bypass. This computerized mapping system has proved to be extremely helpful not only in decreasing the time required for the usual mapping procedures but also in four problematic groups of patients: (1) those with atrial fibrillation and varying degrees of ventricular preexcitation, (2) patients with only intermittent ventricular preexcitation in whom reciprocating tachycardia cannot be induced intraoperatively, (3) patients with concealed accessory pathways (i.e., pathways that conduct in the retrograde [ventricle to atrium] direction only), and (4) patients with multiple accessory pathways.

The precise surgical approach to the accessory pathway depends on its location in one of the four positions around the mitral or tricuspid valve annulus: (1) left free-wall, (2) right free-wall, (3) anterior septum, and (4) posterior septum (Fig. 24–3).[3] Cardiopulmonary bypass is instituted in all patients following completion of the epicardial mapping procedures. In patients with right free-wall, anterior septal, and posterior septal pathways, right atrial *endocardial* mapping with a hand-held electrode is performed during reciprocating tachycardia. Endocardial mapping is not performed in patients with left free-wall pathways.

Following completion of the intraoperative electrophysiologic mapping procedures, a specific surgical technique is applied in each patient, depending on the location of the accessory pathway. In the presence of *left free-wall* pathways, a left atriotomy is performed to expose the mitral valve annulus. A supra-annular incision is placed 2 mm above the posterior mitral valve annulus, extending from the left fibrous trigone to the posterior interventricular septum (Fig. 24–4). A plane of dissection is established between the AV groove fat pad and the top of the posterior left ventricle throughout the length of the supra-annular incision. This plane of dissection is carried down the posterior left ventricular wall until the epicardium can be visualized as it reflects off the posterior left ventricle onto the AV groove fat pad. Because of the possibility that an accessory pathway could still be connecting the atrial rim to the ventricle at the mitral annulus, a sharp nerve hook is used to divide any remaining fibers near the annulus, or the atrial rim is isolated by "squaring off" each end of the supra-annular incision.

Surgical division of *right free-wall* accessory pathways is performed via a right atriotomy, and a supra-annular incision is placed 2 mm above the tricuspid valve annulus from the anterior septum to the posterior septum. The dissection is performed between the underlying AV groove fat pad and the top of the right ventricular free-wall exactly as described above for left free-wall pathways.

Surgical division of *anterior septal* accessory pathways is also performed through a right atriotomy, and a supra-annular incision is placed from the anterior border of the membranous portion of the interatrial septum to the anterior free-wall of the right ventricle. A plane of dissection is established between the underlying AV groove fat pad and the top of the anterior interventricular septum. It is important to be aware that the right coronary artery originates in this region and courses through the substance of this fat pad between the medial base of the right atrium and the root of the aorta. However, if the proper plane of dissection is maintained in the potential space between the AV groove fat pad and the top of the anterior ventricular septum, the right coronary artery usually is not visualized. It is important that the plane of dissection be extended to the level of the epicardial reflection.

Historically, surgical division of *posterior septal* accessory pathways was characterized as being the most difficult.[4] However, since modification of the original surgical approach, these pathways have become perhaps the easiest ones to divide.[3] A right atriotomy is

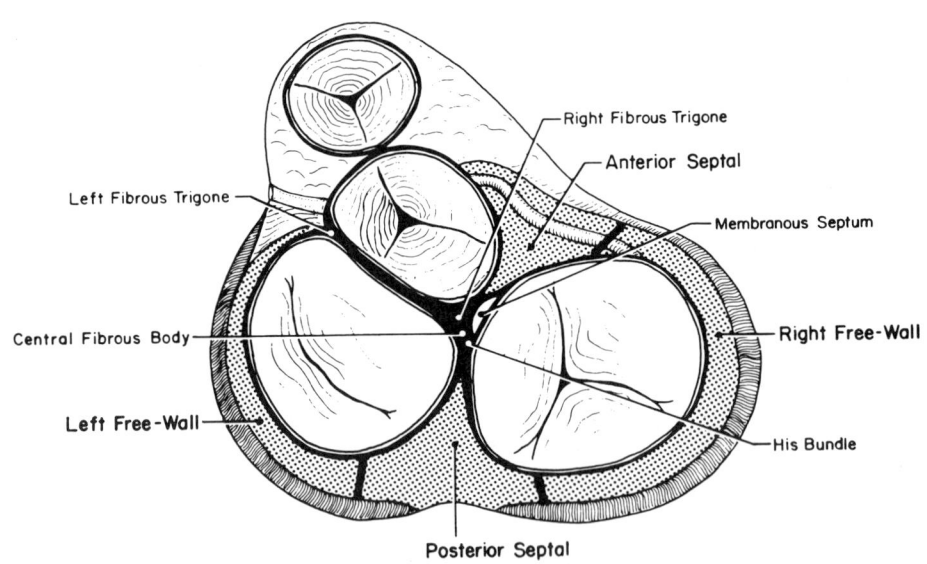

FIGURE 24–3
A diagram of the superior view of the heart with the atria cut away demonstrating the boundaries of each of the four anatomic areas where accessory pathways can occur in the Wolff-Parkinson-White syndrome. The boundaries of the *left free-wall* space are the mitral valve annulus and the ventricular epicardial reflection extending from the left fibrous trigone to the posterior septum. The boundaries of the *posterior septal* space are the tricuspid valve annulus, the mitral valve annulus, the posterior superior process of the left ventricle, and the ventricular epicardial reflection. The boundaries of the *right free-wall* space are the tricuspid valve annulus and the epicardial reflection extending from the posterior septum to the anterior septum. The boundaries of the *anterior septal* space are the tricuspid valve annulus, the membranous portion of the interatrial septum, and the ventricular epicardial reflection. All accessory atrioventricular connections must insert into the ventricle somewhere within these anatomic boundaries. (Reprinted by permission from Cox JL, Gallagher JJ, Cain ME: J Thorac Cardiovasc Surg 90:490, 1985.)

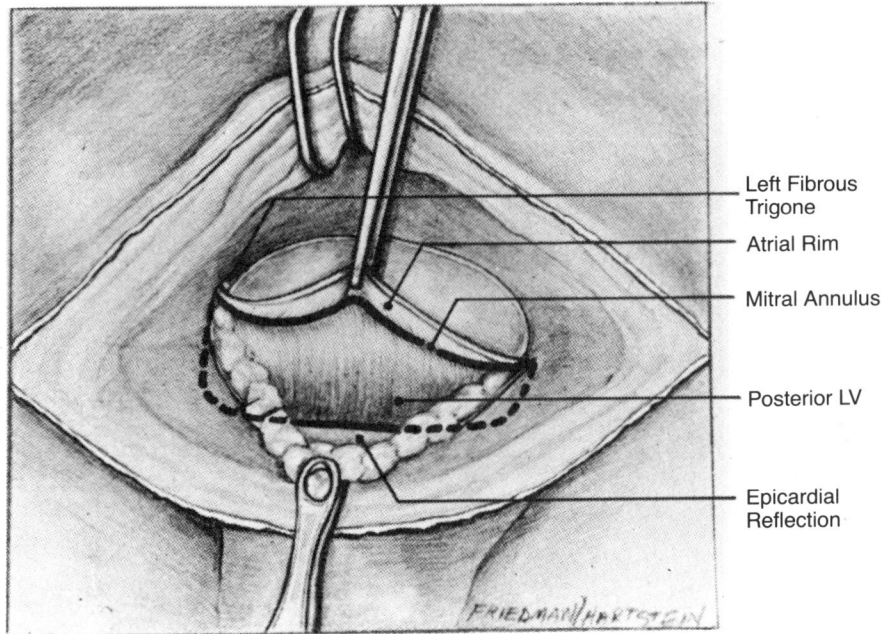

FIGURE 24–4
The anatomic boundaries of the *left free-wall* space. Complete dissection of this space for all free-wall pathways includes exposure of the mitral valve annulus throughout its length between the left fibrous trigone and the posterior ventricular septum. The top of the posterior left ventricle is then exposed underneath the AV groove fat pad all the way to the epicardial reflection off the posterior left ventricle (LV) throughout the length of the supra-annular incision. (Reprinted by permission from Cox JL, Gallagher JJ, Cain ME: J Thorac Cardiovasc Surg 90:490, 1985.)

performed in these patients prior to arresting the heart with cold potassium cardioplegia. The His bundle is identified with the same hand-held probe that is used to map the lower right atrium septum. Once the His bundle is identified, a supra-annular incision is placed just posterior to the site of the His bundle and extended in a counterclockwise direction onto the posterior right atrial free-wall. A plane of dissection is established between the fat pad and the top of the posterior interventricular septum (Fig. 24–5). Dissection in the region of the His bundle is performed during either atrial pacing or reciprocating tachycardia to avoid injury to the AV node–His bundle complex. Once dissection in this area has been completed, the heart is arrested with a cold potassium cardioplegia solution, and the remainder of the posterior pyramidal space overlying the posterior interventricular septum is dissected. This dissection is carried medially to the level of the mitral valve annulus and posteriorly to the epicardial reflection off the posterior ventricular surface. Particular attention is paid to dissection of the left ventricle at the site where the posterior interventricular septum is juxtaposed to the posterior free-wall of the left ventricle. After dissection of the posterior pyramidal space has been completed, the supra-annular incision is closed with a continuous 4-0 nonabsorbable suture.

Using the "endocardial" approach for the surgical division of accessory atrioventricular connections, 137 of 137 accessory pathways were divided successfully in 108 consecutive patients.[3] The re-operation rate was 0%, and the recurrence rate on follow-up (range 1 to 57 months) was 0%.

Klein and colleagues have recently reported an external closed heart approach for the division and/or cryoablation of accessory pathways.[5] Sealy first used a similar approach in the initial patient operated upon at Duke University and, until 1981, both Dr. Sealy and I continued to combine external dissection and cryosurgery with the endocardial technique described above.[6] At that time, the external approach and cryosurgery were abandoned because of difficulties with intraoperative hemorrhage as well as an unacceptable postoperative recurrence rate.[7] The external atrial approach is designed to divide the atrial end of the

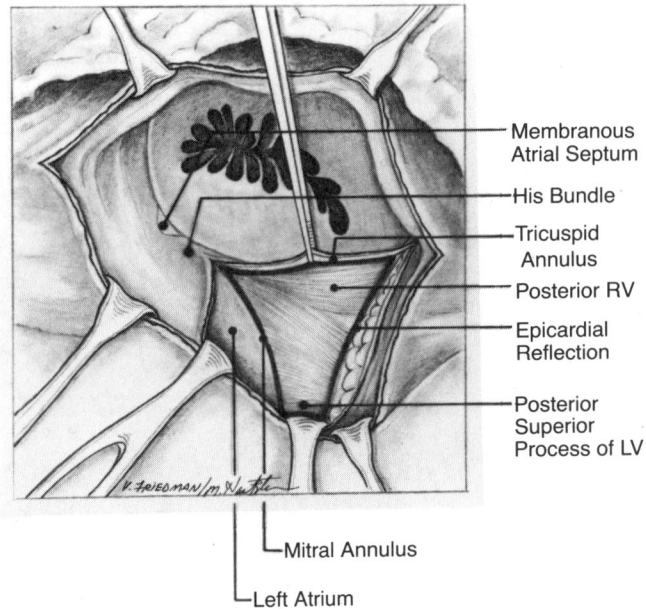

FIGURE 24–5
Completed dissection of the posterior septal space, which is bounded by the tricuspid valve annulus, the mitral valve annulus, and the epicardial reflection. The mitral valve annulus and epicardial reflection are dissected to the left to expose the posterior superior process of the left ventricle (LV), which represents the beginning of the left posterior free-wall. (Reprinted by permission from Cox JL, Gallagher JJ, Cain ME: J Thorac Cardiovasc Surg 90:490, 1985.)

accessory pathway and it continues to represent a satisfactory technique when applied to appropriately selected patients.

Other investigators have reported the use of catheter-delivered electric shocks to accessory pathways for the treatment of the WPW syndrome.[8,9] Although the concept of ablating accessory pathways without resorting to a formal cardiac surgical procedure is attractive, the early results with this technique have been discouraging except when applied for ablation of certain posterior septal accessory pathways.[8]

PAROXYSMAL SUPRAVENTRICULAR TACHYCARDIA (PSVT) DUE TO A CONCEALED ACCESSORY ATRIOVENTRICULAR CONNECTION

Paroxysmal supraventricular tachycardia may be due to either: (1) a concealed accessory atrioventricular connection that conducts in the retrograde (ventricle to atrium) direction only or (2) AV node reentry. Patients who have PSVT due to a concealed accessory atrioventricular connection technically do not have the WPW syndrome, because of lack of antegrade (atrium to ventricle) conduction across the accessory pathway does not preexcite the ventricles, and thus the ECG during sinus rhythm is normal. However, the presence of the anatomic accessory atrioventricular connection and its ability to conduct electrical impulses from the ventricle to the atrium provides the anatomic-electrophysiologic substrate for the development of reciprocating tachycardia that is identical to that which occurs in patients with the classic WPW syndrome. The inability of the accessory pathway to conduct in the antegrade direction means that the intraoperative mapping procedures in these patients is confined to performing retrograde atrial maps during induced reciprocating tachycardia or during ventricular pacing. These intraoperative retrograde atrial maps are performed as described above for patients with the WPW syndrome, and they identify the site of atrial insertion of the accessory pathway. The surgical technique employed to divide these accessory pathways is the same as for patients with the classic WPW syndrome.

PAROXYSMAL SUPRAVENTRICULAR TACHYCARDIA (PSVT) DUE TO AV NODE REENTRY

Prior to 1981, the only surgical therapy available for patients with medically refractory AV node reentry tachycardia was elective cryoablation of the bundle of His.[10] In 1981, a closed-chest technique was developed for permanent His bundle ablation in which 200 to 500 joules are delivered through a His bundle catheter.[11] This procedure effectively replaced cryoablation of the His bundle for the treatment of medically refractory AV node reentry tachycardia, because it did not require a formal cardiac surgical operation. However, because ablation of the His bundle replaces one problem (tachycardia) with another (heart block), we developed and tested a surgical technique capable of interrupting the reentrant circuit responsible for AV node reentry tachycardia without blocking normal AV conduction.

In 1982, we reported that multiple discrete (3-mm) cryolesions placed around the triangle of Koch were capable of altering the input pathways of the AV node, resulting in permanent prolongation of AV conduction in experimental animals.[12] Subsequent studies documented that in the presence of dual AV node conduction pathways, this discrete cryosurgical procedure was capable of selectively ablating only one of the pathways of conduction, thereby leaving normal AV conduction intact while interrupting the anatomic-electrophysiologic substrate responsible for AV node reentry tachycardia.[13-15] After first developing and characterizing the salutory effects of this approach in experimental animals, we applied this procedure in patients with AV node reentry tachycardia.[16]

The heart is exposed through either a median sternotomy or a right anterior thoracotomy in the fourth intercostal space. The aorta and both venae cavae are cannulated for cardiopulmonary bypass, and epicardial plaque electrodes are sutured to the right atrium and right ventricle. Following incremental atrial pacing and induction and termination of AV node reentry tachycardia, normothermic cardiopulmonary bypass is instituted and a right atriotomy is performed. A hand-held probe is used to confirm that the His bundle is in its normal position at the apex of the triangle of Koch (Fig. 24–6). Atrial pacing is then instituted, and the AV interval is monitored on a beat-to-beat basis. A nitrous oxide cryoprobe with a 3-mm diameter tip is then placed over the tendon of Tadaro at the upper edge of the os of the coronary sinus. Cryothermia is applied at a temperature of $-60°$ C for 2 minutes. Three more cryolesions are placed along the tendon of Tadaro, moving sequentially toward the apex of the triangle of Koch near the His bundle (sites 2, 3, and 4 in Fig. 24–7). Cryothermia is applied at each site for a period of 2 minutes or until transient heart block occurs. In our experience, the placement of the first four cryolesions did not result in significant prolongation of the AV interval.

Cryolesions are then placed along the annulus of the tricuspid valve beginning just beneath the os of the coronary sinus (sites 5, 6, 7 and 8 in Fig. 24–7). Prolongation of the AV interval usually occurred first during application of cryothermia at site 7 or 8. It is important to apply cryothermia to each of these sites for the full 2 minutes, if possible, since permanent tissue injury cannot be assured otherwise.[17] Fortunately, the AV interval prolongs in a linear fashion during cryothermia application, allowing the electrophysiologist to notify the surgeon of the degree of AV interval prolongation with each succeeding beat. As the AV interval prolongs to approximately 200 to 300 ms, one can expect complete AV block to occur within the next few beats. Cryothermia is terminated instantly on the development of complete AV block, and the tip of the cryoprobe is irrigated immediately with copious amounts of warm saline. AV conduction invariably resumes within 2 or 3 beats, and the AV

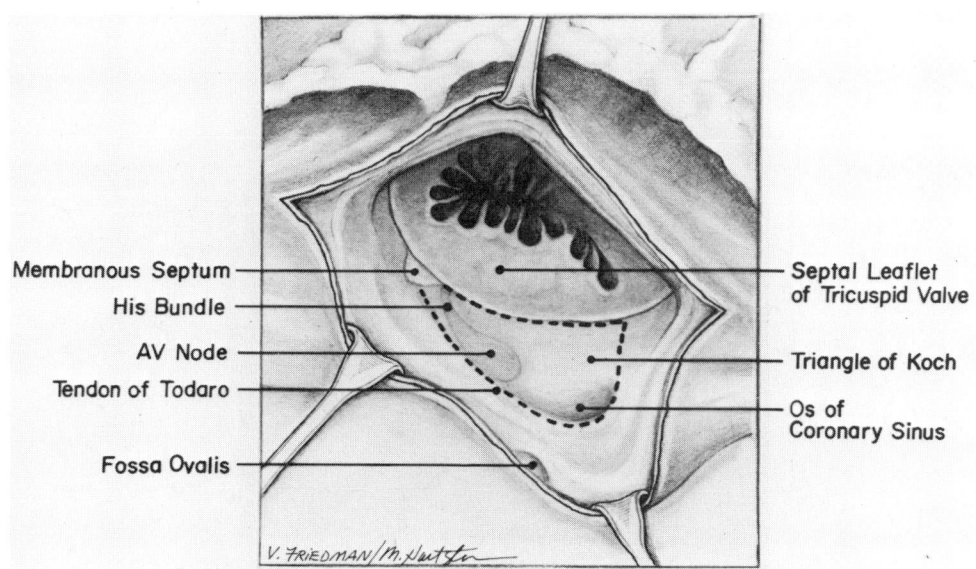

FIGURE 24–6
The right atrial septum viewed through a longitudinal right atriotomy. The patient's head is to the left and feet to the right. The boundaries of the triangle of Koch are the tendon of Tadaro, the tricuspid valve annulus, and a line connecting the two at the level of the os of the coronary sinus. Within the triangle of Koch resides the AV node and proximal portion of the His bundle, which enters the ventricular septum immediately posterior to the membranous portion of the interatrial septum. (Reprinted by permission of the American Heart Association, Inc., from Cox JL, Holman WL, Cain ME: Circulation 76:1329, 1987.)

interval returns to its control value during the ensuing 10 to 15 beats. The cryoprobe is then moved slightly more peripherally until cryothermia can be applied for the full 2 minutes to a given site without causing heart block. In this manner, the cryoprobe serves as a "reversible knife" and permanent AV block is precluded, since the cryothermia would have to be applied for a more protracted interval to result in permanent conduction block.

After placement of cryolesions at sites 1–9 (Fig. 24–7), thus encircling the AV node, cryolesions are also placed at as many sites within the triangle of Koch as possible without creating permanent AV block, using the same end point of temporary block as described above. However, having placed the first nine cryolesions, it is usually impossible to apply cryothermia to additional sites within the triangle of Koch for a full 2 minutes without causing temporary block. In essence, the objective of this operation is to cryoablate as much of the perinodal tissue as possible without causing permanent AV conduction block. This approach is feasible only because of the unique nature of cryosurgery, which allows a definitive end point (complete heart block) to be reached, but only on a temporary, reversible basis.

In patients with AV node reentry tachycardia and concomitant WPW syndrome, the latter problem must be surgically corrected before any attempt is made to treat the AV node reentry. Correction of the WPW syndrome initially is essential because the discrete cryosurgical procedure for AV node reentry depends on the ability to monitor exclusive conduction through the AV node–His bundle complex on a beat-to-beat basis. If the patient has a functioning accessory pathway that conducts in the antegrade direction, it is impossible to monitor the effects of cryosurgical modification of normal AV conduction during atrial pacing, since the atrial impulse travels preferentially across the accessory pathways to the ventricles.

Application of the discrete cryosurgical procedure has resulted in the selective ablation of only one of the two AV node conduction pathways present in all patients and has effected a permanent cure of the AV node reentry tachycardia in all patients. There have been no operative deaths. Results of the immediate and late postoperative electrophysiologic studies have demonstrated smooth AV node conduction curves (Fig. 24–8) and no inducible AV node reentry tachy-

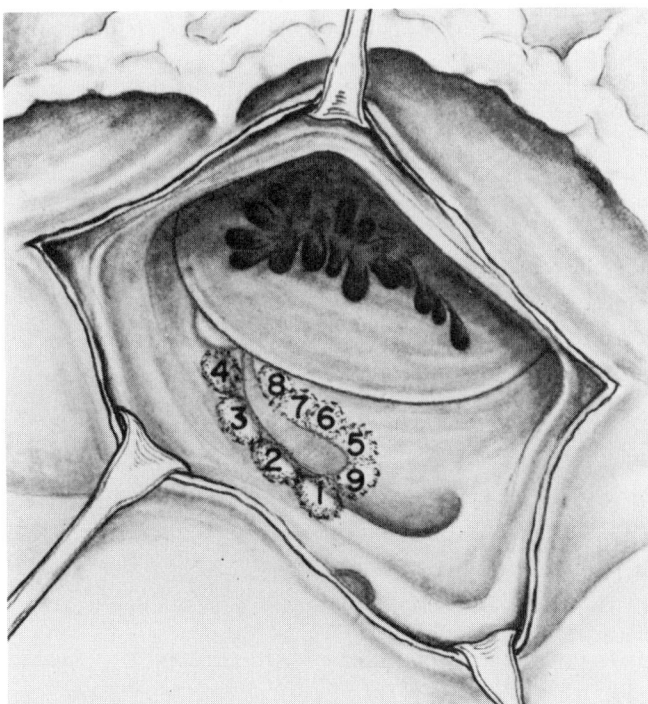

FIGURE 24–7
Cryolesions are placed in positions 1–4 as diagrammed, then in positions 5–8 and finally in position 9. During the application of cryothermia at positions 7 and 8, prolongation of the AV interval usually begins to occur. (Reprinted by permission of the American Heart Association, Inc., from Cox JL, Holman WL, Cain ME: Circulation 76:1329, 1987.)

Surgical Management of Cardiac Arrhythmias

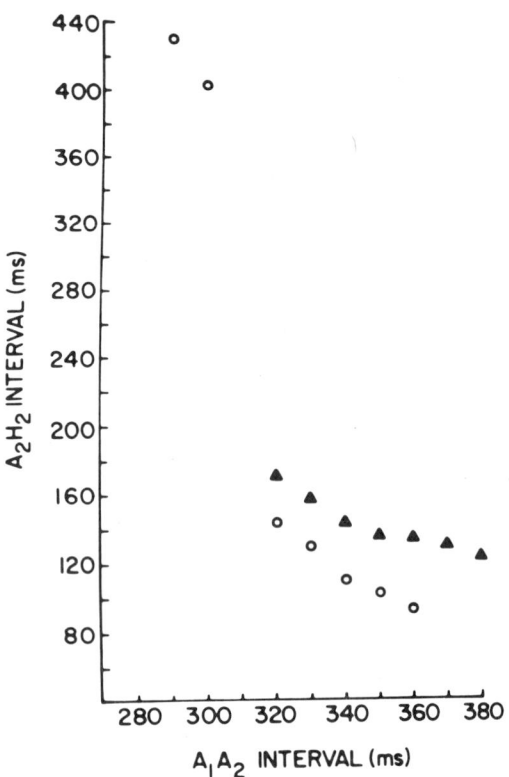

FIGURE 24–8
Comparison of preoperative (open circles) and postoperative (closed triangles) AV node conduction curves obtained during an atrial paced cycle length (PCL) of 400 msec. Dual AV node conduction pathways were no longer demonstrated postoperatively. (Reprinted by permission of the American Heart Association, Inc., from Cox JL, Holman WL, Cain ME: Circulation 76:1329, 1987.)

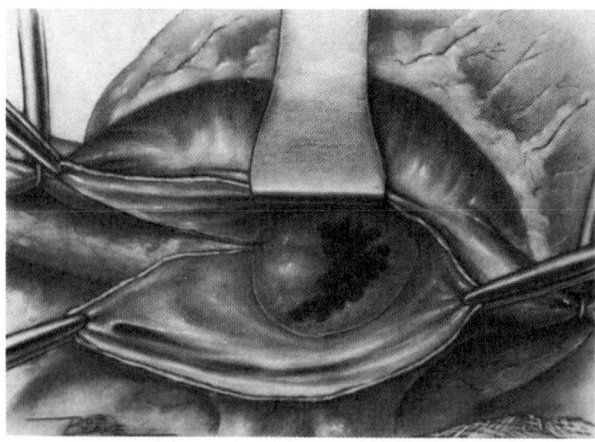

FIGURE 24–9
Left atrial isolation procedure. Following a standard left atriotomy incision, the interatrial septum is retracted gently and the atriotomy is extended anteriorly across Bachmann's bundle to the level of the mitral valve annulus just to the left of the right fibrous trigone. Note that the anterior atriotomy extends across the mitral valve annulus. The posterior portion of the incision is transmural to the level of the coronary sinus. The remaining portion of the incision is made through the endocardium and extends across the mitral valve annulus posteriorly just to the left of the interatrial septum. At this point, electrical activity continues to be propagated in a 1:1 fashion between the right and left atria because of the presence of interatrial muscular connections accompanying the coronary sinus. (Reprinted by permission from Williams JM, Ungerleider RM, Lofland GK, et al.: J Thorac Cardiovasc Surg 80:373, 1980.)

cardia. Moreover, all patients have maintained normal conduction through the AV node–His bundle complex during a 5-year follow-up period.

ECTOPIC (AUTOMATIC) ATRIAL TACHYCARDIA

Automatic atrial tachycardias are frequently suppressed by general anesthesia and, as a result, intraoperative mapping to localize their site of origin may not be possible. However, if the arrhythmia persists intraoperatively so that it can be localized precisely, simple surgical excision or isolation of that part of the atrium or local cryoablation will eliminate the problem.[18] If the arrhythmogenic myocardium cannot be localized intraoperatively, elective cryoablation of the His bundle has been the only alternative in the past. To avoid having to resort to His bundle ablation, we have recently developed alternative surgical techniques that leave normal AV conduction intact while isolating the arrhythmogenic atrial myocardium from the remainder of the heart.

Automatic *left atrial tachycardias* usually originate in the body of the left atrium. Since the sinoatrial node, internodal conduction routes, and AV node–His bundle complex reside either in the right atrium or atrial septum, a technique was developed to isolate the entire left atrium from the remainder of the heart, which then persists in normal sinus rhythm regardless of the presence or absence of tachycardia in the left atrium (Figs. 24–9 and 24–10). After developing the tech-

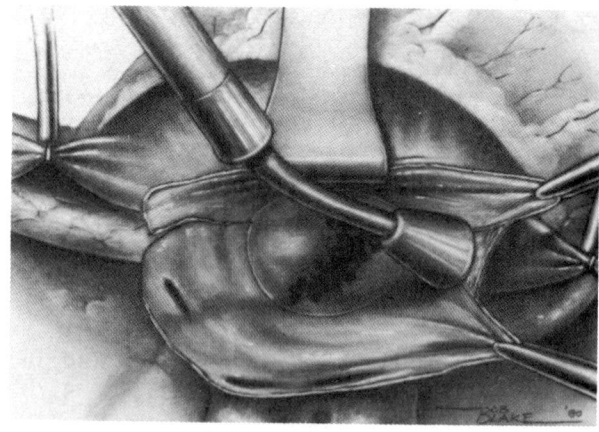

FIGURE 24–10
Left atrial isolation procedure. A cryoprobe is positioned over the endocardial aspect of the posterior atriotomy and its temperature is decreased to −60° C for 2 minutes. This cryolesion ablates the endocardial interatrial fibers accompanying the coronary sinus. A similar cryolesion is created on the epicardial aspect of the atrioventricular groove on the opposite side of the coronary sinus to ablate all remaining interatrial epicardial connections. (Reprinted by permission from Williams JM, Ungerleider RM, Lofland GK, et al.: J Thorac Cardiovasc Surg 80:373, 1980.)

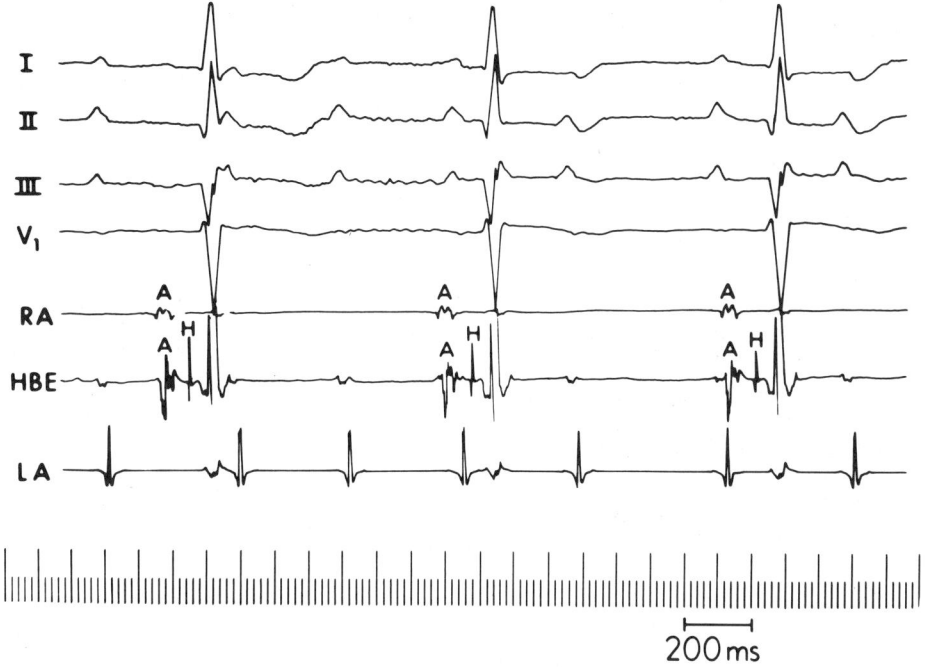

FIGURE 24-11
Postoperative recordings following surgical exclusion of the left atrium. Recordings, from the top down, are surface ECG leads I, II, and III, V₁, bipolar catheter recordings of the right atrium (RA) and the His bundle HBE; and a bipolar recording obtained by permanent electrodes sutured to the left atrial (LA) appendage.

The right and left atria are dissociated. Right atrial activity proceeds from the catheter positioned in the high right atrium to the atrial septum as recorded on the His bundle catheter, followed by conduction to the ventricle. An irregular left atrial tachycardia is present that fails to propagate to either the right atrium or to the ventricles. Note that the surface P wave correlates with left atrial activity although the ventricles are responding to activity initiated in the right atrium. A = atrial, H = His. (Reprinted by permission from Gallagher JJ, Cox JL, German LD, et al.: In Josephson ME, Wellens HJJ (eds.): Tachycardias: Mechanisms, Diagnosis, and Treatment, pp. 271–285. Philadelphia, Lea & Febiger, 1984.)

niques for left atrial isolation in 1979[19] (Fig. 24–11) and evaluating its hemodynamic effects for over three years, we applied it clinically on December 6, 1982. The patient has remained in normal sinus rhythm on no antiarrhythmic medications postoperatively, despite the presence of incessant tachycardia confined to the left atrium. She has suffered no adverse hemodynamic sequelae from the left atrial isolation procedure.

Right atrial tachycardias may occur on the basis of either automaticity or reentry and are usually confined to the body of the right atrium. In our experience, the suppression of these arrhythmias by general anesthesia is somewhat less of a problem intraoperatively than it is with left atrial automatic tachycardias. As mentioned above, if the automatic atrial tachycardias occur spontaneously intraoperatively or if the reentrant atrial

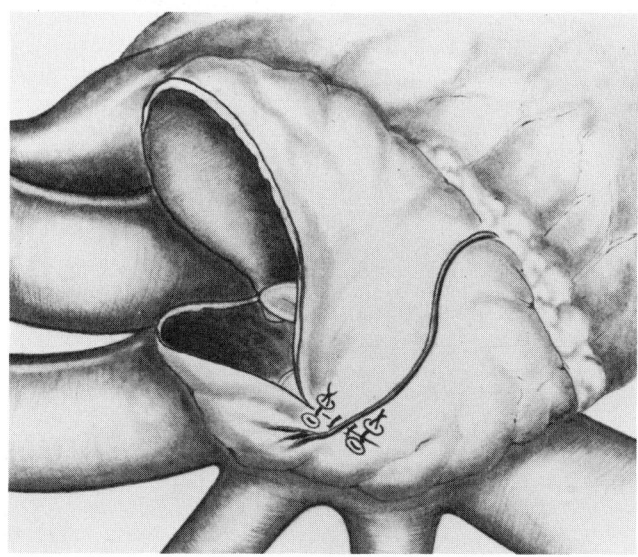

FIGURE 24-12
Right atrial isolation. Initially, the sinoatrial (SA) node artery is dissected free from the atrial tissue 5 mm anterior to the crista terminalis. A 2-cm incision parallel to the crista terminalis is placed beneath the artery. The incision beneath the sinoatrial node artery is closed with a continuous nonabsorbable 5-0 suture, taking care not to damage the artery. Small pledgets are used above and below the artery to reinforce the incision. The right atriotomy is then extended to a point anterior to the junction of the superior vena cava and the base of the right atrial appendage and then along the anterior limbus of the fossa ovalis to the anteromedial tricuspid valve annulus, just anterior to the membranous interatrial septum.

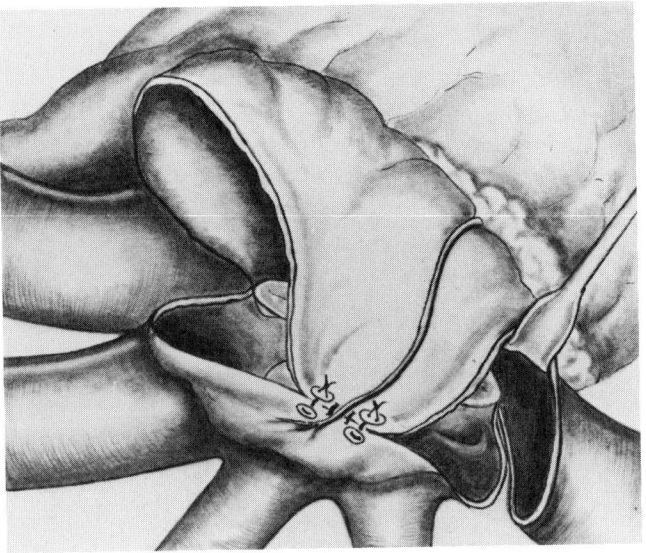

FIGURE 24–13
Right atrial isolation. Caudad extension of the right atriotomy around the posterior right atrial–inferior vena cava junction to the posterior-lateral tricuspid valve annulus. A cryolesion (−60° C for 2 minutes) is placed at the end of the incision to ensure complete interruption of connecting atrial muscle fibers between the body of the right atrium and the remainder of the heart.

tachycardias can be induced intraoperatively, they can be mapped by electrophysiologic means and cryoablated. However, if the tachycardia cannot be induced intraoperatively, the surgeon has, in the past, had to resort to ablation of the His bundle with insertion of a permanent pacemaking system. We have recently developed a procedure to isolate the body of the right atrium while leaving the atrial pacemaker complex in continuity with the atrial septum and the ventricles (Figs 24–12, 24–13, and 24–14).[20] This technique was considerably more difficult to develop than was the left atrial isolation procedure because of the complexities of the atrial pacemaker tissue and the anatomic variability of its blood supply. Nevertheless, we performed isolation of the body of the right atrium exclusive of the atrial pacemaker complex in a 35-year-old woman on November 14, 1986.

ATRIAL FLUTTER/FIBRILLATION

Recent studies by Boineau on atrial flutter[21] and by Allessie on atrial fibrillation[22] have documented that both of these supraventricular tachyarrhythmias most likely occur on the basis of macro-reentrant circuits. This new information provides, for the first time, a "target" for the arrhythmia surgeon and will undoubtedly pave the way for the development of specific surgical procedures to ablate these two arrhythmias. The detrimental hemodynamic effects of atrial flutter and atrial fibrillation, as well as the thromboembolic

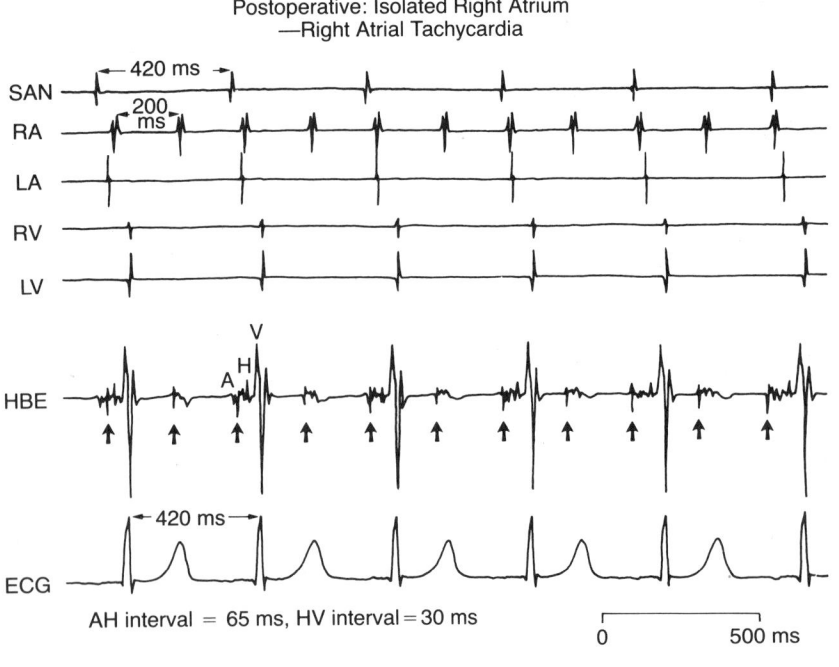

FIGURE 24–14
Postoperative electrograms recorded during simulated tachycardia in the isolated right atrium. Tachycardia is simulated by rapid right atrial pacing at a cycle length of 200 ms and is confined to the isolated right atrium. Moreover, the simulated right atrial tachycardia does not affect sinus rhythm or the normal conduction sequence in the remainder of the heart. Arrows mark right atrial pacing spikes reflected in the His bundle electrogram. SAN = sinoatrial node; RA = right atrium; LA = left atrium; RV = right ventricle; LV = left ventricle; HBE = His bundle electrogram; AH = atrio–His bundle interval.

complications associated with both arrhythmias, would seem to warrant the development of such surgical procedures. Surgical ablation of these arrhythmias appear to be particularly appropriate in patients undergoing isolated mitral valve replacement, 60% of whom suffer from chronic atrial flutter/fibrillation.[23]

Our previous approach to this problem has been to evaluate the potential beneficial effects of either a complete or partial left atrial isolation procedure. Experimentally, the complete left atrial isolation procedure has been shown to ablate chronic atrial flutter/fibrillation, but it results in a loss of synchrony of contraction of the left atrium. Incomplete isolation of the left atrium has proved to be unsatisfactory for the control of atrial flutter/fibrillation (unpublished data). However, the new knowledge and insights gained from the studies by Boineau and Allessie have encouraged the development of intraoperative computerized mapping techniques to identify the reentrant circuits responsible for atrial flutter and atrial fibrillation, and they will almost certainly lead to the development of specific surgical techniques for their ablation.

Ventricular Tachyarrhythmias

All patients who are to undergo surgical therapy for ventricular tachyarrhythmias should first undergo an endocardial catheter electrophysiology study. The objectives of the preoperative study are (1) confirmation that the arrhythmia is ventricular rather than supraventricular in origin, (2) demonstration that the ventricular arrhythmia can be induced and terminated by programmed electrical stimulation techniques (i.e., that it is a reentrant arrhythmia), and (3) localization of the region of origin of the ventricular tachycardia by "catheter mapping" when possible. In addition to the preoperative electrophysiology study, patients with ventricular tachyarrhythmias routinely undergo cardiac catheterization and coronary angiography prior to surgical intervention.

The preoperative electrophysiology study may demonstrate the arrhythmia to be ventricular tachycardia of a single morphologic type, indicating that it is originating from a single region in the left or right ventricle. Following induction, these *monomorphic ventricular tachycardias* are usually sustained for a sufficient length of time to allow endocardial catheter mapping to determine their site of origin. However, monomorphic ventricular tachycardia may be nonsustained, thus precluding adequate mapping during the preoperative electrophysiology study.

The preoperative study may also document the arrhythmia to be *polymorphic ventricular tachycardia.* This term is applied not only to ventricular tachycardia that originates from several different regions of the left ventricle, giving rise to different morphologic types of tachycardia, but it is also applied to tachycardia that originates from one general region of the left ventricle but is characterized electrophysiologically by excessive fragmentation such that individual depolarization complexes may be difficult to identify. Polymorphic ventricular tachycardia may also be either sustained or nonsustained, and it commonly deteriorates rather quickly into ventricular fibrillation. Electrophysiologic deterioration to ventricular fibrillation may be the result of primary electrical instability, or it may occur because of hemodynamic compromise associated with the onset of polymorphic ventricular tachycardia.

The third type of ventricular tachyarrhythmia that may be identified by the preoperative electrophysiologic study is *primary ventricular fibrillation*. This arrhythmia is characterized by the absence of any type of induced ventricular tachycardia prior to the onset of ventricular fibrillation following programmed electrical stimulation.

Indications for Surgery

The major indications for surgical intervention in ventricular tachyarrhythmias include medical refractoriness to ventricular tachycardia, patient intolerance to effective medical treatment, and poor patient compliance. The contraindications to surgical intervention for these arrhythmias are determined by the preoperative electrophysiology study and include noninducible ventricular tachycardia, automatic ventricular tachycardia, and primary ventricular fibrillation. Nonsustained polymorphic ventricular tachycardia was previously considered to be a contraindication to surgical intervention,[24] but the development of computerized intraoperative mapping systems has provided a means of identifying the area or areas of arrhythmogenic myocardium, even with this fleeting, changing type of ventricular tachyarrhythmia.

Intraoperative Electrophysiologic Mapping

In patients undergoing surgery for ventricular tachyarrhythmias, the first step intraoperatively is to perform detailed electrophysiologic mapping procedures to guide the specific surgical technique to be employed. As mentioned in the previous section, all 160 channels of the computerized system are used to map the heart in patients with ventricular tachycardia. The sock electrode array (Fig. 24–15) is first used to determine the epicardial activation sequence during sinus rhythm and during induced ventricular tachycardia. The sock electrode array presently employed contains 96 electrodes. The earliest site of epicardial breakthrough is automatically cursored in red by the computer for rapid detection of the region of most interest (Fig. 24–16). It should be emphasized that the epicardial data are not used to identify the site to be ablated; rather, the data are used to guide the subsequent placement of plunge needle electrodes to further delineate the specific site of arrhythmogenesis. The epicardial map is not only helpful as an initial screening device that can be obtained in 2 to 3 minutes, but also is most useful in characterizing nonclinical arrhythmias that may be induced during programmed electrical stimulation.

Once the epicardial activation sequence during ventricular tachycardia has been established, multiple plunge-needle electrodes containing 4 bipolar pairs of

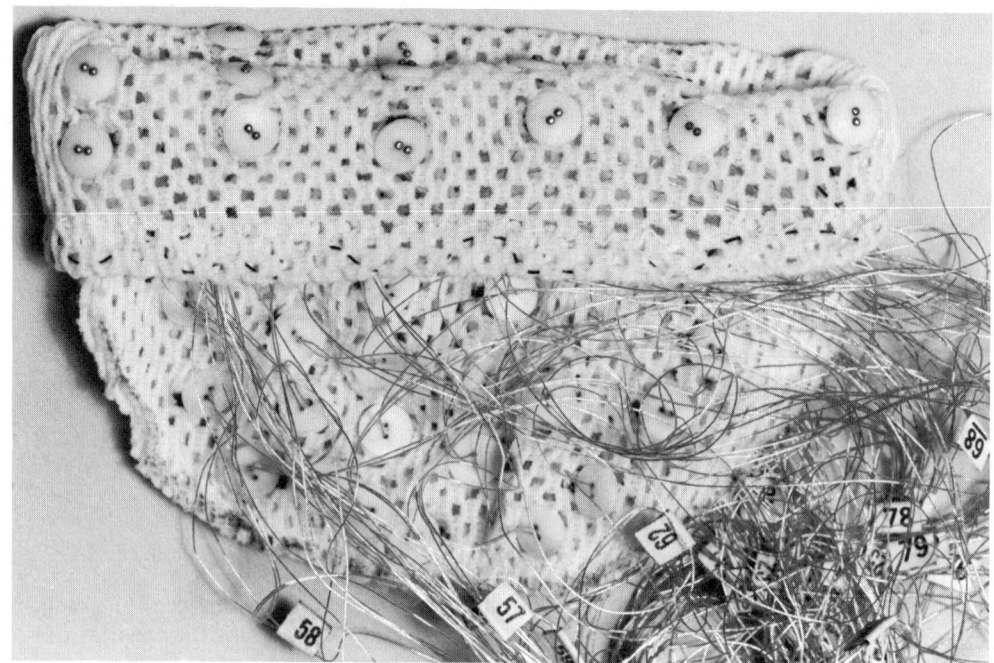

FIGURE 24–15
The sock electrode array. The 96 bipolar electrodes are maintained in contact with the epicardial surface of the ventricles by a nylon mesh stocking.

contacts along the needle shaft are inserted into the ventricle in the region of earliest epicardial activation (Figs 24–17 and 24–18). If the epicardial map has suggested that the tachycardia is arising from the ventricular septum, a right atriotomy is performed, and up to 15 right-angle needle electrodes are inserted into the ventricular septum from the right side, access being gained across the tricuspid valve. This provides up to 60 transmural data points from the ventricular septum without the necessity for performing a ventriculotomy. As many as 25 other needle electrodes can be placed in or near the arrhythmogenic region, yielding a total of 160 endocardial, intramural, and epicardial data points simultaneously from the septum and free-wall without performing a ventriculotomy. It has been demonstrated on many occasions by various investigators that a ventriculotomy frequently alters electrophysiologic milieu sufficiently to prevent further

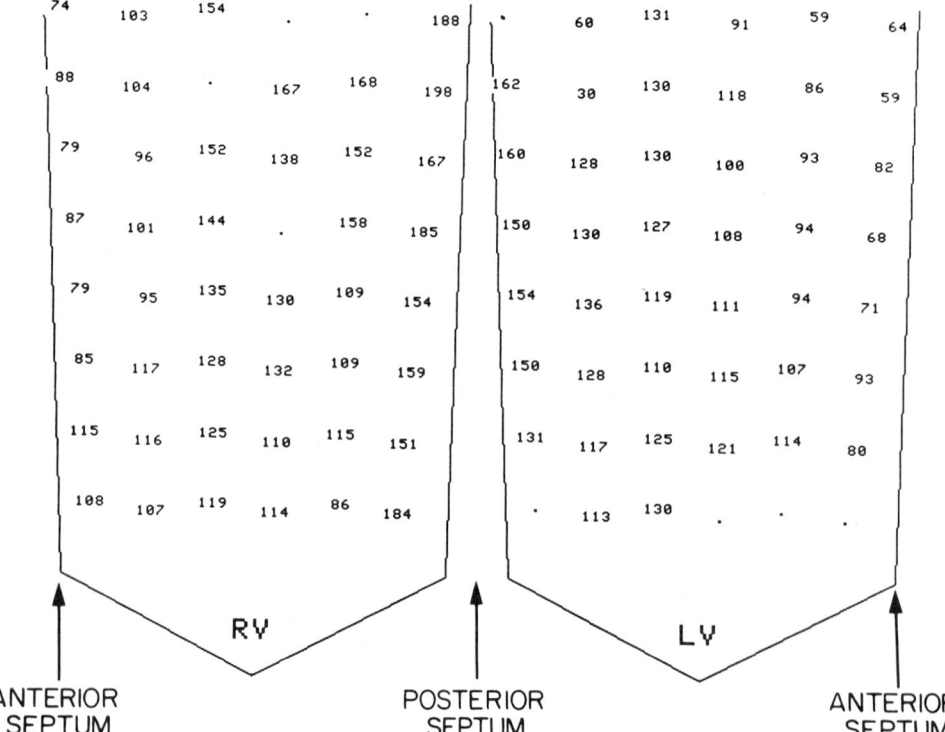

FIGURE 24–16
Hard copy of the color graphics terminal display of data recorded from the 96 epicardial electrodes in the sock electrode array during induced ventricular tachycardia. The epicardial data show that the earliest area of epicardial breakthrough is over the upper anterior ventricular septum. These data were used to guide the subsequent placement of multiple plunge needle electrodes in the ventricular septum and anterior right (RV) and left ventricular (LV) free-wall to obtain data from 160 endocardial, intramural, and epicardial sites in and around this region of early epicardial breakthrough. (Reprinted by permission from Cox JL: In Brugada P, Wellens I (eds.): Proceedings of 20 Years of Programmed Electrical Stimulation of the Heart, pp. 613–637. Mount Kisco, Futura Publishing Co., 1987.)

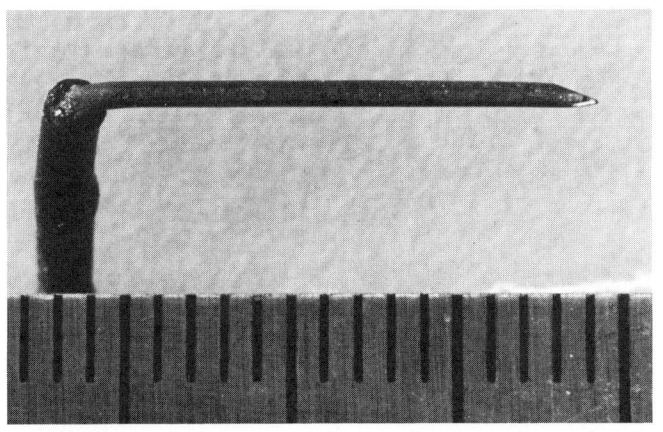

FIGURE 24–17
Close-up view of a single intramural needle electrode. Each needle shaft contains four bipolar electrodes to record data from four different layers of the ventricular free-wall and/or septum.

inducibility of the ventricular tachycardia, thereby preventing further mapping and necessitating a non-guided operation.

NONISCHEMIC VENTRICULAR TACHYARRHYTHMIAS

The majority of ventricular arrhythmias unassociated with coronary artery disease arise in the right ventricular free-wall and are remarkably intractable to medical therapy. As a result, much emphasis has been placed recently on the surgical therapy of these arrhythmias.

Idiopathic ventricular tachycardia refers to tachycardia patients in whom the only clinical manifestation of cardiac disease is the arrhythmia. Both the macroscopic appearance of the heart at operation and the pathologic data acquired at the time of autopsy in such patients fail to show any evidence of primary cardiac disease. The only abnormality noted has been global dilatation of the heart, secondary to functional post-tachycardia heart failure. Surgical approaches have included simple ventriculotomy, isolation procedures, and cryoablation. However, the results have been poor, because many of these arrhythmias arise within the ventricular septum.

A small group of patients have been shown to have ventricular tachycardia due to *nonischemic cardiomyopathy*. This group has angiographic and catheter data indicating some type of abnormal myocardial contractility associated with recurrent ventricular tachycardia. These patients usually have global dilatation of both ventricles, with diffuse patchy myocardial fibrosis. These tachyarrhythmias frequently arise in the right ventricle, and our approach to such patients has been to use a combination of surgical isolation and cryoablation of the origin of the arrhythmia (Fig. 24–19).[26]

In 1978, Fontaine described a previously unrecognized form of cardiomyopathy localized to the right

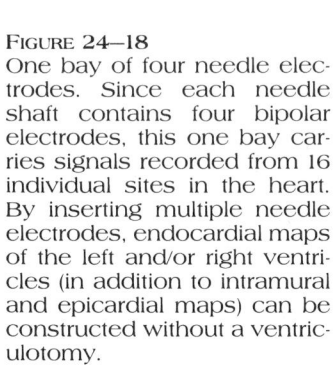

FIGURE 24–18
One bay of four needle electrodes. Since each needle shaft contains four bipolar electrodes, this one bay carries signals recorded from 16 individual sites in the heart. By inserting multiple needle electrodes, endocardial maps of the left and/or right ventricles (in addition to intramural and epicardial maps) can be constructed without a ventriculotomy.

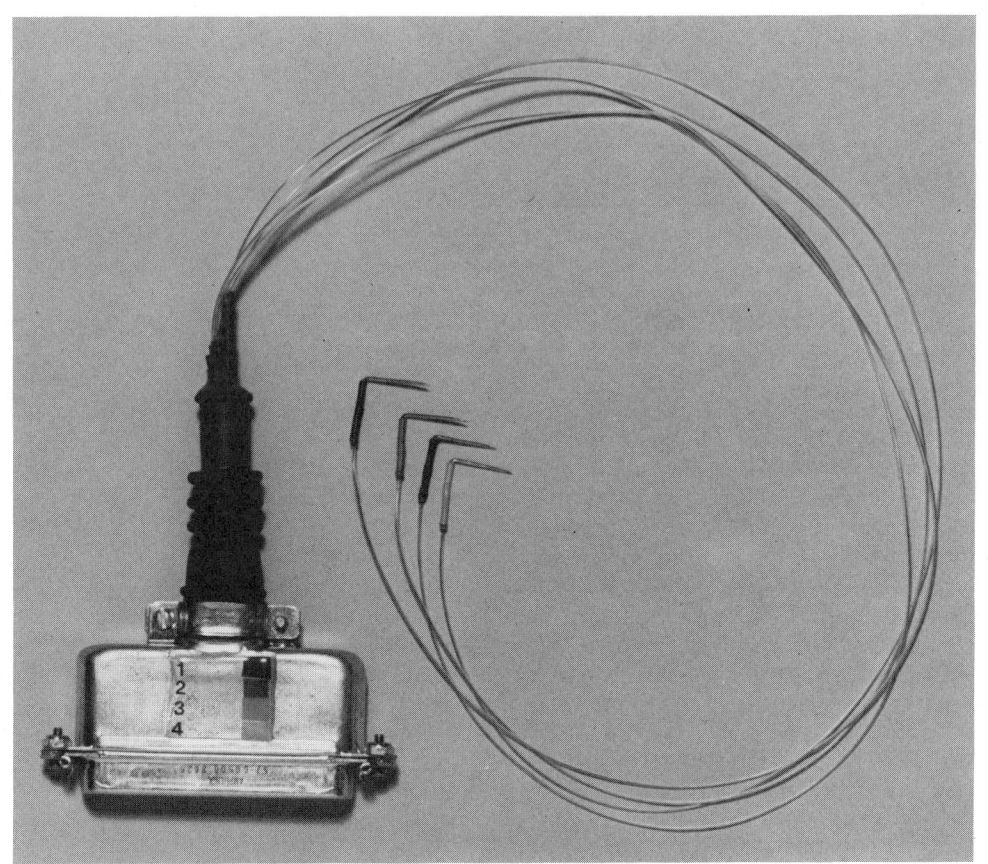

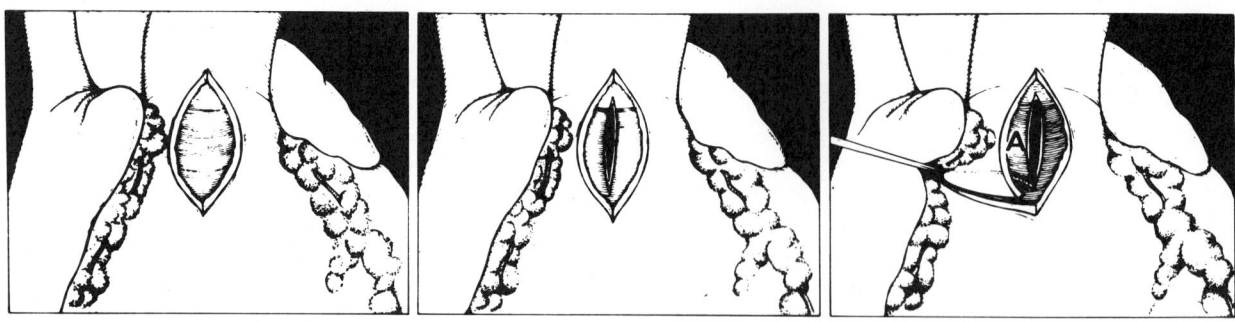

FIGURE 24–19
Localized right ventricular isolation procedure employed for the treatment of ventricular tachycardia arising in the supracristal ventricular septum (A) of a 16-year-old girl with cardiomyopathy. The distal ends of the anterior (left panel) and posterior (middle panel) transmural longitudinal ventriculotomies were extended just beyond the level of the pulmonary valve annulus, and their proximal ends were connected by transmural semicircular ventriculotomy as diagrammed. These incisions totally isolated the arrhythmogenic myocardium (A) from the remainder of the heart (right panel). The isolated segment of the pulmonary outflow tract received its blood supply from the adjacent right coronary artery (being retracted laterally in the right panel), and thus was not subject to ischemic injury. The ventriculotomies were closed with a continuous 3-0 nonabsorbable suture. (Reprinted by permission of F. A. Davis Co. from Cox JL: Cardiovasc Clin 18(1):207, 1987.)

ventricle, which he termed *arrhythmogenic right ventricular dysplasia*.[27] This syndrome appears to be a congenital cardiomyopathy characterized by transmural infiltration of adipose tissue, resulting in weakness and aneurysmal bulging of the infundibulum, apex, and/or posterior-basilar region of the right ventricle. This syndrome is characterized clinically by intractable ventricular tachycardia originating from one or all three of the pathologic areas of the right ventricle. Previous surgical efforts employing simple ventriculotomies, aneurysm excision, or a combination of ventriculotomy and excision have been associated with excessive mortality and recurrence rates.[25] Our initial approach to such patients employed a transmural encircling ventriculotomy that isolated the arrhythmogenic myocardium from the remainder of the heart (Fig. 24–20).[26]

Although Fontaine's original description of arrhythmogenic right ventricular dysplasia suggested that the cardiomyopathy was confined to three discrete areas of the right ventricle, intraoperative mapping of these patients has suggested that the entire right ventricular free-wall may be arrhythmogenic in certain cases. As a result, the localized isolation procedures described above were combined and slightly modified so that the entire free-wall of the right ventricle could be disconnected from the remainder of the heart, in hopes of encompassing all of the multiple sites of arrhythmogenic myocardium and thereby confining the tachycardia to the right ventricle.[14] The right ventricular isolation procedure thus represents a logical extension of the two localized isolation procedures that were first employed in 1979 (Fig. 24–21).[26] The surgical technique for right ventricular disconnection begins with a longitudinal ventriculotomy in the anterior right ventricle parallel to the interventricular septum approximately 5 mm to the right of the septum. This ventriculotomy is extended toward the apex, and several trabeculae, including the moderator band of the right ventricle, are transected sharply. The incision is then carried up to the pulmonary outflow tract just to the right of the interventricular septum, to a point approximately 1 mm across the anterior pulmonic valve annulus. The incision is then carried around the apex of the right ventricle just to the right of the interventricular septum, onto the posterior surface of the right ventricle. The posterior portion of the incision is extended to a point near the base of the heart approximately 1 cm from the posterior tricuspid valve annulus. The re-

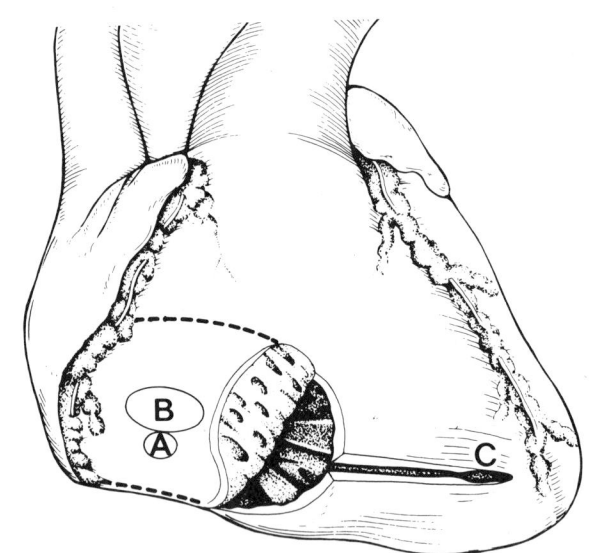

FIGURE 24–20
Localized right ventricular isolation procedure employed for the treatment of ventricular tachycardia due to arrhythmogenic right ventricular dysplasia in a 69-year-old man. The isolated pedicle of right ventricular free-wall encompassed both the apparent site of arrhythmogenesis (A) and an adjacent, electrically silent region (B). Thinning of the right ventricular wall at the site of the small apical aneurysm (C) is apparent. Although no evidence for the occurrence of ventricular tachycardia rising from the apical aneurysm was detected preoperatively or intraoperatively, the anterior incision was made in an effort to decrease the likelihood of development of a second arrhythmogenic focus later at the site of the small apical aneurysm. (Reprinted by permission of F. A. Davis Co. from Cox JL: Cardiovasc Clin 18(1):207, 1987.)

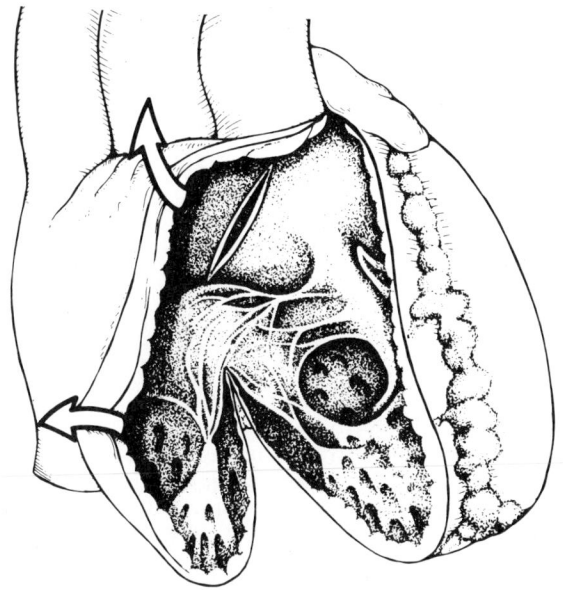

FIGURE 24–21
Right ventricular disconnection procedure performed in two 16-year-old males for polymorphic ventricular tachycardia arising from multiple sites in the right ventricle due to arrhythmogenic right ventricular dysplasia. After completion of the two transmural incisions described in the text, the papillary muscle attached to the anterior leaflet of the tricuspid valve was divided at its base and reimplanted on the lower ventricular septum with interrupted 3-0 pledgeted nonabsorbable sutures. Cryolesions were placed at each end of the anteroposterior ventriculotomy and at each end of the ventriculotomy between the posterior pulmonary valve annulus and the anterior medial tricuspid valve annulus. Both ventriculotomies were closed with continuous 3-0 nonabsorbable sutures. (Reprinted by permission of F. A. Davis Co. from Cox JL: Cardiovasc Clin 18(1):207, 1987.)

maining portion of the posterior incision is made from the endocardial aspect, but it continues to be transmural to the level of the posterior tricuspid valve annulus, sparing only the AV groove fat pad and its encompassed coronary vessels. A cryolesion is placed at the distal extent of the incision at the level of the posterior tricuspid valve annulus.

Attention is then directed to the supracristal ventricular septum between the posterior pulmonic valve annulus and the anterior medial tricuspid valve annulus. The His bundle and right bundle branch are identified with a hand-held electrode, and an incision is placed between the posterior pulmonic valve annulus and the anterior medial tricuspid valve annulus from the endocardial aspect. This incision is transmural, so that the aorta is visualized through the incision. A cryolesion is placed at each end of the incision at the levels of the pulmonic valve annulus and the tricuspid valve annulus. It may be necessary to transplant the anterior papillary muscle to the ventricular septum if evidence of continued electrical conduction exists between the isolated right ventricular free-wall and the remainder of the heart. The anterior papillary muscle may be transected at its base and reimplanted with multiple 3-0 pledgeted nonabsorbable sutures onto the right ventricular septum. The entire right ventricular free-wall is thus disconnected from the remainder of the heart, except for the papillary muscle attachments to the posterior and septal leaflets of the tricuspid valve that are attached to the right ventricular septum. Several cryolesions are placed at the base of these papillary muscles, preventing any possible electrical conduction from the papillary muscles to the right ventricle. The septal ventriculotomy between the posterior pulmonic valve annulus and the anterior medial tricuspid valve annulus is then closed with a continuous 3-0 nonabsorbable suture. The long right free-wall ventriculotomy extending from the anterior pulmonic valve annulus, down the anterior surface of the right ventricle, around the right ventricular apex, and up the inferior right ventricular free-wall to the posterior tricuspid valve annulus is closed with a single layer of 3-0 nonabsorbable suture.

A 6-year follow-up of the localized right ventricular isolation procedures has demonstrated complete success, with no adverse long-term sequelae, no recurrence of ventricular tachycardia, and no need for antitachycardia medications.[26] Although the early results of the total right ventricular isolation procedure

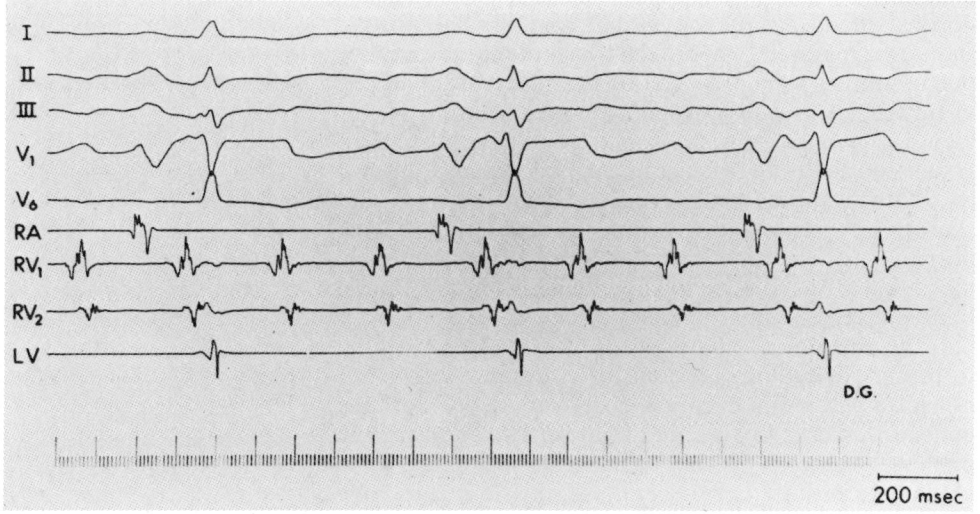

FIGURE 24–22
Surface recordings and intracardiac electrograms in a patient during an episode of right ventricular (RV) tachycardia postoperatively. The limb lead (I–III) and precordial lead (V_1 and V_6) electrograms demonstrated normal sinus rhythm in the remainder of the heart documented by right atrial (RA) activity preceding each left ventricular (LV) complex. (Reprinted by permission from Cox JL: In Cohn LH (ed.): Modern Technics in Surgery, pp. 1–18. Mount Kisco, Futura Publishing Co., 1985.)

were encouraging (Fig. 24–22), a 3-year follow-up of these patients indicates that a progressive dilatation of the right ventricle occurs to such an extent that overall left ventricular function may be compromised because of displacement of the ventricular septum.[26] While the potentially progressive nature of this problem remains unknown, it should be emphasized that the more localized isolation procedures of the right ventricular free-wall should be applied, when possible, and that isolation of the entire right ventricular free-wall should be reserved for only the most serious and complex nonischemic right ventricular tachyarrhythmias.

REFRACTORY ISCHEMIC VENTRICULAR TACHYARRHYTHMIAS

The surgical approach to refractory ischemic ventricular tachycardia should depend upon two factors: (1) the electrophysiologic characteristics of the ventricular tachycardia and (2) the anatomic site of origin of the ventricular tachycardia. Sustained monomorphic ventricular tachycardia can be easily mapped intraoperatively, and its site of origin can be identified without difficulty. Proper localization of the site of origin of nonsustained monomorphic ventricular tachycardia may be difficult intraoperatively unless an electrophysiologic mapping system capable of recording multiple electrograms simultaneously is available.[28] In general, these types of arrhythmias must be treated with a less localized procedure than those employed for tachycardias that are sustained long enough for accurate intraoperative localization of the arrhythmogenic site. Likewise, polymorphic ventricular tachycardia routinely requires one of the less localized procedures.

VENTRICULAR TACHYARRHYTHMIAS ARISING IN THE ANTERIOR OR LATERAL LEFT VENTRICLE

If the anterior left ventricular septum is found to be the arrhythmogenic site, and the tachycardia is sustained and monomorphic so that the site of origin can be precisely identified, resection of the local fibrosis may be sufficient to ablate the tachycardia. If the tachycardia cannot be mapped sufficiently because it is nonsustained, all of the visible endocardial fibrosis should be resected to avoid the likelihood of recurrence postoperatively (Fig. 24–23). If the tachycardia arising in this region is polymorphic, we have found it necessary not only to resect all of the endocardial fibrosis associated with the left ventricular aneurysm, but also to perform endocardial cryoablation in the area that shows the greatest degree of fragmentation during normal sinus rhythm mapping. We approach tachycardias arising in the anterior free-wall and in the lateral free-wall in the same manner.

If the anterior papillary muscle can be demonstrated to be the arrhythmogenic site of either a sustained or nonsustained monomorphic tachycardia, we perform endocardial cryoablation of the lower two thirds of the papillary muscle. If the tachycardia appears to be arising from the anterior papillary muscle but is polymorphic, all of the endocardial fibrosis associated with the aneurysm is resected, and endocardial cryoablation is applied to the lower two thirds of the papillary muscle.

VENTRICULAR TACHYARRHYTHMIAS ARISING IN THE POSTERIOR LEFT VENTRICLE

Ventricular tachyarrhythmias arising in the posterior region of the left ventricle are more difficult to treat surgically than those arising in the anterior or lateral left ventricle, because of two technical problems. The first involves the difficulty in mapping in these patients, even with a sustained ventricular tachycardia, because of the necessity to retract the ventricular apex out of the pericardial sac. A longitudinal left ventriculotomy must be placed between the base of the posterior papillary muscle and the posterior interventricular septum, and the posterior endocardium must then be mapped through this posterior ventriculotomy. Such retraction of the heart frequently induces significant aortic insufficiency, which may preclude one's ability to identify accurately the site of origin of the arrhythmia. The second technical problem in this region involves the potential disruption of either the aortic or

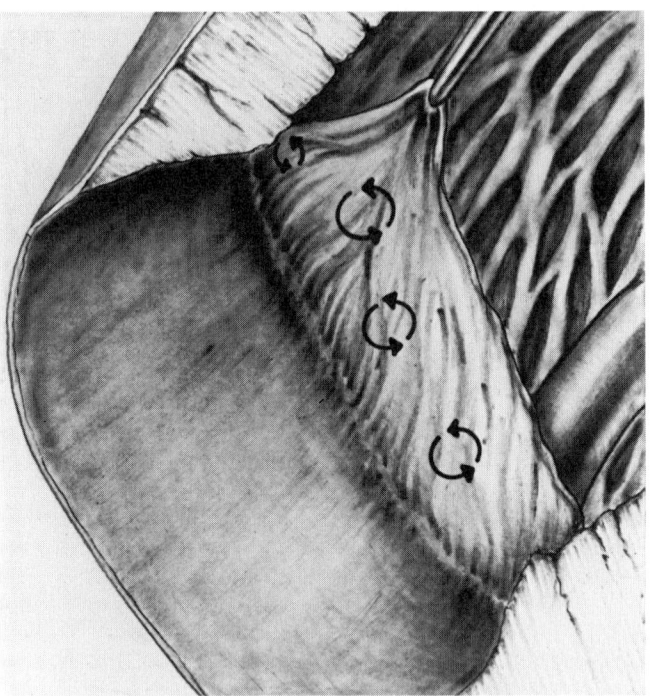

FIGURE 24–23
Diagrammatic sketch of an "extended endocardial resection procedure" in which *all* of the endocardial fibrosis associated with the anterior aneurysm is resected. This procedure is usually employed for the treatment of ventricular tachycardia with multiple sites of origin (polymorphic ventricular tachycardia) or when the site of origin of the tachycardia cannot be adequately localized by intraoperative electrophysiologic mapping. (Reprinted by permission from Cox JL: In Cohn LH (ed.): Modern Technics in Surgery, pp. 1–18. Mount Kisco, Futura Publishing Co., 1985.)

the mitral valve apparatus by the surgical procedure itself. It has been our experience that these tachyarrhythmias usually originate very close to the junction of the aortic and mitral valves and that resection of the endocardial fibrosis to within 3 to 5 mm of the valve annuli frequently does not interrupt the tachycardia. These technical difficulties are magnified if the patient has only a posterior myocardial infarction rather than a posterior left ventricular aneurysm associated with the ventricular tachycardia.

Regardless of whether or not the site of origin of the tachycardia can be identified, we routinely resect all of the fibrosis associated with posterior infarcts or aneurysms except that involving the papillary muscle. In the latter case, we apply endocardial cryosurgery to the base of the papillary muscle in all cases. If the site of origin of the tachycardia can be identified by intraoperative mapping, we apply endocardial cryosurgery to that site (or sites) *after* resection of the endocardial scar. If the tachycardia cannot be localized satisfactorily within the posterior septum or posterior papillary muscle because it is either nonsustained or polymorphic, we resect all of the endocardial fibrosis and apply endocardial cryolesions along the aortic and mitral valve annuli and over the base of the posterior papillary muscle (Fig. 24–24).

It is apparent that the specific surgical procedure applied in a given patient with refractory ischemic ventricular tachycardia must be tailored to the anatomic and electrophysiologic characteristics presented in each individual case. We believe that it is extremely important to perform these surgical procedures during induced ventricular tachycardia, when the arrhythmia is sustained, or to perform the procedures in the beating, nonworking heart in the case of nonsustained ventricular tachycardia. Immediately after performing the specific endocardial surgical procedure, we repeatedly attempt to reinduce the arrhythmia until we are convinced that it can no longer be induced. By performing the procedures without utilizing cardioplegic arrest, the potential temporary salutory effects of hypothermia and of the cardioplegic solution itself are eliminated. It is our belief that the 30% reinducibility rate of ventricular tachycardia at the time of the postoperative electrophysiologic study in most reported series is related to the fact that the surgical procedures were performed during cardioplegic arrest, and that the temporary effects of hypothermia and/or cardioplegia resulted in the lack of inducibility in the operating room immediately following surgery, despite the fact that the tachycardia could be induced 7 to 10 days later in one of every three patients.

A question that should be addressed is whether or not it is necessary to perform intraoperative electrophysiologic mapping to attain satisfactory results with surgical procedures for ventricular tachyarrhythmias. The presence of a visible anatomic substrate (endocardial fibrosis) that is known to harbor all or a portion of the reentrant circuit responsible for ischemic ventricular tachycardia provides the surgeon with a means of focusing the surgical intervention without the assistance of intraoperative mapping techniques. This fact

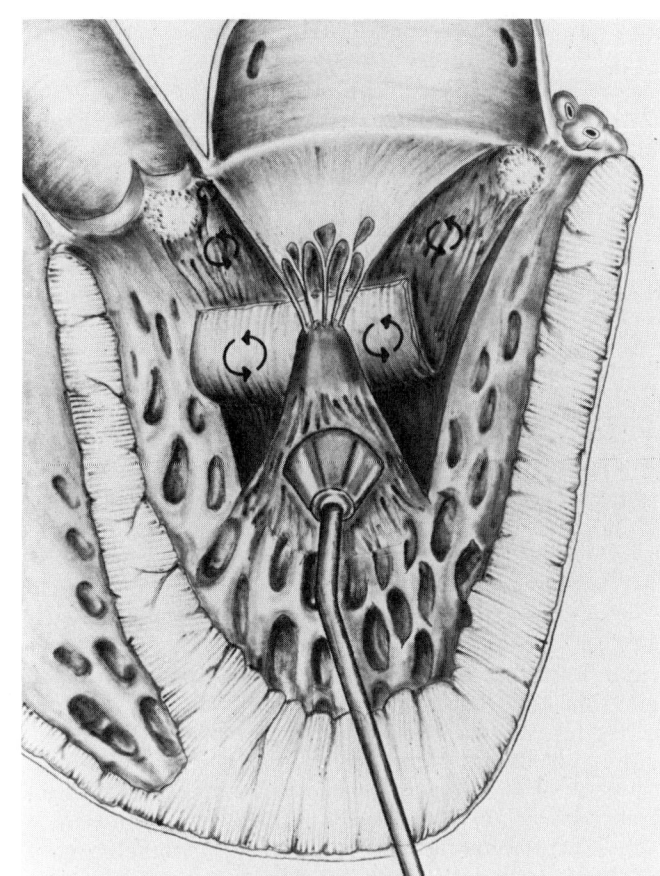

FIGURE 24–24
Extended endocardial resection of the fibrosis associated with a posterior myocardial infarction or aneurysm and cryoablation of the lower two thirds of the posterior papillary muscle. The endocardial fibrosis is resected to within 5 mm of the aortic and mitral valve annuli. Since the site of origin of the ventricular tachycardia is frequently adjacent to the junction of the aortic and mitral valve annuli, endocardial cryolesions (white circles) are applied at the base of the aortic and mitral valve annuli to ablate any reentrant circuits that might reside in the remaining endocardial fibrosis immediately beneath the valve annuli. (Reprinted by permission from Cox JL: In Cohn LH (ed.): Modern Technics in Surgery, pp. 1–18. Mount Kisco, Futura Publishing Co., 1985.)

has led to the increasingly common practice of simply resecting or encircling the fibrotic myocardium for treatment of ischemic ventricular tachycardia, while making no attempt at precise localization of the arrhythmogenic myocardium. These surgical procedures without electrophysiologic guidance, while not as effective as electrophysiologically guided ones, have one major advantage: they can be used, with reasonable results, for urgent or emergent cases to solve a lethal problem in institutions with no electrophysiologic mapping capabilities. Under such circumstances, procedures without electrophysiologic guidance are most appropriate.

If such an approach is taken routinely, however, the surgical treatment of these complex arrhythmias becomes a completely service-oriented exercise. Although delivery of such a service is of undeniable importance, the potential for learning more about these complex and lethal arrhythmias is lost unless each patient is studied as comprehensively as possible. Since 1978, fewer than 1000 patients worldwide have been treated by one of the direct endocardial surgical techniques. If we are going to propose an intelligent approach to the numerically overwhelming problem of sudden death from cardiac causes, it is mandatory that we subject every patient with the unique clinical problem of refractory ischemic ventricular tachycardia to extensive electrophysiologic study.

We must remember that the only true model of ischemic ventricular tachycardia is the human being. The immediate benefits of our present state of knowledge may be offered with gratifying results to a few patients. However, unless these operations are performed in association with the appropriate electrophysiologic studies, we may be doing an immense disservice to a much larger group of future patients. Just as the electrophysiologic expertise and surgical principles learned from the earlier approaches to surgery for the WPW syndrome paved the way for the wider application of ventricular tachycardia surgery, scientific approaches to the latter problem will hopefully guide us toward the development of electrophysiologic predictors of sudden cardiac death. The establishment of such electrophysiologic indexes, based on a more complete understanding of ischemic ventricular tachyarrhythmias, might then lead to the development of pharmacologic and/or nonpharmacologic measures to prevent sudden deaths caused by arrhythmias.

References

1. Witkowski FX, Corr PB: An automated simultaneous transmural cardiac mapping system. Am J Physiol 247:H661, 1984.
2. Kramer JB, Corr PB, Cox JL, et al.: Arrhythmia and conduction disturbances: Simultaneous computer mapping to facilitate intraoperative localization of accessory pathways in patients with Wolff-Parkinson-White syndrome. Am J Cardiol 56:571, 1985.
3. Cox JL, Gallagher JJ, Cain ME: Experience with 118 consecutive patients undergoing surgery for the Wolff-Parkinson-White syndrome. J Thorac Cardiovasc Surg 90:490, 1985.
4. Gallagher JJ, Sealy WC, Cox JL, et al.: Results of surgery for pre-excitation caused by accessory atrioventricular pathways in 267 consecutive cases. In Josephson ME, Wellens HJJ (eds.): Tachycardias: Mechanisms, Diagnosis, Treatment, 1st Ed., pp. 259–269. Philadelphia, Lea & Febiger, 1984.
5. Klein GJ, Guiraudon GM, Perkins DG, et al.: Surgical correction of the Wolff-Parkinson-White syndrome in the closed heart using cryosurgery: A simplified approach. J Am Coll Cardiol 3:405, 1984.
6. Gallagher JJ, Sealy WC, Cox JL, et al.: Results of surgery for preexcitation in 200 cases (Abstract). Circulation 64(Suppl IV):IV-146, 1981.
7. Cox JL: Editorial: Current status of cardiac arrhythmia surgery. Circulation 71:413, 1985.
8. Morady F, Scheinman MM: Transvenous catheter ablation of a posteroseptal accessory pathway in a patient with the Wolff-Parkinson-White syndrome. N Engl J Med 310:705, 1984.
9. Fisher JD, Brodman R, Kim SG, et al.: Attempted nonsurgical electrical ablation of accessory pathways via the coronary sinus in the Wolff-Parkinson-White syndrome. J Am Coll Cardiol 4:685, 1984.
10. Sealy WC, Gallagher JJ, Kasell JH: His bundle interruption for control of inappropriate ventricular responses to atrial arrhythmias. Ann Thorac Surg 32:429, 1981.
11. Scheinman MM, Morady F, Hess DS, et al.: Catheter-induced ablation of the atrioventricular junction to control refractory supraventricular arrhythmias. JAMA 248:851, 1982.
12. Holman WL, Ikeshita M, Lease JG, et al.: Elective prolongation of atrioventricular conduction by multiple cryolesions. J Thorac Cardiovasc Surg 84:554, 1982.
13. Holman WL, Ikeshita M, Lease JG, et al.: Alteration of antegrade atrioventricular conduction by cryoablation of peri-atrioventricular nodal tissue. J Thorac Cardiovasc Surg 88:67, 1984.
14. Cox JL: Surgery for cardiac arrhythmias. In Harvey WP (ed.): Current Problems in Cardiology, pp. 7–60. Chicago, Yearbook, 1983.
15. Holman WL, Ikeshita M, Lease JG, et al.: Cryosurgical modification of retrograde atrioventricular conduction. Implications for the surgical treatment of atrioventricular nodal reentry tachycardia. J Thorac Cardiovasc Surg 91:826, 1986.
16. Cox JL, Holman WL, Cain ME: Cryosurgical treatment of atrioventricular node reentry tachycardia. Circulation 76:1329, 1987.
17. Mazur P: Physical-chemical factors underlying cell injury in cryosurgical freezing. In Rand RW, Rinfret PR, Von Leden H (eds.): Cryosurgery, p. 32. Springfield, Charles C Thomas, 1968.
18. Gallagher JJ, Cox JL, German LD, et al.: Nonpharmacologic treatment of supraventricular tachycardia. In Josephson ME, Wellens HJJ (eds.): Tachycardias: Mechanisms, Diagnosis, and Treatment, 1st Ed. pp. 271–285. Philadelphia, Lea & Febiger, 1984.
19. Williams JM, Ungerleider RM, Lofland GK, et al.: Left atrial isolation: A new technique for the treatment of supraventricular arrhythmias. J Thorac Cardiovasc Surg 80:373, 1980.
20. Harada A, D'Agostino HJ Jr, Schuessler RB, et al.: Right atrial isolation: A new surgical treatment for supraventricular tachycardia. I. Surgical technique and electrophysiologic effects. J Thorac Cardiovasc Surg 95:643–650, 1988.
21. Boineau JP, Wylds AC, Autry LJ, et al.: Mechanisms of atrial flutter as determined from spontaneous and experimental models. In Josephson ME, Wellens HJJ (eds.): Tachycardias: Mechanisms, Diagnosis, and Treatment, pp. 91–111. Philadelphia, Lea & Febiger, 1984.
22. Allessie MA, Lammers WJEP, Bonke IM, et al.: Intra-atrial reentry as a mechanism for atrial flutter induced by acetylcholine and rapid pacing in the dog. Circulation 70:123, 1984.
23. Salomon N, Stinson E, Randall B, et al.: Patient related risk factors as predictors of results following isolated mitral valve replacement. Ann Thorac Surg 24:519, 1977.
24. Cox JL: Surgical treatment of ischemic and non-ischemic ventricular tachyarrhythmias. In Cohn LH (ed.): Modern Technics in Surgery, pp. 1–18. Mount Kisco, Futura, 1985.
25. Guiraudon G, Fontaine G, Frank R, et al.: Surgical treatment of ventricular tachycardia guided by ventricular mapping in 23 patients without coronary artery disease. Ann Thorac Surg 32:439, 1981.
26. Cox JL, Brady GH, Damiano RJ, et al.: Right ventricular isolation procedures for non-ischemic ventricular tachycardia. J Thorac Cardiovasc Surg 90:212, 1985.
27. Fontaine G, Guiraudon G, Frank R: Management of chronic ventricular tachycardia. In Narula OS (ed.): Innovations in Diagnosis and Management of Cardiac Arrhythmias, pp. 516–545. Baltimore, Williams & Wilkins, 1979.
28. Cox JL: Intraoperative computerized mapping techniques: Do they help us to treat our patients better surgically? In Brugada P, Wellens I (eds.): Proceedings of 20 Years of Programmed Electrical Stimultion of the Heart, pp. 613–637. Mount Kisco: Futura, 1987.
29. Cox JL: The surgical management of cardiac arrhythmias. Cardiovasc Clin 18(1) 21:207, 1987.

25

Catheter Ablation Techniques for Supraventricular Tachyarrhythmias

Fred Morady

A relatively recent development in the field of clinical electrophysiology has been the therapeutic application of intracardiac direct-current shocks to eliminate symptomatic, drug-refractory tachycardias. Catheter ablation techniques were first directed toward creating third-degree atrioventricular (AV) block without the need for open heart surgery.[1,2] Subsequently, catheter ablation techniques have also been aimed at ablation of accessory AV connections and atrial and ventricular tachycardias. The purpose of this chapter is to review the catheter ablation techniques that have been used to treat patients who have supraventricular tachyarrhythmias, including ablation of the AV junction, accessory AV connections, and atrial tachycardia foci. Although other forms of energy such as radiofrequency, laser, thermal, and microwave energy recently also have been investigated for their potential use in catheter ablation, the most clinical experience by far has been with the use of direct-current shocks. This chapter will therefore concentrate on the data regarding the use of direct-current shocks for catheter ablation. The current status of radiofrequency and laser energy for use in catheter ablation will also be reviewed. Published data on the use of thermal[3] and microwave[4] energy are scant and will not be reviewed here.

Biophysics of Transcatheter Direct-Current Shocks

In vitro studies have been performed using both clear media and blood to investigate biophysical aspects of direct-current shocks. Although the effects of shocks in clear media such as saline or Ringer's solution may not accurately predict the effects of transcatheter shocks in whole blood, the use of clear media has the advantage of allowing direct observations of the electrode tip.

Studies utilizing a standard defibrillator back paddle and a catheter submerged in a tank of Ringer's solution have demonstrated that delivery of a shock is associated with an intense flash of light and the generation of gas bubbles around the electrode.[5] The size of the flash increases as the energy level of the shock increases and, for shocks of 400 joules, the diameter of the flash is approximately 2 cm (Fig. 25–1). Fine, bright tracks may be observed within the flash. High-speed cinephotography demonstrates an incandescent globe that

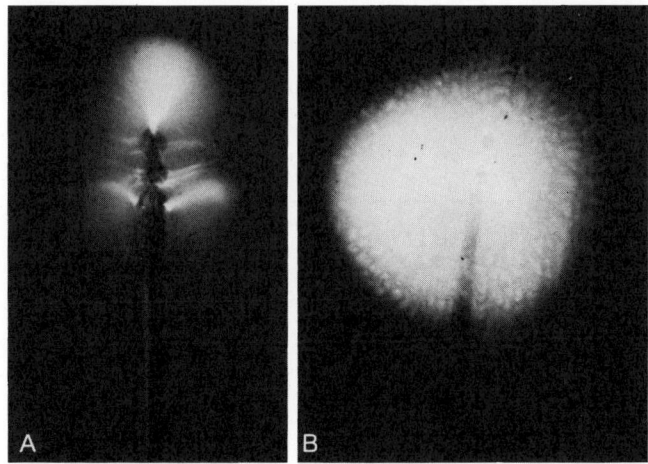

FIGURE 25–1
Time exposures (35 mm) of transcatheter shocks delivered in a tank of Ringer's solution. A, A 400-joule shock delivered through a No. 6 French bipolar electrode catheter. B, A 50 joule shock delivered through an active fixation electrode catheter.
The scalloped surface of the vapor-gas bubble and intrabubble arcing can be seen. (Photographs courtesy of Dr. E. G. C. A. Boyd.) (Reprinted by permission from Boyd EGCA, Holt PM: J Electrophysiol 1:62, 1987.)

453

forms around the electrode tip and subsequently collapses into a fine mist of gas that then condenses into discrete gas bubbles that rise away from the electrode. A pressure wave of over 1 atmosphere can be measured 3 cm from the electrode. The temperature at the time of the electrode during delivery of the pulse exceeds 1700° C. Voltage and current recordings during delivery of the shock generally show a smooth current waveform and a discontinuous and irregular voltage waveform (Fig. 25-2).

Boyd and Holt[6] have explained the sequence of events during delivery of a shock in Ringer's solution in the following fashion. At the onset of current flow, energy dissipated into the medium surrounding the electrode tip results in a rapid rise in temperature and vaporization of the liquid in contact with the electrode. The high current field strength in the last of the vapor film to be formed may initiate ionization, producing streams of ionized particles (arcing) in the vapor volume surrounding the electrode. The arcing phenomenon results in high temperatures, a light flash, and intraelectrode impedance discontinuities that account for the discontinuous voltage waveform. A further increase in current produces more vaporization, and rapid expansion of the bubble generates a positive pressure wave.

In vitro studies of the effects of shocks delivered in tanks of whole blood have provided additional information about the biophysics of transcatheter shocks. Bardy et al.,[7] after immersing an electrode catheter and a 8.5-cm disk representing a chest electrode in a tank of bovine blood, delivered damped sinusoidal shocks, using the electrode catheter as either the anode or cathode. Bubble and gas formation was found to be directly related to the energy delivered, indirectly related to the electrode surface area, and highly dependent on the electrode polarity. At a 200-joule pulse setting, anodal shocks generated approximately 50 times more gas than cathodal shocks. The gas composition included nitrogen, oxygen, carbon dioxide, argon, and hydrogen and could not be explained by simple hydrolysis. The genesis of the gas in the bubbles may be related to high-pressure shock waves, which force gases such as nitrogen out of solution, and to direct thermal dissociation of water.

Bardy and coworkers[7] demonstrated that smooth voltage and current waveforms occurred only in the absence of bubbles, and that the process of bubble formation was associated with distorted voltage waveforms resulting from impedance changes near the electrode (Fig. 25-3). These investigators suggested the following sequence of events. The onset of current flow is associated with hydrolysis that generates enough gas to create a bubble large enough to insulate the electrode from the blood. Current flow to the blood therefore is temporarily interrupted and impedance rises. There is then a rise in voltage between the bubble-insulated electrode and the surrounding blood. As the electric field strength increases, electrons enter the bubble that surrounds the electrode. When the electrode density becomes sufficient, there is arcing of current between the electrode and the surrounding blood. As would occur in a clear medium, arcing is associated with a light flash and a large rise in temperature in the bubble. The high temperature in turn causes the bubble volume to expand rapidly, resulting in a high-pressure shock wave.

Studies of the effects of transcatheter shocks in whole blood have clearly demonstrated that anodal shocks are associated with considerably more hemolysis and gas formation and a larger magnitude high-pressure shock waves than are cathodal shocks (Fig. 25-4).[7, 8] Because complications related to bubble embolization and barotrauma are more likely to occur with shocks delivered in an anodal fashion, it may be preferable to use cathodal shocks for catheter ablation.

Mechanisms of Tissue Injury

The possible mechanisms by which transcatheter shocks result in tissue injury include thermal injury, barotrauma, and the adverse cellular effects of electrical current.

Most of the available data suggest that thermal injury is unlikely to play a major role in the tissue damage caused by catheter ablation procedures. Despite very high temperatures at the tip of the electrode used to deliver a shock, in vitro measurements of the temperature at the endocardium and within the myocardium have indicated that tissue temperatures remain low as long as the endocardium is in contact with blood.[9] It is possible that a gas film adjacent to the endocardial wall provides thermal insulation.[6] A study comparing the thermal effects of laser and direct-current shocks demonstrated that endocardial temperature changes were smaller with the electrical shocks.[10] Nevertheless, tissue temperature 2 mm from the site of delivery of a 200-joule shock increased approximately 15° C imme-

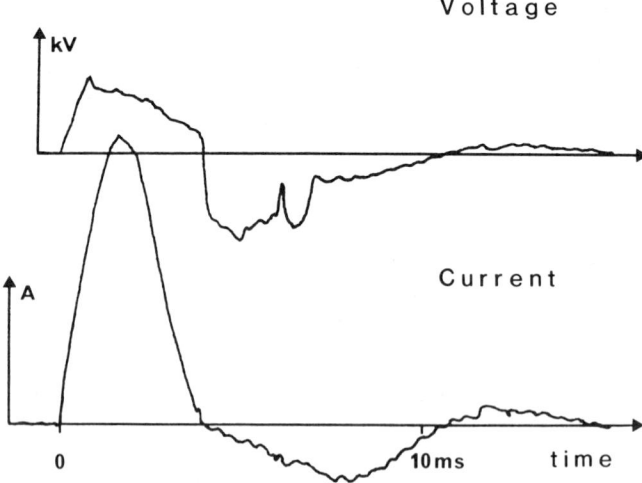

FIGURE 25-2
Voltage and current recordings for a 50-joule shock delivered in a clear medium. The voltage recording is discontinuous, indicating voltage breakdown caused by arcing. (Figure courtesy of Dr. E. G. C. A. Boyd.) (Reprinted by permission from Boyd EGCA, Holt PM: J Electrophysiol 1:62, 1987.)

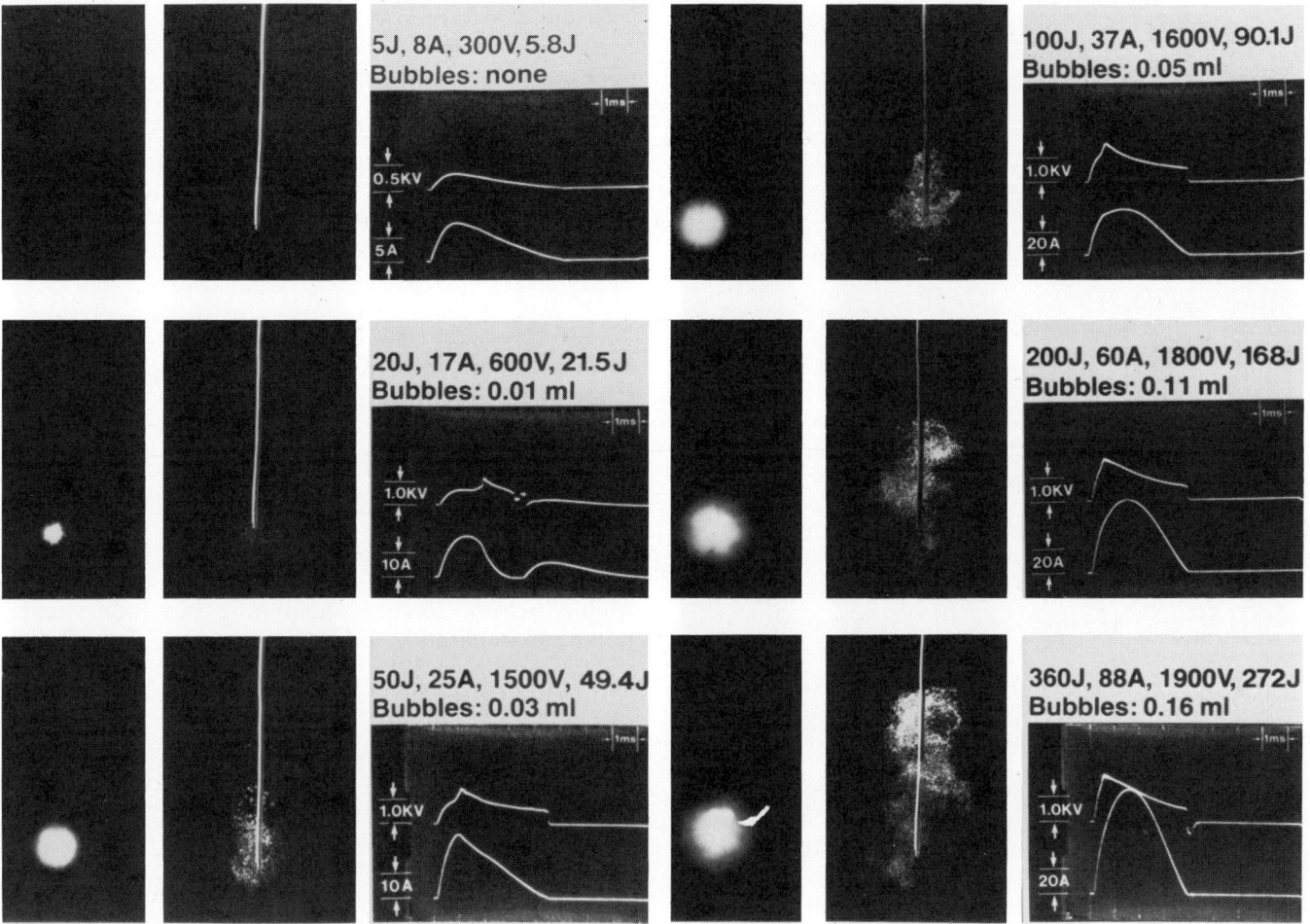

FIGURE 25–3
Flash, bubbles, and voltage and current recordings during anodal shocks of increasing strength in saline. Flashes resulting from arcing are shown on the left; the resulting bubbles seen within 1 second later are shown in the middle; and the voltage and current waveforms are shown on the right. The energy setting, peak delivered current and voltage, delivered energy, and bubble volume are shown for each shock. Note that a 5-joule shock does not cause arcing or gas formation and that the voltage and current waveforms maintain a damped sinusoidal configuration. However, there is arcing and gas formation during 20- to 360-joule shocks, and the amount of arcing and gas formation increases as the energy increases. The voltage waveform shows a rise two thirds to one third of the way through the discharge, probably correlating with a rise in impedance from electrolysis gas insulting the electrode. (Figure courtesy of Dr. G. H. Bardy.) (Reprinted by permission of the American Heart Association, Inc., from Bardy GH, Coltorti F, Ivey TD, et al.: Circulation 73:525, 1986.)

diately after the shock and remained elevated for nearly 1 minute, suggesting that some thermal injury may occur.[10] However, whereas thermal injury would be expected to cause coagulation necrosis, several histologic studies have demonstrated contraction band necrosis at sites of shock delivery.[11–13] Based on these data, thermal injury may not be a major therapeutic mechanism during catheter ablation but nevertheless may contribute to tissue injury.

The role of barotrauma in catheter ablation has remained controversial. On the one hand, pressure recordings from within the myocardium demonstrate that significant pressure pulses occur in response to transcatheter shocks,[9] and barotraumatic damage to cardiac structures can be demonstrated in vitro. For example, a 200-joule shock delivered within the coronary sinus of an isolated sheep heart may rupture the wall of the coronary sinus.[6] Histologic studies in dogs who received 200 to 300-joule shocks at the os of the coronary sinus have consistently demonstrated rupture of the internal elastica of the coronary sinus and displacement of tissue, which is consistent with barotrauma.[14] Furthermore, histologic examination in a patient who died 5 months after undergoing successful catheter ablation of AV conduction with a single 275-joule shock demonstrated selective loss of AV nodal tissue and no damage to the fibrous stroma, vascular system, or endocardium in the vicinity of the AV node.[15] This histologic picture was thought to be consistent with barotrauma.[15]

On the other hand, there are also data that suggest that barotrauma is not an important mechanism of tissue injury during catheter ablation. First, lower-energy non-arcing defibrillator pulses that are not associated with high-pressure shock waves may be successful in ablating arrhythmogenic tissue. Second, although mechanical shock waves can produce myocardial injury due to shearing stresses,[16] the injury

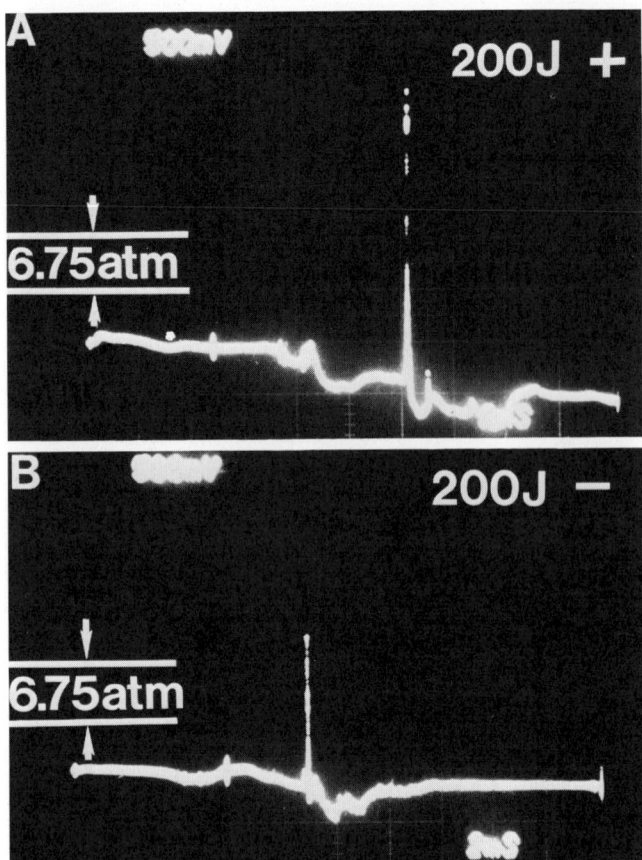

FIGURE 25—4
Shock waves recorded in bovine blood with a pressure transducer positioned 2 cm from the electrode. A, A 200-joule anodal shock. The shock wave measures 38.5 atmospheres, or 29,260 mm Hg. B, A 200-joule cathodal shock, which generates a shock wave of 18.9 atmospheres, or 14,364 mm Hg. These shock waves are responsible for the barotrauma that may be associated with the delivery of intracardiac shocks. (Figure courtesy of Dr. G. H. Bardy. Reprinted by permission of the American Heart Association, Inc., from Bardy GH, Coltorti F, Ivey TD, et al.: Circulation 73:525, 1986.)

occurs not only at the point of impact but also distant from the point of impact.[17] In contrast, the histologic abnormalities in animals that receive transcatheter shocks are localized to the shock site, and usually there are no signs of myocardial cell rupture to suggest barotrauma. Third, an in vitro study demonstrated that myocardial tissue specimens 3 mm and 15 mm thick failed to absorb any energy from the shock wave associated with a high-energy arcing pulse in a tank of saline.[18]

Based on the above observations and data, it appears that barotrauma probably plays an important role in complications of catheter ablation such as coronary sinus rupture; however, it may not be a major mechanism by which transcatheter shocks exert their therapeutic effect.

A likely mechanism of tissue injury during catheter ablation appears to be damage to cells by electrical current. The distribution of histologic and cellular electrophysiologic abnormalities usually corresponds with the distribution of the electric field.[11, 19] In addition, the findings of contraction band necrosis and polarization of cell nuclei are consistent with exposure to electrical current.[11-13] Studies in cultured myocytes exposed to electric field stimulation have suggested that microlesions are produced in the sarcolemma by compression of the membrane by the electric field.[20] These data suggest that catheter ablation procedures may be more likely to be effective if the current density in the target tissue is maximized.

Cellular Electrophysiologic Effects of Direct-Current Shocks

The cellular electrophysiologic effects of direct-current shocks have been studied by Levine et al.[11] These investigators recorded action potentials at varying distances from the site of delivery of 5- to 40-joule shocks in isolated sections of epicardial tissue from normal canine hearts. Resting membrane potential, action potential amplitude, and the rate of rise of the action potential were each decreased after delivery of a shock, with the changes becoming more severe closer to the site of energy delivery.

It is noteworthy that the area of myocardial cell damage, as reflected by action potential abnormalities, was extensive relative to the size of the cathode. Although the cathode was less than 2 mm in diameter, significant abnormalities in the action potential were observed 5 to 10 mm away from the shock site. The extent of the electrophysiologic abnormalities was greater than the extent of histologic abnormalities, implying that there may be a relatively larger border zone of injured but viable myocardium surrounding an ablation site.

Current density and the electrode configuration were found to be important determinants of the extent of injury.[11] Action potential abnormalites were most severe in the myocardial cells that lay between the cathode and the anode, presumably because these cells were subject to a greater current density. The histologic abnormalities were consistent with this observation, with contraction band necrosis being present at a greater distance from the cathode in the direction of the anode than in the opposite direction. These findings suggest that the cathode-anode orientation may influence the outcome of catheter ablation procedures.

The study by Levine and coworkers[11] also demonstrated alterations in conduction and repolarization that might account for the proarrhythmic effects of intracardiac shocks. Non-uniform decreases in conduction velocity and action potential duration were found to occur in the border zone, and these alterations might predispose to reentrant arrhythmias. In addition, secondary depolarizations of varying amplitude were observed during the plateau phase of the action potential, at times associated with the propagation of spontaneous premature responses. It was felt that these secondary depolarizations may have represented true afterdepolarizations or may have resulted from an electrotonic interaction between cells that remained electrically coupled but separated by tissue exhibiting varying degrees of conduction block.

Electrode Catheters Used for Ablation

The majority of catheter ablation procedures have been performed using standard electrode catheters intended for use as temporary pacing leads and not for delivery of high-energy shocks. High-energy shocks of 100 to 300 joules may expose these catheters to an energy level several million times greater than the energy level of the pacing stimuli that the catheters were intended to deliver. Therefore, it is not surprising that these pacing catheters may not be able to withstand high-energy direct-current shocks.

Fisher and colleagues[21] performed in vitro testing of various types and brands of electrode catheters. A series of 25- to 320-joule cathodal shocks were delivered through the catheters in a tank of saline. The catheters were inspected after each shock, and the resistance to the distal and proximal electrodes was measured periodically. Several types of lead failures were observed, including internal wire failure, electrode failure, connector disruption, sheath distortion, separation of the tip electrode, sheath perforations, and interelectrode shredding of the sheath. It is notable that USCI 6 and 7 French standard production catheters, which are the types of catheters that have been most commonly used in catheter ablation procedures, were able to withstand multiple 320-joule shocks. The study demonstrated that there is significant variability in the ability of various types of catheters to withstand high-energy shocks, indicating the importance of in vitro lead testing prior to the use of a particular catheter model for ablation procedures in humans.

It is important to realize that catheter-related problems may arise during ablation procedures even in the absence of any visible catheter defects or abnormalities in lead resistance as measured by an ohmmeter. Bardy et al.[22] measured the dielectric strength (defined as the voltage at which current leakage occurs through the insulation separating the electrodes) of No. 6 French USCI catheters before and after delivery of 200- and 360-joule anodal shocks.[22] The dielectric strength of unused catheters ranged between 2200 and 3500 volts (2780 ± 517 volts, mean + standard deviation). After a single 200-joule shock delivered to the distal electrode of a tripolar catheter, the dielectric strength ranged from 100 to 3500 volts (mean 1325 ± 1320 volts). When shocks were delivered to the two proximal electrodes of a quadripolar catheter, as may be done in posteroseptal accessory pathway ablations, the mean dielectric strength was 1425 ± 826 volts after a 200-joule shock, and only 601 ± 707 volts after a 360-joule shock. These dielectric strengths were often lower than the peak delivered voltage, which ranged from 2300 to 3400 volts for 200-joule shocks and from 3900 to 4400 volts for 360-joule shocks.

These data indicate that there is a high likelihood of current leakage when high-energy shocks are delivered through standard electrode catheters, especially after one shock has already been delivered. The potential for misdirected shocks was confirmed by the observation that electrode pitting, a manifestation of platinum melting that usually occurs on the electrode used to deliver a shock, at times also was found on electrodes that had not been connected to the defibrillator.[22] Current leakage and misdirected shocks may account for failure of an attempted ablation procedure and may also result in complications. The potential for undesired current leakage may be lessened by minimizing the energy level of the shocks and by not using a catheter for delivery of more than one shock.

The development of new types of catheters may result in greater precision of catheter ablation procedures. For example, a suction electrode catheter actively fixed to atrial endocardium at the level of the His bundle may allow better control of energy delivery than when a shock is delivered to a catheter floating near the His bundle. Saksena et al.[23] have demonstrated that successful ablation of the AV junction often can be achieved with relatively low-energy shocks (20–30 joules) when a suction electrode catheter is used. Improved localization of energy delivery to target tissues will allow the use of lower-energy shocks and may reduce the risk of complications. However, clinical experience with the use of suction catheters for ablation procedures has not yet been published.

The problem of plasma arcing during delivery of high-energy shocks has been addressed by alterations in catheter design. Arcing is initiated at the junction of the electrode and insulation, and non-uniform current density at the electrode surface reduces the arcing threshold. Cunningham and coworkers[24] have designed a new catheter in which the electrode and insulation are interfaced at right angles and in which there is uniform current density in the distal electrode. In vitro testing has demonstrated a 73% increase in arcing threshold with this catheter compared to conventional catheters of the same gauge. Although clinical experience with this catheter is very preliminary as yet, it appears that delivery of high-energy shocks may be possible without adverse effects caused by arcing.

Defibrillators Used for Ablation

Standard direct current defibrillators usually have been employed for catheter ablation, and the most commonly used waveform has been a damped sinusoid. Other types of waveforms include the exponential and truncated exponential. Although the form of the pulse may influence the results of catheter ablation, the efficacy of the various waveforms has not been compared in clinical studies.

Modification of the energy source may minimize undesirable arcing. For example, a reduction in shock duration may allow higher current to be delivered without arcing. Accordingly, Rowland and colleagues[25] have developed a new "ablater" capable of delivering stored energy three to four times faster than a standard defibrillator. Their preliminary experience with this energy source suggests that it may allow for successful ablation with low-energy non-arcing shocks.[25]

Catheter Ablation of the AV Junction

INDICATIONS

Potential indications for ablation of the AV junction include the following:

1. Atrial tachyarrhythmias, such as atrial fibrillation, atrial flutter, and atrial tachycardia, in which symptoms are attributable to a rapid ventricular response that results from conduction solely through the AV node–His bundle axis.
2. Any tachyarrhythmia that depends on participation of the AV node–His bundle axis for the initiation or maintenance of the tachycardia such as AV nodal reentrant tachycardia; orthodromic reciprocating tachycardia in which the AV node–His bundle axis serves as the anterograde limb of the tachycardia circuit; the permanent form of AV junctional reciprocating tachycardia; and tachycardias involving an accessory nodoventricular connection, in which the AV node–His bundle axis serves as the retrograde limb of the reentry circuit.[26, 27]

If AV junctional ablation is being performed with the intent of preventing AV reciprocating tachycardia in a patient with an accessory AV connection, anterograde conduction properties of the accessory AV connection must be carefully evaluated, because AV junction ablation would not eliminate the risk of a rapid ventricular rate during atrial fibrillation or flutter.

Ablation of the AV junction will eliminate symptoms caused by these tachycardias, but at the cost of inducing high-degree AV block, necessitating a permanent pacemaker. Therefore, ablation of the AV junction generally is indicated only in patients who are refractory to pharmacologic therapy and who cannot be better managed with other forms of nonpharmacologic therapy.

EXPERIMENTAL BACKGROUND

Gonzalez et al.[28] demonstrated that it was possible to induce complete AV block in dogs by delivering shocks through an electrode catheter positioned across the tricuspid valve. One to four cathodal shocks of 300 joules, delivered between the electrode that recorded the largest unipolar His bundle potential and a back plate, resulted in chronic, complete AV block in nine dogs. Angiographic and hemodynamic evaluation demonstrated no evidence of tricuspid insufficiency. The escape rhythm was infranodal in origin.

In a subsequent study, Gonzalez and coworkers[29] performed detailed histologic studies of the specialized cardiac conduction system 3 months after the induction of complete AV block in the same nine dogs they studied in their first report. Upon gross inspection of the hearts of these dogs, there was no evidence of damage to the heart valves, chordae tendineae, or papillary muscles. In the dogs who had received one shock, fibroelastosis was localized to the AV junction, whereas in the dogs who had received multiple shocks, fibroelastosis was more diffuse, involving not only the AV junction but also the adjacent atrial and ventricular myocardium. Histologic manifestations of injury included fatty infiltration, fibrosis, chronic inflammatory changes, giant cell infiltration, and at times basophilic degeneration and calcification of the conduction system. In all of the dogs there was damage to the approaches to the AV node, the AV node itself, and the penetrating His bundle. In the dogs who had received multiple shocks, there was also damage in the branching portion of the common bundle, the His bundle branches, and the summit of the ventricular septum. This study therefore demonstrated that catheter ablation of the AV junction in dogs was associated with no damage to the tricuspid valve, minimal damage to the myocardium, and extensive damage to the approaches to the AV node, the AV node itself, and the penetrating portion of the common bundle.

Bardy and colleagues[30] also performed a study of the electrophysiologic and histologic changes induced by catheter ablation of the AV junction in dogs. A standard No. 6 French tripolar electrode catheter was used to deliver cathodal shocks through the electrode that recorded the largest unipolar His bundle potential. A back paddle positioned between the spine and left scapula was used as the anode. Ten dogs each received a single shock of 280 joules (delivered). Complete AV block was induced acutely in all dogs; however, over a 4-week observation period, AV conduction returned in five dogs. In the dogs who had persistent, complete AV block, histologic examination 4 weeks after the catheter ablation procedure demonstrated extensive damage to the approaches to the AV node, the AV node itself, the penetrating His bundle, and the branching portion of the His bundle. Histologic evidence of injury included dense fibrosis and, at times, calcium deposits surrounded by granulomatous inflammation and giant cell formation. There was mild fibrosis at the base of the septal tricuspid leaflet; however, in no dog was there perforation or thinning of the atrial or ventricular septum. By planimetry of serial sections, the ventricular volume of injury was estimated to be less than 1% of the total myocardial mass.

Among the five dogs in which AV block was not persistent, only one had histologic evidence of extensive injury to the approaches to the AV node and to the AV node itself, whereas in the other four dogs there was either minimal or no damage noted in the AV node–His bundle axis. Therefore, as expected, there appeared to be an association between the extent of histologic injury to the AV conduction system and the electrophysiologic outcome after catheter ablation of the AV junction.

An additional observation reported in this study was that the ratio of the amplitudes of the atrial and His bundle electrograms recorded by the electrode used as the cathode was between 4 and 10 in the dogs in whom extensive damage to the AV conduction system was produced. In the dogs in whom minimal or no damage was produced, this ratio was usually less than 4 or greater than 10. This suggested that the catheter used to deliver the intracardiac shock could be positioned properly by locating an atrial electrogram which was large relative to the amplitude of the His bundle position. A second factor associated with successful catheter ablation of the AV junction appeared to be the electrode that was used as the cathode. Severe damage to the AV conduction system was produced in five of six dogs who received the shock through the distal electrode, but in only one of four dogs who received the shock through a more proximal electrode. The authors postulated that this might be because current flux is higher from the rounded, free end of a distal electrode than from a more proximal electrode that is adjacent to insulation on both sides.[30]

A study correlating the electrophysiologic and anatomic effects of direct-current shocks was performed by Scheinman et al.[31] In six dogs, a series of cathodal 20- to 240-joule shocks were delivered through barbed tip or screw-in electrode catheters fixated in the region of the AV node. In general, shocks of 20 to 180 joules resulted in damage to the approaches of the AV node, the AV node itself, and the common bundle, whereas shocks of larger energy resulted in diffuse damage involving the His bundle and bundle branches. Only minor functional changes in AV conduction were observed, despite histologic destruction of 50% or more of the AV conduction system. Therefore, there appears to be a large safety margin in AV conduction when shocks are delivered to the AV node.

The results obtained with fixation catheters appear to be very dependent on the location along the AV conduction system where the catheter is fixated. As discussed earlier in the section dealing with electrode catheters, Saksena et al.[23] demonstrated that it is possible to induce complete AV block in dogs by the selective delivery of 20- to 30-joule shocks to the His bundle with the use of a suction electrode catheter. In contrast, in the study by Scheinman et al.,[31] minimal changes in AV conduction were induced when shocks were selectively delivered to the AV node.

TECHNIQUE

A cannula inserted percutaneously into a femoral, brachial, or radial artery is used for continuous monitoring of blood pressure. An electrode catheter is placed in a stable position against the right ventricular apex, to be used for ventricular pacing after AV conduction is interrupted.

The electrode catheter that will be used to deliver the intracardiac shock is inserted percutaneously into a femoral vein and positioned across the tricuspid valve (Fig. 25–5). After a bipolar His bundle recording is obtained, the catheter is maneuvered to find the largest unipolar His bundle deflection possible, preferably recorded by the distal electrode. Because intracardiac shocks delivered to the distal portions of the AV

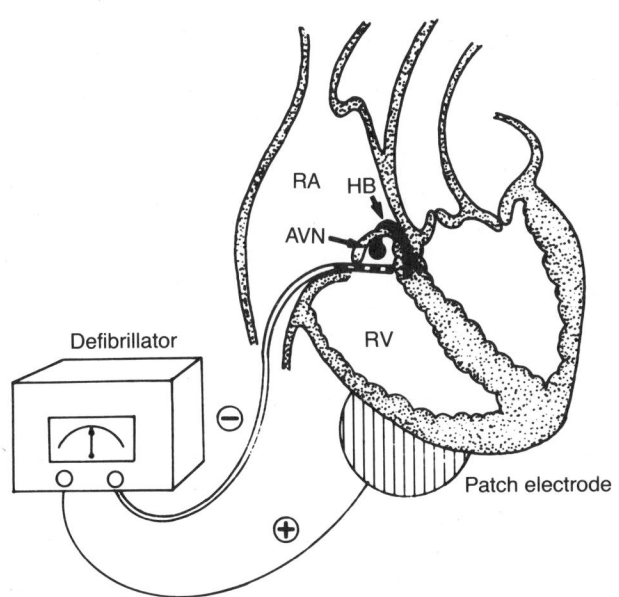

FIGURE 25–5
A schematic illustration of the technique used for ablation of the AV junction. An electrode catheter is positioned across the tricuspid valve such that the largest possible unipolar His bundle potential is recorded, preferably with the distal electrode. The electrode is connected to the cathodal output of a defibrillator, and a patch electrode in the region of the left scapula serves as the anode. Not shown is the temporary pacing catheter that must be in position in the right ventricle before the ablation is attempted.

conduction system are more likely to cause unwanted injury to ventricular myocardium, the catheter should be adjusted such that the largest atrial deflection possible is recorded, indicating a more proximal position. If the patient is in atrial fibrillation, and discrete atrial electrograms are not present, one should search for the longest H-V interval possible, which would also indicate a more proximal position of the catheter. The optimal catheter position should be visualized by fluoroscopy, and the position of the catheter relative to fixed landmarks, such as the vertebral column, should be noted. This is to enable appropriate positioning of the catheter if a second shock is necessary and the His bundle electrogram can no longer be recorded, as may occur after the first shock.

The electrode through which the largest His bundle and atrial electrograms are recorded is then connected by a cable to the cathodal output of a standard defibrillator. A back paddle or patch electrode is positioned adjacent to the left scapula and connected to the anodal sink of the defibrillator. The anesthesiologist who is in attendance then administers a short-acting general anesthetic. Immediately before delivering the shock, adequate ventricular capture by the back-up pacemaker is confirmed, and the position of the ablation catheter is checked by fluoroscopy. The intracardiac shock is then delivered, synchronized to the QRS complex. The optimal energy level of the shock is as yet undetermined but appears to be in the range of 200 to 300 joules. The capability for immediate external direct-current countershock must be available, should ventricular fibrillation or ventricular tachycardia occur as a complication of the intracardiac shock. If complete AV block is successfully induced, temporary pacing is initiated.

The patient is then monitored for 30 to 60 minutes in the electrophysiology laboratory. If AV conduction returns, a second intracardiac shock is delivered in the same manner as the first. As mentioned above, at times only a small or no His bundle electrogram can be recorded after the first shock, even when one-to-one AV conduction is present. If this is the case, the catheter should be positioned under fluoroscopic guidance in the same position that was used for the first shock.

If complete AV block persists for at least 1 hour, a His bundle electrogram is searched for to ascertain the level of block. The patient is then brought to the coronary care unit, where temporary pacing is continued at a rate of 60 to 70 per minute and the patient is monitored for 24 to 48 hours. If complete AV block persists, a permanent pacemaker is then implanted.

Modification of AV Conduction Instead of Ablation

The ideal catheter technique for treating patients who have drug-refractory supraventricular tachycardias would be one that modifies AV conduction and eliminates symptomatic tachycardia without inducing high-degree AV block or myocardial injury. McComb et al. reported that this may be possible in a small number of patients by using low-energy shocks of 20 to 50 joules.[38] However, shocks of this strength also may either result in complete AV block or have no effect at all on AV conduction. Therefore, catheter techniques will require further refinement before modification of AV conduction can be reliably achieved.

RESULTS

The Percutaneous Cardiac Mapping and Ablation Registry has collected data on 499 patients who have undergone catheter ablation of the AV junction at 55 centers.[32-34] Forty-eight percent of the patients did not have structural heart disease, whereas 15% had coronary artery disease, 14% had cardiomyopathy, and 22% had other miscellaneous types of heart disease. All of the patients had symptomatic drug-refractory supraventricular tachycardias, most commonly atrial fibrillation or flutter (60%), AV nodal reentrant tachycardia (22%), atrial tachycardia (13%), and orthodromic reciprocating tachycardia (11%). Prior ineffective antiarrhythmic drug therapy included digitalis in 82% of patients, type I antiarrhythmic drugs in 77%, beta-blockers in 72%, calcium channel blockers in 71%, and amiodarone in 56%. Tachycardia-related symptoms consisted of palpatations in 70% of patients, presyncope in 36%, syncope in 25%, and cardiac arrest in 2%.

The majority of patients received one or two shocks; however, in some patients, three to six shocks were needed to induce persistent complete AV block. The range of stored energy for the individual shocks was 50 to 500 joules, and the most commonly used energy level was 200 joules. The mean cumulative energy used ranged from 50 to 3550 joules, with a mean of approximately 600 joules. The mean amplitudes of the unipolar His bundle potential and atrial deflection were 0.38 ± 0.29 mV and 0.87 ± 0.83 mV, respectively. Complete AV block was present immediately after the shocks in 90% of patients, and the average rate of the escape rhythm was 45 ± 25 beats per minute. The escape pacemaker was infra-His in origin in 58% of patients, supra-His in 32%, and absent in 10%.

The mean duration of follow-up was 12 ± 11 months, with a range of 1 to 52 months. In 64% of patients, AV block was persistent and complete, and no further pharmacologic therapy was necessary to control symptoms (Fig. 25–6). In 9% of patients, the procedure was partially successful, in that AV block was neither complete nor persistent, but, medications were no longer required for control of symptoms. In 12% of patients, AV conduction and symptomatic arrhythmias were still present after the ablation procedure; however, symptoms could be controlled with drug therapy that had been ineffective before the catheter ablation procedure. Fifteen percent of patients continued to have symptomatic, drug-refractory supraventricular tachycardia.

Analysis of several variables in patients who underwent catheter ablation of the AV junction indicated that a successful outcome was associated with a unipolar His bundle deflection greater than 0.3 mV, a left ventricular ejection fraction greater than 0.40, and a shock strength of 300 joules or more.

In summary, among the 499 patients entered into the Percutaneous Mapping and Ablation Registry, persistent complete AV block was induced by catheter ablation in 64%, and the response in regard to control of symptoms was judged to be either excellent or good in 85% of patients.

It is interesting to note that when AV block was transient, AV conduction usually returned within several days after the ablation procedure. However, at times AV conduction did not return until 6 to 8 months later. Therefore, persistence of AV block for more than 3 months unfortunately does not guarantee long-term success.

Conversely, the presence of 1:1 AV conduction several days after catheter ablation may not necessarily imply that the procedure was unsuccessful in inducing high-degree AV block. Bru et al.[35] reported that among 12 patients in whom 1:1 AV conduction resumed after catheter ablation, two (17%) were found to have high-degree AV block 4 to 6 weeks after hospital discharge. It is notable that an infranodal conduction disturbance could not be detected during a predischarge electrophysiology test in one of these two patients. Bru and coworkers suggested that a prophylactic permanent pacemaker may be indicated in patients in whom catheter ablation of the AV junction apparently has been ineffective, because of the possibility of delayed

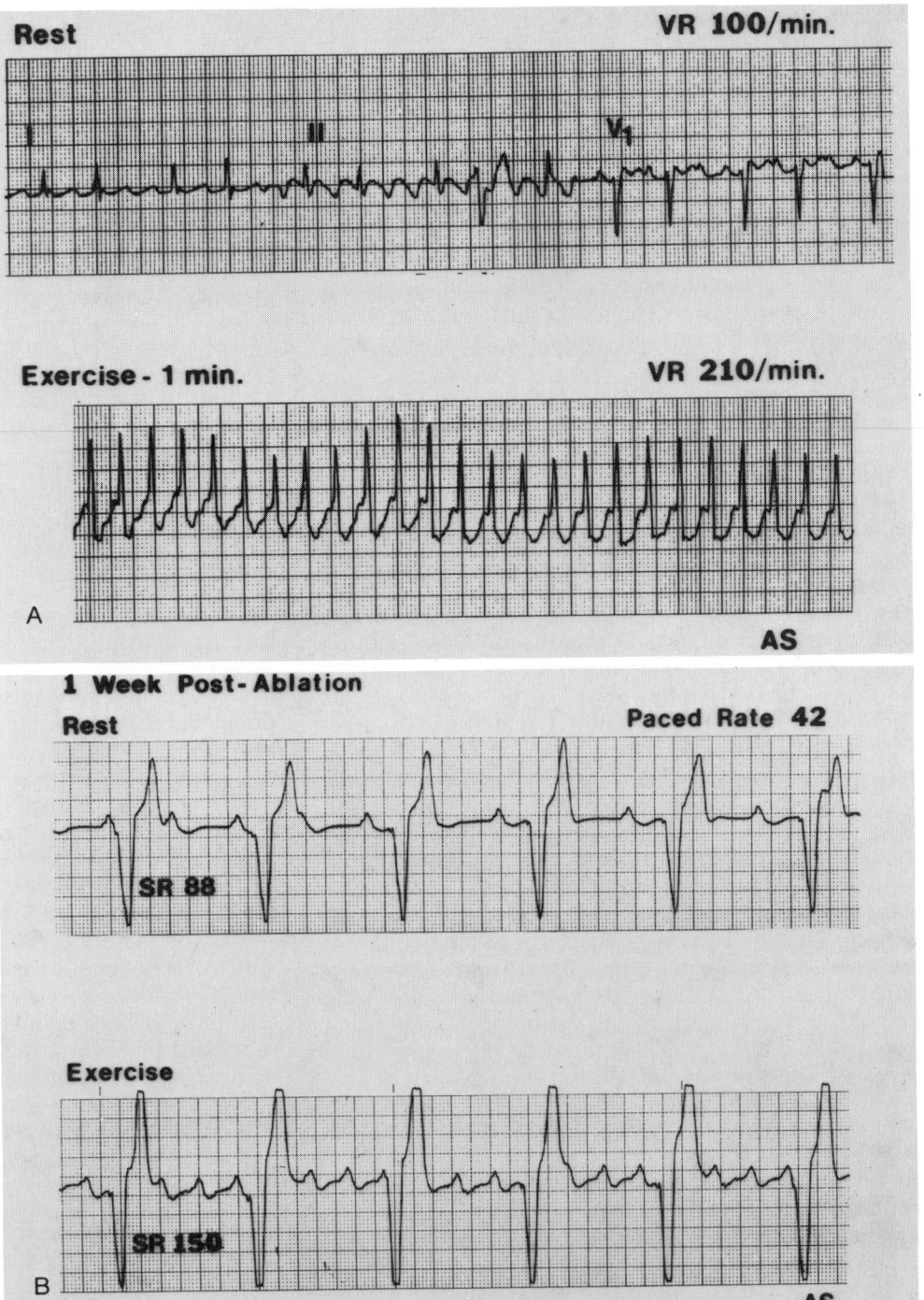

FIGURE 25–6
Example of a patient who underwent catheter ablation of the AV junction. The patient was a 42-year-old man who had, over a period of several years, a history of exertional syncope caused by a rapid ventricular rate during atrial fibrillation/flutter.

A, In the resting state, the ventricular rate was approximately 100 beats/minute. After two months of mild exercise, the ventricular rate was approximately 210 beats/minute and the patient was lightheaded. The atrial fibrillation/flutter and the rapid ventricular rate both were refractory to pharmacologic treatment.

B, One week after catheter ablation of the AV junction, the patient had complete AV block that persisted during exercise. Sinus rhythm was temporarily restored by the ablation shock. The permanent pacemaker was temporarily programmed to a rate of 42 beats/minute to make the underlying sinus rate more apparent. Several days later, atrial fibrillation/flutter recurred, but the patient remained in complete AV block and had no recurrence of tachycardia-related symptoms.

onset of high-degree AV block.[35] Additional experience will be required before it can be determined which patients who apparently have failed an ablation attempt should nevertheless receive a permanent pacemaker.

COMPLICATIONS

Among the more serious early complications of catheter ablation of the AV junction in the 499 patients reported to the Percutaneous Cardiac Mapping and Ablation Registry have been four cases of cardiac tamponade.[34] The source of tamponade has not always been clear, but may include perforation of the right ventricle by the electrode catheter used for temporary pacing. In addition, there has been at least one case of coronary sinus perforation, thought to be caused by movement of the ablation catheter into the coronary sinus.[36]

Other early complications have included sepsis in ten patients, transient hypotension in seven patients, thrombophlebitis in five patients, pericarditis in four patients, hemothorax in two patients, and right atrial thrombus and subclavian vein thrombosis in one patient each[34].

Despite delivery of the shocks in a synchronized fashion, there were six instances of ventricular fibrillation or ventricular tachycardia immediately postshock. In addition, nonsustained ventricular tachycardia was observed as a new arrhythmia within several days of the ablation procedure in 22 patients (4.9%).[34] The risk of new arrhythmias indicates the importance of having the capability for immediate defibrillation at the time of catheter ablation, and the need for continuous electrocardiographic monitoring for several days afterward.

Another source of complications has been the permanent pacemakers that are implanted following catheter ablation of the AV junction. The incidence of pacemaker-related complications has been approximately 4%, and the complications have included pacemaker failure, pacemaker syndrome, diaphragmatic pacing, pacemaker-mediated tachycardia, and myopotential sensing.[34]

It is of concern that eight patients (1.8%) died suddenly from 3 days to 13 months after the ablation procedure.[34] There was no evidence of pacemaker failure in these patients. Seven of the eight patients had organic heart disease and left ventricular dysfunction, and it is possible that the sudden death in these patients was related to the underlying heart disease and not to the ablation procedure. However, it is also possible that these patients died of a malignant ventricular arrhythmia, which occurred as a late complication of myocardial scarring caused by the intracardiac shocks. Consistent with this possibility are the postmortem histologic findings in one of the patients who died suddenly several weeks after the ablation procedure.[37] There was a significant degree of myocardial necrosis in the summit of the ventricular septum.[37] It is possible that this chronic myocardial injury could serve as a nidus of malignant arrhythmias.

Current Status

Based on six years of experience with catheter ablation of the AV junction in a large number of patients, it seems appropriate to conclude that catheter ablation is the procedure of choice in patients who are deemed to be appropriate candidates for ablation of AV conduction. Surgical techniques for ablation of the AV junction probably should be reserved only for patients who fail attempts at catheter ablation. Comparison of catheter and surgical ablation suggests that the efficacy and risk of the two approaches are comparable.[39] However, the catheter approach is less expensive, causes less discomfort, and is associated with a shorter convalescence.

Because catheter ablation of the AV junction results in pacemaker dependency and a possible risk of sudden death, the indications for AV junction ablation should not be broadened simply because of the ease with which catheter ablation can be performed. Catheter ablation of the AV junction should continue to be limited to patients who are refractory to pharmacologic therapy. Consideration should be given to other types of nonpharmacologic therapy before embarking on the irreversible path of the AV junction ablation.

Catheter Ablation of Accessory AV Connections

INDICATIONS FOR NONPHARMACOLOGIC MANAGEMENT

Patients who have either the Wolff-Parkinson-White syndrome or a concealed accessory AV connection may be appropriate candidates for nonpharmacologic treatment for one or more of the following reasons:

1. The occurrence of rapid and potentially life-threatening atrial fibrillation.
2. Inefficacy of antiarrhythmic drugs.
3. Intolerance to antiarrhythmic drugs.
4. Patient preference.

Up till the recent past, if it was decided that a patient was an appropriate candidate for definitive therapy, surgery provided the only means by which an accessory AV connection could be ablated. However, investigational transcatheter ablation techniques may provide a potential alternative to surgical ablation of some types of accessory AV connections.

EXPERIMENTAL BACKGROUND

Because there is no readily available animal model of the Wolff-Parkinson-White syndrome, experimental studies of the effects of intracardiac shocks on accessory AV connections have not been possible. Experimental studies have instead focused on the safety and effects of shocks delivered within the coronary sinus or against the right atrial wall in dogs that did not have an accessory AV connection.

The feasibility of ablating right free-wall accessory AV connections with direct-current shocks was investigated by Ruder et al.[40] Cathodal shocks of 50 to 400 joules were delivered in the right atrium near the tricuspid annulus in dogs. There were no cases of atrial perforation or cardiac tamponade. Anatomic studies 1 to 10 days after the shock demonstrated a circular endocardial lesion whose area correlated with both the strength of the shock and the atrial pacing threshold. When the ratio of the atrial electrogram to the ventricular electrogram was 1:1.5 and the atrial pacing threshold was 1.5 mA, there was always transmural necrosis at the level of the tricuspid annulus. These findings suggested that right free-wall accessory AV connections potentially could be ablated by direct-current shocks.

Brodman and Fisher[41] evaluated the potential applicability of the catheter ablation technique for interrupting conduction in left-sided accessory AV connections by studying the effects of graded shocks delivered within the coronary sinus of dogs. The shocks were delivered through a bipolar or hexapolar electrode catheter positioned inside the coronary sinus, with the distal electrode connected to the cathodal output of a defibrillator, and the proximal electrode connected to the anodal sink. The amount of injury was found to be related to the strength of the shocks. Among five dogs who received a single shock of 35 to 45-joules, gross and microscopic examination 6 hours later demonstrated extensive ecchymosis and edema surrounding the coronary sinus, extending into the adjacent left atrial and ventricular walls and into the coronary sulcus from the mitral annulus into epicardial fat. Perforation of the coronary sinus at the site of the shock was found in one dog. Coronary sinus rupture and perforation occurred in two of three dogs who received two to three 240-joule shocks.

In another 16 dogs, morphologic examination was performed 2 to 11 weeks after one to four shocks of 35 to 45 joules had been delivered in the coronary sinus. Dense scarring of the left atrial wall adjacent to the site where the shocks were delivered was observed in 15 of the 16 dogs. In the remaining dog the area of fibrosis was mottled. The coronary sinus was completely occluded at the shock site in 8 of 16 dogs and was moderately to markedly stenotic in 5. The circumflex coronary artery was found to have mild to marked intimal hyperplasia in 3 dogs.

Brodman and Fisher concluded that multiple 35- to 45-joule shocks in the coronary sinus could cause enough fibrosis of the adjacent left atrial wall to potentially result in ablation of left-sided accessory AV connections.[41] However, their results demonstrated that even low-energy shocks of 35 to 45 joules could result in perforation, occlusion, or stenosis of the coronary sinus.

Transcatheter ablation techniques for posteroseptal accessory AV connections have involved delivery of shocks at the os of the coronary sinus. Electrophysiologic and histologic effects in dogs of shocks delivered to the region of the os of the coronary sinus were studied by Coltorti et al.[14] The proximal two electrodes of a quadripolar electrode catheter were positioned at the os of the coronary sinus and served as the anode, and a disk electrode on the anterior chest wall served as the cathode. A 200-joule shock (stored energy) was delivered in six dogs and a 360-joule shock in another six. Transient AV block and idioventricular rhythms occurred in five and six dogs of each group, respectively. An electrophysiology study made 4 weeks after the shocks showed that AV conduction was normal in all dogs, there was no spontaneous or inducible ventricular tachycardia, and ventricular fibrillation was inducible in only one dog. Histologic examination demonstrated transmural atrial injury at the level of the coronary sinus over a 10 ± 5 mm length with the 200-joule shock and 21 ± 6 mm length with the 360-joule shock. Localized intramural atrial rupture of the endocardial aspect of the coronary sinus wall was found in each dog; however, there were no cases of cardiac tamponade, and there was no evidence of damage to coronary arteries or to the conduction system. The findings demonstrated that it was possible, without serious complications, to produce atrial injury potentially capable of blocking conduction through a posteroseptal accessory AV connection, by delivering a shock at the os of the coronary sinus.

In a later study, Coltorti and colleagues[42] compared the effects of unipolar and bipolar shocks delivered at the os of the coronary sinus. In ten dogs a single 200-joule shock was delivered, with an electrode at the os serving as the anode and a disc electrode on the anterior chest serving as the cathode; in another ten dogs, the 200-joule shock was delivered, with the proximal electrode of a bipolar catheter serving as the anode and the distal electrode serving as the cathode. Transmural atrial scarring occurred in each of the ten dogs that received a unipolar shock but in only two dogs that received a bipolar shock. Therefore, unipolar shocks may be more likely than bipolar shocks to result in transmural atrial injury sufficient to prevent conduction through an accessory AV connection. There was gross rupture of the coronary sinus in two dogs who received a bipolar shock, and also in two dogs who received a unipolar shock. In contrast, in these investigators' prior study, no instances of coronary sinus rupture occurred with shocks of 200 to 360 joules when two electrodes in parallel served as the anode.[14] Coltorti et al. suggested that the use of two electrodes in parallel may avoid the high concentration of energy to a small area that may occur when a single electrode serves as the anode.

Overall, the findings of these experimental studies suggested that it may be possible with intracardiac shocks to cause enough atrial injury to successfully ablate right free-wall and posteroseptal accessory AV connections without a high risk of atrial or coronary sinus perforation. However, shocks within the coronary sinus that results in left atrial injury sufficient to block conduction within a left free-wall accessory AV connection appeared to be associated with a significant risk of coronary sinus injury. Possible long-term deleterious effects of right atrial or coronary sinus shocks on the coronary arteries were not ruled out by these studies.

TECHNIQUE

Many different techniques have been used for attempts at catheter ablation of accessory AV connections. The only technique that will be described in detail here is a technique that has been found to be successful in a series of patients with a posteroseptal accessory AV connection.[43,44] Other techniques will not be described in detail because they have been either unsuccessful or associated with serious complications or were tested in only a small number of patients.

Before an attempt at transcatheter ablation of a posteroseptal accessory AV connection, a detailed electrophysiologic study is necessary to confirm the location of the accessory AV connection, to confirm that the accessory AV connection is involved in the patient's tachycardias, and to rule out a second accessory AV connection.

At the time of the ablation procedure, surgical backup should be arranged in the event of coronary sinus rupture and cardiac tamponade. An electrode catheter is positioned against the right ventricular apex for use as a temporary pacemaker, in case transient AV block occurs after delivery of the shocks. A short arterial cannula is inserted to allow continuous monitoring of the blood pressure. Using a left subclavian approach, a central lumen catheter is positioned within the coronary sinus and contrast material is injected to visualize the location of the coronary sinus os. This catheter is then removed and a new No. 6 or No. 7 French quadripolar electrode catheter (1 cm interelectrode distance) is inserted into the coronary sinus, such that the third electrode from the tip is situated at the os. The proximal two electrodes are made electrically common and connected to the cathodal output of a defibrillator, and a 16-cm patch electrode positioned on the posterior chest is connected to the anodal sink of the defibrillator (Fig. 25–7).

After the induction of general anesthesia by an anesthesiologist, the correct catheter position is verified by fluoroscopy and a 200- to 300-joule shock (stored energy) is delivered. If the patient's hemodynamic status and AV conduction through the AV node–His-Purkinje axis remain normal, a second shock is delivered to minimize the possibility that conduction through the accessory AV connection will return at a later date. After the ablation procedure, the patient should undergo observation and electrocardiographic monitoring. Patients who have an uncomplicated course are generally discharged from the hospital 5 to 7 days after the ablation procedure.

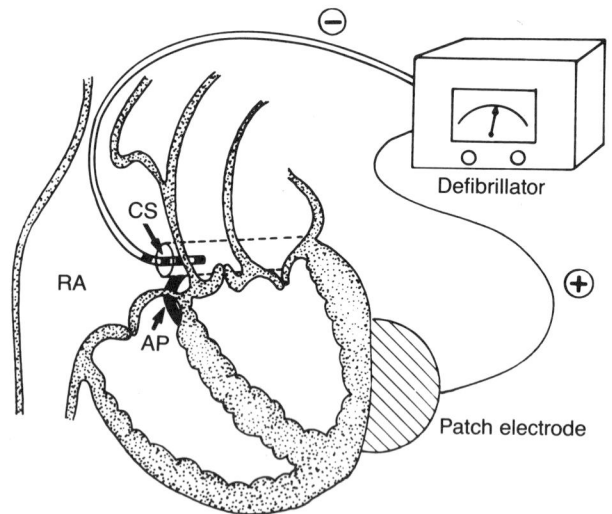

FIGURE 25–7
Schematic illustration of a technique used for catheter ablation of posteroseptal accessory pathways. A No. 6 French quadripolar catheter is positioned within the coronary sinus such that the third electrode from the tip is located at the mouth of the coronary sinus. The third and fourth electrodes from the tip are made electrically common and connected to the cathodal output of a defibrillator. A patch electrode positioned on the back serves as the anode. Not shown is the electrode catheter in the right ventricle that is used for temporary pacing in the event of AV block after delivery of a shock.

CATHETER ABLATION OF POSTEROSEPTAL ACCESSORY AV CONNECTIONS

Results

The results of catheter ablation using the technique described above were reported in 1985 in a series of eight patients who had a posteroseptal accessory AV connection.[44] This series has been expanded to 27 patients and will be described here.

The mean age of the patients was 32 ± 11 years. In 18 patients there was overt retrograde conduction over the posteroseptal accessory AV connection, and in 9 patients the accessory AV connection was concealed. Each of the patients had a history of symptomatic tachycardia and 17 of the 27 patients had a history of atrial fibrillation with a rapid ventricular rate. Follow-up evaluation after the catheter ablation procedure consisted of an electrophysiologic study 4 to 8 months after the shocks in 18 patients; an intraoperative electrophysiology study in 5 patients who underwent an operation, either because of a second accessory AV connection or because of persisting conduction over the posteroseptal accessory AV connection; and clinical evaluation of 4 patients who declined a follow-up electrophysiologic study. The last 4 patients each had overt ventricular preexcitation on their baseline electrograms.

The posteroseptal accessory AV connection was successfully ablated in 19 of 27 patients (70%). These patients have had no recurrence of symptomatic tachycardia involving the accessory AV connection over a mean follow-up period of 22 ± 13 months (Fig. 25–8). In an additional 2 patients (7%), retrograde conduction was slowed; these 2 patients have not had symptomatic tachycardia for 47 to 50 months. Therefore, the catheter ablation procedure was successful in completely eliminating conduction over the accessory AV connection, or modifying conduction such that symptomatic tachycardia no longer occurred, in 77% of patients. The procedure failed to modify significantly conduction over the accessory AV connection in 6 of 27 patients (23%). In 2 of these 6 patients, inefficacy was apparent within 24 hours of the procedure, whereas in 4 patients, evidence of ventricular preexcitation on the electrocardiogram recurred 5 days to 6 weeks after delivery of the shocks.

Comparison of the patients in whom the outcome was and was not successful indicated no significant difference in age, the ventriculoatrial interval at the os of the coronary sinus during orthodromic tachycardia, the number of joules delivered (605 ± 122 joules in patients with successful outcome and 733 ± 250 joules in patients with unsuccessful outcome), or the position of the anode on the anterior or posterior chest. However, the success rate in patients who had a concealed accessory AV connection (9 of 9, 100%) was significantly greater than the 67% success rate among the patients who had an overt accessory AV connection. This observation suggests that there may be an anatomic difference between concealed and overt accessory AV connections that accounts for the higher

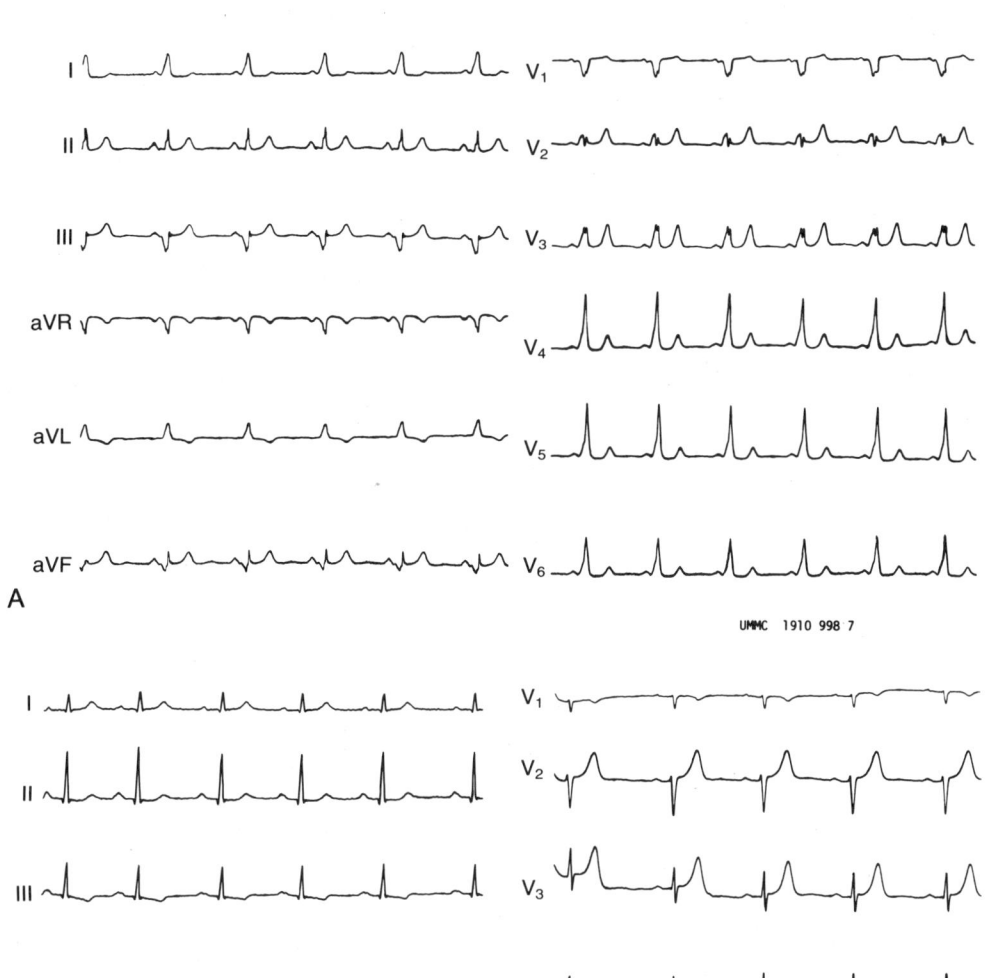

FIGURE 25–8

A, A 12-lead ECG of a patient who had a posteroseptal accessory pathway. The delta waves are inverted in the inferior leads, upright in lead I and aVL, and there is a transition from a small to a large R wave between V_1 and V_2. This pattern is typical of posteroseptal accessory pathways.

B, Four months after catheter ablation of the accessory pathway, there is no longer any evidence on the ECG of an accessory pathway. An electrophysiologic study demonstrated that both anterograde and retrograde accessory pathway conduction were absent, and the patient had no recurrences of symptomatic tachycardia.

success rate in the patients with a concealed accessory AV connection.

Bardy et al.[45] used a modified technique in 19 patients with a posteroseptal accessory AV connection and reported a successful outcome in 13 patients (68%). Between two and five shocks of 150 to 400 joules were delivered at the os of the coronary sinus, just outside the coronary sinus, or 1 cm in from the os. The shocks were delivered through No. 8 French high dielectric-strength catheter in most of the patients. Other reports of catheter ablation for posteroseptal accessory AV connections have included small numbers of patients and will not be described here.

Complications

In the series of 27 patients studied by us, the mean peak creatine kinase MB fraction was 25 ± 13 IU/L after the shocks (normal, 0–10 IU/L). A few minutes of AV nodal block was common immediately after the shocks, but normal AV conduction returned in all patients except one, who was left with persistent AV block. This patient had the sick sinus syndrome and already had a permanent pacemaker in place. Follow-up coronary angiography in seven patients did not demonstrate any coronary artery abnormalities.

The most serious complication was cardiac tamponade in one patient after delivery of a single 300-joule shock. The cardiac tamponade was successfully managed by needle pericardiocentesis, and emergent surgery was not required. Examination of the electrode catheter used in this case revealed breaks in the insulation. It was presumed that some energy was inadvertently delivered through the distal electrode within the coronary sinus, resulting in rupture of the coronary sinus. This was borne out when the patient underwent elective surgical ablation of the posteroseptal accessory AV connection 1 month later and was found to have a small healed perforation of the coronary sinus 2 to 3 cm from the os.

A case of coronary sinus perforation and fatal cardiac tamponade was reported by Ward et al.[46] In addition, coronary sinus rupture and nonfatal cardiac tamponade occurred in 3 of the 19 patients in the series reported by Bardy et al.[45] It is interesting that the ratio of the width of the catheter to the width of the coronary sinus as visualized angiographically was greater than 0.5 in each of the 3 patients who had cardiac tamponade.

The experience cited above suggests that factors that may predispose to coronary sinus rupture may include catheter defects and a small coronary sinus relative to the elective size. A small coronary sinus may be more susceptible to mechanical perforation by the electrode catheter, which may be forced against the wall of the coronary sinus as a result of the shock. The potential risk of cardiac tamponade necessitates the immediate availability of surgical back-up when catheter ablation of a posteroseptal accessory pathway is attempted with direct-current shocks.

Another complication of catheter ablation of a posteroseptal accessory AV connection has been ectopic atrial tachycardia originating at the site of shock delivery.[47]

CATHETER ABLATION OF FREE-WALL ACCESSORY AV CONNECTIONS

Results

The results of transcatheter ablation of ten left-sided AV connections in eight patients were reported by Fisher et al.[48] They used 2 to 26 shocks ranging in strength from 40 to 80 joules, except in one patient, who received shocks of 100 and 150 joules. The electrode configuration used in these patients was variable. In six patients, the shocks were delivered between two adjacent electrodes within the coronary sinus; in two patients, an electrode within the coronary sinus served as the cathode, and an external plate served as the anode. Conduction through the accessory AV connection was eliminated acutely in each patient; however, conduction returned in all patients within 10 days. Only one patient remained asymptomatic without antiarrhythmic medication during the follow-up period; the other patients all required either antiarrhythmic drug therapy or surgical ablation of the accessory AV connection.

The low success rate of catheter ablation of left free-wall accessory AV connections with direct-current shocks delivered within the coronary sinus also is apparent in the experience accumulated in the Catheter Ablation Registry.[49] Permanent ablation was achieved in only one of 15 patients who had a left free-wall accessory AV connection.

A more promising approach for electrical catheter ablation of left free-wall accessory AV connections may be to identify an accessory AV connection potential with a mapping catheter in the coronary sinus, and then to deliver a shock directly to the atrial side of the mitral annulus with an electrode catheter passed through the foramen ovale and positioned as close as possible to the mapping electrodes within the coronary sinus.[50] This technique has been reported to be successful, but the experience to date is far too preliminary to allow any conclusions regarding efficacy or risk.

In regard to right-sided accessory AV connections, Kunze and Kuck[51] reported their experience with attempted transcatheter ablation of a right free-wall accessory AV connection in five patients. The right-sided accessory AV connection was localized by identification of an accessory pathway potential. Four shocks of 80 to 300 joules were then delivered in the right atrium. Persistent conduction block in the accessory AV connection was achieved over the long term in only one of the five patients.

The successful ablation of two concealed right-sided accessory AV connections was reported in a patient who had a pacemaker-mediated tachycardia incorporating these two aberrant pathways as the retrograde limb of the tachycardia circuit.[52] Each of the two right-sided accessory AV connections were successfully ablated with two 200-joule shocks.

Complications

Delivery of shocks within the coronary sinus in an attempt to ablate a left free wall accessory AV connection may result in barotraumatic coronary sinus rupture and cardiac tamponade. Cardiac tamponade occurred in one patient after two shocks of 150 and 100 joules delivered at the junction of the proximal and middle thirds of the coronary sinus[48]; this patient was successfully treated by pericardiocentesis. However, there have been several unpublished cases of fatal cardiac tamponade following the delivery of shocks within the coronary sinus.

Coronary sinus occlusion has also occurred as a complication of shocks delivered within the coronary sinus. Coronary sinus occlusion was found in two patients at the time of surgical ablation 8 to 9 weeks after the delivery of multiple 40- to 500-joule shocks within the coronary sinus.[48]

Although the published experience with transcatheter ablation of the left-sided accessory AV connections is very limited, it is apparent that there is a significant risk of coronary sinus perforation or injury when shocks are delivered directly within the coronary sinus.

In regard to the complications of transcatheter ablation of right-sided AV connections, there were no instances of right atrial performance when shocks of 80 to 300 joules were delivered in the right atrium of five patients.[51] However, one patient with a right septal accessory AV connection developed complete AV block, necessitating implantation of a permanent pacemaker.[51]

CATHETER ABLATION FOR PERMANENT JUNCTIONAL RECIPROCATING TACHYCARDIA

The retrograde limb of the reentry circuit in the permanent form of junctional reciprocating tachycardia has been reported to be a tortuous, slowly conducting posteroseptal accessory AV connection.[53] Attempts to ablate this type of posteroseptal accessory AV connection have generally met with failure. Among a total of 11 patients who had permanent junctional reciprocating tachycardia, catheter ablation by delivery of shocks in the region of the os of the coronary sinus were successful in eliminating conduction through the accessory AV connection in only two patients.[46, 54, 55] The reasons for the low success rate with this type of accessory AV connection are unclear.

OVERVIEW

Catheter ablation of accessory AV connections must still be viewed as an experimental procedure whose success rate cannot yet compete with the success rate of well-established operative techniques. The most promising results have been achieved with posteroseptal accessory AV connections; however, the risk of coronary sinus rupture will have to be greatly minimized before catheter ablation can be considered definitely preferable to surgery. Eliminating the risk of coronary sinus rupture may well require the use of alternative types of energy such as radiofrequency.

Attempts to ablate free-wall accessory connections with transcatheter shocks to date have had a very low success rate and, in the case of left-sided accessory AV connections, have been associated with a significant risk of cardiac tamponade. Therefore, surgical ablation of free-wall accessory AV connections, which has a success rate greater than 95% and a low morbidity rate, remains the procedure of choice for curative treatment. It remains to be determined whether improvements in mapping catheters, refinement of techniques to record accessory AV connection potentials,[56] elimination of barotrauma, and development of techniques to deliver energy directly to the AV annulus will result in catheter ablation techniques that preclude the need for surgery.

Catheter Ablation of Atrial Tachycardias

Few experimental studies have investigated the effects of transcatheter shocks delivered to the free-wall of the atria. Moak et al.[57, 58] studied the electrophysiologic and histologic effects of cathodal shocks of 100 to 400 joules delivered to the right atrial free-wall of puppies. The dogs were not able to tolerate shocks of 200 joules or more because of either refractory ventricular fibrillation or atrial perforation and cardiac tamponade. Transient ventricular arrhythmias and AV block were common after the shocks. Cellular electrophysiologic studies demonstrated marked depression of action potential characteristics in atrial muscle at the shock site acutely, but only mild abnormalities 11 weeks later. Local areas of conduction delay and block were demonstrated by microelectrode mapping in the area of the shock site. Acutely, the shocks caused transmural hemorrhagic necrosis. The area of atrial endocardial necrosis was 56 ± 11 mm^2 and 94 ± 14 mm^2 for shocks of 100 and 150 joules, respectively. The anatomic findings 11 weeks after the shocks were delivered consisted of nonhomogeneous atrial fibrosis. Based on these findings, Moak and coworkers concluded that (1) 150 joules is a safe upper limit for ablative shocks in the right atrium; (2) because the injury is nonhomogeneous, accurate atrial mapping is critical; and (3) local regions of conduction delay and block may provide the substrate for late atrial arrhythmias.

The published clinical experience with catheter ablation of atrial tacycardias also is scanty. Gillette and colleagues[59] reported a series of four children who underwent an attempt at ablation of an atrial automatic tachycardia. One to three cathodal shocks of 50 to 200 joules were delivered in the right atrium. The procedure was successful in two patients whose tachycardia focus was at the tip of the right atrial appendage. These two patients had no recurrence of the atrial tachycardia over a follow-up interval of 14 to 20 months. No complications were observed.

Davis et al.[60] attempted catheter ablation of incessant or recurrent ectopic atrial tachycardia in three patients. Two to five cathodal shocks were delivered, with a total energy of 400 to 800 joules. The procedure was successful in two patients whose tachycardia focus was close to the os of the coronary sinus, but was unsuccessful in a patient whose ectopic focus was in the right atrial appendage. This patient then underwent surgical ablation of the ectopic focus but later had a recurrence of an atrial tachycardia from a new ectopic focus. No complications were encountered.

The limited clinical experience with catheter ablation of atrial tachycardias suggests that successful long-term suppression of the tachycardia is possible, and that the procedure can be carried out safely. The actual efficacy and risk remain to be determined.

Catheter Ablation in the Presence of a Permanent Pacemaker

External defibrillation shocks have been reported to adversely affect permanent pacemakers at times by causing an increase in pacing rate, a decrease in spike amplitude, programming failure, a transient or permanent increase in the stimulation threshold, and sensing failure.[61-65] It is therefore possible that intracardiac shocks may also have adverse effects on a permanent pacemaker. The potential adverse effects of intracardiac shocks on a permanent pacemaker may include damage to the pacemaker generator, reprogramming of programmable pacemakers, myocardial injury at the tip of the pacing lead resulting from current being shunted down the lead, and displacement or direct damage to the lead by the spark and/or high-pressure wave associated with intracardiac direct-current shocks.

There are two clinical situations in which it may be

necessary to attempt catheter ablation of the AV junction in the presence of a permanent pacemaker:

1. Some patients may have a recurrence of AV conduction after undergoing catheter ablation of the AV junction and may undergo a second attempt.
2. Some patients who have undergone implantation of a permanent pacemaker because of the sick sinus syndrome may then develop a drug-refractory supraventricular tachycardia and require catheter ablation of the AV junction.

Reports of patients with a permanent pacemaker who have undergone a catheter ablation procedure have demonstrated that transient pacemaker malfunction is common and that permanent malfunction occasionally may occur. For example, Bowes and Bennett[65] and Fontaine et al.[67] reported several instances of reprogramming of pacing mode or rate and temporary failure to capture or failure to sense for up to 40 minutes. They also reported isolated instances of permanent loss of telemetry function, permanent sensing failure, and a rise in chronic stimulation threshold from 2 to 7 mA.

Because pacemaker malfunction may occur as a result of intracardiac shocks, a temporary ventricular pacemaker should be placed if it is necessary to attempt a catheter ablation procedure in the presence of a permanent pacemaker. If possible, the external indifferent electrode should be positioned such that the electrical field is orthogonal to a line connecting the tip of the pacing lead and the pacemaker generator. In addition, a complete pacemaker analysis should be performed after the ablation procedure to confirm appropriate programming, pacing, and sensing.

Use of Laser Energy for Ablation

Experimental studies have investigated the cellular, electrophysiologic, anatomic, and histologic effects of either argon or neodymium:YAG laser energy on myocardial tissue.[68–70] These studies have demonstrated that laser energy causes focal thermal injury with crater formation, vacuolization, and coagulation necrosis of endocardium and myocardium. Comparisons with direct-current shocks have demonstrated that transcatheter laser ablation produces lesions of comparable size at less than half the energy of the electrical shocks.[68] A lower incidence of arrhythmias and hemodynamic dysfunction has been observed with laser ablation, and this is probably attributable to the more focal nature of the injury with laser energy, compared to direct-current shocks.[68–70] These data suggest that catheter ablation with laser energy may have advantages over the use of electrical shocks.

Applications of laser energy to catheter ablation of supraventricular tachycardias have been very limited to date. Narula et al.[71] used argon laser energy delivered through a quartz fiber positioned within a transvenous guiding lumen catheter to successfully produce complete AV block in an intact dog. Histologic studies demonstrated microtransection of the His bundle by a channel 0.2 to 0.3 mm wide, with no injury to the AV node, proximal and distal His bundle segments, or bundle branches. In a subsequent study, Narula and coworkers[72] demonstrated that laser energy delivered through a transvenous catheter also could result in significant AV nodal delays and AV nodal block in intact dogs.

The results of these experimental studies suggest that transvenous delivery of laser energy may be capable of producing focal injury with minimal injury to surrounding tissues and may have the potential for use in humans to ablate accessory pathways and to modify or ablate AV conduction. However, the only clinical experience to date with the use of laser energy to ablate arrhythmogenic tissue in patients has been by direct application to the endocardium in the operating room,[73–75] and it remains to be determined whether transcatheter laser ablation will be feasible in humans.

Use of Radiofrequency Energy for Ablation

Radiofrequency energy causes cell death by evaporation of intracellular water and dessication, and it can be delivered through a standard electrode without producing barotrauma. Because of possible advantages over direct-current shocks, radiofrequency energy recently has been studied as a potential alternative to electrical shocks in catheter ablation procedures. Huang et al.[76] delivered radiofrequency energy of 750 kHz to the AV junction of dogs through standard transvenous electrode catheters and demonstrated that complete AV block or impaired AV conduction was produced in 10 of 11 dogs. Pathologic examination demonstrated discrete areas of coagulation necrosis at the AV junction without damage to surrounding tissues. The results of this study indicate the feasibility of using radiofrequency energy for transcatheter ablation of AV conduction.

Several experimental studies have investigated the potential for radiofrequency energy to be used for catheter ablation of accessory pathways. In these studies, radiofrequency energy has been delivered through a transvenous catheter to the coronary sinus, mitral annulus, or tricuspid annulus of intact dogs.[77–80] Discrete areas of necrosis extending to the epicardial surface were noted in the atrial and/or ventricular side of the AV sulcus, suggesting that accessory pathways might have been successfully ablated. No instances of atrial perforation, ventricular arrhythmias, or coronary sinus perforation were noted, indicating the safety of radiofrequency energy.

In regard to clinical applications of radiofrequency energy for catheter ablation to treat supraventricular tachycardias, there has been a preliminary report of two patients who underwent catheter ablation of the AV junction using radiofrequency energy.[81] Persistent complete AV block was produced in one of the two patients. Borggrefe et al.[82, 83] have used radiofrequency energy in several types of catheter ablation procedures.

Successful ablation was achieved without complications in three of six patients who underwent ablation of the AV junction and one of five patients who underwent ablation of an accessory AV connection; however, the procedure was unsuccessful in two patients who underwent an attempt at ablation of an atrial tachycardia focus.

In conclusion, radiofrequency catheter ablation has several advantages over the use of direct-current shocks:

1. It does not cause arcing and barotrauma.
2. There is no bubble production or risk of gas embolization.
3. The procedure is painless and therefore general anesthesia is not needed.
4. It does not damage electrode catheters, and therefore there is less likelihood of current leakage and misdirected energy.

However, the initial clinical results with the use of radiofrequency for catheter ablation in patients with supraventricular tachycardias have been only modest, and it may be that the limited lesion size produced by radiofrequency ablation will limit the clinical efficacy of this technique. Further clinical experience is needed to define the role of radiofrequency energy as an ablation tool.

Acknowledgment

The author is grateful to Drs. E. G. C. A. Boyd and G. H. Bardy for providing Figures 25–1 through 25–4, and to Mrs. Lisa Hackbarth for her excellent secretarial assistance.

References

1. Scheinman MM, Morady F, Hess DS, et al.: Catheter-induced ablation of the atrioventricular junction to control refractory supraventricular arrhythmias. JAMA 248:851, 1982.
2. Gallagher JJ, Svenson RH, Kasell JH: Catheter technique for closed-chest ablation of the atrioventricular conduction system. N Engl J Med 306:194, 1982.
3. Narula OS, Narula J, Finzi A, et al.: Electro-thermal catheter modification of atrio-ventricular nodal conduction and automaticity in man (Abstract). J Am Coll Cardiol 9:252A, 1987.
4. Beckman KJ, Lin JC, Wang Y: Production of reversible and irreversible atrio-ventricular block by microwave energy (Abstract). Circulation 76(Suppl 4):IV-405, 1987.
5. Boyd EGCA, Holt P: An investigation into the electrical ablation technique and a method of electrode assessment. PACE 8:815, 1985.
6. Boyd EGCA, Holt PM: The biophysics of catheter ablation techniques. J Electrophysiol 1:62, 1987.
7. Bardy GH, Coltorti F, Ivey TD, et al.: Some factors affecting bubble formation with catheter-mediated defibrillator pulses. Circulation 73:525, 1986.
8. Holt PM, Boyd EGCA: Hematologic effects of the high-energy endocardial ablation technique. Circulation 73:1029, 1986.
9. Boyd E, Holt P: Hematological and tissue effects of high energy ablation (Abstract). Br Heart J 53:99, 1985.
10. Lee BI, Rodriquez ER, Notargiocomo A, et al.: Thermal effects of laser and electrical discharge on cardiovascular tissue: Implications for coronary artery recanalization and endocardial ablation. J Am Coll Cardiol 8:193, 1986.
11. Levine JH, Spear JF, Weisman HF, et al.: The cellular electrophysiologic changes induced by high-energy electrical ablation in canine myocardium. Circulation 73:818, 1986.
12. Westveer DC, Nelson T, Stewart JR, et al.: Sequelae of left ventricular electrical endocardial ablation. J Am Coll Cardiol 5:956, 1985.
13. Lee BI, Gottdiener JS, Fletcher RD, et al.: Transcatheter ablation: Comparison between laser photoablation and electrode shock ablation in the dog. Circulation 71:579, 1985.
14. Coltorti F, Bardy GH, Reichenbach D, et al.: Catheter-mediated electrical ablation of the posterior septum via the coronary sinus: Electrophysiologic and histologic observations in dogs. Circulation 72:612, 1985.
15. Ward DE, Davies M: Transvenous high energy shock for ablating atrioventricular conduction in man. Observations on the histological effects. Br Heart J 51:175, 1984.
16. Cooper GJ, Maynard RC, Pearse BP, et al.: Cardiovascular distortion in experimental nonpenetrating chest impacts. J Trauma 24:188, 1984.
17. Cooper GJ, Pearse BP, Strainer MC, et al.: The biomechanical response of the chest wall to impact with particular reference to cardiac injuries. J Trauma 22:994, 1982.
18. Cunningham D, Rowland E, Rickards A: Lack of shock wave absorption after high energy catheter discharge suggests that direct barotrauma is a myth (Abstract). Circulation 76(Suppl 4):IV-407, 1987.
19. Levine JH, Merillat JC, Stern M, et al.: The cellular electrophysiologic changes induced by ablation: Comparison between argon laser photoablation and high-energy electrical ablation. Circulation 76:217, 1987.
20. Jones JL, Lepeschkin E, Jones RE, et al.: Response of cultured myocytes to countershock-type electric field stimulation. Am J Physiol 235:H214, 1978.
21. Fisher JD, Brodman R, Johnston DR, et al.: Nonsurgical electrical ablation of tachycardias: Importance of prior in vitro testing of catheter leads. PACE 7:74, 1984.
22. Bardy GH, Coltorti F, Ivey TD, et al.: Effect of damped sine-wave shocks on catheter dielectric strength. Am J Cardiol 56:769, 1985.
23. Saksena S, Tarjan PP, Bharati S, et al.: Low-energy transvenous ablation of the canine atrioventricular conduction system with a suction electrode catheter. Circulation 76:394, 1987.
24. Cunningham D, Rowland E, Rickards A: A new non-arcing electrode for catheter ablation—Design and trial performance (Abstract). Circulation 76(Suppl 4):IV-405, 1987.
25. Rowland E, Cunningham D, Rickards AF: Transvenous ablation of AV conduction using a new energy source (Abstract). Circulation 74:II:386, 1986.
26. Bhandari A, Morady F, Shen EN, et al.: Catheter-induced His bundle ablation in a patient with reentrant tachycardia associated with a nodoventricular tract. J Am Coll Cardiol 4:611, 1984.
27. Ellenbogen KA, O'Callaghan WG, Colavita PG, et al.: Catheter atrioventricular junction ablation for recurrent supraventricular tachycardia with nodoventricular fibers. Am J Cardiol 55:1227, 1985.
28. Gonzalez R, Scheinman M, Margaretten W, et al.: Closed-chest electrode catheter technique for His bundle ablation in dogs. Am J Physiol 24:H283, 1981.
29. Gonzalez R, Scheinman M, Bharati S, et al.: Closed chest permanent atrioventricular block in dogs. Am Heart J 105:461, 1983.
30. Bardy GH, Ideker RE, Kasell J, et al.: Transvenous ablation of the atrioventricular conduction system in dogs: Electrophysiologic and histologic observations. Am J Cardiol 51:1775, 1983.
31. Scheinman MM, Bharati S, Wang Y, et al.: Electrophysiologic and anatomic changes in the atrioventricular junction of dogs after direct-current shocks through tissue fixation catheters. Am J Cardiol 55:194, 1985.
32. Scheinman MM, Evans-Bell T, and the Executive Committee of the Percutaneous Cardiac Mapping and Ablation Registry: Catheter ablation of the atrioventricular junction: A report of the Percutaneous Mapping and Ablation Registry. Circulation 70:1024, 1984.
33. Evans GT, Jr., Scheinman MM and the Executive Committee of the Registry: Catheter ablation of the atrioventricular junction: A report of the Percutaneous Cardiac Mapping and Ablation Registry. PACE 10:1026, 1987 (abstr).
34. Evans GT, Jr., Scheinman MM, Zipes DP, et al.: The Percutaneous Cardiac Mapping and Ablation Registry: Summary of results. PACE 10:1395, 1987.

35. Bru P, Levy S, Metge M, et al.: Remote occurrence of high degree heart block following failure of transcatheter AV junctional ablation: Incidence and clinical significance. PACE 10:937, 1987.
36. Feld M, Fisher J, Brodman R, et al.: Coronary sinus rupture complicating catheter ablation of the atrioventricular junction. J Electrophysiol 1:257, 1987.
37. Bharati S, Scheinman MM, Morady F, et al.: Sudden death after catheter-induced atrioventricular junctional ablation. Chest 88:883, 1985.
38. McComb JM, McGovern B, Garan H, et al.: Management of refractory supraventricular tachyarrhythmias using low-energy transcatheter shocks. Am J Cardiol 58:959, 1986.
39. Marchese AC, Pressley JC, Sintetos AL, et al.: Cryosurgical versus catheter ablation of the atrioventricular junction. Am J Cardiol 59:870, 1987.
40. Ruder MA, Davis JC, Eldar M, et al.: Effects of catheter-delivered electrical discharges near the tricuspid anulus in dogs. J Am Coll Cardiol 10:693, 1987.
41. Brodman R, Fisher JD: Evaluation of a catheter technique for ablation of accessory pathways near the coronary sinus using a canine model. Circulation 67:923, 1983.
42. Coltorti F, Bardy GH, Reichenuach D, et al.: Effects of varying electrode configuration with catheter-mediated defibrillator pulses at the coronary sinus orifice in dogs. Circulation 73:1321, 1986.
43. Morady F, Scheinman MM: Transvenous catheter ablation of a posteroseptal accessory pathway in a patient with the Wolff-Parkinson-White syndrome. N Engl J Med 310:705, 1984.
44. Morady F, Scheinman MM, Winston SA, et al.: Efficacy and safety of transcatheter ablation of posteroseptal accessory pathways. Circulation 72:170, 1985.
45. Bardy GH, Coltorti F, Ivey TD, et al.: Catheter mediated electrical ablation of posterior septal accessory pathways: Complications and effectiveness. J Am Coll Cardiol 9:250A, 1987.
46. Ward DE, Rowland E, Camm J: Transvenous ablation of anomalous conduction. J Electrophysiol 1:197, 1987.
47. Borggrefe M, Breithardt G: Ectopic atrial tachycardia after transvenous catheter ablation of a posteroseptal accessory pathway. J Am Coll Cardiol 8:441, 1986.
48. Fisher JD, Brodman R, Kim SG, et al.: Attempted nonsurgical electrical ablation of accessory pathways via the coronary sinus in the Wolff-Parkinson-White syndrome. J Am Coll Cardiol 4:685, 1984.
49. Scheinman MM: Catheter ablation for patients with cardiac arrhythmias. PACE 9:551, 1986.
50. Warin JF, Haissaguerre M, Belhassen B, et al.: Electrical catheter ablation of accessory pathways: Beneficial effects using a direct approach in 10 patients (Abstract). Circulation 74(Suppl 2):II-387, 1986.
51. Kunze KP, Kuck KH: Transvenous ablation of accessory pathways in patients with incessant atrioventricular tachycardia. Circulation 70(Suppl 2):II-412, 1984.
52. Weber H, Schmitz L, Hellberg K: Pacemaker-mediated tachycardias: A new modality of treatment. PACE 7:1010, 1984.
53. Critelli G, Gallagher JJ, Monda V, et al.: Anatomic and electrophysiologic substrate of the permanent form of junctional reciprocating tachycardia. J Am Coll Cardiol 4:601, 1984.
54. Gang ES, Oseran D, Rosenthal M, et al.: Closed chest catheter ablation of an accessory pathway in a patient with permanent junctional reciprocating tachycardia. J Am Coll Cardiol 6:1167, 1985.
55. Smith RT, Jr., Gillette PC, Massumi A, et al.: Transcatheter ablative techniques for treatment of the permanent form of junctional reciprocating tachycardia in young patients. J Am Coll Cardiol 8:385, 1986.
56. Jackman WM, Friday KJ, Scherlag BJ, et al.: Direct endocardial recording from an accessory atrioventricular pathway: Localization of the site of block, effect of antiarrhythmic drugs, and attempt at nonsurgical ablation. Circulation 68:906, 1983.
57. Moak JP, Friedman RA, Garson A Jr: Electrical ablation of atrial muscle. I. Early and late anatomic observations in canine atria. Am Heart J 113:1397, 1987.
58. Moak JP, Friedman RA, Garson A Jr: Electrical ablation of atrial muscle. II. Early and late electrophysiologic observations in canine atria. Am Heart J 113:1404, 1987.
59. Gillette PC, Wampler DG, Garson A Jr, et al.: Treatment of atrial automatic tachycardia by ablation procedures. J Am Coll Cardiol 6:405, 1985.
60. Davis J, Scheinman MM, Ruder MA, et al.: Ablation of cardiac tissues by an electrode catheter technique for treatment of ectopic supraventricular tachycardia in adults. Circulation 74:1044, 1986.
61. Levine PA, Barold SS, Fletcher JD, et al.: Adverse acute and chronic effects of electrical defibrillation and cardioversion on implanted unipolar cardiac pacing systems. J Am Coll Cardiol 1:1413, 1983.
62. Barold SS, Ong LS, Scovil J, et al.: Reprogramming of implanted pacemaker following external defibrillation. PACE 1:1514, 1978.
63. Norman JC, Robinson WJ: Effects of internal and external AC and DC countershock on totally implanted pacemaker function (Abstract). Circulation 32(Suppl 2):164, 1965
64. Aylwards P, Blood R, Tomkin AM: Complications of defibrillation with permanent pacemaker in situ. PACE 2:462, 1979.
65. Bowes RJ, Bennett DH: Effect of transvenous atrioventricular nodal ablation on the function of implanted pacemakers. PACE 8:811, 1985.
66. Bowes RJ: Atrioventricular nodal fulguration in the presence of an implanted pacemaker. J Electrophysiol 1:127, 1987.
67. Fontaine G, Lemoine B, Frank R, et al.: Effects of fulguration on the permanent pacemaker. In Fontaine G, Scheinman MM (eds.): Ablation in Cardiac Arrhythmias, pp. 367–465. Mount Kisco, Futura Publishing Co., 1987.
68. Lee BI, Gottdiener JS, Fletcher RD, et al.: Transcatheter ablation: Comparison between laser photoablation and electrode shock ablation in the dog. Circulation 71:579, 1985.
69. Saksena S, Ciccone JM, Chandran P, et al.: Laser ablation of normal and diseased human ventricle. Am Heart J 112:52, 1986.
70. Levine JH, Merillat JC, Stern M, et al.: The cellular electrophysiologic changes induced by ablation: Comparison between argon laser photoablation and high-energy electrical ablation. Circulation 76:217, 1987.
71. Narula OS, Bharati S, Chan MC, et al.: Microtransection of the His bundle with laser radiation through a pervenous catheter: Correlation of histologic and electrophysiologic data. Am J Cardiol 54:186, 1984.
72. Narula OS, Boveja BK, Cohen DM, et al.: Laser catheter-induced atrioventricular nodal delays and atrioventricular block in dogs: Acute and chronic observation. J Am Coll Cardiol 5:259, 1985.
73. Saksena S, Hussain SM, Gielchinsky I, et al.: Laser ablation of human atrium and accessory pathways: Experimental observations and early clinical experience (Abstract). PACE 10:427, 1987.
74. Saksena S: Laser ablation for tachyarrhythmia control: Development and expectations (Abstract). PACE 10:1027, 1987.
75. Svenson RH, Gallagher JJ, Selle JG, et al.: Photoablation of ventricular tachycardia with Nd:YAG Laser: A two year experience. Circulation 76(Suppl 4):498, 1987.
76. Huang SK, Bharati S, Graham AR, et al.: Closed chest catheter desiccation of the atrioventricular junction using radiofrequency energy—A new method of catheter ablation. J Am Coll Cardiol 9:349, 1987.
77. Jackman WM, Kuck KH, Naccarelli GV, et al.: Catheter ablation at the tricuspid annulus using radiofrequency current in canines (Abstract). J Am Coll Cardiol 9:99A, 1987.
78. Langberg J, Griffin JC, Bharati S, et al.: Radiofrequency catheter ablation in the coronary sinus (Abstract). J Am Coll Cardiol 9:99A, 1987.
79. Jackman WM, Kuck KH, Naccarelli G, et al.: Catheter ablation at the mitral annulus using RF current in canines. PACE 10:410, 1987.
80. Huang SKS, Graham AR, Lee MA, et al.: Closed-chest catheter ablation of the canine coronary sinus using radiofrequency energy. PACE 10:410, 1987.
81. Lavergne T, Guize L, Le Huezey JY, et al.: Transvenous ablation of the atrio-ventricular junction in human with high-frequency energy (Abstract). J Am Coll Cardiol 9:99A, 1987.
82. Borggrefe M, Budde T, Podczeck A, et al.: High frequency alternating current ablation of an accessory pathway in humans. J Am Coll Cardiol 10:576, 1987.
83. Borggrefe M, Budde T, Podczeck A, et al.: Application of transvenous radio-frequency alternating current ablation in humans (Abstract). Circulation 76(Suppl 4):IV-406, 1987.

26

Catheter Ablation Techniques for Ventricular Tachycardia

G. Fontaine
A. Cansell
R. Frank
J. L. Tonet
S. Aaddaj
M. Aldakar
Y. Grosgogeat

Endocardial catheter fulguration (electrode catheter ablation) is an ablative technique that is considered in our group when other methods of treatment, including drugs, anti-tachycardia pacemakers,[1] cardioverter,[2] implantable defibrillator,[3] and surgery are not appropriate. The aim of fulguration is to permanently alter conduction in a limited area of the heart. Surgery has previously demonstrated that at least in some patients, a simple transmural incision can be effective.[4] In other words, a limited procedure precisely directed by activation mapping during VT can modify enough myocardium to prevent relapses of life-threatening arrhythmias.[5–7]

Endocardial catheter fulguration, which uses the effects of a strong electrical shock delivered at the tip of an endocardial catheter positioned in the area to be modified, has been extensively explored as indirect treatment of supraventricular tachycardia by His bundle ablation.[8,9] The same electrical energy applied to the site of origin of abnormal ventricular activation, as determined by electrophysiological parameters, is a more recent and promising development for the treatment of chronic ventricular arrhythmias.[10–13]

The purpose of this chapter is to report the techniques and methods used in fulguration procedures for the treatment of ventricular tachycardia.

MATERIALS

The techniques developed in our department are primarily based on new experimental invasive approaches. The equipment available at Jean Rostand Hospital has been selected for both surgical and nonsurgical basic clinical research. It is therefore important for reasons other than its use in routine clinical applications.

Fluoroscopic Equipment

The patient lies on the fluoroscopic table in the sterile room, which is separated by a large window from the technical room where most of the equipment and controls are located. An arcus structure provides either a posteroanterior view or a left lateral oblique view (Fig. 26–1). In the latter position, the anterior aspect of the septum is clearly suggested by the catheter positioned in the right ventricular apex. It is therefore easy to locate the positions of other catheters during mapping of the left septum and lateral walls.

Catheter Technology and Selection

The first step of the endocardial catheter fulguration procedure is the localization by endocardial mapping

---

Supported in part by grants from: Centre de Recherche sur les Maladies Cardiovasculaires de l'Association Claude Bernard, La Fondation de Cardiologie, and L'Institut National de la Santé et de la Recherche Médicale (INSERM Contrat No. 865005)

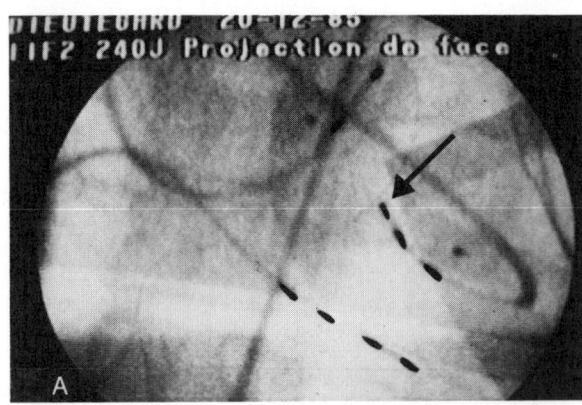

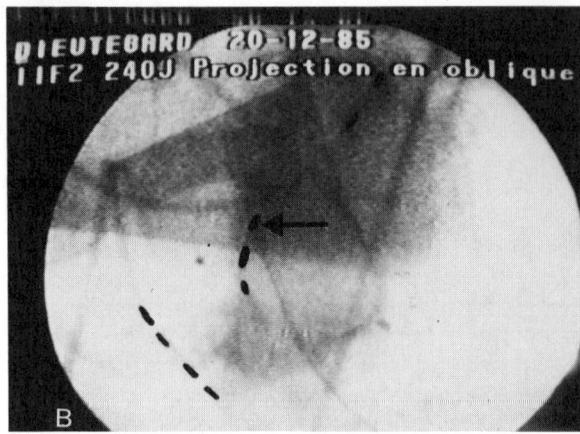

FIGURE 26–1
Anterior (A) and left anterior oblique (B) views of the catheters just prior to fulguration in a patient with right bundle branch block–left axis ventricular tachycardia. The bipolar catheter is located in the coronary sinus, and the quadripolar catheter is located at the apex of the right ventricle. The tripolar fulgurating catheter is positioned in the middle of the left ventricular septum. The shock will be delivered at the catheter tip (arrow).

of the area to be fulgurated. Catheter selection should stress the ability of the catheters to be appropriately positioned inside the cavities. An important prerequisite is the property of torque control. In our experience, USCI catheters are presently the most suitable, probably because of their unique, woven Dacron structure. Problems concerning their steering properties, however, have not been completely solved. Also, their standard length is not sufficient when a femoral approach to the left ventricle is necessary (e.g., for mapping in cases of a large aneurysm or in patients with a dilated aortic arch).

Insulation strength and steering properties of catheters vary with catheter design. The schematic description of the USCI catheter internal structure is related to the number of electrodes (Fig. 26–2). In bipolars, the structure is "coaxial," like a television cable. The conductor connected to the electrode tip consists of a cable of low resistance (about 2 ohms). The other conductor is a shield composed of an interwoven mesh of wires separated and isolated from the cable by the woven Dacron and covered by a layer of plastic. In multipolars, the conductors going to the nondistal electrodes are made of discrete wires that form a long spiral around the woven Dacron axis. Given these designs, it is possible to understand why the steering properties of the different models are not the same. In addition, these design features strongly affect the catheter's insulation properties. It has been demonstrated in our own laboratory and in those of others that ordinary catheters that have been developed for endocardial recording or pacing are for the most part unable to withstand the high peak voltage and/or current used in the fulguration procedure.[14, 15]

The discovery of abnormal catheter behavior had interesting connotations. It was first observed by one of us (G. F.) during fulguration of our second case of reentrant ventricular tachycardia (VT). The excellent results obtained in our first patient with incessant VT prompted us to design a protocol (later abandoned when we observed that in most cases the catheter tip was displaced by the shock) to evaluate the effect of shocks on myocardial tissue. The same approach previously used for the study of other ablative techniques consisted of the recording of both endocardial electrogram and pacing threshold.[16] It was observed after the first shock that bipolar recording and pacing was no longer possible, whereas unipolar recording and pacing were obtained at the same threshold and with the same endocardial signal configuration. To anyone with some expertise in cardiac pacemaker implantation and trouble-shooting, it was obvious that a short circuit had taken place. This result was immediately confirmed by our electronic technician after catheter withdrawal. However, this event was surprising because the endocardial fulgurating catheter was used in the *unipolar* mode, the terminal connector of the unused electrodes being left exposed on a nonconductive material.

Fortunately, instead of rejecting this catheter, we sent it to an electronic engineer (A. C.), the same person who had previously modified a defibrillator to adapt it for the purpose of fulguration. He noticed that the catheter sheath had narrow holes near the catheter tip, almost invisible by direct vision. In addition, smoke

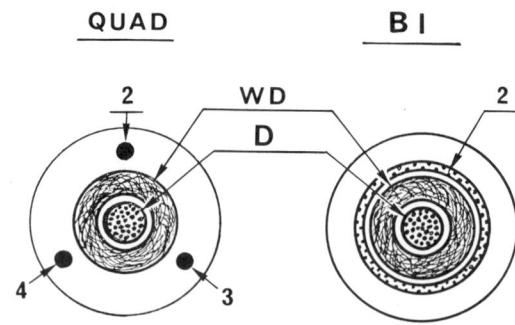

FIGURE 26–2
Internal structure of USCI quadripolar (QUAD) and bipolar (BI) catheters. The conductor going to the distal electrode (D) has the lowest impedance and constitutes the catheter axis. It is surrounded by a sheath of woven Dacron (WD). In the quadripolar structure, isolated copper wires (2, 3, 4) run around the main axis of the catheter; in the bipolar structure, the conductor going to the second electrode (2) constitutes the external shield in an arrangement comparable to that of a television cable.

and flames were abruptly released through these holes when voltages comparable to fulgurating voltages were applied to two adjacent electrodes. However, this occurred using the catheter in a *bipolar* mode.

In order to explain the strange behavior of the catheter used in the unipolar mode during fulguration, the following explanation was proposed. Take, for example, the case of a bipolar catheter in which the distal electrode is connected to one defibrillator terminal, the other being connected to the sink electrode. When a voltage of 2 kV is applied, an approximate resistance of 50 ohms, which constitutes the electric load, is registered by the defibrillator circuit. The second nonconnected electrode is, however, immersed in the blood conductive medium. If we postulate that a second 50 ohm resistor is located between the second electrode and the sink electrode, we are forced to conclude that the potential difference between the two electrodes is equal to the applied voltage of 2 kV. This is due to the fact that no current is flowing inside the second 50 ohm resistor, the circuit being electrically open. However, if a voltage difference of 2 kV is present between two adjacent electrodes, the same voltage will be observed along the wires going to the catheter connectors. The zone with the weakest electric strength will fail and produce the arcing phenomenon within the catheter sheath. Heat produced by the Joule effect will melt the plastic coating of the catheter and some part of the insulating material, and their abrupt destruction will release explosively smoke and gas. This interpretation was, however, not completely satisfactory because no role was given to the shunting effect of blood situated *between* the two electrodes. At the beginning we wrongly assumed that the distribution of resistance was linear along the line situated between the electrode tip and the sink electrode. In that case, when a 2-kV shock is applied for a distance of approximately 10 cm, the voltage between the two catheter electrodes will be, at the most, 200 volts. This difference should not affect catheter behavior. The only possible explanation was that some unexpected phenomenon was occurring in the distribution of resistance within the blood.

To investigate this possibility, we mapped with an electronic alternative bridge (Helwett-Packard 4262A LCR meter) the resistance produced in a saline container. It varied in a nonlinear fashion at the three available testing frequencies of 120 Hz, 1 kHz, and 10 kHz. A similar experiment was later confirmed by investigating the repartition of voltages in saline when 2kV impulses were applied between the terminal electrode and a sink plate at a distance of 10 cm. We observed that the resistance and consequently the voltages were not linearly distributed in the bath but, on the contrary, demonstrated a high concentration around the catheter electrode. The final and, in fact, most simple confirmation was obtained by directly recording the interelectrode potential through a voltage divider probe on an oscilloscope screen.[17] After two weeks of discussion and in vitro experiments the surprising mechanism of catheter failure was clearly understood.[18]

A method for testing catheters by specific, commercially available equipment was demonstrated by the ODAM Company (Wissembourg, France). This led us to design a cheaper device (provided that an oscilloscope is at hand) for selecting catheters before the fulguration procedure.

The first report concerning catheter failure was made at an international meeting held in Florence, Italy, in June 1983. A brief note was published in English in the Stimarec Bulletin,[19] and a paper was published in the Stimucoeur journal.[20] A short time later, an article confirmed the possible problems with catheters used for fulguration.[15]

The method used to select catheters prior to their sterilization proved to be useful in the vast majority of cases.[20] However, it has been observed recently that exceptions do exist. As previously suggested by in vitro studies and confirmed by another group,[14] catheters that pass the test in the electronic laboratory could fail during the actual procedure (Fig. 26–3). A vast spectrum of possibility could exist when an isolation break is observed. These situations could in some cases be determined by an ohmmeter; however, in most cases these problems are observed *only* when voltages comparable to fulguration voltages are used.

More surprisingly, we have recently observed one case in which a catheter which passed the test before and after the procedure manifested abnormal behavior on the voltage curve obtained during the shock (Fig. 26–4). Analysis of the electrode by light microscopy revealed that the distal electrode was pitted (which is normal), and that one of the nondistal electrodes was also pitted. We concluded that internal arcing took place, but that nonconductive material was deposited between the two responsible wires, re-establishing proper insulation. This suggests that recording of the voltage curve is mandatory even when catheters are properly tested. Even more complex is the situation already reported in which the insulation strength decreased progressively from shock to shock, using the same catheter (Fig. 26–5).[21]

The insulation properties of catheters have also changed as modifications have been made in manufacturing. We recently observed that insulation ruptures, which occurred previously at the catheter tip and therefore within a cardiac cavity,[22] are now more frequently observed outside of the body, on the proximal part of the catheter at the connection with the independent wires terminated by connecting plugs.

Proper catheter selection is important because inappropriate material, at the very least, will lead to a decrease of energy at the catheter tip and reduction of the effect of the shock on myocardium. It is our opinion that most cases of ineffectiveness and even major problems with fulguration procedure are related to this situation. It is not uncommon that groups experienced in the field of cardiac electrophysiology are not knowledgeable enough as far as electric circuitry is concerned.

During the 5-year interval between the first report on catheter failure and the time of this writing, an industrial solution has not been found. The fact that

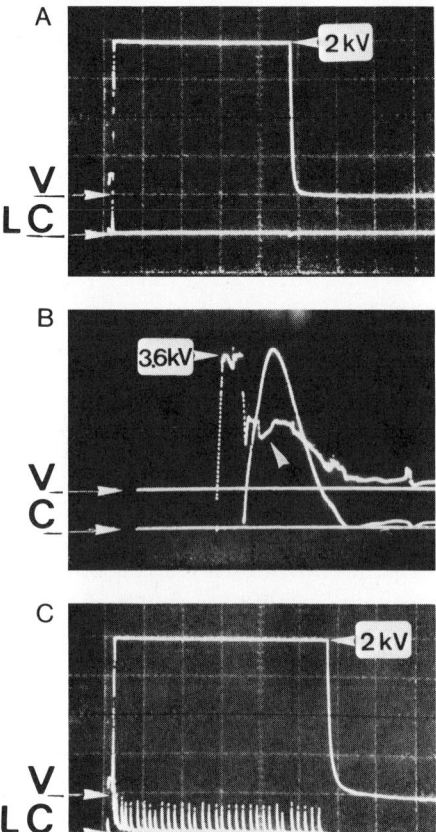

FIGURE 26-3
Abnormal behavior of a USCI catheter that had passed the high-voltage test before the procedure. A, a test voltage of 2 kV is applied on two adjacent electrodes; there is no leakage of current (LC). B, During the procedure, the defibrillator artifact indicates a charging voltage of 3.6 kV, which drops to 1.8 kV when the current is delivered during the shock. However, the voltage curve shows notches (arrowhead) that indicate that something wrong occurred in the catheter. (C) After the procedure, when the catheter is submitted to the same high voltage test of 2 kV, blips occur that indicate the beginning of ionization within the catheter. This catheter should be therefore rejected for the fulguration procedure.

V = The reference zero for the high voltage test (the calibration is 0.5 kV per vertical division for the test and 1 kV per division during the procedure); LC = leakage of current; C = current flow during procedure (10 amperes/div.).

catheters were originally designed for endocardial recording and/or pacing explains their insulation weakness when fulgurating voltages are used. A custom-made No. 7-F quadripolar catheter has been manufactured in small quantities by the USCI Company. We have used this catheter extensively for animal experiments, with good results. However, it is not yet commercially available. Thus, despite its limitations, we continue using the high-potential test to select catheters for the fulguration procedure.

The differences in the catheter internal structures previously described also explain why the insulation properties of multipolar catheters are generally better than those of bipolars. In practice, we generally use either tri- or quadripolar catheters. Fulguration shocks are always delivered through the distal electrode to ensure close contact with the endocardium. The catheters that are used for mapping are also subsequently used for shock delivery.

Catheter introduction and positioning for VT ablation depend on the VT site. In the case of a right-sided VT, catheters are introduced through the femoral vein. Three catheters are used, two of which are positioned in the infundibulum and apex and are introduced for endocavitary recording and pacing, while the third is located in the coronary sinus or the atrial wall. For left-sided VT the catheter used for fulguration and mapping is introduced by a femoral or axillary artery puncture. The use of a guiding tube (98-cm sheath with hemostasis valve and sideport,*) pushed beyond the aortic cusps facilitates catheter positioning within the left ventricle, and prevents inadvertent entry into the ostium of the coronary arteries.

Fulgurator

At the beginning of our experience the fulguration shock was delivered by a modified defibrillator,† in-

---
*Catalog No. 501-617; Cordis, Miami, FL, USA.
†Defigard M; ODAM, Wissembourg, France.

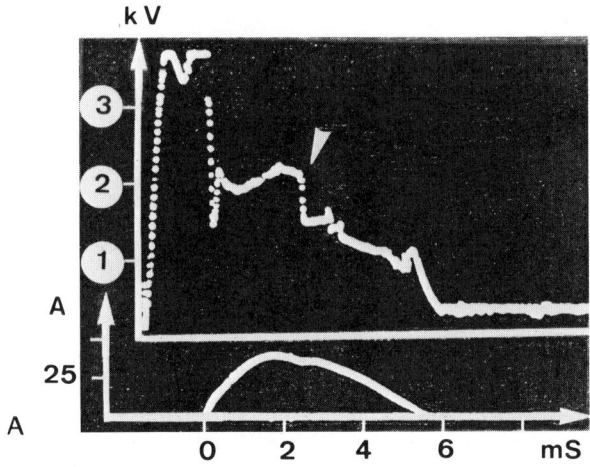

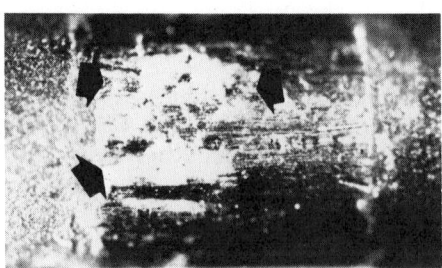

FIGURE 26-4
Another example of abnormal catheter insulation behavior during the fulguration procedure. A, The voltage curve shows abrupt changes in the voltage (arrowhead). The current curve shows two close peaks occurring during the voltage drop and indicates abnormal catheter behavior. B, Careful study of the nondistal electrode No. 3 demonstrates abnormal pittings (arrows).

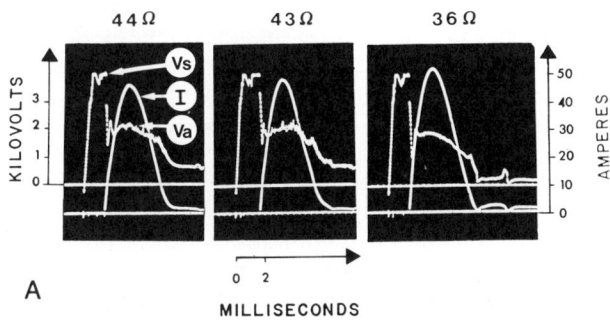

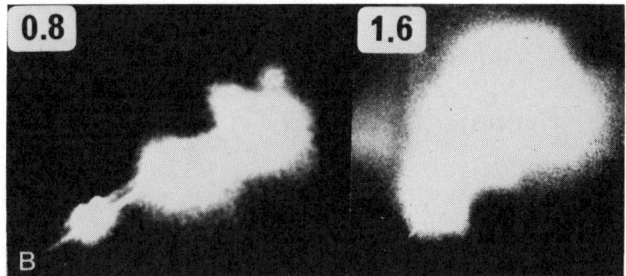

FIGURE 26–5
A, Progressive decrease in impedance due to arcing within the catheter (measurements are made at the peak of current). Vs = stored voltage; I = current curve; Va = Applied voltage.
B, The same energy is delivered to a catheter immersed in saline. High-speed cinematography shows the consequences of internal arcing. Sparks and vapor globes occur at electrode No. 2 or No. 3, which decreases the energy applied to the distal electrode. High-speed cinematography taken at 0.8 and 1.6 ms.

cluding an external electromechanical relay switching automatically to endocardial recording of the flow of the fulgurating impulse, developed for our first His bundle ablation procedure.[12] This equipment had a capacitor of 45 µF, an inductor of 100 mH, and an internal resistance of 16 ohms. The waveform produced by this apparatus was 6 ms in duration, with a peak at 2.5 ms. Later, a new piece of equipment was developed specifically for this application,* incorporating advanced design in defibrillator circuits. This equipment now incorporates a capacitor of 45 µF and an inductor of 45 mH with an internal resistance of approximately 10 ohms; the waveform produced is 4 ms in duration, and its peak is observed at 2 ms. However, the same amount of joules is delivered for the same settings. We have not studied the biologic effects of these changes.

A high-voltage electromechanical relay system has been incorporated in the new equipment, which also includes an electric circuit that measures both the current and voltage applied to the fulgurating catheter.[23] Previous to these measurements, voltage is applied to the measuring circuit before the load. This produces an "artifact" on the voltage curve that indicates the voltage (and subsequently the exact energy) stored in the capacitor. Voltage and current curves are displayed on a 5115 Tektronix oscilloscope with a 5A18

*Fulgucor; ODAM, Wissembourg, France.

vertical amplifier and 5B12N time base plug-in units. Recently, this equipment has been replaced by the 7854 Tektronix* oscilloscope, including a waveform calculator. This oscilloscope is connected to an IBM PCG microcomputer through a general-purpose interface bus (GPIB); its combination with a specialized software package allows the storing of waveforms and programs on diskettes and the print-out of measurements on the oscilloscope screen. Polaroid pictures of the screen are taken when measurements of the significant points have been made on each curve by the use of specially identified cursors (Fig. 26–6).

This oscilloscope digitizes the signals and can perform computations on waveforms stored in its memory. It is therefore possible to develop a computer program to display the evolution of the instantaneous electrical power delivered all along the shock impulse. The surface under the curve indicates the energy delivered. The evolution of impedance is also displayed and demonstrates the complex behavior of the physical phenomenon obtained during the fulguration procedure. This phenomenon is related to various patterns of ionization, which depend on the initial energy stored in the capacitor and the other electrical properties observed during the disruptive nature of the shock. These phenomena have been studied in more details elsewhere; the most important point of practical importance is that during the summit of the current curve,

*Tektronix Inc., Beaverton, Oregon.

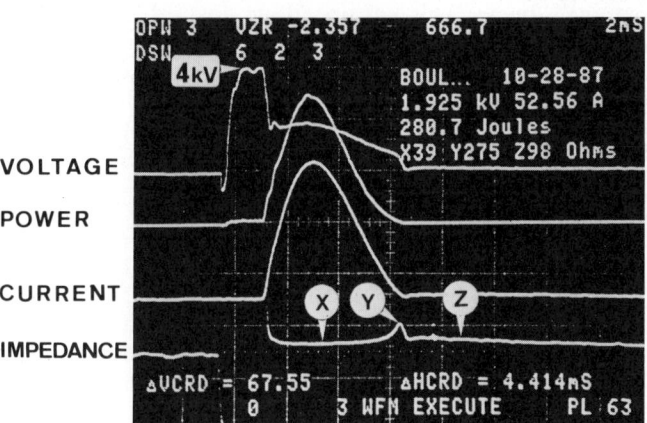

FIGURE 26–6
Improvements in waveform recording and processing during the fulguration procedure. The use of a Tektronix 7854 oscilloscope provides recording of both voltage and current curves. In addition, power and impedance curves are calculated from the digitized previous wave forms and displayed on the screen. The use of a cursor allows precise measurements of all these parameters. The voltage curve is preceded by an artifact indicating the voltage charging of the equipment (4 kV), and the peak voltage on the cardiac load is reduced to 1.9 kV. In this shock, the peak current reaches 52.56 A and the delivered amount of joules is 280.7. The impedance curve, which is also preceded by an artifact, shows an impedance of 39 ohms in the middle of the pulse (X), at 275 ohms (Y) just before the collapse of the cavitation bubble, and finally of 98 ohms (Z). The low value of 39 ohms indicates that the surface of the electrode has been increased by the plasma formed within the cavitation bubble.

impedance is in the range of 40 ohms. This value differs from the nominal impedance (50 ohms) of circuits designed for regular defibrillators. Therefore, the amount of energy spent in the inductor's internal resistance is increased, and the real energy delivered is reduced. This situation is in any case more critical if the internal resistance of the inductor is higher, as it is with the old designs. Another point concerns defibrillator calibration. In many laboratories defibrillator parameters are not periodically recalibrated. It has been our experience that nominal values may change with time in most pieces of equipment, in a range up to 15%. In the ODAM defibrillator, a particular basic circuit design assumes a high level of stability of the charging voltage, assuring constant delivery of energy for each energy setting.

The preselected discharge energy for VT ablation has varied from 160 to 320 joules, with the actual value set at an amount equal to 3 joules per kg of body weight. This equation was determined from animal experiments that indicated it was appropriate with our equipment.[24,25]

A completely independent and electrically isolated defibrillator is located in the same piece of equipment. It is left in a waiting position, charged at 40 to 80 joules (as a first step), on stand-by, connected to an anterior patch-defibrillating electrode.* This patch electrode is positioned on the precordial region. The defibrillator's other electrode is the indifferent electrode used for the fulguration shock, provided that the indifferent electrode is located on the left side of the patient's back. This set-up allows instant reaction to cases of ventricular arrhythmias with hemodynamic deterioration, without requiring the removal of the sterile fields and/or the fluoroscopic equipment (see Fig. 26–6). A back-up independent defibrillator with standard paddles is also available, ready to be charged at 400 joules.

Videotape Recordings

A custom-made video system records either the signal from a camera focused on the areas of catheter entry in the femoral vessels or the video signal generated by the fluoroscopic equipment. Alpha-numeric data concerning the patient's name, the date, and the characteristics of the shocks are superimposed on the video images (see Fig. 26–1).

A videotape recorder is connected to the fluoroscopic equipment to store the data from the video system. During the time that the fluoroscope is turned off, a separate solid-state memory is used to store and display the final image obtained. An electronic arrow provides a manually controlled indication for each point to be mapped. Under our recently modified protocol, videotape recording is done on a JVC U-matic Video cassette recorder during the entire procedure, except for two vital periods: (1) the catheter's final position just prior to the shock and (2) the end of the fulguration countdown. The data from these important periods are stored on a permanent, separate tape kept in the files. The other tape is erased during the following procedure but can be played back if special investigation is required. The fulguration videotape recording is frequently played back during the session to study catheter behavior during the shock. In addition, Polaroid pictures are taken in both the anterior and left anterior oblique views to ascertain catheter position before the shock.

A specially developed software program ("Chronos"), running on the general purpose PDP 11/73 computer (working in RSX 11M), stores the timing and provides a hard copy of important events observed throughout the procedure.

Hemodynamic Monitoring

Radial arterial pressure and pulmonary capillary wedge pressure are continuously monitored using a Swan-Ganz catheter introduced from the internal jugular vein. The cardiac output is also studied by thermodilution. These measurements are taken by the anesthesia team. In addition, in patients with poor cardiac contractility, permanent monitoring of the radial artery blood pressure is done by a dedicated team member located in the technical room. The blood pressure signal is displayed with a slow sweep of 5 s/div on the 5115 storage Tektronix oscilloscope with 5A14N vertical amplifier and a 5B12N time base plug-in unit.

Equipment for Activation Time Measurements

ECG leads I, V_F, V_1, and V_6 (or I, II, III, V_1) are recorded with an Electronics for Medicine machine (VR 12). Activation times are measured on a 12-channel ink jet paper recorder.* Comparison is made with digital measurements from a 5116 digital Tektronix oscilloscope with a 2D10 signal-sampling and storage unit. We store two channels on the screen. The first one is the endocardial mapping signal and the second is derived from the analog summation of the absolute value of 1 to 4 orthogonal surface leads. Prematurity is easily determined on the oscilloscope screen by moving two cursors positioned on the signal's relevant points (Fig. 26–7). Each mapped area is indicated on a schematic representation of the inside of the heart, similar to the classic Josephson's drawing.[26]

ECG and endocardial signals are also amplified by a custom-made piece of equipment incorporating analog low-pass and high-pass filters adapted for both surface ECG and endocardial signals.† The same piece of equipment allows placement of markers to indicate QRS detection and position of the shock in the cardiac cycle (Fig. 26–8). An automatic calibration signal for both amplitude and filtering is delivered every 5 to 30 seconds and is interrupted just before the shock (Fig. 26–9).

---

*R2 Corp., Morton Grove, IL, USA.

*Mingograph; Siemens, Solna, Sweden.
†ODAM, Wissembourg, France.

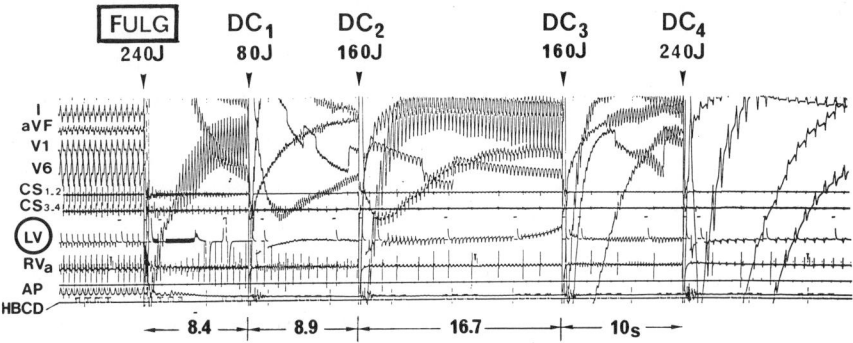

FIGURE 26-7
External shocks of increasing energies delivered in close succession after acceleration of ventricular tachycardia following a fulgurative shock. The drop in blood pressure suggests poor contractility of the underlying myocardium. Cardiac function was restored only after external cardiac massage. A quadripolar catheter with two bipolar leads was used. Leads I, aVF, V_1 and V_6 are shown. FULG = fulguration shock; DC = defibrillation shock (1-2-3-4) at increasing energies, from 80 to 240 joules; CS (1-2, 3-4) = coronary sinus; LV = left ventricle; RVa = right ventricular apex; AP = arterial blood pressure; HBCD = binary coded time marks. The numbers in the lower part of the tracing indicate the second intervals between the shocks.

Study of the endocardial electrogram prior to shock delivery assumes, if the endocardial electrogram remains the same, that the fulgurating electrode tip has not changed its position before transmission of the shock (Fig. 26–10).

Analog Signal Recordings

Surface and endocardial signals are recorded with an EMI SE 7000 14-channel magnetic tape recorder. Time marks generated by the PDP 11/73 Dec computer (program HBCD) are recorded on tape and provide exact timing of the events. The recorded signals can be replayed, filtered, and traced either on the Electronics for Medicine machine or the Mingograph ink jet recorder.

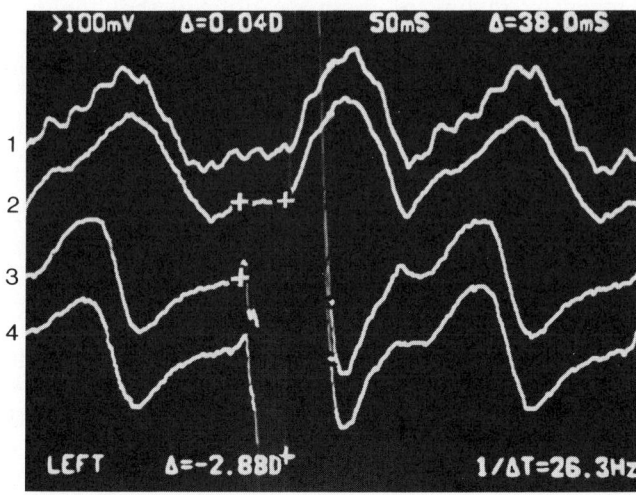

FIGURE 26-8
The top two traces (1 and 2) show the summation of the absolute value of surface leads. The two lower traces (3 + 4) are endocardial signals recorded close to the "site of origin" of ventricular tachycardia. Traces 2 and 4 are stored in the Tektronix 5116 digital sampling oscilloscope; traces 1 and 3 are live-display electronic superposition on top of the stored traces (see text for explanation). Time interval measurements are easily achieved by moving cursors positioned at the beginning of the relevant signals.

Five of the ten people involved in the procedure—three in the technical room and two in the sterile room—wear microphones and headsets; multiplexing allows recording of all the comments on the same voice-recording channel. These comments have proved to be of the utmost importance in the event of major complications.

METHOD

Prior to the fulguration procedure, class I antiarrhythmic drug therapy is interrupted for a period equivalent to 5 half-lives. Amiodarone therapy is not discontinued (about 60% of cases). Protracted general anesthesia is used because of the duration of the procedure and the frequent need to deliver more than one shock in a single procedure.

Endocardial Mapping

Endocardial mapping is used to localize the presumed area of VT origin.[27] In cases in which VT is not incessant, programmed stimulation is used to induce the arrhythmia. In our equipment, remote-controlled electric relays switch catheters from signal-recording amplifiers to a Savita programmed stimulation unit. The protocol includes the introduction of one to three progressively more premature stimuli delivered within a paced basic stimulation with a progressively increasing rate. In some cases isoproterenol is injected to facilitate VT induction. When unstable VT or VF is induced during the pacing protocol, the session is interrupted or postponed and drugs are prescribed. After drug treatment, previously unstable arrhythmias generally become mappable.

Pace-mapping

Identification of the area of origin of VT is also attempted through the use of pace-mapping, in which the ventricle is paced in an effort to exactly reproduce the ECG signals observed during documented episodes

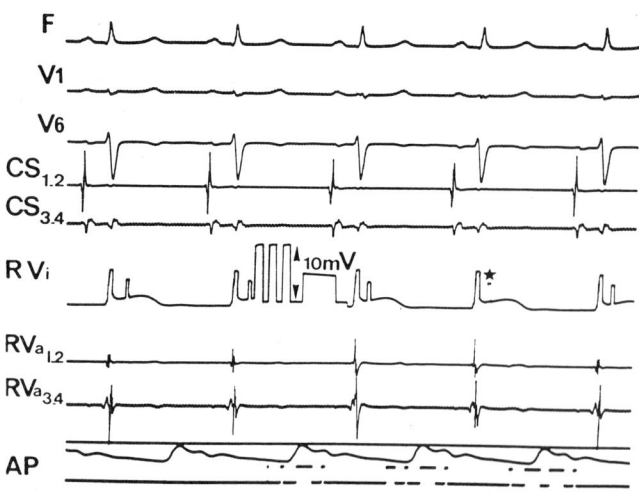

FIGURE 26-9
Recordings prior to the fulguration procedure. Two electronic markers are displayed on the right ventricular infundibulum (RVi) electrogram. The first rectangular pulse indicates detection of the endocardial signal. The leading edge of the second pulse ★, which can be moved to any desired distance from the first one, indicates the exact timing of the shock. Note also the automatic calibrating signal, which indicates the gain and filtering. In this particular example the upper pass filter has a long time constant, allowing proper recording of ST-segment elevation on the endocardial lead (assuming that a good but not strong contact of the catheter tip is exerted against the endocardial wall). Gain of amplifier is indicated by a binary coded signal with a sensitivity of 10 mV for the distance between the two arrowheads.

of VT or episodes induced at the beginning of the procedure.[28, 29] Three methods of ventricular pace-mapping are used: (1) continuous pacing in sinus rhythm at a rate identical to the tachycardia rate, (2) slight overdrive of ventricular tachycardia, and (3) introduction of a premature stimulus during ventricular tachycardia.

Precise comparison between documented arrhythmias and pace-mapping is performed with the previously described equipment. Recently we have introduced the use of 12-lead ECG recordings produced by an independent, battery-operated 3-channel microprocessor-based recorder.

Pacing the Area of Slow Conduction

Because reentry phenomenon is the underlying mechanism of most chronic ventricular arrhythmias, a zone of slow conduction is supposed to be operative in a circus movement involving part of the ventricular myocardium.[30-32] Epicardial data recorded in sinus rhythm and/or during VT in the experimental laboratory,[33] as well as in clinical cases, has substantiated the evidence of zones of slow conduction:

- In sinus rhythm, potentials occurring late in the diastole (up to 300 ms) were observed after the onset of the QRS complex.[34]
- Pacing in the zone of slow conduction induced activation of the remaining part of the ventricle after a certain delay.[35]
- In a patient with Uhl's anomaly, the pathway followed by the circus movement involving a zone of slow conduction was traced. In this patient a two-dimensional clinical model was probable. The spread of activation was therefore delineated without the imprecision that would have been observed in a myocardium of normal thickness.[36, 37]

Recently we have considered concentrating the ablative action on the area of slow conduction because (1) this area was already abnormal, and (2) this could decrease the damage produced on healthy myocardium.

Delay between pacing stimulus and ventricular response was observed in several patients during endocardial mapping preceding the fulguration procedure. However, in one of them we noticed that the morphology of the ventricular responses was *identical* to the morphology of the QRS complexes observed during spontaneous VTs. It was deduced that pacing was achieved in a zone of slow conduction close to the area of the circus movement, or at least in a zone of slow conduction in relation to the exit zone of the circus movement (Fig. 26-11). However, the experience gained during pace mapping and the electrophysiologic study preceding the surgical treatment of VT suggested that zones of slow conduction could be quite diffuse in the myocardium. On the other hand, the fulguration procedure, like other ablative techniques, will modify myocardium in a very restricted area. In order to be effective, the ablative technique should involve the area of slow conduction that is *critical* (or indispensable) for the perpetuation of the arrhythmia. Such a zone should meet the following conditions:

- Stimulation during sinus rhythm at a rate close to the tachycardia rate should induce a ventricular response after a certain *delay*.
- Ventricular response induced by stimulation should have the *same morphology* as the QRS complexes observed during spontaneous VT.
- Presystolic coupling of the local potential during VT

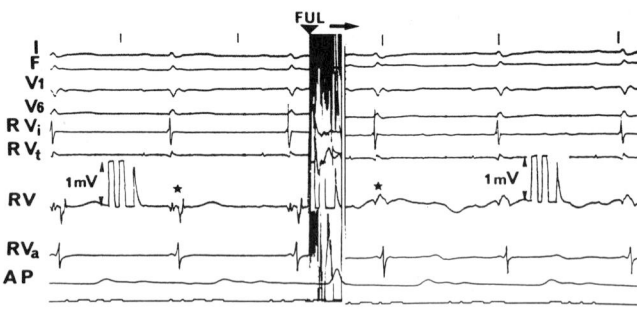

FIGURE 26-10
Recording of endocardial signals before and after shock delivered inside the right ventricle. The endocardial signal is highlighted (stars) before and after the shock. Stability of the electrode is ascertained by the endocardial signal's stability prior to the shock delivery. A few seconds after the shock (at right) a small-amplitude potential is recorded. This feature is observed only on the rare occasions when the catheter has not changed its position during or after the shock.

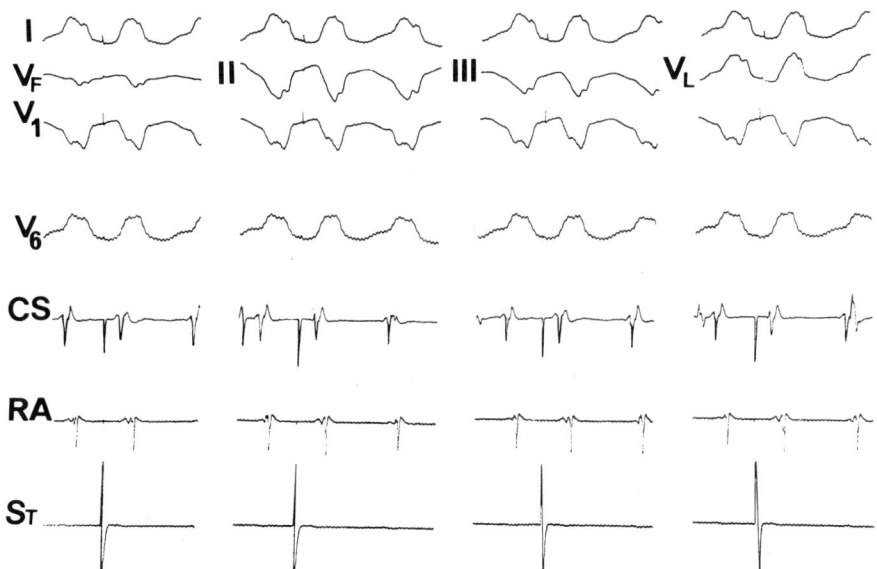

FIGURE 26–11
An example of pacing in a zone of slow conduction during ventricular tachycardia. A stimulation impulse is prematurely delivered within the tachycardia cycle and produces a QRS complex after a delay that is seen in each lead and that is followed by a QRS complex with almost the same QRS morphology as that of the spontaneous ventricular tachycardia. The second trace indicates successively leads VF (V_F) I, II, III, and VL and the good pace-mapping without fusion in seven leads. CS = coronary sinus; RA = right atrium; St = stimulation mark; This illustration shows that pacing has been achieved in the zone of slow conduction in the vicinity of the exit site of the spontaneous ventricular tachycardia.

should be the same as the stimulation-response coupling of the first criterion.[38]

Additional information is provided by pacing during ventricular tachycardia at a rate slightly faster than the spontaneous VT rate obtaining ventricular responses with the same morphology as during VT, and then returning to the spontaneous VT rate at the cessation of pacing.[39] This "entrainment without fusion" suggests that stimulation was achieved in the zone of slow conduction that is critical for the circus movement. This zone could be ablated successfully either in the proximal part of the slow conduction area, as suggested by the initial case,[38] or on its distal part, as suggested in a more recent study.[40] The slow conducting zone seems therefore preferable to the "site of origin" of the ventricular tachycardia. However, this approach needs confirmation, and the frequency with which this new criteria can be obtained remains to be demonstrated.

Fulguration

Fulguration is delivered at the conclusion of a protocol with checklist format (Fig. 26–12; Table 26–1), which is followed by a countdown during which every piece of relevant equipment is put into action. The shock is synchronized with the surface QRS complexes during sinus rhythm[41] or during VT if the arrhythmia is incessant (delivering the shock in sinus rhythm is now preferred). Triggering of the shock can be linked either to the ECG or to an endocardial signal when the surface recording of the QRS complexes shows a smooth rise time. As a last resort if other methods are not possible, a nonsynchronized shock is automatically delivered after 2 seconds. The shock is applied between the distal electrode of the fulgurating catheter, which is used as an anode, and an indifferent electrode, which functions as a cathode, and is positioned under the patient's back. From 1 to 8 shocks are delivered during each session.

In cases in which atrioventricular block occurs, ventricular pacing is performed. A defibrillating external shock is immediately delivered when acceleration of VT or its degradation to ventricular fibrillation (VF) occurs.[42] After completion of the fulguration shock, it is possible to record flattening of the endocardial potential (see Fig. 26–10), provided stability of the fulgurating electrode has been maintained.[23] Programmed stimulation is resumed after a 10-minute rest period to permit electrical and hemodynamic stabilization.

The main end points of a session for VT ablation are:

- Failure to induce a stable, monomorphic VT by a programmed pacing protocol equivalent to or more aggressive than that employed for initiating the VT required for mapping.
- Spontaneous interruption in less than 1 minute of a previously sustained VT.
- Induction of repeated episodes of acceleration of VT or VF after fulguration.
- Repeated induction of VT, leading to hemodynamic deterioration.
- Time limitation due to technical considerations (procedure lasting more than 8 hours or 8 shocks).

Postoperative Surveillance

The patient's radial artery and venous blood pressures are monitored for 24 hours postoperatively. ECG monitoring is achieved by cable or telemetrics (Hewlett-Packard HP 78225 system associated with the NADIA software). All alarm signals are recorded. Graphs indicating trends in cardiac rhythm, extrasystole frequency, tachycardia, and so forth can be printed out, and the data can be corrected when necessary by using the "recall" function.

A left subclavicular catheter is left at the apex of the right ventricle in order to permit reassessment of bedside VT reinduction, which is done at or within 10

```
VT FULGURATION BASIC PROTOCOL JEAN ROSTAND 10–85                         Time
```

 0. CLASS I DISCONTINUATION .... AMIO .... ISOPROT ....
 1. PATIENT SEDATION ....
 2. ECG LEAD I,F, V1,V6 1mV CALIBRATION .... 12 LEAD ....
 3. RADIAL BP .... 0–100 CAL .... RBP ....
 4. SWAN-GANZ CATHETER INSERTION ....
 5. BASIC CARDIAC OUTPUT ....
 6. C.S. CATH. or .... ATRIAL CATH for A record in VT ....
 7. BIPOLAR APEX CATH. FOR POSTSHOCK PACING ....
 8. QUADRIPOLAR CATH. VENTRICULAR APEX RV PACING & SENSING ....
 9. TRI .... QUADRI .... CATH .... FULGURATION ....
10. CHECK LIST: CPK/MB Control sampling ....
        Emergency defibrillator .... FULG DEF ....
        EMI Tape recorder "RECORD"+"ENRGTR" ....
        Computer time marks OK ....
        Computer "Chronos" program ON ....
        FULG AMPLI AUTO CALIB 5s ....
        FULG CATH CONNECTION ....
        FULG SYNCH MARKER ....
11. INDUCTION OF VT BY PROG PACING (UP TO BURST PACING) ....
12. CHECK FOR HEMODYNAMICS AFTER ACCOMMODATION PHASE ....
13. VIDEO TAPE CATHETERS DESCRIPTION AND CONNECTIONS (CHANNELS)
14. PRESYSTOLIC POTENTIALS Premat .... Small .... Large ....
15. PACE-MAPPING SINUS RHYTHM .... EFM .... 12 LEAD ....
        PREMATURE S. DURING VT ....
        Ampli fulgur CALIB ....
        Electrogram fulg Nonfiltered .... Filtered ....
        Lesion Wave .... Filtered .... Filtered ....
        Delay .... Recycling .... QRS-TV ....
        Threshold measurement ....
        Fulgurator synchronisation (comment) ....
        V-I Tektronix Synchro Ext .... Clear Screen ....
        50mm/s SIE, EFM 10mm/s Temp corrected ....
        Image intensifier proper centering ....
        V C R .... M T .... N .... E M I .... M T .... N ...
        Hemodynamic last check OK .... BP on line + + ...
16. COUNT DOWN: Beginning at 25.
        25- Siemens recorder runnning at 50/mm s,
        22- Video tape recorder started,
        16- PRESHOCK SUMMARY: Name of patient, Date,
                • Catheter Type .... Site Selection ....
                • Procedure Number .... Shock Number ....
                • Energy Chosen .... Patch Position ....
        15- Fulgurator charging,
        10- EFM recorder running at 10 mm/s started,
         8- Image intensifier ON,
17. >>>>>>0- QRS SYNCHRONISED SHOCK ...OK ...NONSyn 2 Sec Del ...
18. V. PACING AV BLOCK .... DEFIB VT Acc .... VF ....
19. BLOOD PRESSURE CHECK .... I-V Tektronix check Polaroid ....
20. 10-15 MN. OF REST, COMMENTS ....
21. > GO TO 11.
22. END POINT OF SESSION:
    NON INDUC ... NON SUSTAINED .... NON CLINICAL .... M ... R.... D....
    PACE PROT .... TIME LIMITATION or SHOCK-7 ....

FIGURE 26–12

TABLE 26-1
Interpretation of Protocol Checklist Illustrated in Figure 26-12

0	Time interval between class I drug discontinuation and fulguration.		
1	Calibration leads D1, aV_F, V_1, V_6 for EFM and SIEMENS recorders.		
2	Time at the beginning of general anesthesia.		
3	Verification of the Zero reference and 150 mm Hg of the radial probe for pressure recording.		
4	Time of Swan-Ganz catheter insertion.		
5	Control of thermodilution measurements.		
6	Coronary sinus catheter in place (associated with taking a blood sampling for measuring lactates).		
7	Threshold OK for bipolar catheter, ready for post-shock pacing.		
8	Quadripolar catheter for atrial or ventricular pacing and for sensing before and during the shock.		
9	High-voltage tests for tripolar or quadripolar catheter used for the fulguration procedure.		
10	Recording of the His bundle potentials or coronary sinus potentials by bipolar catheter.		
11	Pre-check list:		

- Verification of control sampling for the CPK MB.
- Emergency defibrillator should be adjusted to 400 Joules.
- EMI tape recorder should be in position of "record" with the position "Enrgtr" for an external device assuming proper switching.
- Computer time marks OK.
- Computer marks OK; marks appearing at the bottom constitute the last trace of the technical track indicating precisely the timing; the reference Zero is also used for blood pressure recording.
- Computer program "Chronos" on: This program generated by the PDP 11/73 is used to indicate the precise timing of the events on the recording equipment.
- Fulg cath connection: This means that the *fulguration director* personally will check that the negative pole of the catheter is securely connected to the appropriate terminal, providing a positive impulse through the catheter. Triggering of VT by programmed pacing or burst of pacing in case of inducible VT. Wait 10 to 15 minutes for accommodation of the hemodynamics after VT induction. Measurements of the rate, looking for tolerance.

14 Recording of the endocardial map for premature presystolic potentials. Pace-mapping during sinus rhythm or by premature stimulation during ventricular tachycardia, recorded in 12-leads.

16 Videotape catheter description and connection: This is made on the videotape in both the anteroposterior and left anterior oblique positions.

17 Check list:
- Energy selected and the reason.
- Calibration of the recording channel that records the electrogram and on which the shock is delivered.
- Same recording without filtering.
- Measurement of lesion waves; recording with the same filter that will be used during the fulguration procedure.
- Pacing threshold measurements by the fulgurating catheter.
- Check for proper synchronization of the fulgurator, as shown by the pulses appearing on the channels used for fulguration and by measurements of the interval between the QRS complex and the shock delivery.
- Voltage and current curves recorded by Tektronix oscilloscope synchronized with the fulgurator.
- Clear the screen of the storage by Tektronix oscilloscope.
- Adust the recording speed of the Siemens and EFM recorders; in this last equipment, temperature should be adjusted for proper contrast.
- Proper centering of the anteroposterior view of the image intensifier. Videotape ready to be started before the shock delivery.
- Systemic blood pressure on line; no more cardiac output measurements are permitted after this time.

18 Countdown:
- At count 25, the Siemens recorder is running at 50 mm/s
- At 22, the videotape recorder is started.
- At 19, there is a brief preshock summary indicating the name of the patient, date, catheter type, site selection, procedure number, shock number, and energy chosen.
- At 15, the fulgurator is put in the charging mode.
- At 10, the EFM recorder, running at 10 mm/s, is started.
- At 8, the image intensifier is ON.
- At 5, the calibrating amplitude and filtering markers are OFF.
- At 0, the fulgurator key is activated. A QRS-synchronized shock will be delivered within 2 seconds.

19 The videotape will continue to run for 5 seconds after shock delivery, or more in case of particular problems; this decision is made by the videotape technician.

20 Ventricular pacing is achieved in case of AV block, or defibrillation in case of acceleration of VT or VF.

21 Blood pressure is checked as well as voltage and current curves; Polaroid pictures are taken of the Tektronix screen.

22 During a rest period of 10 to 15 minutes, comments are made by the director of the procedure.

23 Return to 11 and try to reinduce VT by programmed pacing.

24 End point of study: VT is not inducible, or VT is inducible but nonsustained, or VT is modified and should or should not be refulgurated in terms of morphology, rate, and duration. Pacing protocol used. Session interrupted for time limitation or number of shocks.

days after fulguration, provided that no recurrence has occurred spontaneously. This reassessment is done using a programmed pacing protocol incorporating up to three extrastimuli on basic pacing cycles of 600 to 400 ms.

When VT comparable to previous attacks either occurs spontaneously or is inducible, antiarrhythmic drug therapy is again attempted. If the latter proves effective, drug therapy is reconsidered; if it proves ineffective, a new fulguration session is scheduled.

The effectiveness of the fulguration procedure is reassessed a final time before patient discharge by use of 24-hour Holter monitoring, stress testing on a stationary bicycle, and programmed stimulation.

OVERVIEW

We consider the fulguration procedure to be a definite step forward in the treatment of severe ventricular arrhythmias. However, the recurrence of VT has been observed in some cases, and this fact, along with the need for several shocks or several sessions and the necessity for fulguration in combination with antiarrhythmic therapy, has led us to conclude that improved techniques and methods must be developed for the procedure to achieve optimal results.

Acknowledgment

We are indebted to Mrs. Nicole Proust for her secretarial support.

References

1. Dulk KD, Bertholet M, Brugada P: Clinical experience with implantable devices for control of tachyarrhythmias. PACE 7:548, 1984.
2. Zipes DP, Heger JJ, Miles WM, et al.: Synchronous intracardiac cardioversion. PACE 7:522, 1984.
3. Mirowski M, Reid PR, Mower MM, et al.: The automatic implantable cardioverter-defibrillator. PACE 7:534, 1984.
4. Fontaine G, Guiraudon G, Frank R, et al.: La cartographie épicardique et le traitement chirurgical par simple ventriculotomie de certaines tachycardies ventriculaires rebelles par réentrée. Arch Mal Coeur 68:113, 1975.
5. Garan H, Nguyen K, McGovern BA, et al.: Perioperative and long-term results after electrophysiologically directed ventricular surgery for recurrent ventricular tachycardia. J Am Coll Cardiol 8:201, 1986.
6. Ostermeyer J, Breithardt G, Kolvenbach R, et al.: The surgical treatment of ventricular tachycardias. Simple aneurysmectomy versus electrophysiologically guided procedures. J Thorac Cardiovasc Surg 84:704, 1982.
7. Borggrefe M, Podczeck A, Ostermeyer J, Breithardt G: Presented for the Collaborative Report on Antitachycardiac Surgery. In Non-Pharmacological Therapy of Tachyarrhythmias. Dusseldorf, 1987, pp. 109–132.
8. Scheinman MM, Evans-Bell T: Catheter ablation of the atrioventricular junction: A report of the Percutaneous Mapping and Ablation Registry. Circulation 70:1024, 1984.
9. Gallagher JJ, Svenson RH, Kasell JH, et al.: Catheter technique for closed-chest ablation of the atrioventricular conduction system. N Engl J Med 306:194, 1982.
10. Hartzler GO: Electrode catheter ablation of refractory focal ventricular tachycardia. J Am Coll Cardiol 2:1107, 1983.
11. Puech P, Gallay P, Grolleau R, et al.: Traitement par électrofulguration endocavitaire d'une tachycardie ventriculaire récidivante par dysplasie ventriculaire droite. Arch Mal Coeur 77:826, 1984.
12. Fontaine G, Tonet JL, Frank R, et al.: La fulguration endocavitaire. Une nouvelle méthode de traitement des troubles du rythme? Ann Cardiol Angeiol 33:543, 1984.
13. Fontaine G, Frank R, Tonet JL, et al.: Treatment of resistant ventricular tachycardia with endocavitary fulguration and antiarrhythmic therapy, compared to antiarrhythmic therapy alone: Experience in 111 consecutive cases with a mean follow-up of 18 months. Texas Heart Inst 13:401, 1986.
14. Bardy GH, Coltorti F, Ivey TD, et al.: Effect of damped sine-wave shocks on catheter dielectric strength. Am J Cardiol 56:769, 1985.
15. Fisher JD, Brodman R, Johnson D, et al.: Nonsurgical electrical ablation of tachycardia: Importance of in vitro testing of catheter leads. PACE 7:74, 1984.
16. Fontaine G, Lechat Ph, Cansell A, et al.: Advances in the treatment of cardiac arrhythmias in the last decade. Definition and role of ablative techniques. In Fontaine G, Scheinman MM (eds.): Ablation in Cardiac Arrhythmias. Mount Kisco, Futura Publishing Co., 1987, p. 5.
17. Fontaine G, Cansell A, Lechat Ph, et al.: A nondestructive method to select catheters for ablation techniques (Abstract). Eur Heart J 5(Suppl 1):258, 1984.
18. Fontaine G, Cansell A, Lampe L, et al.: Endocavitary fulguration (electrode catheter ablation): Equipment-related problems. In Fontaine G, Scheinman MM (eds.): Ablation in Cardiac Arrhythmias, pp. 85–100. Mount Kisco, Futura Publishing Co, 1987.
19. Fontaine G, Cansell A: Potential risk of using multipolar catheters for the treatment of tachycardias. Stimarec Bull 5–6:1, 1983.
20. Fontaine G, Cansell A, Lechat Ph, et al.: Method of selecting catheters for endocavitary fulguration. Stimucoeur 12:285, 1984.
21. Fontaine G, Tonet JL, Frank R, et al.: Electrode catheter ablation of resistant ventricular tachycardia by endocavitary fulguration associated with anti-arrhythmic therapy. Experience of 38 patients with a mean follow-up of 23 months. In Brugada P, Wellens HJJ (eds.): Cardiac Arrhythmias. Where to Go From Here, pp. 539–569. Mount Kisco, Futura Publishing Co., 1987.
22. Fontaine G, Volmer W, Nienaltowska E, et al.: Approach to the physics of fulguration. In Fontaine G, Scheinman MM (eds.): Ablation in Cardiac Arrhythmias, pp. 101–116. Mount Kisco, Futura Publishing Co, 1987.
23. Fontaine G, Tonet JL, Frank R, et al.: Traitement des tachycardies ventriculaires rebelles par fulguration endocavitaire associée aux anti-arythmiques. Arch Mal Coeur 79:1152, 1986.
24. Fontaine G: The effects of high energy DC shocks delivered to ventricular myocardium. In Scheinman MM (ed.): Catheter Ablation of Cardiac Anhythmias, pp. 97–114. Boston, Martinus Nijhoff, 1988.
25. Tonet JL, Fontaine G, Frank R, et al.: Treatment of refractory ventricular tachycardias by endocardial fulguration (Abstract). Circulation 72(Suppl 3):388, 1985.
26. Josephson ME, Horowitz LN, Spielman SR, et al.: Role of catheter mapping in the preoperative evaluation of ventricular tachycardia. Am J Cardiol 49:207, 1982.
27. Frank R, Fontaine G, Baraka M, et al.: Catheter endocardial mapping in fulguration. In Aliot E, Lazzara R (Eds.): Ventricular Tachycardia From Mechanism to Therapy, pp. 390–402. Martinus Nijhoff, Dondrecht, 1987.
28. O'Keefe DB, Curry PVL, Prior AL, et al.: Surgery for ventricular tachycardia using operative pace mapping. Br Heart J 43:116, 1980.
29. Holt PM, Smallpeice C, Deverall PB, et al.: Ventricular arrhythmias. A guide to their localisation. Br Heart J 53:417, 1985.
30. Wellens HJJ, Schuilenburg RM, Durrer D: Electrical stimulation of the heart in patients with ventricular tachycardia. Circulation 46:216, 1972.
31. Wellens HJJ, Lie KI, Durrer D: Further observations on ventricular tachycardias as studied by electrical stimulation of the heart. Circulation 49:647, 1974.
32. Wellens HJJ, Duren DR, Lie KI: Observations on mechanisms of ventricular tachycardia in man. Circulation 54:237, 1976.
33. El-Sherif N, Gough WB, Restivo M: Reentrant ventricular arrhythmias in the late myocardial infarction period. 14. Mech-

anisms of resetting entrainment, acceleration, or termination of reentrant tachycardia by programmed electrical stimulation. PACE 10:341, 1987.
34. Fontaine G, Frank R, Vedel J, et al.: La genèse de certains troubles du rythme ventriculaire. Nouv Presse Med 3:2321, 1974.
35. Fontaine G, Guiraudon G, Frank R: Intramyocardial conduction defects in patients prone to ventricular tachycardia. I. The postexcitation syndrome in sinus rhythm. In Sandoe E, Julian DG, Bell JW (eds.): Management of Ventricular Tachycardia. Role of Mexiletine, pp. 39–55. Amsterdam, Excerpta Medica, 1978.
36. Fontaine G, Guiraudon G, Frank R, et al.: Surgical treatment of ventricular tachycardia. In Bayes A, Cosin J (eds.): Diagnosis and Treatment of Cardiac Arrhythmias, pp. 368–390. Oxford, Pergamon Press, 1980.
37. Fontaine G, Guiraudon G, Frank R, et al.: Stimulation studies and epicardial mapping in ventricular tachycardia: Study of mechanisms and selection for surgery. In Kulbertus HE (ed.): Reentrant Arrhythmias, pp. 334–350. Lancaster, MTP Pub., 1977.
38. Fontaine G: Prevention of sudden arrhythmic death. Catheter ablation. In Proceedings of the 1985 Sydney Opera House Symposium, pp. 18–21. Sydney, Telectronics Vectors Pub., October 1986.
39. Waldo AL, Okumura K, Olshansky B, et al.: Use of transient entrainment of tachycardia as an aid to application of fulguration. In Fontaine G, Scheinman MM (eds.): Ablation in Cardiac Arrhythmias, pp. 1–12. Mount Kisco, Futura Publishing Co, 1987.
40. Frank R, Tonet JL, Kounde S, et al.: Localization of the area of slow conduction during ventricular tachycardia. In Brugada P, Wellens HJJ (eds.): Cardiac Arrhythmias. Where to Go From Here, pp. 191–208. Mount Kisco, Futura Pub. Co., 1987.
41. Gallais Y, Touzet M, Gateau O, et al.: Anesthésie et surveillance dans la fulguration endocavitaire pour le traitement radical des tachycardies ventriculaires. Ann Cardiol Angeiol 35:539, 1986.
42. Tonet JL, Baraka M, Fontaine G, et al.: Ventricular arrhythmias during endocardial catheter fulguration of ventricular tachycardias (Abstract). J Am Coll Cardiol 7(No. 2):236A, 1986.

27

Engineering Aspects of Modern Cardiac Pacing

Peter P. Tarjan

Historical Overview

Transistors, which act as low-power electron valves, began to move from laboratories to industrial production in the 1950s. This advance was crucially important for the development of implantable pacemakers. Almost three decades have passed since Elmqvist and Senning[1] announced their implantable pacemaker, a device powered by a rechargeable battery. The development of polymerizable synthetic resins for the encapsulation and protection of electronic circuits and the introduction of synthetic rubbers and noncorrosive, highly fatigue-resistant, flexible conducting wires for leads were similarly important technological advances needed to reach the objectives of the Swedish team. These also enabled Glenn's group[2] to develop a pacemaker whose power was supplied continuously, by noninvasive means, from an externally worn transmitter. Greatbatch's design[3] employed the Rubin or "mercury" cell to provide a truly self-contained design that has remained a basic requirement. The introduction of noninvasive programming in the early 1970s established an optional but very powerful and useful link between the implant and an external instrument to control the implant's functions. In the future this link may become unnecessary for at least some pacemakers, when reliable techniques for self-adjustment for optimal performance are achieved.

By 1960 the foundations of pacemaker engineering and the industry had been established. Bringing this new technology into the clinical stage was possible only through the vision and determination of surgeons and cardiologists who defined the requirements and constructively evaluated the various designs.

The applications for pacemakers and the technologies for their construction have evolved far beyond the dreams of the pioneers, and continuous interaction between clinicians and engineers has remained the key to clinically successful innovation. The dimensions and weight of pacemakers of the late 1980s are a small fraction of those of early implants, which are now museum pieces. Today's pacemakers are hermetically sealed in highly biocompatible metal enclosures. Their realistically expected service life is at least ten times longer, and their functional complexities have increased by about four orders of magnitude, based on the number of electronic gates, or elementary control units, in each implant. The functional capabilities of pacemakers have evolved from uninterrupted preset support of (or "competition" with) the ventricular rate, to sophisticated, "as needed" multichamber electrophysiologic prostheses equipped with sensors through which the device can adequately respond to the continuously changing demands of the body. In addition, some implants can be custom-engineered for the patient, by noninvasive programming, to provide specific ways to recognize and treat arrhythmias. A great many implants are also capable of gathering data regarding their own operation and the dynamic behavior of the heart they are assigned to support. This information can be retrieved by the physician to decide how well the device has served the patient and how, if at all, the functions of the implant should be modified.

Finally, in the last half decade, internal defibrillators have become widely accepted for the prevention of sudden death due to ventricular fibrillation. In the coming years these are expected to be integrated with the established functions of pacemakers and to become widely used for the control of a broad range of arrhythmias.

The future of pacing is expected to combine the best of all presently available functions in reliable and compact configurations, operating as self-regulating systems. Their cost will decline, and their reliability will increase well beyond the reliability expected from the heart. Significant advances are expected in the areas of tachyarrhythmia recognition and their treatment with low-energy stimulation, and in the performance of implantable defibrillators.

This chapter provides an overview of the principles,

applications, technologies and compromises in the design of pacemakers.

Basic Principles

TREATMENT

The working principles common to most implantable pacemakers can be illustrated with an apparatus devised from a partially insulated needle, a flat piece of metal, a battery, a telegrapher's key, and some wire. Once the needle is inserted through the chest wall and into the myocardium, the needle's bare tip, serving as the stimulating electrode, delivers current to the heart each time the circuit is closed. The return path for the current is through a metal plate in contact with the body surface (Fig. 27–1).

The key operator is the true pacemaker. A person who can interpret an ECG "in real time" can also provide *noncompetitive* pacing by keeping track of time after each spontaneous, normal, or premature wave. If the elapsed time is too long, then the operator depresses the key for a brief moment to evoke a response from the heart. With just one needle, at least three pacing methods may be implemented: (1) pace the ventricles, (2) pace the atria, and (3) provide a prosthetic AV node by keeping an eye on the atrial waves on the ECG and, after each of these, depressing the key after a short pause to stimulate the ventricles in case the ventricular wave is delayed. Until about ten years ago, the commonly used pacemakers merely substituted relatively simple electronic circuits for the operator of the telegraph key.

A significant advance evolved about ten years ago with the clinical emergence of dual-chamber stimulation and sensing. Its basic function is illustrated by the addition of a second needle and telegraph key to our previous simple model. An alert operator keeps track of time after each atrial and ventricular ECG complex to provide appropriate control for the heart according to the following simple rules.

1. After each atrial wave wait for T_1 milliseconds (ms). If there is no ventricular activity during this time, then depress the key for ventricular stimulation.
2. After each ventricular wave wait T_2 ms, and if there is no atrial activity, then depress the key for atrial stimulation.

These simple rules will work very well for many patients, but they may create very undesirable situations in others. These problems and their corrections will be discussed in more detail in the section on dual-chamber pacing.

TIMING

In all the early pacemakers, up to the middle of the 1970s, the time intervals between pulses and the duration of the stimuli were determined by the charging or discharging of a capacitor through a resistor. A capacitor stores electrical charges much like a container stores liquid. A pipe that resists the flow of liquids is analogous to an electrical resistor that counters the movement of electrons. The mechanism of the circuits commonly used for setting time intervals is similar to that of the water tank of a toilet that flushes automatically, as shown in Figure 27–2A. When the tank is emptied, a new cycle begins. The electrical equivalent of the automatically flushing toilet is shown in Figure 27–2B.

Resistor-capacitor timers have been replaced by piezoelectric crystals. Their physical principle of operation is identical to that of ultrasonic transducers. The miniature timing crystals used in pacemakers were previously developed for use in electronic clocks and watches. These crystals resonate (naturally oscillate) at an extremely stable rate. They are quite independent of temperature variations and other factors. The frequency of resonance can be set quite precisely by controlling a dimension of the crystal. A commonly selected frequency is 32,768 Hz, because this number is equal to 2^{15}, a number easily handled by digital electronics to generate fractions of a second. Counting the oscillations of the crystal in the binary system produces the intervals needed for pacing. For example, as the count of consecutive oscillations goes from 255 to 256 (binary 1111 1111 + 1 = 1 0000 0000) it yields an interval of about 7.8 ms. Counting 128 (binary 1000 0000) of these larger intervals provides a 1-second interval. Three oscillations provide a pulse duration very close to 0.01 ms, and so on.

Is accurate timing really important? In pacing for bradycardia, it is not, except to protect the patient against significant ($> \pm 5\%$) rate changes due to battery depletion or slow drifts in the electronic circuits. A downward drift in rate was used for many years to detect battery depletion. An anecdote illustrates the point:[4] A woman in complete heart block phoned the head of a London pacemaker clinic with the news, "I think it's time again for another one, luv, the eggs are getting harder. . . . " Every morning she timed her soft-boiled egg by counting 220 of her pulses. She was right, of course; the battery was indeed on its way out,

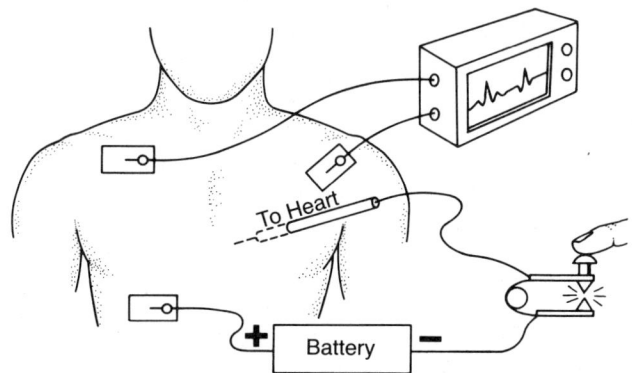

FIGURE 27–1
Diagram of a simple pacemaker. Electric current flows through the heart muscle every time the telegrapher's key is depressed. Noncompetitive pacing is established by monitoring the spontaneous activity of the heart and operating the key so that the pacemaker pulse does not interfere with the spontaneous heart action.

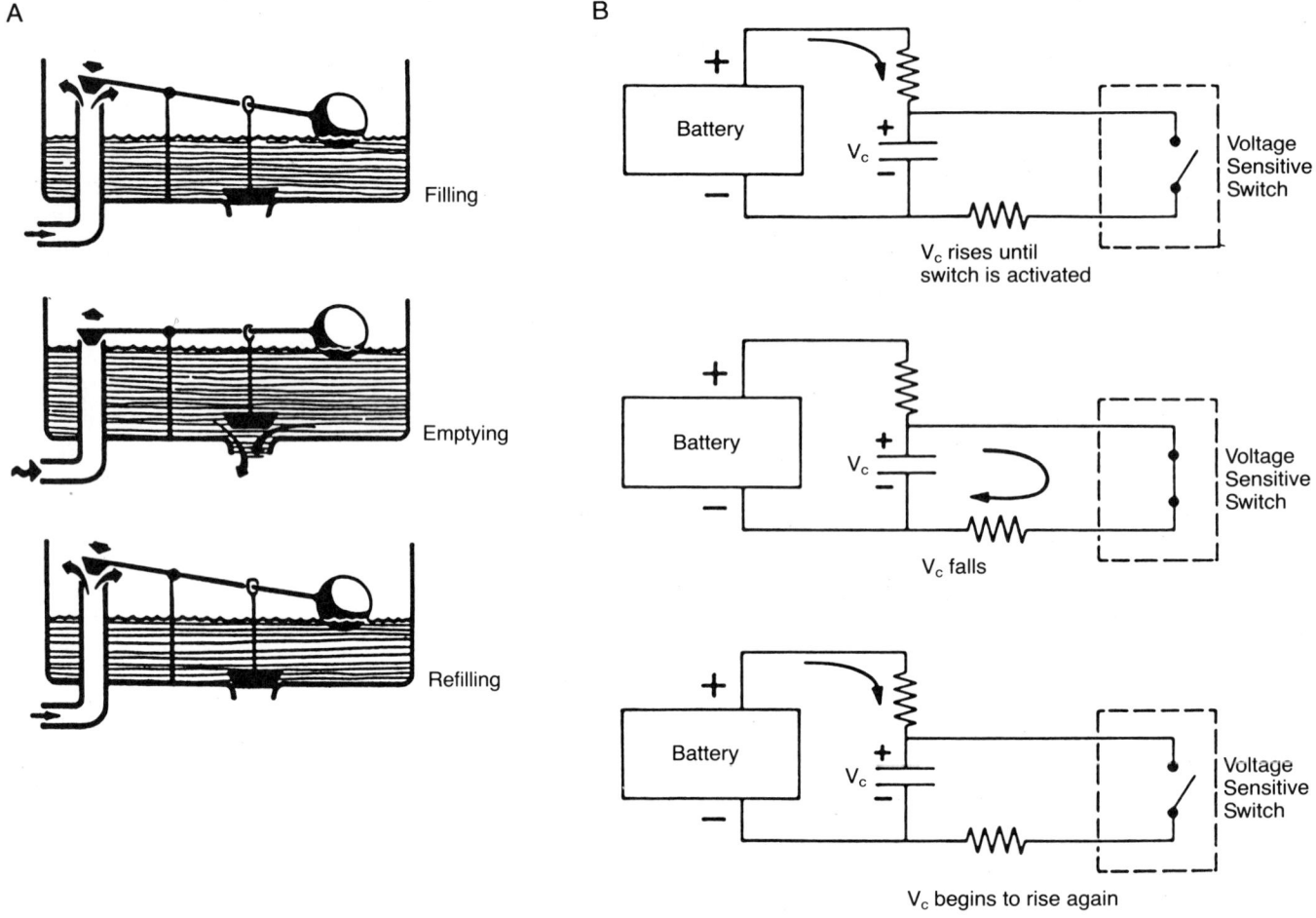

FIGURE 27–2
A, A hydraulic timer. The timer periods for filling and emptying can be adjusted by additional valves on the intake and outflow pipes.
B, An electrical timer. The charging and discharging periods can be adjusted by using different resistors.

causing a decrease in her rate of stimulation. Today, with crystal oscillators stable within a few minutes per year, less direct and more transparent techniques are used to detect impending battery depletion.

STIMULATION

The most fundamental technical issue in cardiac pacing is how to cause the heart to contract with the least expense of energy. This issue really has two distinct aspects:

1. How to design the electrical stimuli and the electrodes to minimize the drain on the power source.
2. How to design the functions and interfaces between the stimulator and the heart to optimize the hemodynamic operation of the heart, over a wide range of demands, with minimal stress on the heart.

The mechanism by which a pacemaker stimulates the heart is quite complex. It may be understood in terms of the spontaneous electrical activity of the tissues involved.

There is a resting potential difference between the exterior and interior of a living cell. This potential difference is greatest in the immediate vicinity of the membrane, with the cell interior being at one equipotential level, and the exterior at another. In a universe that contains only one cell floating in normal saline, a potential difference cannot exist between any two arbitrary points, both either within or outside the cell, as current must flow between two points in a conducting medium in order to maintain the suggested potential difference. While the cell is at rest, there is no source to supply this current. Hence the potential drop must be confined to be across the membrane. This resting potential difference is about 90 mV for the fibers in the heart.

As long as the cell is at rest, the concentration of sodium ions is greater outside the membrane, while the concentration of potassium ions is greater inside. The electric field, caused by the resting potential across the membrane, aids the inward travel of positive ions. The intensity of this field is about 10 million volts per meter. Despite this inward field, sodium ions are kept outside the membrane because the resting membrane is virtually impermeable to them.

Automaticity is an important property of the fibers. While the cell is at rest, there is a slow inward leakage of sodium and calcium ions. This process gradually lowers the potential difference across the membrane and leads to a spontaneous depolarization of the membrane. When this occurs, the permeability of the membrane is dramatically altered to permit the inward flow of Na and the outbound flow of K ions. Certain cells in the heart are dedicated to excelling in starting this process: these are the primary pacemaker cells. After each depolarization the cells recover through the process of pumping sodium and calcium outward through the membrane until the resting state is restored. The processes of depolarization and repolarization are the consequence of the membrane's *field-dependent permeability* to specific ions.

For purposes of this discussion, the cell membrane may be viewed as a capacitor charged to 90 mV. When an electrical stimulus is applied to the cell membrane, its depolarization leads to an *action potential*. This may be viewed as a result of disturbing the charges on the capacitor at some point by superimposing an electrical field on it. In engineering terms, an electrical field must be locally and temporarily imposed on some muscle fibers in the heart to disturb their resting state and cause their depolarization. This is easily done by passing a pulse of current between two electrodes through the desired site of stimulation. If the strength of the pulse is sufficient (i.e., greater than the threshold of response), then this local depolarization can propagate through all excitable fibers in the heart. This ability to propagate local depolarizations to neighboring fibers is a unique property of heart muscle. After the fibers depolarize, they shorten their lengths in an organized sequence to produce a contraction and eject a stroke of blood from the stimulated chamber.

What kind of stimulus is most efficient in producing membrane depolarization—a current pulse that mobilizes ions, or a voltage pulse that changes the potential drop across the membrane? How are these different? The intensity of an ideal *constant current pulse* (Fig. 27-3) remains unchanged regardless of its duration or the resistance of its path (however great that resistance might be). Such a pulse would be issued by an ideal *constant current source*. An ideal *constant voltage pulse* would similarly maintain its level throughout its duration regardless of how low the resistance of the path might be between the delivery points. Such a pulse would be issued by an ideal *constant voltage source*. These terms are often used loosely: in some cases constancy refers to time, in others it refers to the independence of the source regarding its load, the impedance of its path. In a conductive medium, such as living tissue, charged particles must travel between the electrodes regardless of whether the objective of the arrangement is for the electrodes to maintain a potential difference or to inject a certain amount of charges into the tissues. A voltage or potential difference must appear between the electrodes to drive the charged particles, which are ions in all aqueous electrolytes. This is necessary to satisfy Ohm's law, which states that in a resistive medium the voltage between two points is proportional to the net flow of electrical charges between the points. (The word "net" is used to clarify that positive charges moving in one direction have the same contribution to current as negative charges moving in the opposite direction.)

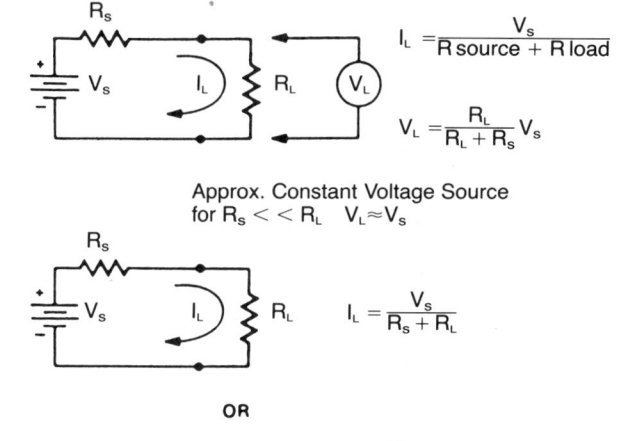

FIGURE 27-3
An ideal voltage source has no internal resistance ($R_s = 0$). An ideal current source has no internal leakage ($R_s = \infty$). V_s is the source voltage, R_s and R_L represent source and load resistances, and I_L is the current through the load.

In excitable tissues a constant current pulse achieves its effect on the membrane by mobilizing a fixed and predetermined number of charges. Its source is able to supply whatever voltage is necessary to maintain this current level between the electrodes. The change in the local electrical field is determined by the product of the local current density and the local value of resistivity; it depends directly on the total current introduced into the tissue between the electrodes. (Current density is defined as the amount of current flowing through a unit cross-sectional area in the direction perpendicular to the area.) A constant voltage pulse achieves its effect a little differently: it changes the local electric field by maintaining a flow of charges sufficient to keep the potential difference between the electrodes at its desired level.

A constant current source is analogous to a huge constant flow pump that is able to maintain flow at a set level in a pipeline even when some obstruction develops in the line. It is able to supply any pressure necessary to keep up the flow. A constant voltage source is analogous to a huge fluid reservoir that can maintain a certain pressure head (potential energy level) regardless of how fast it is being drained through its outflow channels.

Naturally, such ideal constant current and voltage sources do not exist. Constant current sources do become "voltage limited" when the load is too great and the source can no longer increase the voltage at its terminals to maintain steady flow. Constant voltage sources become "current limited" when the load becomes too low in resistance and the source can no longer supply enough current to maintain the set terminal voltage.

Practical stimulators are either voltage-limited constant current sources of "current-limited" constant voltage sources. The difference between their local stimulating action is not significant except when there is a clinical problem regarding the gratuitous stimulation of tissues other than heart muscle.

The site of stimulation is virtually always at the negative electrode. This location is important because in a typical stimulating circuit both electrodes are situated in the extracellular space and cannot *directly* change the potential difference across the fiber membranes. Stimulation may be attributed to the sudden movement of sodium ions from the membrane toward the negative electrode. The movement of other, more mobile ions must also contribute to the local displacement of sodium ions. The membrane potential is thus reduced near the electrode, and the movement of sodium and potassium ions is suddenly facilitated as the membrane becomes more permeable to those ions. These concepts are supported by the well-known strength-duration curves, which show that a given amount of charge (current · time) must be set in motion to depolarize a membrane. These curves typically show that, for *short* pulse durations, the amplitude of a stimulation threshold current pulse (I_{th}) and its duration (T) are inversely proportional:

$$I_{th} = \frac{Q_o}{T} \text{ or } Q_o = I_{th} \cdot T$$

where Q_o is a constant with the dimensions of electrical charge (coulombs), and its value is specific for the characteristics of the electrode-tissue interface. The charge threshold increases as the pulse duration becomes long compared with the chronaxie value (the pulse duration at which the threshold is exactly twice that of an infinitely long current pulse).

$$I_{th} = \frac{Q_o}{T} + I_\infty \text{ or } Q_{th} = I_{th} \cdot T = Q_o + I_\infty \cdot T$$

where Q_{th} is the charge threshold. Chronaxie is

$$T_{chronaxie} = \frac{Q_o}{I_\infty}$$

I_∞ is referred to as the rheobase; its value is also dependent on the physical and chemical properties of the tissue-electrode interface.

The relationship between threshold current and pulse duration may also be fitted to other relationships, such as

$$I_{th} = \frac{I_\infty}{1 - e^{-T/\theta}}$$

where I_∞ is again the rheobase and θ is the time constant of the tissue. (Chronaxie is $\theta \cdot \ln 2$, and the threshold charge for short pulses is $I_\infty \cdot \theta$.)

Constant-voltage thresholds also show an inverse relationship to pulse duration. This is attributed to the fact that a voltage difference in a conducting medium is always accompanied by current flow. If electrical breakdown of the membrane were the mechanism of electrical stimulation, then the threshold strength of the stimulus could reasonably be expected to be dependent on the peak amplitude of the pulse and not on its duration. In fact, voltage strength-duration curves are similar in shape, although not identical, to current curves. It has been claimed that the chronaxie value is shorter for constant voltage strength-duration curves than for constant-current curves.[5]

In summary, a certain amount of positive ionic charge must arrive at the negative electrode surface to elicit a depolarization in the tissue surrounding it. This amount increases as the pulse duration increases.

STIMULATING ELECTRODES

It is generally agreed that resting heart muscle becomes depolarized when a critical threshold current density (J_{th}) is reached for a given pulse duration in accordance with the strength-duration relations. For pulses lasting about 1 ms, this threshold level is about 0.05 mA/mm². As the pulse duration increases, the current density threshold level decreases.

The following discussion is limited to the analysis of spherical electrodes, but it can be extended to any electrode shape. For a spherical electrode (Fig. 27–4), the lowest possible current threshold of stimulation is

$$I_{TH\ acute} = J_{th} \cdot 4\pi \cdot r^2$$

where r is the radius of the electrode. This condition is most likely to exist when the electrode is first introduced into the heart. As a result of motion, reaction to foreign material, and so forth, the healthy muscle tissue in the vicinity of the electrode changes

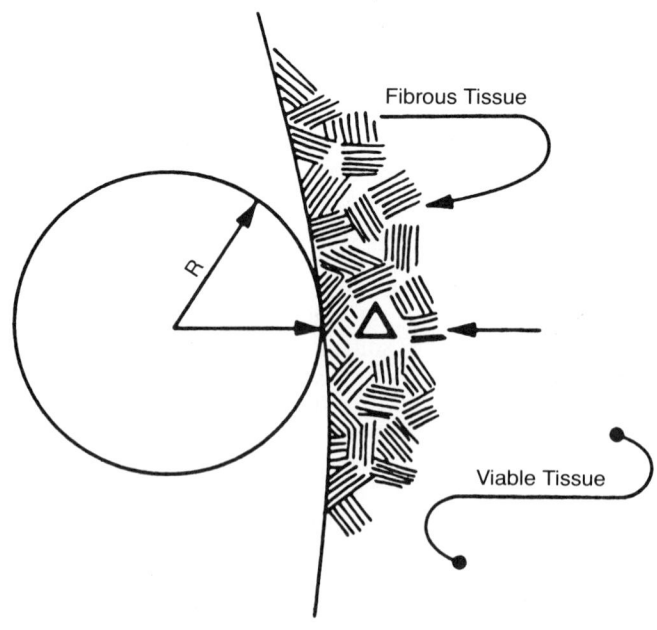

FIGURE 27–4
Spherical stimulating electrode separated from viable tissue by fibrous tissue.

to fibrous tissue. If the shortest distance between the electrode surface and the healthy tissue is δ, then the chronic threshold of stimulation becomes

$$I_{TH\ chronic} = J_{th} \cdot 4\pi \cdot (r + \Delta)^2$$

because the critical current density must now be reached at the surface of a sphere whose radius is r + δ.

A conclusion can be drawn from

$$\frac{I_{TH\ chronic}}{I_{TH\ acute}} = [1 + (\Delta/r)]^2$$

For large electrodes, the thickness of the fibrous layer is small compared to the radius of the electrode; thus the chronic threshold rise is slight. For small electrodes, δ can be larger than r; therefore a severalfold rise in threshold can take place. The current obtainable from presently used pacemakers, I_o, rarely exceeds 10 mA. Such a pulse can stimulate at distances from the center of the electrode not greater than

$$r + \Delta = \text{sqrt}\ [I_o/(J_{th} \cdot 4\pi)]$$

$$= \text{sqrt}\ (10/4\pi \cdot 0.05) \approx 4\ mm$$

That is, an electrode with a radius of 1 mm can stimulate through approximately 3 mm of fibrotic growth with a 1-ms pulse. At shorter pulse durations, the distance decreases for the same current intensity. This distance factor also explains why stimulation can be lost when an endocardial electrode is accidentally displaced a few millimeters in an infarcted region. It also explains why the acute threshold may decrease dramatically when an endocardial electrode is repositioned closer toward normal tissue.

Usually, the smaller the electrode, the more likely it is that capture will be maintained at a given stimulus intensity. This is not always true, however, because the smaller the electrode, the larger the resistive load it presents to the pulse generator and the greater the voltage required to reach the threshold current. The capture capability of a pacemaker is limited by the maximum voltage available for stimulation.

The voltage threshold of stimulation is related to the current threshold through three factors:

1. The resistance of the tissue between the stimulating electrode and the return electrode, often called the spreading resistance. For a spherical electrode its value is $1/(4\pi \cdot \sigma \cdot r)$, where σ is the conductivity of the tissue and r is the radius of the electrode. The conductivities of fibrosed tissues are somewhat lower than that of excitable heart muscle.
2. The voltage at the metal-tissue interface, sometimes called the dipole layer voltage, polarization voltage, or overvoltage. This voltage results from current through the electrode surface when electrons are exchanged between ions in the electrolyte and the metal electrode itself. The magnitude of this voltage depends on the current density at the electrode surface.
3. The resistance of the lead, which creates an additional voltage drop that must be overcome by the battery. This third factor depends on the design of the lead rather than on the design of the electrode; therefore, it need not be considered in determining optimal electrode size.

The voltage threshold is

$$V_{TH} = I_{TH} \cdot R_{tissue} + V_{polarization} + I_{TH} \cdot R_{lead}$$

The first term can be minimized. In the chronic case,

$$I_{TH} \cdot R_{tissue} = J_{TH} \cdot 4\pi\ (r + \Delta)^2/(4\pi\sigma\ r)$$
$$= J_{TH}(1/\sigma)(r + \Delta)^2/r$$

By differentiation, the critical electrode size for which the voltage requirement takes its lowest value can be determined:

$$\frac{d}{dr}(I_{TH} \cdot R_{tissue}) = 0 \quad \text{when } r = \Delta$$

There are probably two main causes for trauma to the tissue:

1. Mechanical irritation, which is proportional to (a) the pressure applied by the electrode to the tissue, and (b) the surface roughness. The force is dependent on the stiffness of the lead, and the pressure is roughly equal to this force divided by the hemispherical contact area:

$$\Delta = f\ (\text{pressure, roughness}) = A \cdot F \cdot g/2\pi r^2$$

   where F is the force resulting from the stiffness of the lead, A is a constant that relates fibrous thickness to pressure and g represents irritation due to surface roughness. The stiffer the lead, the higher the threshold.
2. Irritation due to lack of biocompatibility, which depends on the metal employed in the electrode, its electrical polarity, and the peak current density at the electrode surface. It may also depend on the insulating materials surrounding the electrode. These factors are related to electrochemical and biocompatibility problems.

In summary, an inert and properly prepared electrode can be reduced in size to conserve charge, reduce the voltage requirement, and extend the service life of the power source if the stiffness of the lead is minimal.

There are several ways to minimize the amount of tissue reaction and the required driving voltage for a given electrode size. It is obvious that biocompatible, noncorrosive metal electrodes must be used to prevent the metal ions from entering excitable tissues. Platinum and its alloys are excellent candidates for this. The second approach is *biointegration* through the use of porous surfaced electrodes. The irregularities and interstices of the electrode must be small enough to allow the electrode to arrive at its destination without getting snagged and without damaging the tissues that it contacts, yet the pores and interstices must be large enough to permit tissue to grow into them. This process seems to be self-limiting and results in a mechanically stable electrode with a minimally thick fibrous capsule. The large effective interface between the electrode and the electrolytically conducting tissues helps reduce polarization without decreasing the current density at nearby excitable tissues.

SENSING ELECTRODES

The ability of the system to detect the electrical activity of the heart also depends on the design of the electrodes. The electrode pair connected to an ideal amplifier causes minimal perturbation in its environment, as it neither introduces nor shunts current away from the environment. (An ideal amplifier would exhibit infinite input impedance.) The perturbation is due to the finite size of the electrodes. If the electrodes were tiny points, then they would detect the potential difference that may exist between their sites in the tissue. The resistance of a spherical electrode was given earlier as $1/(4\pi\sigma r)$. As r becomes very small, the *source resistance* of the electrode becomes very large. This source resistance and the finite input impedance of the amplifier form a signal attenuator, a voltage divider. The smaller the electrodes' source impedance, or *series equivalent* impedance, the larger the percentage of amplification of the biological signal. For this reason, as well as for the reasons related to the stimulation functions of the electrodes, their size must not be too small. Electrodes with dimensions much greater than the fiber diameters of cardiac muscle sense the average activity of their surrounding tissues. Their size determines how large a tissue volume is being averaged in space. The sensitivity of the electrode to local activity thus depends on its physical size. It also depends on its proximity to excitable tissue; hence tissue reaction to the electrode plays an important role in the selectivity of the electrode.

The sensitivity and selectivity of a pair of electrodes also depend on the distance between them and on their orientation with respect to the depolarizing tissue. Figure 27–5 illustrates this factor. Closely spaced electrodes are locally sensitive; electrodes with larger spacing are more globally sensitive. The detectable rate of change with time in the signal depends on the distance; hence the *frequency spectrum* of the sensed signal is dependent on the electrode spacing. In addition to the separation between the electrodes, their orientation toward the excitable tissues and toward the preferred direction of propagation of the depolarization activity is an important factor in the frequency spectrum of the signal. For these reasons the sensing amplifier of an implantable pacer should ideally be designed for a specific electrode configuration. As this is not practical, programmable sensitivity and possibly programmable frequency response become very desirable features.

Closely spaced electrodes have a natural insensitivity to distant electromagnetic interference. This advantage is partly offset by the simplicity and inherent reliability of unipolar sensing systems in which the metal encapsulation of the implant serves as the reference electrode.

FUNCTIONS

Assuming that the interfaces between the electrodes and the heart are adequate and reliable, we need to address the control functions of the pacemaker. Specifically, how to optimize the hemodynamic operation of the heart, over a wide range of demands, with minimal stress on the heart?

The simplest function is asynchronous or fixed rate pacing. It carries the risk of arrhythmia induction and it can easily generate hemodynamically inferior performance compared to the patient's existing condition. Ventricular demand pacing is ideal as a back-up or safety measure, but if the patient's condition changes then a more complex function may be needed. The various *modes* of pacing have evolved as technological limitations were cleared away. Demand pacing originally required an increase in electronic complexity that resulted in shorter longevity and reduced reliability. The prosthetic AV node in the form of the atrial triggered ventricular pacer required a more complex connector and eventually two sensing circuits. These enabled a large group of patients with AV nodal disease to receive hemodynamically optimized support.

Dual-Chamber Pacing

Sinus node disease prompted the development of various modes to assure atrial contractions until finally the power requirements could be lowered, by efficient electronics, batteries, and electrodes, to allow the emergence of dual-chamber, dual-demand (DDD) modes. Lithium power sources and complementary metal oxide semiconductor (CMOS) integrated circuits finally cleared the path for DDD pacing at the beginning of the 1980s. The operating rules of DDD pacing have become somewhat complicated to allow the system to deal with spontaneous or pacer-initiated retrograde conduction without causing sustained arrhythmias. The many variations in the rules are amply

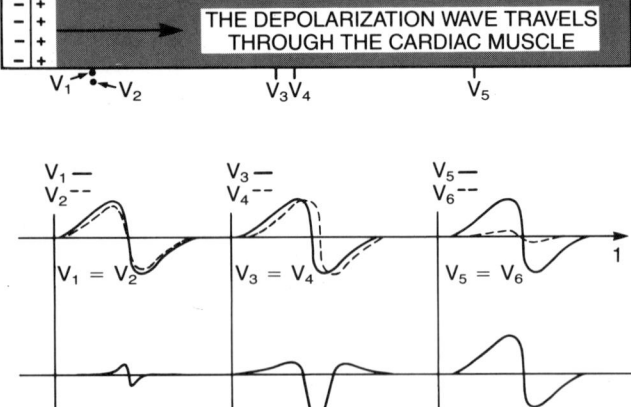

FIGURE 27–5
A model for sensing. A depolarization wave travels past three separate pairs of electrodes. The electric potentials are shown as a function of time as the wave passes each electrode pair. V_1 with V_2 and V_3 with V_4 form bipolar pairs. V_5 and V_6 represent a unipolar pair. The difference between the potentials at the electrodes in each pair is introduced to the pacemaker as the signal to be sensed.

reviewed in the clinical literature. The simple principle, that atrial sensing should be disabled long enough after each ventricular stimulus to prevent reentry via the pacer, was acceptable but not optimal. Variations have emerged, some simple and some hopelessly complicated. The ideal solution seems to be a smarter system that is able to distinguish between retrograde conducted and spontaneously generated atrial depolarizations. This discrimination is possible through space and time factors (which way is the depolarization traveling?), by comparing its shape with templates, or by extracting some important features of the depolarization, such as its path, velocity, and amplitude.

Present solutions of the retrograde problem are adequate. An ideal solution will emerge after some of the discriminating algorithms mature through clinical tests and refinements. Even at that stage, DDD mode pacing with its sophisticated, virtually seamless transitions, from complete inhibition through various single-chamber pacing and AV synchronizing modes to pacing both chambers, remains less than optimal for active patients with sick sinus syndrome who require a dynamic range of heart rates for their activities. These patients cannot rely on the dynamic response of the natural pacemaker.

Rate-Responsive Pacing

The need to adjust dynamically the rate of stimulation for some patients was recognized even before the arrival of the AV synchronizing pacer. The stimulation rate of some early pacemakers could be adjusted by the patient using an external overdriver (e.g., an RF burst generator) that could temporarily increase the patient's heart rate to its own burst rate. This system was used by an elderly grocer who would always reach for it whenever he encountered a cantankerous customer.[6] The need for this dynamic adjustment on a continuous and automatic basis is quite clear, but the method of detecting the need for a change in rate, its extent, and its smooth implementation are serious engineering challenges.

The natural rate is determined by sympathetic and parasympathetic inputs from the central nervous system. Their direct detection and analysis are beyond present day technology. For this reason various indirect indicators have been evaluated and introduced into clinical use. Their review here would be pointless, as the field is evolving rapidly and clinical experience is accumulating to guide the evolution.

It should be stated that chemical sensors have not performed well enough even for short periods of time to be considered seriously for *closed-loop* pacing. (This mode relies on an input fed back to the rate-determining system regarding the effect of its present output on a controlled system, the heart, and the entire organism.) Physical parameters have been more successful, but they reflect the need of the organism less directly.

The possibilities for physical measurements include oxygen saturation (by optical means), mechanical activity of the body, temperature, respiration rate and volume, parameters of blood flow, pressure, and various electrical measurements of muscle activity. It is not enough for a parameter to be measurable, but its value, or its rate of change, must also indicate whether the rate should be increased or decreased. It is clearly not our objective to maximize cardiac output at all times, but rather to adjust the rate until the system is in dynamic equilibrium between its demand for cardiac output and its actual cardiac output. Another objective may be the need to minimize stress in the cardiovascular system as well as in the entire physiologic system while dynamic equilibrium is maintained: Impose a heart rate in response to need but keep the heart minimally stressed.

The most readily available sensors are conventional pacing electrodes. Detection of the time of repolarization after a stimulus was proposed in 1979.[7] This could be achieved with a relatively minor modification of the electrode-sensing amplifier. Detection of the evoked depolarization is technically more difficult, due to electrode polarization. The sensing electrode either must be rapidly restored to its equilibrium after a stimulus is delivered through it, or it must not participate in the stimulation function to be ready for its assigned function. Various studies have been performed to determine the best measure of the evoked response. Some of these are computationally intensive; others are too insensitive or their response does not correlate with the apparent need. It is too early to tell whether the evoked potential can provide the needed feedback information. To achieve greater economy with the power source and minimize interference with the natural activity of the heart while it is performing adequately on its own, it would be desirable to derive the feedback signal for rate control from spontaneously occurring depolarization signals.

The second technical issue is related to the concept of *setpoint*. If a thermostat is set for a preferred room temperature, a good heating-cooling system will maintain it within a narrow range. At certain times the set temperature may become inappropriate. The implantable rate controller is expected to recognize the need for such adjustments without drifting into extremes. The setpoints of physiologic systems tend to drift; this must either be detected or be prevented.

The third issue is the selection of an existing or new pacing mode to be enhanced by rate-responsiveness. It is well known that cardiac output can be stepped up by increasing the heart rate or the stroke volume. The stroke volume can be increased by atrial augmentation; however, this becomes less important at higher rates where atrial filling is inefficient. Because of this, the majority of the present rate-responsive pacers focus on the ventricles. This is a sensible and practical approach in light of the existing technical limitations. However, when the patient is at rest or mildly active, the contributions of the atria are useful and reduce stress on the heart. For this reason, future generations of rate-responsive modes are expected to be derived from dual-chamber pacing modes.

Automatic Self-Adjustment

The rate of stimulation is only one parameter that may need continuous or discrete adjustments to optimize pacing therapy. Mode is already adjusted in response to the heart with DDD and other modes. Stimulation intensity can be adjusted on the basis of the presence or absence of an evoked potential. Automatic sensitivity adjustment calls for more complex algorithms. The delay between atrial and ventricular events may also be optimized with respect to the momentary mode of pacing and its rate.

It is likely that pacemakers in the future will first perform some preliminary setpoint-seeking tests under the supervision of the implanter to be followed by automatic operation with monitoring of the patient's needs through sensors and continuous optimizing of the mode of pacing in response to the patient's activities and changing physiologic parameters.

Technological Limitations

The main advantage of using a stable, crystal oscillator-type time source is that all the functional time intervals (e.g., pulse duration, refractory period, A-V delay, escape interval, monitoring period), are derived from a common reference. The relationships between these (their ratios) remain unchanged and the system can operate indefinitely according to its programmed rules. Automatic adjustments must be based on a stable time reference, otherwise they would tend to drift. The limitations of such a system include the possibility of sudden failure and abrupt change.

Contemporary pacemakers utilize a variety of semiconductor technologies. Semiconductors become electrically unstable when their surfaces carry contamination or moisture. Therefore, semiconductor devices are hermetically sealed in metal or ceramic containers to assure long-term reliable performance. The early pacemakers used two to ten individual transistors in individual hermetically sealed containers. Their functional complexity was greatly limited by the available space in an implant and by their individual reliability. The now ubiquitous integrated circuits (ICs) first became available for pacemaker applications in the early 1970s. Until then, pacemaker circuits were designed with "analog" circuit techniques. The voltage level at the terminal of a semiconductor device may gradually change with time with these techniques. Digital electronic circuits are different, in the sense that the terminals of their devices are at either a low-voltage or a high-voltage level. This offers advantages in terms of speed, reproducibility, cost, and miniaturization. Technology using a type of electronic valve or switch (electronic "gate") made by CMOS was particularly suited for battery-powered digital circuit applications because CMOS ICs consume power only when they are switched from the high- to low-voltage state, or vice versa. To remain in a stable state, the IC "chip" does not require power.

The first CMOS ICs contained only a few switches or gates; yet they made possible the development of the first noninvasively programmable pacemakers. These early chips were not made specifically for pacemaker applications, and several of them had to be combined in a common, hermetically sealed so-called "hybrid" electronic package to achieve the desired circuit functions. Contemporary pacemakers are built with dedicated chips of 10,000 or more gates that can provide virtually all the electronic functions of the implant. The development of these "custom ICs" requires much time, effort, and expense; hence the intent is to build as many functions into each chip as permitted by the compromises between chip size, power consumption, cost, reliability, and foreseeable functional needs.

About 1980, microprocessors were incorporated in some implantable pacemaker designs for the first time. These represented a major step toward the development of present-day pacemakers, because these first implantable computers could be altered by modifying their mode of operation via changing their internal software. In fact, this was a "firmware" change in the design, as the programs were unalterably written in the microprocessor's ROM (read only memory). The evolution has continued toward the use of RAM (random access memory), which permits noninvasive alteration of the pacemaker's mode of operation by entering or "writing," via telemetry, new software into the memory of the pacemaker that determines the operation of the microprocessor. Thus, the implant becomes a microcomputer whose function can be modified as needed.

This functional flexibility is a complex issue. It offers a tremendously broad range of therapies while it carries a major set of limitations because of problems in security, reliability, and human error. For instance, if the contents of the memory may be deliberately altered through electromagnetic means by a specific external instrument, then what are the chances for its accidental alteration by some source of natural or man-made interference? If the functions can be restructured, who may construct such new functions—the original manufacturer, the physician, or a specialist in this type of software? Who is going to keep track of the contents of the memory in case there is some confusion regarding the device's performance? There are no absolute answers to these questions.

The security of a program may be enhanced by several means. For example, access to the code to make changes can be very restricted. Changes in specific memory locations may be caused by radiation. Storing a duplicate of the program in a separate memory area is a possible protective measure. The contents of the two programs may be compared on a step-by-step basis. If there is any difference detected between the two sets, then the system will automatically switch to a nonvolatile program stored in ROM that offers a safe, although suboptimal, alternative. Naturally, the price for this security is paid for by added complexity and power requirements and by a certain reduction in reliability because of the added structural and functional complexities.

The legal issues of responsibility for writing, testing, and individually prescribing programs are intriguing. They may be solved by a modular approach: a finite set of functions may be prescribed for a given patient. These functions can be individually tested rather thoroughly, with the assurance that their interactions with other functions are limited to a minimum. These interactions can be tested by simulating the extreme ranges of operating conditions on the bench. The selection of a relatively small number of functions for a patient may provide a more improved level of integrity than would a broad group of simultaneously available functions in a nonvolatile system, because a complex system is much more difficult to test for interactions than one with a small number of functions.

To illustrate this, an implant for tachycardia termination may have five different pattern recognition programs to offer, together with another five modes to terminate tachycardias. Each of these may have five selectable parameters, with an average of ten values. If we add two channel capabilities to this, the number of combinations is beyond the range of complete testability. There are 25 recognition-termination combinations for each channel, and 625 if each channel has a different combination. Each function may be used with 105 separate parametric configurations. The number of possible sets is in the millions. Each of these would need to be tested in the presence of a broad range of cardiac functions.

In contrast, based on a thorough series of electrophysiologic tests, let us suppose that only a single recognition and termination function were each to be loaded into the memory of the device, with minor adjustability in their operating parameters. Their interactions could be much better understood and tested than those of the previously considered complex configuration, and this second approach might turn out to be safer than the first, nonvolatile system.

The second main area of technological limitation is related to the power source of the pacer. After many unsuccessful attempts to harness biological energy to power pacemakers, the idea seems to be dormant if not abandoned. Contemporary lithium batteries offer high-energy density and excellent reliability. The selection of a specific battery is mainly determined by cosmetic factors related to overall size of the implant, but function, size, and longevity must still be traded against one another.

Noninvasive communication (programming and telemetry) are limited in speed. They also represent a potential source of faulty performance. Training and memorization of the programming functions are time-consuming for the physician. It would be advantageous to allow the physician to assume the role of a monitor rather than of the actuator of adjustments.

Finally, the evolution of new sensors and transducers is expected to remove some existing barriers to open the way for truly automatic and optimized pacing.

References

1. Elmqvist R, Senning A: Implantable pacemaker for the heart. *In* Smyth CM (ed.): Medical Electronics, Proceedings of the Second International Conference on Medical Electronics, Paris, 1959. London, Iliffe and Sons, 1960.
2. Glenn WWL, Mauro A, Longo E, et al.: Remote stimulation of the heart by radio-frequency transmission: Clinical application to a patient with Stokes-Adams syndrome. N Engl J Med 261:948, 1959.
3. Chardack WM, Gage AD, Greatbatch W: A transistorized, self-contained, implantable pacemaker for the long-term correction of heart block. Surgery 48:643, 1960.
4. Personal communication with Mr. Geoffrey Davies of St. George's Hospital, London, UK.
5. Irnich W: The chronaxie time and its practical importance. PACE 3:292, 1980.
6. Personal communication with Mr. L. Wechsler of the General Electric Co., 1962.
7. Rickards AF, Akhras F, Baron DW, et al.: Proceedings of the VIth World Symposium on Cardiac Pacing. Montreal, 1979.

28

Classification of Cardiac Pacemakers

Alan D. Bernstein

Classification is intrinsic to the learning process: it helps in establishing the connections between related concepts and in systematically identifying important differences. In an area as complex as cardiac pacing, even a reasonably comprehensive outline of significant classifications quickly becomes quite lengthy. In this chapter, therefore, some issues will be presented in outline form with relatively little comment in order to permit more thorough consideration of more critical topics or of important concepts less likely to be encountered elsewhere in the pacing literature.

Obviously, cardiac pacemakers can be understood only in the context of cardiac pacing; therefore, it makes sense to begin with the motivation for the application of this form of therapy.

Indications for Pacing

Guidelines have been established for the identification of appropriate electrocardiographic indications for pacing, considered together with related symptomatology.[1] In practice, the criteria actually applied for pacemaker implantation, choice of pacing mode, and adjustment of "programmable" pacing parameters may vary considerably from one institution to another. For completeness, the summary in Table 28–1 includes high-energy interventions that extend beyond the conventional concept of pacing as stimulated cardiac depolarization, partly because more electrical energy is involved and partly because these interventions serve to "reset" the conduction system rather than evoking one or more timed depolarizations.

Power Sources for Implantable Pacemakers

Rechargeable batteries are no longer used in today's implantable pacemakers because the power requirements of the newer implants can be met satisfactorily by nonrechargeable sources, eliminating the need for periodic recharging and the concomitant concern about patient compliance. The remaining power-source types differ most importantly in terms of their discharge characteristics and actuarial survival.

MERCURY-ZINC BATTERIES ■ Early pulse generators, constructed largely with electronic circuitry made from discrete components (in contrast to today's integrated-circuit technology), were often powered by series-wired mercury-zinc batteries. Such batteries, now obsolete as pacemaker power sources, had two major disadvantages. First, the chemical reaction by which they convert chemical potential energy into electrical energy produces gas, which can permeate the epoxy resin that was used in manufacturing the housings of early implantable pulse generators but precludes the use of hermetically sealed housings such as those in common use today. Second, the terminal-voltage decay characteristic of the mercury-zinc battery is such that normal battery depletion results in very little change in the terminal voltage available for pacing until the end of the battery's useful life is reached, when the terminal voltage plummets sharply. This makes pacemaker failure due to normal battery depletion relatively difficult to anticipate, so that actual failure (with clinical consequences) may well take place. Actuarial-survival analysis shows that 50% of mercury-zinc pulse generators failed at approximately 41 months (3.4 years).[2]

LITHIUM-CHEMISTRY BATTERIES ■ Lithium-iodine and other lithium-chemistry batteries represent the vast majority of today's pulse-generator power sources. The chemical reaction produces no gases, and both the batteries and the pulse-generator housing normally are hermetically sealed. The terminal-voltage decay characteristic is well behaved from the standpoint of clinical pacing, falling slowly enough to permit battery end-of-life to be anticipated in routine follow-up so that timely pulse-generator replacement can be planned. The 50% survival point for lithium-chemistry pulse generators

TABLE 28–1
Electrocardiographic (ECG) Indications for Pacing as Interpreted at the Newark Beth Israel Medical Center*

Acceptable (Chronic or Recurrent Conditions)
A. Sinoatrial Node (SN) Disorders
  1. Acceptable (Class I)
    a. Regular sinus bradycardia with (documented) associated symptoms
    b. Regular sinus bradycardia secondary to required drugs
    c. Chronotropic incompetence with (documented) associated symptoms
    d. Bradycardia-tachycardia syndrome with (documented) associated symptoms
  2. Marginally Acceptable (Class II)
    a. Asymptomatic regular sinus bradycardia secondary to required drugs
    b. Hypersensitive–carotid sinus syndrome
B. Atrioventricular (AV) conduction disorders
  1. Acceptable (Class I)
    a. Congenital complete heart block (CHB)
    b. Acquired CHB (age-related or secondary to cardiac surgery or AV-node ablation)
    c. CHB acquired in the course of acute myocardial infarction (AMI), as an indication for prophylactic pacing
    d. Mobitz II with documented symptoms attributable to CHB
  2. Marginally Acceptable (Class II)
    a. Bifascicular block with syncope of undocumented association
    b. Mobitz II, asymptomatic or without documented symptoms associated with CHB
C. Tachyarrhythmias
  1. Supraventricular tachycardia (SVT), after suitable electrophysiologic (EP) evaluation
  2. Frequent ventricular ectopy, manageable by overdrive suppression, after suitable EP evaluation
  3. Ventricular tachycardia (VT) or ventricular fibrillation (VF) (aborted sudden death) after suitable EP evaluation

Questionable or Under Investigation
  1. Asymptomatic regular sinus bradycardia
  2. Asymptomatic sinus pause or arrest
  3. Syncope of undetermined cause
  4. Asymptomatic bifascicular block
  5. Mobitz I with narrow QRS complex
  6. VT manageable by pacing protocols other than overdrive

*Courtesy of V. Parsonnet (private communication, Jan., 1988.)

depends on the battery formulation, as illustrated in Table 28–2.[2-5]

RADIOACTIVE-PLUTONIUM REACTORS ■ "Nuclear" pacemakers have been in use for 15 years. Their triply-encapsulated radioactive plutonium power sources have proven reliable and long-lived. Recent actuarial data indicate that 88% of nuclear pacemakers are still operational after 12 years of use.[5] Their chief drawback is administrative; considerable paperwork is involved in their use, and special precautions must be taken to avoid events that might disrupt the encapsulation of the radioactive material, such as exposure to high temperatures, as in cremation.

Pacing-System Configuration

Electrical stimulation of the heart requires the passage of current through a portion of the myocardium. The pacemaker accomplishes this by establishing a voltage difference between two electrodes, at least one of which is situated in close proximity to susceptible myocardial tissue. It is useful to classify electrode systems in each of three ways: according to (1) electrical configuration, (2) electrode type, and (3) single- and dual-chamber systems.

ELECTRICAL CONFIGURATION

BIPOLAR PACING ■ Bipolar electrodes lie in close proximity to one another and to cardiac tissue. Two conductors are required between the pulse generator and the heart for each chamber paced. Far-field signals, such as myopotentials and ambient electrical "noise," propagate at much higher speeds than cardiac-activation wavefronts, and are sensed with relatively low amplitudes through electrical cancellation. The bipolar configuration is therefore superior for rejection of electrical interference that could be interpreted erroneously as spontaneous cardiac depolarizations by the pacemaker's sensing circuitry. The stimulus artifact at the surface of the body is often only a few millivolts in amplitude; thus it may be difficult to detect and may be unnoticeable on a surface-lead electrocardiogram.

UNIPOLAR PACING ■ In this configuration only one electrode is in contact with cardiac tissue; this is the cathode, or "different" electrode, which provides a negative-going electrical pulse. The second ("indifferent") electrode, or anode, is usually all or part of the metal housing of the pulse generator and is distant from the point of cardiac stimulation. Only one conductor is required between the pulse generator and the heart for each chamber paced. Myopotentials and extracorporeal sources of electrical interference are more likely to interfere with the pacemaker's detection of spontaneous cardiac depolarizations. The stimulus artifact on the surface-lead electrocardiogram is of relatively high amplitude, sometimes approaching 1 volt, and is easily detected. Temporary pacemakers are normally bipolar systems, because the pulse generator remains outside the body, and its housing, even if it were conductive, could not conveniently serve as a reliable electrode.

ELECTRODE TYPE

ENDOCARDIAL ■ The pacing electrode is within the heart, in contact with the interior surface of the atrial

TABLE 28–2
Actuarial Survival of Pacemaker Pulse Generators as a Function of Battery Formulation

Battery Formulation	Approximate 50% Survival	
	Months	Years
Mercury-zinc (HgZn)	41	3.4
Lithium-lead (LiPb)	43	3.4
Lithium–silver chromate (LiAgCrO$_4$)	75	6.3
Lithium–cupric sulfide (LiCuS)	132	11.0*
Lithium-iodine (LiI)	144	12.0

*Projected.

or ventricular wall, or with the atrial or ventricular septum. The electrode is at the tip of a lead that has been inserted *pervenously* (often called a "transvenous" lead even though it goes through the vessel, not across it). The stability of the electrode's position depends in part on the presence or absence of fixation mechanisms. *Active-fixation* electrodes are attached to the endocardial surface or septum by means of hooks or corkscrews that may be advanced during implantation from the pulse-generator end of the lead; a *passive-fixation* electrode is equipped with tines or fins that can engage trebeculae and thus contribute to the stability of the electrode's position in the heart. Some endocardial electrodes are equipped with no means of fixation whatever and depend entirely on the development of a fibrous-tissue sheath at the junction between the electrode and the cardiac tissue to keep the electrode in place.

MYOCARDIAL ■ The electrode is buried within the myocardial wall, having been poked or screwed in from the exterior surface of the heart. Although active-fixation pervenous leads may have electrodes that bury themselves within the myocardial wall from the interior of the heart, they are not commonly referred to as myocardial electrodes. Conductive-suture electrodes, however, which are sometimes implanted during cardiac surgery for temporary pacing, qualify as myocardial electrodes.

EPICARDIAL ■ The electrode is sutured to the epicardial surface of the atrium or ventricle.

SINGLE- AND DUAL-CHAMBER SYSTEMS

SINGLE-CHAMBER PACING ■ In single-chamber pacing, stimulation takes place in either the atrium or the ventricle. There may, however, be electrodes in both chambers, as in atrial-synchronous ventricular pacing, represented as VAT in the NBG Pacemaker Code (described below in the section on "Mode of Pacing"), which will be used throughout this chapter.

DUAL-CHAMBER PACING ■ In dual-chamber pacing, electrodes are placed in (or on) both the atrium and ventricle, and both chambers are stimulated. Depending on the mode of pacing, sensing of spontaneous depolarizations may take place in the ventricle (as in DVI pacing), both the atrium and the ventricle (as in DDD pacing) or in neither chamber (as in DOO pacing).

ALTERNATIVE (SURGICAL) DEFINITION ■ Sometimes the term "single-chamber system" is used to represent a pacing system with a single lead, in the atrium or the ventricle, and the term "dual-chamber system" is used to represent a system with both atrial and ventricular electrodes, even if stimulation takes place in only one of the two chambers.

Lead Construction

In addition to the issue of electrode configuration discussed above, two characteristics of pacing-lead construction are of practical importance.

CONDUCTORS ■ Modern pacing leads are commonly made with multifilar conductors, which are capable of withstanding repeated flexure without breaking, unlike single-strand conductors. (If a patient is paced continuously at 72 beats per minute for 10 years, the lead flexes 378,691,200 times.) This issue is of particular importance in adaptive-rate pacing, where the pacing rate is modulated during exercise or stress by signals derived from measurements of physiologic variables such as right ventricular blood temperature or mixed venous oxygen saturation. Thermistors, phototransistors, or other hardware must sometimes be incorporated in the pacing lead in order to monitor these controlling variables. Auxiliary wires connecting such additional hardware to the pulse generator must also be able to withstand the same amount of repeated flexure.

INSULATION ■ The two materials commonly used in insulating pacing leads have somewhat different properties. *Silicone rubber* is quite flexible, and may be cemented using an appropriate quick-drying adhesive made from the same material. This permits the straightforward splicing of unipolar leads for the repair of extracardiac conductor fractures or insulation ruptures and for the removal of superfluous length.[6] Silicone rubber insulation is soft and can easily be nicked inadvertently during pacemaker implantation. It may be cut by fixation sutures placed around the lead without a strain-relieving collar. *Polyurethane* insulation is tougher and more slippery, facilitating the insertion of two leads through a single vessel. In general, despite problems caused by the chemical degradation of a particular polyurethane formulation, it has proved to be quite reliable over the long term. There is less probability that this material will be damaged inadvertently during implantation, but splices must rely for their long-term integrity upon mechanical pressure (friction fits) because no suitable cement is available that will bond to this material.

Types of Output Circuits

Two output-circuit configurations are encountered in pacing; they too have somewhat different properties.[7]

VOLTAGE-SOURCE PACING ■ This common output-circuit configuration is often misunderstood because it is almost invariably incorrectly referred to as "constant-voltage" pacing. A charged capacitor is permitted to discharge through the cardiac circuit. Both the voltage across the cardiac electrodes and the current passing through the heart decay exponentially during the stimulus. The rate of decay may change markedly in the presence of a pacing lead insulation defect or other pacing system problem, making the examination of stimulation-artifact waveforms a useful technique for detecting incipient lead complications even before clinical consequences become manifest. The effect of battery and electrode system changes on the stimulus-artifact waveform has been well understood for almost two decades.[8]

CURRENT-SOURCE PACING ■ With this circuit configuration, the output current and voltage are almost invariant throughout the stimulus, so that the commonly used term "constant current" pacing is correct. In the presence of an insulation defect in a unipolar system, part of the current supplied by the pulse generator bypasses the heart, and the remaining current may drop below the threshold of stimulation.

Mode of Pacing

In general, it is more useful in clinical practice to classify pacemakers in terms of function than by pacing system structure or technical design. The mode of pacing is much the most important functional classification and is of critical importance in the choice and optimization of the most appropriate pacemaker therapy for each patient.

Much effort has been devoted to the development of the special language by which pacing modes can be described and understood.[9–15] The classification of pacing modes can be accomplished most easily with the aid of the new NASPE/BPEG Generic Pacemaker Code (the "NBG Code"), which is summarized in Table 28–3. Several levels of classification are incorporated into the structure of the NBG Code. For example, the first three positions deal exclusively with antibradyarrhythmia pacing, while the fifth position refers only to antitachyarrhythmia capability.

ANTIBRADYARRHYTHMIA PACING

CHAMBER(S) PACED (POSITION I) ■ The first position of the NBG Code classifies the pacemaker in terms of the four possibilities of stimulation in antibradyarrhythmia pacing (Table 28–4).

CHAMBER(S) SENSED (POSITION II) ■ The second position classifies the pacemaker in terms of its ability to detect spontaneous atrial depolarizations, spontaneous ventricular depolarizations, or both for the purpose of antibradyarrhythmia pacing. This is, of course, a very specific and restricted definition of the term "sensing" (Table 28–5).

RESPONSE TO SENSING (POSITION III) ■ This position classifies what the pacemaker does when it detects a spontaneous depolarization (Table 28–6).

LEVEL OF PROGRAMMABILITY AND RATE MODULATION (POSITION IV) ■ This position serves three purposes. It indicates the presence of *rate modulation* (R), a form of adaptive pacing in which the pacing rate is adjusted automatically by the pacemaker itself on the basis of measured values of physiologic parameters, such as stimulus-to-T-wave interval, right-ventricular blood temperature, or mechanical vibration, to provide suitably faster pacing rates during exercise or stress in the presence of chronotropic incompetence, or the inability of the sinus rate to increase appropriately, in those circumstances. When the rate modulation feature is absent, this position is used to indicate the degree to which the pulse generator's operating parameters can be adjusted *(programmed)* noninvasively. This position also denotes the presence of pacemaker *telemetry*, a concept discussed in greater detail below. What makes position IV able to encompass both rate modulation and programmability is the fact that any adaptive-rate pacemaker may be reasonably assumed to be multiprogrammable and capable of some degree of telemetry (Table 28–7).

ANTITACHYARRHYTHMIA CAPABILITY (POSITION V) ■ This position, if occupied, designates the presence of antitachyarrhythmia pacing, cardioversion, or defibrillation capabilities independent of antibradyarrhythmia pacing function (Table 28–8).

TABLE 28–4
NBG Code, Position I (Antibradyarrhythmia-Pacing Location)

O = None	No antibradyarrhythmia stimulation. This does not preclude the possibility of stimulation for tachyarrhythmia termination.
A = Atrium	
V = Ventricle	
D = Dual	Both atrium and ventricle may be stimulated for control of bradyarrhythmia.
S = A or V	A manufacturer may use "S" to label a single-chamber pacemaker suitable for use in either the atrium or the ventricle.

TABLE 28–3
A Summary of the NASPE/BPEG Generic (NBG) Pacemaker Code*

Position†	I	II	III	IV	V
Category	Chamber(s) paced	Chamber(s) sensed	Response to sensing	Programmability, rate modulation	Antitachyarrhythmia function(s)
	O = None	O = None	O = None	O = None	O = None
	A = Atrium	A = Atrium	T = Triggered	P = Simple Programmable	P = Pacing (antitachyarrhythmia)
	V = Ventricle	V = Ventricle	I = Inhibited	M = Multiprogrammable	S = Shock
	D = Dual (A+V)	D = Dual (A+V)	D = Dual (T+I)	C = Communicating	D = Dual (P+S)
				R = Rate modulation	
Manufacturers' designation only	S = single (A or V)	S = single (A or V)			

*Reproduced by permission from Bernstein AD, et al.: PACE 10:794–799, 1987.
†Note: Positions I through III are used exclusively for antibradyarrhythmia function.

TABLE 28–5
NBG Code, Position II (Sensing Location)

N = None		No sensing capability for bradyarrhythmia management, although the device may be able to detect a tachyarrhythmia.
A = Atrium		Spontaneous atrial depolarizations can be detected.
V = Ventricle		Spontaneous ventricular depolarizations can be detected.
D = Dual		Spontaneous depolarizations can be detected independently in the atrium and the ventricle.
S = A or V		A manufacturer may use "S" in Position II to label a single-chamber pacemaker suitable for use in either the atrium or the ventricle.

A Generic Code for Antitachyarrhythmia Devices

The NBG Code indicates the presence or absence of antitachyarrhythmia capabilities but does not indicate

TABLE 28–6
NBG Code Position III (Response to Sensing)

O = None	No response. This designation is used when the device does not possess sensing capability; it is inappropriate otherwise. Thus "O" in Position II is always accompanied by "O" in Position III.
I = Inhibited	When a spontaneous depolarization is detected, a pending stimulus does not occur. This may be because the pacemaker escape timing is reset by sensing, as in the VVI or AAI modes. A pending atrial stimulus may also be skipped after atrial sensing without affecting the escape timing, as in the DDI mode.
T = Triggered	In single-chamber pacing, sensing immediately produces a stimulus in the same chamber. The stimulus has no effect, of course, if the chamber has just depolarized spontaneously. If what has been sensed is a spurious noise signal, the stimulus may be effective. The single-chamber triggered modes are often used in assessing pacemaker function and in identifying the effects of muscle-potential sensing and extracorporeal electromagnetic interference.
D = Dual	This denotes the simultaneous presence of triggered and inhibited pacing. In the VDD mode, ventricular pacing is inhibited when the escape timing is reset by ventricular sensing. This special use of the "triggering" concept means that ventricular stimulation is evoked, after a suitable atrioventricular interval, upon sensing of a spontaneous atrial depolarization. In the DDD mode, sensing results in inhibition of a pending stimulus in the chamber where the sensing occurs; at the same time, atrial sensing triggers ventricular stimulation after an appropriate interval.

in which chamber a tachyarrhythmia can be detected or in which chamber an antitachyarrhythmia intervention takes place. Although antitachyarrhythmia devices represent a very small percentage of implanted devices for the control of cardiac rhythm disorders, it is easy to see how an auxiliary generic code could be devised to describe antitachyarrhythmia devices conversationally yet in greater detail. Table 28–9 summarizes an experimental code devised by the author for this purpose.[16]

The NASPE Specific Code

Visualization of the pacing modes can often be facilitated by the ratio-format NASPE Specific Code.[13, 14] Based on an earlier code,[12] it is unsuitable for use in conversation but can provide more information about the functions that make up antibradyarrhythmia and antitachyarrhythmia modes. None of the codes presented in this chapter provides details of pacemaker timing.

The numerator and denominator of the ratio format represent the atrial and ventricular channels of the pulse generator, respectively. Capital letters represent basic functions:

$$
\begin{aligned}
O &= \text{None} \\
P &= \text{Pacing} \\
S &= \text{Sensing} \\
I &= \text{Inhibition} \\
T &= \text{Triggering}
\end{aligned}
$$

Thus, an asynchronous ventricular pacemaker (VOO) would be represented as

$$\frac{O}{P} \quad \text{or (to save space)} \quad O / P$$

In this mode, the pacemaker does nothing (O) in the atrium, but paces (P) the ventricle.

Lower-case letters represent the source of a sensed signal that gives rise to inhibition (I) or triggering (T). They include

$$
\begin{aligned}
a &= \text{atrium} \\
v &= \text{ventricle} \\
e &= \text{external}
\end{aligned}
$$

Using these notation conventions, inhibited ventricular pacing (VVI) is represented as

$$O / PSIv$$

In this mode, the pacemaker does nothing (O) in the atrium, but paces (P) and senses (S) in the ventricle. Ventricular pacing is inhibited (I) upon sensing of spontaneous activity in the ventricle (v). Note that this code permits explicit and unambiguous specification of what happens when a VVI pacemaker's sensing circuit is tested by the application of trigger signals (often erroneously called "chest-wall stimuli") to the surface of the body, using a temporary pacemaker or other external source:

$$O / PSIvIe$$

TABLE 28–7
NBG Code Position IV (Programmability and Rate Modulation)

O = None	No rate modulation, no programmability.
S = Simple Programmable	Adjustable rate, output, or both.
M = Multi-programmable	More extensively programmable.
C = Communicating	Multiprogrammable and capable of some degree of pacemaker "telemetry."
R = Rate Modulation	Multiprogrammable, capable of some degree of pacemaker telemetry and capable of automatic control of rate through measurement of one or more auxiliary physiologic variables.

This is the same as VVI pacing, except that ventricular stimuli will also be inhibited upon sensing of an external (e) signal. In practice, *any* VVI pacemaker can be "fooled" into inhibition through sensing an external trigger signal of sufficient amplitude.

As a further example, the mechanism of conventional DDD pacing is represented clearly by the NASPE Specific Code, as follows:

$$PSIaIv \,/\, PSIvTa$$

In the atrium, pacing (P) and sensing (S) take place, with atrial stimuli inhibited by atrial sensing (Ia) and inhibited by ventricular sensing (Iv). Because it does not provide timing details, however, the code does not specify that this inhibition results from resetting of the escape interval. In the ventricle, pacing (P) and sensing (S) take place; however, whereas ventricular pacing is inhibited (Iv) by ventricular sensing, it is triggered (Ta) by atrial sensing. Here again the code does not reflect pacemaker timing, and therefore it makes no explicit reference to the AV interval associated with that triggering.

A final example is provided by DDI pacing, a dual-chamber mode suitable for use in the presence of episodically unstable atrial rhythms such as atrial flutter or atrial fibrillation:

$$PSIaIv \,/\, PSIv$$

TABLE 28–8
NBG Code Position V (Antitachyarrhythmia Function)

O = None	No antitachyarrhythmia capability
P = Pacing	Low-energy stimulation protocol for tachyarrhythmia interruption. There is no mechanism for indicating which chamber is involved, although the ventricle is assumed if the first three positions indicate single-chamber ventricular pacing, and similarly for the atrium.
S = Shock	High-energy antitachyarrhythmia intervention capability; cardioversion or defibrillation.
D = Dual	Both low- and high-energy antitachyarrhythmia intervention capabilities.

This is the same as the DDD example just considered, except that normal sinus activity will not produce properly synchronized ventricular pacing, but inappropriate ventricular stimuli will not be evoked through tracking of unstable atrial activity.

The NASPE Specific Code can be used to classify different types of antitachyarrhythmia pacing. Moreover, unlike the NBG Code, it indicates precisely what functions exist in which channel. Using parentheses to contain the antitachyarrhythmia functions, separating them from the antibradyarrhythmia-pacing descriptors discussed above, one commercially available device can be described by

$$PSIaIV \,(BaBvUv) \,/\, PSIvTa \,(Uv)$$

This device is therefore a conventional DDD pacemaker with the following antitachyarrhythmia capabilities added.

Atrial channel:
Ba = atrial bursts upon atrial-tachyarrhythmia detection

Bv = atrial bursts upon ventricular-tachyarrhythmia detection

Uv = atrial underdrive pacing upon ventricular-tachyarrhythmia detection

Ventricular channel:
Uv = ventricular underdrive upon ventricular-tachyarrhythmia detection

A mechanism for the detailed specification of adaptive pacing, including rate modulation, can be incorporated easily in the NASPE Specific Code, although such incorporation has not been officially adopted (Table 28–10). Adaptive features associated with antibradyarrhythmia pacing can be appended to the antibradyarrhythmia descriptors for the atrial and ventricular channels as suffixes separated by hyphens. For example, capital letters can be used to represent pacing parameters with lower-case letters representing controlling variables.

Pacing Parameters:
E = escape interval
R = refractory period
AV = atrioventricular interval

Controlling Variables:
qt = stimulus–to–T wave interval
act = activity (mechanical vibration)
t = temperature
r = respiration
ps = pace or sense
vpb = ventricular premature depolarization

Using this arrangement, a VVI pacemaker with rate hysteresis can be represented by

$$O \,/\, PSIv - Eps$$

and a vibration-sensing VVIR pacemaker by

$$O \,/\, PSIv - Eact$$

TABLE 28–9
Experimental Generic Code for Antitachyarrhythmia Devices

Position	I	II	III
Category	Chamber(s) where antitachyarrhythmia intervention occurs	Chamber(s) sensed for tachyarrhythmia recognition	Type of antitachyarrhythmia intervention
	A = Atrium	A = Atrium	P = Pacing (antitachyarrhythmia)
	V = Ventricle	V = Ventricle	S = Shock
	D = Dual (A+V)	D = Dual (A+V)	D = Dual (P+S)
Manufacturers' designation only	S = Single (A or V)	S = Single (A or V)	

In the first instance, the code refers specifically to the mechanism of rate hysteresis (different pacemaker escape intervals depending on whether the interval begins with a spontaneous beat or a pacemaker stimulus). Similarly, a DDD pacemaker whose AV interval differs after paced and sensed atrial events (to mimic normal physiology more closely) and whose atrial refractory period is extended after a ventricular premature depolarization to prevent the sensing of an anticipated retrograde atrial activation (which might initiate a pacemaker-reentrant tachycardia) could be described by

$$\text{PSIaIv} - \text{Rvpb} / \text{PSIvTa} - \text{AVps}$$

It should be emphasized that the NBG Code was designed deliberately for conciseness and convenience in conversation. Not surprisingly, therefore, it has certain limitations, among them an inability to classify a pacemaker's behavior beyond identifying the mode.

This limitation can be important in practice, because two pulse generators may behave quite differently in the same mode. Even the NASPE Specific Code does not reflect timing details such as variations in refractory-period structure, which may often explain such differences, as will be illustrated below.

Refractory-Period Classifications

In dual-chamber (DVI, DDI, and DDD) pacing, whether or not the ventricular channel of the pulse generator is refractory throughout the atrioventricular (AV) interval determines a further subclassification of such devices.

"COMMITTED" VENTRICULAR PACING ■ As illustrated in Figure 28–1, if the ventricular channel is refractory throughout the AV interval, a spontaneous ventricular response to a stimulated atrial depolarization cannot

TABLE 28–10
Examples of the NGB and NASPE Specific Codes. The author's "unofficial" technique for amending the NASPE Specific Code to permit the description of adaptive pacing features is used in some of the examples.

NASPE Specific Code	Corresponding NBG Code	Device Description
$\frac{O}{P}$	VOO	Asynchronous ventricular pacemaker.
$\frac{O}{\text{PSIv}}$	VII, VVIM, or VVIMO	Multiprogrammable, inhibited ventricular pacemaker without antitachyarrhythmia capability.
$\frac{O}{\text{PSIv-Eps}}$	VII, VVIC, or VVICO	"Communicating," inhibited ventricular pacemaker with rate hysteresis.
$\frac{O}{\text{PSIv-Et (BXe)}}$	VVIRP	Inhibited ventricular pacemaker with temperature-controlled rate modulation and externally initiated antitachyarrhythmia burst plus extrastimulus.
$\frac{O}{O \text{ (Dv)}}$	OOOPS	Simple programmable automatic defibrillator.
$\frac{\text{PIv (Ba)}}{\text{PSIv}}$	DVIMP	Multiprogrammable atrioventricular-sequential pacemaker with atrial burst pacing upon detection of tachyarrhythmia in the atrium.
$\frac{\text{PSIaIv}}{\text{PSIvTa}}$	DDD, DDDC, or DDDCO	"Communicating" dual-chamber pacemaker capable of atrial-synchronous and atrioventricular-sequential pacing but without antitachyarrhythmia capabilities.
$\frac{\text{PSIaIv-Rvpb}}{\text{PSIvTa-AVps}}$	DDD, DDDC, or DDDCO	"Communicating" dual-chamber pacemaker, as in the previous example, but with automatic PVARP extension and equalization of the mechanical AV interval.
$\frac{\text{PSIaIv (BaBvUv)}}{\text{PSIvTa (Uv)}}$	DDDCP	"Communicating" dual-chamber pacemaker described in text, with automatic burst and underdrive interventions for tachyarrhythmias detected in the atrium or the ventricle.

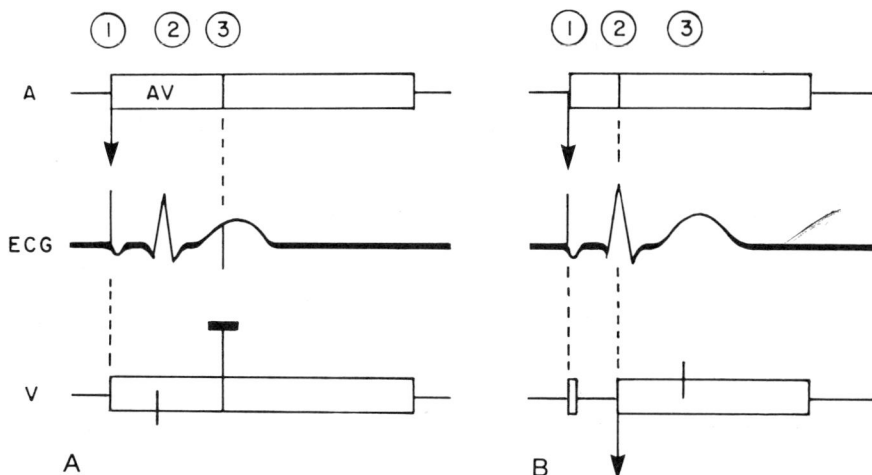

FIGURE 28–1
The refractory-period structure of a dual-chamber pacemaker determines whether the ventricular stimulus is classified as "committed" or "uncommitted," as explained in the text. A, When the ventricular channel is refractory throughout the atrioventricular (AV) interval, the spontaneous ventricular depolarization cannot be sensed; the ventricular stimulus is not inhibited and is therefore inevitable. B, When the ventricular channel can sense spontaneous activity during the AV interval, a spontaneous ventricular response to an atrial depolarization inhibits a pending ventricular stimulus and resets the pacemaker's escape timing.

be detected by the pacemaker. Once the AV interval has begun, therefore, a ventricular stimulus is inevitable. In other words, the pacemaker is "committed" to pace the ventricle whether or not a ventricular stimulus is actually needed. This situation may be more clearly understood with the use of an ECG overlay diagram, as shown in the Figure 28–1, Panel A.[17] An atrial stimulus (Event 1) captures the atrium and initiates refractory periods in both the atrial and ventricular channels. The spontaneous ventricular response to the paced atrial depolarization (Event 2) cannot be sensed by the ventricular channel because the channel is in its refractory period; a ventricular stimulus (Event 3) is therefore inevitable. That stimulus does not capture the ventricle, which has just depolarized spontaneously and is itself refractory, but the stimulus is undesirable because it is released when the ventricle may be particularly vulnerable to the induction of a tachyarrhythmia.

"UNCOMMITTED" VENTRICULAR PACING ■ On the other hand, if the ventricular channel is alert during the AV interval (usually following a short blanking period during which the ventricular sensing amplifier is disabled, or turned off, until the large residual voltages produced by pacing in the atrium have disappeared), a spontaneous ventricular response can be detected, inhibiting the ventricular stimulus and resetting the pacemaker's escape timing. As before, the atrial stimulus (Figure 28–1, Panel B, Event 1) captures the atrium and initiates an atrial refractory period. After a short blanking period, the ventricular channel again becomes alert to spontaneous events, and the spontaneous ventricular depolarization (Event 2) is sensed, which resets the pacemaker's escape timing and inhibits the ventricular stimulus (Event 3) that would otherwise have been released at the end of the programmed AV interval.

Selection of the Appropriate Pacing Mode

As an example of how the classifications of electrocardiographic indications for pacing and of antibradyarrhythmia and antitachyarrhythmia devices can be related, Table 28–11 is a simplified selection table developed to facilitate the identification of possible therapeutic choices in the electrical management of brady- and tachyarrhythmias.[18]

Pacemaker Programming and Telemetry

In pacing, the term "programming" is used to refer to the modification of a pulse generator's operation through the noninvasive transmission of commands from an external device (a pacemaker "programmer"). This usage of the term has nothing to do with "programming" in the computer-science sense, but refers specifically to the digital communication of data and commands between an external or implanted pulse generator and an associated programming device. Such communication is achieved most commonly through radio frequency (RF) communications, but pulsed magnetic fields are also used, and some European devices have been designed to use pulsed electrical voltages applied to the skin, and even bursts of ultrasound.

Pulse generators are classified in terms of their degree of programmability (Table 28–12) as described in the following paragraphs, particularly in the use of the NBG Code discussed earlier (see Table 28–3).

Strictly speaking, telemetry means "measurement at a distance," and the term is used widely in this sense throughout the scientific and engineering literature. In pacing, this term is used more loosely to describe the degree of communications capability a pulse generator may possess. In general, pacemaker telemetry falls into the following four categories.

CONFIRMATION OF PROGRAMMING ■ By sending an appropriate message to its associated external programming device, the pulse generator confirms that it has successfully received a transmission of instructions from the external device.

STATUS REPORTING ■ When the pulse generator is interrogated by means of the external programmer, it

TABLE 28–11
Selection of the Appropriate Pacing Mode

AV Node	Atrial Rhythm			
	Normal	Bradycardia	Unstable or Brady-Tachy Syndrome	Reentrant Tachyarrhythmia
Normal	—	AAIR	—	AAICP
AV Block, VA Intact	DDD	DDDR	DDIR or VVIR VVIR	DDIRP or DDDRP
AV Block, VA Block	DDD or VVI	DDDR or VVIR	DDIR or VVIR	DDIRP or DDDRP

reports the value to which each of its programmable operating parameters has been set.

TELEMETRY OF PARAMETER VALUES AND MEASUREMENT RESULTS ■ Pulse generators with this capability perform true telemetry in that they make it possible to *measure* the actual value of, for example, the stimulus amplitude, instead of merely reporting the theoretical value to which it has been set. Often, through interaction with the programmer, derived variables may be evaluated, such as the electrical resistance of the lead and its cardiac interface (determined from the ratio of measured pacing voltage to measured pacing current at the onset of the stimulus) or the internal resistance of the pulse generator battery.

WAVEFORM TELEMETRY AND TIMING DIAGRAMS ■ Especially in dual-chamber pacing, follow-up and trouble-shooting are greatly simplified by the use of timing diagrams that display clearly the temporal relationships between escape intervals, rate limits, AV intervals, and refractory and blanking periods. The usefulness of such diagrams has been widely recognized, and several specialized diagramming techniques exist in addition to that used in Figure 28–1.[19]

Some microprocessor-based pacemaker systems can assist, together with their associated programming devices, in producing surface electrocardiograms and telemetered intracardiac electrograms annotated with fiduciary markers or fairly complete timing diagrams. This permits the clinician to see exactly what the pacemaker "sees," to interpret its behavior more easily, and to determine with greater confidence whether or not that behavior, however bizarre, is consistent with the pacemaker's design, the mode of pacing, and the programmable parameter settings in effect at the moment. These features can help considerably in the identification of pacemaker "pseudomalfunctions," reducing the likelihood of unnecessary surgical intervention for a nonexistent device problem.[20]

TABLE 28–12
Degree of Programmability

Nonprogrammable	No noninvasive adjustment possible.
Simple programmable	Pacing rate, output, or both may be programmed.
Programmable	Pacing rate, output, and at least one additional parameter may be programmed.
Multiprogrammable	The device is capable of extensive programming, often including refractory-period durations, choice of pacing mode, atrioventricular interval in the case of dual-chamber pacemakers, and special features such as rate hysteresis.
Communicating	In addition to multiprogrammability, the device is capable of transmitting intracardiac electrogram signals, timing-diagram data, or both, noninvasively to an external device for plotting or display. (See discussion of pacemaker telemetry in text.)

References

1. Frye RL, Collins JJ, DiSanctis RW, et al.: Guidelines for permanent cardiac pacemaker implantation. J Am Coll Cardiol 4:434, 1984.
2. Bilitch M, Hauser RG, Goldman BS, et al.: Performance of cardiac pacemaker pulse generators. PACE 5:139, 1982.
3. Bilitch M, Hauser RG, Goldman BS, et al.: Performance of cardiac pacemaker pulse generators. PACE 8:276, 1985.
4. Bilitch M, Hauser RG, Goldman BS, et al.: Performance of implantable cardiac rhythm management devices. PACE 9:256, 1986.
5. Bilitch M, Hauser RG, Goldman BS, et al.: Performance of implantable cardiac rhythm management devices. PACE 10:389, 1987.
6. Parsonnet V, Bernstein AD, Gallagher R, et al.: Preoperative estimation of the proper transvenous lead length (Abstract). PACE 7:475, 1984.
7. Gold RD: Designing output circuits for implantable electronic stimulators. Med Dev Diag Ind 9:61, 1987.
8. Thalen HJTh, Van den Berg J: Follow-up of patients with implanted pacemakers. Israel J Med Sci 5:819–823, 1969.
9. Parsonnet V, Furman S, Smyth NPD: Implantable cardiac pacemakers: Status report and resource guidelines. Pacemaker Study Group, Inter-Society Commission for Heart Disease Resources (ICHD). Circulation 50:A21, 1974.
10. Parsonnet V, Furman S, Smyth NPD: A revised code for pacemaker identification. PACE 4:400, 1981.
11. Parsonnet V, Furman S, Smyth NPD, et al.: Implantable cardiac pacemakers: Status report and resource guidelines, 1982. Pacemaker Study Group, Inter-Society Commission for Heart Disease resources. Circulation 68:227A, 1983.
12. Brownlee RR, Shimmel JB, Del Marco CJ: A new code for pacemaker operating modes. PACE 4:396, 1981.
13. Bernstein AD, Brownlee RR, Fletcher RD, et al.: Report of the NASPE Mode Code Committee. PACE 7:395, 1984.
14. Bernstein AD, Brownlee RR, Fletcher RD, et al.: Pacing mode codes. *In* Barold S (ed.): Modern Cardiac Pacing, pp. 307–322. Mt. Kisco: Futura Publishing Company, 1985.
15. Bernstein AD, Camm AJ, Fletcher RD, et al.: The NASPE/BPEG Generic Pacemaker Code for antibradyarrhythmia and adaptive-rate pacing and antitachyarrhythmia devices. PACE 10:794, 1987.

16. Bernstein AD: A new generic code for antitachyarrhythmia devices. See review by the North American Society of Pacing and Electrophysiology (NASPE), 1984.
17. Bernstein AD, Parsonnet V: Notation conventions and overlay diagrams for analysis of paced electrocardiograms. PACE 6:73, 1983.
18. Parsonnet V, Bernstein AD, Myers MM: Unpublished observations.
19. Lindemans FW: Diagrammatic representation of pacemaker function. *In* Barold S (ed.): Modern Cardiac Pacing, pp. 323–353. Mt. Kisco: Futura Publishing Company, 1985.
20. Parsonnet V, Bernstein AD: Pseudomalfunctions of dual-chamber pacemakers. Proc. Cardiostim 1982. PACE 6:376, 1983.
21. Parsonnet V: Private communication, January, 1988.

29

Multiprogrammability of Modern Cardiac Pacemakers

Jacques Mugica
Pierre Birkui

Definition and Historical Overview

Multiprogrammability in pacing can be defined as the possibility of adjusting, in a noninvasive fashion, the functional parameters of a pacing system. The growing complexity of the new pacing systems (DDD-RR) makes programmability an absolute necessity, with the goal of obtaining "physiologic" pacing tailored to the needs of each individual patient.

The concept of programmability and its clinical application appeared relatively early. In the 1970s the Medtronic Corporation introduced to the market their Model 5842, which was equipped with two accessible contact points with a tri-faced needle, permitting the modification of two parameters, namely the frequency and voltage. In 1972, General Electric introduced their AA 2071 BA, which featured the capability of choosing up to two frequencies by application of a magnet. Ultimately, the Cordis Corporation, with its Omnistanicor model, heralded the era of programmability. By 1978, approximately 36% of all implanted pacemakers in the United States were of the multiprogrammable type. In 1983 and 1984, the North American Society of Pacing and Electrophysiology officially recommended the use of multiprogrammable pacing systems and added that, ". . . solely on the basis of patient safety, there is no indication for the implantations of a single- or dual-chambered pulse generator which is not programmable."[1,2]

The appearance of new generations of DDD, or rate-responsive, systems has underscored the absolute importance of multiple rate programming choices, with the goal of better adaptation to each patient's particular condition, as determined by stress testing or hemodynamic evaluation.

Programming Technologies

Cordis utilized for its multiprogramming purposes magnetic field pulses that activate a reed-switch, according to a code that consists of a certain number of switch openings and closings that allow for adjusting of frequency and current amplitude. This process was followed by other designs, but the limitations of this system (lack of sufficient transmitting speed) became readily apparent. As a result, programming is now performed by means of high-frequency electrical fields emanating from the programmer and received by an antenna system within the pacing device. The multiplicity of programmable parameters, the care taken to prevent programmer crosstalk (between different makes and models), and the potential dangers due to electromagnetic interference led pacemaker designers, at the start of the 1980s,[3] to utilize redundant and sophisticated encoding systems. The speed of these modes of transmission enable multiple commands to be transmitted from the programming device to pacemaker, as well as rapid feedback transmission from the pacemaker to programmer: for example, confirmation of good reception of program commands and feedback information from the pulse generator (voltage, battery current, lead impedance, event markers) and patient information (electrogram and Holter functions).[4]

Multiprogrammability of Classic Single-Chamber Pacemakers

Multiprogramming offers several advantages, some of which are not only theoretical but also practical.

First and foremost, there is the capability to recognize and treat complications (Table 29–1) such as loss

TABLE 29–1
Programming as Treatment of Pacing Complications in Single-Chambered Pacing

Complication	Treatment by Programming
Loss of capture	Increase output: (1) voltage; (2) pulse width
Undersensing	Increase sensitivity Convert from unipolar or bipolar mode
Oversensing	Decrease sensitivity Change the mode (triggered or asynchronous) Increase refractory period if senses T wave Convert from unipolar or bipolar mode
Myopotentials	Convert from unipolar or bipolar mode Reduce sensitivity Convert to triggered mode
Parasitic stimulation (muscle, diaphragmatic..)	Reduce output (mainly voltage) Change the polarity
Atrial or ventricular arrhythmias	Change the rate
Inadequate cardiac output	Change the rate
Pacemaker syndrome	Convert to atrial or DVI-VDD-DDD systems
Noisy leads, or environment	Convert to VVT or VOO
Wire fracture (temporary solutions)	Convert from bipolar to unipolar mode Convert to VOO mode (if not complete fracture)

of capture, undersensing, and extracardiac stimulation (muscular, diaphragmatic). These capabilities are attractive to physicians because they entail simple, noninvasive corrective maneuvers that preclude the need for reintervention.

Another advantage lies in optimizing of the heart rate in a specific clinical situation, such as lowering of the base rate in patients with coronary artery disease (CAD) or, in another case, setting of a better frequency to achieve a maximal cardiac output.

Among the multiple programmable parameters, all are valuable but three are fundamental: output programmability, rate, and sensitivity. These characteristics can be found in the more advanced pacemakers such as the DDD type, which are endowed with further programmable parameters (e.g., programmability of refractory period).

OUTPUT PROGRAMMABILITY

As a rule, all pulse generators should be programmable for pulse amplitude (voltage) as well as for pulse width, which allows for diagnostic as well as therapeutic functions. The diagnostic goal is to determine the pacing safety margin (noninvasive determination of pacing threshold).

The first system, described in 1973 by Meibom,[5-6] is without any doubt still the best: The "Vario" system (Siemens-Elema, Telectronics) will convert to a fixed rate after application of the magnet along with the setting of maximal output voltage for 16 beats, followed by the Vario cycle, in which there is a progressive decrease in output voltage for 16 steps, with a reduction of 0.35 volts per step until 0 voltage occurs (Fig. 29–1). This system permits, in a simple fashion, an accurate, noninvasive means of determining the voltage pacing threshold, allowing for a good pacing margin of safety by, for example, doubling the pacing output to twice threshold given a constant pulse width. On the other hand, if the Vario system is used at the same time as the pulse width programming function, this permits noninvasive construction of a strength-duration curve as well as a precise measurement of the pacing margin of safety. The strength-duration curve can be constructed with a lesser number of measurements than is obtained with the Vario system, but doubling the measured threshold value is recommended to maintain a good margin of safety (Fig. 29–2).[7] The ability to program the output allows monitoring of the evolution of chronic thresholds.

Long-term follow-up data shows that thresholds, particularly in some patients, continue to rise progressively,[8-9] particularly with certain leads.[10] Furthermore, with today's new leads, it has been noted that acute thresholds are very low, rising slightly in the first month, and decreasing later,[10] a phenomenon that should be kept in mind when setting the pulse amplitude at a low-energy level. Setting a low output permits energy conservation and increases the lifetime of the pacemaker. In a series by Hauser,[11] 66% of his patients had output settings lower than the mean, with a consequent increase of 30% in pacemaker longevity.

In a multicenter series using 1000 carbon-tip leads (PMCF) over a 5-year period, Pioger and Mugica[20] reported that 90% of patients equipped with a Vario system demonstrated a threshold value of less than 1 V with a pulse width of 0.8 ms after 12 months from the time of implantation. This allows programming of these pacemakers at 2.5 V and 0.5 ms, with a margin of safety of 100%. In this case, the current drain due to stimulation, which varies as a function of the square root of the voltage, is divided by 4, in contrast to the current drain resulting from programming to 5 V.

Energy conservation becomes all the more important as pacemakers and their lithium batteries become smaller, while at the same time the demand for their energy increases. Current examples include DDD pacemakers, as well as pacemakers with Holter functions, which store data concerning the patient and the pacemaker and can be interrogated.

Lowering of the programmable current output presents us with possible advantages. In certain clinical cases in which it is necessary to elucidate the natural history of conductive disorders, or to diagnose an infarct or digitalis intoxication, it might be necessary to diminish the current output below threshold levels. At times, reducing the pulse width or, more frequently,

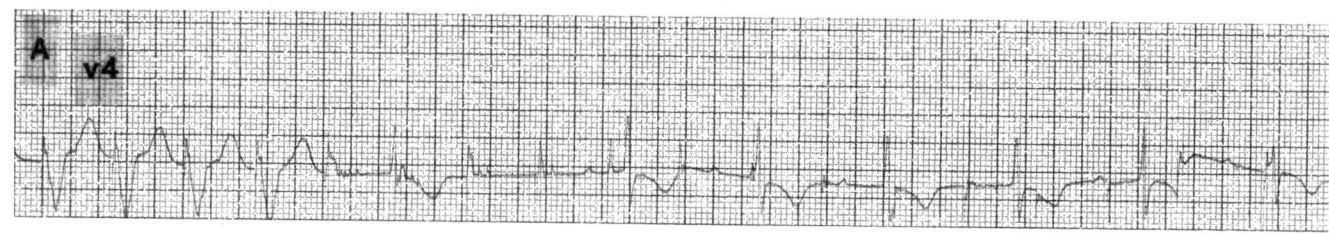

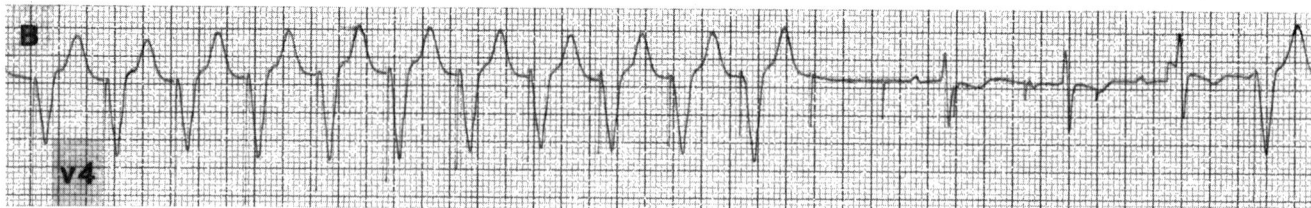

FIGURE 29–1
Noninvasive determination of pacing threshold by the Vario system (Siemens-Elema). Application of the magnet on a Telectronics Optima MPT reverts the pacing rate to 100 bpm (VOO mode). The first 16 impulses are at the program output.

A, The amplitude of the last 16 impulses decreases by step of 0.35 V to 0 V. In this patient, the last 12 spikes are inefficient, which means that the threshold is >4.2 V.

B, The output is reprogrammed to 10 V to increase the safety margin.

lowering the output will suppress muscular or diaphragmatic stimulations. The latter tends to become more frequent with the size reduction of unipolar pulse generators.

Increasing the output voltage may be necessary for a temporary or definitive period following pacemaker implantation or, at times, following infarction, cardioversion, defibrillation, or a hyperkalemic state or when there are high serum levels of a type I antiarrhythmia.[12–14] Last, certain pulse generators are capable of being programmed at a high-energy output level (7.5–10 V).[15, 16] This capability can be of use in an emergency situation or in cases in which chronic, progressive threshold elevations have occurred due to excessive fibrosis surrounding the lead tip (Fig. 29–3). This condition has become less frequent with the advent of modern electrode tips (porous, target, carbon, steroid-eluting).[17–20]

RATE PROGRAMMABILITY

Apart from certain particular indications, the function of rate programmability has been routinely overlooked. In simple VVI pacing, programming of the frequency to improve cardiac output permits the optimal use of these fixed-frequency devices. In our experience, 65% of our patients with implanted pacemakers were reprogrammed in order to achieve improved hemodynamics.

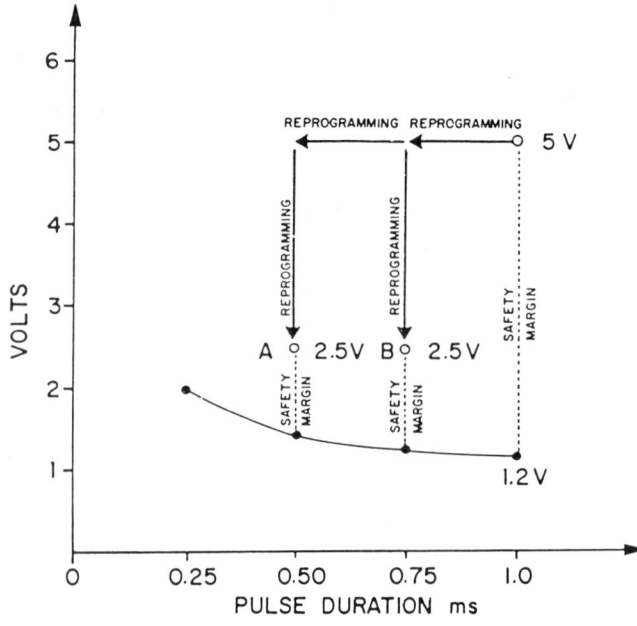

FIGURE 29–2
Energy conservation by reprogramming to a lower output-amplitude. This strength duration curve shows a threshold of 1.2 V at 1-ms pulse duration and 1.4 V at 0.50-ms pulse duration. The safety margin at 5 V and 1-ms pulse width is 3.8 V. At 2.5 V and a pulse width of 0.5 ms, the safety margin is 1.1 V, which is probably still adequate as it represents approximately 75% of the threshold voltage. However, at a pulse width of 0.25 ms, the threshold voltage is 2.0 V. Consequently, it would be appropriate to program the pulse generator to pace at a pulse width of 0.25 ms and output of 5 V, thereby yielding more than a 100% safety margin in terms of voltage. (Reprinted by permission of Futura Publishing Co., Inc., from SS Barold, LS Ong, MD Falkoff, RA Heinle: In SS Barold and J Mugica (eds.): The Third Decade of Cardiac Pacing, p. 27. Mt Kisco, Futura Publishing Co., Inc., 1982.)

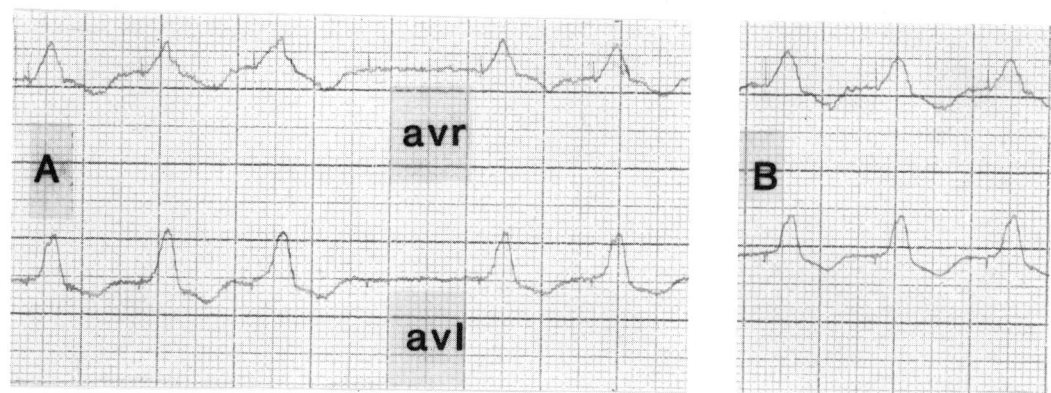

FIGURE 29–3
A, Loss of capture (CPI—ASTRA T6 439); output 5V · 0.5 ms. *B*, Reprogrammed at 7 V at 0.5-ms pulse duration.

Programming Slow Rates

This type of programming is particularly important in patients with CAD and symptomatic angina pectoris. It is preferable in these cases to set the rate at 60 beats per minute (bpm) or lower if the patient is particularly symptomatic. On some occasions, the implantation of a pacemaker at a nominal rate of 70 bpm unmasks previously silent CAD.[21] Setting pacing rates lower than the conventional frequency of 70 bpm is often done, when possible, in patients with intermittent heart block or the sick sinus syndrome. These groups of patients have a good underlying rate most of the time, permitting better cardiac function by maintaining AV synchrony.[22, 23] In certain cases, a low frequency setting can prevent the emergence of retrograde VA conduction that can generate symptoms of the pacemaker syndrome.

Programming Fast Rates

Setting fast pacing rates can be useful in two circumstances. First, in certain arrhythmias such as bigeminy, one extrasystole follows a paced beat; this extrasystole is detected by the pacemaker and the consequence is a low mechanical rate. Increasing the pacing rate can often correct the problem (Fig. 29–4). The second circumstance occurs in patients with congestive heart

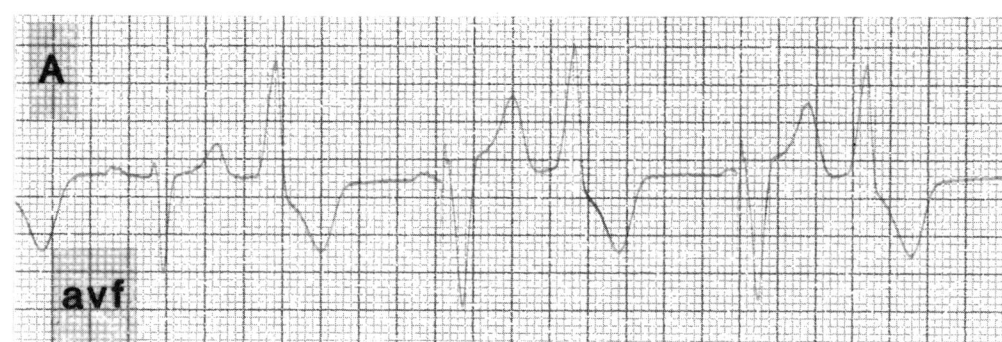

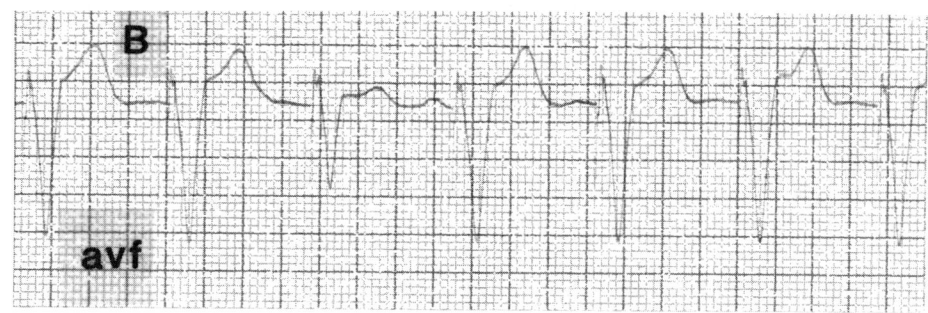

FIGURE 29–4
A, Bigeminy. Pacing rate 70 bpm (Siemens 688). *B*, PVCs disappear after programming the rate to 80 bpm.

failure or in certain patients in need of a higher pacing frequency to improve their hemodynamic condition.[24-26]

The appropriate frequency should be set after determining the patient's ejection fraction and overall cardiac function by nuclear or echo-Doppler studies.[27, 28]

PROGRAMMABILITY OF SENSITIVITY

There is a great variety in electrical characteristics of intracardiac signals, amplitudes from 0.5 mV to 20 mV, slope of detection ranging from 0.1 V to several volts per second.[30] It is necessary to be able to adjust the sensitivity threshold in order to detect the useful signal and to optimize the signal-to-noise ratio. If the slope discriminators are seldom used, programming of sensitivity according to amplitude is extremely useful, particularly for atrial sensing.

It is difficult to define what is "normal" with regard to sensitivity values, because manufacturers use arbitrary, nonstandardized test signals with morphologies that are far removed from the actual electrocardiographic signals.

Undersensing

Undersensing is said to occur when the pacemaker fails to sense an R wave, with the consequent untimely triggering of the pacemaker. The pacemaker spike can fall on a vulnerable period of the T wave, which theoretically can trigger a ventricular tachycardia. At worst, the pulse generator can completely undersense ventricular depolarizations, and the device will function as though it were set in the VOO mode (Fig. 29-5). Problems with undersensing invariably occur if the endocardial signal is less than 5 mv, or if the slow rate is equal or less than 1 volt per second.

An increase in sensitivity can restore correct detection of the R wave (or the P wave) and thereby avoid an operative intervention to reposition an electrode.[30, 31] Too great an increase in sensitivity carries with it the risk of oversensing.

A particularly vexing problem is the failure to detect ventricular extrasystoles. This phenomenon of undersensed ventricular extrasystoles has been seen in 8 to 15% of cases.[29-32] Theoretically, an increase in sensitivity can control this problem, but there are two draw-

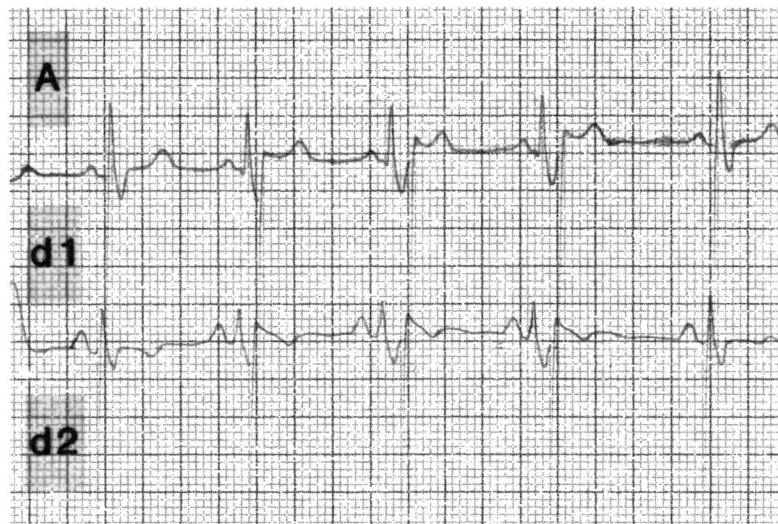

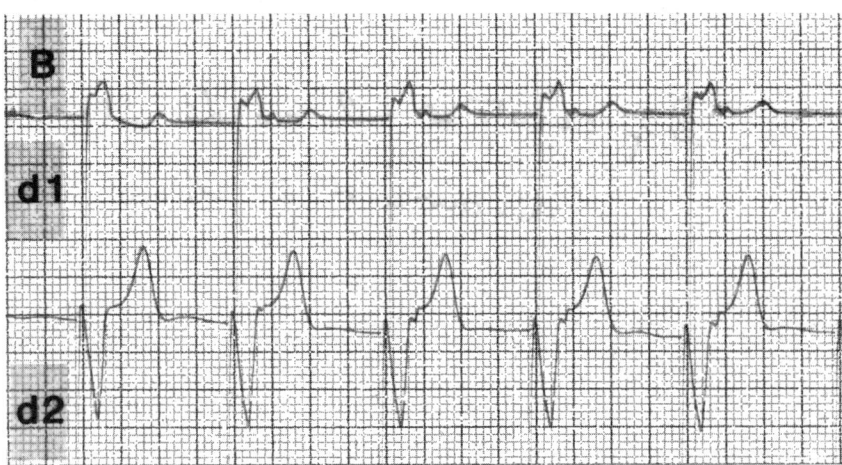

FIGURE 29-5
Undersensing (Pacesetter 2416). *A*, Programmed sensitivity 2 mV. *B*, Programmed sensitivity 1 mV, resulting in correction of the sensing defects.

backs. First, there is an effective slowing of the heart rate, since the extrasystole (with little hemodynamic contribution) will inhibit the appearance of a paced beat at that time. Second, a high sensitivity setting may lead to oversensing of myopotentials and all types of external interference.

Oversensing

At present, the principal problem of oversensing is myopotential inhibition, which is seen frequently with unipolar stimulation. In such cases, the diminution of sensitivity assumes a therapeutic function (Fig. 29–6).[33–38] Moreover, in certain cases programming may not be efficacious and may cause undersensing. Before contemplating a reintervention to change the pulse generator or to implant a Parsonnet pocket, it is necessary to consider programming in the VVT mode or in the bipolar mode.

The problems of oversensing the afterpotential or the T wave have practically disappeared, thanks to the technological advances incorporated in the new pulse generators. Many of these devices can tackle the problem of oversensing by reducing the sensitivity, combined with prolongation of the refractory period and reduction of pulse width or current output.[39–41]

PROGRAMMABILITY OF THE REFRACTORY PERIOD

The refractory period may be defined as the period during which the sensing mechanism becomes "deaf" to electrical signals. This period is necessary to prevent sensing of an afterpotential or a T wave. The ideal refractory period lies somewhere between 200 and 250 milliseconds.[42] Programmability of the refractory period may be useful in the following circumstances.

- Increasing sensitivity in order to correct undersensing may lead to detection of the T wave. Prolongation of the refractory period may correct this problem.
- At times when a pulse generator is programmed with a refractory period of 350 ms or longer, there is failure to sense early ventricular premature contractions (VPCs). These VPCs can be sensed by shortening the refractory period.[43]
- With a synchronous pulse generator (VVT or AAT), the refractory period determines the frequency of maximal stimulation. This is important if cutaneous chest wall stimulation is used for noninvasive electrophysiologic studies or to stop reentrant tachycardias. Shortening of the refractory period permits a maximal triggered frequency.
- Programmability of the refractory period is especially useful in atrial demand pacing. In this instance, because the QRS complex should not be sensed after a pacemaker-induced atrial depolarization, the refractory period should be set close to 400 ms.[43]

PROGRAMMABILITY OF HYSTERESIS

Hysteresis can be said to occur when the escape interval is significantly longer than the automatic interval. Presently, after much discussion,[44–46] the above definition refers to *positive* hysteresis. This concept[44–47] has cer-

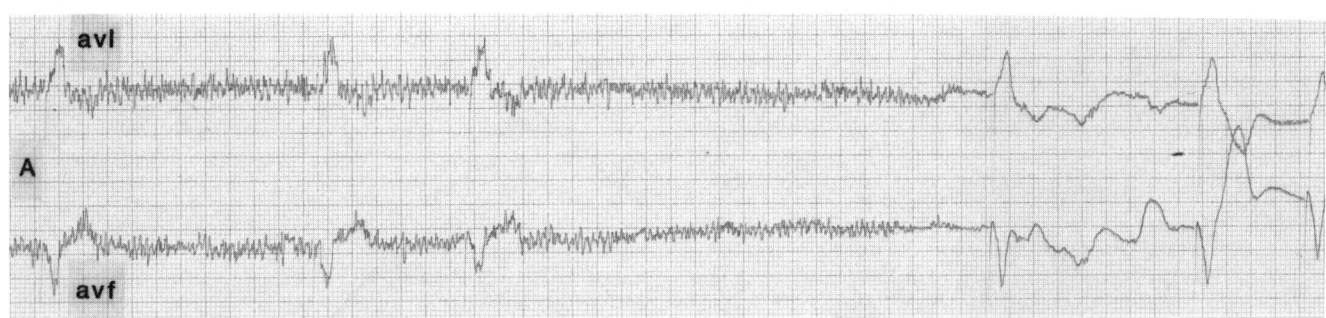

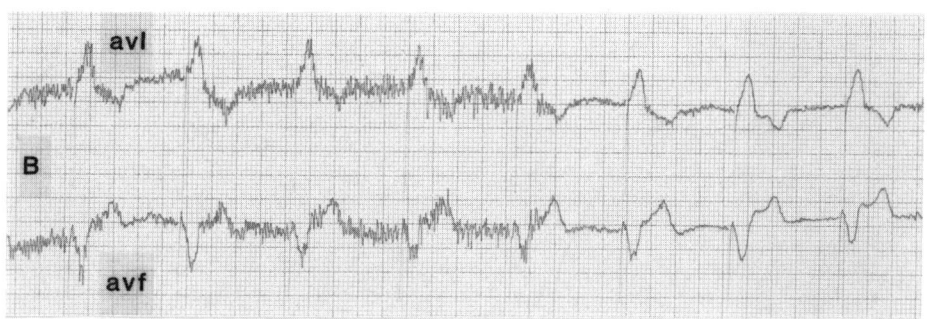

FIGURE 29–6
Oversensing of myopotentials (Siemens 668). A, Programmed sensitivity 2 mV; asystole >3.5 s. B, Programmed sensitivity 4 mV. The myopotentials are as wide as on strip A, but the oversensing is corrected.

tain disadvantages, as it is a frequent source of confusion in the interpretation of electrocardiograms; however, there is renewed interest in its application with programmable pulse generators. For example, a pacemaker setting of hysteresis in patients with the sick sinus syndrome may avoid the use of low pacing rates to take advantage of spontaneous AV synchrony.

Negative hysteresis occurs when the escape interval is significantly shorter than the automatic interval; it can be useful in the prevention of ventricular arrhythmias.

PROGRAMMABILITY OF PACING MODE

The possibility of programming a pacemaker in the unipolar or bipolar mode is already an old concept.[48, 49] It is more useful for DDD devices and also for in-line connectors, which facilitate the introduction of this function. The advantage of switching from a bipolar to a unipolar mode is also useful in certain situations, such as the evaluation of some cases of undersensing or oversensing or in instances of lead fracture. More useful is the possibility of switching from the unipolar to bipolar mode in cases of muscular stimulation.[50–55] The option of programming to asynchronous pacing can avoid some reinterventions, notably in certain cases of oversensing or noisy leads.[56–59]

Finally, conversion of VVI or AAI modes to synchronous VVT or AAT modes can be of use in the following settings:

- Diagnosis or correction of oversensing due to noisy leads or myopotential inhibition.
- Chest wall stimulation for purposes of noninvasive electrophysiologic studies or as a therapeutic tool to stop tachycardias via pacing salvos.[60–63]

Programmability of a DDD Pulse Generator

Today it is inconceivable to imagine a non-multiprogrammable DDD pulse generator. One attempt, made by Intermedics, was cancelled after a small production run. For the present, multiprogrammable pulse generators predominate in clinical use (Table 29–2; Fig. 29–7). In the future, the complexity of such multiprogrammability will be reduced in the "completely automatic" pulse generator.[64]

The programmable parameters in single-chamber pacing are also applicable to dual-chamber DDD pacing. These parameters are set separately for each chamber, and certain ones are of particular importance in pacing the atrium and are almost equally important in AAI pacing.

The pacing thresholds at the level of the atrium are generally higher than in the ventricle, and their values vary more, depending on the lead localization. Furthermore, some sites in the atrium in some patients are totally inexcitable.

The setting of the output (voltage and pulse width) should be carefully adjusted in the upper range to avoid atrial escapes, and also in the lower range to prevent the phenomenon of crosstalk, which may lead to ventricular inhibition.

Above all, the weak amplitude of the electrocardiographic atrial signal, in comparison with the propagated amplitude of a ventricular complex, demands a greater sensitivity of the detection circuits as well as a wider programming range.

TABLE 29–2
Clinical Usefulness of Programming in DDD Pacing

Parameter	Treatment by Programming
Energy (output)	Loss of capture—especially the atrial counter phenomenon of crosstalk
Sensitivity	Undersensing—especially atrial counters against interference (myopotentials, external noise, crosstalk)
Refractory Period/AV interval/Upper Rate	Optimal setting for each patient Counter initiation of tachycardias
Lower Rate	To maintain the spontaneous AV delay for a maximal period
Modes	DDT-AAT-VVT (electrophysiologic studies and treatment of tachycardia) VOO-VDD-DVI (see Fig. 29–7)
Polarity—unipolar/bipolar mode	Prevention of interference improves sensing

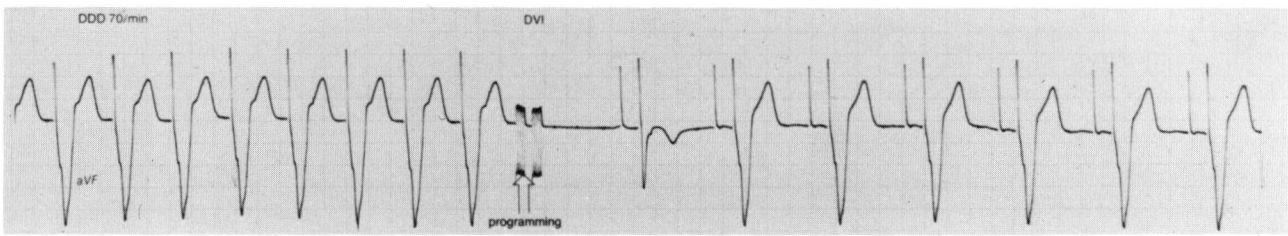

FIGURE 29–7
Reprogramming to stop and prevent recurrent reentrant tachycardia. The pulse generator is reprogrammed to the DVI mode which precludes an endless loop tachycardia, as there is no atrial sensing in this mode. The fixed-rate atrial stimulation in the DVI mode usually stops the continuation of retrograde P waves. (Reprinted by permission from Schuller H, Fähraeus T: Pacemaker Electrocardiograms: An Introduction to Practical Analysis. Solma, Sweden; Siemens Elema AB, 1983.)

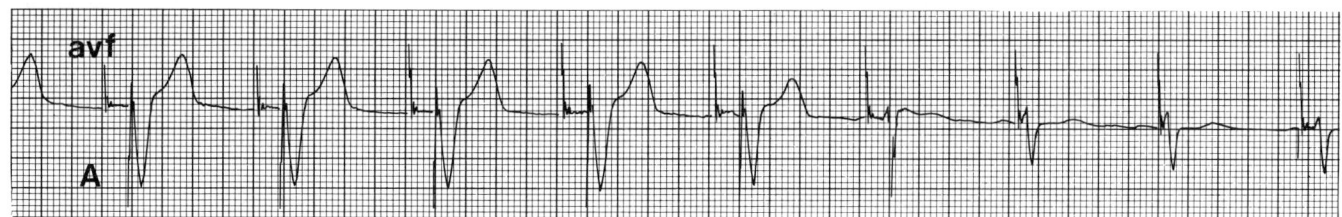

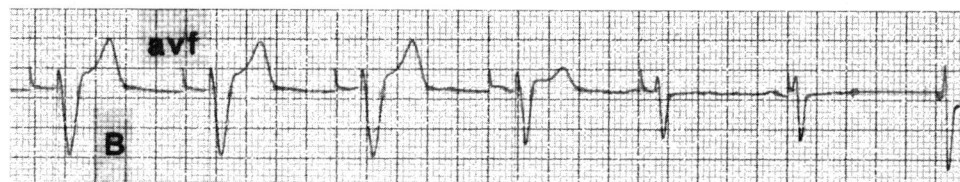

FIGURE 29-8
Intermittent atrial undersensing 5 days after implantation (Pacesetter AFP 283). A, Programmed sensitivity 1 mV. B, Reprogramming 5 days after implantation of 0.5 mV, with intermittent efficacy. The sensing defect will disappear 10 days after implantation.

The possibility of a large range of programming capabilities and fine adjustments allows the physician to better handle the most common problems encountered in DDD pacing.

OVERSENSING (OF MYOPOTENTIALS)[35, 65, 66] AND CROSSTALK ■ (See p. 515 for discussion).

UNDERSENSING ■ This is seen more frequently at the level of the atrium than at the level of the ventricle. Lemke et al.[67] have reported that atrial sensing defects are common in the early postoperative phase in 62.5% of cases. Intermittent sensing defects in the chronic phase are found in 11.1% of cases (Fig. 29-8).

ENDLESS LOOP TACHYCARDIAS ■ Klementowicz and Furman[68] have reported that selective P wave sensing in the DDD mode can abolish endless loop tachycardias if retrograde atrial depolarizations can be distinguished from anterograde depolarizations and if the former is selectively ignored. The introduction of pacemakers with multiple settings can be used to sense selectively the signals of a determined amplitude and to reject the others, such as in discriminating the difference in amplitude and duration of anterograde and retrograde atrial signals. Each pacemaker should have the flexibility to sense and differentiate these anterograde and retrograde signals in patients with endless loop tachycardia. The authors demonstrated that the anterograde signal in half their patients was at least 1.4 times larger than the corresponding retrograde atrial signal.

PROGRAMMABILITY OF THE ATRIAL REFRACTORY PERIOD

This is an essential parameter in DDD pacing and is closely tied to the maximal pacing frequency of the ventricle. The atrial refractory period consists of two parts. The first is that which starts with the beginning of the spontaneous or paced atrial deflection and ends with the R wave. This is the AV delay. The second is the postventricular atrial refractory period.

The AV delay period that exists in all modern DDD pulse generators is programmable, the end point being to obtain the most optimal hemodynamic contribution.[69-75] Moreover, if one wishes to optimize the cardiac output, the AV delay period should be modulated according to what is paced or sensed by the atrium. For example, as shown in Figure 29-9, the

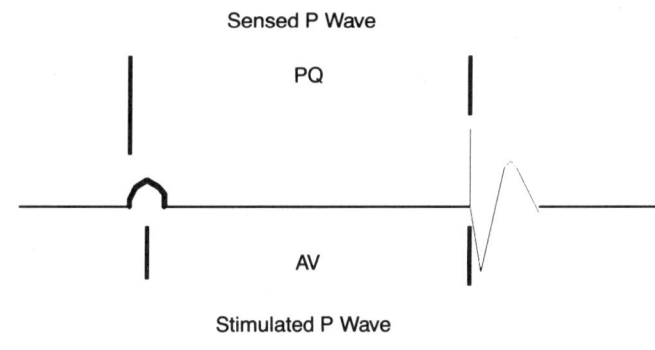

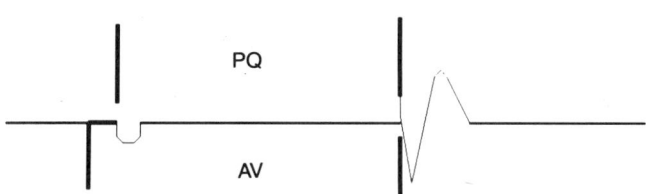

FIGURE 29-9
Optimization of AV delay.
A, Because of the conduction time in the atrium, the spontaneous depolarization is sensed by the atrial electrode a number of milliseconds after it starts at the SA node. The AV delay is shorter than the apparent PQ interval. B, Conversely, the atrial depolarization initiated by a paced event leads to an AV delay longer than the PQ interval.

lead detects the spontaneous atrial depolarization after a delay of several milliseconds or tenths of a millisecond, depending on the lead position in relation to the site of electrical depolarization. The mechanical contraction of the atrium will subsequently follow. On the other hand, when one paces the atrium, there is a functional delay after the atrial impulse before atrial depolarization ensues, and the AV delay period is subsequently longer. If one wishes to maintain, for a given frequency, an AV delay that is "electromechanically" constant, it will be necessary to shorten the post-stimulus AV delay period from the time of atrial depolarization. This can be very important in certain patients in a critical hemodynamic state, and it is in this subset of patients that one would try to optimize the cardiac output (see Fig. 29–9).

For the majority of patients, the AV delay period is shortened with effort, and certainly the cardiac output is modified to a significant degree by high-frequency pacing if the AV delay that is programmed and adjusted at rest is maintained. The automatic shortening of the AV delay period as a function of the heart rate has further hemodynamic benefits with respect to a concomitant shortening of the atrial refractory period and permits a high frequency of AV synchrony.[72–74]

The second part of the atrial refractory period is called the postventricular atrial refractory period, which starts when the paced or spontaneous R wave occurs. Programming of this period is useful in countering retrograde P waves that follow VPCs.[76]

UPPER-RATE LIMIT OF VENTRICULAR STIMULATION

Different systems are utilized to determine the upper-rate limit of ventricular stimulation. One system, already near obsolescence, simply depends on the maximal frequency of the atrial refractory period. The maximal frequency will be lower if the AV delay and the postventricular atrial refractory periods are longer (Fig. 29–10). The disadvantage of this system is the sudden fall in rate that can occur with the development of a Mobitz II block, when the atrial rate reaches the maximal level. If retrograde P waves suddenly appear, it will be necessary to extend the refractory period and to diminish the upper rate.[77, 78]

The sudden and abrupt change to the 2-to-1 mode is quite often felt acutely by the patient, particularly during exercise. The manufacturers have devised methods for controlling the ventricular upper rate independently of the programming of the atrial refractory period. One solution consists of reproducing a pseudo-Wenckebach mode, with a progressive lengthening of the AV delay period and an intermittent passage into the 2-to-1 mode (Fig. 29–11).[29, 79, 80] To further limit the variations of ventricular frequency, some mechanisms that progressively reduce the frequency (fallback, flywheel, rate-smoothing systems) have been proposed for use in modern pacing systems.[81]

The *fallback* response is a programmable option to prevent the tracking of pathologic atrial rates above the maximum atrial tracking rate by switching over to the VVI mode. The ventricular pacing rate is then slowly reduced. In the presence of VA conduction beyond the atrial refractory period,[81, 82] the fallback mode can give rise to intermittent pacemaker mediated tachycardias.

The *rate-smoothing* option in some DDD pacemakers aims at eliminating abrupt rate fluctuations by preventing pacing rate changes by more than a programmed percentage from one cardiac cycle to next. With a bradycardia-tachycardia syndrome, rate smoothing offers the possibility of preventing a rapid deceleration by gradually lowering the rate. The rate-smoothing option can lead to loss of AV synchrony and can thus initiate pacemaker-mediated tachycardias (PMTs).[81–83]

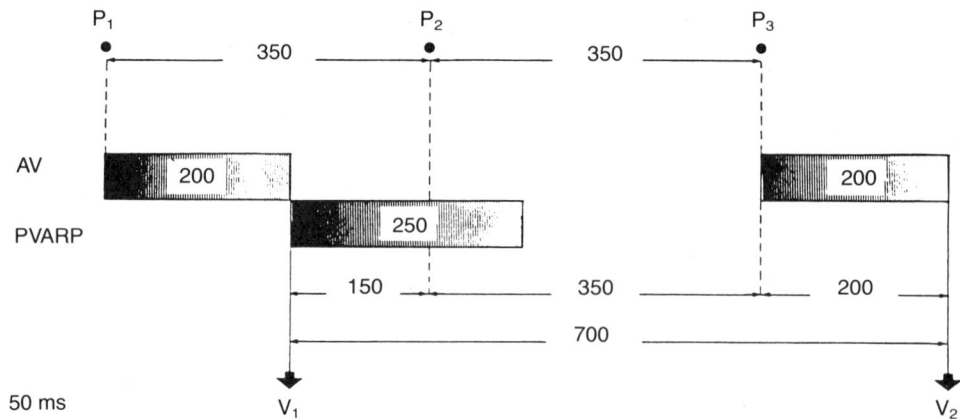

FIGURE 29–10
Limitation of maximal synchronous rate by addition of the AV delay and the postventricular atrial refractory period (PVARP). The pacemaker is set at an AV delay of 200 ms and a PVARP of 250 ms. The P_2 wave follows 350 ms after P_1 and falls in the PVARP and cannot be recognized. The P_3 wave follows 350 ms after P_2. It will be detected and V_2 will follow at 200 ms (AV delay). The V_1-V_2 interval will be double that of the P_1-P_2 interval, or 700 ms. The device has a maximum period of synchronization of 450 ms, which corresponds to an upper rate limit of 133 bpm.

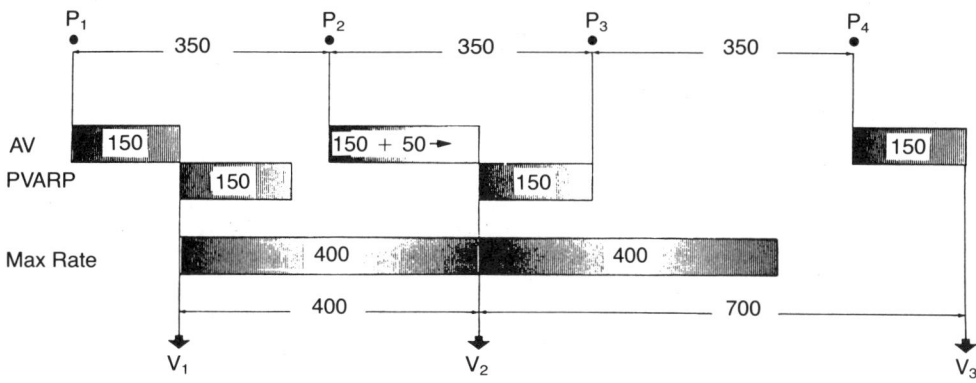

FIGURE 29-11
Upper rate limit. The device is programmed with an AV delay of 150 ms, a short postventricular atrial refractory period (PVARP) of 150 ms, and an upper rate limit of 150 bpm (400 ms). The P_2 wave follows 350 ms after the end of the atrial refractory period (AV delay and PVARP). It is detected by the sensing circuit and it cannot be followed by a ventricular spike after the delay of 150 ms because of the rate limit. The ventricular stimulation is delayed by 50 ms because the V_2 spike cannot follow less than 400 ms after V_1. The V_1-V_2 interval (400 ms) corresponds to the upper rate limit program (150 bpm). The P_3 wave follows 350 ms after P_2. It falls at the end of the atrial refractory period and cannot be sensed. In turn, the P_4 wave, which follows 350 ms after P_3, is sensed by the atrial circuit and will be followed 150 ms later by a V_3 stimulus. The V_2-V_3 interval is double that of the P_2-P_3 (block 2:1).

PROGRAMMING OF THE LOWER RATE

The lower rate programming function is even more useful in dual chamber pacing than in single-chamber pacing, if one wishes to conserve at a maximum the spontaneous atrial to spontaneous or paced ventricular sequences, particularly at rest. One indirect benefit of the conservation of atrial spontaneous activity is the saving of battery capacity.

Principal Problems of DDD Pacing

As mentioned previously, the most common problems encountered with DDD pacing are endless loop tachycardias, PCMTs, and crosstalk.

PREVENTION OF ENDLESS LOOP TACHYCARDIAS

The growth of DDD pacing has been slowed principally by the occurrence of endless loop tachycardias, particularly with first-generation pacemakers (pacemaker-mediated tachycardias). The capability of making fine adjustments of parameters such as the AV delay period and the postventricular atrial refractory period have prevented the recurrence of these tachycardias to a large degree.[81-84] The existence of an artificial system of AV conduction in patients with normal VA conduction can produce the creation of true, sustained reentrant tachycardias (Fig. 29-12). These tachycardias may be induced spontaneously if the patient exhibits constant retrograde P waves during ventricular stimulation, in conjunction with AV dissociation that is real or perceived by the pacing system. Thus, the principal triggering mechanisms are:

- Ventricular extrasystoles (Fig. 29-13)
- Atrial extrasystoles
- Periodic atrial or ventricular undersensing
- Placement or removal of magnet
- Presence of electrical interference
- Myopotential interference
- Chest wall pacing

The induction of tachycardias may be facilitated when the pacemaker is functioning in the pseudo-Wenckeback mode, with artificial lengthening of the AV delay period that favors dissociation. To prevent the onset of such tachycardias, two methods are used in first-generation DDD devices: the programmability of the AV delay and the programmability of the postventricular atrial refractory period (PVARP).

The median value for retrograde VA conduction times is approximately 240 ms, with a maximum value of about 400 ms. The ability to program a long PVARP eliminates the risk of induction of a PMT (Sequicor*).

---

*Telectronics-Cordis, Englewood, CO, USA.

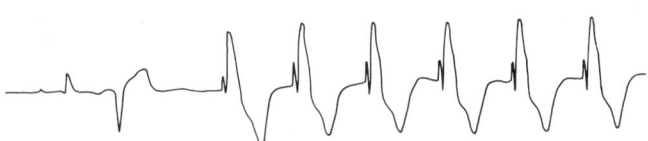

FIGURE 29-12
Pacemaker-mediated endless loop tachycardia induced by an AV desynchronization (ventricular premature contraction).

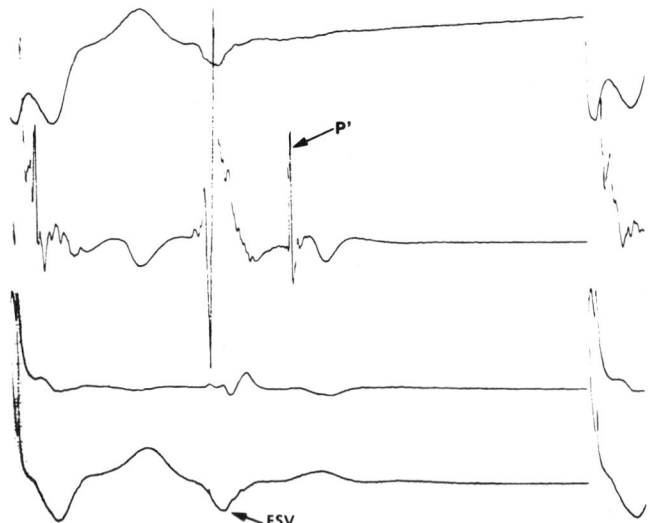

FIGURE 29–13
Retrograde P wave (P′) caused by a premature ventricular contraction (PVC).

This can also lead to an important loss of positive hemodynamic benefit.

Indeed, in an individual patient the VA interval varies in relation to the frequency of ventricular stimulation. Consequently, if, for reasons of security, one programs a permanent PVARP of 400 ms, and if the VA delay is set at 200 ms, the pacing cycle length cannot be less than 600 ms, which corresponds to a heart rate of 100 bpm. Thus a good portion of the theoretical advantage of sequential pacing is lost, particularly in young patients.

Programmability of the AV Delay

By programming permanently a very short AV delay period, one can avoid triggering of the atrium by the retrograde ventricular wave of depolarization, insofar as the wave of depolarization finds the atrial tissue still refractory. One can appreciate the hemodynamic impact of such situations. To overcome such limitations, methods have been devised to automatically lengthen the PVARP when the risk of tachycardias is high—as, for example, when one detects VPCs or APCs, which is what most of today's modern DDD devices are capable of doing (Cosmos,* Symbios,† AFP‡). However in order for this solution to be really effective, the pulse generator must carry out the operation in all cases in which it perceives a situation of AV dissociation (such as ELA is proposing with the Chorus system). A partial solution, implemented in the Quintech 931,§ consists of stimulating the atrium in synchrony with the detection of a VPC. If, despite this precaution,

---

*Intermedics Inc., Freeport, TX, USA.
†Medtronic, Inc., Minneapolis, MN, USA.
‡Siemens-Elema, Sweden.
§Vitatron Medical B. V., Dieren, The Netherlands.

the tachycardia is triggered, it will be detected by the Quintech 931. If the sum of

$$DAV + AV < T\ min$$

that is, if the theoretical frequency of the tachycardia is greater than the maximal programmable frequency, the pulse generator activates a Wenckebach function that will automatically lengthen the AV delay until both limits coincide. The result will be a reentrant tachycardia induced by the pacemaker that is occurring at the maximal allowable frequency and that is easy to detect (Fig. 29–14). (This simple algorithm is a component of the Cosmos system.)

Unfortunately, this type of example is not the one most frequently observed. Let us suppose that the pulse generator has been programmed in the following fashion:

$$\text{Upper rate limit} = 150\ \text{bpm}$$
$$\text{Cycle length} = 400\ \text{ms}$$
$$\text{AVD} = 160\ \text{ms}$$

The tachycardia will be detected only if the retrograde conduction time is less than the tachycardia cycle length: that is:

$$T\ min - DAV = 400\ ms - 160\ ms = 240\ ms$$

That is to say, it will be detected in one of two patients, because we have seen that 240 ms corresponds to the median VA conduction interval. The tachycardia rate can range between 90 bpm and the maximal programmable rate, which in certain models can surpass 150 bpm.

Being able to discriminate this type of tachycardia from a sinus tachycardia or effort-related tachycardia is the goal that we must try to reach. On the other hand, once detected, this phenomenon can be easily terminated by, for example, inhibiting the atrial sensing amplifier.

An interesting algorithm is seen in the Chorus system for correcting this problem. The Chorus pacemaker evaluates permanently the stability of the sinus rhythm. If the variations in rhythm measured in 8 consecutive beats are of a lower value than the pre-set value, the

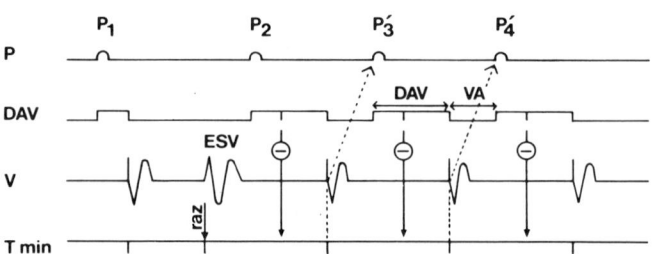

FIGURE 29–14
Endless loop pacemaker-mediated tachycardia. The premature ventricular contraction (PVC) restarts the upper rate limit counter (T min). The P_2 wave that follows triggers an AV delay (DAV), which is enlarged up to T min. The AV desynchronization creates a retrograde P wave (P'_3), which induces a PMT with a T min period equal to DAV + VA.

pacemaker will modify the AV delay period by a few milliseconds.

Two conditions are possible: if the VP interval follows this modification, we know we are dealing with a stable sinus rhythm. In the second case, if the VP interval remains stable, we know that we are dealing with a PMT. The automatic reset of a long refractory period of 450 ms will terminate the tachycardia. In case of an immediate recurrence, the pacemaker will reprogram itself to set a shorter AV delay period, until the minimum of 100 ms is reached; if the tachycardia persists, the pacemaker will lengthen the PVARP to a sufficient width to eliminate the problem. The Chorus pacemaker, therefore, arrives at the best hemodynamic/security compromise.

CROSSTALK

Crosstalk can be defined as the inappropriate sensing of a paced atrial stimulus or atrial depolarization by the ventricular sensing amplifier. This is a problem that is seen almost exclusively with DDD pacing (Table 29–3); however, rare cases have been described with VVI pacing (Fig. 29–15).[85] The result of crosstalk is partial inhibition of ventricular pacing.[86] The definition of crosstalk has been broadened by Levine[87] to pertain to the inappropriate sensing of one phenomenon originating from one chamber or another by the other. This definition is logical because atrial sensitivity is more often programmed at high sensitivities, and dual-chamber pacemakers, particularly the monopolars, are more susceptible to the phenomenon of crosstalk.

Pacemaker designers have struggled with this phenomenon, using their capability to program the ventricular blanking period; the ventricle is rendered "deaf" during a short period that starts with the atrial stimulus and continues for about 10 to 60 ms. into the period of atrial depolarization. The result is that some VPCs may not be sensed and the subsequent paced stimulus may fall in a period of vulnerability. Despite the use of blanking, crosstalk may still exist, due to faulty lead insulation or electrical noise (see Table 29–3).

To avoid these pitfalls, some designers have proposed programming a second parameter such as a nonphysiologic AV delay (Fig. 29–16). The latter is shorter than the true AV delay, and generally its

TABLE 29–3
Causes and Correction of Crosstalk

Principal Causes
- Poorly set programmable parameters, such as a very high ventricular sensitivity, a very short blanking period, or very high atrial output.
- Displacement of the lead toward triscupid valve.
- Loss of integrity of electrode sheath.

Correction
- If due to lead trouble, replace or change the electrode.
- All other cases are amenable to correction by programming: reduction of sensitivity or output; increase of blanking period or nonphysiologic AV delay period; passage from unipolar to bipolar mode; programming to VDD, DVI, DOO, DAT, DAD or AAI, according to the capabilities of the pacing system and the clinical circumstances (for example: AAI in the sick sinus syndrome).

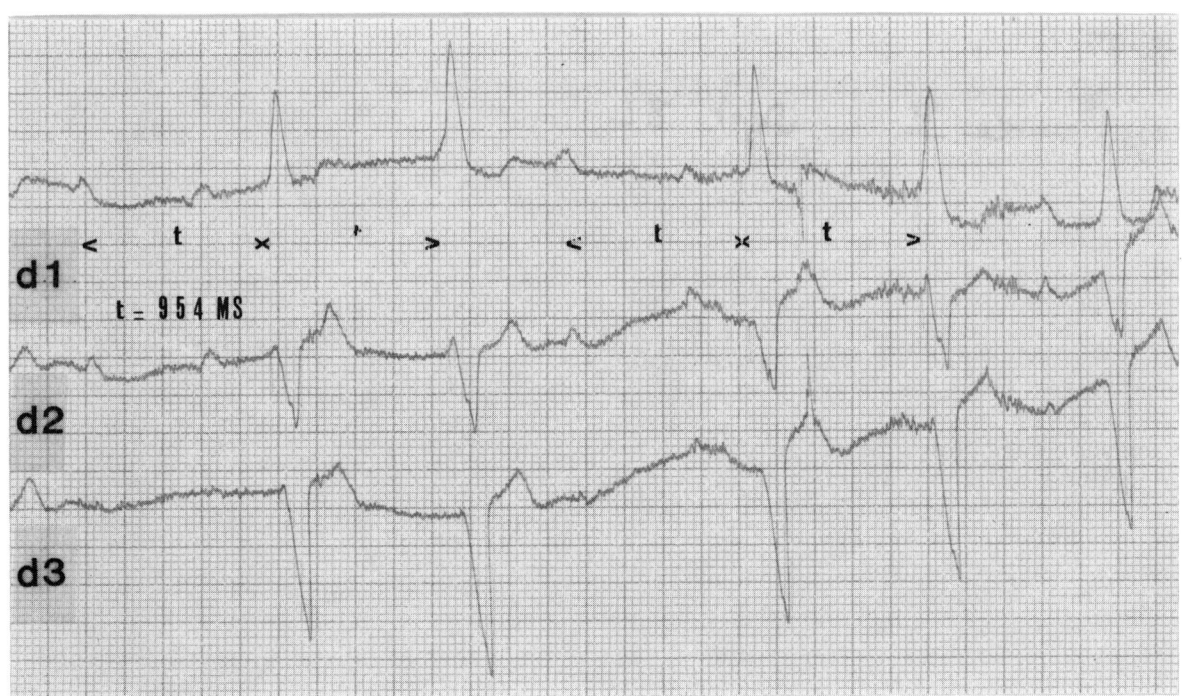

FIGURE 29–15
Inhibition of Medtronic 8422 (subxiphoid approach; 6917 lead) by atrial sensing. Reprogramming of sensitivity from 2.5 mV to 5 mV corrects the recycling.

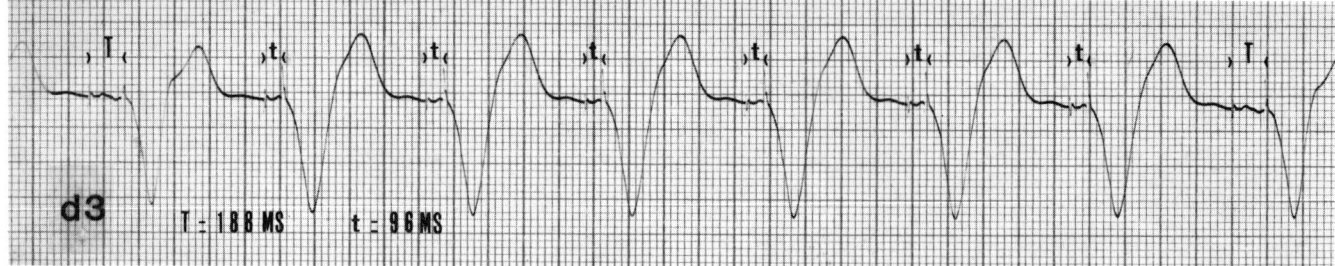

FIGURE 29–16
Nonphysiologic AV delay. The normal AV delay of this device (Sirius, Intermedics) decreases after detection of crosstalk from 188 ms to 96 ms.

duration is around 100 to 110 ms. Several existing pacing systems are capable of programming this delay.

The possibility of crosstalk underscores the need for generous programming capabilities; even so, these problems will not disappear completely.[88, 89] The need for high atrial sensitivity settings to counter the possibility of undersensing favors the appearance of crosstalk by undersensing of spikes or ventricular activity.[90] The programming of a DDD pacing system should include the systematic adjustment of sensitivities at high levels in both chambers. If crosstalk appears, fine adjustments prior to the time of patient discharge will control recurrences, given that the sensing threshold remains stable throughout the useful lifetime of the leads.[17]

To conclude, programming a DDD pacing system is a sophisticated task that in time will become more and more automated.

Programmability of Rate Responsiveness

Rate-responsive pacemakers are all single-chamber devices that share in common the basic parameters of the classic multiprogrammable devices.[91] To these functions is added the particular capability of automatic rate adaptation to a parameter that reflects more or less faithfully the exercise activity or metabolism at a given time. The adaptable capability, even if automatically set, gives way to particular programming applications that will allow the customization of a programming function to the patient's particular physiologic needs and condition (Table 29–4).

Rate-responsive devices that are currently marketed, or are about to be, utilize different parameters to modulate response (e.g., activity, respiratory frequency, volume, variation of QT interval, temperature). Each type of device has its own individually programmed rate response (Table 29–5), but in all of them we found common points:

CAPABILITY OF ACTIVATING OR DEACTIVATING RATE RESPONSIVENESS ■ The rate-responsive pacemaker is delivered to the physician in the VVI mode. The rate-responsive function is usually activated during the course of hospitalization, when the patient can perform a stress test. The rate responsive function can be deactivated at any moment in case of unstable angina pectoris or in case of surgical intervention or for any other valid clinical reason.

PROGRAMMABILITY OF LOWER RATE (FIGS. 29–17 AND 29–18) ■ This is equivalent to the basal resting rate. It is best to set the basal rate in the neighborhood of 60 bpm so that at least three lower values are selectable.

PROGRAMMABILITY OF UPPER RATE (FIGS. 29–17 AND 29–18) ■ This places a limit on the upper rate with exercise. It is particularly important in patients with angina or in other cardiac conditions where exercise places undue demands on the heart. There are also at least three selectable upper values, between 80 and 150 bpm.

SENSING THRESHOLD ■ No matter which parameter modulates rate responsiveness, it is necessary to program a threshold beyond which a variation in a parameter will result in a change in the heart rate. In effect, depending on the particular patient, it is necessary to obtain an increase in heart rate with a given level of activity.

TABLE 29–4
VDD/DDD Pacing: New Technological Progress and Programming*

I. Improvement of Basic Functions
   A. Increase in programming capacity
   B. Help in programming by telemetry
      1. battery to electrode condition
      2. sensing of endocavitary signals
   C. Development of bipolar systems or "switchable" monopolar-bipolar systems
II. More "Physiologic" Functions
   A. Hysteresis of AV delay period
   B. Programmable AV delay period that adapts automatically to rate
   C. Modes of programmable rate decrease (fall-back, rate smoothing)
   D. Rate responsive to one or several factors
III. Diagnostic Aids in Monitoring or Treatment of Arrhythmias
   A. Diagnostic functions
   B. Sensing algorithms and automatic slowing of reentrant ventricular tachycardias
   C. Ability to carry out programmed stimulation
   D. Antitachycardia functions: temporary activation by programming or automatic activation

*Modified from Daubert JC, Rennes, France.

TABLE 29–5
Principal Characteristics of 1987 Commercial VVIR Systems

Number of Programmable Settings	Activitrax (Medtronic)	Sensolog (Siemens/Pace)	TX	Biorate (Biotec)	Meta MV (Telectronics)	Nova MR (Intermedics)	Kelvin 500 (Cook)
Minimum Frequency	60–70–80	60 to 150 in 5-beat steps	30 to 125	50 to 80	50 to 120	45 to 120	50
Maximal Frequency	100–125–150	102–126–150	80 to 142	100 to 123	80 to 180	90 to 175	160
Sensing Threshold	3	16	10	4 levels	Automatic	10	3
Rate-Responsive Slope	10	8	25	8	70	10	3
Programming Aid	0	+	+	0	+		+
Response Time	—	4 values	—	—	—	4 values	2 values
Recovery Time	—	3 values	—	—	—	10 values	3 values

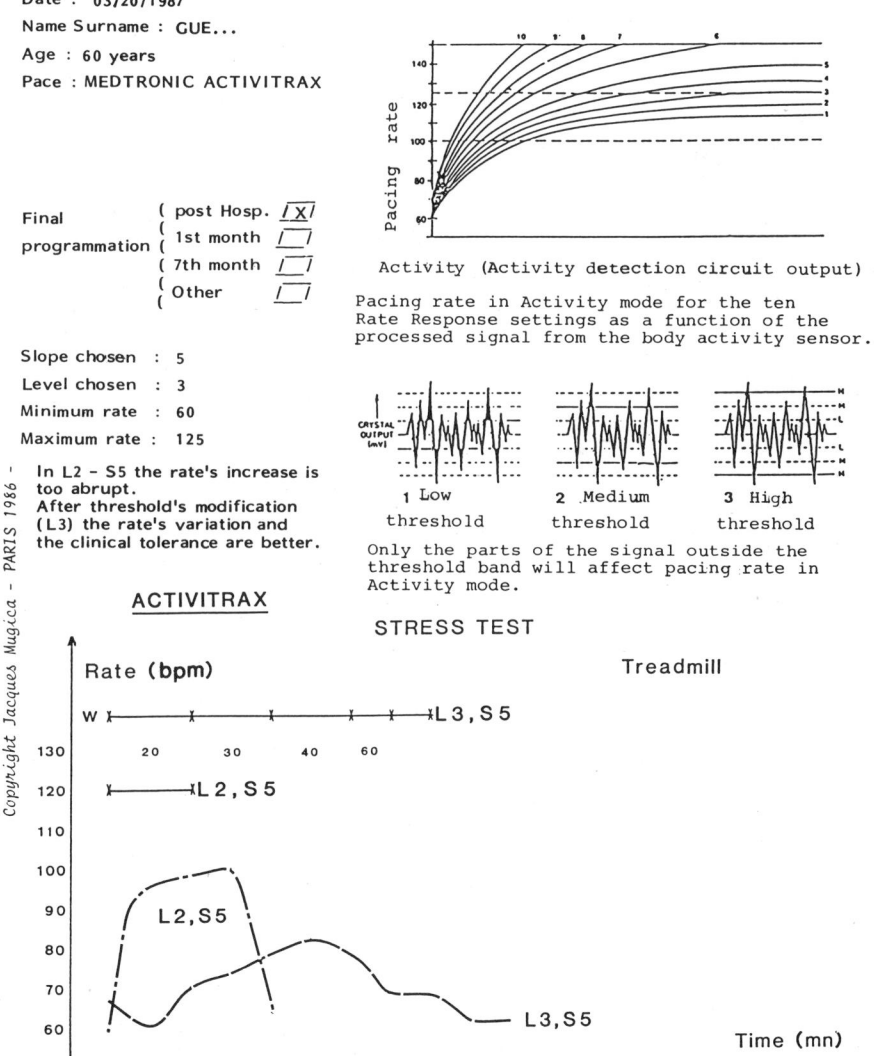

FIGURE 29–17
Follow-up form of the CCVO Center (St-Cloud-F) for Activitrax. Programming to a medium value of sensitivity threshold (L2, S5) gives too fast a rate increase for low exercise grade (25 W). Reprogramming of sensitivity to high threshold (L3) reduces the slope of rate increase but improves the clinical performance (curve L3, S5).

Multiprogrammability of Modern Cardiac Pacemakers 517

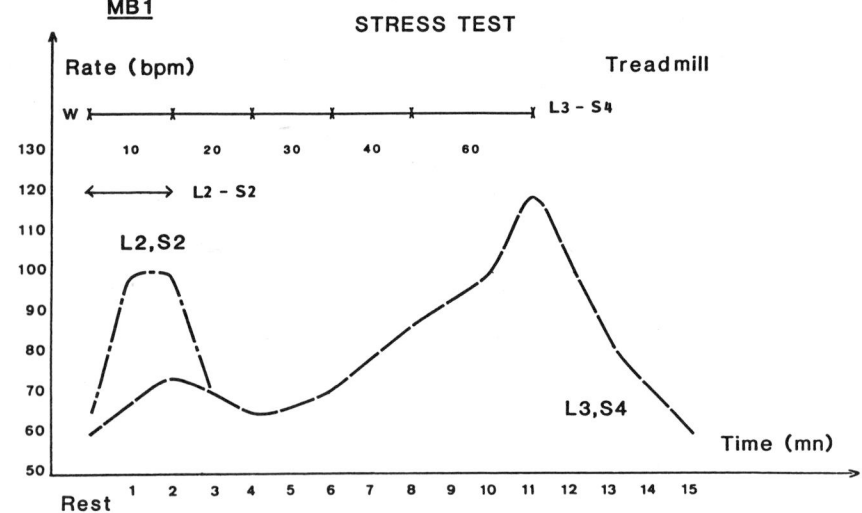

FIGURE 29–18
Follow-up form of the CCVO Center (St-Cloud-F) for Biotec MB1. The initial settings (L2-S2) result in a response that is too fast. Reprogramming to a lower respiratory threshold (L3) and to a higher slope (S4) leads to a more progressive and efficient clinical result (60 W).

THE RATE-RESPONSIVE SLOPE (FIGS. 29–17 AND 29–18) ■ This slope corresponds to the degree of frequency change commensurate with modulation of the parameter that reflects exercise activity. The increase in heart rate will be modest if the slope is shallow, and will be pronounced if the slope is steep.

PROGRAMMABILITY OF REACTION AND RECOVERY TIMES ■ In some recent rate responsive devices, one can program reaction times as well as recovery times. Reaction time refers to the length of time it takes the pacemaker to gear up from its minimal to its maximal frequency once an activity is initiated. Recovery time refers to the time it takes for the pacemaker to return to its minimal frequency once exercise activity ceases.

Programming Aids

Increasingly, the new VVIR devices give the physician programming help. This is a virtual necessity because of the absence of a reliable indicator of the atrial activity. In one system, the Quintech TX* responds to variations in the QT interval, which shortens under the influence of catecholamines or during exercise. With the programmer, one can verify if the T waves are properly sensed. This system calculates the slope by means of continuous measurement of the stimulus to the T wave interval.

The Kelvin 500† is a temperature-responsive device that contains a temperature sensor and can memorize data in its memory for up to 1½ hours. To optimize adjustment of this device, it is necessary to perform a stress test, during which the temperature curves and the frequencies are registered on a small computer screen. The physician can then make adjustments in the slope to better simulate physiologic conditions. The sensing threshold can also be set after taking into account the number of rate responses registered by the counter.

With the Sensolog‡ (activity response), when functioning in the VVI mode, one can know in advance the rate response that the device will recommend if it is set to the standard program. Moreover, the histograms of the frequency can be stored in the memory, and the trigger level of responsiveness function can be adjusted.

In the META* system, the response is related to the minute volume, and the slope is calculated directly by the device at the time of the stress test because of the quasi-linear relationship between heart rate and minute volume. The physician programs the minimum and maximum rates and the device measures the minute volume and suggests a slope of rate responsiveness.

Clinical Value of Programmability

The clinical value of programmable functions in diagnosis is relatively minor, except when it concerns the determination of chronic thresholds and the determination of the safety margin with regard to energy output, and the use of event markers. On the other hand, the therapeutic value is relatively important, but this is a factor that depends on knowledge and motivation of the physician.

The first study dealing with the importance of programmability in avoidance of a second intervention was published by Pannizo and Furman,[92] who compared two series of patients with and without programmable pacemakers. The authors demonstrated that the simple act of programming the output decreased the number of interventions by 50%. Billhardt et al.,[33] Griffin,[34] and Hayes et al.[23] cite figures of 64%, 85%, and 36%, respectively, for successful correction of all types of pacemaker malfunctions by means of programming.

By comparing the programming percentages (Tables 29–5 and 29–6), it is evident that in all these series it is the heart rate parameter that is most often modified. In a series of 3411 cases from 1982 to 1986, reported by Mugica (Table 29–7), the total percentage was 29%; however, the heart rate percentage parameter rose to 60% in the last year of the study, in accordance with data from other authors.[23, 29, 93] During 1986, reprogramming was done in 65% of cases because of the need for frequency modification to optimize cardiac output,[96–97] in 14% of cases because of anginal symptoms, and in 11% of cases because of the presence of

---
*Vitatron.
†ELA Medica.
‡Siemens Elema AB.

*Telectronics.

TABLE 29–6
Frequency of Programming

Authors/Ref.	Year of Publication	Rate	Pulse Width	Amplitude	Output	Sensitivity	Refractory Period	Hysteresis	Mode
Hayes et al.[23]	1981	>65%	16%	1%	—	5%	0	0	0
Parsonnet and Rodgers[95]	1981	37%	—	—	60.5%	1.2%	0.9%	—	—
Tyers et al.[93]	1981	67%	58%	—	—	2%	—	—	33%
Billhardt et al.[33]	1982	40%	—	—	>65%	>33%	0	11%	4%
Elmqvist et al.[15]	1982	24%	32%	26%	—	7%	3%	8%	—
Furman[96]	1982	53%	—	—	13.9%	6%	—	—	<1%
Griffin[34]	1982	46%	27%	18%	—	22%	18%	22%	11%
Barold et al.[30]	1985	>65%	60%	12%	—	10%	0%	1%	1%

TABLE 29–7
Frequency of Programmation from 1982 to 1986*

Mode	No. of Cases	Rate	Duration	Voltage	Output	Sensitivity
VVI	3411	1000 (29.32%)	48 (1.41%)	53 (1.5%)	101 (2.96%)	88 (2.58%)
DDD	80	18 (22.5%)	1 (1.25%)	2 (2.5%)	3 (3.75%)	3 (3.75%)
RR	141	47 (33.33%)	5 (3.55%)	3 (2.13%)	8 (5.67%)	5 (3.5%)

*From series of 3632 cases reported by J. Mugica.

bradycardia. These percentages reflect the general experience with the VVI pacemakers, although reprogramming percentages with rate-responsive devices remain low (33%), and even lower with DDD systems (see Table 29–7). This disparity is due to the fact that the increase in frequency occurs automatically with exercise with the two latter systems.

After the heart rate, the second parameter that is most often modified is the energy output (see Table 29–6). The low percentages of the Mugica series (see Table 29–7) can be explained on the basis of the systematic use of porous or carbon-based lead tips with low capture thresholds.[10, 17–19]

Difficulties, Risks, and Errors of Programming

The inherent difficulties in programming arise not from the multiplicity of programmable parameters with DDD pacing but from the multiplicity of pacemaker and programmer types, which vary widely in complexity, size, design, and speed of operation. The development of a universal programmer[96–99] is a difficult goal for several reasons, among them the current antitrust laws, differences in technologies and their execution, and commercial interests that have long opposed this concept.

A second difficulty is the quality and speed of telemetry.[100] The telemetry probe must be well positioned, as directly as possible over the pacemaker site, because at times feedback data acquisition can be hampered by excessive musculature or subcutaneous fat.

RISKS OF PROGRAMMING ■ Aside from programming errors made by the physician due to the complexity of certain programmers or due to the use of a programmer with another type of pacemaker (cross-programming), the only risks incurred during programming entail the occurrence of more or less long asystolic periods.[101–103] It is recommended and indeed essential for each programmer to be equipped with a "panic button" that will permit, if needed, the device to revert to the VOO mode with an emergency output of 5V.[104–106]

PROGRAMMING FAULTS ■ Spontaneous reprogramming, or rather deprogramming, is a rare occurrence. This spontaneity can be due to unknown causes such as electromagnetic interference or the effects of cold during transport or storage of these devices. An accidental reprogramming can occur as a result of electromagnetic interference, electrocautery, or electrical shock.[107–110] Finally, a breakdown can occur at the moment of programming due to malfunction of the programmer (Fig. 29–19) or the pacemaker itself (Fig. 29–20).

Conclusion

Multiprogrammability is a complex, varied and important part of pacing. Currently, efforts to simplify these new devices are being made, with the goal of reducing multiprogrammable functions controlled by the physician, emphasizing progressive automation of multiple settings. Examples of the latter include automatic measurement of sensing and pacing thresholds; automatic adaptation of the AV delay period with exercise. This automation is leading to keeping as basic controls the minimum and maximum heart rate and the length of time it takes the pacemaker to gear up from minimum to maximum rate. Even today, we can envision a future in which one will be able to change automatically from the DDD to the RR mode.

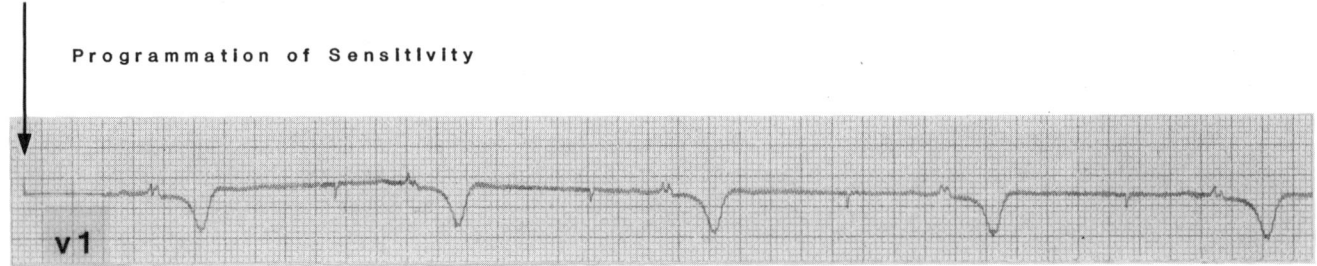

FIGURE 29–19
Programmer dysfunction. Reprogramming of sensitivity (Cordis 337A) for myopotential inhibitions. Now the pacemaker delivers microspikes at a rate of 34 bpm. After changing the programmer, reprogramming was successful.

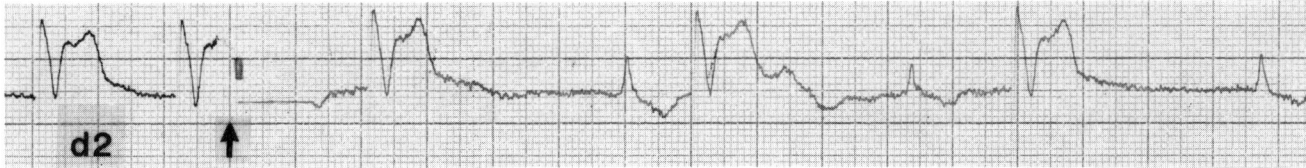

FIGURE 29–20
Pacemaker dysfunction after programming. Reprogramming of sensitivity (Telectronics Optima MPT 5281) for undersensing. At the onset of programming, the asynchronous pulse generator starts pacing at 30 bpm with loss of capture. The replacement of the device was necessary.

Acknowledgments

The authors wish to thank A. RIPART, PhD., of Ela Medical, Montrouge, France, for his technical help.

References

1. Levine PA, Belott PH, Bilitch M, et al.: Recommendations of the NASPE Policy Conference on Pacemaker Programmability and Follow-up. PACE 6:1221, 1983.
2. Levine PA: Proceedings of the Policy Conference of the North America Society of Pacing and Electrophysiology on Programmability and Pacemaker Follow-up Programs. Clin Prog Pacing Electrophysiol 2:145, 1984.
3. Gordon PL, Calfee RV, Baker RG: Multiprogrammable pacemaker technology. A tutorial review and prediction. In Barold SS, Mugica J. (eds.): The Third Decade of Cardiac Pacing, p. 127. Mt. Kisco, Futura Publishing Co., 1982.
4. Ripart A, Jacobson P: Memory technology and implantable Holter systems. In Barold SS, Mugica J (eds.): The Third Decade of Cardiac Pacing, p. 353, Mt. Kisco: Futura Publishing Co., 1982.
5. Meibom J: Vario-pacemaker. An implantable pacemaker especially developed for an easy check. In Thalen HJTH (ed.): Cardiac Pacing: Proceedings of the 4th International Symposium, p. 300. Assen, The Netherlands, Van Gorcum, 1973.
6. Starke ID: Long-term follow-up of cardiac pacing threshold using a noninvasive method of measurement. Br Heart J 40:530, 1978.
7. Astrinsky EA, Furman S: Pacemaker output programming for maximum safety and maximum longevity. Clin Prog Pacing Electrophysiol 1:51, 1983.
8. Luceri RM, Furman S, Hurzeler P, et al.: Threshold behavior of electrodes in long-term ventricular pacing. Am J Cardiol 40:184, 1977.
9. Rossi P, Palma G, Marino B, et al.: Long-term follow-up of myocardial pacing threshold measurement with an external radio frequency transmitter in patients with an implanted pacemaker and an independent radio receiver (Radiocor). In Watanabe Y (ed.): Cardiac Pacing, p. 433. Amsterdam, Excerpta Medica, 1977.
10. Mugica J, Ripart A: Twelve years experience with cardiac pacing leads: Clinical conclusions for 8004 cases. Clin Prog Pacing Electrophysiol 2:513, 1984.
11. Hauser RG: Multiprogrammable cardiac pacemakers: Applications, results and follow-up. Am J Surg 145:740, 1983.
12. Hellestrand K, Nathan A, Bexton R, et al.: The effect of the antiarrhythmic agent flecainide on acute and chronic pacing thresholds (Abstract). PACE, 6:318, 1983.
13. Ohm OJ, Breivik K, Hammer EA, et al.: Intraoperative electrical measurements during pacemaker implantation. Clin Prog Pacing Electrophysiol 2:1, 1984.
14. Nathan A, Hellestrand KJ: Flecainide acetate: A review. Clin Prog Pacing Electrophysiol 2:43, 1984.
15. Elmqvist H, Marco J, Meibom J, et al.: Utilization of programmability. In Feruglio GA (ed.): Cardiac Pacing. Electrophysiology and Pacemaker Technology, p. 769. Padova, Italy, Piccin Medical Books, 1982.
16. Smyth NPD, Sager D, Keshishian JM: A programmable pulse generator with high output option. PACE 4:566, 1981.
17. Mugica J, Henry L, Attuel P, et al.: Clinical experience with 910 carbon tip leads: Comparison with polished platinum leads. PACE 86:1230, 1986.
18. Amundson DC, McArthur W, Mosharrafa M: The porous endocardial electrode. PACE 2:40, 1979.
19. Garberoglio B, et al.: Initial results with an activated pyrolitic carbon tip electrode. PACE 6:440, 1983.
20. Ripart A, Mugica J, Pioger G: Acute and long-term evaluation of a low threshold endocardial carbon tip lead. In Pacemaker Leads, p. 359. New York, Elsevier, 1984.
21. Bodereau P, Calibre A, Kevorkian M, et al.: Entraînement électrosystolique permanent et manifestations cliniques de l'insuffisance coronarienne. Ann Med Interne 129:711, 1978.
22. Sukhum P, Campion BC, McBride JW, et al.: Programmable pacemaker indications and physiologic rate determination during follow-up. PACE 6:A–101, 1983.
23. Hayes DL, Maloney JD, Merideth J, et al.: Initial and early follow-up assessment of the clinical efficacy of a multiprogrammable pulse generator. PACE 4:416, 1981.
24. Davidson DM, Braak CA, Preston TA, et al.: Permanent ventricular pacing: Effect on long-term survival, congestive heart failure and subsequent myocardial infarction and stroke. Ann Intern Med 77:345, 1972.
25. Hamby RU, Aintablian A: Preload reduction with right ventricular pacing: Effect on left ventricular hemodynamics and contractile pattern. Clin Cardiol 3:169, 1980.
26. Narahara KA, Blettel ML: Effect of rate on left ventricular volumes and ejection fraction during chronic ventricular pacing. Circulation 67:323, 1983.
27. Steingart R, Yee C, Wexler J, et al.: Gated radionuclide angiography during upright exercise in patients with programmable pacemakers. Am J Cardiol 47:435, 1981.
28. Romero LR, Haffajee CL, Levin W, et al.: Non-invasive evaluation of ventricular function and volumes during atrioventricular sequential and ventricular pacing. PACE 7:10, 1984.
29. Barold S, Mugica J, Falkoff MD, et al.: Multiprogrammability in Cardiac Pacing. In Barold SS, Mugica J (eds.): The Third Decade of Cardiac Pacing, p. 16. Mt Kisco, Futura Publishing Co., 1982.
30. Barold SS, Ong LS, Heinle RA: Demand pacemakers. Normal and abnormal mechanisms of sensing. In Samet P, El-Sherif N (eds.): Cardiac Pacing, p. 551. New York, Grune and Stratton, 1980.
31. Ohm O: Demand failures occurring during permanent pacing in patients with serious heart disease. PACE 3:44, 1980.
32. Secemsky SI, Hauser RG, Denes P, et al.: Unipolar sensing abnormalities. Incidence and clinical significance of skeletal muscle interference and undersensing in 228 patients. PACE 5:10, 1982.
33. Billhardt RA, Rosenbush SW, Hauser RG: Successful management of pacing systems malfunction without surgery: The role of programmable pulse generators. PACE 5:675, 1982.
34. Griffin JC: Pacemaker programmability. Its role in the maintenance of pacing system function. In Feruglio GA (ed.): Cardiac Pacing. Electrophysiology and Pacemaker Technology, p. 759. Padova, Italy, Piccin Medical Books, 1982.
35. Zimmern SH, Clark MF, Austin WK, et al.: Characteristics and clinical effects of myopotential signals in a unipolar DDD pacemaker population. PACE 9:1019, 1986.
36. Breivik K, Ohm O: Myopotential inhibition of unipolar QRS-inhibited (VVI) pacemakers, assessed by ambulatory Holter monitoring of the electrocardiogram. PACE 3:470, 1980.

37. Daly J, Witte A: Non-invasive analysis of simulated pacemaker failure available in multiprogrammable pulse generators. PACE 5:4, 1982.
38. Halpern J, Camunas G, Stern E, et al.: Myopotential interference with DDD pacemakers: Endocardial electrographic telemetry in the diagnosis of pacemaker-related arrhythmias. Am J Cardiol 54:97, 1984.
39. Barold SS, Caroll M: "Double reset" of demand pacemakers. Am Heart J 84:276, 1972.
40. Gould L, Reddy CVR, Singh BK, et al.: Inappropriate slowing of the pacemaker rate with programmable demand pacemaker. PACE 2:370, 1979.
41. Hauser RG, Susmano A: Afterpotential oversensing by a programmable pulse generator. PACE 4:391, 1981.
42. Barold SS: Clinical significance of pacemaker refractory periods. Am J Cardiol 28:237, 1971.
43. Barold SS, Ong LS, Heinle RA: Demand pacemakers. Normal and abnormal mechanisms of sensing. In Samet P, El-Sherif N (eds.): Cardiac Pacing, p. 551. New York, Grune and Stratton, 1980.
44. Friedberg HD, Barold SS: On hysteresis in pacing. J Electrocardiol 6:1, 1973.
45. Azulay A, Vagnini FJ, Saha CK, et al.: Permanent prophylactic ventricular demand pacing with VVI extended negative rate/hysteresis, p. 5. In Meere C (ed.): Cardiac Pacing, Proceedings of the 6th World Symposium on Cardiac Pacing, Montreal, Pacesymp, 1979.
46. Irnich W, Parsonnet V, Myers GH: Compendium of pacemaker technology II, definitions and glossary (Part II). PACE 2:634, 1979.
47. Thompson ME, Shaver JA: Undesirable cardiac arrhythmias associated with rate hysteresis pacemakers. Am J Cardiol 38:685, 1976.
48. Breivik K, Ohm OJ, Engedal H: Long-term comparison of unipolar and bipolar pacing and sensing using a new multiprogrammable pacemaker system. PACE 6:592, 1983.
49. Smyth NPD, Sager D: A multiprogrammable pacemaker with unipolar or bipolar option. Am Heart J 106:412, 1983.
50. DeCaprio V, Hurzeler P, Furman S: A comparison of unipolar and bipolar electrograms for cardiac pacemaker sensing. Circulation 56:750, 1977.
51. Hauser R: Bipolar leads for cardiac pacing in the 1980s: A reappraisal provoked by skeletal muscle interference. PACE 5:34, 1982.
52. Jacobs L, et al.: Pacemaker inhibition by myopotentials detected by Holter monitoring. PACE 5:30, 1982.
53. Neilsen A, Cashion W, Spencer W, et al.: Long-term assessment of unipolar and bipolar stimulation and sensing thresholds using a lead configuration programmable pacemaker. J Am Coll Cardiol 5:1198, 1985.
54. Fetter J, Hall D, Hoff G, et al.: The effects of myopotential interference on unipolar and bipolar dual chamber pacemakers in the DDD mode. Clin Prog Pacing Electrophysiol 3:368, 1985.
55. Czernin J, Kaliman J, Laczkovics A, et al.: Unipolar versus bipolar pacing—A prospective, intra-patient, long-term study (Abstract). PACE 10:663, 1987.
56. Furman S, DeCaprio V: Electrode causation of pacemaker inhibition. Chest 72:117, 1977.
57. Mugica J, Dubos M, Duconge R, et al.: Arythmies des stimulateurs cardiaques à la demande par défauts du matériel de conduction sonde-électrode. 36 cas—Intérêt de la méthode de Holter. Arch Mal Coeur 73:72, 1980.
58. Coumel Ph, Mugica J, Barold SS: Demand pacemaker arrhythmias caused by intermittent incomplete electrode fracture. Diagnosis with testing magnet. Am J Cardiol 36:105, 1975.
59. Mugica J, Duconge R, Dubos M, et al.: Methods for recording intermittent contact signals in demand pacemaker arrhythmias (11 cases). PACE 1:222, 1978.
60. Fletcher RD, Keimel J, Larca LJ, et al.: Non-invasive serial electrophysiologic testing using an implanted pacemaker to track chest wall stimuli. Am J Cardiol 47:392, 1981.
61. Fletcher RD, Keimel J, Larca LJ, et al.: Non-invasive serial testing using an implanted pacemaker. PACE 4:A-11, 1981.
62. Fletcher RD, Keimel JG, Cohen AI, et al.: Synchronized programming. A new technique for serial non-invasive electrophysiological testing in single and dual chamber implanted pacemaker. J Am Cardiol 1(2):720, 1983.
63. Fletcher RD, Cohen AI, Del Negro AA: Non-invasive electrophysiologic studies using implanted pacemaker. In Barold SS, Mugica J (eds.): The Third Decade of Cardiac Pacing, p. 18. Mt. Kisco, Futura Publishing Co., 1982.
64. Belott PH: Clinical experience with over 250 DDD pacemakers. In Barold SS (ed.): Modern Cardiac Pacing, p. 439. Mt. Kisco, Futura Publishing Co., 1985.
65. Fetter J, Hall DM, Hoff GL, et al.: The effects of myopotential interference on unipolar and bipolar dual chamber pacemakers in the DDD mode. Clin Prog Pacing Electrophysiol 3:368, 1985.
66. Silbergleit A, Frumin H, Kerner NJ, et al.: The incidence of myopotential oversensing in DDD pacemakers: Attention to the predominance of ventricular tracking (Abstract). PACE 10:743, 1987.
67. Lemke B, Höltmann, Lawo Th, et al.: DDD-Schrittmacher: Häufigkeit und relevanz von Vorhofwahrnehmungsstörungen durch Unversensing und AV-Knotenrythmen. Herzschrittmacher 5:3, 1985.
68. Klementowicz PT, Furman S: Selective atrial sensing in dual chamber pacemakers eliminates endless loop tachycardia. J Am Coll Cardiol 7-3-590-4, 1986.
69. Zugibe FT Jr, Nanda NC, Barold SS, et al.: Usefulness of Doppler echovelocity and atrial capture. PACE 6:1350, 1983.
70. Coskey RL, Feit TS, Plaia R, et al.: AV pacing and LV performance. PACE 6:631, 1983.
71. Wish M, Fletcher RD, Gottdiener JS, et al.: Optimal left atrioventricular sequence in dual chamber pacing—Limitations of programmed A-V interval. J Am Coll Cardiol 3:507, 1984.
72. Daubert C, Ritter Ph, Mabo Ph, et al.: Physiological relationship between AV-interval and heart rate in healthy subjects: Applications to dual-chamber pacing. PACE 9:1032, 1986.
73. Daubert C, Ritter Ph, Mabo Ph, et al.: Physiological basis for an automatic adaptation of A-V delay to heart rate in VDD-DDD pacing (Abstract). PACE 10:663, 1987.
74. Ritter Ph, Daubert C, Ollitrault J, et al.: Influence of atrial and ventricular electro-mechanical intervals on effective mechanical A-V interval: Consequences for programming the optimal A-V delay in dual-chamber pacing (Abstract). PACE 10:734, 1987.
75. Daubert JC, Ritter Ph, Mabo Ph: Stimulation séquentielle et délai auriculo-ventriculaire optimal. Stimucoeur 14:79, 1986.
76. Levine PA: Postventricular atrial refractory periods and pacemaker mediated tachycardias. Clin Prog Pacing Electrophysiol 1:934, 1983.
77. Furman S: Dual chamber pacemakers: Upper rate behavior. PACE 8:197, 1985.
78. Stroobandt R, Willems R, Holvoet G, et al.: Prediction of Wenckebach behavior and block response in DDD pacemakers. PACE 9 Cardiostim 86:1040, 1986.
79. Hauser RG: The electrocardiography of AV universal DDD pacemaker. PACE 6:399, 1983.
80. Furman S: Retreat from Wenckebach. PACE 7:1, 1984.
81. Den Dulk K, Lindemans FW, Wellens HJJ: Merits of various antipacemaker circus movement tachycardia features. PACE 9:1055, 1986.
82. Wehr M, Schmitt CG, Peter JH: Irregular pacemaker tachycardia in a patient with WPW syndrome and AV universal pacemaker. PACE 7:320, 1984.
83. van Mechelen R, Ruiter J, de Boer H, et al.: Pacemaker electrocardiography of rate smoothing during DDD pacing. PACE 8:684, 1985.
84. Hayes DL, Holmes DR, Vlietstra RE, et al.: Changing experiences with dual chamber (DDD) pacemakers. J Am Coll Cardiol 4:556, 1984.
85. Mugica J, Podeur H, Bourdarias JP, et al.: Recyclage d'un stimulateur VVI épicardique sur l'onde P. Stimucoeur 12:209, 1984.
86. Furman S, Reichter-Reiss H, Escher DJW: Atrioventricular sequential pacing and pacemakers. Chest 63:783, 1973.

87. Levine PA, Mace RC: Assessment and management of crosstalk. *In* Pacing Therapy, p. 239. Mt. Kisco, Futura Publishing Co., 1983.
88. Stone JM, Bhakta RD, Lutgen J: Dual chamber sequential pacing in the management of sinus node dysfunction: Advantages over single chamber pacing. Am Heart J 104:1319, 1982.
89. Potential crosstalk in early Gemini 415A pacers with dual anodal rings. Product Safety Alert, Cordis Corporation, October 19, 1984.
90. Reynolds D, Combs W, Bennett T: "Crosstalk" in bipolar DDD pacemakers (Abstract). PACE 10:734, 1987.
91. International Congress on Rate Responsive Cardiac Pacing—Munich Oct., 1987 (Abstracts). PACE 10:5, 1203, 1987.
92. Pannizzo F, Furman S: Clinical tests of the effects of simulated inadvertent "cross programming". *In* Meere C (ed.): Cardiac Pacing, Proceedings of the 6th World Symposium on Cardiac Pacing. Montréal: Pacesymp 35-4, 1979.
93. Tyers GFO, Williams EH, Larrieu AJ, et al.: Multiprogrammable pacemakers. Can J Surg 24:252, 1981.
94. Parsonnet V, Rodgers T: The present status of programmable pacemakers. Prog Cardiovasc 10 23:401, 1981.
95. Furman S: Pacemaker programmability. Contemp Surg 20:35, 1982.
96. Furman S: Universal programming. PACE 4:131, 1981.
97. Furman S: Universal programming. PACE 7:163, 1984.
98. Buffet J, Gautier JP, Jacquet JP, et al.: The universal programmer—Feasibility and engineering considerations. *In* Barold SS, Mugica J (eds.): The Third Decade of Cardiac Pacing, p. 115. Mt. Kisco, Futura Publishing Co., 1982.
99. Thakor N: A universal program for fully programmable pacemakers. Comput Biol Med 13:271, 1983.
100. Sholder J, Levine PA, Mann BM, et al.: Bidirectional telemetry and interrogation in cardiac pacing. *In* Barold SS, Mugica J (eds.): The Third Decade of Cardiac Pacing, p. 145. Mt. Kisco, Futura Publishing Co., 1982.
101. Sinnaeve A, Piret J, Stroobandt R: Potential causes of spurious programming: Report of a case. PACE 3:541, 1980.
102. Genovese B, Judge RD: Random reprogramming during pacemaker inhibition. *In* Meere C (ed.): Cardiac Pacing, Proceedings of the 6th World Symposium on Cardiac Pacing. Montréal: Pacesymp, 35–13 1979.
103. Astrinski EA, Furman S, Florio J: Asystolic episodes during pacemaker programming. Circulation 63:379, 1981.
104. Boal Bh: Emergency reprogramming of cardiac pacemakers. PACE 6:651, 1983.
105. Parsonnet V: Editorial. PACE 6:652, 1983.
106. Parsonnet V, Bilitch M, Furman S, et al.: Implantable cardiac pacemakers. Status report and resources guidelines 1982. Intersociety Commission for Heart Disease Resources (ICHD). Circulation 68:227A, 1983.
107. Belott PH, Sands, Warren J: Resetting of DDD pacemakers due to EMI. PACE 7:169, 1984.
108. Dodinot B, Meunier JF: Modifications accidentelles et répétitives des paramètres d'un stimulateur multiprogrammable. Stimucoeur 8:14, 1980.
109. Irnich W: Electrosurgery in pacemaker patients. PACE 10:691, 1987.
110. Irnich W, Lazica M, Gleissner M: Pacemaker patients and extracorporeal shock wave lithotripsy. PACE 10:692, 1987.

30

Rate-Responsive Pacing: Technical and Clinical Aspects

Chu-Pak Lau
A. John Camm

Overview

The normal cardiovascular system can increase the cardiac output by three- to fourfold during maximum exercise.[47] When patients with complete heart block are treated with a constant frequency ventricular pacemaker, the ventricular rate cannot increase during exercise. However, the effects of circulating catecholamines and increased venous return result in an increased stroke volume, such that cardiac output is increased by about 50% during moderate activity.

Most studies have shown that atrial contraction contributes about 20% to cardiac output.[94] An ideal physiologic pacemaker, therefore, must be capable of increasing the pacing rate during exercise and maintaining atrioventricular (AV) synchrony. Dual-chamber pacing improves the cardiac output both at rest and during exercise by over 30%, compared to ventricular constant frequency pacing.[61,79] However, two pacing wires are needed and atrial sensing must be constant. Dual-chamber pacing is only fully functional in patients with intact sinus node activity. Sinoatrial disease has been reported to occur in 30 to 40% of patients with complete heart block.[40,106] In addition, a dual-chamber pacemaker may respond inappropriately to pathologic tachycardias. Atrial fibrillation, flutter, and inexcitable atria pose further difficulties. Finally, endless loop tachycardia can result from such a system.[42] Although to a certain extent this complication can be minimized by suitably adjusting the atrial refractory period, this would necessarily lead to a limitation of the upper rate response.

The deterioration of sinoatrial function with time is slow.[39,72] However, a recent study[82] on the stability of pacing in the DDD mode indicated that after a period of 5 years, about 18% of patients required a change in pacing mode (Fig. 30–1). For these reasons, an alternative method of physiologic pacing is necessary for some patients.

Although AV synchrony can increase the cardiac output by 20 to 30% during exercise by augmenting the stroke volume, its contribution is less important in the face of the 300% increase achieved by an increase in ventricular rate.[17,53] Using external stimulation to vary the ventricular rate of DDD pacemakers, Fananapazir et al,[102] demonstrated similar maximum exercise capacity in patients exercising in the VDD mode and rate-matched VVI mode; both pacing modes were found to be better than ventricular pacing at a constant rate. Similarly, Kristensson and coworkers[59] showed no difference in cardiac output and stroke volume in patients exercising in the atrial synchronous mode, compared to rate matched ventricular pacing during moderate exercise. Although previous studies have shown higher cardiac output during atrial triggered versus ventricular pacing at rest, a more recent study[14] did not show such difference when the study was performed with the patients standing. Thus the contribution of AV synchrony to resting cardiac output is probably limited.

In patients who require permanent pacing, atrial support becomes less important during exercise in patients with impaired left ventricular function and filling pressures that are already high.[45] On this basis, a single-chamber pacemaker that can automatically adjust the pacing rate to metabolic demands is a feasible method for physiological pacing. The prerequisite of such a system is some form of sensor for metabolic needs.

TERMINOLOGY

Variable frequency pacing, adjusted by a sensor of metabolic demand or exercise status, has been var-

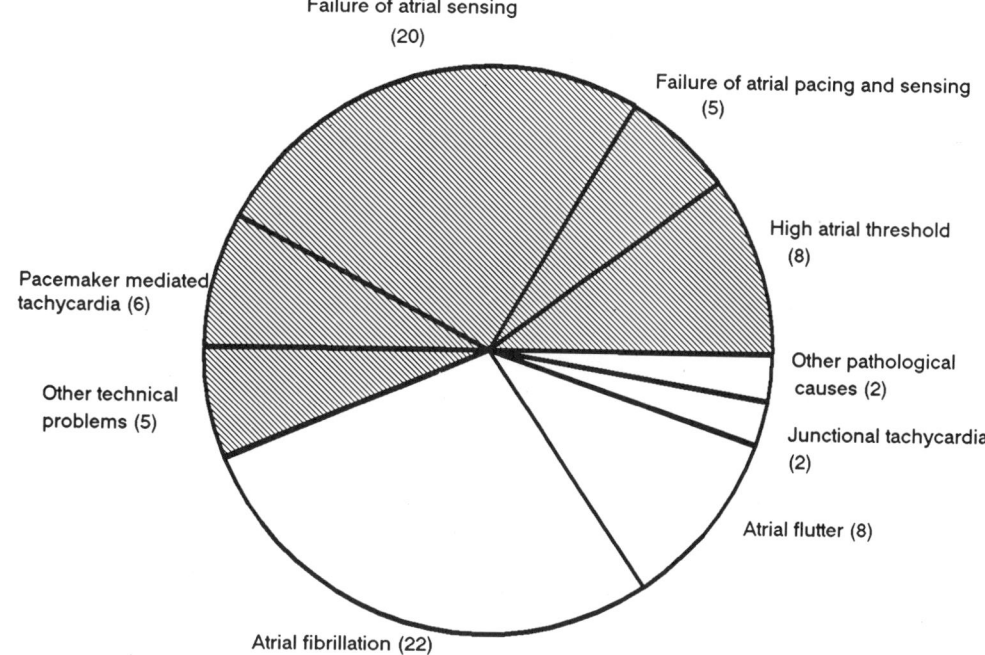

FIGURE 30–1
Indication for a change in pacing mode over a follow-up period of 5 years in 423 patients receiving a DDD pacemaker. Of the 423 patients, 78 required a mode change (18.4%). Technical problems were responsible for 56.4% of pacing mode changes (hatched section of the pie chart), and pathophysiologic reasons for 43.5% (open section of pie chart). (Based on data from Oseroff O, Klementowicz P, Andrews C, et al. (Abstract): PACE 10:1224, 1987.)

iously known as "autoregulatory,"[26] "physiologically adaptive,"[87] and "rate-responsive"[117] pacing; the last term has been widely accepted and seems satisfactory. However, some authorities have pointed out that "rate-adjusted" or "rate-modulated" pacing might be better terms. At the present time, all of these terms are used interchangeably. A recent modification of the five-letter pacemaker code suggests the use of the letter "R" in the fourth position to indicate rate-adaptive function.[20]

THE RATE-RESPONSIVE PHILOSOPHY

Originally rate-responsive pacing was considered as a technique for increasing the pacing rate upward from a basic frequency of 70 beats per minute (bpm) (approximately). This limited view of the possibilities of rate-responsive pacing is now changing. The ability to allow the rate to decrease (for example, to perhaps 30 to 40 bpm) must now be considered. The broader perspective of rate-responsive pacing requires better sensors of physiologic status.

Indicators of Metabolic Demand

The sensors that have been investigated for rate-responsive pacing are listed in Table 30–1. These sensors detect either primary indicators of physiologic needs or secondary indicators that change during physical activity, especially exercise.

CHARACTERISTICS OF AN IDEAL SENSOR

An ideal sensor of physiologic needs should be capable of imitating the normal sinus rate responses during various activities. The following properties should be considered in evaluating a sensor.

- The sensor should be *sensitive* not only to exercise but also to emotional, vasodilatory, and postural stresses and to diurnal rhythm changes.
- The response of the sensor should be *specific*; there should not be inappropriate response to changes either within the body or from the environment.
- The response should be *accurate*; the magnitude of the changes should be proportional to the need.
- The sensor should respond with an appropriate *speed*.
- *Technical factors* should also be considered. A good rate-responsive pacemaker should be reliable and stable over time. Implantation (preferably using only a conventional unipolar or bipolar pacing lead) and programming should be simple.

Table 30–2 summarizes the relative ability of some sensors to meet these specifications. At present, most studies on sensor evaluation have relied on exercise testing, although this is only one aspect of physiologic rate modulation. Other frequent needs for rate modulation are probably sleep, changes in posture, mild Valsalva-like strain, changes in body temperature, and vasodilatation. The usual assessments of rate-responsive function that rely almost exclusively on sustained exercise may give very misleading results. It is now time to break down the investigational perspectives and at least make an assessment of rate modulation during simple and straightforward daily activities.[69, 120] Currently, none of the available sensors is ideal. Specific sensors are discussed individually below.

TABLE 30–1
Possible Sensors of Rate-Responsive Pacing

Indicators of Metabolic Demands	Examples	Manufacturer*
Catecholamine levels		
Autonomic nervous signals		
Q-T interval	TX1 & 2	Vitatron
	Quintech 911 & 915	
	Rhythmyx (new software)	
Average atrial rate	RS4	Cardiac Pacemakers
Body movement	Activitrax	Medtronic
	Synergist I/II (dual-chamber)	Medtronic
	Sensolog 703	Siemens-Elema
	Sensolog P49	
Respiratory control	RDP3/MB-1	Biotec
	Meta	Telectronics-Cordis
Central venous temperature	Nova MR	Intermedics
	Kelvin 500	Cook Pacemakers
	Thermos	Biotronik
Central venous oxygen saturation	Oxytrax	Medtronic
pH		
Stroke volume/pre-ejection interval/right ventricular ejection time	Model 1100 (single-chamber)	Cardiac Pacemakers, Inc.
	Model 1200 (dual-chamber)	
Right atrial pressure	Deltatrax	Medtronic
First derivative of right ventricular pressure		
Evoked QRS response (gradient)	Prism	Telectronics-Cordis

*Addresses of manufacturers: Vitatron Medical B.V., Dieren, The Netherlands; Cardiac Pacemakers, Inc., Minneapolis, MN, USA; Medtronic, Inc., Minneapolis, MN, USA; Siemens-Elema, Sweden; Biotec, S.p.A., Bologna, Italy; Telectronics-Cordis, Englewood, CO, USA; Intermedics Inc., Freeport, TX, USA; Cook Pacemakers Corp., Leechburg, PA, USA; Biotronik GmBH & Co., Berlin, Fed. Rep. of Germany.

TABLE 30–2
Characteristics of Sensors That Have Been Incorporated into Rate-Responsive Pacemakers*

| | Q-T Sensing | Respiration Sensing | | Activity Sensing | Temperature Sensing | dp/dt Sensing |
		RR	MV			
Sensitivity						
Exercise	+	+	+	+	+	+
Emotion	+	−	±	−	±	+
Vasodilation	±	−	±	−	±	+
Posture	±	−	−	−	+	±
Diurnal rhythm	−	±	±	−	+	+
Specificity	Medium; Q-T affected by ischemia, drugs and pacing rate	Medium; respiratory changes may not be related to cardiac needs—e.g., phonation, pneumonia		Low; affected by extraneous vibrations	Medium; affected by internal and external temperature changes	Medium-high
Accuracy	Medium	Medium	Medium-high	Medium-low	Medium-high	Medium-high
Speed of response	Slow*	Medium	Medium	Fast	Slow-medium*	Medium
Reliability/longevity	Medium-low	High	High	High	Uncertain	Uncertain
Programming	Complex	Simple	Simple	Simple	Depends on algorithm	Simple

*Analysis based on early models as outlined in Table 30–1.
†Depending on the algorithm used.
RR = respiratory rate; MV = minute ventilation.

pH SENSING

Principle

A pH sensor was incorporated in the earliest rate-responsive pacemaker. An increase in tissue metabolism results in the production of carbon dioxide, which leads to a fall in pH of the venous blood, because it serves as a carrier of carbon dioxide to the lungs for elimination. In patients with chronotropic incompetence and a resultant inadequate cardiac output, the change in venous pH is more than that in normal individuals. This principle was utilized in the construction of a rate-responsive pacemaker.[26, 27]

The pH sensor consisted of a sensing iridium/iridium oxide (Ir/IrO_2) ring at the atrial level of a "conventional" ventricular lead, with the pacemaker casing serving as the reference electrode (silver/silver chloride). Exercise induced a rapid fall in pH with a corresponding increase in pacing rate (Fig. 30–2). The pH level returned to baseline about 15 minutes after an exercise. The sensor was also reported to respond to cold, pain and emotional changes.[27]

Limitations

Cammilli et al.[27] reported on seven patients with this pacemaker. Four functioned adequately over a 1-year period; three did not respond, probably because of a decline in baseline voltage. Thus the reliability and long-term stability of the sensor were questionable. Furthermore, the biocompatibility of the silver chloride electrode has limited its development. A recent study by Cammilli and coworkers[28] suggested the use of Ir/IrO_2 as the reference electrode in the pacemaker casing to avoid this problem. This works on the assumption that local pH changes are minimal in a chronic pacemaker pocket; thus, changes in the venous pH can be measured by the ring electrode. Further research is awaited.

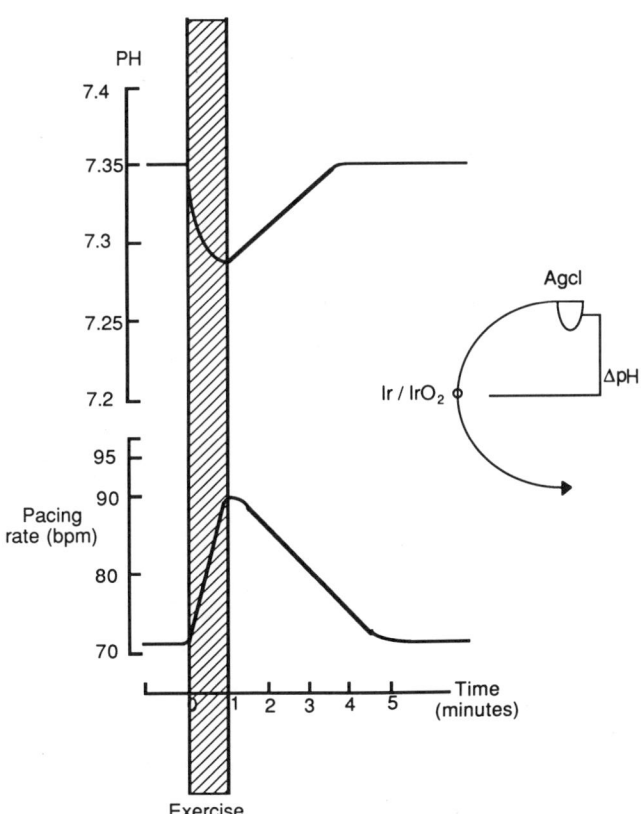

FIGURE 30–2
Schematic representation of the working of a pH-sensing pacemaker. A fall in pH during exercise triggers an increase in pacing rate. pH is sensed between the pacemaker and a ring electrode at the atrial level.

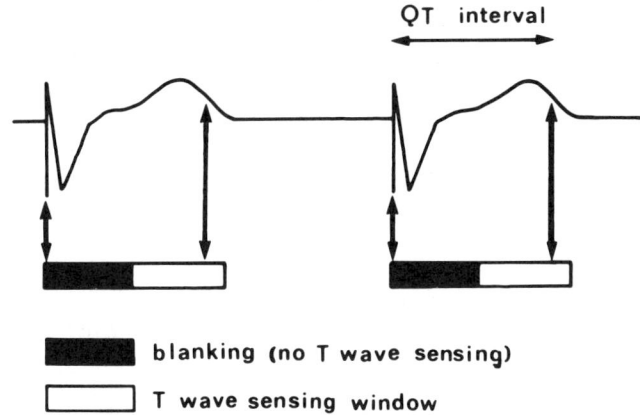

FIGURE 30–3
Principle of T wave detection in a Q-T-sensing pacemaker. Stimulus-evoked T wave response is measured from the pacing spike to the maximum deflection of the first derivative of the T wave. The T wave is detected within a T wave–sensing window after a blanking period for the evoked QRS response.

STIMULUS-EVOKED T INTERVAL

Principle

The Q-T interval shortens during physical exercise and mental stress.[87] Approximately half of this shortening is brought about by an increase in heart rate, but the other half is probably related to the direct effect of catecholamines on myocardial recovery and repolarization.[35, 86] Thus, the ventricular paced Q-T interval during exercise is shorter than when pacing the ventricle at a similar rate at rest,[87] and exercise performed at a fixed ventricular rate in patients with complete heart block results in shortening of the Q-T interval. A biological sensor exploiting the changes in Q-T interval with exercise has been developed.[87]

The endocardial T wave of an evoked (paced) complex can be detected: the paced Q-T (stimulus-T) interval is measured from the pacemaker spike to the maximum negative of first derivative of the T wave. When the stimulus-evoked T interval falls within the T wave sensing window, pacing rate modulation occurs (Fig. 30–3). The stimulus-evoked T interval is used to assess the "expected" pacing rate and thus set the "actual" pacing rate. When the intrinsic heart rate exceeds the pacemaker rate, the pacemaker "tracks" the stimulus–T interval by intermittently effecting an overdrive capture. An algorithm converts the change in stimulus-evoked T interval into a change of pacing rate. Theoretically, fusion beats (simultaneously paced and spontaneous depolarizations) may result in inappropriate stimulus–T interval assessment. This inappropriate and unwarranted ventricular pacing may be sensed by the patient and result in unwanted symptoms.

The TX1 (Vitatron Medical Diagnostic Pulse Generator) was the first in this series.[33] In addition to conventional functions, the programmable parameters and features included (1) upper and lower rate limits, (2) slope or sensitivity of the system to changes in the stimulus–T interval (from 0.5 to 5.0 bpm/ms), (3) T wave sensing window and sensitivities, and (4) slow exponential drift back to the basic rate (nulling, from 85 to 125 bpm/hour). The TX2, a later model, enabled the TX mode (rate-responsive) to function in cases in which the pacemaker was inhibited by acceleration of the spontaneous rhythm (see above). The Quintech pacemaker incorporates the software of the TX2 and has a system of hardware for T wave filtering.

Clinical Performance

When compared with fixed rate pacing, pacing in the TX mode has resulted in a 45% increase in cardiac output and a 57% increase in maximal exercise capacity.[33] Exercise performance was also comparable to that achieved during VAT pacing.[36] Conventional electrodes are used for pacing and sensing, and it has the ability to respond to a non–exercise related increase in circulating catecholamines, such as that due to emotional stress.

Limitations

The Q-T interval can be affected by conditions other than variation in heart rate and exercise. Drugs, myocardial ischemia, and electrolyte changes can vary the duration of the Q-T interval and hence affect the heart rate in the absence of changes of metabolic demand.[36]

Failure of endocardial T wave sensing can occur, especially with chronic leads, and T wave sensing can deteriorate with time,[36, 75] a problem that was reported to occur in 26% of cases in one study.[75] This is related to the effect with repolarization, which is partly overcome by reducing the pulse amplitude (from 5 mV to 2.5 mV). A recent analysis[21] of over 1500 leads showed that the use of an electrode with a small area (<12 mm^2), porous surface structure (preferably carbon), and atraumatic fixation significantly improves T wave sensing. Failure of the Q-T interval to shorten during exercise despite a normal catecholamine response also has been reported,[43, 109] although this is probably a rare event. On the other hand, spontaneous acceleration in rate (known as "oscillation") in the absence of activity can occasionally occur.[116] This may result from a positive feedback generated by Q-T shortening with an increase in pacing rate, especially in conjunction with a sensitive slope.

The heart rate/stimulus–T interval relationship varies significantly in different patients and in the same subject from one occasion to another.[36, 119] Close follow-up and frequent reprogramming, guided by the results of exercise tests and Holter monitoring, may be necessary to adjust for chronic changes in Q-T parameters to ensure that the pacemaker continues to function.

Although the response is related to the work load (good proportionality), it occurs with a delay for exercises lasting for a brief period.[64] This may lead to post-exercise tachycardia (Fig. 30–4). Part of this delay is related to the algorithm used in the early versions of the Q-T sensing pacemaker, which utilizes a constant slope setting for all pacing cycle lengths. It has been observed that the relation between rate and Q-T interval at rest and during exercise is probably not linear as reported by Rickards and Norman[87] but rather follows an exponential curve, with a greater Q-T change at a slower rate.[95] The previously reported linearity of the paced Q-T/heart rate relationship is probably related to the pooling of data, which tends to obscure individual trends. A recent advance in software uses a nonlinear slope adjustment with differ-

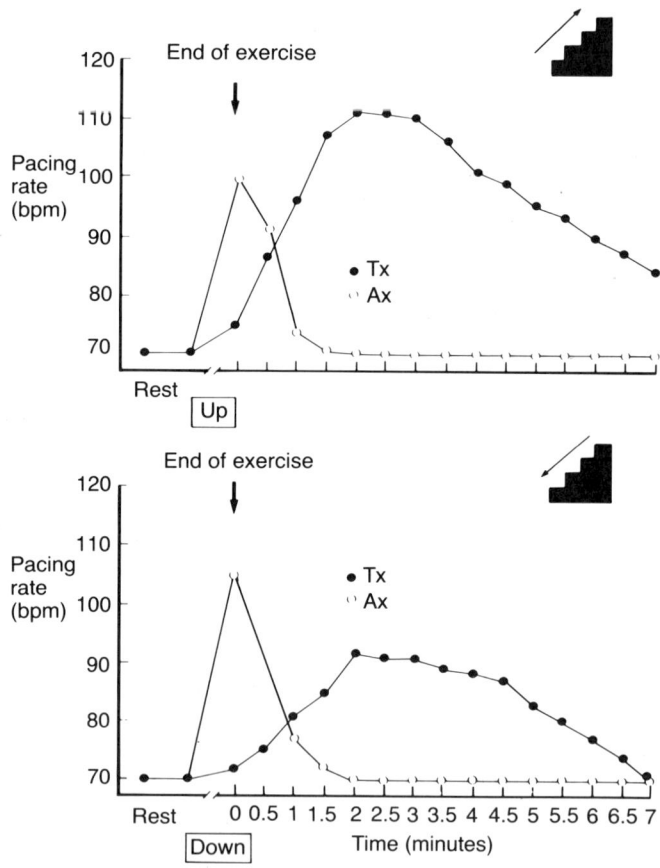

FIGURE 30–4
Comparative rate responses between an activity-sensing (Activitrax, nine patients) and Q-T-sensing pacemaker (TX2, five patients) during climbing stairs. The maximum pacing rate was achieved by the Activitrax pacemakers at the end of the activity, although the pacing rate was higher on descending stairs. On the other hand, the maximum pacing rate was higher on ascending stairs with the QT-sensing pacemakers, although the rate response was delayed.

ent pacing intervals (Fig. 30–5). With this new algorithm,[15, 121] a higher slope is utilized at slow pacing rates (which will therefore speed up the rate response) and a smaller slope at high rates prevents inappropriate rate acceleration that may contribute to the oscillation phenomenon.

To simplify programming and to take into account the variability of heart rate/paced Q-T interval with time, the new software also has improved rate monitoring and automatic slope adjustment capability. A built-in real-time Holter monitor is incorporated, which can be assessed by telemetry. Automatic adjustment of the slope occurs at the lower and the upper rate limits (Fig. 30–6). The pacing rate/Q-T relationship is automatically measured daily at the resting rate (e.g., during sleep) to take into account the long-term changes in this relationship. On the other hand, if further stimulus–T interval shortening occurs at the maximum rate, automatic slope adjustment enables

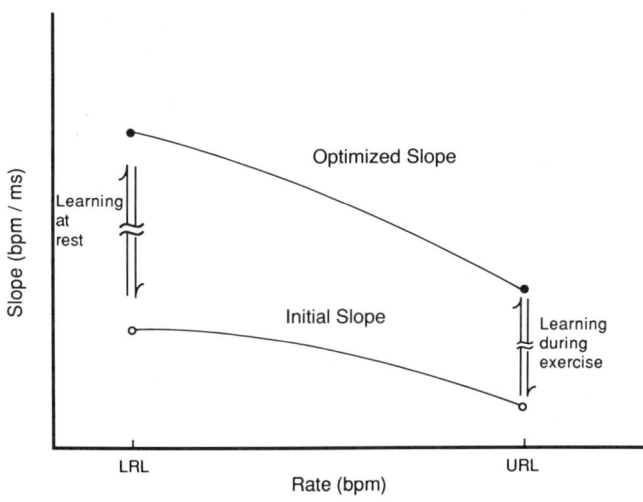

FIGURE 30–6
Automatic slope adjustment in the new software of the Q-T-sensing pacemaker. See text for discussion.

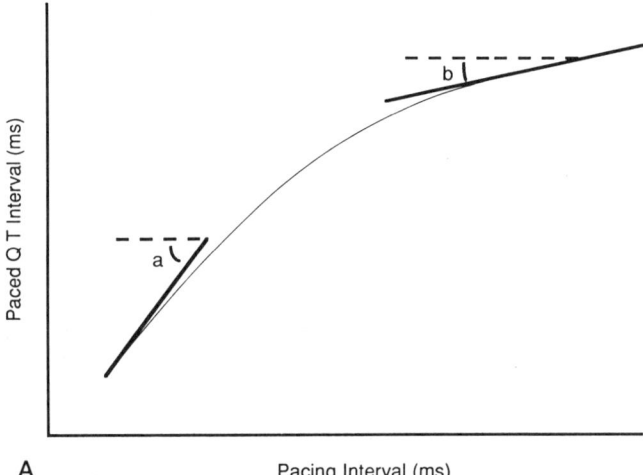

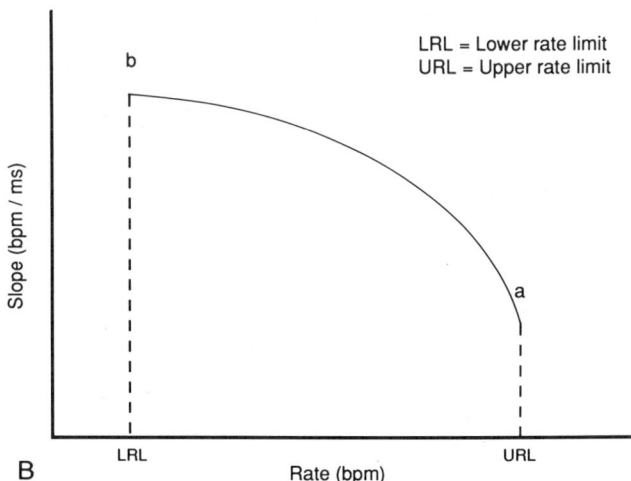

FIGURE 30–5
New algorithm for a Q-T-sensing pacemaker. A, The pacing and Q-T intervals are related by a curvilinear rather than by a linear formula. B, The new algorithm uses a dynamic relation between rate and slope such that a higher rate is associated with a lower slope.

the slope setting to be scaled down for subsequent rate adjustment.

RESPIRATION SENSING

Ventilatory response during exercise parallels the work load up to 70% of maximum oxygen consumption.[8–10, 23] Above this anaerobic threshold,[57, 111] accumulation of lactic acid increases the minute ventilation at a rate far in excess of oxygen uptake. Since oxygen consumption has a linear relationship with heart rate,[11] this suggests that ventilatory changes during exercise can be used to determine an appropriate rate response during submaximal exercise. Currently there are rate-responsive pacemakers that utilize this principle, either by tracking the respiratory rate (RDP3 and MB-1, Biorate*) or by measuring minute ventilation (Meta†).

Biorate

Principle

The idea of linking heart rate to respiratory rate was initially suggested by Funke[41] and others.[49, 58] Rossi and colleagues[88] have shown that changes in the respiratory rate correlate significantly with changes in heart rate during exercise. Furthermore, the correlation is assumed to hold in patients with restrictive or obstructive airways disease.[89] A pacemaker sensing the respiratory rate has been developed.[88]

This respiration-dependent pacemaker (Biorate, RDP3 or MB-1) consists of a demand cardiac pacemaker in which the pacing rate is controlled by an algorithm based on the sensing of respiration rate. This is determined by the changes in thoracic impedance due to respiration (Fig. 30–7). Inspiration leads to

---

*Biotec, S.p.A., Bologna, Italy.
†Telectronics-Cordis, Englewood, CO, USA.

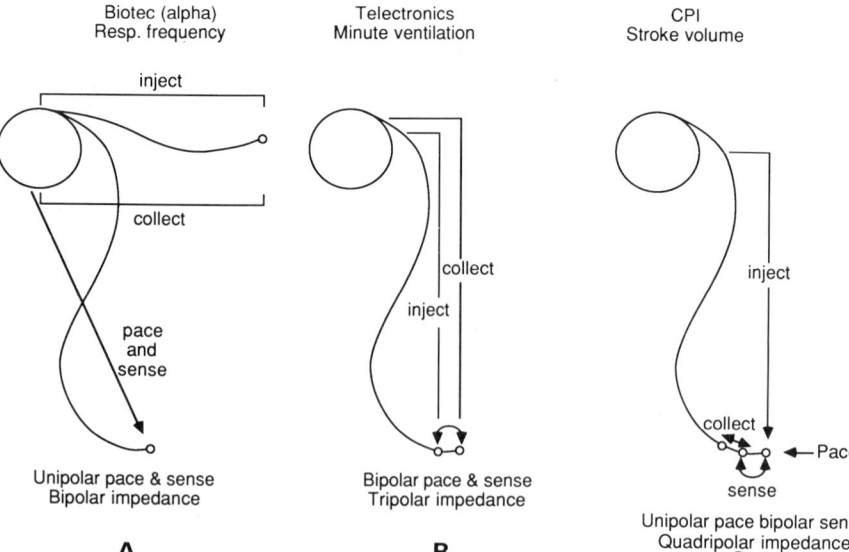

FIGURE 30-7
Schematic representation of three different impedance-measuring rate-responsive pacemakers. A, The principle of respiratory rate sensing in the Biorate pacemaker (RDP3/MB-1). Impedance is measured by a two-electrode configuration between the pacemaker casing and the tip of an auxiliary lead. B, Tripolar electrode configuration in measuring thoracic impedance of Meta, which avoids the use of an auxiliary lead. C, Quadripolar arrangement using a special tripolar electrode for measuring stroke volume Cardiac Pacemakers, Inc., (CPI = 1200).

increased chest volume and increased impedance. In the current version of this pacemaker, impedance variations are detected using a bipolar impedance measuring electrode configuration. The active electrode is the pacemaker casing. The sensing electrode (passive) consists of an auxiliary lead that is tunneled subcutaneously 8 to 10 cm from the pulse generator pocket to a site on the thorax. Programmable parameters include respiratory level, which determines the depth of tidal volume necessary to trigger respiration sensing. The measured respiratory rate is converted into a rate response by a series of programmable slopes (Table 30-3). MB-1 is a more programmable version in which there is the facility to program sensitivity and the provision of limited telemetry function of the basic pacing parameters.

Clinical Performance

A 25% improvement in exercise performance with this pacing system over the VVI mode has been reported.[90] In addition, maximum aerobic and hemodynamic variables were similar to those achieved with dual-chamber pacing.

We[65] and others[113] have observed that arm swinging can lead to an increase in pacing rate (Fig. 30-8). This results from motion artefact generated by the relative displacement between the pacemaker casing and the auxiliary lead.[65] A two-electrode impedance measuring system is particularly prone to motion artifact.[92] We have shown that the rate response is attenuated by swinging both arms, which leads to the displacement of the pacemaker–auxiliary lead unit in the same direction, thus reducing motion-induced impedance changes. Furthermore, the response to arm swinging depends on the position of the auxiliary lead: the rate response is maximal when swinging the arm on the same side as the auxiliary lead if it is laterally situated. In some patients it is possible to program the pacemaker respiratory level so that rate response occurs primarily due to motion artifact, although the rate response is erratic (Fig. 30-9). This may explain the

TABLE 30-3
Rate-Responsive Parameters of Two Forms of Respiratory Controlled Pacemakers*

Parameters	Biorate		Meta
	RDP3	MB-1	
Basic rate (bpm)	65, 75	50–80 (1)	50–150 (5)
Maximum rate (bpm)	Depends on basic rate	100, 123, 145, 163	80–165 (5)
Respiratory level	0–7 (1)	1–4 (1)	—
Slope	0–7 (1)	0–7 (1)	1–60 (1)
Sensitivity (V)	2	1–7 (1) 0 (asynchronous)	0, 7–4, 5
Telemetry function	Not available	Sensitivity, output	Rate-responsive parameters, sensitivity, output, lead and cell impedance

*The Biorate (RDP3 and MB-1) pacemakers detect the respiratory rate as an indicator of increase in physiologic needs. The Meta pacemakers sense the minute ventilation to determine the rate response. Numbers in parentheses = stepping function.

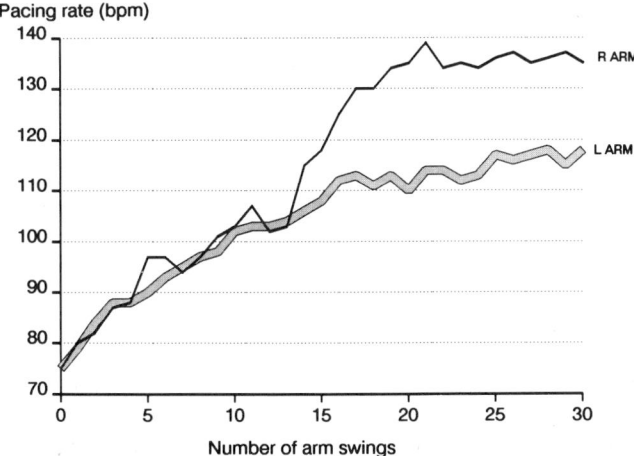

FIGURE 30–8
Effect of swinging arm movement in a patient with an RDP3 pacemaker in the left prepectoral area and the tip of the auxiliary lead in the right second intercostal space lateral to the midclavicular line. The arm swinging was performed during apnea. A higher pacing rate was achieved when the arm on the side of the laterally situated auxiliary lead was swung.

9.3% erratic rate response reported.[80] However, we consider this "dual sensing" ability of the RDP3 to be generally an advantageous combination. It does allow the pacemaker to react quickly to an activity, which would otherwise occur slowly if only respiratory rate were sensed, especially with low work activity when tidal volume increase is the main respiratory change. Furthermore, it may give a rate response in those who have very shallow breathing during exercise (especially elderly subjects). In such patients it is difficult to adjust a respiratory level to discriminate between the minimal tidal volume changes at rest and during exercise. On the other hand, inappropriate rate response possibly can occur if the subject swings one arm. This effect should be considered when programming this pacemaker.[65]

Limitations

The heart rate–respiratory rate correlation coefficient demonstrated (of the order of 0.70), although significant, is not ideal for predicting heart rate from respiratory rate. Theoretically, the physiologic loop between the cardiac output and respiratory rate may complicate the eventual response.[32, 51] In patients with tachypnea due to heart failure, a potential positive feedback may occur, leading to an increase in pacing rate.

The need for an additional electrode is a disadvantage, because electrode erosion can occur, especially if the electrode is tunneled across the chest (Fig. 30–10).[70] With RDP3, which has a fixed sensitivity, myopotential interference is common.[54] This has necessitated the replacement of the unit in some patients.[66] This problem is largely reduced in the more programmable MB-1.

Meta

Principle

Minute ventilation is better correlated with sinus response during exercise than the respiratory rate. At low workloads, a normal subject increases minute ventilation mainly through an increase in tidal volume rather than respiratory rate. At peak exercise, the increase in respiratory rate becomes steeper.[2, 78] Thus the correlation with sinus rate is significantly better

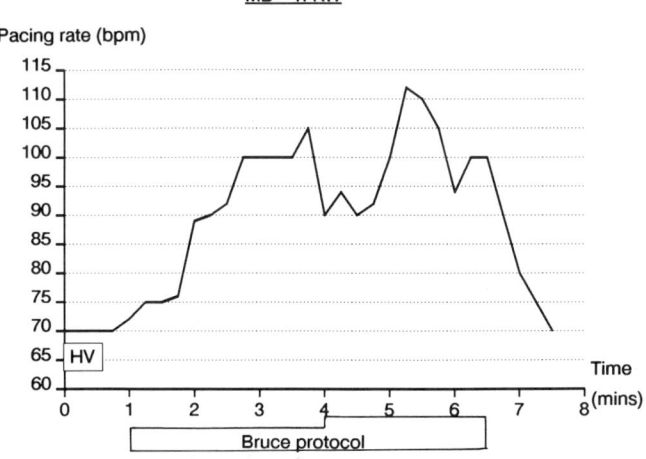

FIGURE 30–9
Rate response of a patient with an MB-1 pacemaker. The following rate-responsive settings were used: pacing range = 70–145 bpm; respiratory level = 2; slope = 1. Hyperventilation (HV) was not detected in this setting. However, during treadmill exercise, rate-responsive pacing occurred primarily by motion-induced artifact associated with arm swinging and walking, although the rate response was erratic.

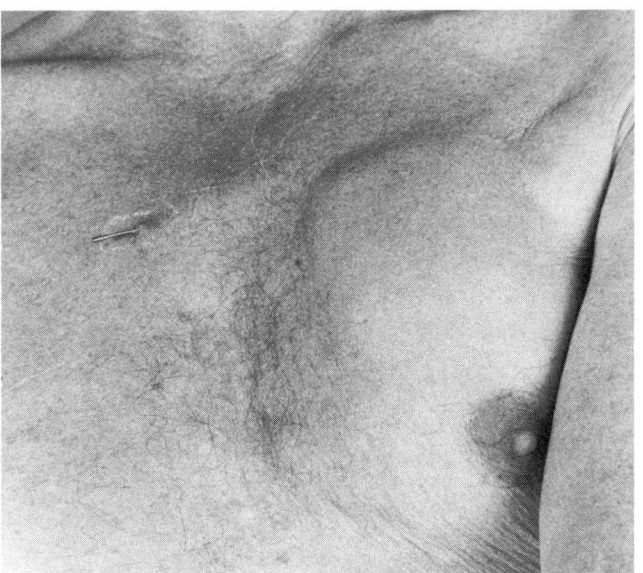

FIGURE 30–10
Erosion of the auxiliary lead in a patient with an RDP3 pacemaker.

when minute ventilation (r = 0.85) is used instead of respiratory rate (r = 0.7).[2, 110]

Minute ventilation can be sensed by measuring impedance changes inside the ventricle, provided that the influence of stroke volume can be filtered. In a study examining the possible electrode configurations suitable for measuring thoracic impedance, Nappholtz et al.[78] found that a bipolar configuration proved unreliable and was affected by postural changes. Although increasing the number of electrodes can improve the quality of the respiratory signal, a tripolar configuration is an appropriate compromise between the complexity of the lead and quality of the signal. In addition, a tripolar configuration has the advantage of being suitable for a standard bipolar pacing lead.

A pacemaker that is based on this principle has been developed (Meta). Minute ventilation is measured by impedance changes using the proximal ring electrode of a bipolar pacing lead and the pacemaker casing as the sourcing electrodes, and the distal pole of the bipolar lead and the pacemaker casing as the sensing electrodes (Fig. 30–7). Any change in minute ventilation is compared with an average minute ventilation over the last hour to avoid artifactual, sudden increase in measured minute ventilation and consequent elevation in pacing rate. In this pacemaker, there are 60 programmable slopes of rate response (see Table 30–3). Programming involves an exercise test in the "minute ventilation adaptive" mode, and a "suggested slope" can be requested at each level of exercise. The pacemaker paces in the constant rate in this pacing mode but senses the minute ventilation changes. Programming the slope value suggested results in the maximal rate at that level of minute ventilation if the exercise is repeated. Figure 30–11 shows the typical rate response in a patient with an implanted Meta. The pacemaker is easy to program and its rate response is workload-related.[71] Our early experience shows a correlation coefficient between the pacing rate and oxygen consumption of 0.85. An improvement in exercise capacity of 39% and in cardiac output of 45% was found in a group of 11 patients tested with this device. In addition, similar to the RDP3, this pacemaker is also sensitive to motion artifact although the response appears to be frequency-dependent (maximum sensitivity at 30 to 40 arm swings per minute).[122] This may confer additional benefits, especially in speeding up the rate responses.

Limitations

Respiratory change is not a fast responding parameter. Respiration is potentially influenced by conditions which may not be of direct relevance to cardiac output. For example, respiration is affected by the needs of phonation and during coughing. Our experience shows a lower pacing rate response during exercise performed with continuous talking than when exercise is performed in silence, indicating safety from undue rate acceleration.[71] The effects of lung disease, e.g. asthma, on rate responses remain to be assessed.

ACTIVITY SENSING

Body movements and vibrations are often associated with physical effort. These parameters can be used to determine the pacing rate of a rate-responsive pacemaker.[6] Vibration can be detected by means of a piezoelectric crystal (Activitrax;* Sensolog 703†), accelerometers,[67] and mechanical sensors (Sensolog P49†).[76]

Activitrax
Principle

The Activitrax is the commonest rate-responsive pacemaker in current use. By means of a piezoelectric crystal, vibrations above a programmable threshold are treated as counts, the frequency of which can then be converted into a pacing rate by a series of programmable slopes of rate response (Fig. 30–12). Table 30–4 summarizes the programmable features of this pacemaker.

Clinical Performance

Humen and coworkers[48] reported the initial clinical experience of six patients implanted with this pacemaker. Improvement in cardiac output was observed in all patients in the rate-responsive mode. However, these investigators were unable to demonstrate improvement in exercise capacity in their patients because some patients were limited by noncardiac factors such as intermittent claudication. In subsequent larger studies, improvement in exercise capacity has been demonstrated.[73] When first released, the rate-responsive

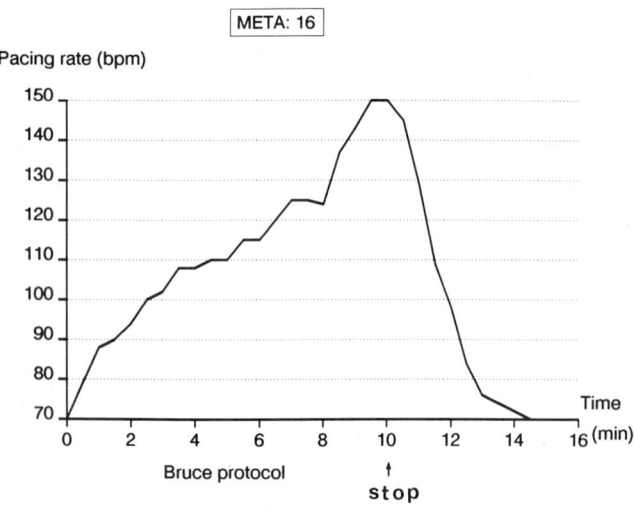

FIGURE 30–11
Rate response of a patient with an implanted Meta pacemaker during treadmill exercise using the Bruce protocol.

*Medtronic Inc, Minneapolis, MN, USA.
†Siemens-Elema, Sweden.

TABLE 30-4
Programmable Rate-Responsive Parameters of Three Different Activity-Sensing Rate-Responsive Pacemakers

Parameters	Activitrax*	Sensolog 703	Sensolog P49
Basic rate (bpm)	60, 70, 80	60 (19 options)	60 (19 options)
Maximum rate (bpm)	100, 125, 150	100, 126, 150	102, 126, 150
Activity threshold	Low, medium, high	0–15	0–15
Slope	1–10	0–7	0–7
RR gain	—	High, low	Very high, high, low, very low
Reaction time	—	Very fast, fast, medium, slow	Fast, medium, slow
Recovery time	—	Fast, medium, slow	Fast, medium, slow
Histograms	—	Long-term, short-term	Long-term, short-term

*Activitrax II has wider programmable rate limits and refractory periods.

setting was set cautiously at a low level (most were programmed at threshold = medium, response = 5) and rate response was reported as "moderate."[73] We[69] and others[101] have shown that a better rate response can be achieved with a more sensitive setting (usually threshold = medium, response = 7–8). Cardiopulmonary testing has confirmed the benefit of this pacemaker in improving maximum oxygen consumption and anaerobic threshold.[19] Symptomatic benefit has also been reported.[73, 74]

Limitations

Body vibration is a by-product of physical exercise, and it has only a loose association with metabolic demand.[67, 103] This pacemaker cannot respond to physiological changes that are associated with minimal body movement, such as the Valsalva maneuver and hand grip.[69] In particular, the rate response does not correlate with the level of exertion; for example, there is no pacing rate change on walking at a high slope on a treadmill (Fig. 30–13).[69] The reason for this behavior is related to the algorithm used for the detection of vibration, which measures the frequency of vibration peaks. We have shown that the pacing rate is dependent on the step frequency (Fig. 30–14).[69] In addition, as vibration ceases at the end of an activity, the pacing rate decays according to an arbitrary curve that bears

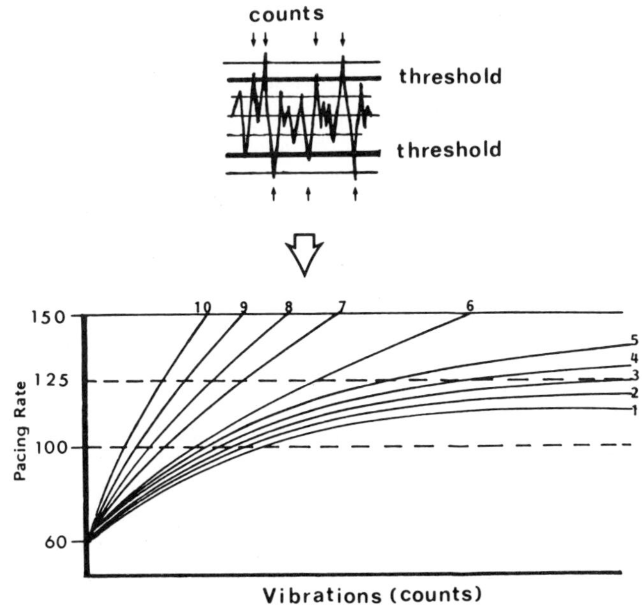

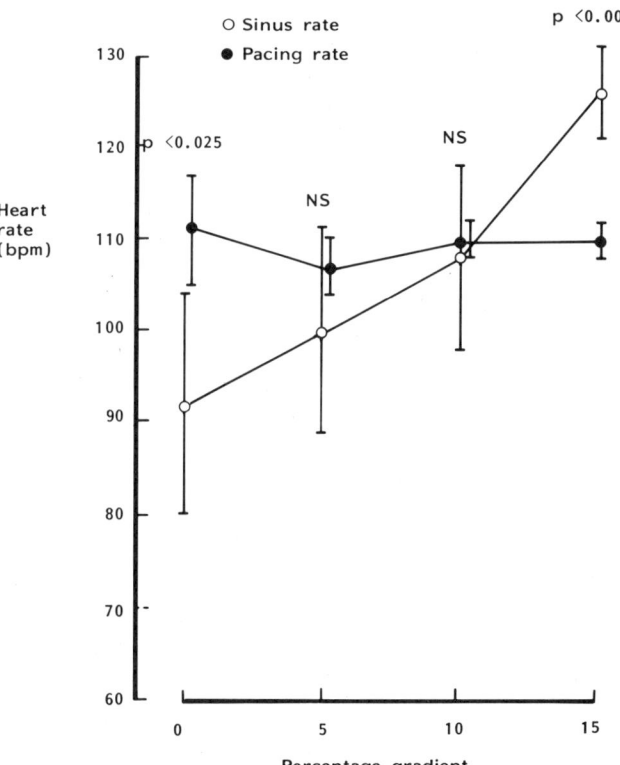

FIGURE 30–13
Rate responses of six volunteers during brief treadmill exercise with the treadmill speed set at 2.5 mph. This graph summarizes the rate responses of four different exercise tests (each lasting for 3 minutes) at each of the four gradients. The pacing rate did not increase on ascending an incline. The pacing rate was faster than the sinus rate at 0% gradient but was too low for a higher workload when the subjects walked at higher gradients. The p values were derived from paired comparisons of the sinus and pacing rates at each level of exercise; each error bar refers to 1 standard deviation. NS = not significant.

FIGURE 30–12
The mechanism of an Activitrax pacemaker. Sensed vibrations (i.e., vibration above a programmable threshold) (arrows, upper panel) are counted. The counts are converted to a rate response by a series of programmable slopes (lower panel).

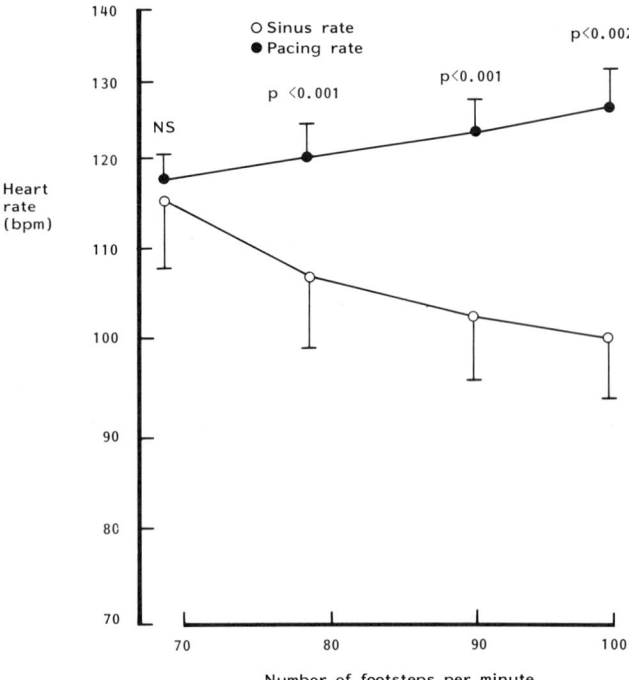

FIGURE 30–14
Pacemaker and sinus rates of eight volunteers during treadmill exercise at 2 mph, walking at different step frequencies governed by a metronome. The pacemaker rate increased when the number of steps was increased, but the sinus rate was lower at a higher stepping frequency, which was the most comfortable stepping frequency for this group of volunteers walking at this speed. Each error bar refers to 1 standard deviation of the mean.

little relationship to the metabolic debt that was incurred during exercise.

Environmental vibrations such as those occurring during many forms of transport can affect the pacing rate (Fig. 30–15).[103, 108] Direct pressure on the pacemaker can also deform the piezoelectric crystal, leading to an increase in the pacemaker rate. This can be of clinical importance during sleep if the subject lies on the pacemaker.[115]

Sensolog

Sensolog 703 uses a piezoelectric crystal sensor for activity sensing similar to that of the Activitrax. The reported algorithm involves the integration of the vibration signal, which is subsequently processed by one of the two gain settings, 16 thresholds, and 8 slopes (see Table 30–4). A special feature of this pacemaker is the provision of rate histograms (Fig. 30–16). The long-term histogram samples a pacing rate every 16 seconds and allocates the rate into one of the four histogram ranges. The short-term histogram measures every pacing rate during an activity and thus allows assessment of the rate changes during brief activities such as walking. These histograms facilitate programming and allow programming to be carried out for daily activities, rather than artificially on a treadmill or cycle ergometer.

Although the rate-responsive behavior of this pacemaker has been shown to be slightly more physiologic than that of the Activitrax pacemaker, it has similar limitations, especially with respect to the influence of external direct pressure and vibration effects on the pacemaker.[68, 105]

The Sensolog P49 is a newer version that utilizes the

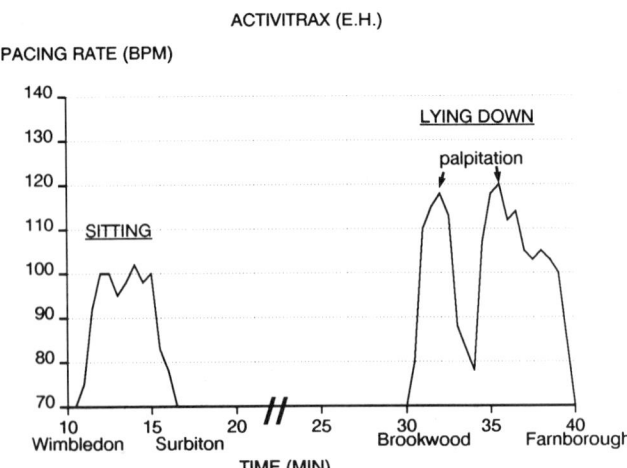

FIGURE 30–15
Rate responses during a train ride in a patient with an implanted Activitrax pacemaker. Pacemaker setting: threshold = medium, response = 7.

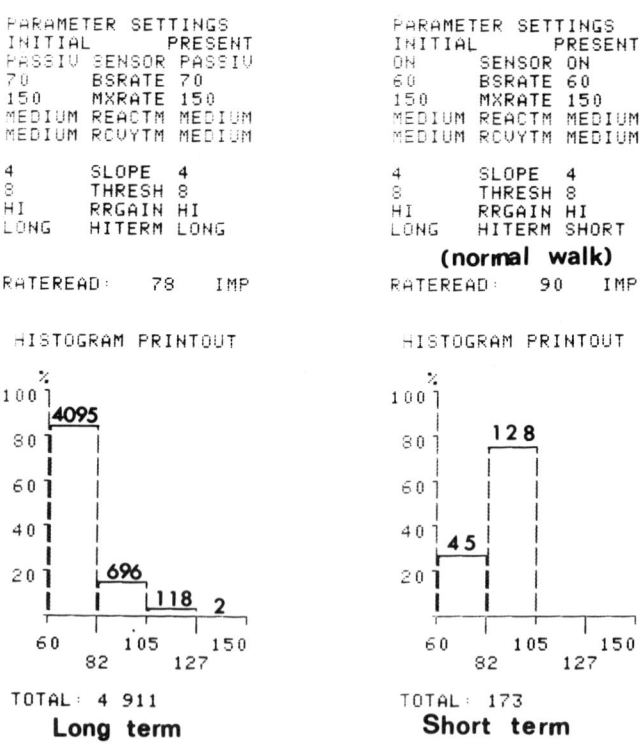

FIGURE 30–16
Long- and short-term histograms of the Sensolog 703. See text for description.

motion inertia of a non-piezoelectric sensor. This system obviates the problem of rate acceleration caused by direct pressure on the pacemaker. Our early experience with six units has shown improved rate response with this device.

Other Methods of Activity Sensing

Using triaxially sensitive accelerometers mounted on the surface of an external Activitrax pacemaker, we have shown that the root mean square value of acceleration (either the vertical or anteroposterior component) correlated better with the workload than the Activitrax pacemaker.[67] Furthermore, the dominant frequencies of acceleration during walking are under 4 Hz, and it is possible to utilize a low-pass filter without affecting the "physiologic" acceleration signals, while reducing the influence of unwanted external vibrations (Fig. 30–17). Alt and coworkers[3] reported the use of a piezo-resistive linear frequency response sensor with a low-pass filter at 3 Hz. The acceleration forces detected by their system were related to the intensity of workload during daily activities, with good discrimination against extraneous vibrations.

By means of a mechanical sensor incorporating a tilt switch principle (Fig. 30–18), postural and activity detection can be achieved by the movement of a mercury ball over a disc of on/off switches.[76] The level of activity is indicated by the rate of opening and closing of the tilt switches, and the site of switches closed by the mercury ball indicates the posture. Postural detection may be useful both to allow a slower pacing rate during sleep and to enable a rapid rate response on adopting an erect posture.

MIXED VENOUS TEMPERATURE

Principle

The changes in mixed venous temperature with exercise as a biosensor of metabolic demand was first suggested by Weisswange et al.[114] Early studies in the development of a temperature-based rate-responsive pacemaker were published by Griffin and colleagues[46] and Jolgren and coworkers.[50] The overall efficiency of the body to perform mechanical work is around 20%. The heat generated by this process is detected first in the working muscle, and soon afterward in the venous blood, which serves as a carrier of heat.[16] Laczkovics et al.,[62] using a thermistor in the right atrium, reported a temperature increase of up to 1.5° C, beginning after a delay of 20 to 40 seconds following the onset of exercise. This temperature change is of sufficient magnitude to control a rate-responsive pacemaker. Pacemakers utilizing a thermistor and algorithm relating pacing rate to temperature were successfully implanted in animal studies.[50]

Extensive studies in humans show good correlation of temperature change with workload.[1] The temperature change in elderly subjects is higher than in those more physically fit, probably due to reduced heat dissipation related to more pronounced reduction of

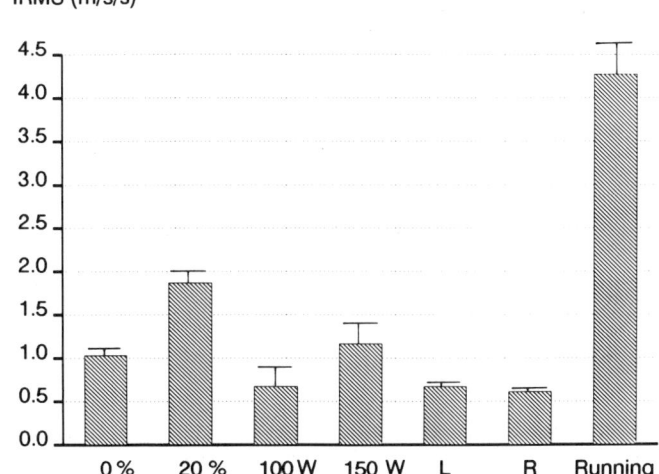

FIGURE 30–17
Low-pass root mean square value of (fRMS) acceleration during a variety of exercises. Note appropriate workload-related responses.

blood flow to the skin during exercise. It is further postulated that the slow circadian change in temperature could be used to simulate the diurnal variation in heart rate. A more recent study by Fearnot and colleagues[37] demonstrates the possible physiologic parameters that can affect central venous temperature (Table 30–5).

Clinical Performance

Three pacemaker companies have brought a temperature-sensing, rate-responsive pacemaker into clinical trials (Nova MR, Intermedics;* Thermos, Biotronik†; Kelvin 500, Cook Pacemaker‡). Each utilizes a different algorithm for processing temperature signals. Characteristic rate-responsive programming parameters are listed in Table 30–6. The Nova MR and Kelvin 500 use the initial temperature "dip" to trigger a rate response, giving an arbitrary rate of 85 bpm. The

---

*Intermedics Inc., Freeport, TX, USA.
†Biotronik GmbH & Co., Berlin, West Germany.
‡Cook Pacemaker Corporation, Leechburg PA, USA.

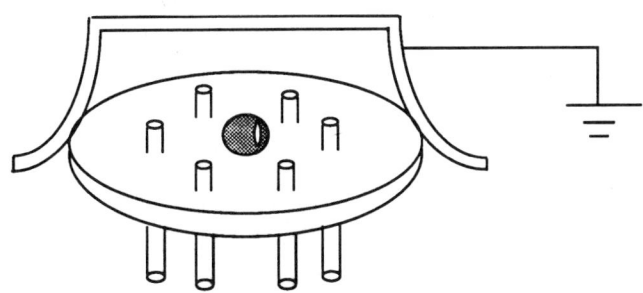

FIGURE 30–18
Schematic representation of a mechanical sensor (See text for description.)[76]

TABLE 30–5
Physiologic Changes That Can Affect Central Venous Temperature*

Variables	Temperature
Vasodilation	−0.24° C
Exercise	0.02 to 1.37° C (depending on level of exercise)
Emotion	Slow increase of central venous temperature
High external temperature	
Hot coffee	0.07 ± 0.09° C
Cold drink	0.06 ± 0.03° C
Warm tub (37.5° C)	0.10 ± 0.42° C
Hot tub (41° C)	0.86 ± 0.61° C
Diurnal changes	Up to 2° C
Cyclic variation during sleep	

*Data compiled from Fearnot NE, Smith HJ: PACE 8:701, 1985; and Alt E, Volker R, Hogl B, et al.: PACE 10:1206, 1987.

Thermos uses this temperature dip to set up a "start interval," and rate response occurs when temperature change subsequently confirms the beginning of exercise. With continued exercise, the increase in temperature is used in an algorithm for a rate response. The response of the Nova MR during exercise is illustrated in Figure 30–19.

Only early clinical results are available. In a study of seven patients with Nova MR, a mean response time of 23 seconds was reported.[4] A sophisticated sensor and algorithm are needed to detect and respond to temperature changes during physical exercise (average 0.3° C) compared with the much higher diurnal variation in temperature (2° C). Similar response times (24.3 s) were reported in patients with the Kelvin 500.[38, 98] These authors also reported improvement in oxygen consumption, exercise performance, and subjective well-being when pacing in the rate-responsive rather than in the VVI mode. Improvement in exercise performance was also demonstrated in patients with Thermos pacemakers.[63] In this study, isolation failure in two thermistor electrodes (in a series of six patients) was also reported.

Limitations

As noted above (see Table 30–5), central venous temperature can be affected by external and internal temperature changes. Environmental changes in temperature, drinking cold liquids, and fever (only partly related to an increase in metabolism) may be expected to cause changes in rate response that are not related to metabolic needs. Acceleration to the upper rate limit can occur during an unusually hot bath.[96] Increase in heat dissipation during exercise (e.g., swimming) may blunt the rate response. At the start of exercise following prolonged rest, the central venous temperature falls when cold peripheral blood reaches the central circulation. Although this drop in temperature has been used to trigger an immediate increase of heart rate, the rate response can only be to an arbitrary value. Also, this response is unpredictable because the initiation of exercise in a patient who is already warmed up by previous exercise does not cause a fall of central temperature.[97] The use of temperature sensing at the atrial level is still under investigation.[99] The temperature response at this level may be affected by inadequate venous mixing.[2, 62]

MIXED VENOUS OXYGEN SATURATION

Principle

Physical activity causes an increase in cardiac output and oxygen extraction from the blood. A prompt drop in the mixed venous oxygen saturation (SO_2) results. The extent of the desaturation depends on the level of activity and on the cardiac performance. Unlike the pH value, or to a lesser extent, central venous temperature (both of which may be "buffered" by the body's regulatory mechanisms), there is no appreciable pool of oxygen in the body, and changes in SO_2 rapidly reflect metabolic needs in response to exercise.[117]

Using a special optical sensor and a light-emitting diode incorporated in the body of an electrode, Wirtzfeld and colleagues[117, 118] measured the changes of oxygen saturation during exercise. Triggered by the intracardiac R wave or pacing spike, the fluctuation in signals received from the sensor during each cardiac cycle can be eliminated. Experiments in humans at rest and during exercise have shown that with the SO_2 sensor working in the "triggered" mode, a reliable reproduction of SO_2 could be obtained. At each level of activity, a new plateau was reached within a period of about 60 seconds. Changes in SO_2 may be used in a closed-loop system, because any change in pacing rate improves the cardiac output, which reduces the arteriovenous oxygen difference, leading to a negative

TABLE 30–6
Comparison of Rate-Responsive Parameters in Three Different Models of Temperature Sensing Rate-Responsive Pacemakers

Parameter	Nova MR (Intermedics)	Thermos (Biotronik)	Kelvin 500 (Cook)
Baseline temperature	36.0 to 38.0 in 0.02° C increment	35 to 41° C in 0.1° C increment	Not programmable
Onset detection	1–10, temperature "dip" increases rate to 85 bpm	"Dip" in temperature results in "start interval"	"Interim" heart rate
Exercise rate response	1–10	1 bpm/0.1° C	Rate ramps, temp-5 or temp-10
Post-exercise rate	1–10	1 bpm/0.1° C	Rate ramps

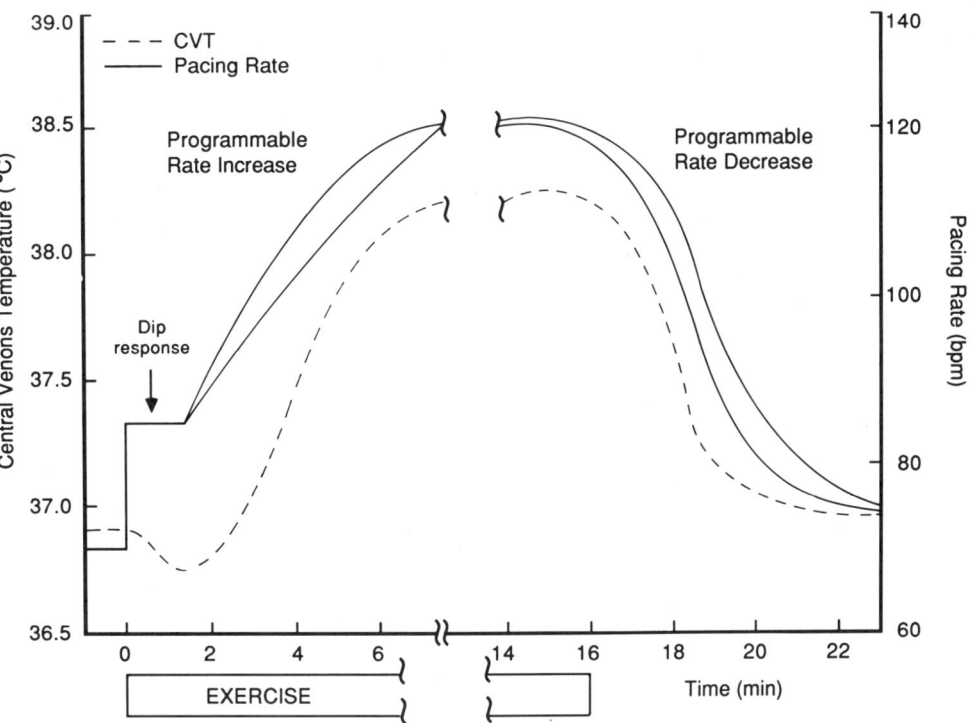

FIGURE 30–19
Rate-responsive features of a temperature sensing rate-responsive pacemaker (Nova MR). At the start of exercise, the temperature dip results in an arbitrary rate response of 85 bpm. Further rate change occurs when the temperature continues to rise during exercise. Both the onset and recovery rate response are programmable. CVT = central venous temperature.

feedback that increases the value of SO_2. Thus, a pacing system can be designed that will automatically adjust the pacing rate to achieve an optimal SO_2, the theoretical advantage being that programming is unnecessary. Whatever the subject's rate/SO_2 relationship, the pacing rate will adjust to give an optimal SO_2. It also follows that any change in the subject's condition over time would be automatically compensated.

Limitations

Besides its complicated technology, fibrin coating and thrombus deposition on the optical sensor cause difficulties with this type of sensor. This problem may be corrected by using differential absorption with two different wavelengths rather than the absolute SO_2 value as measured by one wavelength. Thus, any fibrin coating would "scale down" the values of both wavelengths without affecting the differential value. A variety of chemical coatings designed to prevent fibrin and platelet deposition are also being evaluated.

dp/dt Sensing

Principle

Right ventricular contractile function is determined mainly by the inotropic state of the heart and its preload. The first derivative of the right ventricular pressure (dp/dt) has been suggested as a useful parameter to correlate with the heart rate.[7, 18] Using a piezoelectric crystal attached to a deflectable diaphragm, right ventricular pressure and dp/dt can be measured. During exercise there is an increase in amplitude, decrease in duration, and increase in sharpness of the right ventricular waveform, reflected by an increase in dp/dt maximum. The last effect was found to have a good correlation with the sinus rate (r = 0.83).[18]

An implantable pacemaker (Model 2503, Medtronic) has been used in conjunction with a special pressure-sensing electrode (Model 6220, Medtronic). Each lead is calibrated individually and high-fidelity pressure waveforms can be assessed using telemetry (Fig. 30–20). Implantation of the lead and pacemaker is done by conventional methods; however, recording of the pressure waveform from the lead (either directly or indirectly through telemetry) is necessary to ensure normal functioning of the pressure sensor.

Clinical Performance

Initial experience with the Medtronic 2503 indicates that the rate response is workload-related.[100, 107] By programming the pacemaker to a lower rate of about 50 bpm, the rate-response setting can be adjusted so that the dp/dt maximum while the patient is awake enables a pacing rate of about 70 bpm to be achieved, with the capability of the pacing rate to fall to the lower rate during sleep.

The early prototype unit had technical problems which limited the upper rate response to 100 bpm for some units. This problem is currently being investigated by the manufacturer.

Limitations

The main concern is the longevity of the sensor, which may be affected by the fibrin coating or by the burying

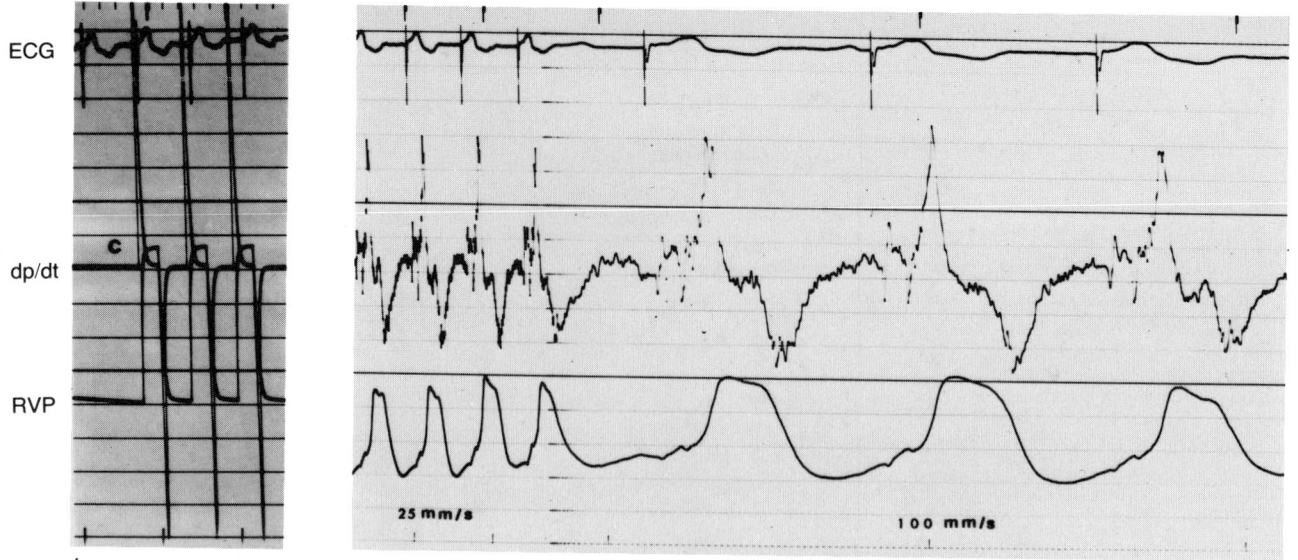

FIGURE 30-20
Telemetry waveform of a patient with a Deltatrax pacemaker. The dp/dt value shown is externally digitized from the right ventricular pressure. Calibrations are shown on the left. RVP = right ventricular pressure.

of the sensor within the cardiac trabeculae. The effect of acutely changing the posture (head-up tilt) results in an increase in pacing rate from 64 to 71 bpm.[107] The potential positive feedback by the Treppe effect[21, 85] (increase in dp/dt as a result of increase in pacing rate) has not been significant.[100] The effects of acute ischemia and heart failure on dp/dt have not been systematically assessed. Drugs with a negative inotropic effect (e.g., beta-blockers) are believed to alter the dp/dt response. Although the prototype unit was beset with technical problems, there is no reason to suppose that dp/dt sensing is not a sound indicator of rate response.

OTHER BIOSENSORS

Goldreyer et al.[44] and Knudson et al.[56] described a pacemaker using the average P wave rate to alter the ventricular rate (maximum 110/min). This avoided the problem of pacemaker-mediated tachycardia, as ventricular pacing was not synchronized to atrial activity. Only the changes in atrial rate were measured; therefore, a pacemaker based on this principle could theoretically be useful in patients with atrial bradycardia and an inadequate but noticeable atrial response to exercise. However, the RS4-SRT pacing system* was shown to be unreliable in atrial sensing.[84] Implantation time was prolonged because of the difficulty in obtaining satisfactory P wave amplitudes, and consistent rate responsiveness was not obtained.

Systolic intervals have also been investigated. The left ventricular pre-ejection interval (PEI) during exercise was found to correlate with the workload. In addition, the PEI also responds appropriately to vasodilatation and does not shorten with an increase in pacing rate.[29] On the other hand, the left ventricular ejection time (LVET) shows more individual variations, is preload-dependent, and can be influenced by rate changes. Klein et al.[55] showed similar PEI changes in the right ventricle but found that the minimum right ventricular PEI occurred after cessation of exercise and lasted for several minutes.

Salo and colleagues[93] measured the alteration of right ventricular stroke volume by means of the changes in electrical impedance. Olson used an electromagnetic flow probe to measure stroke volume.[12] An increase in stroke volume is a marker of increased venous return during exercise without an appropriate increase in rate. This system has the potential for a fast response. However, some investigators have not found the stroke volume changes to be a reliable parameter.[55, 104]

The ventricular depolarization "gradient" describes the spatial distribution of activation times associated with ventricular excitation. The paced ventricular depolarization area is integrated with and is found to decrease with stress and exercise but to increase with increase in pacing rate.[25] This principle has been incorporated in a new rate-responsive pacemaker (Prism*). However, technical problems were encountered in early devices. In our experience with two units, there was a rapid onset of rate response at the beginning of exercise. The gradient sensed by both patients exceeded the available range of the pacemaker (so-called "rate-control parameter"), resulting in failure of rate response on follow-up. Further refinement of the unit and modification of the range of the rate-control parameter is currently being carried out.

Cohen[31] published a theoretical right atrial pressure heart rate control system that utilized the principle of increased right atrial pressure during exercise to determine the pacing rate. Other parameters such as chemical sensors, pacing threshold (falls during exercise), and nervous signals have also been investigated.

*Cardiac Pacemakers Inc., Minneapolis, MN, USA.

*Telectronics-Cordis, Englewood, CO, USA.

Which Sensor?

The myriad of sensors that have been tested and realized as pacemakers means that physicians have to make a choice. The relative merits of some sensors are presented in Table 30–2, and certain limitations of the most commonly used sensors are summarized in Table 30–7. Certain sensors should be avoided in some groups of patients. Experience, especially with certain newer units, is still rudimentary.

In our institution, an activity sensor (which has the best speed of onset of rate response) is currently chosen for elderly patients and for relatively inactive individuals who exercise only for very brief periods. In such cases, a rapid speed of onset of rate response is a particularly desirable feature. On the other hand, a sensor showing better proportionality to workload (e.g., a respiratory sensor) is used in patients who are likely to undertake more prolonged activities, in order to optimize the pacing rate response to the workload.

Sensor Combination

The normal heart rate is controlled by multiple inputs, which act via the autonomic nervous system. It seems appropriate to use several sensors for smoothing rate responses and minimizing the limitations of individual sensors. Among the existing systems, the RDP3/MB-1 and Meta are already dual-sensor pacemakers (by accident rather than design), capable of responding to both activity and respiratory rate.[65, 113] Another useful combination is that of the fast response of an activity sensor with a slow-responding but more accurate parameter, such as the central venous temperature (Fig. 30–21). It has also been suggested that this combination will enable the discrimination of extraneous vibration for the activity sensor.[5] Stangl and coworkers[104] compared S_{O_2}, central venous temperature, stroke volume, and sinus rate, using a novel multisensor catheter. These workers concluded that stroke volume was a fast-responding parameter but was not stress load–related. S_{O_2} was found to be sensitive at low to medium workload, and temperature at a higher workload. Thus, sensor combinations of these parameters are potentially advantageous. However, the drawback of any sensor combination is the need for complex algorithms to discriminate possible contradictory inputs from different sensors, thus possibly adding to the burden of programming. An alternative is to develop and use a better single sensor.

Dual-Chamber Rate-Responsive Pacing

In patients with complete AV block, a dual-chamber pacemaker is the pacemaker of choice. However, if the AV block is associated with sinoatrial disease, especially chronotropic incompetence and paroxysmal

TABLE 30–7
Major Limitations of Some Sensors Used in Rate-Responsive Pacing

		Major Clinical Limitations of			
Q-T Sensing	RR Sensing	MV Sensing	Activity Sensing	Temperature Sensing	dp/dt
Slow response, giving post-exercise tachycardia	Requirement of auxiliary lead	Effect in patients with chest disease not yet assessed	Certain occupations or hobbies	Effect of environmental temperature	Effect of ischemia and heart failure not yet assessed
Easily affected by drugs and ischemia	"Erratic" rate response can occur		Critical and accurate response needed	Accurate rate response to high stress load only	Cannot be used in atrium
Long-term reliability questionable			Rate affected by external vibrations	Use in atrium still under investigation	
Complex programming*					
Cannot be used in the atrium		Cannot be used in children with fast respiratory rate			
Avoid in:					
Patients with major Q-T abnormality	Patients with thin chest wall	Young children	Patients exposed to high vibration levels	Relatively inactive subjects	†
Patients on antiarrhythmic drugs				Patients with severe heart failure	
Atrial pacing					Atrial pacing

*New algorithm will simplify programming.
†Further evaluation needed.
RR = respiratory rate, MV = minute ventilation.

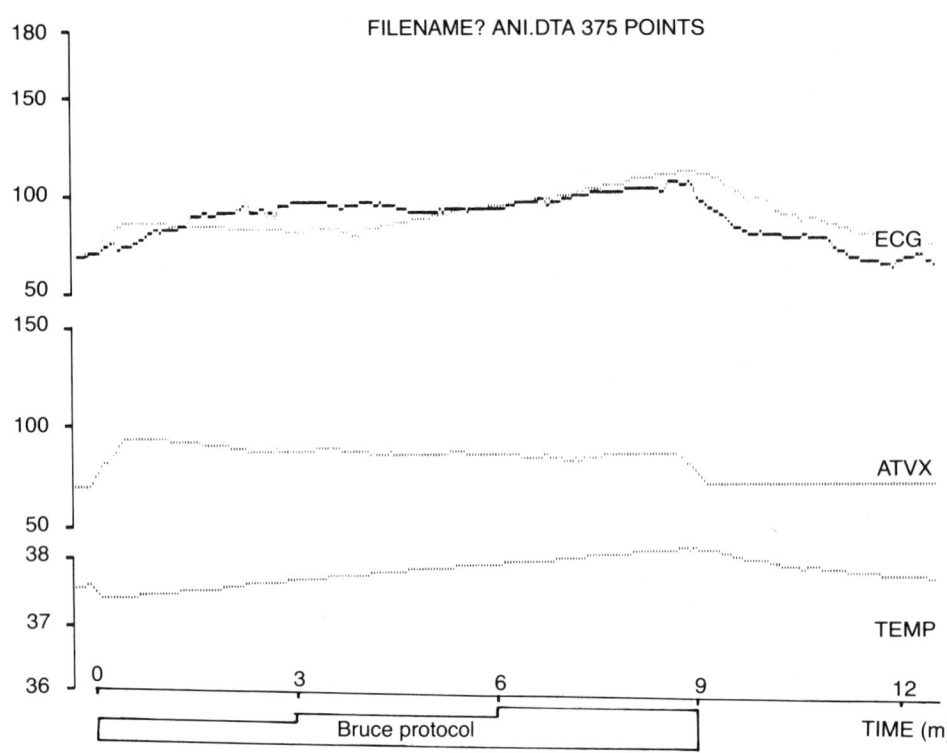

FIGURE 30-21
Combination of activity sensing (using of an externally attached Activitrax) and central venous temperature for rate-responsive pacing. An algorithm developed in our institution compares the rate responses derived from these two parameters. There was a rapid response with activity (ATVX) at the onset of exercise, but the pacemaker rate failed to respond to increasing workload. Central venous temperature (TEMP) responded first with a dip followed by a relatively slow rise. However, it was better correlated with the sinus rate at a higher workload. The combined result (light line, upper graph) resulted in a sensor-derived rate that was more closely related to the sinus rate (heavy line) during the stress test at all levels of workload. The rate decay, as determined by the temperature response, was much more physiologic than the rapid decay as recorded by the Activitrax.

atrial fibrillation, a dual-chamber rate-responsive pacemaker would be a better choice. This combines the benefits of AV synchrony and of an adequate rate response, even during atrial fibrillation or when the sinus response is inadequate.

A prototype unit has been reported,[52] which consists of an Activitrax and a Symbios connected by an interface hybrid (SP 102 BV*), (Fig. 30–22). This device can be programmed as DDD, with and without backup pacing rate control by activity sensing. With activity sensing, the fall-back rate is governed by the Activitrax determined rate, so that in case of chronotropic insufficiency during exercise, the rate response is governed by the activity sensor. Atrial synchronized ventricular pacing (VDD) up to the maximum rate will be obtained only when the activity determined rate corresponds to the sensed atrial rhythm. Using this activity sensor, pathologic atrial tachycardia (which will not be confirmed by the activity sensor) will be discriminated. Doppler study at rest and during isometric exercise in two patients showed improved hemodynamics in the dual-chamber pacing mode. An improved unit has become available for clinical trials (Synergist II*).

The sensing of right ventricular relative stroke volume, pre-ejection interval, and ejection time has been realized using a special tripolar pacing electrode (Model 1200, CPI) (see Fig. 30–7).[81] The first derivative of the relative stroke volume gives the contractility of the right ventricle, which is also a useful parameter for rate-responsive pacing. The unit is capable of pacing in the DDD rate-responsive mode and the DDD mode and is capable of single-chamber rate-responsive pacing with any of the parameters sensed (Fig. 30–23).

Patient Selection; Should All Pacemakers Be Rate-Modulated?

Indications for a rate-responsive pacemaker should take into account the cost of the pacemaker and

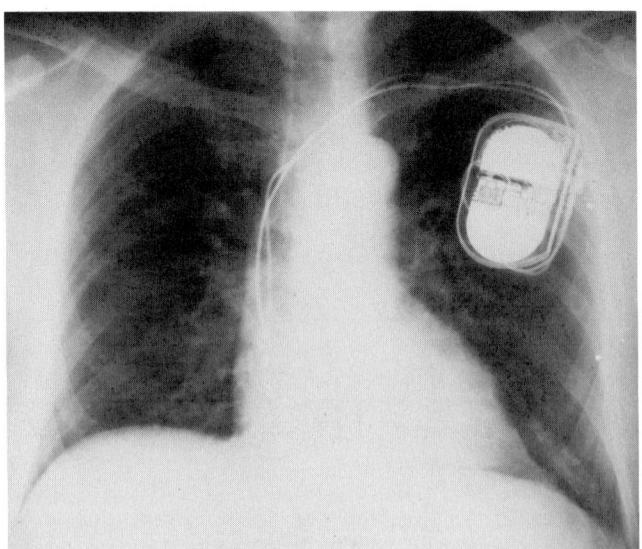

FIGURE 30–22
Chest x-ray of a patient with a dual-chamber Activitrax pacemaker. This represents the side-to-side merging of a Symbios and an Activitrax. (Courtesy of Dr. R. Sutton, Consultant Cardiologist of the Westminster Hospital, London.)

*Medtronic Inc., Minneapolis, MN, USA.

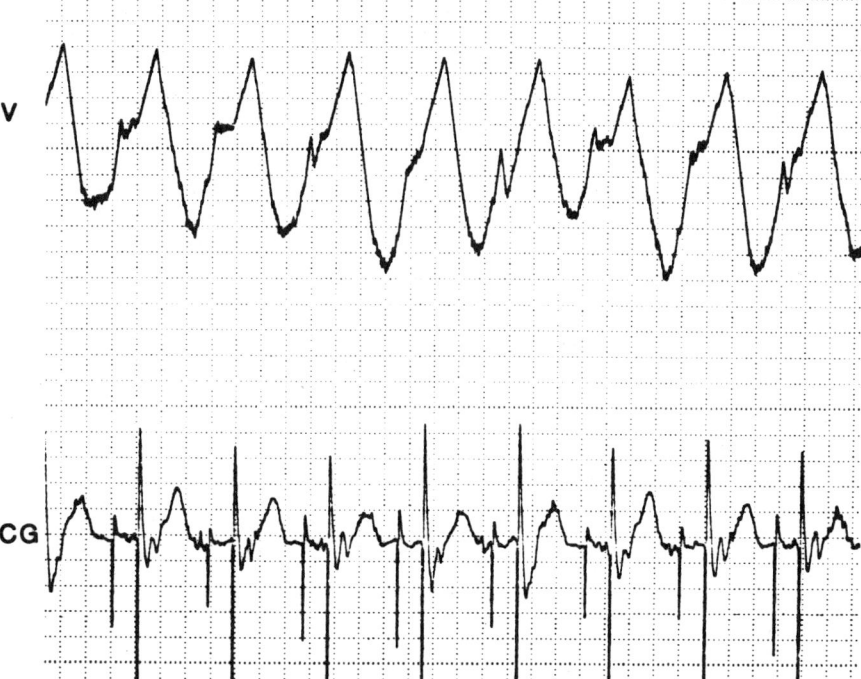

FIGURE 30–23
Relative stroke volume (SV) assessed from telemetry in a patient with a CPI Model 1200 pacemaker in the dual-chamber pacing mode.

possible patient benefit. In addition, it should be kept in mind that all currently available sensors have their limitations (see Table 30–7), and none can imitate perfectly a normal sinus response. Furthermore, many of the earlier systems have had technical problems. Unlike a dual-chamber system, much more programming time is necessary to ensure adequate functioning of these pacemakers.

In patients who have infrequent episodes of bradycardia, an ordinary VVI pacemaker with hysteresis usually will be satisfactory. A rate-responsive unit is inappropriate, not only because of its cost but also because hysteresis and rate-responsive pacing are a difficult combination; ventricular pacing will occur unnecessarily and could result in a fall of blood pressure[34] and produce the pacemaker syndrome in patients with intact ventriculoatrial conduction.[13]

In patients with complete heart block and normal sinus and atrial function, a dual-chamber pacemaker should be the pacemaker of choice because it provides better hemodynamics at rest and reduces the incidence of pacemaker syndrome. Also, programming is easier because the sinus rate determines the ideal chronotropic response. The progression of sinoatrial disease tends to be slow,[39, 72] and it is probably unnecessary to implant a single-chamber rate-responsive pacemaker as a prophylactic measure, given the limited longevity of present pacemaker batteries. In a patient who is inactive or bed-bound (provided the inactivity is not related to bradycardia), only a bradycardia support pacemaker will be necessary.

About half of the patients with sinoatrial disease have chronotropic incompetence during exercise.[83] Overall, one third of these patients have chronotropic insufficiency at submaximal exercise. As most patients do not perform strenuous exercise in everyday life, normal rate response at submaximal workload should be adequate, and chronotropic insufficiency at maximum exercise will seldom become clinically important. In this group of patients, when a rate responsive pacemaker is implanted for an "inadequate" sinus response rather than because of the absence of response, a very accurate sensor will be necessary in order to improve the inadequate sinus response. A too-rapid acceleration of the atrial rate (for example, using an activity-sensing atrial pacemaker) may not be followed by physiologic shortening of the AV interval or reduction of the AV nodal refractory period. Thus, adverse hemodynamics[30, 91] or even AV nodal block[24] may result.

Although single-chamber rate-responsive pacing can result in almost similar cardiac output and exercise tolerance at moderate and maximum exercise, recent evidence[14] suggests that this is achieved only at the expense of contractility reserve. Likewise, arterial lactate and arteriovenous oxygen difference is less at submaximal exercise with atrial synchronous pacing than with rate-responsive pacing.[60] In addition, a recent study suggests that a short AV interval may further increase the cardiac output during exercise in patients with dual-chamber pacemakers programmed with "standard" intervals.[77] Although the clinical significance of these observations awaits further studies, it seems likely that atrial synchronous pacing is the ideal pacing mode. Retrograde conduction, particularly at rest, may induce the pacemaker syndrome in patients paced with rate-responsive ventricular pacing. The possibility of the pacemaker syndrome occurring on exercise with VVI and VVIR pacemakers has not yet been systematically investigated. The pacemaker syndrome is, however, a practical drawback to VVI pacing whether or not rate response is also used.

Conclusion

The normal atrial signal is ideal for physiologic pacing, and a single-chamber sensor-driven pacemaker is no substitute. However, physiologic pacing can be difficult to achieve, and some patients do not have adequate sinus function. Therefore, a certain number of patients who require pacemakers cannot fully benefit from dual-chamber pacing. A single-chamber rate-responsive system, adapting to the metabolic needs of the body, is an attractive alternative for "part-physiologic" pacing, and the prerequisite is some form of sensor of metabolic demand. However, no single sensor has proved ideal. At present, active research is being undertaken to evaluate a better sensor or a combination of several sensors with different characteristics. A completely satisfactory physiologic pacemaker requires better dual-chamber pacing and sensing capacity and adequate rate response to exercise and other metabolic changes.

References

1. Alt E, Hirgstetter C, Heinz M, et al.: Rate control of physiologic pacemakers by central venous blood temperature. Circulation 73:1206, 1986.
2. Alt E, Heinz M, Hirgstetter C, et al.: Control of pacemaker rate by impedance based respiratory minute ventilation. Chest 92:247, 1987.
3. Alt E, Heinz M, Theras H, et al.: A new body motion activity based rate-responsive pacing system (Abstract). PACE 10:422, 1987.
4. Alt E, Volker R, Hogl B, et al.: Function of the temperature-controlled Nova MR pacemaker in patients' everyday life: preliminary clinical results (Abstract). PACE 10:1206, 1987.
5. Alt E, Theras H, Heinz M, et al.: A new rate-responsive pacemaker system optimized by combination of two sensors (Abstract). PACE 10:422, 1987.
6. Anderson K, Humen D, Klein GJ, et al.: A rate-variable pacemaker which automatically adjusts for physical activity (Abstract). PACE 6:A12, 1983.
7. Anderson KM, Moore AA, Bennett TD: Sensors in pacing. PACE 9:954, 1986.
8. Asmussen E: Muscular exercise. In Asmussen E (ed.): Handbook of Physiology and Respiration, p. 939. Washington, DC, American Physiological Society, 1965.
9. Astrand I: Aerobic work capacity in men and women with special reference to age. Acta Physiol Scand (Suppl)169:15, 1960.
10. Astrand PO, Saltin B: Maximal oxygen uptake and heart rate in various types of muscular activity. J Appl Physiol 16:977, 1951.
11. Astrand P, Rodahl K: Textbook of Work Physiology: Physiological Basis of Exercise, 3rd Ed., pp. 365–374. New York, McGraw-Hill, 1986.
12. Olson W: Stroke volume controlled rate responsive pacing in exercise in heart-block canine. Circulation 72:132, 1985.
13. Ausubel K, Furman S: The pacemaker syndrome. Ann Intern Med 103:420, 1985.
14. Ausubel K, Steingart RM, Shimshi M, et al.: Maintenance of exercise stroke volume during ventricular versus atrial synchronous pacing: Role of contractility. Circulation 72:1037, 1985.
15. Baig W, Begemann M, Rickards A, et al.: Automatic adjusting slope setting for the QT sensing pacemaker—initial clinical evaluation (Abstract). PACE 10:1207, 1987.
16. Bazett HO: Theory of reflex controls to explain regulation of temperature at rest and during exercise. J Appl Physiol 4:245, 1951.
17. Benchimol A, Ligget MS: Cardiac dynamics during stimulation of the right atrium, right ventricle and left ventricle in normal and abnormal hearts. Circulation 33:933, 1966.
18. Bennett TD: Dynamic characteristics of alternative physiological pacing (Abstract). PACE 8:294, 1985.
19. Benditt DG, Mianulli M, Fetter J, et al.: Single-chamber cardiac pacing with activity-initiated chronotropic response: Evaluation by cardiopulmonary testing. Circulation 75:184, 1987.
20. Bernstein AD, Camm AJ, Fletcher RD, et al.: NASPE/BPEG generic pacemaker code for antibradyarrhythmia and adaptive-rate pacing and antitachyarrhythmia devices. PACE 10:794, 1987.
21. Boute W, Derrien Y, Wittkampf FHM: Reliability of evoked endocardial T-wave sensing in 1500 pacemaker patients. PACE 9:948, 1986.
22. Bowditch HP: Uber die Eigenthumlichkeiten der Reizacbeit, welche die Muskelfasern des Herzenszeigen. Ber Verh der Kongiglich Sachsischenges Wissenschaften Zu Leipzig 23:652, 1871.
23. Brouha L, Radford EP Jr: The cardiovascular system in muscular activity. In Johnson W (ed.): Science and Medicine of Exercise and Sports, p. 178. New York, Harper, 1960.
24. Butrous GS, Cockrane T, Camm AJ: Rapid autonomic tone regulation of atrioventricular nodal conduction in man. Am Heart J 113:934, 1987.
25. Callaghan F, Camerlo J, Tarjan P: The ventricular depolarization gradient: exercise performance of a closed-loop rate-responsive pacemaker (Abstract). PACE 10:1212, 1987.
26. Cammilli L, Alcidi L, Papeschi G: A new pacemaker autoregulating the rate of pacing in relation to metabolic needs. In Watanabe Y (ed.): Proceedings of the Vth International Symposium, Tokyo, pp. 414–419. Amsterdam, Excerpta Medica, 1976.
27. Cammilli L, Alcidi L, Shapland E, et al.: Results, problems and perspectives with the autoregulating pacemaker. PACE 6:488, 1983.
28. Cammilli L, Alcidi L, Papeschi G, et al.: Blood pH as a signal for rate responsive pacemaker. PACE 10:1209, 1987.
29. Chirife R: Evaluation of systolic time interval as physiologic signals for rate responsive pacing (Abstract). PACE 10:1209, 1987.
30. Clarke M, Allen A: Rate-responsive atrial pacing resulting in pacemaker syndrome (Abstract). PACE 10:1209, 1987.
31. Cohen TJ: A theoretical right atrial pressure feedback heart rate control system to restore physiologic control to the rate-limited heart. PACE 7:671, 1984.
32. Cummin ARC, Iyawe VI, Mehta N, et al.: Ventilation and cardiac output during the onset of exercise, and during voluntary hyperventilation, in humans. J Physiol 370:567, 1986.
33. Donaldson RM, Fox K, Rickards AF: Initial experience with a physiological, rate responsive pacemaker. Br Med J 286:667, 1983.
34. Erlebacher JA, Danner RL, Stelzer PE: Hypotension with ventricular pacing. An atrial vasodepressor reflex in human beings. J Am Coll Cardiol 4:550, 1984.
35. Fananapazir L, Bennett DH, Faragher EB: Contribution of heart rate to QT interval shortening during exercise. Eur Heart J 4:265, 1983.
36. Fananapazir L, Rodemaker M, Bennett DH: Reliability of the evoked response in determining the paced ventricular rate and performance of the QT or rate responsive (TX) Pacemaker. PACE 8:701, 1985.
37. Fearnot NE, Smith HJ: Six components of intracardiac temperature-based rate modulated pacing (Abstract). PACE 10:1211, 1987.
38. Fearnot N, Lee Evans M: A second generation algorithm for temperature-based rate modulated pacing (abstract). PACE 10:1211, 1987.
39. Ferrer I: The sick sinus syndrome. Circulation 47:635, 1973.

40. Fromer M, Kappenberger L, Steinbrunn W: Binodal disease: diseased sinus node and atrioventricular block. Z. Kardiol, 72:410, 1983.
41. Funke HD: Ein Herschrittmacher mit belastung sabhangiger Frequenzregulation. Biomed Tech (Berlin) 20:225, 1975.
42. Furman S: Arrhythmias of dual chamber pacemakers (Editorial). PACE 5:469, 1982.
43. Fyfe T, Robinson JF: Failure of Quintech TX pacemaker caused by loss of stimulus–T interval shortening during exercise. Br Heart J 56:391, 1986.
44. Goldreyer BN, Olive AL, Leslie J, et al.: A new orthogonal lead for P synchronous pacing. PACE 4:638, 1981.
45. Greenberg B, Chatterjee K, Parmley WW, et al.: The influence of left ventricular filling pressure on atrial contribution to cardiac output. Am Heart J 98:742, 1979.
46. Griffin JC, Jutzy KR, Claude JP, et al.: Central body temperature as a guide to optimal heart rate. PACE 6:498, 1983.
47. Hermansen L, Ekblom B, Saltin B: Cardiac output during submaximal and maximal treadmill and bicycle exercise. J Appl Physiol 29:82, 1973.
48. Humen DP, Kostuk WJ, Klein GJ: Activity-sensing, rate responsive pacing: improvement in myocardial performance with exercise. PACE 8:52, 1985.
49. Ionescu VL: An on-demand pacemaker responsive to respiration rate (Abstract). PACE 3:375, 1980.
50. Jolgren D, Fearnot N, Geddes L: A rate-responsive pacemaker controlled by right ventricular temperature. PACE 7:794, 1984.
51. Jones PW, French W, Weissman ML: Ventilatory response to cardiac output changes in patients with pacemakers. J Physiol Resp Environ Exerc Physiol 5:1103, 1981.
52. Kappenberger LJ, Herpers L: Rate responsive dual chamber pacing. PACE 9:987, 1986.
53. Karlof I: Haemodynamic effect of atrial triggered versus fixed rate pacing at rest and during exercise in complete heart block. Acta Med Scand 197:195, 1975.
54. Kingwell S, Lau CP, Butrous GS, et al.: Myopotential interference in rate responsive pacemakers (Abstract). PACE 10:1225, 1987.
55. Klein H, Olive A, Pederson B, et al.: The pre-ejection interval: a reliable biosensor for rate-responsive pacing (Abstract). PACE 10:1215, 1987.
56. Knudson MB, Amundson DC, Mosharrafa M: Hemodynamic demand pacing. In Barold SS, Mugica J (eds.): The Third Decade in Cardiac Pacing: Advances in Technology and Clinical Applications, pp. 249–264. New York, Futura Publishing Co., 1982.
57. Koyal SN, Whipp BJ, Huntsman D, et al.: Ventilatory responses to the metabolic acidosis of treadmill and cycle ergometry. J Appl Physiol 40:864, 1976.
58. Krasner JL, Voukydis PC, Nardella PC: A physiologically controlled cardiac pacemaker. J Assoc Adv Med Instrum 1:14, 1966.
59. Kristensson B-E, Arnman K, Ryden L: The haemodynamic importance of atrioventricular synchrony and rate increase at rest and during exercise. Eur Heart J 6:773, 1985.
60. Kristensson B, Arnman K, Smedgard P, et al.: Physiological versus single-rate ventricular pacing. A double-blind cross-over study. PACE 8:73, 1985.
61. Kruse I, Arnman K, Conradson TB, et al.: A comparison of the acute and long-term hemodynamic effects of ventricular inhibited and atrial synchronous ventricular inhibited pacing. Circulation 65:846, 1982.
62. Laczkovics A, Schlick W, Losert U, et al.: The use of central venous blood temperature (CVT) as a guide for rate control in pacemaker therapy (abstract). PACE 6:46, 1983.
63. Laczkovics A, Laufer G, Ohner T, et al.: First clinical results with a temperature guided rate responsive pacemaker (Abstract). PACE 10:1216, 1987.
64. Mehta DM, Lau CP, Mehta DM, Ward DE, et al.: Comparative evaluation of chronotropic responses of QT sensing and activity sensing rate responsive pacemakers. PACE 11:1405, 1988a.
65. Lau CP, Ritchie D, Butrous GS, et al.: Rate modulation by arm movements of the respiratory dependent rate responsive pacemaker. PACE 11:744, 1988.
66. Lau CP, Camm AJ, Ward DE: A severe case of myopotential interference in a patient with a respiration dependent rate modulated pacemaker. Int J Cardiol, 17:98, 1987.
67. Lau CP, Stott JRR, Toff WD, et al.: Selective vibration sensing: A new concept for activity sensing rate responsive pacing. PACE 11:1299, 1988a.
68. Lau CP, Tse·WS, Kingwell S, et al.: Clinical experience with Sensolog: A new activity sensing rate responsive pacemaker. PACE 11:1444, 1988b.
69. Lau CP, Mehta D, Toff WD, et al.: Limitations of rate response of an activity sensing rate responsive pacemaker to different forms of activity. PACE 10:141, 1988c.
70. Lau CP, Ward DE, Camm AJ: Rate responsive pacing by a pacemaker that detects the respiratory rate (Biorate): Clinical advantages and complications. Clin Cardiol 11:318, 1988d.
71. Lau CP, Antoniou A, Ward DE, et al.: Initial clinical experience with a minute ventilation sensing rate responsive pacemaker: improvements in exercise capacity and symptomatology. PACE 11:1815, 1988e.
72. Lien WP, Lee YS, Chang FZ, et al.: The sick sinus syndrome (natural history of dysfunction of the sinoatrial node). Chest 72:628, 1977.
73. Lindemans FW, Rankin IR, Murtaugh R, et al.: Clinical experience with an activity sensing pacemaker. PACE 9:978, 1986.
74. Lipkin DP, Buller N, Frenneaux M, et al.: Randomised crossover trial of rate responsive Activitrax and conventional fixed rate ventricular pacing. Br Heart J 58:613, 1987.
75. Maisch B, Langenfeld H: Rate adaptive pacing—clinical experience with three different pacing systems. PACE 9:997, 1986.
76. Matula M, Alt E, Theres H, et al.: A new mechanical sensor for the detection of body activity and posture suitable for rate responsive pacing (Abstract). PACE 10:1221, 1987.
77. Mehta D, Gilmore S, Lau CP, et al.: Is the optimal atrioventricular delay the same at rest and during exercise? An assessment in patients with dual chamber pacemakers (Abstract). Br Heart J 59:93, 1988.
78. Nappholtz T, Valenta H, Maloney J, et al.: Electrode configurations for rate responsive pacing. PACE 9:960, 1986.
79. Nathan D, Center S, Wu C, et al.: An implantable synchronous pacemaker for the long-term correction of complete heart block. Am J Cardiol 11:362, 1963.
80. Occhetta E, Prando MD, Perucca A, et al.: Respiratory pacemaker dysfunction: 4 years follow up. In Santini M, Pistolese M, Alliegro A (eds.): Progress in Clinical Pacing, pp. 77–79. Rome: Centro Editoriale Publicitario Italiano, 1986.
81. Olive AL, Pederson BD, Salo RW, et al.: Relative stroke volume (SV) and contractility (CONT) as sensors for rate responsive pacing (Abstract). PACE 10:1223, 1987.
82. Oseroff O, Klementowicz P, Andrews C, et al.: Indications for permanent mode change during DDD pacing (Abstract). PACE 10:1224, 1987.
83. Prior M, Masterson M, Wilkoff B, et al.: Classification of chronotropic incompetence in patients with sinus node dysfunction for requiring a permanent pacemaker (Abstract). PACE 10:1225, 1987.
84. Ramsdale DR, Charles RG: Rate-responsive ventricular pacing: clinical experience with the RS4-SRT pacing system. PACE 8:378, 1985.
85. Ricci D, Orlick A, Alderman E: Role of tachycardia as an inotropic stimulus in man. J Clin Invest 63:695, 1979.
86. Rickards AF, Akhras F, Baron DW: Effects of heart rate on QT interval. In Meere C (ed.): Proceedings of the VIth World Symposium on Cardiac Pacing, pp. 2–7. Montreal, PACE-SYMP, 1979.
87. Rickards AF, Norman J: Relation between QT interval and heart rate. New design of physiologically adaptive cardiac pacemaker. Br Heart J 45:56, 1981.
88. Rossi P, Plicchi G, Canducci G, et al.: Respiratory rate as a determinant of optimal pacing rate. PACE 6:502, 1983.
89. Rossi P, Plicchi G, Canducci G, et al.: Respiration as a reliable physiological sensor for the control of cardiac pacing rate. Br Heart J 51:7, 1984.
90. Rossi P, Rognoni G, Occhetta E, et al.: Respiration-dependent

ventricular pacing compared with fixed ventricular and atrial-ventricular synchronous pacing: Aerobic and hemodynamic variables. J Am Coll Cardiol 6:646, 1985.
91. Ruiter J, Burgersdij K, Zeeders M, et al.: Atrial Activitrax pacing: The atrioventricular interval during exercise (Abstract). PACE 10:1226, 1987.
92. Sahakian AV, Tompkins WJ, Webster JG: Electrode motion artefacts in electrical impedance pneumography. IEEE Trans Bio-Med Eng 32:448, 1985.
93. Salo RW, Pederson BD, Olive AL, et al.: Continuous ventricular volume assessment for diagnosis and pacemaker control. PACE 7:1267, 1984.
94. Samet P, Castillo C, Bernstein WH: Haemodynamic sequelae of atrial, ventricular and sequential atrioventricular pacing in cardiac patients. Am Heart J 72:725, 1966.
95. Sarma JSM, Sarma RJ, Bilitch M: An exponential formula for heart rate dependence of QT interval during exercise and cardiac pacing in humans: Reevaluation of Bazett's formula. Am J Cardiol 54:103, 1984.
96. Seger JJ, Edelman SK, O'Driscoll P: Comparison of the Nova MR temperature-sensing pacemaker and activity rate responsive pacing (Abstract). PACE 10:1227, 1987.
97. Sellers TD, Fearnot N, Dilorenzo D, et al.: Right ventricular blood temperature change during daily activity: Implication for rate responsive pacing (Abstract). PACE 9:286, 1986.
98. Sellers TD, Fearnot N, Smith HJ, et al.: Right ventricular blood temperature profiles for rate responsive pacing. PACE 10:467, 1987.
99. Sellers TD, Fearnot N, Boal B, et al.: Clinical experience and follow-up of a temperature-based rate modulating pacemaker. A multicenter experience of the US Kelvin implants (Abstract). PACE 10:1227, 1987.
100. Sharma AD, Yee R, Bennett T, et al.: The effects of ventricular pacing on right ventricular maximum positive dp/dt: Implications for a rate-responsive pacing system based on this parameter (Abstract). PACE 10:1228, 1987.
101. Smedgard P, Kristensson BE, Kruse I, et al.: Rate responsive pacing by means of activity sensing versus single rate ventricular pacing: a double-blind cross-over study. PACE 10:902, 1987.
102. Fananapazir L, Bennett DH, Monks P: Atrial synchronized ventricular pacing: contribution of the chronotropic response to improved exercise performance. PACE 6:601, 1983.
103. Stangl K, Wirtzfeld A, Heinze H, et al.: Activitrax pacemaker: Physiological rate response with a nonphysiological sensor? In Sartini M, Pistolese M, Alliegro A (eds.): Progress in Clinical Pacing, pp. 124–132. Rome, Centro Editoriale Publicitario Italiano, 1986.
104. Stangl K, Wirtzfeld A, Gobl G, et al.: Development of multisensor-catheter recording mixed venous oxygen saturation, blood temperature and stroke volume. In Sartini M, Pistolese M, Alliegro A (eds.): Progress in Clinical Pacing, pp. 117–123. Rome, Centro Editoriale Publicitario Italiano, 1986.
105. Stangl K, Wirtzfeld A, Lochschmidt O, et al.: Erst klinische erfahrungen mit einem neuen akivitåtsgesteuerten Schrittmachersystem (Sensolog 703)—Vergleich mit dem Activitrax. Herz-Schrittmacher 7:146, 1987.
106. Sutton R: Physiological cardiac pacing. In Meere C (ed.): Proceedings of the VIth World Symposium on Cardiac Pacing, pp. 16–17. Montreal, PACESYMP, 1979.
107. Sutton R, Sharma A, Ingram A, et al.: First-derivative of right ventricular pressure as a sensor for an implantable rate responsive VVI pacemaker (Abstract). PACE 10:1210, 1987.
108. Toff WD, Leeks C, Joy M, et al.: The effect of aircraft vibration on the function of an activity-sensing pacemaker (Abstract). Br Heart J 57:573, 1987.
109. Travill C, Ingram A, Vardas P, et al.: Inadequate rate response of a stimulus–T sensing pacemaker (Abstract). PACE 10:1231, 1987.
110. Valenta H Jr, Nappholz T, Maloney J, et al.: Correlation of heart rate with an intravenous impedance, respiratory sensor. Biomed Sci Instr 22:7, 1986.
111. Wasserman K, Whipp BJ, Koyal SN, et al.: Anaerobic threshold and respiratory gas exchange during exercise. J Appl Physiol 35:236, 1973.
112. Webb SC, Lewis L, Morris-Thurgood JA, et al.: A comparative assessment of rate-responsive pacemakers (Abstract). PACE 10:1232, 1987.
113. Webb SC, Lewis LM, Morris-Thurgood JA, et al.: Rate responsive pacing: Is there already a dual sensor system? (Abstract). Br Heart J 57:585, 1987.
114. Weisswange A, Csapo G, Perach W: Frequenzsteuerung von Schrittmachern durch Bluttemperatur Verh (Abstract). Deutsch Ges Kreislaufforsch 44:152, 1978.
115. Wilkoff BL, Shimokochi DD, Schaal SF: Pacing rate increase due to application of steady external pressure on an activity sensing pacemaker (Abstract). PACE 10:423, 1987.
116. Winter UJ, Behrenbeck DW, Hoher M, et al.: Problems beider slope-Einstellung und der Frequenzanpassung in frequenzvariablen Schrittmachern: Oszillationsphanomene und plotzliche Frequenzlinbruche. Herzschrittmacher 5:50, 1985.
117. Wirtzfeld AL, Goedel-Meinen L, Bock T, et al.: Central venous oxygen saturation for the control of automatic rate responsive pacing. Circulation 64(Suppl IV):299, 1981.
118. Wirtzfeld A, Heinze R, Liess HD, et al.: An active optical sensor for monitoring mixed venous oxygen-saturation for an implantable rate-regulating pacing system. PACE 6:494, 1983.
119. Zegelman M, Cieslinski G, Kreuzer J, et al.: QT-related pacing—point of view after 36 implantations in 4 years (Abstract). PACE 10:1234, 1987.
120. Lau CP, Butrous G, Ward DE, et al.: Comparison of exercise performance of six rate-adaptive right ventricular cardiac pacemakers. Am J Cardiol 63:833, 1989.
121. Boute W, Gebhardt U, Begemann MJS: Introduction of an automatic QT interval driven rate responsive pacemaker. PACE 11:1804, 1988.
122. Lau CP, Ward DE, Camm AJ: Single chamber cardiac pacing with two forms of respiration-controlled rate responsive pacemakers. Chest 95:352, 1989.

31

Hemodynamic Effects of Cardiac Arrhythmias and Pacemakers

Sanjeev Saksena

Overview

Changes in cardiac rhythm can be highly symptomatic and can contribute to major cardiac events. Symptoms can be related primarily to the electrical disturbance, but the more common mechanism underlying both effects is the mechanical sequelae of the cardiac arrhythmia. These result in altered hemodynamic states that produce symptoms and cardio-circulatory disturbances. The clinical effects of heart rate and rhythm have often been mentioned in ancient medical writings. The relationship between the circulation of blood and cardiac rhythm was commented upon by William Harvey in the seventeenth century.[1] Extensive experimental and clinical investigations have been undertaken since the beginning of this century. Thomas Lewis[2] observed changes in blood pressure and cardiac output with the development of atrial fibrillation in experimental studies. The earliest clinical reports on "Stokes-Adams' disease" commented on the association of "epileptiform" attacks, "cardiac asthma," angina pectoris, and "heart shock" with a slow heart rhythm.[3] The development in the last three decades of artificial cardiac pacemakers designed to correct bradyarrhythmias has also resulted in a plethora of iatrogenic cardiac rhythms. It is the purpose of this chapter to review the physiologic basis for the hemodynamic effects of different spontaneous and artificial cardiac rhythms.

Physiologic Effects of Heart Rate and Rhythm

A major determinant of circulatory stability and tissue perfusion is the systemic arterial pressure. Systemic arterial pressure is determined by cardiac output and peripheral vascular resistance. Cardiac output, in turn, is dependent on heart rate and stroke volume. Alterations in cardiac output are frequent and permit the cardiovascular system to meet the changing demands of the human body. The primary mechanism to obtain this responsiveness is the ability to change heart rate. Secondary mechanisms include alterations in stroke volume and peripheral vascular tone. Physiologic increases in circulatory demands such as those seen during exercise are met largely by an increase in heart rate and, to a lesser extent, by increased stroke volume and decreased peripheral resistance. Sinus tachycardia is accompanied by abbreviation of ventricular diastole, and thus filling time. Although this could reduce preload, and secondarily stroke volume, this effect is offset by the maintenance of the rapid filling phase in early diastole and atrial systole and enhanced venous return due to mechanical effects of muscular activity. These effects, coupled along with increased sympathetic activity enhancing cardiac contractility, help to maintain and even augment stroke volume.[4-7] Echocardiographic studies in humans confirm a progressive decrease in end-diastolic and end-systolic left ventricular dimensions with increase in atrial rate from 50 to 150 beats per minute (bpm) with a constant shortening fraction.[8] Cardiac output thus rises, due to a major increase in heart rate. The model of exercise-induced hemodynamic changes is a useful one to dissect the involved parameters, which are common to the physiologic effects of other cardiac rhythms.

Stroke volume dependence on left ventricular filling has been well established in experimental and clinical studies.[4,5] Factors influencing left ventricular filling include preload, diastolic filling time, left ventricular compliance, and atrioventricular synchrony. Decreasing preload and filling time and impaired compliance passively reduce left ventricular filling and thus stroke volume. The atrial contribution to left ventricular filling has been referred to as a "booster pump" and is an active mechanism to enhance left ventricular filling and, secondarily, stroke volume.[9] Gilmore and coworkers[10] demonstrated the importance of atrial filling to ventricular stroke volume in experimental studies and related it to the sequence of atrioventricular contraction. They also noted the role of the specialized conduction system in mediating an optimal sequence of ventricular mechanical contraction, commenting that altered sequence of depolarization may also reduce ventricular stroke volume. Early observations by Wiggers and Meijler as well as subsequent studies on artificial ventricular pacing support a secondary role for this factor.[11-17]

In canine studies, depression of ventricular function is noted with shortening of the interval between atrial and ventricular systole even prior to loss of atrioventricular synchrony. Ventricular pacing without atrioventricular synchrony compounds this deterioration in left ventricular function initially by loss of atrioventricular synchrony. It has also been suggested that left ventricular apical pacing sites have more favorable effects with respect to peak left ventricular pressure and dp/dt developed in an isorhythmic left ventricle than right ventricular apical or basal left ventricular and right ventricular locations.[13] In other studies, the role of this factor has been questioned.[18, 19] Samet and coworkers[19] noted that development of bundle branch block or ventricular premature beats did not necessarily produce mechanical ventricular asynchrony. Clinical studies have been limited but confirm that mechanical ventricular asynchrony does not necessarily result from bundle branch block[20]; however, in individual patients this may be observed.[21] In contrast, ventricular premature beats often produce mechanical ventricular asynchrony.[14] The mechanical consequences of asynchronous contraction can be of varying importance and are often influenced to a great extent by preload, rate, end-diastolic volume, and afterload. This issue will be examined in greater detail in a later section in this chapter dealing with ventricular tachycardia.

The role of atrial contribution to cardiac output has been examined in normal and disease states.[22-26] It is important to understand the varying significance of this factor as a function of overall cardiac status, since this may be a key issue in individual patients. Even in normal subjects, atrial or atrioventricular sequential pacing is associated with improved cardiac output, compared to ventricular pacing at identical rates.[22] This contribution is, however, probably smaller than that observed in certain disease states. Clinical studies have reported variable results on the value of atrial contribution to cardiac output in disease states. Initial reports were contradictory,[9, 23, 27] but physiologic studies in humans have clarified the issues. Greenberg and coworkers[26] examined the relationship between absolute left ventricular filling pressure and the atrial contribution to cardiac output in chronic disease states. Data derived from their studies and inferences with respect to the role of end-diastolic volume suggest that atrial transport is particularly important in patients with chronic heart disease, normal or minimally elevated left ventricular end-diastolic pressure, normal or mildly increased left ventricular end-diastolic volume, and decreased left ventricular compliance.[26, 28] The relative value of atrial filling declines in patients with high left ventricular end-diastolic pressures and markedly increased end-diastolic volumes. In acute myocardial infarction, atrial contribution to left ventricular stroke volume is significant in patients with and without depressed cardiac index and elevated left ventricular end-diastolic volume.[9] In contrast, many patients with primary electrical disturbances such as chronic complete heart block usually have minimal or chronic heart disease with well-preserved left ventricular function, near-normal end-diastolic volume, and absence of congestive heart failure.[29] Atrial synchrony significantly enhances cardiac output in these patients.[29-30] Thus, in analyzing the hemodynamic consequences of dysrhythmias or artificial cardiac pacing in individual patients, the importance of several baseline hemodynamic and disease variables needs to be carefully assessed. These influence the outcome of the rhythm disturbance to a profound extent and determine its clinical sequelae.

Hemodynamic Effects of Bradyarrhythmias

SINUS BRADYCARDIA

The hemodynamic consequences of sinus bradycardia are related primarily to the slow ventricular rate. Ventricular filling is well preserved in most instances, and an adequate or enhanced stroke volume may be present in patients with normal ventricular function. Symptoms are uncommon in patients with resting sinus bradycardia due to lower perfusion demands at rest. Samet[18] reported an average resting cardiac index in one series of patients at 1.9 L/min/m². Similar observations are applicable to patients with atrial fibrillation and conduction system disease with slow ventricular response and good left ventricular function. The response of the sinus rate (or AV conduction, in the case of atrial fibrillation) to exercise usually determines symptomatology. Inadequate heart rate response elicits symptoms of low cardiac output relative to body demands. Easy fatigability, limited exercise tolerance, or even near syncope or syncope at exercise can be observed. In contrast, an adequate response to exercise may be observed in asymptomatic individuals. Figure 31–1 shows electrocardiographic recordings obtained from a 49-year-old asymptomatic executive with coronary artery disease at rest and during exercise. Note that the absence of symptoms can be explained by the good exercise response and absence of myocardial disease. In contrast, patients with poor left ventricular function and congestive heart failure tolerate sinus bradycardia poorly. Symptoms of low cardiac output are common at rest and can be profound in the absence of a heart rate response during exercise.

Sinus bradycardia and arrest can also be a secondary manifestation of vagal stimulation. It can be associated

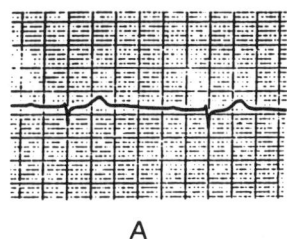
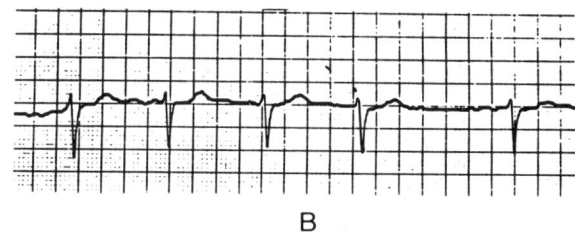
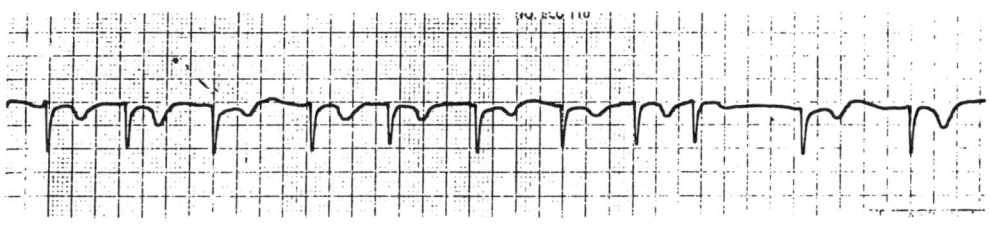

FIGURE 31–1
A, Resting ECG in 1985 of an asymptomatic man with severe sinus bradycardia and first degree atrioventricular block. B, Resting ECG in 1988 of the same patient, showing progression to atrial fibrillation with a slow ventricular rate. C, Exercise ECG in 1988 of the same patient, showing that exercise resulted in acceleration of ventricular rate, precluding significant symptoms of low cardiac output.

with hypotension in normal individuals due to the bradycardia which is accompanied by a loss of peripheral vasomotor tone. Myocardial infarction, particularly inferior wall injury, is associated with this disorder. In this situation, poor left ventricular compliance and depressed systolic function aggravate reduced cardiac output due to the bradycardia.[28] Symptomatic hypotension is common and is usually vagally mediated. Reversal with atropine injection is common and advisable. Failure of atropine response may necessitate temporary transvenous pacing to support heart rate and blood pressure.

ATRIOVENTRICULAR BLOCK

Hemodynamic consequences of atrioventricular block are due to two major pathophysiologic mechanisms. The effects of bradycardia are largely akin to those observed with sinus node dysfunction. These have been detailed in the prior section. In second- and third-degree atrioventricular block, these are compounded by varying atrioventricular relationships. Absence of 1:1 sequential atrioventricular contraction impairs ventricular filling. However, stroke volume is usually preserved, due to prolonged diastole, and may even be increased. The heart rate response to exercise or other stress is usually impaired because of impaired atrioventricular conduction.[32, 33] In specific clinical syndromes (e.g., congenital complete heart block), the lower pacemaker can exhibit a good exercise response and minimize symptoms.[34] Cardiac output in these patients is relatively normal, as are intracardiac pressures.[35] In contrast, elevation of atrial pressures with cannon "a" waves, in conjunction with depressed cardiac output and reduced systemic arterial pressures, are often observed in older patients, particularly when acquired myocardial disease is present.

The effects of alteration in ventricular rate by pacing in complete heart block have been extensively examined. Asynchronous ventricular pacing at rates between 40 and 120 bpm resulted in an increase in cardiac output in two of every three patients studied in one report.[36] Peak cardiac outputs were generally observed at heart rates of 80 to 105 bpm. Stroke volume decreased with increasing ventricular rate in all patients, but this decline was more than offset by the increased heart rate; however, cardiac output did not increase in direct proportion to heart rate for this reason. In another report,[37] atrial synchronous pacing increased cardiac output by 10% in patients with complete heart block. However, ventricular rate was also increased by pacing in this study. Benchimol and coworkers[38] demonstrated that atrioventricular synchrony improved systemic arterial pressure and left ventricular ejection indices in patients with heart block over a wide range of heart rates (20 to 125 bpm). Figure 31–2 is an example of these observations. The second ventricular paced beat is preceded by an appropriately atrial systole and systolic arterial pressure is markedly improved. There is no significant change in pulmonary arterial pressures. The maximal contribution of atrial synchrony was observed at rates of 50 to 80 bpm. These data support the use of atrial synchronous pacemakers for treatment of complete and second-degree atrioventricular block.

Hemodynamic Effects of Tachyarrhythmias

SUPRAVENTRICULAR TACHYCARDIA (SVT)

A variety of supraventricular tachyarrhythmias can be examined for hemodynamic consequences. Pathophysiologically they can be divided into macroreentrant mechanisms, such as atrioventricular reentrant tachycardia in the Wolff-Parkinson-White (WPW) syndrome, localized reentry (e.g., atrioventricular nodal

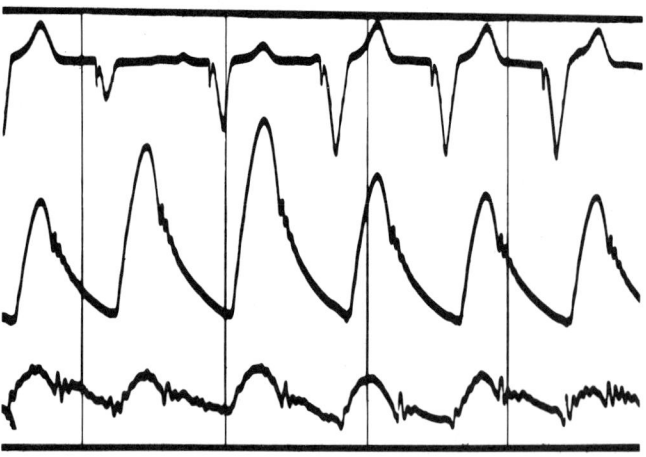

FIGURE 31-2
Ventricular pacing (50 mm/s) in a patient with atrioventricular block: The upper trace is ECG lead V_1, the middle trace is systemic arterial pressure, and the lower trace is pulmonary arterial pressure. Note that the demand ventricular pacing, when clearly preceded by an atrial contraction (third pressure waveform), shows a significantly higher systemic arterial pressure compared to subsequent paced leads that are not preceded by atrial systole. Minimal change is noted in pulmonary arterial pressures.

reentry), atrial flutter, atrial fibrillation, and ectopic atrial tachycardia. The hemodynamic consequences are determined by factors similar to those described earlier, as well as some specific to these arrhythmias. Common factors include heart rate, preload, afterload, atrioventricular relationships, and presence of coexisting cardiac disease. Specific additional factors include the effects of autonomic tone, posture, and valvular function. The role of altered ventricular contraction patterns in the WPW syndrome remains to be examined. Experimental observations are derived largely from pacing studies in anesthetized and, to a lesser extent, conscious animals, and have major limitations in mimicking clinical SVT. Clinical studies are scanty and are lacking particularly in detailed examination of all potential factors affecting the observations.

The classic macroreentrant model for SVT (i.e., atrioventricular reentrant tachycardia in the WPW syndrome) has been studied to a limited extent. It provides a useful model for examining the aforementioned hemodynamic factors. The onset of reentrant SVT in patients is characterized by a small or moderate decline in systolic arterial pressure, with a more limited change in diastolic pressure and a narrower pulse pressure (Fig. 31-3A and B). A significant decline in stroke volume is offset by the increased heart rate to help maintain cardiac output at resting levels, at low normal or mildly depressed levels. It is important to realize that this output is strikingly below expected levels for that heart rate. The onset of SVT is accompanied in some other patients by a decline in systemic arterial pressure, which may recover completely due to increase in peripheral vascular resistance (Fig. 31-4). Alternatively, the tachycardia rate may increase during the course of the episode due to shortening of refractoriness in the tachycardia circuit, producing more pronounced hemodynamic effects after maintenance of the arrhythmia.

The major mechanisms responsible for decline in stroke volume during SVT include abbreviation of diastolic filling time, due to the heart rate, and loss of sequential atrioventricular contraction. AV reentry is thus characterized by little change in left and right ventricular end-diastolic pressure, with an increase in atrial pressures. Unfortunately, in many instances this increased atrial pressure does not translate into improved ventricular filling, due to the timing of atrial contraction secondary to a retrograde P wave. This P wave follows the QRS complex by 100 to 200 ms and may or may not encounter ventricular relaxation. Thus, atrial contraction may occur against partially or completely closed atrioventricular valves, resulting in cannon "a" waves. Mean atrial pressure is further raised by atrioventricular valvular regurgitation that may occur at the onset of ventricular contraction due to the position of the atrioventricular valve leaflets. Tricuspid and mitral valvular regurgitation has been documented and, especially at rapid heart rates, diminishes forward stroke volume and increases mean left and right atrial pressure. Progressive increase in atrial cannon waves also may be due to more forceful atrial contraction as a result of these increased pressures. This, in turn, contributes to symptoms of pulmonary congestion and increased pulmonary capillary wedge pressures, with head and neck pulsations due to cannon "a" waves. This tenuous situation with respect to ventricular filling may be aggravated by a change in posture. Upright posture particularly has been characterized by a fall in blood pressure associated with symptoms due to loss of preload. Waxman and associates[41] noted that hypotension at the initiation of SVT results in sympathetic stimulation to elevate systemic arterial pressure. In some instances this can exceed the resting arterial pressure and result in a vagal discharge that terminates SVT. This effect is most common in the supine as compared to the upright or Trendelenburg positions.[42, 43] The former blunts the sympathetic mediated pressure increase while the latter blunts the initial hypotension. Enhanced peripheral vascular resistance due to sympathetic stimulation may or may not affect these orthostatic changes. Pulsus alternans has been noted.[39] Respiration may also significantly alter filling, and respiratory variations in pulse and blood pressure have been documented.[39, 42]

In patients with atrioventricular nodal reentrant tachycardia, a significant (>30%) decline in systolic brachial artery pressure with a similar (37.5%) decrease in cardiac index was documented during SVT despite a major increase (132%) in heart rate. Pulmonary artery systolic and diastolic pressures rose, as did right atrial pressures in most patients. Fusion of atrial A and V waves was noted, due to simultaneous atrial and ventricular contraction without change in left ventricular end-diastolic pressures (see Fig. 31-4). The role of AV valvular regurgitation remains unsettled in this rhythm. Atrial distention can initiate a vasodepressor response mediated by atrial stretch receptor stimulation,[44] and this can result in peripheral

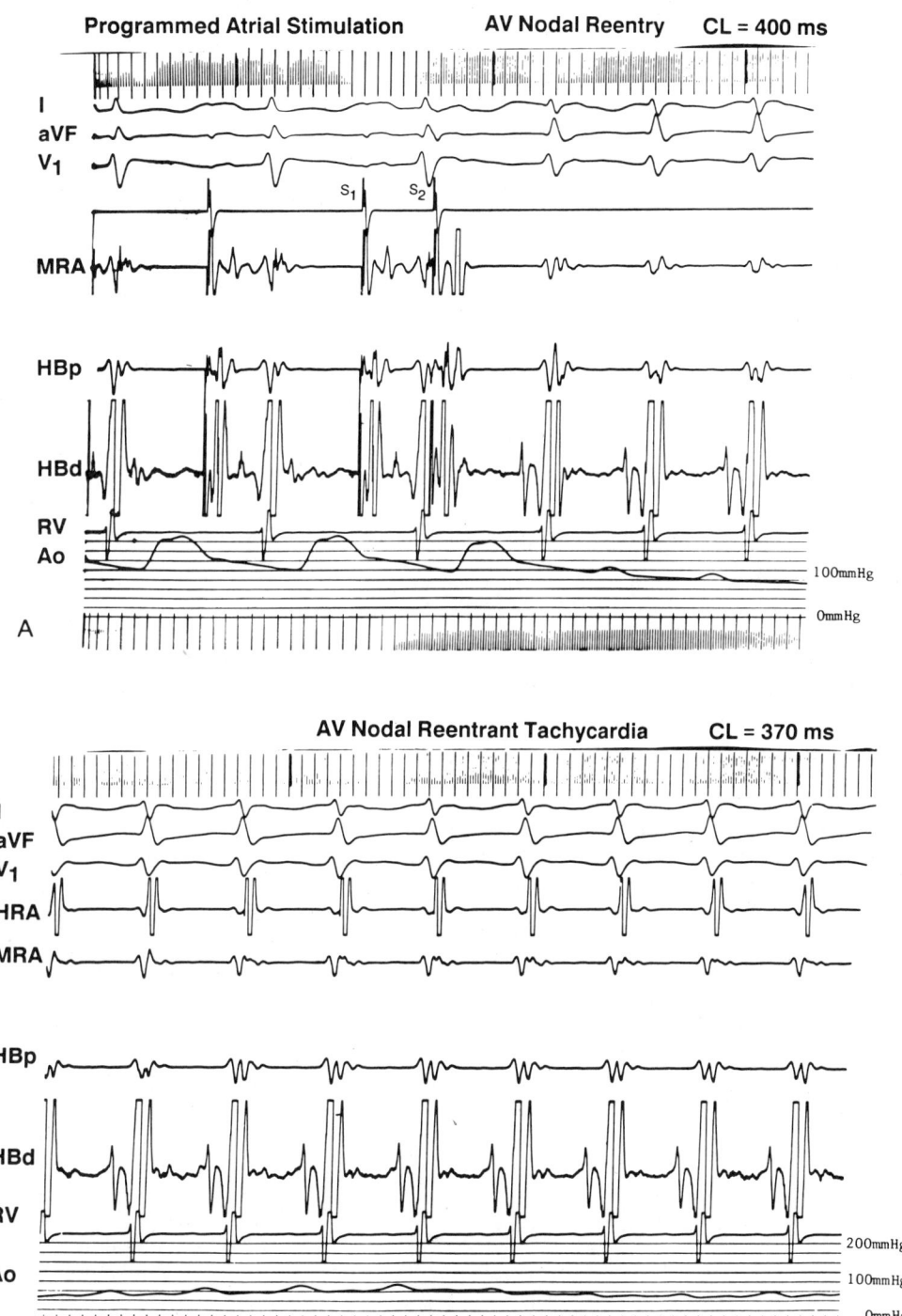

FIGURE 31-3
A, Induction of AV nodal reentrant tachycardia during an electrophysiologic study. ECG leads I, aVF, and V₁ are displayed, along with intracardiac atrial His bundle and ventricular electrograms for simultaneous aortic pressure recordings. Note that programmed atrial extrastimulation induces AV nodal reentrant tachycardia (type I) with a cycle length of 400 ms. Retrograde atrial activation during the tachycardia occurs simultaneously with ventricular systole. Marked decline in systemic arterial blood pressure is apparent.

B, Persistence of hypotension during sustained AV nodal reentrant tachycardia in the same patient as in A. Note that the systolic arterial pressure has declined from 170 mm Hg to 60 mm Hg.

Abbreviations: HRA = high right atrium; MRA = mid right atrium; HBp = proximal His bundle electrogram; HBd = distal His bundle electrogram; RV = right ventricular electrogram; AO = aortic pressure. The heavy vertical line marker at the top of the tracing represents 1-s interval. CL = cycle length.

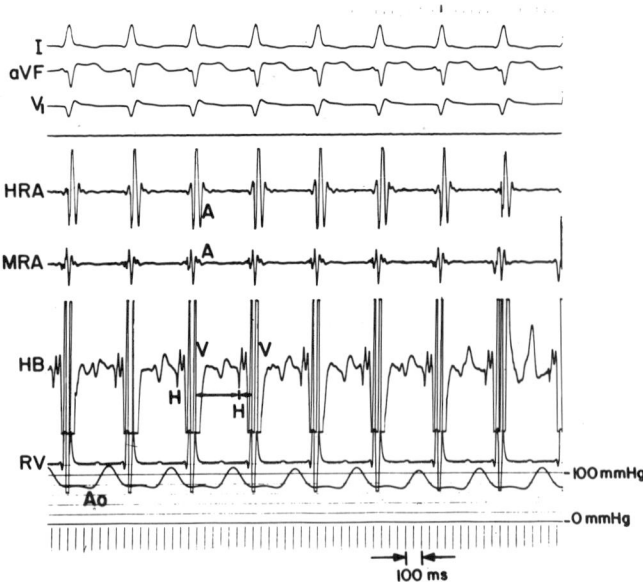

FIGURE 31-4
Maintenance of systemic arterial blood pressure in another patient with type I AV nodal reentrant tachycardia. This patient has a tachycardia with a cycle length similar to that of the patient shown in Figure 31-3; however, systolic arterial blood pressure has been maintained at 110 mm Hg by sympathetic stimulation. Note that retrograde atrial activation occurs simultaneously with ventricular systole. For abbreviations, see legend of Figure 31-3.

vasodilatation. Additional phenomena described in supraventricular tachycardia include polyuria. Clinical observations characterizing this association have been frequent, but the mechanism was unknown until recently.[45, 46] Atrial natriuretic peptide is released from atrial cell granules in response to elevation of atrial pressure,[47–49] which results in sodium excretion with secondary water loss, inhibition of aldosterone secretion, and vasodilatation. Levels of this peptide are increased in AV nodal reentrant tachycardia but not in sinus tachycardia.[50] Chronic supraventricular tachycardia has been associated with the development of a dilated cardiomyopathy.[51] Clinical and laboratory studies document the development of left ventricular dilatation and dysfunction in chronic tachycardia.[52, 53] As a consequence of chronic rapid atrial pacing, systolic left ventricular dysfunction has been documented, and myocardial stores of creatinine phosphokinase and adenosine triphosphate were depleted.[51]

ATRIAL FLUTTER/FIBRILLATION

Mechanical effects of atrial flutter and fibrillation are determined by the ventricular rate and the extent of the atrial contribution to ventricular filling in an individual patient.[54, 55] Rapid ventricular rates are associated with abbreviated diastolic filling, lower preload, and thus stroke volume. Increased cardiac work secondary to this rate, particularly in the presence of coronary artery disease with resulting ischemia, may further impair cardiac output. Antegrade coronary blood flow has been shown to decrease in experimental studies.[56] Contractions are present in atrial flutter and flutter waves at rates of >250 beats per minute are seen in atrial pressure recordings. These are seen in right and left atrial pressure recordings (Fig. 31–5A and B). Thus, some degree of active atrial transport may persist in this disorder. A previous study showed decreased cardiac output during atrial flutter that improved significantly (by 40%) after conversion to sinus rhythm.[57] Atrial flutter is particularly common after cardiac surgical procedures and in chronic lung disease and is occasionally observed in acute myocardial infarction. In the latter condition, it is usually accompanied by extensive myocardial injury and has markedly deleterious effects in previously hemodynamically unstable patients.

Atrial fibrillation has similar effects but has no discernable mechanical atrial contribution. Reversion of atrial fibrillation to sinus rhythm has been reported to produce an average increase in cardiac output ranging from 11 to 140% in different studies.[58–63] The extent of increase varies from patient to patient. In a minority of patients no improvement has been noted.[63] Hemodynamic collapse in both these rhythms is usually observed either in patients with preexisting cardiac disease or at excessively rapid ventricular rates (e.g., in pre-excitation syndromes) and is an indication for direct current cardioversion.

VENTRICULAR TACHYCARDIA (VT)

Intermittent attention has been devoted to the examination of the hemodynamics associated with VT. Carl Wiggers described the altered contraction patterns associated with ectopic ventricular stimulation in experimental studies, and it was suggested that an optimal contraction pattern may be important for the generation of maximal intraventricular pressure.[64] The clinical consequences of VT were considered so dire that the presence of significant hemodynamic stability and patient survival engendered case report material.[65] Corday and coworkers[56] suggested a "benign" versus a "malignant" pattern of ventricular contractility for premature ventricular extrasystoles, based on results of apical versus basal left ventricular pacing. Early experimental studies attempted to replicate these events, using intravenous administration of epinephrine after drug-induced depression of atrioventricular and intraventricular conduction.[66] It was noted that blood pressure was occasionally well preserved even in paroxysmal ventricular tachycardia and ventricular flutter. Imaging studies in humans confirmed the variation in mechanical contraction patterns produced by premature ventricular extrasystoles and ventricular tachycardia.[14, 67–69] Left ventriculography confirmed an "hourglass" type of contraction pattern for ventricular premature beats arising in the apical left ventricle, compared to basilar stimulation, which produced a "teardrop" pattern.[14] Aortic pressure and ejection fraction were better preserved with the former than the latter. Different patterns have been described for other stimulated beats. Mitral regurgitation was observed more often with basilar origin of the premature beats.

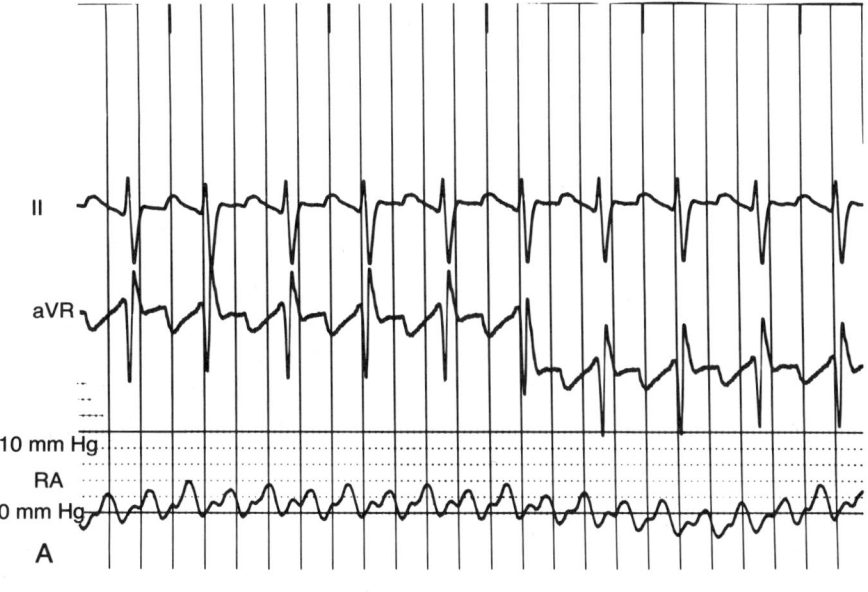

FIGURE 31–5
Pressure recordings from the right atrium (A) and left atrium (B) as seen in the wedge pressure during atrial flutter in a patient with dilated cardiomyopathy. Note the flutter waves in both recordings despite significant AV block. ECG leads II and aVR are shown. AO = aortic pressure; RA = right atrium; PCW = pulmonary capillary wedge pressure.

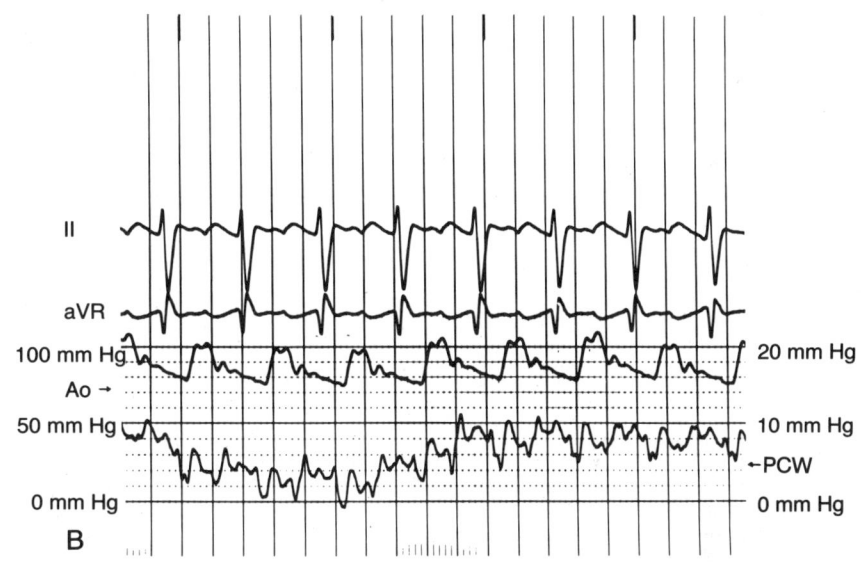

These data supported the viewpoint that site of VT origin may influence hemodynamics, and thus prognosis. Echocardiographic studies lent further credence to this view by demonstrating primary alterations in the pressure-volume relations of the left ventricle.[67] However, some experimental evidence questions the primacy of altered mechanical contraction in the hemodynamic consequences associated with ventricular premature beats and ventricular tachycardia.[13, 70] Canine experiments using areflexic left ventricle preparations demonstrated that AV sequential pacing with a proper AV interval overcame the adverse hemodynamics associated with ectopic activation of the ventricles. However, hemodynamic performance during ventricular pacing varied to a limited extent the site of ventricular pacing. These data could potentially be extrapolated to VT.

Direct measurement of left ventricular hemodynamics during sustained VT were reported from our laboratory in 1984.[71, 72] Altered ventricular contraction patterns during pacing-induced ventricular fusion with a normal atrioventricular relationship resulted in a decline in left ventricular negative dp/dt alone (Fig. 31–6). Impaired left ventricular relaxation was accompanied by preserved left ventricular systolic function, thus illustrating that, even in the diseased human heart, effective ventricular filling can overcome adverse hemodynamic effects of ectopic ventricular contraction. Furthermore, the altered contraction pattern contributes to impaired systolic function via reduced diastolic compliance and a secondary decrease in left ventricular filling. However, loss of atrial filling has a much greater effect on left ventricular systolic and diastolic function (Fig. 31–7). Hemodynamic and echocardiographic studies confirm increasing systolic left ventricular dysfunction with shorter coupling intervals of ventricular premature contractions (Fig. 31–8).[15, 16] During sustained VT left ventricular end-diastolic pressure is artificially maintained by impaired left ventricular relaxation leaving an inaccurate impression of adequate left ventricular filling (Fig. 31–9A and B).[71] However, systolic left ventricular function is primarily dependent

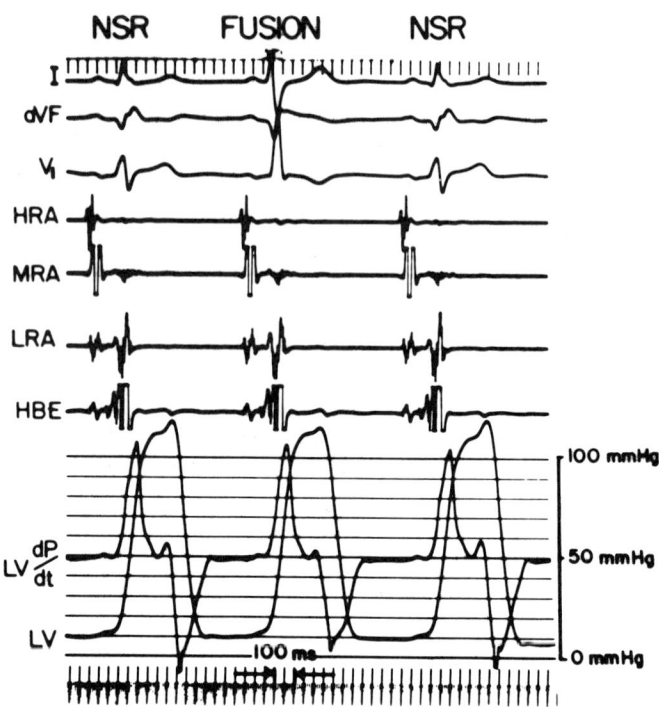

FIGURE 31–6
Effect of alteration of ventricular activation pattern on left ventricular hemodynamic parameters. Pacing-induced ventricular fusion complex is preceded by atrial systole with a near-normal atrioventricular conduction time. Note that left ventricular systolic and diastolic pressure as well as systolic peak dp/dt are unaltered in the fusion beat. Left ventricular negative dp/dt is minimally reduced in the fusion complex. ECG leads I, aVF, and V₁ are shown. NSR = normal sinus rhythm; HRA = high right atrium; MRA = mid right atrium; LRA = lower right atrium; HBE = His bundle electrogram; LV = left ventricular pressure. (Reprinted by permission of the Journal of the American College of Cardiology from Saksena S: J Am Coll Cardiol 4:501, 1984.)

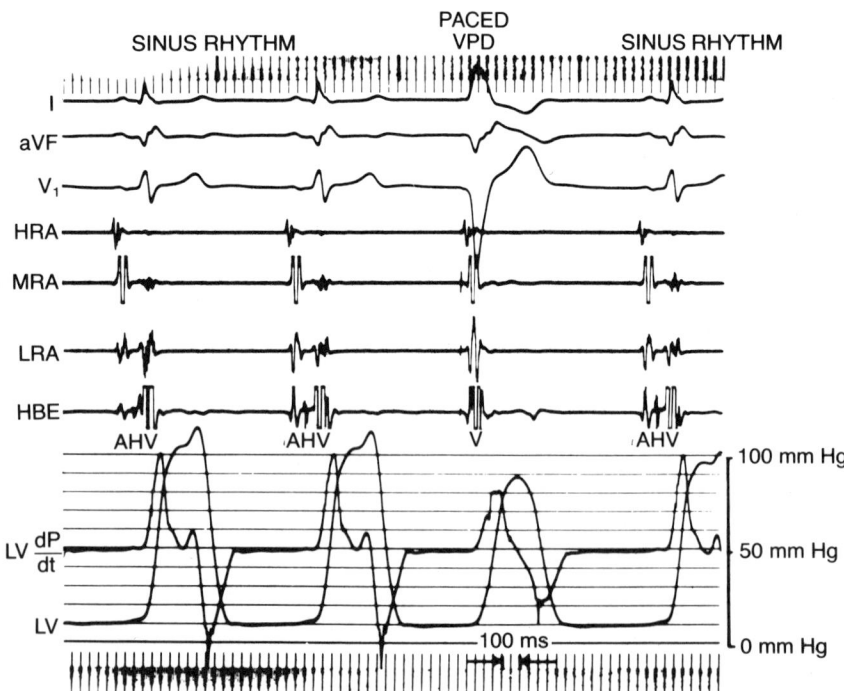

FIGURE 31–7
Effect of increasing prematurity of paced ventricular premature depolarization (VPD). Ventricular paced beats simultaneous with atrial systole result in marked reduction in left ventricular systolic pressure, peak dp/dt, and negative dp/dt. Note that left ventricular end-diastolic pressure is unaltered. Loss of atrial systole contributes to systolic dysfunction. A = atrial electrogram; H = His bundle electrogram; V = ventricular electrogram. For other abbreviations, see legend of Figure 31–6. (Reprinted by permission of the Journal of the American College of Cardiology from Saksena S: J Am Coll Cardiol 4:501, 1984.)

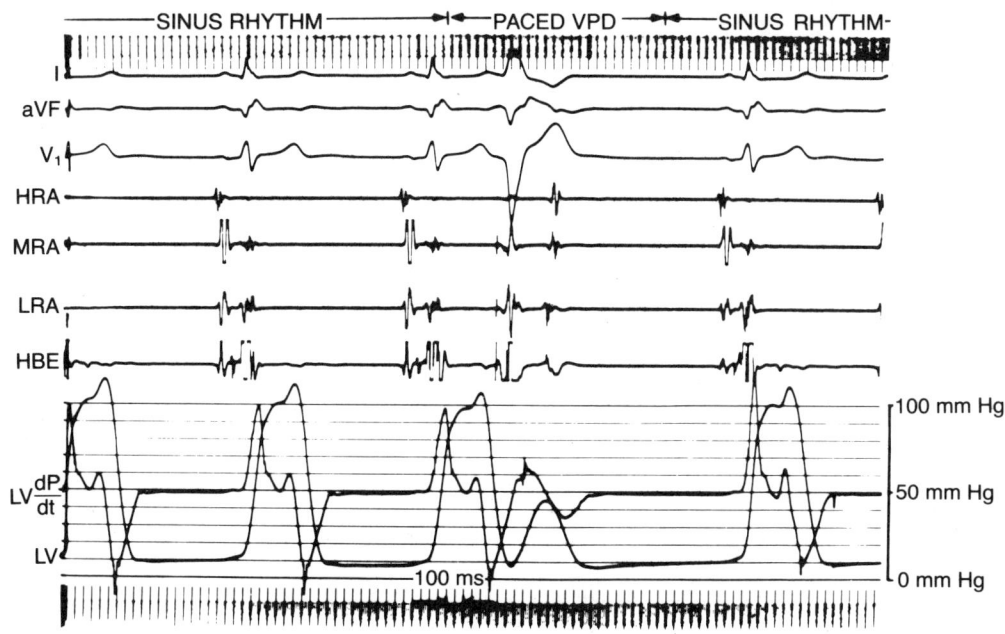

FIGURE 31–8
Effect of increasing prematurity of paced ventricular premature depolarization (VPD) on left ventricular hemodynamic function. Paced ventricular depolarization is induced at a shorter coupling interval compared to Figure 31–7 in the same patient. Note the progressive decrease in left ventricular systolic pressure and peak dp/dt with increase in prematurity as well as in negative dP/dt. Left ventricular end-diastolic pressure is minimally altered. For abbreviations, see legend of Figure 31–6.

on ventricular rate during VT which determines the period of diastolic filling. Left ventricular systolic pressure and ejection indices decline during VT (Fig. 31–9B). Echocardiographic studies show decreased left ventricular wall motion in all segments.[73] Improvement in systolic left ventricular function and systemic arterial pressure has been observed with properly timed atrial contraction during VT.[71, 74] Similar observations are noted during sustained and induced VT.[71] Recent clinical observations have documented that hemodynamic stability during VT is not uncommon and diagnostic differentiation from SVT on this basis is inaccurate.[76] Echocardiography performed during VT has documented hemodynamic stability and atrioventricular dissociation.[76] The primacy of end-diastolic volume in determining the hemodynamic outcome in VT was confirmed in recent studies.[15] Beat-to-beat stroke volume correlates directly with this parameter in patients with premature ventricular contractions. However, the benefits of increased end-diastolic volume have certain limits and postextrasystolic beats do not fully compensate for the loss of stroke volume observed with the premature contraction.[15, 77] Transient bundle branch block and occasional premature beats have little effect on the overall hemodynamic state of a patient but frequent ectopy does adversely impact on this clinical situation. The onset of VT is characterized by a continuously changing end-diastolic volume, stroke volume, and left ventricular systolic and diastolic function and is directly dependent on the effectiveness of ventricular filling. Cardioversion of VT is accompanied by marked improvement in all these variables. Regional wall-motion analysis by echocardiography in experimental studies of ventricular premature beats showed a characteristic pattern of early systolic contraction and wall thickening, followed by paradoxical motion and wall thinning in late systole at the site of inflow.[16] This latter pattern is probably due to earlier relaxation at this site. Analysis of global left ventricular function in patients with VT and heart disease showed decline in overall regional systolic function in multiple segments.[73] Reduced mitral blood flow has been demonstrated in our laboratory by continuous and colorflow Doppler studies in patients during induced VT (Fig. 31–10).[78] Reduced mitral inflow is confirmed by Doppler parameters (Fig. 31–11).[73, 78] Furthermore, mitral regurgitation was quantified in these studies. Patients with pre-existing competent mitral valves develop minimal or no regurgitation during VT, whereas patients with pre-existing mitral regurgitation note significant worsening of this condition, contributing to hemodynamic deterioration. The role of adrenergic reflexes in maintaining hemodynamic stability during VT has been examined. Sympathetic stimulation resulting in norepinephrine release and peripheral vasoconstriction has been noted.[79, 80] Alpha-adrenergic blockade can enhance the hypotensive effects of ventricular tachycardia. Hormonal changes such as release of atrial natriuretic hormone and aldosterone have also been observed.[80] These are particularly important compensatory mechanisms and probably influence the development of a cascade of life-threatening events such as coronary ischemia and degeneration into ventricular fibrillation.

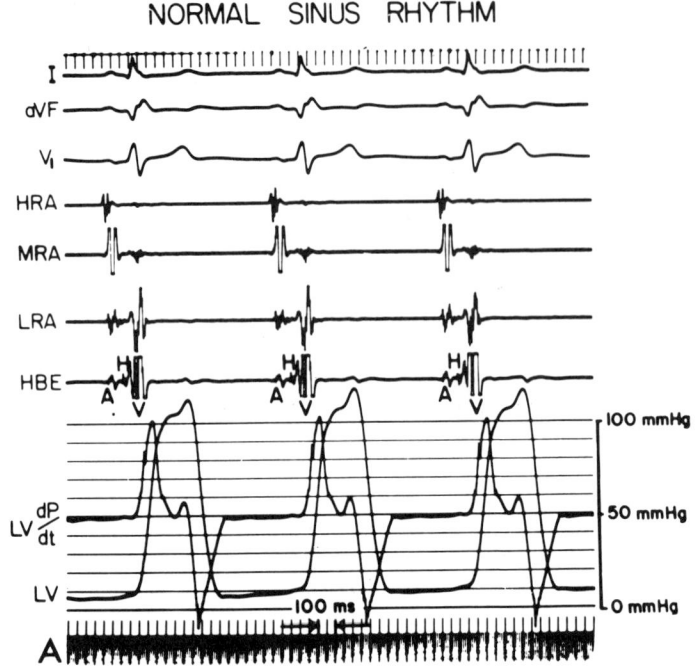
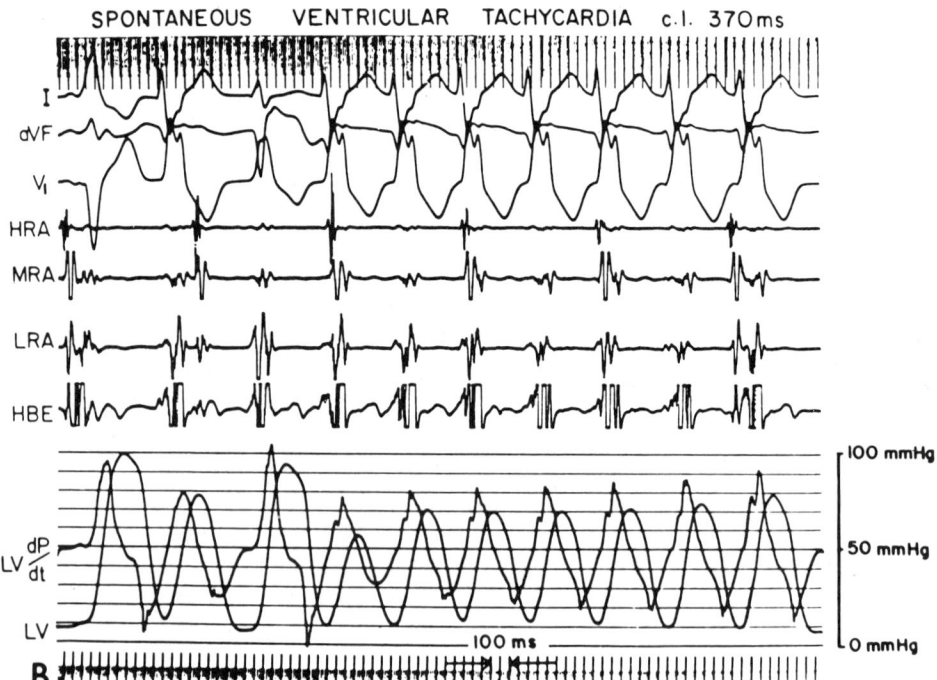

FIGURE 31–9
Left ventricular hemodynamic parameters during sinus rhythm and ventricular tachycardia in the same patient as in Figures 31–7 and 31–8. Sinus rhythm (A) was followed by spontaneous ventricular tachycardia (B) in this patient. Note the decline in left ventricular systolic pressure, peak dp/dt and negative dp/dt, with little change in left ventricular end-diastolic pressure during ventricular tachycardia. c.l. = cycle length; for other abbreviations, see legend of Figure 31–7. (Reprinted by permission of the Journal of the American College of Cardiology from Saksena S: J Am Coll Cardiol 4:501, 1984.)

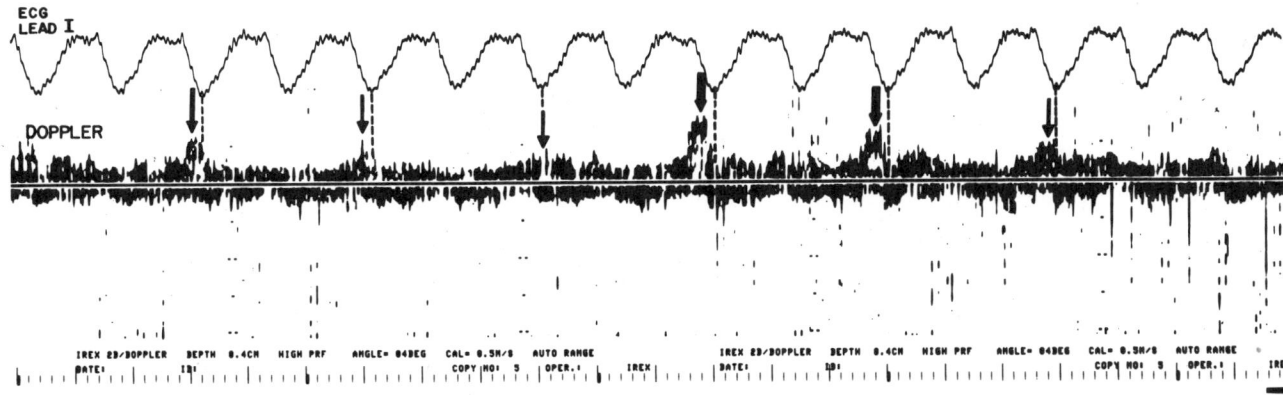

FIGURE 31–10
Pulse Doppler echocardiogram during ventricular tachycardia. Using the Irex phased array imager, the Doppler sample volume was placed in the left ventricle below the level of the mitral valve in the apical four-chamber plane. The flow velocity is considerably greater (maximum 0.9 m/s; thick arrows) when mitral inflow occurs well before the peak of the QRS complex as compared to its occurrence very close to or at the peak of the QRS complex (0.5 m/s; thin arrows). (Reprinted by permission of Futura Publishing Co., Inc., from Switzer D, Saksena S, Nanda N, et al.: PACE 7:136, 1984.)

Hemodynamic Effects of Artificial Cardiac Pacemakers

The hemodynamic consequences of artificial cardiac pacemaker rhythms have been extensively studied. Early reports focused on optimal heart rates in patients with complete heart block who were receiving a ventricular demand or asynchronous pacemaker.[36, 81] Experimental studies had suggested that cardiac output could be maintained over a wide range of heart rates by altering ventricular rate and stroke volume in inverse proportion.[82, 84] Initial ventricular pacemaker implants in complete heart block utilized fixed or variable rate devices in asynchronous or inhibited modes.[85, 86] Hemodynamic studies showed that correction of bradycardia in complete heart block usually improved cardiac output and lowered right atrial pressure.[81, 87–89] The optimal atrial rate varies widely between patients. A variety of rate responses with respect to cardiac output have been observed.[81] A plateau or "flat" rate output curve in which a cardiac output may remain constant ($\pm$ 15%) over a wide or narrow range of ventricular rates has been reported in 50% of patients.[81] An equal number of "peaked" rate output curves in which a particular rate is associated with maximal output have been reported. Atrial rates and pressures were lowest at this rate and an optimal rate with highest cardiac output and lowest atrial rate or pressure can be defined in a majority of patients.[81, 88–90] In one study this ranged from 56 to 90 bpm with a mean of 71 bpm.[81] During exercise, both types of rate output curves can be observed. Peaked rate output curves are particularly associated with presence of myocardial disease.[81] Fixed rate pacing, however, does not preclude increase in cardiac output with exercise.[81] Increased stroke volume during exercise mediates this response. Improved hemodynamics with pacing have translated into resolution of Stokes-Adams' syncopal episodes, refractory congestive heart failure, angina pectoris, and increased exercise/physical work capacity in uncontrolled studies.[88, 89] Subsequent controlled studies in patients with programmable pacemakers confirmed these results.

Experimental studies have documented several hemodynamic advantages of atrial pacing with respect to ventricular pacing. As detailed earlier in this chapter, optimal sequence of AV contraction enhances left ventricular filling and, thus, stroke volume and cardiac

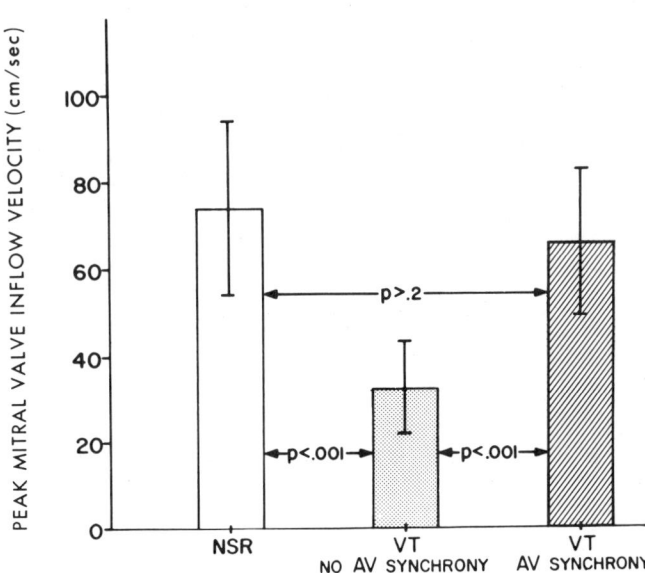

FIGURE 31–11
Mitral valve inflow velocity measured during sinus rhythm (NSR) and ventricular tachycardia (VT) by color Doppler studies. Note the marked decline in mitral flow during VT without atrial synchrony and the improvement with atrial synchrony. (Based on data from Switzer D, Saksena S, Nanda N, et al.: PACE 7:136, 1984.)

output. This "booster pump" effect assumes considerable importance in specific acute and chronic clinical conditions. Acute studies in patients with cardiac disease have confirmed these benefits.[91, 92] The advantages conferred by atrial pacing are largely due to sequential atrioventricular contraction rather than the normal ventricular contraction pattern observed with atrial pacing in contrast to ventricular pacing.[92] Specific clinical situations showing the benefits of atrial pacing in atrioventricular sequential pacing are characterized by impaired left ventricular function and may be accompanied by excessive cardiocirculatory demands. Topol and coworkers[93] noted that atrial or atrioventricular sequential pacing was essential to establish hemodynamic stability in patients with right ventricular injury and volume-refractory hypotension associated with acute myocardial infarction. This could not be achieved with ventricular pacing alone. In patients with left ventricular dysfunction, atrioventricular sequential pacing improved cardiac index 17 to 29% over ventricular pacing alone at paced rates of 75 to 100 bpm.[94] Improved hemodynamics with atrial pacing can be predicted by the clinical observation that significant variations in pulse pressure occur during ventricular pacing. Baseline clinical left ventricular function indexes are not useful in this regard. Postoperative cardiac surgical patients in sinus or junctional rhythm can experience deterioration in left ventricular function during ventricular pacing alone, whereas sequential atrioventricular pacing improves cardiac output in most patients.[95] Temporary pacing in this mode may be particularly important in this clinical scenario. The development of an implantable atrial synchronous pacemaker has spurred interest in long-term use of this mode.[96] Furman[97] initially suggested that indications for atrial pacing alone included bradyarrhythmias due to sinus node dysfunction and overdrive suppression of ventricular arrhythmias, to improve cardiac output and termination of reentrant SVTs.[97] Currently the hemodynamic benefits largely contribute to the use of this mode. It is uncommon to use atrial pacing alone in patients with sinus node disease, because of the frequent occurrence of AV conduction abnormalities. The treatment of ventricular ectopy or sustained supraventricular tachyarrhythmias with atrial pacing is a limited application at best (Fig. 31–12).

The hemodynamic benefits of implanted pacemakers in the AV sequential pacing modes (DDD, VDD, DVI) over ventricular demand pacing (VVI mode) or fixed rate pacing (VOO mode) have been documented in a number of randomized controlled prospective studies. Cardiac output is improved at rest and during exercise in comparison to fixed rate ventricular pacing, whereas stroke volume is comparable at rest but higher during exercise.[98] Left ventricular filling pressure is reduced by atrial triggered pacing at rest, but not during exercise. These advantages were preserved even when ventricular pacing rates were increased during exercise to match atrial rates.[90] Thus, while rate responsive ventricular pacing has significant advantages over VVI and VOO pacing modes, atrial synchronous pacing remains the gold standard if normal sinus pace-

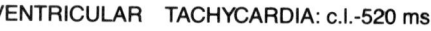
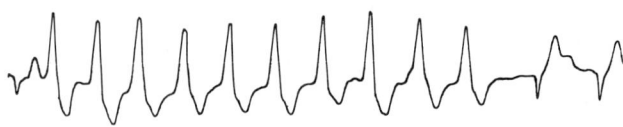
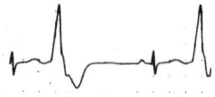
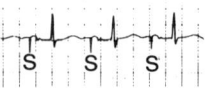

FIGURE 31–12
The results of combined drug therapy and demand atrial pacemaker for suppression of ventricular arrhythmias in a patient with spontaneous ventricular tachycardia and mitral valve prolapse. Verapamil converted ventricular arrhythmia to continuous ventricular bigeminy. Atrial pacing at a rate of 90 bpm suppressed the atrial bigeminy completely, and a demand atrial pacemaker eliminated ventricular arrhythmias on a long-term basis.

maker function is present. This translates into improved physical work capacity during acute and chronic follow-up.[99] Physical performance improves in both young and elderly patients. This is observed in the presence or absence of cardiac disease, although it is most pronounced in the former. The physiologic variables showing significant improvement include cardiac output, and this is associated with lower arteriovenous oxygen content differences and arterial blood lactate. Cardiac size is decreased by physiologic sequential pacing.[100] Patients are symptomatically subjectively improved to a greater extent. Reduced dyspnea and palpitation and a sense of general well-being have been reported.[101, 102]

Ventricular pacing has one additional specific deleterious hemodynamic result. Presence of retrograde ventriculoatrial conduction has been reported.[103, 104] In our and other laboratories' experience, retrograde ventriculoatrial conduction may be present in 33 to 50% of individuals with normal antegrade atrioventricular conduction.[105] It is usually absent in patients with spontaneous AV block. Retrograde ventriculoatrial conduction can result in a specific clinical condition, the pacemaker syndrome, due to its hemodynamic effects. A typical clinical presentation of this disorder usually involves a patient who underwent demand permanent ventricular pacemaker implantation and subsequently presents with continuation of symptoms or development of new cardiac symptoms. These include symptoms of low cardiac output (e.g., fatigue, limited exercise capacity, presyncope or syncope, and

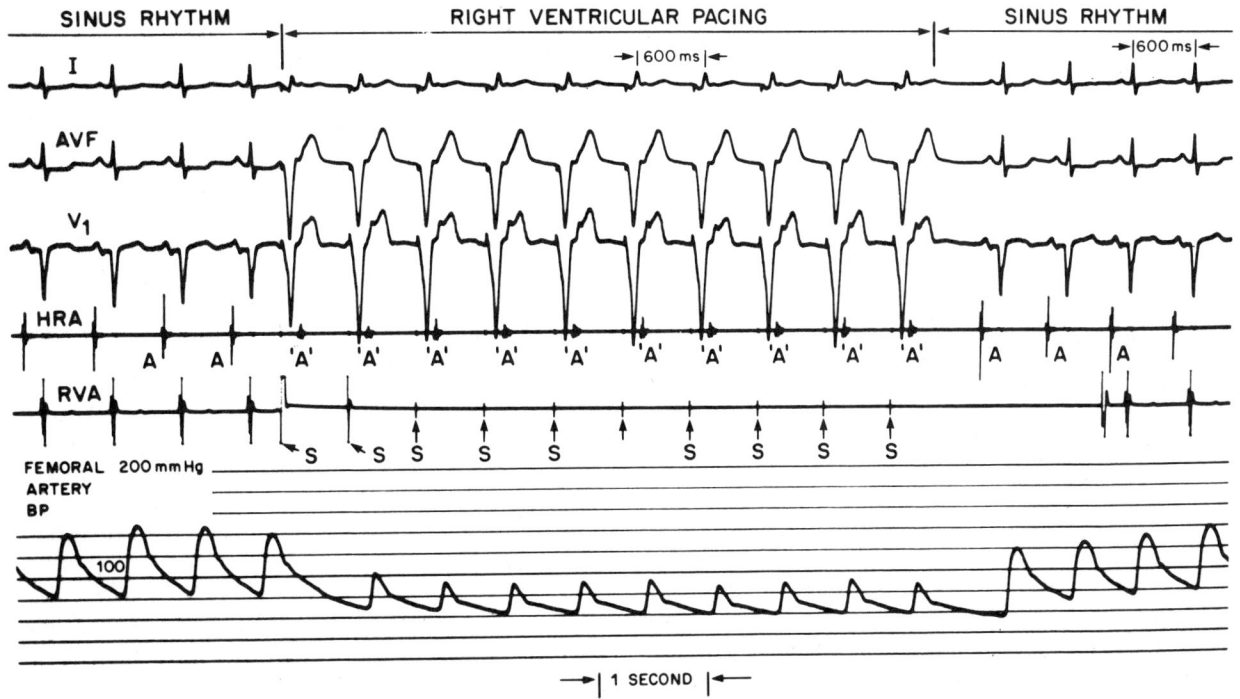

FIGURE 31–13
Hemodynamic consequences of ventricular pacing with retrograde atrial conduction ("pacemaker syndrome") in a patient with hypertensive heart disease. The patient is initially in sinus rhythm at 100 bpm, and ventricular pacing is commenced at the identical rate. Ventricular pacing is associated with retrograde atrial activation ('A'). Despite a constant identical ventricular rate, a marked decline in systemic arterial pressure from 145 mm Hg to 85 mm Hg is observed during ventricular pacing. Cessation of ventricular pacing is associated with recovery of normal arterial pressure. HRA = high right atrium; RVA = right ventricular apical electrogram; A = antegrade atrial activation; S = pacing stimulus; BP = blood pressure.

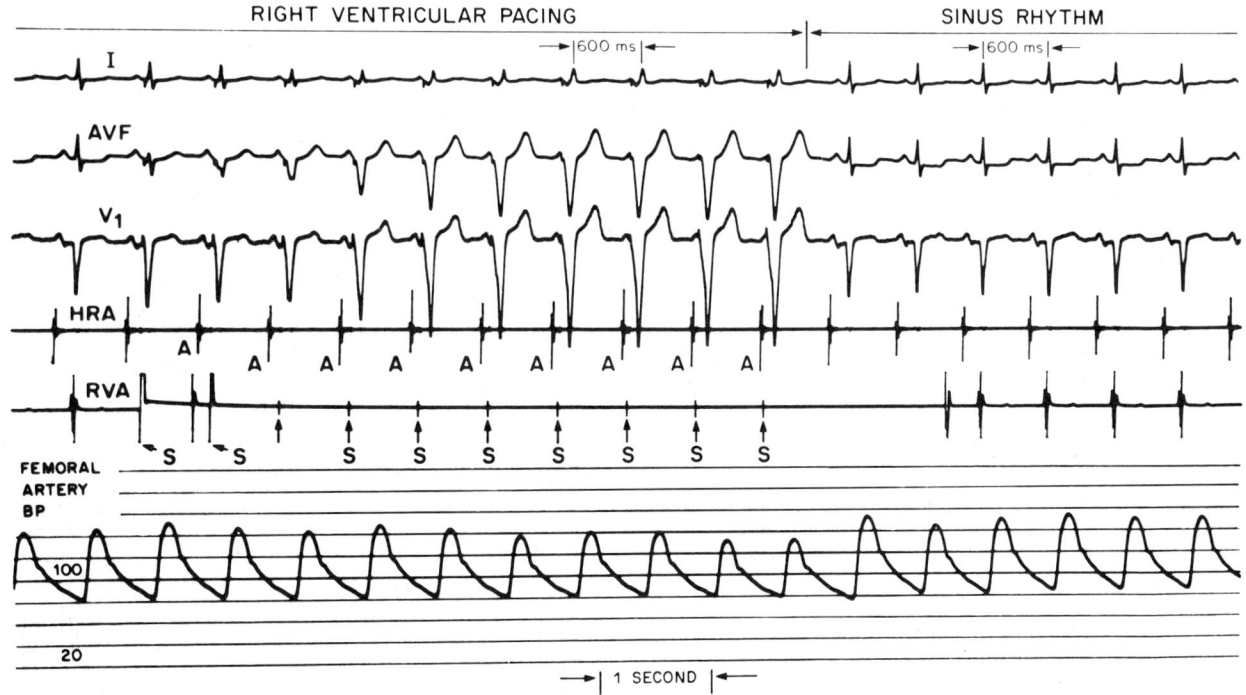

FIGURE 31–14
Maintenance of hemodynamic stability in the same patient as in Figure 31–13 during ventricular pacing with fortuitous antegrade atrial contraction. Ventricular pacing is commenced, and isorhythmic but dissociated atrial activity is present antegrade to the ventricular-paced depolarization for several complexes. Note that the systemic arterial blood pressure (BP) remains unchanged, but a progressively shortening PR interval with a slight decline in arterial pressure is observed toward the end of the pacing sequence. For abbreviations, see legend of Figure 31–13.

Hemodynamic Effects of Cardiac Arrhythmias and Pacemakers

weakness or lassitude) and elevated venous pressure (e.g., dyspnea, chest congestion, head and neck pulsations due to cannon "a" waves, right upper quadrant tenderness due to hepatic congestion, and peripheral edema).[106]

On physical examination, low pulse amplitude, elevated jugular venous pressure with cannon "a" waves, gallop rhythms, pulmonary rales, accentuation of the pulmonic second heart sound, and peripheral edema have been reported. The symptoms can be typically paroxysmal or chronic. The resting ECG during symptoms demonstrates ventricular pacing at an acceptable heart rate with a retrograde P wave. With demand pacing units, 24-hour ambulatory ECG recordings may be necessary to demonstrate ventricular pacing and correlate it with symptoms. This condition should be suspected whenever a patient with an implanted demand ventricular pacemaker presents with symptoms of low cardiac output and cardiac failure. Ventriculoatrial conduction may be either intermittent or present at lower pacing rates and may be absent at high rates due to retrograde decremental AV nodal conduction.

Diagnosis of the pacemaker syndrome is performed by right heart catheterization and measurement of hemodynamics during sinus rhythm and atrial and ventricular pacing. Recording of atrial and ventricular electrograms is useful in this regard (Fig. 31–13). In our laboratory, we typically use a hexapolar Berkovits-Castellanos electrode catheter for atrial and ventricular pacing. Alternatively, the implanted pacemaker may be used at rates above and below the sinus rate to achieve this result. A Swan-Ganz catheter is inserted for pressure measurements. Ventricular pacing demonstrates retrograde atrial activation, with the earliest atrial activity in the low right atrium. Retrograde conduction usually should be 1:1 at the programmed pacemaker rate. Uncommonly decremental retrograde conduction may nevertheless be associated with pacemaker syndrome. Ventricular pacing produces retrograde atrial contraction with elevation in right and left atrial pressures, pulmonary capillary wedge pressure, and cannon "a" waves due to simultaneous atrial contraction during or at completion of ventricular systole. Decreased left ventricular and aortic systolic pressures and systemic arterial pulse pressure may be observed (see Fig. 31–13). A decline in cardiac output, compared to sinus rhythm or atrial pacing at the same rate, is present. Hypotension may be aggravated by initiation of an atrial vasodepressor reflex due to atrial distention. Mitral regurgitation typically is not present. These findings are pathognomonic and are most often observed in patients with prior left ventricular dysfunction or reduced left ventricular compliance. Sinus rhythm or atrial pacing obviates symptoms and negative hemodynamic effects. Thus, treatment of this disorder is directed at achieving this result.

The demand ventricular pacemaker may be programmed to a lower rate to permit emergence of native sinus rhythm in some patients. Infrequent use of demand ventricular pacing may eliminate or minimize symptoms. The definitive treatment, should symptoms or extensive use of demand ventricular pacing persist, is to revise the pacemaker system to an atrial or atrioventricular sequential pacing system (Fig. 31–14). On occasion, ventricular pacing may result in severe mitral insufficiency with similar results to those observed with ventriculoatrial conduction.[107] Color Doppler studies from our laboratory suggest that this is seen only in patients with pre-existing, significant mitral regurgitation.[71] Lowering demand ventricular rate can result in symptomatic improvement.[107] However, revision to a physiologic pacing system is recommended.

Consideration of the hemodynamic impact of permanent pacemaker implantation should be prospective and should influence the process of device selection in each patient. This is particularly important in patients with prior cardiac disease and left ventricular dysfunction. In children, younger individuals, and active patients, if there is concern with respect to this aspect, a combined electrophysiologic and hemodynamic evaluation for optimal pacing mode prior to device implant is recommended. The role of exercise should be adequately considered.[4] The development of single- and now dual-chamber rate-responsive pacing systems should provide the opportunity for optimal device selection for hemodynamic benefit.

References

1. Harvey W: Exercitatio anatomica de motu cordis et sanguinis in animalibus. London, 1628. Translated by Robert Willis, England, Barnes Survey, 1847.
2. Lewis T: Fibrillation of the auricles: Its effects upon the circulation. J Exper Med 16:395, 1912.
3. Osler W: On the so-called Stokes-Adams' disease (slow pulse with syncopal attacks, etc). Lancet 2:516, 1903.
4. Ross J Jr, Linhart JW, Braunwald E: Effects of changing heart rate in man by electrical stimulation of the right atrium—studies at rest, during exercise and with isoproterenol. Circulation 32:549, 1965.
5. Wang Y, Marshall RJ, Shepherd JT: Stroke volume in the dog during graded exercise. Circ Res 8:558, 1960.
6. Braunwald E, Goldblatt A, Harrison DC, et al.: Studies on cardiac dimension in intact unanaesthetised man. IV. Effects of muscular exercise. Circ Res 13:460, 1963.
7. Gorlin R, Cohen LS, Elliott WC, et al.: Effect of supine exercise on left ventricular volume and oxygen consumption in man. Circulation 32:361, 1965.
8. DeMaria AW, Neumann A, Schubart PJ, et al.: Systemic correlation of cardiac chamber size and ventricular performance determined with echocardiography and alterations in heart rate in normal persons. Am J Cardiol 43:1, 1979.
9. Rahimtoola SH, Ehsani A, Sinno EZ, et al.: Left atrial transport function in myocardial infarction: Importance of its booster pump function. Am J Med 59:686, 1975.
10. Gilmore JP, Sarnoff SJ, Mitchell JH, et al.: Synchronicity of ventricular contraction: Observations comparing hemodynamic effects of atrial and ventricular pacing. Br Heart J 25:299, 1983.
11. Wiggers CJ: The muscular reactions of the mammalian ventricles to artificial surface stimuli. Am J Physiol 73:346, 1925.
12. Meijler FF, Weiberdink J, Durrer D: L'importance de la position des électrodes stimulatrices au cours du traitement d'un bloc auriculo-ventriculaire postoperativ total. Arch Mal Coeur 55:690, 1962.
13. Daggett WM, Bianco JA, Powell WJ, et al.: Relative contributions of the atrial systole–ventricular systole interval and of patterns of ventricular activation to ventricular function during electrical pacing of the dog heart. Circ Res 27:69, 1970.
14. Eber LM, Berkovits BV, Matloff JM, et al.: Dynamic charac-

terization of premature ventricular beats and ventricular tachycardias. Am J Cardiol 33:378, 1974.
15. Cohn K, Kryda W: The influence of ectopic beats and tachyarrhythmias on stroke volume and cardiac output. J Electrocardiol 14:207, 1981.
16. Uchiyama T, Corday E, Meerbaum S, et al.: Characterization of left ventricular mechanical function during arrhythmias with two dimensional echocardiography. I. Premature ventricular contractions. Am J Cardiol 48:679, 1981.
17. Torres MAR, Corday E, Meerbaum S, et al.: Characterization of left ventricular mechanical function during arrhythmias by two dimensional echocardiography. II. Location of the site of onset of premature ventricular systoles. J Am Coll Cardiol 1:819, 1983.
18. Samet P: Hemodynamic sequelae of cardiac arrhythmias. Circulation 47:399, 1973.
19. Samet P, Bernstein WH, Litwak RS: Electrical activation and mechanical asynchronism in the cardiac cycle of the dog. Circ Res 7:228, 1959.
20. Braunwald E, Morrow AG: Sequence of ventricular contraction in human bundle branch block: A study based on simultaneous catheterization of both ventricles. Am J Med 23:205, 1957.
21. Bourassa MG, Birteau GM, Allenstein BJ: Hemodynamic studies during intermittent left bundle branch block. Am J Cardiol 10:792, 1962.
22. Samet P, Castillo C, Bernstein WH: Hemodynamic consequences of sequential atrioventricular pacing: Subjects with normal hearts. Am J Cardiol 21:207, 1968.
23. Benchimol A, Ellis JG, Dimond EG: Hemodynamic consequences of atrial and ventricular pacing in patients with normal and abnormal hearts. Effect of exercise at a fixed atrial and ventricular rate. Am J Med 39:911, 1965.
24. Benchimol A, Dimond EG: Cardiac function in man during artificial stimulation of the left ventricle, right ventricle and right atrium. Am J Cardiol 17:118, 1966.
25. Mitchell JH, Gilmore JP, Sarnoff SJ: The transport function of the atrium. Factors influencing the relation between mean left atrial pressure and left ventricular end diastolic pressure. Am J Cardiol 9:237, 1962.
26. Greenberg B, Chatterjee K, Parmley WW, et al.: The influence of left ventricular filling pressure on atrial contribution to cardiac output. Am Heart J 98:742, 1979.
27. Gillespie WJ, Greene DG, Karatzas NB, et al: Effect of atrial systole on right ventricular stroke output in complete heart block. Br Med J 1:75, 1967.
28. DeMaria AN, Miller RR, Amsterdam EA, et al.: Mitral valve early diastolic closing velocity in the echocardiogram. Relation to sequential diastolic flow and ventricular compliance. Am J Cardiol 37:693, 1976.
29. Samet P, Bernstein WH, Nathan DA, et al.: Atrial contribution to cardiac output in complete heart block. Am J Cardiol 16:1, 1965.
30. Samet P, Bernstein W, Levine S: Significance of the atrial contribution to ventricular filling. Am J Cardiol 15:195, 1965.
31. Schneller SJ, Harthorne JW: Carotid sinus hypersensitivity. Clin Prog Pacing Electrophysiol 3:389, 1985.
32. Levinson DC, Gunther L, Mechan JP, et al.: Hemodynamic studies in five patients with heart block and slow ventricular rates. Circulation 12:739, 1955.
33. Stark MF, Rader B, Sobol BJ, et al.: Cardiovascular hemodynamic function in complete heart block and response to isopropylnorepinephrine. Circulation 17:526, 1958.
34. Ikkos D, Hanson JS: Response to exercise in congenital complete atrioventricular block. Circulation 22:583, 1960.
35. Scarpelli FM, Rudolph AM: The hemodynamics of congenital complete heart block. Prog Cardiovasc Dis 6:327, 1964.
36. Samet P, Bernstein WH, Medow A, et al.: Effect of alterations in ventricular rate on cardiac output in complete heart block. Am J Cardiol 14:477, 1964.
37. Samet P, Bernstein WH, Nathan JA, et al.: Atrial contribution to cardiac output in complete heart block. Am J Cardiol 16:1, 1965.
38. Benchimol A, Duenas A, Liggett MS, et al.: Contribution of atrial systole to the cardiac function at a fixed and at a variable ventricular rate. Am J Cardiol 16:11, 1965.
39. Saunders DE, Ord JW: The hemodynamic effects of paroxysmal supraventricular tachycardia in patients with the Wolff-Parkinson-White syndrome. Am J Cardiol 9:223, 1962.
40. Ferrer MI, Harvey RM, Weiner HM, et al.: Hemodynamic studies in two cases of Wolff-Parkinson-White syndrome with paroxysmal AV nodal tachycardia. Am J Med 6:725, 1949.
41. Waxman MB, Sharma AD, Cameron DA, et al.: Reflex mechanisms responsible for early spontaneous termination of paroxysmal supraventricular tachycardia. Am J Cardiol 49:259, 1982.
42. Waxman MB, Bonet JF, Finley JP, et al.: Effects of respiration and posture on paroxysmal supraventricular tachycardia. Circulation 62:1011, 1980.
43. Waxman MB, Wald RW, Huerta F, et al.: Vagal techniques for termination of paroxysmal supraventricular tachycardia. Am J Cardiol 46:655, 1980.
44. Erlebacher JA, Danner RL, Stelzer PE: Hypotension with ventricular pacing: An atrial vasodepressor reflex in human beings. J Am Coll Cardiol 4:550, 1984.
45. Wenkebach KF, Winteberg H: Die Unregel maessige Herztaetigkeit, p. 252. Leipzig, Wilhelm V. Engelmann, 1927.
46. Wood P: Polyuria in paroxysmal tachycardia. Br Heart J 25:273, 1963.
47. Kaye GC, Nathan AW, Camm AJ: Polyuria associated with paroxysmal tachycardia. Clin Prog Pacing Electrophysiol 2:349, 1984.
48. Nicklas JM, DiCarlo LA, Koller PT, et al.: Plasma levels of immunoreactive atrial natriuretic factor increase during supraventricular tachycardia. Am Heart J 112:923, 1986.
49. Bolli P, Muller IB, Linder L, et al.: The vasodilator potency of atrial natriuretic peptide in man. Circulation 75:221, 1987.
50. Canepa-Anson R, William M, Marshall J, et al.: Mechanism of polyuria and natriuresis in atrioventricular nodal tachycardia. Br Med J 289:866, 1984.
51. Coleman HN, Taylor RR, Pool PE, et al.: Congestive heart failure following chronic tachycardia. Am Heart J 81:790, 1971.
52. Gallagher JJ: Tachycardia and cardiomyopathy: The chicken-egg dilemma revisited. J Am Coll Cardiol 6:1172, 1985.
53. Packer DL, Bardy GH, Wosley SJ, et al.: Tachycardia-induced cardiomyopathy: A reversible form of left ventricular dysfunction. Am J Cardiol 57:563, 1986.
54. McIntosh HD, Morris JJ Jr: The hemodynamic consequences of arrhythmias. Prog Cardiovasc Dis 8:330, 1966.
55. DeMaria AN, Vismara LA, Vera Z, et al.: Hemodynamic effects of cardiac arrhythmias. Angiology 28:427, 1977.
56. Corday E, Gold H, DeVera LB, et al.: Effect of the cardiac arrhythmias on the coronary circulation. Ann Intern Med 50:535, 1959.
57. Harvey RM, Ferrer MI, Richards DW, et al.: Cardio-circulatory performance in atrial flutter. Circulation 12:507, 1955.
58. Smith WC, Walker GL, Alt HL: Cardiac output in heart disease. I. Complete heart block, auricular fibrillation before and after restoration to normal rhythm, subacute rheumatic fever and chronic rheumatic valvular disease. Arch Intern Med 45:706, 1930.
59. Kerkhof AC: Minute volume determinations in mitral stenosis during auricular fibrillation and after restoration of normal rhythm. Am Heart J 11:206, 1936.
60. Hecht H, Osher WJ, Samuels AJ: Cardiovascular adjustments in subjects with organic heart disease before and after conversion of atrial fibrillation to normal sinus rhythm. J Clin Invest 30:653, 1951.
61. Oran S, Weingren L, Davis JPH, et al.: Conversion of atrial fibrillation to sinus rhythm by direct current shock. Lancet 2:159, 1963.
62. Gilbert R, Eich RE, Smalyan H, et al.: Effect on circulation of conversion of atrial fibrillation to sinus rhythm. Circulation 27:1079, 1963.
63. Morris JJ Jr, Entman M, North WC, et al.: The changes in cardiac output with reversion of atrial fibrillation to sinus rhythm. Circulation 31:670, 1965.
64. Lester JW, Klotz DH, Jomain SL, et al.: Effect of pacemaker site on cardiac output and ventricular activation in dogs with complete heart block. Am J Cardiol 14:494, 1964.
65. Papadopoulos C, Blazek CJ: Ventricular tachycardia of 70 days' duration with survival. Am J Cardiol 11:107, 1963.
66. Smirk FH, Nolla-Panades J, Wallis T: Experimental ventricular

flutter and ventricular paroxysmal tachycardia. Am J Cardiol 14:79, 1964.
67. Lima JAC, Weiss JL, Guzman PA, et al.: Incomplete filling and incoordinate contraction as mechanism of hypotension during ventricular tachycardia in man. Circulation 68:928, 1983.
68. Swiryn S, Pavel D, Bysom E, et al.: Sequential radionuclide phase mapping of radionuclide-gated ventriculograms in patients with sustained ventricular tachycardias. Close correlation with electrophysiologic characteristics. Am Heart J 103:319, 1982.
69. McFarland TM, McCarthy DM, Makler PT, et al.: Relation between site of origin of ventricular tachycardias and relative left ventricular myocardial perfusion and wall motion. Am J Cardiol 51:1329, 1983.
70. Ueda H, Harumi K, Ueda K: Cineangiographic observations on the asynchronism of cardiac contraction during ventricular pacing. Jpn Heart J 9:295, 1968.
71. Saksena S: Studies on left ventricular function during sustained ventricular tachycardia. J Am Coll Cardiol 4:501, 1984.
72. Saksena S, Craelius W, Pantopoulos D, et al.: Left ventricular function during ventricular pacing and ventricular tachycardia in man. *In* Cardiac Pacing, pp. 683–690. Darmstadt, Steinkopff Verlag, 1983.
73. Rosenbloom M, Saksena A, Rogal G, et al.: Two-dimensional echocardiographic studies in sustained ventricular tachycardia. PACE 7:136, 1984.
74. Hamer WF, Zaher C, Peter CT, et al.: Hemodynamic benefits of sequential atrial pacing during ventricular tachycardia in man (Abstract). J Am Coll Cardiol 1:636, 1983.
76. Manyari DE, Ko P, Gulamhaussein S, et al.: Simple echocardiographic method to detect atrioventricular dissociation. Chest 81:67, 1982.
77. Sakamaki T, Corday E, Meerbaum S, et al.: Relationship between myocardial injury and post extrasystolic potentiation of regional function as measured by two dimensional echocardiography. J Am Coll Cardiol 2:52, 1983.
78. Switzer D, Saksena S, Nanda N, et al.: Color and pulsed Doppler flow mapping of mitral flow during sustained ventricular tachycardia. Clin Res 34:347A, 1986.
79. Feldman T, Carroll JD, Munkenbeck F, et al.: Hemodynamic recovery during stimulated ventricular tachycardia: Role of adrenergic receptor activation. 115:588, 1988.
80. Ikram H, Krozier IG, Nicholls MG: Hemodynamic and hormone changes during ventricular tachycardia in man (Abstract). Eur Heart J 9Suppl 1:15, 1988.
81. Sowton E: Hemodynamic studies in patients with artificial cardiac pacemakers. Br Heart J 26:737, 1964.
82. Warner HR, Toronto AF: Regulation of cardiac output through stroke volume. Circ Res 8:549, 1960.
83. Bristow JD, Ferguson RE, Mintz F, et al.: The influence of heart rate on left ventricular volume in dogs. J Clin Invest 42:649, 1963.
84. Miller DE, Gleason WK, Whalen RE, et al.: Effect of ventricular rate on the cardiac output in the dog with chronic heart block. Circ Res 10:658, 1962.
85. Elmquist R, Landegren J, Patterson SO, et al.: Artificial pacemaker for treatment of Adams-Stokes syndrome and slow heart rate. Am Heart J 65:731, 1963.
86. Chardack WM, Gage AA, Schimert G, et al.: Two years clinical experience with the implantable pacemaker for complete heart block. Dis Chest 43:225, 1963.
87. Samet P, Jacobs W, Bernstein WH, et al.: Hemodynamic sequelae of idioventricular pacemaking in complete heart block. Am J Cardiol 11:594, 1963.
88. Escher DJW, Schwedel JB, Eisenberg R, et al.: Cardiovascular dynamic responses to artificial pacing of patients in heart block. Circulation 24:928, 1961.
89. Muller OF, Bellet S: Treatment of intractable heart failure in the presence of complete atrioventricular heart block by the use of the internal cardiac pacemaker. N Engl J Med 265:768, 1961.
90. Bevegard S: Observation on the effect of varying ventricular rate on the circulation at rest and during exercise in two patients with an artificial pacemaker. Acta Med Scand 172:615, 1962.
91. Samet P, Castillo C, Bernstein WH, et al.: Hemodynamic results of right atrial pacing in cardiac subjects. Dis Chest 53:133, 1968.
92. Samet P, Castillo C, Bernstein WH: Hemodynamic sequelae of atrial, ventricular and sequential atrioventricular pacing in cardiac patients. Am Heart J 72:725, 1966.
93. Topol E, Goldschlager N, Posts TA, et al.: Hemodynamic benefit of atrial pacing in right ventricular myocardial infarction. Ann Intern Med 96:594, 1982.
94. Reiter MJ, Hindman MC: Hemodynamic benefits of acute atrioventricular sequential pacing in patients with left ventricular dysfunction. Am J Cardiol 49:687, 1982.
95. Hartzler GO, Maloney JD, Curtis JJ, et al.: Hemodynamic benefits of atrioventricular sequential pacing after cardiac surgery. Am J Cardiol 40:232, 1977.
96. Nathan DA, Center S, Wu C, et al.: An implantable synchronous pacemaker for the long-term correction of complete heart block. Am J Cardiol 11:362, 1963.
97. Furman S: Therapeutic uses of atrial pacing. Am Heart J 86:835, 1973.
98. Karlof I: Haemodynamic effect of atrial triggered versus fixed rate pacing at rest and during exercise in complete heart block. Acta Med Scand 197:195, 1975.
99. Kruse I, Ryden L: Comparison of physical work capacity and systolic time intervals with ventricular inhibited and atrial synchronous ventricular inhibited pacing. Br Heart J 46:129, 1981.
100. Kruse I, Arnman K, Conradson TB, et al.: A comparison of the acute and long-term hemodynamic effects of ventricular inhibited and atrial synchronous ventricular inhibited pacing. Circulation 65:846, 1982.
101. Perrins EJ, Mosley CA, Chan SL, et al.: Randomized controlled trial of physiological and ventricular pacing. Br Heart J 50:112, 1983.
102. Raza ST, Lajos TZ, Bhayana JN, et al.: Improved cardiovascular hemodynamics with atrioventricular sequential pacing compared with ventricular demand pacing. Ann Thorac Surg 38:260, 1984.
103. Barold S, Linhart J, Samet P: Reciprocal beating induced by ventricular pacing. Circulation 38:330, 1968.
104. Goldreyer BN, Bigger JT: Ventriculo-atrial conduction in man. Circulation 41:935, 1970.
105. Akhtar M: Reentry within the His-Purkinje system. *In* Narula OS (ed.): Cardiac Arrhythmias, pp. 397–418. Baltimore, Williams & Wilkins, 1979.
106. Johnson AD, Laiken SL, Engler RL: Hemodynamic compromise associated with ventriculoatrial conduction following transvenous pacemaker placement. Am J Med 65:75, 1978.
107. Edhag O, Fagrell B, Lagergren H: Deleterious effects of cardiac pacing in a patient with mitral insufficiency. Acta Med Scand 202:331, 1977.

32

Pacemaker Implantation Techniques

Arjun D. Sharma
Gerard M. Guiraudon
George J. Klein
Raymond Yee

The development of percutaneous techniques for permanent endocardial pacemaker lead placement has led to an increase in the number of physicians without surgical training who are performing permanent pacemaker implantation. Further reductions in lead and generator size, and other simplifications in the implant procedures, are likely to perpetuate this trend. This chapter is written with emphasis on techniques performed by physicians who are not surgeons but also discusses potential surgical complications.

Selection of Implantation Site

The commonly used approaches to lead placement can be classified as endomyocardial and epimyocardial. The *endomyocardial* lead placement is the most commonly used method and can be utilized by obtaining venous access at several sites, including the subclavian vein, cephalic vein, and internal jugular and external jugular veins. The techniques using an endomyocardial lead offer the advantages of requiring relatively minor surgical expertise, only local anesthesia, better long-term lead performance than epicardial leads, bipolar electrodes on single leads, and better atrial lead function. Of the endomyocardial lead techniques, the subclavian vein approach offers the advantages of the least surgical dissection, ease of placement of multiple leads, and easy maneuverability of the leads once they are intravascular. However, the subclavian vein approach has the potential for complications with a frequency of 0.5%. This is the major reason why some centers prefer to use the cephalic vein approach. The cephalic vein approach requires more surgical dissection to identify and cannulate the vein, which may on occasion be of insufficient size to permit introduction of two leads for dual-chamber pacemakers. Both jugular vein approaches have the disadvantage of requiring a lead to be either tunneled under the clavicle or passed over the clavicle, increasing the complexity of the surgical approach and the risk of subsequent skin erosion. The internal jugular approach also may potentially result in arterial injury.

Other factors that influence the choice of venous access site include the presence of previously abandoned leads in the cephalic vein, which usually prevent the second use of the same site; a clavicular fracture, which distorts the anatomic localization of the subclavian vein; and the presence of infection or skin erosion, which may necessitate an approach to the contralateral side.

The *epimyocardial* approach is used infrequently ($< 5\%$). In patients who develop heart block as a consequence of cardiac surgery, permanent epicardial leads may be placed at the time of the initial operation. More often, temporary epicardial leads are placed, and if conduction does not recover during the postoperative period, an endomyocardial lead can then subsequently be effectively placed. Epicardial leads are indicated when there is no venous access site available, because of the presence of old leads or subclavian or superior vena caval thrombosis or obstruction; when there is no remaining precordial site for pulse generator placement because of repetitive erosion or infection; and in patients with a prosthetic tricuspid valve or with complex congenital heart disease with septal defects. In rare cases, endomyocardial leads fail to be placed because of inadequate sensing or pacing thresholds; an epicardial lead system can then be used.

Techniques for Endomyocardial Lead Placement

SUBCLAVIAN VEIN

Method

The subclavian vein technique, described in 1977 by Friesen,[8] is now the most commonly used method. The procedure is carried out under sterile conditions in either an operating room or designated procedure room. The patient is positioned on a fluoroscopy table in the horizontal or slight Trendelenburg position with the arms adducted. A sedative may be administered, but generally the procedure is carried out with the patient fully conscious. The implanting physician should inspect the region and identify anatomic landmarks that will enable the subclavian vein to be localized. Any superficial skin infection should be identified and avoided. The skin is prepared, and sterile draping is placed so that the medial two thirds of the clavicle and about 5 inches of the infraclavicular region are exposed. Local anesthesia is infiltrated below the clavicle at a point one third of its length away from the mid line. A small notch or indentation in the clavicle can frequently be palpated at this location. Commercially available kits with a narrow-walled 18-gauge needle, guidewire with deflector, dilator, and sheath are available for lead introduction. The sheath diameter should be chosen to be at least sufficient to pass the lead electrode and tines. However, a larger size such as a No. 12 or No. 14 French may be chosen in order to introduce two leads via one sheath.

The No. 18-gauge needle attached to a fluid-filled syringe is introduced 1 cm below the clavicle at the junction of the medial and center thirds of the length of the clavicle, pointed in the direction of the suprasternal notch. The needle is advanced while maintaining gentle suction in the syringe. The free return of desaturated blood in the syringe indicates puncture of the vein. Suction of air indicates puncture of the apex of the lung, whereas pulsatile high-pressure blood flow on removal of the syringe from the needle suggests subclavian arterial puncture. Dysesthesia or pain radiating down the ipsilateral arm suggests trauma to the brachial plexus. In each of these cases removal of the needle is indicated, followed by gentle pressure. A reassessment of the anatomic landmarks is then indicated prior to repeat puncture. The needle should never be redirected while inside the patient, as this could potentially damage the artery, nerves, and vein.

On successful cannulation of the vein, the guidewire is introduced with the flexible end first. Under fluoroscopic control, the guidewire is advanced to a position in the right atrium. Occasionally the guidewire may tend to advance up the neck veins; it should then be withdrawn and redirected. A J-shaped flexible tip may aid in directing the guidewire. Confirming that the guidewire will reach the right atrium also helps rule out venous anomalies. The needle is then removed, leaving the guidewire in place, taking care not to allow the guidewire to be either retracted or advanced. At this point, the appropriate lead is obtained, tested to ensure that it will pass through the sheath, and placed so that it is readily available. A small incision is made in the skin at the site of the guidewire, and hemostats are used to spread a small superficial tract in order to easily pass the dilator and sheath through the superficial tissues. The dilator and sheath are slipped over the guidewire, ensuring that the guidewire protrudes from the end of the dilator before this assembly is advanced below the skin. This reduces the likelihood of guidewire embolization. A tract is formed by advancing the dilator and sheath through the tissue under the clavicle with a rotating motion and gentle pressure until it slides into the vein.

With the sheath advanced well into the vein, the dilator and guidewire are then removed. The sheath should be either pinched off or covered with the finger in order to prevent air embolism or excessive bleeding. The patient may also be kept in a slight Trendelenburg position to reduce the likelihood of air embolism. The lead can then be advanced through the sheath, with the stylet retracted well away from the tip in order to reduce the likelihood of venous perforation. A guidewire can be introduced through the sheath at this point to permit easy access to the subclavian vein without the need of a second puncture. This guidewire should be fastened to a snap in order to prevent it from accidentally embolizing. This is useful for both dual-chamber pacemaker implants and single-chamber pacemakers because occasionally the initially selected lead may fail to be adequately placed, necessitating a change to an active fixation lead.

Early Complications of Subclavian Vein Cannulation

FAILURE TO LOCATE THE VEIN ■ To facilitate entry into the vein, the Trendelenburg position, a cushion behind the scapula which allows the shoulder to fall back, and a slightly different orientation of the needle may be used. A change in the entry site of the needle to a more lateral location should only be done with the recognition of the increased risk of arterial puncture.

FAILURE TO ADVANCE THE GUIDEWIRE ■ This may occur in the presence of a branch in the vein or angulation of the vein at the point of entry. The position of the guidewire should be verified under fluoroscopy. The intravascular location of the sheath should be confirmed by withdrawing blood. If necessary, a small amount of contrast material can be injected under fluoroscopy to rule out venous anomalies such as a persistent left superior vena cava. Difficulty may also be encountered because the guidewire passes into the jugular vein or across to the contralateral veins. Changing the guidewire to one with a different-size flexible, J-shaped tip or, on occasion, to a flexible straight tip may permit the guidewire to be appropriately directed.

PULMONARY PUNCTURE ■ Suction of air with a needle suggests puncture of the apex of the lung, and the needle should be withdrawn. The fluoroscopic image intensifier can be used to determine if there is evidence of an apical pneumothorax. Only rarely will this develop rapidly enough to be obvious during the implant procedure. However, post-implant chest x-rays should be done routinely in order to monitor the development of a subsequent pneumothorax. The incidence of pneumothoraxes is low, in the order of 1%, when the procedure is properly performed, and most pneumothoraxes are small and spontaneously resolve without requiring a chest tube insertion.

OTHER COMPLICATIONS ■ Arterial puncture usually does not result in severe consequences when only the thin-walled 18-gauge needle is introduced into the artery and then withdrawn. However, significant damage and a hemothorax can result when the dilator and sheath are introduced into the artery. Rarely nerve root damage may occur. Inadvertent puncture of the needle into the clavicle may result in considerable discomfort from hematoma under the periosteum. Inadvertent use of excessive local anesthetic may suppress otherwise stable ventricular escape rhythms rendering the patient asystolic. Patients with vasovagal syncope may respond to pain with hypotension which may necessitate immediate resuscitation.

CEPHALIC VEIN APPROACH

The cephalic vein is a good alternative to the subclavian vein. It can be used for at least one lead in 90% of patients. The cephalic vein is approached via a transverse skin incision astride the deltopectoral groove in the prethoracic region. The vein courses into the groove. It is exposed, tied distally, and snared proximally. After it is opened, a pacing lead can be introduced gently into the superior vena cava. Additional dissection is needed when the lead is trapped into a lateral thoracic vein.

JUGULAR VEIN APPROACH

The internal jugular vein is used only when the other veins are not usable. It is easily exposed via a neck incision. The pacing lead must be tunneled over or under the clavicle, with a consequent increased incidence of lead fracture and skin erosion.

EPIMYOCARDIAL LEAD IMPLANTATION

This approach is no longer used as a primary choice even in patients undergoing combined cardiac surgery. The epicardial leads have a higher pacing threshold and less reliable intraoperative threshold testing. The preferable site of the pacing lead should be the left ventricular apex because of lower pacing thresholds and better sensing. Epicardial lead implantations require general anesthesia and are associated with greater morbidity and mortality.

Two approaches can be selected: transthoracic approaches and the abdominal incision. The median sternotomy is associated with higher morbidity but allows easy access to both ventricles, and choice of optimal site may be associated with a lower pacing threshold. It is used mostly when the pacemaker implantation is combined with another cardiac intervention. The left anterior thoracotomy via the fourth or fifth intercostal space, combined with resection of the cartilage, provides an elective access to the anterior left ventricular wall. It is associated with low morbidity. The midline epigastric incision combined with resection of the xiphoid process provides limited access to the right ventricle. The patient should be prepared for a median sternotomy if an unexpected complication occurs, particularly bleeding and laceration of the right ventricle.

The left subcostal approach is our incision of choice. When the size of the incision is appropriate, this approach provides easy access to both ventricles. A 15-cm skin incision is carried out along the left subcostal edge. The rectus abdominalis is transversally divided. The diaphragm is incised along its attachment onto the cartilage and ribs. The pericardium is incised transversally above its diaphragmatic insertion. The left pleura can be opened without any added morbidity.

Lead Placement

VENTRICULAR PASSIVE FIXATION LEAD

Polyurethane and silastic leads currently used for ventricular pacing are highly flexible and usually require the use of a metal stylet to gain appropriate positioning in the right ventricular apex. Fixation is then dependent on tines or ribs attaching to right ventricular trabeculae. The lead can be advanced to the level of the right atrium following introduction into the vein without the stylet. One technique then employs a stylet that has been bent to produce a smooth 90 degree arc. The stylet is advanced to the tip of the lead, taking care to ensure that no blood makes contact with the stylet, as this may render it impossible to introduce another stylet subsequently. Using fluoroscopy, the lead tip is directed anteriorly and leftward and then advanced through the tricuspid valve orifice. On occasion, the lead will advance directly to the right ventricular apex. However, in the event that the lead curls up toward the right ventricular outflow tract the curved stylet is withdrawn and replaced by a straight stylet. With the lead against the interventricular septum it is then slightly withdrawn; the straight stylet tends to bend the lead toward the apex, after which the stylet can be removed. Passive fixation may be confirmed by gently retracting the lead. This should meet with mild pulsatile resistance. The position of the lead on the fluoroscopic image should be toward the left of the cardiac silhouette in the anterior posterior view, and the lateral view should show the lead sitting anteriorly directed toward the inferior portion of the sternum. The stylet should be removed and sufficient slack allowed in the lead so that it maintains a curvature as it passes from the right atrium to the right ventricle even when the patient takes a deep breath. This additional slack is required to account for the change in diaphragmatic and cardiac position with the upright posture. The adequacy of sensing and pacing thresholds is then determined after a stable satisfactory lead location is obtained.

An alternative technique for lead placement involves forming a gentle bend in the lead with the tip directed laterally in the right atrium and the stylet withdrawn. The lead is then advanced with the loop forming backward through the tricuspid valve. With advancement of the stylet and unfolding of the loop, the lead tends to fall into the right ventricle. Similar techniques may then be used to position the tip in the right ventricular apex.

ATRIAL PASSIVE FIXATION LEAD

The preshaped atrial "J" lead has greatly facilitated the placement of an adequate atrial lead. Usually, the atrial lead is placed as the second lead of a dual-chamber pacing system, and care should be taken to prevent dislodgement of the initially placed ventricular lead. A straight stylet is placed in the atrial lead sufficient to straighten the J-shaped tip. The lead is then advanced toward the orifice of the tricuspid valve. The stylet is withdrawn, allowing the "J" to reform its shape. The J should be oriented anteriorly. The lead is then slowly withdrawn until the tip of the J lead lodges in the right atrial appendage. This is usually demonstrated by fluoroscopy showing an anterior location of the lead tip, with lateral torsion of the lead tip occurring with each cardiac cycle. Again, the stability of the lead should be confirmed by deep respiration and coughing. Gentle tension on the lead should tend to unbend the J shape without immediate dislodgement. The lead should then be given sufficient slack so that the J shape is maintained even with deep inspiration. Finally the adequacy of the sensing and pacing thresholds should be determined.

ACTIVE FIXATION LEADS

In patients with a dilated right ventricle, or an anteroseptal or right ventricular infarct, difficulty may be encountered in either obtaining a stable lead position or adequate pacing or sensing thresholds. An active fixation lead may then be used to obtain a stable lead position in a location other than the right ventricular apex. Most active fixation leads involve a screw mechanism which may be extended beyond the lead tip to enable fixation in the myocardium. This mechanism should be tested prior to introducing the lead and care taken to ensure that the screw is fully retracted before intravascular placement. Some active fixation leads have the screw extended at all times and in these instances care must be taken to rotate the lead only in the opposite direction of the screw until fixation is desired. An atrial active fixation lead may also be required in patients who have had previous cardiovascular surgery, particularly if the right atrial appendage has been removed. In these cases, the lateral right atrial wall may be used as a site for active fixation. At the time of writing, bipolar active fixation leads were just becoming available. Up until this time it was therefore necessary to use unipolar lead systems and to place the active fixation tip well away from the ventricles to prevent oversensing of ventricular activity on the atrial lead.

The active fixation leads are in general traumatic to the tissue. As a result, adequate pacing and sensing thresholds may not be obtained immediately but may improve spontaneously given a 5 to 10 minute wait. In the event that a new pacing site is needed, care should be taken to fully retract (or unscrew) the active fixation lead before attempting to reposition it. This is important as the risk of a pericardial effusion or tamponade is appreciable when this precaution is not observed. Care should also be taken not to exert excessive pressure of the lead tip against the myocardial wall when the screw is extended, as this may result in lead perforation.

Complications of Lead Placement

Complications of lead placement include vascular injury and perforation while advancing the lead; this may be avoided if excessive force is not used. When resistance is met, fluoroscopic imaging should be used in order to redirect the lead tip appropriately. When difficulties are encountered with the lead advancing into the neck veins, a curved stylet may be used to attempt to redirect the lead appropriately. Lead perforation of the myocardium may result in tamponade, diaphragmatic stimulation, or symptoms of pericarditis. In general, a lead that has obviously perforated should be withdrawn into the cavity. In cases of right ventricular perforation, the muscle will frequently seal itself without undue complications. Ventricular tachycardia or ventricular fibrillation may be induced when placing a ventricular pacing lead. This is particularly the case when the stylet is still in place up to the lead tip exerting force against the myocardium. Additionally when the lead is not fixed but mobile within the cavity, it may also be prone to inducing arrhythmias, which may often spontaneously terminate if the lead is withdrawn to the atrium.

Sensing and Pacing Thresholds

The adequacy of the lead position for sensing spontaneous atrial or ventricular activity and the threshold for pacing need to be determined. In general these functions are assessed with the aid of a pacing system analyzer, which should ideally be made by the same manufacturer as the implantable pulse generator. This permits appropriate comparison of sensing and pacing parameters. In practice, the variability between devices is relatively small in most cases, and many implanting centers use a single pacing system analyzer at the time of implant. Bipolar leads have the tip (distal) electrode connected to the negative terminal, and the proximal electrode connected to the positive terminal. For unipolar leads, the lead electrode is connected to the negative terminal, and a plate in the pacemaker pocket is connected to the positive end. As a result, checking a unipolar lead usually necessitates forming a pacemaker pocket first. However, a preliminary impression of the suitability of the lead position can be obtained by connecting the positive end of the pacing system analyzer to an indifferent electrode, such as the guidewire or a skin electrode. Sensing R wave voltage should be monitored during spontaneous, rather than paced ventricular activity. For ventricular leads the acutely measured R wave should be greater than 5 mV, and with atrial electrograms usually greater than 2 mV; however, higher values are preferred, and lower values can be sensed acutely, but often lead to later sensing problems. In fully pacemaker-dependent patients with no spontaneous activity, sensing may not be obtained. Pacing thresholds are usually determined by setting the pulse width and amplitude to the nominal settings of the pulse generator that will be implanted, and at a rate exceeding the spontaneous rhythm. The pulse amplitude (usually voltage, but current in some pulse generators) is then reduced while observing the electrocardiogram until a pacing pulse fails to evoke capture. The voltage, current, and pulse width at threshold are read from the pacing system analyzer. Acceptable thresholds vary with the lead types, but in general a voltage less than 1 volt at 0.5 ms pulse width should be sought for. The lead impedance should also be determined (usually between 300 and 700 ohms, depending on lead type). At our center, bipolar leads are used by preference, but when problems are encountered with appropriate pacing or sensing thresholds, measurements can be made in the unipolar manner, as this will on occasion be adequate without repositioning the lead. In such a case a pulse generator with a bipolar connector and a programmable choice of unipolar or bipolar modes can be selected.

Precautions need to be observed in patients who have an unstable ventricular escape rhythm or who are fully paced. In such patients a temporary pacing electrode may be placed via another venous site in order to easily maintain pacing. Care needs to be taken so that subthreshold pacing does not inhibit a temporary external pacing unit in the demand mode, as this can result in prolonged asystole. Sudden cessation of pacing in a patient following threshold determination may also result in overdrive inhibition of spontaneous rhythms, leading to asystole. This tendency may also be worsened by excessive use of lidocaine as a local anesthetic.

Pacemaker Pocket

PREPECTORAL

The prepectoral location for placement of the pulse generator is used with all the endocardial lead placement techniques on the ipsilateral side. The pacemaker pocket may be fashioned after venous puncture or after lead placement, depending on preference. A local anesthetic without epinephrine is infiltrated superficially in a linear fashion 3 to 4 cm inferior to the clavicle in its mid portion. The length of the skin infiltration should be sufficient to make an incision long enough to insert the pulse generator. Following incision of the skin, blunt dissection to the level of the prepectoral fascia should be carried out. Care should be taken to ligate or cauterize any bleeding at this point. A local anesthetic is again infiltrated along the level of the prepectoral fascia to anesthetize the region where the pacemaker pocket will be formed. Once the pectoral fascia is reached, a good plane of dissection is generally available. The pocket can be formed manually by the physician, using fingers and spreading outward in a fashion to form a pocket about one and a half times the size of the pulse generator. Following formation of the pocket, care should be taken to ensure that sites of bleeding are dealt with. In the most frequently used subclavian vein technique for lead introduction, the lead may then be tunneled into the pacemaker pocket, using blunt dissection. Some physicians prefer to form the pacemaker pocket prior to lead introduction but after introduction of a guidewire into the vein. The guidewire may then be tunneled into the pacemaker pocket, and the lead then subsequently introduced directly from the pacemaker pocket. This latter maneuver reduces the likelihood of traumatic damage to the lead as it is tunneled into the pacemaker pocket. However, the disadvantage is that on occasion it may be slightly more difficult to position a lead.

Following tunneling of the lead into the pacemaker pocket, it is generally advisable to make one last threshold check after the guidewire has been removed. The lead is then actively fixed to the prepectoral fascia, using an attachment provided on the lead. In general, nonabsorbable sutures are used in order to maintain fixation for a prolonged period. The cleaned lead is then connected to the pulse generator, the set screws are tightened and, if necessary, capped or sealed with medical adhesive. The pulse generator is then sutured to the prepectoral fascia in order to prevent it from sliding inferiorly or into the axilla. At our center absorbable suture is used to close the subcutaneous tissue with interrupted inverted mattress sutures. The skin may then be closed, using a subcuticular running absorbable suture. Final apposition of the skin may be maintained, using tape and/or clear plastic adhesive dressing.

On conclusion of the implant, the patient generally requires mild analgesics for the first 24 hours. The patient should be checked frequently for vital signs for 4 to 6 hours and should be checked by the physician later the same day to ensure that there is adequate hemostasis. A chest x-ray series should be obtained to ensure that lead position is maintained and that there is no formation of a pneumothorax or hemothorax. The patient should be on continuous electrocardiographic monitoring for a period of 24 to 48 hours to ensure that the lead maintains capture. The day following implant, sensing and pacing thresholds are checked to determine that they are maintaining a relatively stable value before the patient is discharged from hospital. At our center it is a practice to maintain the pacing parameters at nominal values until the patient returns for subsequent pacemaker follow-up.

In patients who have a temporary pacing wire in place at the time the lead and pulse generator are positioned, a decision needs to be made on when to remove the temporary wire. In patients who are not fully pacemaker-dependent, the temporary lead may be removed at the time of implantation. Also, this may be done in cases where the lead position appears exceedingly stable. In patients who are fully pacemaker-dependent, and who would otherwise be asystolic if there were loss of capture, it is our practice to leave the temporary wire in for 24 hours and then remove it under fluoroscopic imaging to ensure that the removal of the temporary wire does not dislodge the recently placed permanent lead.

THE RETROMAMMARY PACEMAKER POCKET

The retromammary implantation of the pacemaker generator is a good alternative in women for cosmetic reasons, or in thin women to use the breast to protect the implant site. The retromammary pocket requires general anesthesia. After completion of the conventional subclavian lead implantation, an incision is made just over the inframammary fold. The retromammary space anterior to the pectoral fascia is dissected. Then, using a long, smooth forcep, the leads are brought into the pocket. The surgery is completed, and special care is given to hemostasis.

THE ABDOMINAL PACEMAKER POCKET

The pacemaker pocket can be constructed either in the subcutaneous tissue if the patient is obese or within the rectus abdominis sheath if the patient is slim, to prevent skin erosion. In the latter case, the pocket is developed within the rectus abdominis sheath posterior to the muscle. The incision of the sheath is conveniently located at a different site than that of the pocket in order to facilitate closure of the sheath and to prevent pacemaker migration.

Techniques for Pulse Generator Replacement

Prior to embarking on pulse generator replacement, adequate data need to be obtained from the pacemaker follow-up clinic to determine the pulse generator characteristics, type and size of the lead, and the connector type. Data must be obtained on the likely adequacy of this particular lead. This would include the known sensing and pacing thresholds and lead impedance, when this can be obtained by telemetry and programming. When further data from the manufacturer on the longevity of the lead suggests that the lead may have a high failure rate, elective replacement of the lead may also be considered. The chest x-ray should be examined to determine the location of the lead with respect to the pulse generator.

In general, patients are prepared and draped for generator replacement very much the same as they would be for an initial lead implant. However, the local anesthetic is now infiltrated in such a manner as to approach the pulse generator without damaging the lead. Making the incision in the site of a previous incision will produce a better cosmetic result, as the patient will be left with only a single scar. However, this is technically a more difficult approach, as the tissue is extremely fibrotic and generally very vascular. Blunt dissection should be used as much as possible in order to minimize the likelihood of damage to the permanent pacing lead, and electrocautery should be avoided. Most patients form a very firm pocket around the pulse generator. Once this pocket is reached it can be incised, and the pulse generator can be removed from the patient.

In patients who are fully pacemaker-dependent, elective placement of a temporary pacing lead for the procedure may be chosen. This is less of a problem with patients with bipolar pacing systems, as pacing will be maintained even when the pulse generator is removed from the pacemaker pocket. With a bipolar lead, pacing function is lost when the lead is disconnected from the pulse generator. However, it should be noted that, in the case of unipolar pacing systems, at the moment that adequate contact between the pulse generator and the patient is lost, pacing function will also be lost.

When the pulse generator has been removed from the pacemaker pocket, the set screws are unscrewed and the pulse generator is disconnected from the lead. The adequacy of the sensing and pacing thresholds and lead impedance are then determined. In the event that they are inadequate, then a new pacemaker lead also needs to be considered. An attempt should be made to withdraw the old pacemaker lead, but excessive force should never be used, as the lead may break or the insulation may fragment and embolize. Gentle steady traction should be applied in order to slide out the old lead. When this fails, the lead may be cut and a cap placed over the distal end and attached to the deep tissue. A new pacemaker lead will then be placed.

In the event that the old lead was adequate, then a compatible pulse generator can be connected directly to this lead, or if necessary an adaptor may be used to adapt the lead to newer pulse generators. After the lead is appropriately connected to the pulse generator, the pulse generator is placed in the pocket, the pacemaker pocket closed, and then the subcutaneous tissue and skin closed. A chronically placed lead does not need to be reattached to the deep tissue.

Special Considerations Related to Rate-Responsive Pacing

At the time of this writing, several rate-responsive pacemakers based on a parameter measured from the lead were either in clinical trials or development. These devices are dependent on the use of a sensor to determine the variable pacing rates in the rate-responsive mode. Currently, guidelines and techniques are not yet standardized for the assessment of these rate-responsive devices. However, it may be anticipated that there will be specialized assessment to determine the functionality of each of the leads for these rate-responsive pacing systems, particularly when the sensor is placed on the lead. Additional measurements need to be made for these various pacing systems, such as determination of the evoked potential for the QT-dependent pacemaker.

Late Complications of Pacemaker Implantation

Late complications of pacemaker implantations may be classified in terms of problems related to the surgical procedure, the implantation of the device, and problems related to the lead. Surgical complications include infections, which in general are caused by organisms present on the skin and are manifest within a week. Infection is particularly common in diabetics. Because of the presence of a foreign body (pulse generator and lead), acute infections are generally extremely difficult to treat with antibiotics and necessitate removal of the pulse generator and lead.

Infections may also be extremely deceptive because of the presence of the preformed pocket. Superficial inflammation may be minimized and a large quantity of purulent material may be present in the pocket without marked superficial evidence of this. However, fluctuancy of the pacemaker pocket and fever would suggest infection. A needle aspiration may then be performed under sterile conditions in order to obtain a sample for culturing for diagnosis, to determine appropriate antibiotics, and to rule out a sterile abscess.

Another postoperative complication includes hemorrhage, which may be particularly serious in patients who are started immediately after implantation on anticoagulants. Dysesthetic pain and keloid formation may occur as late postoperative complications. Failure to mobilize the patient early may lead to a sympathetic dystrophy producing pain and immobility in the ipsilateral shoulder and arm.

Complications related to the presence of the pulse generator include migration of the pulse generator either inferiorly or into the axilla. This may contribute to the development of another complication, namely skin erosion. The likelihood of migration may be reduced by attachment of the pulse generator to the deep fascia. In addition, placing the pulse generator in a Dacron sack may reduce the likelihood of this problem. Failure to make a sufficiently large pacemaker pocket, or marked debility and emaciation in the patient may also contribute to skin erosion.

Late complications related to the lead include late loss of capture, which is most prevalent within the first 1 to 3 weeks following placement of a new lead. Venous thrombosis may occur, leading to engorgement of the arm veins. Rare cases of endocarditis have been reported, and very rarely pacemakers may induce arrhythmias.

References

1. Belott PH, Bucko D: Inframammary pulse generator placement for maximizing cosmetic effect. PACE 6:1241, 1983.
2. Bisping HJ, Kreuzer J, Birkenheier, H: Three year clinical experience with a new endocardial screw-in lead with introduction protection for use in the atrium and ventricle. PACE 8:424, 1980.
3. Bognolo DA: Recent advances in permanent pacemaker implantation techniques. *In* Barold SS (ed.): Modern Cardiac Pacing, pp. 199–229. Mt. Kisco, Futura Publishing Co., 1985.
4. Bognolo DA, Vijayanagar RR, Eckstein PF, et al.: Two leads in one introducer technique for AV sequential implantations. PACE 5:217, 1982.
5. Bognolo D, Vijay R, Eckstein P, et al.: Technical aspects of pacemaker system upgrading procedures. Clin Prog Pacing Electrophysiol 1:269, 1983.
6. Bognolo DA, Vijayanagar R, Eckstein PF, et al.: Implantation of permanent transvenous atrial "J" lead using lateral view fluoroscopy. Ann Thorac Surg 31:574, 1981.
7. Byrd C: Permanent pacemaker implantation techniques. *In* Samet P, El-Sherif N (eds.): Cardiac Pacing, 2nd Ed, Clinical Cardiology Monographs, p. 232. New York, Grune & Stratton, 1980.
8. Friesen A, Klein GJ, Kostuk WJ, et al.: Percutaneous insertion of a permanent transvenous pacemaker electrode through the subclavian vein. Can J Surg 20:131, 1977.
9. Furman S, Fisher JD: Cardiac pacing and pacemakers. V: Technical aspects of implantation and equipment. Am Heart J 94:250, 1977.
10. Holmes DR Jr: Permanent pacemaker implantation. *In* Furman S, Hayes DL, Holmes DR Jr (eds.): A Practice of Cardiac Pacing, p. 97. Mt. Kisco, Futura Publishing Co., 1986.
11. Kleinert M, Bock M, Wilhemi F: Clinical use of a new transvenous atrial lead. Am J Cardiol 40:237, 1977.
12. Lawrie GM, Scale JP, Morris GC Jr, et al.: Results of epicardial pacing by the left subcostal approach. Ann Thorac Surg 28:561, 1979.
13. Littleford PO, Spector SD: Device for the rapid insertion of a permanent endocardial pacing electrode through the subclavian vein: Preliminary report. Ann Thorac Surg 27:265, 1979.
14. Martinis AJ: Pacemaker insertion. *In* Dillard DH, Miller DW Jr (eds.): Atlas of Cardiac Surgery, pp. 156–163. New York, Macmillan Publishing Co., 1983.
15. Messenger JC, Castellanet MJ, Stephenson NL: New permanent endocardial atrial J lead: Implantation techniques in clinical performance. PACE 5:767, 1982.
16. Smyth NPD: Pacemaker implantation: Surgical techniques. Cardiovasc Clinic 14:31, 1983.

33

Electrocardiography of Single-Chamber Pacemakers

John M. Fontaine
Shantha Ursell
Nabil El-Sherif

Overview

Since the development of the implantable cardiac pacemaker nearly three decades ago, numerous bioengineering and technological advancements have been made. The spectrum of change includes the development of the ventricular demand pacemaker (VVI) from the fixed rate type (VOO) to the development of the more physiologic dual-chamber and rate-responsive pacing systems. The introduction of antitachycardia pacing and the advent of the automatic implantable defibrillator are among the myriad advances in cardiac pacing. In spite of those advances, the understanding of the electrocardiographic manifestation of normal and abnormal function of the basic single-chamber pacemaker remains quintessential and fundamental to pacemaker rhythm analysis and appropriate follow-up care of patients. This knowledge is an important prerequisite for understanding the more complex pacing systems.

The 1986 world survey data, acquired by the International Cardiac Pacing Society and derived from 26 countries at 5500 implanting centers and involving over 230,000 pacemakers, revealed that VVI pacing was the leading mode utilized throughout the world.[1] Within the United States, 67% of all pacemakers were programmed to the VVI mode, whereas the remainder were either DVI, DDD or VAT. The single chamber atrial pacing mode (AAI) accounted for approximately 1% of the pacing modalities utilized in North America.

The purpose of this chapter is to review the various electrocardiographic patterns of the basic single-chamber pacemaker and to distinguish the electrocardiographic manifestations of pacemaker malfunction from pseudo-malfunction and other variations of normal. The predominant emphasis will be placed on the single-chamber ventricular pacemaker, with only brief mention of the single-chamber atrial pacemaker. Because of the existence of many pacemaker manufacturers and a legion of pacemaker models, it is extremely difficult to memorize all of the individual pacemaker specifications and their idiosyncrasies. In view of this, pacemaker rhythm analysis should be ideally performed with the full knowledge of the manufacturer and model number of the pacemaker undergoing evaluation. In addition, since programmability has become a feature of all current pacemakers, it is important that an accurate record of the programmed parameters be maintained for follow-up and detection of pacemaker malfunction.

The pacemaker study group in 1974 recommended a three-position code to describe pacemaker function.[2] This code has recently been modified to a five-position code to include programmability, rate modulation and antitachyarrhythmia functions (Table 33–1).[3,4] The electrocardiography of dual-chamber, rate-responsive, and antitachycardia pacemakers will be discussed in subsequent chapters. Since this chapter will deal only with single-chamber antibradyarrhythmia pacing, the first three positions of the recent five-position NASPE/BPEG generic pacemaker code will be appropriately descriptive and sufficient in a general discussion. A specific pacemaker will be described using the five-position code.

The Pacemaker Stimulus Artifact

The stimulus artifact or pacemaker spike represents electrical energy generated from the power source of the pacemaker and stored in the capacitor until the pacemaker's timely discharge. Its successful delivery is

TABLE 33–1
Five-position Pacemaker Identification Code of the North American Society of Pacing and Electrophysiology (NASPE) and the British Pacing and Electrophysiology Group (BPEG)

Position/Category	I Chamber(s) Paced	II Chamber(s) Sensed	III Response to Sensing	IV Programmability, Rate Modulation	V Antitachy- arrhythmia Function(s)
Letter Codes	O = None V = Ventricle A = Atrium D = Dual (A + V)	O = None V = Ventricle A = Atrium D = Dual (A + V)	O = None T = Triggers pacing I = Inhibits pacing D = Dual (T + I)	O = None P = Simple programmable M = Multi programmable C = Communicating (telemetry) R = Rate Modulation	O = None P = Pacing (antitachy-arrhythmia) S = Shock D = Dual (P + S)

NOTE: Positions I through III are used exclusively for antibradyarrhythmia pacing.
Manufacturers may use "S" in Positions I and II to indicate single chamber (A or V).
A minimum of 4 positions is required to describe a pacemaker.

dependent on an intact pulse generator and lead system. The characteristics of the stimulus artifact are dependent on the strength of the power source, lead position, and polarity, as well as the method of signal processing used during electrocardiographic recording. Precise analysis of the stimulus artifact can be performed via oscilloscopic analysis of the output pulse.[5] The use of the conventional scalar electrocardiograph (ECG) equipped with analog signal processing may be useful in assessing pacing system malfunction. Noted changes in the amplitude or frontal plane axis of the stimulus artifact during held respiration may be an early sign of insulation breakage.[6] A considerable change in the stimulus amplitude, documented in three or more ECG leads, from a bipolar pacing system provides evidence suggestive of insulation breakage.

In addition to the stimulus artifact, a voltage exponential decay curve is often seen immediately following it. The typical ECG stimulus artifact is usually ≤1 ms in duration and possesses an amplitude of 2 to 3 mV. The voltage exponential decay curve represents the dissipation of that energy through the body tissues. Its amplitude is directly proportional to the amount of voltage delivered from the pulse generator. On rare occasions complete obliteration of the subsequent QRS complex may occur.[7] The frontal plane vector of the decay curve (in a unipolar system) will yield information regarding directionality of current traveling from the pulse generator site to the electrode tip.[8] The dipole of the unipolar system is dependent on the orientation of the anode to the cathode; hence, the frontal plane of the stimulus artifact parallels that of dipole orientation, since the indifferent electrode or ground is often the titanium case of the pulse generator and opposite the anodal pole.

Using an analog ECG, the vector of the decay curve can be used to confirm the site of the pulse generator or diagnose ECG lead reversal errors. Utilizing frontal plane bipolar leads, right and left infraclavicular and abdominal site pacemakers can be electrocardiographically located. A positive vector is obtained if the flow of current is parallel to the lead orientation. A left infraclavicular pulse generator position yields a positive decay curve vector in leads 2, 3, aVF, and aVR, and a negative vector in lead 1 (Fig. 33–1). A lead 1 reversal error leads to a positive decay curve vector in

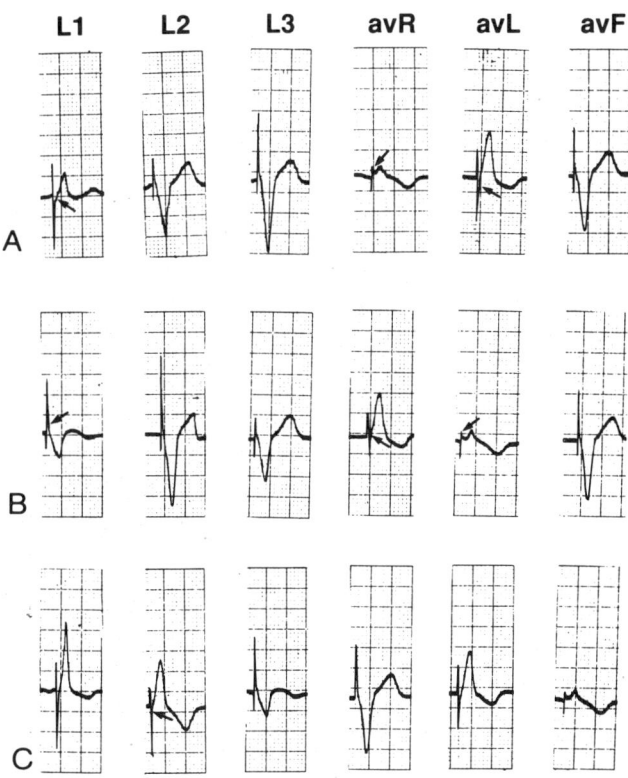

FIGURE 33–1
Analog 12-lead ECG from a patient with a left infraclavicular site pulse generator. In A (unipolar pacing), the vector of the exponential decay curve is negative in leads 1 and aVL, and positive in lead aVR (see arrows). In B, a lead 1 reversal error can be recognized when the vector becomes positive in leads 1 and aVL and negative in lead aVR. The vector of the exponential decay curve remains unchanged in leads 2, 3, and aVF. In C, a lead 2 reversal error results in an isolated change in the vector of lead 2 from positive to negative.

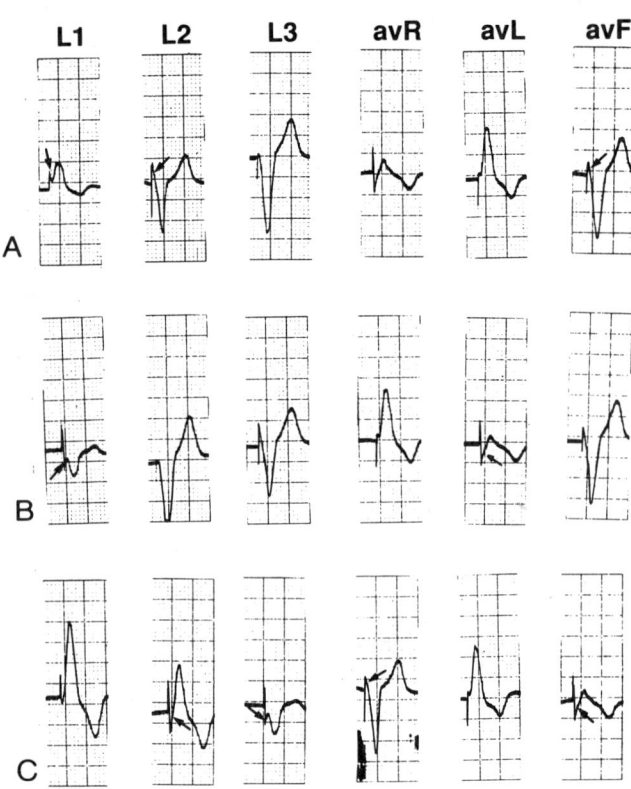

FIGURE 33–2
Analog 12-lead ECG from a patient with a right infraclavicular site pulse generator. In A (unipolar pacing), the vector of the exponential decay curve is positive in leads 1, 2, 3, aVL, and aVF and negative in lead aVR (see arrows). In B, a lead 1 reversal error results in a change from a positive to a negative vector in leads 1 and aVL, and from a negative to a positive vector in lead aVR. Leads 2, 3, and aVF remain essentially unchanged. In C, a lead 2 reversal error results in a change from a positive to a negative vector in leads 2, 3, and aVF, whereas lead aVR becomes positive.

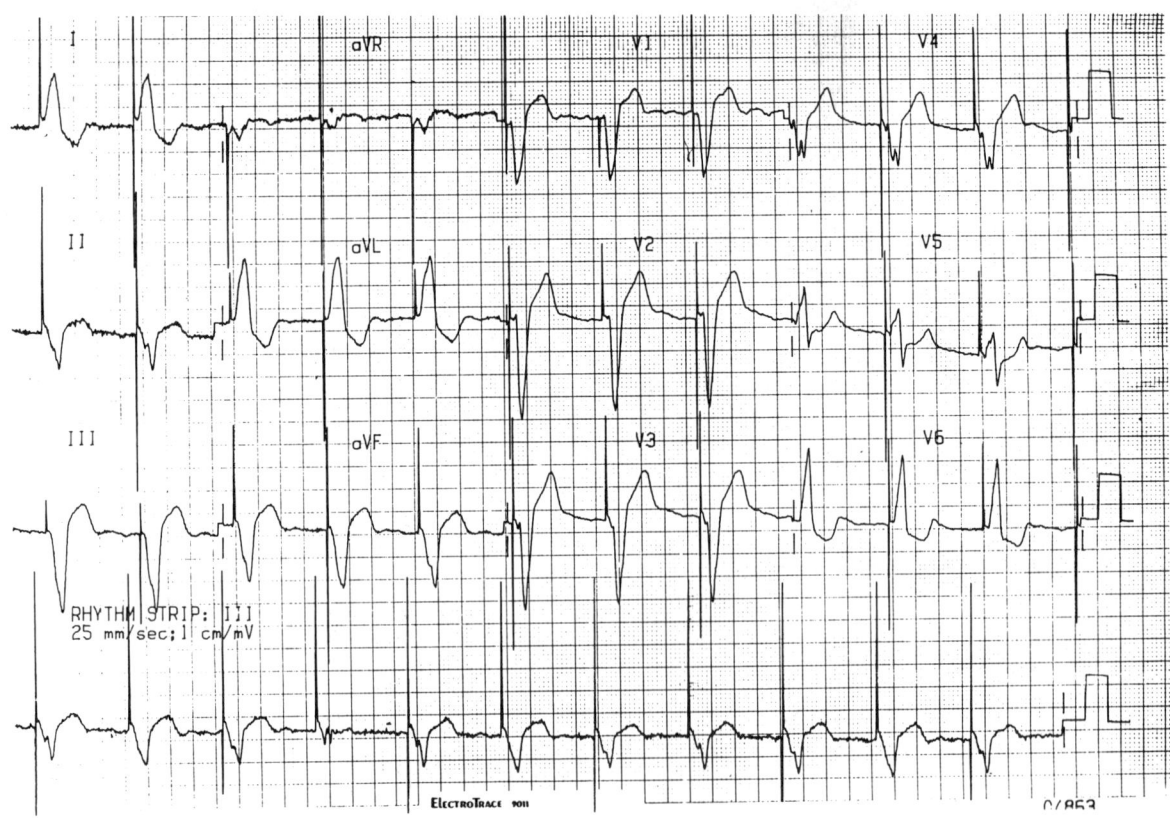

FIGURE 33–3
Digital processing artifact of the pacemaker output pulse. The marked variation in the pacemaker spike amplitude and vector is a common occurrence in digital electrocardiographic recordings. Note regular alternation of amplitude and configuration of the stimulus artifact in the rhythm strip.

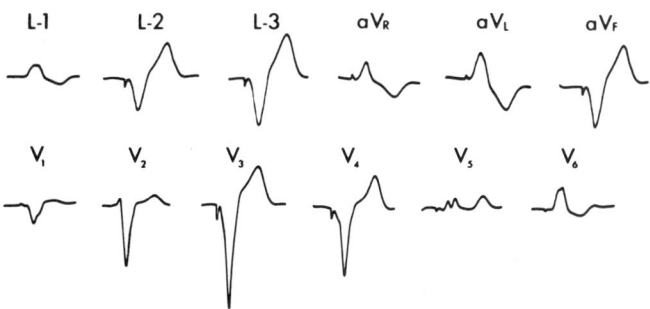

FIGURE 33–4
Electrocardiographic pattern of left bundle branch block and left axis deviation noted during endocardial pacing at the right ventricular apex. The relatively small pacemaker spikes are secondary to bipolar pacing.

lead 1, whereas a lead 2 reversal error produces a negative lead 2 vectorial change. Lead 1 and 2 reversal errors for a right infraclavicular pulse generator site are shown in Figure 33–2.

Alterations in the amplitude or axis of the stimulus artifact itself are not always evidence of pacing system malfunction. The advent of digital electrocardiography has made this a common finding (Fig. 33–3).[9–12] The digital ECG usually processes the analog signal at a sampling rate of 250 Hz, which is ample for recording the ECG signal but may not adequately detect all of the stimulus artifact. This is so because the duration of this signal is generally ≤1 ms, whereas the sampling rate is once every 4 ms. As a result, the stimulus artifact will vary in amplitude depending upon how much of this high-frequency signal is detected. This can sometimes result in regular alternation of amplitude and/or configuration of the stimulus artifact (see Fig. 33–3, rhythm strip). On occasion the signal may be completely missed, thus simulating pacemaker artifact failure. Standard analog electrocardiography is preferred when monitoring patients with suspected wire fracture or pulse generator failure. Marked attenuation of the stimulus artifact noted in several monitoring leads during held respiration is suggestive of such malfunction.

QRS Patterns Associated with Ventricular Pacing

The QRS morphology during pacing depends on the site of stimulation. Right ventricular stimulation usually results in a left bundle branch block (LBBB) pattern, whereas left ventricular stimulation results in a right bundle branch block (RBBB) pattern. The frontal plane QRS axis is determined by the stimulation site in the ventricle. Right ventricular apical stimulation, commonly seen with transvenous endocardial stimulation, results in an LBBB pattern associated with abnormal left axis deviation (−30° to −90°) due to apex-to-base activation of the ventricles (Fig. 33–4). Left ventricular epicardial implantation is usually applied close to the base of the left ventricle (as shown in Fig. 33–5). The paced QRS complexes, therefore, show an RBBB pattern with right axis deviation (Fig. 33–6). Rarely is the right ventricular outflow tract used for permanent pacing, if so, the resulting QRS complex will have an LBBB pattern with a normal axis or, uncommonly, a right axis deviation (Fig. 33–7).

Although transvenous right ventricular apical stimulation produces an LBBB pattern, RBBB morphology is occasionally seen (Fig. 33–8). If there is a change from an LBBB to an RBBB pattern, myocardial perforation by the electrode catheter producing left ven-

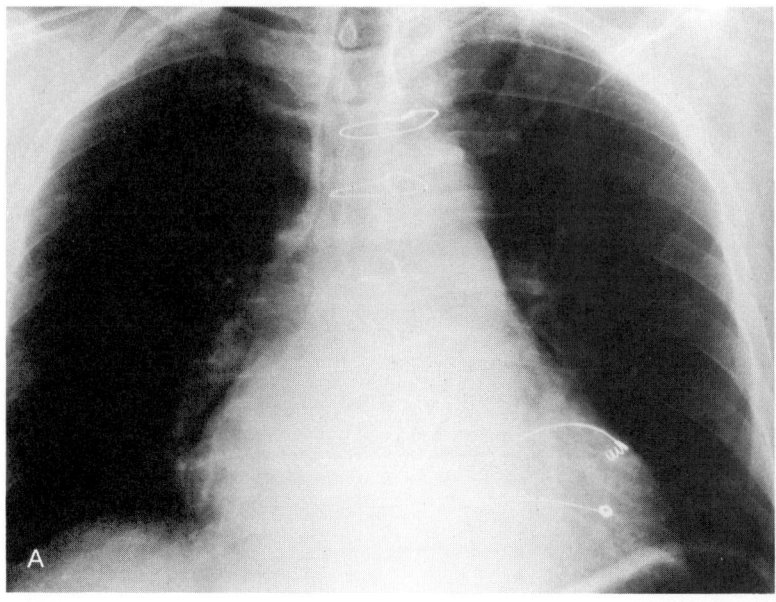
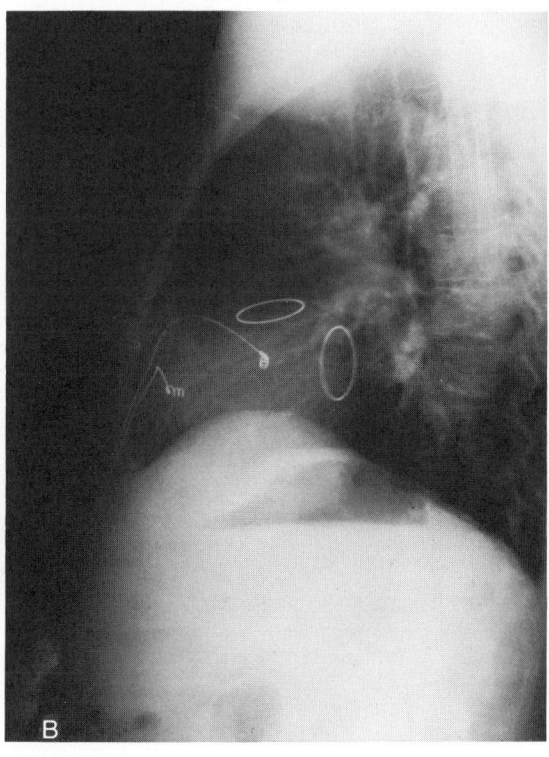

FIGURE 33–5
Posteroanterior (A) and lateral (B) chest radiographs of normal epicardial lead placement. Screw-in epicardial leads are properly positioned toward the base of the heart in a patient with both aortic and mitral valve bioprostheses.

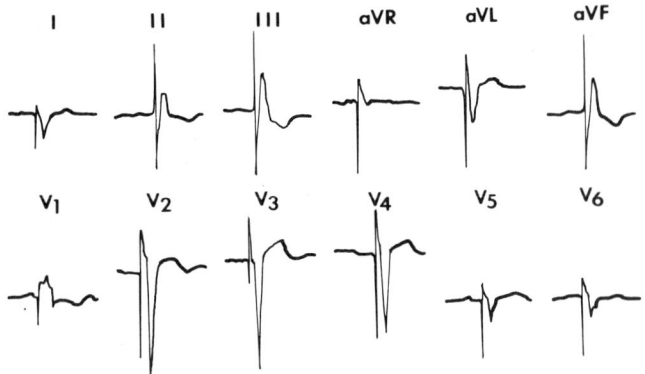

FIGURE 33–6
Electrocardiographic pattern of right bundle branch block and right axis deviation during left ventricular epicardial pacing close to the basal portion of the left ventricle. The relatively large pacemaker artifacts are secondary to unipolar pacing.

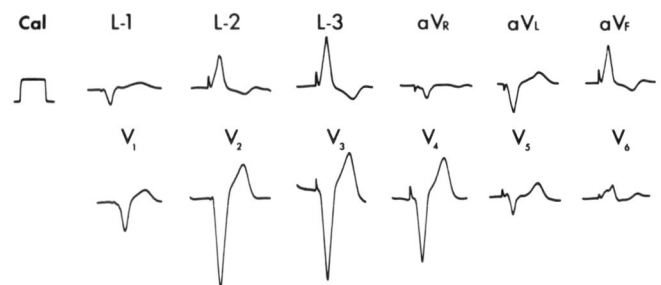

FIGURE 33–7
Uncommon frontal plane axis during epicardial stimulation of the right ventricular outflow tract. The ECG reveals a left bundle branch block pattern and right axis deviation.

tricular stimulation should be considered.[13, 14] However, there are several theoretical mechanisms by which an RBBB pattern can be produced by right ventricular septal stimulation. Mower et al.[15] attributed it to direct selective stimulation of the right bundle branch with retrograde conduction to the His bundle and subsequent activation of the left bundle branch. Sodi-Pallares,[16] on the other hand, suggested that the anatomic left septum can extend to the right ventricular endocardium, and stimulation of this area could therefore produce an RBBB pattern.

Others have postulated that a delay in right ventricular activation exists, which allows the left ventricle to be depolarized first.[17] One other explanation suggests that rapid conduction from right to left occurs through Purkinje bridges between the right and left bundle branches, thus producing an RBBB pattern.[18]

The presence of a dominant R wave in leads V_1 and V_2 or an RBBB pattern during right ventricular apical pacing may also reflect altered ECG lead placement. It is possible to record a dominant R wave when those leads are placed in the fourth intercostal space. Repositioning V_1 and V_2 to the fifth intercostal space will abolish the dominant R wave pattern if displacement of the electrode catheter has not occurred (Fig. 33–9). The dominant R wave pattern infrequently noted in V_1 and V_2 may reflect partial anterior direction of vectorial forces; however, the presence of a dominant R wave in V_5 or V_6 or the loss of the dominant R wave in V_2 positioned at the 5th interspace suggests that the predominant terminal vectorial forces are directed posteriorly.

Occasionally, during implantation of a transvenous electrode catheter, inadvertent placement in the coronary sinus or in one of its tributaries may occur and give rise to an RBBB pattern.[19] More often, migration or displacement of the catheter into the coronary sinus from its original position in the right ventricular apex can result in stimulation of the left ventricle and an RBBB pattern. Spontaneous displacement of the pacemaker lead from the right ventricular apex to the middle cardiac vein is shown in Figure 33–10. An RBBB pattern may also be seen when a pacemaker lead is positioned directly into the left ventricle via a patent foramen ovale or an atrial septal defect. X-rays of the chest, both posteroanterior and lateral views,

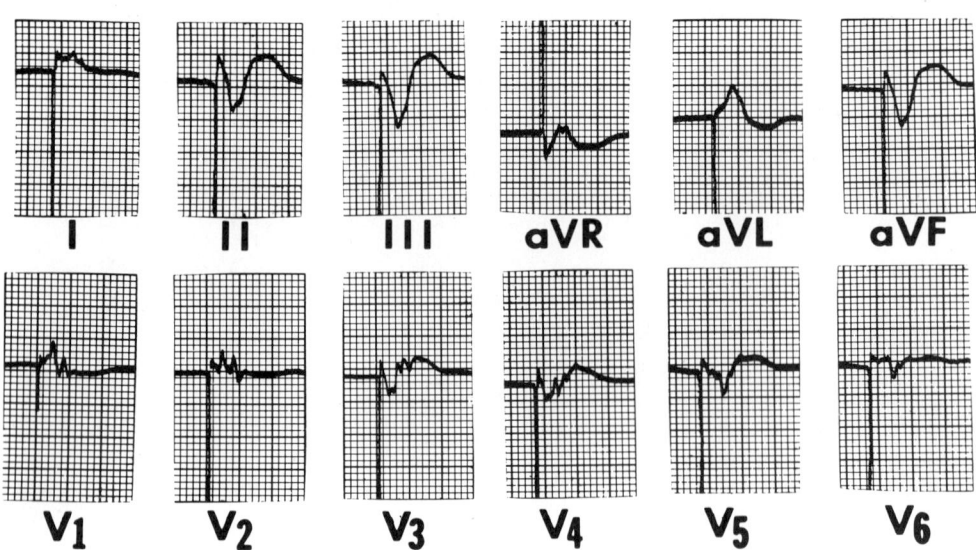

FIGURE 33–8
Uncommon electrocardiographic pattern during endocardial stimulation of the right ventricular apical region, showing an atypical right bundle branch block pattern and left axis deviation. See text for possible explanations.

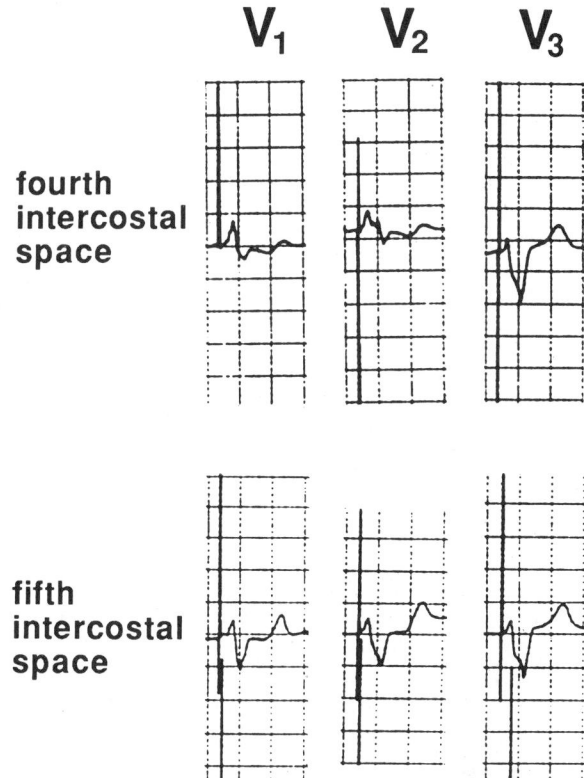

FIGURE 33-9
Pseudo–right bundle branch block during right ventricular apical pacing. Shown is a dominant R wave pattern in precordial leads V_1-V_2 positioned at the fourth intercostal space. The V_3 lead positioned in the same interspace demonstrates posterior-directed terminal forces (loss of R wave). Repositioning the same leads to the fifth intercostal space fails to show persistence of anterior-directed terminal forces that would be expected to be present during true right bundle branch block. See text for explanation.

will aid in making the diagnosis. When the catheter tip is in the right ventricular apex, the lateral chest x-ray should show the lead to be directed anteriorly (Fig. 33-11), whereas a posterior location of the tip suggests displacement to the coronary sinus. A posteroanterior chest x-ray alone cannot distinguish a right ventricular apical position of the catheter from one in which the electrode was introduced into the coronary sinus.

Figure 33-12 illustrates pacing from a lead in the middle cardiac vein resulting in an RBBB pattern associated with left axis deviation. A unique feature of this electrocardiogram is the fact that the paced QRS

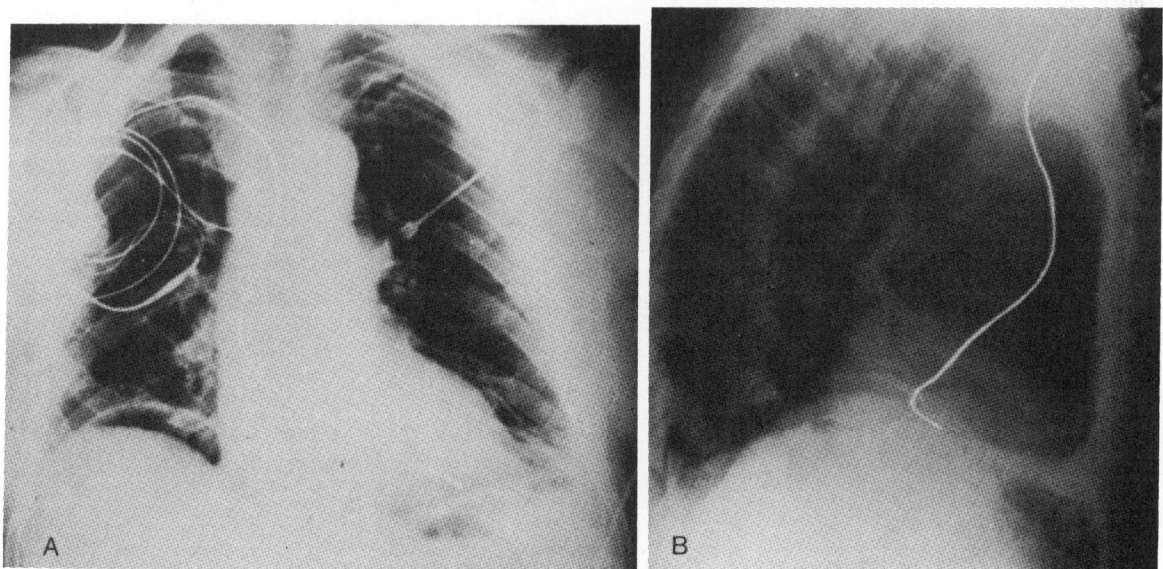

FIGURE 33-10
Posteroanterior (A) and lateral (B) chest radiographs illustrating a pacing lead in the middle cardiac vein—a tributary of the coronary sinus vein. Note the posterior displacement of the electrode in the lateral view.

Electrocardiography of Single-Chamber Pacemakers

complexes are almost identical to the patient's conducted supraventricular beats in all 12 ECG leads.[20] An RBBB pattern plus left axis deviation during sinus rhythm suggests conduction delay and/or block in both the right bundle and the anterior division of the left bundle. The supraventricular impulse would reach the ventricles through the posterior division of the left bundle. Epicardial stimulation of the posterior septal portion of the left ventricle by a pacing lead in the middle cardiac vein presumably resulted in early activation of the posterior fascicular system, thus simulating the normal spread of the supraventricular impulse. This observation lends credence to the anatomically distinct trifascicular nature of the atrioventricular (AV) conduction system.

PACEMAKER FUSION AND PSEUDOFUSION BEATS

True fusion beats occur when the ventricles are simultaneously activated by a spontaneous depolarization and a paced impulse.[21] The spontaneous depolarization can be either a conducted supraventricular beat or an ectopic ventricular impulse. Pseudofusion, on the other hand, refers to the superimposition of an ineffectual pacemaker spike on a QRS complex originating from a single focus.[22] This occurs because the pacemaker emits discharges after the onset of ventricular depolarization and within the absolute refractory period of the myocardium, but before the intrinsic ventricular depolarization has reached adequate voltage and slew rate (dv/dt) to activate the sensing circuit, thus inhibiting pacemaker output. A varying portion of the QRS complex may be inscribed on the surface ECG before the superimposition of the pacemaker spike. When the rate of the spontaneous cardiac rhythm is nearly identical to the pacemaker rate, regular alternation of a spontaneous beat and a pseudofusion beat may be seen (Fig. 33–13). This probably occurs because of the slight difference between the pacemaker escape and automatic intervals.

POSTPACING ST-T WAVE CHANGES

Chatterjee et al.[23] first described the frequent occurrence of ST-T wave changes in the unpaced ECG, subsequent to right ventricular endocardial pacing, that persist for varying lengths of time depending on the duration of pacing (Fig. 33–14). Similar changes were later reported with intermittent LBBB.[24] Rosenbaum and associates[25] noted that the T wave changes in normally conducted beats have a similar direction to that of the QRS complex of the abnormally conducted beats in each of the 12 ECG leads. The recovery time of the ST-T wave changes seems to depend on the magnitude of the change attained during the pacing period. During continuous right ventricular pacing, marked ST-T wave changes are induced in a gradually cumulative fashion. After the provoking stimulus is discontinued and its effects are no longer apparent, the heart seems to retain a "memory" of the previous effect so that reintroduction of the stimulus will result in redevelopment of the ST-T wave changes in a much shorter time span.[25]

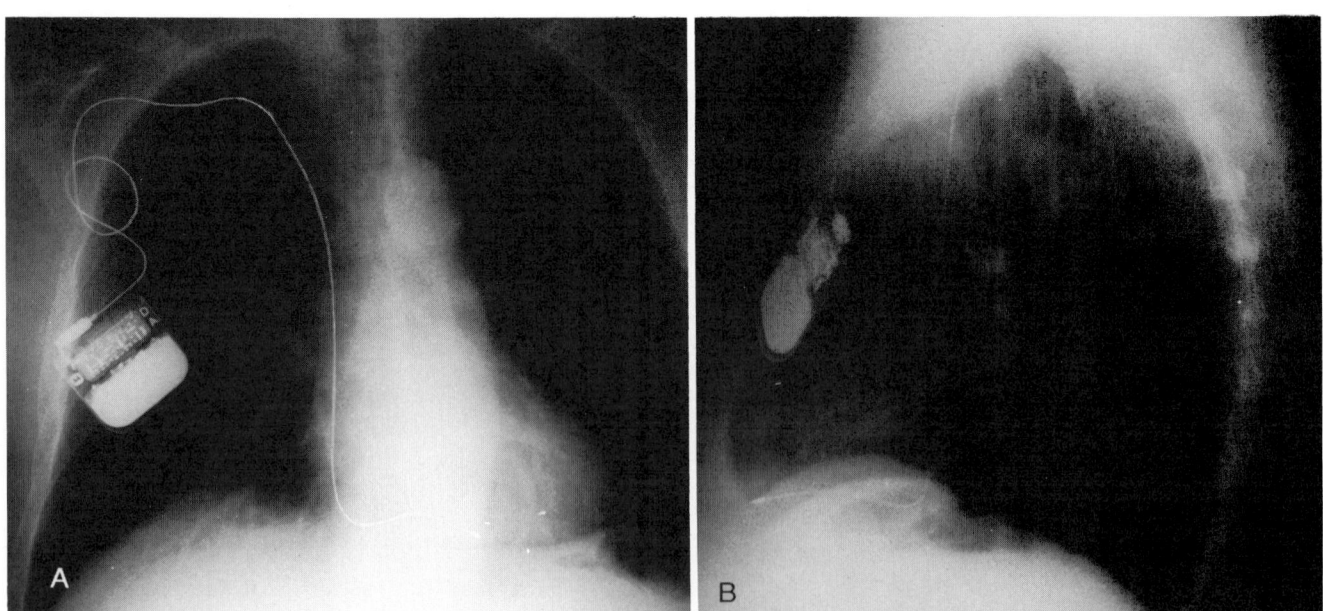

FIGURE 33–11
Posteroanterior (A) and lateral (B) chest radiographs demonstrating the normal position of a right ventricular pacing lead. Confirmation that the lead is positioned at the apex of the right ventricle is evident on the lateral view, which reveals that the lead is located in the anterior ventricular chamber.

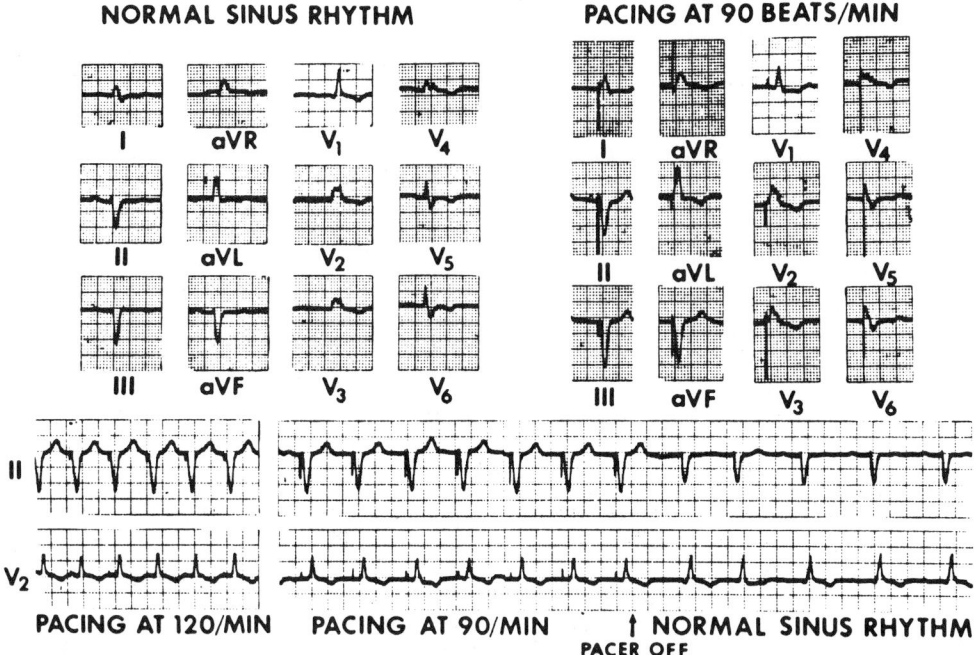

FIGURE 33–12
ECG recorded during pacing from a lead located in the middle cardiac vein. A unique feature of this ECG is the almost identical electrocardiographic pattern during both conducted sinus beats and ventricular paced beats. See text for information.

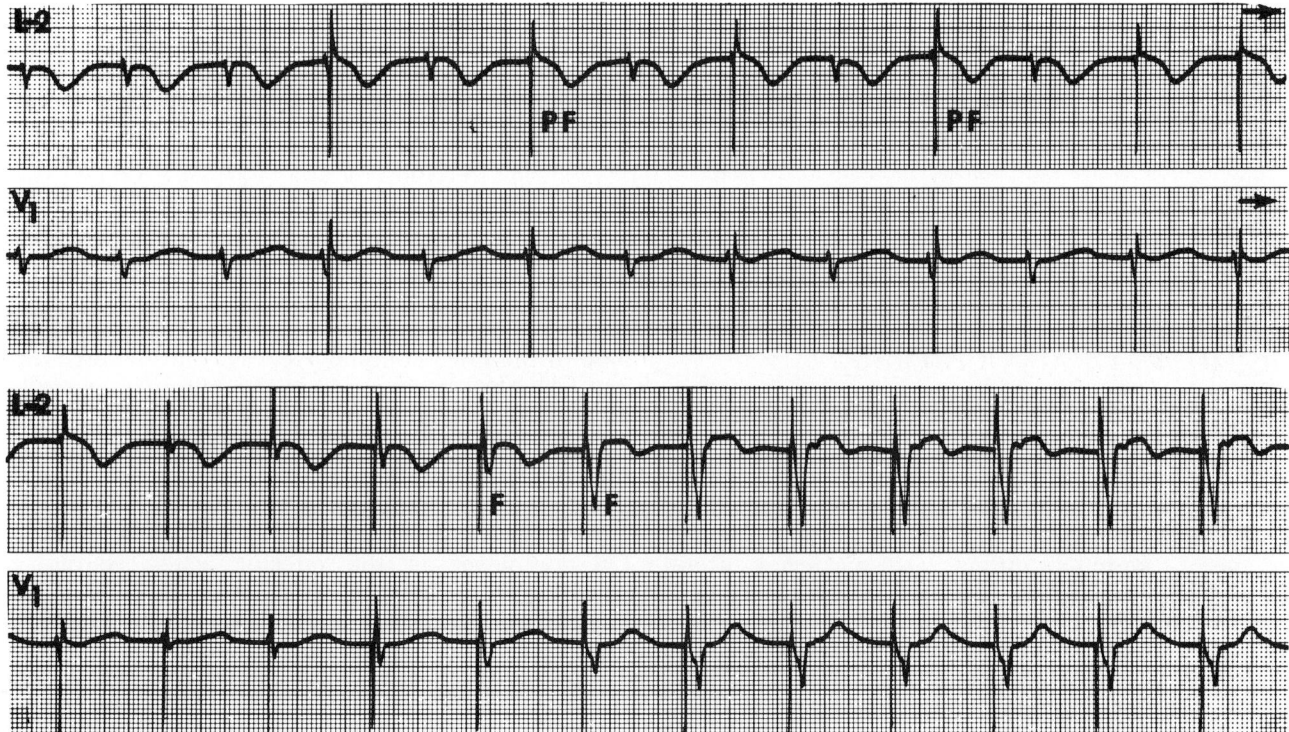

FIGURE 33–13
Simultaneous continuous rhythm strip of leads 2 and V_1 in a patient with accelerated junctional rhythm and a VVI pacemaker. The rate of the spontaneous rhythm is almost identical to the pacemaker rate, resulting in alternation of a paced beat and a pseudofusion beat (PF) before consecutive discharge of the pacemaker occurs at the end of the upper rhythm strip. This initially results in the inscription of several pseudofusion beats in succession before the pacemaker spike starts to contribute to ventricular depolarization giving rise to true fusion beats (F). In the second half of the lower rhythm strip, pure paced beats are seen. Note that in pseudofusion beats, the large (unipolar) pacemaker artifact significantly distorts the spontaneous QRS complex.

Electrocardiography of Single-Chamber Pacemakers

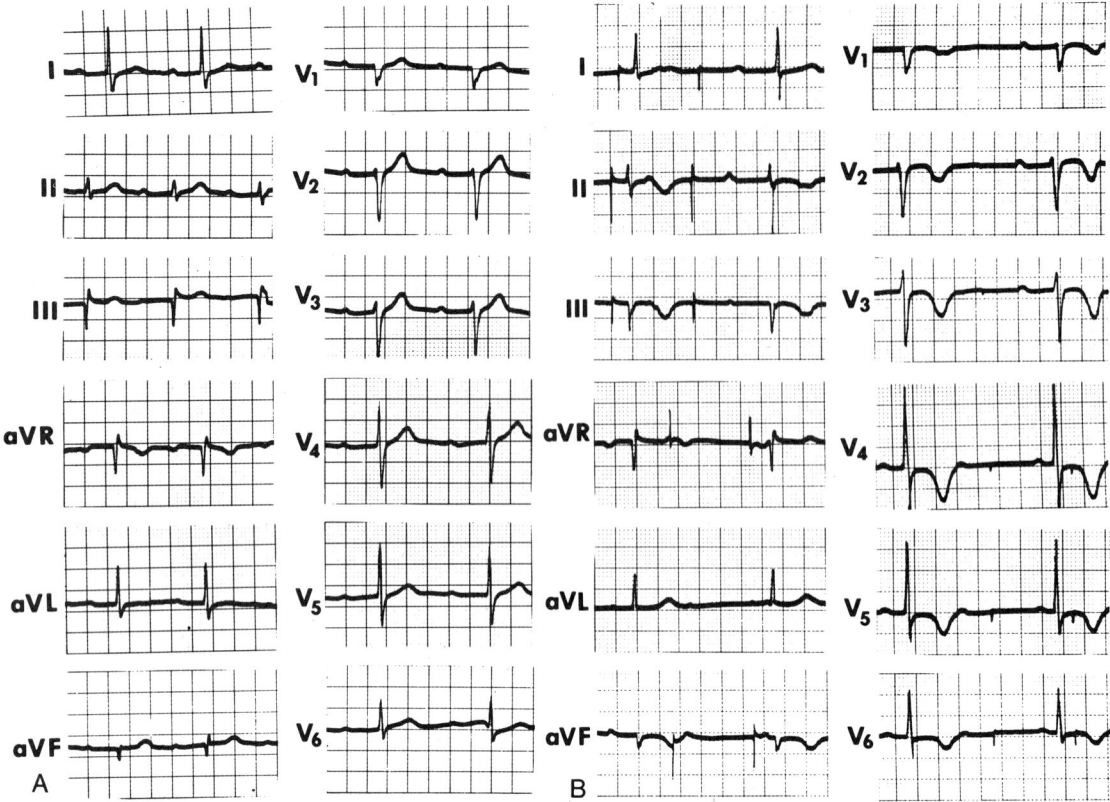

FIGURE 33-14
Postpacing ST-T wave changes.

A, Pre-pacing 12-lead ECG from a 41-year-old man with myotonic dystrophy and both AV nodal and intra–His bundle conduction delay that was confirmed in an electrophysiologic study. The ECG shows normal sinus rhythm and first-degree AV block. Other records, however, showed periods of an AV nodal Wenckebach block and 2:1 AV block. A transvenous right ventricular apical VVI pacemaker was implanted because of symptoms of dizziness and near-syncope that were thought to be related to AV conduction abnormality.

B, A 12-lead ECG from the same patient as in *A*, obtained 6 months after pacemaker implantation. The VVI pacemaker was suppressed by chest wall stimuli. The underlying spontaneous cardiac rhythm alternated between 2:1 AV block and complete AV dissociation with a supraventricular escape focus. The QRS configuration of escape beats was similar to that of conducted beats, as shown in *A*. However, there is marked symmetric inversion of T waves in the inferior leads and all precordial leads in the post-pacing tracing, compared to the pre-pacing recording.

Diagnosis of Myocardial Infarction During Ventricular Pacing

Since ventricular pacing results in altered activation and repolarization patterns, the diagnosis of acute ischemia or infarction during VVI pacing is often difficult. The pacing artifact, particularly with unipolar pacing, frequently distorts the initial part of the QRS complex, thus making the presence of Q waves difficult to discern.

Marked ST segment elevation, especially when associated with T wave inversion, indicates underlying myocardial ischemia or infarction. This is true of changes seen in the anterior or inferior leads. Serial changes in the ST-T segment are very important in the diagnosis of acute ischemia. During right ventricular endocardial pacing, the initial vectorial forces, due to septal activation from right to left, cause initial positive deflections in leads 1, aVL, V_5, and V_6. With an anteroseptal infarction these leads usually develop abnormal q waves (Fig. 33-15). Notching in the ascending limb of the QRS complex (R wave) in the left precordial leads has been noted in the majority of patients with LBBB and acute anteroseptal infarction.[26] Similar findings during pacing-induced LBBB have been mentioned in the literature.[27]

Inferior wall infarction is more difficult to diagnose during pacing, since right ventricular pacing produces QS complexes in the inferior leads. Barold and coworkers[28] have described a QR or Qr pattern in the inferior leads as being specific for inferior wall infarction.

Modes of Cardiac Pacing

ASYNCHRONOUS PACEMAKER (VOO)

This was the first type of pacemaker implanted in the early 1960s to provide antibradycardia support for patients with complete heart block, the predominant indication for pacing at that time.[29] Since this pace-

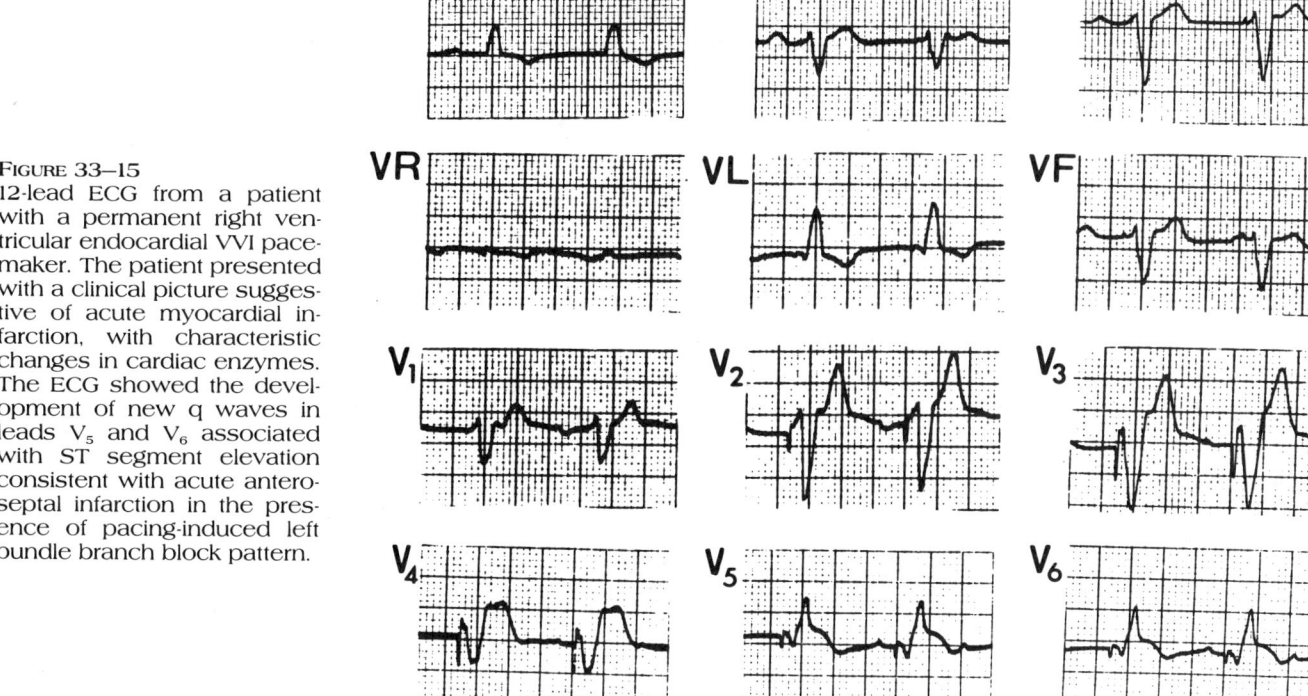

FIGURE 33–15
12-lead ECG from a patient with a permanent right ventricular endocardial VVI pacemaker. The patient presented with a clinical picture suggestive of acute myocardial infarction, with characteristic changes in cardiac enzymes. The ECG showed the development of new q waves in leads V_5 and V_6 associated with ST segment elevation consistent with acute anteroseptal infarction in the presence of pacing-induced left bundle branch block pattern.

maker lacks a sensing circuit, the pulse generator is expected to deliver stimuli at a preset constant rate independent of the spontaneous rhythm of the patient. The pacemaker stimuli will capture the ventricle only if and when they fall outside of the ventricular refractory period following spontaneous beats. Nowadays, since VOO pacemakers are obsolete, an ECG that shows asynchronous ventricular pacing is almost always caused by loss of the sensing function of a ventricular inhibited pacemaker (Fig. 33–16). Competition between the asynchronous pacemaker and the spontaneous cardiac rhythm may cause serious ventricular tachyarrhythmias if the pacemaker stimulus interrupts the T wave of a previous spontaneous or conducted beat and captures the ventricle during the vulnerable period.[30] Ventricular fibrillation induced by a pace-

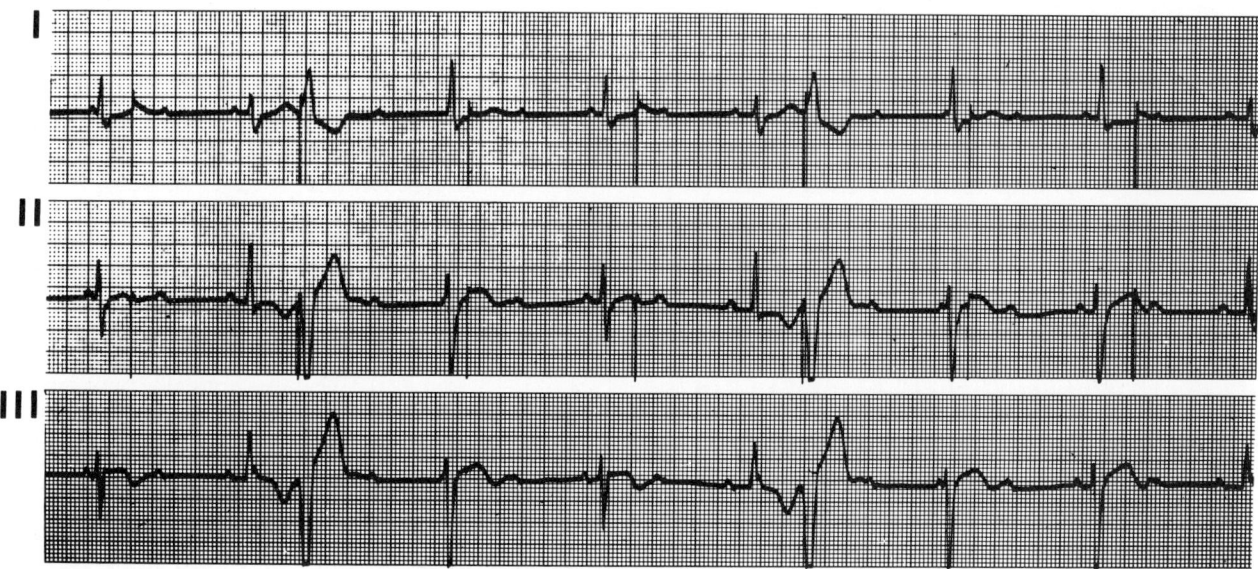

FIGURE 33–16
Asynchronous ventricular pacing (VOO mode). The spontaneous cardiac rhythm is sinus with incomplete AV dissociation and a slow idioventricular escape rhythm. The pacemaker stimuli appear at a constant rate regardless of the spontaneous cardiac rhythm and capture the ventricles only when they fall outside the refractory period of the preceding spontaneous beat. Note the numerous pacemaker spikes that fall on the T wave of the preceding QRS complex.

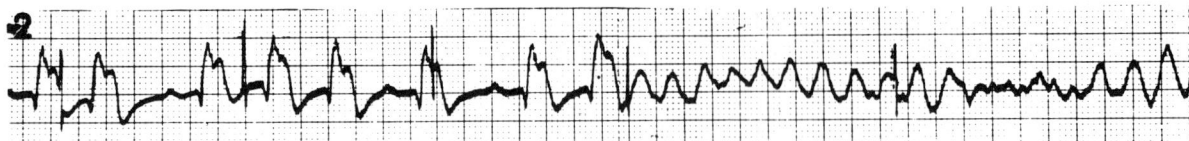

FIGURE 33-17
Recording obtained from a 62-year-old patient with a malfunctioning VVI pacemaker that was firing asynchronously at an irregular slow rate. The patient was admitted to the coronary care unit with an acute anterior wall myocardial infarction and developed a right bundle branch block and left posterior hemiblock. This tracing shows the presence of frequent atrial premature beats and the sudden onset of ventricular fibrillation that was probably related to the pacemaker spike falling on the early ST-T segment of the preceding spontaneous beat. The apparently long latency between the stimulus and the first induced ventricular beat is probably related to the occurrence of the spike during the relative refractory period. In this particular example, the fortuitous occurrence of the arrhythmia cannot be excluded.

maker stimulus falling in the vulnerable period has been reported.[31] However, its incidence is much less common than theoretically anticipated. Ventricular fibrillation rarely occurs in the absence of an abnormally enhanced ventricular vulnerability. The latter may be due to myocardial ischemia (Fig. 33-17), electrolyte abnormalities, or autonomic imbalance.

VENTRICULAR TRIGGERED PACEMAKER (VVT)

The ventricular triggered or QRS triggered pacemaker is also referred to as an R wave synchronous pacemaker, since it has both sensing and pacing mechanisms. Unlike the VVI pacemaker, the R wave synchronous pacemaker emits a nonstimulating pulse with every sensed intrinsic ventricular depolarization. However, since the pacemaker artifact or spike occurs within the QRS complex or during the absolute refractory period of the ventricle, it is ineffective. In addition, the pacemaker fires on demand after an escape interval during which the patient's intrinsic ventricular depolarization is not sensed. All sensed QRS complexes with a VVT pacemaker show a spike after the onset of the QRS complex, and all paced QRS complexes show a pacemaker artifact preceding the complex (Fig. 33-18). Since the pulse generator emits an impulse continuously, its longevity is abbreviated.

During spontaneous cardiac rhythm, the timely delivery of a spike in the early portion of the QRS complex indicates that the sensing function of the pacemaker is intact. However, whether the output of the pacemaker is effective in capturing the ventricle can be established only by placing an external magnet and converting the pacemaker to the asynchronous mode. External chest wall stimulation can also be used to evaluate the integrity of the pacemaker. The external stimuli will usually be sensed by the VVI pacemaker in a 1:1 fashion until limited by the refractory period of the pacemaker (Fig. 33-19). The VVT pacemaker will sense every external stimulus, emit a spike of its own, and capture the ventricle. Impending failure of the pulse generator of a VVT pacemaker usually results in slowing of the automatic rate. Concomitantly, the normal response to chest wall stimulation is frequently lost (Fig. 33-19).

VENTRICULAR (DEMAND) INHIBITED PACEMAKER (VVI)

The ventricular inhibited pacemaker, also called the R wave inhibited pacemaker, is the commonest type of pacemaker in use today (Fig. 33-20). The generator has a sensing circuitry, which senses the intrinsic R wave of the patient and inhibits the pulse generator output. The pacemaker spike will be delivered on demand if no spontaneous R wave is sensed for a preset interval. Three pacing intervals describe the

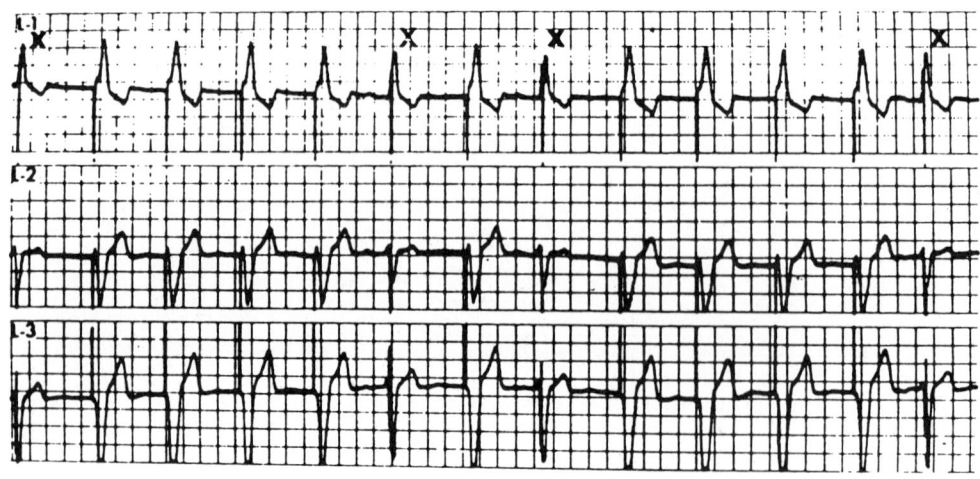

FIGURE 33-18
Simultaneous 3-lead electrocardiographic recording from a ventricular triggered pacemaker (VVT). All beats are paced except those marked X, which are spontaneous conducted beats. All spontaneous beats fall outside the refractory period of the pacemaker (400 ms) and trigger the pacemaker to fire a spike within the QRS complex.

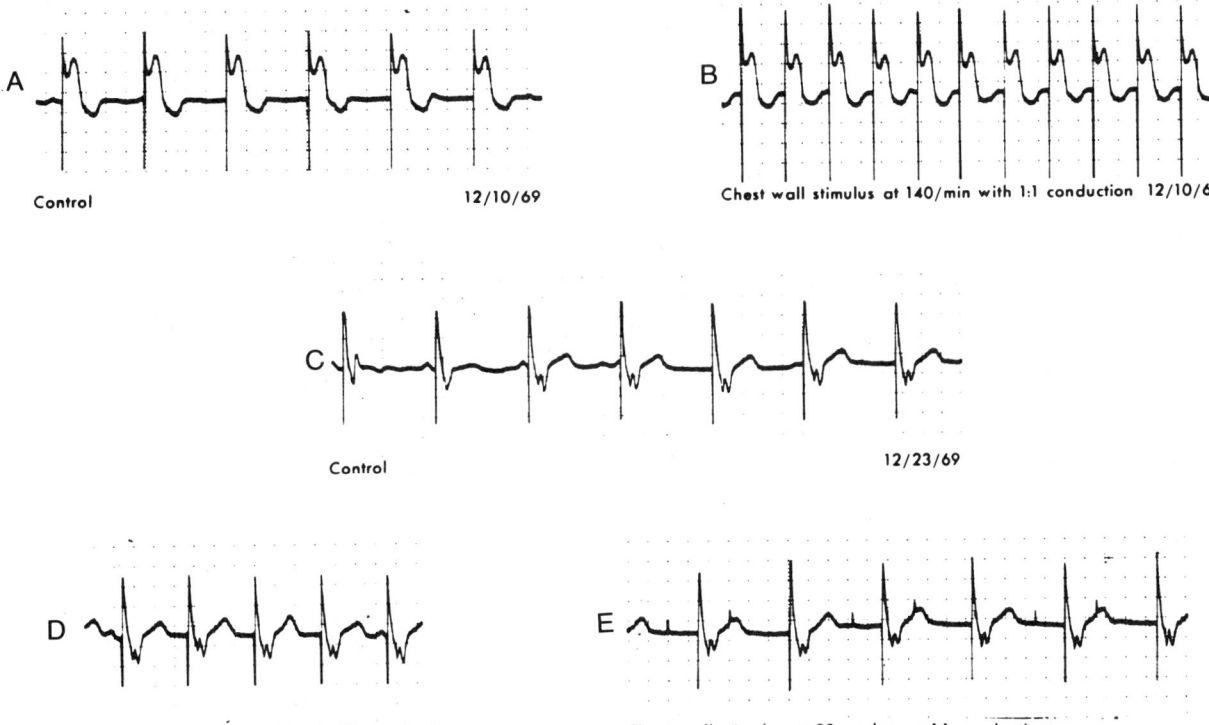

FIGURE 33–19
Normal response of a ventricular triggered pacemaker (VVT) to chest wall stimuli (B). A 1:1 response is usually maintained up to rates of 150 bpm (the pacemaker's refractory period is 400 ms). C illustrates impending failure of the pulse generator, resulting in slowing of the automatic rate from 72 to 66 bpm. E shows loss of normal response to chest wall stimuli, with 1:1 response maintained only up to a rate of 92 bpm (D).

pacing function of a demand R wave inhibited pacemaker: (1) the automatic pacing interval, (2) the pacemaker escape interval, and (3) the magnet mode rate or fixed rate pacing interval.

The *automatic pacing interval* is the time between two consecutive pacemaker stimuli during demand pacing. *The pacemaker escape interval* is measured from a sensed spontaneous ventricular depolarization to the subsequent escape pacemaker spike. In most VVI pacemakers, these two intervals are identical. On the surface ECG, however, the escape interval, which is measured from the spontaneous sensed QRS complex to the next pacer spike, may be slightly longer compared to the automatic pacing interval. This occurs because one cannot precisely determine the moment within the QRS complex when the intrinsic ventricular depolarization at the site of the pacemaker sensing electrode has reached adequate voltage and slew rate (dv/dt) to activate the sensing mechanism and initiate a new escape interval.

Occasionally the pacemaker is designed to have an escape interval longer than the automatic pacing inter-

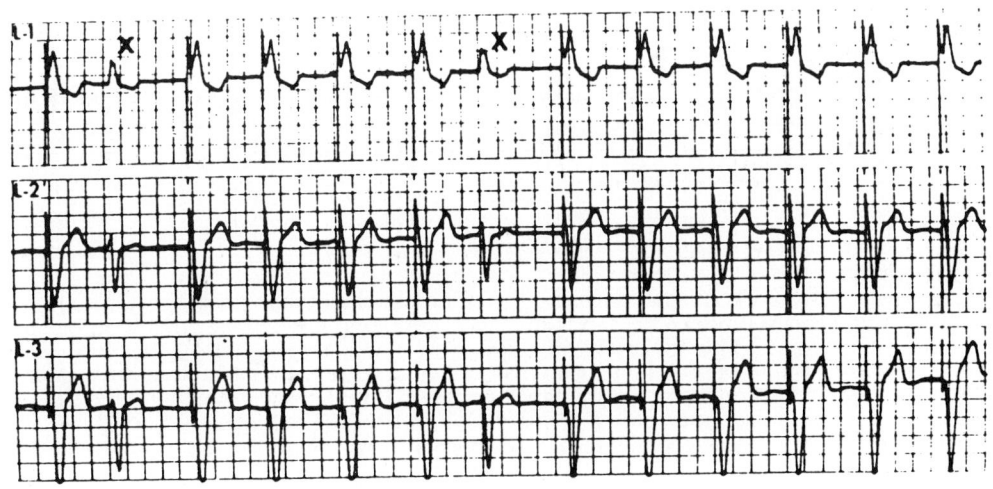

FIGURE 33–20
Ventricular inhibited pacemaker (VVI) in the same patient as in Figure 33–18. The VVT pacemaker has been replaced by a VVI unit. In contrast to the VVT pacemaker, spontaneous beats that are successfully sensed by the VVI pacemaker (marked X) inhibit the spike and recycle the pacemaker to discharge after a set interval.

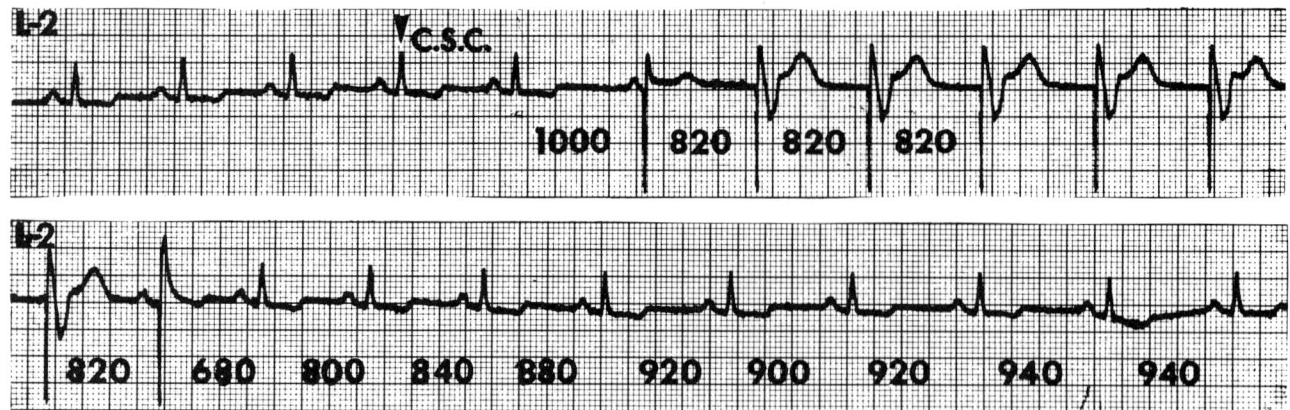

FIGURE 33–21
VVI pacemaker with positive rate hysteresis. In the upper rhythm strip, carotid sinus compression (C.S.C.) resulted in slowing of the sinus rate and escape of the pacemaker after an interval of 1000 ms. This is followed by automatic pacing at a shorter interval of 820 ms. The lower rhythm strip shows sinus arrhythmia. The relatively short sinus cycles resulted in inhibition of demand pacing. However, the sinus interval later lengthened to well beyond the pacemaker's automatic interval without pacemaker escape. This illustrates a paradoxical situation in which a slower spontaneous rhythm inhibits a faster pacemaker rhythm.

val. This pacemaker is said to have a *positive rate hysteresis* (Fig. 33–21).[32, 33] The rationale behind this design is to maintain spontaneous sinus rhythm with its known hemodynamic advantage (AV synchrony), in comparison to the ventricular paced rhythm, at cycle lengths longer than the pacemaker automatic cycle length but shorter than the patient's intrinsic escape rhythm.

The *magnet mode rate*, or *fixed rate pacing interval*, is the rate obtained during placement of a magnet over the implanted generator. All VVI pacemakers have a magnetic reed switch that is activated by the application of a test magnet, allowing the generator to operate in a fixed rate mode.[34, 35] This rate is the most stable and reliable pacemaker rate and is the recommended rate to follow for detection of impending battery failure.[35] In contrast, the automatic or pacing interval can change by up to 40 ms in most normally functioning pacemakers.

In some pacemakers, the magnet rate is the same as the automatic pacing rate. In this case, the function of the magnetic reed switch will be difficult to ascertain in the presence of an exclusive paced rhythm, and chest wall stimulation may be necessary to assess sensing function. In other pacemakers in which the magnet rate is faster than the automatic pacemaker rate, an increase in rate with the application of the magnet can be discerned in an ECG rhythm strip (Fig. 33–22). In some VVI pacemakers, when the magnet is waved over the pulse generator, prolonged inhibition

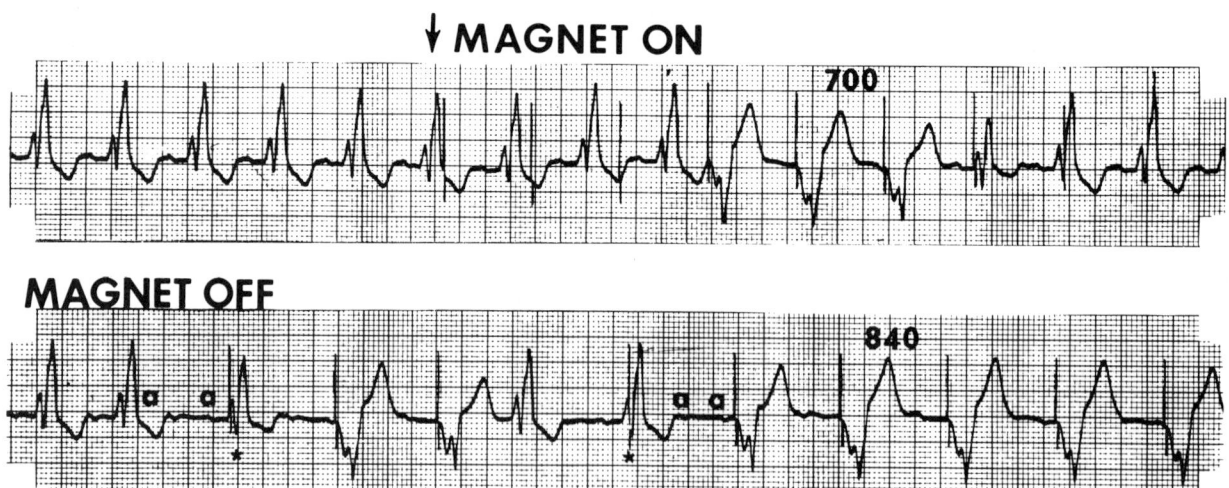

FIGURE 33–22
VVI pacemaker with the magnet-fixed rate faster than the automatic pacing rate. The pacemaker was implanted in a patient with the tachycardia-bradycardia syndrome. The spontaneous cardiac rhythm is an atrial tachycardia with AV block ("a" refers to atrial waves). The first half of the upper rhythm strip shows atrial tachycardia with 2:1 AV block simulating a regular sinus rhythm at a rate of 95 bpm and no paced beats. Application of the magnet (arrow) resulted in fixed rate pacing at an interval of 700 ms. The lower rhythm strip illustrates the occurrence of a higher-degree AV block, resulting in a pacemaker escape at an automatic interval of 840 ms. Beats marked by asterisks are conducted supraventricular beats with a right bundle branch block configuration and a pacemaker spike within the QRS complex during demand pacing (pseudofusion beats).

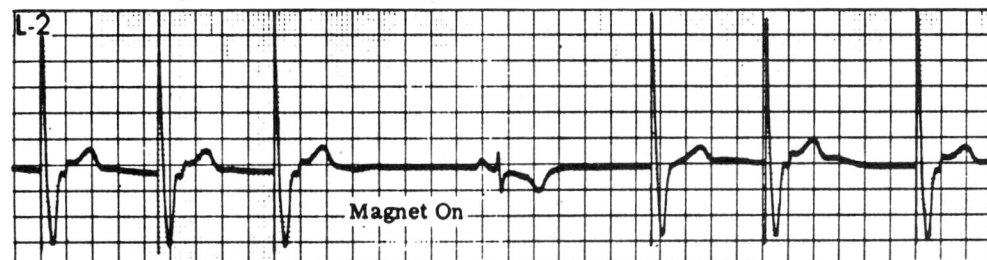

FIGURE 33-23
Magnet waving in front of a VVI pulse generator, causing inhibition of the pacemaker discharge.

may occur[35-37] (Fig. 33–23). A possible explanation is that changes in the electrochemical potential difference between the ground plate and the intracardiac electrode may be shorted out each time the reed switch is in operation. The voltage change is sensed by the pacemaker and inhibition may occur.[35] This can occur in VVI pacemakers in which the reed switch is connected to the sensing circuit. In models where the reed switch is isolated from the sensing circuit, magnet application or removal cannot produce inhibition. Malfunction of the reed switch as a result of mechanical failure can rarely occur.[34, 35] The reed switch may stay in either the open or closed position regardless of the external magnetic field. This is generally referred to as a *sticky reed switch*.

PACEMAKER REFRACTORY PERIODS

There are generally two pacemaker refractory periods:

1. *The delivery (paced) refractory period*: the pacemaker refractory period following the emission of a pacing pulse.
2. *The sensing (sensed) refractory period*: the pacemaker refractory period following sensing of either a spontaneous or artificial electrical signal. Although usually similar, the delivery and sensing refractory periods may differ in some VVI pacemakers.

The relative refractory period of the pacemaker is defined as the period immediately following the delivery refractory period, during which the demand mechanism has not regained its full sensitivity. During the relative refractory period, some generators require a larger signal to activate the sensing mechanism; others can be only partially recycled by a signal capable of completely recycling the generator outside this period.

Chest Wall and Esophageal Stimulation

The VVI pacemaker functions as a demand unit by sensing the intrinsic QRS complex. The pacemaker can also be suppressed by an external electrical field.[38, 39] Chest wall stimulation can be performed by using two suction cups or electrode pads applied to the chest and connected to an external pacemaker that is set at a higher rate to override that of the implanted device. The suction cups or chest wall electrode pads are usually positioned such that the negative terminal is placed over the heart and superimposed on the intracardiac electrode, whereas the positive terminal overlies the pulse generator. The implanted pacemaker senses the external electrical field and is inhibited (Fig. 33–24). The underlying rhythm can then be identified and monitored during the pacemaker follow-up. If, during chest wall stimulation, the patient is shown to have a markedly slow or unreliable intrinsic rhythm, more frequent monitoring may be necessary.

In a unipolar lead system, chest wall stimulation is generally effective in entering the sensing milieu of the pacemaker and in eliciting an inhibitory or triggered response. However, in the case of a bipolar system, chest wall stimulation may prove incapable of being sensed, and thus will be unable to influence the implanted pacemaker. Hence, information regarding the sensing function of the pacemaker in a predominantly pacemaker-dependent individual may not be amenable to this diagnostic modality. In that situation esophageal stimulation via the pill electrode may prove helpful.* The use of the pill electrode will allow closer application of electrical stimuli to both the heart and pacemaker sensing electrode(s), thereby enabling either cardiac stimulation if necessary or electrical signal detection by the implanted pacemaker.[40, 41]

Pacemaker Malfunction

The causes of pacemaker malfunction can be broadly classified as:

1. Abnormalities related to the pacemaker stimulus and or capture.
2. Abnormalities related to sensing.

MALFUNCTION RELATED TO PACEMAKER STIMULUS AND CAPTURE

The various causes of abnormal activation or failure to capture are

1. Battery/component failure resulting in slow or fast rates.
2. Lead displacement, perforation, or failure.
3. Pacemaker exit block.
4. Changes in cardiac pacing mode.

---
*Arzco Medical Electronics, Inc., Chicago, IL.

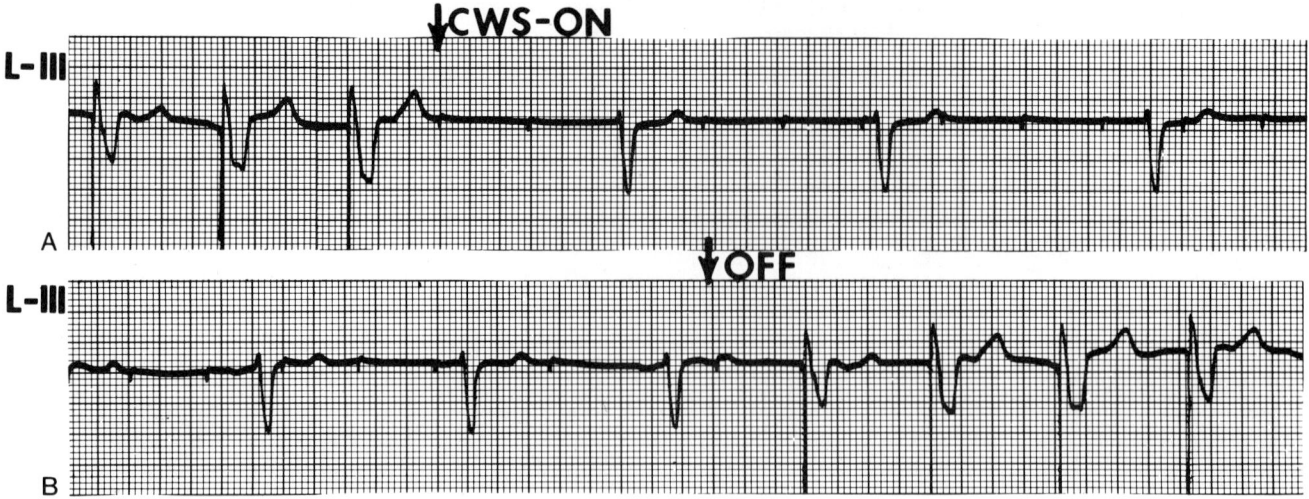

FIGURE 33–24
Inhibition of a VVI pacemaker by external chest wall stimuli (CWS). Note the emergence of an underlying slow junctional rhythm (A) that gradually increased its rate (B), illustrating the phenomenon of overdrive suppression by the faster pacemaker rhythm. The pacemaker was implanted in a patient with symptomatic sick sinus syndrome.

Changes in Rate Due to Battery Depletion

Battery longevity is directly proportional to its capacity and inversely proportional to the current drain. The battery capacity measured in ampere-hours is a function of the number of electrons delivered by the battery cell into an external load.[42–43] The current drain, usually measured in microamperes (μA) is dependent on factors such as electrode size, the impedance within the circuit, and percentage of time the pulse generator is inhibited or pacing. The average current drain is approximately 20 to 25 μA during pacing and 5 to 10 μA during the inhibited mode. The beginning of life (BOL) status for the lithium iodine battery is usually 2.8 volts; with passage of time the cell impedance tends to rise and the battery capacity will predictably decrease. A greater diminution in battery capacity occurs when iodide accumulates, and the battery will then approach its end of life (EOL) status.[44, 45] Most manufacturers usually link voltage changes to the pulse repetition rate. This rate (magnet rate) usually serves as a reliable indicator of battery depletion. Since the typical voltage capacity of the lithium iodine battery is 2.8 V, voltage multipliers are commonly used to enable the 5 to 10 V output capable of being discharged from the pulse generator.

Small variations in the pacemaker automatic rate can be seen with all pacemakers and are based on changes in ambient body temperature[46] and the associated changes in internal battery impedance that occur. However, the magnet rate of the pacemaker is stable and is a sensitive indicator of battery depletion.[34] In earlier pacemaker models, battery depletion resulted in rate increases and pacing rates of 100 to 400 per minute.[47, 48] This condition was called *runaway pacemaker* and occasionally resulted in fatal pacemaker tachyarrhythmias. With the current lithium anode source generator, battery depletion most often leads to a decrease in pacing rate. Eventually, battery depletion will result in totally ineffective stimuli. Since rate is often a programmable parameter, magnet rate should always be checked before diagnosing battery depletion.

Lead Displacement, Perforation, or Failure

Gross displacement of a bipolar lead may be evident in the chest x-ray or may be suggested when a change occurs in the frontal plane QRS axis of the ECG. Similarly, perforation of the septum may result in stimulation of the left ventricle and a change in the QRS pattern from LBBB to RBBB.

Right ventricular lead tip perforation into the pericardial sac[49] is an uncommon complication of perven-

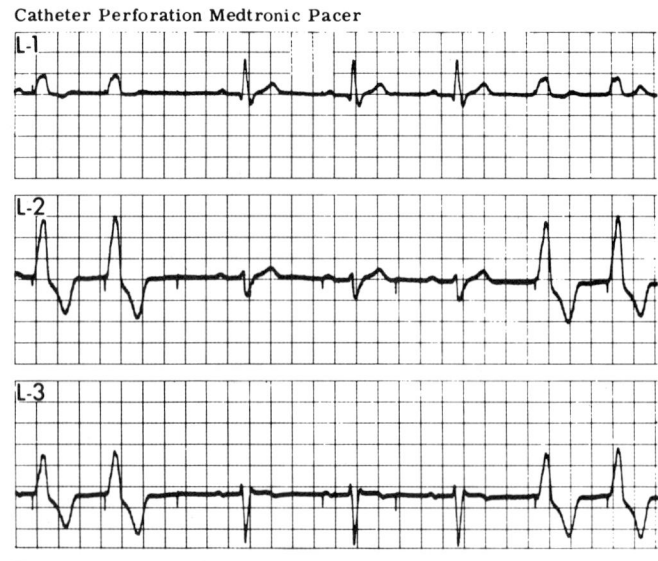

FIGURE 33–25
A VVI pacemaker with lead tip perforation into the pericardium. Both pacing and sensing are intermittent.

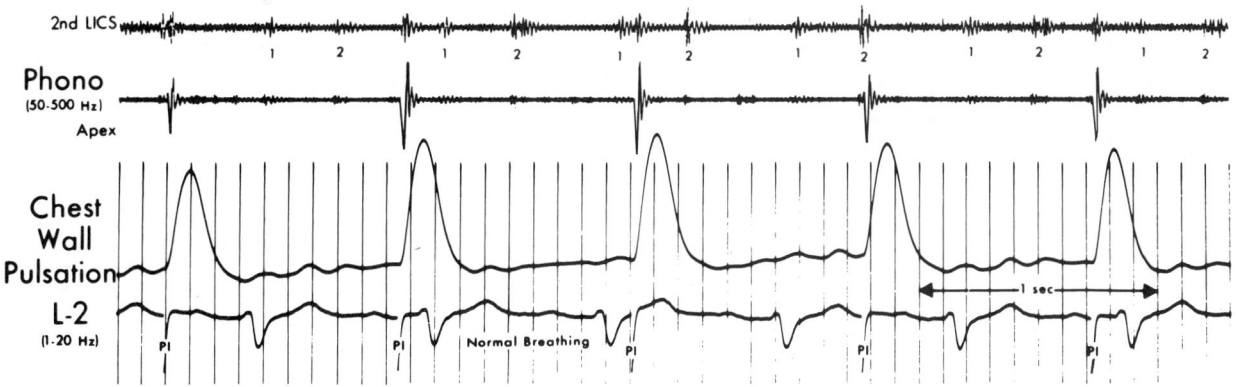

FIGURE 33-26
Right ventricular lead tip perforation into the pericardial sac. The pacemaker spikes were ineffective (PI). However, a loud clicking sound occurred with each spike (prior to S_1) and was associated with an abnormal chest wall pulsation. This probably resulted from stimulation of the overlying intercostal muscles. LICS = left intercostal space.

ous pacing, resulting in characteristic findings. When cardiac perforation by the pacemaker electrode occurs, pacing may be intermittent, especially if a bipolar electrode catheter is utilized (Fig. 33–25). Sensing may also be intermittent (see Fig. 33–25) but is usually intact. A pacemaker sound is commonly heard regardless of whether the pacing stimuli are effective (Figs. 33–26 and 33–27). The pacemaker click is characteristically presystolic in timing, occurring 0.08 to 0.12 seconds before the first heart sound, and is virtually coincident in time with the pacemaker spike recorded in the ECG.[50-52] The sound is probably caused by contraction of intercostal muscles stimulated by current leaking from the catheter tip.[49-51] Abnormal apex cardiograms or chest wall pulsations are usually noted and can be recorded (see Figs. 33–26 and 33–27). A chest radiograph reveals the catheter tip to be outside of the cavity and within the pericardium (Fig. 33–28).

Loss of pacing lead insulation will lead to the creation of an alternate pathway of lower electrical resistance for current to flow. There is usually an increase in the amplitude of the pacemaker spike in the case of a bipolar lead system. Pacing and sensing may continue in the presence of insulation breaks; however, excessive current drain will result in premature battery depletion and failure. Occasionally, sensing abnormalities and extracardiac muscle stimulation can occur due to insulation break (Fig. 33–29). Serial measurements of the amplitude of the pacemaker spike, using an analog electrocardiograph recording during held respiration, may show diminution in size and can be used to predict lead failure months before it is clinically manifested.[53]

Pacemaker Exit Block

Exit block can be defined as failure of an impulse falling outside of the refractory period of the surrounding tissue to elicit a propagated response.[54] The failure of the tissue to respond may be caused either by an alteration of the stimulus intensity or by failure of conduction from the site of the pacemaker lead. In the case of the cardiac artificial pacemaker, exit block describes the clinical condition in which a normal

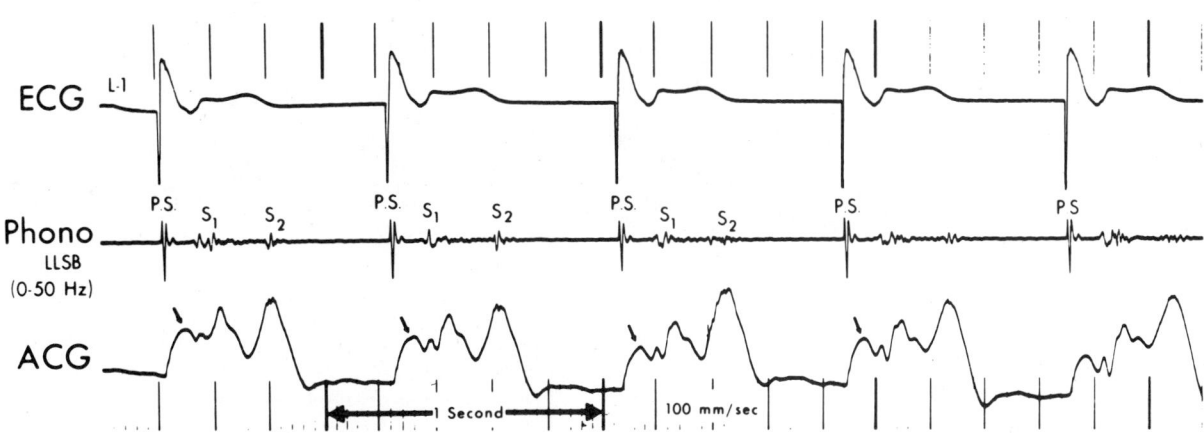

FIGURE 33-27
Pacemaker sound in a patient with effective pacemaker stimuli. The sound was presystolic and temporally related to the timing of an S_4 sound. The apexcardiogram (ACG) was abnormal, probably secondary to intercostal muscle stimulation. PS = pacing sound; LLSB = lower left sternal border.

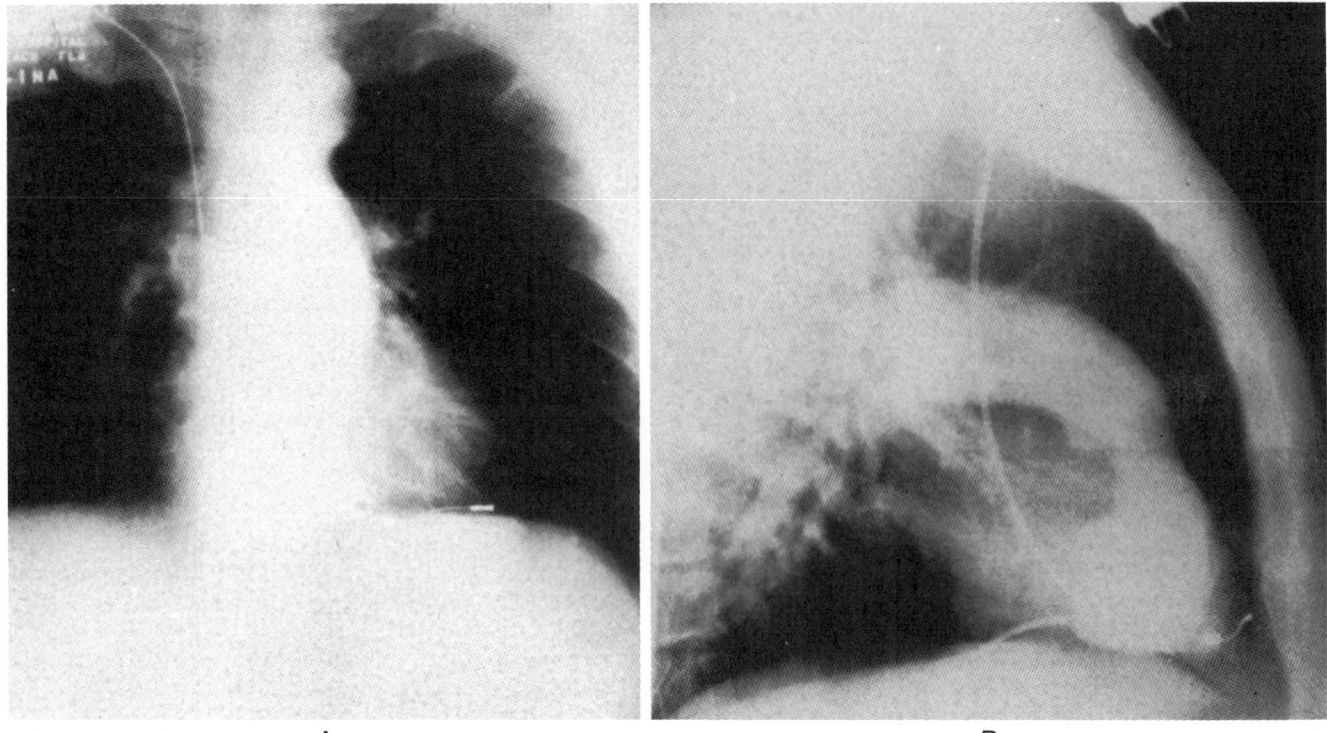

FIGURE 33–28
Posteroanterior (A) and lateral (B) chest radiographs of the same patient as in Figure 34–26 reveal that the lead tip lies well outside the right ventricular cavity and is probably in the pericardium.

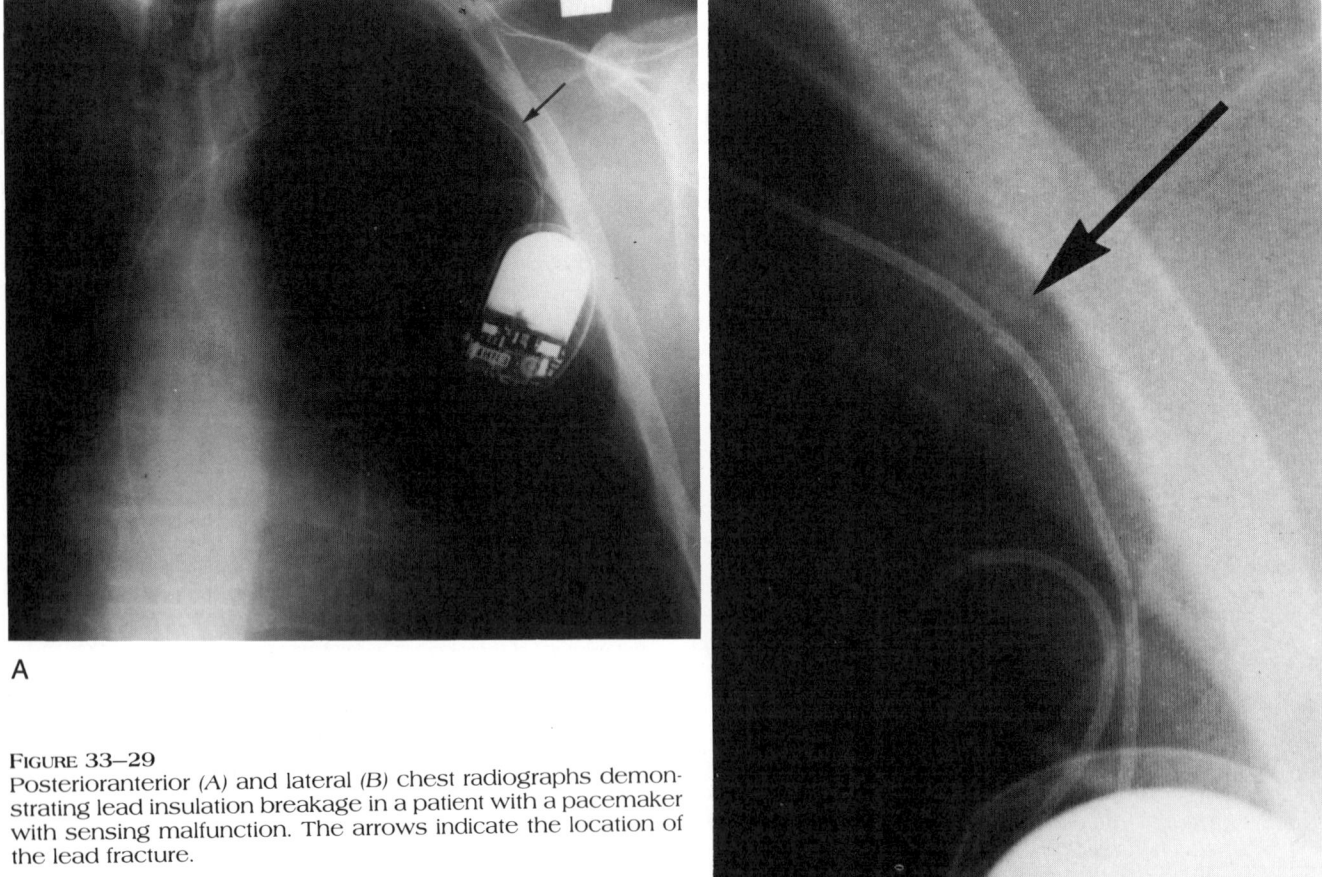

FIGURE 33–29
Posterioranterior (A) and lateral (B) chest radiographs demonstrating lead insulation breakage in a patient with a pacemaker with sensing malfunction. The arrows indicate the location of the lead fracture.

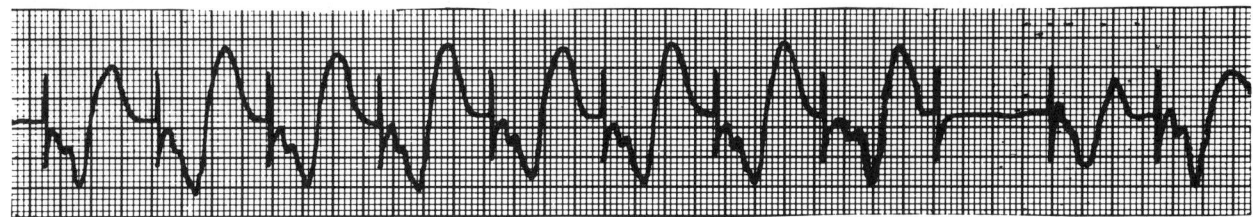

FIGURE 33-30
Pacemaker exit block of the Wenckebach type in a patient with marked hyperkalemia. Note the presence of a slight but definite, gradual increase of the spike-to-QRS interval prior to failure to capture, followed by shortening of the interval in the beat subsequent to the ineffective spike.

pacemaker stimulus fails to excite the heart because of an abnormally high threshold.[55] A normal increase in pacing threshold often occurs after initial placement of the lead. Alterations of pacemaker threshold by physiologic factors, drugs, and electrolyte changes have been extensively studied.[55, 56] Type I antiarrhythmic drugs have been shown to increase the pacing threshold.[57, 58] Although modest elevation of the serum potassium level may decrease the pacemaker threshold,[55] a marked elevation may be associated with a significant increase in threshold[56] and pacemaker exit block[59] (Fig. 33–30). An example of a two-to-one pattern of pacemaker exit block is shown in Figure 33–31.

Occasionally, following direct current (DC) cardioversion or defibrillation, the pacing threshold may increase and result in non-capture of the pacemaker stimuli.[60] Levine et al.[61] described patients in whom transient or chronic rise in the stimulation threshold of the permanently implanted unipolar pacing lead resulted in loss of effective pacing after therapeutic defibrillation or cardioversion. They recommend that the defibrillator paddles be placed at least 5 inches from the pulse generator, or as far as possible in the case of a right infraclavicular implantation site. In patients with permanent pacemakers, an anteroposterior paddle placement is ideal when defibrillation is necessary. Stimulation threshold should be checked in all patients after defibrillation. Similarly, after transvenous catheter countershock, the pacing threshold has been shown to increase.[62]

Changes in Cardiac Pacing Mode

Changes in the electrical output and mode of operation (e.g., change from VVI to VVT) can occur if defibrillation paddles are placed directly over the pacemaker generator.[60, 61] Similar problems have been noted following therapeutic radiation.[63] It is recommended that pulsed x-ray radiation should be avoided even at therapeutic levels.[63] Electromagnetic interference from numerous sources is also known to alter the cardiac pacing mode.[64] Rarely, a malfunctioning programmer or the attempted use of a different manufacturer's programmer, unwittingly, to program a specific parameter may lead to inadvertent re-programming of the pacemaker mode (personal communication).

ABNORMALITIES RELATED TO SENSING IN VVI PACEMAKERS

The various problems related to sensing in VVI pacemakers can be classified as

1. Failure to sense or undersensing
2. Apparent or pseudo-failure to sense
3. Oversensing
4. Partial sensing (partial recycling)

Undersensing

Excluding both temporary reversion of a VVI pacemaker to the VOO mode as a result of electromagnetic

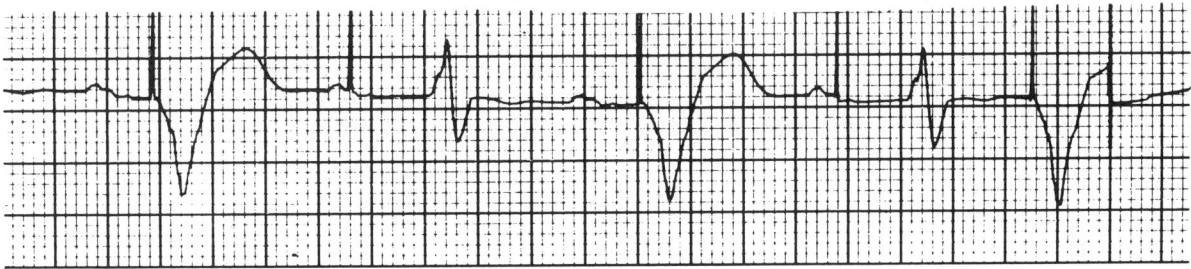

FIGURE 33-31
Exit block during VVI pacing. VVI pacing at 80 per minute with pulse width and amplitude settings of 1.0 ms and 5 volts, respectively. The rhythm strip reveals pacemaker exit block with a 2-to-1 pattern. After the first paced complex, only every other pacemaker output captures the ventricle. The underlying rhythm is a sinus mechanism with marked first-degree AV block. Failure to sense the QRS complex immediately preceding the last paced beat is demonstrated, signifying combined sensing and pacing failure in this patient.

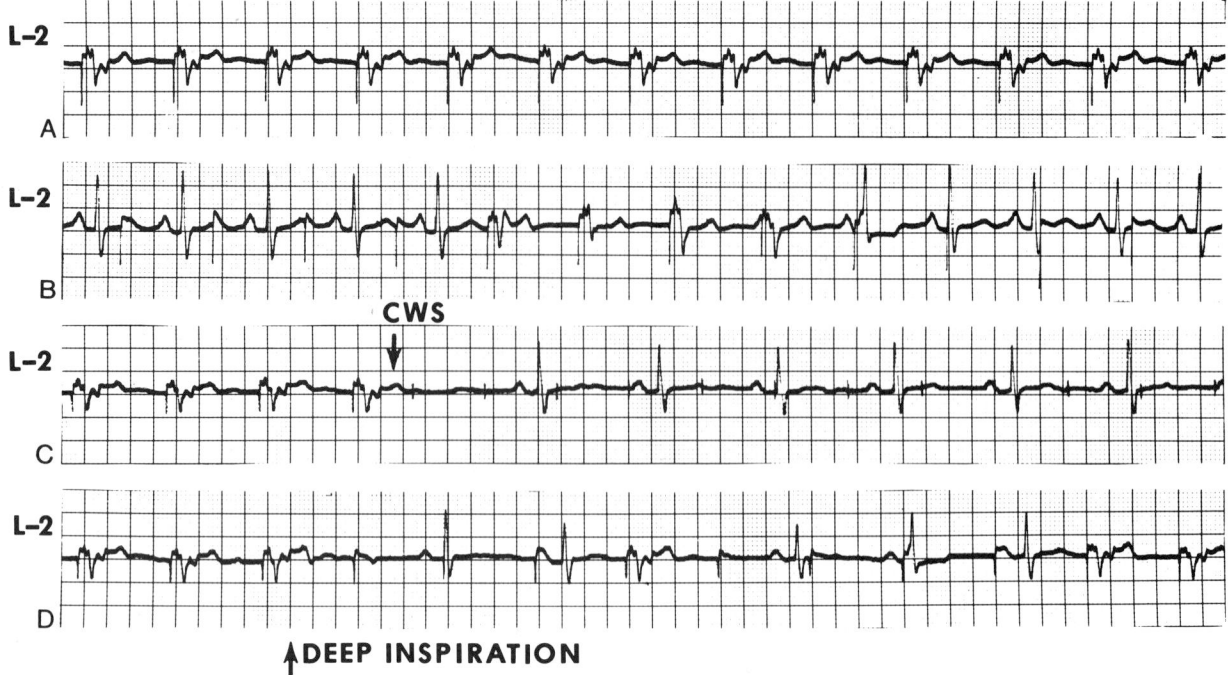

FIGURE 33–32
Rhythm strips from a patient with a VVI pacemaker implanted 6 months previously for symptomatic sick sinus syndrome. On chest x-ray, the electrode tip was found to be displaced close to the tricuspid valve. A was obtained during normal respiration and shows continuous pacing. B was recorded following the administration of 0.6 mg of atropine, which resulted in modest acceleration of the sinus rate. This rhythm strip shows failure of sensing, resulting in asynchronous ventricular pacing. C shows that the pacemaker could be successfully inhibited by external chest wall stimulation (CWS). D was obtained during deep inspiration and shows transient loss of both sensing and pacing.

interference and the falling of a ventricular depolarization in the pacemaker refractory period, failure of a VVI pacemaker to sense a spontaneous QRS results either from the delivery of an inadequate ventricular depolarization to a normally functioning pacemaker or from the delivery of an adequate QRS signal to a malfunctioning pacemaker. Analysis of both the unipolar and bipolar electrograms recorded from the pacing electrode is sometimes essential to evaluate the adequacy of the QRS signal. Normally, a unipolar ventricular electrogram measures 5 to 15 mV,[65] which is more than adequate for sensing by a VVI pacemaker. Most units usually require a minimum signal of 2 to 3 mV for proper sensing. However, marked diminution of the intracardiac ECG may occur as a result of excessive fibrosis at the tip of the lead and may result in inadequate sensing as well as pacing.[66] An acute myocardial infarction can result in a decrease in size of the intracardiac electrogram and predisposes to undersensing.[67] Drug toxicity with type 1A or 1C antiarrhythmic agents, as well as hyperkalemia, may also cause problems with sensing, although these are more often associated with failure to capture. A bipolar signal may occasionally be much smaller than either of its two component unipolar signals.[68] In this case, unipolarization usually restores normal sensing.

Displacement of the pacing electrode with loss of intimate contact with the endocardium may be associated with loss of sensing or failure of both sensing and pacing. This is sometimes intermittent and may only be elicited by deep respiratory or bodily movements (Fig. 33–32). Intermittent pacing and sensing failure can also occur if the lead connector pins are not properly positioned in the generator or because of loose contact. The diagnosis can be confirmed by moving the generator gently in its pocket or by movement of the shoulder, which will result in sensing failure. A normally functioning VVI pacemaker may occasionally be able to sense conducted supraventricular beats but fail to sense certain ventricular ectopic beats (Fig. 33–33). This is usually explained by failure of the ectopic depolarization to generate an adequate dv/dt for proper sensing.

In some instances an adequate signal from a ventric-

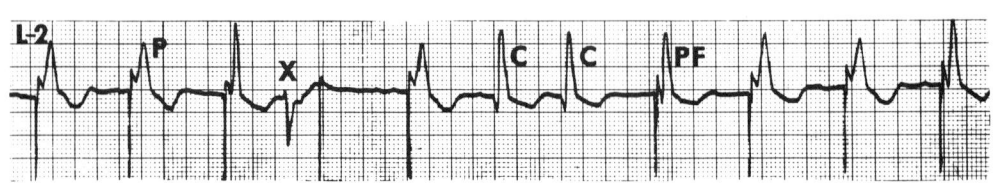

FIGURE 33–33
Failure to sense a ventricular ectopic beat (X) by an otherwise normally functioning VVI pacemaker. Note that conducted supraventricular beats (C) are normally sensed. P = paced beat; PF = pseudofusion beat.

ular depolarization may not be sensed because the signal occurred during the refractory period of the pacemaker. With present-day pacemakers, the refractory period is programmable, and this can be modified so as to sense early signals.

Apparent Failure to Sense

A normally functioning VVI pacemaker may fail to sense late-occurring spontaneous ventricular beats, thus resulting in the pacemaker spike being delivered into the QRS complex and giving rise to pseudofusion beats. This is explained by failure of a late-occurring intrinsic ventricular depolarization to reach adequate voltage and slow rate (dv/dt) at the site of the sensing electrode to activate the sensing circuit before the time of the next pacemaker automatic cycle. An exaggerated form of this phenomenon occurs with right ventricular endocardial VVI pacemakers in the presence of an RBBB pattern of conducted supraventricular beats (see Fig. 33–22) as well as in cases of left ventricular ectopic beats (Fig. 33–34). Both types of QRS complexes will be associated with delayed arrival of the ventricular depolarization at the site of the sensing electrode. These cases may be misinterpreted as failure to sense by the VVI pacemaker. It should be stressed, however, that a pacemaker spike that falls clearly outside of the QRS complex would obviously indicate failure of sensing.

Another reason for apparent undersensing is due to circuit designs of the pacemaker, such as those seen in the new Activitrax rate-responsive pacemaker. In the activity mode, the pacemaker's stimulation rate is controlled by an activity-sensing detector and circuitry.[69] The sensor, a piezoelectric crystal located within the pulse generator, transforms the mechanical vibrations of the body resulting from physical activity into an electrical signal that is further processed for rate control. Occasionally a single output pulse may be emitted at the programmed maximum activity rate when a sensed ventricular event occurs within 8 ms after the pacemaker activity detection/rate circuit is triggered.[70] Such an output pulse will be noted on the ECG at intervals of 400, 480, or 600 ms after the sensed event corresponding to the programmed maximum activity rate of 150, 125, or 100 beats per minute (bpm), respectively. This pulse as observed clinically can be mistaken for sensing malfunction of the device. It usually occurs following a run of sensed intrinsic rhythm and is the result of the normal pacemaker circuitry (Fig. 33–35).

Abnormal Sensing (Oversensing)

Oversensing should be considered in the presence of irregular lengthening of the automatic interspike interval. Abnormal sensing can occur as a result of either extrinsic or intrinsic signals.

Abnormal Sensing Caused by Extrinsic Signals

Both VVT and VVI pacemakers can be modified by external electromagnetic interference.[71, 72] Although less frequent with present-generation pacemakers, electrical appliances that emit continuous wave energy with a frequency of 50 to 60 Hz can interfere with pacemaker function. Such interference can occur with household appliances and electrocardiographic recording equipment.

Following exposure to a 50-Hz electrical field, Butrous and colleagues[74] found that some pacemakers showed normal function, some reverted to a fixed rate mode, some showed irregular pacing, and others showed a mixed response.[74] In general, the interference threshold depended on the magnitude and distribution of the electric field and varied with the patient's height, build, and posture. Interference has been reported to occur if the pacemaker is in the vicinity of pulsed energy sources, such as radio[75] or television transmitters,[76] radar,[77] auto ignition systems or arc welders,[78]

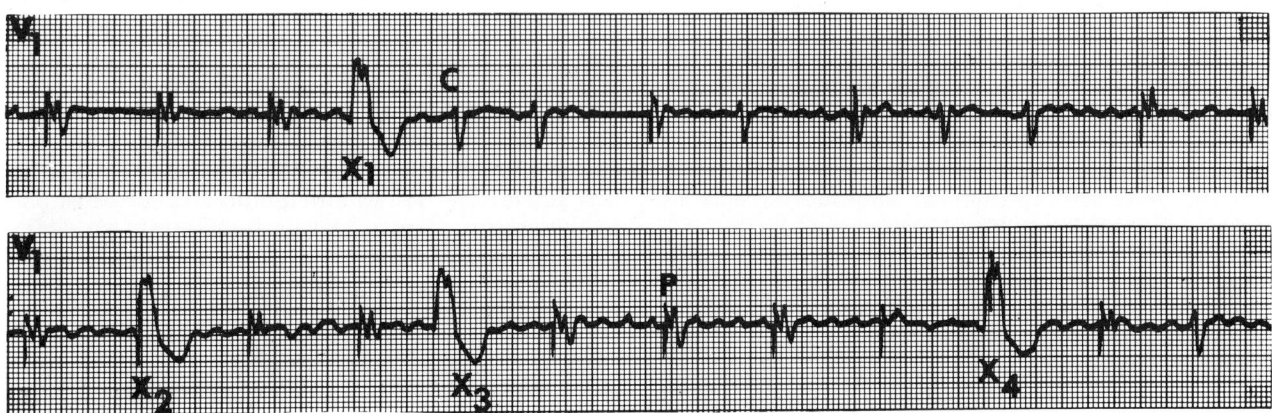

FIGURE 33–34
Apparent failure to sense left ventricular ectopic beats by a transvenous VVI pacemaker. Note the presence of atrial fibrillation, paced beats (P), conducted supraventricular beats (C), and ventricular ectopic beats (X), probably of left ventricular origin, as suggested by the right bundle branch block configuration in lead V_1. Ectopic beats marked X_2 and X_4 have late coupling intervals, and a pacemaker spike is inscribed within the QRS complex as late as 60 ms after the onset of the QRS complex in the ectopic beat marked X4. See text for explanation.

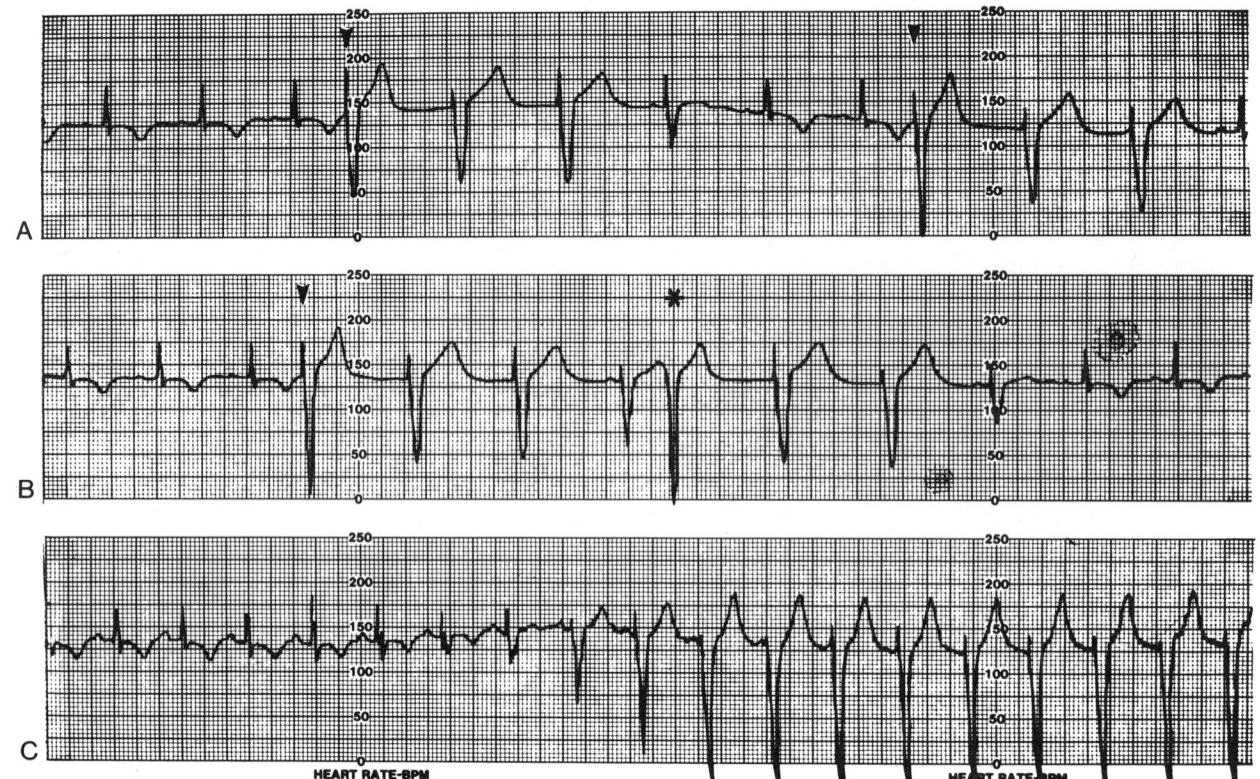

FIGURE 33–35
Selected rhythm strips from a 24-hour Holter recording in a patient with an Activitrax pacemaker (VVIR).
A and *B* were recorded during sleep and show sinus rhythm alternating with a ventricular paced rhythm. The first paced beat follows the last sensed spontaneous beat by 480 ms (arrowheads). This apparent failure to sense is the result of the pacemaker circuitry (see text for details). The sensing mechanism is intact, as shown by proper sensing of the ventricular premature contraction marked by an asterisk.
C was obtained during the morning hours and shows sinus tachycardia followed by ventricular pacing at a rate of 105 bpm. The programmed maximum activity rate was 125 bpm. Note several pseudofusion and true fusion beats during the transition from sinus to paced beats.

or by direct contact with electric razors,[79] electric toothbrushes,[80] or other household appliances. Pulsed energy signals may mimic the R wave potential and inhibit a VVI pacemaker or initiate asynchronous pacing as its noise reversion mode of response.[40, 81, 82] Conversion of a VVI pacemaker to the VOO mode in the vicinity of microwave radio transmitters[83] or microwave ovens has been reported. Electrical interference may be caused by poor grounding or by close contact with the apparatus.[84] Current leakage is particularly dangerous in the presence of diathermy and electrocautery equipment.[85] Interference from external signals is less common with the newer pacemakers, due to better shielding of the pulse generator with a stainless steel or titanium capsule.

Another extrinsic signal commonly associated with oversensing and inhibition is myopotential. Myopotential inhibition is more common with unipolar rather than bipolar pacing systems.[86] This phenomenon, first reported in 1972,[87] has been related to the difficulty in discriminating skeletal muscle potentials from myocardial potentials. Dizziness and lightheadedness during active exercise may occur due to inhibition of the pacemaker output in the presence of an inadequate intrinsic cardiac rhythm (Fig. 33–36). Inhibition during active exercise involving the pectoralis muscle can be reproduced or provoked during routine evaluation in the pacemaker clinic. Although abdominal implantation of the pulse generator has been reported to decrease the incidence of myopotential inhibition,[88] other studies have shown that both the rectus abdominis and pectoralis muscles can be a source of myopotentials.[89] Bipolar units, by virtue of the rejection of far field interference and superior signal-to-noise ratio, are not influenced by myopotentials. Thus conversion of a unipolar system to a bipolar system may be a solution for myopotential inhibition. Also with present-day generators, programming the R wave sensitivity to a higher setting (i.e., lower sensitivity) may prevent oversensing. The presence of myopotential inhibition in a bipolar pacing system is highly suggestive of a lead insulation break.

Abnormal Sensing Caused by Intrinsic Signals

Oversensing of intrinsic signals from the atrium or ventricle can result in inhibition of VVI pacemakers. P wave sensing was described in cases of epicardial leads positioned near the AV groove[22, 90] and displacement of a right ventricular endocardial electrode near

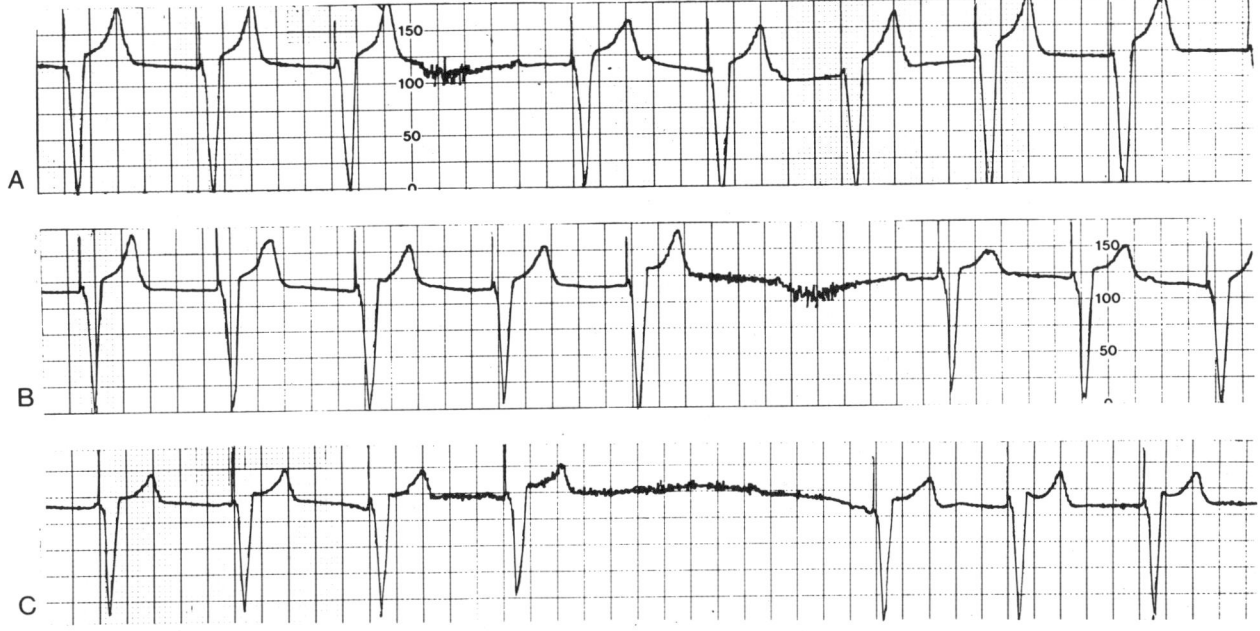

FIGURE 33-36
Inhibition of a VVI pacemaker by musculoskeletal potentials. The recording was obtained from a 65-year-old patient who had a unipolar transvenous VVI pacemaker implanted subcutaneously in the right infraclavicular region for symptomatic complete AV block. Eighteen months following implantation the patient had a recurrence of symptoms of dizziness. A routine ECG showed evidence of power source depletion (lengthening of the interspike interval from 840 to 1020 ms). The patient noted that symptoms only occurred when he used his right arm, especially when the arm was maintained in a forceful abducted position. The tracing was obtained while the patient was asked to exert intermittent pressure medially against resistance with the right hand, causing tensing of the pectoral muscles. This resulted in intermittent inhibition of the pacemaker, with prolonged asystolic intervals. Note the occurrence of baseline artifact from interference during the maneuver. Panels A, B, and C illustrate progressive lengthening of the asystolic intervals.

the tricuspid valve or into the coronary sinus.[91] If the atrial rate is faster than the pacemaker's automatic rate, constant P wave sensing will result in total suppression of a VVI pacemaker.[91]

T wave sensing abnormalities are more common than P wave sensing abnormalities,[22, 92–95] and may occur with pacemakers programmed to have a long pulse width, especially when the ventricular refractory period is short and the sensitivity is high. Sensing of the T wave of paced ventricular beats is far more common than sensing of the T wave of spontaneous beats (Fig. 33–37), probably because the voltage contribution from the pacemaker "afterpotential" following a paced beat tends to generate a larger T wave signal. Abnormal sensing of the pacemaker afterpotential has also been described.[22, 96] Oversensing can be corrected by using a bipolar system or by decreasing the sensitivity (i.e., increasing the sensitivity voltage setting).

Concealed extrasystole has been suggested as a possible reason for oversensing-induced inhibition,[97] although this phenomenon has not been adequately

FIGURE 33-37
An example of probable T wave sensing. Note that the VVI pacemaker escape interval following the ectopic beat marked X_2 is shorter than the pacemaker's normal escape interval of 820 ms. This suggests that complete recycling occurred after sensing of the T wave of the ectopic beat marked X_1. An alternative explanation would be partial sensing of the ectopic beat marked X_2, resulting in partial recycling and an abbreviated escape interval.

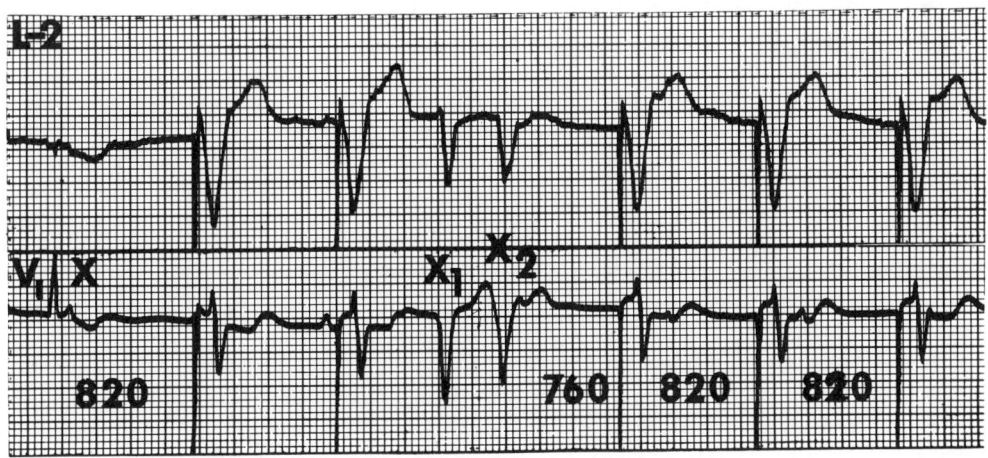

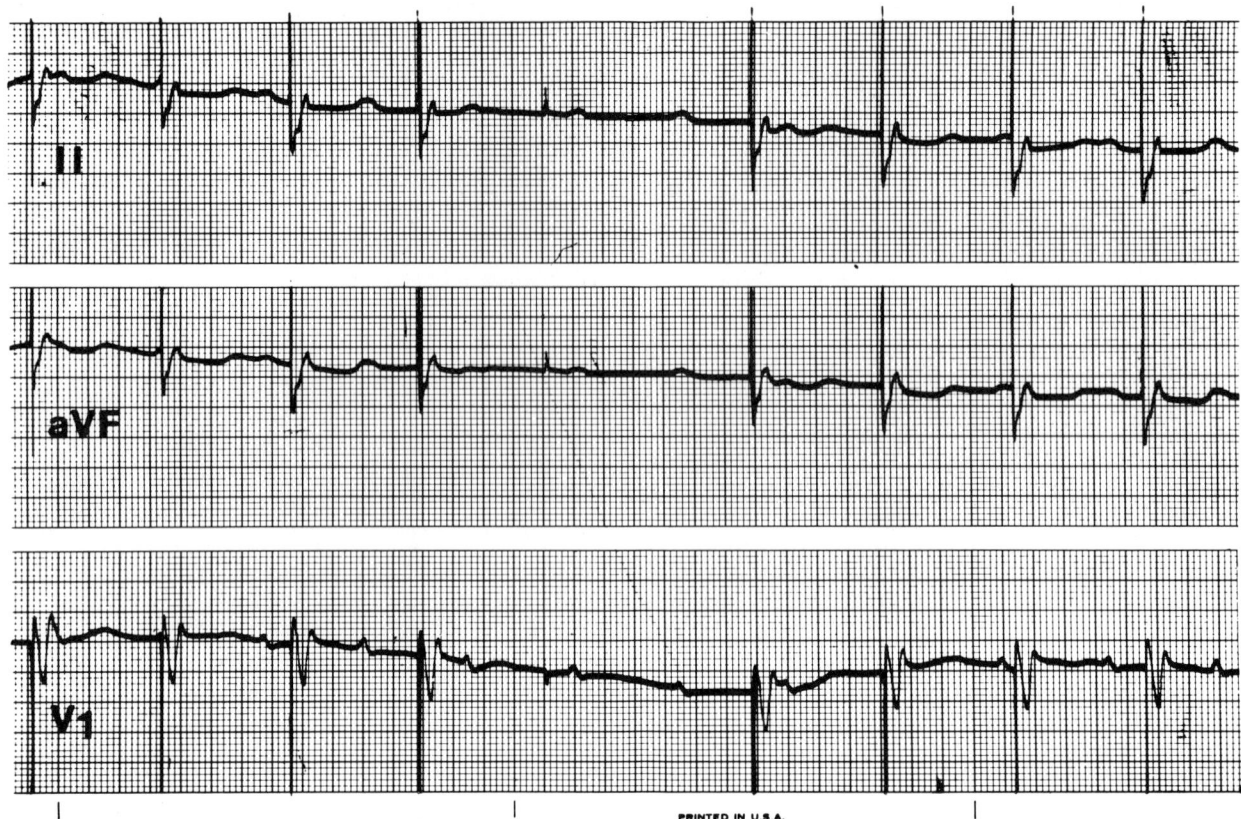

FIGURE 33–38
A characteristic ECG of partial lead fracture showing sudden diminution of the amplitude of the pacemaker artifact, associated with loss of ventricular capture. In this case, partial lead fracture also generated false signals, resulting in abnormal sensing. This explains the abnormally long pacemaker interval following the ineffective pacemaker artifact.

documented. Rarely, auto-interference of demand generators could be due to signals originating within a pulse generator itself.[98] The absence of any visible interference on the surface ECG and the relatively late appearance of auto-interference in the life of a pulse generator may mimic insulation defect or intermittent pulse generator failure.

Partial electrode fracture may generate false potentials, due to changes in electrode resistance and may result in oversensing.[99, 100] The characteristic finding on a surface ECG is marked variation in the amplitude of the pacemaker artifact with intermittent loss of ventricular capture (Fig. 33–38). The diagnosis of electrode fracture can be ascertained by analysis of the

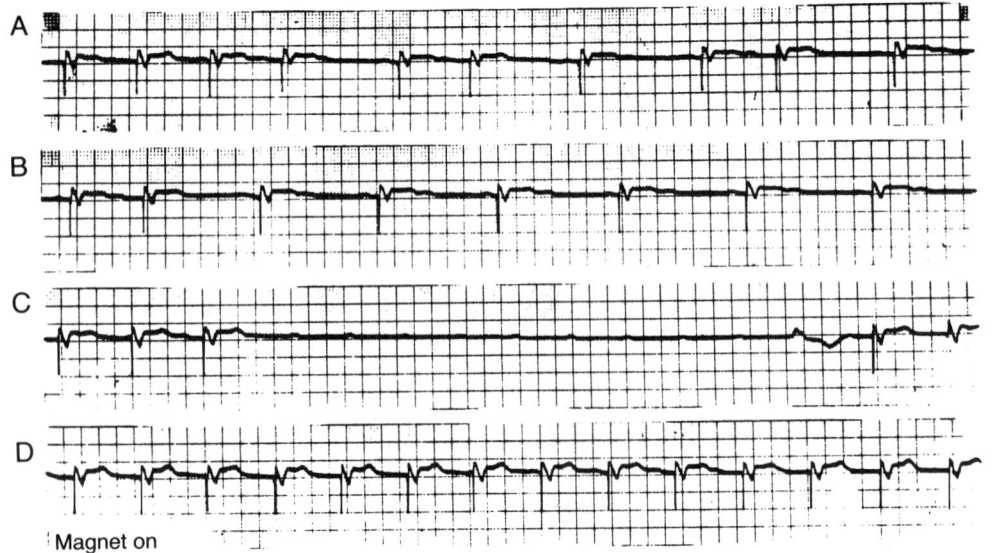

FIGURE 33–39
Abnormal sensing caused by spurious potentials generated by contact between two endocardial electrodes. Panels A–C illustrate irregular function of the VVI pacemaker, resulting in a pseudo-bigeminal pattern in A; an almost regular pattern at a much slower rate than the set discharge rate of the VVI pacemaker (B); and complete suppression of the VVI pacemaker, causing a long period of asystole, in C. Panel D shows normal function in the fixed-rate mode following the application of an external magnet. Note that the fixed rate is slightly faster than the automatic rate, as seen in the first part A.

stimulus artifact as displayed on an oscilloscope. Distortion of the stimulus artifact may be the only sign present, even in the absence of radiologic evidence of lead fracture.[101]

The interaction between two pacing catheters within the heart may also generate false signals when functional and inactive electrodes make intermittent contact.[101–103] An illustrative example is shown in Figures 33–39 and 33–40. The recordings were obtained from a 79-year-old man who was admitted because of intermittent pacing failure of a permanent VVI unit, which was attributed to partial fracture of the epicardial lead.

The patient gave a history of dizziness and syncopal episodes for 1 month prior to admission. Because of his symptoms, he was admitted to the intensive care unit, and a temporary transvenous VVI pacemaker was placed. He was later transferred to the operating room, where a permanent transvenous VVI pacemaker was implanted. The patient returned to the intensive care unit for monitoring with both the temporary and permanent transvenous electrodes in place but was noted to have frequent intermittent inhibition of his permanent pacemaker (see Fig. 33–39). No external electrical interference was found.

The temporary pacemaker, still in place, was activated and similarly demonstrated frequent inhibition. Both pacemakers functioned normally in the fixed-rate mode, however. Oscilloscopic recordings from the cathodal (distal) electrode of the temporary pacing catheter demonstrated spurious potentials with an amplitude of about 169 mV and a very rapid slew rate which inhibited the permanent pacemaker (see Fig. 33–40).

Fluoroscopy and chest x-ray demonstrated the two endocardial electrodes to be in intimate contact. The temporary wire was withdrawn about 2 cm, and similar recordings revealed absence of the spurious potentials with normal function of the pacemaker in the demand mode (see Fig. 33–40). After complete withdrawal of the temporary wire, the permanent pacemaker functioned properly.

Partial Sensing

As a rule, VVI pacemakers respond to sensed signals in an all-or-none fashion, resulting in full recycling of automatic and escape intervals. Certain VVI pacemaker models exhibit partial sensing in response either to borderline signals falling anywhere outside of their refractory period or to large signals—otherwise capable

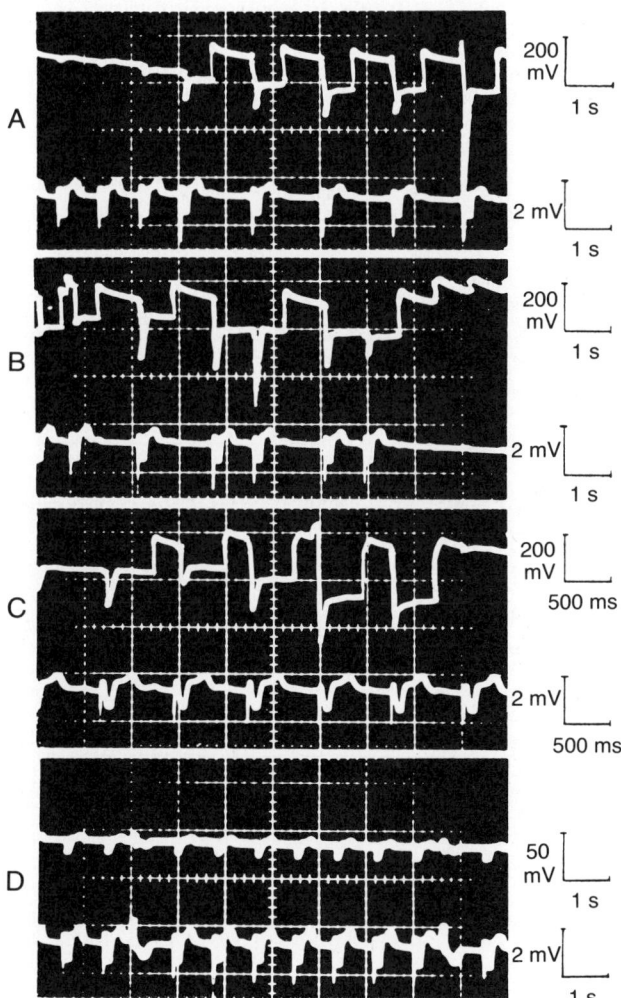

FIGURE 33–40
Oscilloscopic recordings from the cathodal electrode of the temporary wire (from the same patient shown in Figure 33–39) illustrates the presence of spurious potentials (upper tracings in panels A–D). The simultaneously recorded lower tracing in each panel is standard lead 2.

The first part of A shows the absence of spurious potentials that later appear at regular intervals, causing fairly regular pacemaker firing at a slower rate than the set discharge rate. Note that the interval from the onset of the spurious potential to the following pacemaker spike is exactly equal to the escape interval of the VVI pacemaker.

In the first part of B, the spurious potentials occur during every other paced beat, giving rise to a pseudo–bigeminal pattern. The second part of B shows repetitive generation of spurious potentials, resulting in total pacemaker inhibition.

In C, the pacemaker was placed in the fixed-rate mode by application of an external magnet. Note that the spurious potentials failed to affect the pacemaker function.

D was obtained after partial withdrawal of the temporary electrode and shows absence of the spurious potentials and normal function of the VVI pacemaker (the two ventricular premature beats resulted in appropriate inhibition).

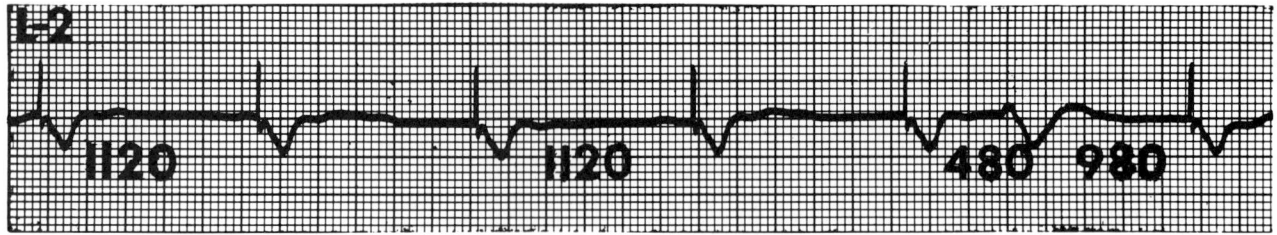

FIGURE 33–41
Partial sensing of a ventricular premature beat, resulting in a shortened escape interval. See text for details.

of recycling the generator completely—that fall within their short relative refractory period.[93] This would result in partial recycling, leading to an abbreviated escape interval. Figure 33–41 illustrates an example of partial sensing of a ventricular ectopic beat that probably generated a borderline electrical signal, resulting in a shortened escape interval.

Value of Holter Monitoring for Follow-Up of Pacemaker Patients

Ambulatory long-term ECG monitoring is valuable for follow-up of pacemaker patients.[104] The recording is well suited to document bradyarrhythmic and tachyarrhythmic events accompanied by conspicuous changes in cardiac rhythm (Fig. 33–42). The ambulatory ECG should be analyzed with care, because of the not uncommon occurrence of recording artifacts (Fig. 33–43). While commercial Holter recorder/scanner systems can faithfully reproduce ordinary ECG waveforms whose major frequency components lie below 50 Hz, they severely attenuate signals of high frequency. Thus pacing spikes, typically 0.5 ms in duration, with very rapid rise time, may sometimes be attenuated and slurred beyond recognition on the scanner oscilloscope or paper print-out. The ability to monitor an amplified pacemaker stimulus on a dedicated channel was first introduced by Kelen et al.[105] This "marker" channel, with various degrees of sophistication, has resulted in marked improvement in the diagnosis of pacemaker malfunctions.[106] Subtle and/or intermittent failure to sense (Fig. 33–44) or failure to capture (Fig. 33–45) can be easily detected. The system can also be used to evaluate dual-chamber pacemaker programming and to assess programming efficacy of antitachycardia pacemakers.[107]

Atrial Pacing (AAI)

Nowadays, sinus node dysfunction is the indication for pacing in approximately half of all patients with per-

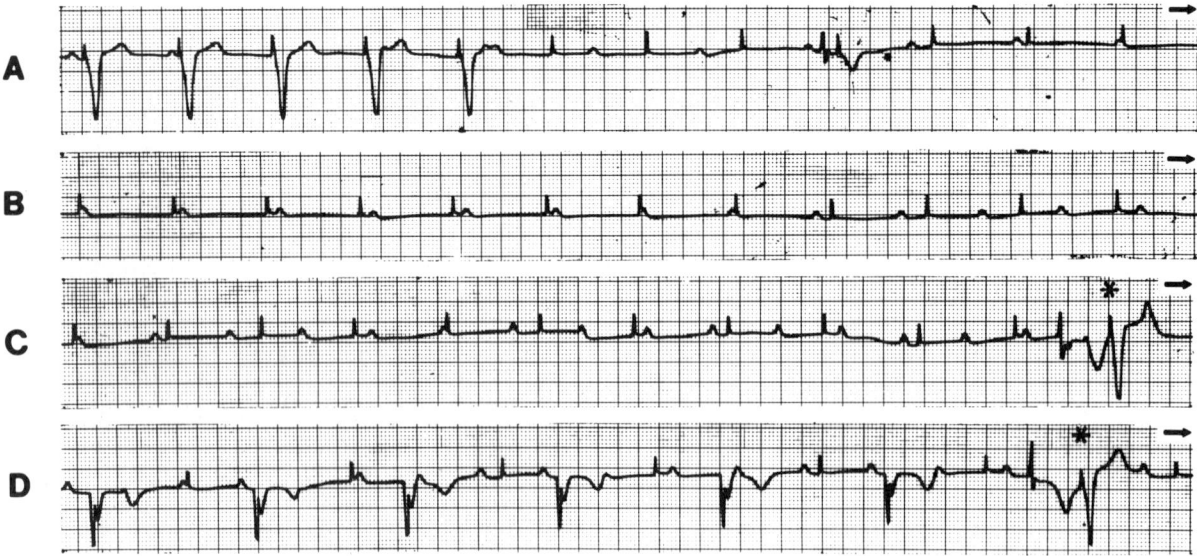

FIGURE 33–42
Ambulatory Holter recording from a patient with a VVI pacemaker, showing intermittent failure to capture. The first half of A shows a regular paced rhythm followed by abrupt loss of capture. This resulted in a prolonged period of asystole (B and C) before the escape of a fairly regular idioventricular rhythm (D). Note the presence of two effective pacemaker stimuli (marked by asterisks). These are a manifestation of the supernormal phase of cardiac excitation and occur only when the spike falls on or close to the end of the T wave of a preceding spontaneous depolarization. The presence of these two paced beats suggests that the intermittent failure to pace was caused by the presence of subthreshold pacemaker stimuli.

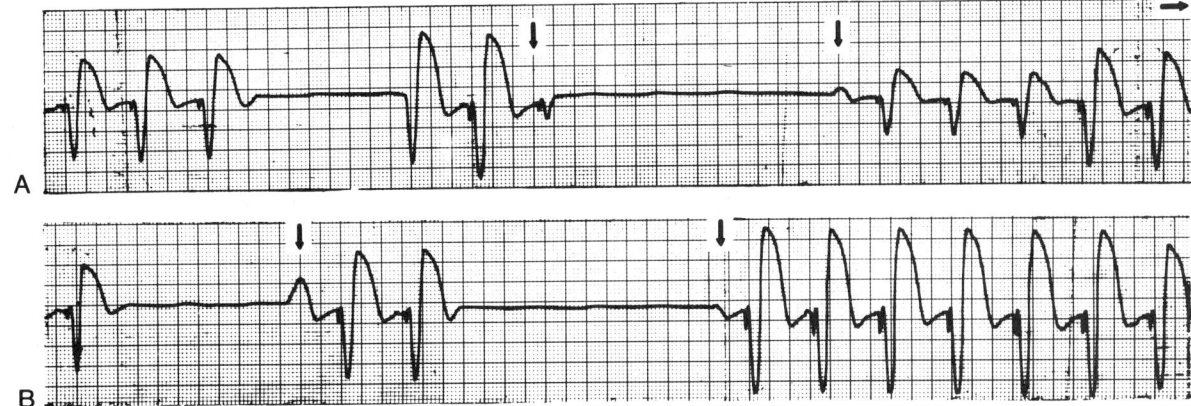

FIGURE 33—43
Ambulatory Holter monitor recording from a patient with a VVI pacemaker, revealing ECG artifact. The recording was obtained from a 69-year-old man with a VVI pacemaker implanted 6 months previously for symptomatic high-degree AV block. The patient presented with symptoms of lightheadedness, and routine ECG examination showed normal pacing and sensing functions. However, the 24-hour Holter monitor recording was interpreted as indicating intermittent pacemaker malfunction. This prompted the change of the pulse generator. A thorough examination later failed to show any evidence of malfunction of the pulse generator, including both batteries and electronic components. A re-examination of the Holter recording clearly unravelled the artifactual nature of the tracing.

The representative tracings shown in the figure illustrate a paced rhythm with intermittent isoelectric pauses that are exact multiples of the pacemaker automatic interval. The artifact should have been readily identified by the deflections marked by arrows, which represent partial inscription of paced QRS-T complexes, and by the obvious variation in the amplitude of the recorded ECG complexes. The artifact was probably related to intermittent loss of contact between a loose recording electrode and the magnetic tape recorder. Panels A and B represent a continuous recording.

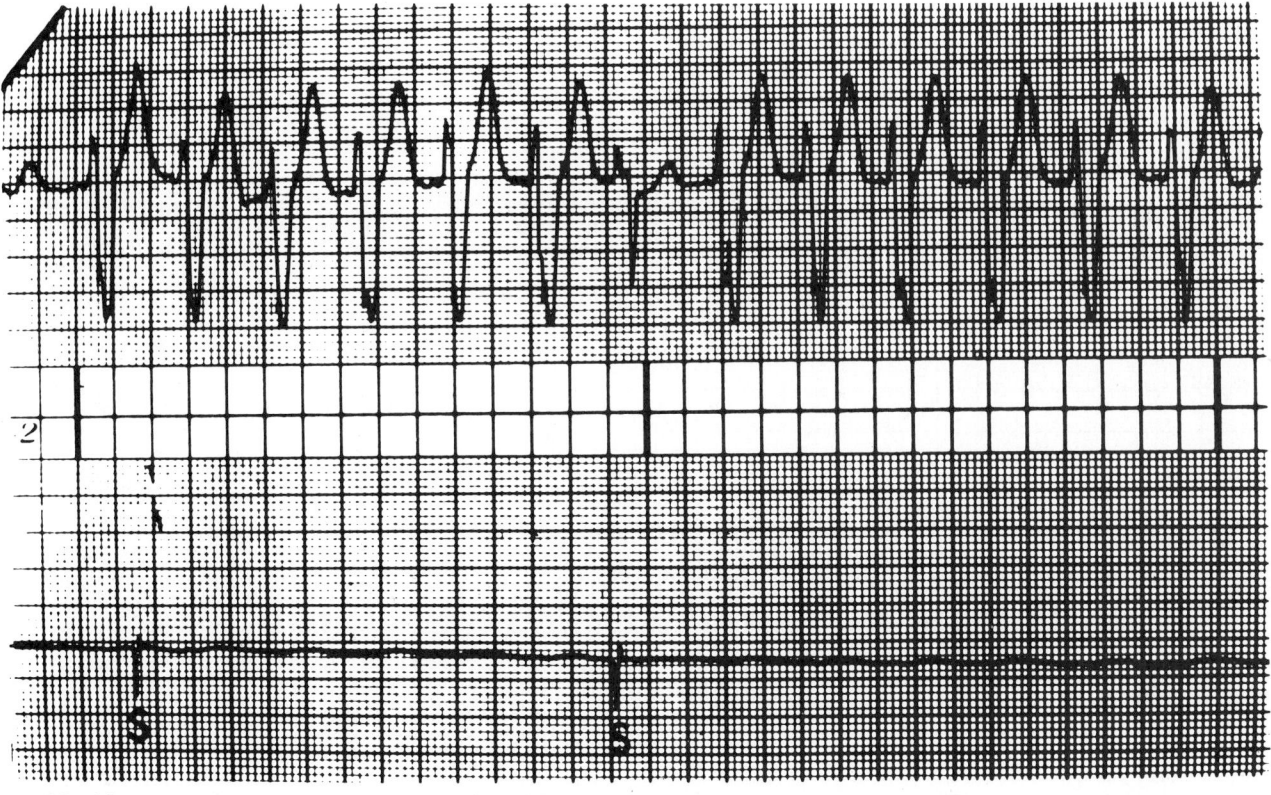

FIGURE 33—44
Ambulatory Holter monitor recording using the marker channel. The intermittent inscription of pacing spikes (s), clearly seen only on the marker channel, represents sensing failure during supraventricular tachycardia.

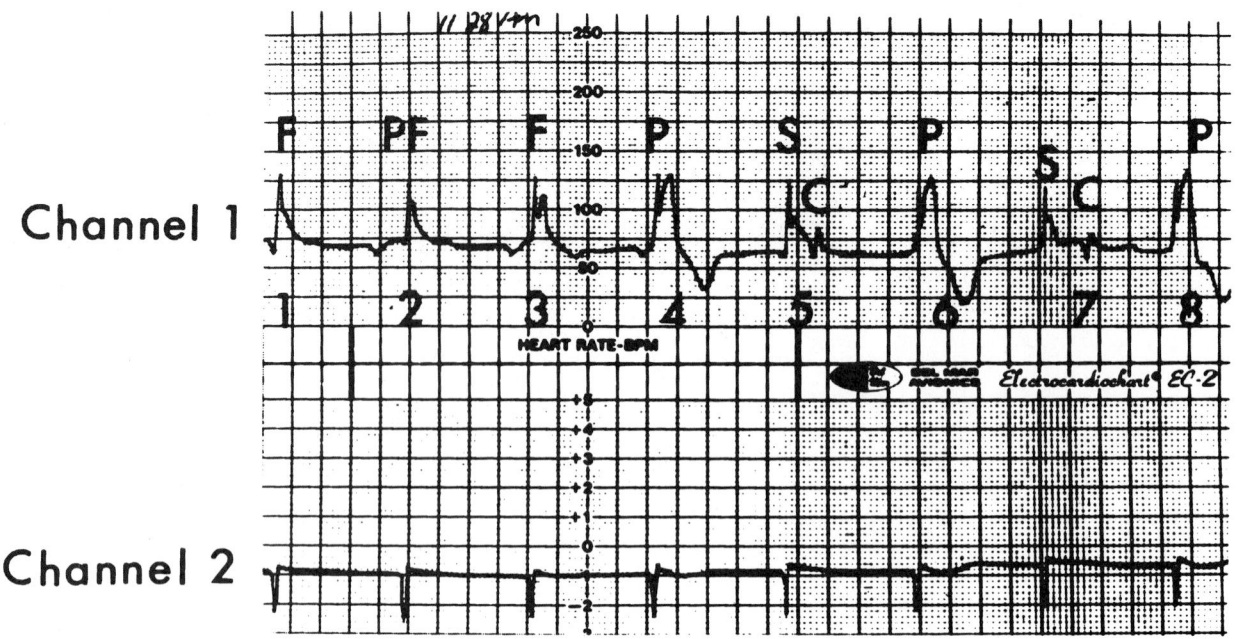

FIGURE 33-45
Ambulatory Holter monitor recording using the marker channel. The recording was obtained from a 70-year-old patient with presyncopal symptoms and illustrates the problem of beat classification when multiple QRS morphologies occur. Beat 2 is a pseudofusion beat (PF); beats 1 and 3 are true fusion beats (F); beats 4, 6, and 8 are normally paced (P); and beats 5 and 7 are spontaneously conducted beats (C). The fifth and seventh pacemaker spikes (S) failed to capture. Sensing failure is also suggested by failure of recycling of the pacemaker following the spontaneously conducted beat 7, although it falls outside the known pacemaker sensing refractory period. Because of the slurring of the trailing edge of the pacing spike in channel 1 (large exponential decay curve), the noncapturing spikes could also be easily mistaken for QRS complexes were the ambiguity not resolved by the marker channel 2.

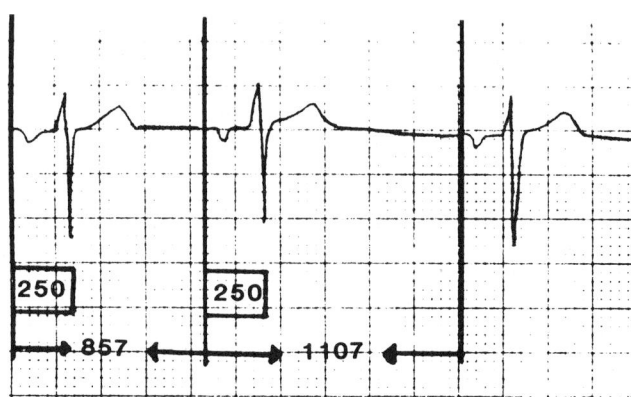

FIGURE 33-46
Sensing malfunction during AAI pacing. Shown is a diagrammatic representation of abnormal sensing of the QRS complex by the atrial lead. During atrial pacing at a rate of 70 bpm (cycle length 857 ms), a prolongation of the pacemaker escape interval to 1107 ms occurs. This prolongation is equal to that of the atrial refractory period and represents recycling of the escape interval as a result of QRS signal sensing in a unipolar pacing system. See text for discussion.

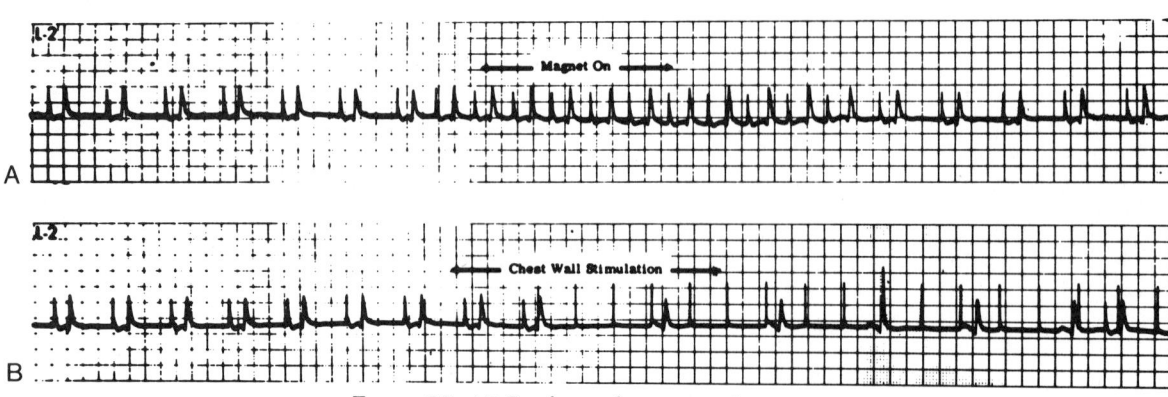

FIGURE 33-47 See legend on opposite page

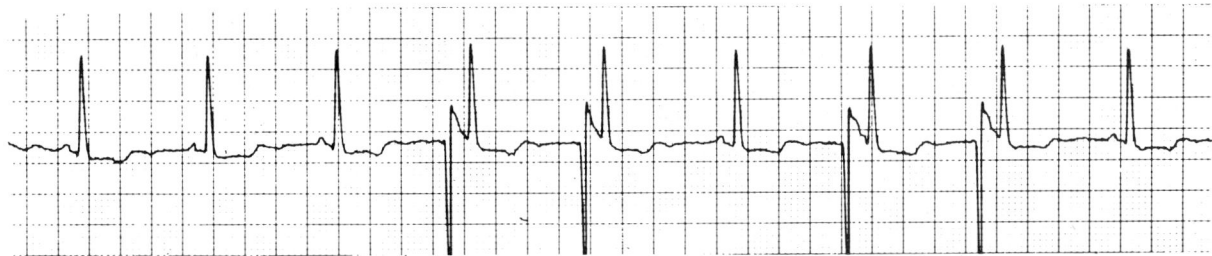

FIGURE 33–48
Normal AAI pacing. During unipolar atrial pacing in a patient with sick sinus syndrome, the exponential decay curve completely obliterates the paced P wave. Confirmation of atrial capture can be achieved by demonstrating 1-to-1 conduction after reprogramming to a faster rate.

manent pacemakers. Single-chamber atrial pacing is generally indicated in patients with sinus node dysfunction who otherwise have an intact AV conduction system. However, since up to one third of patients with the sick sinus syndrome have associated AV conduction system disease at the time of pacemaker implantation, and since an unpredictable small number of patients will develop AV conduction disease, VVI and dual-chamber pacing systems are often implanted in lieu of the single-chamber atrial pacemaker.[108, 109] Consequently, the atrial demand pacemaker (AAI pacing) is responsible for less than 1% of all pacing modalities utilized in the United States today.

The advantages of atrial pacing include (1) preservation of atrial transport and its contribution to improved hemodynamics, and (2) maintenance of AV synchrony, thus preventing retrograde conduction and the possible adverse hemodynamic effects of ventricular pacing and the pacemaker syndrome.[110-112] The sensing and pacing abnormalities seen with AAI pacing are similar to those previously enumerated for the single-chamber ventricular pacemaker.

Sensing malfunctions such as QRS or T wave sensing in an AAI pacemaker with a relatively short atrial refractory period may lead to abnormal prolongation of the escape interval. The subsequent bradycardia has been termed *refractory period bradycardia*.[113, 114] In this situation, the pacemaker's escape interval is recycled, and the prolonged interval is equal to the atrial refractory period plus the programmed escape interval (Fig. 33–46).

In the AAI pacemaker, the duration of the paced refractory period determines whether the QRS complex will be sensed after a pacemaker-induced atrial depolarization. It is advantageous to have the paced atrial refractory period at approximately 400 ms in order to avoid intermittent sensing of the QRS complex after paced atrial beats. An example of QRS sensing during atrial pacing from the coronary sinus is shown in Figure 33–47. The response of the AAI pacemaker to magnet application and chest wall stimulation is qualitatively similar to that of the VVI pacemaker. (see Fig. 33–47).

Lengthening of the automatic interval may also be seen when nonconducted atrial premature depolarizations or retrograde P waves generated by ventricular extrasystoles occur occasionally. These P waves may not be evident on the surface ECG and can lead to the misdiagnosis of abnormal T wave sensing. Undersensing of the atrial signal may also occur and may be diagnosed by utilizing the AAT mode.

Not infrequently, loss of atrial capture may be difficult to recognize on the surface ECG or ambulatory monitor particularly in a unipolar pacing system in which large pacemaker afterpotentials (exponential decay curve) are present (Fig. 33–48). By programming the atrial rate to one higher than the sinus rate and allowing 1:1 AV conduction, the proof of atrial capture can be easily obtained.

FIGURE 33–47
An example of atrial demand (AAI) pacing from the coronary sinus, illustrating an inappropriately slow pacemaker rate due to abnormal sensing of the conducted QRS complex. The pacemaker was implanted for the management of sick sinus syndrome and the demand rate was set at 115 bpm, with the escape interval at 540 ms. As shown in A, the actual pacing rate was 85 bpm (spike-to-spike interval of 750 ms). The demand unit was an old model with a standard refractory period of 200 to 240 ms. Since the combined duration of the P-R interval and the conducted QRS complex was greater than the pacemaker refractory period, the unit sensed its own generated QRS and was recycled by the ventricular deflection. This resulted in an inappropriately slower pacing rate.

A shows that when a magnet was applied over the demand unit, converting the pacemaker to the asynchronous pacing mode, the pacing rate increased to the originally set rate of 115 beats per minute. B illustrates the effect of external chest wall stimulation, which resulted in inhibition of the demand pacemaker, revealing the underlying spontaneous rhythm of sinus bradycardia.

References

1. Feruglia GA, Richards AF, Steinbach K, et al.: Cardiac pacing in the world: A survey of the state of the art in 1986. PACE 10 (Part II):768, 1987.
2. Parsonet V, Furman S, Smyth NPD: Implantable cardiac pacemakers: Status report and resource guidelines. Pacemaker study group, Intersociety Commission for Heart Disease Resources (ICHD). Circulation 50:A21, 1974.
3. Parsonnet V, Furman S, Smyth NPD: Revised code for Pacemaker identification. PACE 4:400, 1981.
4. Bernstein AD, Camm AJ, Fletcher RD, et al.: The NASPE/BPEG Generic Pacemaker Code for Antibradyarrhythmia and adaptive-rate pacing and antitachyarrhythmia devices. PACE 10:794, 1987.
5. Green GD: Assessment of cardiac pacemakers: Frontal plane vector. Am Heart J 81:1, 1971.
6. Mond H, Slowman G: The malfunctioning pacemaker system. PACE Vol 4 (Part I):49, 1981.
7. Gersony WM, Geisler GF, Webb WR: Ventricular fibrillation masked by the unipolar pacemaker. Chest 55:503, 1969.
8. Mond HG: Pacemaker electrocardiography. In Mond HG (ed.): The Cardiac Pacemaker: Function and Malfunction, pp. 93–117. New York, Grune and Stratton, 1983.
9. Murdock DK, Moran JF, Staffor M, et al.: Pacemaker malfunction: Fact or artifact? Heart Lung 15:150, March 1986.
10. Operator's Manual for Microcomputer Augmented Cardiograph (MAC) II. Milwaukee, Marquette Electronics, Inc, 1984.
11. Engler RL, Goldberger AL, Bhargava V: Pacemaker spike alternans: An artifact of digital signal processing. PACE 5:748, 1982.
12. Webster JG, (Ed.): Basic Concepts of Instrumentation. In Medical Instrumentation, pp. 23, 286. Boston, Houghton Mifflin Co, 1978.
13. Castellanos A Jr, Maytin O, Lemberg L, et al.: Unusual QRS complexes produced by pacemaker stimuli. Am Heart J 77:732, 1969.
14. Barold SS, Center S: Electrocardiographic diagnosis of perforation of the heart by pacing catheter electrode. Am J Cardiol 24:274, 1969.
15. Mower MM, Aranaga CE, Tabatznik B: Unusual patterns of conduction produced by pacemaker stimuli. Am Heart J 74:24, 1967.
16. Sodi-Pollares D, Calder RM: New Bases of Electrocardiography. St. Louis, C. V. Mosby Co., 1956.
17. Barold JJ, Narula OS, Javier RP et al.: Significance of right bundle branch block patterns during pervenous ventricular pacing. Br Heart J 31:286, 1969.
18. Hoffman BF, Cranefield PF, Stuckey JH, et al.: Direct measurement of conduction velocity in in situ specialized conduction system of mammalian heart. Proc Soc Exp Biol (NY) 102:155, 1959.
19. Kemp A, Kjersgard J, Kjoegard E: Malplacement of endocardial pacemaker electrodes in the middle cardiac vein. Acta Med Scand 199:7, 1976.
20. Waxman HJ, Lazzara R, Castellanos A, et al.: Ventricular pacing from the middle cardiac vein mimicking supraventricular morphology. PACE 2:203, 1979.
21. Castellanos A Jr, Ortiz JM, Pastis N, et al.: The electrocardiogram in patients with pacemakers. Prog Cardiovasc Dis 13:190, 1970.
22. Barold SS, Gaidula JJ: Evaluation of normal and abnormal sensing functions of demand pacemakers. Am J Cardiol 28:201, 1971.
23. Chatterjee K, Harris A, Davies G, et al.: Electrocardiographic changes subsequent to artificial ventricular depolarization. Br Heart J 31:770, 1969.
24. Denes P, Pick A, Miller RH, et al.: A characteristic precordial repolarization abnormality with intermittent left bundle branch block. Ann Intern Med 89:55, 1978.
25. Rosenbaum MB, Blanco HH, Elizari MV, et al.: Electronic modulation of the T wave and cardiac memory. Am J Cardiol 50:213, 1982.
26. Carrera E, Friedland C: La onda de activación ventricular en el bloqueo de rama izquierda caon infarcto: Un nuevo signo electrocardiografico. Arch Inst Cardiol Mex 23:441, 1953.
27. Dodinot B, Kubler L, Aliot E, et al.: Electrocardiographic diagnosis of myocardial infarction and coronary insufficiency in the pacemaker patient. In Thaleuand HJ Th, Harthrone JW (eds.): To Pace or Not to Pace. Controversial Subjects on Cardiac Pacing, pp. 295–301. The Hague, Martinus Nijhoff, 1978.
28. Barold SS, Ong LS, Banner RL: Diagnosis of inferior wall myocardial infarction during right ventricular apical pacing. Chest 69:232, 1976.
29. Zoll PM: Resuscitation of the heart in ventricular standstill by external electric stimulation. N Engl J Med 247:768, 1952.
30. Wiggers CJ, Wegria R: Ventricular fibrillation due to single, localized induction and condensor shocks applied during the vulnerable phase of ventricular systoles. Am J Physiol 128:500, 1940.
31. Bilitch M, Cosby RS, Cafferky EA: Ventricular fibrillation and competitive pacing. N Engl J Med 276:598, 1967.
32. Furman S, Escher DJW: Arrhythmias associated with hysteresis ventricular inhibited pacing. Chest 64:666, 1973.
33. Castellanos A Jr, Lemberg L: Pacer arrhythmias and electrocardiographic recognition of pacemakers. Circulation 47:1382, 1973.
34. Driller J, Barold SS, Parsonnet V: Normal and abnormal function of the pacemaker magnetic reed switch. J Electrocardiol 9:283, 1976.
35. Barold SS, Gaidula JJ, Castillo R: Unusual response of demand pacemakers to magnets. Br Heart J 35:353, 1973.
36. Voukydis PC, Shulman AN, Cohen ST: Unmasking of slow intrinsic ventricular excitation by magnet inhibition of R wave inhibited demand pacemakers. Chest 67:304, 1975.
37. Sinnaeve A, Williams R, Stroobandt R: Inhibition of the demand pacemakers by magnet waving. PACE 5:878, 1982.
38. Samet P, Abbas SZ, Hildner FJ, et al.: Effect of chest wall stimulation on cardiac pacemaker function. Am J Med Sci 260:285, 1970.
39. Barold SS, Gaidula JJ, Castillo R, et al.: Evaluation of demand pacemakers by chest wall stimulation. Chest 63:598, 1973.
40. Fontaine JM, Perri CA, El-Sherif N: DDD pacemaker pseudo malfunction during supraventricular tachycardia. PACE 11:1380, 1988.
41. Jenkins JM, Dick M, Collins S, et al.: Use of the pill electrode for transesophageal atrial pacing. PACE 8(4):512, 1985.
42. Greatbatch W, Lee JH, Mathias W, et al.: The solid state lithium battery: A new improved chemical power source for implantable cardiac pacemakers. IEEE Trans Biomed Eng BFME 18:317, 1971.
43. Greatbatch W: A new pacemaker system utilizing a long life lithium cell. In Digest of 9th International Conference on Medical and Biological Engineering, Melbourne, Australia, 1971, p. 277.
44. Lehman G, Bussillet H, Dodimot B, et al.: Projected behavior of the first lithium iodine powered pulse generators, pp. 76–81. In Meese C (ed.): Proceedings of the VIth World Symposium on Cardiac Pacing, Montreal, 1979.
45. Mond H, Cole P, Slomon G: Long term experience with early lithium iodine powered pulse generators, pp. 123–127. In Meese C (ed.): Proceedings of the VIth World Symposium on Cardiac Pacing, Montreal, 1979.
46. Furman S: Cardiac pacing and pacemakers. VIII. The followup clinic. Am Heart J 94:795, 1977.
47. Bramowitz AD, Smith JW, Eber LM, et al.: Runaway pacemaker: A persisting problem. JAMA 228:340, 1974.
48. Nasrallah A, Hall RJ, Garcia E, et al.: Runaway pacemaker in seven patients: A persisting problem. J Thorac Cardiovasc Surg 69:365, 1975.
49. Barold SS, Center S: Electrocardiographic diagnosis of perforation of the heart by pacing catheter electrode. Am J Cardiol 24:274, 1969.
50. Korn M, Schoenfeld CD, Grahramani A, et al.: The pacemaker sound. Am J Med 49:451, 1970.
51. Harris A: Pacemaker "heart sound." Br Heart J 29:608, 1967.
52. Murdock ML, Myers BA, Bacos JM: Auscultatory clicks produced by pacemaker catheters. Ann Intern Med 68:1320, 1968.

53. Van Beck GW, Den Dulk K, Lindemans FW, et al.: HJJ detection of insulation failure by gradual reduction in noninvasively measured electrogram amplitudes. PACE 9:772, 1986.
54. Fisch C, Greenspan K, Anderson GJ: Exit block. Am J Cardiol 28:402, 1971.
55. Preston TA, Judge RD: Alteration of pacemaker threshold by drug and physiological factors. Ann NY Acad Sci 167:689, 1969.
56. Gettes LS, Shabetai R, Downs TA, et al.: Effect of changes in potassium and calcium concentrations on diastolic threshold and strength-interval relationship of the human heart. Ann NY Acad Sci 167:693, 1969.
57. Gray RJ, Brown DF: Pacemaker failure due to procainamide toxicity. Am J Cardiol 34:728, 1974.
58. Hellestrand KH, Burnett PJ, Milne JR, et al.: Effect of antiarrhythmic agent flecainide acetate on acute and chronic pacing thresholds. PACE 6:892, 1983.
59. O'Reilley MV, Murnaghan DP, Williams MB: Transvenous pacemaker failure induced by hyperkalemia. JAMA 228:236, 1974.
60. Das G, Eaton J: Pacemaker malfunction following transthoracic countershock. PACE 4:487, 1981.
61. Levine PA, Barold SS, Fletcher RD, et al.: Adverse acute and chronic effects of electrical defibrillation and cardioversion on implanted unipolar cardiac pacing systems. J Am Coll Cardiol 1(6):1413, 1983.
62. Yee R, Jones DL, Klein GJ: Pacing threshold changes after transvenous catheter countershock. Am J Cardiol 53:503, 1984.
63. Adamec R, Haefliger JM, Killiseh JP, et al.: Damaging effect of therapeutic radiation on programmable pacemakers. PACE 5:146, 1982.
64. Irnich W: Interference in pacemakers. PACE 7:1021, 1984.
65. Gordon AJ, Vagueiro MC, Barold SS: Endocardial electrograms from pacemaker catheters. Circulation 38:82, 1968.
66. Walls JT, Maloney JD, Pluth JR: Clinical evolution of a sutureless cardiac pacing lead: Chronic threshold changes and lead durability. Ann Thorac Surg 36(3):328, 1983.
67. Chatterjee K, Sutton R, Davis JG: Low intracardiac potentials in myocardial infarction as a cause of failure of inhibition of demand pacemakers. Lancet 1:511, 1968.
68. Barold SS, Gaidula JJ: Failure of demand pacemaker from low bipolar electrograms. JAMA 215:923, 1971.
69. Lindemans FW, Rankin IR, Murtaugh R, et al.: Clinical experience with an activity sensing pacemaker. PACE 9:978, 1986.
70. Medtronic Activitrax I Technical Manual, p 20.
71. Michaelson EM, Moss AJ: Environmental influences on implanted cardiac pacemakers. JAMA 216:2006, 1971.
72. Walter WH, Mitchell JC, Rustan PL, et al.: Cardiac pulse generators and electromagnetic interference. JAMA 224:1628, 1973.
73. Ohm OJ: Interference with cardiac pacemaker function. Acta Med Scand 596(Suppl):86, 1976.
74. Butrous GS, Male JC, Webber RS, et al.: The effect of power frequency high intensity electronic field on implanted cardiac pacemakers. PACE 6:1282, 1983.
75. Pickers BA, Goldberg MJ: Inhibition of a demand pacemaker and interference with monitoring equipment by radio frequency transmission. Br Med J 2:504, 1969.
76. b'Cunha GF, Nicoud T, Pemberton AH, et al.: Syncopal attacks arising from erratic demand pacemaker function in the vicinity of a television transmitter. Am J Cardiol 31:789, 1973.
77. Yatteau RF: Radar-induced failure of a demand pacemaker. N Engl J Med 283:1447, 1970.
78. Furman S, Parker B, Krauthamer M, et al.: The influence of electromagnetic environment on the performance of artificial cardiac pacemakers. Ann Thorac Surg 6:90, 1968.
79. Crystal RG, Kastor JA, DeSanctis RW: Inhibition of discharge of an external demand pacemaker by electric razor. Am J Cardiol 28:695, 1971.
80. Escher DJW, Parker B, Furman S: Pacemaker triggering (inhibition) by electric toothbrush. Am J Cardiol 38:126, 1976.
81. Falkoff M, Ong S, Heinle RA, et al.: The noise sampling period: A new cause of apparent sensing malfunction of demand pacemakers. PACE 1:250, 1978.
82. Cordis Model 415A (Theta) Gemini (Physician's Manual). Miami, Cordis Co., 1984.
83. King GR, Hamburger AC, Parsa F, et al.: Effect of microwave oven on implanted cardiac pacemaker. JAMA 212:1213, 1970.
84. Ali N, Bhatia S: Pseudomalfunction of pacemaker due to a defective electrocardiograph. Am J Cardiol 53:373, 1984.
85. Wajszczuk WJ, Mowry FM, Dungan NF: De-activation of a demand pacemaker by transurethral electrocautery. N Engl J Med 230:34, 1969.
86. Hauser RG: Bipolar leads for cardiac pacing in the 1980's: A reappraisal provoked by skeletal muscle interference. PACE 5:34, 1982.
87. Wirtzfeld A, Lampadius M, Ruprecht EO: Unterdruckung von Demand-Schritt machern durch Muskelpotentiale. Dtsch Med Wochenschr 97:61, 1972.
88. Rosenquist M, Norlander R, Anderson M, et al.: Reduced incidence of myopotential pacemaker inhibition by abdominal generator implantation. PACE 9:417, 1986.
89. Gialafos J, Maillis A, Kalogeropoulos C, et al.: Inhibition of demand pacemakers by myopotentials. Am Heart J 109:984, 1985.
90. Tabesh E: Intermittent P- and T-wave sensing in demand pacemakers. J Electrocardiol 5:295, 1972.
91. Weinstock M, De Guiaaa R, Daniell M, et al.: Inhibition of transvenous pacing through the coronary sinus by the atrial P wave: Diagnosis with the aid of isoproterenol. Chest 59:563, 1971.
92. Cheng TO, Chaithiraphan S, Baltazarn A, et al.: Suppression by a prominent T-wave: An unusual cause of malfunction of a transvenous demand pacemaker. Chest 60:502, 1971.
93. Barold SS, Gaidula JJ, Lyon JL, et al.: Irregular recycling of demand pacemakers from borderline electrographic signals. Am Heart J 82:477, 1971.
94. Yokoyama M, Wada J, Barold SS: Transient early T wave sensing by implanted programmable demand pulse generator. PACE 4:68, 1981.
95. Furman S, Huang WM: Pacemaker recycle from repolarization artifact. PACE 5:927, 1982.
96. Keller JW, Gosselin AJ, Nathan DA, et al.: Rhythm anomalies in contemporary demand pacing. Am J Cardiol 29:527, 1972.
97. Massumi RA, Mason DT, Amsterdam EA, et al.: Apparent malfunction of demand pacemaker caused by nonpropagated (concealed) ventricular extrasystoles. Chest 61:426, 1972.
98. Barold SS, Levine PA: Auto interference of demand pulse generators. PACE 4:274, 1981.
99. Nevins MA, Landau S, Lyon LJ: Failure of demand pacemaker sensing due to electrode fracture. Chest 59:110, 1971.
100. Coumel P, Mugica J, Barold SS: Demand pacemaker arrhythmias caused by intermittent incomplete electrode fracture. Diagnosis with testing magnet. Am J Cardiol 39:105, 1975.
101. Widmann WD, Mangiola S, Lubow LA, et al.: Suppression of demand pacemaker by inactive pacemaker electrodes. Circulation 45:319, 1972.
102. Johansen JK: Disturbance in rhythm in 2 patients with a permanent pacemaker and two endocardial electrodes. Acta Med Scand 596(Suppl):80, 1976.
103. Waxman HL, Lazzara R, El-Sherif N: Apparent malfunction of demand pacemaker due to spurious potentials generated by contact between two endocardial electrodes. PACE 1:531, 1978.
104. Furman S: Cardiac pacing and pacemakers. VI. Analysis of pacemaker malfunction. Am Heart J 94:378, 1977.
105. Kelen GJ, Bloomfield DA, Hardage M, et al.: Clinical evaluation of an improved Holter monitoring technique for artificial pacemaker function. PACE 3:192, 1980.
106. Famularo MA, Kennedy HL: Ambulatory electrocardiography in the assessment of pacemaker function. Am Heart J 104:1086, 1982.
107. Casey TP, Miyasaki P, Kylarsdam A, et al.: Holter monitoring of pacemaker patients. Cardiology Jan 1988, pp. 47–52.

108. Rosen KM, Loeb HS, Sinna MZ, et al.: Cardiac conduction with symptomatic sinus node disease. Circulation 43:836, 1971.
109. Narula OS: Atrioventricular conduction disturbance in patients with sinus bradycardia. Circulation 44:1096, 1971.
110. El Gamel, Van Gelder LM: Long term advantages of atrial versus ventricular pacing with V-A conduction. PACE 4:A43, 1981.
111. Cohen SI, Frank HA: Preservation of acute atrial transport: An important clinical consideration in cardiac pacing. Chest 81:51, 1982.
112. Samet P, Castillo, Bernstein WH: Hemodynamic sequellae of atrial, ventricular and sequential atrioventricular pacing in cardiac patients. Am Heart J 2:725, 1966.
113. Barold SS, Falkoff MD, Ong LS, et al.: Electrocardiographic diagnosis of pacemaker malfunction. *In* Wellens HJJ, Kulbertus HE (eds.): What's New in Electrocardiography?, p. 236. The Hague, Martinus Nijhoff, 1981.
114. Barold SS, Falkoff MD, Ong LS, et al.: Electrocardiographic analysis of normal and abnormal pacemaker function. *In* Dreifus LS (ed.): Pacemaker Therapy, p. 127. Philadelphia, FA Davis Co., 1983.

34

Electrocardiography of Dual-Chamber Pacemakers

Richard M. Luceri
Agustin Castellanos

For more than a decade, dual-chamber pacemakers have played an increasingly important role in cardiac pacing. The ability to consistently and chronically pace the atrium, as well as to sense its intrinsic activity, has been the key to the success of dual-chamber pacemaking. In addition to advances in lead technology, miniaturization of internal circuitry and the use of microprocessors within the pulse generator have enabled the introduction of advanced pacemaker functions previously unavailable for general use. The internal pacemaker clock, a marvel of modern engineering, is able to track multiple events occurring within milliseconds in both chambers.

This transition toward pacemaker sophistication, however, has imposed additional burdens on the clinical electrocardiographer. Traditionally, the interpretation of a pacemaker electrocardiogram (ECG) required relatively few skills, provided that a minimum amount of information was known regarding a specific pulse generator. With the multiplication of features, including complex timing cycles and so forth, the task of electrocardiographic interpretation has become increasingly difficult.[1-4] Although computer-assisted interpretational aids (including channel markers and ECG telemetry) will continue to proliferate, most clinicians and other potential "interpreters" of pacemaker electrocardiography will continue to use simple and easily available aids such as calipers and rulers. In this chapter, the basics of dual-chamber electrocardiography will be presented in a "generic" manner such that the interpreter of ECG recordings will have a foundation based on common performance characteristics of these pacemakers. However, this can in no manner replace the necessary manuals and feature charts of individual manufacturers' products.

Classification of Dual-Chamber Pacemakers

DVI PACEMAKERS

Dual-chamber pacemakers have been available in one form or another for many years. Several types of dual-chamber units were utilized more than others, depending on their performance, ease of insertion, and programmability. Additionally, the era of dual-chamber pacemakers reached its first peak with the advent of the so-called AV sequential pulse generators (DVI), which provided pacing in both chambers, with sensing only in the ventricle. The success of these pulse generators was largely due to the long-sought stability and quality of the atrial electrode. Additionally, many of these pulse generators were of the unipolar type and were therefore relatively easy to implant, to the extent that both leads could even be inserted into the same subclavian vein site.

From an electrocardiographic point of view, DVI pacemakers provided both clinicians and industry with the first large experience with dual-chamber pacemakers, and set the stage for progression to the more widely used DDD units.[5]

Electrocardiography of DVI Pacemakers

The timing cycles, and thus the electrocardiographic findings, of DVI pacemakers can be summarized as follows.[6]

LOW RATE LIMIT ■ The low rate limit is that predetermined by programming. The low rate in this case is the escape rate of the pacemaker, which results in the emission of an atrial stimulus.

AV Delay ■ This is the interval between the atrial stimulus artifact and the delivery of the ventricular stimulus. It may be programmable or fixed, depending on the type of DVI pacemaker. In either case, the atrium is never sensed and the timing cycle begins with either a ventricular paced or sensed event. Since atrial sensing does not occur, there is no atrial refractory period to consider.

VA Interval ■ This is the period that encompasses both the ventricular refractory and ventricular alert periods. In the absence of ventricular sensed events during this period, the pacemaker responds with the emission of an atrial output. If, however, a native ventricular event is sensed prior to timing out of the VA interval, the pacemaker recycles and emits no output stimuli.

Committed DVI Pacemakers

This variety of DVI pacemaker is the unipolar version that gained widespread utilization a decade ago. The ventricular sensing function is temporarily inhibited during the AV delay (after the atrial stimulus), thus resulting in the mandatory release of a ventricular stimulus. On the ECG the only options one may observe with normal function is the appearance of either two output stimuli (A and V) or none. The committed DVI pacemaker has a fixed, nonprogrammable AV delay, so that inopportune ventricular output stimuli are theoretically not released into the vulnerable period after ventricular depolarization. However, it has been demonstrated that committed ventricular stimulation may result in repetitive ventricular response and, in one reported case, in ventricular fibrillation.[7] The fact is, any time one interrupts ventricular sensing there is the possibility of triggering repetitive ventricular responses (see Ventricular Blanking).

Noncommitted DVI Pacemakers

These pulse generators are usually of the bipolar type and permit ventricular sensing to occur during the AV delay. Thus the ventricular stimulus may be inhibited if a native QRS is sensed during this period. From an electrocardiographic perspective, the possibilities are therefore several: one may observe one stimulus (always atrial), two stimuli, or none in the presence of normal function.

Summary

In both types of DVI pacemakers, atrial competition is possible and may result in the onset of atrial fibrillation or flutter if the stimulus falls within the vulnerable period of the atrial cycle.[8] Thus arrhythmias observed with DVI pacemakers may be initiated by the pulse generator but never participate in the propagation of the arrhythmia, as is commonly observed in the dual-sensing DDD pacemakers.

DDI PACEMAKERS

The DDI mode of pacing, which was developed more or less as an offshoot of DDD pacemakers, provided a needed addition to the function of the DVI pacemaker; that is, atrial sensing capability. In DDI pacemakers, the atrium is sensed but does not "drive" the ventricle (absence of rate response), since the upper rate limit is equal to the lower, or programmed, rate. Sensing in the atrial channel may inhibit atrial output stimuli but does not reset the AV delay.[9] Thus there is no rate response, and only one ventricular rate is possible. The major advantage of the DDI mode of pacing is that it theoretically prevents competitive atrial pacing. As the native atrial rate increases, AV synchrony is diminished but atrial competition is less likely to occur.

VDD PACEMAKERS

The VDD mode is considered a dual-chamber mode in that ventricular pacing occurs in response to sensed atrial activity.[10] The pulse generator is inhibited by spontaneous ventricular activity. Its back-up low rate function results solely in ventricular pacing. The characteristics of VDD pacemakers are similar to many of those observed with DDD pacemakers. The AV delay is initiated by a sensed atrial event. Ventricular output is dictated by the absence of a native QRS complex. The next VA interval begins; this ends with a sensed atrial complex or with a spontaneous ventricular event. In the VDD mode, there is a distinct difference between the low rate limit and the upper rate limit. For low rate ventricular pacing to occur, there is no sensed atrial activity and therefore no initiation of an AV delay. On the other hand, the upper rate limit represents the maximal ventricular pacing rate in response to sensed atrial activity. The upper rate limit is the result of separate programmed parameters, depending on the model of pacemaker chosen. The specific details of the upper rate limit in dual-chamber pacemakers are discussed later in this chapter.

DDD PACEMAKERS

The DDD pacemaker incorporates virtually all of the preceding features of VDD pacemakers, with one major addition: the ability to pace atrially as well as to sense. From an electrocardiographic point of view, the DDD most closely approximates normal cardiac function, provided there is adequate atrial rate response (chronotropic competence). The DDD pacemaker has revolutionized cardiac pacing by its enormous adaptability and programmability.

The choice of the optimal DDD pacemaker mode will result in maximal hemodynamic benefit (Fig. 34–1) and further reduce the potential for pacemaker-related complications.[11,12]

In essence, this type of pacemaker operates in the following four different modes automatically, while maintaining AV synchrony throughout.

Dual-Chamber (Low Rate) AV Sequential Mode

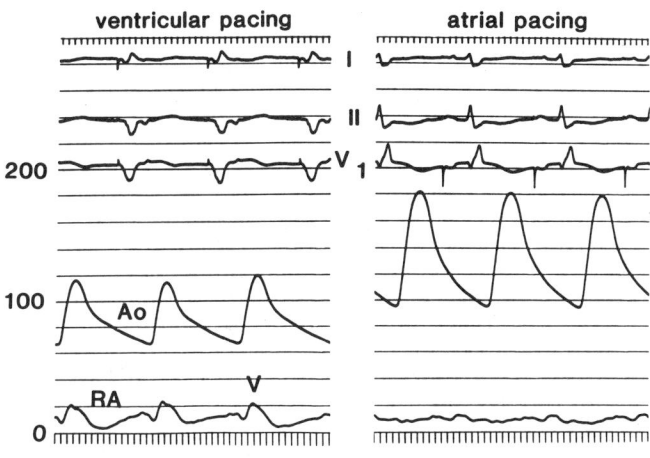

FIGURE 34–1
Hemodynamic comparison of atrial and ventricular pacing. Leads I, II, and V₁ of a surface ECG are shown. Aortic (Ao) and right atrial (RA) pressure tracings appear with the calibration scale in mm Hg. Note the drop in aortic pressure with ventricular pacing and the regurgitant "V" wave due to retrograde conduction to the atrium. Improved hemodynamics occur when atrial pacing is initiated with intact AV conduction.

- Both chambers are paced in the absence of spontaneous atrial or ventricular activity; this is usually associated with antegrade conduction block. The rate is the programmed low rate limit, and the AV delay is programmed as well.

ATRIAL PACING MODE ■ In this case there is atrial bradycardia with generally intact AV conduction, which results in straight atrial pacing with inhibition of ventricular output. There is no added benefit of rate modulation, although AV synchrony is preserved. The newer, rate-modulated systems incorporating sensor technology will allow other parameters to "drive" the pacemakers when there is definite chronotropic incompetence.

ATRIAL TRACKING MODE ■ This is the most beneficial aspect of the DDD system and provides rate modulation between the programmed low rate limit and upper rate limit. In this mode, the spontaneous sinus rate determines the degree of ventricular pacing by "tracking," or following atrial activity, through a wide rate range. Each sensed P wave triggers an AV delay, at the end of which the ventricle is paced if no intrinsic ventricular activity has been sensed.

INHIBITED MODE ■ The DDD pacemaker can be totally quiescent in the presence of an atrial rate above the low rate limit along with appropriate conduction to the ventricles. The inhibition of both atrial and ventricular channels is therefore dependent on several programmed settings, such as the low rate limit (governing either atrial or ventricular activity) and the AV delay. Programming of the latter will control whether intrinsic AV conduction is allowed to occur. This particular subject has generated considerable interest in the past several years and will be addressed separately in this text.

DDDR PACEMAKERS

The newest types of dual-chamber pacemakers that are currently undergoing clinical trials in the United States have succeeded in combining the characteristics of traditional DDD (or other dual-chamber mode) pacemakers with a separate rate modulator. This modulator may be an activity sensor, temperature sensor, or one of many other types that "drive" the pacemaker in addition to the intrinsic atrial rhythm. These combination pacemakers will require sophisticated knowledge of the operational characteristics of both the DDD parameters and the sensor. The ECG tracings will undoubtedly be more difficult to interpret, since at any given point in time dual-chamber pacing may be initiated by the sensor rather than by the intrinsic atrial rate. Thus considerable overlap will occur between these two drive mechanisms. Accurate ECG interpretation will be somewhat dependent on built-in telemetric systems, which will be required to provide the observer with key data regarding specific device functions.

Dual-Chamber Pacemaker Timing Cycles

In order to fully appreciate the electrocardiography of dual-chamber pacemakers, a basic understanding of the timing cycles is necessary. Timing cycles regulate pacemaker function as it applies to the interaction between natural cardiac activity and artificial pacing.[13]

LOWER RATE LIMIT ■ The lower rate limit is the longest allowable interval between two atrial or ventricular events.

UPPER RATE LIMIT ■ This is the maximum pacing rate, which reflects the shortest pacing interval between a sensed or paced ventricular complex.

AV DELAY ■ The AV delay timing cycle is comparable to the natural P-R interval. It represents the interval between an atrial sensed or paced event, and the ensuing ventricular paced or sensed event. Therefore, the AV delay may consist of (1) a sensed P wave–paced QRS pair, (2) a paced atrial stimulus-sensed QRS pair, or (3) two paced stimuli (A and V). The AV delay is programmable (by most dual-chamber pacemakers with the exception of the committed DVI generators); some newer models incorporate AV interval hysteresis, which provides variable AV delays in the presence of sensed versus paced atrial events.

ATRIAL REFRACTORY PERIOD ■ The atrial refractory period is the interval occurring after a sensed or paced atrial event, during which time atrial sensing does not occur; it consists of the AV delay and the postventricular atrial refractory period.

VENTRICULAR REFRACTORY PERIOD ■ This is the interval occurring after a sensed or paced ventricular event, during which time ventricular sensing does not occur.

BLANKING PERIOD ■ This is a brief period of electronic refractoriness imposed on one channel immediately following a stimulus in order to prevent sensing of that stimulus by the other channel. Practically speaking, the blanking period in DDD pacemakers begins with the atrial stimulus and ends shortly thereafter. In some models, this is a programmable feature, lasting on the average of 15 to 25 ms.

UPPER RATE LIMIT AND ITS VARIATIONS

In general, two principles govern the calculation of the upper rate limit.[14, 15]

The *period of total atrial refractoriness* is calculated as the sum of the AV delay plus the postventricular atrial refractory period (PVARP). This total (in milliseconds) represents the duration of mechanical (programmable) refractoriness imparted to the pacemaker system at that particular moment. An example of such a calculation would be the following: an AV delay of 150 ms is programmed with a postventricular atrial refractory period of 300 ms. Thus the total (AV + PVARP) is equal to 450 ms (133 bpm). In some pacemakers this period of total atrial refractoriness is equal to the upper rate limit. Therefore, an atrial sensed event would fall either in or out of this period of refractoriness, allowing no other choice to occur. This is in direct contrast to the second type of upper rate behavior described below.

Many other dual-chamber pacemaker models have the capability to independently program the upper rate limit to a level that is lower (in bpm) than the sum of AV + PVARP. The difference between these two figures is represented by the pseudo-Wenckebach interval, which imposes a temporary prolongation of the AV delay to account for the difference between the two. Thus, the AV delay may become artificially prolonged to account for the difference in time between total refractoriness (AV + PVARP) and the independently programmed upper rate limit. In either case, the upper rate limit cannot be exceeded under normal conditions and, therefore, controls the maximal pacing rate of the system.

A unique method of managing the upper rate limit is that described as the *fallback* response. In this case, when the atrial intrinsic rate exceeds the upper rate limit, atrial tracking is stopped and the pacemaker switches to QRS-inhibited ventricular pacing at a slope that is predetermined. When the atrial rate falls once again below the upper rate limit, atrial tracking resumes.

Arrhythmias of Dual-Chamber Pacemakers

The arrhythmias associated with dual-chamber pacemakers can be conveniently divided into two major categories: (1) those initiated by a pacemaker stimulus but not requiring further participation of the pulse generator and (2) those induced and sustained by pacemaker participation. In this chapter we will focus primarily on the latter type of pacemaker-associated arrhythmia, since it has direct implications for, and is part and parcel of, dual-chamber pacemaker electrocardiography.[16, 17]

ENDLESS LOOP OR PACEMAKER-MEDIATED TACHYCARDIA

The addition of atrial sensing to modern pacemakers has provided the potential for creating an artificial bypass track or accessory pathway that may become operative in the presence of retrograde or ventriculoatrial (VA) conduction. Classically, a ventricular complex (paced or spontaneous) triggers retrograde atrial activation (retrograde limb of the circuit); this is sensed by the atrial electrode, initiating an AV delay. A ventricular stimulus (antegrade limb of the circuit) follows and the process repeats itself (Fig. 34–2). This artificial arrhythmia has been called an "endless loop" tachycardia, referring to a computer program that repeats itself ad infinitum.[18] The basic requirements for pacemaker-mediated tachycardia are not unlike those for the natural reentry phenomenon. They require an antegrade and retrograde limb and a retrograde (VA) conduction time that exceeds the PVARP of the dual-chamber pacemaker. The pacemaker-mediated tachycardia may also be triggered by a premature ventricular extrasystole with VA conduction (Fig. 34–3); by electromechanical interference, whereby noise or myopotentials are inadvertently interpreted as an atrial event by the pacemaker; and by intermittently dissociated P waves, resulting in temporary undersensing. Atrial premature complexes may also result in abnormally prolonged AV delays, thus favoring the occurrence of VA conduction during the subsequent cycle. The electrophysiologic characteristics and hemodynamic consequences of VA conduction have been known for years and once more have played a role in current pacemaker technology.[19, 20]

During a pacemaker-mediated tachycardia, it is assumed that retrograde activation is required to reach the atrium in order to mediate the tachycardia. Spontaneous tachycardia termination usually results from "fatigue" (block) of the retrograde limb. However, the tachycardia may remain incessant so long as retrograde conduction is operative, and in the absence of any termination algorithm intrinsic to the particular pacemaker model.

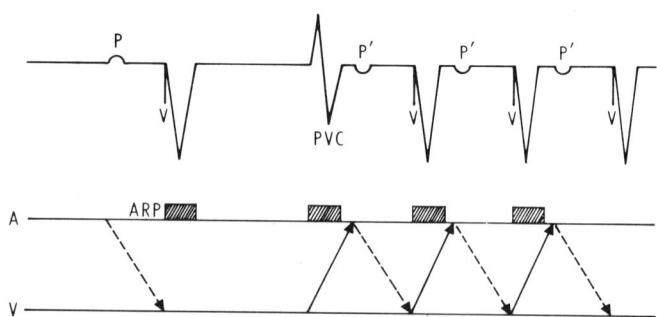

FIGURE 34–2
Schematic diagram of the mechanism of pacemaker-mediated tachycardia initiated by a ventricular extrasystole (PVC). A retrograde P wave (P') falls outside the atrial refractory period of the pacemaker (ARP), is sensed by the ventricular channel, and initiates a pacemaker tachycardia. The retrograde limb is assured by the continuing retrograde conduction following each ventricular paced beat. A = atria, V = ventricles.

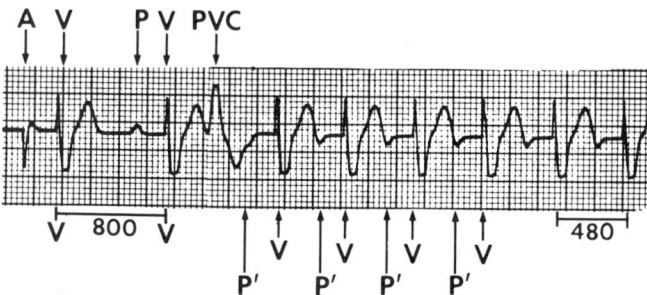

FIGURE 34-3
Actual tracing from a patient in whom a ventricular extrasystole initiates pacemaker-mediated tachycardia. A = atrial stimulus; P = native P wave; V = ventricular stimulus; P' = retrograde P wave. The tachycardia cycle length is 480 ms.

The prevention of pacemaker-mediated tachycardia is generally accomplished by setting the PVARP to extend beyond the VA conduction time, thus rendering the retrograde P wave refractory (to the pacemaker), eliciting no response from the pulse generator (Fig. 34-4).

The maximum tachycardia rate of a pacemaker-mediated tachycardia generally equals the sum of the retrograde VA conduction time and the antegrade AV delay. This is controlled by the programmable upper rate function of the pacemaker and mediated through the AV delay or the atrial refractory period.

WENCKEBACH AND OTHER UPPER RATE RESPONSES

As previously mentioned, the mode of upper rate response will dictate the type of "arrhythmia" one will observe electrocardiographically. Thus, in the pseudo-Wenckebach type of upper rate response, there is progressive prolongation of the AV delay until a sensed atrial event occurs within the atrial refractory period and results in a "dropped" beat. In the AV block type of upper rate response, the atrial event is either sensed or not. If it is the result of atrial (or sinus) tachycardia, the P wave occurring in the atrial refractory period of the pacemaker will not be sensed; therefore, it will not generate an AV delay and the cycle will be "dropped" (Fig. 34-5).

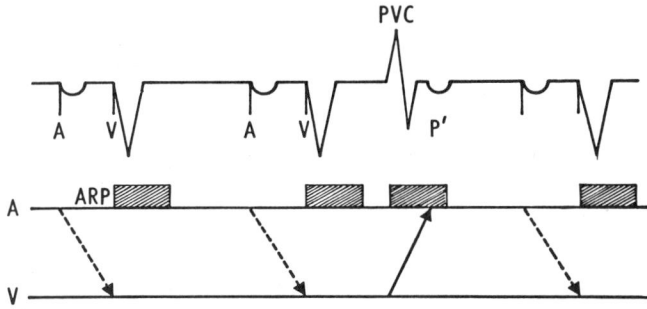

FIGURE 34-4
Diagram representing the usual means of protecting against pacemaker-mediated tachycardia by prolonging the atrial refractory period of the pacemaker (ARP) so that retrograde P waves (P') fall within the ARP and are not sensed by the pulse generator. A = atria, V = ventricles.

Electrocardiographic Correlates of Dual-Chamber Pacing

AV DELAY PROGRAMMING

Optimal AV delay programming will depend on a variety of situations, both clinical (cardiac output, atrial size, etc.) and electrical (status of AV conduction). In the example shown in Figure 34-6, a common situation relating to the AV delay is depicted. In Figure 34-6A, the AV delay of the pacemaker is programmed to 200 ms. After appropriate P wave sensing, the ventricular output occurs but does not "capture" the ventricle, which already has generated a relatively normal QRS complex in the presence of intact AV conduction. This phenomenon is known as *pseudofusion*.[21] It may be avoided by increasing the programmed AV delay to extend beyond this period of natural AV conduction, as shown in Figure 34-6B. In this example, by setting the AV delay at 240 ms, the unnecessary ventricular output stimulus is eliminated, enabling the measurement of the true PR interval, in this case 220 ms. Battery energy is conserved, in addition to the avoidance of ventricular pseudofusion.

ATRIAL UNDERSENSING

One of the most frequently observed electrocardiographic phenomena in DDD pacing is atrial undersensing. Figure 34-7 illustrates intermittent atrial undersensing and its potential consequences. This pacemaker is programmed to the DDD mode, with AV delay of 220 ms and atrial sensitivity of 4.0 mV. The first three P waves appear to be appropriately sensed and generate a normal AV delay, followed by a ventricular output stimulus for each cycle. The fourth P wave, although similar in morphology to the first three, fails to be sensed and is followed by an atrial output stimulus that occurs at the programmed low rate minus the AV delay (otherwise described as the VA interval).

Two potentially deleterious consequences may arise from atrial undersensing. First, the inappropriate atrial stimulus that follows the non-sensed P wave may occur during a period of *atrial* vulnerability and therefore may trigger the onset of atrial repetitive response in the form of atrial flutter or atrial fibrillation. This has been well documented in the DVI mode, which continuously ignores (as part of normal function) atrial activity, thus promoting competition between the natural P waves and the atrial stimuli. Second, the resultant AV delay in the cycle when the P wave is not sensed is abnormally prolonged. This finding is similar to the pseudo-Wenckebach type of upper rate limit. In this case, the marked prolongation of the AV delay allows for recovery of the His bundle. Following the ventricular output, retrograde conduction to the atrium is thus enhanced (P') and may result in the onset of a pacemaker-mediated tachycardia if the retrograde P wave falls outside the PVARP and is appropriately sensed. Although occasional atrial undersensing is probably clinically inconsequential, the initiation of a

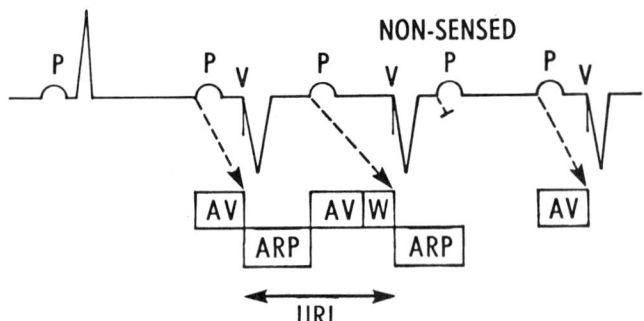

FIGURE 34–5
Schematic of the pseudo-Wenckebach type of upper rate response. The pacing rate is governed by the upper rate limit (URL). The third P wave initiates an AV delay, but ventricular pacing is delayed for a period of time (W) so that the URL may time out. The next P wave falls within the atrial refractory period of the pacemaker (ARP), is not sensed, and therefore is not followed by a ventricular stimulus. The last P wave represents the start of another cycle. See text for further details.

FIGURE 34–6
AV delay programming. As shown in A, a pseudofusion beat occurs if the ventricular stimulus occurs slightly after the normal QRS complex (AV delay = 200 ms). This can be avoided, as shown in B, by programming the AV delay beyond the duration of normal AV conduction (AV delay = 240 ms; PR interval = 220 ms). See text for details.

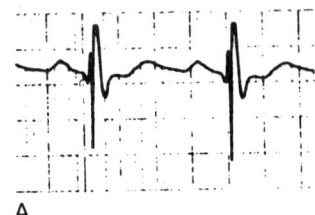
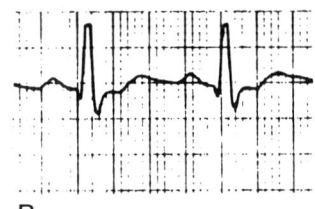

A   B

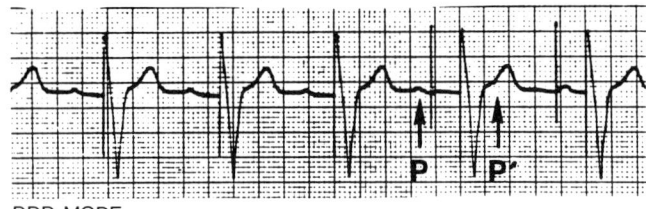

DDD MODE

FIGURE 34–7
Atrial undersensing: the P wave (P, arrow) not sensed is followed by an atrial stimulus. The AV delay is prolonged to such an extent that the AV node–His axis has recovered and is capable of conducting retrograde to the atrium (P', arrow) following the ventricular stimulus. This may commonly cause a pacemaker-mediated tachycardia. AV delay = 220 ms; atrial sensitivity = 4.0 mV.

FIGURE 34–8
Atrial channel oversensing of myopotentials. A, the pacemaker (DDD mode) is triggered by myopotentials to pace at the upper rate limit (URL) of 150 bpm. (AV delay = 150 ms; atrial sensitivity = 0.5 mV). In B, the native underlying rhythm is depicted and shows complete heart block without retrograde conduction. The treatment of oversensing of this nature is to decrease the sensitivity in the atrial channel (P rate = 90 bpm; V rate = 50 bpm).

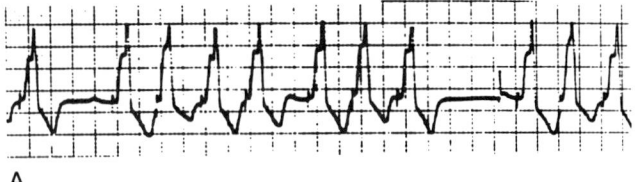

A

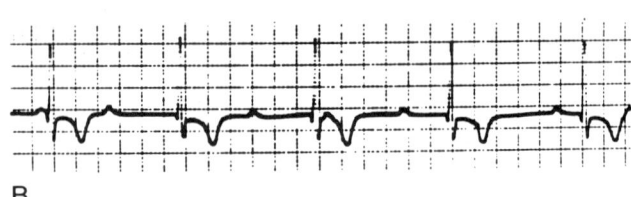

B

pacemaker-mediated tachycardia may not be as well tolerated. The management of this type of problem would be to increase the sensitivity in the atrial channel.

ATRIAL OVERSENSING

Since P waves have generally lower amplitudes than normal QRS complexes, situations may often occur in which the ideal setting for P wave sensing may be too sensitive to exclude extraneous noise or muscle potentials from triggering the tracking state of a DDD pacemaker.[22] An example of this is shown in Figure 34–8. This patient is a 17-year-old male with a history of symptomatic congenital heart block. He was implanted with a DDD pacemaker of the unipolar type, after having undergone electrophysiologic testing. Throughout the testing period, he was incapable of conducting any beats retrograde to the atrium. Figure 34–8B reveals his underlying rhythm.

He was observed to have the tracing in Figure 34–8A during exercise. In this tracing, a P wave, which is appropriately tracked, is followed by a series of five additional ventricularly paced complexes that are not preceded by clearly discernible P waves. Upon closer scrutiny, slight variation can be detected in some of the paced intervals. Most, however, are occurring at the upper rate limit of 150 bpm.

In this case, the atrial channel was programmed to a very high sensitivity (0.5 mV). Since this is a unipolar pacemaker, the sensing "antenna" encompasses the distal pole in the heart and the proximal pole in the pacemaker can. Muscle artifact during exercise was generated in the pectoral area, the site of the pacemaker implant. These muscle potentials reached sufficient amplitude to be sensed by a highly sensitive atrial channel. They "tricked" the pacemaker into tracking them, their frequency resulting in upper rate tracking at 150 bpm. The solution to this problem requires reprogramming to a less sensitive setting. The fact that this patient was known to be incapable of retrograde conduction gave little support to the theory that retrogradely sensed P waves triggered an endless loop tachycardia.

ATRIAL NON-CAPTURE

Atrial capture in DDD pacing is often difficult to verify on standard ECG tracings. This is most commonly encountered in bipolar systems but is prevalent in unipolar systems as well. In the example shown in Figure 34–9, the first two atrial paced complexes do not appear to result in any visible depolarization. On the contrary, retrograde P waves are easily identified. The retrograde P wave following the third ventricular complex falls outside the period of atrial refractoriness (PVARP), is sensed by the pacemaker, and generates an AV delay followed by a ventricular stimulus. This occurs exactly at the upper rate limit of 150 bpm. Although in this case a pacemaker-mediated tachycardia was not initiated, the substrate was present. The appropriate maneuver in this case would be to increase atrial output and verify adequate lead placement.

ATRIAL UNDERSENSING

P waves commonly may be undersensed in normally functioning DDD pacemaker systems. Although the exact mechanisms of P wave undersensing in an otherwise "tuned" system are unknown, it is speculated that small changes in P wave amplitude and morphology occur with a relatively high frequency. These variations may in fact be pseudo-variations—that is they may represent waveform changes due to respiration, movement, and so forth. This problem is certainly less encountered in the ventricle, where the margins between sensing threshold and R wave amplitudes are often superior.

In Figure 34–10, atrial undersensing is occurring for no discernible reason. Full programming of this pacemaker revealed no specific abnormalities, and all the operational characteristics were otherwise normal. This is a Holter monitor tracing, and this phenomenon was observed to occur at least ten times in a 24-hour period.

MYOPOTENTIAL INHIBITION

The interpretation of myopotentials for biological signals is a well-known phenomenon in pacemakers. This is most commonly observed with unipolar systems, in which the pacemaker can represents one pole of the dipole, and the electrode tip the other. This large "antenna" effect is such that pectoral muscle potentials generated near the site of the pacemaker can achieve amplitudes greater than the biological signals, rendering this pattern of interference in the sensing system.[23] Ventricular inhibition is the most serious consequence in VVI systems. In DDD systems, P-wave tracking is commonly observed, as demonstrated in Figure 34–8. However, rarely inhibition occurs in both channels; an example is shown in Figure 34–11. This is a unipolar DDD pacemaker system with very limited programming capability (one of the older DDD models). Frequent inhibition by myopotentials of both chambers necessitated the explantation of this unit and its replacement with a more versatile DDD system.

VENTRICULAR BLANKING

All dual-chamber pacemakers require a brief period of ventricular refractoriness immediately following an atrial output stimulus. The purpose of this is to avoid a phenomenon known as *cross-talk* inhibition, which can be defined as the inhibition of pacemaker output in the opposite chamber of the origin of the stimulus artifact.[24] Otherwise stated, this is an example of cross-sensing (that is, sensing at a distance). The blanking periods are generally brief (12 to 40 ms) and in some DDD pacemaker models are programmable. Figure 34–12 demonstrates one potential effect of even this short period of refractoriness to ventricular sensing. A PVC occurs during the blanking period (arrows) and is therefore, by definition, not sensed by the ventricular

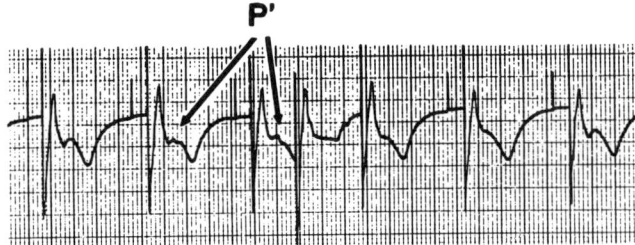

FIGURE 34-9
Atrial non-capture; intermittent sensing. There is no atrial capture on this tracing. Fortuitous retrograde P waves (P′) are a clue to the non-capture of the atrial stimulus. Atrial refractory period = 240 ms; upper rate limit = 150 bpm.

FIGURE 34-10
Atrial undersensing. In this tracing (DDD mode pacemaker), the P wave (arrow) is not sensed although it has the same morphology and timing as the other P waves on the tracing. Low rate = 55 bpm; AV delay = 200 ms; atrial refractory period = 240 ms. See text for details.

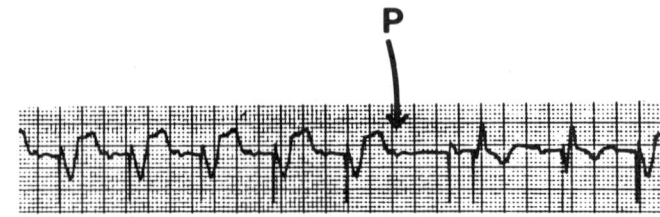

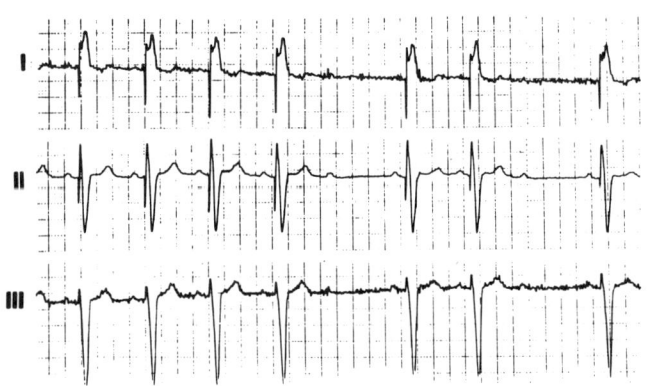

FIGURE 34-11
Myopotential inhibition. An example of myopotential inhibition in both channels of a unipolar DDD pacing system. AV delay = 150 ms; ventricular sensitivity = 3.5 mV; atrial sensitivity = 2.0 mV. See text for details.

FIGURE 34-12
Ventricular blanking period. Note the occurrence of a ventricular extrasystole (PVC) that occurs exactly during the ventricular blanking period (39–47 ms). It is by definition not sensed and therefore is followed by a normal ventricular stimulus after an appropriate AV delay (200 ms). This may initiate ventricular arrhythmias if the ventricular stimulus occurs during a period of ventricular vulnerability.

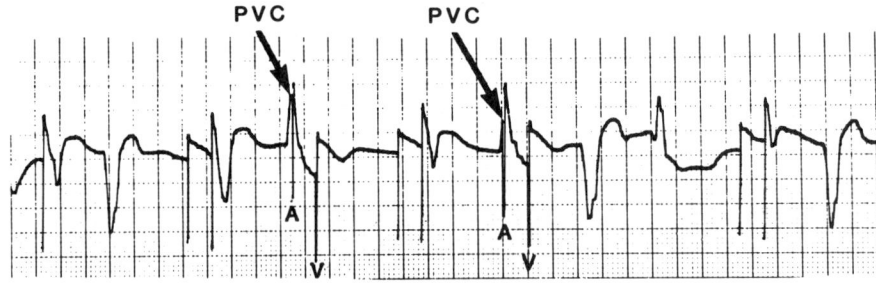

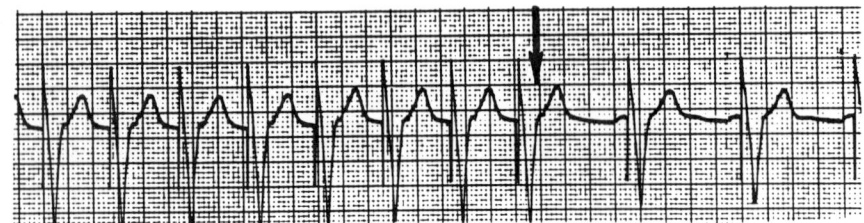

FIGURE 34-13
Termination of DDD pacemaker–mediated tachycardia. Magnet application (arrow) immediately terminates a pacemaker-mediated tachycardia by inhibiting sensing and initiating a DOO type response. Upper rate limit = 110 bpm; atrial refractory period = 150 ms; VA conduction time = 220 ms; AV delay = 125 ms.

channel. The ensuing ventricular output stimulus occurs at the end of the QRS complex and has the potential for triggering ventricular arrhythmias in certain clinical conditions.

TERMINATION OF PACEMAKER-MEDIATED TACHYCARDIA

In many cases, as previously mentioned, pacemaker-mediated tachycardias will continue ad infinitum unless either there is fatigue in the retrograde circuit or a maneuver or termination algorithm[25] is initiated. One simple, effective procedure for terminating a pacemaker-mediated tachycardia is to apply a magnet directly over the pulse generator. Since the magnetic mode inhibits sensing, the pacemaker will revert to a DOO mode (for DDD pacemakers) or VOO mode (for VDD pacemakers). In Figure 34–13, magnet application (arrow) immediately interrupts the pacemaker-mediated tachycardia.

Conclusions

The complexities of dual-chamber cardiac pacemaker electrocardiography are directly related to the type and model of the individual pacemaker. In most cases, a generic approach to the analysis of dual-chamber tracings is often adequate for trouble-shooting even the most complex situations. However, since there is no real uniformity among the various models, each pacemaker will have its own intricacies (often referred to as eccentricities), which can only be known to the observer astute enough to read the particular manufacturer's manual.

With the advent of dual-chamber rate-responsive pacemakers, the ECG interpretations will again require knowledge not only of the standard operating characteristics but also of the sensor algorithms for the specific model (its rate of response, range, limits, etc.). It is assumed that the observer will be aided in this task by advanced telemetric features, capable of "labeling" the tracings by interpreting the pulse generator's functions.

References

1. Hauser RG: The electrocardiography of AV universal DDD pacemakers. PACE 6:399, 1983.
2. Barold SS, Ong LS, Falkoff MD, et al.: Programmable pacemakers: Clinical indications, complications and future directions. *In* Barold SS, Mugica J (eds.): The Third Decade of Cardiac Pacing, pp. 27–77. Mt. Kisco, Futura Publishing Co., 1982.
3. Furman S, Hayes DL, Holmes DR: A Practice of Cardiac Pacing, pp. 159–217. Mt. Kisco, Futura Publishing Co., 1986.
4. Luceri RM, Hayes DL: Follow-up of DDD pacemakers. PACE 7:1187, 1984.
5. Levine PA, Mace RC: Pacing Therapy: A Guide to Cardiac Pacing for Optimum Hemodynamic Benefit, pp. 105–129. Mt. Kisco, Futura Publishing Co., 1983.
6. Barold SS, Falkoff MD, Ong LS, et al.: Interpretation of electrograms produced by a new unipolar multiprogrammable "committed" AV sequential (DVI) pulse generator. PACE 4:692, 1981.
7. Luceri RM, Ramirez AV, Castellanos A, et al.: Ventricular tachycardia produced by a normally functioning A-V sequential demand (DVI) pacemaker with "committed" ventricular stimulation. J Am Coll Cardiol 1:93, 1983.
8. Furman S, Cooper JA: Atrial fibrillation during A-V sequential pacing. PACE 5:133, 1982.
9. Furman S, Hayes DL, Holmes DR: A Practice of Cardiac Pacing, p. 238. Mt. Kisco, Futura Publishing Co., 1986.
10. Kruse IB, Ryden L, Duffin E: Clinical evaluation of atrial synchronous ventricular inhibited pacemakers. PACE 3:641, 1980.
11. Hauser RG: Techniques for improving cardiac performance with implantable devices. PACE 7:1234, 1984.
12. Levine PA, Mace RC: Pacing therapy: A Guide to Cardiac Pacing for Optimum Hemodynamic Benefit, pp. 3–19. Mt. Kisco, Futura Publishing Co., 1983.
13. Furman S, Hayes DL, Holmes DR: A Practice of Cardiac Pacing, pp. 159–219. Mt. Kisco, Futura Publishing Co., 1986.
14. Furman S: Dual chamber pacemakers: Upper rate behavior. PACE 8:197, 1985.
15. Luceri RM, Parker M, Thurer RJ: Particularities of management and follow-up of patients with DDD pacemakers. Clin Prog Pacing Electrophysiol 2:261–271, 1984.
16. Luceri RM, Castellanos A, Zaman L, et al.: The arrhythmias of dual chamber cardiac pacemakers and their management. Ann Intern Med 99:354, 1983.
17. Castellanos A, Lemberg L: Pacemaker arrhythmias and electrocardiographic recognition of pacemakers. Circulation 42:1381, 1973.
18. Furman S, Fisher JD: Endless-loop tachycardia in an A-V universal (DDD) pacemaker. PACE 5:486, 1982.
19. Perrins EJ, Sutton R: Arrhythmias in pacing. Med Clin North Am 68(5):1111, 1984.
20. Sutton R, Perrins EJ, Duffin E: Interpretation of dual chamber pacemaker electrocardiograms. PACE 8:6, 1985.
21. Barold SS: Fusion, pseudofusion and confusion beats. *In* Impulse, pp. 1–6. St. Paul, Minn., Cardiac Pacemakers Inc., 1977.
22. Levine PA, Pirzada FA: Pacemaker oversensing: A possible example of concealed ventricular extrasystoles. PACE 4:199, 1981.
23. Berger R, Jacobs W: Myopotential inhibition of demand pacemakers: Etiologic, diagnostic and therapeutic considerations. PACE 2:596, 1979.
24. Batey RL, Calabria DA, Shewmaker S, et al.: Cross-talk and blanking periods in a dual chamber (DDD) pacemaker: A case report. Clin Prog Pacing Electrophysiol 3:314, 1985.
25. Papp MA, Mason T, Gallastegui J: Use of rate smoothing to treat pacemaker-mediated tachycardias and symptoms due to upper rate response of a DDD pacemaker. Clin Prog Pacing Electrophysiol 2:547, 1984.

35

Interference in Cardiac Pacemakers: Exogenous Sources

S. Serge Barold
Michael D. Falkoff
Ling S. Ong
Robert A. Heinle

Overview

Despite the long list of potential sources of interference, reports of clinical events from oversensing extracorporeal signals outside the hospital setting are now rare and limited to a relatively small number of environmental situations.[1-4] In contrast, endogenous myopotential interference of unipolar pulse generators has defied a definitive solution and still remains an important clinical problem. Over the past 20 years, developments in circuit design have rendered pulse generators relatively immune to domestic and industrial electromagnetic interference.[5-12] Indeed, review of the literature indicates that most cases of interference involved earlier generations of pulse generators without metal encapsulation or sophisticated sensing and rejection circuitry.[13-25] The effect of irradiation from microwave ovens on implanted pacing systems has generated much interest and concern.[26-28] Although pacemaker manufacturers still warn physicians and patients of potential oversensing, clinically significant cases are exceedingly rare with modern pulse generators in the environment of a normally functioning microwave oven. In 1982 Sowton emphasized that the interference problem with pacemakers should be put into its proper perspective and suggested that "it is impractical to advise patients to avoid all of them [sources of interference] even if it were possible to identify them in advance. The patient should be told in general terms about the possibility of interference, but assured that the risks are extraordinarily low."[3]

Interference may enter the pacing system either directly through the pulse generator or indirectly through the electrode, which acts as an aerial or antenna. Ultra high-frequency devices (megahertz range) may bypass the high-frequency noise protection system by taking erratic pathways. Unipolar pacing systems are far more susceptible to interference than bipolar systems, simply because the amplitude of extraneous signals sensed by a pulse generator depends on the geometry (i.e., separation) of the sensing electrodes.[8,29-31] Filtering and processing of a sensed signal by a pulse generator provide an important but not uniformly successful way for discriminating the intracardiac electrogram from extraneous voltages. In this respect, Sowton stated that "all pacemaker manufacturers have designed their product with input filters that reject unwanted frequencies, but it is clearly impossible to reject interference signals that have the same characteristics as a signal from the heart."[3] As most interference signals cover a wide range of frequencies, the input filter of a pacemaker will allow the passage of frequencies normally received from the heart. However, it is usually possible for the pacemaker to recognize these unwanted signals as interference by the *repetition rate*.[4, 8, 10, 32, 33] For this reason, pulse generators contain a specific noise detection circuit that continuously monitors the electrode system for the presence of noise signals generally defined as repetitive signals occurring at a certain rate. When signals are received above a predetermined rate, the pacemaker identifies them as being due to interference and not from the heart. Instead of being inhibited, the pacemaker will then revert to the asynchronous or interference rate. Reversion to the asynchronous mode presents little risk when it occurs for brief periods, although competitive pacing may be hazardous in those situations in which the ventricular fibrillation threshold is markedly decreased, such as in acute myocardial infarction or severe electrolyte imbalance.

PACEMAKER REFRACTORY PERIOD ■ The pacemaker refractory period (RP) was in the past defined as the interval when the pulse generator is insensitive to any incoming signals and cannot respond in any way.[34] With the advent of sophisticated pulse generators with complex circuitry, the definition of the RP has changed, and it is now known as the period during which the basic lower rate timer cannot be reset or restarted. Therefore, a pulse generator may actually recognize signals during part of the RP often called the noise-sampling period, but these detected signals are used only to reset timing intervals other than the inviolable lower rate interval.[35-39]

Pacemaker Response to Interference

Understanding the mechanisms involved in interference protection is important because they may also come into play under certain circumstances in the absence of actual extracorporeal interference. The noise-sampling (or noise-interrogation) period (NSP) may be considered as a relative refractory period (usually in the terminal part of the RP) with design, function, and duration varying from manufacturer to manufacturer. There are at least three types of responses when a signal is sensed within the NSP.

1. The sensed signal may reset the entire RP (retriggerable RP). Conceptually this design is similar to that of the automatic antitachycardia "dual demand" mode of pacing, with overlapping RPs and activation of the pulse generator to pace during both bradycardia and tachycardia (Fig. 35–1*A* and *B*).[40, 41] Reversion to the asynchronous mode occurs when the interval between sensed events becomes shorter than the programmed refractory period. For example, with an RP of 300 ms in the VVI mode, a sensed rate of 200 pulses per minute (ppm) or faster would cause reversion to asynchronous pacing.
2. The sensed signal resets only the NSP rather than the entire RP. Repetitive retriggering of the NSP eventually leads to asynchronous pacing.[9, 10, 33]
3. The sensed signal may cause reversion to asynchronous pacing for one full cycle (i.e., the RP is extended for the duration of one pacing cycle).[42]

EXTENSION OF THE COMPLETE REFRACTORY PERIOD

The behavior of the Medtronic DDD pulse generators may be taken as an example of this particular response (Fig. 35–2).[39, 43, 44] The ventricular RP of the Medtronic Symbios DDD pulse generator (7005 and 7006) lasts for 225 ms (235 ms for Models 7000 and 7000A) from the onset of a ventricular event defined as a paced ventricular stimulus or a sensed QRS complex (i.e., preceded by a sensed P wave) (Fig. 35–3). The ventricular RP of each model under these circumstances is composed of an initial 125 ms absolute RP (also called the ventricular blanking period by Medtronic, Inc.) followed by the NSP constituting the terminal part of the ventricular RP. This terminology is potentially misleading, because this particular blanking period may be confused with the brief ventricular blanking period that occurs coincidentally with the atrial stimulus designed to prevent cross-talk. When the Symbios DDD pulse generator senses a ventricular extrasystole (defined by the pacemaker as two successive ventricular events without any sensed intervening atrial activity), the NSP is automatically lengthened to 220 ms, giving a total ventricular RP of 345 ms (340 ms for Models 7000 and 7000A).

A signal detected during the NSP of a Symbios pulse generator is represented by a telemetered marker pulse indicating a ventricular "sense refractory" (SR) event. Although such a signal does not reset the lower rate timer, it will reset (restart) other intervals in the Symbios pulse generator as follows:

1. A new 345 ms ventricular RP, with the first 125 ms, consisting of the absolute refractory (blanking) period because the signal is interpreted by the pulse generator as a sensed ventricular extrasystole, or ventricular premature contraction (VPC).
2. A new postventricular atrial refractory period (PVARP) together with its automatic extension. The latter occurs because the pulse generator interprets the sensed signal as a VPC, thereby automatically lengthening the duration of the PVARP to 400 ms (to prevent sensing of retrograde P waves). When the extension comes into play, the total duration of the PVARP is always increased automatically to 400 ms, and this is not programmable.
3. A new upper rate limit interval. By design, the upper rate limit circuit governs only the rate of atrial triggered ventricular pacing.

All these considerations have important implications. When a ventricular signal is detected during the NSP, it retriggers another complete ventricular RP. If this occurs continually, the pulse generator will eventually time out at the lower rate interval and will appear to be pacing asynchronously. This RP design (also called retriggerable) is particularly effective in preventing inhibition of the pacing output by the electromagnetic or skeletal muscle interference (Fig.

FIGURE 35–1
A, Effect of atrial premature beats in a patient with an implanted Siemens 668B bipolar VVI pulse generator with a retriggerable ventricular refractory period. The ventricular refractory period was programmed to 437 ms so that the pulse generator could be used on a dual-demand basis for the treatment of supraventricular tachycardia that was easily terminated by a single premature ventricular paced beat. Thus, at a heart rate of 133/min or faster (cycle length≤437 ms), asynchronous ventricular pacing occurs at the programmed lower rate (70 pulses per minute (ppm)). (a): Beat 2 is unsensed because it falls within the pacemaker refractory period generated by beat 1. (b): Beat 2 also falls in the refractory period generated by beat 1. Beat 2 does not reset the lower rate timer of the pulse generator; rather, it reinitiates a complete ventricular refractory period of 437 ms, so that beat 3 is also unsensed. A pacemaker stimulus (solid circle) terminates the escape interval started by sensing beat 1 (outside the refractory period) so that pacing is asynchronous for one cycle. (c): The 1-2-3 sequence is identical to that in (b). In these sequences, if beat 2 had not retriggered another complete refractory period (437 ms), beat 3 would have been sensed and able to initiate a new escape interval. Solid black circles indicate pacemaker stimuli.

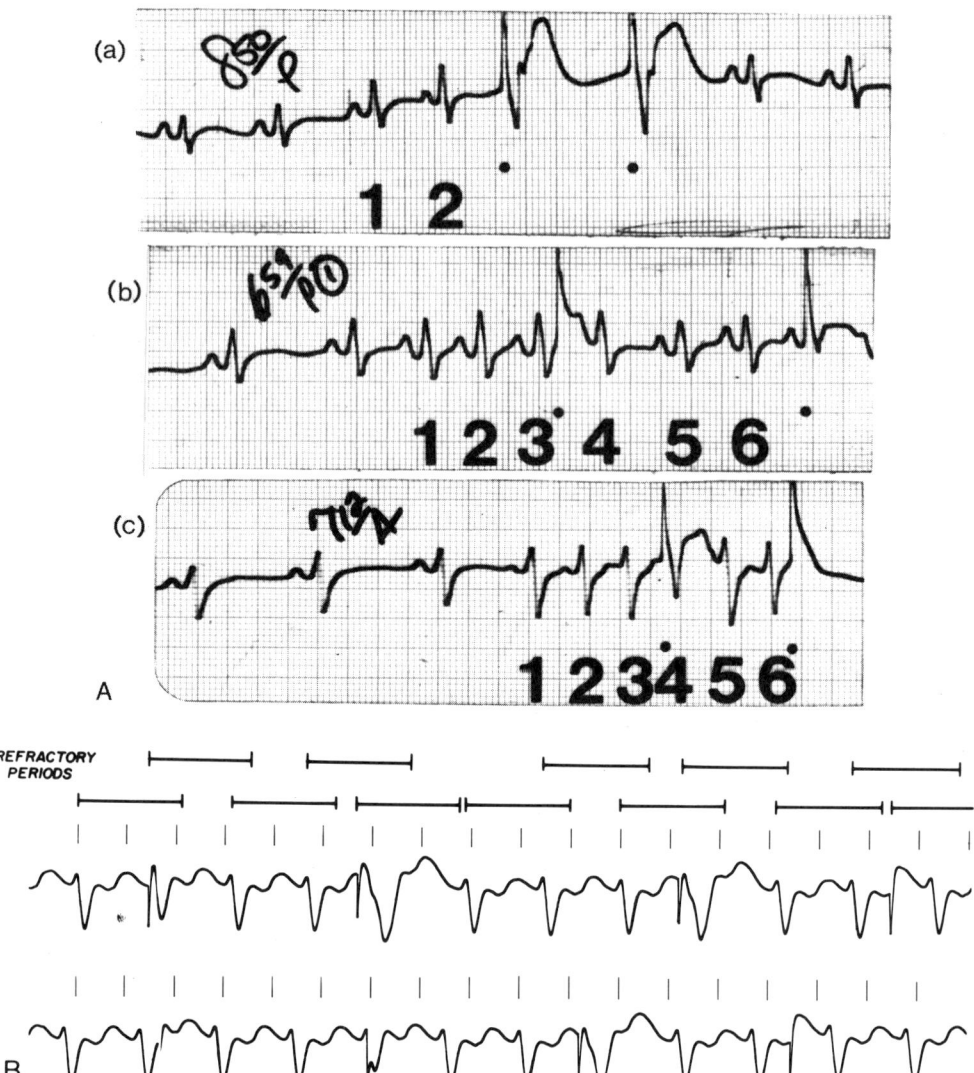

B, Same patient as in A. Dual-demand function of Siemens 668 pacemaker with the capability of retriggering the entire pacemaker refractory period. The horizontal bars represent the duration of the refractory period (437 ms). The first spontaneous QRS complex occurs within the relative refractory period (noise-sampling period occupying the last 312 ms of the refractory period) of the pulse generator and therefore does not reset the lower rate timer, and the next pacemaker stimulus occurs as expected, causing what appears to be a pseudofusion beat. The second QRS complex also initiates a new pacemaker refractory period. The overlap of these retriggered refractory periods causes the pulse generator to revert to its asynchronous mode. Slight fluctuations of the spontaneous rate may alter these interlocking time relationships, allowing a QRS to be sensed just beyond the relative refractory period of the pulse generator (sixth QRS top portion). The second pacemaker stimulus captures the ventricle (fifth QRS on top) and resets the supraventricular tachycardia (SVT) so that the succeeding spontaneous QRS complex falls outside the pacemaker refractory period and resets both the lower rate and refractory period timers (sixth QRS on top). In contrast, all the other QRS complexes or pacemaker stimuli reset the refractory period timer only. The SVT was terminated by right ventricular pacing about 15 seconds (not shown) after this recording was obtained. The horizontal bars over the ECG show how each refractory period would have terminated if it had not been reinitiated by a subsequent pacing stimulus or QRS complex in the relative refractory (noise sampling) period.

(Reprinted by permission from Barold SS, et al.: *In* Feruglio GA (ed.): Cardiac Pacing. Electrophysiology and Pacemaker Technology, pp. 285–288. Padova, Italy, Piccin Medical Books, 1982.)

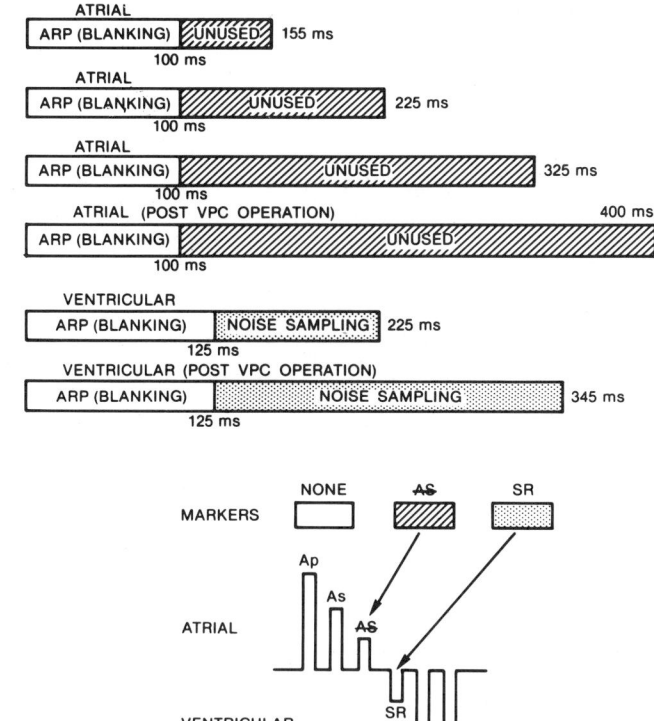

FIGURE 35–2
Diagrammatic representation of the atrial and ventricular refractory periods of the Medtronic Symbios (7005, 7006) DDD pulse generator. The blanking period refers to the absolute refractory period of the pacemaker and not to the ventricular blanking period that occurs coincidentally with the atrial stimulus for the prevention of crosstalk. Sensing can occur in the noise-sampling period of the ventricular channel, and such a sensed event is sometimes labeled as SR or VR. The lower portion depicts the corresponding telemetered markers. Ap = atrial paced beat; As = atrial sensed beat, A̶s̶ = unused sensed atrial event; Vp = ventricular paced beat; Vs = ventricular sensed event; SR = ventricular sensed event in the ventricular refractory (noise-sampling) period; VPC = ventricular extrasystole. See text for details.

(Reprinted by permission of Futura Publishing Co., Inc., from Barold SS, et al.: In Barold SS, Mugica J (eds.): New Perspectives in Cardiac Pacing, pp. 69–119. Mt. Kisco, NY, Futura Publishing Co., 1988.)

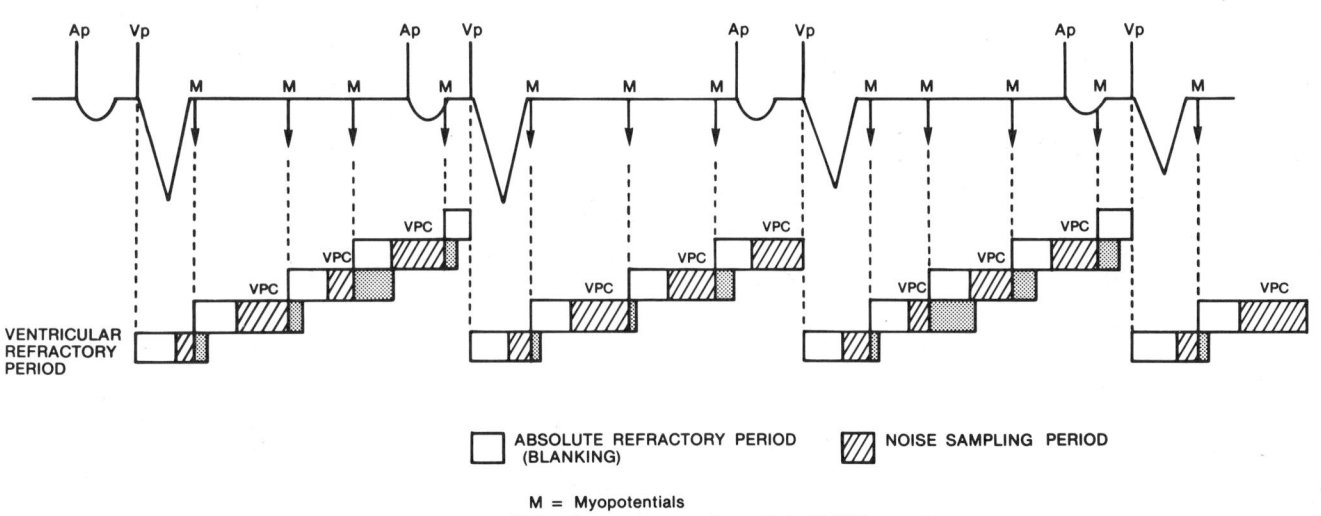

FIGURE 35–3
Diagrammatic representation of the response of a Medtronic Symbios 7005 unipolar DDD pulse generator to myopotential (M) oversensing by the ventricular channel.

When M signals are sensed by the ventricular channel in the noise-sampling period (i.e., beyond the absolute refractory period), a new and complete ventricular refractory period is restarted. The noise-sampling period (and therefore the ventricular refractory period) is automatically extended when the pulse generator detects two ventricular events without an intervening P wave (i.e., the so-called ventricular extrasystolic (VPC) extension, as shown in Figure 35–2. Continual overlap of pacemaker refractory periods forces the pulse generator to pace asynchronously (DOO mode) at the programmed lower rate (i.e., interference or noise reversion rate). The stippled sections indicate how the pacemaker refractory period would have terminated had sensing not occurred in the noise-sampling period. Ap = atrial paced beat; Vp = ventricular paced beat.

(Reprinted by permission of Futura Publishing Co., Inc., from Barold SS, et al.: In Barold SS, Mugica J (eds.): New Perspectives in Cardiac Pacing, pp. 69–119. Mt. Kisco, NY, Futura Publishing Co., 1988.)

35–4 and 35–5). A relatively long NSP permits continuous resetting of the ventricular RP in the presence of rapidly recurring signals, resulting in asynchronous DOO pacing (interference mode). The same response can also be initiated by intrinsic cardiac activity if the cycle length is short enough to allow sensing within the NSP. This may be seen during ventricular tachycardia with a cycle length less than 345 ms[45] or during atrial fibrillation with a rapid ventricular rate and numerous RR intervals shorter than 345 ms (Fig. 35–6).[46] During atrial fibrillation, asynchronous pacing may be intermittent depending on interplay between the constantly varying R-R intervals and the timing intervals of the pulse generator.[43] Therefore in the case of the Medtronic DDD pulse generators, undersensing due to a signal detected in the NSP should not be attributed to a low electrographic signal or misinterpreted as pulse generator malfunction.

Atrial Refractory Period

The Siemens 674 DDD pulse generator possesses an NSP in both the atrial and ventricular channels capable of retriggering the entire refractory periods.[38, 47] With regard to the atrial channel of the 674 DDD pulse generator, a sensed event in the atrial NSP is actually used to restart another entire PVARP (Fig. 35–7). Because this particular pacemaker has a separately programmable upper rate interval and total atrial refractory period, it will exhibit a Wenckebach upper rate response when the upper rate interval is longer than the total atrial RP, provided the P-P interval is longer than the total atrial RP. When the P-P interval becomes shorter than the total atrial RP, the pulse generator will revert to asynchronous atrial pacing at the programmed lower rate.[43] Thus, in the case of this generator, the overlapping RPs cause the atrial channel to revert to its asynchronous mode, so that the pulse generator functions in the DVI mode (and can never develop so-called fixed ratio block) whenever the P-P interval is less than the total atrial RP.[43] This response is similar to the behavior of the ventricular RP of the Medtronic Symbios DDD pulse generator when presented with repetitive ventricular signals within the NSP.

PARTIAL EXTENSION OF REFRACTORY PERIOD

In the case of the Pacesetter AFP DDD pulse generator,[35] the NSP occupies the terminal 100 ms of the RP in the atrial and ventricular channels. A sensed signal within the ventricular NSP resets it for another 100 ms. At the end of the new NSP, the pulse generator can sense again and inhibit the next ventricular output. When signals are continually sensed, the pulse generator continues to overlap the NSPs on one another until it reaches its maximum number of extensions and reverts to asynchronous (DOO) pacing. With the Pacesetter AFP DDD pulse generator, when noise is continually sensed only by the atrial channel, according to the circumstances and amplitude of the noise signals, the atrial tracked signals may induce ventricular pacing at or near the upper rate, or the atrial channel may function asynchronously (in the DVI mode) when the amplitude of the sensed signals exceeds the sensing threshold by about 25% (Fig. 35–8). Simultaneous detection of noise in both channels leads to DOO pacing. In other pulse generators, such as the Intermedics Cosmos, the detection of noise by either the atrial or ventricular channel causes DOO pacing at the programmed lower rate (Fig. 35–9).

EXTENSION OF THE REFRACTORY PERIOD FOR A FULL PACING CYCLE

In the case of the Cordis DDD pulse generator, a sensed signal including the QRS complex or a P wave in the NSP causes the pulse generator to be refractory for the entire cycle, so that it functions in the DOO mode for one cycle (Figs. 35–10 and 35–11).[42, 48, 49]

Automatic Conversion of Pacing Mode

Automatic conversion to another mode of pacing or pacemaker reset may be defined as the automatic conversion of a pulse generator from the programmed mode (e.g., DDD) to another preset mode (usually VVI or VOO).[50–53] The phenomenon of resetting to another pacing mode involving another chamber is presently unique to DDD pulse generators. Single-chamber rate-responsive pacemakers (AAIR or VVIR) such as the Medtronic Activitrax may also be reset under certain circumstances from the VVIR mode to the VVI (non–rate-responsive) mode.[54]

The end-of-service (EOS) point of a DDD pulse generator is triggered by a fall in the battery voltage to a predetermined point. In many DDD pulse generators, the EOS point causes automatic conversion to a relatively simpler, less demanding mode such as the VVI or VOO mode. The reset mode should be considered as a protective mechanism designed to conserve energy and allow basic functions to continue for some time. In the simple VVI (VOO) mode, the reduced battery current drain increases available battery voltage, resulting in conservation of energy. The pulse generator may continue to function in the VVI (VOO) mode for approximately 6 months after the EOS point has been reached. In this way, the circuit voltage is prevented from falling too rapidly to the end-of-life (EOL) point, when the pacemaker can no longer function reliably even in the VVI or VOO mode. The EOL point should not be confused with the EOS indicator. In the latter, the pulse generator functions normally, but in the reset VVI or VOO mode. As a rule, a change in the magnet rate occurs before the reset or EOS point.

A DDD pulse generator may reset to the EOS indicator (or the backup mode in other pulse generators) when exposed to fields of high-strength electromagnetic interference (EMI). Exposure to powerful

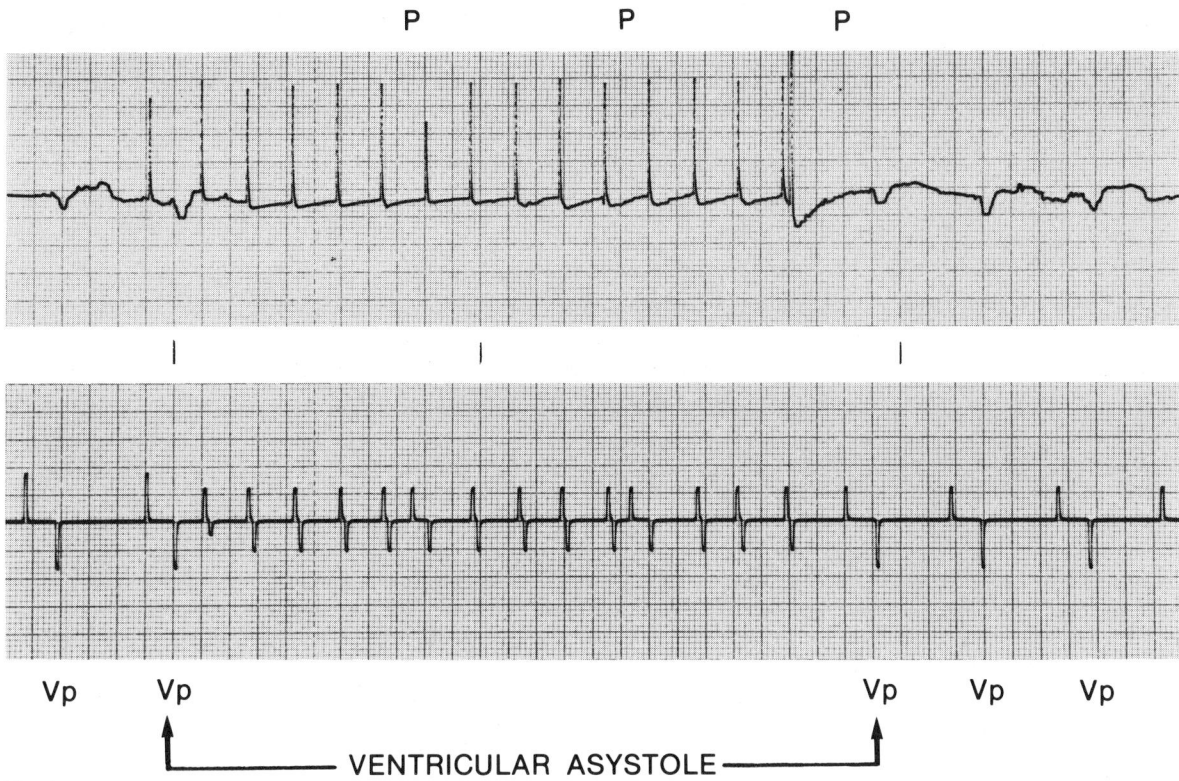

FIGURE 35-4
Response of a Medtronic Symbios 7006 bipolar DDD pulse generator to chest wall stimulation (CWS) delivered at a rate of about 190/min (cycle length = 320 ms). Programmed parameters: lower rate = 70 ppm; AV interval = 200 ms; upper rate = 125 ppm; postventricular atrial refractory period = 155 ms. P = P wave sensed by the atrial channel; Vp = ventricular paced beat.
Real-time markers were recorded simultaneously with the ECG. The pulse generator senses CWS simultaneously in both channels. There is a long period of ventricular asystole due to the relatively long interval between sensed ventricular events causing pacemaker inhibition. When the rate of CWS was increased (see Fig. 35-5), the shorter intervals between sensed ventricular events produced asynchronous DOO pacing (interference or noise reversion rate). The external pulse generator delivering CWS emitted an additional stimulus when it was turned off (preceding the third sensed P wave), but this stimulus falls in the ventricular refractory period initiated by the preceding sensed CWS. The amplitude and direction of markers identify events in the atrial and ventricular channels, as shown in Figure 35-2. Note that the atrial channel does not identify any unused atrial events (i.e., AS).

EMI causes a transient dip in battery voltage as seen by the logic circuitry. The drop in battery voltage triggers the EOS indicator by activating a special switch in the pacemaker circuitry. Once the switch is thrown, regardless of the cause, the pacemaker will remain in its EOS or backup mode until a programming command returns it to the DDD mode. In the case of DDD pulse generators with programmable polarity, the reset mode is always unipolar. In some pulse generators, such as the Intermedics Cosmos DDD unit, a two-stage system responds to a transient drop in voltage by first triggering the EOS mode, and subsequently, with more drop in voltage, the backup mode becomes activated. In the reset VVI mode, some pulse generators may not respond to application of the magnet by conversion to asynchronous pacing, as in the CPI Delta in the reset mode[55] and the Intermedics Cosmos in the backup mode.[36] This should not be misinterpreted as a "no output" situation or component failure.

The use of electrocautery during surgery is probably the most common cause of reset in DDD pulse generators.[50-52, 56] Defibrillation may also reset a DDD pulse generator.[52, 57] Each DDD pulse generator has a characteristic EOS indicator (or backup mode) and reprogramming sequence to reestablish normal function. In the pulse generators of one manufacturer, electrocautery may erase the serial and model number. This "loss of identity" may be corrected by a programming command only from a special programmer not generally available but supplied by the manufacturer on request.[50] Resetting as such does not represent malfunction because the pulse generator itself is not damaged. However, it should be remembered that both electrocautery and defibrillation may occasionally cause permanent damage to a pulse generator if the procedure is not performed according to suggested guidelines.

The importance of the reset phenomenon resides in its ability to avoid the misdiagnosis of pacemaker malfunction or EOS state resulting in inappropriate pacemaker removal. All patients with DDD pulse generators demonstrating EOS characteristics (or backup mode) should therefore be considered reset from a cause other than battery depletion until proved otherwise. Reprogramming to the desired parameters should always be attempted before considering pulse generator replacement. The significance of the EOS

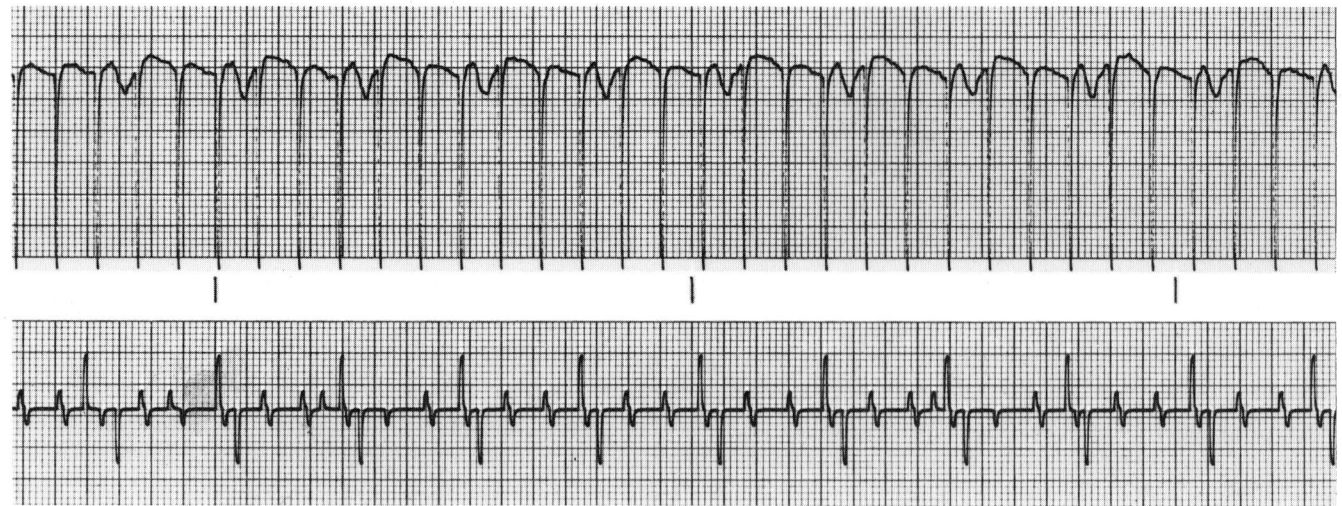

FIGURE 35–5
ECG from the same patient as in Figure 35–4, showing the response of a Medtronic Symbios 7006 bipolar DDD pulse generator (same programmed parameters as in Figure 35–4, except for a postventricular atrial refractory period of 225 ms) to chest wall stimulation (CWS) faster than in Figure 35–4 at a rate of approximately 230/min. (cycle length = 260 ms).

The first AV interval measures 200 ms because the ventricular channel senses CWS beyond the ventricular safety pacing period of 110 ms. This signal is sensed in the noise-sampling period of the ventricular channel (VR) engendered by the previous ventricular signal, itself also sensed within the noise-sampling period. Sensing during the noise-sampling period does not reset the lower rate timer, so that the ventricular stimulus is issued on time at the completion of the AV interval. All other AV intervals are abbreviated because VR events occur during the ventricular safety pacing period, thereby triggering an early release of a ventricular stimulus at the completion of the ventricular safety pacing period. The ventricular channel senses CWS only in its noise-sampling period (as indicated by the small downward deflections in the marker channel, i.e., VR; see Fig. 35–2).

CWS is mostly sensed simultaneously by both channels, but at times stimuli are unsensed by the atrial channel. CWS sensed by the atrial channel occurs in the noise-sampling period and is therefore unused (i.e., events cannot cause ventricular triggering or reset any timing cycles). The repetitive occurrence of VR events causes the asynchronous noise or interference DOO mode of pacing. If no P wave occurs following a paced or sensed ventricular event, the pulse generator interprets the next ventricular sensed event as a ventricular extrasystole with consequent automatic prolongation of the ventricular refractory period. This extension also contributes to the noise reversion mechanism, because a long noise-sampling period favors continuous resetting and overlap of the ventricular refractory periods.

point should be evaluated by first reprogramming the pulse generator to the DDD mode. An attempt to provoke the EOS point should then be made by reprogramming the output to maximum as well as increasing the pacing rate. In the absence of telemetered battery voltage, this battery "stress test" gives an idea of battery reserve and optimum time for pulse generator replacement.[53] In other words, it allows postponement of elective replacement. Thus at the EOS point, the pulse generator reprogrammed to a lower output and rate will require less current drain and may continue to function in the new programmed condition for hours, days, or weeks until such time that the battery voltage again drops below the EOS. If the power cell is indeed depleted (i.e., battery voltage permanently below the EOS point), a reprogramming command may only be able to return the pacemaker to normal operating conditions momentarily. Once the circuitry detects a low battery voltage, it will revert on the very next cycle to the EOS (reset) mode. With a battery voltage indicator, one can easily differentiate between the EOS indicator activated by a true and permanent fall in battery voltage from one activated by EMI, thereby avoiding more frequent follow-up or worse, the early unnecessary replacement of the device. In the presence of significant fall in battery voltage due to depletion of the battery, telemetry (if available) shows a marked increase in battery impedance corroborating the presence of a depleted lithium-iodine battery. Depletion increases the internal resistance and lowers the available battery voltage secondarily.

Electrocautery

Electrocautery is the best known and commonest form of interference in the hospital environment.[58–64] Intraoperative pacemaker complications due to interference produced by electrocautery were first reported in the late 1960s.[19, 62, 64, 65] Twenty-five years later, despite the remarkable technologic progress in cardiac pacing, the problem has become even more important because of different circuit designs.[66–69] Pacemaker malfunction during transurethral prostatectomy has received the most attention in the literature. However, electrocautery during any operation is a potential hazard to the pacemaker patient. Electrocautery uses radio frequency current to sever tissue and achieve hemostasis. A high frequency is used to reduce the possibility of muscle and nerve stimulation. The coagulation and cutting circuits of electrocautery systems may affect pacemakers differently. With bipolar coagulation cautery, the current flow is localized across the two poles of the instrument and so far has caused no problems

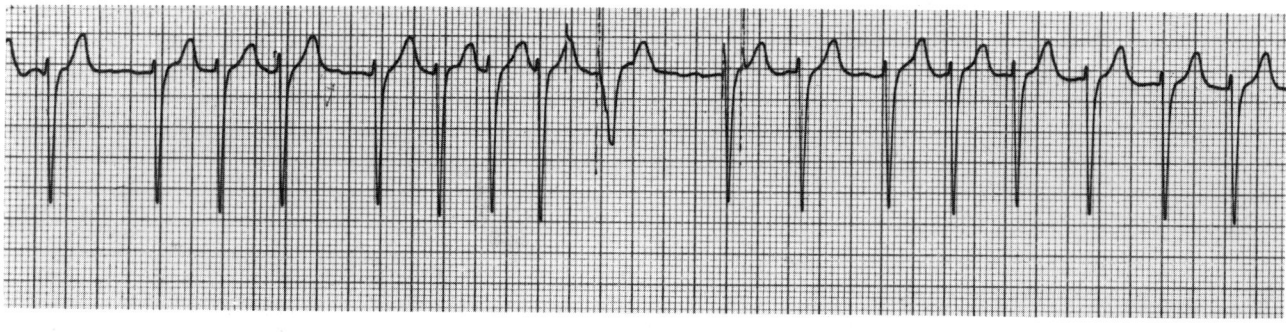
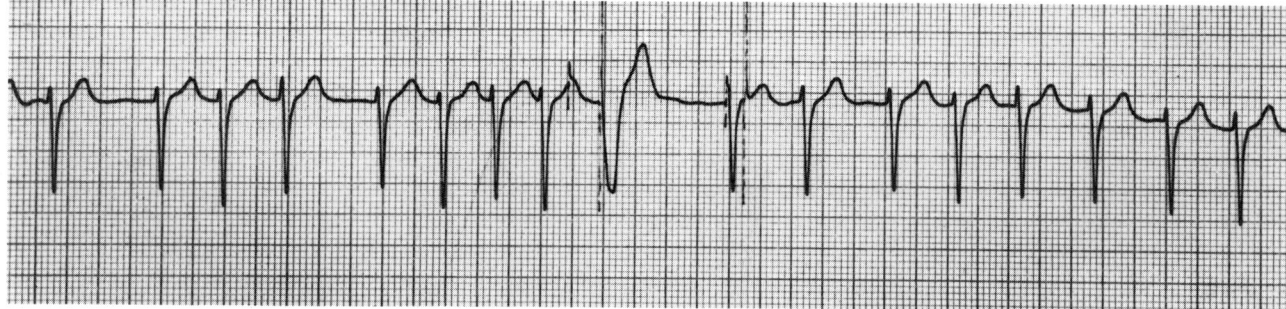

FIGURE 35–6
Atrial fibrillation in a patient with a Medtronic 7000 DDD pulse generator. Programmed parameters: lower rate = 60 ppm (1000 ms); upper rate = 125 ppm (480 ms); AV interval = 250 ms.

The beat labeled 1 is sensed by the ventricular channel and initiates an atrial escape (pacemaker VA) interval of 750 ms. The pulse generator interprets this QRS as a ventricular extrasystole (VPC) because the atrial fibrillatory waves are unsensed by the atrial channel. The ventricular refractory period initiated by sensing QRS labeled 1 therefore lengthens to 340 ms (from 235 ms, because of VPC extension). The QRS complex labeled 2 therefore falls within the noise-sampling period of the extended refractory period generated by the preceding QRS complex (No. 1). The pulse generator also interprets QRS No. 2 as a VPC. Thus, QRS No. 3 is also unsensed because it falls within the extended ventricular refractory (noise-sampling) period generated by QRS No. 2. The overlapping refractory periods therefore cause asynchronous DOO pacing at the lower rate interval (i.e., noise or interference response). The QRS complex that follows the ventricular paced beat falls within the ventricular safety pacing period with resultant abbreviation of the AV interval to 110 ms. Two ECG leads were recorded simultaneously.

(Reprinted by permission of Futura Publishing Co., Inc., from Barold SS, et al.: In Barold SS, Mugica J (eds.): New Perspectives in Cardiac Pacing, pp. 69–119. Mt. Kisco, NY, Futura Publishing Co., 1988.)

with pacemakers. However, bipolar electrosurgery is valuable only for small areas of coagulation, but not for cutting. During unipolar electrocautery (used for cutting), the electric current is not restricted to the tissue interposed between the two electrodes, but spreads out and penetrates the entire body of the patient. Obviously this stray current may be interpreted by an implanted pulse generator as a signal originating in the heart.

Myocardial electrical burns (where none was intended) due to concentration of current at the myocardial-electrode interface may occur when there is conductivity between the pacing electrode and the indifferent (return) electrode of the electrocautery instrument.[51, 70] A pacing electrode with a small surface area may be associated with a high current density and a higher incidence of burns. Furthermore, protective circuitry shunting energy away from the pacemaker may also contribute to the development of burns at the electrode-myocardial interface.

Geddes et al.[70] have shown that, by disconnecting the indifferent electrode from the electrocautery circuit, the pacing electrode becomes the active electrode in the cautery circuit and may create burns and fatal ventricular fibrillation[19, 51, 64, 70–74] because of energy delivered directly into the heart via a low-resistance electrode. Indeed, electrocautery has been reported to cause ventricular fibrillation even in the absence of a pacing electrode.[74] Theoretically in patients with atrial or dual-chamber pulse generators, atrial fibrillation could also be induced by energy transmitted to the atrium via an atrial lead.[75] Electrical and thermal burns at the electrode-myocardial interface may lead to chronic elevation of pacing thresholds, as recorded by Shepard and colleagues,[76] who observed an increased incidence of exit block developing in pacing systems exposed to electrocautery. There are as yet no reported cases of an acute increase in the pacing threshold leading to loss of capture.

Electrocautery, by generating high-strength electromagnetic fields, may occasionally cause random component failure[75] or damage the pulse generator irreversibly with permanent loss of output.[77, 78] Application of the magnet does not prevent current pickup by the electrode and does not protect against ventricular fibrillation. There may be some disturbance of pace-

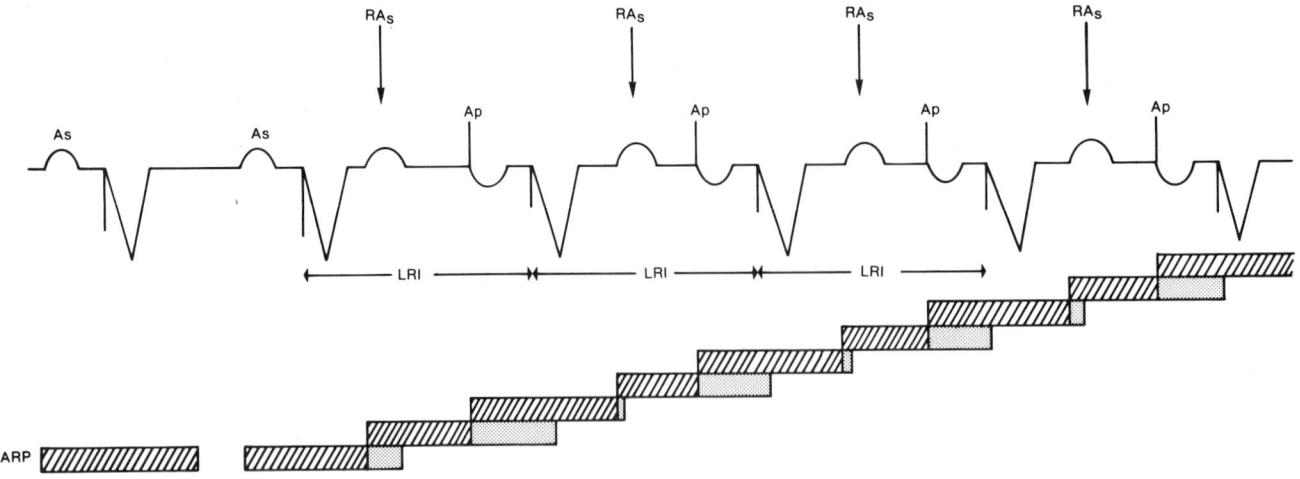

FIGURE 35–7
Diagrammatic representation of the retriggerable atrial refractory period (ARP) of the Siemens 674 DDD pulse generator. As=atrial sensed event outside ARP; RAs=atrial sensed event within the ARP; Ap=atrial paced event; LRI=lower rate interval.

The first 125 ms of the postventricular atrial refractory period (PVARP) consists of the absolute refractory period during which signals cannot be sensed. The second part of the PVARP (and AV interval) consists of the noise-sampling period. P waves falling within the noise-sampling period are sensed by the atrial channel, but they cannot initiate a new AV interval; instead they retrigger a new and complete ARP. Continual retriggering of the ARP causes the pulse generator to operate asynchronously in the atrial channel at the noise reversion rate (equal to the lower rate) so that the pulse generator now functions in the DVI mode if no ventricular signals are sensed. A P wave can initiate an AV interval only when sensed outside the noise sampling period. The stippled bars indicate how the ARP would have terminated had sensing or an atrial stimulus not occurred in the noise-sampling period. This behavior precludes the pulse generator from responding to a fast atrial rate by the development of fixed ratio block (e.g., 2:1, 3:1, etc.).

(Reprinted by permission of Futura Publishing Co., Inc., from Barold SS, et al.: In Barold SS, Mugica J (eds.): New Perspectives in Cardiac Pacing, pp. 121–172. Mt. Kisco, NY, Futura Publishing Co., 1988.)

maker programming, and the new programmed parameters may be unpredictable.[79, 80] There may also be alteration in the random access memory (RAM) as reported with the early generation of Pacesetter AFP DDD pulse generators.[50, 78] These pulse generators lost their RAM register so that the RAM required reloading via a special programmer not generally available. These pulse generators were also prone to irreversible damage by electrocautery.[78] The new generation of Pacesetter DDD pulse generators (Genisis) appears to be refractory to this type of interference.[78]

A VVI pacemaker or the ventricular channel of a dual-chamber pacemaker may be inhibited by electrocautery when the pulse generator picks up electrocautery artifacts.[58, 59, 61, 63, 65, 69, 81, 82] This may occur if multiple bleeding sites are cauterized in a short period of time. Sensing of intermittent electrical interference may cause long periods of asystole, whereas the application of cautery for longer periods may revert the pulse generator to its asynchronous interference (noise) mode. The interference mode of pacing will continue until electrical interference has disappeared, whereupon the pulse generator will automatically revert to its previous mode and function. This type of inhibition from intermittent electrocautery may be prevented by conversion to the asynchronous mode with application of the magnet over the pulse generator. It should be remembered that in pulse generators with a Vario system to test the threshold (with a gradual reduction of the voltage amplitude of pacemaker stimuli over a period of 16 pulses), the application of the magnet may cause long pauses if the pacing threshold is relatively high.

Electrocautery may activate the reset or backup pacing circuit of a DDD pacemaker normally activated by low battery voltage, giving rise to VOO or VVI pacing at lower rates than programmed.[50–53, 56, 66, 67, 78, 83, 84] The reset (backup) mode does not revert back when electrocautery is discontinued. Thus a DDD pulse generator may be converted to the reset or backup mode in the VOO or VVI mode when it might cause hypotension in selected patients,[67] particularly those with a pacemaker syndrome. Rate-responsive single-chamber pacemakers such as the Medtronic Activitrax may be reset to the ordinary VVI mode without rate responsiveness. Bipolar pacemakers have a lower susceptibility to reset than do unipolar ones.[66]

MANAGEMENT OF PACEMAKER PATIENTS DURING ELECTROCAUTERY

- Determine preoperatively whether the patient is pacemaker-dependent. Pacing and sensing thresholds must be documented. In particular, with DDD pulse generators it is important to determine whether the patient can tolerate the VOO or VVI pacing mode hemodynamically.
- In selected patients, the pulse generator could be programmed to the VOO mode or the VVT mode if tolerated hemodynamically during preoperative evaluation. The VOO or VVI mode produced by application of the magnet or by programming, or occurring automatically with reset, may not be tolerated in patients with the pacemaker syndrome.
- Electrocautery distorts the ECG and it may be

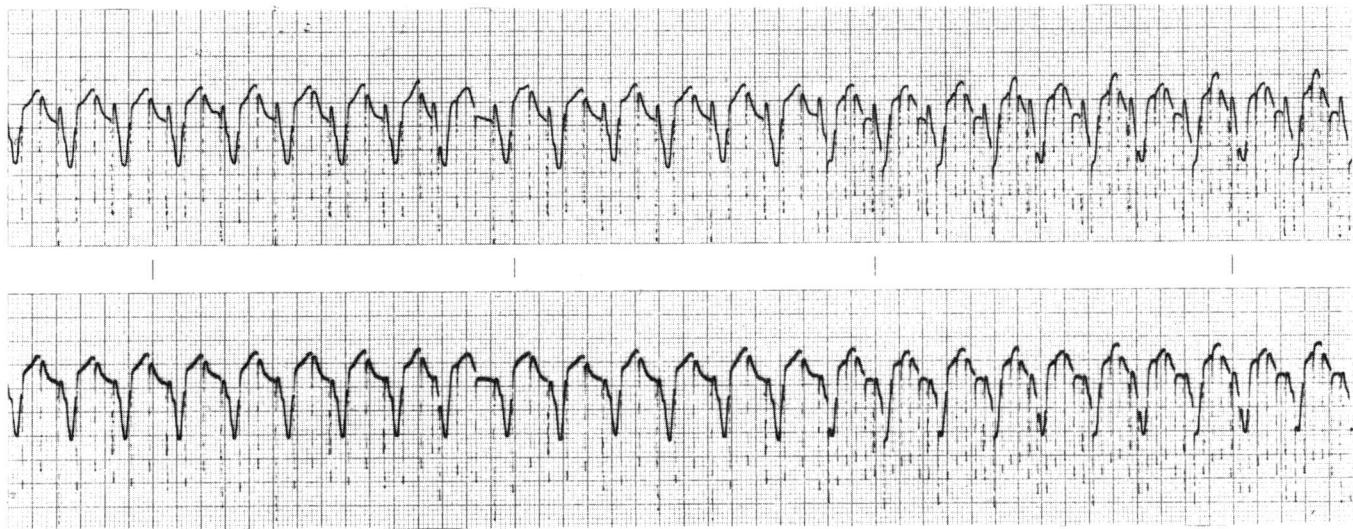

FIGURE 35–8
Response of a Pacesetter-Siemens AFP unipolar DDD pulse generator to rapid chest wall stimulation (CWS) delivered so as to be sensed selectively by the atrial channel. Programmed parameters: lower rate=70 ppm; AV interval=140 ms; upper rate=150 ppm; postventricular atrial refractory period=250 ms. Published specifications by the manufacturer indicate a noise-sampling period of 100 ms, so that repetitive signals occurring at a frequency of 10 Hz or above should be interpreted as interference and activate the noise reversion mode. On the left, CWS was applied at a rate of approximately 375/min (cycle length=160 ms). On the right, the rate of CWS was increased to approximately 800/min (cycle length=80 ms). CWS signals are tracked by the atrial channel so that the ventricular pacing rate is close to the programmed upper rate of 150 ppm. Two ECG leads were recorded simultaneously. The same protocol was repeated with identical rates of CWS but with tripling of the mA output of the external pulse generator delivering CWS. CWS at 375/min was still tracked by the atrial channel, leading to ventricular pacing near the upper rate. However, with CWS delivered at 800/min, the pulse generator reverted to the DVI mode (the DOO mode could not be ruled out because there was no spontaneous ventricular activity).

This sequence illustrates some of the pitfalls of testing the response of pulse generators to interference with CWS and the importance of knowing pacemaker specifications. For this pulse generator, atrial signals occurring with a frequency of 10 Hz or above do not force the atrial channel to pace asynchronously if the amplitude of the atrial signals does not exceed the sensing threshold by 15–25%. The same signals will cause reversion to the noise or interference mode only when they exceed the sensing threshold by 15–25%.

impossible to determine whether pacemaker inhibition occurs. Arterial pressure monitoring may be invaluable in this situation.[85, 86]

- Avoid unipolar electrocautery if the operating field is close to the electrode or pulse generator. In all cases, bipolar electrosurgery is always preferable.
- If unipolar cautery must be used, the ground plate should be positioned so that the current pathway does not pass through or near the pacemaker system. The unipolar or indifferent plate of the equipment should be as close as possible to the operating site and as far away as possible from the pulse generator and the pacing lead, so that the electrical pathway between the electrocautery probe and the ground plate is directed away from the pacemaker lead system.[51, 81] This pathway should be perpendicular to the line joining the two pacing electrodes so as to decrease transmitted interference. The unipolar probe should not be used within 15 cm of the pulse generator or lead. The electrocautery ground plate should not be located between the active electrode and the pulse generator. For transurethral resection of the prostate, the unipolar patch should be on the lower leg.
- Good contact of the indifferent electrode of electrocautery equipment is mandatory, because with poor contact the pulse generator becomes the anode for the electrocautery current. Improper function of the electrocautery plate due to drying out of conductive paste may provide an alternate path for the flow of current via the pacing lead, because electricity seeks the path of least resistance.
- The patient's body should not come in contact with any grounded electrical device that might provide an alternate pathway for current flow during electrocautery. Proper grounding of all electronic equipment used near the patient is essential.[68]
- Electrocautery time should be as short as possible with the lowest feasible energy level.[85] If electrocautery causes inhibition of an implanted pacemaker, it should be used in short bursts so as to produce only one to two dropped beats at a time.[51] If there is no underlying rhythm, only brief bursts of electrocautery (less than 1 second) should be used, followed by 5- to 10-second periods free from electrocautery to allow resumption of rhythm and normal hemodynamics.
- Do not apply the magnet prophylactically in all pulse generators. There is no consistent, industry-wide response of a pacemaker to a magnet.[56, 86] When magnet application forms part of the programming procedure, it may allow inappropriate random reprogramming by electrocautery in certain pulse generators.[80] As a rule, it is preferable to program the pulse generator preoperatively to the VOO mode rather than doing it by application of the magnet.

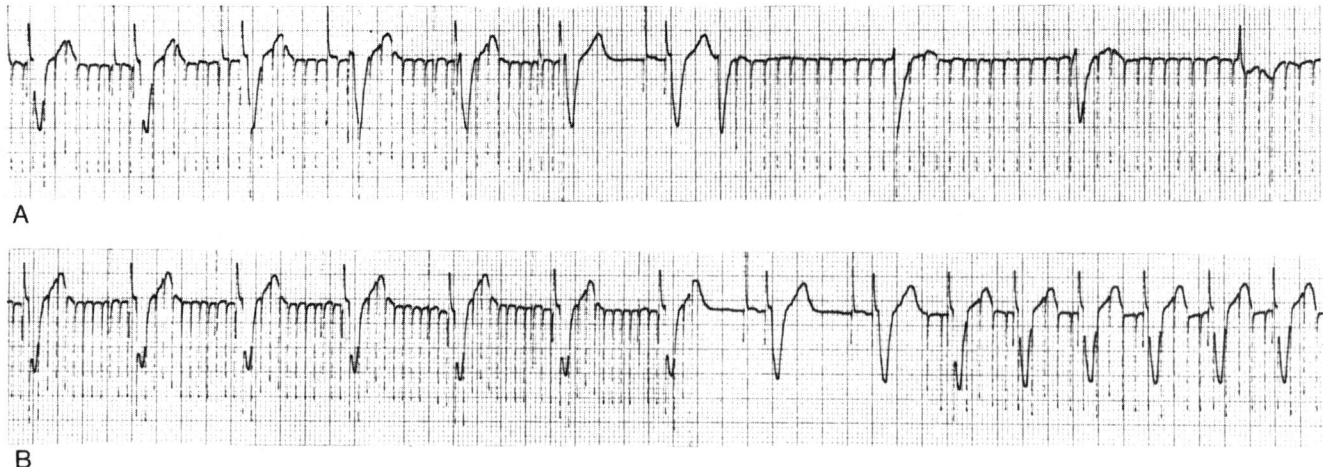

FIGURE 35–9
Response of an Intermedics Cosmos 283-01 unipolar DDD pulse generator to rapid chest wall stimulation (CWS).

A, CWS was delivered so as to be sensed selectively by the ventricular channel. On the left, CWS at a rate of about 750/min (cycle length = approximately 80 ms) forces the pulse generator into its noise reversion mode (DOO). On the right, the rate of CWS was reduced to 600/min (cycle length = 100 ms, frequency >7 Hz), causing inhibition of the pulse generator.

B, CWS was delivered so as to be sensed selectively by the atrial channel. On the left, CWS at a rate of 800/min (cycle length = 75 ms) causes reversion to the DOO noise mode. On the right, the rate of CWS was reduced to 545/min (cycle length = 110 ms, frequency >7 Hz). The atrial channel now tracks CWS and causes ventricular pacing at a rate close to the programmed upper rate (115/min).

According to the technical manual, when the pulse generator senses extraneous electrical (noise) signals occurring at a rate faster than 7 events per second (7 Hz), it should revert to asynchronous pacing at the programmed rate (DOO mode). According to these specifications, the response to CWS shown in the above ECGs suggests abnormal function. However, the specifications reflect the response of a 40-ms sinusoidal waveform, each possessing two signals (positive and negative) capable of triggering the noise response. The 7 Hz refers to continuous interference with a sinusoidal waveform. Thus, for the equivalent response, the pulse generator should sense a repetitive pulsed waveform of 14–15 Hz. This corresponds roughly to the duration of the noise-sampling period occupying the last 64 ms of the programmed refractory period in either the atrial or ventricular channel (i.e., a repetitive signal occurring every 64 ms is equal to approximately 15 Hz, or about double the 7-Hz sinusoidal frequency). These arguments explain the response of the pulse generator to rapid CWS. With CWS delivered at a cycle length of 80 ms and allowing some degree of variance, this comes close to 64 ms. For the lower ECG (B), in which CWS cycle length was 75 ms, this also comes close to 64 ms. This example illustrates the difficulties, limitations, and pitfalls of evaluating the interference response of a pulse generator with CWS.

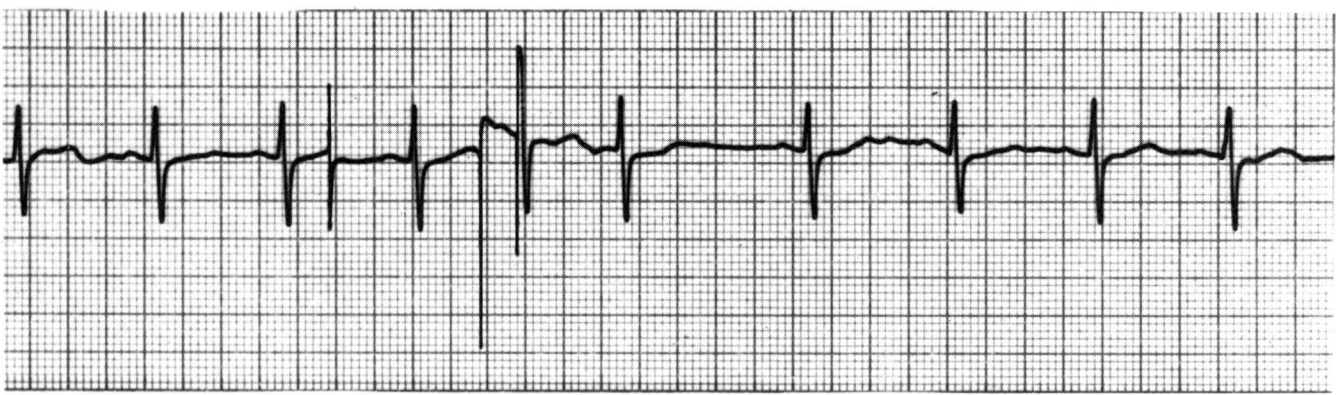

FIGURE 35–10
Behavior of the noise-sampling period of the Cordis Gemini DDD pulse generator. Both ventricular refractory and postventricular atrial refractory periods were programmed to 300 ms. A chest wall stimulus (previously shown to be sensed only by the atrial channel) falls within the noise-sampling period of the atrial channel occupying the last 100 ms of the refractory period (solid black circle). This results in asynchronous (DOO) pacing for one cycle at the lower rate interval of 1000 ms. (Reprinted by permission of Futura Publishing Co., Inc., from Barold SS, et al.: In Barold SS, Mugica J (eds.): New Perspectives in Cardiac Pacing, pp. 69–119. Mt. Kisco, NY, Futura Publishing Co., 1988.)

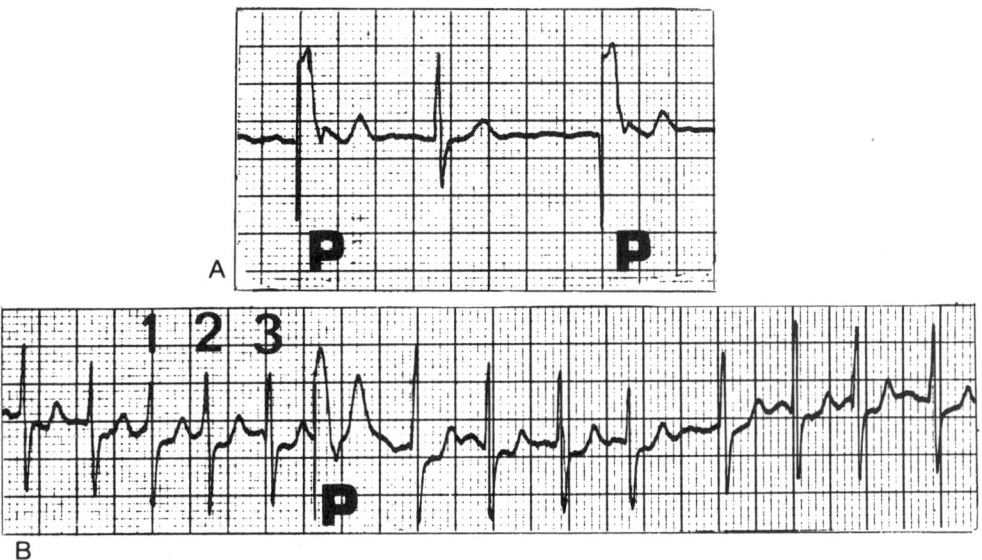

FIGURE 35–11
Cordis Omni-Stanicor pulse generator programmed at 70 ppm (refractory period=322 ms, noise-sampling period=54 ms (i.e., the last 54 ms of the refractory period). A, Normal pacing and sensing. B, Atrial fibrillation with a rapid ventricular rate. The pacemaker senses beat 1. Beat 2 falls in the noise-sampling period initiated by beat 1. This disables the sensing function of the pacemaker so that the refractory period is extended for the entire duration of the escape interval started by beat 1. Beat 3 is unsensed as it occurs in the extended refractory period. The mechanism of asynchronous pacing differs from that shown in Figure 35–1A, but the end result is identical. (Reprinted by permission from Falkoff MD, et al.: PACE 1:250, 1978.)

- Since damage of the pulse generator or pacing system may occur, the capability of instituting emergency pacing must be present. An external transcutaneous pulse generator (and defibrillator) should be available.
- A physician familiar with pacemaker magnets and programmers should be available within the hospital whenever a pacemaker patient is being operated on with electrocautery.[84]
- If a pulse generator has been reprogrammed by electrocautery and the pacing rate is inappropriate or fast, apply the magnet, because the magnet rate usually varies from 70 to 100/min.[79] The pulse generator must then be reprogrammed as soon as possible.
- If application of the magnet does not slow the rate to a tolerable level or there is true pulse generator damage and it cannot be reprogrammed, the pacemaker should be removed and replaced.[52]
- The pulse generator must be carefully tested after the operation, because reprogramming may be inapparent, especially if the spontaneous rhythm is faster than the lower rate of the pulse generator. The pulse generator should be tested immediately after the operation, and then 24 to 48 hours later. Parameters may be different if the pulse generator has been damaged or reprogrammed. Endocardial burns should be suspected if the capture and sensing thresholds have increased. Follow-up is then required until stability can be demonstrated. Occasionally a rise in threshold may need a higher-output pulse generator or a new electrode.[51]

Defibrillation and Cardioversion

Defibrillation, cardioversion, discharge from an automatic implanted cardioverter/defibrillator, and electrical catheter ablation for the treatment of cardiac arrhythmias involve a large amount of energy delivered to the heart during a relatively brief period. Recent pacemaker design with large-scale integrated circuits and microprocessors have made pulse generators more susceptible to these electrical disturbances than in the past.[87, 88]

Most pacemaker malfunctions following D/C shock have occurred in unipolar pacing systems, and it appears that pulse generators implanted in the right pectoral fossa are more susceptible.[89–99] Bipolar units with a short antenna are less vulnerable because they limit current entry into the pulse generator. The incidence of pacemaker malfunction following defibrillation and cardioversion is probably under-reported, because severe and often terminal arrhythmias are being treated.[87, 88]

Pacemakers are generally protected from the high current flow used in defibrillation through a Zenner diode that limits the current allowed to enter the pacemaker circuitry through the lead.[99] With the Zenner diode, the pulse generator can easily withstand a 400-watt · second discharge at a distance of 2 to 4 inches from the pulse generator or lead. When a high external voltage is sensed, the switch in the diode closes to protect pacemaker circuitry. Thus, the Zenner diode behaves as a short circuit as soon as the voltage exceeds a certain value, such as 10 to 15 volts, substantially above the output voltage of the pulse generator. The Zenner diode protects the pulse generator by shunting a large current away from the pulse generator. The shunted current in the lead and electrodes concentrate energy at the electrode-myocardial interface, where burns and local electrical trauma may occur in addition to the myocardial damage produced by transthoracic defibrillation itself.[89, 100] Although the applied energy is brief, the surge of energy is sufficient to produce temporary or permanent alterations of the electrode-myocardial interface. The most important complication of defibrillation (cardioversion) is an increase in the stimulation threshold. According to Fontaine et al.,[96] the damage is related to the current density at the tip electrode, so that older electrodes with large surface areas would be less susceptible than the newer ones with smaller surface areas.

EFFECTS OF DEFIBRILLATION

Damage to Circuitry

Partial or complete destruction of the pulse generator output circuitry,[89, 92, 94–96, 98] decrease in voltage output by destruction of the voltage doubler,[97] runaway state,[96] induction of EOL behavior,[89] and reversible or irreversible alteration of the microprocessor program[57, 96] may occur.

Acute or Chronic Increase in the Pacing Threshold

The myocardium surrounding the electrodes may be injured, causing a transient rise in stimulation threshold. The threshold rise is usually temporary, lasting a few seconds or minutes (Fig. 35–12), but occasionally the pacing threshold may be elevated permanently.[89, 90, 96, 98, 99]

Undersensing

Sensing abnormalities are usually temporary (minutes)[98] but sometimes may last as long as 10 days.[96]

Reprogramming

Electrostatic discharges from the paddles of a defibrillator generated *before* the actual discharge may reprogram certain pulse generators.[101] Reprogramming to another model number may occur even with different parameters.[57] In this situation, the pulse generator cannot be reprogrammed unless one is familiar with this problem.

Reset to the VOO or VVI Mode

(EOS or backup mode.)[53]

Change in Mode from VVI to VVT

Conversion of CPI Model 607 nonprogrammable bipolar VVI pacemaker to R-triggered mode rather than the VVI design has been reported.[97] In this respect, late failure 13 days after multiple shocks has been described with conversion of VVI to the VVT mode with CPI Model 0503.[95]

Lead Displacement

This may be secondary to intense muscle contraction with defibrillation and may require repositioning. This is a rare problem that may occur only with recently implanted electrodes, because old ones have fibrosis around them.[102]

Induction of Ventricular Fibrillation

Thermal and electrical burns at the electrode-myocardial interface may theoretically precipitate ventricular fibrillation. However, in the two cases of ventricular fibrillation reported by Fontaine et al.[96] one was due to a runaway phenomenon and the other was due to temporary pacemaker arrest caused by a high pacing threshold. So far as complications are concerned, Furman has emphasized the importance of determining "whether the episode of ventricular fibrillation was the result of pacemaker malfunction or pacemaker malfunction the result of defibrillation."[88]

MECHANISMS OF PACEMAKER MALFUNCTION AFTER DEFIBRILLATION

Myocardial burns from thermal energy delivered to the heart by the lead appear to be the most important cause of malfunction after defibrillation.[89, 100, 103, 104] Other mechanisms include destruction or reprogramming of the pulse generator, obvious or inapparent displacement of a lead[102] and capacitive coupling of the energy delivered by the defibrillator directly to the pacing lead and hence the heart.[90, 99] The latter mechanism was suggested by Levine and coworkers,[90, 99] based on the observations of Shepard and associates[76] with electrocautery in patients with epicardial pacing electrodes. Shepard et al.[76] postulated that capacitive coupling may cause a high incidence of exit block in patients with permanent pacemakers who underwent open heart surgery during which electrocautery was used. Reiter and coworkers[105] recently presented evidence that the increase in pacing threshold may be related to the duration of ventricular fibrillation (before defibrillation) rather than to the energy of the shock. These interesting observations should be further evaluated, as they have important clinical implications.

Taub et al.[103] demonstrated transient increase in threshold (1–80 min) in dogs with implanted unipolar pulse generators when subjected to D/C countershock. Chronic increase in the pacing threshold was also observed. This disturbance was a function of the delivered energy, the number of shocks, and the type of lead. Lesions at the electrode-tissue interface were observed at autopsy. These consisted of endocardial burn injuries because of the high current transmitted to the leads. Endocardial fibrosis was also observed. The fibrosis often extended through the entire thick-

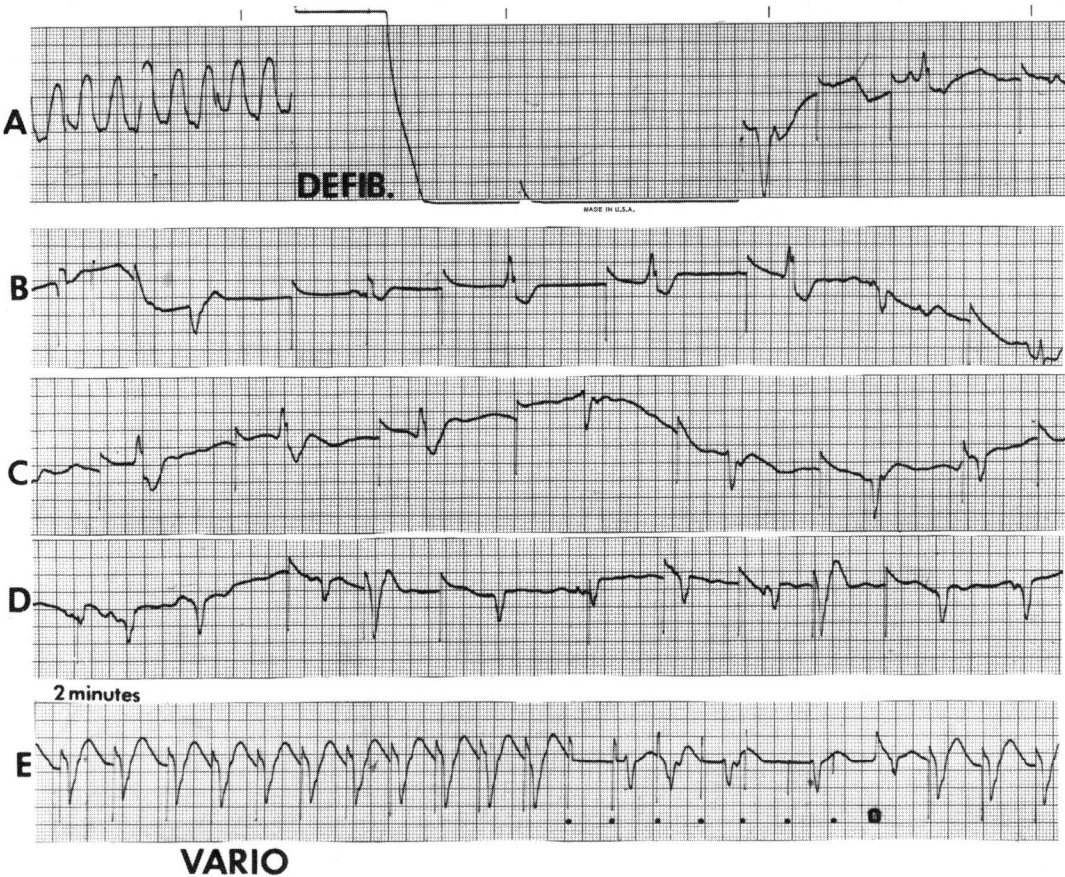

FIGURE 35–12
A–C, Serial electrocardiograms showing transient loss of capture after defibrillation (DEFIB) in a patient with a Siemens 668 pacemaker. The loss of capture is followed by intermittent capture first demonstrated in the supernormal zone of the native beats *(D)*. Sensing function is normal, as the refractory period of this pacemaker was programmed to 437 ms.

E, Demonstration of the stimulation threshold testing using the Vario function of this pacemaker. This is initiated by placing a test magnet over the implanted pulse generator. This starts a test cycle with two phases repeating themselves as long as the magnet remains in place. The first part of the test cycle consists of 16 impulses at the magnetic rate of 100 ppm delivered at the full output (5 V) of the pulse generator. At the end of the 16 impulses, the Vario mechanism comes into play at a rate slightly faster than the preceding magnetic rate. In a conventional 5-V pulse generator, the output voltage is decreased successively by approximately 0.35-V steps during the 16 impulses, down to 0 amplitude (shown at 0). The threshold can then be calculated by counting the number of ineffectual pacing stimuli from right to left. At the end of the test cycle, the pacemaker automatically returns to its programmed voltage output.

(Reproduced by permission of the American College of Cardiology from Levine PA, Barold SS, Fletcher RD, et al.: J Am Coll Cardiol 1:1413, 1983.)

ness of the myocardium and was grossly visible in the epicardial surface overlying the electrode. Such myocardial necrosis has also been reported following external defibrillation.

GUIDELINES FOR DEFIBRILLATION AND CARDIOVERSION IN PACEMAKER PATIENTS

- Use anterior-posterior paddles, if possible (their availability is not universal).
- Do not put the paddle over the pulse generator. When using only anterior paddles, place them along a line perpendicular to the line joining the pulse generator to the tip of the ventricular pacing lead. The upward vector of the defibrillator discharge should be perpendicular to the sensing vector of the pulse generator-lead (line). In a dual-lead system in which the electrodes are roughly perpendicular to each other, give preference to the ventricular system.
- Place the paddles at least 10 cm from the pulse generator or lead. (This may be difficult for a right pectoral implant.)
- Use the lowest possible defibrillator energy.
- A programmer and a transcutaneous external pacemaker should be readily available. Be prepared to increase the output of the implanted pulse generator immediately by programming.
- Carefully monitor the patient for 24 hours. Repeated testing of threshold is important. Because of possible late malfunction, follow-up for several weeks is necessary.

TRANSVENOUS CARDIOVERSION AND DEFIBRILLATION

Yee et al.[106] studied the change in pacing threshold in humans after transvenous catheter countershock for the termination of ventricular tachycardia and ventricular fibrillation, using a catheter with two pairs of electrodes along its length (one pair at the apex of the right ventricle and the other pair at the superior vena cava–right atrial junction). During countershock, the two ventricular electrodes became common (cathode) and the two proximal atrial electrodes served as the anode. Immediately after synchronous cardioversion, the amplitude of unipolar and bipolar ventricular electrograms was significantly reduced and the stimulation threshold was increased (between the two ventricular electrodes). However, all values returned to the baseline about 5 minutes after the shock. One patient could not be paced at 20 volts, 0.5 ms, for 5 minutes after the shock (10–40 joules). Initial changes were probably due to a local phenomenon at the catheter-myocardial interface.

Yee and associates[107] also evaluated the same catheter in dogs and found significant increases in pacing threshold and decreases in the bipolar and unipolar electrograms, as recorded from the distal pair of ventricular electrodes. These abnormalities were still evident 10 minutes after the shock; they were greater when increased energy was used in any given shock, but basically similar after repeated shocks. These investigators also positioned the second electrode catheter in the right ventricle, distant from the defibrillating catheter, in five pigs. Increases in the stimulation threshold were observed only at the countershock catheter, suggesting that changes were secondary to local changes at the electrode-myocardial interface. No changes in pacing or sensing threshold occurred at the second catheter in the right ventricle. In addition, transthoracic shocks of 60 to 250 joules did not cause any significant changes in pacing function from both right ventricular electrodes not participating in defibrillation.[107] This lack of abnormalities may be related to the relatively low amplitude of the shocks, and to the fact that only three pigs were studied.

When the same transvenous electrodes are used for both defibrillation and pacing, pathologic studies in experimental animals support the hypothesis that electrical energy concentrated in the zone of the high-current density at the electrode-myocardial interface is the most important factor in raising the pacing threshold and reducing the amplitude of the ventricular electrogram available for sensing by a pacemaker. The damage due to the defibrillating shocks and not to the presence of the electrode itself is concentrated in the ventricular septum and the right ventricular free-wall adjacent to the transvenous electrodes.[108, 109] Despite their effect on pacemaker function, this focal area of necrosis appears too small to cause hemodynamic complications.[108, 109] Barker-Voeltz and coworkers[109] also examined the damage done 48 hours after transvenous defibrillation in beagles and found that the degree of myocardial necrosis was directly related to the shock strength and not to the cumulative effect of shocks of lesser amplitude. However, Rubin et al.,[110] using a transvenous catheter with a much smaller surface area (1.2 cm^2), found that there was no correlation in dogs of the defibrillation energy with the time of return to the prefibrillation pacing threshold.

Winkle et al.[111] recently evaluated a new tripolar catheter for transvenous defibrillation in humans. The distal tip and the middle electrodes are in the right ventricular apex, and the proximal electrode is at the superior vena cava–right atrial junction. The middle electrode lies 4 mm from the distal tip electrode. Bipolar pacing and sensing were accomplished by using the distal and middle pair of electrodes (tip electrode as cathode, and middle electrode as anode), and defibrillation was accomplished using the middle (cathode) and proximal (anode) pair of electrodes. After the shock, pacing threshold and bipolar ventricular electrograms were basically unchanged compared to preshock levels, because the defibrillating shock did not involve the distal (pacing) electrode.

ELECTRICAL CATHETER ABLATION IN PATIENTS WITH IMPLANTED PACEMAKERS

In catheter ablation techniques, 150 to 500 joules of energy are delivered to the tip of a temporary endocardial electrode that may be quite close to the permanent electrode of an implanted pulse generator. Electrical ablation in patients with implanted pacemakers may cause transient loss of pacing (2–4 min) because of a short-lived increase in the pacing threshold. Theoretically the chronic threshold may also increase. There may be transient loss of sensing function (2–30 min), presumably related to the injury of the myocardial-electrode interface.[112-115] Rarely the pulse generator may be reprogrammed or reset, or permanent malfunction may occur requiring replacement.[112, 114-116] Thus, the pacing and sensing function of the pulse generator must be carefully tested before and after electrical catheter ablation.

INTERACTIONS OF THE AUTOMATIC CARDIOVERTER/DEFIBRILLATOR (AICD) AND IMPLANTED PACEMAKERS

These interactions[117] may be classified as follows:

1. Non-detection of ventricular fibrillation.
2. False shocks due to pacing stimuli or paced QRS causing double or triple counting by the AICD.
3. Increase in the pacing and sensing threshold secondary to the shock.
4. Effect on the pacemaker and the leads, e.g., resetting to the VVI or VOO backup mode.
5. Potential interaction of an AICD device and an antitachycardia pacemaker.

As yet, the discharge of an AICD has not been reported to cause permanent pacemaker malfunction or destruction.

During ventricular fibrillation, a unipolar pacemaker may not be inhibited and large pacemaker stimuli may occur regularly or irregularly. An AICD device may sense these large-amplitude stimuli and interpret them as organized ventricular electrograms, with the result that it ignores the underlying tachyarrhythmia and does not discharge appropriately.[118-123] This response is related to the automatic gain control circuitry of the

AICD, which detects the largest-amplitude signals and ignores the relatively smaller signals.

False or inappropriate discharges may occur because the AICD device senses one or more pacemaker stimuli and ventricular depolarization.[117, 121, 122] A VVI pulse generator may cause "double counting" by the AICD. Dual-chamber pacemakers may cause double or triple counting by the AICD (atrial and ventricular stimuli and QRS complex). These problems are far more common with unipolar pacemakers. Therefore, unipolar single- or dual-chamber pulse generators are contraindicated in patients with an AICD. A pre-existing unipolar pacing system should be converted to a bipolar one. The AICD may occasionally sense stimuli from bipolar single- or dual-chamber pulse generators[120, 121] with consequent inhibition of the AICD[121] or the delivery of inappropriate shocks according to the circumstances. Discharge of the AICD may also occur upon application of the magnet over a pulse generator if the rate of the pacing stimuli (in single- or dual-chamber pulse generators) and the spontaneous QRS complex exceed the rate limit of the AICD.[120, 124] The AICD device can also be triggered by pacemaker programming signals unrelated to subsequent pacemaker function.[125]

During pacing, one can determine what the AICD senses by placing the magnet over it. The tones emitted by the AICD clearly indicate whether there is double or triple counting, and the data may be recorded phonocardiographically. Triple counting may occur with an AV sequential pacemaker if the implanted pulse generator senses the atrial stimulus, ventricular stimulus, and the paced QRS complex. This is important because the refractory period of the AICD is only 150 ms. Drugs that prolong the QRS complex such as amiodarone and flecainide may predispose to double counting of the ventricular stimulus and its accompanying paced QRS complex of long duration.

Guanieri and associates[126, 127] studied the effect of defibrillation from an AICD device in dogs with implanted defibrillating patches, two sets of bipolar pacing electrodes and one bipolar transvenous electrode at the right ventricular apex. A 30-joules shock was delivered to the patches 15 s after the induction of ventricular fibrillation. With the pacemaker set at a baseline threshold value to capture, the time to capture before and after the administration of flecainide was lengthened to 4.9 ± 1.9 s and to 14.9 ± 2.2 s, respectively. At twice the threshold for cardiac pacing, the time to capture after defibrillation was 2.2 ± 0.9 s and 5.6 ± 2.1 s before and after the administration of flecainide, respectively. No significant difference was seen between epicardial and endocardial thresholds. These observations suggest that the pacing threshold immediately after defibrillation may be increased in all patients but, for reasons as yet unknown, may be clinically important with loss of capture in only a certain proportion of patients.

After the delivery of the defibrillating shock, sensing and pacing function may fail. The latter is due to a transient change of excitability at the electrode-myocardial interface. Cohen et al.[121] recently reported their experience with the combination of AICD and pacemakers in nine patients. They found lack of QRS sensing in 11 of 20 analyzable episodes for 9.1 ± 11.6 s. There was lack of capture in 8 of 22 analyzable episodes for 4.9 ± 5.07 s.[121] One patient showed no capture up to 16 s after discharge of the AICD. When tested within 3 months, there was no change in the chronic pacing threshold.[121]

Failure to pace or sense after an AICD shock has important clinical implications, because a substantial number of patients with an AICD have sinus bradycardia,[128, 129] and the pacing threshold may already be elevated by flecainide therapy.[130] In contrast to experimental data in dogs,[110] it appears that in humans the higher the defibrillation energy, the longer the period of pacemaker failure to capture.[129] Transient loss of sensing due to AICD discharge may cause asynchronous pacing. The bipolar rate sensing lead of the AICD may then sense the unsensed spontaneous QRS complexes and the pacemaker stimuli. In this situation, if the rate threshold is met, the AICD will interpret the sequence as ventricular tachycardia and deliver an inappropriate defibrillating shock.

MANAGEMENT OF PATIENTS WITH AN AUTOMATIC IMPLANTED CARDIOVERTER/ DEFIBRILLATOR AND PERMANENT PACEMAKER[122]

- Unipolar pacemakers are contraindicated. If there is a unipolar pacemaker, it should be replaced with a bipolar unit.
- The pacing electrodes should be located as far as possible from the rate-sensing electrode of the AICD.
- Closely spaced (1.0 cm) bipolar electrodes should be used for AICD sensing to avoid detecting pacemaker stimuli. In some cases, this may require epicardial mapping at the time of implantation.
- The capability of the AICD to sense bipolar pacemaker stimuli should be tested thoroughly at the time of implantation. When ventricular tachycardia and ventricular fibrillation are induced, arrhythmia detection by the AICD should not be inhibited by the action of the pulse generator.
- At implantation, convert the AICD to the electrophysiology test mode with the device being inhibited. Increase the output of the pacemaker stimuli to maximum and listen to the audible tones of the AICD reflecting each sensed signal. During induced ventricular fibrillation, verify that the AICD does not sense stimuli from the implanted pulse generator in the asynchronous mode (VOO or DOO) at the maximum programmed output, with the magnet over the pulse generator.[131]
- During follow-up, deactivate the AICD during the magnet test of the pulse generator if there is any doubt that the magnet procedure might cause discharge of the AICD.
- The combination of an antitachycardia pulse generator and AICD is very complex and requires detailed investigation for possible interactions.[132, 133]

Radiation

Contemporary advanced pulse generators with complementary metal oxide semiconductors (CMOSs) are more sensitive to the effects of ionizing radiation, compared with the semiconductor circuits used in old pulse generators.[134–149] This damage is variable and may be serious because life-threatening arrhythmias may be produced. The damage to pacemaker electronics may be transient but often is permanent, and it is dependent on the type of radiation, total dose, type of device, and details of its fabrication. The phenomenon is cumulative. Thus, the effect would be similar whether the same dose is given at one time or spread over several episodes. Given a sufficiently high cumulative absorbed dose, all pulse generators ultimately will fail catastrophically.[139]

Altered function secondary to damage by radiation may produce spontaneous reprogramming in the form of a change in rate, voltage, pulse width, runaway characteristics (in one channel or both in the case of dual-chamber pacemakers), abnormal sensing, failure to reprogram, output failure, and unusual responses to application of the magnet. Because of the complexity of circuit design, the mode of failure cannot be predicted. In pulse generators tested in vitro, transient recovery of function followed by total failure suggests that even transient loss of function must be regarded as the precursor to permanent damage.[143]

In patients requiring irradiation to a particular part of the body other than the site of the pulse generator, a low dose of standard radiation should not cause any problems. Radiation doses used in routine diagnostic x-ray procedures do not produce sufficient radiation to affect pulse generators either immediately or with small cumulative doses.

MANAGEMENT OF PACEMAKER PATIENTS REQUIRING RADIOTHERAPY

- Every attempt should be made to avoid direct irradiation of the pulse generator. If this is not possible, serious consideration should be given to moving the pulse generator to another site.
- The pulse generator should be shielded during radiotherapy.
- Continuous ECG monitoring is required during treatment to detect transient disturbances so that they can be recorded. Transient malfunction should be regarded as a precursor of more serious permanent damage.
- The pulse generator should be tested frequently during and after radiation therapy. Any unexpected behavior should be considered as pacemaker failure until proved otherwise. However, during radiation therapy the pulse generator may also be influenced by EMI from a linear accelerator; such transient malfunction is benign and does not necessitate pacemaker replacement, and it should be differentiated from more serious radiation damage.[148]

Magnetic Resonance Imaging

Despite the apparent lack of biological effects, magnetic resonance imaging (MRI) may have important effects on pacemaker function.[139, 150–157] This is related to the development of strong static and time-varying magnetic fields as well as pulsed radio frequency (RF) fields. Although no apparent damage to pacemaker components has thus far been reported, damage to the reed switch remains a theoretical danger. During MRI, the ECG may be extremely difficult or impossible to interpret because of (1) asynchronous pacing from exposure to the magnetic field and (2) artifacts due to pulsing of the RF field superimposed on the ECG. These artifacts occur irrespective of their effect on pacemaker function.

When an individual with an implanted pacemaker approaches the MRI system, the static or constant magnetic field may eventually become strong enough to close the reed switch even outside the tunnel (approximate average distance of 2 meters from the tunnel[151]). Inside the tunnel, several possibilities may occur.[151]

1. Asynchronous pacing regardless of pulse generator position.
2. Asynchronous pacing only in certain positions according to the alignment of the magnetic field. Some pulse generators tested in vitro remained on demand in a vertical position, but such a position would not be encountered in the pacemaker patient.
3. Several seconds may pass before asynchronous pacing occurs.
4. No effect may occur with preservation of normal demand pacing.
5. Transient reed switch inhibition may occur after the pulsed frequency sequence is turned off.[155]

As a rule, conversion to asynchronous pacing should pose no problem in virtually all the patients with permanent pacemakers. However, RF pulsing may cause an induced voltage across the pacemaker electrodes that may be strong enough to pace the heart. Chauvin et al.[151] observed, in vitro, the existence of an induced current in the electrode synchronous with pulsed RF, of 1 to 4 volts and about 2 ms in duration. This induced current has the characteristics of a current likely to stimulate the myocardium. The ultimate capability of this induced current to pace the myocardium appears to depend on the type of MRI equipment.

CONSEQUENCES OF RADIO FREQUENCY PULSING DURING MRI

Rapid Pacing

Pacing may occur at the same rate as the RF modulation (pulse period), as demonstrated in dogs.[153–155] The mechanism of rapid pacing at the RF pulse period is unknown. Somehow RF energy is coupled with the output circuit of the pulse generator; if the induced voltage across the pacemaker electrodes is strong enough, pacing will occur.[152–155] In this respect, Hayes and colleagues[155] showed that with a DDD pulse generator programmed to the AAI mode, rapid ventricular pacing could still occur. When the ventricular lead was physically disconnected, rapid pacing did not occur. Thus, this effect requires a pulse generator connected to a lead and does not seem to occur with a lead alone (without a pacemaker). Rapid pacing may depend on the polarity of the pulse generator. Hayes et al.[155] described rapid pacing of a VVI pulse generator in the bipolar, but not in the unipolar, mode with the same parameters. Rapid pacing may occur in single- and dual-chamber pulse generators and may exceed the upper rate or runaway rate protection limit. Rapid pacing may also occur even if the magnetic field has converted the pulse generator to the asynchronous mode. MRI requires a pulsing rate usually with a cycle length of 200 to 1000 ms. Thus, cardiac stimulation may occur at the frequency of the RF pulsing (e.g., 200 ms = 300 ppm). In the case of a DDD pulse generator, this may affect the atrial channel or the ventricular channel or both. Rapid atrial pacing may be impossible to detect on the surface ECG. However, atrial arrhythmias and atrial triggering of rapid ventricular rates are possible.[152]

Inhibition

Total inhibition by the RF pulses may occur if the reed switch is not affected by the magnetic field. Despite the fact that magnetic fields may be strong enough to close the reed switch, and the pulse generator is switched to the asynchronous mode, it may still respond to interference with inhibition of the atrial or ventricular output, because interference may pass directly through the circuitry to affect pacemaker function.[152]

Resetting of DDD Pulse Generators

MRI may also cause conversion to the reset or backup mode of DDD pulse generators because the circuit is activated by the high RF pulse repetition rate, interpreted as interference by the implanted pulse generator.[152]

Transient Reed Switch Malfunction

Hayes et al.[155] showed that when RF pulsing is terminated, there may be missing pacemaker artifacts despite a strong magnetic field. This was interpreted as signifying reed switch malfunction that was transient, because asynchronous pacing returned about 15 seconds after RF pulsing was discontinued.

The various effects of MRI on pacemakers described in the literature may vary according to the power of the MRI unit, and this may explain the discrepancies in published data.[155] Further studies are required to determine why specific pulse generators respond with rapid pacing during MRI. A pulse generator exposed to MRI has not yet been shown to alter its programmed parameters (except for reset to the VVI or VOO mode) or impair the ability to reprogram the pulse generator after RF pulsing in dogs (i.e., no damage is produced).

In conclusion, MRI with strong magnetic fields should be avoided in all pacemaker patients. No recommendations can be made as yet.[155] Serious malfunction with no output or rapid pacing may occur. If MRI is deemed essential for the patient, a similar pulse generator should first be tested (without the patient) prior to scanning the patient. Patients undergoing MRI with a pulse generator programmable to the "magnet off" function should have this feature programmed so as to avoid the asynchronous effect during MRI.[154]

Lithotripsy

Extracorporeal shock wave lithotripsy is a noninvasive method for disintegrating renal stones. The procedure generates electromagnetic and mechanical forces that may influence pacemaker function. In vitro testing has demonstrated that this therapy is generally safe with regard to pacemaker function, especially in single-chamber devices.[158, 159] The release of shock waves is triggered by the patient's R wave to prevent ventricular arrhythmias seen during early use of lithotripsy. When lithotripsy is operated in the asynchronous mode, signals may be sensed and may inhibit a single-chamber pulse generator. If the shocks are delivered synchronously with the QRS complex, the likelihood of false inhibition should be quite low in single-chamber pulse generators. Occasionally, lithotripsy may cause intermittent inhibition of VVI or DDD pulse generators or triggering of the ventricular output of DDD pulse generators by electromechanical interference.[160, 161] A DDD pulse generator may reach the upper rate or show irregularities in the pacing rate.[162] Lithotripsy may induce supraventricular tachyarrhythmias that may cause triggering of the ventricular output of a DDD pulse generator, with consequent increase in the ventricular pacing rate.[163] Therefore, a DDD pulse generator should be programmed to the VVI or DOO mode during lithotripsy.

Intermittent reversion to the magnet mode and rate during lithotripsy has been reported due to transient closure of the reed switch by high-energy vibration.[161, 162] During in vitro testing of a relatively large number of pulse generators exposed to lithotripsy, there was an increase in rate in some pulse generators, malfunction of the reed switch and, rarely, failure of output (internal mechanical failure with no output has been reported in 2 of 9 cases in one series,[164] and 1 of 29 cases in another series[165]). However, as yet no permanent damage has been reported with implanted pulse generators in humans. Additionally, no reprogramming abnormalities or conversion to the reset or backup mode have so far been reported. A case of intermittent pacemaker failure has been reported as being possibly due to a loose contact that was unmasked during lithotripsy.[165]

If there are any doubts about the response of a

pacemaker during lithotripsy, an unknown pacemaker should be tested in vitro before treatment. Rate-responsive pulse generators utilizing activity (piezoelectric crystal) as a sensor should have the activity mode programmed off during lithotripsy in order to avoid an increase in rate to the maximum programmed value[159] and also because of the possibility that the piezoelectric element may be shattered when it is situated in the focal point of the lithotripsy system.[159] Patients with piezoelectric activity-sensing rate-responsive pacemakers implanted in the thorax can probably undergo lithotripsy safely, provided the activity mode is deactivated.[159] Patients with such pacemakers implanted in the abdomen should not undergo lithotripsy because of potential damage to the piezoelectric crystal.[159]

MANAGEMENT OF PACEMAKER PATIENTS UNDERGOING LITHOTRIPSY

- An unfamiliar pulse generator should be tested in vitro first.
- Synchronization of the lithotripsy should be with the QRS complex and not the pacemaker artifacts (i.e., shock waves should be triggered by the heartbeat and not the pacemaker stimuli).
- An external transcutaneous cardiac pacemaker should be available in the rare instance of pacemaker malfunction.
- The patient should be followed up closely for the first 6 months after lithotripsy to ensure no latent pulse generator damage, particularly the function of the reed switch.[165]
- ECG monitoring is essential during the procedure.
- A DDD pulse generator should be programmed to the VVI or VOO mode for the procedure.

Diathermy

Short-wave diathermy consists of therapeutic application of current directly to the skin. Diathermy can be a source of high-frequency interference. Diathermy should not be used in patients with pacemakers because of possible effects in the pulse generator and at the implant site and because of the potential for inhibition.[9, 139, 166, 167] Diathermy too close to the pulse generator may damage its circuitry by heating. Selective localized heating of the metal case of the pulse generator may be so intense as to cause burning of the tissues. Signals from ultra high-frequency devices may bypass the noise protection mechanisms and enter the circuitry directly. This may occur even if the pacemaker is programmed to the asynchronous (AOO, VOO, DOO modes). Short-wave or microwave diathermy is therefore definitely contraindicated in patients with pacemakers.

Transcutaneous Electrical Nerve Stimulation (TENS)

Electrical stimulating techniques such as transcutaneous electrical nerve stimulation (TENS) and acupuncture may interfere with pacemaker function by virtue of pulsed or nonpulsed electrical current in contact with body tissues.[168, 169] TENS is often indicated in patients with chronic pain due to muscular or neurologic problems and in some patients with acute pain. Pain is relieved by electrical stimulation of peripheral nerves. Many patients who are candidates for TENS are also in the age range in which pacemakers are commonly used. Rasmussen et al.[170] studied the effect of TENS at four sites in 51 patients with 20 different models of permanent pacemakers and found no episodes of interference, inhibition, or reprogramming. A study by Jones[171] documented the adverse effect of TENS on pacemakers, but this occurred with early pacemakers that are more susceptible to EMI than are contemporary devices. Ross and coworkers[172] found interference in one of six patients, and Ericksson et al.[168] found interference in all of the four patients they studied. Aida and associates[173] suggested that EMI was most likely to occur when TENS electrodes were placed parallel to the vector of the pacemaker stimulus. In this respect, Rasmussen et al.[170] did not place electrodes parallel to the above vector. Wicks and colleagues[174] reported that phrenic nerve stimulation may interfere with unipolar or bipolar pacemaker function. However, LaBan et al.[169] recently demonstrated the safety of peripheral nerve conduction studies in patients with implanted pacemakers.

In conclusion, therefore, it appears that TENS is safe to use in pacemaker patients, provided the electrodes are not placed parallel to the vector of the pacemaker stimulus. So far as other methods of electrical stimulation are concerned, stimulation of muscle appears to be safe, but each case should be assessed individually.[175] Low-frequency currents delivered with acupuncture carry the potential of pacemaker inhibition.[176]

Interference From Equipment Used to Test Pacemakers

INTERFERENCE RELATED TO MAGNET APPLICATION

Inhibition

If the reed switch is connected to the sensing circuit, application or removal of the magnet causes a sudden change in voltage that may be detected by the sensing amplifier if the pulse generator has already come out of its refractory period. This may be due to a direct action on the reed switch, provoking transients within the sensing circuit. In some pulse generators, unduly long pauses may occur.[177–182] Indeed, when the magnet is waved in a certain way to and fro over some pulse generators, sustained inhibition may occur. Although magnet waving may be useful for unmasking the underlying rhythm, other methods are preferable, such as chest wall stimulation or a decrease in the output and/or rate in programmable devices. Activation of the programmer from one manufacturer may sometimes inhibit an implanted pulse generator from a different manufacturer.[183]

Triggering

After interrogation, all Pacesetter AFP DDD pulse generators are automatically programmed to the "magnet-off" function.[35, 184] In this state, the pacemaker will not revert to the DOO mode upon application of the magnet (also present in the programming head). Interrogation is usually the last task of pacemaker evaluation, because it records the final programmed parameters and other data transmitted by telemetry. Thus, an AFP pulse generator may be inadvertently left in the permanent magnet-off function because interrogation automatically reverts it to that function. Moving the magnet or programming head (containing a magnet) toward a unipolar AFP pulse generator in the magnet-off function creates a voltage capable of being sensed only by the atrial channel, thereby triggering a ventricular stimulus after the programmed AV interval.[184]

Removal of the magnet or programming head from the AFP pulse generator may also generate an identical signal capable of triggering ventricular stimulation. Opening and closure of the reed switch by magnet movement creates small voltages varying from 0.5 to 1.0 mV only in the atrial circuit. Continuous waving of the magnet over an AFP pulse generator in the magnet-off function may cause a rapid ventricular response (near or at the upper rate) from the continual detection of signals by the atrial channel. In the magnet-off function, the creation of magnet-induced signals in the atrial channel may precipitate endless loop tachycardia[184] (Fig. 35–13). The tachycardia cannot be terminated by application of the magnet unless asynchronous response to the magnet (DOO mode) is restored by reprogramming the pulse generator back to the "magnet-on" function.

Interference During Programming

Interaction of the programmer and pulse generator during programming may cause a variety of signals

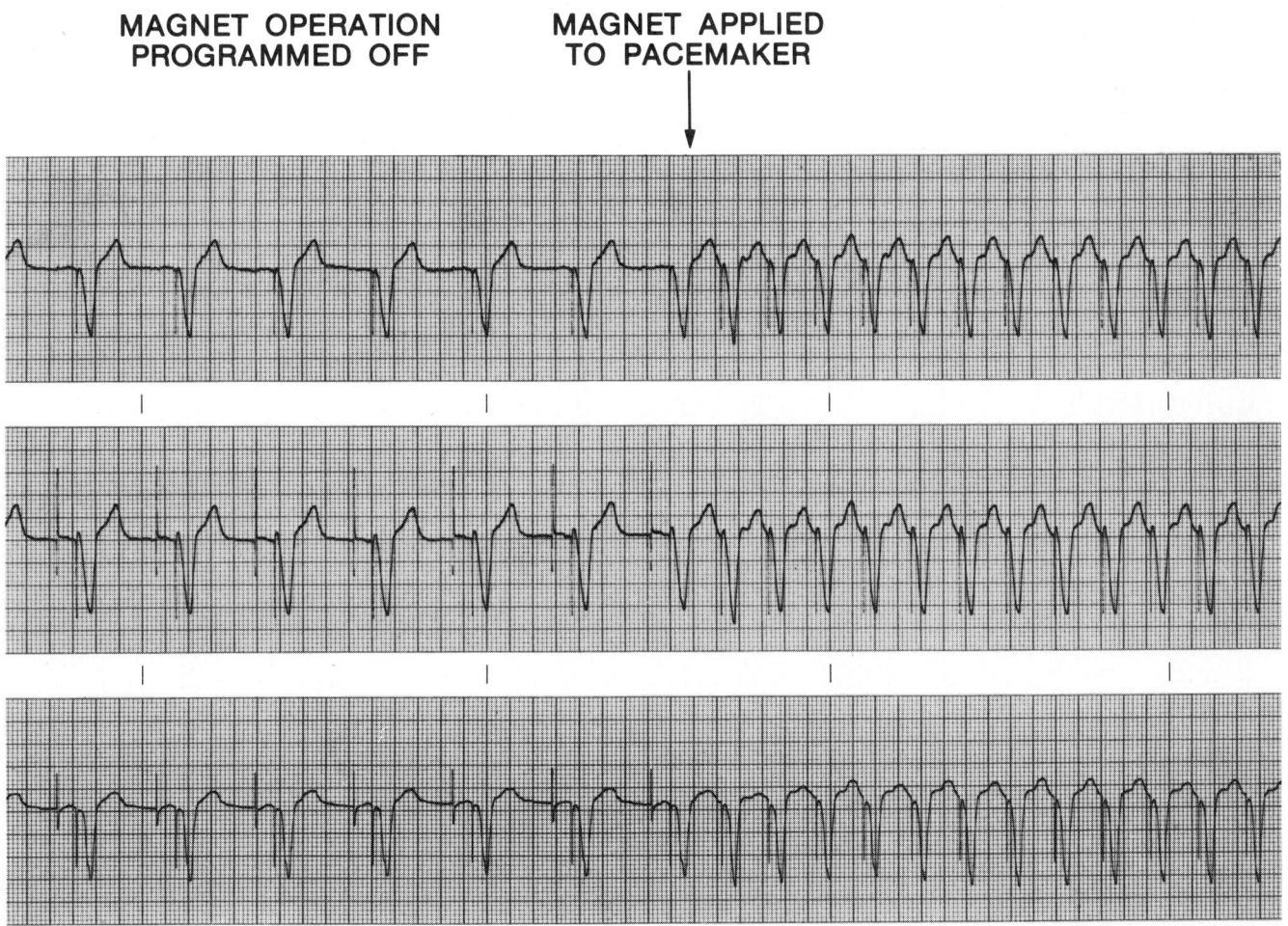

FIGURE 35–13
Three-lead ECG recorded in a patient with a Pacesetter AFP DDD pulse generator with the magnet function programmed off. The atrial sensitivity was programmed to 0.5 mV. Application of the magnet over the pulse generator creates a signal sensed by the atrial circuit, whereupon triggered premature ventricular stimulation is delivered at the end of the AV interval. This leads to retrograde ventriculoatrial conduction and initiation of endless loop tachycardia at a rate of 145/min. Removal of the magnet and its reapplication did not influence the tachycardia. (Reproduced by permission from Barold SS, et al.: PACE 9:503, 1986.)

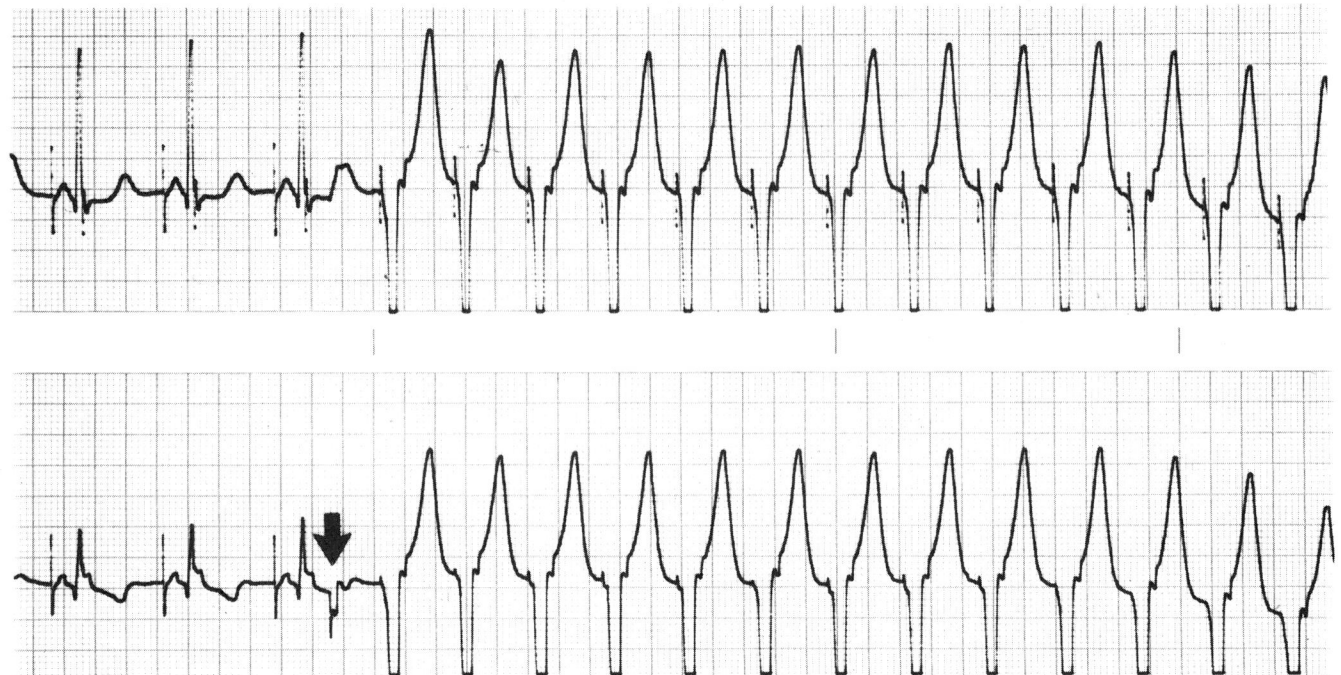

FIGURE 35–14
Induction of endless loop tachycardia in a patient with a Symbios 7006 DDD pulse generator during programming the "cancel magnet" function. This command restores the sensing function of the pulse generator, whereupon the atrial channel then picks up a signal related to the programming procedure (arrow). This causes AV dissociation, leading to retrograde ventriculoatrial conduction and the initiation of endless loop tachycardia.

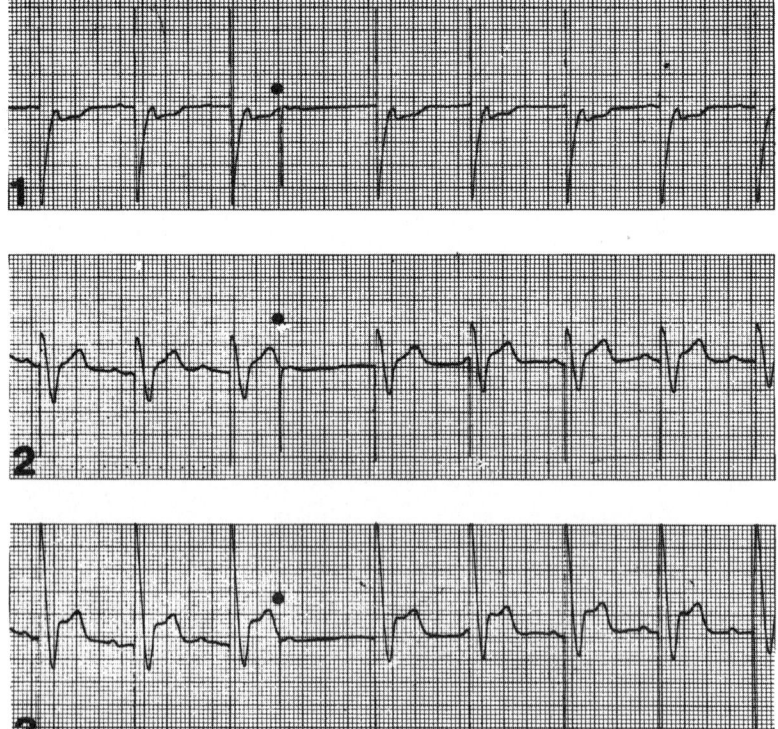

FIGURE 35–15
Simultaneous recording in leads 1, 2, and 3 showing triboelectric inhibition (black dot) by touching the patient's skin over an implanted unipolar pulse generator. (Reproduced by permission from Barold SS, et al.: In Meere C (ed.): Cardiac Pacing: Proceedings of the Sixth World Symposium on Cardiac Pacing, Chap. 18–1, Montreal, PACESYMP, 1979.)

sensed by the pulse generator.[185, 186] Depending on the manufacturer and the position of the programming head over the pulse generator, inhibition, triggering of a ventricular output (if signals are sensed by the atrial channel of a DDD pulse generator), asynchronous pacing or rate change may occur. This response is of no clinical importance, although interference sensed by the atrial channel (in systems not requiring application of a magnet for reprogramming or in other systems with the magnet function turned off) may cause AV dissociation and initiation of endless loop tachycardia (Fig. 35–14).

Triboelectric Phenomena

Triboelectric phenomena may inhibit implanted unipolar pulse generators. An observer may gather considerable static electricity, especially when wearing rubber soles and standing/walking on a carpet.[187] Touching the patient's skin over the unipolar pacemaker may release sufficient static voltage to inhibit the ventricular channel of a unipolar pacemaker (Fig. 35–15). Alternatively, triboelectric signals may be sensed by the atrial channel of a DDD pulse generator, with resultant triggering of the ventricular output.

Electroconvulsive Therapy

During electroconvulsive therapy (ECT) used in psychiatry, only a minimum amount of electricity reaches the heart because of the high resistance of body tissues. ECT appears safe, but little has been published on this subject.[183–191] ECG monitoring is advisable during the procedure, because seizure activity during ECT may generate myopotentials theoretically capable of inhibiting a unipolar pulse generator. Probably a very small number of patients require conversion to the asynchronous mode of pacing during ECT.

Dental Treatment

Some models of ultrasound scalers used to remove calculus from tooth enamel may cause pacemaker inhibition.[192] This can occur if the handle of the instrument comes in close proximity to the patient's neck. A lead apron on the patient does not give protection from this type of interference. The less common type of piezoelectric scaler appears to be without effect on implanted pacemakers. Electric pulp testers also appear to have no effect on implanted pacemakers.[192] If there is any doubt, application of a magnet over the pulse generator (or temporary reprogramming) to produce the asynchronous mode offers a simple solution. Vibrations during dental treatment may increase the rate of activity-sensing rate-responsive pacemakers such as the Medtronic Activitrax.[193] The activity mode should therefore be programmed to "off" during dental treatment.

References

1. O'Brien E: Environmental dangers for the patient with a pacemaker. Br Med J 285:1677, 1982.
2. Sager DP: Current facts on pacemaker electromagnetic interference and their application to clinical care. Heart Lung 6:211, 1987.
3. Sowton E: Environmental hazards for pacemaker patients. J R Coll Physicians Lond 16:159, 1982.
4. Warnowicz-Papp MA: The pacemaker patient and the electromagnetic environment. Clin Prog Electrophysiol Pacing 1:166, 1983.
5. Butrous GS, Meldrum SJ, Barton DG, et al.: Effects of high-intensity power-frequency electric fields on implanted modern multiprogrammable cardiac pacemakers. J R Soc Med 75:327, 1982.
6. Butrous GS, Male JC, Webber RS, et al.: The effect of power frequency high intensity electric fields on implanted pacemakers. PACE 6:1282, 1983.
7. Furman S: Electromagnetic interference. PACE 5:1, 1982.
8. Irnich W: Interference in pacemakers. PACE 7:1021, 1984.
9. Irnich W, deBakker JMT, Bisping HJ: Electromagnetic interference in implantable pacemakers. PACE 1:52, 1978.
10. Irnich W, Barold SS: Interference protection in cardiac pacemakers. In Barold SS (ed.): Modern Cardiac Pacing, p. 839. Mt. Kisco, NY, Futura Publishing Co., 1985.
11. Sowton E, Gray K, Preston T: Electrical interference in non-competitive pacemakers. Br Heart J 32:626, 1970.
12. Kaye GC, Butrous GS, Allen A, et al.: The effect of 50 Hz. external electrical interference on implanted cardiac pacemakers. PACE 11:999, 1988.
13. Carleton RA, Sessions RW, Graettinger JS: Environmental influence on implantable cardiac pacemakers. JAMA 190:160, 1964.
14. Crystal RG, Kastor JA, DeSanctis RW: Inhibition of discharge of an external demand pacemaker by an electric razor. Am J Cardiol 27:695, 1977.
15. Elmqvist H: Pacemakers and external interference. Acta Med Scand 87(Suppl):596, 1976.
16. Furman S, Parker B, Krauthamer M, et al.: The influence of electromagnetic environment on the performance of artificial cardiac pacemakers. Ann Thorac Surg 6:90, 1968.
17. Furman S: Electric razor interference with cardiac pacemakers. JAMA 222:1658, 1972.
18. Bilitch M, Lau FVK, Cosby RS: Demand pacemaker inhibition by radio-frequency signals. Circulation 35(Suppl. 2):II–68, 1967.
19. Lichter I, Borrie J, Miller WM: Radio-frequency hazards with cardiac pacemakers. Br Med J 1:1513, 1965.
20. Meibom J, Andersen JD: Inhibition of demand pacemakers by leakage current from electrocardiographic recorder. Br Heart J 33:326, 1971.
21. Parker B, Furman S, Escher DJW: Input signals to pacemakers in a hospital environment. Ann NY Acad Sci 167:823, 1969.
22. Smyth NPD, Keshishian JM, Hood OC, et al.: Effect of an active magnetometer on permanently implanted pacemakers. JAMA 221:162, 1972.
23. Starmer CF, McIntosh HD, Whalen RE: Electrical hazards and cardiovascular function. N Engl J Med 284:181, 1971.
24. Walter WH, Mitchell JC, Rustan PL, et al.: Cardiac pulse generators and electromagnetic interference. JAMA 224:1628, 1973.
25. Walter WH III, Mitchell JC, Rustan P, et al.: Cardiac pulse generators and electromagnetic interference. JAMA 45:189, 1974.
26. King GR, Parsa F, Heller SJ, et al.: Effect of microwave oven on implanted cardiac pacemaker. JAMA 212:1213, 1970.
27. Medical News—Microwaves and Pacemakers. Just how well do they go together? JAMA 221:957, 1972.
28. Rustan PL, Hurt WD, Mitchell JC: Microwave oven interference with cardiac pacemakers. Med Instrum 7:185, 1973.
29. Hauser RG, Edwards LM, Stafford JL: Bipolar and unipolar sensing. Basic concepts and clinical applications. In Barold SS (ed.): Modern Cardiac Pacing, p. 137. Mt. Kisco, NY, Futura Publishing Co., 1985.

30. Berkovits BV: Advantages of bipolar over unipolar pacing. Medtronic News 15:5, 1985.
31. Baker RG, Falkenberg EN: Bipolar versus unipolar issues in DDD pacing. PACE 7:1178, 1984.
32. Castellanos A, Bloom MG, Sung RJ, et al.: Mode of operation induced by rapid external chest wall stimulation in patients with normally functioning QRS-inhibited (VVI) pacemakers. PACE 2:2, 1979.
33. Hewson JJ, Redding VJ: Correlation between interference response and noise reversion mechanism in VVI pacemakers. In Pérez Gómez F (ed.): Cardiac Pacing. Electrophysiology. Tachyarrhythmias, p. 1110. Mt. Kisco, NY, Futura Publishing Co., 1985.
34. Barold SS: Clinical significance of pacemaker refractory periods. Am J Cardiol 28:27, 1971.
35. AFP Model 283 Cardiac Pacing System, Technical Manual. Sylmar, CA, Pacesetter Systems, Inc., 1984.
36. Cosmos Models 283-01 and 284-02, and Galaxy Model 271-03, Technical Manuals. Freeport, TX, Intermedics, Inc., 1986.
37. Cordis Model 415A Gemini Automatic Universal DDD Cardiac Pacer, Technical Manual. Miami, FL, Cordis Corp., 1984.
38. Siemens 674 DDD Pulse Generator, Technical Manual. Solna, Sweden, Siemens-Elema AB, 1984.
39. Symbios 7005/7006 Universal A-V Telemetric Pacemaker, Technical Manual, Minneapolis, Medtronic, Inc., 1984.
40. Curry PVL, Rowland E, Krikler DM: Dual demand pacing for refractory atrioventricular reentry tachycardias. PACE 2:137, 1979.
41. Barold SS, Falkoff MD, Ryan GF, et al.: Multiprogrammable dual demand pulse generator for the treatment of supraventricular tachycardia. In Feruglio G (ed.): Cardiac Pacing. Electrophysiology and Pacemaker Technology, p. 283. Padova, Italy, Piccin Medical Books, 1982.
42. Falkoff MD, Ong LS, Heinle RA, et al.: The noise sampling period. A new cause of apparent sensing malfunction of demand pacemakers. PACE 1:250, 1978.
43. Barold SS, Falkoff MD, Ong LS, et al.: Timing cycles of DDD pacemakers. In Barold SS, Mugica J (eds.): New Perspectives in Cardiac Pacing, p. 69. Mt. Kisco, NY, Futura Publishing Co., 1988.
44. Fetter J, Hall DM, Hoff GL, et al.: The effects of myopotential interference on unipolar and bipolar dual chamber pacemakers in the DDD mode. Clin Prog Electrophysiol Pacing 3:368, 1985.
45. DelNegro A, Cohen A, Miller F, et al.: Automatic extension of the ventricular refractory period. A cause of sensing failure during tachycardia in dual-chamber pacemakers. PACE 9:304, 1986.
46. Fröhlig G, Dyckmans J, Doenecke P, et al.: Noise reversion of a dual chamber pacemaker without noise. PACE 9:690, 1986.
47. Schüller H, Fåhraeus T: Pacemaker electrocardiograms. An introduction to practical analysis, p. 116. Solna, Sweden, Siemens-Elema AB, 1983.
48. Sudduth BK, Morris DL, Gertz EW: Noise mode response at peak exercise in a DDD pacemaker. PACE 8:746, 1985.
49. VanMechelen R, Hart CT, DeBoer H: Failure to sense P waves during DDD pacing. PACE 9:498, 1986.
50. Belott PH, Sands S, Warren J: Resetting of DDD pulse generators due to EMI. PACE 7:169, 1984.
51. Levine PA, Balady GJ, Lazar HL, et al.: Electrocautery and pacemakers. Management of the paced patient subject to electrocautery. Ann Thorac Surg 41:313, 1986.
52. Lamas GA, Antman EM, Gold JP: Pacemaker backup mode reversion and injury during cardiac surgery. Ann Thorac Surg 41:155, 1986.
53. Sanders R, Barold SS: Understanding elective replacement indicators and automatic parameter conversion mechanisms in DDD pacemakers. In Barold SS, Mugica J (eds.): New Perspectives in Cardiac Pacing, p. 203. Mt. Kisco, NY, Futura Publishing Co., 1988.
54. Activitrax Models 8400/8402/8403 Technical Manual. Minneapolis, MN, Medtronic, Inc., 1986.
55. Delta Model 925 Technical Manual, Type DDD dual chamber pulse generator. St. Paul, MN, Cardiac Pacemakers, Inc., 1985.
56. Shapiro WA, Roizen MF, Singleton MA, et al.: Intraoperative pacemaker complications. Anesthesiology 63:319, 1985.
57. Fernando B, Emery RW, Copeland JG, et al.: Direct current cardioversion. Ann Thorac Surg 37:521, 1984.
58. Greene LF, Merideth J: Transurethral operations employing high frequency electrical currents in patients with demand cardiac pacemakers. J Urol 108:446, 1972.
59. Lerner SM: Suppression of a demand pacemaker by transurethral electrocautery. Anesth Analg 52:703, 1973.
60. McCormack J: Electrosurgical equipment and pacemakers: A potential hazard. Br Dent J 139:221, 1975.
61. O'Donoghue JK: Inhibition of a demand pacemaker by electrocautery. Chest 64:664, 1973.
62. Fein RL: Transurethral electrocautery procedures in patients with cardiac pacemakers. JAMA 202:7, 1967.
63. Smith R: Pacemaker malfunction from urethral electrocautery. JAMA 218:256, 1971.
64. Titel JH, El Etr AA: Fibrillation resulting from pacemaker electrodes and electrocautery during surgery. Anesthesiology 29:845, 1968.
65. Wajszczuk WJ, Mowry FM, Dugan NL: Deactivation of a demand pacemaker by transurethral electrocautery. N Engl J Med 280:34, 1969.
66. Hayes DL, Trusty J, Christiansen J, et al.: A prospective study of electrocautery's effect on pacemaker function. PACE 10 (Part II):686, 1987.
67. Goldberg ME, McSherry RT, O'Connor ME: Electrocautery and pacemaker reprogramming. Anesth Analg 63:541, 1984.
68. Erdman S, Levinsky L, Servadio C, et al.: Management of pacemaker patients while using electrocautery in surgical procedures. PACE 10 (Part II):672, 1987.
69. Batra YK, Bali IM: Effect of coagulating and cutting current on a demand pacemaker during transurethral resection of the prostate. A case report. Can Anaesth Soc J 25:65, 1978.
70. Geddes LA, Tacker WA, Cabler P: A new electrical hazard associated with the electrocautery. Med Instrum 9:112, 1975.
71. Recker S, Gebhart-Seehausen U, Merx W, et al.: The origin of ventricular fibrillation from pacemaker patients during electrocauterization. PACE 6 (Part II):A 54, 1983.
72. Orland HJ, Jones D: Cardiac pacemaker induced ventricular fibrillation during surgical diathermy. Anesth Intensive Care 3:321, 1975.
73. Protin F, Dodinot B, Lefevre JC, et al.: Interférences néfastes entre stimulation cardiaque prophylactique pré-opératoire et bistouri electrique. A propos d'une observation. Ann Anesth Fr 2:127, 1979.
74. Hungerbuhler RF, Swope J, Reves JG: Ventricular fibrillation associated with the electrocautery. A case report. JAMA 230:432, 1974.
75. Levine PA: Electrocautery and pacemakers (letter). PACE 7:925, 1984.
76. Shepard RV, Russo AG, Breland VC: Radiofrequency electrocoagulator hemostasis in chronically elevated pacing thresholds in cardiopulmonary bypass procedure patients. In Meere C (ed.): Proceedings of the VIth World Symposium on Cardiac Pacing, Chap. 35–2. PACESYMP, Montreal, 1979.
77. Dehumeau A, Ronceray S, Moreau X, et al.: Arrêt définitif d'un stimulateur cardiaque après utilisation du bistouri électrique (irreversible damage to a pacemaker by electrocautery). Ann Fr Anesth Reanim 7:162, 1988.
78. Byrd CL, Schwartz SJ, Byrd CB, et al.: Electrocautery and dual chamber cardiac pacemakers. PACE 11 (June Suppl):854, 1988.
79. Caramella JP, Mentre B, Jattiot F, et al.: Reprogrammation d'un stimulateur cardiaque induite pas le bistouri électrique. Ann Fr Anesth Reanim 6:214, 1987.
80. Domino KB, Smith TC: Electrocautery-induced reprogramming of a pacemaker using a precordial magnet. Anesth Analg 62:609, 1983.
81. Richard JP, Conil JM, Antonini A, et al.: Interaction entre bistouri électrique et stimulateur cardiaque. Ann Fr Anesth Reanim 5:72, 1986.
82. Dresner DL, Lebowitz PW: AV sequential pacemaker inhibition by transurethral electrosurgery. Anesthesiology 68:599, 1988.
83. Barold SS, Falkoff MD, Ong LS, et al.: Resetting of DDD pulse generators due to cold exposure. PACE 11:736, 1988.
84. Irnich W: Electrosurgery in pacemaker patients. PACE 10 (Part II):691, 1987.

85. Zaidan JR: Pacemakers. Anesthesiology 60:319, 1984.
86. Parsonnet V, Furman S, Smith NPA, et al.: Optimal resources for implantable cardiac pacemakers. Special report by the intersociety commission for heart disease resources. Circulation 68:226A, 1983.
87. Owen PM: The effects of external defibrillation on permanent pacemakers. Heart Lung 12:274, 1983.
88. Furman S: External defibrillation and implanted cardiac pacemakers. PACE 4:485, 1981.
89. Aylwards P, Blood R, Tonkin A: Complications of defibrillation with permanent pacemaker in situ. PACE 1:1514, 1978.
90. Levine PA, Barold SS, Fletcher RD, et al.: Adverse acute and chronic effects of electrical defibrillation and cardioversion on implanted unipolar cardiac pacing systems. J Am Coll Cardiol 1:1413, 1983.
91. Giedwoyn JO: Pacemaker failure following external defibrillation. Circulation 44:293, 1971.
92. Gould L, Patel S, Gomes GI, et al.: Pacemaker failure following external defibrillation. PACE 4:575, 1981.
93. Hauser RG, McKeever WP, Sweeny MB, et al.: Clinical pulse generator malfunction after DC countershock. In Meere C (ed.): Proceedings of the VIth World Symposium on Cardiac Pacing, Chap. 35-5. PACESYMP, Montreal, 1979.
94. Lau FYK, Bilitch M, Wintraub HJ: Protection of implanted pacemakers from excessive electrical energy of DC shock. Am J Cardiol 23:244, 1969.
95. Palac RT, Hwang MH, Klodnycky ML, et al.: Delayed pulse generator malfunction after DC countershock. PACE 4:163, 1981.
96. Fontaine G, Touil F, Frank R, et al.: Defibrillation, fulguration et cardioversion effets sur les pacemakers. Stimucoeur 12:91, 1984.
97. Das G, Eaton J: Pacemaker malfunction following transthoracic countershock. PACE 4:487, 1981.
98. Levine PA, Seltzer JP, Barold SS: Adverse interaction between cardiac pacing systems and defibrillation. PACE 6:315, 1983.
99. Levine PA: Effect of cardioversion and defibrillation on implanted cardiac pacemakers. In Barold SS (ed.): Modern Cardiac Pacing, p. 875. Mt. Kisco, NY, Futura Publishing Co., 1985.
100. Warner ED, Dahl C, Ewy GA: Myocardial injury from transthoracic defibrillation countershock. Arch Path 99:55, 1975.
101. Barold SS, Ong LS, Scovil J, et al.: Reprogramming of an implanted pacemaker following external defibrillation. PACE 1:514, 1978.
102. Wehr M, Schmitt CG, Kohler F, et al.: Abnormal pacing following defibrillation. Exit block after micro-dislocation of the electrode. Z Kardiol 12:840, 1980.
103. Taube MA, Elsberry DD, Exworthy KW: Physiological effects of DC defibrillation on pacemaker function. In Meere C (ed.): Proceedings of the VIth World Symposium on Cardiac Pacing, Chap. 35-6. PACESYMP, Montreal, 1979.
104. Dahl CF, Ewy GA, Warner ED, et al.: Myocardial necrosis from direct current countershock. Effect of paddle size and time interval between discharges. Circulation 50:956, 1974.
105. Reiter MJ, Lindenfeld J, Breckinridge S, et al.: Does defibrillation raise the ventricular pacing threshold? (Abstract). J Am Coll Cardiol 11:144A, 1988.
106. Yee R, Jones DL, Klein GJ: Pacing threshold changes after transvenous catheter countershock. Am J Cardiol 53:503, 1984.
107. Yee R, Jones DL, Jarvis E, et al.: Changes in pacing threshold and R wave amplitude after transvenous catheter countershock. J Am Coll Cardiol 4:543, 1984.
108. Kallok MJ, Wibel FH, Bourland JD, et al.: Catheter electrode defibrillation in dogs. Threshold dependence on implant time and catheter stability. Am Heart J 109:821, 1985.
109. Barker-Voeltz MA, VanVleet JF, Tacker WA, et al.: Alterations induced by a single defibrillating shock applied through chronically implanted catheter electrode. J Electrocardiol 16:167, 1983.
110. Rubin L, Hudson P, Driller J, et al.: Effect of defibrillation on pacing threshold. Med Instrum 17:15, 1983.
111. Winkle RA, Bach SM, Mead HR, et al.: Comparison of defibrillation efficacy in humans using a new catheter and superior vena cava spring–left ventricular patch electrodes. J Am Coll Cardiol 11:365, 1988.
112. Fontaine G, Lemoine B, Frank R, et al.: Effects of fulguration on the permanent pacemaker. In Fontaine G, Scheinman MM: Ablation in Cardiac Arrhythmias, p. 365. Mt. Kisco, NY, Futura Publishing Co., 1987.
113. Drummer E, Maloney JD, Castle LW, et al.: Catheter ablation of the atrioventricular conduction system to treat patients with atrial tachyarrhythmias including patients with pacemakers. Cleve Clin Q 53:151, 1986.
114. Bowes RJ: Atrioventricular nodal fulguration in the presence of an implanted pacemaker. J Electrophysiol 1:127, 1987.
115. Bowes RJ, Bennett DH: Effect of transvenous atrioventricular nodal ablation on the function of implanted pacemakers. PACE 8:811, 1985.
116. Nathan AW, Bennett DH, Ward DE, et al.: Catheter ablation of atrioventricular conduction. Lancet 1:1280, 1984.
117. Singer I, Guarnieri T, Kupersmith J: Implanted automatic defibrillators. Effects of drugs and pacemakers. PACE 11:2250, 1988.
118. Kim SG, Furman S, Waspe LE, et al.: Unipolar pacer artifacts induced failure of an automatic implantable cardioverter/defibrillator to detect ventricular fibrillation. Am J Cardiol 57:880, 1986.
119. Bardy GH, Ivey TD, Stewart R, et al.: Failure of the automatic implantable defibrillator to detect ventricular fibrillation. Am J Cardiol 58:1107, 1986.
120. Chapman PD, Troup P: The automatic implantable cardioverter-defibrillator. Evaluating suspected inappropriate shocks. J Am Coll Cardiol 7:1075, 1986.
121. Cohen AI, Wish MH, Fletcher RD, et al.: The use and interaction of permanent pacemakers and the automatic implantable cardioverter defibrillator. PACE 11:704, 1988.
122. Platia EV, Watkins L Jr, Mower MM, et al.: Automatic implantable defibrillators. In Platia EV (ed.): Management of Cardiac Arrhythmias: The nonpharmacologic approach, p. 272. Philadelphia, J B Lippincott Co., 1987.
123. Winkle RA, Stinson ED, Echt DS, et al.: Practical aspects of automatic cardioverter defibrillator implantation. Am Heart J 108:1335, 1984.
124. Kim SG, Furman S, Matos JA, et al.: Automatic implantable cardioverter/defibrillator. Inadvertent discharges during permanent pacemaker magnet tests. PACE 10:579, 1987.
125. Gottlieb C, Miller M, Rosenthal ME, et al.: Automatic implantable defibrillator discharge resulting from routine pacemaker programming. PACE 11:336, 1988.
126. DaTorre S, Bondke H, Brinker J, et al.: Increased pacing threshold after an automatic defibrillator shock: Effects of antiarrhythmic drugs. Circulation 76(Suppl. IV):IV–310, 1987.
127. Guanieri T, Datorre SD, Bondke H, et al.: Increased pacing threshold after an automatic defibrillator shock in dogs. Effect of Class I and Class II antiarrhythmic drugs. PACE 11:1324, 1988.
128. Platia EV, Griffith LSC, Reid RR, et al.: Post-defibrillation bradycardia following implantable defibrillator discharge. J Am Coll Cardiol 7:144A, 1986.
129. Slepian M, Levine JH, Watkins L Jr, et al.: Automatic implantable cardioverter defibrillator/permanent pacemaker interaction. Loss of pacemaker capture following AICD discharge. PACE 10:1194, 1987.
130. Hillenstrand KJ, Nathan AW, Bexton RS, et al.: Electrophysiologic effects of flecainide acetate on sinus node function anomalous atrioventricular connections and pacemaker thresholds. Am J Cardiol 53:308, 1984.
131. Ruffy R, Lal R, Kouchoukos NT, et al.: Combined bipolar dual chamber pacing and automatic implantable cardioverter/defibrillator. J Am Coll Cardiol 7:933, 1986.
132. Lüderitz B, Gerckens U, Manz M: Automatic implantable cardioverter/defibrillator (AICD) and antitachycardia pacemaker (Tachylog). Combined use in ventricular tachyarrhythmias. PACE 9(Part II):1356, 1986.
133. Manz M, Gerckens U, Funke HD, et al.: Combination of antitachycardia pacemaker and automatic implantable cardioverter defibrillator for ventricular tachycardia. PACE 9:676, 1986.
134. Adamec R, Haefliger JM, Killisch JP, et al.: Damaging effect of therapeutic radiation on programmable pacemakers. PACE 5:146, 1982.

135. Blamires NH, Myatt J: X-ray effects on pacemaker type circuits. PACE 5:151, 1982.
136. Calfee RF: Therapeutic radiation and pacemakers. PACE 5:160, 1982.
137. Glace C: Influence of ionizing radiation on pacemaker circuits. Stimucoeur Med 11:29, 1983.
138. Glace C, Dodinot B, Godenir JP: Influence of ionizing radiation on pacemaker circuits. In Feruglio GA (ed.): Cardiac Pacing. Electrophysiology and Pacemaker Technology, p. 935. Padova, Italy, Piccin Medical Books, 1982.
139. Hardage ML, Marbach JR, Winsor DW: The pacemaker patient in the therapeutic and diagnostic device environment. In Barold SS (ed.): Modern Cardiac Pacing, p. 857. Mt. Kisco, NY, Futura Publishing Co., 1985.
140. Katzenberg CA, Marcus FI, Heusinkveld RS, et al.: Pacemaker failure due to radiation therapy. PACE 5:156, 1982.
141. Lee RW, Huang SK, Mechling E, et al.: Runaway atrioventricular sequential pacemaker after radiation therapy. Am J Med 81:833, 1986.
142. Lewin AA, Serago CF, Schwade JG, et al.: Radiation induced failure of complementary metal oxide pacemakers. A potentially lethal complication. Int J Radiat Oncol Biol Phys 10:1967, 1984.
143. Maxted KJ: The effects of therapeutic X-radiation on a sample of pulse generators. Phys Med Biol 29:1143, 1984.
144. Marbach JR, Meoz-Mendez RT, Huffman JK, et al.: The effects on cardiac pacemakers of ionizing radiation and electromagnetic interference from radiotherapy machines. Int J Radiat Oncol Biol Phys 4:1055, 1978.
145. Pourhamidi AH: Radiation effect on implanted pacemakers. Chest 84:499, 1983.
146. Quertermonus T, Megahy SM, DasGupta DS, et al.: Pacemaker failure resulting from radiation damage. Radiology 145:257, 1983.
147. Shehata WM, Daoud GL, Meyer RL: Radiotherapy for patients with cardiac pacemakers. Possible risks. PACE 9:919, 1986.
148. Venselaar JLM: The effects of ionizing radiation on eight cardiac pacemakers and the influence of electromagnetic interference from two linear accelerators. Radiother Oncol 3:81, 1985.
149. Venselaar JLM, VanKerkoerle HLMJ, Vet AJTM: Radiation damage to pacemakers from radiotherapy. PACE 10:538, 1987.
150. Agarwal A, Hewson J, Redding VJ: Pacemaker patients and NMR imaging. PACE 11 (June Supplement):853, 1988.
151. Chauvin M, Baruthio J, Wolff F, et al.: Influences de la résonance magnétique nucléaire sur les stimulateurs cardiaques implantables. Stimucoeur 14:205, 1986.
152. Erlebacher JA, Cahill PT, Pannizo F, et al.: Effect of magnetic resonance imaging on DDD pacemakers. Am J Cardiol 57:437, 1986.
153. Fetter J, Aram G, Holmes DR Jr, et al.: The effects of nuclear magnetic resonance imagers on external and implantable pulse generators. PACE 7:720, 1984.
154. Holmes DR, Hayes DL, Gray JE, et al.: The effects of magnetic resonance imaging on implantable pulse generators. PACE 9:360, 1986.
155. Hayes DL, Holmes DR Jr, Gray JE: Effect of 1.5 Tesla nuclear magnetic resonance imaging scanner on implanted permanent pacemakers. J Am Coll Cardiol 10:782, 1987.
156. Pavlicek W, Geisinger M, Castle L, et al.: The effects of nuclear magnetic resonance on patients with cardiac pacemakers. Radiology 147:149, 1983.
157. Zimmerman BH, Faul DD: Artifacts and hazards in NMR imaging due to metal implants and cardiac pacemakers. Diagn Imaging Clin Med 53:53, 1984.
158. Webb CR, Lynch JS, Littleton RH, et al.: Effects of extracorporeal shock wave lithotripsy on cardiac pacemakers. PACE 10:444, 1987.
159. Cooper D, Wilkoff B, Masterson M, et al.: Effects of extracorporeal shock wave lithotripsy on cardiac pacemakers and its safety in patients with implanted cardiac pacemakers. PACE 11:1607, 1988.
160. Fetter J, Hayes D, Aram G, et al.: Electrohydraulic shock wave lithotripsy effects on cardiac pulse generators. PACE 10:674, 1987.
161. Langberg J, Aber J, Thuroff JW, et al.: The effects of extracorporeal shock wave lithotripsy on pacemaker function. PACE 10:1142, 1987.
162. Markewitz A, Weber W, Wildgans H, et al.: Does extracorporeal shock wave lithotripsy affect pacemaker function? PACE 10(Part II):711, 1987.
163. Steinbeck G, Lehman P, Weber W, et al.: Cardiac pacing and induction of arrhythmias by extracorporeal shock wave lithotripsy. PACE 10(Part II):711, 1987.
164. Garza J, Tansey M, Florio J, et al.: The effect of extracorporeal shock wave lithotripsy in implantable cardiac pacemakers. PACE 10(Part II):675, 1987.
165. Irnich W, Lazica M, Gleissner M: Pacemaker patients and extracorporeal shock wave lithotripsy. In Belhassen B, Feldman S, Cooperman Y (eds.): Cardiac Pacing and Electrophysiology. Proceedings of the VIIIth World Symposium on Cardiac Pacing and Electrophysiology, p. 221. Jerusalem, R&L Creative Communications, 1987.
166. Feldman RM: The use of diathermy in the presence of metal implants and cardiac pacemakers. Can Med Assoc J 122:276, 1980.
167. Effert S, Irnich W: Schrittmacherrasen unter holchfrequenztherapie. Dtsch Med Wochenschr 102:909, 1977.
168. Erikson M, Schüller H, Sjölund B: Hazards from transcutaneous stimulation in patients with pacemakers. Lancet 1:1319, 1978.
169. LaBan MM, Petty D, Hauser AM, et al.: Peripheral nerve conduction stimulation. Its effects on cardiac pacemakers. Arch Phys Med Rehabil 69:358, 1988.
170. Rasmussen MJ, Hayes DL, Vliestra RE, et al.: Can transcutaneous electrical nerve stimulation be safely used in patients with permanent cardiac pacemakers? Mayo Clin Proc 63:443, 1988.
171. Jones SL: Electromagnetic field interference and cardiac pacemakers. Phys Ther 56:1013, 1976.
172. Ross C, Black C, Ormerod D, et al.: The use of transcutaneous nerve stimulation (TENS) in the relief of post-op pain in patients receiving a pacemaker by thoracotomy. PACE 3:385, 1980.
173. Aida H, Shimiza T, Fukunaga T: Susceptibility of unipolar demand pacemakers to electromagnetic interference (EMI). PACE 6:A-55, 1983.
174. Wicks JM, Davison R, Belic N: Malfunction of a demand pacemaker caused by phrenic nerve stimulation. Chest 74:303, 1978.
175. Volosin KJ, Dworkin G, Greenberg RM, et al.: Use of external muscle stimulation in a patient with a unipolar DDD pacemaker. PACE 10:958, 1987.
176. Fujiwara H, Taniguchi K, Takeuchi J, et al.: The influence of low frequency acupuncture on demand pacemakers. Chest 78:96, 1980.
177. Hepburn F: Effects of transient magnetic fields on simple demand pacemakers. In Feruglio G (ed.): Cardiac Pacing. Electrophysiology and Pacemaker Technology, p. 923. Padova, Italy, Piccin Medical Books, 1982.
178. Sinnaeve A, Willems R, Stroobandt R: Inhibition of on demand pacemakers by magnet waving. PACE 5:878, 1982.
179. Sakadamis G, Pagonis A, Boudonas G, et al.: The magnetic field changes influence on pacemaker function. PACE 10(Part II):737, 1987.
180. Thorman J, Schwarz F, Ensslen R: Evaluation of implanted faulty demand pacemakers by magnet waving and electrical chest wall stimulation. Eur J Cardiol 5:139, 1977.
181. Voukydis PC, Shulman AN, Cohen SI: Unmasking of slow intrinsic ventricular excitation by magnet inhibition of R wave inhibited demand pacemakers. Chest 67:304, 1975.
182. Sheares R, Wenger NK: The case of the incorrect magnet. Am J Cardiol 62:171, 1988.
183. Latif P, Ewy GA: Temporary inhibition of permanently implanted pacemakers. Circulation 55:27, 1977.
184. Barold SS, Falkoff MD, Ong LS, et al.: Paradoxical induction of endless loop tachycardia by magnet application over a DDD pacemaker. PACE 9:503, 1986.
185. Hardage, Barold SS: Pacemaker programming techniques. In Barold SS, Mugica J (eds.): The Third Decade of Cardiac Pacing. Advances in Technology and Clinical Applications, p. 1. Mt. Kisco, NY, Futura Publishing Co., 1982.

186. Belott PH: Clinical experience with over 250 DDD pacemakers. *In* Barold SS (ed.): Modern Cardiac Pacing, p. 439. Mt. Kisco, NY, Futura Publishing Co., 1985.
187. Barold SS, Falkoff MD, Ong LS, et al.: Differential diagnosis of pacemaker pauses with new observations on triboelectric inhibition of demand pacemakers. *In* Meere C (ed.): Proceedings of the VIth World Symposium on Cardiac Pacing, Chapter 18–1. PACESYMP, Montreal, 1979.
188. Gibson TC, Leaman DM, Devors J, et al.: Pacemaker function in relation to electroconvulsive therapy. Chest 63:1025, 1973.
189. Blitt CD, Kirschrink LJ: Electroconvulsive therapy with a cardiac pacemaker. Anaesthesiology 45:580, 1976.
190. Alexopoulos GS, Frances RJ: ECT and cardiac patients with pacemakers. Am J Psychiatry 137:1111, 1980.
191. Abiuso P, Dunkelman R, Proper M: Electroconvulsive therapy in patients with pacemakers. JAMA 240:2459, 1978.
192. Adams D, Fulford N, Beechy J, et al.: The cardiac pacemaker and ultrasonic scalers. Br Dental J 152:171, 1982.
193. Rahn R, Zegelman M, Kreuzer J: The influence of dental treatment on the Activitrax. PACE 11(June Suppl):852, 1988.

36

Interference in Cardiac Pacemakers: Endogenous Sources

S. Serge Barold
Michael D. Falkoff
Ling S. Ong
Robert A. Heinle

MYOPOTENTIALS

Wirzfeld and coworkers[1] first described the inhibition of unipolar demand pulse generators by skeletal muscle potentials in 1972. Many reports have since documented this form of inhibition in unipolar single- and dual-chamber pacemakers, with an incidence varying from 12 to 85%.[1-20] No unipolar pacemaker is totally immune to myopotential oversensing (Fig. 36–1). The advent of unipolar dual-chamber pacemakers and the need for high sensitivity to sense atrial activity have not reduced the incidence of myopotential oversensing seen with earlier generations of unipolar single chamber pacemakers.[9, 12-20] In our pacemaker clinic, myopotential interference can be demonstrated in about 50% of patients with unipolar pulse generators by a variety of isometric exercise maneuvers involving pushing and pulling, although inhibition may not be consistently reproducible. A small percentage of our patients are actually symptomatic from this type of interference. Probably only 10% of patients with demonstrable myopotential inhibition will be symptomatic and require an intervention such as reprogramming.

The varying incidence of myopotential inhibition reported in the literature may be related to implantation technique, different characteristics of sensing circuits, programmed sensitivity, size and type of pulse generator, coating, method of provocation or detection, and patient population. Myopotential signals may vary according to the patient, proximity of the pacemaker to the active muscle group, site of implant, and depth of the pocket. The amplitude of myopotential signals decreases rapidly with distance and is also influenced by fatigue occurring during the testing procedure.[9] Myopotential inhibition occurs rarely, under special circumstances, in bipolar pacing systems.

Two relatively recent reports serve as reminders that the myopotential problem still exists with contemporary pacemakers. On routine testing, Levine and associates[6] found myopotential inhibition in 33% of patients with unipolar pacemakers, who were totally paced, with a range of 10 to 70% depending on the pacemaker model. They claimed that presyncopal symptoms had occurred in 50% of these patients, but were not mentioned before testing because they were transient and believed to be inconsequential. Dizziness and lightheadedness are frequent symptoms in the elderly, and we wonder whether these so-called "presyncopal" symptoms can be correlated with the presence of myopotential interference. In an evaluation of the performance of 228 unipolar pacing systems by Secemsky and colleagues,[10] 86 patients (38%) exhibited oversensing of myopotentials with pectoral muscle exercises or 24-hour Holter recordings or both. Twelve of these 86 patients (14%), or about 5% of all patients, had symptoms ranging from mild dizziness to syncope during one or more episodes of myocardial inhibition, and 7 required corrective action.

Effects of Myopotential Interference

SINGLE-CHAMBER PACEMAKERS

Myopotential interference may cause various combinations of over- and undersensing. Pacemaker pauses

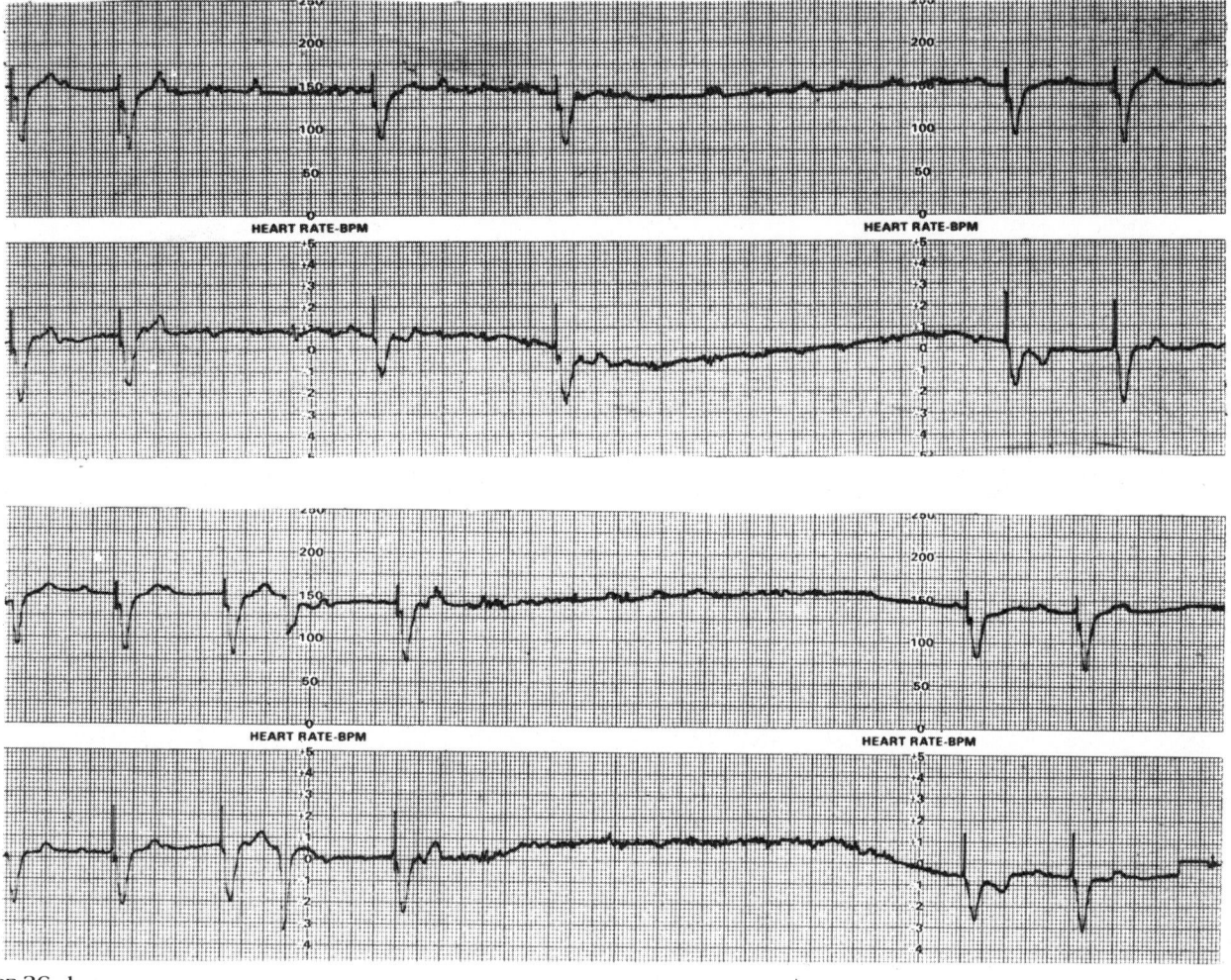

FIGURE 36–1
Representative tracings from a two-channel Holter recording showing marked myopotential inhibition in a unipolar VVI pulse generator in a patient who presented with near-syncope. The pauses were eliminated by reducing the sensitivity of the pacemaker. (Reprinted by permission of Futura Publishing Co., Inc., from Barold SS, et al.: In Barold SS (ed.): Modern Cardiac Pacing, pp. 587–613. Mt. Kisco, NY, Futura Publishing Co., 1985.)

due to oversensing may occasionally be accompanied by periods of undersensing as a consequence of oversensing rather than of pacemaker malfunction or an electrographic signal below the sensitivity of the pulse generator. This type of undersensing is caused by one of two mechanisms:

1. A sensed signal generates a new pacemaker refractory period. If a spontaneous signal (for example, a QRS complex) then falls within the newly generated refractory period, undersensing may occur.[21, 22]
2. Repetitive signals may cause reversion of the pacemaker to its interference (noise) asynchronous mode.[23]

The reversion circuit depends on continuous and rapid sensing of myopotentials for the conversion to the asynchronous interference (noise) mode (Figs. 36–2 and 36–3). Reversion to the interference (noise) mode of unipolar rate-responsive pacemakers (VVIR) may produce a complex response (Fig. 36–4). If the amplitude of myopotential signals is rapidly changing, sensing may be intermittent and the sensed rate may not exceed the reversion limit. In such a case, inhibition occurs rather than asynchronous pacing. The reversion circuit does not always safeguard the pulse generator from continuous inhibition.

DDD PACING

The amplitude of myopotential signals is similar on the atrial and ventricular channels because the myopotentials may be assumed to arise from the same pectoral site. According to the programmed atrial and ventricular sensitivities, the following manifestations may occur:

1. Inhibition of the ventricular channel.
2. Sensing by the atrial channel with consequent triggering of a ventricular output and an increase in the pacing rate. This pacemaker tachycardia is usually irregular, but it may be regular and occur often at or near the programmed upper rate of the pulse generator (Figs. 36–5 and 36–6). During DDD

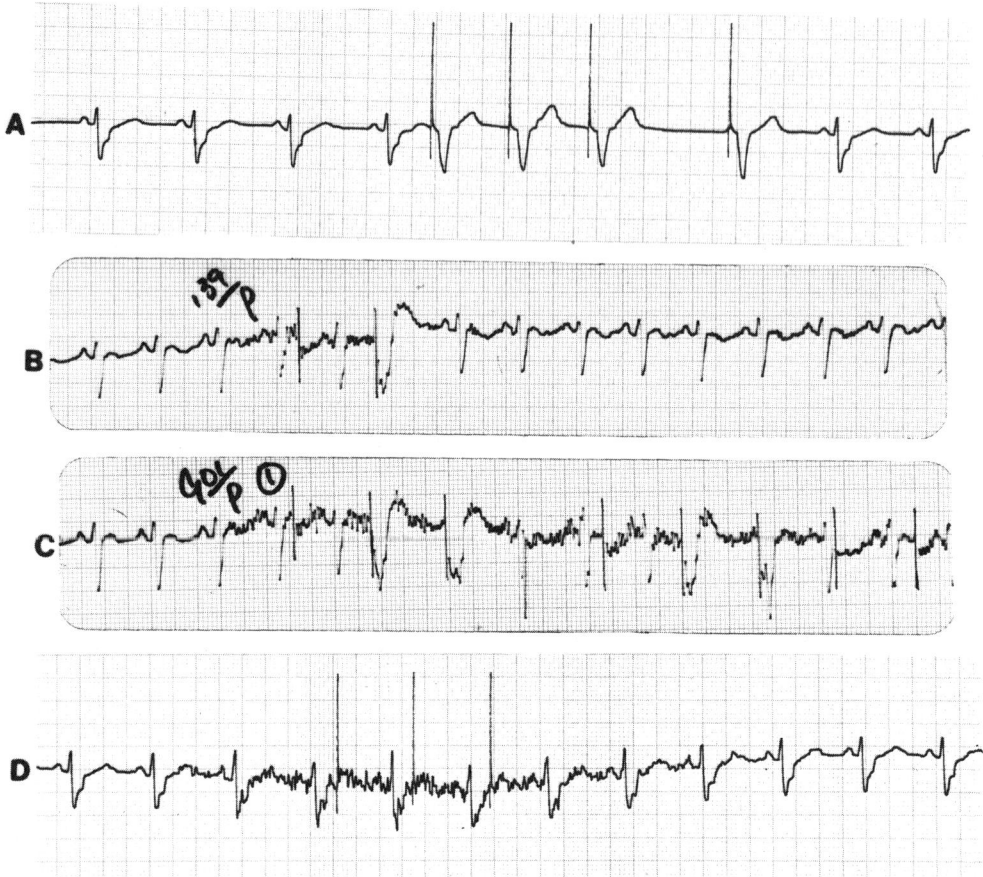

FIGURE 36-2
Undersensing secondary to oversensing by a unipolar Cyberlith (Intermedics) multiprogrammable pulse generator. The pacemaker was implanted in a patient with complete AV block secondary to an acute anteroseptal myocardial infarction. The largest obtainable endocardial signal measured 2 mV. The sensitivity of the pacemaker was programmed to 0.8 mV and the rate to 50/min.

A, Momentary application of the magnet yields the faster magnetic rate of 90/min. Upon withdrawal of the magnet, the spike-to-spike interval lengthens to 1200 ms, corresponding to the programmed rate of 50/min. B and C, Representative rhythm strips from 24-hour Holter recording showing undersensing secondary to oversensing of skeletal myopotentials. Oversensing of myopotentials (note disturbance of baseline) causes reversion to the VOO interference mode at the faster magnet rate of 90/min. D, This response was reproduced in the pacemaker clinic with isometric exercise only at sensitivities of 0.6 and 0.8 mV.

(Reprinted by permission of Futura Publishing Co., Inc., from Barold SS, et al.: In Barold SS, Mugica J (eds.): The Third Decade of Cardiac Pacing, pp. 27-76. Mt. Kisco, NY, Futura Publishing Co., 1982.)

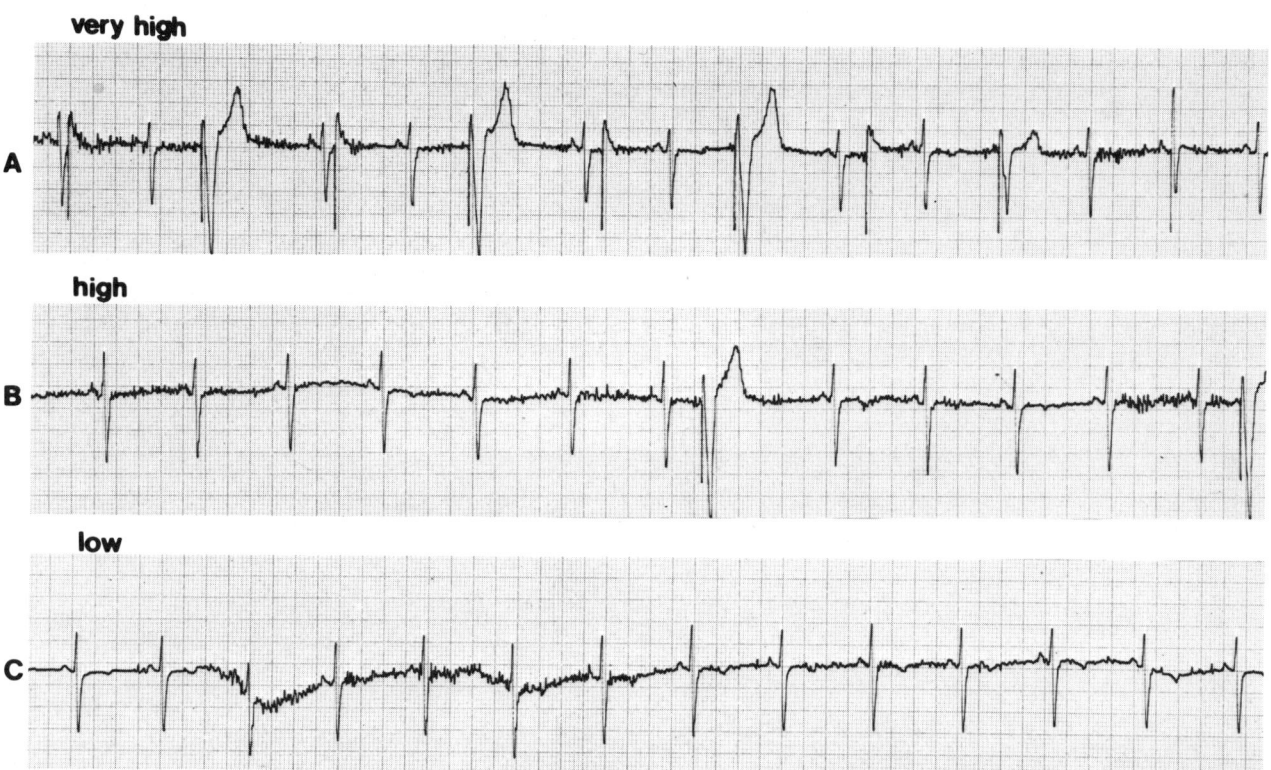

FIGURE 36–3
Undersensing secondary to oversensing by a Siemens-Elema 668 unipolar multiprogrammable pulse generator. The unipolar electrogram exceeded 12 mV. A 24-hour Holter recording revealed periods of undersensing with stimuli falling on the T wave when the sensitivity was programmed at the high setting (selection consists of very high, high, low, and very low, as well as asynchronous mode).

A, When the sensitivity was programmed to the very high setting (most sensitive), isometric exercise produced long periods of asynchronous pacing at the programmed lower rate of 50/min. Sensed myopotentials restart a complete refractory period. The overlapping refractory periods cause reversion to the interference mode at the programmed lower rate of 50/min.

B, At high sensitivity setting (less sensitive than A), isometric exercise caused intermittent undersensing. The unsensed QRS complexes are secondary to oversensing of myopotentials.

C, At the lower sensitivity setting (less sensitive than B), isometric exercise does not cause oversensing of myopotentials and there is no resultant undersensing. Note the apparent paradox of undersensing in B (at the high sensitivity setting) being corrected by reprogramming to a lower sensitivity in C.

(Reprinted by permission of Futura Publishing Co., Inc., from Barold SS, et al.: *In* Barold SS, Mugica J (eds.): The Third Decade of Cardiac Pacing, pp. 27–76. Mt. Kisco, NY, Futura Publishing Co., 1982.)

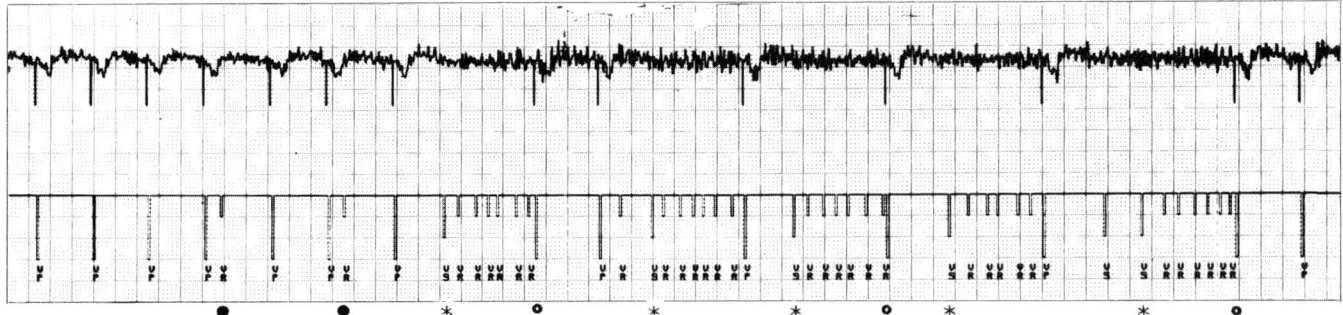

FIGURE 36-4
Myopotential oversensing by a Medtronic Activitrax 8403 unipolar VVIR pulse generator (lower rate = 70 ppm; upper rate = 150 ppm). The ECG (top) was recorded simultaneously with a real-time marker channel. In the following discussion, VP = ventricular paced event; VS = ventricular sensed event; VR = ventricular sensed event in the noise sampling (refractory) period.

The open circles represent a VP event without a corresponding VP printout by the marker channel because of its close proximity to the preceding VR printout. The pacing rate is faster than the programmed lower rate because pressure from the programming head applied over the pulse generator increases the pacing rate. This mimics pacemaker behavior during activity. The total refractory period of 225 ms consists of the absolute refractory period and the noise-sampling period (125 ms). When myopotential oversensing occurs in the noise-sampling (refractory) period (VR), the pulse generator exhibits partial recycling, so that the escape interval initiated by VR (solid circles) is shorter than the sensor-driven VP-VP interval. Actually the VP-VP intervals containing the sensed VR signal (solid circles) lengthen only by 80 ms. Each asterisk represents a VS signal initiating an escape interval that terminates with a VP event so that the VS-VP interval is now equal to the programmed lower rate interval rather than the sensor-driven VP-VP interval (interference or noise rate = programmed lower rate). This is related to the continual sensing of myopotential signals (VR) in the noise-sampling period. Each VR event reinitiates a complete refractory period (i.e., absolute refractory and noise-sampling period), thereby forcing the pulse generator to deliver VP at the end of its programmed lower rate interval.

This tracing illustrates the following points: (1) The concept of overlapping refractory periods as a response to interference; (2) partial recycling of the Activitrax VVIR pulse generator whenever a signal (VR) is sensed within the noise sampling period when the pacing rate is sensor-driven; (3) reversion to asynchronous pacing occurs at the interference or lower rate and not at the prevailing sensor-driven rate at any given time; (4) the valuable information provided by the real-time marker channel in the evaluation of pacemaker function.

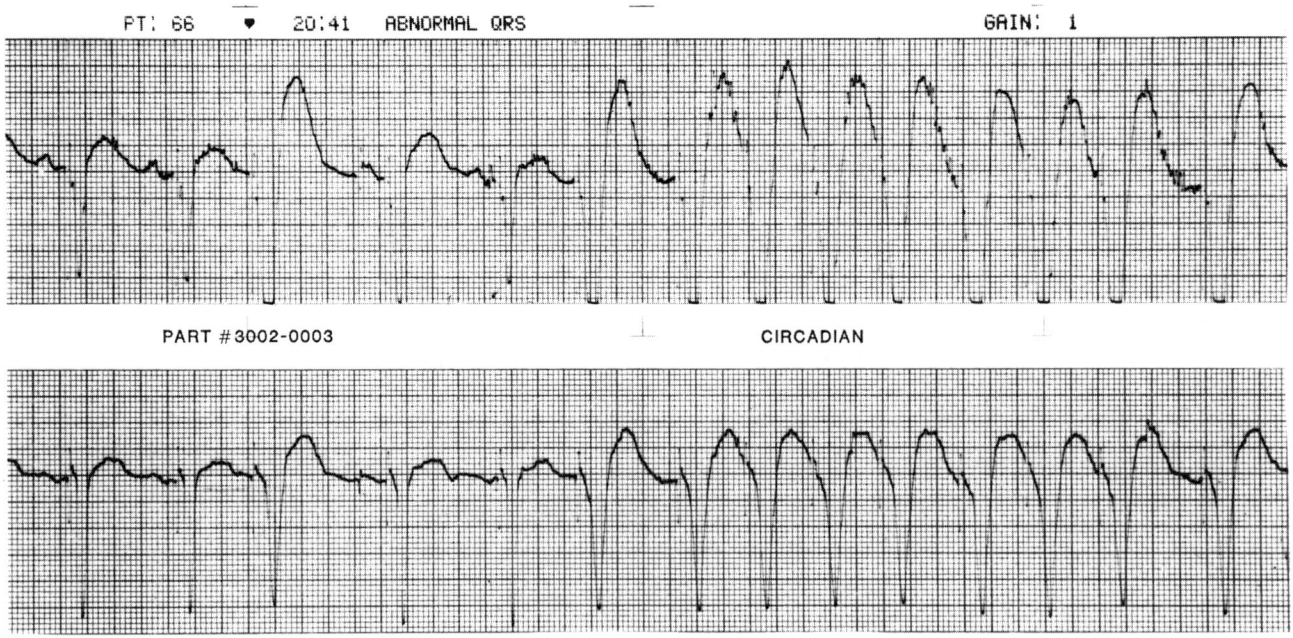

FIGURE 36-5
Two-channel Holter recording in a patient with an Intermedics Cosmos unipolar DDD pulse generator. The patient complained of palpitations. Programmed parameters: lower rate = 60 ppm (1000 ms); upper rate = 125 ppm (480 ms); AV interval = 250 ms; postventricular atrial refractory period = 200 ms; atrial sensitivity = 0.8 mV; ventricular sensitivity = 4 mV. An irregular pacemaker tachycardia is present. The differential diagnosis includes myopotential triggering, atrial fibrillation, and false signals from a defective atrial electrode.

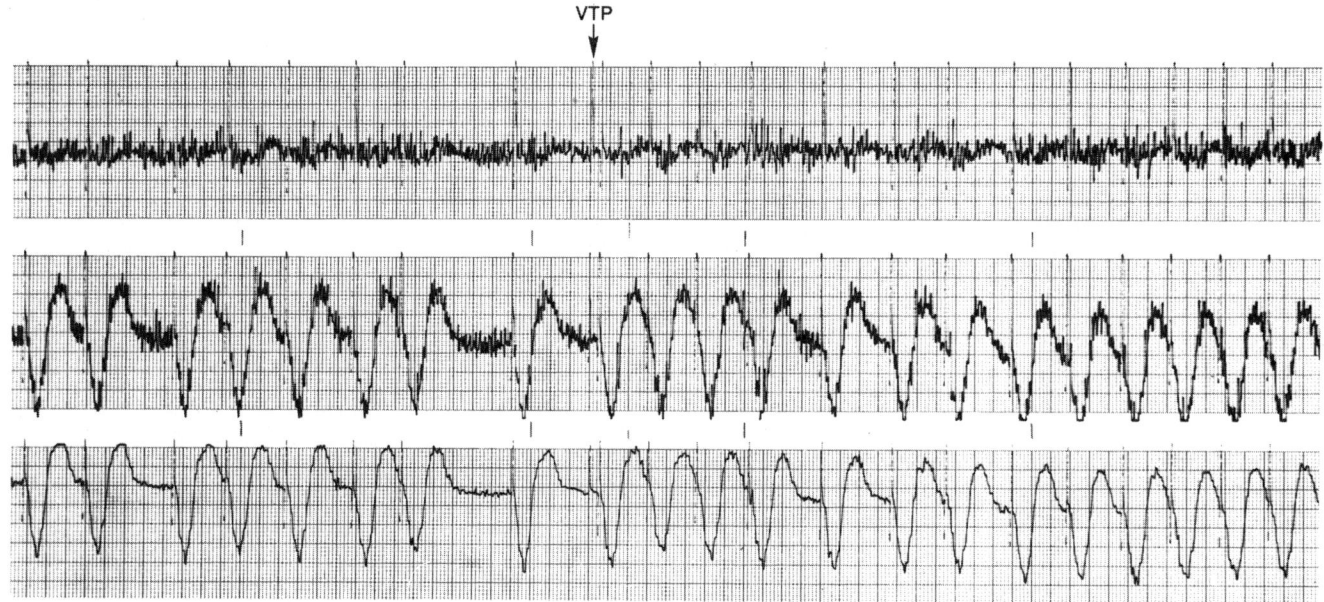

FIGURE 36–6
Same patient as in Figure 36–5 with identical programmed settings. Myopotential sensing was deliberately induced by isometric pectoral exercise. Myopotential sensing by the atrial channel triggers ventricular pacing at a rapid and irregular rate. Myopotential signals are also sensed by the ventricular channel because the interval between the 7th and the 8th ventricular paced beats lengthens to approximately 1120 ms (longer than the lower rate interval of 1000 ms). At the arrow, myopotential signals are sensed by the ventricular electrode within the ventricular safety pacing period (ventricular triggering period=VTP), with resultant abbreviation of the AV interval to 100 ms. Myopotential oversensing was still present when the atrial sensitivity was decreased to 2 mV, but absent at 2.4 mV. Consistent P wave sensing was present when the sensitivity of the atrial channel was decreased to 2.8 mV. Consequently the atrial sensitivity was left at 2.4 mV. At this new setting, myopotential triggering could not be induced. Repeat Holter recordings demonstrated normal P wave sensing and the absence of myopotential triggering.

pacing, rapid ventricular pacing may cause uncomfortable palpitations, angina, dyspnea, and hypotension if rapid pacing occurs for more than a brief period.
3. Mixed response of alternating triggering and ventricular inhibition.[20]
4. Reversion to interference (noise) asynchronous pacing for one or more cycles[16, 20] (Figs. 36–7 and 36–8)
5. Precipitation of endless loop tachycardia by myopotential sensing by the atrial channel (or inhibition of the ventricular channel allowing ventricular escape beats to conduct retrogradely to the atrium) (Fig. 36–9).[19]
6. Single missing stimulus. Oversensing by the atrial channel may prevent the delivery of an atrial stimulus with apparent VVI pacing. Conversely, a ventricular stimulus may not succeed an atrial one if myopotential sensing occurs during the AV interval, a situation that may mimic cross-talk (Fig. 36–10).
7. Abbreviation of the AV interval if myopotentials are sensed in the ventricular safety pacing period

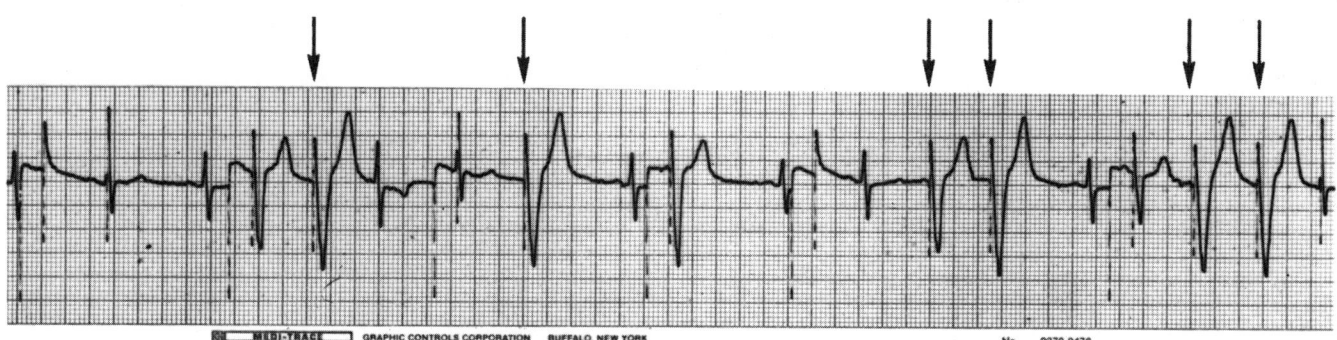

FIGURE 36–7
Activation of the noise-sampling period of the Cordis Gemini DDD pulse generator secondary to myopotential oversensing. The ECG shows (1) atrial triggering of the ventricular stimulus by oversensing of myopotentials by the atrial channel (arrows) and (2) asynchronous DOO cycles due to myopotential sensing within the noise sampling period. (Reprinted by permission of Futura Publishing Co., Inc., from Barold SS, et al.: In Barold SS, Mugica J (eds.): New Perspectives in Cardiac Pacing, pp. 69–119. Mt. Kisco, NY, Futura Publishing Co., 1988.)

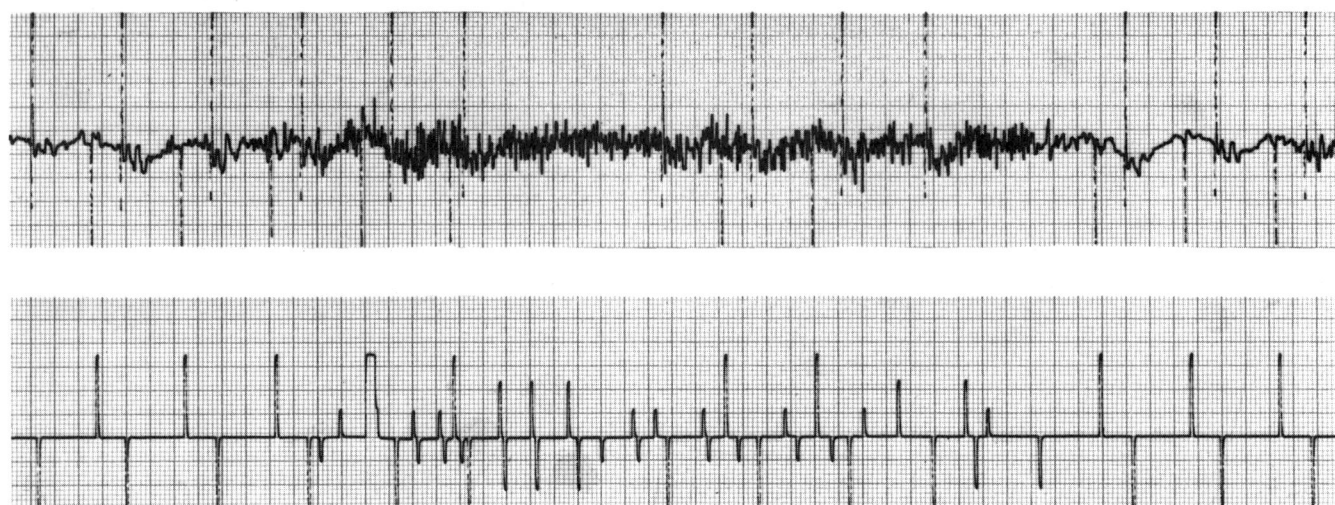

FIGURE 36–8

Myopotential interference in a patient with a Medtronic Symbios 7005 unipolar DDD pulse generator. Programmed parameters: lower rate = 80 ppm (750 ms); upper rate = 100 ppm (600 ms); AV interval = 250 ms; VA interval = 500 ms; postventricular atrial refractory period = 225 ms. LRI = lower rate interval; D = artifactual deformity of the atrial marker; VTP = ventricular triggering period or ventricular safety pacing period. Real-time markers (upper strip) were recorded simultaneously with the ECG (lower strip).

For the atrial channel, the markers point upward: largest size = atrial paced event; intermediate = atrial sensed event; smallest = atrial sensed event in the atrial refractory period (this signal is not used for starting any timing intervals). For the ventricular channel, the markers point downward: largest size = ventricular paced event; intermediate = ventricular sensed event; smallest = ventricular sensed event in the noise-sampling (refractory) period. The solid black circles depict a ventricular paced or ventricular sensed event outside the refractory period. Consequently, all downward deflections without solid black circles represent ventricular sensed events within the ventricular noise-sampling (refractory) period. Ventricular sensed events in the noise-sampling period do not reset the pulse generator and force it to pace at the lower rate interval, as shown in the middle of the tracing (two cycles between the 10th and 12th solid black circles). Myopotentials also inhibit the ventricular channel (7th, 8th, 9th, 14th, and 15th solid black circles) and myopotentials sensed by the atrial channel trigger a ventricular output (13th solid black circle). The 6th solid black circle represents a ventricular stimulus delivered prematurely because of a myopotential signal sensed within the ventricular safety pacing period (or ventricular triggering period = VTP). The 10th solid black circle represents a ventricular paced event not preceded by an atrial paced or sensed event (the atrial markers preceding this particular ventricular stimulus depict atrial sensing in the atrial noise sampling period. In contrast to the ventricular channel, such atrial sensed events do not influence any of the pacemaker timing cycles). The missing atrial stimulus between the 9th and 10th solid black circles is related to the presence of an atrial upper rate interval for this particular pulse generator. The atrial upper rate interval is equal to the ventricular upper rate interval (600 ms). The emission of an atrial stimulus between the 9th and 10th solid black circles would have occurred less than 600 ms from the preceding atrial sensed event. The pulse generator therefore omits this atrial stimulus to conform to its atrial upper rate interval.

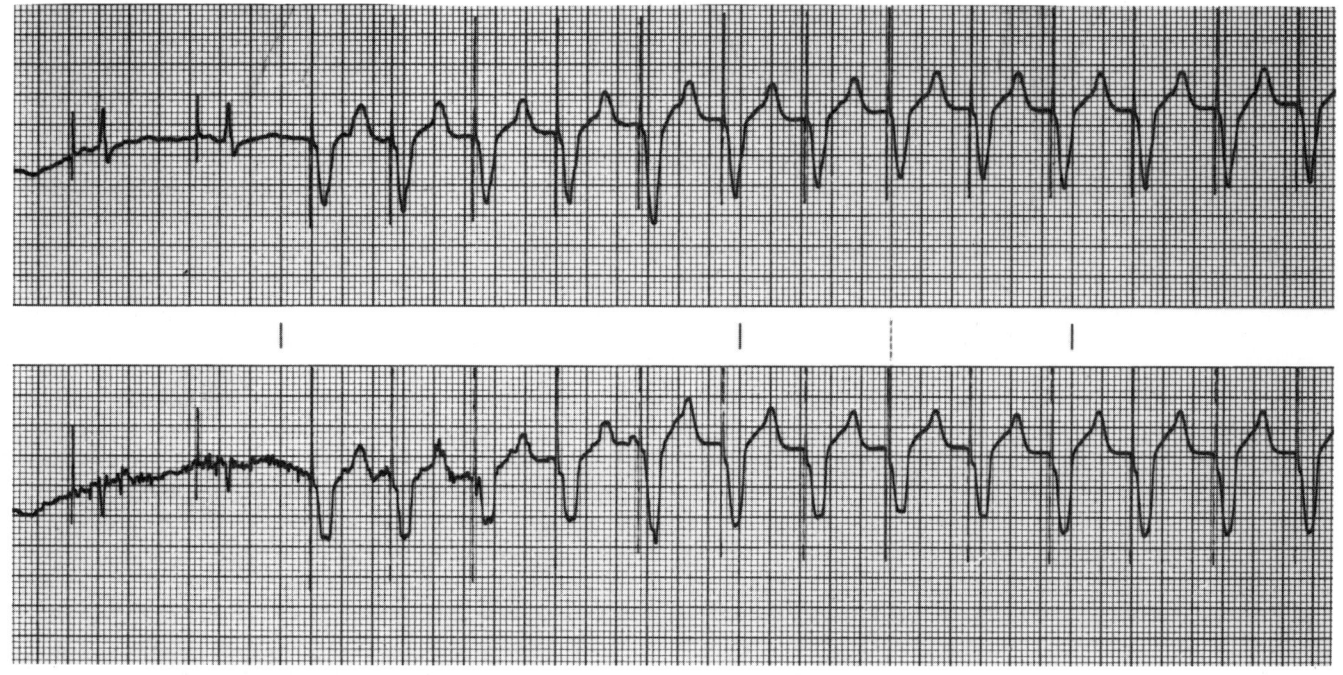

MYOPOTENTIALS

FIGURE 36–9
Initiation of endless loop tachycardia by myopotential oversensing in a patient with a Medtronic 7000 unipolar DDD pulse generator. Programmed parameters: lower rate = 70 ppm; upper rate = 125 ppm; AV delay = 250 ms. Isometric exercise causes myopotential sensing by the atrial channel, thereby triggering a ventricular stimulus independent of atrial activity. This form of AV dissociation leads to retrograde VA conduction, with the retrograde P wave falling beyond the nonprogrammable 155-ms postventricular atrial refractory period. (Reprinted by permission of Futura Publishing Co., Inc., from Barold SS, et al.: In Barold SS (ed.): Modern Cardiac Pacing, pp. 645–675. Mt. Kisco, NY, Futura Publishing Co., 1985.)

(ventricular triggering period) of a pulse generator possessing this characteristic (see Fig. 36–6).[24]

INDUCTION OF VENTRICULAR ARRHYTHMIAS

Myopotential sensing may precipitate ventricular tachyarrhythmias by several mechanisms. These include:

1. Inhibition of the ventricular channel resulting in escape or bradycardia-dependent ventricular arrhythmias (Fig. 36–11).[25]
2. Myopotential oversensing, which may cause rapid (burst) pacing in the VVT or DDD mode capable of inducing ventricular tachycardia in susceptible individuals (Fig. 36–12).
3. Reversion to VOO or DOO (noise) pacing, which may produce ventricular arrhythmias by firing a stimulus in the vulnerable period in predisposed patients with acute myocardial infarction or electrolyte imbalance.

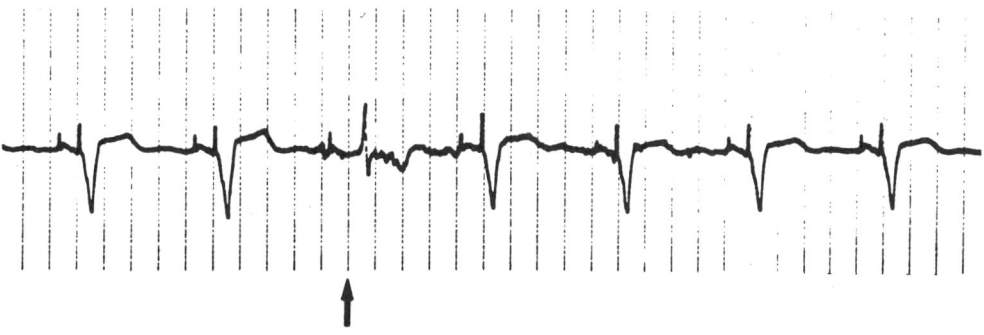

FIGURE 36–10
Myopotential oversensing mimicking crosstalk in a unipolar DDD pulse generator without a ventricular safety pacing period. The 3rd atrial stimulus is followed by unexpected prolongation of the AV interval (arrow) due to oversensing myopotentials. (Reprinted by permission of Futura Publishing Co., Inc., from Barold SS, et al.: In Barold SS (ed.): Modern Cardiac Pacing, pp. 615–623. Mt. Kisco, NY, Futura Publishing Co., 1985.)

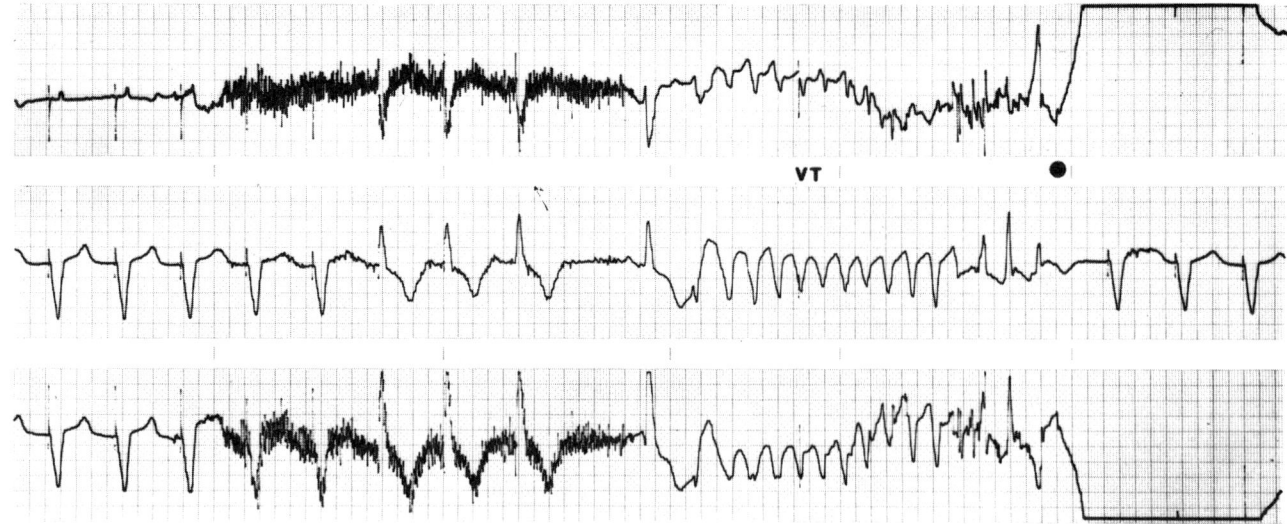

FIGURE 36–11
Myopotential inhibition of unipolar VVI pulse generator (lower rate = 70 ppm) causing bradycardia-dependent polymorphic ventricular tachycardia (VT). A chest thump was delivered at the time indicated by the solid black circle, resulting in resumption of normal ventricular pacing. Three ECG leads were recorded simultaneously.

Sources of Myopotentials

Pectoralis major myopotentials have been traditionally considered as the main source of pacemaker inhibition, but the rectus abdominis, diaphragm, and intercostal muscles may also contribute myopotentials capable of being sensed by pulse generators.

RECTUS ABDOMINIS

Gialafos and coworkers[26] studied the role of the rectus abdominis muscle in connection with the inhibition of unipolar pulse generators implanted in the pectoral and abdominal regions. These workers demonstrated that the rectus abdominis may contribute significantly to myopotential inhibition under certain circumstances. This source of myopotentials should be considered in patients exhibiting symptoms of dizziness during postural changes that may be erroneously attributed to labyrinthine vertigo.[26] Gialafos et al.[26] tested the role of the rectus abdominis during certain maneuvers, such as rising from a supine position or reclining backward to the supine position and also lifting and holding the legs about 20 degrees to the horizontal without support and/or against resistance. Certain conclusions may be drawn from the observations of these investigators,[26] as they pertain to unipolar pacing:

- The rectus abdominis may be an important source of myopotential interference in about 40% of pacemakers implanted in the abdominal wall.
- Myopotentials from the pectoralis and rectus abdominis may act synergistically and, indeed, in some

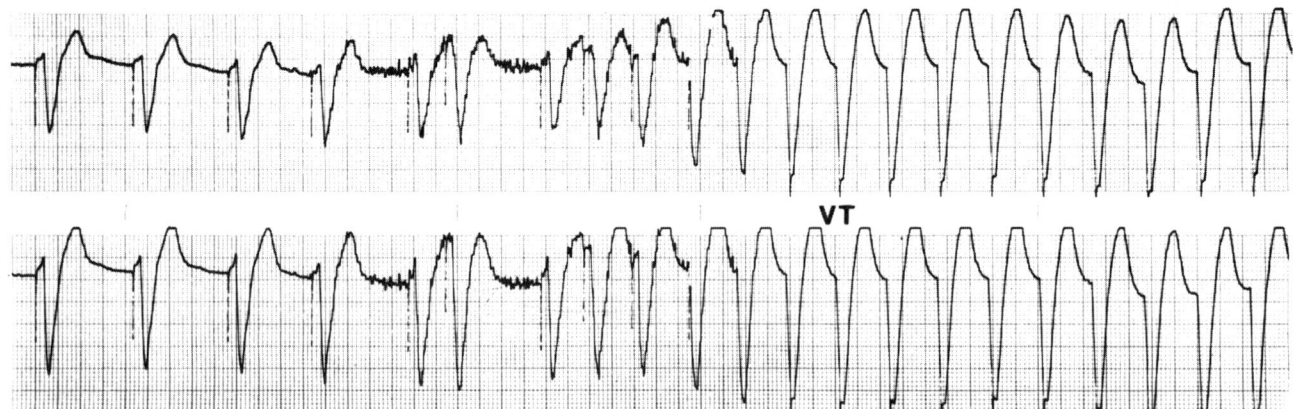

FIGURE 36–12
Induction of ventricular tachycardia (VT) by myopotential oversensing in a patient with a unipolar VVT pulse generator. Programmed parameters: lower rate = 70 ppm; upper limit = approx. 160 ppm; ventricular sensitivity = 2 mV. Myopotential triggering causes a short burst of ventricular pacing (three ventricular stimuli at a rate of approximately 150/min) that precipitates VT (cycle length = 460 ms). Pacemaker stimuli deform the QRS complexes during VT. Two ECG leads were recorded simultaneously.

cases this synergy is required to provoke pacemaker inhibition irrespective of the location of the pacemaker.
- Inhibition of pulse generators implanted over the pectoral region may be uninfluenced by local potentials but may be inhibited only by the rectus abdominis myopotentials.

Consequently, the rectus abdominis should always be considered as a potentially important source of myopotentials that may interfere with the function of unipolar demand pacemakers, irrespective of their location on the abdominal or thoracic wall. As a rule, contraction of the abdominal muscles has the greatest effect on pulse generators implanted over the abdominal wall, an important site in children. Some workers have found a significantly lower incidence of myopotential inhibition in patients with a unipolar VVI pulse generator implanted at an abdominal site in comparison with the conventional pectoral site.[17, 27, 28] The difference may be due to testing techniques, because some workers have not found a lower incidence of myopotential interference with an abdominal site of implantation.[29, 30]

DIAPHRAGMATIC MYOPOTENTIALS

Oversensing of diaphragmatic myopotentials is generally considered rare but is well documented in isolated cases with unipolar or bipolar VVI pulse generators (Fig. 36–13).[31–35] Transient inhibition of a pacemaker by diaphragmatic myopotentials may be provoked by deep respiration and active contraction of the diaphragm during straining, Valsalva maneuvers, coughing, sneezing, and laughing (Fig. 36–14).

We recently evaluated the incidence of oversensing of diaphragmatic myopotentials in 119 patients with multiprogrammable pulse generators from six different manufacturers. There were 105 VVI pulse generators (46 bipolar and 59 unipolar) and 14 unipolar DVI pulse generators.[33] Diaphragmatic myopotential inhibition was evaluated by observing the effect of maximal deep inspiration in the supine position with the pulse generator programmed at various sensitivities. Diaphragmatic inhibition was demonstrated in 4 of 46 bipolar VVI units (8.7%) and in 12 of 59 unipolar VVI units (20.3%). Inhibition also was demonstrated in 4 of 14 unipolar DVI systems from one manufacturer (28.6%). Diaphragmatic myopotential inhibition was observed at sensitivities higher than nominal value in all cases, except in two pulse generators (a unipolar VVI pulse generator and a bipolar VVI pulse generator) that were inhibited when programmed at nominal sensitivity.

Our observations in 119 patients suggest that diaphragmatic myopotential inhibition may not be uncommon when pulse generators are programmed to a high

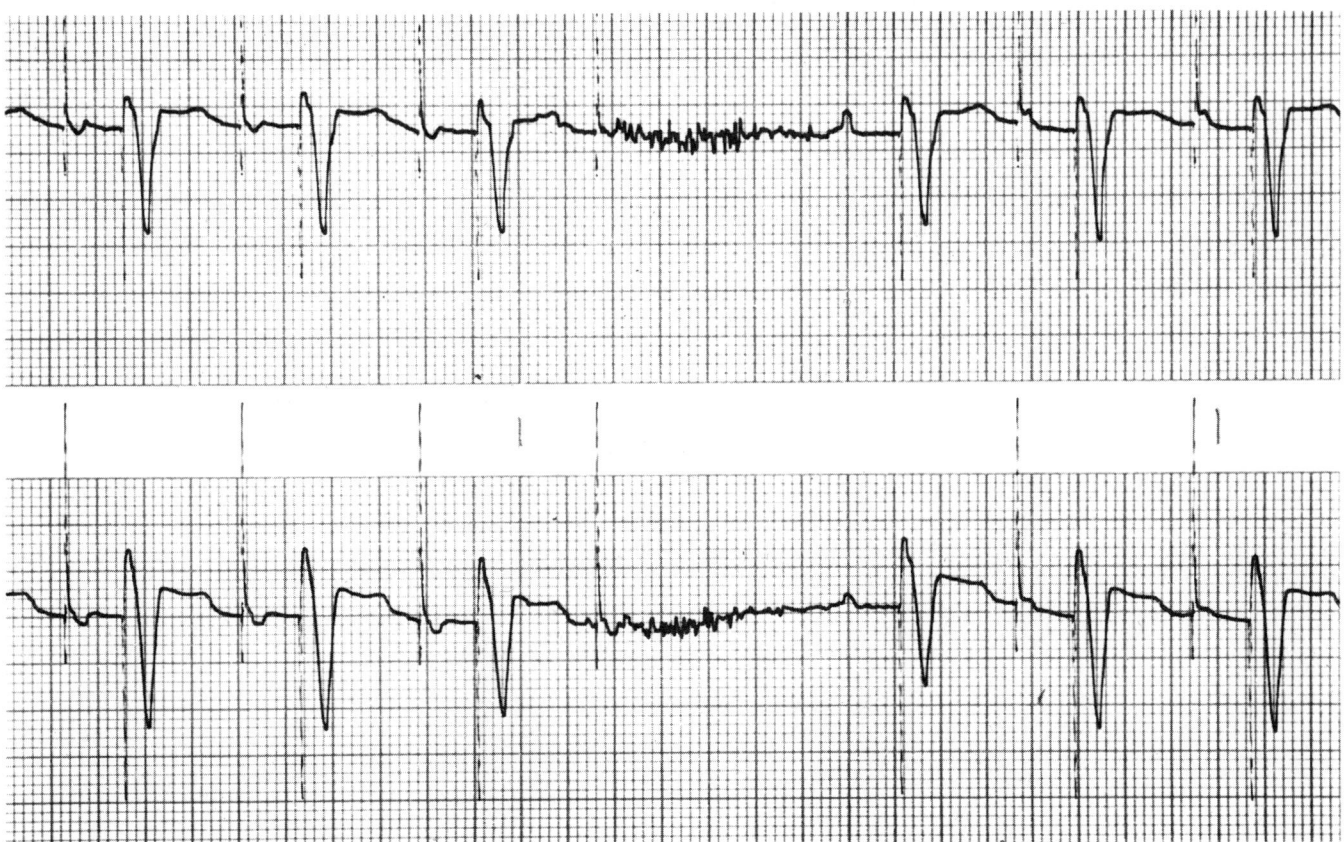

FIGURE 36–13
Oversensing of diaphragmatic myopotentials by a Pacesetter AFP 283 DDD pulse generator. Programmed parameters: lower rate = 80 ppm; AV delay = 240 ms; ventricular sensitivity = 1 mV. Inspiration causes inhibition of the ventricular channel from diaphragmatic myopotential oversensing.

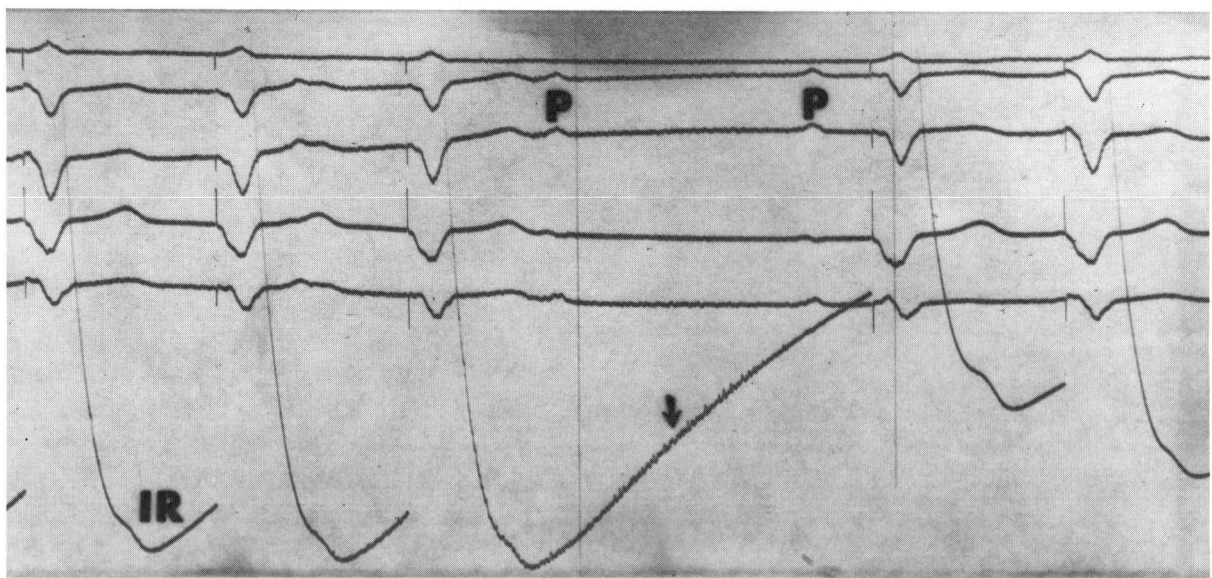

FIGURE 36–14
Diaphragmatic myopotential inhibition of a bipolar VVI pulse generator. The bipolar intracardiac electrogram (IR) was recorded (simultaneously with the surface ECG) from the bipolar ventricular lead during VVI pacing. The baseline of the intracardiac recording (IR) shows disturbance in the baseline consistent with myopotential noise. On deep inspiration, myopotentials (arrow) inhibit the pulse generator, with a resultant pause. No standardization is available. P = P wave.

sensitivity and may not necessarily be related to right ventricular perforation, as proposed previously.[34] Our observations suggest that diaphragmatic myopotential inhibition is more common with unipolar VVI pulse generators than with bipolar VVI pulse generators. We therefore disagree with Gialafos and associates,[26, 29] who challenged the validity of our findings because they were unable to reproduce our relatively high incidence of diaphragmatic myopotential inhibition. The discrepancy may be related to methodology and type of pulse generators, and perhaps these investigators did not test the pulse generators at the highest sensitivity, as we did.

In any case, oversensing of diaphragmatic myopotentials is an unimportant clinical problem because the pauses are relatively short and are always correctable by appropriate programming of sensitivity. Nevertheless, one should be cognizant of this abnormality for the proper interpretation of pacemaker function, bearing in mind that the maneuvers used to detect oversensing of diaphragmatic myopotentials may also unmask a lead fracture or insulation break that may be impossible to differentiate from myopotential inhibition, even with adjustment of sensitivity.

INTERCOSTAL MYOPOTENTIALS

We have observed myopotential triggering of unipolar DDD pulse generators with a J lead in the right atrial appendage, during deep inspiration at a very high sensitivity of the atrial channel (Fig. 36–15). In contrast, with the same or even higher sensitivity, diaphragmatic inhibition of the ventricular channel could not be demonstrated both in the DDD and VVI mode. We believe that sensing of intercostal myopotentials by the atrial channel is possible with both unipolar and bipolar atrial electrodes, although bipolar detection of intercostal myopotentials has not yet been reported. Such sensed intercostal myopotentials may be easily mistaken for other signals sensed by the atrial channel, such as atrial extrasystoles or myopotentials originating from the pectoral area. An intercostal source sensed by the atrial channel of a DDD pulse generator could explain reported cases of myopotential triggering of a ventricular output in the case of bipolar devices.[36]

Myopotential Sensing During Bipolar Pacing

Skeletal myopotential interference in bipolar pacing systems cannot be demonstrated under ordinary circumstances, and the geometry of the sensing electrodes makes its occurrence difficult to understand. However, myopotential sensing by a bipolar device may occur in the following situations.

1. Diaphragmatic inhibition of the ventricular channel of a single or dual-chamber device.
2. Insulation leak of a bipolar system.[37, 38] An insulation leak of the pacing lead relatively close to a pulse generator may detect myopotentials and inhibit the bipolar pulse generator that has essentially been converted to a unipolar-bipolar system.
3. Intercostal myopotentials (as discussed above).
4. Pseudointerference. During testing for myopotential oversensing, if the baseline of the ECG becomes grossly blurred, transient acceleration of the spontaneous rhythm with the occurrence of ventricular extrasystoles may be invisible and, if sensed, the resultant pauses may be attributed to myopotential inhibition.

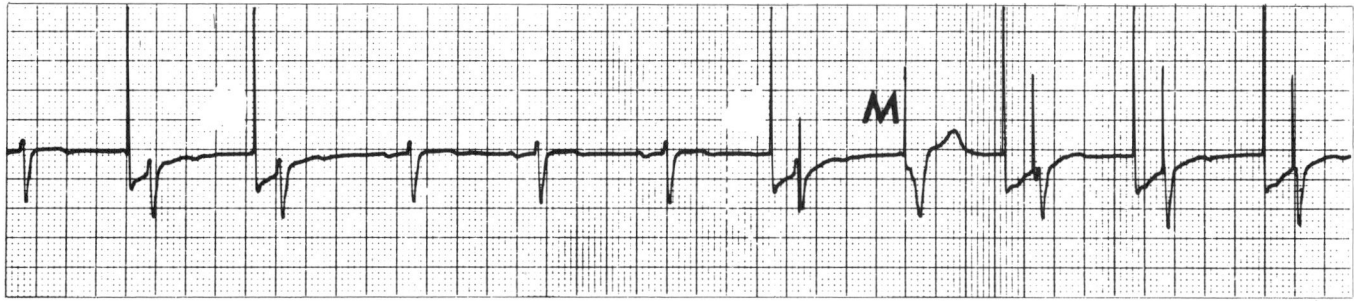

FIGURE 36–15
ECG showing intercostal myopotential oversensing by the atrial channel of a unipolar Cordis 233F DDD pulse generator. Programmed parameters: lower rate = 70 ppm; AV delay = 200 ms; atrial sensitivity = 0.5 mV; postventricular atrial refractory period (PVARP) = 300 ms; ventricular refractory period = 300 ms. The ECG was recorded during normal respiration with the patient otherwise motionless.

It appears that a signal (M) was sensed by the atrial electrode, thereby triggering a ventricular output. A local source of myopotentials was ruled out because there was no myopotential inhibition of the ventricular channel at sensitivities of 0.5, 1.3, and 2.5 mV during deep respiration. However, oversensing by the atrial electrode could be demonstrated at sensitivities of 0.5 and 1.3 mV during normal and deep respiration. Because both channels share the same anode, this ruled out well-known sources of myopotential interference such as pectoral, diaphragmatic, and rectus abdominis sites. There was no evidence of atrial lead malfunction such as an insulation break. Far-field atrial sensing of ventricular activity could be ruled out because of the relatively long PVARP.

This form of oversensing has persisted for 4 years and we believe that it is caused by atrial oversensing of myopotential interference arising from the intercostal muscles, because of the anterior location of the atrial lead in the atrial appendage.

Recently Binner et al.[36] reported that 4 of 18 patients with bipolar DDD pulse generators exhibited myopotential interference. In the bipolar mode, myopotential triggering by the atrial channel was noted in 4 patients at a programmed atrial sensitivity of 0.5 mV, but not at 1.25 mV. In 4 of 18 patients, myopotential inhibition of the ventricular channel was also demonstrated at 1.25 mV sensitivity. The authors did not elaborate on the source of myopotential interference during bipolar DDD pacing. We believe that intercostal myopotentials probably generated sufficient voltage for the atrial J electrode to trigger a ventricular output, and that the ventricular channel was probably inhibited by diaphragmatic potentials.

Testing Maneuvers for Myopotential Interference

During testing for myopotential interference, a high programmed sensitivity may favor reversion to the asynchronous mode. When the patient's spontaneous rhythm is present, there will be competitive asynchronous pacing. However, during continuous pacing, conversion to the asynchronous noise reversion mode may not be detected if the pacing rate during noise is similar to the programmed (lower) rate of the pulse generator. This may be misinterpreted as representing the absence of myopotential oversensing. In this situation, when the sensitivity is reduced, myopotential inhibition should become obvious, giving rise to the paradox of no apparent myopotential inhibition at high sensitivity and the presence of myopotential inhibition at lower sensitivity. For this reason, we suggest that testing for myopotential interference should be performed with the implanted pulse generator programmed at various sensitivities.

The following maneuvers may cause myopotential inhibition (Table 36–1): hand pressing, reaching, pulling interlocking hands apart at the mid chest, pushing against the observer's hand, pushing the fist on the implanted side vigorously into the opposite hand, hand clapping, hyperadduction of the ipsilateral arm, reaching as far as possible around the chest, coupled with pressure on the contralateral shoulder or vigorous scratching by the ipsilateral arm across the abdomen.[15] Occasionally symptomatic myopotential inhibition can occur while brushing teeth.[39] The hyperadduction maneuver is the most sensitive test for myopotential interference.[13]

To test for myopotential interference during DDD pacing, the pulse generator is first programmed to the

TABLE 36–1
Common Testing Maneuvers for Myopotential Interference

Deltopectoral Muscles
 Pressing palm of hand against that of observer or against wall
 Pressing one hand against the other
 Pushing hand against contralateral shoulder
 Lifting or flexing arm against resistance
 Adduction of arm against resistance
 Hyperadduction reach test
 Isometric handgrip
 Treadmill stress test

Rectus Abdominis Muscles
 Trunk lifting from or reclining backward to supine position
 Lifting and holding legs 20 degrees to the horizontal against resistance
 Treadmill stress test

Diaphragm
 Deep inspiration
 Valsalva maneuver, straining, coughing, laughing, sneezing

highest ventricular sensitivity, and the lower rate is increased to ensure continuous pacing. For tracking of myopotentials by the atrial channel, the highest atrial sensitivity should be used.

TREADMILL EXERCISE TESTING

Occasionally, myopotential interference may be observed during exercise and may be reproducible on the treadmill, especially if pacemaker sensitivity is high. Bricker et al.[40] studied the effect of treadmill exercise testing in 24 children from 4.5 to 18 years of age (mean 15 years) with DDD or VDD unipolar pulse generators, with 20 implanted in the pectoral region, three by the subxiphoid approach, and one by thoracotomy. Seven of the 24 patients exhibited reversion to the noise mode during exercise. Systematic comparison with the effect of isometric exercise was not performed, but the authors mentioned that, in one case, conversion to the noise mode during treadmill testing was not observed during arm isometric exercise. Thus, in selected patients with symptoms on exercise, myopotential interference should be tested during treadmill testing.[41]

HOLTER RECORDINGS

Some workers claim that Holter documentation of myopotential inhibition correlates more closely than other methods with the likelihood of symptoms and demonstrable interference by a variety of maneuvers.[9, 10] However, others believe that most patients who display myopotential inhibition during Holter recordings have the same tendency during testing with provocative maneuvers.[42] In contrast, some investigators comparing the efficacy of 24-hour Holter recordings with provocative maneuvers for the detection of myopotential inhibition have shown that the Holter recording offers few advantages over the routine provocative tests for the detection of myopotential inhibition.[27, 43]

TELEMETRY OF THE ELECTROGRAM

The capability of telemetric transmission of intracardiac electrograms has added a new dimension to the diagnosis and treatment of myopotential oversensing. In particular, it allows determination of the signal amplitude to guide programmability of the atrial or ventricular sensitivity to eliminate oversensing while maintaining P wave or QRS complex sensing or both in AAI, VVI, and DDD pacing systems (Fig. 36–16).[16, 44, 45]

Management of Myopotential Interference

Before the advent of multiprogrammability, symptomatic myopotential inhibition required replacement of the pulse generator with an asynchronous or triggered unit or conversion from a unipolar to a bipolar system. Today, with multiprogrammability, several options are available:

- Reduction of the input sensitivity. In some pulse generators, not even programming the lowest sensitivity may correct the problem, and it may lead to undersensing of the QRS complex (or P wave, in the case of AAI or dual-chamber pacing).
- Conversion to the triggered or VVT (AAT) mode with nominal sensitivity. In the case of VVT pace-

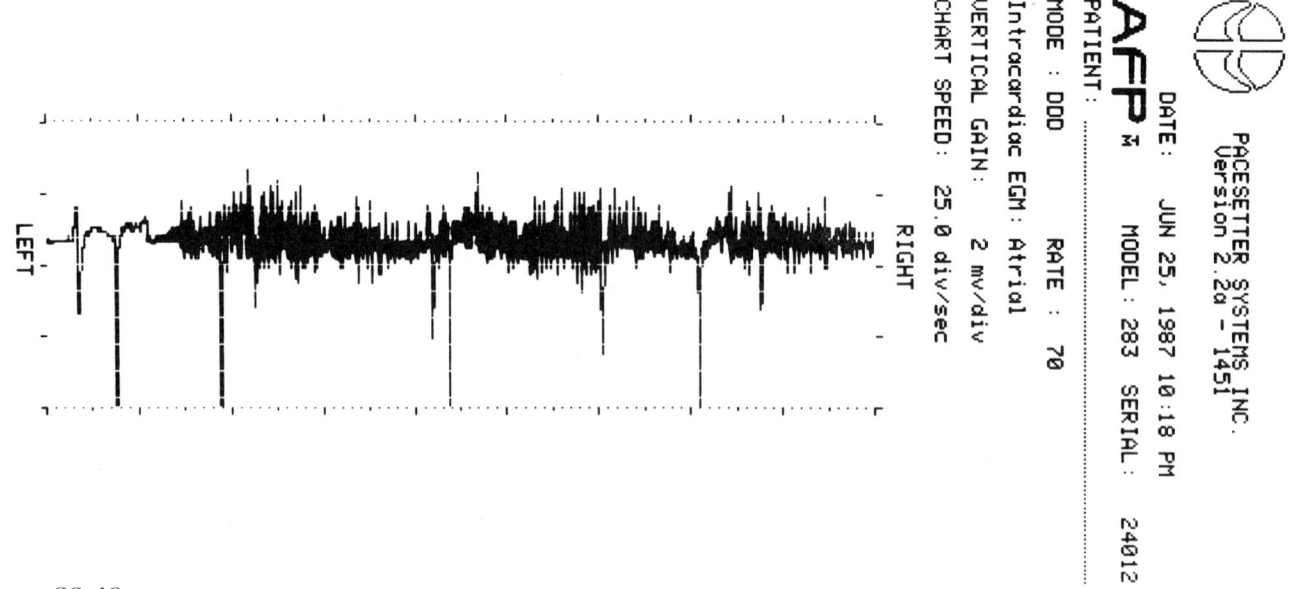

FIGURE 36–16
Myopotential interference recorded on the telemetered atrial electrogram in a patient with a Pacesetter 283 AFP unipolar DDD pulse generator. Note the relatively large amplitude of myopotential interference, at times exceeding 2 mV.

makers, this may allow optimal sensing of the QRS complex; however, there may be periods of undesirable increase in the pacing rate, and the VVT mode may not always prevent firing on the T wave (see Fig. 36–12). Some VVT pulse generators possess a short inhibitory window beyond the refractory period, in which sensed signals including myopotentials may inhibit rather than trigger the pulse generator (Fig. 36–17).[46] As a rule, this occurs when the upper rate interval is longer than the programmed refractory period (Fig. 36–18).[47–49]

- Programmability from the unipolar to the bipolar mode in some pulse generators.
- Conversion to the asynchronous VOO, AOO, or DOO mode.
- If the problem is not severe, the patient may be advised to avoid those body movements that cause myopotential interference.
- A silicone rubber boot may be placed around the back of the pulse generator to prevent detection of myopotential signals.
- The pulse generator may be replaced with one less

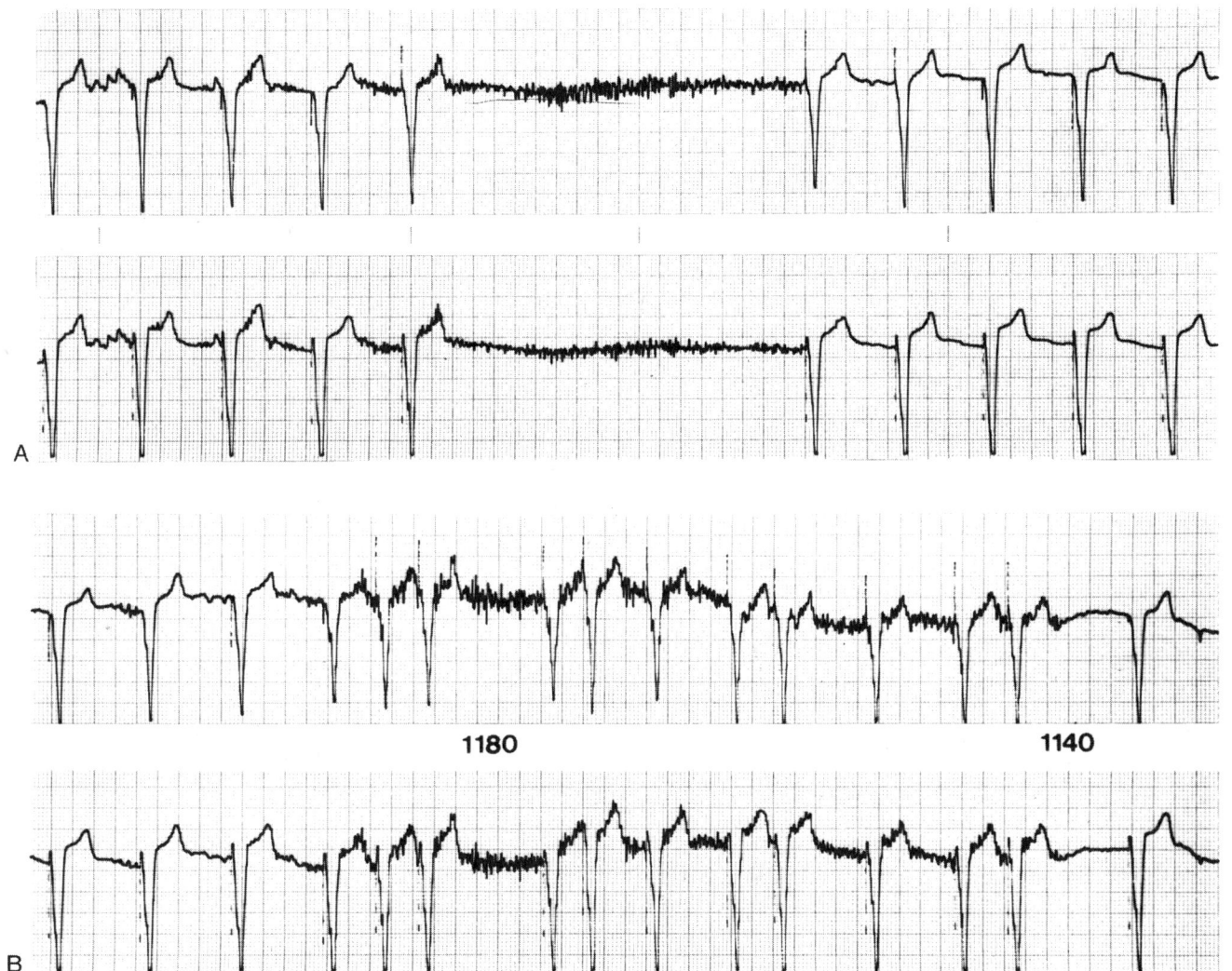

FIGURE 36–17

A, Pacesetter AFP unipolar DDD pulse generator programmed to the VVI mode. Programmed parameters: lower rate = 70 ppm; ventricular sensitivity = 2.0 mV; ventricular refractory period = 250 ms. Isometric pectoral exercise causes prolonged myopotential inhibition (3.9 s). Two ECG leads were recorded simultaneously.

B, Same patient as in A with a Pacesetter AFP DDD pulse generator programmed to the VVT mode (rate = 70 ppm; ventricular sensitivity = 2 mV; ventricular refractory period = 250 ms). Myopotential oversensing causes triggered ventricular pacing with an irregular increase in the pacing rate except for the two interstimulus intervals of 1180 and 1140 ms, both exceeding the lower rate interval of 857 ms. During the VVT mode, the maximum pacing rate is limited to approximately 160 ppm and fixed by design. With a programmed refractory period of 250 ms, a ventricular signal 250 ms beyond a paced event must be sensed, but it does not trigger a ventricular stimulus in order to avoid violating the upper rate interval of approximately 360 ms. Thus, a ventricular signal in the 110-ms window extending from the end of the refractory period (250 ms) to the completion of the upper rate interval (360 ms) inhibits the ventricular channel. The interstimulus interval may therefore lengthen to any value between the lower rate interval and the lower rate interval plus the upper rate interval (i.e., between 857 ms and 857 + 360 = 1217 ms, approximately).

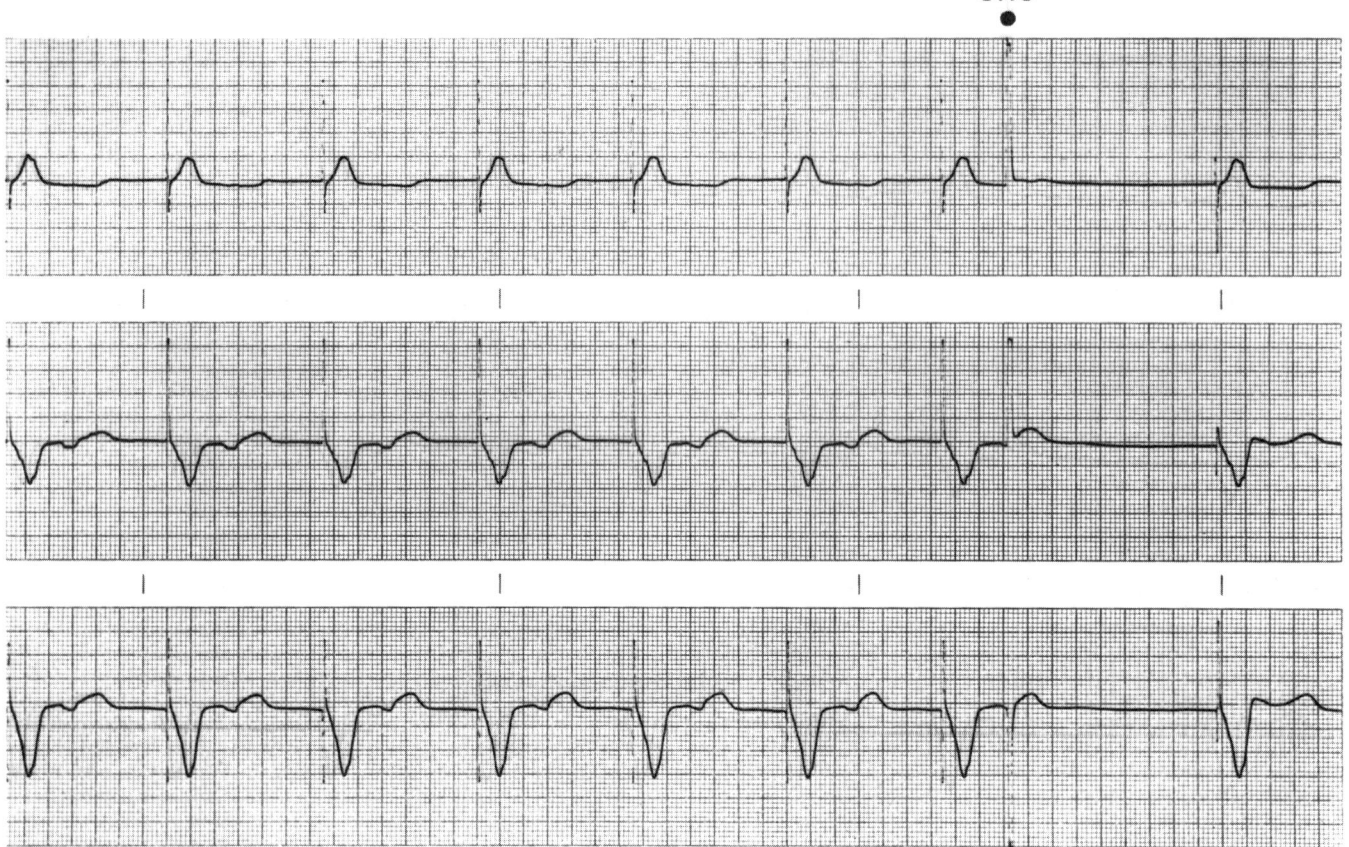

FIGURE 36–18
Chest wall stimulation (CWS) in a patient with a Medtronic Spectrax 8423 single-chamber pulse generator programmed to the VVT mode. Programmed parameters: lower rate=80 ppm; refractory period=220 ms. The maximum pacing (tracking) rate is not programmable and is approximately 150/min by design (upper rate interval=400 ms). Thus, a ventricular signal occurring 220 ms after a ventricular stimulus can be sensed, but it cannot trigger a ventricular stimulus because that would violate the upper-rate interval of approximately 400 ms. The sensed CWS signal therefore causes inhibition of the ventricular channel rather than triggering a ventricular output.

sensitive to myopotentials (smaller, thinner pulse generators have less anodal surface area) or one with an insulative coating. The latter reduces muscle contact around the back and side of the pulse generator.[50, 51] The selection of the replacement pulse generator may be quite difficult and should be based on a thorough review of the literature concerning the response of pulse generators to interference. As shown by Irnich,[52] only certain unipolar pulse generators are capable of rejecting muscle noise with proper circuit design, even when the sensitivity is 2 mV.

- Repositioning the pulse generator to a less active muscle site may eliminate myopotential sensing. When pacemaker sensitivity cannot be altered, reimplantation in the abdominal region may be considered; however, this requires a new incision and a subcutaneous tunneling procedure.
- As suggested by Redding and Lochan,[53] myopotential inhibition may be avoided by implanting the pulse generator away from the muscle mass, in the axilla. In their experience with 150 cases of unipolar pulse generators, none exhibited symptomatic inhibition with isometric exercise and only a few exhibited asymptomatic inhibition.
- Occasionally spontaneous rotation of a unipolar pulse generator in an excessively large pocket may produce previously absent myocardial inhibition (and direct muscle stimulation).[54, 55] Chiu[55] indicated that it is possible to flip these pacemakers back into their normal position blindly, and he mentioned two such cases successfully treated by manipulation through the flaccid skin. We have also used this internal version technique successfully in four such cases, without recurrence over a period of 3 years or longer.

Myopotential interference provides an opportunity to evaluate the usefulness of programmability in the prevention of secondary invasive interventions because of pacemaker malfunction. Billhardt and colleagues[56] studied 295 unipolar pulse generators with a follow-up period of 1 day to 38 months. Twenty-five of these pulse generators (8.5%) exhibited malfunction. Nine required invasive procedures for correction, and 16 of these (64% of all malfunctions and 5.4% of total implants) were corrected by multiprogrammability. In this respect, there were four cases that required reprogramming of the pacemaker because of myopotential inhibition, with two cases requiring conversion to the synchronous or triggered mode (VVI to VVT). This represents 1.4% of the total implants. When considered in terms of problems related to unipolar stimulation and sensing, there were nine cases with abnormalities (five local muscle stimulation and four myopotential inhibition), representing 36% of all malfunctions. These could have been avoided by the implantation of bipolar leads. Griffin[57] followed 83 pulse generators (83% unipolar and 17% bipolar) over a period of 0.1 to 22.5 months. Twenty-four pulse generators (29%) exhibited malfunction, and three required invasive procedures. Twenty-one malfunctions were corrected by programmability (85% of all malfunctions and 29% of total implants). Myopotential inhibition was responsible for malfunction in three cases (4% of total implants). One case required reprogramming to the asynchronous mode (VOO). With regard to problems related to unipolar stimulation, there were five cases (two muscle stimulation and three myopotential inhibition), constituting 20% of all malfunctions. Again, these could have been avoided by the implantation of bipolar systems.

Is Unipolar Pacing Obsolete?

Despite spectacular improvements in pacemaker technology, the incidence of myopotential interference has remained unchanged over the last 17 years. Engineering efforts and surgical techniques have not resolved the myopotential problem during unipolar pacing. Absolute discrimination between the cardiac electrogram and skeletal muscle potentials is difficult and probably impossible in some circumstances, because the frequency spectrum of the myopotential signal overlaps that of the P wave and QRS complex. The amplitude of myopotentials may be as high as 4.5 mV. Myopotential inhibition became an important clinical problem only because of the popularity of unipolar pulse generators. Sensing and stimulating characteristics of unipolar and bipolar pacing systems are basically similar. Many workers have demonstrated that there is no significant difference between unipolar and bipolar electrograms for sensing purposes, and indeed bipolar sensing may actually be superior.[58–65] Bipolar pulse generators provide a superior signal-to-noise ratio and better rejection of far-field interference. The previous advantages of unipolar pacing (for example, smaller electrode size) have disappeared with the advent of multiprogrammability and the recent development of smaller leads because of changes in insulating material and the introduction of coaxial conductors.

With smaller leads and the development of positive fixation bipolar leads, bipolar dual-chamber systems offer the same options as the unipolar configuration. With bipolar dual-chamber pacemakers, the potential for cross-talk is diminished, and a very high sensitivity may be used without the fear of interference from myopotentials or other extraneous noise. Myopotential interference of rate-responsive pulse generators (e.g., VVIR) on exercise may negate the beneficial increase in the pacing rate provided by sensor activity. Oversensing of myopotentials may cause inhibition and/or reversion to the interference or noise mode so that the pacing rate may fall abruptly to the interference (noise) rate, often the lower rate of the pulse generator.[66] Automatic tachycardia-terminating pulse generators should be bipolar in order to avoid inappropriate delivery of stimulation from sensing musculoskeletal potentials.[67]

It appears likely that bipolar systems will regain their previous preeminence, mainly because of their immunity from myopotential inhibition and their capability of providing a greater range of sensitivity settings for optimal sensing.[59, 68–74] Should unipolar systems still be used for primary implantations? Probably not, despite Irnich's plea that the unipolar pacing system must not be abandoned because of muscle noise (at least for ventricular application).[52] Irnich[3] has demonstrated that most pulse generators are much more sensitive than they need to be. Furthermore, the filter characteristics of pulse generators are quite variable, and some have inadequate filter circuits.[75, 76] Irnich[52] has also emphasized that it would be technically possible to reject muscle noise, although he admits that a very sensitive pulse generator for atrial application, with a sensitivity of 0.5–1.0 mV, would always be influenced by muscle noise.

References

1. Wirzfeld S, Lampadius M, Ruprecht EO: Unterdruckung von Demand-Schrittmachern durch Muskelpotentials. Dtsch Med Wochenschr 97:61, 1972.
2. Anderson ST, Pitt A, Whitford JA, et al.: Interference with function of unipolar pacemakers due to muscle potentials. J Thorac Cardiovasc Surg 71:698, 1976.
3. Breivik K, Ohm OJ: Myopotential inhibition of unipolar QRS-inhibited (VVI) pacemakers, assessed by ambulatory Holter monitoring of the electrocardiogram. PACE 3:470, 1980.
4. Furman S: Electromagnetic interference. PACE 5:1, 1982.
5. Gialafos J, Maillis A, Basiakos L, et al.: Rectus abdominis as a source of myopotentials inhibiting demand pacemakers. PACE 6:887, 1983.
6. Levine PA, Caplan CH, Klein MD, et al.: Myopotential inhibition of unipolar lithium pacemakers. Chest 82:461, 1982.
7. Levine PA, Klein MD: Myopotential inhibition of unipolar pacemakers. A disease of technologic process. Ann Intern Med 98:101, 1983.
8. Piller LW, Kennelly BM: Myopotential inhibition of demand pacemakers. Chest 66:418, 1974.
9. Watson WS: Myopotential sensing in cardiac pacemakers. In Barold SS (ed.): Modern Cardiac Pacing, p. 813. Mt. Kisco, NY, Futura Publishing Co., 1985.
10. Secemsky SI, Hauser RG, Denes P, et al.: Unipolar sensing abnormalities: Incidence and clinical significance of skeletal muscle interference and undersensing in 228 patients. PACE 5:10, 1982.
11. Mymin D, Cuddy TE, Sinha SN, et al.: Inhibition of demand pacemakers by skeletal muscle potentials. JAMA 223:527, 1973.
12. Chomka E, Edwards-Strauss L, Papp MA, et al.: Myopotential oversensing in DDD pacemakers. PACE 8:295, 1985.

13. Fetter J, Hall DM, Hoff GL, et al.: The effects of myopotential interference on unipolar and bipolar dual chamber pacemakers in the DDD mode. Clin Prog Electrophysiol Pacing 3:368, 1985.
14. Fröhlig G, Sen S, Blank W, et al.: Susceptibility of a unipolar dual chamber pacemaker to chest wall myopotentials. In Pérez-Gómez F (ed.): Cardiac Pacing. Electrophysiology. Tachyarrhythmias, p. 698. Mt. Kisco, NY, Futura Publishing Co., 1985.
15. Gabry MD, Behrens M, Andrews C, et al.: Comparison of myopotential interference in unipolar-bipolar programmable DDD pacemakers. PACE 10:1322, 1987.
16. Halpern JL, Camunas JL, Stern EH, et al.: Myopotential interference with DDD pacemakers. Endocardial electrographic telemetry in the diagnosis of pacemaker-related arrhythmias. Am J Cardiol 54:97, 1984.
17. Michalik RE, Williams AH, Hatcher CR Jr: Myopotential inhibition of unipolar pacing in children. PACE 8:25, 1985.
18. Quintal R, Dhurandhar RW, Jain RK: Myopotential interference with a DDD pacemaker. Report of a case. PACE 7:37, 1984.
19. Rozanski JJ, Blankstein RL, Lister JW: Pacer arrhythmias. Myopotential triggering of pacemaker mediated tachycardia. PACE 6:795, 1983.
20. Zimmern SH, Clark MF, Austin WK, et al.: Characteristics and clinical effects of myopotential signals in a unipolar DDD pacemaker population. PACE 9:1019, 1986.
21. Irnich W, Barold SS: Interference protection in cardiac pacemakers. In Barold SS (ed.): Modern Cardiac Pacing, p. 839. Mt. Kisco, NY, Futura Publishing Co., 1985.
22. Warnowicz MA, Goldschlager N: Apparent failure to sense (undersensing) caused by oversensing. Diagnostic use of noninvasively obtained intracardiac electrogram. PACE 6:1341, 1983.
23. Erkkila K, Singh J: Reversion mode activation by myopotential sensing in a ventricular inhibited demand pacemaker. PACE 8:50, 1985.
24. Barold SS, Belott PH. Behavior of the ventricular triggering period of DDD pacemakers. PACE 10:1237, 1987.
25. Iseka Y, Pinakatt T, Gosselin A, et al.: Bradycardia dependent ventricular tachycardia facilitated by myopotential inhibition of a VVI pacemaker. PACE 5:23, 1982.
26. Gialafos J, Maillis A, Kalogeropoulos C, et al.: Inhibition of demand pacemakers by myopotentials. Am Heart J 109:984, 1985.
27. Rosenqvist M, Nordlander R, Andersson M, et al.: Reduced incidence of myopotential pacemaker inhibition by abdominal generator implantation. PACE 9:417, 1986.
28. VanGelder L, ElGamal M: Influence of myopotentials on implanted DDD-M pacemakers. PACE 6:A-52, 1983.
29. Gialafos J, Maillis A, Kandilas J: Pacemaker inhibition by myopotentials associated with motion and exercise. Eur Heart J 8(Suppl. D):149, 1987.
30. Ramella I, Oseroff O, Cresimone H, et al.: Myopotential inhibition in patients with unipolar pacemakers. Detection recognition and management. PACE 6:A-53, 1983.
31. Baggioni GF, Antonioli GE: Cause apparentemente isolite di inibizione dei pacemakers unipolari a domanda. G Ital Cardiol 8:61, 1978.
32. Barold SS, Ong LS, Falkoff MD, et al.: Inhibition of bipolar demand pacemakers by diaphragmatic myopotentials. Circulation 56:679, 1977.
33. Barold SS, Falkoff MD, Ong LS, et al.: Diaphragmatic myopotential inhibition in multiprogrammable unipolar and bipolar pulse generators. In Steinbach K (ed.): Cardiac Pacing. Proceedings of the VIIIth World Symposium on Cardiac Pacing, p. 537. Darmstadt, Germany, Steinkopff Verlag, 1983.
34. ElGamal M, VanGelder B: Suppression of an external demand pacemaker by diaphragmatic myopotentials: A sign of electrode perforation. PACE 2:191, 1979.
35. Peter R, Harper R, Sloman G: Inhibition of demand pacemakers caused by potentials associated with inspiration. Br Heart J 38:211, 1976.
36. Binner L, Richter P, Wieshammer S, et al.: Bipolar versus unipolar mode in dual chamber pacing. Comparison of myopotential interference acute and long term pacing and sensing thresholds. PACE 10(Part II):646, 1987.
37. Amikam S, Preleg H, Lemer L, et al.: Myopotential inhibition of a bipolar pacemaker by skeletal muscle insulation defect. Br Heart J 39:1279, 1977.
38. Widlansky S, Zipes DP: Suppression of a ventricular-inhibited bipolar pacemaker by skeletal muscle activity. J Electrocardiol 7:371, 1974.
39. Ito H, Iesaka Y, Taniguchi K, et al.: Comparison of susceptibility of myopotential inhibition between AAI and VVI pacemakers. Jpn Heart J 28:157, 1987.
40. Bicker JT, Garson A Jr, Traweek MS, et al.: The use of exercise testing in children to evaluate abnormalities of pacemaker function not apparent at rest. PACE 8:656, 1985.
41. Harthorne JW, Eisenhauer AC, Steinhaus DM: Pacemaker mediated tachycardias: An unresolved problem. PACE 7(Part II):1140, 1984.
42. Janosik DL, Redd RM, Buckingham TA, et al.: Utility of ambulatory electrocardiography in detecting pacemaker dysfunction in the early post-implantation period. Am J Cardiol 60:1030, 1987.
43. Gaita F, Asteggiano R, Bocchiardo M, et al.: Holter monitoring and provocative maneuvers in assessment of unipolar demand pacemaker myopotential inhibition. Am Heart J 107:925, 1984.
44. Levine PA, Sholder J, Duncan JL: Clinical benefits of telemetered electrograms in assessment of DDD function. PACE 7 (II):1170, 1984.
45. Levine PA: The complementary role of electrogram, event marker, and measured data telemetry in the assessment of pacing system function. J Electrophysiol 1:404, 1987.
46. Furman S: Inhibition of a ventricular synchronous pacemaker. Am Heart J 93:581, 1977.
47. Edwards LM, Hauser RG: Dual mode sensing by a variable cycle ventricular synchronous pulse generator. PACE 4:309, 1981.
48. Lazar AV, Massumi A, Hall RJ: Myopotential inhibition of ventricular synchronous pacemaker. Clin Cardiol 10:535, 1982.
49. VanGelder LM, ElGamal MIH: Prolongation of pacing intervals in triggered pacing systems (AAT, VVT). PACE 10(Part II):757, 1987.
50. Fetter J, Bobeldyk GL, Engman FJ: The clinical incidence and significance of myopotential sensing with unipolar pacemakers. PACE 7:871, 1984.
51. Vrints C, Lambrecht A, Bossaert L, et al.: Myopotential inhibition of unipolar pacemakers. Prevention by an insulating sheath. Acta Cardiol 3:167, 1981.
52. Irnich W: Muscle noise and interference behavior in pacemakers: A comparative study. PACE 10:125, 1987.
53. Redding VJ, Lochan RG: Successful avoidance of electromyopotential inhibition with nonprogrammable ventricular-inhibited pacing via axillary implant. Circulation 70(Suppl. II):432, 1984.
54. Simonsen E, Skov Jensen B: Spontaneous rotation of permanent pacemaker—a cause of muscle stimulation and myopotential inhibition. Scand J Thor Cardiovasc Surg 18:223, 1984.
55. Chiu RCJ: The flipping-pacemaker phenomenon. N Engl J Med 311:602, 1984.
56. Billhardt RA, Rosenbush SW, Hauser RG: Successful management of pacing systems malfunction without surgery. PACE 5:675, 1982.
57. Griffin JC: Pacemaker programmability. Its role in the maintenance of pacing system function. In Feruglio GA (ed.): Cardiac Pacing, Electrophysiology and Pacemaker Technology, p. 759. Padova, Italy, Piccin Medical Books, 1982.
58. DeCaprio V, Hurzeler P, Furman S: A comparison of unipolar and bipolar electrograms for cardiac pacemaker sensing. Circulation 56:750, 1977.
59. Berkovits BV: Advantages of bipolar over unipolar pacing. Medtronic News 15:5, 1985.
60. Hughes HC, Tyers GFO, Brownlee RR, et al.: A comparison of peak QRS potential detection using unipolar and bipolar cardiac pacemaker lead systems. J Surg Res 25:31, 1978.
61. Nielsen AP, Cashion WR, Spencer WH, et al.: Long-term assessment of unipolar and bipolar stimulation and sensing thresholds using a lead configuration programmable pacemaker. J Am Coll Cardiol 5:1198, 1985.
62. Smyth NPD, Sager D: A multiprogrammable pacemaker with unipolar or bipolar option. Am Heart J 106:412, 1983.

63. Breivik K, Ohm O, Engedal H: Long-term comparison of unipolar and bipolar pacing and sensing using a new multiprogrammable pacemaker system. PACE 6:592, 1983.
64. Bagwell P, Pannizo F, Furman S: Unipolar and bipolar right atrial appendage electrodes. Comparison of sensing characteristics. Med Instrum 19:132, 1985.
65. Griffin JC: Sensing characteristics of the right atrial appendage. PACE 6:22, 1983.
66. Lau CP, Camm AJ, Ward DE: A severe case of myopotential interference in a patient with a respiratory-dependent rate modulated pacemaker. Int J Cardiol 17:98, 1987.
67. Sowton E: Clinical results with the Tachylog antitachycardia pacemaker. PACE 7 (Part II):1313, 1984.
68. Baker RG, Falkenberg EN: Bipolar versus unipolar issues in DDD pacing. PACE 7:1178, 1984.
69. Hauser RG: Bipolar leads for cardiac pacing in the 1980's: A reappraisal provoked by skeletal muscle interference. PACE 5:34, 1982.
70. Hauser RG, Edwards LM, Stafford JL: Bipolar and unipolar sensing. Basic concepts and clinical applications. *In* Barold SS (ed.): Modern Cardiac Pacing, p. 137. Mt. Kisco, NY, Futura Publishing Co., 1985.
71. Furman S: Bipolar pacing. PACE 9:619, 1986.
72. Scallhorn R, Markowitz T: Bipolar dual chamber pacemakers: Is myopotential sensing still a problem? PACE 11:852, 1988.
73. Griffin JC, Spencer W, Cashion WR, et al.: Unipolar or bipolar pacing? A rational basis for choice. PACE 6:318, 1983.
74. Beyler M, Edwards L, Espe K, et al.: Adverse effects of unipolar pacing: A clinical comparison of bipolar and unipolar leads. PACE 6:314, 1983.
75. Watson W: Discriminating sense amplifier. A method for dealing with muscle noise. PACE 6:A-114, 1983.
76. Kaye GC, Butros G, Allen A, et al.: The effect of 50 Hz. external electrical interference on implanted cardiac pacemakers. PACE 11:999, 1988.

37

Indications for Cardiac Pacing in Bradyarrhythmias

Alfonso O. Tolentino
Roger P. Javier
Philip Samet

In 1952, Zoll[1] successfully treated a patient in ventricular standstill by external transcutaneous cardiac stimulation. This report was followed by another describing temporary, direct epicardial stimulation by Lillehei and co-workers[2] in 1957 and subsequently by a report on transvenous endocardial pacing for Stokes-Adams seizures by Furman[3] in 1959. These events led to the beginning of the modern era of cardiac pacing. In the early 1960s, symptomatic complete heart block was the sole indication for permanent cardiac pacing, and it still remains a primary indication; however, at present, symptomatic patients with sick sinus syndrome comprise approximately half of the pacemaker population.[4-12]

According to a recent world survey of cardiac pacing,[13] the average number of first implants in the United States has shown a steady decline, from 516 devices per million population in 1981 to 359 implants per million population in 1986. Sinus node dysfunction was the primary indication in 52%; conduction disturbances of the atrioventricular node and His-Purkinje system accounted for 41%, and ventricular tachyarrhythmias for 2%. Advances in pacemaker technology have further broadened the indications for cardiac pacing, which at present include the use of antitachycardia devices and the automatic implantable cardioverter defibrillator. In addition, sensor-triggered, rate-adaptive, antibradycardia pulse generators capable of modulating the pacing rate independently of the atrial activity are currently being employed with increasing frequency.[15, 16]

In 1984, the Joint American College of Cardiology/American Heart Association Task Force on Assessment of Cardiovascular Procedures issued guidelines for permanent pacemaker implantation.[17] A principal criterion used in the guidelines is the presence or absence of documented bradycardia occurring concurrently with symptoms prior to pacemaker implantation. Symptomatic bradycardia is a term generally used to describe clinical manifestations that are directly attributable to the slow heart rate: transient dizziness, lightheadedness, near-syncope or frank syncope as manifestations of transient cerebral hypoperfusion, and more generalized symptoms such as marked exercise intolerance and frank congestive heart failure. The committee further categorized the indications for pacemaker implantation into three classes: class I, those conditions wherein permanent pacemaker implantation is definitely indicated; class II, those conditions wherein pacemaker implantation is debatable or equivocal; and class III, those conditions wherein permanent pacemaker insertion is definitely not indicated.

This chapter reviews the role of cardiac pacing in patients with bradyarrhythmias associated with various degrees of acquired atrioventricular block, congenital complete heart block, paroxysmal atrioventricular block, exercise-induced atrioventricular block, atrial fibrillation with slow ventricular rate, postsurgical atrioventricular block, chronic fascicular block, sick sinus syndrome, hypersensitive carotid sinus syndrome, and other specific clinical entities such as Lyme myocarditis, cardiac transplantation, and cardiac catheterization procedures. The indications for temporary and permanent cardiac pacing in the setting of acute myocardial infarction are discussed in Chapter 7.

Pacing in Acquired Atrioventricular Block

FIRST-DEGREE ATRIOVENTRICULAR BLOCK

First-degree atrioventricular (AV) block is defined as prolongation of the P-R interval beyond 0.20 s without failure of ventricular conduction. In general, if the QRS complex is narrow (≤0.08 s), there is a 90% chance that the delay occurs within the AV node; whereas with a wide QRS complex (≥0.12 s), there is a 50% possibility that at least part of the delay is below the AV node.[18] First-degree AV block, by itself, is not an indication for permanent pacing regardless of the site of block. However, in the rare patient with unexplained syncope and with a normal P-R interval and a narrow QRS complex, electrophysiologic study may demonstrate either a split His bundle deflection or a prolonged H-V interval ≥70 ms.[19] This finding indicates conduction abnormality in the main His bundle proximal to the bundle branches. Progression to second- or third-degree AV block has been reported;[20] therefore, prophylactic pacing is recommended especially after other causes of syncope have been eliminated.

SECOND-DEGREE ATRIOVENTRICULAR BLOCK

Second-degree AV block has been traditionally classified into two types: type I and type II. Type I (AV Wenckebach) is characterized by a progressive lengthening of the P-R interval with progressive decrease of the R-R interval until a sinus P wave is blocked or nonconducted. The site of block is usually within the AV node. Type I AV Wenckebach is most often associated with acute inferior wall myocardial infarction.[21]

Chronic, isolated type I second-degree AV block is relatively infrequent, with an estimated prevalence of 0.003%.[22] Type I AV block has been demonstrated in approximately 9% of asymptomatic athletes who were found to have increased vagal tone.[23] In nonathletes, type I AV Wenckebach caused by hypervagotonia is usually transient and related to specific maneuvers such as swallowing, yawning, micturition, and defecation. Occasionally, atropine-responsive vagotonic AV block is observed in the absence of these vagal maneuvers.[24] The incidence of type I AV Wenckebach block was 6% among 50 healthy medical students without apparent cardiac history and was observed mostly during sleep.[25]

Type I second-degree AV block usually has a benign clinical course in patients without documented organic heart disease.[26] Prophylactic pacing is generally not indicated unless the patient is symptomatic from the bradycardia, and/or the ventricular rate is less than 40 beats per minute. Reversible causes of AV block such as drug toxicity, electrolyte abnormality, transient ischemia, rheumatic inflammation, and myocarditis (Lyme disease) must be carefully excluded before considering permanent pacer insertion.[27]

Type II (Mobitz II) second-degree AV block is characterized by a constant P-R interval before and after the blocked or nonconducted sinus P wave. The site of block is localized within the His-Purkinje system (infranodal); approximately 35% are located in the main His bundle and 65% in the distal His-Purkinje system.[28] Mobitz II AV block associated with a wide QRS complex (≥0.12 s) strongly suggests infranodal conduction block; whereas in Mobitz II AV block with a narrow QRS complex (≤0.08 sec) and a normal P-R interval during 1:1 conduction, the block occurs within the main His bundle (intra-His) and accounts for about 16% to 29% of patients with advanced or third-degree heart block.[29] Patients with this conduction abnormality are often elderly with advanced atherosclerotic cardiovascular disease.[19] Electrophysiologic study is recommended in these patients to confirm the diagnosis. Demonstration of a split His bundle deflection in the presence of a normal QRS complex is considered pathognomonic for intra-Hisian disease.[28] Mobitz II AV block usually has an unreliable escape rhythm and may progress to third-degree heart block.[30] The majority of patients with Mobitz II AV block are symptomatic, and the risk of sudden death is relatively high. For these reasons, permanent pacing is definitely recommended regardless of the presence or absence of symptoms.[31]

Atrial pacing to stress the conduction system during electrophysiologic studies may demonstrate intra-His conduction delay. Block distal to the His bundle deflection during atrial pacing at rates of less than 150 per minute is an abnormal response and implies severe disease of the His-Purkinje system. Induced atrial premature beat with block distal to the His bundle deflection with an H_1-H_2 interval of ≥400 ms has the same clinical significance as atrial-paced infra-His block.[19] Permanent pacemaker therapy should be considered in this group of patients.[32]

PAROXYSMAL ATRIOVENTRICULAR BLOCK

Paroxysmal atrioventricular block is manifested by an abrupt and persistent AV block in the presence of an otherwise normal AV conduction.[33] The block may be initiated by a conducted or nonconducted atrial premature beat or ventricular premature beat or by acceleration or slowing of the sinus rate.

Paroxysmal Vagally Mediated "Mobitz II" Atrioventricular Block

A subgroup of patients with paroxysmal Mobitz II AV block was reported by Huang[34] and Nakagawa.[35] In this group of symptomatic patients, the episodes of AV block were described as paroxysmal; vagally mediated; associated with cough, hiccups, micturition, digitalis toxicity, or acute myocardial infarction; and provokable by vagal maneuvers that were reversible with atropine. In addition, the P-R intervals of several beats preceding the block remained constant, whereas the P-R interval following the block was unchanged or prolonged. The QRS complex during episodes of AV block were usually narrow unless pre-existing bundle branch block was present; and the site of block was localized within the AV node, as documented by electrophysiologic studies. The natural history of this subset of Mobitz II AV block is not known. Since most of the patients have their underlying provokable symptoms corrected, the role of permanent pacing is not clear.

Pseudo Mobitz II Atrioventricular Block

Paroxysmal vagally mediated second-degree Mobitz II AV block should be differentiated from pseudo second-degree Mobitz II AV block. The latter condition is characterized by electrophysiologic demonstration of concealed His bundle extrasystoles, which are not apparent on the surface ECG; also, when conducted retrogradely but not propagated antegradely, the premature His bundle potentials may block the subsequent sinus P waves and thus manifest as Mobitz II AV block on the electrocardiogram.[36] Patients with concealed His bundle extrasystoles usually have prolonged H-V conduction time. Their prognosis may be similar to that of patients true Mobitz II AV block.[19] The incidence of pseudo Mobitz II second-degree AV block is rare; however, pacemaker implantation should be considered once the diagnosis is established.

EXERCISE-INDUCED ATRIOVENTRICULAR BLOCK

The significance and natural history of exercise-induced second- or third-degree AV block are not well known.[37, 38] In a prospective study of 11 symptomatic patients followed from 12 to 68 months, Petrac and coworkers[39] observed the following: the incidence of second-degree block induced by exercise is relatively small; the site of block is localized within the His-Purkinje system; and second-degree block induced by exercise may progress to complete heart block. They recommend prophylactic permanent pacing in patients with documented exercise-induced second-degree AV block.

THIRD-DEGREE (COMPLETE) ATRIOVENTRICULAR BLOCK

Third-degree or complete AV block implies total failure of conduction of atrial impulses to the ventricles. The rate of the subsidiary pacemaker is slow, approximately 40 to 50 beats per minute in the presence of a junctional pacemaker or approximately 30 beats per minute if the impulse originates from the His-Purkinje fibers. Complete heart block may be acquired or congenital.

Acquired Complete Heart Block

Before pacemaker therapy became available, the first-year mortality of patients with acquired complete heart block was 50%.[40, 41] The etiology of chronic, acquired complete AV block is either primary (sclerodegenerative) or secondary to ischemia. Sclerodegenerative disease of the cardiac skeleton (Lev's disease)[42] or of the conduction system itself (Lenegre's disease)[43] is often preceded by bifascicular blocks.[42, 43] Acquired complete heart block may be transient or permanent and may be associated with hypertension, calcific aortic valve disease, syphilis, collagen vascular disease, rheumatic heart disease, Lyme disease, chest trauma, metabolic disorders (myxedema or thyrotoxicosis), and tumor metastasis.[44]

Mesothelioma of the AV node is a rare, benign primary tumor that occurs predominantly in females and is frequently associated with high degrees of heart block and with sudden death. Although permanent pacing may be effective in alleviating the symptoms from bradycardia, mortality remains high. It has been postulated that ventricular tachyarrhythmias may play a role in the mechanism of sudden death in this group of patients.[45]

Acquired complete heart block may be localized anywhere in the AV node, His bundle, or His-Purkinje system, but the most common site of conduction delay is below the AV node (infranodal) in 70% to 88% of patients.[18, 19, 46, 47] The most common etiology of acquired complete heart block is bilateral bundle branch block, and the escape rhythm manifests as a wide QRS complex with rates from 25 to about 60 beats per minute. The subsidiary pacemakers do not accelerate with atropine, are easily suppressed by ventricular stimulation, and are prone to prolonged periods of asystole.[47] These abnormalities in conduction often lead to Stokes-Adams attacks, which occur in approximately 50% of patients with acquired third-degree AV block.[48] Other related symptoms include dizziness, weakness, congestive heart failure, and low cardiac output syndrome.[49]

A permanent pacemaker is definitely recommended for all symptomatic patients with acquired complete heart block after reversible causes have been ruled out. Prophylactic pacing is also indicated in asymptomatic patients with acquired complete AV block especially if the QRS complex is wide and the ventricular rate is less than 40 beats per minute. The clinical course is often unpredictable and a substantial number of these patients die suddenly.[50] Asymptomatic patients with acquired third-degree heart block and ventricular rates over 40 beats per minute should undergo electrophysiologic evaluation to assess the site of block. Neither heart rate nor duration of the QRS complex can be used as a completely reliable guide in the localization of the site of block.[46, 51] Prognosis depends on whether impairment of conduction is in the AV node (intranodal) or within the His-Purkinje system (infranodal). The incidence of syncope is much higher in infranodal blocks (either intra-His or distal to the His bundle).[47] Therefore, permanent pacer implantation is recommended in this group of patients.[49] Asymptomatic patients with acquired complete heart block localized in the AV node, with ventricular rates above 40 beats per minute and a stable subsidiary pacemaker, are not candidates for permanent pacing. These patients should be followed carefully both clinically and with periodic, ambulatory Holter monitoring.

Congenital Complete Heart Block

Congenital complete heart block may occur as an isolated abnormality or associated with other cardiovascular anomalies such as transposition of the great vessels and ventricular septal defects.[53] Patients with congenital complete AV block usually have a narrow QRS complex with the block localized in the AV node in the majority of patients.[52,53] The heart rate is relatively faster compared with patients with acquired complete heart block and may even increase to some extent, with exercise.[53,54] In neonates with congenital complete heart block, the risk of death is much higher if the ventricular rate is less than 55 beats per minute.[55] The majority of deaths occur during the first year of life in infants with associated congenital cardiac defects.[54] Karpawich and associates[53] prospectively studied 24 children with congenital complete heart block for up to 19 years. They found that a resting heart rate of 50 beats per minute or less was predictive of subsequent Stokes-Adams syncope and that other clinical and electrophysiologic factors had little prognostic value. Permanent pacemakers were implanted in ten of the 24 children who remained asymptomatic on follow-up. Besley[56] and Reid[57] also reported improvement of symptoms after pacemaker implantation in patients with congenital complete heart block. In a selected group of patients without symptoms and in whom the QRS complex is wide or the ventricular rate is persistently at or below 50 beats per minute, electrophysiologic studies have been helpful in decision-making. If the block is infranodal, permanent pacemaker implantation is recommended; if the block is intranodal, follow-up observation without pacing is advised.[49]

Congenital complete AV block without congenital malformation of the heart or great vessels is usually discovered accidentally because of inappropriately slow heart rates in otherwise asymptomatic children or young adults. Diagnosis is confirmed on the basis of electrocardiography. The ventricular rate is relatively faster than in acquired complete heart block, since the depolarization focus is often above the His bundle. Accordingly, the QRS complex has normal or near-normal configuration. Familial occurrence is well known, and a history of maternal lupus is of diagnostic importance. Stokes-Adams attacks are uncommon, and adult survival without cardiac pacing is expected.[58]

FIXED 2:1 OR 3:1 ATRIOVENTRICULAR BLOCK

These atrioventricular blocks cannot be classified as to either type I or type II second-degree AV block unless the P-R intervals are observed during periods of changing conduction ratios (3:2, 1:1, 3:1). A change in conduction ratio from 2:1 to 3:2 with a constant P-R interval indicates type II, whereas a changing P-R interval is compatible with type I AV block. Fixed-ratio 2:1 and 3:1 AV blocks are either intranodal (35%) or infranodal (65%) and may be associated with either a normal or a wide QRS complex.[19] Permanent pacemaker implantation is recommended depending on the site of block, presence or absence of symptoms, and overall ventricular rate.[49]

ATRIAL FIBRILLATION WITH SLOW VENTRICULAR RATE

Some patients with atrial fibrillation manifest a very slow ventricular rate in the absence of cardioactive drugs such as digitalis glycosides, beta adrenergic blockers, and calcium channel blockers. This usually indicates impaired AV nodal conduction or probable high-degree atrioventricular block. Prophylactic pacer implantation is recommended in those symptomatic patients with a ventricular rate of less than 40 beats per minute or in those who need drugs, which could further depress the ventricular rate. The latter clinical condition should be properly documented before considering permanent pacing.[49]

Pacing for Postsurgical Atrioventricular Block

Conduction disturbances are relatively frequent after surgery for repair of ventricular septal defect (VSD) or tetralogy of Fallot.[59] Right bundle branch block has been reported in about 80% of children in whom septal defects were repaired via a right ventriculotomy.[60] The right bundle branch block results from damage to the right bundle during surgical closure of the interventricular septum. A small proportion of patients develop right bundle branch block with left anterior hemiblock[61] which has been correlated with the risk for late occurrence of complete heart block, Stokes-Adams attacks, and sudden death.[62] However, other studies have shown no evidence of late complications or further deterioration in conduction abnormality among children followed for 10 years after repair of the VSD.[63,64,65] This discrepancy in results has been attributed to the difference in surgical technique and extent of trauma to the right bundle. Accordingly, electrophysiologic studies have been proposed for localization of the site of block in order to distinguish which patient will benefit from permanent pacing.[66] Previous studies have also shown that complete AV block following cardiac surgery for congenital heart defects implies a poor prognosis.[67] However, improvements in surgical techniques have significantly reduced the incidence of postoperative complete heart block.[68] Furthermore, advancement in pacemaker technology along with a decrease in pulse generator size and increase in battery longevity have helped establish the role of permanent cardiac pacing in the management of children with persistent postsurgical complete AV block.[69,70] The time interval of observation before a permanent pacer is implanted varies from 2 weeks[71] to 4 or 6 weeks.[72]

Bradycardia due to sinus node dysfunction is the most frequently seen arrhythmia after the Mustard operation for transposition of the great arteries.[73] The indications for permanent pacemaker in this group of patients include syncope or near-syncope due to the bradycardia, need for drugs other than digitalis, and bradycardia of less than 40 beats per minute while awake or less than 30 beats per minute while asleep.[74]

The incidence of permanent pacing following valvular heart surgery is extremely small and occurs predominantly in calcified aortic stenoses.[75] Trauma involving the septal area has been implicated as the cause of the bradyarrhythmia. Persistent complete heart block is the primary indication for pacing in this group of postvalvular surgery patients.

Pacing for Chronic Fascicular Block

The distal conduction system includes the right bundle and the two divisions of the left bundle, the anterosuperior and the posteroinferior fascicles. Impairment of conduction within each individual fascicle of the left bundle is referred to as a hemiblock. A right bundle branch block and left anterior or posterior hemiblock constitute a bifascicular block, whereas an additional conduction delay within the remaining fascicle results in a trifascicular block. In patients with such conduction abnormalities, there is convincing evidence that chronic bundle branch block and organic heart disease have an increased incidence of progression to high-degree AV block and sudden death.[76, 77, 78]

Bundle branch block occurs in approximately 0.6% of the general population and in 1% to 2% of the population over 60 years of age.[79] The incidence of organic heart disease among hospitalized patients with bundle branch block is approximately 80%, with coronary artery disease being present in up to 50% of patients.[80] Most patients with chronic bundle branch block who die suddenly have coronary artery disease as the cause of sudden death. Dhingra and coworkers[82] found that patients with chronic left bundle branch block and marked left axis deviation had worse left ventricular function, more advanced conduction disease, and a higher cardiovascular mortality than those with left bundle branch block and a normal frontal QRS axis.

Syncope is relatively common among patients with chronic bifascicular block, but syncope is not necessarily associated with an increased incidence of sudden death.[84] Although pacing has been observed to relieve transient neurologic symptoms, it does not necessarily reduce the mortality from sudden death.[81] Complete heart block is most often preceded by bifascicular block, but studies have shown that the rate of progression to complete heart block is low.[76–78]

Earlier studies by Narula[85] and Vera[86] have shown that prolongation of the H-V interval during electrophysiologic evaluation of symptomatic patients with bundle branch block was associated with progression to higher degrees of AV block. However, subsequent prospective studies by other investigators[76–78] have confirmed that although the prevalence of a prolonged H-V interval is high among patients with chronic bundle branch block, the 5-year cumulative incidence of progression to complete heart block is low (4.9% in those with an H-V interval ≥55 ms, and 1.9% for those with a normal H-V interval of ≤55 ms).[77]

Similar results were reported by Scheinman and associates,[78] of spontaneous progression to second-degree or complete AV block (4% in patients with an H-V interval of ≤55 ms, and 2% in patients with an H-V interval of 55 to 69 ms). The risk of progression appears to be quantitatively related to the degree of H-V prolongation, once a critical H-V interval of 70 ms is exceeded. Scheinman and colleagues found a fourfold increase in the risk of progression to complete AV block among patients with an H-V interval of ≥100 ms, compared with patients who had either a normal or slightly increased H-V interval of 35 to 69 ms. Furthermore, these studies have shown that the mortality in patients with chronic bundle branch block is due to the underlying heart disease (ventricular tachyarrhythmia and myocardial infarction) and not to complete heart block.[77] These investigators concluded that the prolongation of the H-V interval is not an independent risk factor for sudden death when the H-V interval is markedly prolonged, and that electrophysiologic studies in symptomatic patients with chronic bundle branch block should include programmed ventricular stimulation.[87]

Patients with right bundle branch block or those with bifascicular block (right bundle branch block and left anterior or posterior hemiblock, or left bundle branch block) who also have symptoms of syncope or near-syncope with 1:1 AV conduction should have a complete medical and neurologic evaluation including at least two 24-hour, ambulatory Holter recordings. If intermittent second- or third-degree AV block is documented during monitoring, prophylactic pacing is recommended. Symptomatic patients without documentation of second- or third-degree AV block should undergo electrophysiologic studies including assessment of intracardiac conduction, sinus node function, and programmed ventricular stimulation. Documentation of a prolonged H-V interval of ≥70 ms in a patient with unexplained syncope is a probable indication for permanent pacemaker insertion. Demonstration of a prolonged H-V interval of ≥100 ms is a definite indication for permanent pacemaker therapy.[85] If the H-V interval is less than 70 ms, pacing is not usually recommended, and these patients should be followed clinically. Pacing-induced infra-His block in symptomatic patients with chronic bifascicular block and 1:1 AV conduction is another indication for permanent pacer insertion.[87]

Asymptomatic patients with bifascicular block with 1:1 conduction are not investigated. However, demonstration of spontaneous intermittent second- or third-degree AV block in these asymptomatic patients requires electrophysiologic evaluation to determine the site of the block.[49] If the block occurs distal to the His bundle deflection or within the main His bundle, prophylactic pacing is recommended. If the block is intranodal and the heart rate is above 40 beats per minute during periods of AV block, careful follow-up observation is recommended.

GENERALIZED INTRAVENTRICULAR CONDUCTION DEFECTS

Abnormally wide QRS complexes that do not meet the criteria of either right or left bundle branch block have been classified as generalized intraventricular conduction defects (IVCD).[88] The mean QRS frontal axis may be normal or slightly shifted to the left. In most of the cases, the H-V interval is prolonged with a left axis deviation. In all probability, the generalized IVCD is a form of partial bilateral bundle branch block and carries the same clinical significance as right bundle branch block with left axis deviation. Symptomatic patients with these conduction abnormalities may progress to complete heart block; therefore, prophylactic pacing is indicated.[88]

Pacing for the Sick Sinus Syndrome

The sick sinus syndrome is a descriptive term that refers to a constellation of signs, symptoms, and electrocardiographic manifestations of sinus node dysfunction.[89] The syndrome is characterized by syncope or other manifestations of cerebral hypoperfusion, such as light-headedness, dizziness, and near-syncope, in association with sinus bradycardia (usually with rates of less than 50 beats per minute), sinus arrest, sinoatrial block, and alternating tachycardia and bradycardia (tachy-brady syndrome). One or more of these electrocardiographic abnormalities may occur in 38% to 100% of patients with the sick sinus syndrome. In the tachy-brady syndrome, the tachycardia component is usually atrial fibrillation or at times atrial flutter. It is the bradycardia component that results in light-headedness or syncope, whereas the tachycardia component may manifest as palpitations, fluttering in the chest, or angina pectoris in those patients with coronary artery disease.[90] The syndrome may coexist with other abnormalities of AV conduction, such as atrioventricular block and bundle branch block.[91, 92, 93]

Pharmacologic therapy for the bradycardia in the sick sinus syndrome, using atropine, belladonna alkaloids, and sympathomimetic agents, has been tried with unsuccessful results.[94] Permanent pacing remains the definitive treatment for symptomatic patients. Symptomatic patients with unexplained syncope and with a negative medical and neurologic workup should have one or more 24-hour, ambulatory Holter monitoring. If sinus pauses with asystolic periods of more than 2.5 to 3 seconds, or persistent sinus bradycardia below 40 beats per minute, are correlated with the symptoms, then permanent pacemaker insertion is recommended. If the ambulatory recording is inconsistent or if the patient remains asymptomatic throughout the 24-hour recording period, then electrophysiologic evaluation should be performed. An abnormal corrected sinus node recovery time of more than 525 ms before or after the administration of intravenous atropine sulfate (0.04 mg/kg body weight) and propranolol (0.2 mg/kg body weight) and/or the escape of a junctional focus with a rate of less than 80 beats per minute after atrial overdrive pacing are indicative of a diseased sinus node and suggest the need for permanent pacing.[95]

In asymptomatic patients with transient sinus pauses of 1.5 to 2.5 seconds or sinus bradycardia with rates between 40 to 45 beats per minute, the role of prophylactic pacing remains controversial. Therapy for these patients is individualized, and reversible causes of the bradycardia should be carefully ruled out. Persistent sinus bradycardia below 40 beats per minute, especially during sleep, in an otherwise asymptomatic individual is not an indication for pacemaker implantation.[49]

It should be emphasized that certain cardioactive drugs such as digitalis glycosides, beta-adrenergic blockers, calcium channel blockers, and class IA antiarrhythmic agents may induce or unmask an underlying sinus node dysfunction. Prophylactic pacing may be indicated if persistent bradycardia below 40 beats per minute as a result of the necessary drug therapy is properly documented.

The various pacing modalities such as atrial, ventricular, and dual chamber pacing as well as sensor-driven, rate-responsive devices in the treatment of patients with the sick sinus syndrome are presented elsewhere in this book.

Pacing for the Hypersensitive Carotid Sinus Syndrome

Hypersensitive carotid sinus syndrome is clinically composed of excessive slowing of the heart rate and/or a profound decrease in systemic arterial pressure induced by mechanical stimulation of the carotid sinus.[96] Weiss[97] originally described three types of carotid sinus hypersensitivity: (1) cardio-inhibitory or vagal type, associated primarily with bradycardia or asystole with varying degrees of sinoatrial or atrioventricular block; (2) vasodepressor type, characterized by a fall in arterial pressure induced by abrupt decrease in peripheral resistance; and (3) a primary cerebral type, which is not accompanied by either bradycardia or hypotension, is poorly characterized, and is extremely rare.[98] The cardio-inhibitory type is the most common form; a combination of cardio-inhibitory and vasodepressor types (mixed type) may be encountered.

The diagnosis of hypersensitive carotid sinus syndrome is often limited by a lack of standardized techniques for stimulation of the carotid sinus reflex. The reliability and reproducibility of symptoms may be subject to errors because of the variable response and spontaneous remission of the hypersensitive carotid sinus reflex even in the same individual.[99] Multiple studies have defined carotid sinus hypersensitivity as a manifestation of ventricular asystole of more than 3 seconds in duration (cardio-inhibitory type) and/or a fall in systolic arterial pressure of 30 to 50 mm Hg (vasodepressor type) during carotid sinus stimulation from 3 to 8 seconds. The cardio-inhibitory response may be accompanied by a fall in systolic blood pressure; whereas the vasodepressor response may occur in the absence of bradycardia or asystole.[100]

Approximately 10% of the general population demonstrate hyperactive carotid sinus.[101] An abnormal response to carotid sinus stimulation occurs in about one third of elderly men with coronary atherosclerosis and hypertensive heart disease.[102] Syncope is a common manifestation among patients with the cardio-inhibitory response or in the mixed form, but syncope is uncommon in the vasodepressor type. When spontaneous syncope and hypersensitive carotid sinus coexist, it is tempting to assume that the hyperactive carotid sinus reflex is the cause of the syncope. However, most patients with a hypersensitive carotid sinus are often asymptomatic, and its presence may be coincidental.[103]

Permanent pacing eliminates the symptoms in patients with the cardio-inhibitory response to carotid massage, but treatment of patients with the isolated vasodepressor type or mixed response is often difficult.[104] Patients with recurrent unexplained syncope documented to be associated with spontaneous events capable of stimulating the carotid sinus and in whom carotid sinus massage induces 3 or more seconds of asystole are candidates for permanent pacing. Asymptomatic patients with a positive response to carotid sinus stimulation do not require prophylactic pacing.[17]

Pacing for Other Clinical Entities

LYME MYOCARDITIS

Lyme disease is a tick-borne spirochetal infection characterized by fever, myalgia, and a peculiar skin rash—erythema chronicum migrans—that appears at the site of the bite.[105] Transient myocarditis occurs in approximately 4% to 10% of patients and is manifested as varying degrees of atrioventricular block, arrhythmias, and left ventricular dysfunction. The diagnosis of Lyme disease is based on a strong clinical index of suspicion and the presence of the characteristic skin rash, which is pathognomonic. Infrequently, high-grade AV block may require temporary pacer insertion, but resumption to a normal sinus rhythm is excellent. The site of block has been localized above the His bundle in those few patients who have had electrophysiologic studies. Although temporary pacing may be required, especially if the ventricular rate is extremely slow, permanent pacer implantation is not recommended.[106]

CARDIAC TRANSPLANTATION

Cardiac transplantation is now a well-accepted form of treatment for end-stage heart disease.[107] Available data from 528 patients from Stanford, California and 401 patients from Pittsburgh, Pennsylvania have shown that bradyarrhythmias may occur in approximately 6% to 18% of cardiac transplant recipients.[108,109] Sinus bradycardia and junctional bradycardia comprised the majority (80%) of post-cardiac transplant arrhythmias. Permanent pacemakers were inserted in 36 (6%) of patients from Stanford and in 17 (24%) of patients from Pittsburgh. Follow-up at 1 year showed restoration to a normal sinus rhythm in the majority of these patients. The investigators postulated that sinus bradycardia may be related to donor ischemic time or compromise of the blood supply to the sinus node. However, the exact mechanism of the bradyarrhythmia and the role of cardiac pacing are not yet fully understood.

CARDIAC CATHETERIZATION PROCEDURES

The Society for Cardiac Angiography and Intervention has recently issued a recommendation that temporary prophylactic pacemaker insertion should not be done routinely during retrograde left heart catheterization and selective coronary arteriography.[110] Catheter-induced atrioventricular blocks have been demonstrated in certain selected patients undergoing right heart catheterization.[111-113] These conduction abnormalities result from direct catheter trauma to the affected structures and are usually transient, lasting from a few seconds to at most a few days. However, in the occasional patient with pre-existing left bundle branch block who undergoes right heart catheterization, induction of a concomitant right bundle branch block may result in high-degree AV block.[113] Prophylactic temporary pacemaker insertion should be considered in this group of patients.

The use of prophylactic pacemakers during diagnostic cardiac catheterization, percutaneous coronary angioplasty and percutaneous balloon valvuloplasty was retrospectively studied by Baim and associates.[114] The incidence of significant bradycardia requiring initiation of immediate temporary pacing during cardiac catheterization was 0.06% during diagnostic cardiac catheterization, 0.4% during coronary angioplasty, and 2.5% during balloon valvuloplasty. Baim and colleagues concluded that prophylactic temporary pacing is not indicated during either diagnostic cardiac catheterization or coronary angioplasty but should be used routinely during percutaneous balloon valvuloplasty. Persistent complete heart block requiring permanent pacing recently has been reported in another patient who had prior aortic valvuloplasty.[115]

References

1. Zoll PM: Restoration of the heart in ventricular standstill by external electrical stimulation. N Engl J Med 247:768, 1952.
2. Weirich WL, Gott VL, Lillehei CW: Treatment of complete heart block by combined use of myocardial electrode and artificial pacemaker. Surg Forum 8:360, 1957.
3. Furman, S, Schwedel JB: An intracardiac pacemaker for Stokes-Adams seizures. N Engl J Med 261:94, 1959.
4. Chokshi DS, Mascarenhas E, Samet P, et al.: Treatment of sinoatrial rhythm disturbances with permanent cardiac pacing. Am J Cardiol 32:215, 1973.
5. Radford DJ, Julian DG: Sick sinus syndrome: Experience of a cardiac pacemaker clinic. Br Med J 3:504, 1974.
6. Hartel G, Talvensaari T: Treatment of sinoatrial syndrome with permanent cardiac pacing in 90 patients. Acta Scand 198:341, 1975.

7. Krishnaswami V, Geraci AR: Permanent pacing in disorders of sinus node function. Am Heart J 89:579, 1975.
8. Aroesty JM, Cohen SI, Morkini E: Bradycardia-tachycardia syndrome: Results in twenty-eight patients treated by combined pharmacological therapy and pacemaker implantation. Chest 66:257, 1975.
9. Skagen K, Fisher T, Hansen JF: The long-term prognosis for patients with sinoatrial block treated with permanent pacemaker. Acta Med Scand 199:13, 1976.
10. Wohl AJ, Laborde NJ, Atkins JM, et al.: Prognosis of patients permanently paced for sick sinus syndrome. Arch Intern Med 136:250, 1977.
11. Kaul TK, Kumar EB, Thomson RM, et al.: Sick sinus syndrome: Experience with implantable cardiac pacemakers. J Cardiovasc Surg 19:261, 1978.
12. Harthorne JW: Indications for pacemaker insertion: types and modes of pacing. Prog Cardiovasc Dis 23:393, 1981.
13. Feruglio GA, Rickards AF, Steinbach K, et al.: Cardiac pacing in the world: A survey of state of the art. PACE 10:768, 1987.
14. Parsonnet V, Bernstein AD, Galasso D: Cardiac pacing practices in the United States. Am J Cardiol 62:71, 1988.
15. Benditt DG, Milstein S, Buetikofer J, et al.: Sensor-triggered, rate-variable cardiac pacing. Ann Intern Med 107:714, 1987.
16. Goldman BS: Selection of the optimal pacing mode: Modes of pacing. In Belhassen B, Feldman S, Copperman Y, (eds.): Cardiac Pacing and Electrophysiology, p. 3. Tel Aviv, Israel, Creative Communications Ltd. 1987.
17. Joint American College/American Heart Association Task Force on Assessment of Cardiovascular Procedures (Subcommittee on Pacemaker Implantation): Guidelines for permanent pacemaker implantation. J Am Coll Cardiol 4:434, 1984.
18. Puech P, Wainright RJ: Clinical electrophysiology of atrioventricular block. Cardiol Clin 1:209, 1983.
19. Narula OS: Current concepts of atrioventricular block. In Narula OS (ed.): His Bundle Electrocardiography and Clinical Electrophysiology, p. 139. Philadelphia, FA Davis, 1975.
20. Lister JW, Ilsaka Y, Pinakatt T, et al.: An indication for His bundle study: Syncope, a normal P-R interval and a narrow QRS. PACE 4:443, 1981.
21. Goldschlager N: Permanent cardiac pacing for bradyarrhythmia. Postgrad Med 83:156, 1988.
22. Hiss RG, Lamb LE: Electrocardiographic findings in 122,043 individuals. Circulation 25:947, 1962.
23. Meyles I, Kaplinsky E, Yakini JH, et al.: Wenckebach AV block: A frequent feature following heavy physical training. Am Heart J 90:426.
24. Strasberg B, Lam W, Swiryn S, et al.: Symptomatic spontaneous paroxysmal AV nodal block due to localized hyperresponsiveness of the AV node to vagotonic reflexes. Am Heart J 103:795, 1982.
25. Brodsky M, Wu D, Denes P, et al.: Twenty-four hour continuous electrocardiographic monitoring in fifty male medical students without apparent heart disease. Am J Cardiol 39:390, 1977.
26. Strasberg B, Amat-Y-Leon F, Dhingra RC, et al.: Natural history of chronic second-degree atrioventricular nodal block. Circulation 63:1043, 1981.
27. Phibbs B, Friedman HS, Graboys TB, et al.: Indications for pacing in the treatment of bradyarrhythmias. JAMA 252:1307, 1984.
28. Narula OS, Samet P: Wenckebach and Mobitz II A-V block within the His bundle and bundle branches. Circulation 41:947, 1970.
29. Amat-Y-Leon F, Dhingra RC, Denes P, et al.: The clinical spectrum of chronic His bundle block. Chest 70:747, 1976.
30. Dhingra RC, Denes P, Wu D, et al.: The significance of second degree atrioventricular block and bundle branch block: observations regarding site and type of block. Circulation 49:638, 1974.
31. Moses HW, Taylor GJ, Schneider JA, et al.: Indications for pacing. In Moses HW, Taylor GJ, Schneider JA, Dove JT (eds.): A Practical Guide to Cardiac Pacing, p. 1. Boston, Little, Brown and Company, 1983.
32. Dhingra RC, Wyndham C, Bauernfeind R, et al.: Significance of block distal to the His bundle induced by atrial pacing in patients with chronic bifascicular block. Circulation 60:1455, 1979.
33. Rosenbaum MB, Elizari MV, Levi RJ: Paroxysmal atrioventricular block related to hyperpolarization and spontaneous diastolic depolarization. Chest 63:678, 1973.
34. Huang SK: A subset of "Mobitz II" atrioventricular block: role of vagal influence (Letter). PACE 11:472, 1988.
35. Nakagawa S: Vagally mediated paroxysmal atrioventricular block presenting as "Mobitz II" block (Letter). PACE 11:471, 1988.
36. Rosen KM, Rahimtoola SH, Gunnar RM: Pseudo A-V block secondary to premature non-propagated His bundle depolarization by His bundle electrocardiography. Circulation 42:367, 1970.
37. Bakst A, Goldberg B, Schamroth L: Significance of exercise induced atrioventricular block. Br Heart J 37:984, 1975.
38. Woelfel AK, Simpson RJ, Gettes LS, et al.: Exercise induced distal atrioventricular block. J Am Coll Cardiol 2:578, 1983.
39. Petrac D, Gjurovic J, Vukosavic D, et al.: Clinical significance and natural history of exercise-induced atrioventricular block. In Belhassen B, Feldman S, Copperman Y (eds.): Cardiac Pacing and Electrophysiology, p. 265. Tel Aviv, Israel, Creative Communications Ltd., 1987.
40. Johnson BW: Longevity in complete heart block. Ann NY Acad Sci 1967:1031, 1969.
41. Friedberg CK, Donoso E, Stein WG: Non-surgical acquired heart block. Ann NY Acad Sci 111:835, 1964.
42. Lev M: Anatomic basis for atrioventricular block. Am J Med 37:742, 1964.
43. Lenegre J: Etiology and pathology of bilateral bundle branch block in relation to complete heart block. Prog Cardiovasc Dis 6:409, 1964.
44. Peters RW, Scheinman MM: Bundle branch block atrioventricular conduction disorders. In Parmley WW, Chatterjee K (eds.): Cardiology. Physiology, Pharmacology, and Diagnosis, Chapter 68. Philadelphia, J.B. Lippincott, 1988.
45. Strauss WE, Asinger RW, Hodges M: Mesothelioma of the AV node: Potential utility of pacing. PACE 11:1296, 1988.
46. Narula OS, Scherlag BJ, Samet P, et al.: Atrioventricular block: Localization and classification by His bundle recordings. Am J Med 50:146, 1971.
47. Narula OS: Clinical concepts of spontaneous and induced atrioventricular block. In Mandel WJ (ed.): Cardiac Arrhythmias: Their Mechanism, Diagnosis, and Management, p. 321. Philadelphia, JB Lippincott, 1987.
48. Pomerantz B, O'Rourke RA: The Stokes-Adams syndrome. Am J Med 46:941, 1969.
49. Gann D, El-Sherif N, Samet P: Indications for cardiac pacing. In Samet P, El-Sherif N (eds.). Cardiac Pacing, 2nd ed. New York, Grune and Stratton, Inc., 1980.
50. Hollingsworth HJ, Muller WH, Beckwith JR: Patient selection for permanent cardiac pacing. Ann Intern Med 70:263, 1969.
51. Rosen KM, Dhingra RC, Loeb HS, et al.: Chronic heart block in adults: Clinical and electrophysiological observations. Arch Intern Med 131:663, 1973.
52. Pinsky WW, Gilette PC, Garson A, et al.: Diagnosis, management and long term results of patients with congenital complete heart block. Pediatrics 69:728, 1982.
53. Karpawich PP, Gilette PC, Garson A, et al.: Congenital complete atrioventricular block: clinical and electrophysiologic predictors of need for pacemaker insertion. Am J Cardiol 48:1098, 1981.
54. Chawla K, Suratto M, Cruz J, et al.: Response to maximal and submaximal exercise testing in patients with congenital complete heart block (Abstract). Circulation 56:171, 1977.
55. Michaelson M, Engle M: Congenital complete heart block: An international study on the natural history. Cardiovasc Clin 4:85, 1972.
56. Besley DC, McWilliams GJ, Moodie DS, et al.: Long-term follow-up of young adults following permanent pacemaker placement for complete heart block. Am Heart J 103:332, 1982.
57. Reid JM, Coleman EN, Doig W: Complete congenital heart block: Report of 35 cases. Br Heart J 48:236, 1982.
58. Perloff JK: Congenital complete heart block. In Perloff JK (ed.): Clinical Recognition of Congenital Heart Disease, p. 49. Philadelphia, W.B. Saunders, 1987.
59. Krongrad E, Hefler SE, Bowman FO, et al.: Further observations on the etiology of right bundle branch block following right ventriculotomy. Circulation 50:1105, 1975.

60. Boxer R, Krongrad E, Bowman FO, et al.: Conduction defects following ventricular septal defect closure with and without a right ventriculotomy. Pediatr Res 11:386, 1977.
61. Gelband H, Waldo AL, Kaisser GA, et al.: Etiology of right bundle branch block in patients undergoing total correction of tetralogy of Fallot. Circulation 44:1022, 1971.
62. Wolff GS, Rowland TW, Ellison RC: Surgically induced right bundle branch block with left anterior hemiblock: An ominous sign in postoperative tetralogy of Fallot. Circulation 46:587, 1972.
63. Downing JW, Kaplan S, Bove KE: Postsurgical left anterior hemiblock and right bundle branch block. Br Heart J 34:263, 1972.
64. Godman MJ, Roberts NK, Isukawa T: Late post-operative conduction disturbances after repair of ventricular septal defect and tetralogy of Fallot. Circulation 49:214, 1974.
65. Cairns JA, Bobell ARC, Gibbons JE, et al.: Prognosis of right bundle branch block and left anterior hemiblock after intracardiac repair of tetralogy of Fallot. Am Heart J 40:549, 1975.
66. Sung RJ, Tamer DM, Garcia OL, et al.: Analysis of surgically induced right bundle branch block pattern using intracardiac recording technique. Circulation 54:442, 1976.
67. Zion MM, Marchand PE, Obel IWP: Long-term prognosis after cardiac pacing in atrioventricular block. Br Heart J 35:359, 1973.
68. Kirklin JW, Barratt BG: Late results, conduction disturbances, ventricular septal defect. In Kirklin JW, Barratt BG (eds.): Cardiac Surgery, p. 640. New York, John Wiley & Sons, 1986.
69. Driscoll DJ, Gilette PC, Hallman GL, et al.: Management of surgical complete atrioventricular block in children. Am J Cardiol 43:1175, 1979.
70. Beder SD, Hanisch DG, Cohen MH: Cardiac pacing in children: A 15 year experience. Am Heart J 109:152, 1985.
71. Benrey J, Gilette PC, Nasrallah AT, et al.: Permanent pacemaker implantation in infants, children and adolescents: Long-term follow-up. Circulation 53:245, 1976.
72. Hofschire PJ, Nicoloff DM, Moller JH: Postoperative complete heart block in 64 children treated with and without cardiac pacing. Am J Cardiol 39:559, 1977.
73. Hayes CJ, Gersony WM: Arrhythmias after the Mustard operation for transposition of the great arteries: A long-term study. J Am Coll Cardiol 7:133, 1986.
74. Gilette PC, Wampler DG, Shannon C, et al.: Use of cardiac pacing after the Mustard operation for transposition of the great arteries. J Am Coll Cardiol 7:138, 1986.
75. Gaillard P, Lespinasse P, Vanetti A: Cardiac pacing and valvular surgery. PACE 11:2142, 1988.
76. Dhingra RC, Palileo E, Strasberg B, et al.: Significance of HV interval in 517 patients with chronic bifascicular block. Circulation 64:1265, 1981.
77. McAnulty JH, Rahimtoola SH, Murphy E, et al.: Natural history of "high risk" bundle branch block: Final report of a prospective study. N Engl J Med 307:137, 1982.
78. Scheinman MM, Peters RW, Sauve MJ, et al.: The value of HQ interval in patients with bundle branch block and the role of prophylactic pacing. Am J Cardiol 50:1316, 1982.
79. Cohen HC, Singer DH: Bundle branch block and other forms of aberrant intraventricular conduction: Clinical aspects. In Mandel WJ (ed.): Cardiac Arrhythmias: Their Mechanisms, Diagnosis and Management, p. 413. Philadelphia, J.B. Lippincott, 1987.
80. McAnulty J, Rahimtoola SH: Prognosis in bundle branch block. Ann Rev Med 32:499, 1981.
81. Peters RW, Scheinman MM, Modin GM, et al.: Prophylactic permanent pacemakers for patients with chronic bundle branch block. Am J Med 66:978, 1979.
82. Dhingra RC, Amat-Y-Leon F, Wyndham C, et al.: Significance of left axis deviation in patients with chronic left bundle branch block. Am J Cardiol 42:551, 1978.
83. Fisch GR, Zipes DP, Fisch C: Bundle branch block and sudden death. Prog Cardiovasc Dis 23:187, 1980.
84. Dhingra RC, Denes P, Wu D, et al.: Syncope in patients with chronic bifascicular block: Significance, causative mechanisms, and clinical implications. Ann Intern Med 81:302, 1974.
85. Narula OS, Samet P: Right bundle branch block with normal, left or right axis deviation: Analysis by His bundle recordings. Am J Med 51:432, 1971.
86. Vera Z, Mason DT, Fletcher RD, et al.: Prolonged H-Q interval in chronic bifascicular block: Relation to impending complete heart block. Circulation 53:46, 1976.
87. Scheinman MM, Peters RW, Morady F, et al.: Electrophysiologic studies in patients with bundle branch block. PACE 6:157, 1983.
88. Narula OS: Intraventricular conduction defects: Current concepts and clinical significance. In Narula OS (ed.): Cardiac Arrhythmias. Electrophysiology, Diagnosis and Management, p. 114. Baltimore, Williams & Wilkins, 1979.
89. Ferrer MI: Sick sinus syndrome in atrial disease. JAMA 206:645, 1968.
90. Gomes JA: The sick sinus syndrome and evaluation of the patient with sinus node dysfunction. In Parmley WW, Chatterjee K (eds.): Cardiology. Physiology, Pharmacology, and Diagnosis, Chapter 67. Philadelphia, J.B. Lippincott, 1988.
91. Rosen KM, Loeb HS, Sinno MZ, et al.: Cardiac conduction in patients with symptomatic sinus node disease. Circulation 43:843, 1971.
92. Narula OS: Atrioventricular conduction defects in patients with sinus bradycardia. Circulation 44:1104, 1974.
93. Rubenstein JJ, Schulman CL, Yurchak PM, et al.: Clinical spectrum of sick sinus syndrome. Circulation 46:6, 1972.
94. Scarpa, WJ: The sick sinus syndrome. Am Heart J 92:648, 1976.
95. Gann D, Tolentino AO, Samet P: Electrophysiologic evaluation of elderly patients with sinus bradycardia: A long-term follow-up study. Ann Intern Med 90:24, 1979.
96. Wenger TL, Dohrmann ML, Strauss HC: Hypersensitive carotid sinus syndrome manifested as cough syncope. PACE 3:332, 1980.
97. Weiss S, Baker JP: The carotid sinus reflex in health and disease. Medicine 12:297, 1933.
98. Gurjidan ES, Webster JE, Herday WG, et al.: Non-existence of the so-called cerebral form of carotid sinus syncope. Neurology 8:818, 1958.
99. Huang SKS, Ezri MD, Hauser RG, et al.: Carotid sinus hypersensitivity in patients with unexplained syncope: clinical, eletrophysiologic, and long-term follow-up observations. Am Heart J 116:989, 1988.
100. Thomas JE: Hyperactive carotid sinus reflex and carotid sinus syncope. Mayo Clin Proc 44:127, 1969.
101. Heidorn GH, McNamara AP: Effect of carotid sinus stimulation on electrocardiograms of clinically normal individuals. Circulation 14:1104, 1956.
102. Thomas JE: Disease of the carotid sinus syncope. In Vinken PJ, Bruyn GU (eds.): Handbook of Clinical Neurology, p. 532. Amsterdam, North Holland Publishing Co., 1972.
103. Walter PF, Crawley IS, Dorney ER: Carotid sinus hypersensitivity and syncope. Am J Cardiol 42:396, 1978.
104. Keating EC, Burks JM, Calder JR: Mixed carotid sinus hypersensitivity: Successful therapy with pacing, ephedrine and propranolol. PACE 8:356, 1985.
105. Steere AC, Botsford WP, Weinberg M, et al.: Lyme carditis: Cardiac abnormalities of Lyme disease. Ann Intern Med 93:8, 1980.
106. Hayes DL: Indications for permanent pacing. In Furman S, Hayes DL (eds.): A Practice of Cardiac Pacing, p. 3. Mount Kisco, NY, Futura Publishing Co., 1989.
107. Pennock JL, Dyer PE, Reitz BA, et al.: Cardiac transplantation in perspective for the future. J Thorac Cardiovasc Surg 83:168, 1982.
108. Miyamoto Y, Curtiss EI, Koymos RL, et al.: Bradyarrhythmia after heart transplantation: Incidence, time course, and outcome (Abstract). Circulation 80:642, 1989.
109. DiBiase A, Tse CT, Schnittger I, et al.: Indications for permanent pacemaker implantation in cardiac transplant patients (Abstract). Circulation 80:527, 1989.
110. Greene DG: Right heart catheterization and temporary pacemaker insertion during coronary arteriography for suspected coronary artery disease. Cathet and Cardiovasc Diagn 10:429, 1984.
111. Peters RW, Nussbaum S, Mailhot J, et al.: Catheter-induced A-V nodal block occurring during electrophysiologic study. PACE 7:248, 1984.
112. Jacobson LB, Scheinman MM: Catheter-induced intra-Hisian

and intrafascicular block during recording of His bundle electrogram. Circulation 49:579, 1974.
113. Stein PD, Mathos VS, Herman MV, et al.: Complete heart block induced during cardiac catheterization of patients with pre-existing bundle branch block. Circulation 34:783, 1966.
114. Harvey JR, Wyman RM, McKay RG, Baim DS: Use of balloon flotation pacing catheters for prophylactic temporary pacing during diagnostic and therapeutic catheterization procedures. Am J Cardiol 62:941, 1988.
115. Plack RH, Porterfield JK, Brinker JA: Complete heart block developing during aortic valvuloplasty. Chest 96:1201, 1989.

# 38

Pacemaker Follow-Up

Konrad K. Steinbach

Follow-up of patients in the pacemaker clinic permits the evaluation of the efficacy of therapeutic intervention, especially its adverse effects and complications. The efficacy of the specific treatment can be measured by the increase in life expectancy of the treated patient compared with a group of untreated patients. The fact that certain symptoms do not occur in the treated group also enhances the value of a specific therapeutic method.

The follow-up of pacemaker patients is much more labor-intensive than the follow-up of other patient groups, as one has to collect and document clinical information as well as the technical data of the implanted pacemaker. Table 38–1 lists general guidelines for the organization, equipment, and responsibilities of a follow-up pacemaker clinic.

TABLE 38–1
The Follow-up Pacemaker Clinic

Staff
1 cardiologist, 1 nurse, 1 technician, 1 secretary

Equipment
ECG, external pacemaker, programmer, defibrillator, radiograph, long-term ECG recorder, event recorder, transtelephonic monitoring

Operation of Clinic
At least once a week with set schedules for each patient

24-Hour Emergency Service

Schedule of Pacemaker Checks
1. At discharge of the patient
2. 6 weeks after discharge
3. Until 4 years after implantation every 6–9 months
4. After 4 years every 3–6 months

Routine Pacemaker Checks
1. Pacemaker patient
2. ECG
3. Pacemaker stimulus
4. Pacemaker rate (free-running and magnet mode)
5. Pacing and sensing threshold

Optional Pacemaker Checks
1. Other programmable functions
2. Pacemaker dependency
3. X-ray studies
4. Long-term ECG recording

Control of Pacemaker/Electrode Function

For an adequate control of the pacemaker/electrode function it is absolutely essential to know the model of the implanted pacemaker and electrode and to have an appropriately equipped laboratory. The following equipment should be available.

ELECTROCARDIOGRAPHY

The recording of at least a 3-lead ECG is mandatory. In patients with spontaneous heart rhythm at the time of the control, a regular 12-lead ECG should be recorded. In addition to the usual interpretation of the ECG, the efficacy of the pacemaker stimulus and the sensing function can be evaluated. As a specific finding in patients with a VVI pacemaker, the existence or absence of retrograde ventriculoatrial (VA) conduction should be examined. A criterion for retrograde VA conduction is a P wave that follows the pacemaker-induced QRS complex in most cases within a fixed time interval (Fig. 38–1). Usually P waves are best visible in lead V_1. It is clinically relevant that retrograde VA conduction is not a constant finding. In patients who are suspected to suffer from the so-called pacemaker syndrome—palpitation, dizziness, and general discomfort—frequent ECG recordings are necessary to exclude or document retrograde VA conduction as the cause of these conditions. Partial electrode breakage shows a decrease of the amplitude of the pacemaker spike, which expresses the decrease of voltage caused by an increase of the resistance in the electrode patient circuit (Fig. 38–2). Absence of the pacemaker spike (in cases in which the spontaneous heart rate is lower than the pacemaker-induced rate) can be caused by total electrode breakage, disconnection of the electrode and the pacemaker, or dysfunction of the pacemaker.

Proper evaluation of the pacing function is prevented in patients who experience intermittent bradycardia and in whom spontaneous heart rhythm is present

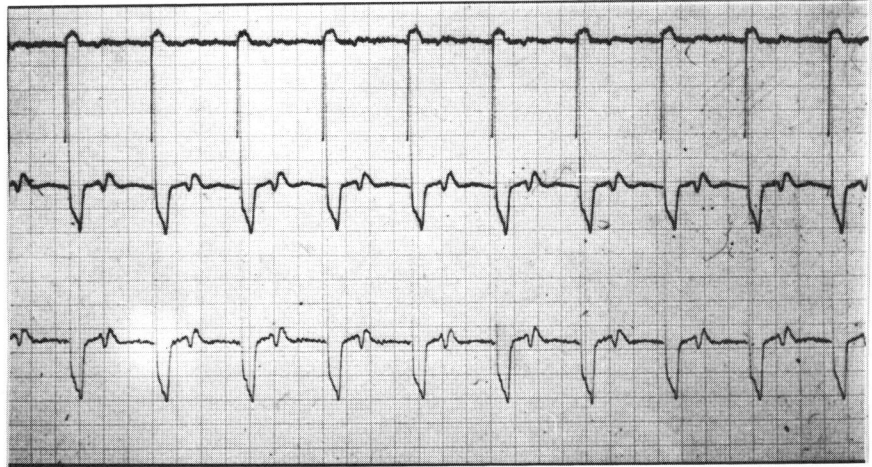

FIGURE 38–1
Retrograde VA conduction. Each pacemaker-induced ventricular complex is followed by a P wave.

while being tested at a pacemaker clinic. By switching off the sensing function by applying a magnet above the pacemaker pocket, or by lowering the heart rate by carotid sinus massage, the pacemaker rhythm can be made visible and the pacing function can be evaluated (Fig. 38–3). The sensing function in patients with continuous pacemaker-induced QRS complexes on the ECG can be evaluated in programmable units only by decreasing the stimulation rate.

PROGRAMMER

At present, each pacemaker manufacturer provides a programmer that can be used only for the units of the specific company. A pacemaker should only be programmed if the pacemaker type is known from the pacemaker passport or if the pacemaker type can be identified by x-ray. By using an inappropriate programmer, the electronic part of the unit can be destroyed, which is extremely dangerous for pacemaker-dependent patients. As a minimal requirement, in SSIPO units one should evaluate the stimulation threshold as well as the sensing threshold in SSIMO units at every patient visit. The programming of the other functions, such as stimulation-rate AV interval in dual-chamber pacemakers, hysteresis refractory period, and so forth, depends on the individual need of the patient. By taking an adequate safety margin into account, the evaluation of the pacing threshold allows one to reduce the output and to adjust the energy to the individual need of the patient. A safety margin of 25 to 30% between threshold and output is adequate. In a voltage pacemaker with an amplitude of 5 volts, an impulse duration of 0.3 ms is adequate if the stimulation threshold is below 0.1 ms. In patients with a low stimulation threshold, replacement of the implanted unit by a VVIOO system or by a DDDMO system (upgrading) is necessary only in rare cases (e.g., elective replacement of a VVIOO system). (See also Chapter 29, "Multiprogrammability of Modern Cardiac Pacemakers.")

EQUIPMENT FOR THE MEASUREMENT OF IMPULSE INTERVAL AND IMPULSE DURATION

The measurement of the impulse interval informs us about the change of the capacity of the pacemaker battery. An increase of the battery impedance causes an increase of the impulse interval. Improvement of the electronic design prevents a decrease of the stimulation rate in the free-running mode. In these pacemakers the depletion of the battery can be detected in the magnet mode. In some pacemaker models this magnet mode shows a gradual decrease in the stimulation rate; in other models the decrease is stepwise. The measurement of the impulse duration provides information about the function of the electronic circuit; however, in contrast to the pacemakers of the 1960s and 1970s, this is of no value for the detection of battery depletion. Equipment for measurement of impulse interval and impulse duration is mainly used for the control of nonprogrammable pacemakers in the private office. In pacemaker clinics, these measurements are performed by the specific programmer that includes these options.

24-HOUR ECG MONITORING

Long-term ECG monitoring is the most important diagnostic method for the evaluation of patients with

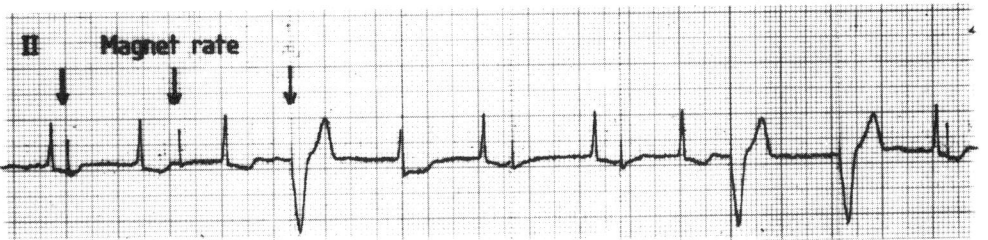

FIGURE 38–2
Partial lead fracture. The amplitude of the pacemaker spike differs between 0.6 (first arrow) and 2.8 mV (third arrow) (magnet rate).

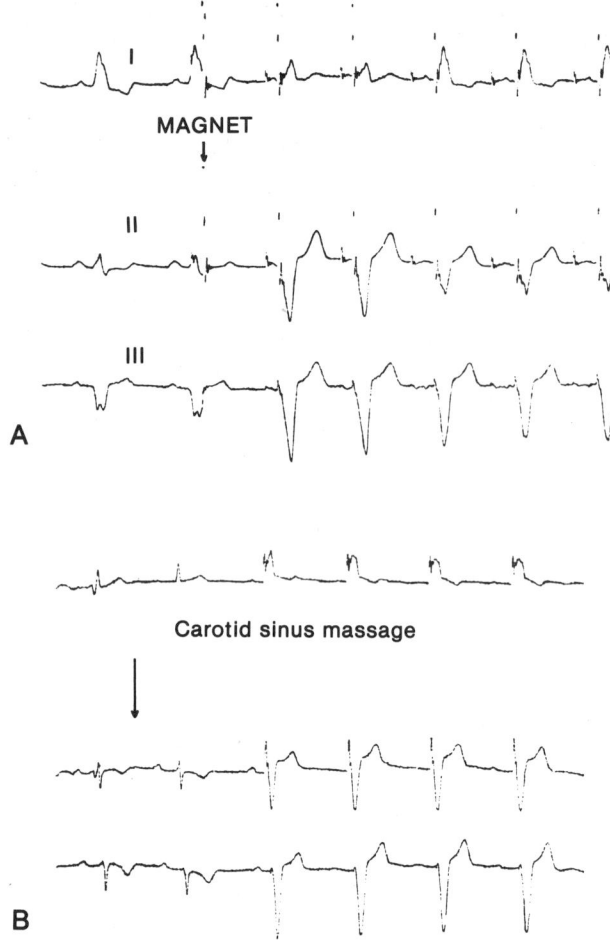

FIGURE 38-3
A, The sensing function is switched off by magnet application (arrow). B, Vagal stimulation by carotid sinus massage (arrow) causes a decrease in spontaneous heart rate below the lower stimulation rate of the pacemaker.

symptoms of a possible pacemaker/electrode failure who did not show any abnormalities at time of checkup at the pacemaker clinic. The analysis of the ECG at the time when these symptoms occur allows the exclusion or the confirmation that failure of the pacemaker/electrode system is the cause of these symptoms (Fig. 38–4). The disadvantage of this method is the limited time of recording—usually 24 hours. For patients with rare events, ECG transmission by telephone or self-recording of the ECG is preferable. Both methods can only be used if the symptoms last at least 5 minutes, or long enough to facilitate connection with the pacemaker clinic, or until connection of the electrodes and activation of the recorder can be accomplished.

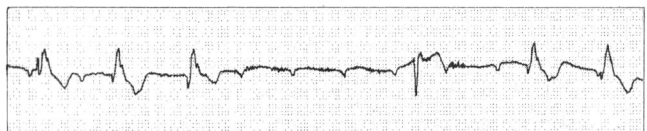

FIGURE 38-4
Suppression of the pacemaker by muscle sensing. The patient-activated marker function during 24-hour ECG recording, when he became symptomatic.

RADIOGRAPHY

X-ray studies allow the identification of the pacemaker model if the pacemaker passport is not available. The position of the lead and especially a displacement in connection with pacing failure can be detected. In most cases the electrode model and a breakage of the insulation cannot be seen on the x-ray. Careful inspection of the electrode allows localization of the lead fracture—in most cases. Incomplete fracture, at least in unipolar pacing, can be easily detected by the decrease of the amplitude of the pacing stimulus in the surface ECG.

EXTERNAL PACEMAKER AND CHEST WALL ELECTRODES

The external pacemaker in the pacemaker clinic can be used for two purposes: (1) inhibition of the implanted pacemaker and (2) termination of tachyarrhythmias.

Inhibition of the Implanted Pacemaker

Inhibition of the implanted pacemaker is used to evaluate the patient's pacemaker dependency. The output of the external unit is set to maximal value and is delivered via chest wall electrodes positioned over the pacemaker pocket and the apex. Stimuli that are recognized by the implanted pacemaker as an intrinsic R wave inactivate the unit (Fig. 38–5A). In some of the new generation pacemakers an inhibition option is implemented (Fig. 38–5B). This method inhibits the pacemaker. The patient is classified as pacemaker dependent if no escape rhythm occurs during the inhibition of the implanted unit until the patient becomes symptomatic. Different methods of pacemaker inhibition are used, and this may explain why the figure for pacemaker dependency varies between 4% and 40% (Fig. 38–6).

These differences are also explained by the fact that the result of pacemaker inhibition—especially in patients with AV block—shows a substantial day-to-day variation. It is recommended that programmable pacemakers should be programmed to work at the minimal rate to aid evaluation of pacemaker dependency of all patients. If no escape rhythm is observed after a period of 1 to 2 minutes, the pacemaker is inhibited until a spontaneous rhythm or symptoms occur. It is well known that in patients in whom instantaneous cessation of pacing causes symptomatic asystole, a gradual decrease of the stimulation rate permits restoration of spontaneous heart rate.

Pacemaker dependency is of practical importance because cessation of pacing caused by pacemaker or electrode dysfunction is extremely dangerous for the patient and can lead to syncope or death. The fact that a patient is pacemaker-dependent should be documented in the patient's file and pacemaker passport.

Termination of Tachyarrhythmias

The VVT mode in programmable pacemakers can be used to terminate ventricular tachycardias by triggering

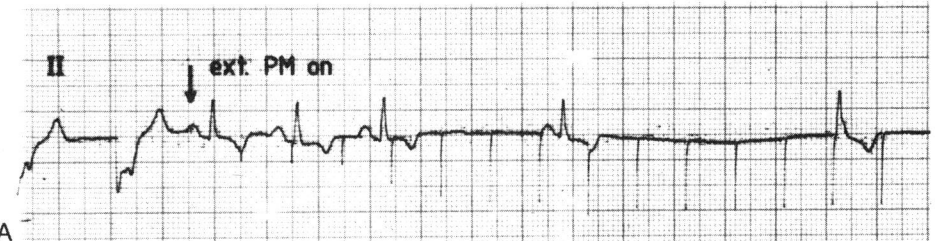
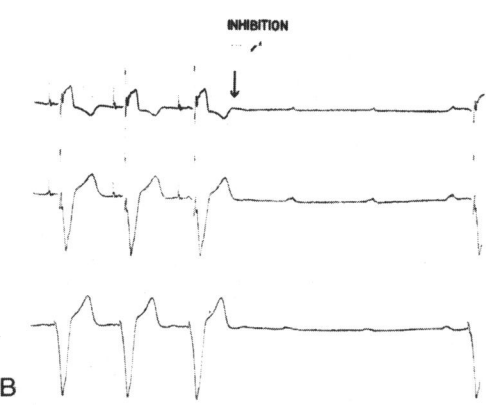

FIGURE 38–5
A, Inhibition of a VVI unit by an external pacemaker (ext PM) (150 bpm, output 20 mA) in a patient with sick sinus node syndrome. Sinus arrest occurred after 3 sinus node induced atrial depolarization. B, Activation of the inhibition option causes asystole.

the implanted unit with an external pacemaker via chest electrodes. In the 1970s when implantable cardioverter/defibrillators were not available this method was the first attempt to terminate ventricular tachycardias by implanting an electrical device.

DEFIBRILLATOR

Immediate cardioversion/defibrillation has to be available in the pacemaker clinic. Magnet-induced inactivation of the sensing function can cause the occurrence of life-threatening ventricular tachyarrhythmias through competition between spontaneous and pacemaker rhythm. Although this is a rare event, magnet application should only be used with continuous ECG monitoring and in the presence of a person trained in resuscitation techniques.

PATIENT RECORD

The organization of a documentation system for patient and pacemaker data is extremely important for patient follow-up. A computerized system enables the person responsible for the patient's follow-up to have all relevant data available whenever needed in the pacemaker clinic or on request of the private physician. The information stored in the patient's file should also be recorded in the pacemaker passport. This is especially important for the data obtained at follow-up controls, such as pacing and sensing thresholds, programmed parameters, and magnet rate. (See also the section on "The European Pacemaker Registration Card.")

PACEMAKER LIBRARY

The specifications of the pacemaker used in a specific center have to be available 24 hours a day. This can be accomplished by a pacemaker library which can be organized by storing special information provided by the manufacturers or as a computerized data base. In most recent-generation pacemakers, this information can be obtained from the data base included in the programmer.

It is also important to have information available concerning the specifications of pacemakers that are not used in the specific pacemaker center. Appropriate documentation of pacemaker data can help to avoid

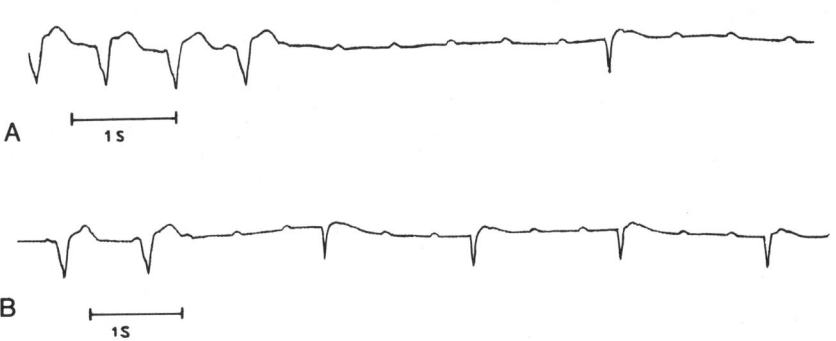

FIGURE 38–6
A, Stimulation of the heart during 2 minutes at a rate of 90 bpm causes asystole when the pacemaker is switched off. B, Using a stimulation rate of 70/min during 2 minutes allows restoration of the spontaneous heart rate (40 bpm).

problems—especially with patients who are not regularly controlled at the pacemaker clinic (e.g., tourists). It can be expected that in the near future smart cards together with a software program that runs with every personal computer will solve the problem.

TRANSTELEPHONIC MONITORING SYSTEM

Transtelephonic monitoring was extremely useful in the early 1970s when the longevity of pacemaker batteries necessitated monthly controls starting 2 years after the implantation of the pacemaker. At the beginning, only transmission of the ECG was possible. Battery depletion could be detected in the ECG by a change of the stimulation rate and/or loss of effective pacing by the stimulus. Systems that were able to transmit and analyze the pulse duration made it possible to detect early battery depletion, thus preventing emergency situations (Fig. 38–7).

Nowadays the value of transtelephonic monitoring is decreasing, as the reliability of the pacemaker and pacemaker electrode has reduced the number of required visits to the pacemaker clinic to two per year. The advantage of a personal visit to the pacemaker clinic is that, in addition to the technical check of the pacemaker/electrode system, the history of the patient and the physical examination can provide useful information concerning further management.

In any case patients with programmable pacemakers have to visit the pacemaker clinic for an evaluation of the pacing and sensing threshold. According to the measurement results, the patient's need for reprogramming of the unit is determined. At present transtelephonic monitoring can be used for patients with nonprogrammable pacemakers who are unable to visit a clinic twice a year or in whom dysfunction of the pacemaker or symptomatic arrhythmias are suspected.

HOLTER FUNCTION IMPLEMENTED IN THE PACEMAKER

A Holter function is already implemented in some single-chamber pacemakers. It can be expected that in the near future sophisticated recordings of arrhythmia events and histograms of spontaneous and paced heart rate will be available. This method will replace 24-hour ECG monitoring as well as transtelephonic monitoring. This new option is of special importance for proper programming of rate-responsive devices.

Goals of Follow-Up of Pacemaker Patients

EVALUATION WHEN THE INDICATION FOR PACEMAKER IMPLANTATION IS APPROPRIATE

It has been shown that in patients with symptomatic third-degree AV block, pacemaker implantation has improved life expectancy. Based on the results of follow-up studies of paced and unpaced patients with sick sinus syndrome, it was concluded that pacing does not improve the prognosis in terms of an increased life expectancy. Furthermore, it was discovered that in some patients with sick sinus syndrome, symptoms are not relieved by the implantation of a pacemaker. Nowadays, as a result of these follow-up studies of patients with sick sinus syndrome, one attempts to record an ECG when the patient becomes symptomatic. Pacemaker implantation is indicated if the symptoms and bradycardia coincide (Table 38–2).

Patients with hypersensitive carotid sinus reflex represent another group in whom follow-up studies have changed the attitude concerning pacemaker implantation. An asystole with a duration of more than 3 seconds caused by mechanical irritation of the carotid sinus in patients more than 70 years of age is a rather frequent finding. Follow-up studies have documented that asymptomatic patients with prolonged asystole during carotid sinus massage have no syncope for years, even if they have a positive response during follow-up. This is also true for patients with a positive response and rare syncopes. Sometimes these patients do not have further events for years. On the other hand, follow-up of patients with hypersensitive carotid sinus

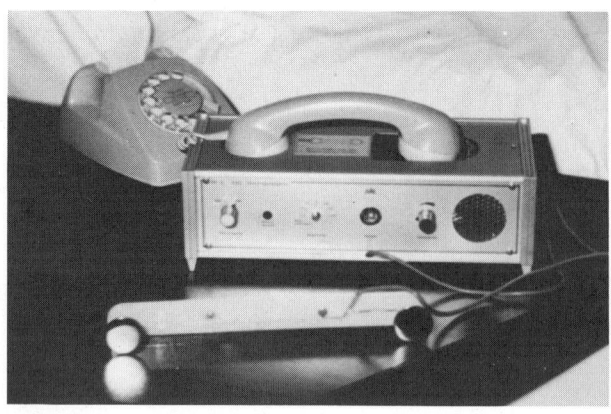
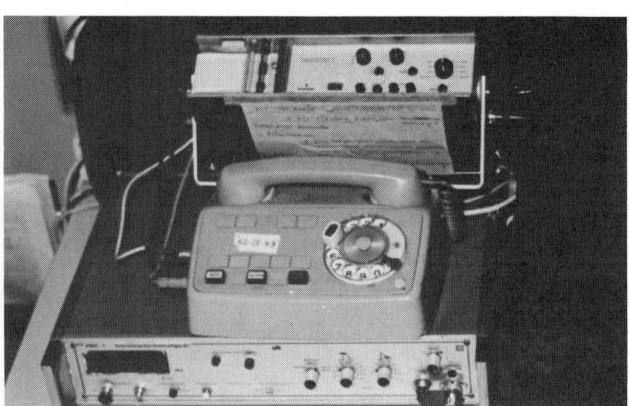

FIGURE 38–7
Telephone transmission system for pacemaker stimuli and ECG. This unit was used from 1971 to 1978 in the Pacemaker Clinic of the Cardiac Department of the University of Vienna.

TABLE 38-2
Clinical Indications for Pacemaker Implantation*

Indication	No.	%
Not stated	107	5.1
Syncope	780	37.1
Lightheadedness	457	21.7
Bradycardia	472	22.4
Tachycardia	14	0.7
Prophylactic	37	1.8
Heart failure	204	9.7
Cerebral dysfunction	20	1.0

*Selected from data on 2091 first implants in Austria in 1986.

reflex and frequent syncopes has proven the efficacy of pacemaker treatment in the prevention of further syncopes.

In an unknown number of patients, especially those with sick sinus syndrome or hypersensitive carotid sinus reflex, inappropriate indications have caused unnecessary implantation of pacemakers (overpacing). Based on the available follow-up data, pacemaker treatment of this group could be terminated. In many cases, however, the pacemaker treatment cannot be stopped—mainly for psychologic reasons. For each patient for whom battery depletion makes it necessary to replace the pacemaker, it should be evaluated if a continuation of the pacemaker treatment is advisable. A specific example is the occurrence of chronic atrial fibrillation in patients with the sick sinus syndrome. This arrhythmia represents the end point of sick sinus syndrome. Usually the heart rate of the patient with atrial fibrillation is normal.

A criterion for the appropriate indication for pacemaker implantation is the efficacy of pacemaker treatment in terms of increased life expectancy and/or quality of life. To facilitate this, pacemaker patients with a specific condition (e.g., sick sinus syndrome) should be pooled in a national (or, better, continental) data base. A prerequisite for data collection of a pacemaker center is a unified registration system. This system, however, is still in the developmental stage. In a few European countries, a representative percentage of pacemaker centers participate in a program with centralized computerized storage of data on pacemakers and pacemaker patients.

EVALUATION WHEN THE APPROPRIATE PACEMAKER MODEL HAS BEEN IMPLANTED

At follow-up of pacemaker patients, it should be determined whether a change of system (e.g., from VVIO to VVIMO, VVIRO, or DDDMO [upgrading]) is indicated. This may be necessary in patients in whom symptomatic retrograde VA conduction is detected and also in patients with VVIMO pacemakers who suffer from inadequate exercise tolerance. For this purpose the behavior of the heart rate over a period of 24 hours should be monitored, especially during exercise; the maximal exercise tolerance can be used for the decision. In patients with an inadequate increase of the heart rate, the replacement of a simple VVI unit by a DDD or VVIR pacer should be considered (Fig. 38-8).

CONTROL OF BATTERY FUNCTION

The function time of the different lithium batteries varies considerably. One of the purposes of the regular check-up of the patient is to detect battery depletion before the pacemaker fails; on the other hand, the implanted pacemaker should stay in place as long as possible. In the 1970s decrease in the stimulation rate following an increase in battery impedance indicated impending battery depletion. The use of digital circuits in newer-generation pacemakers prevents the decrease in the spontaneous stimulation rate, and currently the decrease in the magnet rate is used to indicate the drop in battery capacity, which necessitates replacement of the unit. The percentage of decrease in the magnet rate, which is the indication for replacement, differs from model to model.

This underlines the necessity of a well-organized pacemaker library and continuous training of the pacemaker clinic staff. Information about battery failure should be collected in a national and/or continental registry to allow early warning of the pacemaker centers in the area (see the section on "European Pacemaker Registry"). The control of battery function of reused pacemakers, which is possible without any risk to the patient, is performed as in "first hand" units. The function time in the first patient should be documented in the patient file. The intervals between two controls in the pacemaker clinic have to be fixed according to the period of time that the pacemaker has already been used by the previous patient and according to the expected overall function time.

CONTROL OF PACING THRESHOLD

The function time of the battery depends less on the capacity than on the impedance of the electrode/patient circuit relation between spontaneous and pacemaker-induced beats and, in programmable units, on the programmed impulse duration and/or impulse amplitude. Thus, at each visit to the pacemaker clinic, the stimulation threshold in programmable pacemakers has to be evaluated and has to be compared with the pacing threshold of the previous controls (Fig. 38-9). According to the measured threshold, the output has to be adapted. The safety margin between threshold and programmed output depends on the pacemaker dependency of the patient and the stability of the threshold.

In pacemaker-dependent patients with stable pacing thresholds in the right ventricle during follow-up, the programmed energy should be in a range of 100%; in other patients, it should be 50 to 80% above the pacing threshold. Because of variation of the threshold in the early phase after pacemaker implantation, the output should be set 100 to 150% above the actual threshold, and continuous adaptation is necessary. Programming of the atrial output 50% above the pacing threshold is appropriate in stable conditions.

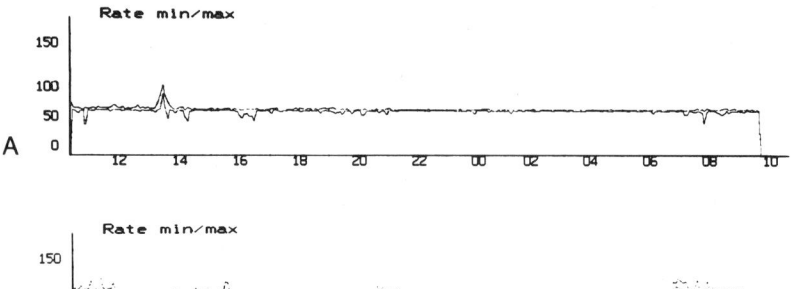
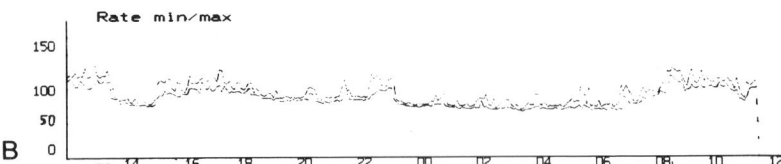

FIGURE 38–8
24-hour transcription of the heart rate of a patient with a VVI pacemaker (A) and after replacement of the VVI pacemaker by a DDD pacemaker (B).

CONTROL OF THE SENSING THRESHOLD

Control of the sensing threshold is possible only in multiprogrammable pacemakers. The sensing threshold should but does not have to be evaluated if the pacing threshold is consistently low.

Evaluation and reprogramming is mandatory if a variation of the pacing threshold is detected or an overt sensing failure is documented in the ECG or, in case of pacemaker-mediated tachycardia in DDDMO units, as an alternative to a prolongation of the refractory period of the atrium. (See Chapter 29, "Multiprogrammability of Modern Cardiac Pacemakers.") A decrease in the atrial sensing threshold enhances the risk of atrial fibrillation caused by the competition of spontaneous and pacemaker-induced atrial depolarization (Fig. 38–10).

REPROGRAMMING OF THE PACEMAKER

In multiprogrammable pacemakers, continuous adaptation of their functions to the needs of the patient is possible. In daily practice, the exercise tolerance as evaluated by ergometry and, even more often, the patient's subjective sense of well-being are used for optimal programming.

Reprogramming is of special importance in rate-responsive pacemakers to ensure maximal benefit for the patient. Optimal programming is a very time-consuming task. Because of lack of time and/or experience the implanted unit often doesn't provide the optimal exercise tolerance in an unknown number of patients. (See also Chapter 29, "Multiprogrammability of Modern Cardiac Pacemakers," and Chapter 30, "Rate-Responsive Cardiac Pacing.")

DETECTION OF FAILURE OF ELECTRONIC COMPONENTS

In recent years, dangerous failures such as no output and runaway have become rare events. When they do occur, immediate replacement of the pacemaker is mandatory. More often, in programmable pacemakers instability of the programmed parameters or inability of reprogramming is observed. In this case the physician has to decide, for each individual patient, whether immediate replacement is necessary or control of the pacemaker function at shorter intervals is advisable. Information concerning electronic failure should be collected in a national and/or continental registry to allow early warning of the pacemaker centers in the area. (See also section on "European Pacemaker Registration Card.")

DETECTION OF ELECTRODE FAILURE

Incomplete or complete lead fractures are rare events. Incomplete lead fractures can be diagnosed from the ECG recording by a decrease in the amplitude of the spike, or by direct evaluation of the impedance of the electrode patient circuit with the pacemaker system analyzer after disconnection of the pacer. In units with the option of telemetric measurement of voltage and current, detection of electrode failure is possible while the unit is in place. Complete lead fracture leads to cessation of pacing.

Insulation defects in most instances are caused by placement of the ligature directly on the lead. It has been reported that polyurethane leads have a higher percentage of insulation defects caused by fatigue of material. In voltage pacemakers, this will cause rapid battery depletion. Stimulation of the muscle, the phrenic nerve and undersensing may indicate the insulation defect. This diagnosis can be made by direct measurement with a pacemaker system analyzer and by telemetry in pacemakers with the option of telemetric evaluation of voltage and current.

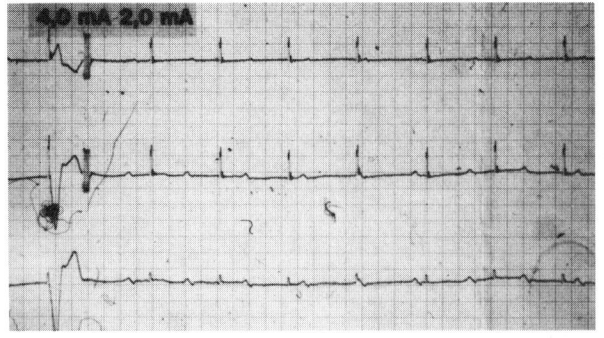

FIGURE 38–9
Reduction of the output to 2 mA (second pacemaker spike) causes ineffective stimulation. The stimulation threshold ranges between 2 and 4 mA.

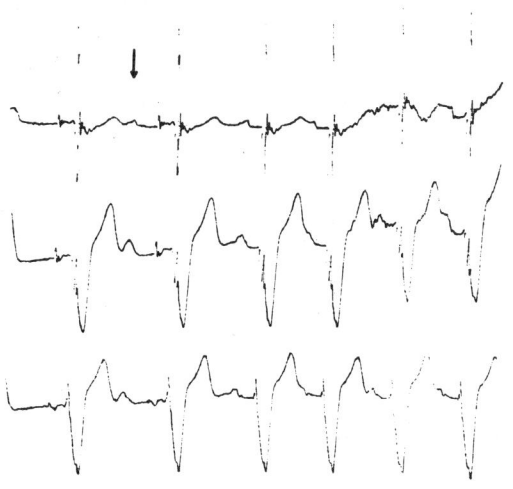

FIGURE 38–10
Sensing failure in the atrium (arrow) of a DDDMO pacemaker.

INSPECTION OF THE PACEMAKER POCKET

Erosion of the skin over the pacemaker or pacemaker infection is a possible complication of pacemaker implantation. The patient should be advised to inspect the skin over the pacemaker and should visit the pacemaker clinic if there is thinning of the skin and/or discoloration. If the skin is still intact, revision of the pacemaker pocket while leaving the same unit in place is possible. When skin erosion is already present, in most instances replacement of the whole system is necessary. Also, late infections require pacemaker explanation and implantation of a new pacemaker/electrode system at the other side of the thorax.

Radiography is able to detect the so-called twiddler syndrome, which is caused by manipulation of the pacemaker by the patient. This is possible if the pacemaker pocket is too large. The twiddler syndrome can cause electrode fracture or dislodgement. The pacemaker pocket should be revised to prevent this complication.

Thrombotic complications of the vein used for introduction of the pacemaker lead during late follow-up is rare. In the acute phase it can cause edema of the involved upper extremity and later subcutaneous venous collaterals. The prognosis of this complication is good.

EVALUATION OF CARDIAC STATUS AND ARRHYTHMIAS

About 20% of the patients visiting a pacemaker clinic experience cardiac and general medical problems. In principle, the pacemaker center should at least take care of the cardiac problems. Depending on the organization of the pacemaker center, cardiac care is provided in the pacemaker clinic or in another outpatient department. The physician responsible for the pacemaker clinic should be involved in the management of cardiac problems because, in some cases (e.g., patients with programmable pacemakers), reprogramming can solve the problem. Reprogramming of the basic heart rate and variation of the AV interval in DDD pacemakers can change the pacing mode and this influences left ventricular performance, which consequently improves the exercise tolerance.

In patients with nonprogrammable pacemakers cardiac symptoms necessitate a decision by the cardiologist responsible for the pacemaker clinic—for example, whether change of pacing mode (AAIMO or DDDMO) is indicated in patients with a pacemaker syndrome caused by retrograde VA conduction.

The relatively high frequency of arrhythmias—both pacemaker-induced and independent of pacemaker treatment—is another argument for including cardiac care in the pacemaker clinic.

Evaluation of patients with respect to complex ventricular arrhythmias is important, since 14% of pacemaker patients die suddenly. Autopsy studies revealed that most of these patients had severe three-vessel disease but no acute thrombosis or subintimal bleeding and no myocardial necrosis. Pacemaker/electrode dysfunction could be excluded. Thus a primary arrhythmogenic event or fatal arrhythmia caused by interference of pacemaker stimulus and spontaneous heart rate has to be suspected.

Interpretation of ECG studies of pacemaker patients, especially 1-lead recordings of 24-hour ECG monitoring, and subsequent decisions concerning further management require special expertise by the physician. Thus, pacemaker treatment should be an integrated part of the division responsible for rhythmology in the specific institution. In Europe the majority of pacemaker clinics also provide cardiologic and especially rhythmologic follow-up, whereas in the United States there is a tendency to separate pacemaker follow-up from medical follow-up.

Requirements for a Pacemaker Center and Follow-Up Clinic

Only an appropriate number of first implants per year justifies the organization of a specialized pacemaker clinic for follow-up. However, it is widely accepted that a pacemaker center should meet the following requirements:

- All pacing modes in use.
- A minimum of 50 first implants per year.
- Serving an area with a certain number of inhabitants.
- Pacemaker clinic at least once a week.
- 24-hour service for emergency cases.
- Regular training of the staff.
- Availability of the most frequently used programmers.
- Documentation of data of pacemaker and pacemaker patients.

In the 1970s, when the reliability of pulse generators and the longevity of batteries increased, pacemaker implantation and follow-up were decentralized. At this time almost all implanted pacemakers were nonprogrammable. With the development of more sophisticated units, the selection of the appropriate unit and the necessity to implant a second electrode in dual-chamber pacemakers made the procedure more complicated. In many hospitals, especially in hospitals with a low number of first implants, physicians were not adequately trained in implantation techniques and follow-up methods. Many hospitals continue to use only nonprogrammable pacemakers because of lack of training and of adequate follow-up facilities.

The appropriate use of sophisticated pacemakers, including prepacing diagnostic procedures and proper selection of the pacemaker model, is a strong argument for concentrating pacemaker implantation and follow-up in a certain number of hospitals, depending on the number of pacemaker patients in the region. For a better comparability between different regions, countries, and continents the so-called implantation ratio (i.e., number of first implants per million inhabitants) is used. Assuming an implantation ratio of 200, one pacemaker center could serve an area with 500,000 to 1,000,000 inhabitants. (See section on "European Pacemaker Registration Card.")

During recent years, international standards for certain special diagnostic and therapeutic interventions in cardiology, such as echocardiography, nuclear cardiology, and coronary angiography, have been worked out. This is also necessary for pacemaker treatment. The requirements listed above (accepted by the European Working Group on Cardiac Pacing) could be adopted by institutions in other countries.

Documentation of Data on Pacemakers and Pacemaker Patients

The data on implanted pacemakers and pacemaker patients should be stored on several levels, such as those outlined below.

IMPLANTING HOSPITAL ■ Patient records have to be available at any time, and not only in the pacemaker clinic (e.g., in case of emergency).

REGIONAL OR NATIONAL DATA BASE ■ Depending on the number of first implants and replacements per year, the data should be stored in a central computerized data base. A minimum of 1000 first implants per year would justify a central data base. There is no absolute upper limit in terms of number of first implants. In regions with more than 20,000 first implants per year, collection of implantation and replacement data—especially collection of follow-up data—is very difficult to accomplish. Until now, only a few countries in Europe have national data bases in operation.

CONTINENTAL DATA BASE ■ A continental data base can be easily organized if regional and national bases exist, because data do not have to be recalled on a daily basis. The stored data need be processed only once or twice a year, and the respective printouts can be distributed among the participating national or regional data bases.

Purpose of Data Collection

SURVEY OF TRENDS IN CARDIAC PACING

EPIDEMIOLOGY ■ Information about the epidemiology of bradyarrhythmias is still lacking. This is true for the frequency of bradyarrhythmias in different areas and the correlation between age, sex, climate, other diseases, and the socioeconomic situation. This is also true for the evaluation of the influence of cardiac pacing on the prognosis in terms of life expectancy and symptoms before pacemaker implantation. At the moment, only data concerning paced patients with bradyarrhythmia are available. These data show a remarkable variation between countries and continents. At present an exact epidemiologic explanation is lacking.

PACING MODE ■ Currently in many patients with the same symptoms and the same prepacing ECGs, different pacing modes are employed at different centers. Comparing data of different centers might lead to an answer to the question of which pacing mode in a specific indication and/or prepacing ECG is superior, or whether two or three different pacing modes are equivalent.

LONGEVITY OF PACEMAKER BATTERIES ■ Even if the longevity of pacemaker batteries depends more on the resistance of the electrode/patient circuit, on the percentage of pacemaker induced beats, and, in programmable units, on the programmed output than on the capacity of the battery, the collection of data of a specific pacemaker model yields valuable information concerning the approximate function time of a specific pacemaker model. In the case of early battery depletion, the function time of the pacemaker, pacing threshold, impedance, and, in programmable units, the programmed output should be documented.

RECALL ■ A well-organized data base is necessary to allow recall of defective pacemakers and electrodes within an appropriate time. A functional recall system is of special importance for pacemaker-dependent patients.

CALCULATION OF COSTS OF PACEMAKER TREATMENT

The financial aspect of pacemaker treatment has become more important during the last few years. With respect to economic pressures, an exact budgeting in the medical field is mandatory. Experience collected from existing data bases indicates that the variation in the number of first implants rarely exceeds 10 to 15% in comparison with the previous year, and that the number of replacements decreases annually by 10 to 20%. Also, the percentage of single- and dual-chamber units remains rather constant. By using the figures from a national data base, the amount of money that will have to be spent for pacemakers and electrodes can be calculated in advance.

OVER- AND UNDERPACING

As a result of the reliability of the pacemaker and electrode, and the simplification of the implantation technique, the indications for pacemaker implantation have been broadened. During the last 10 years the implantation ratio in Europe and the United States has increased by 100 to 200%. Retrospective studies have documented cases in which pacemaker implantation has proved to be unnecessary. Continuous data collection and comparison of clinical indications and of prepacing ECGs can help to identify centers with a marked implantation ratio deviation from the average. The existence of follow-up data is a prerequisite for identification of centers in which possible unnecessary pacemaker implantation has occurred (overpacing).

On the other hand, when the number of first implants are significantly below the average, underpacing is indicated. Possible causes of underpacing are improper training of physicians and/or socioeconomic factors; the exact causes have yet to be established.

The European Pacemaker Registry

In 1979, the European Working Group on Cardiac Pacing (EWGCP) introduced a unified documentation system for pacemaker patients. This system includes:

1. An early warning system
2. A unified pacemaker registration card
3. A continental data base

EARLY WARNING SYSTEM

In the event of battery or pulse generator failure in a pacemaker series, the implantation center and the pacemaker patient must be informed in due time. Essential for an early warning system is the establishment of a central office (e.g., Stimarec, Paris) which collects and verifies incoming information from the pacemaker centers linked with it. In turn, these centers are informed about failures regularly through monthly bulletins or, in the future, via telecommunication facilities (Table 38–3).

THE EUROPEAN PACEMAKER REGISTRATION CARD

The installation of a central data base necessitates the use of a unified documentation system of data collected about patient and pacemaker. At the present time, the identification cards provided by pacemaker manufacturers are widely used. The unified European Registration Card (Fig. 38–11), introduced in 1979 by the EWGCP, is a primary step in the implementation of a centralized data base and an early warning system.

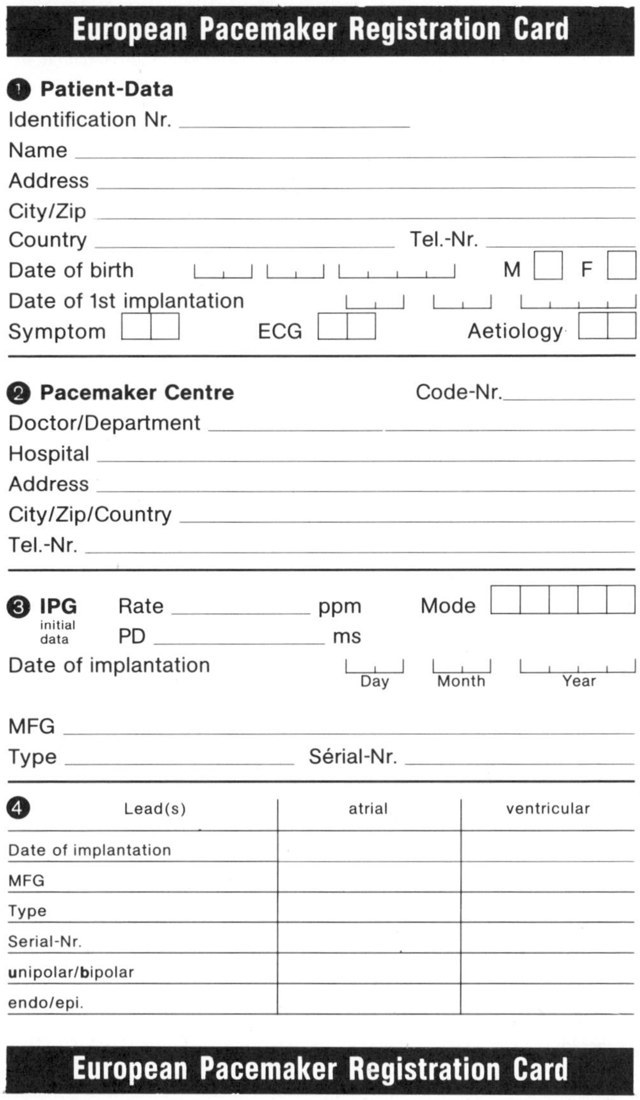
European Pacemaker Registration Card

1 Patient-Data
Identification Nr.
Name
Address
City/Zip
Country Tel.-Nr.
Date of birth M F
Date of 1st implantation
Symptom ECG Aetiology

2 Pacemaker Centre Code-Nr.
Doctor/Department
Hospital
Address
City/Zip/Country
Tel.-Nr.

3 IPG (initial data) Rate ppm Mode
PD ms
Date of implantation Day Month Year
MFG
Type Sérial-Nr.

4 Lead(s)	atrial	ventricular
Date of implantation		
MFG		
Type		
Serial-Nr.		
unipolar/bipolar		
endo/epi.		

European Pacemaker Registration Card

FIGURE 38–11
The European Pacemaker Registration Card. (Copyright © 1985 by IAPM/ EWGCP.)

Both can work properly only if documentation of data is standardized for all pacemaker centers.

The card consists of six parts:

1. Passport—delivered to the patient.
2. Implantation report No. 1—to be sent to the National Registry at the time of implantation of pacemaker.
3. Implantation report No. 2—to be sent to the pacemaker manufacturer.
4. Explantation report No. 1—to be sent to the National Registry at the time of explantation of pacemaker.

TABLE 38–3
Cumulative STIMAREC Report on Cases of Pacemaker Failure (1980–1986)

No. of Case Reports	1980	1981	1982	1983	1984	1985	1986
Received	392	355	265	245	219	168	137
Published	314	272	171	167	151	143	107
Potentially Dangerous	125	92	91	95	99	80	75

CODE EXPLANATION FOR IMPLANTATION

Clinical Indication for pacing

Symptom
- 01 = Unspecified
- 02 = Uncoded
- 03 = Syncope
- 04 = Dizzy spells
- 05 = Bradycardia
- 06 = Tachycardia
- 07 = Prophylactic
- 08 = Heart failure
- 09 = Cerebral dysfunction

ECG = Indication for pacing
Pre-pacing ECG
- 01 = Rhythm unspecified
- 02 = Rhythm uncoded
- 03 = Normal sinus rhythm
- 04 = 1' heart block
- 05 = 2' heart block - Unspecified
- 06 = 2' heart block - Wenckebach
- 07 = 2' heart block - Mobitz
- 08 = CHB - QRS unspecified
- 09 = CHB - Narrow QRS
- 10 = CHB - Wide QRS
- 11 = Bundle branch block - Unspecified
- 12 = RBBB - Incomplete
- 13 = RBBB - Complete
- 14 = LBBB - Complete
- 15 = Left anterior hemi-block
- 16 = Left posterior hemi-block
- 17 = RBBB + LAHB + Normal PR
- 18 = RBBB + LPHB + Normal PR
- 19 = RBBB + LAHB + long PR interval
- 20 = RBBB + LPHB + long PR interval
- 21 = LBBB + long PR interval
- 22 = SSS - Unspecified
- 23 = SSS - SA exit block
- 24 = SSS - SA arrest
- 25 = SSS - Bradycardia
- 26 = SSS - Brady-Tachy
- 27 = SSS + AV block
- 28 = Ventricular extrasystoles
- 29 = Ventricular tachycardia
- 30 = Paroxysmal VF
- 31 = A. Flutter/Fib. + bradycardia
- 32 = Atrial tachycardia
- 33 = Pre-excitation

Aetiology
- 01 = Aetiology unspecified
- 02 = Aetiology uncoded
- 03 = Aetiology unknown
- 04 = Conduction tissue fibrosis
- 05 = Ischaemic
- 06 = Post-infarction
- 07 = Surgical
- 08 = Congenital
- 09 = Cardiomyopathy
- 10 = Myocarditis
- 11 = Valvular heart disease
- 12 = Carotid sinus syndrome

CODE EXPLANATION FOR EXPLANTATION

Indication for generator change
- 01 = Unspecified
- 02 = Uncoded
- 03 = Elective
- 04 = Elective for system change
- 05 = Elective with electrode problem
- 06 = Mechanical protrusion
- 07 = Infection-ulceration
- 08 = Electromyographic inhibition
- 09 = Extracardiac stimulation
- 10 = Failure - Unspecified
- 11 = Failure - Low output
- 12 = Failure - Slow rate
- 13 = Failure - Slow magnetic rate
- 14 = Failure - Fast rate
- 15 = Failure - Fast magnetic rate
- 16 = Failure - Connector fault
- 17 = Failure - Encapsulation
- 18 = Failure - Undersensing
- 19 = Failure - Oversensing
- 20 = Failure - Magnetic switch
- 21 = Failure - Programming
- 22 = Failure - Battery depletion (E.O.L.)
- 23 = Failure - Battery depletion (Premature)

Manufacturer verification
- 01 = Not tested
- 02 = Tested, findings not confirmed
- 03 = Tested, findings confirmed

Indication for electrode change
- 01 = Unspecified
- 02 = Uncoded
- 03 = Elective
- 04 = Displacement
- 05 = Exit block
- 06 = Connector failure
- 07 = Infection-ulceration
- 08 = Electromyographic inhibition
- 09 = Extracardiac stimulation
- 10 = Perforation
- 11 = Undersensing
- 12 = Insulation break
- 13 = Conductor break

Indication for file closure
- 01 = Uncoded
- 02 = Death-cause unknown
- 03 = Death unrelated to pacemaker
- 04 = Generator related death
- 05 = Electrode related death
- 06 = Pacemaker removed
- 07 = Lost to follow-up
- 08 = Sudden death

FIGURE 38–12
Code used for recording pacemaker implantation and explantation. Data include clinical indication, prepacing ECG, etiology, indication for explantation of pacemaker/electrode and file closure (approved by the European Working Group on Cardiac Pacing).

5. Explantation report No. 2—to be sent to the pacemaker manufacturer.
6. Copy for the patient's file.

The EWGCP has agreed upon a code for clinical indications; prepacing ECGs; and indications for pacemaker replacement, electrode replacement, and file closure (Fig. 38–12).

At the time of this writing (1987), the pacemaker registration card is in use in 22 European countries. In about 60% of first implants and replacements, this card is used to document data about the pacemaker patient and pacemaker. In seven countries, a computerized national data base exists. In these countries each center receives an annual report pertaining to the specific center and to other centers in the same nation. These reports include the number of first implants, replacements, clinical indications, prepacing ECGs, age and sex of patient, implanted pacemaker model, and pacing electrode.

In addition, a name list of the pacemaker patients is delivered. This list contains the implantation date and the date of the check-up; it is continuously updated by the pacemaker center. In this way, follow-up data of patients also are available.

The practicality of the European Pacemaker Registry has been demonstrated in a 7-year experience with this system in Austria. All pacemaker centers participate in this program, allowing an overview of trends concerning indications and pacemaker models, as well as follow-up (e.g., complication rate, survival rate).

Preparations have begun to accumulate pacemaker data from different countries in a central European registry. Since a unified documentation system has been employed, data from different countries are comparable. (An example is given in Table 38–4.)

EXAMPLE FOR THE USE OF POOLED DATA

Documentation of data can reveal the divergencies between pacemaker centers. The underlying causes, such as inadequate indication for pacemaker implantation (overpacing), lack of training of physicians (underpacing, high complication rate), and nonmedical reasons (unavailability of pacemakers), must be investigated individually.

The statistical evaluation requires verification of the reliability of the submitted data. The credibility factor "α" defines the systematic deviation of the individual medical center's data from the overall collective data. The numeric quantity of α depends on the constancy

TABLE 38–4
Comparison of Prepacing ECG Studies, Using the European Pacemaker Registration System*

Implantation Ratio	Austria	Belgium	Switzerland	GDR†
Overall	257	359	218	226
Second-degree AV block	22.1	34.5	22.0	63.0
Third-degree AV block	71.9	78.3	47.7	56.9
Bifascicular block	5.4	9.0	5.5	?
Sick sinus syndrome	56.8	64.6	51.4	66.0
Atrial fibrillation + bradycardia	40.3	28.0	22.0	23.9

*In addition to the overall implantation ratio, the ratios for five different ECG indications are shown.
†GDR = German Democratic Republic.

TABLE 38–5
Credibility Factor for Seven Pacemaker Centers in Austria

	Pacemaker Center No.						
	1	4	7	18	19	21	22
Bifascicular block	0.776	0.606	0.620	0.561	0.483	0.521	0.601
Sick sinus syndrome	0.851	0.717	0.729	0.678	0.607	0.643	0.714
Atrial fibrillation + bradycardia	0.817	0.664	0.677	0.621	0.545	0.583	0.659
	0.868	0.744	0.755	0.708	0.639	0.673	0.741

of the figures and the number of first implants performed in the medical center in question:

$$\alpha_j = \frac{w}{\frac{v}{p_j} + w}$$

where

- α = credibility factor
- W = interhospital variance of the mean value of a specific indication within the collective
- V = intrahospital variance of the mean value of a specific indication within the collective
- P = number of patients
- j = symbol of the medical center in question

The parameters W and V are calculated from the stored data. From the implantation figures over a period of 6 years, a trend may be calculated for each individual center:

$$mc_j = \alpha_j x_j + (1 - \alpha_j)m$$

where

- mc_j = expected mean value in the year following the calculation
- x = number of implantations for a certain indication
- m = mean value for the region considered in the calculation

Within this formula the trend for an individual medical center, a region, or an entire country may be calculated in advance. Table 38–5 compares seven centers. It is striking that Center No. 19 has a credibility factor below 0.64 for all investigated indications, whereas the credibility factor for Center No. 1 is around 0.8. The underlying causes of these divergencies will only be determined through comparison of patient data.

A CONTINENTAL DATA BASE

The continental data base is scheduled to operate in 1990. It is expected that, as a first step, seven countries will pool their data in this base.

Bibliography

Adler S, Whistler S: Advances in single-chamber pacemaker diagnostic data. PACE 9:1141, 1986.
Alpert MA, Curtis JJ, Sanfeldippo JF, et al.: Comparative survival after permanent ventricular and dual chamber pacing for patients with chronic high degree atrioventricular block with and without preexistent congestive heart failure. J Am Coll Cardiol 7:925, 1986.
Beaudry PR, Rosengarten MD, Nadeau L: Termination of ventricular tachycardia with transcutaneous cardiac pacing. Can Med Assoc J 134:145, 1986.
Benedek M, Furman S: Semiautomatic computer follow-up for transtelephone patients. PACE 6:316, 1983.
Bernstein AD, Parsonnet V: Computer-assisted measurements in pacemaker follow-up. PACE 9:392, 1986.
Brevik K, Ohm OJ: Myopotential inhibition of unipolar QRS-inhibited (VVI) pacemakers assessed by ambulatory Holter monitoring of the electrocardiogram. PACE 3:470, 1980.
Dreifus LS, Zinberg A, Hurzeler P, et al.: Transtelephonic monitoring of 25,919 implanted pacemakers. PACE 9:371, 1986.
Feruglio GA, Steinbach K: Cardiac pacing in Europe after two decades: A comprehensive survey. In Feruglio GA (ed.): Cardiac Pacing, pp. 1–13. Padova, Piccin Medical Books, 1983.
Feruglio GA, Steinbach K: Pacing in the world today. World survey on cardiac pacing for the years 1979 to 1981. In Steinbach K (ed.): Cardiac Pacing, pp. 963–967. Darmstadt, Steinkopff Verlag, 1983.
Feruglio GA, Rickards AF, Steinbach K, et al.: Cardiac pacing in the world: A survey of the state of the art in 1986. In Bellassen B, Feldman S, Copperman Y (eds.): Cardiac Pacing and Electrophysiology, pp. 563–564. Jerusalem, Creative Communications, 1987.
Furman S: Pacemaker infection. PACE 9:779, 1986.
Furman S: Cardiac pacing and pacemakers VIII. The pacemaker follow-up clinic. Am Heart J 94:795, 1977.
Goldman B, MacGregor D: Management of infected pacemaker system. Progr Clin Pacing Electrophysiol 2:220–235, 1984.
Gould L, Patel C: Long-term threshold stability with porous tip electrodes. PACE 9:1202, 1986.
Hanson J: Sixteen failures in a single model of bipolar poyurethane-insulated ventricular pacing lead. PACE 7:389, 1984.
Hauser RG, Wimer EA, Timmis GC, et al.: Twelve years of clinical experience with lithium pulse generators. PACE 9:277, 1986.
Hoffman A, Jost M, Pfisterer M: Persisting symptoms despite permanent pacing. Incidence, causes and follow-up. Chest 5:207, 1984.
Kaliman J, Scheibelhofer W, Steinbach K: Follow-up of patients with hypersensitive carotid syndrome. In Feruglio GA (ed.): Cardiac Pacing, pp 1–13. Padova, Piccin Medical Books, 1983.
Kristensson BE, Karlsson O, Ryden L: Holter-monitored heart rhythm during atrioventricular synchronous and fixed-rate ventricular pacing. PACE 9(4):511, 1986.
MacGregor DC, Covvey HD, Noble EJ: Computer-assisted reporting system for the follow-up of patients with cardiac pacemakers. PACE 3:568, 1980.
Markewitz A, Hemmer W, Weinhold C: Complications in dual chamber pacing: A six-year experience. PACE 9:1014, 1986.
Mast EG, van Hemel NM, Bakema L, et al.: Is chronic atrial stimulation a reliable method for single chamber pacing in sick sinus syndrome? PACE 9:1127, 1986.
Mugica J, Henry L, Rollet M, et al.: The clinical utility of pacemaker follow-up visits. PACE 9:1249, 1986.
Pfundner P, Steinbach K: Die EKG-Überwachung des Patienten außerhalb des Krankenhauses. Z Inere Med 53:343, 1972.
Platia EV, Brinker JA: Time course of transvenous pacemaker stimulation impedance, capture threshold and electrogram amplitude. PACE 9:620, 1986.
Pless P, Simonsen E, Arnsbo P, et al.: Superiority of multiprogrammable to nonprogrammable VVI pacing: A comparative study with special reference to management of pacing system malfunctions. PACE 9:739, 1986.
Podczeck A, Unger G, Meisl F, et al.: Effect of carotid sinus

massage (csm) on arterial blood pressure in patients with hypersensitive carotid sinus reflex and syncope. *In* Steinbach K (ed.): Cardiac Pacing, pp. 937–941. Darmstadt, Steinkopff Verlag, 1983.

Rosengarten MD: Reuse of permanent cardiac pacemakers. Can Med Assoc J 133:279, 1985.

Rosenqvist M, Edhag O: Pacemaker dependance in transient high-grade atrioventricular block. PACE 7:63, 1984.

Scheiblhofer W, Laczkovics A, Kaliman J, Steinbach K: Complications of physiological pacing. *In* Feruglio GA (ed.): Cardiac Pacing, pp. 1–13. Padova, Piccin Medical Books, 1983.

Simon AB, Jancz N: Symptomatic bradyarrhythmias in the adult. Natural history following ventricular pacemaker implantation. PACE 5:372, 1982.

Steinbach K, Joskowicz G: Erfahrungen mit einem zeitgesteuerten Schrittmachersystem. Wien klin Wochenschrift 87:371, 1975.

Steinbach K, Joskowicz G: Verkürzung der Impulsdauer zur Energieinsparung bei der Schrittmachertherapie. Acta Med Austriaca 3:13, 1976.

Steinbach K, Buchelt N, Frohner K, et al.: Präsynkope und Synkope. *In* Deutsch E (ed.): Vom Symptom zur Diagnose, pp 24–30. Vienna, Verlag Robidruck, 1987.

Steinbach K, Thalen B: World Survey on Cardiac Pacing: Europe. *In* Meere C (ed.): International Cardiac Pacing Society: State of the Art, Montreal, Chap. 41:3, 1979.

Steinbach K, Frohner K, Meisl F, et al.: Atrial stimulation. *In* Perez-Gomez F (ed.): Cardiac Pacing, pp. 629–633. Madrid, Verlag Grouz, 1985.

Steinbach K, Ettl W, Joskowicz G: Can indications for permanent pacing be controlled? Stimulation 5:13, 1986.

Steinbach K: Gutachterliche Beurteilung von Patienten mit Herzschrittmacher. Forschung und Praxis der Begutachtung 29:73–80, 1986.

Steinbach K, Laczkovics A, Mohl W: Plötzlicher Herztod bei Schrittmacherpatienten. Acta Med Austriaca 5:1, 1978.

Steinbach K: Experience with the European Registration Card in Austria. *In* Feruglio GA (ed.): Cardiac Pacing, pp. 519–522. Padova, Piccin Medical Books, 1983.

Stokes KB, Church T: Ten-year experience with implanted polyurethane lead insulation. PACE 9:1160, 1986.

Stryjer D, Friedensohn A, Schlesinger Z: Ventricular pacing as the preferable mode for long-term pacing in patients with carotid sinus syncope of the cardioinhibitory type. PACE 9:705, 1986.

Timmis GC, Westveer DC: Permanent pacemakers and their complications in perspective. Int J Cardiol 13:105, 1986.

Weber H, Glogar D, Joskowicz G, et al.: Computer-assisted long-term ECG analysis of atrial paced patients and the AV conduction. PACE 4:242, 1981.

39

Noninvasive External Cardiac Pacing

Rodney H. Falk

Historical Background

The era of cardiac pacing is generally considered to have begun in 1952 when Zoll[1] published his landmark paper describing two patients resuscitated from ventricular asystole by external cardiac stimulation. Remarkably, this technique, which was considered revolutionary in its time, had been demonstrated to be effective 70 years previously in a patient whose heart had been chronically exposed following a chest wall resection.[2] Von Ziemssen, a German physiologist, was able to stimulate the heart by direct application of an electrode, through which he delivered a rapid series of electrical impulses. Von Ziemssen extended his observations to normal subjects and was able to increase their heart rates by external stimulation, but he appears to have been more interested in the physiology than in clinical applications, as he did not attempt to study patients with bradycardia.

In 1889, in a series of elegant animal experiments, McWilliam[3] of Aberdeen University, Scotland, described a method of pacing the asystolic animal heart using an induction current applied to the ventricular apex. Extrapolating from his experience, he predicted the feasibility of external cardiac pacing in man some fifty years before its development.

> An effective therapy in man would be . . . to send stimulating shocks through the whole heart. In order to do this, one electrode should be applied in front over the area of the cardiac impulse and the other over the region of the fourth dorsal vertebra behind, so that the induction shocks may traverse the organ. *The electrodes should be of considerable extent (for example, large sponge electrodes)* and the skin should be moistened with salt solution. The shocks employed should be strong, sufficient to excite powerful contraction in the voluntary muscle.[3] [italics added]

Unfortunately, McWilliam's suggestions were not put into clinical practice, possibly in part because the contemporary interest was in the role of the nervous system in cardiac acceleration, and further experiments on electrical stimulation concentrated on attempts to stimulate sympathetic nerves.[4]

Attempts at resuscitation using transthoracic stimulation did, however, continue, and a successful case of resuscitation of a patient with an opiate overdose was reported in 1908.[5] The device used was able to produce rhythmic electrical stimuli to the chest wall through large, posteriorly applied electrodes. From the description of the case it is probable that the electric shocks produced diaphragmatic stimulation, enabling some semblance of breathing in this patient with severe respiratory depression. Nevertheless, the author noted that cardiac stimulation sometimes occurred and even proposed the use of this device in ambulances—probably the earliest reference to a mobile intensive care unit!

Development of Modern Transcutaneous Pacing Devices

A major drawback to acceptance of external cardiac pacing was the pain associated with stimulation. In an attempt to modify this discomfort Zoll and coworkers[6,7] increased the electrode size, resulting in a reduced threshold for cardiac stimulation and a consequent improved tolerability of external pacing. Further improvement was gained by the development of a high-impedance electrode gel that abolished the stinging sensation previously associated with cutaneous nerve stimulation. Increasing the pulse width of external pacemakers was found to further reduce the threshold required for cardiac stimulation, with an optimal pulse width of 20 to 40 ms (Fig. 39-1).

Animal experiments evaluating the safety and efficacy of external pacing have confirmed the value of a prolonged stimulus duration in reducing threshold.[8] The relative safety of the technique is indicated in several studies that fail to show repetitive ventricular

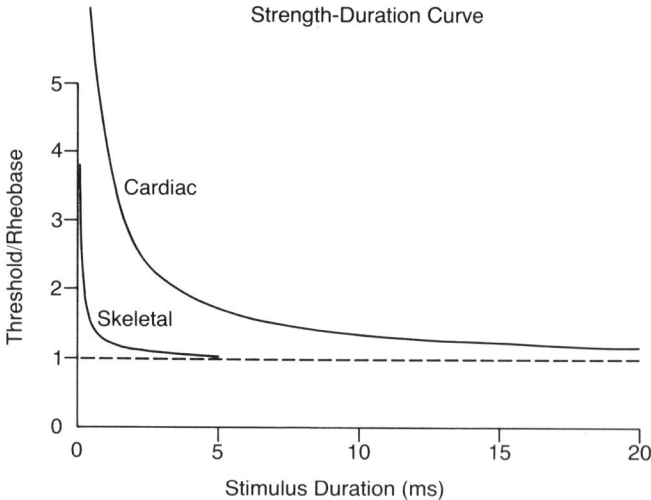

FIGURE 39–1
Strength-duration curve for cardiac and skeletal muscle contraction during external pacing. Maximal skeletal muscle contraction occurs with 5-ms duration stimuli whereas the threshold for cardiac pacing is still falling above 20 ms. (Reprinted by permission from Zoll PM, Zoll RH, Belgard AH: In Cardiac Pacing. Electrophysiology and Pacemaker Technology, pp. 593–595. Padova, Piccin Medical Books, 1980.)

arrhythmias with asynchronous pacing or during suprathreshold stimuli in hypoxic animals.[6,8] Syverud et al.[9] demonstrated a small rise in creatine phosphokinase (CPK) levels following prolonged pacing in dogs, all of which was of the MM component, compatible with skeletal muscle origin. Pathologic examination of the hearts in these animals did not reveal any damage attributable to external pacing.

The effect of transvenous right ventricular pacing, external transthoracic pacing, and external pacing via a tongue-epigastric route have been studied in chronically instrumented anesthetized dogs with complete heart block.[10] Successful ventricular capture was achieved with all three modes, although pacing thresholds for external pacing were, as expected, much higher than those required for transvenous pacing. Cardiac output with transthoracic pacing (4.2 L/min) was significantly greater than with transthoracic pacing (3.2 L/min). Mean arterial pressure was also greater with transthoracic pacing than with transvenous or tongue-epigastric pacing. The authors suggest that simultaneous activation of atria and ventricles may be present with transthoracic pacing, and that the improved hemodynamics may result from a more physiologic sequence of cardiac activation than that produced by right ventricular pacing.

Although external pacing may stimulate both atria and ventricles in dogs, such stimulation is simultaneous[8] and thus is unlikely to contribute to an improved cardiac output in comparison with right ventricular pacing. A more likely explanation of Varghese's data[8] is that the skeletal muscle stimulation associated with pacing results in vasodilation with concomitant improvement of cardiac output by afterload reduction. It is thus unlikely that there is significant advantage of external pacing over transvenous right ventricular pacing, as any increased cardiac output merely goes to skeletal muscle.

EXPERIMENTAL STUDIES IN HUMANS

The feasibility of external cardiac pacing in normal subjects was initially established in 16 normal men in

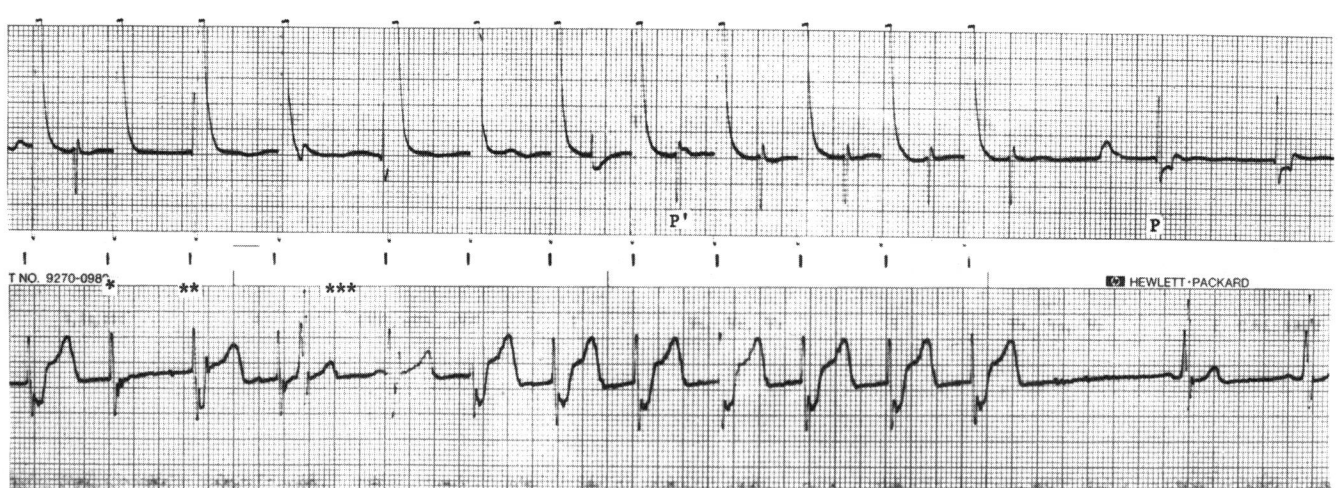

FIGURE 39–2
Representative esophageal and surface tracings from a subject during external pacing. The upper tracing shows the esophageal recording and the lower tracing shows the corresponding tracing from the pacemaker oscilloscope. The first beat is paced with retrograde atrial stimulation. Beat 2 (*) represents a stimulus with no response. Beat 3 (**) presents a pacing stimulus falling just after the P wave (faint, initial upward deflection in upper tracing) and failing to capture the ventricle. The subsequent two beats (***) are also unpaced and are followed by 7 paced beats, the last 5 of which demonstrate retrograde (downward) P wave activity (P'). The small upright P wave following the second paced beat may represent a fusion beat between sinus and retrograde atrial activation. In the final 2 beats of the tracing, the pacemaker is switched off and normal sinus rhythm resumes, with an upright atrial deflection in the esophageal lead. The additional deflection on the surface ECG (lower tracing) during sinus rhythm is a marker indicating pacemaker sensing. (Reprinted by permission from Falk RH, Ngai STA, Kumaki DJ, et al.: PACE 10:503, 1987.)

whom pacing thresholds were found to range from 42 to 60 mA.[11] No evidence of pacing-induced arrhythmias occurred in these subjects, and no relationship was found between body weight and pacing threshold; the heaviest subject paced weighed 125 kg and had a pacing threshold of 56 mA. Other than transient, painless skin erythema in most subjects, there were no adverse sequelae of external pacing. In a study of 10 normal volunteers paced externally for 30 minutes, Meibom and associates[12] showed no alteration in blood pressure during pacing. Serial total CPK measurements and isoenzyme assays were performed during and up to 24 hours following pacing and failed to show any change from baseline, confirming the safety of moderately prolonged external cardiac pacing.

In a study to determine the sequence of cardiac activation during external pacing in humans, atrial activity was recorded with an esophageal electrode.[13] External pacing was associated with ventricular capture only with either atrioventricular dissociation or retrograde ventriculoatrial conduction (Fig. 39–2). These results have been confirmed by other investigators, even when the pacemaker was used at the maximal tolerated output.[14] Thus in humans, as opposed to dogs, external pacing only stimulates the ventricles.

ECHOCARDIOGRAPHY DURING EXTERNAL PACING

A distinctive pattern of septal motion resembling that seen in left bundle branch block is usually seen during transvenous right ventricular pacing.[15] Interestingly, this pattern is rarely seen during external pacing during which echocardiographic parameters of left ventricular function seem relatively normal,[12] thus suggesting that simultaneous right and left ventricular contraction may occur during external pacing (Fig. 39–3). Theoretically, this may have some advantage in maintaining cardiac output, because the abnormal septal motion seen during transvenous pacing may be associated with a mild reduction in cardiac output.[16] However, the predominant determinant of preservation of cardiac output and blood pressure during either transvenous or external pacing is preservation of atrioventricular synchrony at a given heart rate, and susceptible patients may develop the "pacemaker syndrome" during external pacing in the same way that they do during transvenous pacing. This is illustrated in Figure 39–4.

EFFECT OF ELECTRODE POSITION ON PACING THRESHOLD

In temporary transvenous pacing, variations in electrode position may affect pacing threshold, although the major consideration is for stability of electrode position. External pacing thresholds in some individuals vary considerably with changes in anterior electrode position (we have seen a twofold increase in threshold with minor position change), but this is the exception rather than the rule. In a study performed in six normal subjects, using a prototype external pacemaker (Physio Control), three electrode positions were compared.[17]

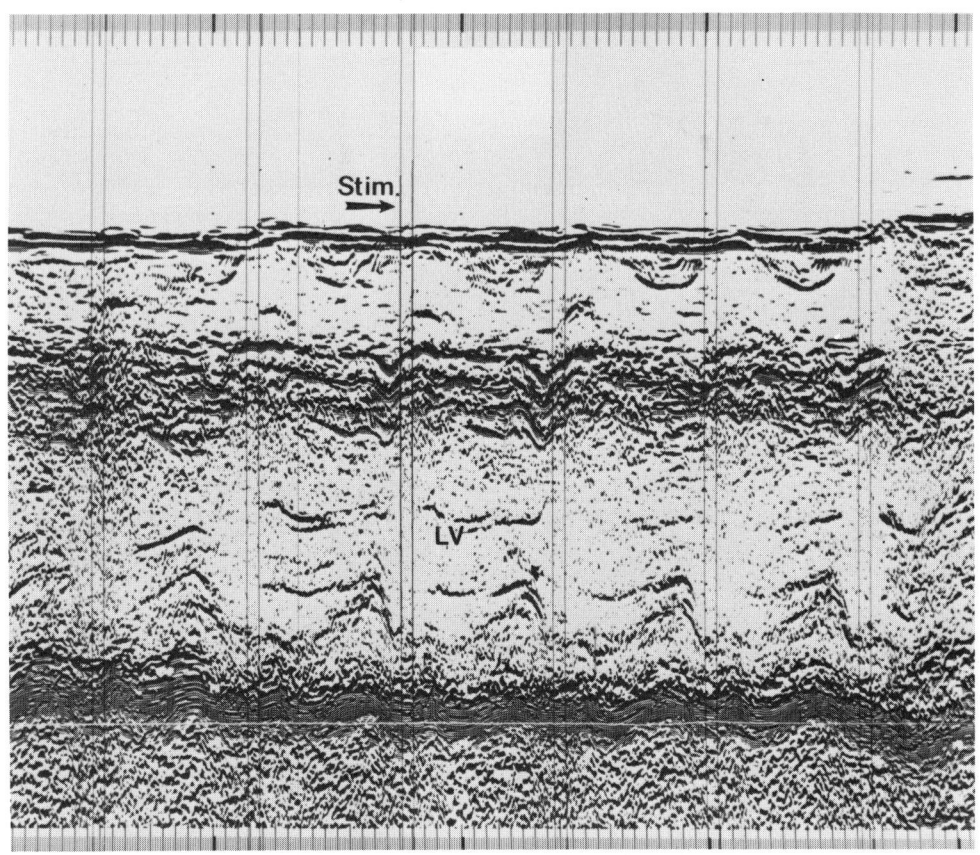

FIGURE 39–3
M-mode echocardiogram during external pacing in a normal volunteer. The stimulus (arrow) is followed by a normal downward septal motion and upward posterior wall motion. The prolonged electromechanical delay following the stimulus artifact (250 ms) typically is seen during external pacing.

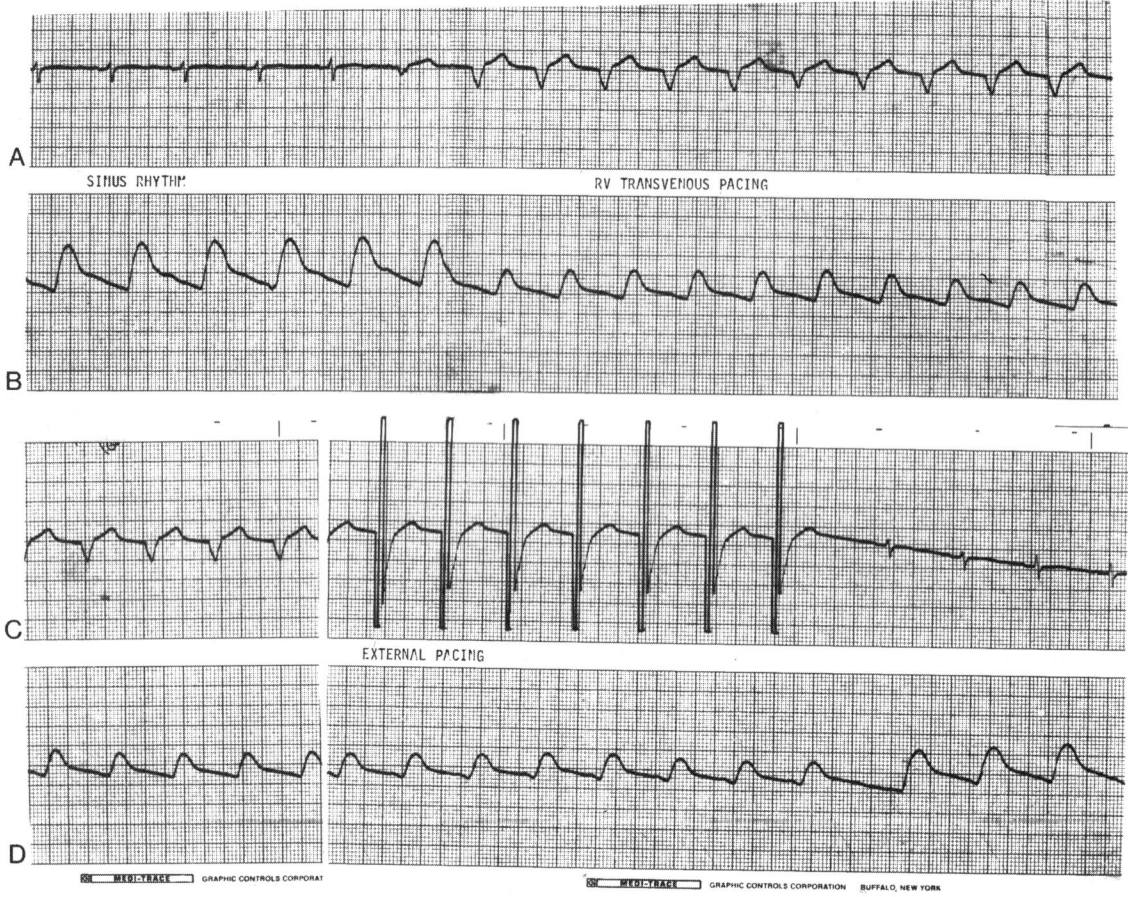

FIGURE 39–4
Comparison of blood pressure response to sinus rhythm, transvenous temporary right ventricular pacing, and external pacing. A and C show surface ECGs, and B and D show simultaneous blood pressure tracings recorded from an arterial line. The blood pressure falls to equivalent levels with both right ventricular and external pacing, compared to sinus rhythm.

When the electrodes were in the anterior-posterior position (i.e., negative electrode in the anterior left parasternal area centered approximately over the third or fourth intercostal space, positive electrode at the lower scapular border) the threshold was approximately 15% higher when the posterior electrode was at the right subscapular area, compared to the left.

However, this difference was not statistically significant. Positioning both electrodes on the anterior chest wall (i.e., negative electrode at apex, positive electrode in right parasternal area) resulted in thresholds no different from those in the direct anteroposterior position. Reversal of polarity increased pacing thresholds to levels greater than most subjects were able to tolerate. Thus, in an emergency, exact positioning of electrodes does not generally appear to be crucial, providing that the negative electrode is over the left anterior chest wall. Nevertheless, since the discomfort of external pacing is primarily related to skeletal muscle stimulation, it is advisable to alter the anterior electrode in conscious patients to obtain the most comfortable position (often the position associated with the least pectoral muscle twitching).

Clinical Applications of External Cardiac Pacing

At the time of this writing there are two commercially available external cardiac pacemakers which are used widely in the United States: the ZMI Noninvasive Transcutaneous Pacemaker (NTP) (Fig. 39–5) and the

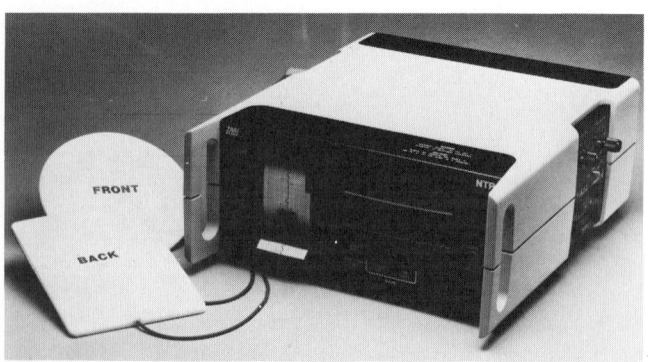

FIGURE 39–5
The noninvasive transcutaneous external pacemaker (NTP) (ZMI Corp.). The electrodes are pre-gelled sponge electrodes, and the pacemaker is combined with its own oscilloscope and a digital readout of heart rate and current.

PhysioControl LifePak 8 (Fig. 39–6). The former is a stand-alone pacemaker monitor; the latter is incorporated into a defibrillator-monitor. A smaller, stand-alone version of the PhysioControl device is currently undergoing clinical testing. The characteristics of the two devices are similar. Both utilize large adhesive electrodes and are capable of delivering a current of up to 200 mA. The pulse width of the PhysioControl pacemaker is 20 ms, and that of the Zoll NTP is 40 ms.

The characteristics of external pacing electrodes differ considerably from those used for defibrillation, predominantly by virtue of their higher impedance. Thus, pacing and defibrillating electrodes are not interchangeable. The delivered energy of the external pacing stimulus is very small compared to that required for defibrillation. For a pulse width of 40 ms and assuming a transthoracic plus electrode resistance of 500 ohms, a 50-mA pacing stimulus delivers 0.05 J (current^2 × resistance × time). For a 100-mA stimulus, the delivered energy increases fourfold to 0.2 J. It can be seen that this is a tiny fraction of the energy required for defibrillation. Despite this low energy, external pacing is usually uncomfortable for the conscious patient, predominantly due to skeletal muscle stimulation. Reassurance does much to assuage the anxiety associated with this unusual sensation, but mild sedation may be required if pacing is to be prolonged.

FACTORS INFLUENCING SUCCESS OF EXTERNAL PACING

External cardiac pacing does not differ from transvenous pacing in the factors influencing its success. Attempts at emergency transvenous or transthoracic needle pacing in asystolic cardiac arrest have been almost universally unsuccessful because of delay in application and associated hypoxia, acidosis, and metabolic disturbance.[18, 19] A similarly poor result is seen if attempts at external pacing are delayed until late in the course of cardiac arrest. Of 20 patients undergoing external cardiac pacing during an out-of-hospital cardiac arrest or following a prolonged emergency room resuscitation attempt, eight had electrical evidence of ventricular capture but only two patients had a palpable pulse with pacing, one of whom survived.[20] The survivor was a woman with a witnessed bradycardic arrest. A similar series of 108 patients paced out-of-hospital for idioventricular rhythm or asystole had no survivors.[20a] The prolonged delay in applying external pacing (in excess of 25 minutes) makes it hardly surprising that the outcome was so poor.

In an attempt to define whether the early application of external pacing may be beneficial in cardiac arrest, we studied the value of external pacing during 58 in-hospital cardiac arrests (55 patients).[21] External cardiac pacing was attempted in 26 patients (45%), and the remainder were either resuscitated without pacing or considered nonresuscitable after failure of initial attempts. Although half the group receiving external pacing had ECG evidence of ventricular capture, palpable pulses occurred in only two patients, one of whom survived. The poor survival in the paced group contrasts with a short-term survival of 38% in patients with bradycardia/asystole, who did not receive external pacing. This result, which initially seems paradoxical, is explained by the fact that paced patients had previously failed to respond to adequate oxygenation and/or pharmacologic therapy (e.g., epinephrine, isoproterenol), whereas survivors in the unpaced group were responders to these therapies. Thus, in an in-hospital population experiencing cardiac arrest, outcome in patients with bradycardia or asystole as the initial rhythm is relatively poor and is usually reflective of

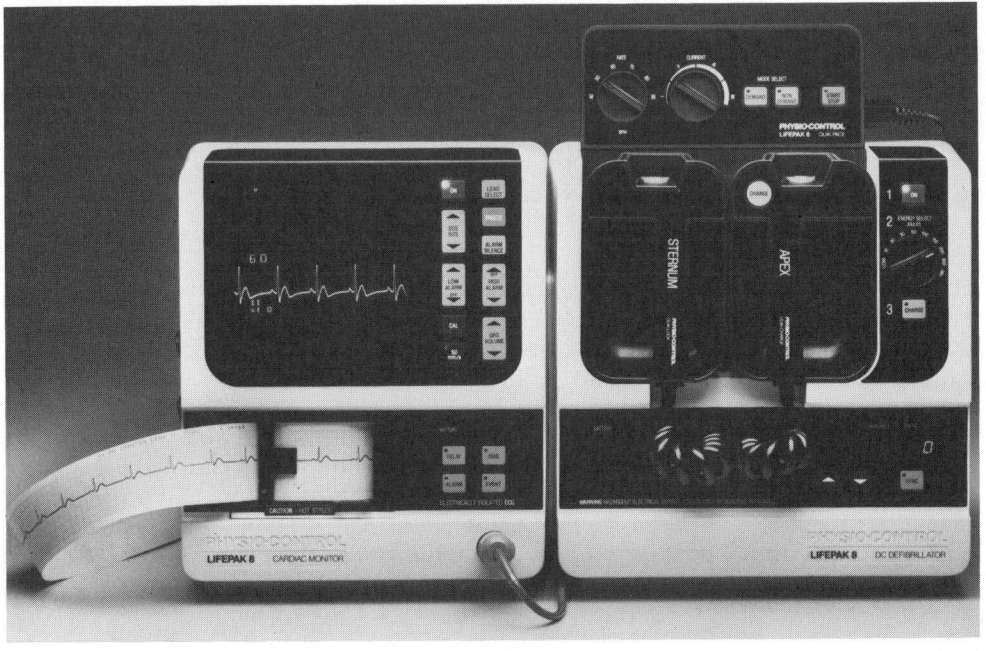

FIGURE 39–6
PhysioControl LifePak 8 defibrillator-pacemaker-monitor. Pacing is performed through specifically designed electrodes, and the output is controlled by a removable module that is slotted into the top of the defibrillator.

generalized noncardiac disease. Furthermore, if the rhythm is unresponsive to initial pharmacologic measures, it is unlikely to respond to cardiac pacing. It is important to note that these results do not reflect a failure of the technique of external pacing, but rather a failure of the hypoxic human heart to respond to pacing with mechanical contractions, despite electrical activity.[22]

MAXIMUM BENEFIT OF EXTERNAL PACING

If cardiac pacing (external or transvenous) is ineffective in the majority of cases of cardiac arrest, whether in-hospital or out-of-hospital, does it have any role as an emergency procedure? The answer is most certainly affirmative, provided that patients are appropriately selected. It is in the subgroup of patients with a primary conduction disturbance (sinus arrest or high degree atrioventricular block) that external pacing is of greatest value. In the original series of patients reported by the author, three patients had sudden ventricular asystole or symptomatic bradycardia, all of whom responded promptly to external pacing with return of blood pressure and improved conscious level.[11] This was confirmed in a larger multicenter trial.[23] Personal experience and review of published cases of successful resuscitation with external cardiac pacing indicates the profile of the type of patient likely to respond to external cardiac pacing: namely, a patient with a primary bradycardia due to conduction system failure in whom external pacing is promptly applied. Unfortunately, initial hopes that pacing (external or transvenous) may be of value in post-defibrillation asystole have not been borne out by either clinical experience or experimental trials.[22, 24, 25]

ELECTROCARDIOGRAPHY OF EXTERNAL PACING

Because of the extremely large, wide pacemaker impulse, recognition of a paced impulse from a standard ECG is virtually impossible (Fig. 39–7). The two major commercially available external pacemakers (ZMI and PhysioControl) incorporate special damping circuits in their oscilloscopes that permit visualization of the paced beats (Fig. 39–8). Nevertheless, certain artifacts may occur, causing misinterpretation of a nonpaced trace as pacing. Since arterial pulses may be difficult to distinguish from the movement produced from skeletal muscle contraction, the correct recognition of pacing on the ECG is crucial.

Several confusing appearances may occur during external pacing. In patients with an intrinsic rhythm, subthreshold stimulation in the demand mode at a rate slightly higher than the intrinsic rate will result in a nonconducted pacing spike occurring just before the native QRS. Failure to recognize this may lead to misinterpretation as a paced rhythm. This is particularly important in patients in whom a pacing threshold is being established with a view to standby pacemaker use (Fig. 39–9).

The ZMI NTP pacemaker has a damping circuit which extends past the visible pacing artifact on the oscilloscope. On occasion this results in the damping or abolition of the QRS, resulting in a paced spike followed by a T wave (Fig. 39–10). Failure to recognize this as the normal functioning of the pacemaker may lead to erroneous interpretation of a sinus beat as a paced beat. Pseudo–T waves following a nonconducted pacing spike have been described in patients undergoing emergency pacing (Fig. 39–11A). These are low-amplitude, prolonged deflections and differ from the clearly visualized T wave of an appropriately paced beat (Fig. 39–11B).

Once these concepts of external pacing are understood, interpretation of the paced ECG is quite simple. Nevertheless, the paced QRS configuration varies considerably from patient to patient, and in doubtful cases a very careful assessment of arterial pulses may be necessary, as well as a trial of increased output to determine whether subthreshold stimuli were being delivered.

PROPHYLACTIC USE OF EXTERNAL PACING

Prophylactic temporary pacemakers are frequently requested for use preoperatively in patients with significant bradycardia, prior to cardioversion in suspected sinus node disease, or in myocardial infarction when a new conduction disorder is considered likely to progress. The availability of external pacing in these circumstances offers an attractive alternative to an invasive procedure, which has a small but significant complication rate.[26, 27] In the large series by Zoll et al,[23] 40 patients received a test of "standby" external pacing with a 100% ability to capture and, presumably, avoidance of the need for transvenous pacing. In a small series by Sharkey and coworkers[28] of patients undergoing cardioversion in whom post-conversion bradycardia was feared, all nine had a successful trial of external pacing pre-cardioversion. One patient developed prolonged sinus arrest post-cardioversion with successful external pacing.

The efficacy of external pacing in patients undergoing general anesthesia for surgical procedures was assessed in 21 subjects by Berliner et al.[29] Although the authors did not determine pre- and post-anesthetic pacing thresholds, all subjects were successfully paced while under anesthesia, confirming the utility of external pacing in this setting and suggesting that anesthetic agents may have little significant effect on pacing thresholds.

The effect of drugs and hypoxia on pacing threshold is of particular importance when external pacing is being considered, since the procedure is uncomfortable, and discomfort may increase considerably in individuals with a relatively small increase in pacemaker output. Hypoxia, hyperkalemia, antiarrhythmic drugs, beta-blockers and calcium channel blockers have all been reported to increase pacing thresholds during transvenous pacing,[30, 31] and thresholds for external pacing are higher during cardiac arrest than during

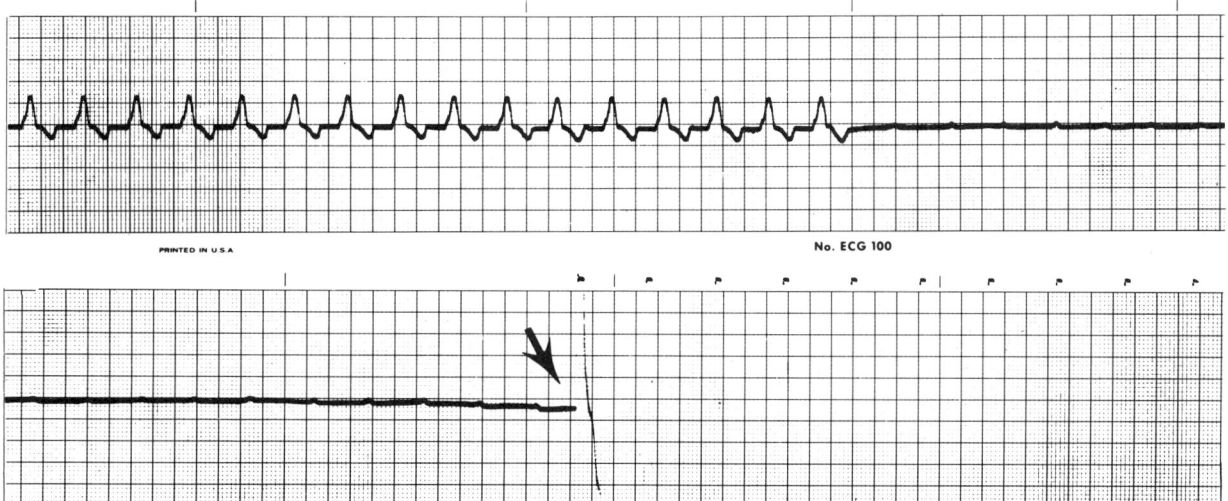

FIGURE 39–7
Standard ECG tracing made during sudden onset of ventricular asystole in a patient with sinus tachycardia, left bundle branch block, and acute anterior infarction. The bottom tracing shows onset of external pacing (arrow), with loss of ECG signal due to the high current of external pacing stimuli.

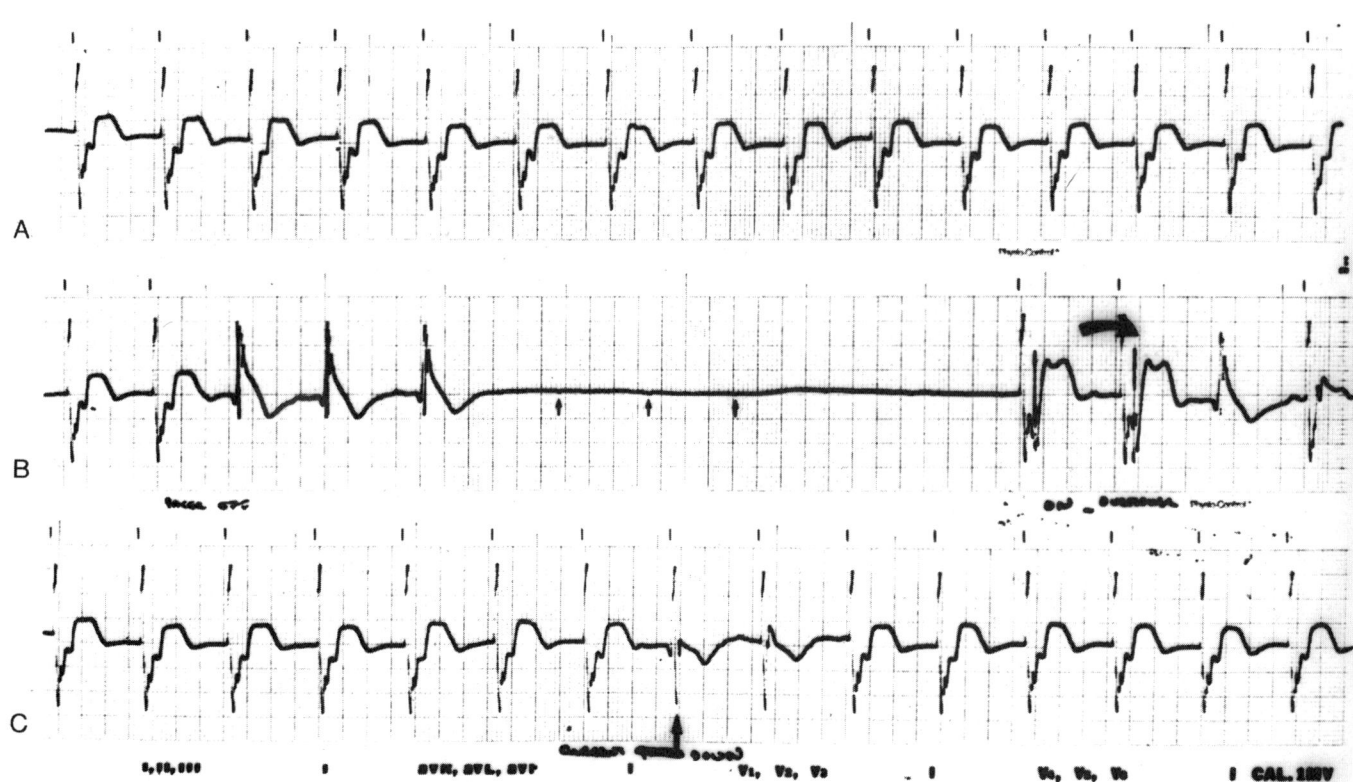

FIGURE 39–8
Recording of external pacing from a PhysioControl pacemaker-monitor. A shows successful pacing, with spike followed by a paced QRS complex (visible mainly as a T wave). B, The current is reduced to below threshold (beats 3–5), and pacer is briefly switched off, revealing low-voltage P waves (small arrows). Pacing is then reinstituted. Large, curved arrow indicates a second pacer spike artifact caused by oversensing of paced QRS complex. This was overcome by reducing the ECG gain (C).

Noninvasive External Cardiac Pacing 681

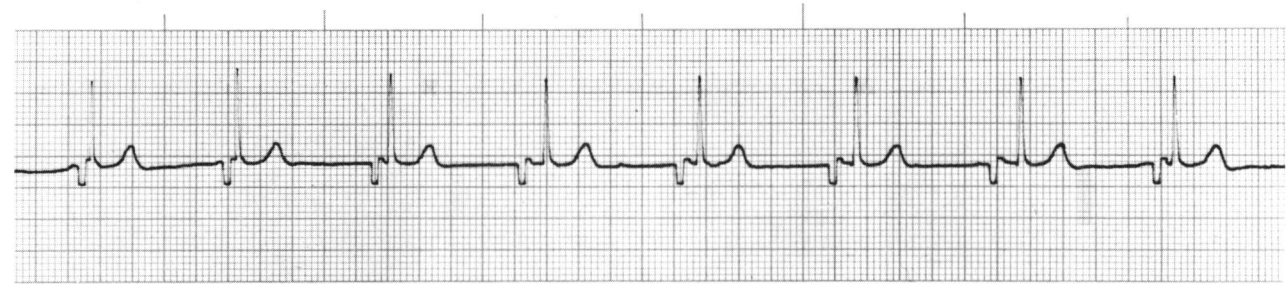

FIGURE 39–9
Tracing from a ZMI pacemaker, showing an example of stimulus artifact at subthreshold levels at a rate minimally faster than the subject's heart rate. The stimulus (downward deflection) appears immediately before the native QRS complex, obliterating the P wave. However, there is no ventricular capture.

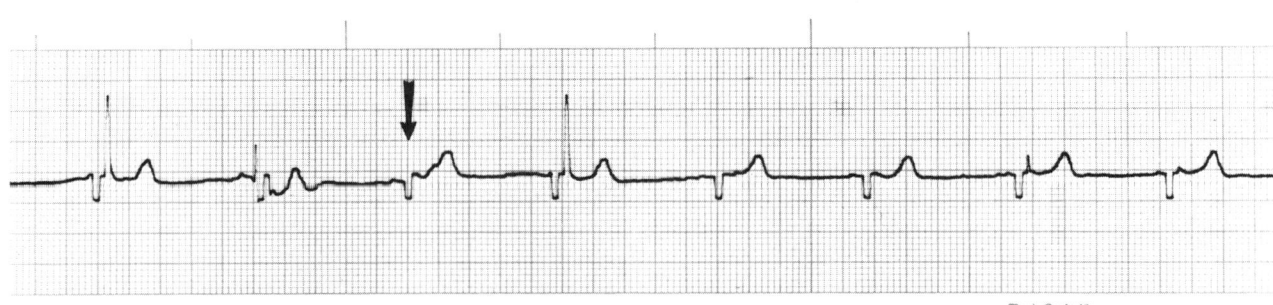

FIGURE 39–10
Minimal acceleration of intrinsic heart rate, causing superimposition of a subthreshold pacing stimulus on the native QRS complex (arrow). The QRS complex is obliterated by the damping circuit, leaving only the T wave visible, thus mimicking a paced beat.

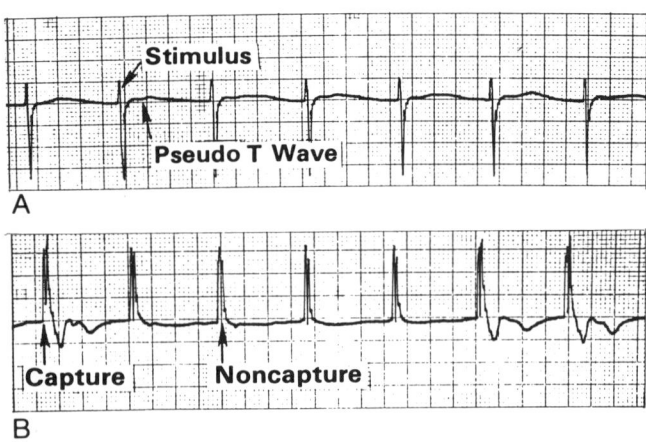

FIGURE 39–11
A, Example of ECG artifact mimicking a T wave in a patient whose heart has been stimulated but not paced. The pseudo–T wave is of a much lower amplitude than a true paced T wave. No QRS is seen. B, Example of true pacing, with reduction of current below threshold to show unpaced stimuli. The first and second arrows indicate a captured and noncaptured pacing stimulus, respectively. (B reprinted by permission from Knowlton AA, Falk RH: Am J Cardiol 57:1295, 1986.)

prophylactic pacing.[10] To date, no study has analyzed whether patients receiving cardiac drugs have higher pacing thresholds (and thus, possibly, less tolerance to external pacing) than normal. However, incidental data gleaned from the literature suggest that this is probably not a major problem.

The pacing thresholds determined by Sharkey and colleagues[28] in their cardioversion study described above were in the usual range despite procainamide use in all but one patient.[28] We have studied six normal subjects, each receiving intravenous propranolol, verapamil, or placebo in a double-blind fashion on separate occasions and could find no drug effect on pacing threshold.[32] While investigators using external pacing for attempted tachycardia termination have not described any increased pacing thresholds with antiarrhythmic drug use, it is prudent to retest external pacing thresholds after any change in cardiac medications in patients for whom external pacing is being held on standby.

TERMINATION OF TACHYARRHYTHMIAS

External pacing preferentially stimulates the ventricles and might be expected to be of value in overdrive pacing of ventricular tachycardia. Isolated case reports of successful tachycardia conversion have appeared,[33-35] including one case in which retrograde atrial activation both induced and terminated a supraventricular arrhythmia.[35] Systematic studies of tachycardia induction and termination in the electrophysiology laboratory, using a modified external pacing device, have confirmed the utility of this approach in a small proportion of patients.[14, 36] In most patients, however, arrhythmia induction/termination is not feasible, either because of intolerable discomfort or because of inability to select multiple stimulation sites.

EXTERNAL PACING IN CHILDREN

Almost all clinical trials of external pacing have been performed in adults. An exception is the study by Beland and colleagues,[37] who paced 22 anesthetized children, 11 months to 18 years of age, a total of 56 times. The mean pacing threshold of 63 mA (range 42–98 mA), using standard adult electrodes, did not differ from that reported for adults. A 60% reduction in electrode area resulted in a threshold reduction of approximately 15%, but with a corresponding increase in current density. Of interest was the lack of correlation between pacing threshold and age, weight, chest circumference, and body surface area. The authors conclude that, in the anesthetized child, external pacing is safe and effective and may be useful in a variety of situations otherwise requiring transvenous temporary pacing.

Summary

External cardiac pacing is a safe and effective method for stimulating the heart in an emergency. Although occasional patients have been externally paced for several hours, most patients find the procedure quite uncomfortable and may require mild sedation. If long-term temporary pacing is required, the transvenous approach is still the procedure of choice; however, in an emergency the availability of an external pacemaker allows a more leisurely and controlled situation for transvenous pacemaker placement.

Since external pacing is not associated with mechanical stimulation of the ventricle it may be safer than transvenous pacing in terms of arrhythmia provocation. Nevertheless, reports of arrhythmia provocation in highly susceptible patients as well as one report of external pacing induced ventricular tachycardia[37] mandate the availability of a defibrillator. Although the results of external pacing in bradyasystolic cardiac arrest have been disappointing, this represents a failure of the heart to respond rather than a failure of the technique, and the rapid and early application of pacing may be life-saving for the occasional patient.

The major application of external cardiac pacing is in the emergency treatment of sudden primary conduction disturbances, and it is useful as a standby measure in patients who would otherwise require prophylactic transvenous pacing for various indications. There is little doubt that this technique, which was the precursor of modern transvenous pacing and once considered obsolete, has resumed an important and well-deserved place in emergency cardiac care.

References

1. Zoll PM: Resuscitation of the heart in ventricular standstill by external electric stimulation. N Engl J Med 247:768, 1952.
2. Schechter DC: Background of clinical cardiac electro-stimulation. Part 1. Responsiveness of quiescent, bare heart to electricity. NY State J Med 71:2794, 1971.
3. McWilliam JA: Electrical stimulation of the heart in man. Br Med J 1:348, 1889.
4. Schechter DC: Background of clinical cardiac electro-stimulation. Part IV. Early studies on feasibility of accelerating heart rate by means of electricity. NY State J Med 72:395, 1971.
5. Robinovitch LG: Resuscitation of a woman in profound syncope caused by chronic morphine poisoning: Means used: rhythmic excitation with an induction current; the author's method and model of a coil. J Ment Pathol 8:180, 1908.
6. Zoll PM, Zoll RH, Belgard AH: Noninvasive cardiac stimulation. In (ed.): Cardiac Pacing: Electrophysiology and Pacemaker Technology, pp. 593–595. Padova, Piccin Medical Books, 1980.
7. Zoll PM, Zoll RH, Belgard A: External non-invasive electrical stimulation of the heart. Crit Care Med 9:393, 1981.
8. Varghese PJ, Bren G, Ross A: Electrophysiology of external pacing: A comparative study with endocardial pacing (Abstract). Circulation 66:II–349, 1982.
9. Syverud SA, Dalsey WC, Hedges JP, et al.: Transcutaneous cardiac pacing: Determination of myocardial injury in canine model. Ann Emerg Med 12:745, 1983.
10. Niemann JT, Rosborough JP, Gardner D, et al.: External noninvasive cardiac pacing; A comparative hemodynamic study of two techniques with conventional endocardial pacing. PACE 7:230, 1984.
11. Falk RH, Zoll PM, Zoll RH: Safety and efficacy of noninvasive cardiac pacing: A preliminary report. N Engl J Med 309:1166, 1983.
12. Meibom J, Madsen K, Pedersen F, et al.: Noninvasive transcutaneous pacing does not traumatize the heart or affect left ventricular function. PACE 10:716, 1987.

13. Falk RH, Ngai STA, Kumaki DJ, et al.: Cardiac activation during external cardiac pacing. PACE 10:503, 1987.
14. Klein LS, Miles WM, Heger JJ, et al.: Transcutaneous pacing: Strength-interval curves and feasibility for programmed electrical stimulation. Circulation 76:IV–84, 1987.
15. Ishikawa K, Yanagisawa A: Evaluation of unusual QRS complexes produced by pacemaker stimuli with special reference to the vectorcardiographic and echocardiographic findings. J Electrocardiology 13:409, 1980.
16. Askenazi J, Alexander JH, Koenigsberg DI, et al.: Alteration of left ventricular performance by left bundle branch block simulated with atrioventricular pacing. Am J Cardiol 53:99, 1984.
17. Falk RH, Ngai STA: External cardiac pacing: Influence of electrode placement on pacing threshold. Crit Care Med 14:931, 1986.
18. Roberts JR, Greenberg MI: Emergency transthoracic pacemaker. Ann Emerg Med 10:600, 1981.
19. Ornato JP, Carveth WL, Windle JR: Pacemaker insertion for prehospital bradyasystolic cardiac arrest. Ann Emerg Med 13:101, 1984.
20. Falk RH, Jacobs L, Sinclair A, et al.: External noninvasive cardiac pacing in out-of-hospital cardiac arrest. Crit Care Med 11:779, 1983.
20a. Paris PM, Stewart RD, Kaplan R, et al.: Transcutaneous pacing for bradyasystolic cardiac arrests in prehospital care. Ann Emerg Med 14:320, 1985.
21. Knowlton AA, Falk RH: External cardiac pacing during in-hospital cardiac arrest. Am J Cardiol 57:1295, 1986.
22. Niemann JT, et al.: Endocardial and transcutaneous pacing, calcium chloride, and epinephrine in postcountershock asystole and bradycardias. Crit Care Med 13(9):699, 1985.
23. Zoll PM, Zoll RH, Falk RH, et al.: External noninvasive temporary cardiac pacing: Clinical trials. Circulation 71:735, 1985.
24. Niemann JT, Haynes KS, Garner D, et al.: Postcountershock pulseless rhythms: Response to CPR, artificial cardiac pacing and adrenergic agonists. Ann Emerg Med 15:112, 1986.
25. Hedges JR, Syverud SA, Dalsey WC, et al.: Prehospital trial of emergency transcutaneous cardiac pacing. Circulation 76:1337, 1987.
26. Austin JL, Preis LK, Crampton RS, et al.: Analysis of pacemaker malfunction and complications of temporary pacing in the coronary care unit. Am J Cardiol 49:301, 1982.
27. Hynes JK, Holmes DR Jr, Harrison CE: Five-year experience with temporary pacemaker therapy in the coronary care unit. Mayo Clin Proc 58:122, 1983.
28. Sharkey SW, Chafee V, Kapsner S: Prophylactic external pacing during cardioversion of atrial tachyarrhythmias. Am J Cardiol 55:1632, 1985.
29. Berliner D, Okun M, Peters RW, et al.: Transcutaneous temporary pacing in the operating room. JAMA 254:84, 1985.
30. Kubler W, Sowton E: Influence of beta-blockade on myocardial threshold in patients with pacemaker. Lancet 2:67, 1970.
31. Dohrmann ML, Goldschlager NF: Myocardial stimulation threshold in patients with pacemakers. Cardiol Clin 3:527, 1985.
32. Falk RH, Knowlton AA, Battinelli NJ: Effect of propranolol and verapamil on pacing threshold during external cardiac pacing—randomized double blinded study. PACE 10:673, 1987.
33. Rosenthal ME, Stamato NJ, Marchlinski FE, et al.: Noninvasive cardiac pacing for termination of sustained, uniform ventricular tachycardia. Am J Cardiol 58:561, 1986.
34. Barold SS, Falkoff MD, Ong LS, et al.: Termination of ventricular tachycardia by transcutaneous cardiac pacing. Am Heart J 114:180, 1987.
35. Luck JC, Davis D: Termination of sustained tachycardia by external noninvasive pacing. PACE 10:125, 1987.
36. Estes NAM, Deering TF, Manolis AS, et al.: External cardiac programmed stimulation for noninvasive termination of sustained supraventricular and ventricular tachycardia. Am J Cardiol 63:177, 1989.
37. Beland MJ, Hesslein PS, Finlay CD, et al.: Noninvasive transcutaneous cardiac pacing in children. PACE 10:1262, 1987.

40

Antitachycardia Pacing: Electrophysiologic Mechanisms

Mark Restivo
William B. Gough
Nabil El-Sherif

Electrical therapy of ventricular tachycardia can be accomplished by high-energy transthoracic electrical shocks, by low-energy transvenous shocks delivered through catheter electrodes,[1,2] or by one or more paced beats, also delivered through catheter electrodes and utilizing energy as low as twice the threshold for stimulation.[3] A pacing stimulus captures locally and generates an activation wavefront that propagates to the rest of the ventricles, including the "site" of ventricular tachycardia. Experimental[4] and clinical observations[5] have recently shown that very low-energy transvenous shocks may resemble a pacing stimulus by inducing a relatively localized depolarization, whereas the rest of the ventricles will be activated by a propagating depolarization wavefront. A high-energy transvenous shock, however, usually results in immediate depolarization of all or major portions of both ventricles and thus resembles a high-energy transthoracic electrical shock.

To understand the electrophysiologic mechanisms of electrical therapy of ventricular tachycardia, one must analyze the mechanism by which a paced wavefront interacts with the tachycardia site. These data may also explain the mechanism of action of low-energy transvenous shocks. Detailed analysis of ventricular activation patterns requires extensive mapping techniques that are more suitably applied to experimental models of ventricular tachycardia. In this chapter, we describe the effects of programmed electrical stimulation on reentrant ventricular tachycardia in the canine post-

---

This work was supported by Grant HL 36680 from the National Institutes of Health and by the Veterans Administration Medical Research Funds.

infarction model. It is generally believed that a majority of recurrent sustained monomorphic ventricular tachycardias in the clinical setting are due to reentrant excitation rather than abnormal pacemaker activity. The role of cycle length of stimulation, number of stimulated beats and site of stimulation, as well as the mechanisms of termination, resetting, entrainment or acceleration of reentrant ventricular tachycardia, are critically analyzed.[6] Also discussed are novel approaches by which electrical stimulation can prevent the initiation of reentrant tachycardia.

EXPERIMENTAL MODELS OF REENTRANT VENTRICULAR TACHYCARDIA

The electrophysiologic characteristics of the reentrant circuit in clinical ventricular tachycardia are not yet well defined. Experimentally, three types of circus movement reentry have been described.[7] These are (1) the ring model, (2) the figure-eight model, and (3) the leading circle model.

Ring Model of Reentry

In this model, originally described in rings of cardiac and other tissue cut from a variety of animals, a fixed anatomic obstacle is required around which the activation wavefront circulates.[8,9] The only two proven examples of ring model reentry in the intact mammalian heart are (1) circus movements involving the AV node and AV nodal accessory pathways and (2) those involving both bundle branches.[10] Clinical ventricular tachycardia due to bundle branch reentry, however, is rare.

Figure-Eight Model of Reentry

In this model, a functional rather than a fixed anatomic obstacle is necessary for the occurrence of circus movement. This model was originally described in the electrophysiologically abnormal, surviving ischemic epicardial layer overlying myocardial infarction in the dog's heart.[11, 12] Ischemia results in nonhomogeneous lengthening of refractoriness with a graded increase in refractoriness going from the border zone toward the center of the ischemic zone.[13] A critically timed premature beat that succeeds in inducing reentry results in a functional arc of unidirectional conduction block around which the reentrant wavefront circulates. The arc of conduction block occurs between adjacent sites of short and long refractoriness with the sites of longer refractoriness distal to the arc of block.

Reentrant activation continues as a figure-eight activation pattern, whereby two circulating wavefronts advance in clockwise and counterclockwise directions, respectively, around two zones (arcs) of functional conduction block. The two wavefronts coalesce into a common reentrant wavefront that conducts slowly between the two arcs of functional conduction block. This wavefront represents the slow zone of the figure-eight reentrant circuit (Fig. 40–1). During a monomorphic reentrant tachycardia, the two arcs of block and the two circulating wavefronts remain fairly stable. During a polymorphic reentrant rhythm, however, both arcs of block and the circulating wavefronts change their geometric configurations while maintaining their synchrony.

We have recently argued that the figure-eight model of reentry may be more representative of reentry in the human ventricle.[15]

Leading Circle Model of Reentry

In this model, originally described in small pieces of atrial myocardium of the rabbit,[14] the center of the circuit or the vortex is made of excitable tissue that is rendered functionally inexcitable by invasion of the center by multiple centripetal wavelets from the leading circuit outside the vortex. The leading circle model of reentry may represent a special modification of the figure-eight model.[15]

MECHANISMS OF TERMINATION OF REENTRANT TACHYCARDIA BY PROGRAMMED STIMULATION

In the figure-eight reentrant circuit, the two arcs of conduction block and the slow common reentrant wavefront are functionally determined and cycle length–dependent. A tight fit exists during the reentrant tachycardia, with the circulating wavefront closely following the refractory tail of the previous revolution. This is particularly significant in the zone of the slow common reentrant wavefront. The total activation time of the reentrant circuit is determined by the area with the longest refractoriness in the zone of the slow common reentrant wavefront. Myocardial refractoriness tends to shorten gradually to a new steady level in response to successive short cardiac cycles.[16] A sustained reentrant tachycardia represents a succession of short cardiac cycles. It is safe to assume that the duration of refractoriness in the zone with the longest refractoriness probably cannot shorten any further. This is not the case, however, with the rest of the reentrant pathway including both the normal zone and the remainder of the ischemic zone. Normal myocardium shows more shortening of refractoriness in response to successive short cardiac cycles compared with ischemic myocardium.[13] A stimulated wavefront at a cycle length shorter than the tachycardia cycle length can still conduct in these zones. In other words, these zones have a window of excitability.

For stimulated termination of the reentrant tachycardia (Fig. 40–2), the stimulated wavefront must arrive at the area with the longest refractoriness in the zone of the slow common reentrant wavefront before refractoriness expires, thus resulting in conduction block. If this area is strategically located between the two arcs of functional conduction block, reentrant

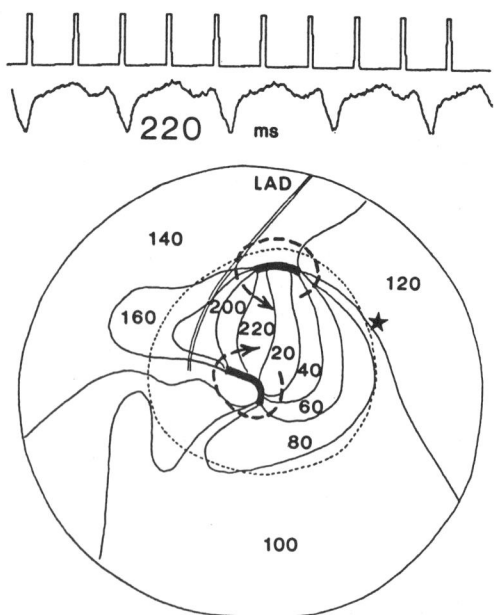

FIGURE 40–1
A lead II electrocardiographic recording and a polar projection of epicardial activation during reentrant ventricular tachycardia in the canine post-infarction heart. In this and subsequent maps, the heart is viewed from the cardiac apex located at the center of the circular map, and the perimeter of the circuit represents the AV junction. The dotted line represents the epicardial outline of the ischemic zone. The isochronal lines are drawn at 20-ms intervals; the time lines represent 100-ms intervals. The reentrant circuit has a characteristic figure-eight configuration in the form of clockwise and counterclockwise circulating wavefronts around two arcs of functional conduction block (represented by the heavy solid lines). The two wave fronts coalesce into a common reentrant wavefront that conducts slowly between the two arcs of block. This wavefront represents the slow part of the reentrant circuit. LAD = left anterior descending artery. (Reprinted by permission from El-Sherif N, Gough WB, Restivo M: PACE 10:341, 1987.)

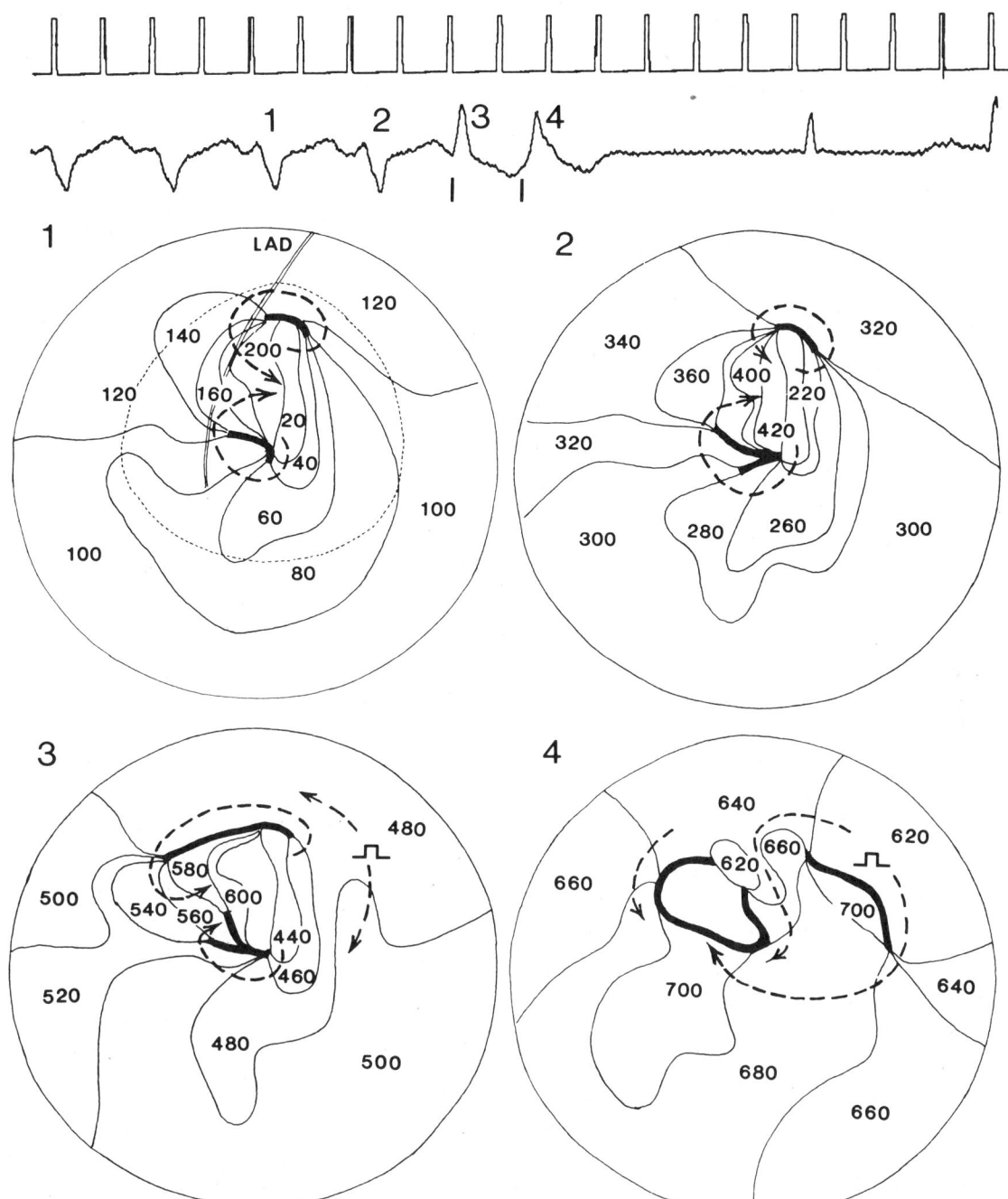

FIGURE 40–2
Tachycardia termination by programmed electrical stimulation. The figure shows epicardial activation maps from the same experiment shown in Figure 40–1 during termination of reentrant ventricular tachycardia by two stimulated beats at a cycle length of 155 ms. The reentrant tachycardia has a cycle length of 220 ms. Control maps are labeled 1 and 2; the maps of the first and second stimulated beats are labeled 3 and 4, respectively.

In this experiment, the reexcitation site was in the lower anterolateral portion of the left ventricle with activation proceeding in an apical-to-basal direction, which explains the negative QRS configuration in surface lead II. Electrical stimulation was applied to the normal zone close to the border of the ischemic zone and distal (downstream) to the slow common reentrant wavefront. The first stimulated beat preexcited normal myocardium and resulted in extension of the basal arc of functional conduction block. However, the slower, common reentrant wavefront could still conduct and reexcite normal myocardium. Thus, a single stimulated beat at a cycle length of 155 ms failed to terminate reentry.

On the other hand, the second stimulated beat resulted in a shift of the arc of functional conduction block to the border between the normal and ischemic zones close to the stimulated site. The two activation wavefronts around this arc of block invaded the distal part of the original site of the common reentrant wavefront and coalesced. However, the wavefronts failed to activate the proximal part of the zone of slow conduction, creating an island of functional conduction block. The last activation isochrone at 700 ms blocked at the proximal side of the original site of the common reentrant wavefront. LAD = left anterior descending artery.

(Reprinted by permission from El-Sherif N, Gough WB, Restivo M: PACE 10:341, 1987.)

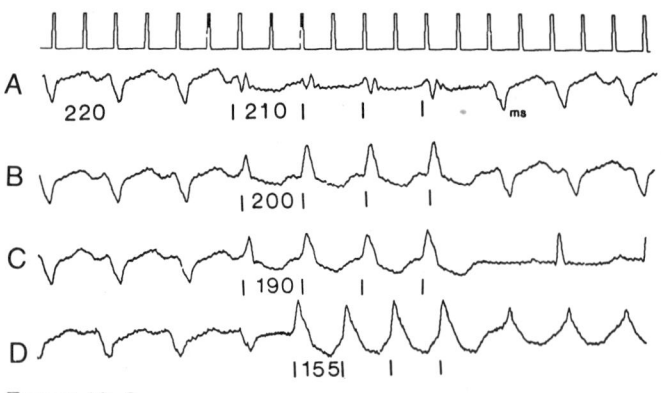

FIGURE 40-3
Effects of the cycle length of stimulation. Selected electrocardiographic recordings, from the same experiment shown in Figures 40-1 and 40-2, illustrate the effects of varying the cycle length of stimulation while the number of beats in the stimulated train was kept constant at 4.

A shows pacing at a cycle length 10 ms shorter than the tachycardia cycle, resulting in fusion complexes. The tachycardia resumed at the control cycle length on cessation of pacing. B, A similar effect occurred when the cycle length of pacing was 20 ms shorter than the tachycardia cycle. C, When the same train of stimulation was applied at a cycle length 30 ms shorter than the tachycardia cycle, it resulted in termination of the tachycardia. D, A much faster train resulted in tachycardia acceleration.

The numbers in the figure are in ms; the time lines represent 100 ms. (Reprinted by permission from El-Sherif N, Gough WB, Restivo M; PACE 10:341, 1987.)

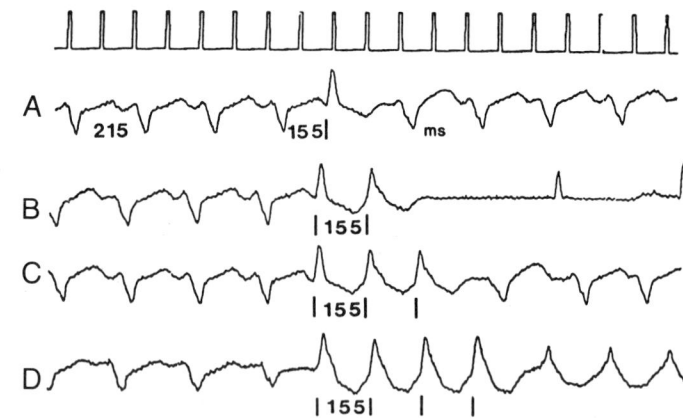

FIGURE 40-4
Effects of the number of stimulated beats. Selected electrocardiographic recordings, from the same experiment shown in Figures 40-1 through 40-3, illustrate the effects of the number of stimulated beats.

In A, during the reentrant tachycardia a single stimulated beat at a coupling interval of 155 ms resulted in resetting of the tachycardia by 20 ms. B shows that the tachycardia could be terminated by a train of two stimulated beats at a cycle length of 155 ms. In C, a train of three stimulated beats at the same cycle length again resulted in resetting of the tachycardia. On the other hand, in D, a train of four stimulated beats induced a new tachycardia (positive QRS in lead II) at a shorter cycle length (170–180 ms) compared with the original tachycardia cycle length (205–230 ms).

(Reprinted by permission from El-Sherif N, Gough WB, Restivo M: PACE 10:341, 1987.)

excitation will be terminated. Otherwise, conduction block in this area may only result in a narrowing of the zone of the slow common reentrant wavefront and/or a change of its configuration. The strategic zone for conduction block was found to be consistently located at the proximal part of the slow zone and never at its distal side.[6]

There are three variables that determine, singly or in combination, whether the stimulated wavefront can reach the strategic zone for conduction block and terminates reentry:

1. The degree of premature stimulation (i.e., the coupling interval of the first stimulated beat as well as the cycle length of a stimulated train) (Fig. 40-3).
2. The number of stimulated beats (Fig. 40-4).
3. The site of stimulation.

When a single premature stimulated wavefront fails to reach the strategic zone with the longest refractoriness early enough, a subsequent stimulated wavefront may succeed. Successive premature stimulated wavefronts can conduct, probably at a control speed or only slightly slower, in the normal zone and part of the ischemic zone but still arrive early enough at the

FIGURE 40-5
Resetting of reentrant tachycardia. Epicardial maps from the same experiment shown in Figures 40-1 through 40-4 illustrate resetting of the tachycardia by two stimulated beats at a cycle length 30 ms shorter than the tachycardia cycle.

The control map is labeled 1; the maps of the two stimulated beats are labeled 2 and 3, respectively. The first stimulated beat preexcited normal myocardium, and the stimulated wavefront arrived approximately 20 ms earlier at the proximal side of the zone of slow conduction. This resulted in relatively slower conduction in this zone. However, the stimulated wavefront could still traverse this zone to reexcite normal myocardium at the distal side of the zone of slow conduction. The second stimulated wavefront also arrived earlier to the proximal side of the zone of slow conduction. This resulted in extension of the arcs of functional conduction block into this zone, with narrowing of the slow common reentrant pathway. The stimulated wavefront also showed further slowing at the proximal side of the slow zone before it could successfully traverse the zone to reexcite normal myocardium and perpetuate the reentrant excitation, as shown in map 4.

The asterisks in the four maps represent the same epicardial site in the posterobasal portion of the left ventricle. If the reentrant tachycardia had continued unperturbed by the two stimulated beats at the original cycle length of 220 ms, this site would have been activated at the 760-ms isochrone rather than at the 740-ms isochrone as shown in map 4. Thus, the two premature stimulated beats resulted in advancing, or resetting, of the tachycardia cycle by 20 ms. The two stimulated wavefronts were each introduced at a cycle length 30 ms shorter than the intrinsic tachycardia cycle. However, the tachycardia was only reset by 20 ms. This was due to the fact that the stimulated wavefronts that arrived earlier to the proximal side of the slow zone showed relatively slow conduction in this zone compared to control. However, the degree of prematurity of the two stimulated beats still outweighed the further slowing of conduction and resulted in advancing the tachycardia cycle by 20 ms.

(Reprinted by permission from El-Sherif N, Gough WB, Restivo M: PACE 10:341, 1987.)

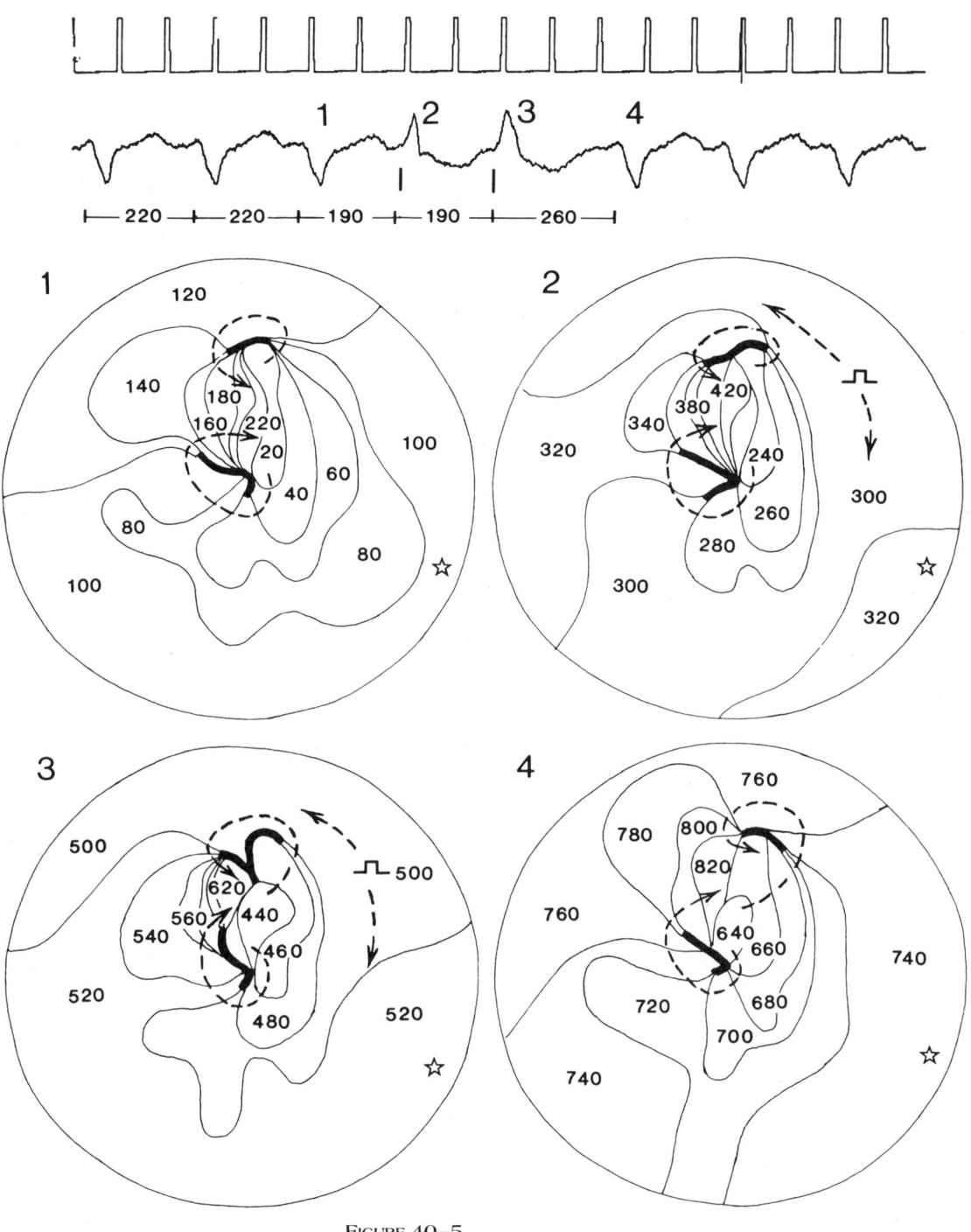

FIGURE 40–5
See legend on opposite page

Antitachycardia Pacing: Electrophysiologic Mechanisms 689

strategic zone with the longest refractoriness to result in conduction block.

MECHANISMS OF TACHYCARDIA RESETTING

Reentrant excitation can be advanced or reset by one or two premature stimuli (Fig. 40–5) or by a train of stimulated beats. A single premature stimulated beat can arrive earlier at the proximal side of the zone of the slow common reentrant wavefront, resulting in further slowing of conduction in this zone, but still succeeds in traversing the zone to perpetuate the reentrant process. If the degree of prematurity outweighs the further slowing of conduction in the slow zone the next reentrant cycle will be reset. On the other hand, there are two different mechanisms for resetting of reentrant tachycardia by a train of stimulated beats at a cycle length shorter than the tachycardia cycle length (i.e., overdrive stimulation): (1) tachycardia termination followed by reinitiation and (2) entrainment.

Tachycardia Termination Followed by Reinitiation

When a train of two or more stimulated beats are required to terminate reentry, the stimulated train must end following the beat that interrupts reentry. Otherwise, a subsequent stimulated beat may reinitiate the same reentrant circuit (one form of resetting) (Fig. 40–6) or induce a different, and possibly faster circuit (tachycardia acceleration; see further on). Similar observations have been previously reported during the initiation of reentrant excitation by burst pacing.[17]

Overdrive Entrainment and Termination of Tachycardia

Entrainment represents another mechanism for resetting of the tachycardia. During entrainment, the stimulated wavefront collides with the reentrant wavefront distal to the slow zone. The site of collision varies according to the site of stimulation in relation to the slow zone. The stimulated wavefront will also arrive earlier at the proximal part of the slow zone. This is consistently associated with a change in the conduction pattern in this zone (Fig. 40–7). A new balance of refractoriness and conduction velocity could develop in the different zones along the reentrant pathway, which would perpetuate the reentrant process at the shorter cycle length of the stimulated train. Following termination of the stimulated train, reentrant excitation continues and the first post-overdrive reentrant cycle is usually shorter than the control reentrant cycle. As shown in Figure 40–7, this is explained by improvement of conduction at the zone that was showing the slowest conduction during the stimulated train.

If a number of stimulated beats entrain the reentrant tachycardia, as described above, the same number of beats at a critically shorter cycle length could terminate the tachycardia. This will occur if a new balance of refractoriness and conduction velocity in the different parts of the reentrant pathway could not be established. In this case, the stimulated wavefront could arrive early enough at the strategic zone with the longest refractoriness, resulting in conduction block and termination of reentry (Fig. 40–8).

The term *entrainment* denotes any stable condition with definable periodicity resulting from the interaction of two rhythms. The term has been usually utilized to denote interaction between automatic pacemakers.[18, 19] However, some authors have used the term to describe the increase in the rate of a reentrant tachycardia with rapid pacing, with resumption of the control rate on cessation of pacing.[20, 21] When overdrive stimulation succeeds in perpetuating the reentrant process, some modification of the activation pattern of the common reentrant pathway always takes place. In other words, there is a change in the reentrant pathway. The modifications in the common reentrant pathway will not be detected in the absence of detailed mapping which is not available in clinical studies of entrainment. The use of the term entrainment in this situation raises at least two questions: First, could the term be applied if there is a subtle but definite change in part of the reentrant circuit? (Compare the control reentrant circuit and the entrained circuit in Fig. 40–7). Second, assuming a reentrant circuit with a tight fit of activation and refractoriness and possibly no gap of excitability in the regions with the longest refractoriness, could this circuit be entrained at a shorter cycle length without causing conduction block in these regions with redirecting, and thus changing, the reentrant pathway?

MECHANISMS OF TACHYCARDIA ACCELERATION AND PRECIPITATION OF VENTRICULAR FIBRILLATION BY ELECTRICAL STIMULATION

Tachycardia acceleration and precipitation of ventricular fibrillation is considered a major limiting factor of stimulated termination of reentrant tachycardia.[3, 22–25] Our recent studies have shown that tachycardia acceleration by overdrive stimulation is always due to interruption of the original reentrant circuit by the first one or few stimulated beats followed by initiation of a different circuit by subsequent stimulated beats.[6] If the new circuit has a shorter revolution time, tachycardia acceleration is said to have been induced. The new circuit may last for one or more cycles before it spontaneously terminates, or it may become sustained. The induction of a new reentrant circuit that fails to be sustained for more than one or a few cycles is not uncommonly observed following overdrive stimulation.[6] In a study that correlated activation and refractory maps, we have shown that an induced reentrant circuit can terminate after one cycle and block if the circulating wavefront, entering the slow zone, encounters a gradient of refractoriness that provides a sufficient barrier to cause conduction block.[13] This was usually caused by non-uniform shortening of refractory periods in the pathway of the circulating wave front.

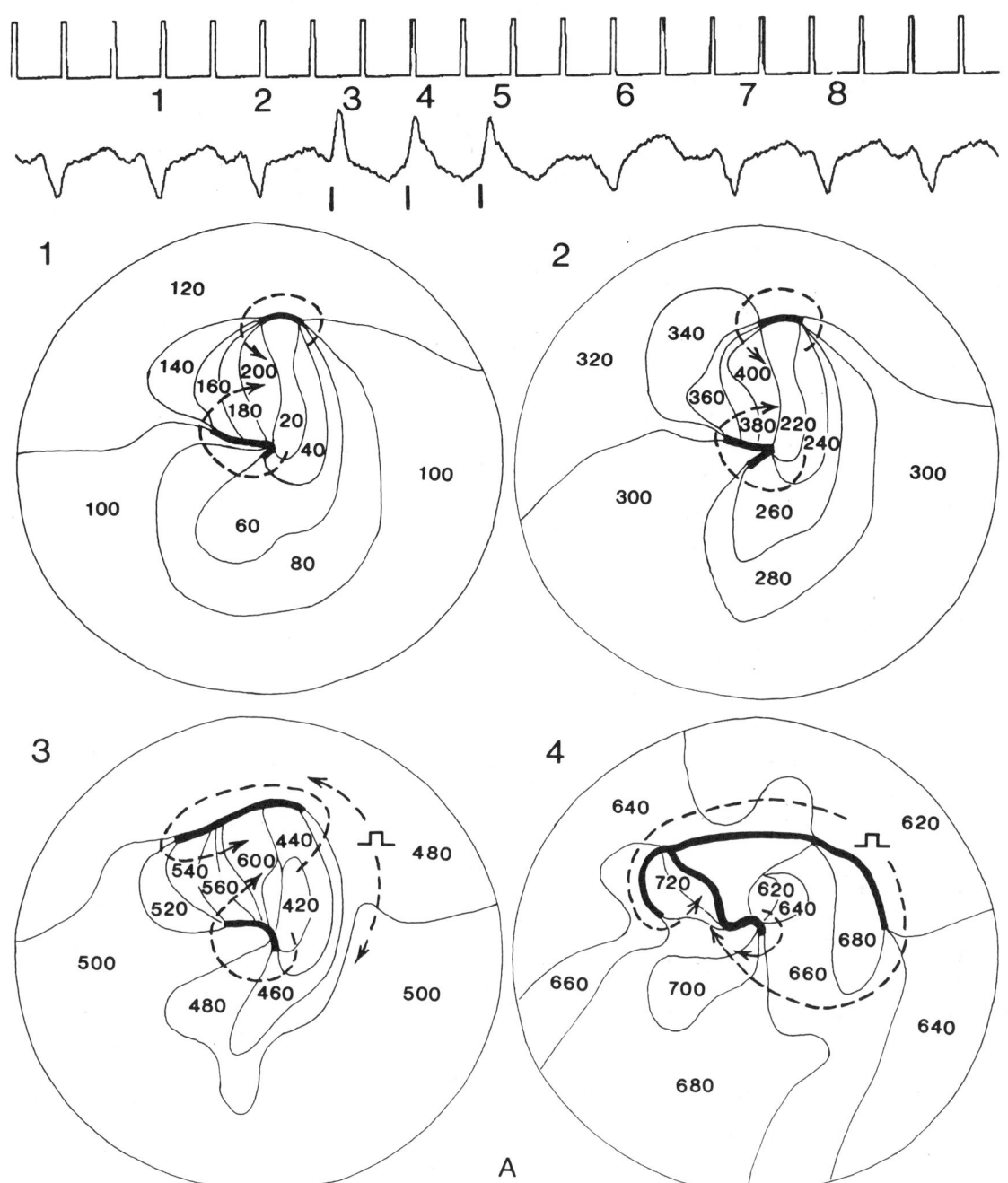

FIGURE 40–6
Tachycardia termination followed by reinitiation. Recordings were obtained from the same experiment shown in Figures 40–1 through 40–5. The figure shows that a train of three stimulated beats at a cycle length of 155 ms failed to terminate the tachycardia but resulted in resetting of the tachycardia cycle. The epicardial activation maps illustrate that the tachycardia was actually terminated by the second stimulated beat as in Figure 40–2 but was reinitiated by the third stimulated beat.

A, Control maps are labeled 1 and 2. As shown in Figure 40–2, the first stimulated beat (map 3) preexcited normal myocardium, which resulted in extension of the basal arc of conduction block and in slower conduction of the common reentrant wavefront. The second stimulated beat (map 4) resulted in marked extension of the basal arc of block into lateral and septal directions. The two circulating wavefronts coalesced with the lingering wavefront of the first stimulated beat. On the other hand, the last isochrone of the second stimulated beat at 740 ms arrived much earlier to the proximal side of the zone of slow conduction, resulting in conduction block and termination of reentry. The site of conduction block in the proximal part of the slow zone of reentry was slightly different from that shown in Figure 40–2.

Illustration continued on following page

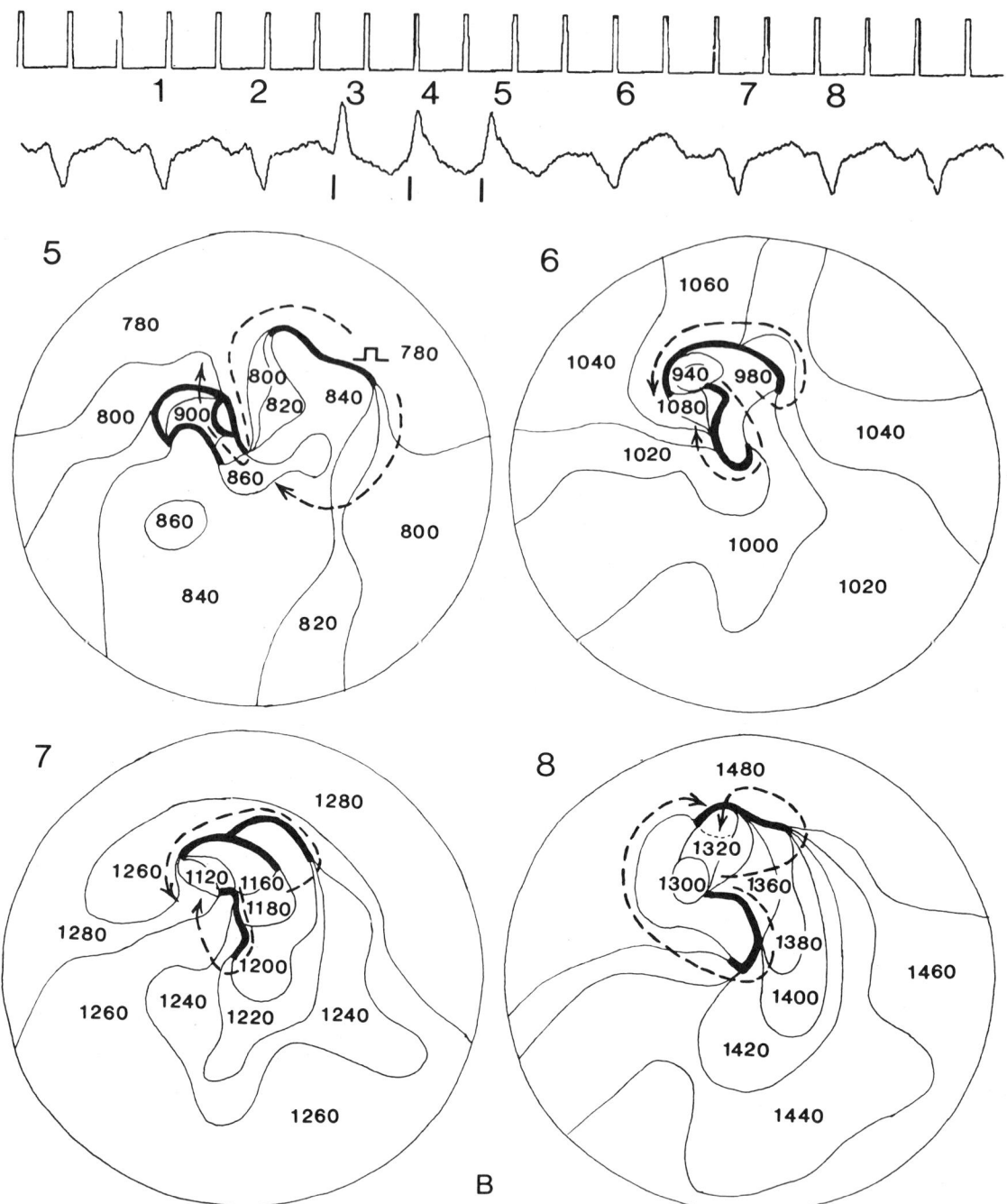

FIGURE 40–6
Continued B, Following termination of reentry at the 740-ms isochrone, the third stimulated beat (map 5) activated normal myocardium at the 780-ms isochrone. The new activation wavefront reinitiated reentrant excitation in the ischemic zone. With the exception of the first beat, the QRS configuration of the tachycardia following the stimulated train was similar to control, reflecting a similar pattern of activation of the normal zone. However, the activation pattern in the ischemic zone and the configuration of the arcs of functional conduction block differed from control for the first few beats following stimulation (see maps 6 and 7). Only the activation pattern in map 8 started to resemble the control reentrant circuit. Following the stimulated train, reentrant excitation was advanced (reset) by 100 ms.
(Reprinted by permission from El-Sherif N, Gough WB, Restivo M: PACE 10:341, 1987.)

Analysis of the ischemic zone activation pattern during the fast reentrant circuit induced by overdrive pacing in Figure 40–9 illustrates why fast reentrant excitation can rapidly degenerate into ventricular fibrillation. During a fast reentrant excitation pattern, several parts of the ischemic zone may fail to activate in a 1:1 fashion. This can result in the fractionation of a regular figure-eight reentrant pattern into multiple asynchronous wavefronts circulating around changing functional arcs of conduction block. A pattern akin to ventricular fibrillation may be confined briefly to the ischemic zone before the involvement of the normal zone.[11] However, as shown in Figure 40–9, a similar complex activation pattern may remain confined to the ischemic zone during a fast regular reentrant circuit without degenerating into ventricular fibrillation.

Figure 40–10 is a diagrammatic illustration of the various effects of overdrive stimulation on reentrant tachycardia. Overdrive stimulation can result in entrainment, termination, or acceleration of reentrant tachycardia, depending on the length of the drive and the cycle length of stimulation.

ROLE OF SITE OF STIMULATION

Reentry could be terminated by fewer stimulated beats when stimulation is applied to the normal zone closer to the proximal side of the slow zone (Figure 40–11B) than to its distal side (Figure 40–11A). When stimulation is applied closer to the distal side of the slow zone, the prematurely stimulated wavefront frequently induces extension of the functional arcs of conduction block, resulting in lengthening of the reentrant pathway. In this case, one or more stimulated beats may fail to reach the strategic zone with the longest refractoriness early enough to result in conduction block. There is thus a better chance for entrainment of the reentrant tachycardia from sites closer to the distal side of the slow zone. On the other hand, the most optimal site for stimulated termination of reentrant tachycardia is the ischemic zone close to the proximal side of the slow zone (Figs. 40–11C and 40–12). At this site, a critically coupled stimulus could capture locally and conduct prematurely to the proximal side of the slow zone resulting in conduction block and termination of reentry. The site of stimulation in the ischemic zone does not have to be very close to the proximal side of the slow zone. However, it has to be able to conduct slightly prematurely to the strategic zone with the longest refractory period. The stimulus does not have to capture the normal zone, and therefore the QRS configuration of the last reentrant beat will not change. The altered activation pattern in the ischemic zone has a negligible effect on the surface QRS configuration.

In the figure-eight reentrant circuit, one or more sites could usually be identified in the ischemic zone where a premature stimulus could terminate the reentrant tachycardia by capturing locally and conducting prematurely to the proximal side of the common reentrant wavefront.[6] On the other hand, only a few clinical examples of ventricular tachycardia have been reported in which the arrhythmia could be terminated by a single stimulus that did not seem to capture the ventricles.[26-28] This underscores the fact that the site for stimulated termination is less than optimal in the overwhelming majority of clinical cases.

PREVENTION OF INITIATION OF REENTRANT TACHYCARDIA BY ELECTRICAL STIMULATION

Prevention of the initiation of reentrant tachyarrhythmias by appropriate electrical stimulation is a more appealing concept than current antitachycardia stimulation techniques.[25] One possible method has been reported.[29, 30] The authors showed that a subthreshold preconditioning stimulus can inhibit capture of a subsequent premature stimulus. As a result, there is an increase in the effective refractory period of the preconditioned tissue. We have recently shown that appropriate stimulation at two selected sites during the basic rhythm (i.e., dual S_1 stimulation) can modify the spatial distribution of recovery of excitability in a way that prevents the initiation of reentrant excitation in response to premature stimulation (S_2).[31] In all instances which resulted in the prevention of reentry, the secondary site was distal to the arc of block that formed following the control S_2 stimulation. The secondary site should be in an area of long refractoriness that activates late during the basic beat. Properly applied dual stimulation differentially peels back recovery time (defined as S_1 conduction time + effective refractory period) in the ischemic zone. Successful dual stimulation depends on the reduction of two factors: (1) The spatial gradient of recovery time and (2) the dispersion of recovery time across the arc. The former determines the extent and location of the continuous arc of conduction block. The latter determines when areas distal to block are recovered during the premature stimulation. Reducing the difference in activation time across the arc of block to a value less than the effective refractory period of the premature stimulus (ERP_2) proximal to the arc is the mechanism by which dual S_1 stimulation can prevent the initiation of reentry.

If dual simultaneous stimulation fails to prevent the initiation of reentry, preexcitation of the ischemic zone may succeed. Asynchronous dual stimulation was successful at a greater number of sites (34% vs. 9%) than was simultaneous dual stimulation.[31] In the same fashion that dual simultaneous stimulation peels back refractoriness in the ischemic zone, asynchronous excitation of the ischemic zone further peels back refractoriness and can significantly reduce the dispersion of recovery time. Asynchronous stimulation has been used for the treatment of supraventricular reentrant tachyarrhythmias in humans.[32] Permanent atrioventricular sequential pacemakers have been successful in treating atrioventricular nodal reentrant tachycardias and those involving accessory pathways. The proposed

Text continued on page 700

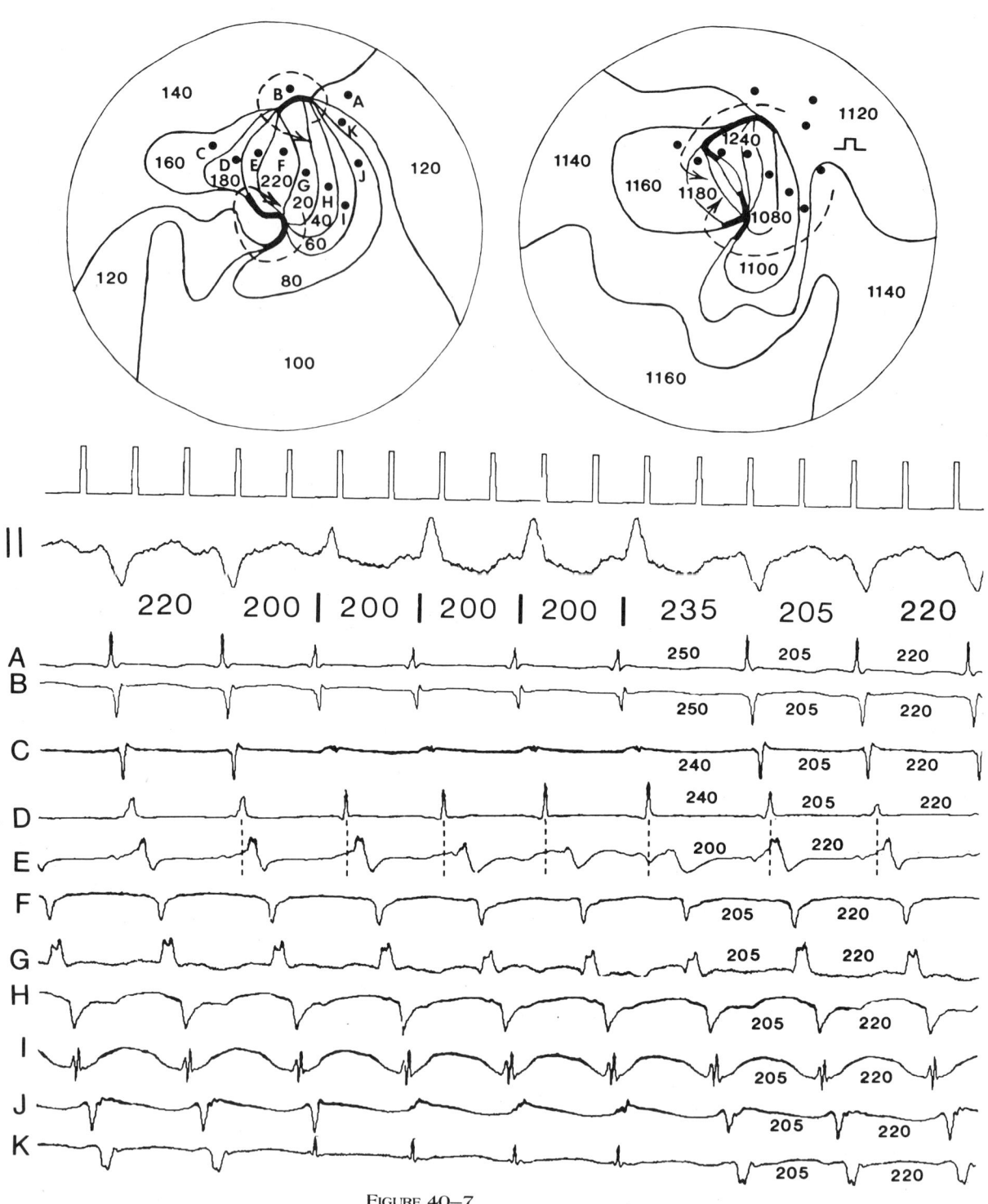

FIGURE 40–7
See legend on opposite page

694 Antitachycardia Pacing: Electrophysiologic Mechanisms

FIGURE 40–7
Entrainment of reentrant tachycardia by a run of four stimulated beats (marked by vertical bars in the lead II electrocardiogram). The cycle length of stimulation was 20 ms shorter than the tachycardia cycle. Recordings were obtained from the same experiment shown in Figures 40–1 through 40–6. The control reentrant circuit map is shown at top left; the map of the last stimulated beat is shown at top right. The electrograms labeled A–K represent each of the 11 20-ms isochrones in the control reentrant circuit and their sites on the maps are marked by solid circles.

During the four-beat stimulated train, electrograms A–D, J, and K, which represented activation of the normal and border zones, had changed their configuration, denoting that these sites were activated by the stimulated wavefronts. On the other hand, electrograms F–I, which represented conduction in the middle and distal parts of the slow zone, did not change their configuration, denoting that the pathway of the activation wavefronts in these zones was similar to the control reentrant wavefront. The collision of the stimulated and reentrant wavefronts probably occurred between sites I and J.

Electrograms D and E were recorded from the proximal part of the slow zone and represented the sites where most of the conduction delay during the stimulated run took place (highlighted by the vertical dashed lines). The degree of conduction delay between these two sites gradually increased during the first three stimulated beats but remained constant during the third and fourth stimulated wavefronts. On cessation of the stimulated train, conduction between sites D and E improved to a degree better than control for the first post-overdrive reentrant cycle before returning to control values during the second post-overdrive cycle. The changes in the conduction pattern in the proximal part of the slow zone both during and following overdrive stimulation resulted in characteristic changes in the cycle length of the first two post-overdrive reentrant cycles.

At sites distal to the zone of marked conduction delay (electrograms E–I), the first post-overdrive cycle was shorter than control at 200 to 205 ms. On the other hand, at sites proximal to this zone (A–D and K) as well as in the surface electrocardiogram, the cycle was longer than control at 235 to 350 ms. At these sites, however, the second post-overdrive reentrant cycle was shorter at 205 ms. Analysis of the surface electrocardiogram also reveals that the four-beat overdrive train advanced (reset) the reentrant tachycardia by approximately 65 ms (measured from the pre-overdrive to the first post-overdrive QRS complexes) or by 80 ms (measured from the pre-overdrive to the second post-overdrive QRS complex).

(Reprinted by permission from El-Sherif N, Gough WB, Restivo M: PACE 10:341, 1987.)

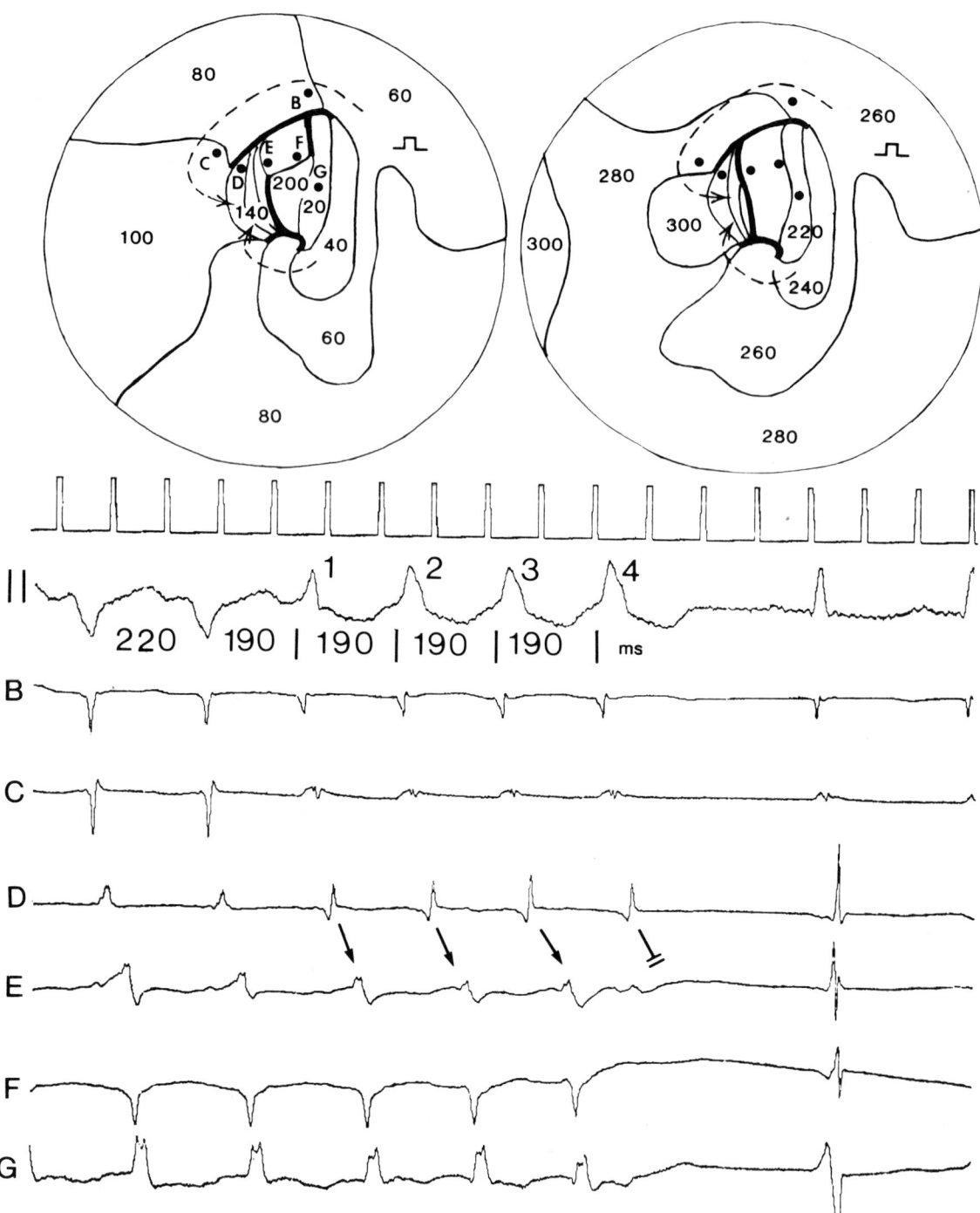

FIGURE 40–8
Overdrive termination of reentrant tachycardia. The figure illustrates the mechanism of overdrive termination of reentrant tachycardia by a train of four stimulated beats at a cycle length of 190 ms (30 ms shorter than the tachycardia cycle length). Recordings were obtained from the same experiment shown in Figures 40–1 through 40–7. Maps of the third and fourth stimulated beats are labeled 3 and 4, respectively. Selected electrograms along the activation wavefront are labeled B–G.

As was shown during the entraining train in Figure 40–7, the major conduction delay of the stimulated wavefronts occurred between sites D and E. However, in contrast to the entraining train when conduction delay between the two sites remained constant after the second stimulated beat, here the conduction delay gradually increased during successive stimulated beats until conduction block between the two sites developed following the fourth stimulated beat. This resulted in extension of the arc of functional conduction block across the proximal part of the slow zone and in termination of reentrant excitation. Note the electrotonic deflection in electrogram E during conduction block.

(Reprinted by permission from El-Sherif N, Gough WB, Restivo M: PACE 10:341, 1987.)

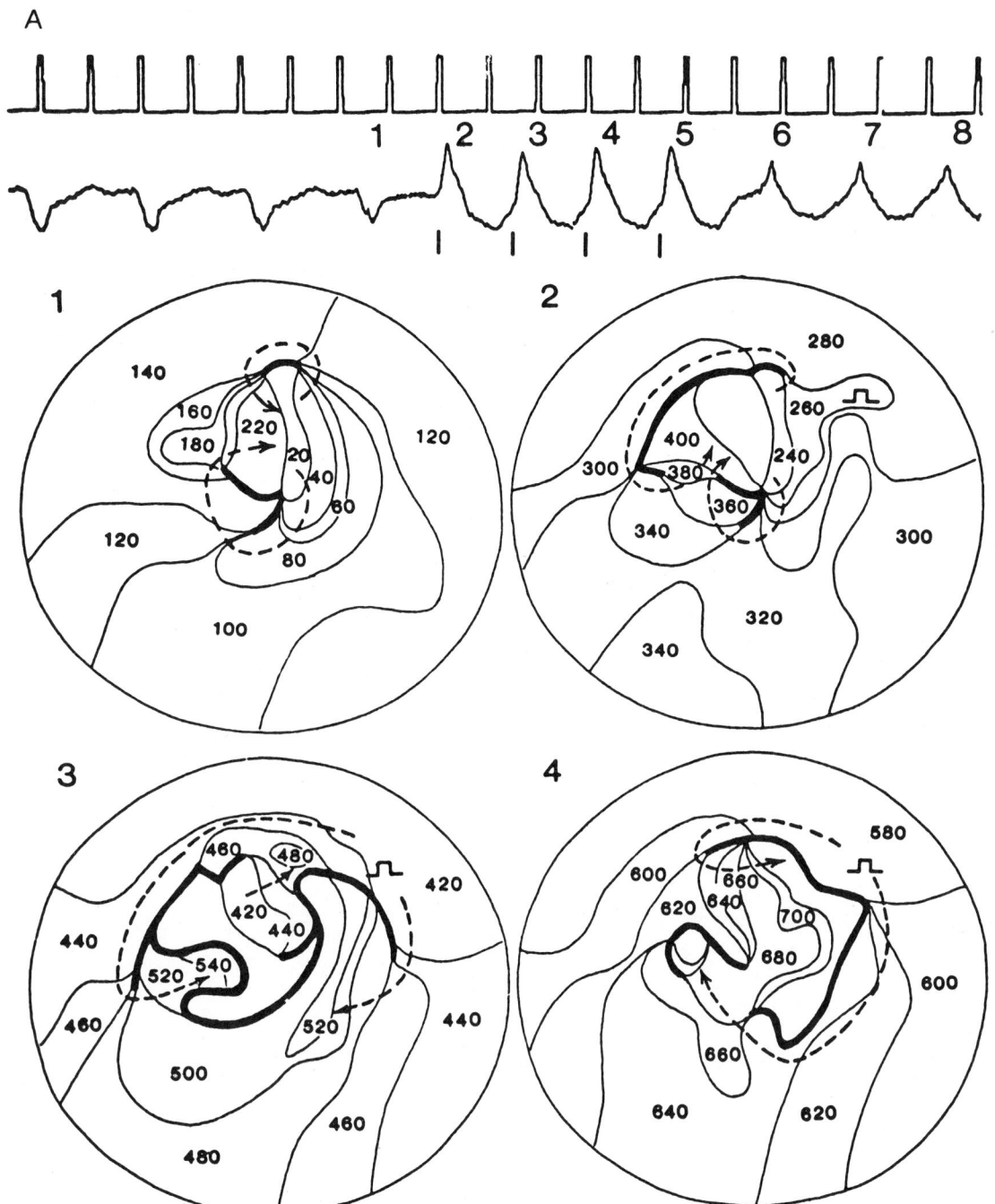

FIGURE 40–9
Tachycardia acceleration. The recordings obtained from the same experiment shown in Figures 40–1 through 40–8 illustrate acceleration of reentrant tachycardia by a train of four stimulated beats at a short cycle length of 155 ms.

A, Control map is labeled 1. As shown in Figures 40–2 and 40–5, the first two stimulated beats (maps 2 and 3) resulted in termination of the original reentrant tachycardia. The last isochrone of the second stimulated beat arrived relatively early at the proximal side of the common reentrant wavefront, resulting in conduction block and termination of reentry. The activation pattern in the ischemic zone of the second stimulated beat and the exact site of conduction block were different in Figures 40–2, 40–5, and 40–9. However, in all instances, reentry terminated due to conduction block in the proximal portion of the zone of slow conduction, and never at its distal side. Following termination of the original reentrant circuit, the third and fourth stimulated beats (maps 4 and 5) initiated a different reentrant circuit. The new circuit was located close to the lateral border of the ischemic zone at the 2 o'clock position on the polar map. The circuit had a shorter pathway and a faster circulation time (170–180 ms). The new reentrant wavefront circulated in an opposite direction to the original reentrant wavefront, resulting in positive QRS configuration in surface lead II.

Illustration continued on following page

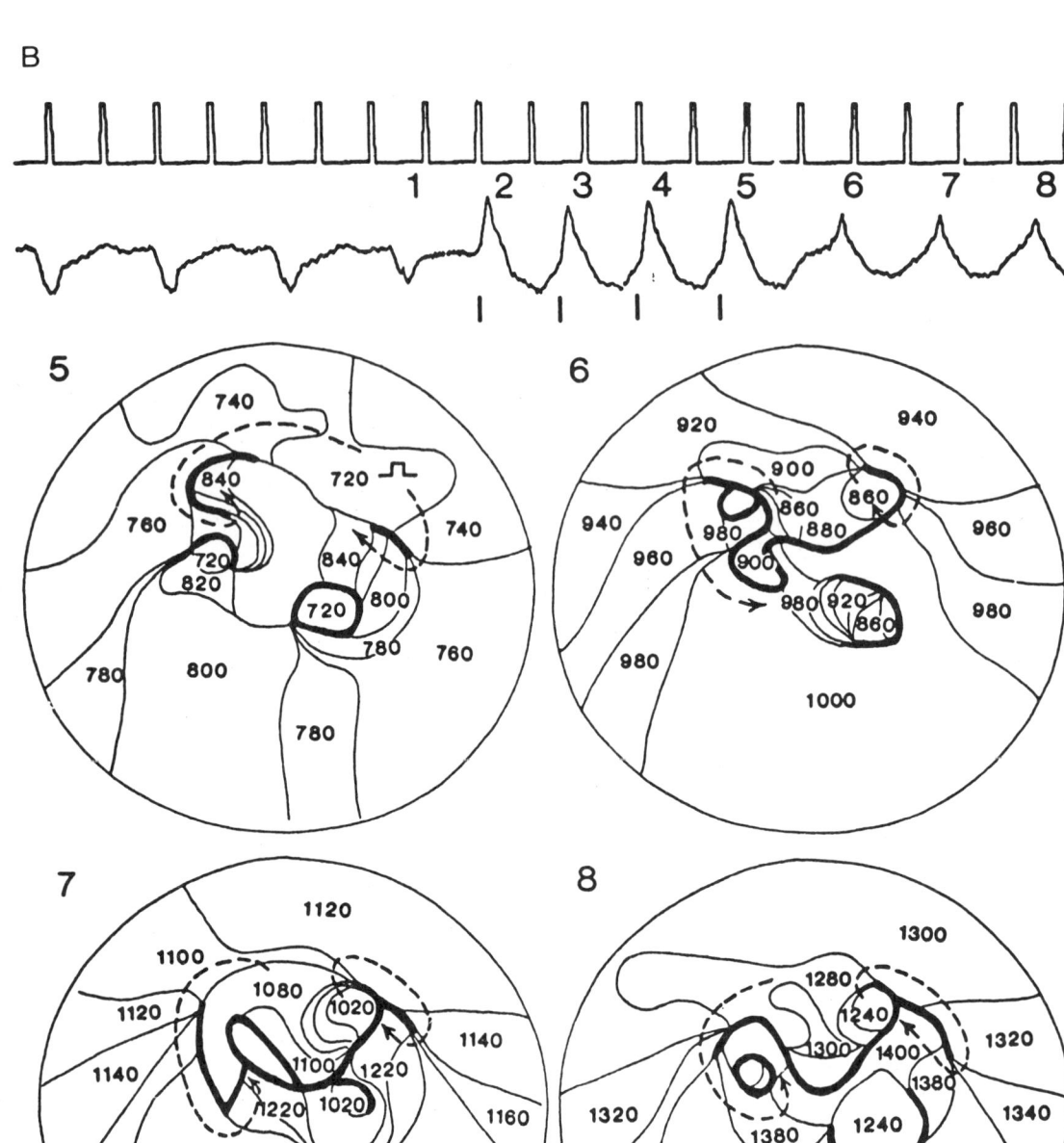

FIGURE 40–9
Continued B, Because of the faster circulation time of the new reentrant circuit, several parts of the ischemic zone failed to activate in a 1:1 fashion. Instead, a Wenckebach-type conduction and/or a 2:1 block developed, resulting in a complex activation pattern for the rest of the ischemic zone that varied from beat to beat (see maps 6–8). Because of this complex activation pattern, the classic figure-eight reentrant pattern could not be established. In spite of the complex activation pattern in the ischemic zone, the reentrant pathway remained stable, and ventricular fibrillation did not develop.

In other experiments, however, a train of stimulated beats could induce a different, faster reentrant excitation that could rapidly degenerate into ventricular fibrillation because of fractionation of activation in the ischemic zone into multiple asynchronous reentrant circuits.

(Reprinted by permission from El-Sherif N, Gough WB, Restivo M: PACE 10:341, 1987.)

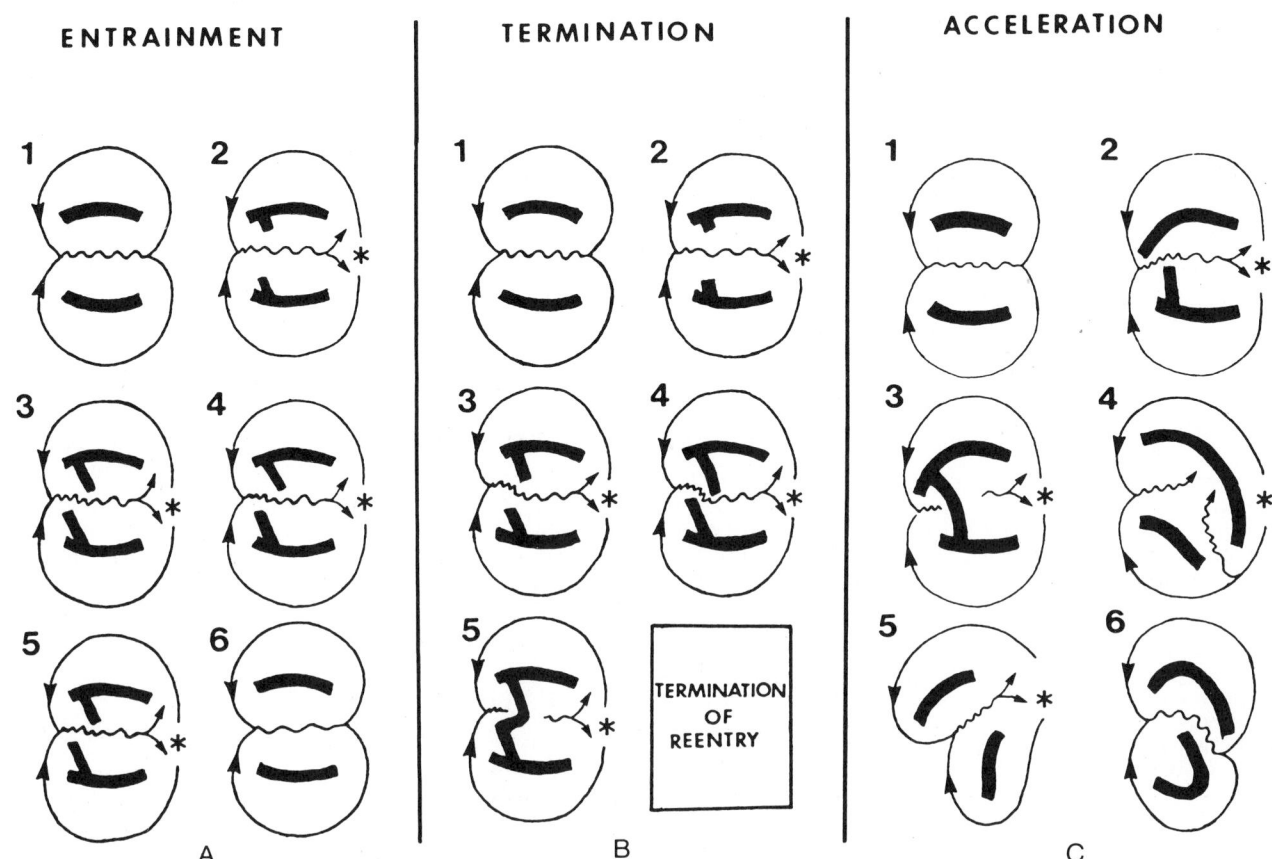

FIGURE 40–10
Diagrammatic illustration of the mechanisms of entrainment, termination, and acceleration of reentrant tachycardia by overdrive stimulation.

In each panel (A–C), the control reentrant circuit is labeled 1 and the four beats of the stimulated train are labeled 2–5. The control circuit has a figure-eight configuration, and conduction in the slow zone of reentry proceeds from left to right. The heavy solid lines represent arcs of functional conduction block. Stimulation is applied at the distal side of the slow zone (asterisks).

A, During entrainment, the stimulated wavefront collides with the emerging slow reentrant wavefront. It then circulates and arrives earlier to the proximal part of the slow zone of reentry. This is consistently associated with a change in the slow zone with the development of new functional arcs of block and much slower conduction in parts of this zone. However, a new equilibrium quickly develops in which successive stimulated beats, represented by cycles 3, 4, and 5, maintain the same new conduction pattern at the shortest cycle length of stimulation, thus entraining the tachycardia. On cessation of stimulation, reentry will resume, as shown in cycle 6.

B, For termination reentry, on the other hand, successive stimulated beats, now applied at a shorter cycle compared with A, will result in gradually more conduction delay. Eventually, conduction block develops at the proximal part of the slow zone of reentry, as shown in cycle 5.

In C, the same four-beat stimulated train is applied at a still shorter cycle length. In this case, and because of the short cycle length of stimulation, the second stimulated beat, represented by cycle 3, has already blocked in the proximal part of the slow zone of reentry. If stimulation is stopped at this point, the reentrant tachycardia will terminate. However, if stimulation is continued, the third and fourth stimulated beats, represented by cycles 4 and 5, will initiate new arcs of block and different reentrant pathways, so that on termination of the stimulated train, a new and possibly faster reentrant circuit will occur.

(Reprinted by permission from El-Sherif N, Gough WB, Restivo M: PACE 10:341, 1987.)

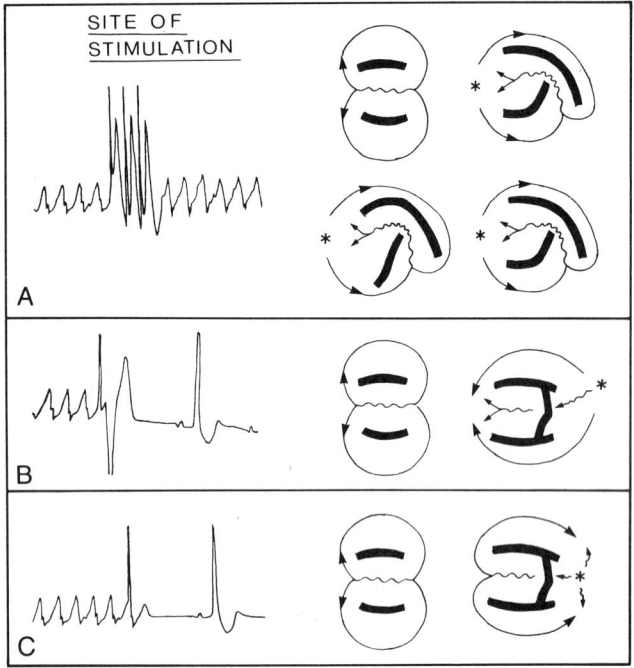

FIGURE 40-11
Diagrammatic illustration of the role of the site of stimulation in relation to the slow zone of reentry on termination of reentrant tachycardia by programmed stimulation. The control reentrant circuit shows conduction in the slow zone moving in the right to left direction.

A, Three stimulated beats applied at a site distal to slow zone of reentry (asterisk), failed to terminate reentry. The stimulated wavefront collided with the reentrant wavefront as it emerged from the slow zone. It then circulated around much longer functional arcs of block, compared with control. This resulted in lengthening of the stimulated wavefront pathway. Thus, even though the stimulated wavefront still arrived earlier at the proximal part of the slow zone, it failed to arrive early enough to result in conduction block and to terminate reentry. In other words, the stimulated run resulted in entrainment of the tachycardia.

In B and C, on the other hand, reentry terminated when stimulation was applied at sites proximal to the slow zone of reentry. In B, stimulation was applied to the border of the ischemic zone at some distance from the proximal part of the slow zone. The stimulated wavefront arrived early enough at this site, resulting in conduction block and termination of reentry. The stimulated wavefront also activated most of the ventricles and collided with the emerging wavefront of the last reentrant cycle at the distal side of the slow zone. In C, stimulation was applied in the ischemic zone much closer to the proximal part of the slow zone. The stimulated wavefront arrived prematurely at the slow zone, resulting in conduction block, but failed to conduct outside the ischemic zone. In this case, the ventricles were activated by the last reentrant cycle. The electrocardiogram could be misinterpreted as showing that the stimulus artifact failed to capture and that the reentrant tachycardia terminated spontaneously; in fact, however, the stimulus artifact did capture locally, resulting in concealed conduction.

(Reprinted by permission from El-Sherif N, Gough WB,

mechanism of the technique is that preexcitation of a limb of the circuit will render it refractory to the returning impulse. In reentry of this type, the critical zone may be situated such that preexcitation ensures that recovery time in the entire zone is sufficiently reduced. Conduction block still occurs, but without the presence of alternate reentrant exits. Success in these cases is possible with less attention having to be given to location of the stimulating sites. This differs from the model of reentrant activation in the canine postinfarction heart. In the figure-eight model, suppression of one reentrant pathway does not preclude the appearance of an alternate pathway.[6] Preexcitation has been used in a similar fashion either to reduce or to abolish the window of premature coupling that induced ventricular macroreentry.[33] Increasing the degree of atrioventricular delay forces preexcitation of the critical zone for reentry. After premature ventricular stimulation, the window of reentry is reduced due to enhanced conduction in the His-Purkinje system.

In the same way that dual S_1 stimulation reduced the spatial dispersion of recovery, dual stimulation during a sensed premature beat may also prove to be helpful in preventing reentry. It is possible to envision a strategically positioned electrode that senses a spontaneous premature beat, which may initiate a reentrant tachyarrhythmia, and soon thereafter stimulate the underlying myocardial zone. Thus, dual premature stimulation can possibly prevent the perpetuation of reentry and have an even wider application than dual S_1 pacing.

Conclusion

The relevance of studies of electrophysiologic mechanisms of programmed electrical stimulation in an experimental model of reentrant ventricular tachycardia depends on whether the figure-eight model is representative of reentry in the human ventricle. However, the experimental data provide several guidelines:

1. The role of the site of stimulation cannot be overemphasized. Innovative techniques for more precise localization of the reentrant circuit, particularly the slow zone of reentry and the direction of the activation front in this zone, should be searched out.
2. Protocols for pacing termination of reentrant tachycardias should utilize a stepwise increase of the number of paced beats, a stepwise decrease of the cycle length of stimulation, or a combination of both (see Fig. 40-16). The last is best exemplified by the technique of autodecremental pacing.[34-36] In this technique, the coupling interval of the first stimulated beat is only slightly shorter than the tachycardia cycle, and both a stepwise decrement of consecutive cycle lengths and a stepwise increase of the number of stimulated beats are introduced as required.
3. Electrical stimulation techniques for prevention of the initiation of reentrant tachyarrhythmias are feasible and should be explored more actively in the clinical setting.

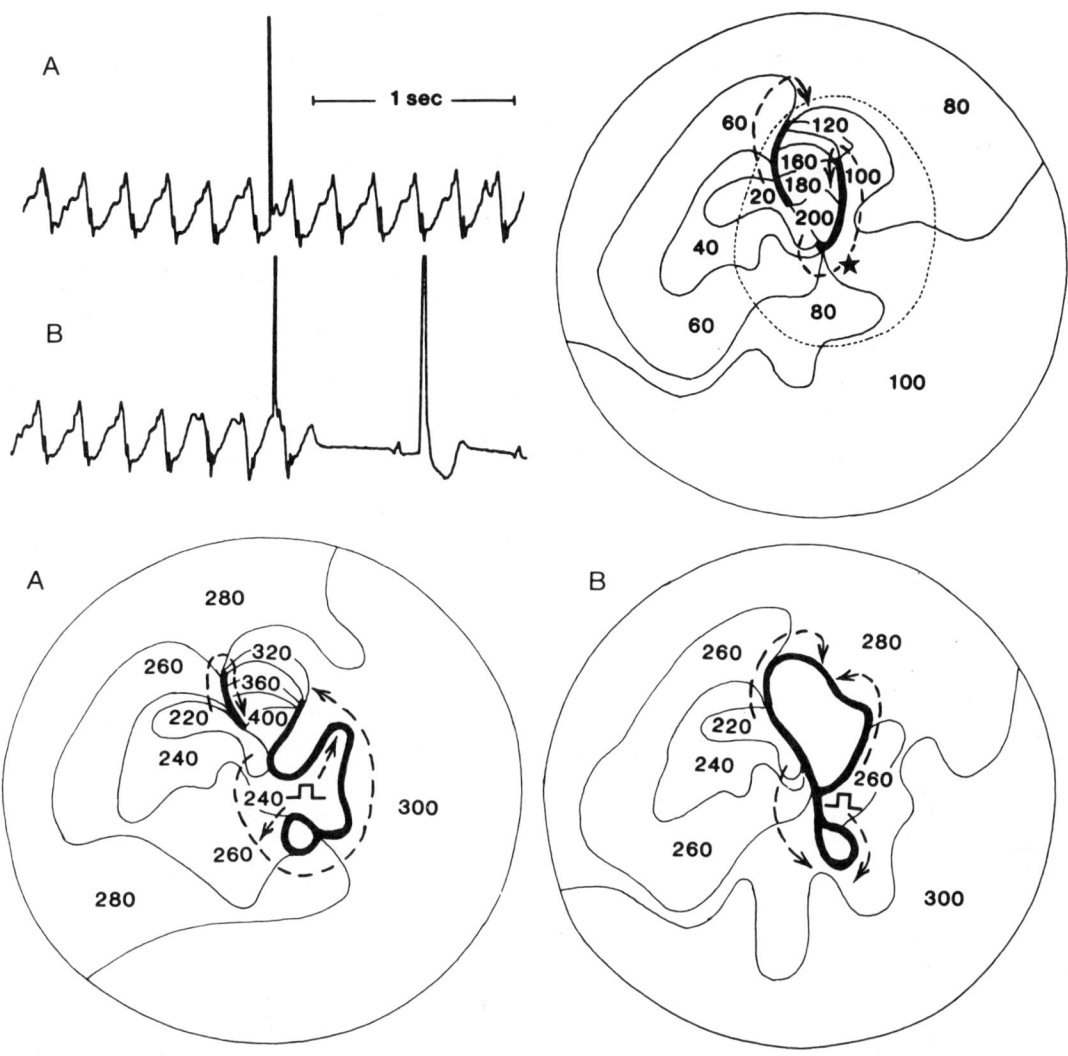

Restivo M: PACE 10:341, 1987.)
FIGURE 40–12
Termination of reentrant tachycardia by a single stimulus (asterisk) applied to the ischemic zone (outlined by dotted line). Control map is shown at top right. In this experiment, a trial was made to stimulate from different sites in the ischemic zone. A stimulus, applied to the site indicated by the asterisk on the control map, failed to capture less than 160 ms following activation of this site.

In A (see electrocardiogram and map), a stimulus applied 160 to 170 ms following activation of the site captured locally but failed to conduct to the rest of the ischemic zone.

In B (see electrocardiogram and map), on the other hand, a stimulus applied 175 ms following activation of the site not only captured locally but also conducted in the ischemic zone and prematurely excited myocardial zones at the proximal side of the slow zone, resulting in conduction block and termination of reentry. The tachycardia terminated with the reentrant QRS that immediately followed the pacing stimulus. This is explained by the fact that the pacing stimulus did not capture the normal zone and therefore did not change the overall ventricular activation pattern and the QRS configuration.

(Reprinted by permission from El-Sherif N, Gough WB, Restivo M: PACE 10:341, 1987.)

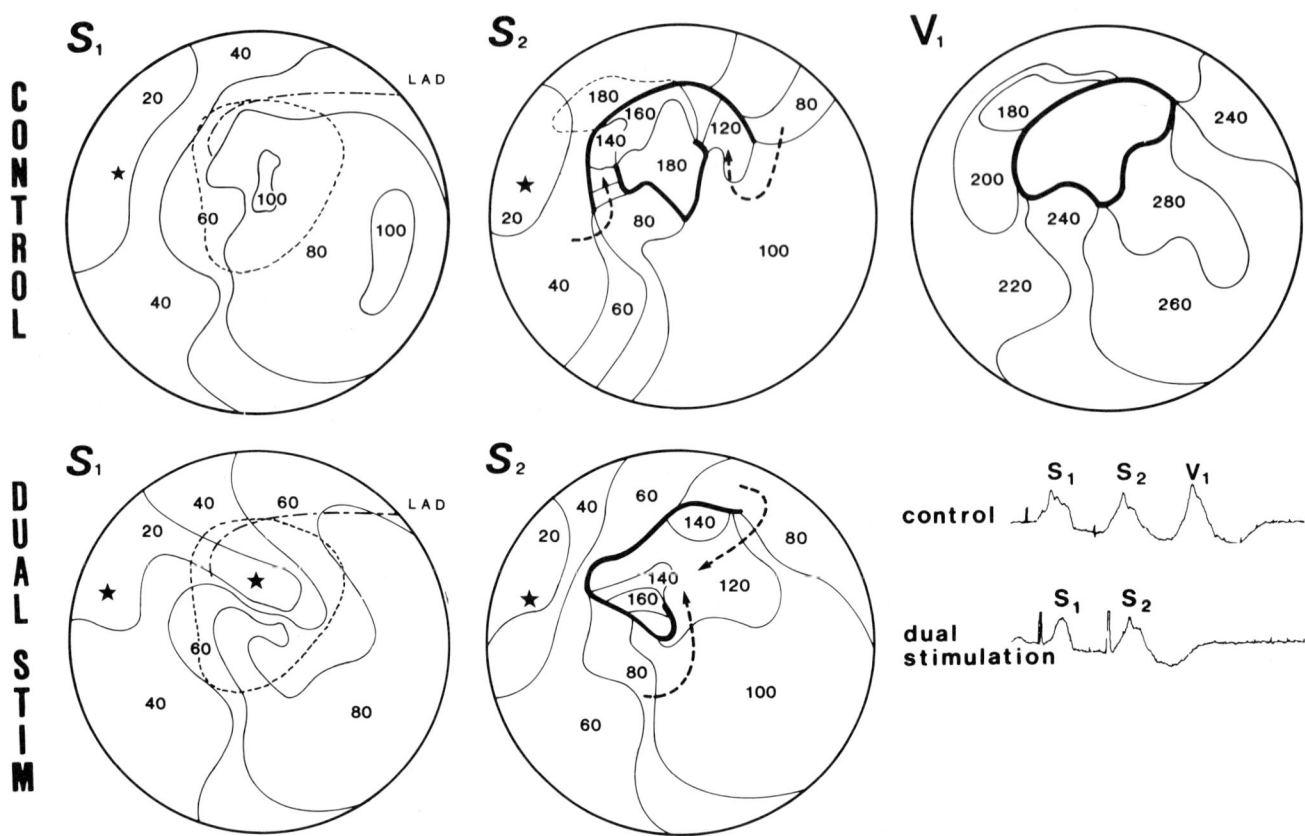

FIGURE 40–13
Prevention of initiation of reentrant excitation by dual S_1 stimulation.

During control, following an S_1 drive at 380 ms, a premature stimulus, S_2 delivered from the same site (asterisk), gave rise to an unstimulated beat, V_1. The premature coupling interval was 180 ms. Within 40 ms the S_2 activation wavefront encountered an arc of functional unidirectional conduction block. Two circulating wavefronts traveled clockwise and counterclockwise around the arc of conduction block, joined distal to the arc and conducted slowly through the ischemic region. The common reentrant wavefront reexcited a region on the proximal border of the arc 180 ms later. The difference in conduction time across the arc, in the region of reactivation, was 120 ms.

In the dual-stimulation mode, a second site was selected and paced simultaneously with the control site during the basic driven beats (both sites are marked by asterisks in the S_1 map below). The secondary site was located distal to the arc of block shown on the control S_2 map. After dual stimulation, the length of the arc of block was reduced, and the position of the arc, opposite the control stimulation site, receded toward the core of the infarct. Although the entire epicardial surface was again activated in 180 ms, the maximum difference in activation time across the arc of block was reduced to only 80 ms. The difference in activation time across the arc at the site of reactivation during control was reduced to less than 60 ms. Therefore, reactivation was impossible at any site proximal to the arc of conduction block.

LAD = left anterior descending artery. (Reprinted by permission of the American Heart Association, Inc., from Restivo M, Gough WB, El-Sherif N: Circulation 77:429, 1988.)

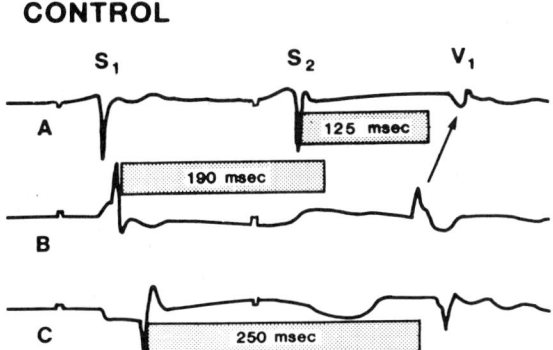
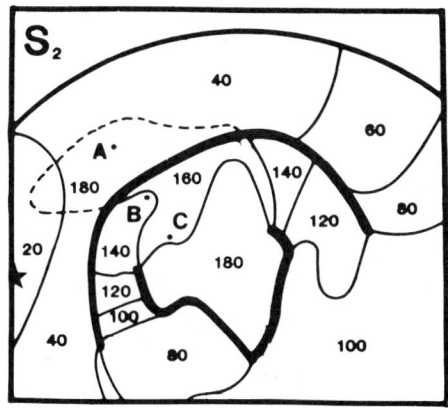
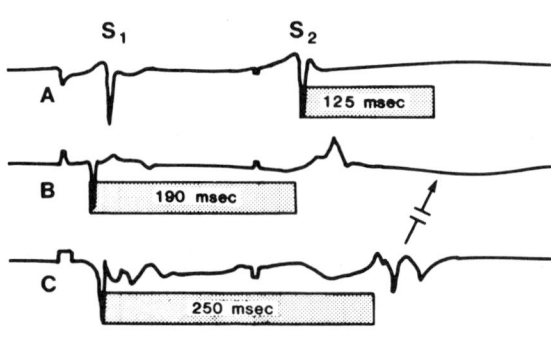
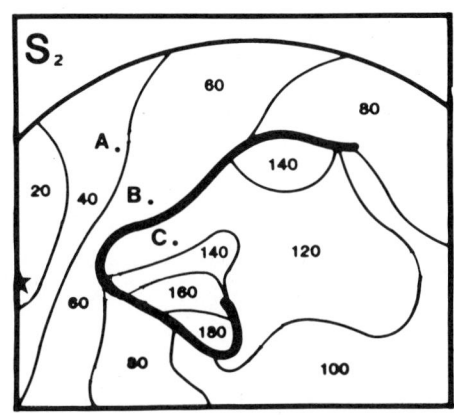

FIGURE 40–14

Recordings obtained from the same experiment shown in Figure 40–13. Electrograms from sites that traversed the arc of block during control and dual-site stimulation are shown on the left. Expanded views of the same S_2 activation sequences shown in Figure 40–13 are shown on the right. Effective refractory periods are indicated by shaded boxes.

The response interval for site A during control was equal to the S_1–S_2 interval of 180 ms. The refractory period at site A was 160 ms. Site B was activated 62 ms after the onset of the S_1 stimulus artifact. Coupled with a refractory period of 190 ms, the expiration of refractoriness, or the recovery of excitability, for site B was 252 ms after S_1. S_1 activation at site A was 34 ms. This interval, added to the S_1–S_2 interval of 180 ms, corresponds to S_2 activation at site A 214 ms after S_1. Therefore, site B had not recovered excitability from the previous S_1 stimulation at the time that site A was activated by the S_2 wavefront. As a result, unidirectional conduction block occurred between the two sites. The activation wavefront circumvented the arc of block and activated site B 120 ms later. The effective refractory period of S_2 (ERP_2) measured at site A was 125 ms. As shown by the electrograms activation at site B followed upon the expiration of ERP_2 for site A. The reentrant wavefront was able to reactivate a region proximal to the arc, in the vicinity of site A.

When dual stimulation was applied, the S_1 activation sequence was modified such that S_1 activation at site B preceded that at site A by 16 ms. S_1 activation at site B was 17 ms, a reduction of 45 ms from control. As a result, the recovery of excitability for site B, relative to the S_1 stimulus, was reduced to 207 ms. S_1 activation at site A was 33 ms, a reduction of only 1 ms from control. Therefore, dual stimulation shifted the expiration of refractoriness at site B leftward in time, relative to site A.

The same S_1–S_2 coupling interval of 180 ms was applied from the control site. Conduction from site A now proceeded antegradely to site B. However, the activation wavefront arrived at site B before recovery of excitability at site C. An arc of block formed between sites B and C. The reentrant wavefront traveled around the arc of block and activated site C 47 ms after activation at site B. This interval was far too short to permit reactivation of site B. Dual stimulation prevented reentry by shifting the arc of conduction block and allowing sites distal to the arc to activate before recovery of excitability proximal to the arc.

(Reprinted by permission of the American Heart Association, Inc., from Restivo M, Gough WB, El-Sherif N: Circulation 77:429, 1988.)

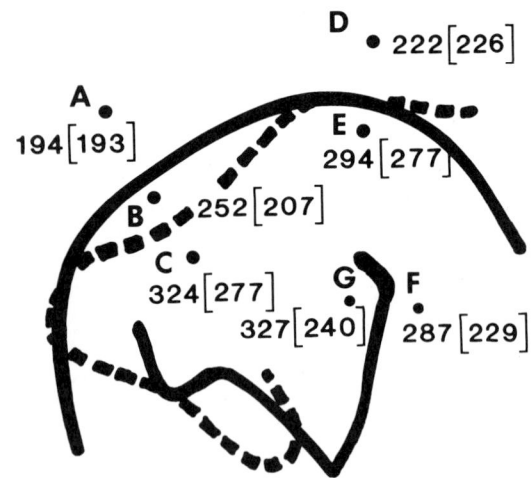

FIGURE 40–15
Recordings were obtained from the same experiment shown in Figures 40–13 and 40–14. Correlation of changes in recovery times (i.e., S_1 activation plus effective refractory period) and modification of the arc of block after dual S_1 stimulation. Recovery time values of several sites are shown with the value after dual stimulation in brackets. The control arc of block is depicted by the solid line; the dashed line represents the arc after dual stimulation.

During control, conduction block occurred between sites A and B, D and E, and F and G. The difference in recovery time between the three pairs was 58, 72, and 40 ms, respectively. After dual stimulation, the difference was 14, 51, and 11 ms, respectively. After dual stimulation, conduction block did not occur between sites A and B, and the arc shifted toward the ischemic core, between sites B and C where the recovery difference was 60 ms. There was no shift in the arc of block between sites D and E.

Since the recovery time difference between sites D and E was sufficiently long during control (72 ms), the 21-ms reduction in recovery time difference to 51 ms induced by dual stimulation was able to eliminate conduction block when the recovery differences between adjacent sites were smaller than during control, as between sites F and G. The 40-ms recovery time difference between these sites during control was reduced to only 11 ms after dual stimulation. Most of the arc that passed between sites F and G during control disappeared after dual stimulation.

(Reprinted by permission of the American Heart Association, Inc., from Restivo M, Gough WB, El-Sherif N: Circulation 77:429, 1988.)

FIGURE 40–16
Diagrammatic illustration of three different stimulation protocols (A–C) for termination of reentrant ventricular tachycardia.

In A, the extrastimulus technique is utilized with the first stimulated beat falling just outside the refractory period at the site of stimulation. Additional stimuli are added, as required, in a stepwise fashion at a cycle length equal to the coupling interval of the first stimulated beat. In B, a fixed train of stimuli is utilized. The cycle length of the first train is only slightly shorter than the tachycardia cycle. The cycle length of subsequent trains is shortened in a stepwise fashion until the tachycardia is terminated. C shows autodecremental pacing. In this protocol, the coupling interval of the first stimulated beat is only slightly shorter than the tachycardia cycle, and both a stepwise decrement of consecutive cycle lengths and a stepwise increase of the number of stimulated beats are utilized as required.

(Reprinted by permission from El-Sherif N, Gough WB, Restivo M: PACE 10:341, 1987.)

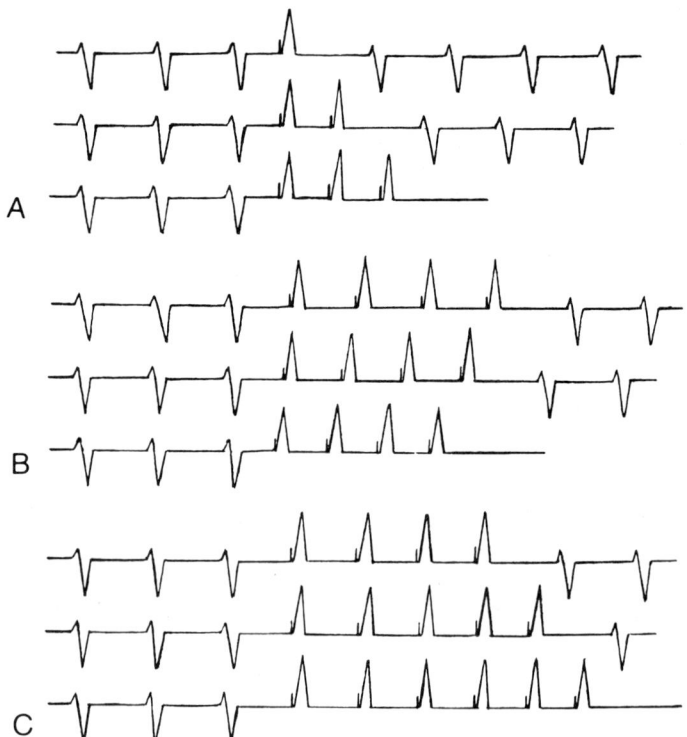

References

1. Jackman WM, Zipes DP: Low-energy synchronous cardioversion of ventricular tachycardia using a catheter electrode in a canine model of subacute myocardial infarction. Circulation 266:1982.
2. Zipes DP, Jackman WM, Heger JJ, et al.: Clinical transvenous cardioversion of recurrent life threatening ventricular tachyarrhythmias: Low energy synchronized cardioversion of ventricular tachycardia and termination of ventricular fibrillation in patients using a catheter electrode. Am Heart J 103:789, 1982.
3. Fisher JD, Mehra R, Furman S: Termination of ventricular tachycardia with bursts of rapid ventricular pacing. Am J Cardiol 41:94, 1978.
4. Colavita PG, Wolf P, Smith WM, et al.: Determination of the effects of interval countershock by direct cardiac recordings during normal rhythm. Am J Physiol 250:H376, 1986.
5. Saksena S, Pantopoulos D, Hussain SM, Gielchinsky I: Mechanisms of ventricular tachycardia termination and acceleration during transverse cardioversion as determined by cardiac mapping in man. Am Heart J 113:1495, 1987.
6. El-Sherif N, Gough WB, Restivo M: Reentrant ventricular arrhythmias in the late myocardial infarction period: 14: Mechanisms of resetting, entrainment, acceleration or termination of reentrant tachycardia by programmed electrical stimulation. PACE 10:341, 1987.
7. El-Sherif N: Reentry revisited. PACE 11:1358, 1988.
8. Mines GR: On dynamic equilibrium in the heart. J Physiol 46:350, 1913.
9. Mines GR: On circulating excitations in heart muscles and their possible relation to tachycardia and fibrillation. Trans R Soc Can 8 (Ser 3, Sect IV):43, 1914.
10. Moe GK, Mendez C, Han J: Aberrant AV impulse propagation in the dog heart: a study of functional bundle branch block. Circ Res 16:261, 1965.
11. El-Sherif N, Mehra R, Gough WB, Zeiler RH: Ventricular activation patterns of spontaneous and induced ventricular rhythms in canine one-day-old myocardial infarction. Evidence for focal and reentrant mechanisms. Circ Res 51:152, 1982.
12. Mehra R, Zeiler RH, Gough WB, El-Sherif N: Reentrant ventricular arrhythmias in the late myocardial infarction period. 9. Electrophysiologic-anatomic correlation of reentrant circuits. Circulation 67:11, 1983.
13. Gough WB, Mehra R, Restivo M, et al.: Reentrant ventricular arrhythmias in the late myocardial infarction period in the dog. 13. Correlation of activation and refractory maps. Cir Res 57:432, 1985.
14. Allessie MA, Bonke FIM, Schopman FJG: Circus movement in rabbit atrial muscle as a mechanism of tachycardia. III. The "leading circle" concept: A new model of circus movement in cardiac tissue without the involvement of an anatomical obstacle. Circ Res 41:9, 1977.
15. El-Sherif N, Gough WB, Zeiler RH, Hariman R: Reentrant ventricular arrhythmias in the late myocardial infarction period. 12. Spontaneous versus induced reentry and intramural versus epicardial circuits. J Am Coll Cardiol 6:124, 1985.
16. Janse MJ, Van derSteen ABM, Van Dam RT, Durrer D: Refractory period of dog's ventricular myocardium following sudden changes in frequency. Circ Res 24:251, 1969.
17. El-Sherif N, Mehra R, Gough WB, Zeiler RH: Reentrant ventricular arrhythmias in the late myocardial infarction period. 11. Burst pacing versus multiple premature stimulation in the induction of reentry. J Am Coll Cardiol 4:295, 1984.
18. Jalife J, Moe GK: Effect of electrotonic potentials on pacemaker activity of canine Purkinje fibers in relation to parasystole. Circ Res 39:801, 1976.
19. Ypey DL, Van Meerwijk WPM, Ince C, Gross G: Mutual entrainment of two pacemaker cells. A study with an electronic parallel conductance model. J Theor Biol 86:731, 1980.
20. Waldo AL, MacLean WAH, Karp RB, et al.: Entrainment and interruption of atrial flutter with atrial pacing. Studies in man following open heart surgery. Circulation 56:737, 1977.
21. Waldo AL, Henthorn RW, Plumb VJ, MacLean WAH: Demonstration of the mechanism of transient entrainment and interruption of ventricular tachycardia with rapid atrial pacing. J Am Coll Cardiol 3:422, 1984.
22. Fisher JD, Kim SG, Matos JA, Ostrow E: Comparative effectiveness of pacing techniques for termination of well-tolerated sustained ventricular tachycardia. PACE 6:915, 1983.
23. Naccarelli GV, Zipes DP, Rahilly TG: Influence of tachycardia cycle length and antiarrhythmic drugs on pacing terminations and accelerations of ventricular tachycardia. Am Heart J 105:1, 1983.
24. Roy D, Waxman HL, Buxton AE, et al.: Termination of ventricular tachycardias: Role of tachycardia cycle length. Am J Cardiol 50:1346, 1982.
25. Fisher JD, Kim SG, Matos JA, Waspe LE: Pacing for tachycardias: clinical translations. In Zipes DP, Jalife J (eds.): Cardiac Electrophysiology and Arrhythmias, pp 507–511. New York, Grune and Stratton, 1985.
26. Wellens HJJ, Lie KI, Durrer D: Further observations on ventricular tachycardia as studied by electrical stimulation of the heart. Chronic recurrent ventricular tachycardia and ventricular tachycardia during acute myocardial infarction. Circulation 49:647, 1974.
27. Ruffy R, Friday KJ, Southworth WP: Termination of ventricular tachycardia by single extrastimulation during the ventricular effective refractory period. Circulation 67:457, 1983.
28. Podczeck A, Borggrefe M, Martinez-Rubio A, Breithardt G: Termination of reentrant ventricular tachycardia by subthreshold stimulus applied to the zone of slow conduction. Eur Heart J 9:1146, 1988.
29. Prystowsky EN, Zipes DP: Inhibition in the human heart. Circulation 68:707, 1983.
30. Windle JR, Miles WM, Zipes DP, Prystowsky EN: Subthreshold conditioning stimuli prolong human ventricular refractoriness. Am J Cardiol 57:381, 1986.
31. Restivo M, Gough WB, El-Sherif N: Reentrant ventricular rhythms in the late myocardial infarction period: Prevention of reentry by dual stimulation during basic rhythm. Circulation 77:429, 1988.
32. Medina-Ravell V, Castellanos A, Portillo-Acosta B, et al.: Management of tachyarrhythmias with dual chamber pacemakers. PACE 6:333, 1983.
33. Mahmud R, Tchou PJ, Denker ST, et al.: Functional characteristics of human macro-reentry: A study of pre-excited circuits by extrastimulus method. J Am Coll Cardiol 8:1073, 1986.
34. Ward DE, Camm AJ, Gainsborough J, Spurrell RAJ: Autodecremental pacing—a microprocessor base modality for termination of tachycardia. PACE 3:178, 1980.
35. Nathan A, Hellestrand K, Ward DE, et al.: Rate-related accelerating (auto-decremental) atrial pacing. J Electrocardiol 15:77, 1982.
36. Charos GS, Haffajee CI, Gold RL, et al.: A theoretically and practically more effective method for interruption of ventricular tachycardia: Self-adapting auto-decremental overdrive pacing. Circulation 73:307, 1986.

41

Antitachycardia Pacing: Clinical Aspects

Christopher R. C. Wyndham

Chapter 40 has laid the basis for the use of pacing therapy for paroxysmal tachycardias. This chapter will review the techniques and indications for temporary and permanent antitachycardia pacing for selected patients with tachyarrhythmias. The application of pacing in these clinical situations should be considered carefully in relation to the nature of the arrhythmia, including its frequency, rate, and duration; the degree of hemodynamic compromise, types of alternative and adjunctive therapies and their effects on the tachycardia and its response to pacing; and, finally, with an appreciation of the risks and adverse effects of pacing. For a few arrhythmias, pacing may be the treatment of choice; more usually it represents one of several effective therapies and sometimes will be frankly contraindicated, either because of inefficacy or clinical risk. As in every area of medicine, treatment should be chosen based on the specific conditions present in the individual patient.

HISTORICAL ASPECTS

The earliest observations on the effects of pacing on tachyarrhythmias were concerned with the ability of normal-rate pacing to prevent tachyarrhythmias. For example, in 1951 Pick et al.[1] noted suppression of ventricular premature beats by ventricular pacing; in 1960 Zoll and associates[2] reported on the prevention of ventricular tachycardia and fibrillation in patients with complete atrioventricular (AV) block; Sowton and colleagues,[3] in 1965, reported on studies on the prevention of ventricular fibrillation in patients with bradyarrhythmias accompanying myocardial infarction; and in 1970, Goel and Han[4] noted the suppression of atrial ectopy and atrial fibrillation by atrial pacing.

Nowadays, the use of pacemakers to prevent tachycardias is relatively limited, more effort being expended on the more fruitful modality of interruption of tachycardias by pacing. Haft et al.[5] showed that atrial flutter could successfully be terminated by rapid atrial pacing, and Lister and coworkers[6] documented the interruption of reentrant supraventricular tachycardias by rapid atrial pacing. The use of single stimuli to interrupt reentrant tachycardias was found to be effective in selected patients, especially those with relatively slow tachycardias. By pacing at a rate slower than the tachycardia, various authors have documented that random stimuli might, at critical coupling intervals, successfully interrupt tachycardias.[7-10] This principle was later incorporated in an implantable automatic pacemaker that scanned diastole with extrastimuli, seeking a "window of termination" of tachycardia.[11]

Rapid pacing at rates faster than the tachycardia was introduced in the treatment of ventricular tachycardia by Fisher et al.[12] The automatic detection and termination of ventricular tachycardia by an implantable device was described in 1980 both by Fisher and colleagues[13] and by Griffin et al.[14] Implantable pacemakers for the control of atrial flutter were described in six patients by Wyndham and coworkers[15] and Barold and associates.[16]

The introduction into clinical use of the automatic implantable defibrillator by Mirowski et al.[17] in 1980 ushered in a new era of antitachycardia device therapy. With increasing experience with programmable antitachycardia pacemakers, the dream of implanting a fully automatic device capable of delivering a variety of programmable modes of antitachycardia pacing therapies, backed up by low- or high-energy DC shocks is now being realized. A number of such devices are currently being planned for clinical trials.

Finally, renewed interest in the idea of tachycardia prevention by pacing has been pursued. It is hoped that subthreshold stimulation may one day be utilized to render tissue critical to the maintenance of tachycardia sufficiently refractory that reentry may be prevented.

Coincident with the development of hardware for antitachycardia pacing has been an ongoing study of monitoring of electrograms and the development of reliable algorithms for the detection of tachycardia and differentiation of paroxysmal from physiologic tachycardias and of ventricular tachycardia from supraventricular arrhythmias. An important further line of investigation is a by-product of the rate-responsive pacemaker development: namely, the perfection of sensors of biologic variables. Thus, newer antitachycardia pacemakers will be able to detect not only the presence of tachycardia by analysis of electrograms, but also something of the physiologic impact of the arrhythmia by measuring such variables as right ventricular impedance, systolic time intervals, respiratory function, blood pH, and oxygen saturation. In this way, these devices will then be able to organize the order, duration, and complexity of pacing and shock therapies, based on whether there is serious hemodynamic compromise as a result of the tachycardia.

Modalities of Antitachycardia Pacing

TERMINOLOGY

In an attempt to characterize descriptively an increasingly complex array of modes of programmed stimulation, a profusion of terms that apply to antitachycardia pacing has grown up within the more generalized jargon of cardiac pacing. This section will define more commonly encountered terms and attempt to simplify an unnecessarily complicated terminology.

There are really only three types of fundamental pacing modes used in antitachycardia pacing: extrastimuli, continuous pacing, and burst pacing.

EXTRASTIMULI ■ Extrastimuli are defined as single or multiple (a few) premature stimuli, in which the coupling interval of each stimulus is individually controlled. As shown in Table 41–1, these may be asynchronous or synchronous. When synchronous, the extrastimuli may be introduced at pre-programmed intervals or be timed according to "adaptive" behavior—that is, as a percentage of prevailing cycle length. Subsequent iterations of extrastimuli may be unchanged in coupling intervals or else may scan diastole by decrementing the first or all coupling intervals of the extrastimuli. Since multiple extrastimuli are usually introduced at progressively shorter coupling intervals, it should be apparent that a series of many extrastimuli will often be synonymous with a short decremental burst of pacing (see below).

CONTINUOUS PACING ■ This term is usually reserved for pacing used for the *prevention* of tachycardias.[1-4] Continuous pacing may be further classified into normal rate and overdrive pacing (Table 41–2). A standard VVI pacemaker will be capable of the former modality and often (in the magnet mode) also the latter. In the magnet (asynchronous) mode, such a pacemaker will also be delivering random extrastimuli if used during a tachycardia whose rate is faster than the magnet rate of the pacemaker.

BURST PACING ■ Burst pacing is the term used for pacing for a limited period of time whether the rate be fast or relatively slow. Some authors have used the term "overdrive pacing" for burst pacing at relatively slow rates (e.g., up to 140% tachycardia rate) and the term burst pacing only for faster rates. This distinction seems highly arbitrary to this author. It is more widely accepted to reserve the term overdrive for use in continuous pacing, as defined above. Burst pacing, then, encompasses any brief period of pacing above the rate of the tachycardia that is designed to interrupt rather than to prevent tachycardia. The duration of burst pacing is variable but essentially exceeds three stimuli, since one to three stimuli are more properly termed extrastimuli. A form of burst pacing known variously as ultrafast train pacing or ultrarapid pacing is designed to ensure a single capture at the earliest possible moment in diastole. Thus, although the technology delivers a burst of pacing above diastolic threshold, only a single stimulus actually captures. The physiologic result is a single premature beat. Finally, another form of burst pacing which has not, as yet, been employed extensively in clinical settings, is subthreshold stimulation with a single stimulus or a train of stimuli, designed to alter local refractoriness to inhibit impulse formation or conduction.

TABLE 41–1
Extrastimuli

Definition
Timing of each stimulus is individually controlled.

Number
Single or multiple.

Asynchronous
Random timing, as in "underdrive" pacing.

Synchronous
First extrastimulus is coupled to a beat of tachycardia.

Preprogrammed Coupling Interval
All coupling intervals (ms) are controlled by programming.

Adaptive
Coupling interval of first extrastimulus is some percentage of tachycardia cycle length.

Scanning
Each iteration of the extrastimulus or extrastimuli decrements the first coupling interval with or without decrementing subsequent coupling intervals of multiple extrastimuli.

TABLE 41–2
Classification of Continuous Pacing

Normal Rate Pacing
Pacing above the rate of spontaneous normal rhythm (but not above, e.g., 85 bpm), designed to prevent the arrhythmogenic effects of bradycardia.

Overdrive Pacing
Pacing at rates above approximately 85 bpm, designed to suppress atrial or ventricular ectopy or runs of tachycardia occurring at normal heart rates but demonstrably suppressed at higher than normal heart rates.

Whenever burst stimulation is performed, this may be delivered in one or more of three fundamental modes, as shown in Table 41–3: namely, fixed rate, scanning, and decremental pacing. All three modes may be introduced either at preprogrammed cycle lengths or as adaptive pacing (i.e., beginning at some percentage of prevailing cycle length). Adaptive behavior is synonymous with "orthorhythmic" pacing cited by French authors. It should also be noted that the term "autodecremental burst" is used synonymously with "decremental burst" when employed by implanted pulse generators. A variety of scanning burst pacing known as incremental-decremental burst or "centripetal" burst pacing is designed to search for an effective pacing rate by starting at an arbitrary rate, and then successively increasing and decreasing the rate with each successive burst, each of which has a fixed rate.

LEAD SYSTEMS FOR TEMPORARY PACING

Noninvasive transcutaneous pacing has been discussed in Chapter 39. Although largely employed for bradyarrhythmias, experience is increasing in the use of transcutaneous pacing for the termination of tachycardias.[18]

Transesophageal pacing has been advocated by Kerr et al.[19] as a relatively noninvasive way of investigating certain patients with or without arrhythmias—for example, with asymptomatic Wolff-Parkinson-White (WPW) syndrome. Usually it is possible to capture only the atria, and this necessitates pacing with relatively high amplitude (10–30 mA) and pulse width (10–60 ms) using special pacing equipment. These energies frequently result in esophageal spasm and chest discomfort requiring parenteral analgesics or sedatives. However, the technique has the advantage of being quickly instituted in an emergency without the use of fluoroscopy, and it can be facilitated by a "pill electrode."

Transthoracic pacing employs a small-diameter, bipolar electrode or two individual plunge electrodes advanced through a large-bore needle into the right or left ventricle by transthoracic cardiac puncture. As a temporary measure in patients unconscious from bradysystolic arrest, it is sometimes life-saving while more formal transvenous electrodes are being advanced. This author has never used this technique for tachycardia termination.

Temporary epicardial leads in postoperative open-heart patients are of proven value in the diagnosis and treatment of postoperative arrhythmias, as investigated by Waldo.[20] It is recommended that two wires be used for the atria and two for the ventricles to facilitate bipolar recording of electrograms, avoid sensing problems (cross-talk, myopotential inhibition), and provide fail-safe backup in the event that one of the wires becomes nonfunctional in the postoperative period. The method of attachment of the epicardial lead is a matter of judgment on the part of the surgeon but has been variously achieved by simply suturing the wire electrode itself directly into the myocardium, by forming a tunnel for the lead on the epicardial surface, and by using temporary extension adaptors in order to exteriorize standard permanent epicardial screw-in electrodes. When properly managed, the risks of bleeding, infection, erosion, and lead failure are minimal.[21]

Transvenous atrial and ventricular leads are most frequently employed for temporary pacing. In general, a quadripolar lead is preferred for atrial pacing in order to provide electrograms for diagnosis of wide-QRS tachycardias and confirmation of atrial capture during pacing. Such a lead also permits more options in lead selection, should there develop a problem in reliably capturing the atria after implantation. Temporary leads should always be inserted under fluoroscopic control for maximum stability. It is this author's preference to utilize a subclavian or internal jugular approach when possible, for patient comfort, enhanced lead stability, and freedom from infection and thrombophlebitis relative to antecubital or femoral routes. The three most important elements in preventing infection of an indwelling transvenous electrode are scrupulous sterile procedure in the insertion of the lead, elimination of the introducer sheath as a route for intravenous therapy, and good wound care—either with an occlusive dressing or careful daily redressing of the wound.

Concerning the type of electrode for atrial pacing, there is a great need for a reliable, temporary, quadripolar atrial appendage lead. Temporary "basket" or other atrial leads have not gained wide acceptance. Occasionally a coronary sinus lead will be preferred, either because of enhanced lead stability or capture threshold or because of better access to the reentrant circuit in an individual case. Whenever an atrial lead is used for pacing termination of a supraventricular tachycardia or atrial flutter, it should first be ascertained that the lead has not inadvertently migrated to the right ventricle. This can be determined by preliminary underdrive pacing at high output to document the absence of direct ventricular pacing before the rapid pacing modality is instituted.

PULSE GENERATORS FOR TEMPORARY CARDIAC PACING

Burst pacing can be accomplished by all standard external pacemakers. The efficacy in capturing the

TABLE 41–3
Fundamental Modes of Burst Stimulation, Introduced at Either Preprogrammed or Adaptive Rate

---

Fixed Rate
Cycle length of pacing is constant both within and between successive bursts.

Scanning
Cycle length of pacing decrements automatically between successive bursts.

Decremental
Cycle length of pacing decrements within each burst.

Incremental Burst Pacing
A subvariety in which the cycle length increases within a given burst.

chamber paced is limited by the integrity and stability of the lead system used and by the output, pulse width, and maximum rate of the pacemaker. Occasionally, to overcome high capture thresholds on temporary leads, change in polarity or lead combinations will be effective. Otherwise, high-output generators capable of high current or increased pulse width will assist. As a general rule, capture threshold is somewhat higher during paroxysmal tachycardias than during sinus rhythm.

Extrastimulation can be performed randomly by underdrive pacing with any external pacemaker, but it is rarely efficacious in terminating any but the slowest tachycardias. Programmed extrastimulation is available in a number of custom and commercial external stimulators. All such devices should be operated only by experienced personnel, fully familiar with the safety precautions and the risks of their use. Whenever pacing of the ventricles or atrial pacing is used in a patient with the WPW syndrome or enhanced AV nodal conduction, the possibility of induction of rapid ventricular tachycardia or fibrillation always demands the proximity of a DC cardioverter and full emergency resuscitation equipment.

Clinical Application and Mechanism of Pacing Techniques

PACING TERMINATION OF PAROXYSMAL SUPRAVENTRICULAR TACHYCARDIA

Temporary Pacing

Temporary pacing in the control of paroxysmal supraventricular tachycardia (PSVT) is indicated when the mechanism is known or thought to be reentrant and when initial vagal maneuvers performed before and after administration of AV nodal blocking agents have failed to convert the tachycardia. It is also the preferred method in patients in the postoperative period, when epicardial atrial or ventricular wires are present, and in patients undergoing cardiac catheterization with venous access. One to three extrastimuli delivered into the atrium or ventricle seeking a termination "window," or short bursts of rapid pacing approximately 20 to 30% faster than the tachycardia, will generally interrupt PSVT when the mechanism involves reciprocation via an accessory pathway or AV nodal reentrance. Similar pacing methods may produce transient slowing of automatic tachycardias by the mechanism of transient "overdrive suppression," but this is rarely of sustained therapeutic benefit. If a tachycardia were to occur on the basis of triggered activity (as postulated in digitalis toxicity, for example), pacing may only accelerate the tachycardia.

Under any circumstances, all forms of atrial pacing may sometimes induce atrial flutter or atrial fibrillation when used for interruption of PSVT. If atrial flutter or fibrillation is nonsustained, or if a slower ventricular response is thereby obtained, this will itself impart clinical benefit. On the other hand, some patients will develop further hemodynamic embarrassment from the induction of atrial fibrillation or flutter and require DC cardioversion (in the case of atrial fibrillation) or use of more rapid pacing (in the case of atrial flutter).

Permanent Pacing

Permanent pacing for PSVT was once heralded as a major advance over chronic drug therapy in patients with occasional albeit highly symptomatic episodes, or even in patients with relatively frequent episodes. Several factors have prevented the widespread use of automatic implanted antitachycardia pacemakers in patients with PSVT. Among these are loss of chronic lead stability, rising capture threshold, deterioration in electrogram voltage interfering with appropriate sensing, the effects of modulation of tachycardia rate, and the timing of the termination window by changes in autonomic tone, physical activity, and the effects of concomitant antiarrhythmic drugs or autonomically active drugs such as bronchodilators. Induction of atrial fibrillation is a further limitation.

Before implantable antitachycardia devices are prescribed for patients with PSVT, prolonged testing with a temporary pacing lead under a variety of conditions is necessary to demonstrate the reliability of the method. These conditions may include testing in the supine, sitting, or standing posture or during upright tilt; during sleep; and certainly under the conditions of any adjunctive drug therapy chosen. Prior detailed electrophysiologic testing should be a prerequisite, in order to ascertain the tachycardia mechanism and to determine if operative or catheter ablation of the reentrant or automatic mechanism might be the preferred therapy. Detailed atrial mapping and repeated terminations of PSVT from multiple atrial and ventricular sites also allows the choice of the most advantageous site for permanent pacing.

Follow-up of patients with a variety of permanent pacing devices for the control of PSVT has shown good short-term results. However, the problems alluded to above have weighed against truly satisfactory long-term results in all patients. To date, only about 300 patients worldwide have been reported with a variety of pacing devices implanted for PSVT. These include radio-frequency pacemakers, ventricular demand pacemakers, dual-demand pacemakers, dual-chamber pacemakers, and sophisticated multiprogrammable single- and dual-chamber devices capable of a wide range of antitachycardia and backup pacing modes.

PACING TERMINATION OF PAROXYSMAL ATRIAL FLUTTER

Temporary Pacing

Temporary pacing for the termination of atrial flutter was introduced by Haft and associates[5] in 1967 and has been extensively reviewed and studied by Waldo and colleagues.[20, 21] The phenomenon of *transient entrainment* of tachycardias was first described in the setting of atrial flutter,[22] providing important evidence of the reentrant nature of atrial flutter. Transient entrainment is the continuous capture of all elements of a reentrant circuit by rapid pacing impulses, resulting in repeated resetting but not termination of the tachycardia. Entrainment is usually manifested by increasing degrees of fusion in the chamber paced as the rate is progressively increased, but by a constant degree of fusion at any given pacing rate. This is the case in "manifest," or classical entrainment. Detectable fusion may be absent, as in "concealed," or atypical entrainment. In both varieties, the hallmark is reproducible resetting of tachycardia by all paced beats yielding, after cessation of pacing, a return cycle that varies with the pacing cycle length. In the case of manifest entrainment, this is a direct relationship; in concealed entrainment the return cycle varies inversely with the pacing cycle length. In atrial flutter the observation of progressive fusion requires a multiple lead recording and careful inspection of flutter wave morphology during pacing. Whether fusion will be seen depends, in part, on the site of pacing (e.g., right atrial appendage or coronary sinus) and on the direction of rotation of the reentrant wavefront in the right atrium, as shown by Beckman and coworkers.[23]

The importance of transient entrainment during attempts at pacing termination of tachycardias is that it implies a reentrant basis for the arrhythmia and, further, that there is an excitable gap in the tachycardia circuit. In atrial flutter, as in other tachycardias, the atrial pacing must be at a sufficient rate with sufficient current to achieve reliable atrial capture long enough to invade and finally block in the reentrant circuit without re-initiating the tachycardia. If all these conditions are met, then the flutter will be terminated. This will often require pacing at rates of 330 to 400 beats per minute (bpm), using amplitudes of 5 to 20 mA at pulse widths of 2 to 5 ms for 10 to 60 seconds.

Following termination of atrial flutter, three types of rhythm may develop: sinus, atrial fibrillation, or a second form of atrial flutter (type II). Type II flutter is characterized by rates in excess of 300 bpm, generally with upright flutter waves in lead II and sometimes with a visible isoelectric interval between flutter complexes. This rhythm has a tendency not to respond similarly to pacing as does classical (type I) atrial flutter and also has a tendency to be unstable, usually resulting in atrial fibrillation. If atrial fibrillation is also an unstable arrhythmia, sinus rhythm will often follow after seconds to hours.

In any event, the induction of atrial fibrillation in a patient with atrial flutter and normal AV conduction (e.g., with a 2:1 AV ratio) will usually result in hemodynamic benefit because of a slowing of net ventricular response. This reflects the faster atrial rate and the effects of anterograde concealed conduction in the AV node. In fact, the deliberate induction of atrial fibrillation is a legitimate method of management of otherwise uncontrollable atrial tachycardias, especially incessant "multifocal" atrial tachycardia. This is only achievable in practice for temporary pacing methods, because of inordinate battery drain at the high rates employed. Finally, because of the rather frequent occurrence of sinus node dysfunction in patients prone to atrial flutter and fibrillation, one should always be prepared to provide backup atrial pacing in the event of prolonged post-conversion pauses from overdrive suppression of the sinus node.

TEMPORARY PACING IN THE MANAGEMENT OF ATRIAL FIBRILLATION

Although atrial fibrillation is resistant to atrial pacing, judicious use of ventricular pacing techniques can sometimes yield important hemodynamic benefit by slowing the mean ventricular response. This can be achieved by simple demand ventricular pacing at rates somewhat *less* than that of the conducted atrial fibrillation, or by arranging coupled or paired ventricular pacing (i.e., the induction of paced ventricular bigeminy "coupled" either to conducted beats or "paired" to paced ventricular beats). In either case, the net slowing of ventricular response is attributed to the effects of retrograde concealed conduction of ventricular impulses to the AV node. Hemodynamic improvement then may reflect both the slower mean rate and the inotropic stimulus of post-extrasystolic pauses. These techniques are only applicable to temporary methods while drug therapy or cardioversion is being instituted or arranged. Programmable implanted ventricular pacemakers could also, in theory, be used for "normal rate" ventricular pacing or asynchronous pacing in the magnet mode as a temporary measure.

PACING TERMINATION OF VENTRICULAR TACHYCARDIA

Temporary Pacing

Temporary pacing techniques are extremely valuable in two situations in patients with paroxysmal ventricular tachycardia (VT). The first relates to the emergency management of patients with recurrent torsades de pointes in the setting of drug-induced QT prolongation. This has been discussed in Chapter 14 and will not be further elaborated here. The second is as a temporary measure to control episodes of sustained monomorphic VT under the following situations: during washout of arrhythmogenic drugs, during the course of serial evaluation of antiarrhythmic drugs by electrophysiologic techniques, during the loading phase with long-acting drugs like amiodarone, and in postoperative patients after heart surgery. As mentioned above, only the slowest VTs respond to the introduction of one or two extrastimuli or, indeed, to any form of atrial stimulation, for reasons of limited access of the paced beats to the site of reentrance. The most consistently effective termination mode is brief burst ventricular pacing of 5 to 20 beats in duration at rates about 20 to 40% faster than the tachycardia. Prerequisites for successful termination of VT include (1) demonstrable capture of the ventricle paced; (2) entry into the presumed reentrant circuit, sometimes manifested by features of transient entrainment;[22] and (3) block of a paced impulse probably within the slow limb of the reentrant process.[23]

As with atrial pacing for PSVT, it is very helpful to be able, with a quadripolar electrode, to record ventricular electrograms during attempts at pacing. This will assist in identifying ventricular capture. In the absence of electrograms, capture by pacing stimuli will be documented by progressive fusion of the QRS complex if the tachycardia has a stable QRS morphology and if the tachycardia has a different QRS complex from that of pacing. Thus, a tachycardia activating the apex of the right ventricle initially, with a superior, leftward, and posterior vector, may not show detectable fusion when pacing is also performed from this common site. Acceleration of the QRS complex and local electrograms to the paced rate will of course be observed. It is in this situation that the "concealed" form of transient entrainment of VT may occur: namely, entrainment and resetting of the tachycardia without fusion.[24,25] Conversely, when a site distant from the pacing site is the site of earliest activation of the ventricles during tachycardia, pacing above the tachycardia rate will frequently show all the familiar features of manifest entrainment: that is, progressive and constant fusion at different paced rates and a direct relationship between the post-pacing return cycle and pacing cycle length.

As demonstrated by Mann et al.,[24] termination of tachycardia may be heralded by an abrupt change in the fused QRS complex to that of a pure paced beat (as defined by pacing during sinus rhythm). This event seems to represent block of the paced impulse in the slow limb of the circuit in an "orthodromic" direction, followed by activation of the entire ventricle from the paced site without fusion. Experience has shown, however, that this otherwise reliable sign of impending termination of tachycardia is fairly uncommon. Perhaps this is a consequence of virtually complete capture of the ventricular mass by pacing impulses at rates fast enough to terminate the tachycardia. Thus, the abrupt change in activation of the ventricles may be subtle when using only QRS morphology as a guide. Use of electrograms from the pacing catheter may shed further light on the direction of depolarization near the exit site from the slow limb, provided that the catheter is close to that site.

As always, when pacing the ventricles for termination of a tachycardia, full preparations for cardiopulmonary resuscitation and DC cardioversion or defibrillation are mandatory. As a practical, humanitarian consideration, transthoracic shock should be delayed until full loss of consciousness has occurred or until adequate general anesthesia has been achieved. When hemodynamic compromise occurs as a result of induction of a new, more rapid tachycardia (so-called "acceleration"), it is frequently best to continue pacing attempts at increasing rates either until loss of consciousness occurs, allowing painless cardioversion, or until sinus rhythm is restored by pacing. One should, of course, limit this (iatrogenic) period of dangerous instability of rhythm and hemodynamics to an absolute minimum in order to avoid the generalized consequences of prolonged hypotension and acidosis. For these reasons, these methods of termination of ventricular tachycardia should be performed only by thoroughly experienced personnel who are intimately familiar with the hazards of these techniques and constantly mindful of the safety and comfort of the patient.

Permanent Pacing

Permanent pacing for VT has been attempted in various modalities since about 1975, when the reports of Fisher and colleagues[13] and Griffin et al.[14] indicated the feasibility of these techniques in selected patients; however, these authors (at this early stage of the application of these techniques) were unable to address the important issue of the general applicability of implantable ventricular pacing devices to patients with paroxysmal VT as a group. It now seems clear that the hazard of induction of unstable VT or ventricular fibrillation (VF) is such that automatic methods of termination of VT can be generally acceptable only in the presence of backup defibrillation capability (see in Chapter 46).

On the other hand, physician-interactive permanent pacing devices have been relatively widely employed as adjunctive therapy for sustained VT. In this mode, the pacing device lies in a dormant state during VT until external programming, activation by a magnet, or activation by radio-frequency (RF) stimulation by an external transmitter is performed. For example, Herre et al.[26] described 28 patients with implanted devices, of whom nine had 133 episodes of spontaneous sustained VT. All but six of these episodes were successfully terminated by pacing. The pacing devices employed included RF devices in ten patients, a unipolar VVI device in which magnet-induced VVT sensing allowed induced pacing during skin stimulation in 16 patients, and in two patients a programmable bipolar pacemaker in which antitachycardia pacing was initiated by a temporary programming sequence.

These systems have the advantage that their termination of tachycardias are always physician-supervised, minimizing the risk of accidental iatrogenic death due to pacemaker-initiated VF. However, these systems suffer from the serious limitation that they are applicable only to patients with very well-tolerated tachycardia that never leads spontaneously to VF or cardiovascular collapse. In addition, the tachycardia must be reliably detected by the patient so that he or she can present quickly for pacing intervention. With the advent of transtelephonic ECG monitoring and of transtelephonic defibrillation, these devices may have wider application in the future. However, for the majority of patients with VT who are candidates for permanent pacing, the newer devices combining antitachycardia pacing with low- and high-energy shock will be more applicable.

USE OF TEMPORARY TRANSVENOUS LEADS FOR CARDIOVERSION OR DEFIBRILLATION

Occasionally, when in the electrophysiology laboratory, it will seem to be impossible to defibrillate a patient in induced VF. Mann and associates[27] described a patient with congestive cardiomyopathy in whom intractable VF during the course of an electrophysiologic study could not be reverted using conventional transthoracic shock, despite repositioning of defibrillating paddles, use of an auxiliary defibrillator, and administration of antiarrhythmic drugs and membrane-stabilizing electrolytes. Finally a 360-joule shock delivered via an electrode catheter in the right ventricular apex was successful in restoring sinus rhythm. A second transvenous shock was again successful in a subsequent spontaneous episode of VF also resistant to transthoracic shock. We have since experienced a 300-pound patient whose induced VF could be converted only by a transvenous high-energy shock of 500 joules through four intracardiac electrodes as a common cathode and with a posterior thoracic paddle as the anode. Both patients recovered promptly from cardiopulmonary arrest of 50 minutes and 45 minutes, respectively, without neurologic sequelae.

Conclusion

The role of temporary pacing for a variety of reentrant tachycardias is now well established. The place for permanent pacemakers in patients with recurrent drug-resistant supraventricular and ventricular tachycardias is still undergoing re-examination after a period of initial popularity. Undoubtedly, the availability of highly sophisticated devices capable of a wide range of sensing and pacing behaviors, backed up by cardioversion and defibrillation, will greatly expand the applicability of implantable devices for ventricular tachycardia. One of the most exciting prospects is the application of biosensor technology to antitachycardia devices, whereby the hemodynamic impact of the tachycardia can be closely monitored, allowing rapid cycling past the available pacing modes to shock therapy if the imminent collapse of the patient demands this.

The author acknowledges the expert preparation of the manuscript by Kalene Farley.

References

1. Pick A, Langendorf R, Katz LN: Depression of cardiac pacemakers by premature impulses. Am Heart J 41:49, 1951.
2. Zoll PM, Linenthal AJ, Zarsky LRN: Ventricular fibrillation treatment and prevention by external electric currents. New Engl J Med 262:105, 1960.
3. Sowton E, Leatham A, Carson P: The suppression of arrhythmias by artificial pacemaking. Lancet 2:1098, 1965.
4. Goel BG, Han J: Atrial ectopic activity associated with sinus bradycardia. Circulation 42:853, 1970.
5. Haft JI, Kozowsky BD, Lam SH, et al.: Termination of atrial flutter by rapid electrical pacing of the right atrium. Am J Cardiol 20:239, 1967.
6. Lister JW, Cohn LS, Bernstein WH, et al.: Treatment of supraventricular tachycardias by rapid atrial stimulation. Circulation 38:1044, 1988.
7. Hunt NC, Cobb FR, Waxman MB: Conversion of supraventricular tachycardias with atrial stimulation, evidence of reentry mechanisms. Circulation 38:1060, 1968.
8. Ryan GF, Easley RM, Zaroff LI: Paradoxical use of a demand pacemaker in treatment of supraventricular tachycardia due to the Wolff-Parkinson-White syndrome. Circulation 38:1037, 1968.
9. Urbaszek W, Gunther K, Trenckmann H: Zur therapie tachycarder rhythmusstorungen mit der intermittenden electrostimulation dez herzens nach dem sender-empfarger-prinzip. Z Gesamte Inn Med 26:475, 1971.
10. Moss AJ, Rivers RJ: Termination and inhibition of recurrent tachycardias by implanted pervenous pacemakers. Circulation 50:942, 1974.
11. Spurrell RAJ, Nathan AW, Bexton RS, et al.: Implantable automatic scanning pacemaker for termination of supraventricular tachycardia. Am J Cardiol 49:753, 1982.
12. Fisher JD, Furman S, Mehra R: Ectopic ventricular tachycardia treated with bursts of pacing at 300 per minute from an implanted ventricular pacer. Circulation 52(II):182, 1975.
13. Fisher JD, Furman S, Kim SG: Implanted automatic burst pacemakers for termination of ventricular tachycardia. Am J Cardiol 45:458, 1980.
14. Griffin JD, Mason JW, Calfee RV: Clinical use of an implantable automatic tachycardia terminating pacemaker. Am Heart J 100:1093, 1980.
15. Wyndham CRC, Wu D, Denes P, et al.: Self-initiated conversion of paroxysmal atrial flutter utilizing a radio-frequency pacemaker. Am J Cardiol 41:1119, 1978.
16. Barold SS, Wyndham CRC, Kappenberger LL, et al.: Implanted atrial pacemakers for paroxysmal atrial flutter. Long-term efficacy. Ann Intern Med 107:144, 1987.
17. Mirowski M, Reid PR, Mower MM, et al.: Termination of malignant arrhythmias with an implantable automatic defibrillator in human beings. N Engl J Med 303:322, 1980.
18. Luck JC, Grubb BP, Artman SE, et al.: Termination of sustained ventricular tachycardia by external noninvasive pacing. Am J Cardiol 61:574, 1988.
19. Kerr CR, Gallagher JJ, Smith WM: The induction of atrial flutter and fibrillation and the termination of atrial flutter by esophageal pacing. PACE 6:60, 1983.
20. Waldo AL: Some observations concerning atrial flutter in man. PACE 6:1181, 1983.
21. Waldo AL, MacLean WAH, Cooper TB, et al.: The use of temporarily placed epicardial atrial wire electrodes for the diagnosis and treatment of cardiac arrhythmias following open heart surgery. J Thorac Cardiovasc Surg 76:500, 1978.
22. Waldo AL, MacLean WAH, Karp RB, et al.: Entrainment and interruption of atrial flutter with atrial pacing: studies in man following open heart surgery. Circulation 56:737, 1977.
23. Beckman KJ, Lin HT, Krafchek J, Wyndham CRC: Classic and concealed entrainment of typical and atypical atrial flutter. PACE 9:826, 1986.
24. Mann DE, Lawrie GM, Luck JC, et al.: Importance of pacing site in entrainment of ventricular tachycardia. J Am Coll Cardiol 5:781, 1985.
25. Lin HT, Mann DE, Luck JC, et al.: Two different patterns of entrainment of ventricular tachycardia. J Electrocardiol 20:55, 1987.
26. Herre JM, Griffin JC, Nielsen AP, et al.: Permanent triggered antitachycardia pacemakers in the management of recurrent sustained ventricular tachycardia. J Am Coll Cardiol 6:206, 1985.
27. Mann DE, Inouye IK, Sakun V, et al.: Emergency defibrillation using a temporary pacing electrode catheter. PACE 8:753, 1985.

42

Ventricular Defibrillation: Basic Concepts

Raymond E. Ideker
Anthony S.L. Tang
David W. Frazier
Nitaro Shibata
Peng-Sheng Chen
J. Marcus Wharton

Overview

The automatic implantable cardioverter-defibrillator[1-4] has engendered a renewed interest in the basic mechanisms of defibrillation. In this chapter we will review some of the recent findings about how a shock succeeds or fails in halting ventricular fibrillation. We will also present possible mechanisms for the increased defibrillation efficacy of biphasic waveforms.

The first theories of defibrillation focused on the termination of activation fronts by the shock. In 1940, Wiggers et al.[5] proposed the "total extinction" hypothesis, which states that, to defibrillate, the shock must halt all of the activation fronts present throughout the ventricles during fibrillation. In 1975, this explanation was supplanted by the "critical mass" hypothesis of Zipes and coworkers.[6] The critical mass mechanism postulates that activation fronts must be halted only within a certain critical mass of the myocardium, thought to be about 75% of the ventricular mass in the dog. Activation fronts in the remaining 25% are thought to be insufficient to maintain fibrillation and soon die out. More recently, as discussed later, proposed mechanisms of defibrillation have focused on the ability of the shock (1) to initiate new activation fronts, (2) to alter refractoriness, and (3) to cause electrophysiologic abnormalities and damage in myocardial regions where the shock field is strong.

The development of computer-assisted cardiac mapping techniques[7] has led to the acquisition of much new information about the initiation and maintenance of cardiac arrhythmias.[8-10] Computer-assisted mapping has recently been applied to the study of ventricular defibrillation by extending the technique so that recordings of shock potentials of hundreds of volts can be made, followed a few milliseconds later by recordings of the millivolt signals generated by cardiac activation.[11,12] Much of the following information about the mechanism of defibrillation was learned using such mapping techniques.

Electrophysiologic Mechanisms of Defibrillation

Earliest activations following a subthreshold defibrillation shock occur in regions of low-potential gradient generated by the shock. Activation fronts after subthreshold shocks are not continuations of fronts present just before the shock. An upper limit exists to the strength of shocks that induce fibrillation during the vulnerable period of regular rhythm and correlates with the defibrillation threshold. To defibrillate, a shock must halt the activation fronts of fibrillation without giving rise to new activation fronts that reinduce fibrillation.

Supported in part by the National Institutes of Health Research Grants HL-28429, HL-33637, and HL-17670; National Science Foundation Engineering Research Center Grant CDR-8622201; and by CPI Inc. and Physio-Control Corp. Dr. Tang is the recipient of a Canadian Heart Foundation Fellowship.

The response to shocks during regular rhythm just below the upper limit of vulnerability is similar to the response to subthreshold defibrillation shocks. Shocks during regular rhythm initiate reentry when a critical point is formed at which a certain critical value of shock field strength intersects with a certain critical degree of myocardial refractoriness. This critical point may explain the existence of the upper limit of vulnerability. The critical point may also partially explain the probability function of defibrillation.

Biphasic waveforms, with the first phase larger or equal to the second phase, are more efficacious for defibrillation than monophasic waveforms of the same total duration. The reason for the increased efficacy of biphasic waveforms is not yet known. Very high-potential gradients have detrimental effects on the heart, including conduction block, decreased wall motion, arrhythmogenesis, and necrosis.

ACTIVATIONS FOLLOWING SUBTHRESHOLD SHOCK

Regions in Which Earliest Activations Occur

With several different configurations of epicardial or catheter defibrillation electrodes, recordings in dogs have been made of cardiac activation immediately before and after a defibrillation shock as well as of the potentials caused by the shock itself at 56 to 120 electrodes placed on or in the ventricles.[13-15] An example of the potential distribution is shown in Figure 42–1 for a 500-V shock delivered via a catheter electrode in the right ventricular apex and a cutaneous patch electrode over the left thorax.[15] Potentials were recorded from 52 plunge needles inserted within the right and left ventricular free walls. Each plunge needle contained two electrodes, one to record from the subepicardium, the other from the subendocardium. Another 18 electrodes were placed to record potentials from the ventricular septum and the atria.[15] The most negative potentials are in the posterolateral right ventricle, adjacent to the catheter cathode electrode. The potentials change rapidly in this region (high-potential gradient), as indicated by the closely spaced isopotential lines. Distant from the catheter electrode, in the anterior left and right ventricles, the potentials change more slowly (low-potential gradient). The least negative potentials are in the left ventricular apex, the portion of the heart closest to the cutaneous anode electrode. In all regions, the subendocardial potentials are more negative than the subepicardial potentials, indicating a transmural component to the potential gradient field.

The extracellular potential gradient field created throughout the ventricles by the shock is thought to be a determining factor for the threshold of defibrillation.[16] The potential gradient field can be calculated from the shock potentials and the locations of the recording electrodes.[13] At the end of the study, the animal heart was cut into slices approximately 2 mm thick and, with a hand-held digitizer, the locations of the recording electrodes were entered into a computer

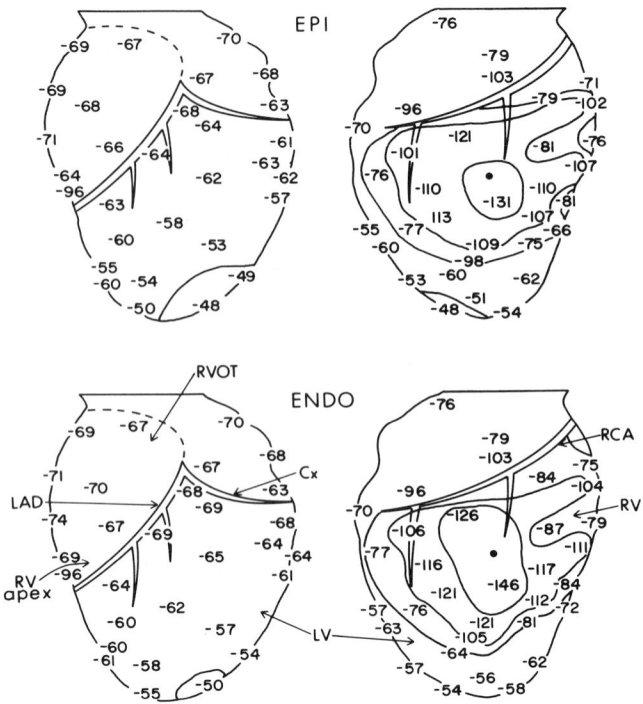

FIGURE 42–1
The potential field from an unsuccessful 500-V, 6-ms monophasic truncated exponential defibrillation shock. A catheter in the right ventricular apex was the cathode, and a cutaneous patch over the left lower thorax was the anode. Potentials were recorded from subepicardial (EPI) and subendocardial (ENDO) electrodes within plunge needles in the ventricles and from epicardial electrodes in the atria. The top two panels show the subepicardial potentials and the bottom two panels the subendocardial potentials. All panels show the potentials superimposed on the epicardial surface. The two panels on the left represent the left anterolateral cardiac surface, and the two panels on the right the right posterolateral surface. Numbers denote the location of the recording electrodes and the potential in volts recorded at each site referenced to the left leg. Isopotential lines are drawn 25 V apart. Solid circles represent unsatisfactory electrode recordings. The dashed line indicates the upper border of the right ventricular outflow tract. LV = left ventricle; RV = right ventricle; RVOT = right ventricular outflow tract; LAD = left anterior descending coronary artery; RCA right coronary artery; Cx = left circumflex coronary artery. (Reprinted by permission from Tang ASL, et al.: Proc IEEE. In press.)

from the individual slices.[15, 17] The potential gradient distribution was very uneven for all configurations in which at least one defibrillation electrode was in or on the heart, with high gradients near these electrodes and much weaker gradients on portions of the heart distant from these electrodes. For example, Figure 42–2 shows the magnitude of the potential gradient field for the same shock for which the potentials are shown in Figure 42–1. Although not shown, the X, Y, and Z components of the gradient were also calculated. The highest gradients are in the posterolateral right ventricular apex around the catheter, as suggested by the closely spaced isopotential lines in Figure 42–1. The lowest gradients are in the anterobasal right and left ventricular free-walls, distant from the catheter. The

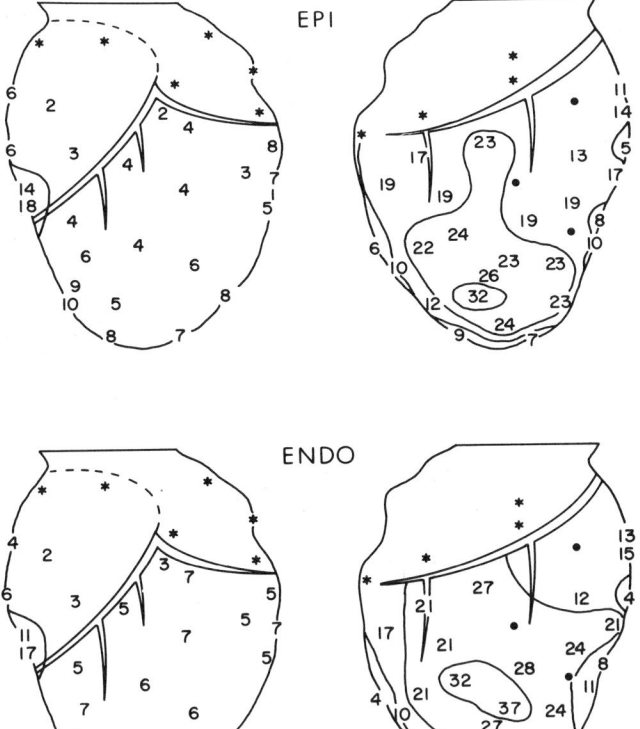

FIGURE 42–2
The potential gradient field calculated from the potentials shown in Figure 42–1 and from the locations of the recording sites. The numbers are the potential gradients at each recording site in V/cm. Asterisks represent the top row of electrodes on the atria and on the right ventricular outflow tract where potential gradients are not calculated because no recording sites are above them. Isogradient lines are drawn 10 V/cm apart. (Reprinted by permission from Tang ASL, et al.: Proc IEEE. In press.)

gradient field is very uneven, with the highest gradient (37 V/cm) over 18 times larger than the lowest gradient (2 V/cm).

After unsuccessful shocks slightly weaker than the defibrillation threshold, earliest activation leading to the resumption of fibrillation arose in a region of low-potential gradient for each defibrillation electrode configuration tested. Figure 42–3 illustrates the first three post-shock cycles of activation leading to the resumption of fibrillation after the shock for which the gradient field is shown in Figure 42–2. The shock was administered 10 seconds after the electrical induction of ventricular fibrillation. Earliest recorded activation occurs in the subepicardium of the anterobasal left ventricular free-wall, within the low gradient region shown in Figure 42–2. The activation front arising in this region conducts only for a short distance before blocking, as indicated by the wide black line for the first post-shock beat in Figure 42–3. The front is able to conduct to the subendocardium, however (long arrow in first post-shock beat of Fig. 42–3). From there activation spreads caudally toward the apex but cannot spread to the adjacent basal regions because of block, as shown by the wide black lines on the endocardium for the first post-shock beat in Figure 42–3. Instead, the front curves around the line of block to activate the adjacent basal region. By this time, the tissue first activated after the shock has had time to recover, so that it is re-excited by the fronts curving around both lines of blocks (second post-shock beat). Activation then spreads caudally along the subendocardium and to the anterior subepicardium. The fronts then form two mirror-image rotors, clockwise on the right ventricular side and counterclockwise on the left ventricular side, in both the subepicardium and subendocardium. This pair of rotors then continues (third post-shock beat), forming a figure-of-8 reentrant pattern.[18]

ACTIVATION FRONTS OF FIBRILLATION

One possible explanation for the finding that earliest post-shock activation occurs in low gradient regions is that the gradient field is too weak to halt the activation fronts of fibrillation present in these regions at the time of the shock. These fronts then spread, causing disorganization of activation in the remainder of the ventricles, so that fibrillation continues. Thus, to defibrillate, the shock must either halt all activation fronts[19, 20] or halt those activation fronts within a certain critical mass.[6] Mapping results do not support this explanation, however.[21–23] Excitation following subthreshold shocks appears to occur via new activation fronts rather than via continuation of fronts present just before the shock.[23] Post-shock activation is first recorded after a long pause called the isoelectric window, which is tens of times longer than any pauses observed during fibrillation just before the shock.[21, 24] For example, earliest activation in Figure 42–3 is recorded 37 ms after the beginning of the shock. As shock strength decreases, the post-shock isoelectric window shortens, and at fractions of a joule, can no longer be detected (Fig. 42–4), suggesting that unsuccessful defibrillation shocks of very low strength do not halt the activation fronts of fibrillation.[22] For stronger shocks slightly below the defibrillation threshold, the isoelectric window shortens as the recording electrodes are placed closer together,[21, 23] suggesting that very slow conduction is the cause of the isoelectric window, perhaps because of the latency associated with stimulation of highly refractory tissue.[25]

UPPER LIMIT OF VULNERABILITY

The above findings suggest the possibility that the new activation fronts leading to the resumption of fibrillation after a subthreshold defibrillation shock are initiated by the stimulation of highly refractory tissue by the shock itself. This possibility raises the question of how a shock ever succeeds in defibrillating. Since activation occurs continuously during fibrillation, repolarization should also occur continuously, so that at any time some portion of myocardium should be in the vulnerable period of refractoriness, during which a stimulus of sufficient strength can induce fibrillation. The fact that it is possible to defibrillate with a large shock implies that there is an upper limit of strength

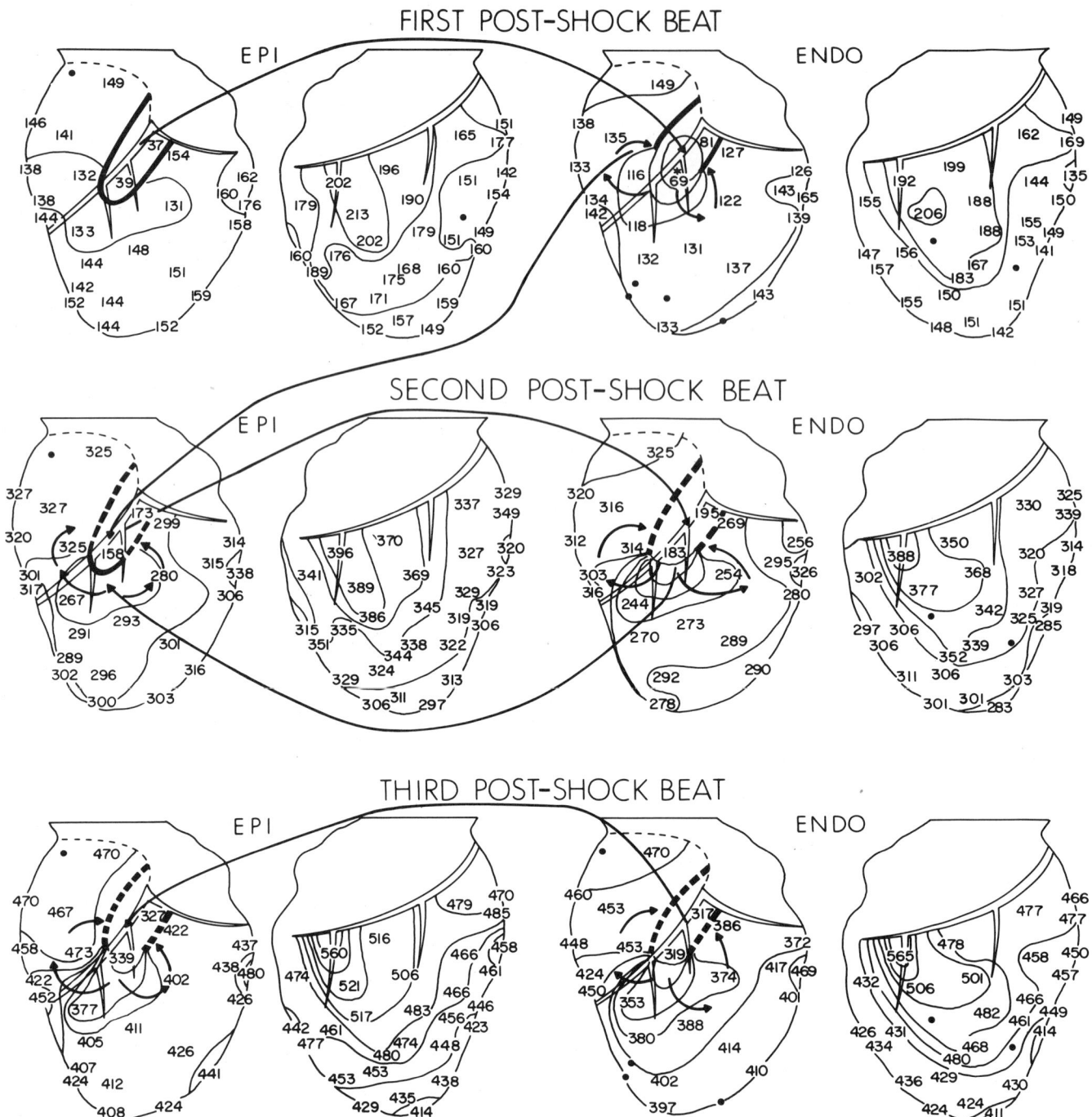

FIGURE 42–3
The first three cycles of activation leading to the resumption of fibrillation after an unsuccessful 500-V shock. The numbers are the times in ms of local activations at each recording site, timed from the beginning of the shock. Isochronal lines are drawn 20 ms apart. The heavy solid lines signify conduction block; the heavy dashed lines indicate a frame shift from one isochronal map to the next. Such frame lines are necessary whenever a continuous process such as reentrant activation is illustrated by a series of static maps. (Reprinted by permission from Tang ASL, et al.: Proc IEEE. In press.)

above which a shock will not induce fibrillation during the vulnerable period. Such a limit has been found and correlates strongly with the defibrillation threshold (Fig. 42–5).[26–28] This upper limit of vulnerability should not be confused with the finding that still higher-strength shocks can induce fibrillation at any time during the cardiac cycle, probably by causing cardiac damage.[26–27]

Correlation with Defibrillation Threshold

The existence of an upper limit of vulnerability and the high correlation between this upper limit and the defibrillation threshold are consistent with the hypothesis that successful defibrillation requires a shock strength that reaches or exceeds the upper limit of ventricular vulnerability.[28] This hypothesis implies that, following unsuccessful shocks just below the defibril-

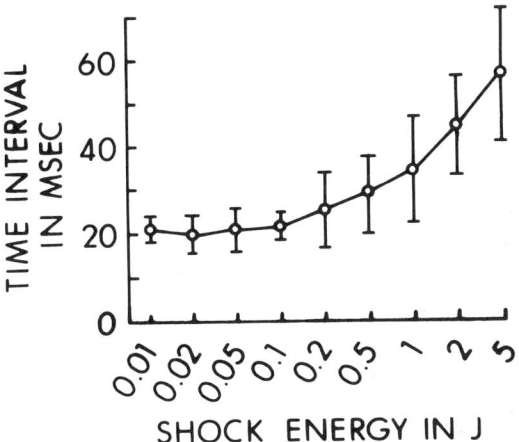

FIGURE 42–4
Effect of shock energy on the time of earliest recorded post-shock activation. Mean values are shown for unsuccessful defibrillation shocks given via electrodes on the left ventricular apex and right atrium to seven dogs 10 s after the electrical induction of fibrillation. Standard deviations are indicated by brackets. The shortest time interval following the beginning of the shock for which activations could be reliably detected is about 20 ms. The time until earliest recorded activation shortens as shock energy decreases. (Reprinted by permission from Shibata N, et al.: Am J Physiol 255:H902, 1988.)

lation threshold, earliest post-shock activation sequences should be similar to activation sequences at the start of fibrillation induced by shocks of the same energy during the vulnerable period of regular rhythm. Cardiac mapping has shown that the responses to both types of shocks are similar in many respects.[22, 29] Excitation following both types of shocks usually follows a pause (the isoelectric window) of 30 to 50 ms, begins from a few early sites in regions of low gradient, and spreads over the rest of the ventricles as large, coherent activation fronts (Fig. 42–6). No significant differences are present in the time from the shock until earliest activation, the number of early sites, the location of the earliest site, or the total time for the first post-shock activation fronts to traverse the ventricles.[22]

CRITERIA FOR DEFIBRILLATION

The above results are consistent with the existence of two criteria that must be met for defibrillation:

1. The shock field must abolish the activation fronts of fibrillation throughout all or a critical mass of myocardium.[6, 19, 20] This criterion is met by shocks well below the defibrillation threshold, but fibrillation is still not halted. Thus, this criterion may be a necessary but not a sufficient condition for defibrillation.
2. The shock field must not give rise to new activation fronts that reinitiate fibrillation. This criterion is important at higher shock field levels and is responsible for most of the energy required for defibrillation.

The mechanism by which a shock just below the defibrillation threshold fails to halt fibrillation is similar to that by which a shock of the same strength initiates fibrillation during the vulnerable period of regular rhythm, and the long pause following both types of shocks is caused by the latency of stimulation of relatively refractory tissue.

CRITICAL POINT HYPOTHESIS

Based on the phase-resetting patterns of various periodic oscillators such as cardiac pacemakers,[30–35] Winfree[36] has developed a topological model demonstrating the unavoidable existence of a critical point where the interaction of a specific stimulus at a certain point in time within the natural cycle of the oscillator causes the timing, or resulting latency, to become undefined. In this topological model, a continuous

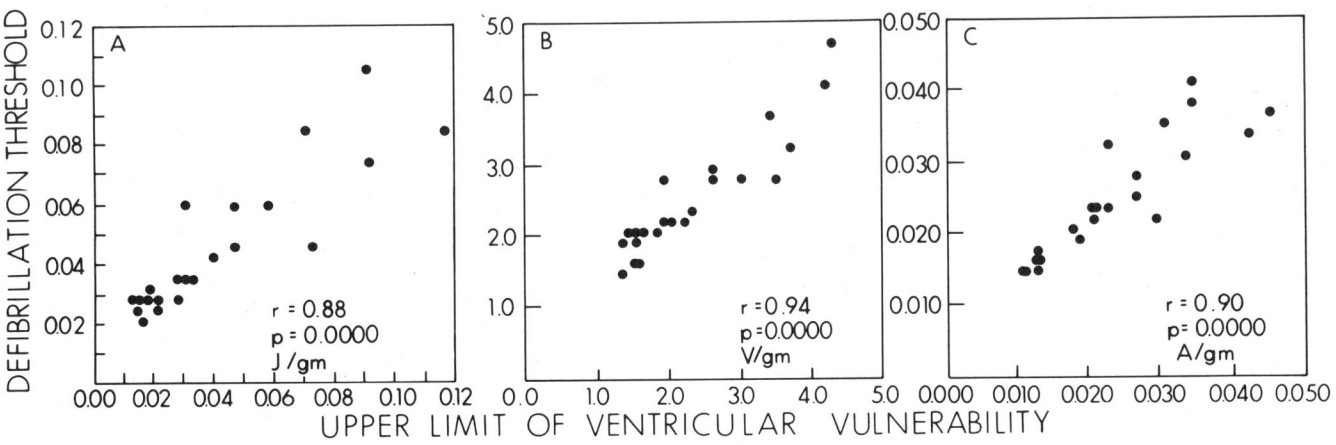

FIGURE 42–5
Correlation of the defibrillation threshold and the upper limit of vulnerability for defibrillation electrodes on the right atrium (anode) and the left ventricular apex (cathode) in 22 dogs. The defibrillation threshold was determined by a modified Bourland technique. The upper limit of vulnerability was determined by scanning in 5-ms increments to determine within 10% the largest shock energy that induced fibrillation during the vulnerable period. Results are expressed in units of energy (A), voltage (B), and current (C). All units are expressed per gram of heart weight. (Reprinted by permission of the American Heart Association, Inc., from Chen P-S, et al.: Circulation 73:1022, 1986.)

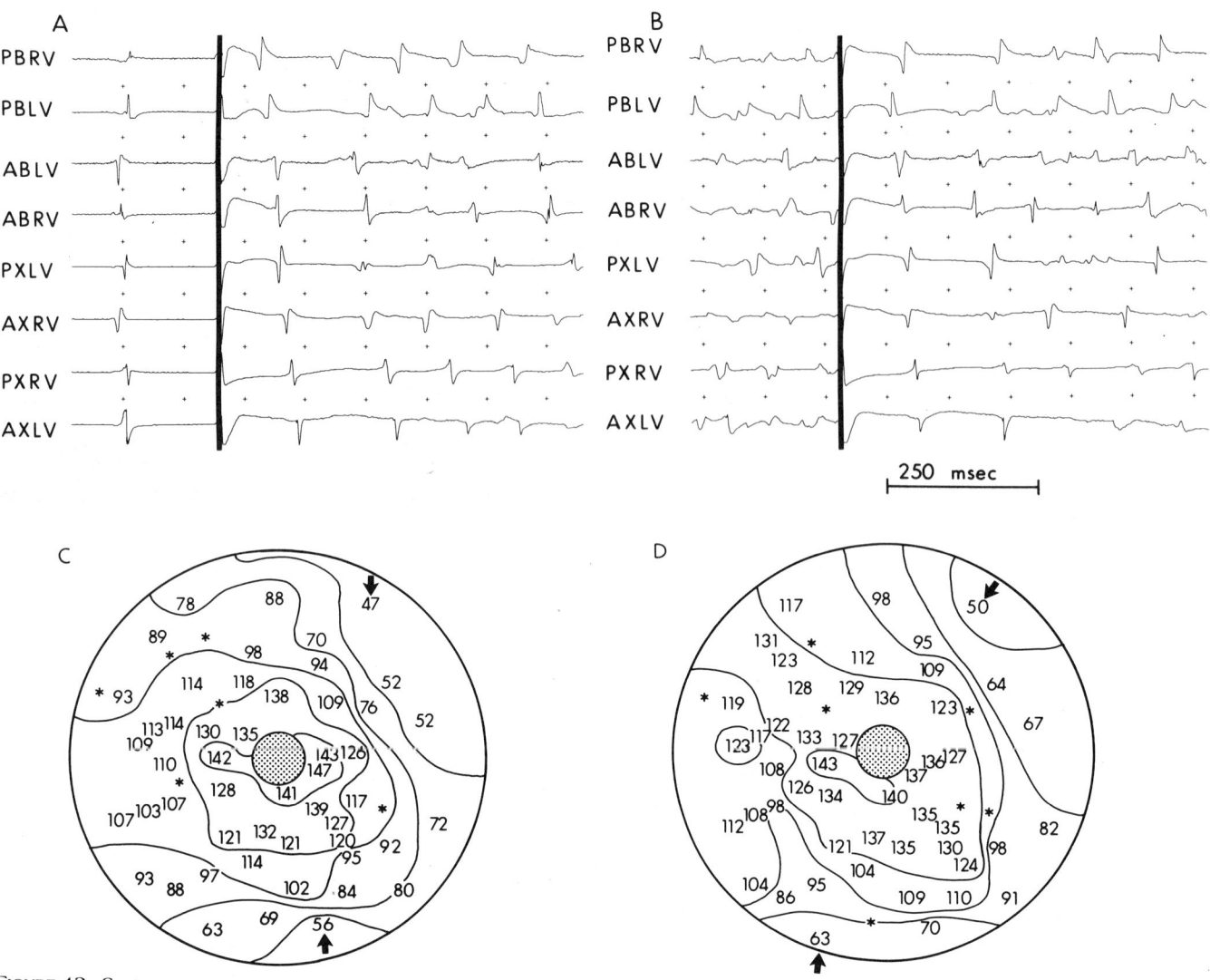

FIGURE 42–6
Examples of recordings and isochronal maps following the largest shock (2 J) that induced fibrillation during the vulnerable period of normal rhythm and the largest shock that failed to defibrillate (2 J) 10 s after the electrical induction of fibrillation in the same dog. Shocks were delivered via electrodes on the left ventricular apex (cathode) and the right atrium (anode). Epicardial electrode recordings taken over both ventricles are shown in A and B. A pause in activation followed both the shock during the vulnerable period (A) and the unsuccessful defibrillation shock (B). Epicardial maps from 56 electrodes are shown in C and D. Polar projections of the ventricles are shown with the stippled apical defibrillation electrode in the center and the atrioventricular groove at the periphery. Numbers represent the locations of electrodes with satisfactory recordings and give the time of activation for those locations in ms from onset of the shock. Asterisks indicate electrode sites where adequate recordings were not obtained. The isochronal lines are 20 ms apart. Earliest activation (arrows) was in the base of the ventricles following the shock during the vulnerable period (C) as well as following the unsuccessful defibrillation shock (D). In both cases, activation conducted toward the apex as large, coherent activation fronts. A = anterior; P = posterior; B = base; X = apex; R = right; L = left; V = ventricle; Lat = lateral. (Reprinted by permission from Shibata N et al.: Am J Physiol 255:H902, 1988.)

graded cycle of latencies surrounds the critical point (which he calls a phase singularity), similar to isochrones spiraling around the center of leading circle reentry. Winfree has used these concepts to explain the behavior of chemical waves that propagate through an excitable medium, the Belousov-Zhabotinsky reagent,[36] and the behavior of cardiac activation following a shock with the Fitzhugh-Nagumo model.[30]

The experimental findings of Frazier et al.[37] closely correspond to the modeling results of Winfree. A leading circle reentry rotor[38] is produced when refractoriness is dispersed uniformly through a myocardial region and a shock is given that creates a range of potential gradients dispersed at an angle to the dispersion of refractoriness. Reentry is thought to be induced because potential gradients higher than a certain critical value cause unidirectional block and prolongation of refractoriness. The center of the reentry rotor is reliably formed where a critical degree of refractoriness intersects this critical level of potential gradient (Fig. 42–7). For a 3-ms monophasic shock of low tilt, this critical point is formed where a shock field of 5 V/cm intersects tissue just coming out of its effective refractory period as determined by a 2-mA stimulus.[37] The

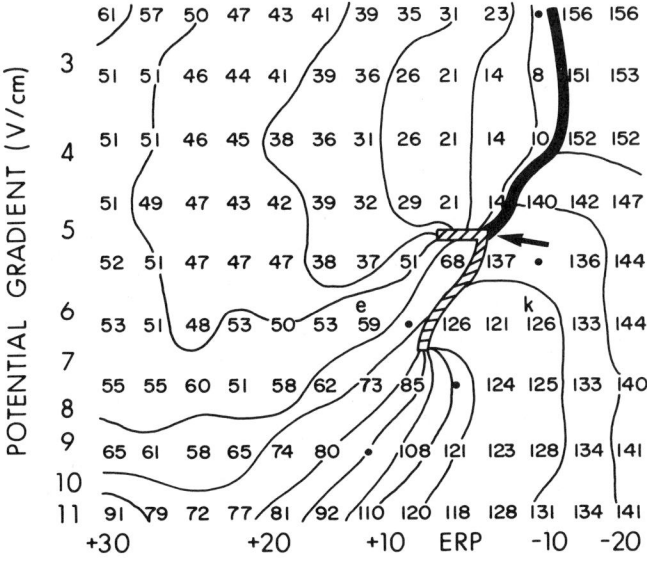

FIGURE 42–7
Isochronal map demonstrating the initiation of reentry and fibrillation around a critical point formed by the orthogonal interaction of refractoriness and the potential gradient field created by a shock. Numbers represent the locations of 117 epicardial recording electrodes covering a 30- by 32-mm area of canine right ventricle and give the time of activation at each electrode in milliseconds after the shock. Tissue refractoriness was uniformly dispersed horizontally, as determined at multiple sites using 2-mA cathodal stimulation. The stage of refractoriness at the time of the shock is given at the bottom of the figure with respect to the effective refractory period (ERP) for the 2-mA stimulus. Tissue to the right is least refractory, tissue to the left is most refractory. The potential gradients created by the 3-ms monophasic shock were uniformly dispersed vertically, as shown to the left of the figure. The thin solid lines represent isochrones after the shock and are spaced 10 ms apart. A rotor of reentry leading to fibrillation was induced, of which only the first cycle is shown. The reentrant circuit was centered about a critical point (arrow) in which refractoriness was approximately equal to the effective refractory period of the tissue and shock strength was approximately 5 V/cm. The thick dashed line represents an area of temporary conduction block, and the thick solid line represents the end of the first cycle of reentry.

critical values will probably be different for other shock waveforms.

Relation to Upper Limit of Vulnerability

The vulnerable region of fibrillation includes all of the S1-S2 intervals and S2 strengths that induce fibrillation.[39-41] The upper limit to the vulnerable region can be explained by the existence of the critical point[30, 31] and by the fact that the potential gradient field decreases with increased distance from the defibrillation electrodes.[13, 14] At the lower limit of vulnerability (i.e., the ventricular fibrillation threshold), fibrillation will be induced when the stimulus becomes so strong that the critical level of potential gradient is just far enough away from the S2 electrode to form the minimum length of block necessary for the induction of reentry (Fig. 42–8, isogradient line a). The formation of a critical point will occur when the critical degree of refractoriness intersects the critical isogradient line. As the stimulus strength is increased, the critical isogradient line moves farther away from the S2 electrode and so increases in length (Fig. 42–8, isogradient line, for example). Because reentry will be induced at all places where the critical isorecovery and isogradient lines intersect, fibrillation can then be induced over a wider range of intervals at sites more distant from the S2 electrode, as previously shown.[28, 42] Stimulation at very long or short coupling intervals will fail to induce fibrillation because the critical isogradient and critical isorecovery lines will not intersect; rather, the critical isogradient line will fall entirely within excitable or refractory tissue. When the S2 strength is further increased so that the critical isogradient line is moved off the base of the ventricles, fibrillation will not occur at any interval, because no critical point will be created (Fig. 42–8, isogradient line i). Thus, an upper limit of vulnerability occurs.

The induction of fibrillation as is normally done with stimulating wires or small catheter electrodes will not show an upper limit of vulnerability, since the stimulus currents are not usually increased so greatly that the potential gradients exceed the critical isogradient level over all of the ventricles. Such extremely high currents from point sources would probably induce severe myocardial damage close to the stimulating wires.[43] The vulnerable region therefore appears open at the top for point stimulation, the pattern traditionally reported.[39, 44]

According to the critical point hypothesis,[30, 31] all S2 strength and S1-S2 interval combinations that result in fibrillation or repetitive responses occur as a result of the intersection of approximately the same critical isorecovery and isogradient lines. Therefore, the sites at which reentry is induced should vary for different S2 strengths and S1-S2 intervals as shown by Shibata et al.[22] This hypothesis accounts for the induction of reentry and the existence of the vulnerable region; however, it does not explain why some reentrant circuits lead to fibrillation while others cause only a few repetitive responses.

Relation to Probability Function of Defibrillation

The defibrillation threshold is not a discrete value; instead, a sigmoidal relationship usually exists between the shock strength and the probability of successful defibrillation (Fig. 42–9).[45, 46] Nonetheless, a single threshold value is frequently used in the study of defibrillation and, depending on chance and on the manner in which it is determined, may be markedly different from the 50% success point of the probability function.[47] A potential gradient of approximately 6 V/cm has been postulated as the minimal field strength required for defibrillation with a 14 ms truncated exponential monophasic waveform.[14] Increasing the shock voltage so that this critical field strength is exceeded over the entire heart produces defibrillation in most cases, whereas decreasing this voltage yields a

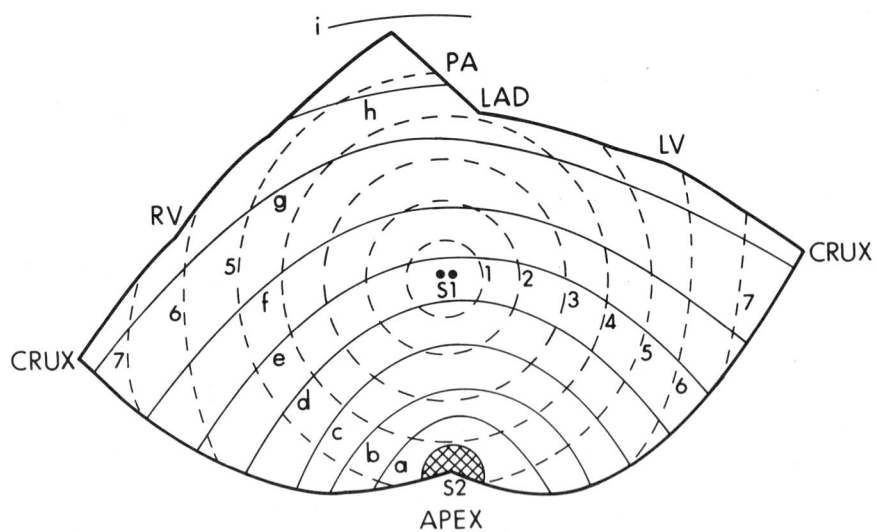

FIGURE 42–8
Critical points, vulnerability, and defibrillation. The epicardial surface of the canine heart is depicted as if the ventricles were folded out after an imaginary cut was made from the crux to the apex. Isorecovery lines (dashed lines 1–7) radiate outward from the site labeled S1. S2 stimuli, or defibrillation shocks, are delivered from the apex of the heart. Isogradient lines (solid lines a–i) radiate outward from the S2 electrode with minimal ventricular values occurring in the small region representing the pulmonary outflow tract. The isogradient line i is located outside the ventricles in the atria. When the S2 voltage is low, so that the critical isogradient line is located at a, a critical point (and thus reentry) will occur near the apex of the heart for those S1-S2 intervals for which the critical isorecovery line crosses line a. When the S2 strength is increased so that the critical isogradient line is at f, a wider range of S1-S2 intervals can create critical points. Increasing the S2 strength so that the critical isogradient line is at i moves all critical points off the ventricles regardless of the S1-S2 interval; thus, an upper limit to vulnerability exists. See text for further discussion. RV = right ventricle; LV = left ventricle; PA = pulmonary artery; LAD = left anterior descending coronary artery.

greater percentage of unsuccessful defibrillation episodes, with earliest activation arising from areas of low-potential gradient. As the shock strength is decreased further, the probability of successful defibrillation continues to decrease in an approximately sigmoidal relationship.[46]

The concept of a critical point, although demonstrated only for the electrical induction of reentry, can be used to explain these findings in a fashion similar to the explanation for the upper limit of ventricular vulnerability. Multiple wavefronts occur on the myocardium at all times during fibrillation,[48] presumably due to the presence of multiple shifting reentrant circuits.[49] Thus, at any one time the critical isorecovery line should also exist in multiple regions. When the shock voltage is high enough that the critical gradient is exceeded over the entire myocardium, a critical point should not occur, regardless of the locations of the critical isorecovery lines (Fig. 42–8, isogradient line i). Because excitation does not conduct away from tissue directly excited by potential gradients greater than the critical gradient,[37] all activation fronts will be halted, no new fronts will be created by the shock field, and defibrillation will occur. Thus, 100% successful defibrillation should occur when the potential gradients over both ventricles exceed the critical gradient.

Decreasing the shock voltage so that the critical isogradient line occurs on the ventricles creates the possibility that, depending on the distribution of refractoriness at the time of the shock, the critical isogradient line can intersect a critical isorecovery line, creating a critical point. Thus, reentry rotors can be induced and lead to refibrillation, even though all fibrillatory activation fronts are extinguished by the shock. For shocks of slightly lower energy than the 100% successful shock, a high probability of success continues to exist. These shocks presumably produce the critical isogradient line in very small areas of myocardium in which the probability that the critical degree of refractoriness will be present is small (Fig. 42–8, isogradient line h).

As the shock voltage is further decreased, progressively larger areas of myocardium will contain the critical isogradient value, yielding a higher probability that the critical isogradient line will intersect myocardium at the critical degree of refractoriness, creating a critical point and, hence, reentry. Low probabilities of successful defibrillation occur when the critical isogradient line falls in such a large volume of myocardium that it usually intersects the critical isorecovery line (Fig. 42–8, isogradient line g). Thus, successful defibrillation depends on avoidance of the creation of critical points, best accomplished by increasing the shock

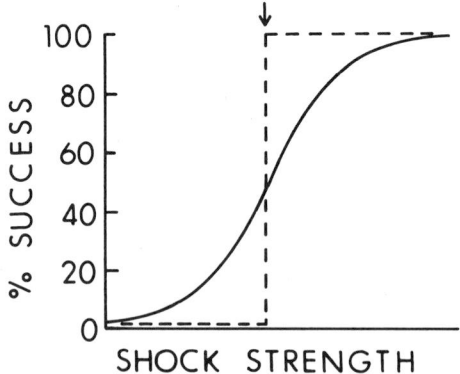

FIGURE 42–9
The probability curve for defibrillation. There is not a discrete defibrillation threshold (dashed line), above which all shocks succeed and below which all shocks fail. Rather, a dose-response type of curve usually exists (solid line), in which greater shock strengths are associated with greater percentages of success. (Modified by permission of the C.V. Mosby Co. from Davy JM, et al.: Am Heart J 113:77, 1987.)

voltage to exceed the critical potential gradient over the entire myocardium.

This explanation may not hold true for infarcted, ischemic, or diseased myocardium. In these instances anatomic obstacles or inherent disparities in refractoriness may exist prior to the application of the stimulus and may create the conditions necessary to initiate reentry independent of the interaction of critical isorecovery and isogradient lines. However, although some controversy exists, defibrillation thresholds appear to be similar for normal, acutely ischemic, and chronically infarcted myocardium,[3, 50, 51] suggesting that the critical point concept applies also to abnormal myocardium. Further studies are necessary to validate this concept for the induction of fibrillation as well as defibrillation in normal, ischemic, and infarcted myocardium. The critical point concept, by itself, does not totally account for the probability function for defibrillation, because it does not explain why a few cycles of rapid activation frequently follow successful defibrillation shocks.[6, 21, 52] The reason why these activation fronts sometimes stop spontaneously and at other times continue on to reinduce fibrillation may be similar to the reason why activation following shocks during the vulnerable period of normal rhythm sometimes stops following a few repetitive responses and other times lead to fibrillation. An additional point not explained by the critical point concept is why only a portion of the activation sequences seen after the initiation of fibrillation during the vulnerable period[22] and after unsuccessful defibrillation shocks[23, 29] demonstrate reentry rotors; the majority appear focal.

BIPHASIC WAVEFORMS

Many different waveforms have been tested for defibrillation.[53] Several investigators have found that biphasic waveforms, in which polarity is reversed during the shock (Fig. 42–10), are more efficient for defibrillation than monophasic waveforms of the same (or for one half of the) total duration in both animals and humans.[4, 54–62] Some biphasic waveforms are much better for defibrillation than others. Schuder et al.[63] were able to defibrillate calves with symmetric biphasic shocks (Fig. 42–10B) at a lower range of energy and current and to achieve a higher percentage of successful first-shock defibrillations than with monophasic waveforms. The same investigators found that asymmetric biphasic waveforms in which the amplitude of the second phase was smaller than the first (Fig. 42–10C) defibrillated at lower energy than waveforms with the second phase larger than the first.[58] Jones and Jones[59] reported that biphasic waveforms with the second phase smaller than the first also decreased post-shock dysfunction in cultured myocardial cells. Biphasic waveforms have been tested in which the duration of the two phases is asymmetric.[4, 62] Waveforms in which the second phase is shorter than or equal to the first (Fig. 42–10D) defibrillate at much lower energy, current, and voltage than waveforms in which the second phase is longer than the first. In fact, biphasic waveforms with the second phase longer than the first are frequently worse for defibrillation than monophasic waveforms of the same total duration. It has recently been suggested that triphasic waveforms (Fig. 42–10E) are even better for defibrillation than biphasic waveforms.[64] Thus, the number, amplitude, and duration of the phases of a shock waveform may all influence defibrillation efficacy.

Role of Decreased Impedance

There are several possible reasons why some biphasic waveforms are more efficacious than a monophasic waveform of the same total duration. For truncated exponential waveforms, impedance across the defibrillation electrodes increases throughout a monophasic shock and throughout both phases of a biphasic shock, whereas impedance decreases immediately following the switch in polarity of the biphasic waveform.[62] Hence, one possible explanation for the increased efficacy of the biphasic waveform could be decreased impedance. However, the decrease of impedance is not sufficient to account for all of the improved efficacy of biphasic compared to monophasic waveforms. The increased efficacy of the biphasic waveform in terms of voltage and energy is greater than that caused by the decrease in impedance, and the biphasic waveform also requires less current for defibrillation,[62] which should be independent of impedance.[65] Decreased impedance also cannot explain why biphasic waveforms with the second phase longer than the first are less effective than monophasic waveforms of the same total duration in spite of the decrease in impedance.

Effect on Sodium Channel Reactivation

Another possible reason for the increased efficacy of biphasic waveforms is that the first phase reactivates sodium channels in the myocardial membrane so that the cells can be excited by the second phase. Jones et al.[66] compared biphasic to monophasic waveforms and found that biphasic waveforms exhibited a lower exci-

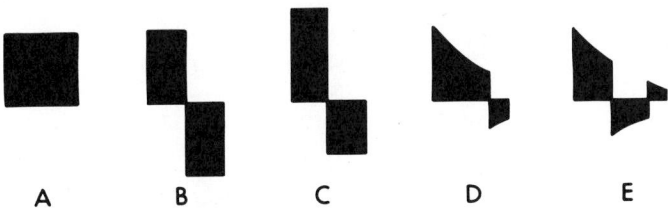

FIGURE 42–10
Biphasic waveforms. Time is plotted horizontally and shock strength is plotted vertically. A shows a monophasic rectangular waveform. B illustrates a symmetrical biphasic rectangular waveform of the same duration. C shows an asymmetric biphasic rectangular waveform in which the amplitude of the first phase is greater than that of the second, with both phases of the same duration. D shows an asymmetric truncated exponential biphasic waveform in which the first phase is both longer and higher than the second. E illustrates a triphasic rectangular waveform in which the amplitude of the third phase is smaller than that of the first two.

tation threshold in chick embryo myocardial cells bathed in a high potassium solution to inactivate sodium channels. Sodium channels may be totally or partially inactivated during fibrillation, because the resting potential has been reported to be reduced to about minus 60 mV during ventricular fibrillation induced by reperfusion.[67] Jones and coworkers[66] hypothesized that the first phase of the biphasic waveform acts as a "conditioning" pulse, causing hyperpolarization of some portions of the heart. The first pulse may reactivate the sodium channels by bringing the transmembrane potential in these portions of the heart closer to the normal resting potential. The second phase, which depolarizes these portions of the heart, may then be able to excite the cells, thus lowering the excitation threshold. If excitation of myocardium is the determining factor for defibrillation as hypothesized by the total extinction and critical mass theories, then the defibrillation threshold should also be lowered.

This explanation for the increased efficacy of bipolar defibrillation waveforms can be extended to incorporate the concept of discontinuous intracellular conductivity. The presence of discontinuous intracellular conductivity implies that when an extracellular current is applied to the heart, cells more than a few space constants away from the electrodes experience both positive and negative transmembrane potentials, the end closer to the anode being hyperpolarized while the end closer to the cathode being depolarized.[68, 69] Thus, according to the explanation of Jones et al., the first or conditioning phase will hyperpolarize one end of most cells, bringing the transmembrane potential of that end of the cell to a more normal value. The second phase, which will depolarize that portion of the cell, will then be more likely to excite it.

Effect on Refractory Period Duration

A third possible mechanism for the increased efficacy of biphasic shocks is shortening of the refractory period due to the hyperpolarization of the transmembrane potential caused by the first phase. Cells that are refractory at the time of the shock may not be depolarized by the first phase of the waveform. Nonetheless, the first phase may still affect the cells by changing the duration of their refractory periods, as described by Cranefield and Hoffman.[70] A hyperpolarizing pulse during phase 2 of the action potential shortens the refractory period, so that a depolarizing pulse applied immediately afterward can activate the cell. The biphasic waveform may have the same action.

As discussed previously, the first phase of the biphasic shock may hyperpolarize one end of most cells and depolarize the other end.[68, 69] At the hyperpolarized end, refractoriness may be decreased sufficiently so that the second phase, which depolarizes this end of the cell, may then cause excitation. Cranefield and Hoffman[70] also showed that a depolarizing pulse during some portions of the refractory period had an effect opposite to that of a hyperpolarizing pulse, (i.e., prolonging refractoriness). Therefore, at the other end, where the depolarizing effect is maximum during the first phase of the biphasic shock, refractoriness may be prolonged. Thus, the effect of the biphasic shock on refractoriness is complex and may or may not be the reason for the improved defibrillation efficacy.

Critical Point for Biphasic vs. Monophasic Waveforms

Yet a fourth possible explanation for the increased defibrillation efficacy of biphasic waveforms is that the critical point is different than for monophasic waveforms. As previously discussed, the minimum potential gradient for 100% successful defibrillation should be slightly higher than the critical point; otherwise, critical points could occur in the ventricles and reinitiate reentry and fibrillation. It has been shown that the upper limit of vulnerability is lower for a biphasic truncated exponential waveform with both phases equal than for a monophasic waveform of the same total duration.[72] Based on the critical point concept, the increased efficacy of biphasic shocks may be due to (1) differences in the strength-interval curves for biphasic and monophasic waveforms,[71–73] (2) different locations of critical points for biphasic and monophasic waveforms on the strength-interval plot, or (3) changes in the characteristics of the reentrant circuits caused by differences in the durations of prolongation of refractoriness and block and by differences in conduction velocity.

Strength-Duration Curves of Biphasic vs. Monophasic Waveforms

Depending on the wave shape of the shock, the strength-duration curve in terms of current for defibrillation with a monophasic waveform is hyperbolic for shock durations ranging from 12 to 40 ms (Fig. 42–11),[74–77] similar to the shape of the strength-duration curve for stimulation of nonfibrillating, fully recovered

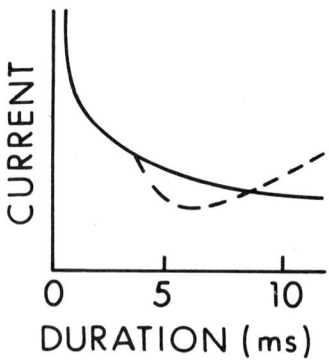

FIGURE 42–11
Strength-duration curves for defibrillation. Current requirements for defibrillation with rectangular monophasic waveforms are very high for shocks of short duration but rapidly decrease toward an asymptote as shock duration is increased up to 40 ms (solid line). For defibrillation with a truncated exponential biphasic waveform in which the first phase is held constant at 3.5 ms, current decreases as shock duration is increased until the second phase approximately equals the first (7 ms), but then increases (dashed line).

myocardium.[78] For monophasic shocks longer than 12 to 40 ms, the strength required for defibrillation increases, causing Schuder and colleagues[79] to hypothesize that these longer shocks, particularly when the tail has low-amplitude (e.g., untruncated exponential or negatively ramping triangular) pulses, are more likely to reinduce fibrillation.[79] In contrast, for biphasic shocks, as shock duration is increased by prolonging the second phase while holding the first phase constant at 3.5 ms, the shock current required for defibrillation first decreases, as for the monophasic waveform, but soon begins to increase (see Fig. 42–11).[62]

There are several possible reasons for this shape of the strength-duration curve. One possible explanation is that the trailing edge of the second phase activates fibrillating myocardium by "break" excitation.[80, 81] Since the trailing edge of the second phase of a truncated exponential waveform becomes smaller with increasing duration of this phase, the shock strength required for defibrillation should increase, as has been observed. While break excitation is most commonly discussed for hyperpolarizing stimulation, under certain conditions depolarizing break stimulation can also occur.[82] Thus, this explanation may not necessarily conflict with the concept that the second phase activates tissue by depolarization, which, as discussed above, is an integral part of the hypotheses of sodium channel reactivation or of refractory period shortening by a hyperpolarizing first phase.[66]

Biphasic waveforms in which the first phase is longer than the second phase defibrillate much more efficiently than waveforms with the first phase shorter than the second when both waveforms are of the same total duration.[4, 62] Therefore, other factors besides the trailing edge of the second phase must also be important for defibrillation, since the two biphasic waveforms have the same total duration and, hence, the same trailing edge voltage for the second phase. These two waveforms also have the same leading edge voltage for the first phase and both deliver the same total amount of charge. The charge delivered during each polarity of the two phases is different, however. When the duration of the first phase is held constant while the duration of the second phase is lengthened, the charge delivered by the second phase is increased. If the total charge delivered is more important than the size of the trailing edge for the excitation of fibrillating myocardium, then, as the second phase is lengthened, the ability of the shock to activate tissue should increase, not decrease. Although the previous statements in this paragraph are paradoxical with respect to the total extinction and critical mass hypotheses of defibrillation, they are consistent with the upper limit of vulnerability hypothesis. Even though biphasic shocks with a longer second phase may be better able to halt the activation fronts of fibrillation, they may also be better able to give rise to new activation fronts that reinitiate fibrillation. This argument suggests that for less efficient biphasic waveforms with a longer second phase duration, the upper limit of vulnerability (i.e., the highest shock strength giving rise to activation fronts that induce fibrillation) should be greater than for biphasic shocks with a shorter second phase. Thus, biphasic waveforms with a shorter second phase would have lower defibrillation thresholds than biphasic waveforms with a longer second phase. This suggestion has not yet been tested experimentally.

EFFECTS OF VERY HIGH-POTENTIAL GRADIENTS ON THE HEART

In addition to the salubrious effects of stimulation, defibrillation, and cardioversion, electrical fields can have detrimental effects on the heart if the potential gradient is too high. If a very strong shock is given that is much greater than the upper limit of vulnerability, ventricular fibrillation can be induced at any time during the cardiac cycle, not just during the vulnerable period.[26, 27] This response is probably due to myocardial damage caused by the large magnitude of the shock field.[83] Strong shocks can produce loss of potassium from myocardial fibers, decrease conduction velocity, prolong depolarization, and cause neurostimulation of both cholinergic and adrenergic fibers.[84-87] At slightly higher levels of shock strength, decreased cardiac function, cessation of conduction, and inhibition of pacemaker cells occur.[85, 88, 89] At still higher strengths, frank necrosis of myocardium is observed.[90]

The potential gradient and current density levels have been determined at which some of these detrimental effects occur. Niebauer and associates[91] have reported that, for a 10-ms truncated exponential monophasic waveform, a 50% decrease in left ventricular systolic pressure is caused by a shock field strength of approximately 200 mA/cm^2. Jones et al.[88] found that inhibition of pacemaker cells in clusters of chick embryo cells occurs for 4 seconds with monophasic waveforms at approximately 80 V/cm. This value is different for different types of biphasic waveforms.[59] Conduction block occurs at approximately 70 V/cm for a monophasic waveform.[92] Ventricular tachycardia arises from regions with gradients of 100 to 200 V/cm.[14]

Strong defibrillation shocks can prolong depolarization and prevent activation for seconds to minutes.[86, 93] Dudel[93] has hypothesized that this paralysis of myocardium is the mechanism of defibrillation. This prolonged depolarization may be caused by alterations in intracellular ionic concentrations created by holes in the cell membrane, which Jones et al.[83] found to occur at potential gradients of 200 V/cm applied to in vitro chick embryo myocytes. Since defibrillation requires a much smaller potential gradient than this,[14, 94] and since activation is normally observed within a fraction of a second following a defibrillation shock,[21] electrical paralysis is not the usual mechanism of defibrillation. In fact, electrical paralysis is probably harmful, decreasing wall motion and possibly inducing arrhythmias. Assuming such paralysis is detrimental, Jones and coworkers[64] proposed use of a triphasic waveform for defibrillation, in which the third phase is smaller than the first two, since this third "healing" phase reduces the duration of electrical quiescence of high gradient shocks. Limited studies to date have not found that the defibrillation threshold is lower for triphasic shocks than for biphasic shocks.[4, 95] However, this does not rule out the possibility that suprathreshold defibrillation shocks are less likely to induce tachyarrhythmias or refibrillate the heart if they are triphasic.

Conclusions

Many of the ideas discussed in this chapter are speculative. The true mechanism of defibrillation is not yet definitely known. Knowledge is advancing quickly about defibrillation, and the information in this chapter probably will soon be out of date. Adding to the excitement of this area is the steady improvement being made in the shock strength required for defibrillation with implantable devices.[2-4]

Acknowledgment

This chapter is an expanded version of a paper presented at the Tenth Annual Conference of the IEEE Engineering in Medicine and Biology Society.[96]

References

1. Mirowski M: The automatic implantable cardioverter-defibrillator: An overview. J Am Coll Cardiol 6:461, 1985.
2. Jones DL, Klein GJ, Guiraudon GM, et al.: Internal cardiac defibrillation in man: Pronounced improvement with sequential pulse delivery to two different lead orientations. Circulation 73:484, 1986.
3. Chang MS, Inoue H, Kallok MJ, et al.: Double and triple sequential shocks reduce ventricular defibrillation threshold in dogs with and without myocardial infarction. J Am Coll Cardiol 8:1393, 1986.
4. Dixon EG, Tang ASL, Wolf PD, et al.: Improved defibrillation thresholds with large contoured epicardial electrodes and biphasic waveforms. Circulation 76:1176, 1987.
5. Wiggers CJ: The physiologic basis for cardiac resuscitation from ventricular fibrillation—Method for serial defibrillation. Am Heart J 20:413, 1940.
6. Zipes DP, Fischer J, King RM, et al.: Termination of ventricular fibrillation in dogs by depolarizing a critical amount of myocardium. Am J Cardiol 36:37, 1975.
7. Smith WM, Ideker RE: Computer techniques for epicardial and endocardial mapping. Prog Cardiovasc Dis 26:15, 1983.
8. El-Sherif N, Gough WB, Restivo M: Reentrant ventricular arrhythmias in the late myocardial infarction period: 14. Mechanisms of resetting, entrainment, acceleration, or termination of reentrant tachycardia by programmed electrical stimulation. PACE 10:341, 1987.
9. Wit AL, Allessie MA, Bonke FIM, et al.: Electrophysiologic mapping to determine the mechanism of experimental ventricular tachycardia initiated by premature impulses: Experimental approach and initial results demonstrating reentrant excitation. Am J Cardiol 49:166, 1982.
10. Pogwizd SM, Corr PB: Reentrant and nonreentrant mechanisms contribute to arrhythmogenesis during early myocardial ischemia: Results using three-dimensional mapping. Circ Res 61:352, 1987.
11. Wolf PD, Rollins DL, Smith WM, et al.: A cardiac mapping system for the quantitative study of internal defibrillation. Proceedings of the Tenth Annual Conference of the IEEE Engineering in Medicine and Biology Society. 1988, pp. 208–209.
12. Witkowski FX, Penkoske PA: Simultaneous cardiac potential field and direct cardiac recordings during ventricular defibrillation (DF) (Abstract). Circulation 76:IV-108, 1987.
13. Chen P-S, Wolf PD, Claydon FJ, et al.: The potential gradient field created by epicardial defibrillation electrodes in dogs. Circulation 74:626, 1986.
14. Wharton JM, Wolf PD, Chen P-S, et al.: Is an absolute minimum potential gradient required for ventricular defibrillation? (Abstract). Circulation 74:II-342, 1986.
15. Tang ASL, Wolf PD, Claydon FJ III, et al.: Measurement of defibrillation shock potential distributions and activation sequences of the heart in three dimensions. Proc. IEEE 76:1176, 1988.
16. Lepeschkin E, Jones JL, Rush S, et al.: Local potential gradients as a unifying measure for thresholds of stimulation, standstill, tachyarrhythmia and fibrillation appearing after strong capacitor discharges. Adv Cardiol 21:268, 1978.
17. Laxer C, Ideker RE, Smith WM, et al.: Computer acquisition of a database for relating myocardial infarct geometry to cardiac electrical potentials. In Ripley KL, Ostrow HG (eds.): Proceedings of Computers in Cardiology, pp. 339–342. Los Angeles, IEEE Computer Society, 1980.
18. El-Sherif N, Smith RA, Evans K: Canine ventricular arrhythmias in the late myocardial infarction period. 8. Epicardial mapping of reentrant circuits. Circ Res 49:255, 1981.
19. Wiggers CJ: The mechanism and nature of ventricular defibrillation. Am Heart J 20:399, 1940.
20. Lown B: Electrical reversion of cardiac arrhythmias. Br Heart J 29:469, 1976.
21. Chen P-S, Shibata N, Dixon EG, et al.: Activation during ventricular defibrillation in open-chest dogs: Evidence of complete cessation and regeneration of ventricular fibrillation after unsuccessful shocks. J Clin Invest 77:810, 1986.
22. Shibata N, Chen P-S, Dixon EG, et al.: Influence of shock strength and timing on induction of ventricular arrhythmias in dogs. Am J Physiol 255:H891, 1988.
23. Chen P-S, Wolf PD, Bowling SD, et al.: Mechanism of failure of subthreshold defibrillation shocks (Abstract). J Am Coll Cardiol 9:94A, 1987.
24. Chen P-S, Shibata N, Wolf PD, et al.: Epicardial activation during successful and unsuccessful ventricular defibrillation in open chest dogs. Cardiovasc Rev Rep 7:625, 1986.
25. Orias O, Brooks CM, Suckling EE, et al.: Excitability of the mammalian ventricle throughout the cardiac cycle. Am J Physiol 163:272, 1950.
26. Fabiato A, Coumel P, Gourgon R, et al.: Le seuil de reponse synchrone des fibres myocardiques. Application à la comparaison expérimentale de l'efficacité des différentes formes de chocs électriques de défibrillation. Arch Mal Coeur 60:527, 1967.
27. Lesigne C, Levy B, Saumont R, et al.: An energy-time analysis of ventricular fibrillation and defibrillation thresholds with internal electrodes. Med Biol Eng 14:617, 1976.
28. Chen P-S, Shibata N, Dixon EG, et al.: Comparison of the defibrillation threshold and the upper limit of ventricular vulnerability. Circulation 73:1022, 1986.
29. Shibata N, Chen P-S, Dixon EG, et al.: Epicardial activation following unsuccessful defibrillation shocks in dogs. Am J Physiol 255:H902, 1988.
30. Winfree AT: When Time Breaks Down: The three-dimensional dynamics of electrochemical waves and cardiac arrhythmias, pp. 261–288. Princeton, Princeton University Press, 1987.
31. Winfree AT: Sudden cardiac death. Sci Am 248:144, 1983.
32. Winfree AT: Unclocklike behavior of biological clocks. Nature 253:315, 1975.
33. Jalife J, Slenter VAJ, Salata JJ, et al.: Dynamic vagal control of pacemaker activity in the mammalian sinoatrial node. Circ Res 52:642, 1983.
34. Jalife J, Antzelevitch C: Phase resetting and annihilation of pacemaker activity in cardiac tissue. Science 206:696, 1979.
35. Antzelevitch C, Moe GK: Electronic inhibition and summation of impulse conduction in mammalian sinoatrial node. Am J Physiol 245:H42, 1983.
36. Winfree AT: Spiral waves of chemical activity. Science 175:634, 1972.
37. Frazier DW, Wolf PD, Wharton JM, et al.: A stimulus induced critical point: A mechanism for electrical initiation of reentry in normal canine myocardium. J Clin Invest 83:1039, 1989.
38. Allessie MA, Bonke FIM, Schopman FJG: Circus movement in rabbit atrial muscle as a mechanism of tachycardia. III. The "leading circle" concept: A new model of circus movement in cardiac tissue without the involvement of an anatomical obstacle. Circ Res 41:9, 1977.

39. Hoffman BF, Gorin EF, Wax FS, et al.: Vulnerability to fibrillation and the ventricular-excitability curve. Am J Physiol 167:88, 1951.
40. King BG: The effect of electric shock on heart action with special reference to varying susceptibility in different parts of the cardiac cycle. PhD Thesis, Columbia University, 1934.
41. Wiggers CJ, Wegria R: Ventricular fibrillation due to single, localized induction and condenser shocks applied during the vulnerable phase of ventricular systole. Am J Physiol 128:500, 1940.
42. Shibata N, Chen P-S, Dixon EG, et al.: Epicardial mapping of the initiation of ventricular fibrillation by shocks during the vulnerable period (Abstract). J Am Coll Cardiol 7:183A, 1986.
43. Gaum WE, Elharrar V, Walker PD, et al.: Influence of excitability on the ventricular fibrillation threshold in dogs. Am J Cardiol 40:929, 1977.
44. Hoffman BF, Suckling EE, Brooks CM: Vulnerability of the dog ventricle and effects of defibrillation. Circ Res 3:147, 1955.
45. Gold JH, Schuder JC, Stoeckle H: Contour graph for relating per cent success in achieving ventricular defibrillation to duration, current, and energy content of shock. Am Heart J 98:207, 1979.
46. Davy JM, Fain ES, Dorian P, et al.: The relationship between successful defibrillation and delivered energy in open-chest dogs: Reappraisal of the "defibrillation threshold" concept. Am Heart J 113:77, 1987.
47. McDaniel WC, Schuder JC: The cardiac ventricular defibrillation threshold: Inherent limitations in its application and interpretation. Med Instrum 21:170, 1987.
48. Ideker RE, Klein GJ, Harrison L, et al.: The transition to ventricular fibrillation induced by reperfusion following acute ischemia in the dog: A period of organized epicardial activation. Circulation 63:1371, 1981.
49. Moe GK, Rheinboldt WC, Abildskov JA: A computer model of atrial fibrillation. Am Heart J 67:200, 1964.
50. Jones DL, Sohla A, Klein GJ: Internal cardiac defibrillation threshold: Effects of acute ischemia. PACE 9:322, 1986.
51. Wharton JM, Richard VJ, Murray CE, et al.: Effect of chronic myocardial infarction on defibrillation (Abstract). Circulation 76:IV-108, 1987.
52. Mower MM, Mirowski M, Spear JF, et al.: Patterns of ventricular activity during catheter defibrillation. Circulation 49:858, 1974.
53. Tacker WA Jr, Geddes LA: Electrical Defibrillation, pp. 59–89. Boca Raton, Florida, CRC Press, 1980.
54. Jude JR, Kouwenhoven WB, Knickerbockir GG: An experimental and clinical study of a portable external cardiac defibrillator. Surgical Forum 13:185, 1962.
55. Gurvich NL, Markarychev VA: Defibrillation of the heart with biphasic electrical impulses. Kardiologiia 7:109, 1967.
56. Schuder JC, Stoeckle H, Dolan AM: Transthoracic ventricular defibrillation with square-wave stimuli: one-half cycle, one cycle, and multicycle waveforms. Circ Res 15:258, 1964.
57. Jones JL, Jones RE: Improved defibrillator waveform safety factor with biphasic waveforms. Am J Physiol 245:H60, 1983.
58. Schuder JC, McDaniel WC, Stoeckle H: Defibrillation of 100-kg calves with asymmetrical, bidirectional, rectangular pulses. Cardiovasc Res 18:419, 1984.
59. Jones JL, Jones RE: Decreased defibrillator-induced dysfunction with biphasic rectangular waveforms. Am J Physiol 247:H792, 1984.
60. Winkle RA, Mead RH, Ruder MA, et al.: Improved low energy defibrillation efficacy in man using a biphasic truncated exponential waveform (Abstract). J Am Coll Cardiol 9:142A, 1987.
61. Chapman PD, Wetherbee JN, Vetter JW, et al.: Comparison of monophasic, biphasic, and triphasic truncated pulses for nonthoracotomy internal defibrillation (Abstract). J Am Coll Cardiol 11:57A, 1988.
62. Tang ASL, Yabe S, Wharton JM, et al.: Ventricular defibrillation using biphasic waveforms: The importance of phasic duration. J Am Coll Cardiol 13:207, 1989.
63. Schuder JC, Gold JH, Stoeckle H, et al.: Transthoracic ventricular defibrillation in the 100 kg calf with symmetrical one-cycle bidirectional rectangular wave stimuli. IEEE Trans Biomed Eng BME-30:415, 1983.
64. Jones JL, Balasky G, Jones RE: Triphasic defibrillator waveforms decrease arrhythmias in myocardial cells (Abstract). Circulation 74:II-185, 1986.
65. Lerman BB, Halperin HR, Tsitlik JE, et al.: Relationship between canine transthoracic impedance and defibrillation threshold: Evidence for current-based defibrillation. J Clin Invest 80:797, 1987.
66. Jones JL, Jones RE, Balasky G: Improved cardiac cell excitation with symmetrical biphasic defibrillator waveforms. Am J Physiol 253:H1418, 1987.
67. Akiyama T: Intracellular recording of in situ ventricular cells during ventricular fibrillation. Am J Physiol 140:H465, 1981.
68. Plonsey R, Barr RC: Effect of microscopic and macroscopic discontinuities on the response of cardiac tissue to defibrillating (stimulating) currents. Med Biol Eng Comput 24:130, 1986.
69. Krassowska W, Pilkington TC, Ideker RE: Periodic conductivity as a mechanism for cardiac stimulation and defibrillation. IEEE Trans Biomed Eng BME-34:555, 1987.
70. Cranefield PF, Hoffman BF: Propagated repolarization in heart muscle. J Gen Physiol 41:633, 1958.
71. Kavanagh KM, Duff HJ, Clark R, et al.: Decreased energy requirements for cardiac pacing using biphasic stimulation (Abstract). Circulation 76:IV-242, 1987.
72. Wharton JM, Frazier DW, Ideker RE: Electrophysiologic effects in vivo of biphasic and monophasic stimuli (Abstract). J Am Coll Cardiol 11:144A, 1988.
73. Daubert JP, Frazier DW, Tang ASL, et al.: Biphasic shocks excite refractory myocardium less effectively than monophasic shocks (Abstract). PACE 11:503, 1988.
74. Geddes LA, Tacker WA Jr, McFarlane J, et al.: Strength-duration curves for ventricular defibrillation in dogs. Circ Res 27:551, 1970.
75. Bourland JD, Tacker WA Jr, Geddes LA: Strength-duration curves for trapezoidal waveforms of various tilts for transchest defibrillation in animals. Med Instrum 12:38, 1978.
76. Koning G, Schneider H, Hoelen AJ: Amplitude-duration relation for direct ventricular defibrillation with rectangular current pulses. Med Biol Eng 13:388, 1975.
77. Chapman PD, Wetherbee JN, Vetter JW, et al.: Strength-duration curves of fixed pulse width variable tilt truncated exponential waveforms for nonthoracotomy internal defibrillation in dogs. PACE 11:1045, 1988.
78. Brooks CM, Hoffman BF, Suckling EE, et al.: Excitability of the Heart, pp. 66–97. New York, Grune and Stratton, 1955.
79. Schuder JC, Rahmoeller GA, Stoeckle H: Transthoracic ventricular defibrillation with triangular and trapezoidal waveforms. Circ Res 19:689, 1966.
80. Cranefield PF, Hoffman BF, Siebens AA: Anodal excitation of cardiac muscle. Am J Physiol 190:383, 1957.
81. Negovsky VA, Gurvich NL, Tabak VY, et al.: The nature of electric defibrillation of the heart. Resuscitation 2:255, 1973.
82. Dekker E: Direct current make and break thresholds for pacemaker electrodes on the canine ventricle. Circ Res 27:811, 1970.
83. Jones JL, Proskauer CC, Paull WK, et al.: Ultrastructural injury to chick myocardial cells in vitro following "electric countershock." Circ Res 46:387, 1980.
84. Arnsdorf MF, Rothbaum DA, Childers RW: Effect of direct current countershock on atrial and ventricular electrophysiological properties and myocardial potassium efflux in the thoracotomised dog. Cardiovasc Res 11:324, 1977.
85. Koning G, Veefkind AH, Schneider H: Cardiac damage caused by direct application of defibrillation shock to isolated Langendorff-perfused rabbit heart. Am Heart J 100:473, 1980.
86. Moore EN, Spear JF: Electrophysiologic studies on the initiation, prevention, and termination of ventricular fibrillation. In Zipes DP, Jalife J (eds.): Cardiac Electrophysiology and Arrhythmias, pp. 315–322. Orlando, Grune and Stratton, 1985.
87. Peleska B: Cardiac arrhythmias following condenser discharges and their dependence upon strength of current and phase of cardiac cycle. Circ Res 13:21, 1963.
88. Jones JL, Lepeschkin E, Jones RE, et al.: Response of cultured myocardial cells to countershock-type electric field stimulation. Am J Physiol 235:H214, 1978.
89. Pansegrau DG, Abboud FM: Hemodynamic effects of ventricular defibrillation. J Clin Invest 49:282, 1970.
90. Dahl CF, Ewy GA, Warner ED, et al.: Myocardial necrosis from direct current countershock. Effect of paddle size and time interval between discharge. Circulation 50:956, 1974.

91. Niebauer MJ, Babbs CF, Geddes LA, et al.: Efficacy and safety of the reciprocal pulse defibrillator current waveform. Med Biol Eng in Comput 22:28, 1984.
92. Yabe S, Daubert JP, Wolf PD, et al.: Effect of strong shock fields on activation propagation near defibrillation electrodes (Abstract). Circulation 78:II-154, 1988.
93. Dudel J: Elektrophysiologische grundlagen der defibrillation und künstlichen stimulation des herzens. Med Klin 52:2089, 1968.
94. Zhou X, Daubert JP, Wolf PD, et al.: The potential gradient for defibrillation (Abstract). Circulation 78:II-645, 1988.
95. Chapman PD, Wetherbee JN, Vetter JW, et al.: Comparison of monophasic, biphasic, and triphasic truncated pulses for nonthoracotomy internal defibrillation (Abstract) J Am Coll Cardiol 11:57, 1988.
96. Ideker RE, Wharton JM, Shibata N, et al.: The mechanism of ventricular defibrillation. Proceedings of the Tenth Annual Conference of the IEEE Engineering in Medicine and Biology Society, 1988, pp. 210–211.

43

Cardioversion and Defibrillation: Clinical Aspects

William M. Miles
Douglas P. Zipes

A variety of cardiac tachyarrhythmias can be safely terminated using a transthoracic electrical discharge,[1-3] offering obvious advantages over drug therapy to terminate tachycardias in many situations. Under conditions optimal for close supervision and monitoring, a regulated "dose" of electricity can restore sinus rhythm immediately and safely. The distinction between supraventricular and ventricular tachyarrhythmias, crucial to the proper medical management of arrhythmias, becomes less significant, and the time-consuming titration of drugs with potential side effects is abolished. In addition, defibrillation can be performed by paramedical personnel with relatively little training. Rapid defibrillation of patients with out-of-hospital cardiac arrest has been associated with their increased survival in reaching the hospital and being discharged.[4-6] The dramatic impact of the automatic internal cardioverter defibrillator on survival emphasizes the importance of rapid electrical defibrillation of ventricular tachyarrhythmias.[7,8] Electrical defibrillation has allowed the evolution of a variety of invasive cardiac procedures (including diagnostic cardiac catheterization, electrophysiologic testing, coronary arteriography, and angioplasty) that could not be performed safely if rapid defibrillation were not available.

Mechanism of Cardioversion and Defibrillation

A defibrillator is a device that stores electrical charge on a capacitor and, when activated, delivers voltage and current via electrodes that are placed on the chest wall or in direct contact with the heart. External defibrillators most commonly deliver dampened sinusoidal waveforms, but trapezoidal waveforms are sometimes employed. Neither waveform is clearly superior for transthoracic defibrillation,[9] but trapezoidal waveforms are employed in implantable cardioverter/defibrillators. The product of the instantaneous voltage (E) and current (I, in amperes) delivered by a defibrillator is a measure of power (in watts). If the area under this sinusoidal or trapezoidal power curve is integrated, the energy (in watt seconds or joules) can be derived. The output of most defibrillators is selected in terms of stored energy. Because the energy actually delivered to the patient is approximately 20% less than that stored by the capacitors, many defibrillators indicate their energy settings both in stored joules and as an estimate of delivered joules. It is important to distinguish stored from delivered energy when interpreting studies involving measurement of defibrillation thresholds. Even though the defibrillator output is measured in joules, the current density delivered by the defibrillator is probably related most closely to the efficacy of cardiac defibrillation.[10] Since voltage is the product of current and resistance ($E=IR$, Ohm's law), the amount of current delivered by the defibrillator is inversely related to the resistance (or impedance, in ohms) between the two electrode paddles. Therefore, both current and voltage delivered by external defibrillators depend on the transthoracic impedance. The factors influencing impedance and its importance in ventricular defibrillation will be discussed below.

The term cardioversion refers to a capacitor discharge that is synchronized to the patient's QRS complex. Lower-energy direct current discharges that are timed to occur during ventricular depolarization (i.e., the QRS complex) are unlikely to result in ventricular fibrillation, compared with discharges occurring during repolarization (i.e., during inscription of the T wave).

Supported in part by the Herman C. Krannert Fund, by Grants HL-06308 and HL-07182 from the National Heart, Lung, and Blood Institute of the National Institutes of Health, U.S. Public Health Service, the American Heart Association, Indiana Affiliate, Inc.; by the Attorney General of Indiana Public Health Trust; and by the Roudebush Veterans Administration Medical Center, Indianapolis.

However, there is an upper limit of shock energy that can induce ventricular fibrillation during repolarization,[11] and therefore it is not as critical that high-energy shocks be synchronized to the QRS. Capacitor discharges that do not require synchronization are used to terminate ventricular fibrillation and sometimes ventricular flutter.

Electrical cardioversion terminates most effectively those tachycardias presumed to be due to reentry, including atrial flutter and atrial fibrillation, AV nodal reentry, reciprocating tachycardia associated with the Wolff-Parkinson-White syndrome, most forms of ventricular tachycardia, ventricular flutter, and ventricular fibrillation. The electrical shock, by depolarizing all or very large portions of excitable myocardium, interrupts reentrant circuits, discharges foci, and establishes electrical homogeneity that terminates reentry. A shock that does not end a tachycardia may fail to depolarize critical areas involved in the maintenance of the tachycardia.[12] Successful shocks, however, may not necessarily depolarize all myocardium, and a critical mass of ventricular myocardium may have to be depolarized for defibrillation to be accomplished (Fig. 43-1).[13, 14] Alternatively to this "critical mass" hypothesis of defibrillation, other investigators have demonstrated that shocks of at least 1 joule can extinguish all cardiac activations for a mean of 64 ms[15] but fail to defibrillate because of the reinitiation of ventricular fibrillation. They postulate that, since repolarization occurs at all times during ventricular fibrillation, the shock always occurs when a portion of the myocardium is "vulnerable" and reinitiates fibrillation. There appears to be an upper limit of energy above which the shock will not reinduce fibrillation during the vulnerable period, correlating with the defibrillation threshold.[11, 16]

A tachycardia that terminates for a few seconds and then restarts may be reinitiated by factors provoking the tachycardia in the first place. If the precipitating factors are no longer present, interrupting the tachyarrhythmia by the shock may prevent its return for a long duration even though the anatomic and electrophysiologic substrates required for the tachycardia are still present.

General Indications and Contraindications

Before considering electrical cardioversion as a therapeutic option, the likelihood of establishing and maintaining sinus rhythm using electrical countershock should be weighed against risks of other forms of therapy. As a rule, any tachycardia that produces hypotension, congestive heart failure, or angina and that does not respond promptly to medical management should be terminated electrically.

Tachycardias thought to be due to disorders of impulse formation (automaticity) rather than to reentry include parasystole, some forms of atrial tachycardias

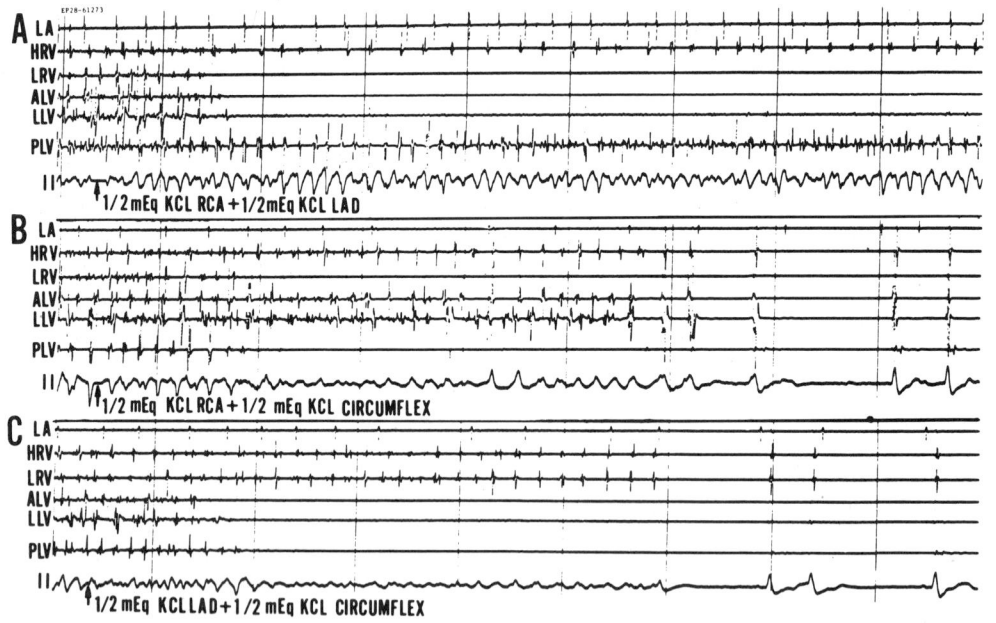

FIGURE 43-1
Termination of ventricular fibrillation in a dog by selective potassium chloride infusion. Potassium chloride injections into the right, left anterior descending, or circumflex coronary artery individually depolarized the limited portions of the ventricle supplied by these vessels but did not terminate ventricular fibrillation (not shown). LA = left atrium; HRV = high right ventricle near the outflow tract; LRV = low right ventricle along the inferior border; ALV = apex of the left ventricle, reflecting distribution of left anterior descending artery; LLV = free wall of the lateral left ventricle adjacent to the interventricular septum, reflecting distribution of the left anterior descending artery; PLV = posterior left ventricle reflecting distribution of the circumflex coronary artery; II = lead II of the electrocardiogram.

A, Potassium chloride was injected simultaneously into both the right (RCA) and left anterior descending (LAD) coronary arteries at arrow. Electrical activity at the LRV, ALV and LLV electrodes became suppressed but ventricular fibrillation continued, presumably because the remaining excitable mass was large enough to support continued fibrillation. B, Potassium chloride was injected simultaneously into both the right and circumflex coronary arteries. Electrical activity recorded at the LRV and PLV electrodes became suppressed and ventricular fibrillation was terminated, implying that the remaining number of excitable cells represented a critical mass insufficient to maintain fibrillation. C, Potassium chloride was injected simultaneously into both the left anterior descending and circumflex arteries. Electrical activity recorded at the ALV, LLV and PLV electrodes became suppressed and ventricular fibrillation was terminated.

(Reprinted by permission from Zipes DP, Fischer J, King RM, et al.: Am J Cardiol 36:37, 1975.)

with or without AV block, nonparoxysmal AV junctional tachycardia, and accelerated idioventricular rhythms. These tachycardias do not respond to electrical cardioversion in most instances. It is possible that a shock can terminate tachycardias due to enhanced automaticity or triggered activity, but this notion is conjectural at present.

Digitalis intoxication is a relative contraindication to direct current shock because refractory ventricular fibrillation may occur after the shock.[17, 18] However, if hemodynamically intolerated ventricular tachycardia or fibrillation occurs in a patient with digitalis intoxication, emergency direct current (DC) shock may be necessary. The severity of complicating arrhythmias after cardioversion in patients with digitalis intoxication may be a function of the energy level, and therefore electrical cardioversion of these arrhythmias, if absolutely necessary, should be titrated starting at lower energy levels. If electrical cardioversion cannot be avoided, lidocaine may be used as a pretreatment. It is not necessary to withhold digitalis prior to elective cardioversion in patients without evidence of digitalis toxicity;[19, 20] instead, only the dose of digitalis on the morning of cardioversion needs to be withheld.

An arrhythmia that terminates spontaneously for a brief period and then resumes should not be cardioverted, since electrical termination is also likely to be followed by spontaneous reinitiation. An example would be a patient with frequent paroxysms of atrial fibrillation alternating with short periods of sinus rhythm after cardiac surgery. In this and similar situations, the therapeutic objective would be to remove any precipitating causes for the arrhythmia and/or initiate pharmacologic antiarrhythmic therapy. If one is preparing to cardiovert a sustained atrial or ventricular tachyarrhythmia that is likely to recur, the patient should receive oral or intravenous antiarrhythmic drug therapy prior to cardioversion in an attempt to maintain sinus rhythm after the shock.

Technique of Elective Cardioversion

After the procedure has been explained to the patient, a careful physical examination should be performed prior to elective cardioversion. This should include palpation of all pulses, because of the potential complication of peripheral embolism. A 12-lead electrocardiogram (ECG) is obtained before and after cardioversion, as well as a rhythm strip during the electrode shock. The patient should be in a fasting state, overnight if possible. The oxygenation, acid-base status, and serum electrolytes should be normal and there should be no evidence of drug toxicity (especially digitalis). The room should be equipped with an oxygen source and suction and resuscitation equipment. Adequate intravenous access should be obtained, and the blood pressure should be measured at baseline and at intervals throughout the procedure. The largest QRS deflection should be obtained for synchronization, taking care that double sensing of the T wave does not occur. A short-acting barbiturate such as methohexital in intravenous doses of 25 to 75 mg, or an amnesic such as diazepam given in incremental intravenous doses of 2.5 to 5 mg at 30-second intervals may be used. A physician skilled in airway management should be in attendance. Before cardioversion, 100% oxygen may be administered for 5 to 15 minutes and is continued throughout the procedure. Manual ventilation of the patient may be necessary to avoid hypoxia during periods of deepest sleep. Routine endotracheal intubation is not necessary unless the patient had ingested a meal within the previous 4 hours. Fear and discomfort from inadequate anesthesia during elective or semi-elective cardioversion may cause the patient to refuse necessary electrophysiologic testing with arrhythmia induction in the future.

The electrode paddles should have a good cover of conductive gel or paste to prevent skin burns. Commercially available conductive electrode pads are also available. Correct electrode paddle placement is important to ensure that maximal current density is delivered through myocardial tissue and that current does not shunt through conductive paste or gel bridging the two paddles on the chest surface. In the anteroapical paddle configuration, one electrode is placed just to the right of the upper sternum below the clavicle and the other electrode is placed in the left midaxillary line lateral to the cardiac apex. In the anteroposterior paddle configuration one electrode is placed in the fourth intercostal space to the left of the sternum anteriorly and one to the left of the spine posteriorly. This electrode location is more clumsy than the anteroapical and does not clearly reduce cardioversion or defibrillation energy requirements. If the electrodes are placed over bony prominences (for example, the sternum, spine, or scapula), transthoracic impedance may be increased. Pre-applied self-adhesive electrode patches (R2 Inc.) have impedance characteristics similar to conventional paddles and may be more useful than paddles in a setting in which the likelihood of inducing arrhythmias is relatively high (e.g., in the electrophysiology laboratory).[21] In this situation, defibrillation can be accomplished by operating a defibrillator connected to the R2 patches on the patient's chest without having to contaminate sterile drapes or struggle to apply electrode paddles to a patient who is losing consciousness.

If, after the first or second shock, reversion to sinus rhythm does not occur, a higher energy level should be tried (see section on Defibrillation Energy Requirements below). If sinus rhythm returns only transiently and is promptly supplanted by the tachycardia, a repeat shock may be tried, depending on the tachyarrhythmia being treated and its consequences. Administration of an antiarrhythmic agent intravenously may be useful prior to delivering the next cardioversion shock but may facilitate the development of post-shock bradyarrhythmias.[22, 23] After cardioversion, the patient should be monitored at least until full consciousness has been restored and preferably for several hours thereafter. Maintenance of sinus rhythm, once established, is often the difficult problem, and not the immediate termination of the tachycardia, and depends on the particular arrhythmia, the presence of underlying heart disease and the adequacy of antiarrhythmic drug therapy.

Cardioversion of Atrial Tachyarrhythmias

Favorable candidates for electrical cardioversion of atrial fibrillation include

- Patients with symptomatic atrial fibrillation of less than 12 months duration and who derive significant hemodynamic benefits from sinus rhythm.
- Patients with a history of embolic episodes.
- Patients who continue to have atrial fibrillation after the precipitating cause has been removed (e.g., following treatment of thyrotoxicosis).
- Patients with a rapid ventricular rate that is difficult to slow.

Unfavorable candidates include patients with:

- Digitalis toxicity.
- No symptoms and a well-controlled ventricular rate without therapy.
- Sinus nodal dysfunction and various unstable supraventricular tachyarrhythmias or bradyarrhythmias (often the bradycardia-tachycardia syndrome), and who finally develop and maintain atrial fibrillation (which in essence represents a "cure" of the sick sinus syndrome).
- Little or no benefit from normal sinus rhythm, and prompt reversion to atrial fibrillation after cardioversion despite drug therapy.
- A large left atrium and long-standing atrial fibrillation.
- Infrequent episodes of atrial fibrillation that revert spontaneously to sinus rhythm.
- No mechanical atrial systole after the return of electrical atrial systole.
- Atrial fibrillation and advanced heart block.
- Plans for cardiac surgery in the near future.
- Antiarrhythmic drug intolerance.

Atrial fibrillation is likely to recur after cardioversion in patients who have significant chronic obstructive lung disease, congestive heart failure, or mitral valve disease. Maintenance quinidine or other type I antiarrhythmic agent administration 1 to 2 days before electrical cardioversion of patients with atrial fibrillation may revert 10 to 15% to sinus rhythm and help prevent recurrence of atrial fibrillation once sinus rhythm is restored. Since quinidine increases digoxin levels, digoxin dosage should be reduced by approximately one half if quinidine is added.

In general, atrial fibrillation requires more energy than atrial flutter or ventricular tachycardia, usually 50 to 100 joules for the initial shock. The discharge should always be synchronized to the QRS complex to prevent induction of ventricular fibrillation. Even though cardioversion restores sinus rhythm in the majority of patients (75–95%), sinus rhythm remains after 12 months in less than one third to one half of patients with chronic atrial fibrillation. Patients with mitral valvular disease and/or large left atria are less likely to have atrial fibrillation successfully cardioverted or to be maintained in sinus rhythm. However, most of these patients deserve one attempt at restoring sinus rhythm. After cardioversion of atrial fibrillation, a junctional rhythm, sinus bradycardia, first-degree AV block, frequent atrial extrasystoles, paroxysms of atrial fibrillation, or an atrial rhythm with differing P waves may occur. These rhythms are often transient and gradually disappear, although atrial ectopic activity may reinitiate atrial fibrillation.

Blood flow in portions of the atria is stagnant during atrial fibrillation, and clots from the left atrial appendage may be dislodged by the vigorous atrial contraction upon resumption of sinus rhythm. Embolic episodes occur in 1 to 3% of patients converted to sinus rhythm, whether accomplished by DC shock or by pharmacologic means. Emboli can occur late (days to weeks) after cardioversion and may reflect delayed return of atrial systolic contractile function. In patients with atrial fibrillation, prior anticoagulation for 1 to 2 weeks should be considered for those who have no contraindication to such therapy and who are at high risk for emboli such as those with mitral stenosis and atrial fibrillation of recent onset, a history of recent or recurrent emboli, a prosthetic mitral valve, enlarged heart (including left atrial enlargement), congestive heart failure, or a clot visualized by echocardiography. Anticoagulation with warfarin for several weeks afterward is recommended to prevent late embolization, especially if paroxysms of atrial fibrillation recur. However, it must be emphasized that few controlled studies to support this approach have been published.

In patients with atrial flutter, slowing the ventricular rate by administering digitalis or terminating the flutter with quinidine may be difficult, so that electrical cardioversion is often the initial treatment of choice. Low energies (10–50 J) are usually effective. Anticoagulation may not be necessary prior to cardioversion in patients with atrial flutter, because atrial contraction is more vigorous than during atrial fibrillation, decreasing the risk of clot formation. For the patient with other types of supraventricular tachycardia, electrical cardioversion may be employed when maneuvers to enhance vagal tone or simple medical management (e.g., intravenous verapamil) has failed to terminate tachycardia, and the clinical setting indicates that fairly prompt restoration of sinus rhythm is desirable because of hemodynamic decompensation or electrophysiologic consequences of the tachycardia. Except for atrial fibrillation, shocks in the range of 25 to 50 joules successfully terminate most supraventricular tachycardias and should be tried initially. If unsuccessful, a second shock of higher energy may be delivered. If the patient has nonparoxysmal junctional tachycardia from digoxin excess, electrical cardioversion is contraindicated.

Cardioversion of Ventricular Tachycardia

In patients with ventricular tachycardia, the hemodynamic and electrophysiologic consequences of the arrhythmia determine the need and urgency for direct current cardioversion. If the ventricular tachycardia is stable, a trial of medical therapy (e.g., intravenous lidocaine or procainamide) may be warranted. A chest thump is useful on rare occasions for terminating ventricular tachycardia.[24, 25] Its mechanism of termination probably relates to a mechanically induced premature atrial or ventricular complex that interrupts tachycardia. The thump cannot be timed very well and is probably effective only when delivered during a nonrefractory part of the cardiac cycle. In addition to being uncomfortable, the thump can alter a ventricular tachycardia[26] and may possibly induce ventricular flutter or fibrillation.[27, 28, 29] For patients with stable ventricular tachycardia, synchronized energies in the range of 25 to 50 joules may be employed initially.[30] If there is some urgency to terminate the tachyarrhythmia one can begin with higher energies.

An occasional patient has recurrent ventricular tachycardia requiring multiple cardioversions before effective antiarrhythmic drug therapy can be found. In addition to transvenous pacing techniques, another useful alternative to repeated transthoracic cardioversion in this situation is low-energy (0.2–2.0 J) temporary transvenous cardioversion, using a special electrode catheter (Medtronic 6880) with two large distal electrodes in the right ventricular apex serving as a cathode, and two proximal electrodes in the region of the superior vena caval right atrial junction serving as anode.[31] These low-energy shocks are well tolerated by patients, are usually perceived as large "hiccups," and are appreciated by the patient who had previously required multiple transthoracic cardioversions.

Defibrillation

Early defibrillation is the most important factor in increasing survival in patients with out-of-hospital cardiac arrest. Most episodes of ventricular fibrillation can be terminated if shocked immediately, but the success rate decreases in patients with ventricular fibrillation of longer duration, leading to hypoxia and acid-base imbalances,[32] in patients with hypotension or shock prior to ventricular fibrillation, and in patients with extensive myocardial damage. Thus, emergency personnel trained to defibrillate early at the scene of cardiac arrest have made an impact on both immediate survival and survival to hospital discharge.[4–6]

Automatic external defibrillators have been developed that can detect ventricular fibrillation using an algorithm applied to the surface ECG recorded with the defibrillating electrodes and can be employed successfully by emergency personnel with minimal training.[33–35] This device may be especially useful in rural areas, where defibrillation is not commonly needed and ambulance personnel may have difficulty maintaining their defibrillation skills. Similar devices may be useful in large public areas such as shopping centers or sporting arenas.

A portable (approximately 7 pounds) defibrillator (Physiocontrol, Inc.) is available for home use by spouses or friends of patients at high-risk for recurrent cardiac arrest.[36] This device analyzes the electrocardiogram from the defibrillating electrode patches using an algorithm to determine whether ventricular fibrillation is present. If ventricular fibrillation is detected, the device questions the operator, using an LED display, as to whether the patient is unconscious; if so confirmed, it will allow a 180-joule shock to be delivered. This device has the advantage of being immediately available before emergency medical personnel can arrive, but the disadvantages of having to be kept close to the patient and operated by another person; the patient must always be observed, and a cardiac arrest during sleep may be missed.

More recently, a system has been developed whereby a physician can establish voice contact with the spouse, interpret the electrocardiogram, and control defibrillation if needed via a telephone connection.[9, 37] The unit consists of a microprocessor, microphone, defibrillator, and patient electrodes. Once connected to a telephone line, the unit automatically dials a remote station, and the ECG monitored from the defibrillating electrodes can be interpreted, the positioning of the electrodes confirmed by transthoracic impedance measurement, and defibrillation activated, if necessary, by a physician.

The ultimate device at present to effect immediate defibrillation in high-risk patients is the automatic implantable cardioverter defibrillator.[7, 8] This device senses ventricular tachyarrhythmias automatically and delivers a shock(s) via chronically implanted epicardial electrodes (see Chapters 44 and 45). The major disadvantages of the currently available device is that it requires major surgery to implant the epicardial leads and arrhythmia detection is imperfect.

"Blind" defibrillation in an unmonitored, unconscious patient is recommended if a defibrillator is available and the cardiac rhythm is unknown. However, this is usually not necessary, because most defibrillators allow display of the rhythm recorded from the paddle electrodes on an oscilloscope prior to delivering a shock. Ventricular fibrillation may occasionally mimic asystole if only one ECG lead is available; therefore, it may be advisable to deliver at least one shock to an unconscious patient with apparent asystole.[38] Likewise, artificial pacemakers may continue to discharge regularly and obscure the electrocardiographic diagnosis of ventricular fibrillation.

TRANSTHORACIC IMPEDANCE

Myocardial current density, the major determinant of defibrillation efficacy, depends on paddle placement, and every effort should be made to include as much of the heart as possible between the two paddles during the discharge. If the paddles do not bridge the heart or are too close together, energy may be shunted through other tissues, with the result that the current density is insufficient to defibrillate.

Likewise, the current delivered from a defibrillator discharge is inversely related to the impedance or resistance across the thorax at the time of the shock (Ohm's law; $E = IR$); in other words, when a defibrillator discharges its capacitor through a low impedance circuit, current flow is higher than when the same energy is discharged through a circuit with a higher impedance. Human transthoracic impedance has been reported to range between 15 and 143 ohms, with a mean of 67 to 75 ohms if standard 8-cm diameter paddles were used or approximately 20% lower if one of the paddles were larger (13 cm).[39, 40] If the transthoracic resistance is high, a lower-energy shock may be unable to generate sufficient current to defibrillate the heart. In animals, the success of defibrillation has been related to transthoracic impedance, as one would predict.[41] By optimizing the impedance, lower energies may successfully defibrillate, preventing myocardial damage and arrhythmias that may occur from repetitive shocks at higher energies.

Several determinants of transthoracic impedance have clinical importance:

1. Impedance is decreased by a highly conductive interface between the patient's chest wall and the defibrillating electrodes.[42] If there is no interface, the skin/electrode impedance is very high. This resistance can be decreased markedly by using an electrode cream or gel or electrode pads.
2. The size of the defibrillating electrode paddle is inversely related to impedance, (i.e., the larger electrodes having the lower impedance).[39, 41–45] However, when the electrode diameter is increased beyond 12 to 13 cm, the current density delivered to the myocardium decreases and defibrillation efficacy diminishes.[43, 44] In practice, nevertheless, an advantage of this larger paddle size over 8-cm paddles has not been clearly established.[45, 46]
3. The impedance decreases with successive shocks and is dependent on the time interval between shocks.[39, 47, 48] In humans, however, the impedance decreases by only 8% between first and second shocks having the same energy.[39] Thus, an initial discharge close to the defibrillation threshold that fails to defibrillate may decrease impedance sufficiently that a second shock may be effective. The mechanism of this phenomenon is unclear but may be related to alterations in skin resistance.
4. Impedance varies inversely with the amount of energy delivered; that is, the higher the energy, the lower the transthoracic impedance.[44, 49] Thus, it is more important to minimize other impedance factors if lower defibrillation energies are being used.
5. The distance between the defibrillating electrodes (chest width) is a major determinant of impedance.[39, 50] The lowest impedance occurs during expiration, when the distance and the amount of air (a good insulator) between the defibrillation electrodes is at a minimum. There is a significant improvement in defibrillation efficacy when subjects are shocked during expiration, compared with inspiration.[51] The amount of pressure on the defibrillating paddles alters impedance, with heavy pressure producing better skin contact and possibly forcing air from the thoracic cavity, allowing for better defibrillation.[39]

MYOCARDIAL DAMAGE

Epicardial necrosis was described in early studies when defibrillation electrodes were applied directly to the heart.[52] In animals given ten direct current discharges of 240 joules, no immediate damage was seen, but animals sacrificed 4 days later had areas of subepicardial necrosis.[53] In another study, animals that received energies less than twice the defibrillation threshold showed no evidence of myocardial necrosis, but animals that received shocks 2.3 and 5.5 times their defibrillation threshold had transmural necrosis, being most severe in those animals receiving the largest shocks.[54] Myocardial damage in animals is more likely to occur with smaller (8-cm) than larger (12.8-cm) paddles, and it is more difficult to produce damage if the shocks are delivered at longer time intervals (i.e., greater than 3 minutes apart).[55]

In humans, epicardial necrosis from defibrillation has not been reported. ST segment elevation may occur with direct current cardioversion,[22, 56, 57] although cardiac enzymes and myocardial scintigraphy may be unremarkable.[57] Serum creatine phosphokinase (CPK) and glutamic oxaloacetic transaminase levels may be increased but may originate from chest wall muscle injury.[58, 59] However, two of 30 patients undergoing elective cardioversion had modest elevation of the CPK-MB isozyme.[60] These two patients both received more than one shock with a cumulative dose greater than 425 joules. CPK-MB was not elevated in any of 27 patients who received a cumulative energy of less than 425 joules. These data suggest that a cumulative delivered energy of greater than 425 joules over a short period of time can produce mild myocardial necrosis in humans.

DEFIBRILLATION ENERGY REQUIREMENTS

The optimum energy for ventricular defibrillation is controversial.[32, 61–69] It would seem that the minimum consistently effective energy should be used to prevent myocardial damage and possibly arrhythmias after the shock. In animals of markedly different size, the energy necessary for defibrillation increases with weight;[10, 70] in human infants and small children, the energy requirement for defibrillation is less than that in adults.[71] However, in adult humans, factors other than weight may be more important; for example, causes of excessive impedance such as faulty electrode position or poor chest wall contact. Although it has been suggested that very high-output defibrillators may be needed for obese patients,[62] most studies have shown that almost all patients can be defibrillated with devices that store energies up to 400 joules.[63–68] Higher-energy defibrillation could result in myocardial damage in some patients.

Weaver et al.[72] tested the energy necessary for out-of-hospital defibrillation in 249 patients by instructing ambulance personnel to alternate 175- and 320-joule (delivered energy) shocks every other day.[72] The efficacy of defibrillation and the number of patients resuscitated and subsequently discharged from the hospital were similar in each group. AV block occurred more often in patients receiving high-energy than in those receiving low-energy defibrillation, especially in patients receiving two or three shocks. Kerber and associates[46] also demonstrated that initial shocks above 200 joules did not result in any added efficacy. These data are especially relevant because current versions of automatic defibrillation systems for home and paramedic use store only 200 joules to allow greater portability.

Therefore, it appears reasonable that the first shock for out-of-hospital ventricular fibrillation should be 200 joules. If defibrillation is accomplished but ventricular fibrillation recurs, 200 joules can again be employed. If ventricular fibrillation persists after the first shock, Kerber[73] suggests that the next shock can also be 200 joules, although others recommend an increase to 300 joules.[69] There is a reasonable chance that a shock of similar energy may defibrillate on the second occasion because (1) transthoracic impedance will be lowered somewhat after the first shock,[39] facilitating defibrillation by a second shock of similar energy; and (2) there is a specific probability at any given energy that defibrillation will occur (defibrillation is a probability function—see below), and thus a second shock at 200 joules may be successful when the initial shock was not. If ventricular fibrillation persists, the next shock should be 300 to 360 joules (maximal output).

There is insufficient data on shocks of even lower energies for defibrillation in adult humans, and currently these energies are not recommended for initial defibrillation of out-of-hospital cardiac arrest patients. However, in controlled situations in which defibrillation is immediately available after the onset of ventricular fibrillation (e.g., in the electrophysiology laboratory) energies as low as 50 joules can commonly defibrillate. Defibrillators that can measure impedance by passing a small current through the electrode paddles prior to delivering the shock and thereby adjust the energy may be useful for minimizing defibrillation energy.[74-76]

DEFIBRILLATION THRESHOLDS

Defibrillation threshold has become an even more important clinical concept upon the introduction of lower-energy implantable devices to terminate ventricular fibrillation. Defibrillation thresholds are usually measured by determining the lowest energy that consistently defibrillates. In reality, though, there is not a distinct energy above which defibrillation is always accomplished and below which it is not. Rather, the energy required for successful defibrillation may be described as a sinusoidal dose-response relationship.[77]

In any particular patient, lower energies may never defibrillate and higher energies may always defibrillate. Intermediate energies, though, will successfully defibrillate only a percentage of the VF episodes (range of intermediate success), illustrating why a second shock at the same energy may defibrillate when the first shock did not (Fig. 43–2). Even though it is useful conceptually, determination of this sinusoidal curve is time-consuming and impractical in humans. Whether the traditional defibrillation threshold determinations relate consistently to the "dose-response" curve is controversial.[77, 78]

The effect of antiarrhythmic drug therapy on defibrillation thresholds is also of greater importance when lower-energy defibrillation is contemplated. Lidocaine has been reported to increase the energy necessary for transthoracic[79-80] and internal[81] defibrillation, although the clinical importance of this effect for transthoracic cardioversion is probably minimal.[46] Bretylium has been reported to either decrease[79, 82] or have no effect[80] on the transthoracic defibrillation threshold. Using the implantable automatic cardioverter/defibrillator electrodes, amiodarone has been reported to both increase[83] and decrease[84] the defibrillation threshold, and encainide (a drug prone to cause refractory incessant ventricular tachycardia) markedly increased the energy required for successful defibrillation.[85] Beta-adrenergic stimulation appears to decrease defibrillation threshold.[86]

Complications

Arrhythmias induced by direct current shock are usually caused by inadequate synchronization with the shock occurring during the ST segment or T wave. Occasionally a properly synchronized shock may produce ventricular fibrillation (Fig. 43–3).[87] Other postshock arrhythmias usually are transient and do not require therapy. They may be due to either transient injury from the shock or possibly simultaneous cholin-

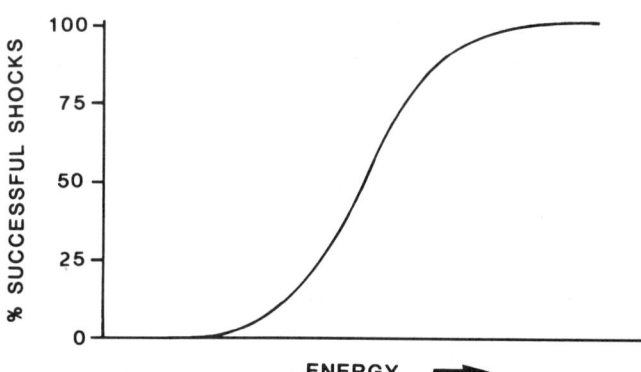

FIGURE 43–2
Schematic representation of the sinusoidal dose-response curve relating delivered energy to defibrillation efficacy in any given patient. Lower energies never defibrillate, higher energies always defibrillate, and over a range of intermediate values the curve defines the probability of successful defibrillation at any given energy.

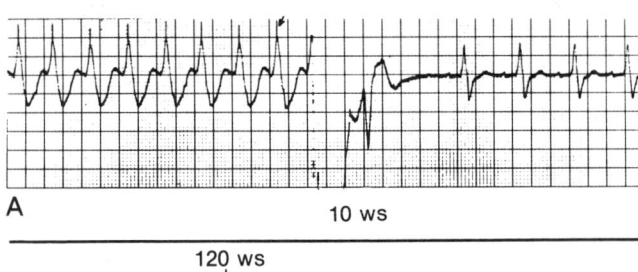
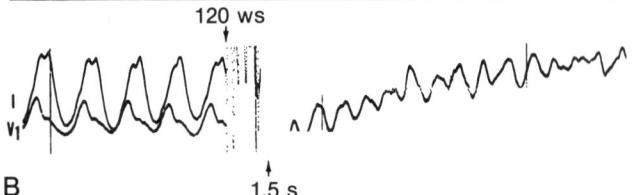

FIGURE 43-3
A, A synchronized shock (note synchronization mark in the apex of the QRS complex; diagonal arrow) during ventricular tachycardia is followed by a single repetitive ventricular response and then by normal sinus rhythm. B, A shock synchronized to the terminal portion of the QRS complex in a patient with atrial fibrillation and conduction to the ventricle over an accessory pathway results in ventricular fibrillation that was promptly terminated by a 120-ws shock. Recording was lost for 1.5 s owing to baseline drift after the shock.

(Reprinted by permission from Zipes DP: In Braunwald E (ed.): Heart Disease—A Textbook of Cardiovascular Medicine, pp. 642–645. Philadelphia, W.B. Saunders Co., 1988.)

ergic and adrenergic discharge caused by the shock.[88] Arrhythmias more commonly complicate cardioversion or defibrillation when digitalis toxicity is present, including ventricular fibrillation that is difficult to terminate. Atrial arrhythmias or atrial fibrillation may occur, as may cardiac standstill, especially in patients with the sick sinus syndrome. Worse arrhythmias can occur with repeated high-energy discharges, digitalis excess, severe heart disease, or electrolyte disorders.

An occasional patient may develop hypotension, reduced cardiac output, or congestive heart failure following the shock,[89] possibly related to complications of the cardioversion, such as embolic events, myocardial depression resulting from the anesthetic agent, hypoxia, lack of restoration of left atrial contraction despite return of electrical atrial systole, or post-shock arrhythmias.[22,23] Although most commonly associated with atrial fibrillation, systemic embolism can also occur after electrical termination of ventricular tachycardia or fibrillation.

Defibrillation shocks do not damage permanent pacemakers unless the shock is delivered directly over the pulse generator. Therefore, paddle positions should be adjusted to be at least 5 inches away from the pulse generator. A shock directly over the generator may cause generator malfunction or elevated pacing threshold, and some authors recommend that the pacing threshold be checked at frequent intervals for 6 weeks after the shock.[90] If a transthoracic shock is necessary in a patient who has epicardial defibrillation, leads for the automatic implantable cardioverter defibrillator, transmyocardial impedance, and current flow may theoretically be different between the anteroapical and anteroposterior paddle positions; in this situation, if the anteroapical electrode configuration does not defibrillate, the anteroposterior position should be tried.

Direct current cardioversion in pregnant patients does not appear to harm the fetus. Nevertheless, it is advisable to monitor the fetal heart rate and rhythm during cardioversion.

References

1. Beck CS, Pritchard WH, Feil HS: Ventricular fibrillation of long duration abolished by electric shock. JAMA 135:985, 1947.
2. Zoll PM, Linenthal AJ, Gibson W, et al.: Termination of ventricular fibrillation in man by externally applied countershock. N Engl J Med 254:727, 1956.
3. Lown B, Amarasingham R, Neuman J: New method for terminating cardiac arrhythmias. Use of synchronized capacitor discharge. JAMA 182:548, 1962.
4. Eisenberg MS, Copass MK, Hallstrom AP, et al.: Treatment of out-of-hospital cardiac arrests with rapid defibrillation by emergency medical technicians. N Engl J Med 302:1379, 1980.
5. Stults KR, Brown DD, Schug VL, et al.: Prehospital defibrillation performed by emergency medical technicians in rural communities. N Engl J Med 310:219, 1984.
6. Weaver WD, Copass MK, Bufi D, et al.: Improved neurologic recovery and survival after early defibrillation. Circulation 69:943, 1984.
7. Mirowski M, Reid PR, Mower MM, et al.: Termination of malignant ventricular arrhythmias with an implanted automatic defibrillator in human beings. N Engl J Med 303:322, 1980.
8. Echt DS, Armstrong K, Schmidt P, et al.: Clinical experience, complications and survival in 70 patients with the automatic implantable cardioverter/defibrillator. Circulation 71:289, 1985.
9. Dalzell GWN, Cunningham SR, Wilson CM, et al.: Ventricular defibrillation: The Belfast experience. Br Heart J 58:441, 1987.
10. Geddes LA, Tacker WA, Rosborough JP, et al.: Electrical dose for ventricular defibrillation of large and small animals using precordial electrodes. J Clin Invest 53:310, 1974.
11. Chen P-S, Shibata N, Dixon EG, et al.: Comparison of the defibrillation threshold and the upper limit of ventricular vulnerability. Circulation 73:1022, 1986.
12. Garrey WE: The nature of fibrillatory contraction of the heart—its relation to tissue mass and form. Am J Physiol 33:397, 1914.
13. Mower MM, Mirowski M, Spear JF, et al.: Patterns of ventricular activity during catheter defibrillation. Circulation 49:858, 1974.
14. Zipes DP, Fischer J, King RM, et al.: Termination of ventricular fibrillation in dogs by depolarizing a critical amount of myocardium. Am J Cardiol 36:37, 1975.
15. Chen P-S, Shibata N, Dixon EG, et al.: Activation during successful and unsuccessful ventricular defibrillation in open-chest dogs: Evidence of complete cessation and regeneration of ventricular fibrillation after unsuccessful shocks. J Clin Invest 77:810, 1986.
16. Chen P-S, Wolf PD, Claydon FJ, et al.: The potential gradient field created by epicardial defibrillation electrodes in dogs. Circulation 74:626, 1986.
17. Kleiger R, Lown B: Cardioversion and digitalis. II. Clinical studies. Circulation 33:878, 1966.
18. Ten Eick RE, Wyte SSR, Ross SM, et al.: Postcountershock arrhythmias in untreated and digitalized dogs. Circ Res 21:375, 1967.
19. Ditchey RV, Karliner JS: Safety of electrical cardioversion in patients without digitalis toxicity. Ann Intern Med 95:676, 1981.
20. Mann DL, Maisel AS, Atwood JE, et al.: Absence of cardioversion-induced ventricular arrhythmias in patients with therapeutic digoxin levels. J Am Coll Cardiol 5:882, 1985.
21. Kerber RE, Martins KB, Kelly KJ, et al.: Self-adhesive preapplied electrode pads for defibrillation and cardioversion. J Am Coll Cardiol 3:815, 1984.
22. Eysmann SB, Marchlinski FE, Buxton AE, et al.: Electrocardiographic changes after cardioversion of ventricular arrhythmias. Circulation 73:73, 1986.

23. Waldecker B, Brugada P, Zehender M, et al.: Dysrhythmias after direct-current cardioversion. Am J Cardiol 57:120, 1986.
24. Pennington JE, Taylor J, Lown B: Chest thump for reverting ventricular tachycardia. N Engl J Med 283:1192, 1970.
25. Caldwell G, Millar G, Quinn E, et al.: Simple mechanical methods of cardioversion: Defence of the precordial thump and cough version. Br Med J 291:627, 1985.
26. Sclarovsky S, Kracoff O, Arditi A, et al.: Ventricular tachycardia. "Pleomorphism" induced by chest thump. Chest 81:97, 1982.
27. Cotoi S: Precordial thump and termination of cardiac reentrant tachyarrhythmias. Am Heart J 101:675, 1981.
28. Krijne R: Rate acceleration of ventricular tachycardia after a precordial chest thump. Am J Cardiol 53:964, 1984.
29. Ewy GA: Electrical therapy for cardiovascular emergencies. Circulation 74(Suppl IV):IV-111, 1986.
30. Geuze RH, deFeijter PJ: Evaluation of transthoracic countershock with initial energy levels up to 200 J in a coronary care unit. J Electrocardiol 18:251, 1985.
31. Zipes DP, Jackman WM, Heger JJ, et al.: Clinical transvenous cardioversion of recurrent life-threatening ventricular tachyarrhythmias: Low energy synchronized cardioversion of ventricular tachycardia and termination of ventricular fibrillation in patients using a catheter electrode. Am Heart J 103:789, 1982.
32. Kerber RE, Sarnat W: Factors influencing the success of ventricular defibrillation in man. Circulation 60:226, 1979.
33. Stults KR, Brown DD, Kerber RE: Efficacy of an automated external defibrillator in the management of out-of-hospital cardiac arrest: Validation of the diagnostic algorithm and initial clinical experience in a rural environment. Circulation 73:701, 1986.
34. Stults KR, Brown DD: Special considerations for defibrillation performed by emergency medical technicians in small communities. Circulation 74(Suppl IV), IV-13, 1986.
35. Weaver WD, Copass MK, Hill DL, et al.: Cardiac arrest treated with a new automatic external defibrillator by out-of-hospital first responders. Am J Cardiol 57:1017, 1986.
36. Moore JE, Eisenberg MS, Anderson E, et al.: Home placement of automatic external defibrillators among survivors of ventricular fibrillation. Ann Emerg Med 15:811, 1986.
37. Dalzell GWN, Cunningham SR, Pruznia S, et al.: Remote telephonic control of defibrillation (Abstract). Circulation 76(Suppl IV):IV-464, 1987.
38. Ewy GA, Dahl CF, Zimmerman M, et al.: Ventricular fibrillation masquerading as ventricular standstill. Crit Care Med 9:841, 1981.
39. Kerber RE, Grayzel J, Hoyt R, et al.: Transthoracic resistance in human defibrillation. Influence of body weight, chest size, serial shocks, paddle size and paddle contact pressure. Circulation 63:676, 1981.
40. Ewy GA, Ewy MD, Silverman J: Determinants of human transthoracic resistance to direct current discharge. Circulation 46(Suppl II):II-150, 1972.
41. Thomas ED, Ewy GA, Dahl CF, et al.: Effectiveness of direct current defibrillation: Role of paddle electrode size. Am Heart J 93:463, 1977.
42. Connell PN, Ewy GA, Dahl CF, et al.: Transthoracic impedance to defibrillation discharge: Effect of electrode size and electrode-chest wall interface. J Electrocardiol 6:313, 1973.
43. Ewy GA, Horan WJ: Effectiveness of direct current defibrillation. Role of paddle electrode size II. Am Heart J 93:674, 1977.
44. Hoyt R, Grayzel J, Kerber RE: Determinants of intracardiac current in defibrillation. Experimental studies in dogs. Circulation 64:818, 1981.
45. Kerber RE, Jensen SR, Grayzel J, et al.: Elective cardioversion: Influence of paddle-electrode location and size on success rates and energy requirements. N Engl J Med 305:658, 1981.
46. Kerber RE, Jensen SR, Gascho JA, et al.: Determinants of defibrillation: Prospective analysis of 183 patients. Am J Cardiol 52:739, 1983.
47. Geddes LA, Tacker WA, Cabler DP, et al.: Decrease in transthoracic resistance during successive ventricular defibrillation trials. Med Instrum 9:179, 1975.
48. Dahl CF, Ewy GA, Ewy MD, et al.: Transthoracic impedance to direct current discharge: Effect of repeated countershocks. Med Instrum 10:151, 1976.
49. Ewy GA, Ewy MD, Nuttall AJ, et al.: Canine transthoracic resistance. J Appl Physiol 32:91, 1972.
50. Kerber RE, Klein S, Kouba C, et al.: Evaluation of a new defibrillation pathway: Tongue-epigastric/tongue-apex route. II. Impedance characteristics in human subjects. J Am Coll Cardiol 4:253, 1984.
51. Ewy GA, Hellman DA, McClung S, et al.: Influence of ventilation phase on transthoracic impedance and defibrillation effectiveness. Crit Care Med 8:164, 1980.
52. Tedeschi CG, White CW Jr: Morphologic study of canine hearts subjected to fibrillation, electrical defibrillation and manual compression. Circulation 9:916, 1954.
53. Warner ED, Dahl C, Ewy GA: Myocardial injury from transthoracic defibrillation countershock. Arch Pathol 99:55, 1975.
54. Davis JS, Lie JT, Bentinck DC, et al.: Cardiac damage due to electric current and energy, p. 27. In Proceedings of the Cardiac Defibrillation Conference. Purdue University, 1975.
55. Dahl CF, Ewy GA, Warner ED, et al.: Myocardial necrosis from direct current countershock. Effect of paddle electrode size and time interval between discharges. Circulation 50:956, 1974.
56. Tacker WA, Van Vleet JF, Geddes LA: Electrocardiographic and serum enzymic alterations associated with cardiac alterations induced in dogs by single transthoracic damped sinusoidal defibrillation shocks of various strengths. Am Heart J 98:185, 1979.
57. Chun PK, Davia JE, Donohue DJ: ST segment elevation with elective cardioversion. Circulation 63:220, 1981.
58. Slodki SJ, Falicov RE, Katz MJ, et al.: Serum enzyme changes following external direct current shock therapy for cardiac arrhythmias. Am J Cardiol 17:792, 1966.
59. Konttinen A, Hulpi V, Louhija A, et al.: Origin of elevated serum enzyme activity after direct current countershock. N Engl J Med 281:231, 1969.
60. Ehsani A, Ewy GA, Sobel BE: Effects of electrical countershock on serum creatine phosphokinase (CPK) isoenzyme activity. Am J Cardiol 37:12, 1976.
61. Lown B, Crampton RS, DeSilva RA, et al.: The energy for ventricular defibrillation—too little or too much. N Engl J Med 298:1252, 1978.
62. Tacker WA, Galioto FM, Giuliani E, et al.: Energy dosage for human trans-chest electrical defibrillation. N Engl J Med 290:214, 1974.
63. Pantridge JR, Adgey AAJ, Webb SW, et al.: Electrical requirements for ventricular defibrillation. Br Med J 2:313, 1975.
64. Campbell NPS, Webb SW, Adgey AAJ, et al.: Transthoracic ventricular defibrillation in adults. Br Med J 2:1379, 1977.
65. Gascho JA, Crampton RS, Sipes JN, et al.: Energy levels and patient weight in ventricular defibrillation. JAMA 242:1380, 1979.
66. Gascho JA, Crampton RS, Cherwek ML, et al.: Determinants of ventricular defibrillation in adults. Circulation 60:231, 1979.
67. De Silva RA, Lown B: Energy requirement for defibrillation of a markedly overweight subject. Circulation 57:827, 1978.
68. Adgy AAJ: Electrical energy requirements for ventricular defibrillation. Br Heart J 40:1197, 1978.
69. Standards and Guidelines for Cardiopulmonary Resuscitation and Emergency Cardiac Care. JAMA 255:2905, 1986.
70. Gold JH, Schuder JC, Stoeckle H, et al.: Scaling current and energy with body weight: Requirements for the transthoracic ventricular defibrillation of calves as they grow from 50 to 150 kg. Circulation 60:187, 1979.
71. Gutgesell HP, Tacker WA, Geddes LA, et al.: Energy dose for defibrillation in children. Pediatrics 58:898, 1978.
72. Weaver WD, Cobb LA, Kopass MK, et al.: Ventricular defibrillation—A comparative trial using 175J and 320J shocks. N Engl J Med 307:1101, 1983.
73. Kerber RE: Energy requirements for defibrillation. Circulation 74(Suppl IV):IV-117, 1986.
74. Geddes LA, Tacker WA, Schoenlein W, et al.: The prediction of the impedance of the thorax to defibrillating current. Med Instrum 10:159, 1976.
75. Kerber RE, Kouba C, Martins J, et al.: Advance prediction of transthoracic impedance in human defibrillation and cardioversion: Importance of impedance in determining the success of low energy shocks. Circulation 70:303, 1984.
76. Kerber RE, McPherson D, Charbonnier F, et al.: Automated

impedance-based energy adjustment for defibrillation: Experimental studies. Circulation 71:136, 1985.
77. Davy J-M, Fain ES, Dorian P, et al.: The relationship between successful defibrillation and delivered energy in open-chest dogs: Reappraisal of the "defibrillation threshold" concept. Am Heart J 113:77, 1987.
78. Rattes MF, Jones DL, Sharma AD, et al.: Defibrillation threshold: A simple and quantitative estimate of the ability to defibrillate. PACE 10:70, 1987.
79. Babbs CF, Yim GKW, Whistler SJ, et al.: Elevation of ventricular defibrillation threshold in dogs by antiarrhythmic agents. Am Heart J 98:345, 1979.
80. Kerber RE, Paudian NG, Jensen SR, et al.: Effect of lidocaine and bretylium on energy requirements for transthoracic defibrillation: Experimental studies. J Am Coll Cardiol 7:397, 1986.
81. Dorian P, Fain ES, Davy J-M, et al.: Lidocaine causes a reversible, concentration-dependent increase in defibrillation energy requirements. J Am Coll Cardiol 8:327, 1986.
82. Tacker WA, Niebauer MJ, Babbs CF, et al.: The effect of newer antiarrhythmic drugs on defibrillation threshold. Crit Care Med 8:177, 1980.
83. Troup PJ, Chapman PD, Olinger GN, et al.: The implanted defibrillator: Relation of defibrillating lead configuration and clinical variables to defibrillation threshold. J Am Coll Cardiol 6:1315, 1985.
84. Fain ES, Lee JT, Winkle RA: Effects of acute intravenous and chronic oral amiodarone on defibrillation energy requirements. Am Heart J 114:8, 1987.
85. Fain ES, Dorian P, Davy J-M, et al.: Effects of encainide and its metabolites on energy requirements for defibrillation. Circulation 73:1334, 1986.
86. Ruffy R, Schechtman K, Monje E, et al.: Adrenergically mediated variations in the energy required to defibrillate the heart: Observations in closed-chest, nonanesthetized dogs. Circulation 73:374, 1986.
87. Zipes DP: Management of cardiac arrhythmias: Pharmacological, electrical, and surgical techniques. In Braunwald E (ed.): Heart Disease—A Textbook of Cardiovascular Medicine, pp. 642–645. Philadelphia, W.B. Saunders Co., 1988.
88. Cobb FR, Wallace AG, Wagner GS: Cardiac inotropic and coronary vascular responses to countershock. Evidence for excitation of intracardiac nerves. Circ Res 23:731, 1968.
89. Resnekov L, McDonald L: Complications in 220 patients with cardiac dysrhythmias treated by phased direct current shock and indications for electroversion. Br Heart J 29:926, 1967.
90. Levine PA, Barold SS, Fletcher RD, et al.: Adverse acute and chronic effects of electrical defibrillation and cardioversion on implanted unipolar cardiac pacing systems. J Am Coll Cardiol 1:1413, 1983.

44

The Automatic Implantable Cardioverter-Defibrillator (AICD): Clinical Experience

Enrico P. Veltri
Morton M. Mower
M. Mirowski

Sustained ventricular tachyarrhythmias are the predominant cause of sudden cardiac death, a leading cause of cardiovascular mortality in the world.[5, 9, 18] An estimated 400,000 individuals in the United States alone succumb to life-threatening ventricular arrhythmias annually.[6] Prompt and accurate recognition of sustained ventricular tachyarrhythmias followed by effective administration of a cardioverting or defibrillating electrical countershock is required to rescue such individuals from sudden death. Optimal circumstances for delivering emergent electrical therapy are lacking, however, in the vast majority of instances, due to the fact that life-saving intervention requires immediate availability of bystanders trained in cardiopulmonary resuscitation and of reliable defibrillating equipment.

Historical Background

The concept of automatic electrical defibrillation by an implanted device was first proposed in 1970 by Mirowski et al.[10] and Schuder and coworkers.[21] The evolution of technology, coupled with a decade of bench and animal testing, led to the first human implant in February, 1980 at The Johns Hopkins Hospital in Baltimore.[14] The key developments leading to human implantation included experimental models consisting initially of a transvenous catheter paired to a prepectoral plate[11] and testing of a single transvenous catheter[12] and culminating in the discovery of a more efficient and effective energy delivery system using two transcardiac electrodes, one placed in the superior vena cava and the other directly on the left ventricle.[13]

The initial implanted human device identified only ventricular fibrillation or sinusoidal ventricular tachycardia greater than 200 beats per minute (bpm). This device was termed the automatic implantable defibrillator (AID).* Further technological developments resulted in modifications of the device resulting in the automatic implantable cardioverter-defibrillator (AICD).† These advances were in large part due to the addition of an R wave sensing lead, allowing sensing and R wave synchronous cardioversion of ventricular tachycardia.[28] Clinical trials using this device commenced in 1982, and more recently a hybridized microcomputer-processed AICD has been in clinical use.[16]

Based on extensive clinical trials demonstrating impressive reduction in the expected arrhythmic mortality in high risk patients,[1, 15, 21, 23] the United States Food and Drug Administration‡ approved the AICD for broad clinical use in patients with refractory sustained ventricular tachyarrhythmias. Over 6000 patients have received this therapy worldwide.

The Device

The device is composed of two systems: a pulse generator and electrode leads. The newest generation of the AICD in clinical use (Ventak) is shown in Figure 44–1. The pulse generator, a hermetically sealed titanium can, houses specially designed lithium batteries, capacitors, and electronic logic circuits. It measures

---
*Intec Systems, Pittsburgh, PA.
†Cardiac Pacemakers, Inc., St. Paul, MN.
‡Fed. Reg. (50) 4727, November 15, 1985.

10.8 cm in length, 7.6 cm in width, and 2 cm in depth, weighs 250 grams, and has a volume of 148 cubic centimeters.

The electrode leads serve for (1) sensing rate and morphology of cardiac electrical activity and (2) delivery of R wave synchronized cardioverting/defibrillating electrical pulses. Rate sensing and R wave synchronization are performed by either right ventricular endocardial (tined) or left ventricular epicardial (intramural screw-in) bipolar leads. The cardiac electrical morphology sensing function and electrical pulse delivery are performed by an anode-cathode pair. Anode-cathode electrode pairs may consist of a titanium spring electrode (placed at the junction of the superior vena cava and right atrium), serving as an anode, and a left ventricular patch (flexible rectangular titanium mesh placed at the left ventricular apex), serving as cathode, or alternatively two patches (right ventricular/left ventricular or anterior/posterior left ventricular).

ARRHYTHMIA RECOGNITION

Cardiac electrical activity is continuously monitored by the device via the implanted electrode leads. Arrhythmia recognition is based on two parameters: signal morphology and rate.

The *morphology parameter,* known as the probability density function (PDF), is based on the derivative of the input signal as a function of the amount of time spent near a zero-potential (isoelectric) baseline. Most sustained ventricular tachyarrhythmias exhibit sinusoidal morphologic patterns spending relatively little time near the isoelectric potential. Supraventricular tachyarrhythmias without underlying intraventricular conduction delay, on the other hand, spend a relatively greater amount of time at the isoelectric baseline. The *rate parameter* is based on the R wave input signal and allows recognition of arrhythmias above a predetermined rate level.

The arrhythmia recognition algorithm for any given patient may be based on both parameters (morphology and rate) or on rate alone. Such algorithms are fixed by the given model of the device and are not programmable. The implanting physician therefore must choose an algorithm based on the needs of the individual patient (based on pre-implantation evaluation). Dual recognition parameters allow higher specificity for ventricular tachyarrhythmias; however, "spiky" ventricular tachycardias, which are typically nonsinusoidal and thus unlikely to satisfy morphology (PDF) criteria, may be missed. The "rate-only" devices use only the rate recognition criteria and thus these models provide higher sensitivity with faster arrhythmia recognition time. Specificity is lower, however, since any tachycardia above the rate cut-off would satisfy arrhythmia detection criteria of the device.

ARRHYTHMIA TERMINATION

Once arrhythmia recognition parameters are satisfied (5–20 s), the device's arrhythmia termination cycle is initiated. The capacitors charge to approximately 720

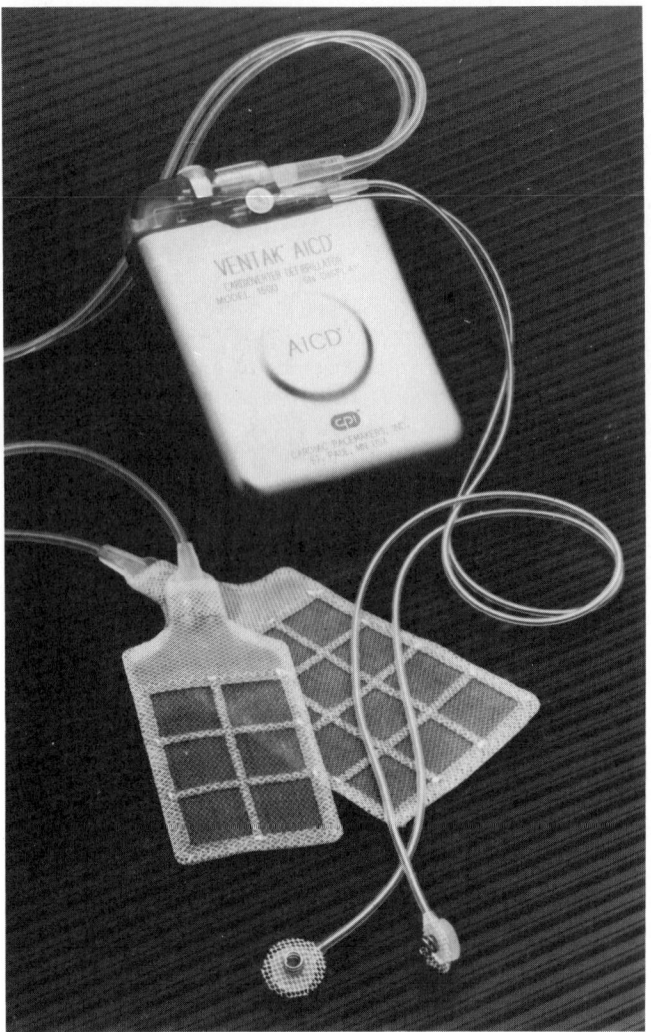

FIGURE 44–1
The newest-generation AICD (Ventak) pulse generator with two patch leads and epicardial bipole screw-in leads. (Reprinted by permission of Cardiac Pacemakers, Inc., St. Paul, Minn.)

volts in 7 to 9 seconds. A truncated exponential pulse of 25 to 35 joules (4–6 ms duration) is delivered through the anode-cathode electrode pair. For any persistent ventricular tachycardia/fibrillation episode meeting recognition criteria, the device is capable of recycling three times. Each post-discharge period requires 35 seconds of a rhythm other than ventricular tachycardia/fibrillation in order to reset for another four discharges. All discharges are synchronized to the onset of ventricular depolarization (R wave). The device is designed to deliver approximately 200 pulses.

Implantation

CRITERIA FOR IMPLANTATION

AICD implantation at our institution requires the following:

1. History of documented or presumed ventricular

fibrillation (cardiac arrest) or sustained hypotensive ventricular tachycardia (presyncope or syncope).
2. Absence of an identifiable correctable cause for ventricular tachyarrhythmia (e.g., acute myocardial infarction, electrolyte imbalance, drug toxicity).
3. Failure of antiarrhythmic drug therapy to suppress spontaneous or inducible ventricular tachycardia/fibrillation.
4. Absence of medical disease processes limiting survival to less than 6 months.
5. Ability to obtain informed consent.
   Of note, reimbursement for AICD implantation by Medicare (Health Care Financing Administration guidelines) requires inducible sustained ventricular tachyarrhythmia.* This latter prerequisite is controversial in light of recent information, however.[24]

PRE-IMPLANTATION EVALUATION

Patients with sustained ventricular tachyarrhythmias manifesting cardiac arrest or hypotensive symptoms (e.g., presyncope, syncope) should undergo extensive evaluation in an effort to exclude potentially correctable causes of arrhythmias, define the pathophysiologic substrate, assure an attempt to adequately control the arrhythmia with pharmacologic therapy, and identify additional surgical interventions which may be indicated, such as coronary artery bypass or angioplasty, valve replacement, subendocardial resection, or aneurysmectomy. Evaluation should include the following:

1. History and physical examination.
2. Blood work-up, including electrolytes (potassium, magnesium), arterial blood gases, and antiarrhythmic drug levels (digoxin, class I antiarrhythmic drugs).
3. Electrocardiogram.
4. Noninvasive assessment of spontaneous supraventricular and ventricular arrhythmias on 24 to 72-hour Holter monitoring (preferably off all antiarrhythmic drugs).
5. Exercise stress testing with or without radionuclide imaging.
6. Noninvasive assessment of left ventricular function (echocardiography or radionuclide).
7. Coronary angiography.
8. Electrophysiologic testing at baseline and with serial antiarrhythmic drugs to assess inducibility and suppression of the clinical arrhythmia.

Prior to AICD implantation, the detection of supraventricular tachyarrhythmias, frequent spontaneous nonsustained ventricular tachycardia, sinus node dysfunction, or high grade distal conduction disease will identify the need for concomitant antiarrhythmic drug or pacemaker therapy. Certainly potential interactions of AICD and other concomitant antiarrhythmic therapies must be addressed prior to implantation, for these factors may impact on the AICD model chosen and on the operative approach.

OPERATIVE APPROACH

A review of the four AICD surgical approaches has been previously published.[27] Basically these include median sternotomy, left thoracotomy, subcostal, and subxiphoid. The selection of approach is based on the surgeon's preferences, the need for concomitant cardiac surgery (median sternotomy preferred), and the patient's history of previous cardiac surgery (left thoracotomy preferred). In these latter instances, a total epicardial lead system (intramural screw-in rate-sensing leads and two ventricular patches) is placed. At our institution, whenever implantation of the AICD alone is required in a patient without prior cardiac surgery, a subcostal approach is used.

INTRAOPERATIVE TESTING

Intraoperative electrophysiologic testing is necessary to confirm adequate AICD function. This includes determination of defibrillation threshold (DFT) and assessment of the device's ability to detect and terminate ventricular fibrillation. DFT is defined as the least amount of energy needed to defibrillate the heart.

DFT testing is performed intraoperatively (or postoperatively in patients undergoing coronary artery bypass, subendocardial resection, or aneurysmectomy) by applying AC current to the heart[17] and using a standby external cardioverter-defibrillator (ECD),* which delivers decremental (1–5 J) amounts of energy after 10 to 15 seconds of ventricular fibrillation. These energy pulses are identical in waveform to the AICD. In general, DFT ≤ 20 joules is acceptable, thereby allowing an approximate 10-joule margin of safety at the minimum output of the AICD.

The patch-patch lead system has been the preferred lead configuration, given that energy requirements can usually be diminished by approximately 50% compared with superior vena cava–left ventricular patch lead configuration.[22] Of note, however, persistently high DFTs despite optimum lead configuration may be secondary to underlying cardiac substrate or effects of antiarrhythmic drugs.[2, 4, 8] In such patients, AICD implantation should not be performed until a satisfactory DFT is confirmed.

Having determined a satisfactory DFT, the leads are connected to the AICD pulse generator, the device is activated, and ventricular fibrillation is induced to ensure proper performance. Patients whose clinical arrhythmia is sustained ventricular tachycardia should also have the arrhythmia induced, either intraoperatively, or postoperatively in the electrophysiology laboratory prior to hospital discharge to assure detection and termination by the AICD. In patients undergoing concomitant coronary artery bypass or "ablative" arrhythmia surgery (subendocardial resection/aneurysmectomy or cryoablation) the entire AICD system may

---

*U.S. Department of Health and Human Services, Health Care Financing Administration: Section 35–85, Implantation of Automatic Defibrillators, Jan. 1986.

*Cardiac Pacemakers, Inc., St. Paul, MN.

be implanted at the time of surgery.[19] Alternatively, some centers prefer to implant "leads only" with or without a "dummy box" in such cases, delegating AICD pulse generator implantation for cases in which persistently inducible ventricular tachycardia/fibrillation is found at postoperative electrophysiologic study.

NONINVASIVE MONITORING

An external detection system (AID Check)* is used to noninvasively interrogate the AICD (Figure 44–2).

The AICD can be tested noninvasively prior to, during, and after implantation. Application of a "donut" magnet over the pulse generator for approximately 30 seconds activates or inactivates the device. A piezoelectric crystal emits audible tones synchronous to the R wave of the ECG during the implanted activated mode, ensuring adequate R wave sensing. A monotonous tone during magnet application confirms the inactivated mode.

The AID Check is used to determine the number of pulses delivered to the patient and the capacitor charging time. A brief application of the donut magnet over the activated pulse generator initiates the capacitor charging cycle: however, the energy pulse is delivered into a test load resistor rather than through the leads to the patient. Prolongation of the charge time during routine follow-up (serial 1- to 3-month intervals) generally indicates battery depletion and, if exceeding the elective replacement indicator (ERI), usually requires generator replacement. Ambulatory monitoring of the AICD has recently been reviewed.[25]

PATIENT POPULATION

During a 7-year cumulative experience (1980–1987), 198 patients underwent AID and/or AICD implantation at The Johns Hopkins and Sinai Hospitals in Baltimore.[26] The clinical characteristics of the patient population are summarized in Table 44–1.

Coronary artery disease, the predominant underlying substrate in these patients, was found in 74%. The mean ejection fraction was 35%. Patients had survived a mean of 3 previous cardiac arrests and failed a mean of 3.8 antiarrhythmic drugs prior to implantation.

Thirty-three patients received the AID as the first device, and 174 patients received the AICD (including nine patients with cross-over from AID to AICD when the latter technology became available); 147 patients (74%) underwent implantation without associated surgical procedures. Twenty-five patients (13%) underwent subendocardial resection (associated with aneurysmectomy in 24 patients and coronary artery bypass in 17), and 26 patients (13%) underwent associated coronary artery bypass surgery as the sole concomitant surgical procedure.

OPERATIVE COMPLICATIONS

Operative death (defined as death prior to hospital discharge or 30 days postoperatively) occurred in nine

*Cardiac Pacemakers, Inc., St. Paul, MN.

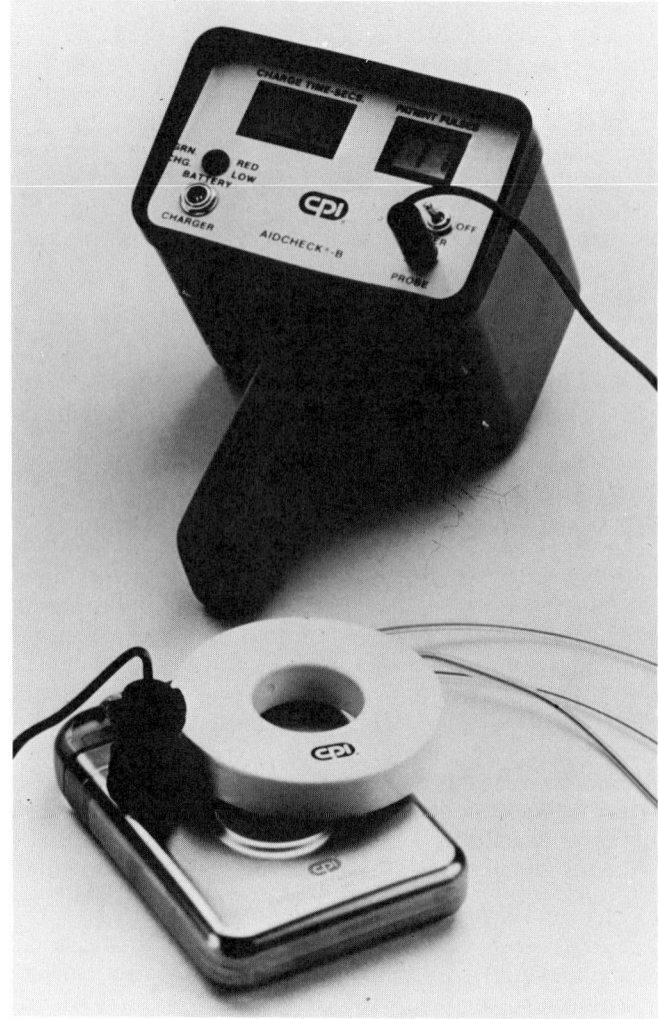

FIGURE 44–2
The AID Check system consists of an interrogator, probe, and donut magnet. The digital charge time (seconds) is displayed on the left-hand side and the patient pulse count is displayed on the right-hand side of the interrogator. (Reprinted by permission of Cardiac Pacemakers, Inc., St. Paul, Minn.)

patients (4.5%). Six patients died from incessant ventricular tachycardia/fibrillation and one death each occurred from acute myocardial infarction, refractory congestive heart failure, and vascular tears. Other

TABLE 44–1
Characteristics of Patient Population with AID and/or AICD Implantation*

Characteristic	No. of Patients
Male/female	157/41
Underlying disease	
Coronary disease	147
Cardiomyopathy	33
Primary electrical	7
Mitral valve prolapse	7
Prolonged Q-T interval	3
Coronary spasm	1

*A total of 198 patients were followed, with a mean age of 56 years. See text for discussion.

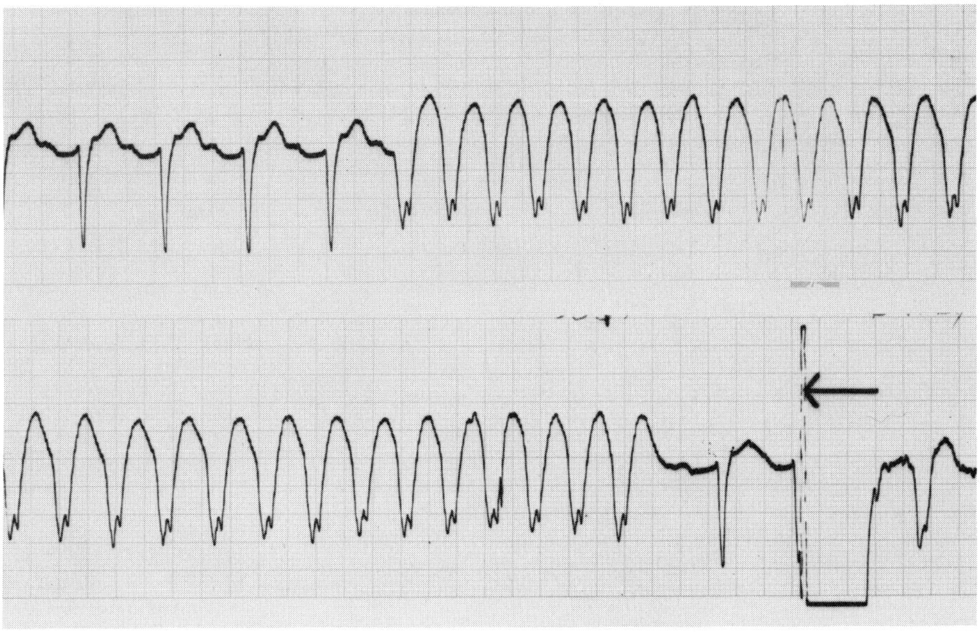

FIGURE 44–3
Continuous electrocardiographic tracing of spontaneous nonsustained ventricular tachycardia (9-s duration) triggering AICD discharge (arrow) in sinus rhythm.

major, but nonfatal, operative complications included infection in 12% (i.e., pulse generator pocket, pneumonia, thoracotomy site), blood transfusion requirements in 10%, pneumothorax in 5% (related to superior vena cava lead insertion), pericardial tamponade necessitating pericardiocentesis in 2%, and cardiogenic shock in 2%. Sixty-five percent of patients were free from any operative complication.

CLINICAL OUTCOME

At long-term follow-up (mean 22 months) after hospital discharge, 98 patients (52%) had at least one "appropriate" AID or AICD discharge. Appropriate discharges were defined as those occurring with premonitory symptoms of presyncope or syncope, or during sleep. "Asymptomatic" discharges occurred in 23% of patients. It is important to note that although asymptomatic discharges may occur secondarily to supraventricular tachyarrhythmias above the rate cut-off of the device or to nonsustained ventricular tachycardia, a substantial proportion (20–50%) of such discharges are indeed for sustained ventricular tachycardia.[3, 8] AICD discharges during asymptomatic nonsustained ventricular tachycardia and sustained pleomorphic ventricular tachycardia are depicted in Figures 44–3 and 44–4, respectively.

During our 7-year cumulative experience, 142 patients (75%) were alive, and 47 patients (25%) died (excluding operative deaths). Deaths included documented or presumed ventricular tachycardia/fibrillation in 19 patients (10%), refractory heart failure in 18 (9.5%), myocardial infarction in four, bradyarrhythmia in one, and noncardiac in five patients.

Kaplan-Meier survival curves for the AICD patient group are depicted in Figure 44–5. Actuarial incidence of out-of-hospital sudden cardiac death (death within 1 hour of symptoms from documented or presumed

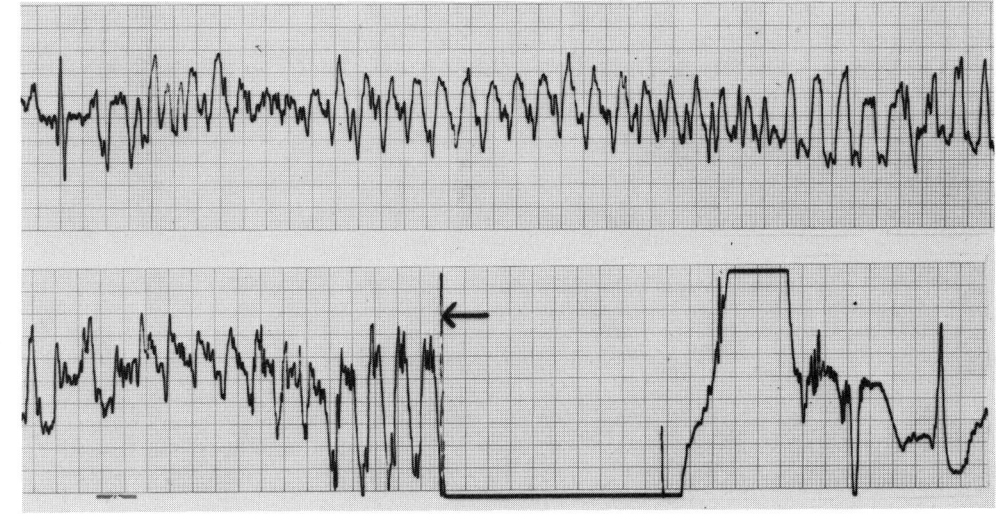

FIGURE 44–4
Continuous electrocardiographic tracing of spontaneous sustained pleomorphic ventricular tachycardia/fibrillation terminated by AICD discharge (arrow) after 12-s duration.

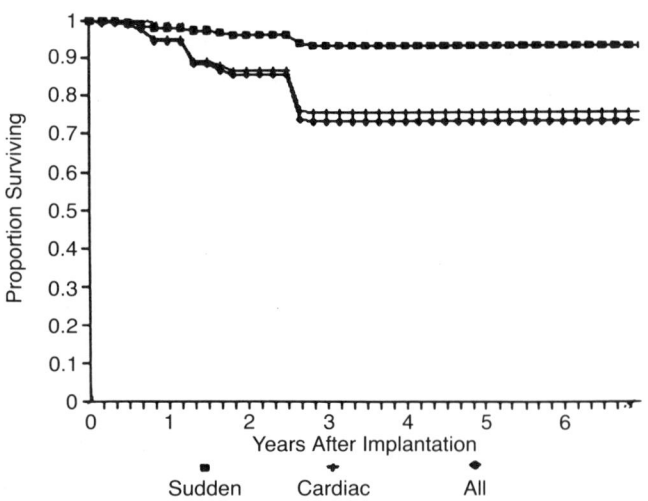

FIGURE 44—5
Kaplan-Meier survival curves for the AICD patient population depicting actuarial incidence of sudden, cardiac, and all-cause deaths.

ventricular tachycardia/fibrillation, unwitnessed or unexpected death, or death during sleep) was 1.5% and 4.1% at 1 and 2 years, respectively. Actuarial incidence of cardiac death was 8.2% and 17.4% at 1 and 2 years, respectively.

Summary

The impressive reduction in the expected sudden death incidence of high-risk patients following AICD therapy has clearly been demonstrated. Undoubtedly, nonpharmacologic electrical therapy for ventricular tachyarrhythmias will be further refined. Specifically, further developments in technology will include addition of pacing capability (both bradycardia and antitachycardia modes), graded energy delivery (low-energy cardioversion), rate and morphology sensing function programmability, incorporation of other electrical (atrial) or hemodynamic sensing functions to better delineate supraventricular from ventricular tachyarrhythmias, more efficient modes of defibrillation (alternate lead configuration, pulse characteristics), smaller-size units with greater battery longevity, and nonthoracotomy approaches. These advances will hopefully enhance physician acceptance and improve patient comfort, management, and survival.

References

1. Echt DS, Armstrong K, Schmidt P, et al.: Clinical experience, complications and survival in 70 patients with the automatic implantable cardioverter-defibrillator. Circulation 71:289, 1985.
2. Guarnieri T, Levine JH, Veltri EP, et al.: Success of chronic defibrillation and the role of antiarrhythmic drugs with the automatic implantable cardioverter-defibrillator. Am J Cardiol 60:1061, 1987.
3. Guarnieri T, Strickberger A, Magiros E, et al.: Is an asymptomatic automatic implantable cardioverter-defibrillator discharge a false positive? PACE 1:983, 1987.
4. Haberman R, Veltri EP, Mower MM: The effect of amiodarone on defibrillation threshold. PACE 10:406, 1987.
5. Kempf FC, Josephson ME: Cardiac arrest recorded on ambulatory electrocardiograms. Am J Cardiol 53:1577, 1984.
6. Kuller L: Sudden death in arteriosclerotic heart disease: The case for preventive medicine. Am J Cardiol 24:617, 1969.
7. Marinchak RA, Friehling TD, Kline RA, et al.: Effect of antiarrhythmic drugs on defibrillation threshold: Case report of an adverse effect of mexiletine and review of the literature. PACE 11:7, 1988.
8. Masterson M, Maloney JD, Wilkoff B, et al.: Clinical performance of automatic implantable cardioverter-defibrillator: Electrocardiographic documentation of 82 spontaneous discharges. J Am Coll Cardiol 11:18A, 1988.
9. Milner PG, Platia EV, Reid PR, et al.: Holter monitoring recording at the time of sudden cardiac death. Circulation 68:III-106, 1983.
10. Mirowski M, Mower MM, Staewen WS, et al.: Standby automatic defibrillator—an approach to prevention of sudden coronary death. Arch Int Med 126:158, 1970.
11. Mirowski M, Mower MM, Staewen WS, et al.: Ventricular defibrillation through a single intravascular catheter electrode system. Clin Research 19:328, 1971.
12. Mirowski M, Mower MM, Staewen WS, et al.: The development of the transvenous automatic defibrillator. Arch Int Med 129:773, 1972.
13. Mirowski M, Mower MM, Langer A, et al.: A chronically implanted system for automatic defibrillation in active conscious dogs: Experimental model for treatment of sudden death from ventricular fibrillation. Circulation 58:90, 1978.
14. Mirowski M, Reid PR, Mower MM, et al.: Termination of malignant ventricular arrhythmias with an implanted automatic defibrillator in human beings. N Engl J Med 303:322–324, 1980.
15. Mirowski M, Reid PR, Winkle RA, et al.: Mortality in patients with implanted automatic defibrillators. Ann Intern Med 98:585, 1983.
16. Mirowski M: The automatic implantable cardioverter-defibrillator: An overview. J Am Coll Cardiol 6:461, 1985.
17. Mower MM, Reid PR, Watkins L, Jr, et al.: Use of alternating current during diagnostic electrophysiologic studies. Circulation 67:69, 1983.
18. Nikolic G, Bishop RL, Singh JB: Sudden death recorded during Holter monitoring. Circulation 66:218, 1982.
19. Platia EV, Griffith LSC, Reid PR, et al.: Treatment of malignant arrhythmias with endocardial resection and implantation of the automatic cardioverter-defibrillator. N Engl J Med 314:213, 1986.
20. Reid PR, Mirowski M, Mower M, et al.: Clinical evaluation of the internal automatic cardioverter-defibrillator in survivors of sudden cardiac death. Am J Cardiol 51:1608, 1983.
21. Schuder JC, Stoeckle H, Gold JH, et al.: Experimental ventricular fibrillation with an automatic and completely implanted system. Trans Am Soc Artific Intern Organs 16:207, 1970.
22. Troup PJ, Chapman P, Olinger GN, et al.: The implanted defibrillator: Relation of defibrillating lead configuration and clinical variables to defibrillation threshold. J Am Coll Cardiol 6:1315, 1985.
23. Veltri EP, Mower MM, Guarnieri T, et al.: Clinical efficacy of the automatic implantable defibrillator: 6 year cumulative experience. Circulation 74:II-109, 1986.
24. Veltri EP, Mower MM, Mirowski M, et al.: Clinical outcome of patients with noninducible ventricular tachyarrhythmias and the automatic implantable defibrillator. Circulation 74:II-109, 1986.
25. Veltri EP, Mower MM, Mirowski M: Ambulatory monitoring of the automatic implantable cardioverter-defibrillator: A practical guide. PACE 11:315, 1988.
26. Veltri EP, Mower MM, Guarnieri T, et al.: Clinical efficacy of the automatic implantable defibrillator: 7 year cumulative experience. Chest 92:975, 1987.
27. Watkins L, Jr, Guarnieri T, Griffith LSC, et al.: Implantation of the automatic defibrillator: Current surgical techniques. Clin Prog Electrophysiol Pacing 4:286, 1986.
28. Winkle RA, Bach SM, Echt DS, et al.: The automatic implantable defibrillator: Local ventricular bipolar sensing to detect ventricular tachycardia and fibrillation. Am J Cardiol 52:265, 1983.

45

The Automatic Implantable Cardioverter Defibrillator (AICD): Follow-Up and Complications

Francis E. Marchlinski
Alfred E. Buxton
Belinda Flores

The process of developing the "perfect" antitachycardia device is in an exponential growth phase. Many of the changes in technology have been triggered by the recognition of the complications and limitations associated with the use of the commercially available automatic implantable cardioverter defibrillator (Ventak—AICD*) and its immediate predecessors, models AID-B and AID-BR, over the last 6 years. With over several thousand devices implanted in the United States, multiple centers involved with the initial clinical investigation of the device have reported on their short- and long-term experience.[1-9] Results of the overall clinical experience are summarized in Chapter 44. This chapter will focus on the type of follow-up required in patients with the AICD, the timing of generator replacement, and the complications that have been observed. We will use, as a focal point for our discussion, our own experience in using 108 AICD generators in 77 patients over the last 6 years. Emphasis will be placed not only on the recognition of the potential complications but also on suggestions for avoiding adverse effects.

Description of AICD System

Any discussion of the AICD follow-up and associated complications should be preceded by a brief description of the AICD generator and system. As will be evident later, many of the observed complications and limitations of the AICD are related to (1) the nature of the implantation technique and the lead system used, (2) the sensing algorithm used for ventricular tachycardia and ventricular fibrillation detection, (3) the absence of programmability, and (4) the absence of antitachycardia and backup bradycardia pacing capabilities.

The currently available AICD system has three components:

1. The battery operated pulse generator
2. Defibrillating leads
3. Rate-sensing lead(s)

The generator (Ventak AICD) is rectangular with dimensions of 10.8 by 7.6 by 2.0 cm. Its weight is approximately 250 grams. The dimensions of the AICD-B and AICD-BR systems are slightly larger, with a weight of approximately 290 grams. The rate-sensing electrodes consist of an endocardial bipolar lead positioned at the right ventricular apex, or two closely spaced epicardial screw-in leads.

The transcardiac energy delivery system is composed of an epicardial patch placed over the apex of the left ventricle used in combination with either a spring-lead that is positioned at the junction of the superior vena cava and right atrium or a second patch. The flexible patches are either approximately 14 or 28 cm² square

---

*Cardiac Pacemakers, Inc., Minneapolis, MN.

Supported in part by grants from the American Heart Association, Inc., Southeast Pennsylvania Chapter, Philadelphia, PA; and Grant No. HL24278, from the National Heart, Lung, and Blood Institute, Bethesda, Maryland.

centimeters in size. The spring electrode (12.2 F) is approximately 8 cm in length and 4.1 mm in diameter and consists of approximately 60 turns of titanium. If two patches are used, one is routinely placed over the anterior right ventricle or anterior intraventricular septum while the other is secured on the posterolateral surface of the left ventricle. Placement of the patch(es) requires entering the thoracic cavity.

We and others have noted that a two-patch lead system appears to be associated with a lower defibrillation threshold in patients in whom the spring-patch system was incapable of reliably terminating ventricular fibrillation within the energy output of the AICD device.[10-12] Troup et al.[13] demonstrated that the lowest defibrillation threshold was obtained with patch-patch combinations using at least one large patch. Experimental work has confirmed the efficacy of a larger patch size in effecting lower defibrillation thresholds.[14, 15] A two-patch lead system has become the preferred system for energy delivery at many AICD implantation centers, including our own (see below).[10]

Sternotomy, lateral thoracotomy, subxyphoid, and subcostal approaches have all been used to gain access to the thoracic cavity and allow patch placement. Of note, the subcostal approach has been reported to be well tolerated, to be associated with a decreased risk of postoperative pulmonary complications (see below), and to permit sufficient access such that two patch leads can be placed without difficulty.[16]

The two basic types of AICD devices are differentiated based on the sensing criteria used for arrhythmia detection. The first type of device requires only a certain rapid rate for arrhythmia detection (i.e., mean electrogram-to-electrogram interval as recorded by the bipolar rate-sensing electrode, which is less than a preset value). The second type of device uses heart rate and the probability density function (PDF) as rate detection criteria. The PDF is a morphologic sensing criterion that assesses the amount of time the QRS waveform (as indexed by the recording from the two energy delivering leads) spends away from the isoelectric baseline. The QRS waveform in supraventricular rhythms without associated ventricular conduction abnormalities spends most of the time on the isoelectric baseline. Ventricular tachycardia, ventricular fibrillation, and any supraventricular rhythm of a sufficiently rapid rate, or those with associated QRS widening, will in general easily satisfy the morphologic sensing criteria.

The AICD in general requires 5 to 30 s (mean of 13 ± 8 s in our experience) for recognition of ventricular tachycardia and 5 to 25 s (mean of 11.5 ± 6 s) for recognition of ventricular fibrillation. Devices that have both rate and PDF sensing criteria are associated with a longer arrhythmia detection time. Once the AICD recognizes the arrhythmia, the pulse generator's capacitor is charged usually within 5 to 10 s, and the device is *committed* to discharge even if the arrhythmia has spontaneously terminated (Fig. 45–1). The AICD delivers a shock of 25 ± 5 J (normal energy device) or 30 ± 3 J (high-energy device) synchronous with the sensed electrogram. If the tachycardia persists, three additional shocks at a slightly increased energy level will be delivered after brief periods required for arrhythmia recognition and capacitor charging. After the fourth countershock, the AICD requires 35 seconds of a rhythm other than one that would normally trigger the device in order to again recognize the tachyarrhythmia and discharge appropriately. This period of time was designed to eliminate the chance of multiple shocks

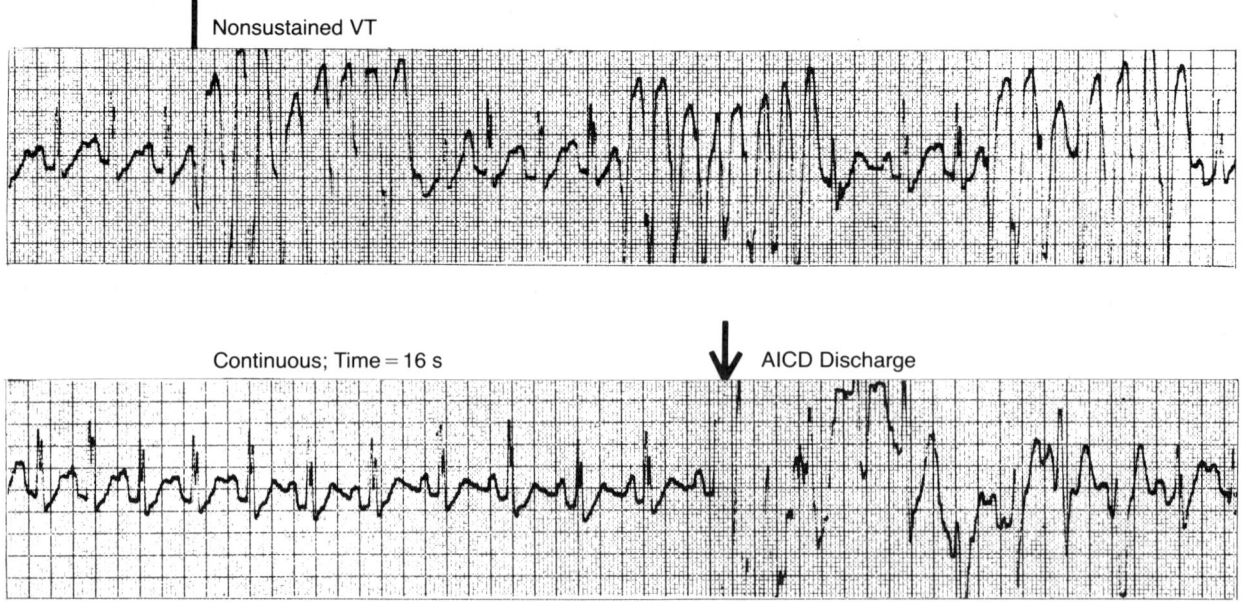

FIGURE 45–1
Nonsustained ventricular tachycardia (VT) triggering the AICD. Once arrhythmia is sensed, the AICD is committed to discharge even if arrhythmia spontaneously terminates. (Reprinted by permission from Marchlinski FE, Flores BT, Buxton AE, et al.: Ann Intern Med 24:481, 1986.)

for a misdiagnosed supraventricular rhythm with a maintained rate above the cut-off for the AICD.

Reference AICD Study Population

In order to use our own experience in 77 patients as a reference, a brief description of our patient population, device and lead selection, and implantation technique follows. A detailed report of our early experience in the first 26 patients has been previously reported.[4] Our patient population consisted of 65 men and 12 women with a mean age of 57 years (range 24–78 years). Forty-eight of the patients had coronary artery disease, 28 had cardiomyopathies of unknown cause or, less commonly, valvular or congenital heart disease, and one patient had a primary electrical abnormality. The mean ejection fraction was 32 ± 12%. Nearly all patients (91%) had at least one documented cardiac arrest. Six of the remaining seven patients had syncope with inducible sustained ventricular arrhythmias which were poorly tolerated hemodynamically and refractory to antiarrhythmic therapy. One patient had recurrent episodes of a hemodynamically tolerated ventricular tachycardia that did not respond to antiarrhythmic agents. Twenty (26%) of the patients had no inducible arrhythmias in the baseline state, using our standard stimulation protocol, which included up to three extrastimuli introduced during at least two paced cycle lengths from at least two right ventricular sites. All antiarrhythmic therapy planned for chronic administration was begun prior to AICD implantation. Fifty one (66%) of our patients were treated with antiarrhythmic therapy at the time of AICD implantation, and approximately 50% (28 patients) of these patients were treated with amiodarone. All patients treated with amiodarone had at least 10 days of antiarrhythmic therapy, with a loading dose of 1400 mg per day administered during the first week prior to implantation.

A left lateral thoracotomy (49 patients) or a sternotomy (27 patients) was used for patch lead placement in all cases, except for a subcostal approach used in one patient. A total epicardial lead system was used in 57 patients (74%), and a two-patch lead system was used in 61 (79%) of patients. Forty-four patients had two large patches used for energy delivery. The patches were placed intrapericardially unless placed in approximation to coronary artery bypass grafts (four patients), at which time they were placed extrapericardially. The AICD generator was positioned subcutaneously in the left upper abdominal quadrant in all patients. All but five AICD generators were high-energy units delivering between 28 and 33 joules on the first discharge. Sensing criteria for arrhythmia recognition were rate-only in 38 patients and rate plus PDF sensing in 39 patients. The mean rate cut-off for arrhythmia detection was 167 beats per minute (bpm), with a range of 143 to 203 bpm.

As part of the routine evaluation of our patients, the defibrillation threshold was determined intraoperatively and the AICD documented intraoperatively to sense and terminate ventricular fibrillation. In patients with documented ventricular tachycardia, the threshold energy value for ventricular tachycardia termination was assessed also, and the AICD was demonstrated to be capable of sensing and terminating all ventricular tachycardia. All but 15 of our patients also underwent postoperative electrophysiologic study aimed at reconfirming normal AICD function in sensing and terminating ventricular tachycardia and ventricular fibrillation.

Our patients have been followed for a mean of 14 ± 13 months (range 1 to 48 months). Twenty-one of the patients have had their AICD pulse generator replaced once during follow-up and seven patients have had a second generator replacement. It is noteworthy that only one of our 77 patients with an activated AICD died suddenly during 1050 patient-months of total follow-up (Fig. 45–2). The AICDs of 29 patients (37%) discharged for an electrocardiographically documented or suspected (symptoms of syncope or presyncope with palpatations) ventricular arrhythmia, including two patients whose first discharge occurred following their second generator replacement at 43 and 39 months, respectively, following the initial AICD implant.

Procedure for Follow-Up

FOLLOW-UP GUIDELINES

In general it has been recommended that patients be seen in follow-up at a minimum of every 2 months during the first year following AICD implantation and subsequently every month.[17–19] The physician following the patient must be vigilant to identify early mechanical

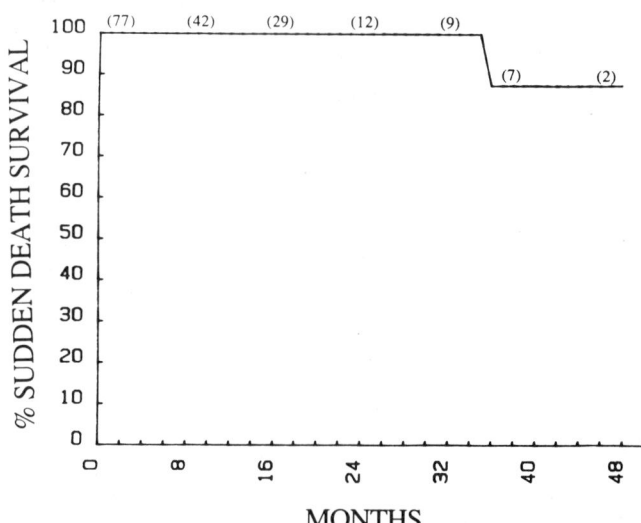

FIGURE 45–2
Sudden death survival in 77 patients who underwent AICD implantation at the Hospital of the University of Pennsylvania.

malfunction and/or battery depletion (see below). Frequent follow-up also affords the patient and his family the opportunity to be re-educated about normal device function and the use of a magnet to activate and deactivate the device. Patients have the opportunity to have all questions related to the device answered and any fears allayed.

At each follow-up visit, historical information related to device discharge is obtained. In addition, the AICD generator and sensing leads are evaluated using a magnet and a noninvasive, hand-held analyzer (AIDCHECK*). The AICD device is activated and/or deactivated (if previously activated) by placing a donut-shaped magnet over the upper right corner of the device for 30 seconds. When activated with the magnet left in position, an R wave synchronous tone is emitted. Oversensing of myopotentials and pacemaker signals, or intermittent lead breaks, may be recognized by comparing the timing of the emitted signals with the simultaneously recorded QRS complexes.[20]

AICD MAGNET TESTING

A donut-shaped magnet is also used to activate the telemetry of the AICD and to initiate a charging cycle. The magnet is placed over the device for 2 to 25 s and abruptly removed to initiate the test. When performing this magnet test, a monitoring probe, attached to the hand-held external AIDCHECK device is positioned over the upper left corner of the AICD generator. The AIDCHECK device displays (1) the time required to charge the unit's capacitor and (2) the number of pulses that have been discharged externally to the patient. The number of discharges displayed can be correlated with the patient's symptoms and reports of device discharge. The magnet test capacitor charge is delivered to an internal resistor and is not recorded as a shock by the telemetry circuit, although the energy used to initiate the charge does decrease the battery energy source. In rare instances, the stored energy may be inadvertently delivered to the patient during the baseline rhythm.[21] This phenomenon has been termed "magnet misdirect." Because of the potential for arrhythmia induction with shock, all magnet testing should be performed with an external cardioverter defibrillator device available for arrhythmia termination.

The charge time recorded during the magnet test is an indicator of battery life (see below). Unfortunately, the first measured charge time can be influenced by the interval between magnet tests. During an inactive period, a passivation layer accumulates on the battery, which reduces voltage for the initial period of charging. In addition, dielectric deformation of the capacitor occurs with periods of inactivity, resulting in an increased leakage current and a longer charge time. The first magnet test will eliminate any increase in charge time due to deformation of the capacitor. A second magnet test charge time assessed between 10 and 30 minutes after the first will accurately reflect battery condition, and thus the approaching end of battery life. Winkle et al.[22] documented in a clinical trial that the second magnet test charge time shows a slow and predictable linear increase over time and is not influenced by the interval between magnet tests and/or spontaneous shocks. Unless the first charge time is repeatedly and dramatically prolonged (>28 s), a second magnet test charge time is routinely assessed during follow-up.

TIMING OF AICD PULSE GENERATOR REPLACEMENT

Guidelines for replacing the AICD generator have been established by the manufacturer. Unfortunately, confirmation of the guidelines based on detailed clinical evaluation has not yet been reported. The average time to elective replacement has been reported to be between 20.4 and 24.8 months.[7,19] Our own time for electively replacing the pulse generator has varied between 19 and 25 months, with a mean of 22 months. It is currently suggested that the most precise indicator for elective device replacement is a second magnet test charge time that is 1.2 times greater than the second magnet test charge time measured at 8 months. When this value is reached, the AICD pulse generator has approximately 3 months of monitoring time remaining or approximately 200 seconds of remaining cumulative (including magnet testing) charging time. If a second magnet test charge time at 8 months is not available, it has been suggested that a second charge time greater than 12 seconds be used as an index for elective device replacement. A more detailed discussion of guidelines for elective or immediate device replacement are provided by the manufacturer in the physician's manual for the currently commercially available AICD.[18]

STABILITY OF RECORDINGS AND DEFIBRILLATION THRESHOLDS

The bipolar electrical signal recorded from the rate-sensing leads and the bipolar signal recorded from the energy-delivering leads have been reported to remain stable over time with respect to the signal amplitude.[8,19,23] Guarnieri and colleagues[19] reported no significant difference in the amplitude of the signals recorded from bipolar endocardial rate sensing lead and from a patch-spring lead bipolar pair when signals recorded at the time of generator replacement were compared with those obtained at the time of original implantation.[19] Our own experience, using primarily a two-patch lead system and epicardial screw-in leads, also demonstrates that there is no significant change in signal amplitude at the time of generator replacement. The mean rate-sensing signal amplitude was 10.5 ± 2.9 mV at initial implantation and 9.8 ± 4.5 mV at the time of replacement. Similarly, the bipolar signal recorded from energy-delivering leads measured 5.5 ± 3.2 mV at initial implantation and 4.9 ± 3.2 mV at the time of generator replacement. Of note, in our experience there was an occasional marked disparity in the signal size between

---

*Cardiac Pacemakers, Inc.

the recordings obtained at the time of the generator replacement versus that noted at original implantation, R wave amplitude changes as much as 10 mV for the rate-sensing leads and 6 mV for the energy-delivering leads were noted. Of note, at the time of initial implant we registered a signal amplitude >5–6 mV for the rate-sensing leads and >3 mV for the energy-delivering leads. In all but one patient (in whom the rate-sensing lead was replaced), the rate-sensing lead signal amplitude was >4 mV at the time of generator replacement. In addition, the energy-delivering lead signal recording was always greater than 2 mV at the time of generator replacement. All of our patients demonstrated normal AICD sensing function of induced ventricular arrhythmias at the time of AICD replacement.

STABILITY OF DEFIBRILLATION THRESHOLDS

The stability of the defibrillation thresholds over time has been addressed by several investigators. Guanieri and associates[19] noted that in patients not treated with amiodarone, the defibrillation threshold using a spring-patch energy delivering lead system remained remarkably constant after a mean generator replacement time of 24 months. They noted, however, that in a subgroup of eleven patients treated with amiodarone at the time of both implantation procedures or in whom amiodarone was added after the implantation (three patients), the defibrillation threshold rose significantly from 10.9 ± 4.3 J at initial implant to 20.0 ± 2.7 J at replacement ($p < .05$). In contrast, Meade and coworkers[23] noted in their preliminary report that the defibrillation thresholds appeared to decrease or remain stable with time, and that antiarrhythmic drugs including amiodarone had no systematic effect on chronic defibrillation thresholds. Both Kadri and colleagues[24] and Chapman et al.[25] noted in preliminary reports that the defibrillation thresholds using a two-patch lead system remained remarkably constant when the initial implantation values were compared with those measured at the time of device replacement. According to Kadri et al.,[24] amiodarone withdrawal in five patients and continuation in five patients had no consistent effect on the defibrillation threshold.

Our own experience with 17 patients also confirms the stability of the defibrillation threshold over time in the majority of patients. The defibrillation threshold changed by greater than 5 joules in only three of 17 patients. In one patient the threshold decreased 10 J, and in two patients there was an increase of 10 and >15 J, respectively. Unfortunately, in the last two patients, the resultant defibrillation threshold exceeded the energy output of the available AICD device. Neither patient had experienced a device discharge for an arrhythmia during the life span of their initial AICD pulse generator; in both patients, a spring and patch lead combination was used for energy delivery. An additional surgical procedure to alter lead type to a two-patch system in an attempt to lower the defibrillation threshold was declined. Of note, both of these patients were being treated with amiodarone. However, an additional 11 patients, who were also treated with amiodarone at both initial and replacement generator implantation, were not noted to have a significant (>5 J) change in defibrillation threshold (mean defibrillation threshold was 19.1 ± 7.6 J at initial implantation and 18.6 ± 8.6 J at the time of replacement). Five of these additional 11 patients had a spring patch energy-delivering lead system, whereas the remaining six patients had a two-patch energy-delivering lead system. Thus, the defibrillation threshold, in general, appears to remain remarkably stable over time. Individual exceptions have been noted however, and repeat threshold determination should be documented at the time of device replacement.

The influence of antiarrhythmic drugs on the defibrillation threshold in humans has not been clearly established (see below). Data published by Guarnieri et al.,[19] and Troup and coworkers,[26] isolated case studies,[27] and data published from animal experiments[28] suggest that amiodarone may increase the defibrillation threshold, although a consistent effect has not been observed in humans.[23–25] Nevertheless, until more information is accumulated in man, any antiarrhythmic drug change should be considered to have the potential to alter the defibrillation threshold (see below). In patients with documented defibrillation thresholds that approached the maximum energy output for the AICD device, a change in drug therapy should be accompanied by a demonstration of the AICD's efficacy in terminating ventricular fibrillation.

ELECTROCARDIOGRAPHIC, HEMODYNAMIC, AND PATHOLOGIC EFFECTS OF PATCH LEADS AND INTERNAL DEFIBRILLATION

Significant bradyarrhythmias and primary induction of sustained ventricular arrhythmias (Fig. 45–3) appear, fortunately, to be unusual electrocardiographic effects associated with the AICD discharge.[29–31] (See section on Complications below.) Eysmann et al.[32] assessed serial 12-lead electrocardiograms at 1, 3, 5, 10, and 15 minutes following AICD discharge. Transient ST segment elevation and/or depression of 1 mm or more in amplitude was observed in approximately 25% of discharges. In all cases, ST segment changes returned to baseline within 3 to 5 minutes following device discharge (Fig. 45–4).

The effects of repeated internal defibrillator discharges on the human myocardium was recently reported by Singer and coworkers.[32] These investigators assessed the pathologic consequences of short- and long-term placement of the intravascular and intrapericardial leads of the AICD in 25 patients. They noted that pathologic changes related to defibrillation via the patch electrode consisted of contraction band necrosis and loss of myocytes confined to the myocardium directly under the patch lead. Pathologic changes were estimated to affect less than 2% of the total myocardial mass. Also of note, these same investigators noted that large venous thrombi, confirmed by autopsy, occurred in 20% of patients in association with the intravascular spring lead.

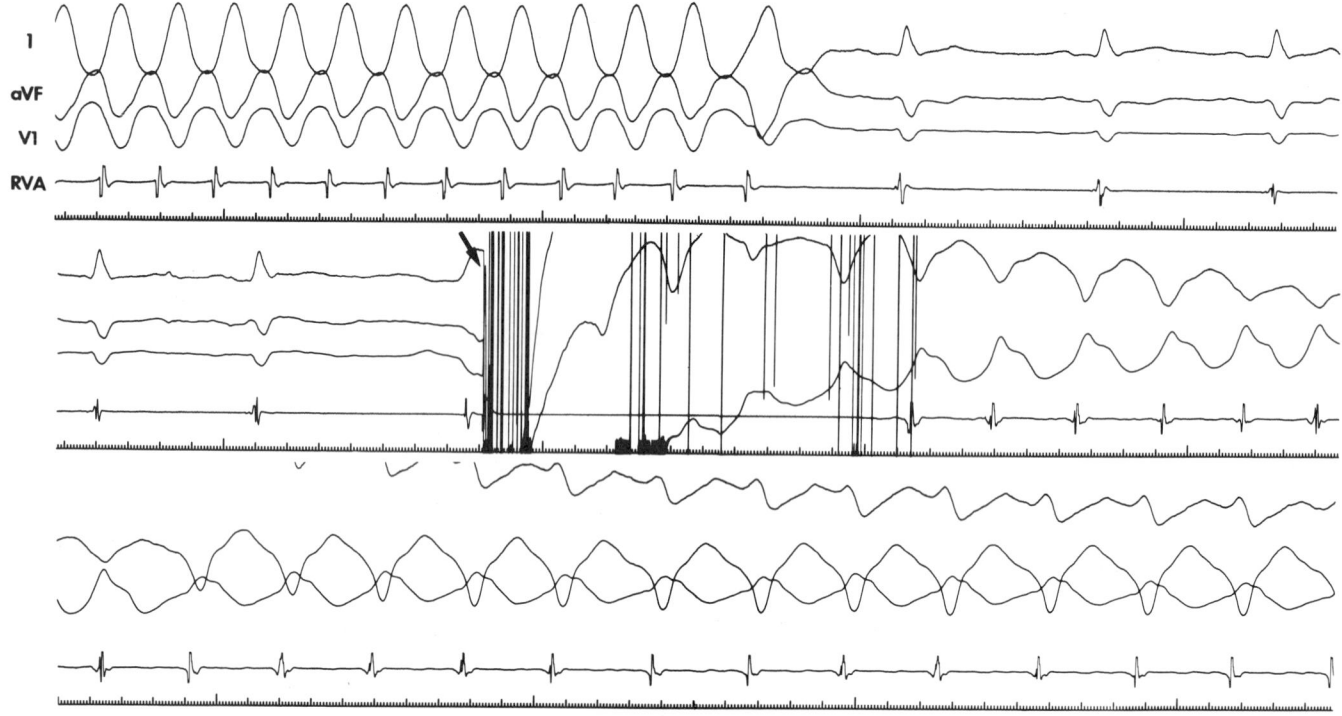

FIGURE 45-3
Ventricular tachycardia initiation following AICD discharge. Surface ECG leads I, avF, and V₁ are shown, as well as a recording from the right ventricular apex (RVA) and 10-ms time lines.

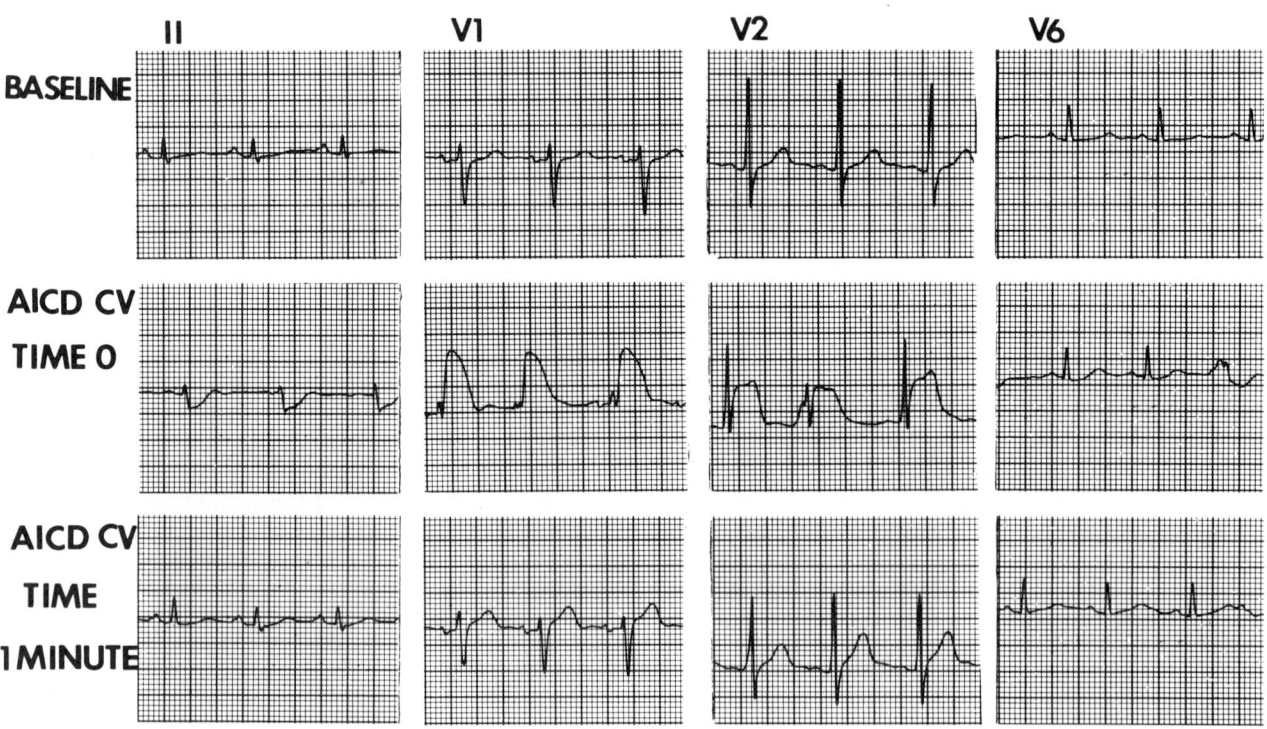

FIGURE 45-4
ST segment elevation following AICD discharge and cardioversion (CV) of ventricular tachycardia. Dramatic ST elevation in the precordial leads, seen immediately after AICD discharge, rapidly resolve. (Reprinted by permission of the American Heart Association, Inc., from Eysman SB, Marchlinski FE, Buxton AE, et al.: Circulation 73:73, 1986.)

With respect to the hemodynamic effects of defibrillation testing, Antunes et al.[33] in a preliminary report, noted no significant effect on the myocardial ejection fraction assessed by intraoperative two-dimensional (2-D) echocardiography in six patients undergoing AICD implantation. Finally, Trappe and associates[34] determined whether the patch electrodes of the implantable defibrillator impaired left ventricular function, as assessed by pre- and postoperative (1.5 months) 2-D and M-mode echocardiograms. Using fibrin glue, patch electrodes were attached to the epicardium after determination of the defibrillation threshold. No significant impairment of global or regional left ventricular function was observed. No significant differences between the pre- and postoperative end-diastolic cross-sectional area (16.3 ± 3.7 cm^2 versus 15.6 ± 3.4 cm^2, respectively) nor between the pre- and postoperative end-systolic areas (11.3 ± 2.7 cm^2 versus 12.5 ± 3.4 cm^2, respectively) were noted. Of note, a single case of constriction pericarditis associated with the patch electrodes has been reported by Almassi and coworkers.[35]

Thus, in general the AICD energy-delivering leads plus repeated defibrillation during testing and/or following spontaneous arrhythmias do not appear to be associated with persistent or significant electrocardiographic or hemodynamic effects. With the exception of the frequent autopsy finding of endovascular thrombus formation associated with the spring coil lead, myocardial pathologic changes related to AICD patches and defibrillation appear minimal. Although the chronic hemodynamic sequelae of a two-patch lead system does not seem to be significant, a longer duration of follow-up and a more rigorous assessment of the hemodynamic effects of this type of lead system is needed.

Complications of AICD Implantation

Although the AICD has been demonstrated to dramatically reduce the risk of sudden cardiac death,[4, 37, 38] numerous complications have been reported in association with implantation and during follow-up.[2, 4, 7-9, 29, 39] Of note, despite the increased risk of associated morbidity, the incidence of intraoperative or perioperative mortality appears to be low. Those centers reporting on their results with 50 or more patients note an operative mortality of 1 to 4%.[2, 40, 41] In our experience, there were two early (<1 month) postoperative deaths out of 77 patients (3%) undergoing generator implantation. Failure to achieve a lead position or type which will result in a defibrillation threshold that is less than the energy output of the currently available AICD device also appears to be low.[41] Winkle and coworkers[41] reported that in only three of 157 patients was defibrillation ineffective with any lead type or configuration. Similarly, we observed only one out of 77 (1%) patients in whom the intraoperative defibrillation threshold was greater than the maximum output for the AICD device after adjusting lead position and polarity and implanting two large patches.[42]

Reports of overall complication rates vary dramatically. We observed complications in approximately 60% of our 77 patients (Fig. 45–5), whereas Luceri et al.[5] reported complications in only 14% of 20 patients. The variation in the incidence of complications is partly related to the recognition and/or development of implantation techniques with decreased operative risk and technical improvements in the device and to differences in opinion as to what constitutes a complication.

In our study, we elected to define a complication as any untoward effect experienced by the patient related to the AICD implantation and function. Admittedly many of the untoward effects are related to the surgical procedure involved with the implantation process and not to the AICD itself, or they may result in symptoms that are minimal but that nevertheless are quite alarming to the patient (e.g., large seroma at the generator site). In addition, some of the adverse effects represent appropriate device function (e.g., AICD discharge during hemodynamically well-tolerated ventricular tachycardia). However, for the patient and the physician orchestrating his care, this normal function creates a problem that has, on occasion, forced explantation or deactivation of the device. Thus, for the purpose of providing the physician who is or will be involved in the implantation and follow-up of the AICD with the necessary information to permit optimum patient management, we will present a detailed compendium of problems encountered.

We have divided our discussion of complications that are seen in association with the AICD into two major categories: (1) early (operative and perioperative) complications and (2) late complications noted during follow-up. We have also elected to discuss as a separate category the problem of the AICD discharge in the absence of symptoms. We address the latter subject separately because of its magnitude. Of note, it is

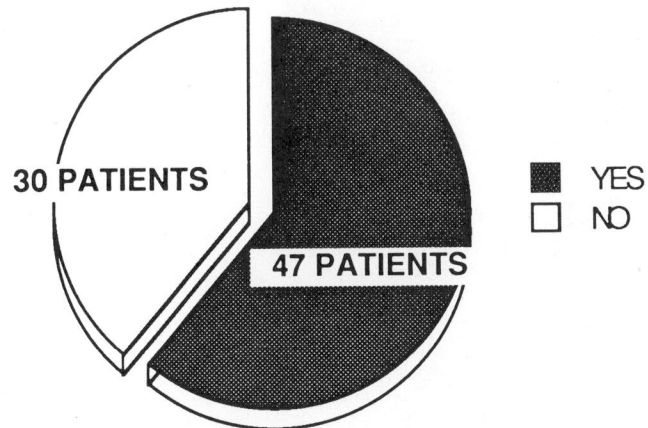

FIGURE 45–5
Number of patients with at least one complication following AICD implantation from representative study population (see text). Complication was defined as any adverse effect including discomfort due to AICD discharge in the absence of arrhythmia symptoms.

obvious that some problems such as generator failure or malfunction can occur soon after implantation. However, for the sake of simplifying the presentation and categorizing complications reported by others, these complications have been reported as occurring late (see below). Suggested strategies for avoiding or managing the complications encountered are also discussed.

EARLY POSTOPERATIVE COMPLICATIONS

Complications reported to occur in the early postoperative period, along with their estimated incidence, are listed in Table 45–1. Many of the problems encountered early are clearly related to the surgical technique and the extent of the tissue dissection required for implantation of the AICD generator and lead system and to the size and number of leads used. A subcostal approach for epicardial lead placement, which appears to provide adequate exposure for two-patch lead placement, is accompanied by much less pain and may help obviate some of the pulmonary complications noted.[16] Rarely, subclavian vein thrombosis and large seromas at the generator pocket site have been seen with implantation of standard bradycardia pacing devices. Because of the size of the AICD leads (spring lead, No. 12.2 French) and the amount of tissue dissection, these problems are more common with the AICD system (Fig. 45–6).[4, 7, 29] The risk of subclavian vein thrombosis appears to be less if the spring lead, used as part of the energy-delivering system, and the endocardial rate-sensing lead are implanted in the opposite subclavian veins. A total epicardial approach with respect to lead placement will obviously eliminate the risk of endovascular complications. This policy is now advocated by a number of institutions, including our own.[10, 39, 41] The large fluid accumulation that can develop at the generator pocket

TABLE 45–1
Early Postoperative Complications of AICD Implantation*

Complications	Estimate of Incidence (%)
Death (intra- or early postoperative)	<1–8
High defibrillation threshold—AICD not implanted	1–4
Vascular erosion	<1–2
Arterial embolic events	
Intraoperative myocardial infarction	<1–4
Vascular thrombosis (usually subclavian vein)†	2–10
Infection	1–5
Atelectasis/pneumonia	<1–10
Pneumothorax	<1–4
Large symptomatic pleural effusion	<1–10
Large seromas (generator pocket)	2–5
Subcutaneous hematoma	1–2
Bradycardia (post-shock) requiring pacing	<1–4
Failure to terminate VT/VF during postoperative testing	3–6
Early reoperation (change lead or generator)	<1–5

*Does not include AICD discharge when asymptomatic. Based on data compiled from references 2–9, 20, 30, 37, and 39–41.
†Seen exclusively with endovascular spring lead.

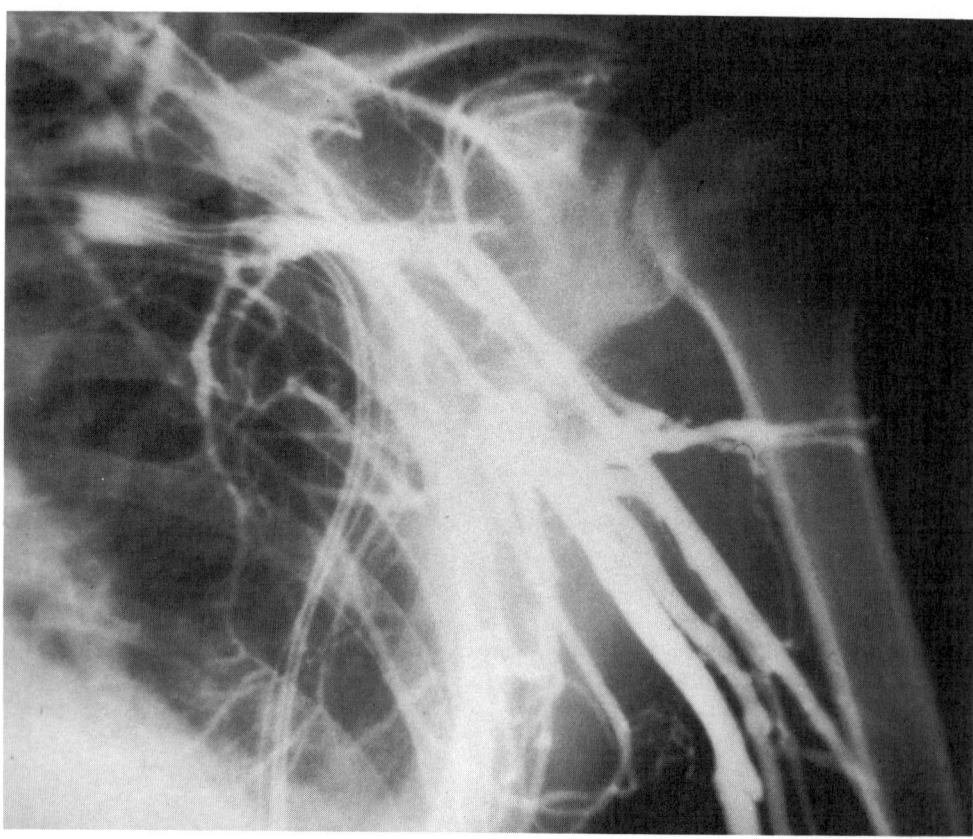

FIGURE 45–6
Left subclavian vein thrombosis at site of insertion of rate-sensing lead and energy-delivering spring lead.

site is usually asymptomatic and generally resolves spontaneously. There does not appear to be an associated increase risk of infection with the seromas; thus, needle aspiration to rule out infection in the absence of significant tenderness or evidence of inflammation is not advocated. Needle aspiration itself has the potential for seeding the generator pocket site.

One of the most serious complications that we have observed in the early postoperative period has been vascular erosion or disruption due to the AICD patch leads. Because this complication, to our knowledge, has not been noted by others, we believe that the risk of this problem is low. Placement of the flexible patch electrode in approximation to an aortic anastomosis site of a coronary artery bypass graft led to early graft dehiscence during the postoperative period in one of our patients and required emergent reoperation. Care should be taken to place the epicardial patches away from coronary artery bypass grafts and preferably outside the pericardium if in approximation to a bypass graft.

Arterial embolic phenomena occurred in two (3%) of our 77 patients. One patient was documented to have an embolus of the left femoral artery, noted at the end of the implantation procedure. The second patient had acute onset of a cerebral vascular accident in the left parietal lobe 48 hours after device implantation. This patient had a history of atrial fibrillation for more than two years. During interoperative device testing, atrial fibrillation was converted to normal sinus rhythm. Of note, the risk of embolic phenomena following routine electrophysiologic testing is extremely low.[43] Because the episodes of embolic phenomena that we noted are the only ones reported to date,[4] the use of anticoagulation therapy immediately before and after AICD implantation should be considered with caution. This is especially true in light of the large amount of serosanguineous pleural fluid accumulation/drainage that has been documented following AICD lead placement.[3]

Bradyarrhythmias following AICD discharge appear to be common.[32] However, severe bradycardia (>6–10 s of asystole) is rather uncommon (see Table 45–1).[29,30] We have implanted a backup bradycardia pacing device to manage post-shock bradyarrhythmias in only two of 77 patients.

Although it is recommended, postoperative electrophysiologic testing to evaluate AICD function is not routinely performed at all institutions. As noted previously, we attempt to test AICD function in terminating ventricular fibrillation in all our patients. At the time of postoperative testing in our first 34 patients, we noted the inability to terminate ventricular fibrillation with two to four AICD discharges in five patients.[43] In two of these five patients, the AICD terminated ventricular tachycardia. Of note, all five patients had defibrillation thresholds that approached the energy output of the AICD device (less than 10-J difference). In two of the five patients (both with a clinical history of ventricular fibrillation), the findings at postoperative testing led us either to modify the lead position or to replace the generator with one capable of delivering a higher output.

Echt et al.[2] noted findings similar to ours. They reported that in two of their 70 patients (both with "increased" defibrillation thresholds during intraoperative testing), the AICD device failed to terminate their arrhythmia during postoperative testing. In fact, because of ventricular tachycardia acceleration noted in these patients, the AICD was explanted. Because of the findings of these investigators and our own experience, we now modify patch position, polarity, or type to achieve a defibrillation threshold that is less than the energy output of the AICD by at least 10 J.[42,44]

LATE COMPLICATIONS

The most frequent serious late complication is infection (Table 45–2). Pocket infection usually requires explantation of the entire AICD lead system.[29,41] We have had noted two (3%) such infections. The seeding process in one patient, we believe, occurred at the time of repositioning of a migrated spring lead. Winkle and colleagues[40] reported a similar incidence of serious infection with five (3.2%) of 157 patients requiring removal of the entire AICD system. Of note, Platia et al.[29] reported that of seven patients with generator pocket infections (6% incidence), only two required explantation of the lead system. The remaining five patients were adequately treated by removal of the generator alone and by antibiotic therapy.

Lead migration was frequently experienced early in the clinical trials involving the AICD (Fig. 45–7).[4,38] Three of our first 15 patients and four of the initial nine implants by Kadri et al.[38] were associated with spring lead migration during follow-up. Many institutions, including our own, have switched to a two-patch lead system in part to avoid this complication.[13,39] As suggested by Mower and coworkers,[45] all endovascular leads should be secured with a Silastic anchor at the point of entry into the vein.

Early generator failure related to battery or component failures has not been uncommon, especially in the early experience with the device. Kadri and

TABLE 45–2
Late Complications of AICD Implantation*

Complications	Estimate of Incidence
Infection	1–6
Lead migration†	10–40
Early generation failure/malfunction	5–8
Lead fracture/insulation break	<1–2
Skin erosion	<1–3
Need for acute psychiatric support	2–10
Failure to sense VT above rate cut-off	<1–2
Constrictive pericarditis	<1

*Does not include AICD discharge without symptoms. Based on data compiled from references 2–9, 29, 30, 37, and 39–41.
†Prior to use of Silastic anchor.

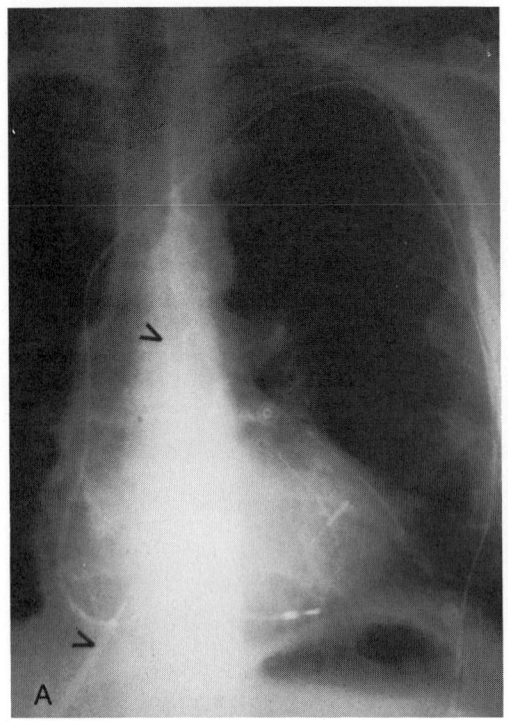
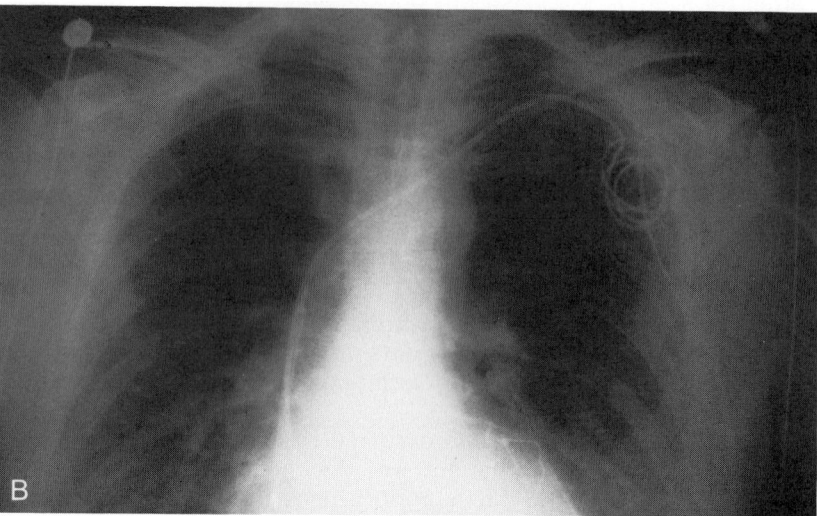

FIGURE 45-7
A, Migration of spring lead and bipolar rate-sensing leads (arrowheads). The spring lead has migrated to the level of the liver from its normal position at the superior vena cava and right atrial junction. The bipolar rate-sensing lead has formed a loop that extends out of the right ventricular outflow tract. B, After pulling back the leads, normal positioning can be seen. The extra lead wire is coiled and secured in the subcutaneous tissue just below the venous insertion site.

coworkers[38] reported nine such failures in the first 25 devices implanted at their institution.[39] The manufacturer recently reported 118 (6%) confirmed pulse generator failures in 2120 device implants for the AID-B, AID-BR, and Ventak AICD.[46] Lead problems related to fracture or insulation break have been remarkably uncommon. Life expectancy of the patch and spring leads remain to be determined in humans, but durability testing suggests a long life expectancy for these leads.[45] As noted previously, the patch leads placed over the epicardium do not appear to be associated short-term with significant hemodynamic effects. However, a case report by Almassi et al.[25] demonstrated that constrictive pericarditis can develop many months (i.e., 15) following patch placement. The frequency of this problem during long-term follow-up remains to be determined.

Skin erosion by the large AICD generator has been documented by several investigators.[5, 8] This problem may be aggravated by generator placement at the belt line in male patients. Reconstruction of the generator pocket is necessary. Close observation for this adverse affect is necessary to avoid contamination from a skin break and serious infection.[8]

Severe psychiatric disturbances have been documented during long-term follow-up.[3, 29, 47] Discharge of the device in the absence of significant symptoms (see below) can lead to extreme avoidance of activity in which the patient was engaged at the time of discharge. In one of our patients, discharges during teeth brushing had dire consequences with respect to oral hygiene. Frequent discharge of the device for symptoms consistent with an arrhythmia may lead to an inordinate fear concerning device malfunction. We now advocate professional psychiatric support for all of our patients. Just as important as the need for formal psychiatric support is the effort spent by the electrophysiologist/cardiologist in educating the patient on normal function of the device and its potential for dysfunction.

AICD DISCHARGE IN THE ABSENCE OF SYMPTOMS

AICD discharge in the absence of symptoms has been the most common problem encountered during follow-up.[3-10, 48, 49] In our experience and that of other investigators, discharge in the absence of symptoms occurs as commonly as or more commonly than discharge in association with arrhythmia symptoms.[2, 48] Of our 77 patients, 35 experienced discharge of the AICD without symptoms (Fig. 45–8). Echt et al.[2] noted that only a minority of the 37 patients in their study who experienced device discharge had prior symptoms consistent with an arrhythmia. We were able to document electrocardiographically at least one episode of asymptomatic discharge in 24 of these 35 patients (Fig. 45–9). In over one third of these patients the ECG demonstrated a sustained, ventricular tachycardia with uniform morphology prior to AICD discharge. The absence of significant symptoms has occurred even in association with a ventricular tachycardia cycle length of 260 ms and an arrhythmia duration of 16 s prior to

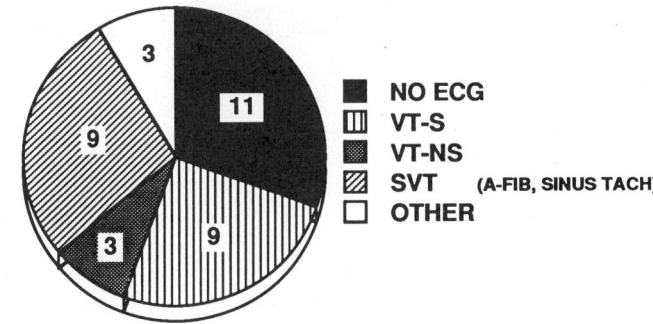

FIGURE 45–8
ECG diagnosis of 35 patients at the time of AICD discharge in the absence of significant symptoms. See text for discussion. VT-S = sustained ventricular tachycardia; VT-NS = unsustained ventricular tachycardia; SVT = supraventricular tachycardia.

device discharge (Fig. 45–9). Clearly, as suggested by Echt and associates[2] and Masterson and coworkers,[49] many asymptomatic shocks are actually for sustained ventricular arrhythmias.

Of note, however, in 17 patients (20%) we documented AICD discharge during rhythms other than sustained ventricular tachycardia or ventricular fibrillation. In three patients, the rhythm was nonsustained ventricular tachycardia (see Fig. 45–1) and in nine patients the rhythm was supraventricular in origin (Fig. 45–10). One patient with nonsustained ventricular tachycardia and three patients with documented atrial fibrillation did have palpitations prior to the AICD discharge, suggesting that the development of symptoms does not always indicate that the device discharged for sustained ventricular arrhythmia, as is frequently assumed. In the remaining patients in our study, the AICD discharged in the absence of symptoms due to (1) misdirection of the energy to the patient during magnet testing, (2) sensed myopotentials during arm movement or shivering, and (3) electromagnetic signals emitted during initiation of the "stat" VVI mode during routine pacemaker programming (Fig. 45–11).[50]

Additional causes for inappropriate shocks that have been reported include sensing-lead insulation breaks or intermittent fracture and double counting due to sensed atrial pacing stimuli or ventricular pacing stimulus and the local ventricular electrogram during atrial and/or ventricular pacing (see below).[3, 20] Winkle et al.[41] noted that 23 out of their 157 patients (15%) experienced problematic inappropriate shocks, an incidence which is similar to ours.

It is obvious that electrocardiographic monitoring just prior to the device discharge is the best way to document the appropriateness of the device discharge and the rhythm responsible for triggering the AICD device. Unfortunately, because the episodes of asymptomatic shocks may be separated by months or may occur as isolated events in selected patients, long-term electrocardiographic monitoring is frequently not productive. If electrocardiographic monitoring is available at the time of AICD discharge, a comparison should be made between the heart rate and the AICD rate cut-off. It should be recognized that the surface electrocardiogram does not always reflect the recording registered by the defibrillating leads. Rhythms that result in a relatively narrow QRS width on a single surface lead electrocardiogram may be of a sufficient width on the recording from the energy delivering leads such that the PDF sensing criteria may be fulfilled.

Many of the shocks can be avoided by proper preoperative and intraoperative evaluation. Documentation of (1) the maximum sinus rate with exercise, (2) the presence of episodes of nonsustained ventricular tachycardia or paroxysmal supraventricular tachyarrhythmias, and (3) the rates and hemodynamic tolerance of all ventricular tachycardias should be part of the routine evaluation. The use of an antitachycardia pacemaker for tolerated ventricular tachycardia in conjunction with an AICD for backup management of accelerated arrhythmias should be considered.[51, 52]

If the rate-sensing criteria are not fulfilled and/or if electrocardiographic documentation of the rhythm prior to AICD discharge is not available, then several

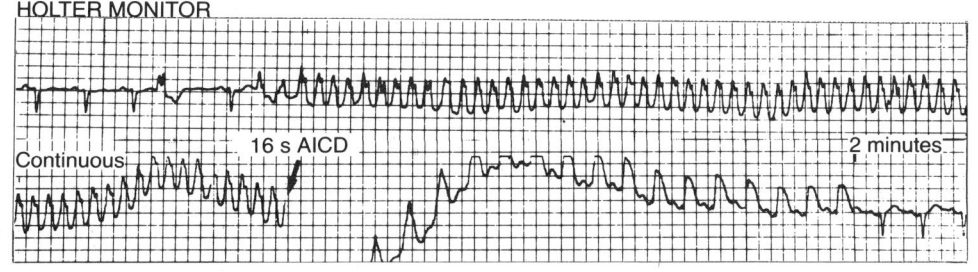

FIGURE 45–9
Holter monitor recording demonstrating AICD termination of spontaneous ventricular tachycardia. Rapid recognition and AICD discharge by the AICD resulted in no or minimal symptoms despite the rapid ventricular rate. (Reprinted by permission from Marchlinski FE: In Zipes DP, Rowlands DJ (eds.): Progress in Cardiology, pp. 231–253. Philadelphia, Lea & Febiger, 1988.)

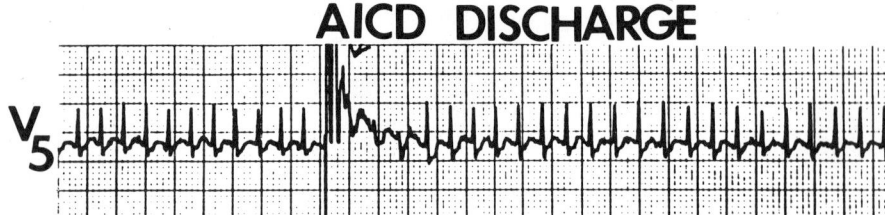

FIGURE 45-10
AICD discharge during sinus tachycardia (rate = approximately 170 bpm). ECG recording of lead V_5 was obtained at 50% of normal speed (12.5 mm/s).

additional steps should be carried out to attempt to document the basis for the AICD discharge by placing and holding a magnet over the upper right-hand corner of the pulse generator, the piezoelectric device in the generator emits a tone synchronous with each sensed event. To evaluate the tones, and therefore the sensed events, the AICD device is deactivated and then reactivated, leaving the magnet in place. Chapman and Troup[20] have suggested obtaining simultaneous surface electrocardiographic and phonographic recordings of the emitted tone to document whether "double beeping" occurs due to oversensing of P or T wave or pacing stimulus (Fig. 45–12).

Because oversensing sometimes is related to sensed myopotentials, it is always appropriate to evaluate beeping tones at rest and with at least upper extremity exercise or movement.[53] Counting of P waves or T waves or double counting of R waves can occur when (1) epicardial rate-sensing electrodes are in proximity to the atrium or have a wide interelectrode spacing and (2) in association with a bradycardia, during which the automatic gain control is increased in an attempt to identify presumed ventricular fibrillation that may be associated with a small signal amplitude. Radiographic evaluation of the AICD generator and leads should be performed to identify possible lead fracture or migration.

A poorly inserted lead pin at the site of the pulse generator may also be documented. Frequent AICD discharges in the absence of a heart rate which is above the rate cut-off for the AICD device may necessitate opening the generator pocket to see that the AICD set screw caps are intact. In addition, evaluation of electrograms from both the rate- and morphology-sensing leads can be performed. Leads should be inspected for damage or fracture. Finally, the leads should be disconnected from the header and unipolar and bipolar resistances, pacing thresholds, and R wave amplitude and duration should then be measured directly from the rate-sensing electrodes and compared with baseline measurements obtained at the time of initial implantation.

If the discharge occurred during exercise or physical activity, a formal exercise test should be performed with the AICD maintained in an active state.[53] Triggering of the device by a rhythm other than a ventricular tachycardia or ventricular fibrillation during exercise can be dumped internally by placing the magnet over the generator for 2 seconds after the initiation of the charging cycle.[53] Unfortunately, despite all these evaluation techniques, the basis for a large number of AICD discharges cannot be determined. We have observed a greater risk of AICD discharge in the absence of symptoms or ECG-documented ventricular tachycardia in patients with AICD devices that have rate only–sensing criteria (Fig. 45–13). Patients with frequent short-lived episodes of nonsustained ventricular tachycardia or with atrial fibrillation that cannot be suppressed by antiarrhythmic drug therapy should have AICD devices with both rate- and PDF-sensing

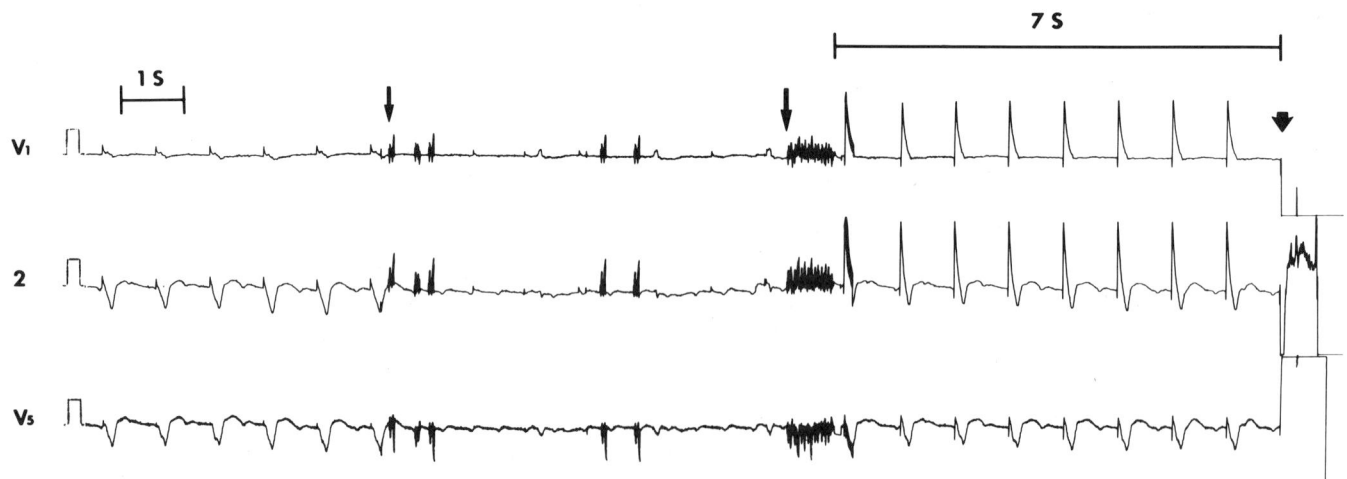

FIGURE 45-11
AICD discharge during pacemaker threshold determinations (first arrow). Initiation of "STAT" VVI mode produced an electromagnet signal that contributed to fulfillment of rate-sensing criteria and AICD discharge (broad arrow). (Reprinted by permission from Gottlieb C, Miller J, Rosenthal ME, et al.: PACE 11:336–338, 1988.)

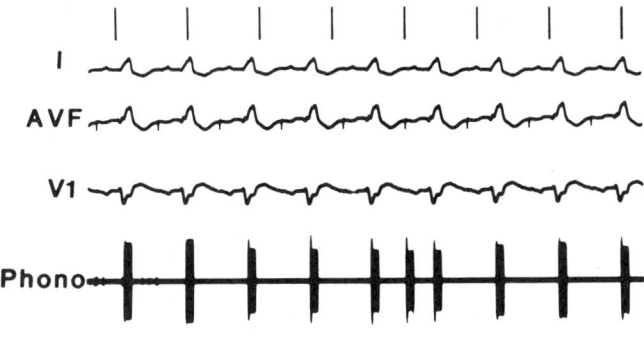

FIGURE 45–12
Simultaneous surface ECG (leads I, avF, and V₁) and surface phonocardiographic (Phono) recordings demonstrating continuous sensing of the QRS complex and intermittent sensing of atrial pacemaker stimuli (sixth atrial stimulus from the left). Paper speed is 25 mm/s. Time lines (T) are shown with the interval between longer lines equal to 1 s. (Reprinted by permission of the American College of Cardiology from Chapman PD, Troup P: J Am Coll Cardiol 7:1075, 1986.)

criteria, which necessitate a longer duration of arrhythmia.

FAILURE OF THE AICD TO RECOGNIZE VENTRICULAR TACHYCARDIA OR VENTRICULAR FIBRILLATION

The most common cause for failure of the AICD to sense a sustained ventricular arrhythmia is a tachycardia rate that falls below the rate cut-off of the device. This can happen due to inadequate pre- and intraoperative evaluation and documentation of tachycardia rates or due to the addition of an antiarrhythmic agent that slows the rate of the tachycardia (see below).[4] Occasionally, episodes of ventricular tachycardia or fibrillation that should satisfy the rate criteria for the AICD device are not sensed. Bardy et al.[54] reported a case in which excessive variability in the electrogram size (2–39 mV) during ventricular fibrillation prevented the automatic gain of the AICD to adjust rapidly enough to sense the low-amplitude signals that occurred following the large-amplitude electrograms. Occasionally very narrow complex sustained ventricular tachycardia will not fulfill the PDF-sensing criteria. Symptomatic arrhythmias may require a change to a generator with a rate only–sensing criterion.

AICD AND PACEMAKER INTERACTIONS

Conduction system disease and/or sinus node dysfunction with symptomatic bradyarrhythmias are frequently found in the same patients who experience life-threatening sustained ventricular arrhythmias. Ten (13%) of our 77 patients who received the AICD also had a pacemaker implanted for bradyarrhythmias. Signals produced by pacemakers implanted to manage bradyarrhythmias may affect adversely the function of the AICD. Oversensing, leading to inappropriate AICD discharge, or undersensing of life-threatening ventricular arrhythmias can occur. Specifically, atrial and ventricular pacemaker stimulus artifacts may be inappropriately sensed as a ventricular electrogram, resulting in a sensed rate that is above the rate cut-off.[20]

The sensing of a large-amplitude atrial pacing spike during atrial pacing with intact atrioventricular conduction is also possible, resulting in a doubling counting of the true rate.[20] Double counting may also occur when excessive latency exists between the pacemaker stimulus artifact and the evoked ventricular electrogram. Since the nominal value for the refractory period of the AICD sensing circuit is 150 ms, a stimulus to the electrogram interval exceeding this duration potentially can lead to sensing of both the ventricular stimulus artifact and the ventricular electrogram as separate signals. The problems of double counting can be potentiated by increasing the spacing of the interelectrode distance of the AICD sensing system and/or by recording from myocardium demonstrating abnormal multicomponent electrograms. Sensing electrodes should be implanted with a very narrow (> 1 cm) interelectrode distance. A large-amplitude single component signal should be documented during sinus rhythm and during ventricular pacing. Other steps to reduce the risk of double counting include (1) placement of the bradycardia pacing lead at a maximum distance from the AICD rate-sensing lead, (2) use of the smallest effective pulse amplitude during pacing and, most important, (3) use of a bipolar pacing system to avoid large-amplitude unipolar pacing spikes. Of note, at the time of AICD implantation, recordings from the AICD sensing electrodes during fixed-rate atrial and/or ventricular pacing should be documented. It is recommended that the maximum current output of the pacemaker device be used when these recordings are obtained. In addition, the interval from the ventricular pacing stimulus, if identifiable, to the end of the ventricular electrogram recorded by the AICD rate-sensing lead should be documented not to exceed 140 ms.

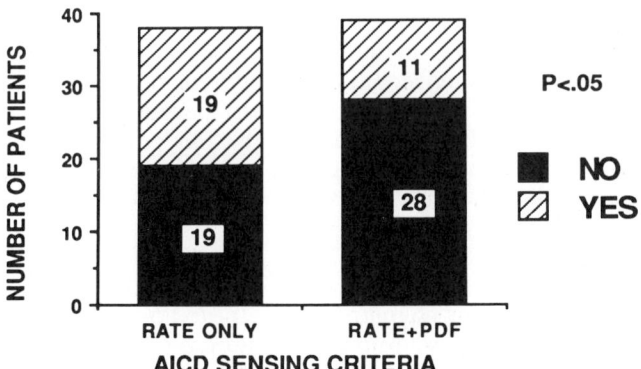

FIGURE 45–13
Relationship between (1) AICD discharge in the absence of symptoms consistent with a sustained ventricular arrhythmia and (2) the sensing criteria used by the AICD device. AICD discharge in the absence of symptoms or ECG-documented ventricular tachycardia appeared more commonly in patients with AICD that used rate only–sensing criteria. PDF = probability density function.

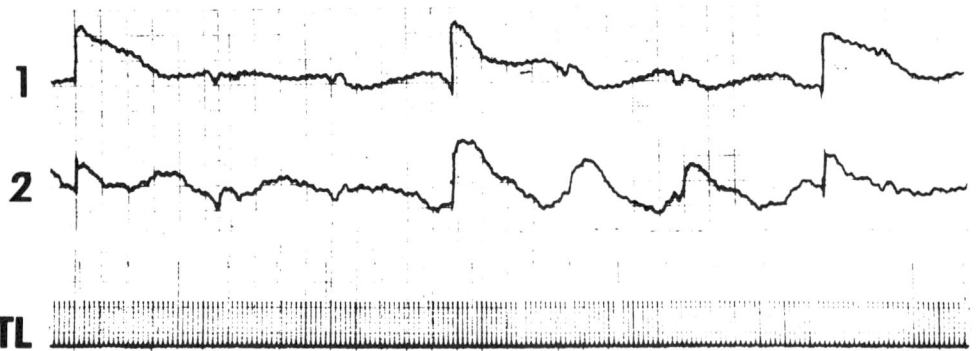

FIGURE 45–14
Failure of pacemaker to sense ventricular fibrillation, leading to large unipolar pacing stimulus signals. Large-amplitude signals delayed sensing of ventricular fibrillation by the AICD device. Surface ECG leads (1 and 2) are shown with 10-ms time lines (TL).

It is possible for the pacemaker to fail to sense ventricular tachycardia or fibrillation and to produce asynchronous atrial and/or ventricular pacing during these arrhythmias (Fig. 45–14). The potential exists for the large-amplitude pacing stimulus signals to be sensed by the AICD device. Because of the automatic gain of the AICD, the large-amplitude signals would prevent the device from being able to adjust rapidly enough to sense the lower-amplitude signal produced by ventricular fibrillation before the next large-amplitude pacing spike occurs. Thus, large-amplitude pacing spikes during ventricular arrhythmias can inhibit appropriate sensing function of the AICD device, leading to disastrous consequences. In order to prevent this potential problem, not only should the amplitude of the pacemaker signal be minimized and the distance between pacemaker and AICD sensing leads maximized, but also the sensitivity setting of the pacemaker should be at the highest setting to increase the chance of arrhythmia detection by the pacemaker.

The final AICD-pacemaker interaction with the potential to precipitate problems is related to transient undersensing and failure to capture that occur in pacemakers following AICD discharge. Cohen et al.[57] reported pacemaker failure to capture for 6.8 ± 5.3 s following 8 of 35 AICD discharges, and failure to sense for 4.7 ± 5.6 s following 10 of 35 AICD discharges. Failure in pacemaker sensing may result in the large pacemaker spikes being sensed as additional ventricular electrograms, leading to inappropriate retriggering of the AICD device. It is quite obvious that, given the multitude of problems related to pacemaker AICD interactions, future developments that permit the incorporation of backup pacing capabilities following AICD discharge are advisable.

AICD DRUG INTERACTIONS

Throughout this chapter we have noted potential ways by which antiarrhythmic drug therapy can interfere with optimal function of the AICD device. To summarize, antiarrhythmic drugs may

- result in a proarrhythmic effect and increase the frequency of AICD discharge leading to early battery depletion and increased patient discomfort;
- alter morphologic characteristics of the arrhythmia, with the potential for the new morphology not to be sensed by the AICD device or to produce aberrant conduction during supraventricular tachyarrhythmias, leading to triggering of the device;
- slow the tachycardia rate below the cut-off for the device[3, 57];
- transiently depress excitability following AICD discharge, potentiating the failure of pacemaker capture[58];
- alter the defibrillation threshold.

The effect of antiarrhythmic drugs on the defibrillation threshold in humans is still unknown. Animal studies suggest that antiarrhythmic drugs such as amiodarone, type IC agents, and lidocaine may produce significant elevations in defibrillation thresholds.[59–61] It would seem prudent until additional information is available to consider that all changes in antiarrhythmic drug therapy can significantly alter optimal AICD function. Documenting the ability of the AICD to sense and terminate all symptomatic arrhythmias should be considered following any change in antiarrhythmic therapy.

Future Considerations

There is little doubt the development of the "perfect" device for managing ventricular arrhythmias is still in its infancy. Many of the aforementioned adverse effects doubtlessly will be eliminated as the device is modified. A reduction in the physical size of the generator and the development of an effective transvenous lead system will eliminate the need for, and thus the risks involved with, thoracotomy. Programmability of the sensing criteria and the amount of energy delivered would clearly be advantageous, especially in those patients requiring changes in antiarrhythmic therapy. Incorporation of backup bradycardia pacing capabilities and antitachycardia pacing capabilities will obviate the need for two separate generators in a significant number of patients and may eliminate the frequent episodes of symptomatic device discharge for hemodynamically tolerated sustained ventricular tachycardia.

Finally, telemetry with memory to document the electrocardiographic signal prior to device discharge will clearly enhance our ability to determine the etiology of both asymptomatic or symptomatic discharges.

Appropriate therapy can then be instituted that can prevent frequent additional discharges. With the advances in technology, a compact, multipurpose antitachycardia pacing/cardioverting/defibrillating system will find increasing application in the management of sustained ventricular arrhythmias.

References

1. Mirowski M, Marton MM, Reid PR, et al.: The automatic implantable defibrillator: New modality for treatment of life-threatening ventricular arrhythmias. PACE 5:384, 1982.
2. Echt DS, Armstrong K, Schmidt P, et al.: Clinical experience, complications, and survival in 70 patients with the automatic implantable cardioverter/defibrillator. Circulation 71:289, 1985.
3. Reid PR, Morowski M, Mauer MM, et al.: Clinical evaluation of the internal automatic cardioverter-defibrillator in survivors of sudden cardiac death. Am J Cardiol 51:1608, 1983.
4. Marchlinski FE, Flores BT, Buxton AE et al.: The automatic implantable cardioverter-defibrillator: Efficacy, complications, and device failures. Ann Intern Med 104:481, 1986.
5. Luceri RM, Thurer RJ, Palatianos GM, et al.: The automatic implantable cardioverter-defibrillator: Results, observations, and comments. PACE 9:1343, 1986.
6. Vetri EP, Mower MM, Guarnieri T, et al.: Clinical efficacy of the automatic implantable defibrillator: Six-year cumulative experience (Abstract). Circulation 74:109, 1986.
7. Gabry MD, Brodman R, Johnston D, et al.: Automatic implantable cardioverter defibrillator: Patient survival, battery longevity and shock delivery analysis. J Am Coll Cardiol 9:49, 1987.
8. Borbola J, Denes P, Ezri MD, et al.: The automatic implantable cardioverter defibrillator: Clinical experience, complications and followup. Arch Intern Med 148:70, 1988.
9. Fogoros RN, Fiedler SB, Elson JJ: The automatic implantable cardioverter-defibrillator in drug-refractory ventricular tachyarrhythmias. Ann Intern Med 107:637, 1978.
10. Troup PJ: Lead system selection, implantation, and testing for the automatic implantable cardioverter defibrillator. Clin Prog Electrophysiol Pacing 4:260, 1986.
11. Winkle RA, Bach SM, Echt DS: The automatic implantable defibrillator: Local bipolar sensing to detect ventricular tachycardia and fibrillation. Am J Cardiol 52:265, 1983.
12. Reid PR, Griffith LSC, Mower MM, et al.: Implantable cardioverter-defibrillator: Patient selection and implantation protocol. PACE 7:1338, 1984.
13. Troup PJ, Chapman PD, Olinger GN, et al.: The implantable defibrillator: Relation of defibrillating lead configuration. J Am Coll Cardiol 6:1315, 1985.
14. Rubin L, Hudson P, Snively S, et al.: Defibrillation threshold energy and epicardial electrode size. Med Instrum 14:58, 1984.
15. Dixon EG, Tang ASL, Wolf PD, et al.: Improved defibrillation threshold with large contoured epicardial electrodes and biphasic waveforms. Circulation 76:1176, 1987.
16. Lawrie GM, Griffin JC, Wyndham CRC: Epicardial implantation of the automatic implantable defibrillator by left subcostal thoracotomy. PACE 7:1370, 1984.
17. Winkle RA, Stinson EB, Echt DS, et al.: Practical aspects of automatic cardioverter/defibrillator implantation. Am Heart J:1335, 1984.
18. Cardiac Pacemakers, Inc. (CPI): Physicians manual for the automatic implantable cardioverter defibrillator. Minneapolis-St. Paul, Minn: August, 1986.
19. Guarnieri T, Levine JH, Veltri EP, et al.: Success of chronic defibrillation and the role of antiarrhythmic drugs with the automatic implantable cardioverter/defibrillator. Am J Cardiol 60:1061, 1987.
20. Chapman PD, Troup P: The automatic implantable cardioverter-defibrillator: Evaluating suspected inappropriate shocks. J Am Coll Cardiol 7:1075, 1986.
21. Kim SG, Furman S, Matos JA, et al.: Automatic implantable cardioverter/defibrillator: Inadvertent discharges during permanent pacemaker magnet tests. PACE 10:579, 1987.
22. Winkle R, Schmidt P, Mead RH, et al.: Magnet test charge times to predict end of life of the automatic implantable defibrillator (Abstract). Circulation 74:II-110, 1986.
23. Mead RH, Ruder M, Schmidt P, et al.: Improved defibrillation efficacy with chronically implanted defibrillation leads (Abstract). Circulation 74:II-110, 1986.
24. Kadri N, Niazi I, Caceres J, et al.: Electrical stability of chronically implanted lead systems in patients with automatic cardioverter defibrillators (Abstract). Circulation 9:IV-461, 1987.
25. Chapman PD, Troup PJ, Wetherbee JN, et al.: The implanted defibrillator: Defibrillation threshold stability over time (Abstract). J Am Coll Cardiol 9:186A, 1987.
26. Troup PJ, Chapman PD, Olinger GN, et al.: The implanted defibrillator: Relation of defibrillating lead configuration and clinical variables to defibrillation threshold. J Am Coll Cardiol 6:1315, 1985.
27. Fogoros RN: Amiodarone-induced refractoriness to cardioversion. Ann Intern Med 100:699, 1984.
28. Frame LH, Hoffman N, Kolenik SA, et al.: Oral loading with amiodarone increases ventricular defibrillation threshold with implanted electrodes in dogs (Abstract). J Am Coll Cardiol 7:82A, 1986.
29. Platia EV, Veltri EP, Griffith LSC, et al.: Post defibrillation bradycardia following implantable defibrillator discharge (Abstract). J Am Coll Cardiol 7:73A, 1986.
30. Niazi I, Tchou P, Mahmud R, et al.: Significance of post defibrillation bradyarrhythmias in patients with automatic implantable defibrillators (abstract). Circulation 74:II-109, 1986.
31. Gottlieb C, Rosenthal M, Marchlinski F: Initiation of a sustained ventricular arrhythmia resulting from an R wave synchronous AICD discharge. Am Heart J 115:915–917, 1988.
32. Eysmann SB, Marchlinski FE, Buxton AE, et al.: Electrocardiographic changes after cardioversion of ventricular arrhythmias. Circulation 73:73, 1986.
33. Singer I, Hutchins GM, Mirowski M, et al.: Pathologic findings related to the lead system and repeated defibrillations in patients with the automatic implantable cardioverter defibrillator. J Am Coll Cardiol 10:382, 1987.
34. Antunes ML, Spotnitz HM, Livelli FD, et al.: Effect of electrophysiologic testing on ejection fraction during cardioverter defibrillator implants (Abstract). Circulation 76:IV-310, 1987.
35. Trappe HJ, Daniel WG, Klein H, et al.: Do patch electrodes of the implantable defibrillator impair left ventricular function? (Abstract) Circulation 74:II-111, 1986.
36. Almassi GH, Chapman PD, Troup PJ, et al.: Constrictive pericarditis associated with patch electrodes of the automatic implantable cardioverter-defibrillator. Chest 92:369, 1987.
37. Mirowski M, Reid PR, Mower MM, et al.: Clinical performance of the implantable cardioverter-defibrillator. PACE 7:1345, 1984.
38. Mirowski M: The automatic implantable cardioverter-defibrillator: An overview. J Am Coll Cardiol 6:461, 1985.
39. Kadri N, Niazi I, Elkhatib I, et al.: Automatic implantable cardioverter defibrillator: Problems and complications (Abstract). J Am Coll Cardiol 9:142A, 1987.
40. Singer I, Reid PR, Griffith LSC, et al.: Causes of death in patients with the internal defibrillator: Analysis of 188 patients at 60 months follow-up (Abstract). J Am Coll Cardiol 7:200A, 1986.
41. Winkle RA, Mead RH, Ruder MA, et al.: Five-year experience with the automatic implantable defibrillator in 157 patients (Abstract). J Am Coll Cardiol 9:167A, 1987.
42. Marchlinski F, Gottlieb C, Miller J, et al.: Effect of lead polarity on defibrillation threshold (Abstract). PACE 11:182A, 1988.
43. Horowitz LN, Kay HR, Kutalek SP, et al.: Risks and complications of clinical cardiac electrophysiologic studies: A prospective analysis of 1,000 consecutive patients. J Am Coll Cardiol 9:1261, 1987.
44. Marchlinski FE, Flores B, Miller JM, et al.: Is postoperative testing of the automatic implantable defibrillator necessary? (Abstract). PACE 10:438, 1987.
45. Mower MM, Reid PR, Watkins L, et al.: Automatic implantable cardioverter-defibrillator structural characteristics. PACE 7:1331, 1984.
46. Cardiac Pacemakers, Inc.: U.S. Experience with the AICD:

AICD Technology and Therapy Advances. Minneapolis-St. Paul, Minn: July, 1987.
47. Cooper DK, Luceri RM, Thurer RJ, et al.: The impact of the automatic implantable cardioverter defibrillator on quality of life. Clin Prog Electrophysiol Pacing 4:306, 1986.
48. Wetherbee JN, Chapman PD, Troup PJ, et al.: Relationship of automatic implantable cardioverter-defibrillator shocks to arrhythmia characteristics (Abstract). J Am Coll Cardiol 11:18A, 1988.
49. Poole JE, Troutman CL, Anderson J, et al.: Inappropriate and appropriate discharges of the automatic implantable cardioverter defibrillator (Abstract). J Am Coll Cardiol 11:210A, 1988.
50. Gottlieb C, Miller J, Rosenthal ME, et al.: Automatic implantable defibrillator discharge resulting from routine pacemaker programming. PACE 11:336–338, 1988.
51. Luderitz H, Gerckens U, Manz M: Automatic implantable cardioverter/defibrillator (AICD) and antitachycardia pacemaker (Tachylog): Combined use in ventricular tachyarrhythmias. PACE 9:1356, 1986.
52. Masterson M, Maloney JD, Wilkoff B, et al.: Automatic antitachycardia pacemaker and the automatic implantable cardioverter defibrillator as therapy for recurrent drug refractory ventricular tachycardia (Abstract). J Am Coll Cardiol 11:17A, 1988.
53. DeBorde R, Levine JH, Griffith LSC, et al.: Exercise testing in patients with automatic implantable cardioverter defibrillators (Abstract). J Am Coll Cardiol 2:169A, 1987.
54. Bardy GH, Evey TD, Steward R, et al.: Failure of the automatic implantable defibrillator to detect ventricular fibrillation. Am J Cardiol 58:1107, 1986.
55. Kim SG, Furman S, Waspe LE, et al.: Unipolar pacer artifacts induced failure of an automatic implantable cardioverter/defibrillator to detect ventricular fibrillation. Am J Cardiol 57:880, 1986.
56. Cohen C, Wish M, Miller F, et al.: Interactions between the automatic implantable defibrillator and implanted pacemakers (Abstract). Circulation 74, 1986.
57. Kadish AH, Marchlinski FE, Josephson ME, et al.: Amiodarone: Correlation of early and late electrophysiologic studies with outcome. Am Heart J 112:1134–1140, 1986.
58. DaTorre S, Bondke H, Brinker J, et al.: Increased pacing threshold after an automatic defibrillator shock: Effects of antiarrhythmic drugs (Abstract). Circulation 76:IV-310, 1987.
59. Black JN, Barbey JT, Echt DS: Modulation of lidocaine effects on ventricular defibrillation (Abstract). J Am Coll Cardiol 9:166A, 1987.
60. Arredondo MT, Guillen SG, Quinteiro RA: Effect of amiodarone on ventricular fibrillation and defibrillation thresholds in the canine heart under normal and ischemic conditions. Eur J Pharmacol 125:23, 1986.

46

The Future of Electrical Devices in the Chronic Treatment of Tachyarrhythmias

Ed Duffin
Earl Bakken

Overview

Innovations are successful, usually, because they meet user *wants* (which may differ from the designing technologists' perceptions of user *needs*). Predictions for the future role and characteristics of electrical devices in the chronic control of cardiac tachyarrhythmias can best be developed by considering the expressed desires of the physicians who prescribe them. Estimations of the timing of these advances, however, must be made in light of available and evolving technologies and the status of on-going electrophysiologic research.

Currently, technology and our understanding of electrophysiology equip us to produce devices capable of terminating tachyarrhythmias, once in progress. Thus, the immediate future will see significant development directed toward improving tachyarrhythmia-terminating devices. The first portion of this chapter describes the likely progress of devices designed to terminate malignant ventricular tachyarrhythmias. The second section describes devices designed to treat the less threatening supraventricular tachyarrhythmias.

Prevention of tachyarrhythmias is the preferred approach, but electrophysiologic research has yet to reach the point where practical devices with widespread applicability can be designed. Current efforts to reach this goal are discussed next, along with the prediction that neurocardiology, a multidisciplinary effort involving cardiac and neural medical specialists and engineers, may well provide the needed breakthroughs.

In the far distant future it is highly probable that multiple "smart" devices, each dealing with a specific aspect of arrhythmia management, may be implanted and interlinked via telemetry to provide an extremely powerful "rhythm governor." Such integrated systems are the subject of the final portion of this chapter.

Devices for the Termination of Ventricular Arrhythmias

The future of devices designed to terminate ventricular arrhythmias is probably easiest to predict in light of a 1986 survey conducted by the North American Society for Pacing and Electrophysiology (NASPE), of users of the automatic implantable cardioverter-defibrillator (AICD*), regarding their experiences with these first-generation devices. The respondents ranked the clinical limitations of these units in descending order of significance as follows:

1. Lack of programmability
2. Dependence on rate or rate/PDF for rhythm detection
3. Limited battery longevity
4. Lack of antitachycardia pacing
5. Need for major surgery to implant system
6. Lack of antibradycardia pacing
7. High cost
8. Large pulse generator
9. Problematic elective replacement indicator
10. Limited output energy (25–30 J)

Newly emerging devices are beginning to address many of these problems.[35] One unit now in clinical

---
*Cardiac Pacemakers, Inc., St. Paul, MN.

trials, the implantable pacemaker/cardioverter/defibrillator (PCD)* is highly programmable, allowing the user to noninvasively alter detection criteria, therapy sequencing, and monitoring capabilities. Detection of tachyarrhythmias is accomplished with two levels of criteria, one for tachycardia and a second for fibrillation. Rate of arrhythmia onset and rhythm stability are evaluated in addition to conventional rate and event counting, helping to minimize false detections due to atrial fibrillation or rapid sinus rhythms. The inclusion of pacemaker circuitry allows the PCD to integrate single-chamber antibradycardia pacing, multiple antitachycardia pacing therapies, and noninvasive electrophysiologic stimulation sequences. Sequential pulse delivery via three epicardial electrodes contributes to greater efficiency in defibrillation, thereby lowering energy requirements,[5, 20] and allowing a 30% reduction in generator size.

One can certainly expect to see a continuing series of rapidly improving PCDs over the next decade. Certainly there will be substantial gains in efficiency. Researchers are already reporting multiple sequential shocks,[8] biphasic pulse waveforms,[9, 14, 37, 42] bidirectional shocks,[33] and revised electrode configurations[11, 18, 19, 25, 26] that appear to reduce defibrillation energy requirements. These, in turn, will allow designers to further decrease pulse generator size and to increase device longevity. As devices become more flexible and longer-lasting, the annual cost of therapy for the electrical approach should decrease substantially.

Detection of tachyarrhythmias has historically been a problem for implantable devices. (Lerman, 1983)[22] Although the latest devices have substantially enhanced detection capabilities, they still leave considerable room for improvement. Ideally, such devices should not only detect but also classify arrhythmias. This will then make it possible for the devices to deliver therapies uniquely suited for each of multiple specific rhythms and to withhold therapies when they would be inappropriate. Various detection and classification strategies are currently being developed, including:

- Multichamber sensing for the evaluation of atrial and ventricular timing[28]
- Measurement of electrogram phase angles to distinguish among ventricular tachycardia, ventricular fibrillation, and normal sinus rhythm[38]
- Measurement of hemodynamic parameters such as right ventricular stroke volume,[1] right ventricular pressure,[3] and right ventricular dp/dt[40]
- Evaluation of electrogram waveform morphology[10, 23, 29]
- As algorithms using the more successful of these techniques are incorporated into newer devices, one can expect to see greater efficacy, less patient trauma due to inappropriate delivery of therapies, and fewer device-induced rhythm accelerations.

One of the most frequently voiced wants is for a defibrillator that can be implanted without a thoracotomy. Much research is being devoted to developing efficient defibrillation electrodes that do not require epicardial placement. One AICD implant was successfully achieved using a combination of two transvenous leads and a submuscular patch electrode in the mid-axillary line, delivering energy simultaneously over dual pathways.[34] This system resulted in defibrillation thresholds of roughly 10 joules. Ultimately, designers should be able to develop a completely transvenous system.[20, 41] This will have a significant positive effect on the level of acceptance of PCDs. Some clinicians speak of the possibility of prophylactic implantation of defibrillators in post–myocardial infarction patients who appear to be at high risk of malignant ventricular arrhythmias—*if* the system is reliable, small enough, transvenous, and cost-effective.

Although a great deal of development remains before we have a truly practical PCD, the task is not insurmountable. Looking back two and a half decades, similar problems were encountered with the early pacemakers. Figure 46–1 illustrates how far pacemaker technology has advanced in 25 years. There is little

DEFIBRILLATORS AND PACEMAKERS

Early Defibrillators

Intec AID
250 grams
Non-programmable
Epicardial leads
Thoracotomy required
Approximate 15 mos life
"Last resort" approach
Asynchronous operation
Single mode of operation
30 Joules output

Early Pacemakers

Medtronic Model 5850
250 grams
Non-programmable
Epicardial leads
Thoracotomy required
Approximate 15 mos life
"Last resort" approach
Asynchronous operation
Single mode of operation
600 microJoules output

25 YEARS

Future Defibrillators

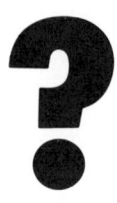

Modern Pacemakers

Medtronic Classix
26 grams
Multiprogrammable with Telemetry
Transvenous steroid lead with <1 microJoule threshold
10 year longevity
First resort therapy
Demand mode
Multimodal operation
25 microJoules output

FIGURE 46–1
Bradyarrhythmia pacemakers have undergone significant changes since 1959. Tachyarrhythmia devices should undergo equally significant and more rapid changes, since they will draw upon technology that has been developed for conventional pacemakers.

---

*Medtronic, Inc., Minneapolis, MN.

reason to doubt that PCDs will achieve comparable gains in less time in the future, since they can draw upon many of the technologies that have been pioneered with antibradycardia pacemakers. Indeed, in just 7 years, implantable defibrillators have advanced to a degree that required nearly 15 years for pacemakers.

Devices for the Termination of Atrial Arrhythmias

Electrical devices for the termination of supraventricular tachyarrhythmias have not received widespread acceptance despite having been available since the early 1970s. This, in part, is attributable to the availability of acceptable alternative therapies, including drugs, ablation, and various surgical techniques, that can prevent arrhythmia onset. Moreover, atrial tachyarrhythmias usually are not life-threatening and, therefore, do not justify unorthodox procedures. Nevertheless, numerous pioneering physicians have reported significant success with antitachycardia pacing to terminate supraventricular tachycardia (SVT), and a number of manufacturers have produced patient-activated and automatic devices for this application.[12, 17]

Looking to the future, it seems possible that these atrial devices may ultimately be embraced by users if suitable controlled studies are conducted to compare the electrical and pharmacologic approaches. There is reason to believe that the electrical systems can be superior to pharmacology, offering higher patient compliance, fewer side effects, and greater cost-effectiveness. Moreover, implantable devices are beginning to offer increasingly powerful patient monitoring capabilities that can help to establish the true efficacy of a particular therapeutic regimen. Positive user experiences with the evolving implantable defibrillators could well create a halo effect, increasing the acceptance of electrical therapies for supraventricular tachyarrhythmias.

One atrial arrhythmia that currently frustrates most clinicians is atrial fibrillation. A successful chronic electrical approach would be readily accepted, should one evolve. Also, because implantable ventricular defibrillators are capable of inducing atrial fibrillation, there is a need to find means to avoid this side effect. In the future, it seems likely that ventricular arrhythmia devices will ultimately be enhanced to include facilities for detecting and treating naturally occurring and iatrogenic atrial fibrillation.

Tachyarrhythmia Prevention

The preferred operating mode for antitachycardia devices is arrhythmia prevention rather than termination. Conventional pacing systems have been used with some success to prevent tachyarrhythmias, using the following techniques:

1. Rate support to prevent tachycardias secondary to bradycardia.
2. Overdrive pacing to prevent emergence of tachycardia.
3. Rapid atrial stimulation to create AV block.
4. Dual-chamber pacing to prevent accessory pathway reentry and to ensure normal atrial-ventricular sequencing.

A recent retrospective Swedish study compared AAI and VVI pacing in sizable matched patient groups and found substantially higher rates of congestive heart failure and atrial fibrillation in patients with ventricular pacemakers.[32] Atrial pacing appears, in these patients, to have played a significant role in preventing the onset of atrial fibrillation. Other researchers have reported beneficial effects of VVI pacing in the prevention of ventricular tachyarrhythmias.[16] As dual-chamber adaptive rate pacemakers become commonly available, it seems likely that they will demonstrate even greater ability to prevent arrhythmias; controlled studies are certainly needed to validate this hypothesis.

Some currently available dual-chamber pacemakers offer unique operating modes designed specifically for tachyarrhythmia prevention.[7] These devices prevent sudden rate changes, acting as though the rate-determining mechanism had high inertia. Clinical studies to substantiate efficacy are not yet conclusive, although the technique seems promising.

A number of preventive pacing techniques are being investigated by electrophysiologists in the hope that practical devices can be developed for chronic application. These techniques include

- Precisely timed single and multiple subthreshold stimuli[31, 44]
- Simultaneous stimulation at multiple sites to prevent reentry[27]
- Pacing at the site of spontaneous tachycardia initiation with elevated energies, as shown in Figure 46–2[24]
- Dual-chamber pacing with flexible upper rate behavior[15]
- Train stimulation at the atria[35]
- Precisely timed atrial-triggered ventricular stimulation[2]

Because practical implementation of any of these methods presents a difficult challenge, it seems unlikely that they will become commercially available in the immediate future.

A particularly promising area of research in arrhythmia prevention is that of neurocardiology, the study of the interactions between the heart and the nervous system. Ventricular tachycardia or fibrillation may be due to chronic electrophysiologic abnormalities (e.g., damage resulting from infarction), acute and transient ischemia serving as a primary induction mechanism or as a trigger in the presence of chronic electrophysiologic abnormalities, or transient disturbances in neural innervation, which may act alone or in conjunction with the former mechanisms.[6, 30]

Schwartz and coworkers[36] have been systematically

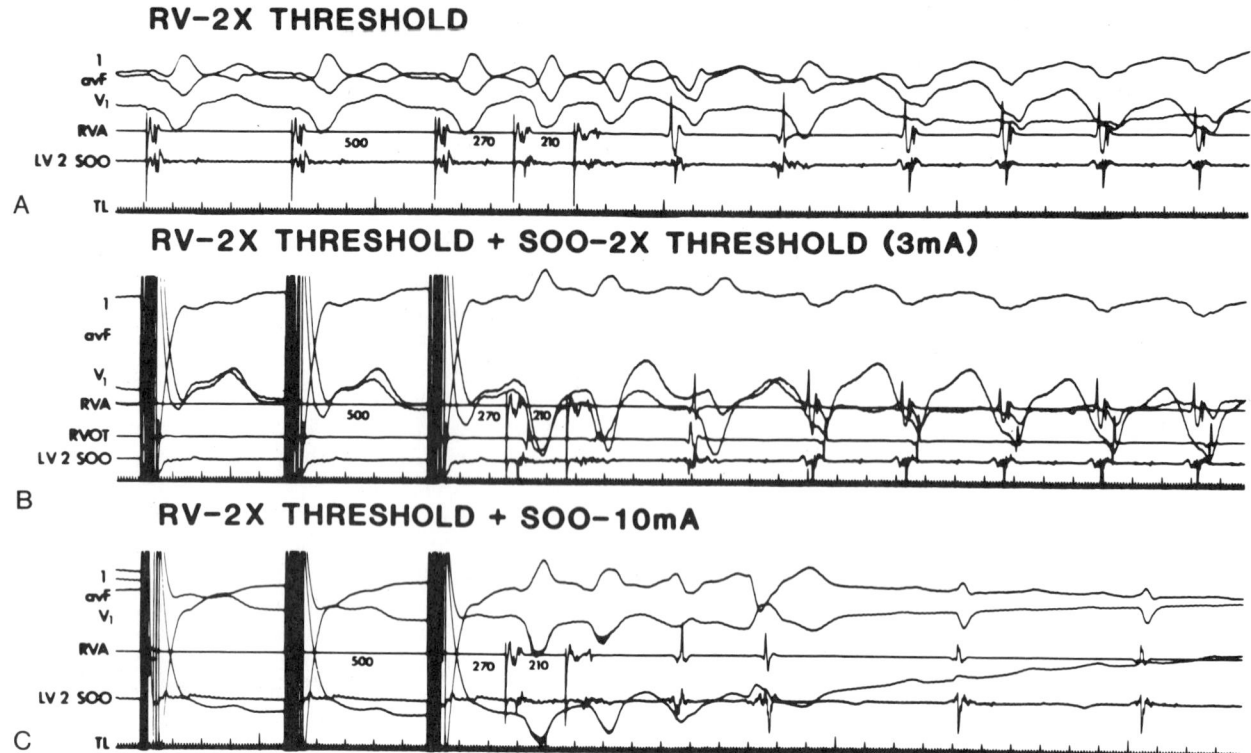

FIGURE 46–2
The influence of current strength on prevention of ventricular tachycardia induction with pacing at the left ventricular site of origin (LV 2 SOO).
 Ventricular tachycardia is induced during right ventricular apex (RVA) stimulation only (A) and when the RVA and LV 2 SOO are both paced at 2 times threshold (B). C, VT induction by extrastimuli from the RVA was prevented only when pacing the LV 2 SOO at 10 mA during the drive train. Distortions of surface ECGs are observed with LV pacing and in this patient are related to poor surface ECG isolation. Recording from the right ventricular outflow tract (RVOT) is demonstrated only in B. TL = time line.
 (Reprinted by permission of the American Heart Association, Inc., from Marchlinski, FE, Buxton AE, Miller JM, et al.: Circulation 76:336, 1986.)

studying the role of autonomic innervation in malignant ventricular arrhythmias and have shown that a high level of left sympathetic activity is associated with a poor prognosis following circumflex coronary artery occlusion in previously infarcted (anterior) canines.[4, 36, 39] Inducible animals were particularly susceptible when the occlusion occurred during exercise. In these animals, parasympathetic activity seemed protective, and, if not sufficient initially, could be enhanced by exercise regimens. The expected reduction in susceptibility to arrhythmias accompanied the increase in tone. Left stellectomy also afforded significant protection to the canine models. Schwartz has shown that this procedure increases ventricular refractory periods, myocardial reactive hyperemia, and fibrillation thresholds.

It may well be that neural pacemakers serving as governors of autonomic tone and balance may provide a more flexible and powerful tachyarrhythmia preventative than can a surgical approach such as stellectomy. Technology developed for adaptive rate cardiac pacemakers could conceivably be used to monitor autonomic balance without the need for neural sensing electrodes. The baroreflex slope, an indicator of such balance, may be obtainable from an implanted pressure sensor incorporated in a standard pacing lead (Fig. 46–3). Such a system could monitor variations in heart rate and right ventricular pressure throughout the respiratory cycle, providing a reasonable approximation of the baroreflex slope. Variations in this slope might herald ominous changes in autonomic status prior to the onset of tachyarrhythmias thereby allowing a neural pacemaker to correct autonomic balance before an arrhythmia can evolve.

As the science of neurocardiology advances, it will surely yield a multitude of approaches to a host of cardiac and cardiovascular malfunctions. Clinicians faced with managing tachyarrhythmias are likely to be the early beneficiaries of this rapidly evolving field.

Integrated Systems

As our approach to tachyarrhythmias becomes increasingly multidisciplinary, it is unlikely that a single device

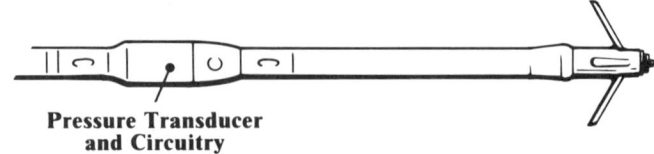

FIGURE 46–3
A chronically implantable pressure sensor developed by Medtronic, Inc., for use with rate-adaptive antibradycardia pacemakers. This technology may be directly applicable to antitachycardia applications.

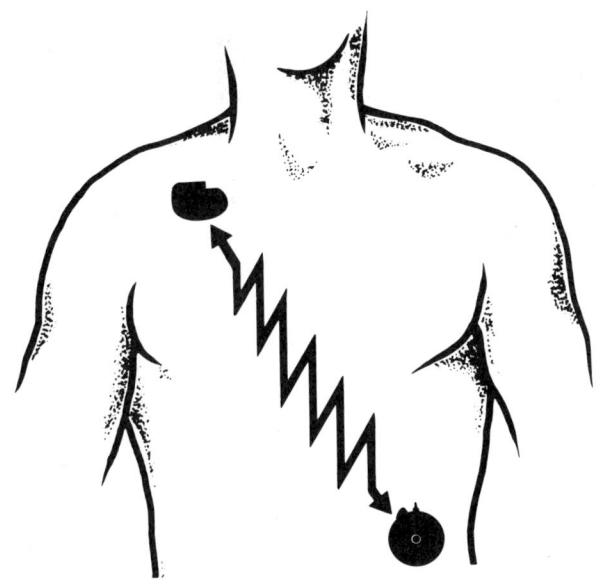

FIGURE 46—4
The integration of multiple "smart" devices is a likely development for a future tachyarrhythmia management system. In this illustration, an antitachycardia pacing system is linked via telemetry to an implantable drug infusion device.

will be capable of providing a completely satisfactory therapy. Most current electrical antitachycardia systems are used in conjunction with some pharmacologic agents (1) to make an arrhythmia less frequent or easier to terminate, (2) to reduce symptoms during the brief termination period, and (3) to slow the arrhythmia in order to simplify automatic detection by the implantable stimulator. Although the link has yet to be established, it is highly likely that electrical stimulators and triggered implantable drug infusion pumps will eventually be combined to accomplish similar goals, while eliminating the need for continuous medication and its attendant side effects. A simple system of this type is shown in Figure 46–4.

Eventually these systems may become far more elaborate. One can envision multiple remote sensor modules transmitting hemodynamic and neural status to a central "smart" administrative device, which would then control the operation of numerous effector systems such as neural stimulators, myocardial stimulators, and infusion pumps via bidirectional telemetry.

Epilogue

And now, ". . . we come into those realms of conjecture where the most logical minds may be at fault: each may form its own hypothesis upon the present evidence, and yours is as likely to be correct as mine."
—Sherlock Holmes, in The Adventures of the Empty House by A. Conan Doyle.

References

1. Bardy GH, Olson WH, Fishbein DP, et al.: Transvenous right ventricular impedance during spontaneous ventricular arrhythmias in man (Abstract). Circulation 72:III-474, 1985.
2. Begemann MJS, Bennekers JH, Kingma JH, et al.: Prevention of tachycardia initiation by programmed stimulation. J Electrophysiol 1:350, 1987.
3. Bennett T, Beck R, Erickson M: Right ventricular dynamic pressure parameters for differentiation of supraventricular and ventricular rhythms (Abstract). PACE 10:415, 1987.
4. Billman GE, Schwartz PJ, Stone HL: The effects of daily exercise on susceptibility to sudden cardiac death. Circulation 69:1182, 1984.
5. Bourland JD, Tacker WA, Wessale JL, et al.: Sequential pulse defibrillation for implantable defibrillators. Med Instrum 20:138, 1986.
6. Breithardt G, Borggrefe M, Haerten K, et al.: Mechanisms of sudden cardiac death and of syncope, In Proceedings of the XVth Tromso Seminar in Medicine, p. 24. Tromso, Norway, University of Tromso, 1987.
7. Brottier L, Bricaud H, Derrien Y: Antiarrhythmia pacing using the Quintech DPG 921. A case report. In Vitatext, pp. 14–17. Dieren, The Netherlands; Vitatron Medical, 1981.
8. Chang MS, Inone H, Kallok MJ, et al.: Double and triple sequential shocks reduce ventricular defibrillation thresholds in dogs with or without myocardial infarction. J Am Coll Cardiol 8:1393, 1986.
9. Chapman PD, Wetherbee JN, Vetter JW, et al.: Nonthoracotomy internal defibrillation: Improved efficacy with biphasic shocks (Abstract). Circulation 76:IV-312, 1987.
10. Davies DW, Tooley MA, Cochrane T, et al.: Real time automatic tachycardia diagnosis and treatment from analysis of electrogram morphology. In Proceedings, Xth World Congress of Cardiology, p. 971. Washington, DC, 1986.
11. Dixon EG, Tang ASL, Wolf PD, et al.: Decreased defibrillation thresholds with large contoured patch electrodes in dogs (Abstract). J Am Coll Cardiol 9:143A, 1987.
12. Duffin EG, Zipes DP: Chronic electrical control of tachyarrhythmias. In Mandel W (ed.): Cardiac Arrhythmias: Their Mechanisms, Diagnosis, and Management, 2nd Ed., pp. 764–781. Philadelphia, J. B. Lippincott, 1987.
13. Echt DS: Potential hazards of implanted devices for the electrical control of tachyarrhythmias. PACE 7:580, 1984.
14. Fain ES, Sweeney MB, Franz MR: Improved internal defibrillation efficacy using a biphasic waveform (Abstract). Circulation 76:IV-312, 1987.
15. Friedman PL, Berkovits B: Prevention of reentrant supraventricular tachycardia with a new antitachycardia pacemaker (Abstract). PACE 10:609, 1987.
16. Fisher JD, Teichman SL, Ferrick A, et al.: Antiarrhythmic effects of VVI pacing at physiologic rates: A crossover controlled evaluation. PACE 10:822, 1987.
17. Fisher JD, Johnston DR, Furman S, et al.: Long-term efficacy of antitachycardia pacing for supraventricular and ventricular tachycardias. Am J Cardiol 60:1311, 1987.
18. Hannekum A, Dalichau H, Kochs M, et al.: Sequential or single pulse defibrillation? Investigations towards energy reduction in experimental animals. Thorac Cardiovasc Surg 35:270, 1987.
19. Jones DL, Klein G, Kallok MJ: Improved internal defibrillation with twin pulse sequential energy delivery to different lead orientations in pigs. Am J Cardiol 55:821, 1985.
20. Kallok MJ, Marcaccini S: Efficacy of two transvenous electrode systems for sequential pulse defibrillation. In Gomez FP (ed.): Cardiac Pacing, pp. 1497–1504. Mount Kisco, Futura Publishing Co., 1985.
21. Kallok MJ, Bourland JD, Tacker WA, et al.: Optimization of epicardial electrode size and implant site for reduced sequential pulse defibrillation threshold. Med Instrum 20:36, 1986.
22. Lerman BB, Waxman HL, Buxton AE, et al.: Tachyarrhythmias associated with programmable automatic atrial antitachycardia pacemakers. Am Heart J 106:1029, 1983.
23. Lin DL, Jenkins JM, Wiesmey MD, et al.: Endocardial electrogram analysis: Techniques for distinguishing ventricular tachycardia from sinus rhythm. In Proc. AAMI 22nd Annual Meeting, p. 41. Los Angeles, CA, May 16–20, 1987.

24. Marchlinski FE, Buxton AE, Miller JM, et al.: Prevention of ventricular tachycardia induction during right ventricular programmed stimulation by high current strength pacing at the site of origin. Circulation 76:332, 1987.
25. Mead RH, Echt DS, Stinson EB, et al.: The automatic implantable defibrillator: Improved defibrillation and lowered impedance using two large patch leads (Abstract). J Am Coll Cardiol 5:455, 1985.
26. Mead RH, Ruder M, Schmidt P, et al.: Improved defibrillation efficacy with chronically implanted defibrillation leads (Abstract). Circulation 74:II-110, 1986.
27. Mehra R, Gough WB, Zeiler R, et al.: Dual ventricular stimulation for prevention of reentrant ventricular arrhythmias (Abstract). J Am Coll Cardiol 3:472, 1984.
28. Mercando AD, Vincenti A, Furman S, et al.: Tachycardia differentiation using one atrial and two ventricular electrodes (Abstract). PACE 10:998, 1987.
29. Pannizzo F, Amikam S, Bagwell P, et al.: Discrimination of antegrade and retrograde atrial depolarization by electrogram analysis. Am Heart J 112:780, 1986.
30. Priori SG, Schwartz PJ: Sympathetic nervous system and sudden cardiac death. In Proceedings of the XVth Tromso Seminar in Medicine, p. 63. Tromso, Norway, University of Tromso, 1987.
31. Prystowsky E, Zipes DP: Inhibition in the human heart. Circulation 68:707, 1983.
32. Rosenqvist M, Brandt J, Schüller H: Atrial versus ventricular pacing in sinus node disease: A treatment comparison study. Am Heart J 111:292, 1986.
33. Saksena S, Parsonnet V, Pantopoulos D, et al.: Transvenous cardioversion and defibrillation of ventricular tachyarrhythmias using bidirectional shocks: Acute feasibility studies and chronic device implant (Abstract). Circulation 76:IV-311, 1987.
34. Saksena S, Parsonnet V: Implantation of a cardioverter/defibrillator without thoracotomy using a triple electrode system. JAMA 259:69, 1988.
35. Schlüter M, Kunze KP, Kuck KH: Train stimulation at the atria for prevention of atrioventricular tachycardia: Dependence on accessory pathway location. J Am Coll Cardiol 9:1288, 1987.
36. Schwartz PJ: The rationale and the role of left stellectomy for the prevention of malignant arrhythmias. Ann NY Acad Sci 427:199, 1984.
37. Tang ASL, Dixon EG, Frazier DW, et al.: Comparison of contoured and patch electrodes for defibrillation with monophasic and biphasic waveforms (Abstract). Circulation 76:IV-311, 1987.
38. Tronstad A, Hoff PI, Ohm OJ: A new method for automatic detection of ventricular tachyarrhythmias (Abstract). PACE 10:754, 1987.
39. Vanoli E, Stramba-Badiale M, de Ferrari G, et al.: Baroreflex sensitivity and sudden death in conscious dogs before and after myocardial infarction (Abstract). J Am Coll Cardiol 9:80A, 1987.
40. Wasty N, Pantopoulos D, Rothbart SL, et al.: Detection of sustained ventricular tachyarrhythmias using right ventricular hemodynamic parameters. A prospective study (Abstract). J Am Coll Cardiol 9:141A, 1987.
41. Winkle RA, Mead RH, Echt DS, et al.: Automatic implantable defibrillator: Comparison of catheter defibrillation and defibrillation using superior vena cava spring-patch electrodes (Abstract). J Am Coll Cardiol 5:457, 1985.
42. Winkle RA, Mead RH, Ruder MA, et al.: Improved low energy defibrillation efficacy in man using a biphasic truncated exponential waveform (Abstract). PACE 9:142A, 1987.
43. Yee R, Klein G, Guiraudon GM, et al.: Initial clinical experience with the pacemaker/cardioverter/defibrillator. Can J Cardiol 6:147-156, 1990.
44. Zipes DP, Prystowsky EN, Miles WM, et al.: Future directions: Electrical therapy for cardiac tachyarrhythmias. PACE 7:606, 1984.

INDEX

Note: Page numbers in *italics* refer to illustrations; page numbers followed by t refer to tables.

Abdominal pacemaker pocket, 566
Ablative surgery, sudden cardiac arrest management with, 343
Absolute refractory period, inactivation of, with maximum diastolic potential (MDP), 10
Absorption mechanism, of antiarrhythmic agents, 409–410
 presystemic elimination and, 411
Accelerated idioventricular rhythms, in sustained ventricular tachycardia (VT), 252, *252*
Accessory pathways, catheter ablation of, 462–467
 complications following, 465–466
 experimental background on, 462–463
 for free-wall connections, 466
 for permanent junctional reciprocating tachycardia, 466–467
 for posteroseptal connections, 464–466, *465*
 indications for, 462
 techniques for, 463–464, *464*
 concealed connections in, paroxysmal supraventricular tachycardia due to, 440
 pre-excitation syndrome and, 192
 for surgical management of Wolff-Parkinson-White syndrome, 437–440, *438–439*
  division of anterior septal pathway during, 438
  division of posterior septal pathway during, 438–439, *439*
  electrocardiographic patterns in, 195, *195*
  left free-wall pathways for, 438, *439*
  right free-wall pathways for, 438
 in pre-excitation syndrome, 192–193
  evaluation of multiple pathway patients and, 205–206, *206*
  supraventricular tachycardias and, in infants, 286, *287*
 with decremental properties, 192–193
N-Acetylprocainamide (NAPA), long QT–torsades de pointes syndrome and, 271–273
 procainamide and, 416–417
Acid-base imbalance, sinus node automaticity and, 123
Action potential, abnormal electrophysiology and, 9–12
 cardiac pacing and, 487
 in ischemic epicardium, *37, 38*
 of atrial muscle, 7
 of atrioventricular node, 7–8
 of Purkinje fiber, 8
 of sinoatrial node, 7
 of ventricular muscle, 8–9

Action potential *(Continued)*
 prolongation mechanism of, in torsades de pointes, 274–275
 with acute myocardial infarction, 57
 with chronic myocardial infarction, 57
Action potential duration (APD), changes in, with MDP reduction, 11
 refractoriness and, 12
Activation fronts of fibrillation, defibrillation electrophysiology and, 715, *716–717*
Activation time measurements, during catheter ablation, 476, *477–478*
Active-fixation electrodes, 496
 implantation techniques for, 564
Activitrax device, activity sensing with, 532–533, *533–534*, 533t
Activity sensing, rate-responsive pacemakers and, 532–534
 Activitrax device as, 532–533, *533–534*, 533t
 Sensolog device as, 534–535, *534–535*
Acute coronary thrombosis, as cause of sudden cardiac death, 333–334
Acute drug testing, arrhythmia evaluation for, 103, *104*
Adams-Stokes attacks, hemodynamic effects of, 545
 Mobitz II AV block as sign of, 148
 paroxysmal AV block and, 156, *159*
Adenosine, role of, in treatment of SVT, 209–210
Adenosine diphosphate (ADP), basal energy utilization of, in heart, 58–59, *59*
Adenosine monophosphate (AMP), basal energy utilization of, in heart, 58
Adenosine triphosphate (ATP), basal energy utilization of, in heart, 58–60, *59*
 metabolism of, during myocardial ischemia, 69–73
Adrenergic receptor subtypes, cardiac arrhythmogenesis and, 77–79, *78*
Adrenergic stimulation, of repetitive monomorphic ventricular tachycardia, extrasystoles and heart rate with, 235, *236*
 repetitive response and, 238, *239–240*
Afterpolarizations. See *Delayed afterdepolarizations (DADs); Early afterdepolarizations (EADs).*
A-H interval, evaluation of patients with Mahaim fibers and, 206–207, *207*
 in atrioventricular nodal reentry, 174, *174*
 in first-degree AV block, 142, *143*
 in normal AV conduction, 141, *141*
AIDCHECK device, for automatic implantable cardioverter/defibrillator (AICD), 746

Alpha-adrenergic receptors, role of, in early myocardial ischemia, reperfusion arrhythmias and, 23–24
 sympathetic nervous system and cardiac arrhythmogenesis, 79, *80*
Alternate Wenckebach periodicity, 149–150, *151–152*
Ambulatory monitoring, for evaluation of antiarrhythmic drug therapy, 101–104, *102*, 102t–103t, *104*
 for evaluation of sudden cardiac death, 334–336
 for repetitive monomorphic ventricular tachycardia, 234–245
  extrasystoles and heart rate in, 235, *236*
 prevalence of arrhythmias on, 93–95, 93t, *94*
 risk of cardiac death and, 95–98, 96t–98t
 sustained ventricular tachycardia (VT) and, 258
Amiodarone, adverse effects of, 426–427
 as sudden cardiac arrest therapy, 342–343
 clinical pharmacokinetics of, 425, *426*
 dosage and plasma concentrations of, 425–426
 drug interactions with, 426
 electrophysiologic effects of, 425
 hemodynamic effects of, 425
 indications for use of, 426
 long QT–torsades de pointes syndrome and, 271
Amphipathic lipid metabolites, role of, in early myocardial ischemia, 22–23
Amplifier noise, in electrophysiologic signals, 350
Amygdala, cardiac arrhythmias and, 88, *88*
Analog signal recordings, during catheter ablation, 477
Anesthetic antiarrhythmics, 404–406, *404–405*
Anion-coupled potassium efflux, action of, during acute myocardial ischemia, 62–63, *63*
Anisotropy, abnormal impulse conduction and, 14
Annulus fibrosus, role of, in pre-excitation syndrome, 191
Antiarrhythmic agents, action of, on late potentials, 393–394
 on reentry arrhythmias, 47, 50
 aggravation of arrhythmia and, 105–106, *106*, 107t
 AICD interaction with, 756
 as sudden cardiac death risk factor, 218–219, 229, 336

765

Antiarrhythmic agents *(Continued)*
  cell membrane function and ion selective channels with, 401–404, *401–404*
  channel-blocking drugs as, 406, 407t
  classification of, 412–413
  clinical pharmacology of, 409–429, 414t, 415t
    absorption of, 409–411
    administration procedures for, 411–412, *412*
    bioavailability of, 409–410
    clearance of, 410, 411
    distribution of, 410–411, *411*
    drug release mechanism and, 409
    half-life and steady state of, 410, *410*
    of amiodarone, 424–427
    of bretylium tosylate, 427–428
    of combined agents, 429
    of disopyramide, 417–418
    of encainide, 421–422
    of flecainide, 420–421
    of lidocaine, mexiletine and tocainide, *418*, 418–419
    of procainamide, 416–417
    of propafenone, 422–424
    of quinidine, 414–416
    plasma concentrations of, 412, 413t
    presystemic elimination of, 411
    protein binding by, 410–411, *411*
  combinations of, for arrhythmia therapy, 104–106, *105*
  complex ventricular arrhythmia and, 218–219
  electrophysiologic studies (EPS) of, 296
  for atrial flutter, with cardiac pacing, 188–189
  for evaluation of pre-excitation syndrome patients, 207–208, 208t, 210–212
  for repetitive monomorphic ventricular tachycardia, 242–245
    beta blockers for, 242, *244*
    calcium antagonists for, 242, 244–245, *245*
    type I drugs for, 242, *243*
  for sustained ventricular tachycardia, 257–258, 257t
    precipitation with, 248
  in vitro studies of triggered activity and, 30, 32
  local anesthetic agents as, 404–406, *404–405*
  noninvasive techniques for, 101–104, *102*, 102t–103t, *104*
  prevention of sudden death with, 106–110, 342–343
    guided techniques for, 108–109, *109*
    non-guided techniques for, 106–108, 107t
    noninvasive techniques for drug selection, 109–110
    results of guided therapy, 108–109, *109*
    results of non-guided therapy, 106–108, 107t
  programmed electrical stimulation (PES) studies of, 229
  therapy objectives with, 413
  torsades de pointes and. See *Torsades de pointes*.
Antibiotics, torsades de pointes and, 270
Antibradyarrhythmias, pacing devices for, 497, 497t
Anticoagulation therapy, in patients with sick sinus syndrome, combined with pacemaker therapy, 134–135, *135*
Antitachycardia pacing, 497, 499t

Antitachycardia pacing *(Continued)*
  clinical applications of, 709–712
    atrial fibrillation management with, 710
    cardioversion/defibrillation transvenous leads and, 711–712
    paroxysmal atrial flutter termination with, 709–710
    paroxysmal supraventricular tachycardia termination with, 709
    ventricular tachycardia termination with, 710–711
  electrophysiologic mechanisms of, 685–704
    in reentrant ventricular tachycardia prevention, 693, 700, *702–704*
    models for, 685–686
    termination of, with programmed electrical stimulation (PES), 686, *687*, 688, *688*, 690
    overdrive entrainment and, 690, *694–696*
    site of simulation and, 693, *700–701*
    tachycardia acceleration and ventricular fibrillation, precipitation with, 690, 693, *697–699*
    tachycardia resetting mechanisms for, *689*, 690
    tachycardia termination followed by reinitiation, 690, *691*
  generic code for, 498, 500t
  historical aspects of, 706–707
  lead systems for, 708
  modalities of, 707–709
  pulse generators for, 708–709
  terminology for, 707t, 707–708
Antitachycardia surgery. See *Surgery*.
Arrhythmia(s). See also specific arrhythmias.
  aggravation of, with drug therapy, 105–106, *106*, 107t
  alterations in myocardial perfusion and, 82–83, *83*
  behavioral stress and, 83–87, *85*, 86t
    post-stress ischemia and, 84, *85*, 86, 86t
  effects of sleep on, 86–87
  exercise testing and, 98–100, *99*
  hemodynamic effects of, 545–554
    bradyarrhythmias and, 546–548
    heart rate and rhythm effects and, 545–546
    in tachyarrhythmias, 547–554
  prevalence of, with ambulatory monitoring, 93–95, 93t, *94*
  risk of cardiac death and, 95–98, 96t–98t
  sinus node dysfunction and, 117
  sympathetic nervous system and, 77–80, *78*
    adrenergic receptor subtypes in, 77–79, *78*
    alpha-adrenergic receptors, role of, 79, *80*
    cyclic nucleotides and, 79–80
  sympathetic-parasympathetic interactions during, 80–82, *81*
  in ischemic and infarcted heart, 81–82, *81–82*, 82t
Arrhythmogenesis, during acute myocardial ischemia, 60–61
  right ventricular dysplasia and, surgical management of, 448–450, *448–449*
Arterial emboli, with AICD implantation, 751

Arteriosclerotic heart disease (ASHD), 333–334
Asynchronous cardiac pacing. See *VOO cardiac pacing*.
ATP-sensitive potassium channel, action of, during acute myocardial ischemia, 65–66
  ischemia-induced increase of, 22, *22*
Atrial arrhythmias, evaluation of, with ambulatory monitoring, 95
  in sustained ventricular tachycardia (SVT), 252–253, *253–255*
  termination of, electrical devices for, 761
Atrial conduction, electrophysiologic studies (EPS) of, 296
Atrial fibrillation, after cardioversion, 730
  characteristics of, 177
  effect of antiarrhythmic drugs on, 208, 210–212
  hemodynamic effects of, 550, *551*
  in Wolff-Parkinson-White syndrome, *191*, 191–192
  surgical management of, 444–445
  temporary pacing for, 710
  torsades de pointes syndrome and, 272, *272*
  with slow ventricular rate, 655
Atrial flutter, cardiac pacing therapy for, 187–189, *185–188*
  cardioversion and, 730
  characteristics of, 176
  future research trends for, 189
  hemodynamic effects of, 550, *551*
  in infantile tachycardia, 286–287
  mechanism of, 185–187, *185–186*
  paroxysmal form of, 709–710
  reentry circuit characteristics in, 187
  surgical management of, 444–445
  types of, 184–185, *184–185*
Atrial muscle, action potential and conduction in, 7
Atrial non-capture, dual-chamber electrocardiography and, 605, *606*
Atrial oversensing, dual-chamber electrocardiography and, *604*, 605
  sinus node dysfunction evaluation with, 122–126, *123*, *125*, *126*
Atrial pacing (AAI), DDD pacemaker and, 601
  electrocardiography of, 592, *594–595*, 595
  of repetitive monomorphic ventricular tachycardia, extrasystoles and, distribution with, *236*, 236–238, *237*, *240*
  heart rate in, 235, *236*
Atrial passive fixation lead, techniques for, 564
Atrial premature depolarizations (APDs), 126–129, *127–128*
Atrial refractory period, dual-chamber pacemaker timing cycles and, 601
  exogenous pacemaker interference and, 612, *616*
  in DDD mode programmability, *511*, 511–512
Atrial tachyarrhythmias, cardioversion for, 730
Atrial tachycardia, catheter ablation for, 467
  characteristics of, 176
  drug therapy for, 178, *178*
  ectopic (automatic), left atrial tachycardias and, *442–443*, 442–443

Atrial tachycardia *(Continued)*
    right atrial tachycardias and, 443–444, *444*
    surgical management of, 182, 442–444, *442–444*
Atrial undersensing, dual-chamber electrocardiography and, 603–605, *604, 606*
Atrioventricular (AV) block. See also *Mobitz II atrioventricular (AV) block; Pseudo Mobitz atrioventricular (AV) block.*
    acquired, indications for cardiac pacing in, 652–655
    complete AV block classification of, 152–156, *153, 156*
        acute acquired type of, 152, 154
        chronic acquired type of, 154
        congenital type of, 152
        electrophysiologic evaluation of, 154–156, *155*
    exercise-induced, indications for cardiac pacing in, 654
    first-degree form of, 142–144, *142–144*
        age-related prevalence of, 142, 144
        indications for cardiac pacing in, 652–653
        prognosis and therapy for, 144
    fixed 2:1 or 3:1 form of, indications for cardiac pacing in, 655
    hemodynamic effects of, 547, *548*
    high-degree classification of, 152
        alternate Wenckebach periodicity with, 150, *151*
        characteristics of, 152
        paroxysmal AV block and, 157, *161*
    His bundle electrocardiogram of, 376
    history of research on, 140
    incidence of, in myocardial infarction, 163, 165
    induction of, with catheter ablation, 458–462
        techniques for, 459–460, *459*
    paroxysmal classification of, 156–158, *157–160*
        indications for cardiac pacing in, 653
    postsurgical, indications for cardiac pacing in, 655–656
    second-degree classification of, 144–152
        alternate Wenckebach periodicity, 149–150, *151–152*
        indications for cardiac pacing in, 653–654
        Mobitz II AV block as, 148
            indications for cardiac pacing, 653–654
        pseudo-AV block as, *146,* 149, *151*
            indications for cardiac pacing in, 654
        unified hypothesis of (Mobitz II/Wenckebach), 148–149, *150*
        Wenckebach AV block as, 144–148
            distal to His bundle, 147–148, *147–150*
            in AV node, 144–147, *145–146*
            in His bundle system, 147, *147*
    third-degree classification of, indications for cardiac pacing in, 654
        pacemaker follow-up procedures and, 666–667, 667t
Atrioventricular (AV) conduction, anatomy of, 140–141, *141*
    disorders of. See *Atrioventricular (AV) block; Bundle branch block; Fascicular block.*
    normal rates of, 141, *141*
    pre-excitation syndrome and, 190

Atrioventricular (AV) conduction *(Continued)*
    repetitive concealed conduction in paroxysmal AV block, 156
Atrioventricular (AV) delay, cardiac pacemaker programmability of, 514–515, *514*
    dual-chamber pacing and, programming for, 603, *604*
    timing cycles and, 601–602
    in DVI pacemakers, 600
Atrioventricular (AV) dissociation, differentiation of VT and SVT with, 255, *256*
Atrioventricular (AV) groove, and cardiac arrhythmogenesis, 82, *82*
    band electrode placement in, 437, *437*
Atrioventricular (AV) junction, anatomy of, 140
    catheter ablation of, 458–462
        complications of, 461–462
        current status of, 462
        experimental background on, 458–459
        indications for, 458
        results of, 460–461, *461*
        techniques for, 459–460, *459*
        vs. modification procedures, 460
    tachycardia in, 170–176
        automatic form of, 176
        AV nodal reentry linked to, 170–175, *171–172*
        drug therapy for, 178, *179, 181,* 182
        electrophysiologic and electrocardiographic features of, 170–173, *171–173*
        nonparoxysmal form of, 175
Atrioventricular (AV) nodal reentrant tachycardia, 170–175, *171–173,* 548, *549–550*
    conduction pathways for, *171,* 173–175, *173–175*
    diagnostic criteria for, 200–201
    documentation of reentry site for, *172–174,* 174
    drug therapy for, 178, *179, 181,* 182
    electrophysiologic/electrocardiographic features of, 170–173, *171–173*
    incessant form of, 204–205, *205–206*
    induction methods for, 201
    intranodal pathways for, 174–175
    paroxysmal supraventricular tachycardia and, 440–442, *441–442*
    surgical therapy for, 182
    uncommon patterns of, 175
Atrioventricular node (AVN), action potential and conduction in, 7–8
    electrocardiography for, 377–378, *378*
    in electrophysiologic studies (EPS), 296
    anatomy of, 140, *141*
    midnodal or compact node zone (N region) of, 140, *141*
    nodo-Hisian or penetrating bundle zone (NH region) of, 140, *141*
    pre-excitation syndrome and, 190–191
    transitional cell zone (AN region) of, 140, *141*
Atrioventricular (AV) synchrony, hemodynamic effects of, 546
Atropine, impact on sinus node recovery time, 124–125
Automated discrimination circuit, signal-averaging technique for, 375
Automatic conversion of pacing mode, with exogenous pacemaker interference, 612–614

Automatic implantable cardioverter/defibrillator (AICD), clinical aspects of, 737–742
    arrhythmia recognition with, 738
    arrhythmia termination with, 738
    components of, 737–738, *738*
    historical background on, 737
    implantation techniques for, 738–742
        clinical outcome of, 741–742, *741–742*
        complications of, 740–741
        criteria for implantation, 738–739
        intraoperative testing of, 739–740
        noninvasive monitoring of, 740, *740*
        patient population for, 740, 740t
        pre-implantation evaluation, 739
        surgical approach to, 739
    complications of, *749,* 749–756
        antiarrhythmic agents and, 756
        discharge in absence of symptoms, 752–755, *753–755*
        early postoperative complications of, *750,* 750t, 750–751
        failure to recognize ventricular arrhythmias and, 755
        late complications of, 751t, 751–752, *752*
        pacemaker interactions with, 755–756, *756*
    components of, 743–745, *744*
    follow-up procedures for, 743–757
        defibrillation threshold (DFT) stability, 747
        electrocardiographic, hemodynamic and pathologic effects of, 747, *748,* 749
        guidelines for, 745–746
        magnet testing for, 746
        patch leads and internal defibrillation and, 747, *748,* 749
        pulse generator replacement timing and, 746
        recording stability, 746–747
        reference study population for, 745, *745*
    future research trends and, 756–757
    management of sudden cardiac arrest with, 339–340
    pacemaker interference with, 622–623
    sudden cardiac arrest management with, 344–345
Automatic junctional tachycardia, 175
Automatic pacing interval, definition of, 579
Automatic self-adjustment, in cardiac pacing, 492
Automaticity, abnormal, 12–13
    as mechanism of sustained ventricular tachycardia (VT), 248–249
    in vitro studies of triggered activity, 24, 26–27, *27*
    cardiac pacing and, 486–487
    changes in, with MDP reduction, 10–11
    enhanced, as arrhythmia mechanism, 98–100, *99*
    Na^+-K^+ ATPase pump and, 5
    triggered, as arrhythmia mechanism, 98–100, *99*
    as mechanism of sustained ventricular tachycardia (VT), 249
Autonomic nervous system, long QT syndrome and, 278–279
    modification of sinus node with, 115

Index   767

Autonomic nervous system *(Continued)*
  sinoatrial conduction time (SACT) in, modification of, 129
  sinus node responsiveness to, 121
    subset of testing, 121
  tachyarrhythmia prevention and, 761–762
  ventricular arrhythmias and, after myocardial infarction, 317–318, *318*

Band electrodes, for surgical management of Wolff-Parkinson-White syndrome, 437, *437*
Bandpass filters, in signal-averaged electrocardiography, 352–354, *353–354*
Barotrauma, in catheter ablation procedures, 455–456
Basal energy utilization, *58–59*, 58–59
Batteries, control of function in, 667
  failure of, in pacemaker malfunction, 582
  for implantable pacemakers, 494–495, 495t
  longevity of, 670
Beat-to-beat electrocardiography, for His bundle recordings, 376–377, *377*
  in high-resolution electrocardiography, 362–364, *365–366*
  of ventricular late potentials, 382–383
  pre-atrial activity (sinus node potential), 373, *374*
Behavioral stress, and cardiac arrhythmias, 83–87, *85*, 86t
  post-stress ischemia and, 84, *85*, 86, 86t
Bepridil, for repetitive monomorphic ventricular tachycardia, 242, 244, *245*
Bernstein hypothesis, for resting membrane potential, 4
Beta Blocker Heart Attack Trial, ventricular arrhythmia increase after infarction and, 310, 310t
Beta blockers, antiarrhythmic therapy combined with, 104–105, *105*
  cardiac arrhythmogenesis and, 77–79, *78*
  for repetitive monomorphic ventricular tachycardia, 242, *244*
  management of long QT–torsades de pointes syndrome and, 269, 273–274
Beta-adrenergic receptor antagonists, as antiarrhythmic agents, 413
  cardiac arrhythmogenesis and, 77–79, *78*
  effects of, as antiarrhythmic agents, 428
Beta-endorphins, cardiac arrhythmias and, 88, *88*
Bifascicular block, chronic form of, 165
  definition of, 163
  electrophysiologic studies (EPS) of, 294–295
  in acute myocardial infarction, 163, 165
  indications for cardiac pacing with, 656
  prolonged H-V interval and, 165
Bioavailability mechanism, in antiarrhythmic agents, 409–410
Biointegration, cardiac pacing and, 489–490
Biorate device, respiration sensing with, 529–531, 530t, *530–532*
Biosensors, rate-responsive pacing and, 538
Biphasic waveforms, defibrillation electrophysiology and, *721*, 721–723
Bipolar catheters, for catheter ablation, 473
Bipolar pacemakers, in implantable pacemakers, 495
  myopotential sensing during, 644–645
Blanking period, dual-chamber pacemaker timing cycles and, 601

Bradyarrhythmias, hemodynamic effects of, 546–548
  in atrioventricular block, 547, *548*
  in sinus bradycardia, 546–547, *547*
  in patients with cerebrovascular disease, 133–134
  indications for cardiac pacing in, 652–658
    for acquired atrioventricular (AV) block, 652–655
    for cardiac catheterization, 658
    for cardiac transplantation, 658
    for chronic fascicular block, 656–657
    for hypersensitive carotid sinus syndrome, 657–658
    for Lyme myocarditis, 658
    for postsurgical atrioventricular (AV) block, 655–656
    for sick sinus syndrome, 657
  pacemakers for, *760*, 760–761
  with AICD implantation, 751
Bradycardia, rate-responsive pacing and, 541–542
  refractory period, *594*, 595
Bradycardia-dependent arrhythmias, paroxysmal AV block and, 157, *161*
  torsades de pointes models and, 276–277
Bradycardia-tachycardia syndrome, management of, 134
  sinus node dysfunction and, 118, *119*
Brain-heart interactions, cardiac arrhythmias and, 88, *88*
Bretylium tosylate, effects of, as antiarrhythmic agent, 427–428
Bundle branch block, in acute myocardial infarction, 163, 165
  indications for cardiac pacing in, 656
  intermittent type of, 161–162, *162*
    bradycardia-dependent, 161–162
    tachycardia-dependent, 161
  left branch form of, bifascicular or trifascicular block and, 163
    characteristics of, 158
    QRS pattern with ventricular pacing in, *571–572*, 571–572
    longitudinal dissociation pattern in His bundle and, 162–163, *164*
  right branch form of, as bifascicular or trifascicular block, 163
    characteristics of, 158–159
    QRS pattern with ventricular pacing in, 571–574, *572–575*
  transient type of, 161–162, *162*
Burst pacing technique, for nonsustained ventricular tachycardia, 221

Ca^{2+}-ATPase pump, in ischemic myocardium, 59–60
Caffeine, suppression of delayed afterdepolarizations (DADs) with, 30, *31*
Calcium, and cardiac arrhythmogenesis, 79, *80*
  during myocardial infarction, 37
  in vitro studies of triggered activity, 28, 30, *31*
  ischemia-induced increase of, 22
  overload during acute myocardial ischemia, 66
  sinoatrial node action potential and, 7
Calcium channel, antiarrhythmic agents and, 401–404
  blocking drugs for, 406, 407t

Calcium channel *(Continued)*
  in vitro modulation of triggered activity, in torsades de pointes syndrome, 276
  L-type, reduction of, with maximum diastolic potential (MDP), 10, *10–11*
  resting membrane potential and, 5–6
Calcium channel blockers, definition of, 413
  effects of, as antiarrhythmic agent, 428
  for repetitive monomorphic ventricular tachycardia, 242, 244–245, *245*
  ventricular arrhythmia suppression with, 30, 32, *32*
Capture beats and fusion (Dressler beats), in sustained ventricular tachycardia (SVT), 253, *255*
Cardiac Arrhythmia Pilot Study (CAPS), of antiarrhythmia drug therapy, 108
  of sudden cardiac death risk factors, 336
Cardiac Arrhythmia Suppression Trial (CAST), of antiarrhythmia drug therapy, 108
  complex ventricular arrhythmia and sudden death in, 218–219
Cardiac output, atrial contribution to, 546
  dual-chamber pacing and, 524
  hemodynamic effects of, 545
Cardiac pacing. See also *Antitachycardia pacing*; specific types of pacemakers.
  catheter ablation for, 467–468
  endogenous interference in, 634–649
    from myopotentials, 634–642, *635–638*
      during bipolar pacing, 644–645
      in DDD pacemakers, 635, *638–641*, 639, 641
      in single-chamber pacemakers, 634–635, *636–638*
    management of, 646–649, *647–648*
    sources of, 642–644
    testing maneuvers for, 645t, 645–646
    ventricular arrhythmia induction and, 641, *642*
  engineering aspects of, 484–493
    automatic self-adjustment in, 492
    basic principles of, 485–490
      electrode selection for, 488–490, *488*
      functions of, 490
      sensing electrodes for, 490, *491*
      stimulation mechanisms of, 486–488, *487*
      timing of, 485–486, *486*
    treatment methods for, 485, *485*
    dual-chamber pacing and, 490–491
    historical overview of, 484–485
    rate-responsive pacing techniques and, 491
    technological limitations of, 492–493
  exogenous interference in, 608–629
    automatic conversion of pacing mode and, 612–614
    catheter ablation and, 622
    dental treatment and, 629
    from automatic cardioverter/defibrillator (AICD), 622–623
    from cardioversion, guidelines for, 621
      transvenous cardioversion and, 621–622
    from defibrillation, 619–623
      circuitry damage with, 620
      guidelines for, 621
      lead displacement and, 620
      malfunction mechanisms after, 620–621
      mode change from VVI to VVT, 620

Cardiac pacing (Continued)
    reprogramming and, 620
    threshold increase and, 620
    transvenous cardioversion and, 621–622
    undersensing and, 620
    ventricular fibrillation induction with, 620
  from electrocautery, 614–619
  from electroconvulsive therapy, 629
  from pacemaker testing equipment, 626–629, 627–628
  lithotripsy and, 625–626
  magnetic resonance imaging and, 624–625
    radio frequency pulsing during, 624–625
  pacemaker response to, 609–612, 610
    atrial refractory period as, 612, 616
    partial refractory period extension as, 612, 617
    refractory period extension as, 609, 611, 612, 613–615, 618–619
  radiation and, 624
  transcutaneous electrical nerve stimulation (TENS), 626
  triboelectric phenomena as, 628, 629
follow-up procedures for, 662–673
  data collection for, 670–671
  documentation requirements and, 670
  European pacemaker registry, 671–673
  goals of, 666–669
    battery function control as, 667
    indications for pacemaker and, 666–667, 667
    electrode failure detection as, 668–669
    electronic component failure as, 668
    evaluation of cardiac status and arrhythmias as, 669
    pacemaker pocket inspection as, 669
    pacemaker selection criteria and, 667, 668
    reprogramming as, 668
    sensing threshold control as, 668, 669
    threshold control as, 667–668, 668
  pacemaker/electrode function control and, 662–666
    defibrillator for, 665
    documentation procedures for, 665
    electrocardiography for, 662–663, 663–664
    external pacemaker and chest wall electrodes for, 664–665, 665
    Holter monitoring for, 666
    impulse interval and duration measurement for, 663
    pacemaker library for, 665–666
    programming requirements for, 663
    radiography for, 664
    transtelephonic monitoring system for, 666, 666
    24-hour monitoring for, 663–664, 664
  requirements for pacemaker center and follow-up clinic, 669–670
for atrial flutter, 185–188, 187–189
for atrioventricular (AV) block, 140
  for complete block, 154–156, 155–156
for infantile supraventricular tachycardia, 290–291
for sick sinus syndrome, 134–135, 135
for pre-excitation syndrome, 212

Cardiac pacing (Continued)
  for sustained ventricular tachycardia (VT), 259, 260
    induction of, during, 249–250, 250t, 254–255
    therapy with, 257
  generic code for, 498, 500t
  hemodynamic effects of, 555–558, 557
    "booster pump" effect, 555–556
  implantation techniques for, 561–567
    endomyocardial lead placement and, 562–563
    in rate-responsive pacing, 566–567
    late complications of, 567
    lead placement and, 563–564
      complications of, 564
    pacemaker pocket, 565–566
    pulse generator replacement techniques for, 566
    sensing and pacing thresholds of, 564–565
    site selection for, 561–562
  indications for, 494, 495t
  integrated systems for, 762–763, 763
  interaction with AICDs and, 755–756, 756
  lead construction for, 496
  long QT–torsades de pointes syndrome and, 271
  modes of pacing in, 497, 497t
    selection criteria for, 501, 502t
  multiprogrammability of, 504–521
    clinical value of, 517t, 519t, 519–520, 520t
    definition and history of, 504
    difficulties, risks and errors of, 520, 520–521
    of DDD pulse generator, 510–513, 510, 510t
      lower-rate limit of ventricular stimulation, 513
      of atrial refractory period, 511, 511–512
      principal problems of, 513–516
      upper-rate limit of ventricular stimulation, 512, 512–513
    of single-chamber pacemakers, 504–513, 505t
      hysteresis programmability of, 509–510
      output programmability of, 505–506, 506–507
      rate programmability of, 506–508
      refractory period programmability, 509
      sensitivity programming for, 508–509
    programming aid for, 519
    rate responsiveness programmability and, 516–519, 516t, 517t, 517–518
    technologies for, 504
  Na$^+$-K$^+$ ATPase pump and, 5
  NASPE specific code for, 498–500, 499t
  noninvasive external type of, 675–683
    clinical applications of, 678–683
    current developments in, 675–678, 676
    echocardiography during, 677, 677–678
    electrode position and pacing threshold, 677–678
    experimental human studies in, 676–677, 677
    historical background on, 675
  output circuits for, 496–497
  pacing modes in, 497, 497t
  power sources for, 494–495, 495t

Cardiac pacing (Continued)
    programming and telemetry for, 501–502, 502t
    refractory-period classifications in, 500–501, 501
    sustained ventricular tachycardia and, 259, 260
    future of, 759–763
    system configuration for, 495–496
    thresholds for, control of, 667–668, 668
      defibrillation (DFT) form of, 733, 733
        for automatic cardioverter/defibrillator (AICD), 739–740
        stability of, 747
      in external cardiac pacing, electrode placement and, 677–678
      increase in, with defibrillation interference, 620, 621
    torsades de pointes models and, 276–277
    transplants and, 658
    unipolar pacing obsolescence and, 649
Cardiac tamponade, as complication of catheter ablation, 465–466
Cardiac transplantation, indications for cardiac pacing with, 658
Cardioinhibitory carotid sinus hypersensitivity, 132
Cardiomyopathy, 94
  hypertrophic, 98
  infantile tachycardia with, 288, 288
  nonischemic, surgical management of, 447, 447
  sustained ventricular tachycardia (VT) and, 248
  ventricular arrhythmias and, 97–98
Cardioversion. See also Defibrillation; Direct-current shock.
  clinical aspects of, 727–734
    complications of, 733–734, 734
    for atrial tachyarrhythmias, 730
    for ventricular tachycardia, 731
    indications and contraindications for, 728–729
    mechanism of, 727, 728
    technique for, 729–730
  definition of, 727–728
  for sustained ventricular tachycardia, 256–257
  infantile supraventricular tachycardia management with, 289–290
  long QT–torsades de pointes syndrome and, 273–274
  pacemaker interference with, 619–623
  transvenous form of, 621–622
  transvenous leads for, 711–712
Carotid sinus hypersensitivity. See Hypersensitive carotid sinus syndrome.
Catecholamines, atrial overdrive and sinus node dysfunction and, 122–126, 123, 125, 126
  automaticity enhanced by, 99
  myocardial ischemia and, 66, 86
Catheter ablation, for atrial tachycardias, 467
  for permanent junctional reciprocating tachycardia, 466–467
  for pre-excitation syndrome patients, 212
  for supraventricular tachycardia (SVT), 182
    cellular electrophysiologic effects of direct-current shocks in, 456–457
    defibrillators for, 457–458
    electrode catheters for, 457
    of accessory AV connections, 462–467
    of free-wall connections, 466

Catheter ablation *(Continued)*
    of posteroseptal accessory connections, 464–466, *465*
    of atrioventricular (AV) junction, 458–462
    tissue injury mechanisms in, 454–456
    transcatheter direct-current shock biophysics and, 453–454, *453–455*
    for ventricular late potentials, 396
    for ventricular tachycardia (VT), 471–482
        activation time measurement equipment for, 476, *477–478*
        analog signal recordings during, 477
        endocardial mapping for, 477
        fluoroscopic equipment for, 471, *472*
        fulgurator for, 474–476, *475*, 479, *480*, 481t
        hemodynamic monitoring for, 476
        materials for, 471–477
        pace-mapping for, 477–478
        pacing for slow conduction area, 478–479, *479*
        postoperative surveillance with, 479, 482
        technology and selection procedures for, 471–474
        videotape recordings during, 476
    laser energy for, 468
    pacemaker interference with, 622
    radiofrequency for, 468–469
    with permanent pacemakers, 467–468
Catheter mapping, for pre-excitation syndrome, 201
    of atrial flutter mechanisms, *185–186*, 186–187
Catheterization procedures, in electrophysiologic studies (EPS), 253–255, *254–255*
    indications for cardiac pacing with, 658
    sudden cardiac death evaluation with, 338–339
Cation activity values, for resting membrane potential, 4, 4t
Cell membrane function, antiarrhythmic agents and, 401–404, *401–404*
Cell-to-cell coupling, long QT syndrome and, 278–279
Cellular model of resting membrane potential, 2–4
Cephalic vein cannulation, endomyocardial lead placement techniques and, 563
Channel gate structure, antiarrhythmic agents and, 402
Channel-blocking drugs, 406, 407t
Chest wall stimuli, in pacemaking electrocardiography, 581, *582*
CHF. See *Congestive heart failure (CHF)*.
Children. See also *Infantile tachycardia*.
    external cardiac pacing in, 683
Cimetidine, encainide interaction with, 422
    procainamide clearance and, 417
Circadian rhythms, ventricular premature beats (VPBs) and, *94*, 94–95
Clearance mechanism, in antiarrhythmic agents, 410–411
Clinical pharmacology, concepts of, 409–412
    absorption and bioavailability as, 409–410
    distribution as, 410
    drug release mechanism as, 409
    factors influencing drug disposition, 411–412
    half-life and steady state as, 410, *410*
    plasma concentrations as, 412
    protein binding as, 410–411

Clofilium, action of, on Purkinje fibers, 32, *33–34*
Closed-loop cardiac pacing, 491
Cold pressor test, coronary artery spasm and, 83
"Committed" ventricular pacing, 500–501, *501*
Compartmentalized metabolism, during myocardial ischemia, 69–73
Compensatory pause phenomenon, sinoatrial conduction time and, 126–127, *127–128*
Computers, and cardiac pacing, 492–493
    programming and telemetry for, 501–502, 502t
Conduction. See also *Atrioventricular (AV) conduction; Impulse conduction*.
    abnormal electrophysiology and, 9–12
    delay of, bifascicular or trifascicular block and, 163
        with reentrant ventricular tachyarrhythmias, 323–325, *324–325*
    disorders of, during early myocardial ischemia, 19–20
    of atrial muscle, 7
    of atrioventricular node, 7–8
    of Purkinje fiber, 8
    of ventricular muscle, 8–9
    pathways for, electrophysiology and, 7–9
    slowing of, with maximum diastolic potential (MDP), 9–12
Conductors, in implantable pacemakers, 496
Congestive heart failure (CHF), effects of disopyramide on, 417
    in sick sinus syndrome patients, pacemaker therapy for, 133
    risk of sudden cardiac death and, 96–97, 218
    sinus node recovery time (SNRT) and, 124
    ventricular arrhythmias and, 97, 98t
    complex arrhythmias in, 218
Constant current pulse, in cardiac pacing, 487, *487*
Constant current source, in cardiac pacing, 487
Constant voltage pulse, in cardiac pacing, 487
Constant voltage source, in cardiac pacing, 487
Continuous pacing techniques, calculation of sinoatrial conduction time with, 129, *130*
    definition of, 707, 707t
Coronary angiography, left ventricular function evaluation with, 307
Coronary artery bypass graft surgery, for sustained ventricular tachycardia (VT), 258
Coronary artery disease, as sudden cardiac death risk factor, 333–334
    multiprogrammability of cardiac pacemakers and, 505
    neurogenic aspects of, 82–83, *83*
    surgical correction of, 338–339
    sustained ventricular tachycardia (VT) and, 247–248
    ventricular arrhythmias following, 18–19
Coronary heart disease, incidence of sustained ventricular tachycardia (VT) and, 259–260
    ventricular late potentials in, 379
Coronary sinus, anatomy of, 140, *141*

Coronary sinus *(Continued)*
    perforation of, with catheter ablation, 466
Corrected sinus node recovery time (CSNRT), calculation of, 123–124
    in electrophysiologic studies (EPS), 295
Coupling interval, in repetitive monomorphic ventricular tachycardia, extrasystole mechanism and distribution and, *236*, 237–238
    of initial beat, *239*, 239, *241*, 241–242
Creatine kinase, actions of, during acute myocardial ischemia, *68*, *69*
    infarct size and, 304
Creatine phosphate, basal energy utilization in heart and, 58–59, *59*
Creatine phosphokinase (CPK), levels of, with external cardiac pacing, 676
Critical point hypothesis, defibrillation electrophysiology and, 717–721, *719–720*
    biphasic vs. monphasic waveforms and, 722
    upper limit of vulnerability and, 719, *720*
Cross-talk phenomenon, cardiac pacemaker programmability and, 515–516, 515t, *515–516*
    ventricular blanking in dual-chamber pacemakers and, 605, *606*, 607
Cryolesions, in surgical management of PSVT, 440–442, *441–442*
Cryothermal ablation, in surgical management of Wolff-Parkinson-White syndrome, 439–440
    sudden cardiac arrest management with, 343–344
Current-source pacing, 497
Cyclic AMP (cAMP), and cardiac arrhythmogenesis, 79–80
    elevated levels during acute myocardial ischemia, 66
Cyclic nucleotides, sympathetic nervous system and, 79–80
Cytochrome P-450, in antiarrhythmic agents, 426, 429

Data base, for pacemaker follow-up, 670–673
DDD pacemakers, defibrillation interference with, 613
    dual-chamber (low rate) sequential mode of, 600–601
    electrocardiography of, 600–601, *601*
    electrocautery interference with, 613, 616
    end-of-service (EOS) point in, 612
    exogenous interference with, pacing mode conversion and, 612–614
    refractory period extension and, 609, *611*, 611–612, *613–615*
    intercostal myopotential interference in, 644, *645*
    magnetic resonance interference (MRI) with, 625
    myopotential inhibition in, 605, *606*, 635, *638–641*, 639, 641
    principal problems of, 513–516
    crosstalk in, 515–516, 515t, *515–516*
    prevention of endless loop tachycardia, 513–515, *513–514*
    programmability of, 510–513, 510t, *510*
DDDR pacemakers, electrocardiography of, 601

DDI pacemakers, electrocardiography of, 600
Deafness, long QT syndrome and, 265
Defibrillation. See also *Ventricular defibrillation*.
  clinical aspects of, 727–734
    energy requirements for, 732–733
    indications and contraindications for, 728–729
    mechanisms of, 727, *728*
    myocardial damage and, 732
    techniques for, 731–733
  complications of, 733–734, *734*
  definition of, 727, *728*
  electrophysiologic mechanisms of, 713–724
    activation points of, 715, *716–717*
    biphasic waveforms and, *721*, 721–723
      critical point, vs. monophasic waveforms, 722
      decreased impedance and, 721
      refractory period duration and, 722
      sodium channel reactivation and, 721–722
      strength-duration curves, vs. monophasic waveforms, 722, *722–723*
    criteria for, 717
    critical point hypothesis of, 717–722, *719–720*
    probability function and, 719–721, *720*
    subthreshold shock and, 714–715, *714–716*
    upper limit vulnerability and, 715–717, *717*
      correlation with threshold and, 716–717, *718*
      critical point hypothesis and, 719, *720*
      very high-potential gradients and, 723–724
  for catheter ablation, 457–458
  interference with pacemakers from, 613, 619–623
    circuitry damage from, 620
    guidelines for, 621
    lead displacement and, 620
    mechanisms of, 620–621
    reprogramming, 620
    reset phenomenon and, 620
    threshold increase and, 620, *621*
    transvenous cardioversion and, 621–622
    undersensing and, 620
    ventricular fibrillation induction and, 620
  pacemaker control with, 665
  transvenous leads for, 711–712
Defibrillation threshold (DFT), for automatic implantable cardioverter/defibrillator (AICD), 739–740
  stability of, 747
Delayed afterdepolarizations (DADs), during action potential plateau, 13, *13*
  in vitro studies of triggered activity with, 24–32, *25–26*
    antiarrhythmic agents and, 30, 32
    diastolic potentials and, 27–28, *28–29*
    ionic mechanisms of, 28, 30, *31*
    lysophosphatidylcholine and, 30
    subthreshold, 24, *26*
      diastolic potentials and, 27–28, *29*
    suprathreshold, 24, *25*
"Delayed myocardial ischemia," 84, *85*, 86

Delayed potentials, prognostic implications of, 328–329, 329t, *330*
  signal-averaged electrocardiograms and, 328, 329t
Delivery (paced) refractory periods, 581
Dental treatment, pacemaker interference from, 629
Diabetes mellitus, as sudden cardiac death risk factor, 333–334
Diagnostic-related groups (DRGs), economics of sustained ventricular tachycardia (VT) and, 259
Diaphragmatic myopotentials, pacemaker interference and, 643–644, *643–644*
Diastolic potentials, in vitro studies of triggered activity and, 27–28, *28–29*
Diastolic tension, energy utilization in ischemic myocardium and, 60
Diathermy, pacemaker interference with, 626
Digital electrocardiography, stimulus artifacts in pacemakers and, *570*, 571
Digitalis, intoxication from, cardioversion and defibrillation contraindicated in, 729
  management of ventricular tachycardia with, 289
Digoxin, quinidine interactions with, 415–416
Direct-current shock, biophysics of, 453–454, *453–455*
  cellular electrophysiologic effects of, 456–457
  complications of, 733–734, *734*
  in single-chamber pacemaker malfunction, 585
  interference with pacemakers from, 619–623
Disopyramide, adverse effects of, 418
  arrhythmia evaluation with, 101, *102*
  clinical pharmacokinetics of, 417
  dosage and plasma concentrations of, 417–418
  drug interactions with, 418
  electrophysiological effects of, 417
  hemodynamic effects of, 417
  indications for use of, 418
"Dispersion" hypothesis, for torsades de pointes, 274
Distribution mechanism, in antiarrhythmic agents, 410–411
Diving reflex, for management of infantile supraventricular tachycardia, 289–290
Documentation system for pacemaker follow-up, 665, 670–673
  pacemaker library for, 665–666
Doppler parameters, hemodynamic effects of, 553, *555*
Doxorubicin, suppression of delayed afterdepolarizations (DADs) with, 30, *31*
dp/dt sensing, rate-responsive pacing and, 537–538, *538*
Dressler beats, in sustained ventricular tachycardia (VT), 253, *255*
Drug release mechanism, with antiarrhythmic agents, 409
Drug therapy, effects of on sinus node function, 132–133
Dual-chamber pacemakers, configurations for, 496
  development of, 485
  electrocardiography of, 599–607
    arrhythmias of, 602–603
    atrial non-capture in, 605, *606*

Dual-chamber pacemakers (*Continued*)
    atrial oversensing in, *604*, 605
    atrial undersensing in, 603–605, *604*, 605, *606*
    AV delay programming in, 603, *604*
    DDD pacemakers, 600–601, *601*
    DDDR pacemakers as, 601
    DDI pacemakers as, 600
    DVI pacemakers as, 599–600
    myopotential inhibition of, 605, *606*
    termination of pacemaker-mediated tachycardia in, 607
    timing cycles for, 601–602
    VDD pacemakers as, 600
    ventricular blanking in, 605, *606*, 607
  endless-loop tachycardia with, 602–603, *602–603*
    termination of, 607
  techniques for, 490–491
  Wenckebach and other upper rate responses to, 603, *604*
Dual-chamber rate-responsive pacing, 539–540, *540–541*
DVI pacemakers, diaphragmatic myopotential interference with, 643–644, *643–644*
  electrocardiography of, 599–600

Early afterdepolarizations (EADs), during action potential plateau, *12*, 12–13
  torsades de pointes and, 274, *274*
  transmembrane action potentials, 32, *33–34*
Ebstein's anomaly, incidence of pre-excitation syndrome with, 191, 194
  multiple accessory pathways with, 205–206, *206*
Echocardiography, during external cardiac pacing, 677, *677–678*
  left ventricular function evaluation with, 306–307
Economics of pacemaker treatment, 670
  sustained ventricular tachycardia and, 259
Ectopic (automatic) atrial tachycardia, surgical management of, 442–444, *442–444*
Effective refractory period (ERP), reexcitation studies of, 43, *46*
Electrocardiography, for sustained ventricular tachycardia (VT), 251–253
  sinus node dysfunction monitoring and, 120
  with external cardiac pacing, 680, *681–682*
Electrocautery procedures, interference with pacemakers from, 613–619
  patient management during, 616–617, 619
Electroconvulsive therapy, pacemaker interference with, 629
Electrode catheters, for catheter ablation, 457
Electrodes, chest wall type of, 664–665, *665*
  control of function in, 662–666
    with electrocardiography, 662–663, *663–664*
  endocardial type of, 495–496
  epicardial type of, 496
  failure detection in, 668–669
  for cardiac pacing, 488–490, *488*, 495–496

Index 771

Electrodes (Continued)
    fracture of, and sensing abnormalities, in VVI pacemakers, 590, *590*
    myocardial type of, 496
    placement of, in external cardiac pacing, 677–678
    sensing and, 490, *491*
Electrode-tissue interface noise, in electrophysiologic signals, 350
Electrogenic pump current, resting membrane potential and, 4–5
Electromagnetic interference (EMI), with pacemakers, 612–614
Electromyographic potentials, in electrophysiologic signals, 350–351
Electrophysiologic studies (EPS), for repetitive monomorphic ventricular tachycardia, 234–245
    drug therapy and, 242–245
        with beta blockers, 242, *244*
        with calcium antagonists, 242, 244–245, *245*
        with type I drugs, 242, *243*
    extrasystole distribution and mechanism, 236–237, 236–238, *240*
        adrenergic and rate dependence and, 235–236, *236–237*
    repetitive activity in, 238–242
        adrenergic dependence and, 238, *239–240*
        coupling interval of initial beat and, *239*, 239, *241*, 241–242
        determinants of, 241, *241*
        mechanisms of, 241–242
        R-R interval and rate dependence, 238–239, *240–241*
    for surgical management of Wolff-Parkinson-White syndrome, 436
    for sustained ventricular tachycardia (VT), 249–250, 250t
        effects of therapy assessed with, 258
    for syncope of unknown origin (SUO), 293
        abnormal and positive findings, 297t, 297
        borderline and clearly abnormal findings in, 297, 298t
        comparison of findings in, 298, 299t
        comparison of induced VTs in, 298, 299t
        diagnostic criteria for, 296–297, 297t, 298t
        grading of results in, 297
        indications for, 294–295
        predictors of outcome in, 300t
        risks and complications of, 301–302
        technique and study protocol in, 295–296
        therapy and prognosis of, 300–301
    for ventricular arrhythmias, 311–314, 313t
    noise sources in, 350–351
    sudden cardiac arrest evaluation with, 338–342, *341*
Electrophysiology, abnormal, signs of, 9–12
    atrial muscle action potential and conduction and, 7
    atrioventricular (AV) node potential and conduction and, 7–8
    during acute myocardial ischemia, 61–69, 63t
    Purkinje fiber action potential and conduction and, 8
    resting membrane potential and, 1–7
        basis of, 6–7

Electrophysiology (Continued)
    calcium and, 5–6
    hypothetical cellular model of, 2–4
    Na^+-Ca^{2+} exchange and, 6
    Na^+-K^+ ATPase pump and, 4–5
    origin of, 1–2
    sinoatrial node action potential and, 7
    ventricular muscle action potential and conduction and, 8–9
Embolic events, in patients with sick sinus syndrome, 134–135, *135*
Encainide, adverse effects of, 422
    clinical pharmacokinetics of, 421–422, *422*
    dosage and plasma concentrations of, 422
    drug interactions with, 422
    electrophysiologic effects of, 421
    hemodynamic effects of, 421, *421*
    indications for use of, 422
    metabolic pathways of, *423*
    prevention of sudden death with, 109
Encircling endocardial ventriculotomy, for sustained ventricular tachycardia (VT), 259
End point, in programmed stimulation protocols, 326
    sudden cardiac death as, 318–320, 319t
Endless loop (pacemaker-induced) tachycardia, DDD mode programmability and, 511–512
    dual-chamber pacemakers and, 602–603, *602–603*
    from pacemaker testing equipment, 627, *627*
    prevention of, 513–515, *513–514*
    termination of, 607
End-of-life point, in pacemakers, 612–614
End-of-service point, in pacemakers, 612–614
Endocardial mapping, during catheter ablation, 477
    for surgical management of Wolff-Parkinson-White syndrome, 438–439
Endocrine system, modification of sinus node with, 115
Endomyocardial lead placement, indications for, 561
    techniques for, 562–563
Energy utilization, basal, in the heart, *58–59*, 58–59
    compartmentalized metabolism and, 69–73
    during acute myocardial ischemia, 59–60, *60*
Ensemble averaging. See Signal-averaged electrocardiography (SAECG).
Entrainment, in sustained ventricular tachycardia (VT), 250, *251*
    tachycardia termination and, 690, *694–696*
    transient, pacing termination of atrial flutter and, 709–710
Epicardial activation patterns, of reentrant excitation, 38–40, *39*
Epicardial leads, implantation techniques for, 563
    indications for, 561–562
    temporary, clinical applications of, 708
Epicardial mapping, for sustained ventricular tachycardia (VT), 259
Epicardial necrosis, from defibrillation, 732
Epicardium, ischemic, action potentials in, *36–37*, 38
Epinephrine, and cardiac arrhythmogenesis, 80, *81*

Equilibrium potential, during acute myocardial ischemia, 63–65, *64–65*
    cellular model for, 2–3, *3*
Esophageal electrocardiography, cardiac pacing and, 581, *582*
    for sustained ventricular tachycardia (VT), 253
    His bundle electrocardiography, signal-averaging technique for, 375–376
Ethmozin, in vitro studies of triggered activity and, 30, 32
    ventricular arrhythmia suppression with, 30
European Pacemaker Registry, *671–672*, 671t–672t, 671–673
Excitation-contraction coupling, calcium channel and, 5–6
Exercise testing, AICD discharge and, 754–755
    arrhythmias during, exposure of, 98–100, *99*
        incidence of, 99–100
    antiarrhythmic drug therapy evaluation with, 101–104, *102*, 102t–103t, *104*
    for myopotential interference in pacemaker function, 646
    for pre-excitation syndrome patients, 198–199
    for repetitive monomorphic ventricular tachycardia, 235
    sinus node dysfunction evaluation with, 120
    sudden cardiac death risk factors and, 336–337
    ventricular arrhythmias and, after myocardial infarction, 310–311
        induction of, 100–101
        safety of, 101
Exit block, pacemaker malfunction and, 583, 585, *585*
External closed heart approach, for surgical management of Wolff-Parkinson-White syndrome, 439–440
Extracellular potential recordings of sinus node function, 131–132, *132*
Extrastimuli, definition of, 707, 707t
Extrasystoles, in repetitive monomorphic ventricular tachycardia, adrenergic and rate dependence and, 235–236, *236–237*
    distribution and mechanisms of, *236*, 236–238, *237*, *240*
    in vitro studies of triggered activity and, 24, *26*
    sensing abnormalities and, in VVI pacemakers, 589–590
Extrinsic signals, as cause of abnormal sensing, 587–588, *589*

Fallback response, in DDD mode programmability, 512
Fallot's tetralogy, postsurgical AV block with, 655–656
    ventricular late potentials in, 383
Fascicular block, chronic, indications for cardiac pacing in, 656–657
    left anterior, as bifascicular or trifascicular block, 163
        characteristics of, 159
    left posterior, as bifascicular or trifascicular block, 163
        characteristics of, 159

Fasciculoventricular fibers. See *Mahaim fibers*.
Fast Fourier transform analysis (FFTA), for ventricular late potentials, 383–384, 389–390
  incidence of ventricular tachycardia and, 390–391, 391t
  of signal-averaged electrocardiograms, 359–360, *360–361*
Fatty acid esters, alterations in, during acute myocardial ischemia, 66–67
Fiber orientation, refractoriness and, 43, 47
Field-dependent ion permeability, cardiac pacing and, 487
Figure-eight circuit, around functional conduction block, 47, *49*
  interruption of, *42*, 43
  reentrant activation and, 40, *41*
  model of, 686, *686*
Fixed rate pacing interval, defined, 580, *580*
Flecainide, adverse effects of, 421
  clinical pharmacokinetics of, 420
  dosage and plasma concentrations of, 420
  drug interactions with, 420–421
  electrophysiologic effects of, 420
  hemodynamic effects of, 420
  indications for, 420
Fluoroscopic equipment, for catheter ablation, 471, *472*
Framingham Heart Study, atrial arrhythmias in, 95
  ventricular arrhythmias in, 94
Free fatty acids, alterations in, during acute myocardial ischemia, 66–67
Free radicals, alterations in, during acute myocardial ischemia, 67–68, *67–69*
  role of, in early myocardial ischemia, 23
Free water loss, during acute myocardial ischemia, 62–63
Frequency-domain signal-averaged electrocardiography, 359–360, *360–361*
  for ventricular late potentials, 389–390
Frequency spectrum, cardiac pacing and, 490, *491*
Fulguration for catheter ablation, development of, 474–476, *475*
  protocol for, 479, *480*, 481t
Fusion beats, in ventricular pacing, 574, *575*

Glycolysis and metabolism compartmentalization, during myocardial ischemia, 69–71, *70–71*
  potassium efflux and, 72–73, *73*
Glycolytic pathways, during acute myocardial ischemia, 59–60, 64, 65, 68
Glycolytic substrates (GSS), in myocardial ischemia, 71–72, *72*
Glycosides, inotropic effects of, 6
Goldman-Hodgkin-Katz equation, calcium channel and, 5–6
  for resting membrane potential, 3–4

H-A interval, in AV nodal reentry, 174, *175*
Half-life of antiarrhythmic agents, 410, *410*
Health Care Financing Administration, 259
Heart block. See also *Atrioventricular (AV) block*.

Heart block *(Continued)*
  acquired complete, cardiac pacing for, 654
  congenital complete, cardiac pacing for, 654–655
Heart rate. See also *Intrinsic heart rate; Resting heart rate*.
  hemodynamic effects of, 545
  risk stratification with, of myocardial infarction, 317–318, *318*
  of sudden cardiac death, 97, 97t
Hemodynamic effects of automatic implantable cardioverter/defibrillator (AICD), 747, *748*, 749
Hemodynamic monitoring, during catheter ablation, 476
  of left ventricular function, 305, 305t
Hexokinase (HK), compartmentalization of metabolism and, 71–72, *72*
High-resolution electrocardiogram. See also *Signal-averaged electrocardiography (SAECG)*.
  beat-to-beat recording of, 362–364, *365–366*
  clinical aspects of, 372–384
    AV nodal potentials and, 377–378, *378*
    His bundle potential recordings and, 374–377, *375–377*
    pre-atrial activity and, 372–374, *373*
    ventricular late potentials and, 378–384
  electrophysiologic substrate of, 364, 367–369, *367–368*
  history of, 372
  noise sources in signal measurements, 350–351
    amplifier noise as, 350
    electrode-tissue interface noise as, 350
    electromyographic potentials as, 350–351
    power frequency noise as, 350
  periodicity analysis of late potentials and, *368*, 369
  spatial averaging type of, 349
  technical and basic aspects of, 349–369
  temporal signal averaging (ensemble) type of, 349, 351–359
    bandpass filtering in, 352–354, *353–354*
    from Holter tape recordings, 354, 356, *356*
    lead systems for, 352
    quantitative analysis of time-domain SAECGs, 356–359, *357–358*
    signal alignment for, 351–352, *352*
His bundle recordings, of atrioventricular (AV) block, complete, 154, *155*
  first-degree, 142, *142*
  second-degree, 148–149, *149–150*
  of sick sinus syndrome patients, 133
  signal-averaging technique for, 374–377, *375–377*
  sustained ventricular tachycardia (VT), 254
  unified hypothesis and, 148–149, *149–150*
His bundle system, action potential and conduction in, 8
  anatomy of, 141
  bundle branch block in, 162–163, *164*
  paroxysmal AV block and, 156
  Wenckebach block in, 147–148, *147–150*
His-Purkinje potential, beat-to-beat recordings and, 362–364, *365–366*
  definition of, 349
His-Purkinje system, bradycardia-dependent bundle branch block in, 162
  complete AV block in, 154

His-Purkinje system *(Continued)*
  electrophysiologic studies (EPS) of, 296
  first-degree AV block associated with, 142, *144*
  paroxysmal AV block and, 156–158, *159–161*
  unified hypothesis of second-degree AV block and, 149
Holter monitoring, for myopotential interference in pacemaker function, 646
  for pacemaker followup, 592, *592–594*, 666
  for repetitive monomorphic ventricular tachycardia, 233–234
  for sinus node dysfunction, 120–121
  signal-averaged electrocardiograms from, 354, 356, *356*
H-V interval, evaluation of patients with, 206–207, *207*
  His bundle electrocardiography and, 374, *376–377*
  in complete AV block, 154, *155*
  in first-degree AV block, 142, *142*
  in normal AV conduction, 141, *141*
  with bifascicular and trifascicular block, 163
    prognostic significance of, 165
  with Wenckebach AV block, distal to His bundle, 147, *147–148*
Hydrogen peroxide, alterations in, during acute myocardial ischemia, 67, *67–68*
Hypersensitive carotid sinus syndrome, diagnosis of, 132
  electrophysiologic studies (EPS) of, 296
  indications for cardiac pacing with, 657–658
  pacemaker follow-up procedures and, 666–667
Hypertensive heart disease, as sudden cardiac death risk factor, 333–334
Hypocalcemia, long QT–torsades de pointes syndrome and, 271
Hypokalemia, sustained ventricular tachycardia (VT) and, 248
Hypothalamic control centers, cardiac arrhythmias and, 88, *88*
Hypothermia, modification of sinus node with, 116
Hysteresis, in ventricular pacing, 580, *580*
  programmability of, in single-chamber pacemakers, 509–510

ICI 118,551, and cardiac arrhythmogenesis, 80, *81*
  sympathetic nervous system and, 78, *79*
Impedance, defibrillation electrophysiology and, 721
  respiration sensing with, 529, *530*
Implantation devices. See *Cardiac pacing* and specific types of pacemakers.
Impulse conduction, abnormalities in, 13–14
  reentrant arrhythmias and, 14
  tissue anisotropy and, 14
Impulse initiation, abnormal, 12–13
Impulse ringing distortion, in signal-averaged electrocardiography, 352
Infantile tachycardia, atrial flutter and, 286–287
  cardiac pacing for, 290–291
  cardiomyopathy with, 288, *288*
  cardioversion and, 289–290
  myocardial tumors and, 291

Index 773

Infantile tachycardia *(Continued)*
  propranolol for, 290
  QRS complex and, 286–287
  sudden infant death syndrome (SIDS) and, 285
  surgery for, *290–291*, 291
  verapamil for, 290
Infection, with AICD implantation, 751
Insulation, of leads, in implantable pacemakers, 496
Intercellular coupling, reentrant ventricular tachyarrhythmias and, 323
Intercostal myopotentials, pacemaker interference with, 644, *645*
  paroxysmal AV block and, 157
Intracardiac pacing, sinus node dysfunction and, 123
Intracellular acidosis, during acute myocardial ischemia, 66
Intracoronary platelet aggregation, myocardial perfusion and, 83
Intra-Hisian block, first-degree AV block with, 142
Intraoperative electrophysiologic mapping, for Wolff-Parkinson-White syndrome management, 436–437, *437*
  of ventricular tachyarrhythmias, 445–447, *446–447*
Intraventricular conduction defects (IVCD), 158–165. See also *Bundle branch block; Fascicular block.*
  indications for cardiac pacing in, 657
Intrinsic heart rate (IHR), sinus node evaluation with, 121–122
  sinus node recovery time (SNRT) and, *125*, 125–126
Intrinsic signals, as cause of abnormal sensing, in VVI pacemakers, 588–591, *589–591*
Ion cotransport pump, for resting membrane potential, 2
Ionic mechanisms, antiarrhythmic agents and, 401–404, *401–404*
  in vitro studies of triggered activity and, 28, 30, *31*

Jugular vein cannulation, endomyocardial lead placement techniques and, 563
Junctional recovery time, evaluation of complete AV block with, 154–156, *155–156*
Junctional tachycardia, atrioventricular (AV) type of, drug therapy for, 178, *179*, *181*, 182
  nonparoxysmal AV form of, 175
  automatic form of, 176
  in infants, 286
  reciprocating form of, 466–467

Kelvin 500 temperature-response pacemaker device, 519
Koch, triangle of, 140, *141*

Lactate accumulation, during myocardial ischemia, 66
LAS40 parameter, in signal-averaged electrocardiography, 353
  from Holter monitors, 356
  in time-domain signal-averaged electrocardiograms, 357–358

Laser energy for catheter ablation, 468
Late potentials. See also *Ventricular late potentials.*
  analysis of periodicity in, *368*, 369
  beat-to-beat recordings and, 362–364, *365–366*
  definition of, 349
  electrophysiologic substrate of, 364, 367–369, *367–368*
  in signal-averaged electrocardiography, 224–227
  frequency characteristics of, 354
  in time-domain signal-averaged electrocardiograms, 356–359, *357–358*
  programmed electrical stimulation (PES) results and, 224
  ventricular type of, 387–398
    high-resolution electrocardiography for, 378–384, *380–383*
Leads, displacement of, defibrillation interference and, 620
  in single-chamber pacemakers, 582–583, *582–584*
  with AICD implantation, 751, *752*
  for automatic implantable cardioverter/defibrillator (AICD), 739–740
  for signal-averaged electrocardiography, 352
  for temporary antitachycardia pacing, 708
  placement techniques for, complications of, 564
  ventricular passive fixation lead, 563–564
Leading circle mechanism, reentrant arrhythmias and, 14
Left stellate ganglionectomy, long QT–torsades de pointes syndrome and, 273–274
Left ventricle, aneurysmectomy for sustained ventricular tachycardia (VT) in, 258–259
  anterior or lateral, 450, *450*
  dysfunction in, after myocardial infarction, 303–307
    effects of disopyramide on, 417
    infarct size and, 303–305
    invasive hemodynamic evaluation of, 305, 305t
    noninvasive evaluation of, 305–307
      echocardiographic methods for, 306–307
      radionuclide methods for, 305–306, *306*
    ventricular arrhythmias and, 307–309, 309t, *310*
  hemodynamic effects of, 545–546
  programmed electrical stimulation (PES) and, 224
  posterior, 450–452, *451*
Left ventricular ejection fraction (LVEF), arrhythmia suppression and, 339
  evaluation of, with ambulatory monitoring, 96–97
  hemodynamic effects of, 553, *554*
  predictive value of, 379–381
  programmed electrical stimulation of, 227, 228t
  risk stratification with, 334, 339–342, *341*
Left ventricular ejection time (LVET), rate-responsive pacing and, 538
Lenegre's disease, indications for cardiac pacing with, 654
Lev's disease, indications for cardiac pacing with, 654

Lidocaine, action of, on reentry arrhythmias, 50, *51*
  adverse effects of, 419
  clinical pharmacokinetics of, 419
  dosage and plasma concentrations of, 419
  drug interactions with, 419
  effects of, on membrane potentials, 405, *406*
  electrophysiologic effects of, *418*, 418
  hemodynamic effects of, 418
  indications for, 419
  prevention of sudden death with, 107
  ventricular arrhythmia suppression with, 30
Lithium-chemistry batteries, 494–495, 495t
Lithotripsy, pacemaker interference with, 625–626
Local anesthetics, as antiarrhythmic agents, 413
Long QT syndrome. See also *Torsades de pointes.*
  electrocardiographic features of, 265–269, *265–270*
  etiologies and clinical findings of, 269–273, 271t
  history of, 265
  ventricular late potentials in, 382–383
Longitudinal dissociation, bundle branch block pattern due to, 162–163, *164*
Lower rate limit, dual-chamber pacemaker timing cycles and, 601
  in DDD mode programmability, 513
  in DVI pacemakers, 599
Lown grading system, for arrhythmia evaluation, 102–103, 102t–103t
Lyme myocarditis, indications for cardiac pacing with, 658
Lysophosphatidylcholine (LPC), alterations in, during acute myocardial ischemia, 66–67
  in vitro studies of triggered activity and, 30
  role of, in early myocardial ischemia, 22–23
Lysophosphoglycerides, 66–67

Magnet mode rate, defined, 580, *580*
Magnet testing, for automatic implantable cardioverter/defibrillator (AICD), 746
Magnetic resonance imaging (MRI), pacemaker interference and, 624
Mahaim fibers, evaluation of patients with, 206–207, *207*
  pre-excitation syndrome and, 191, 193, *193*
Maintenance drug testing, arrhythmia evaluation for, 103–105, *104*
Mapping studies. See also *Catheter mapping; Endocardial mapping; Epicardial mapping; Intraoperative electrophysiological mapping.*
  in vivo triggered activity studies and, 34
  neurocardiology research and, 87, 88t
  of reentrant excitation, 37, *39*
  of refractoriness, 43, *44*
  of ventricular arrhythmias, 20–21, *21*
Maximum diastolic potential (MDP), automaticity changes due to, 10–11, *12*
  definition of, 1, *2*
  L-type Ca^{2+} current inactivation with, 10, *10–11*
  Na^+ current inactivation with, 9–10, *9–10*

Maximum diastolic potential (MDP) *(Continued)*
  primary and secondary reduction of, 11
  repolarization with reduction of, 11
Membrane active drugs, antiarrhythmic therapy with, 104–105, *105*
Membrane potential, definition of, 1
Mercury-zinc batteries for implantable pacemakers, 494, 495t
Mesothelioma of AV node, indications for cardiac pacing with, 654
Meta device, 519
  respiration sensing with, 531–532, *532*
Metabolic demand in rate-responsive pacing, 525–539, 526t
  activity sensing in, 532–535
  biosensors for, 538
  ideal sensor characteristics for, 525, 526t
  mixed venous oxygen saturation and, 536–538
  mixed venous temperature and, 535–536, 536t, *537*
  pH sensing for, 527, *527*
  respiration sensing in, 529–532
  stimulus-evoked interval in, 527–529, *527–529*
Metabolic inhibitors, alterations in, 68
Metaprolol, propafenone interaction with, 424
Methacholine, and cardiac arrhythmogenesis, 80, *81*
Mexiletine, adverse effects of, 419
  clinical pharmacokinetics of, 419
  dosage and plasma concentrations of, 419
  drug interactions with, 419
  electrophysiologic effects of, *418*, 418
  hemodynamic effects of, 418
  indications for, 419
  prevention of sudden death with, 107, 109
Mitochondrial metabolism, during acute myocardial ischemia, 64, *65*, 68
Mitochondrial substrates (MSS), during myocardial ischemia, 71–72, *72*
Mixed venous oxygen saturation, rate-responsive pacing and, 536–538
Mixed venous temperature, rate-responsive pacing and, 535–536, 536t, *537*
Mobitz II atrioventricular (AV) block, characteristics of, 148
  indications for cardiac pacing in, 653
  paroxysmal AV block and, 156, *159*
  similarities with Wenckebach AV block, 144–145, *146*
  unified hypothesis for, 148–149
Modulated receptor hypothesis, for antiarrhythmics, *405*, 405–406
Molecular defects, long QT syndrome and, 278
Molecular weight, local anesthetic antiarrhythmics and, 405, *406*
Monophasic waveforms, defibrillation electrophysiology and, *722*, 722–723
Morphology parameter, of automatic implantable cardioverter/defibrillator (AICD), 738
Multicenter Investigation of the Limitation of Infarct Size (MILIS), complex ventricular arrhythmias and sudden death in, 218
  left ventricular dysfunction and, 308, 309t, *310*
Multicenter Post-Infarction Program (MPIP), left ventricular dysfunction evaluation in, 305–306, *306*

Multicenter Post-Infarction Program (MPIP) *(Continued)*
  ventricular arrhythmias and, 308, 309t, *310*
  sudden cardiac death classification in, 319
Multiprogrammability of pacemakers, 504–521
  clinical value of, 517t, 519t, 519–520, 520t
  definition and history of, 504
  difficulties, risks and errors of, 520, *520–521*
  of DDD pulse generator, 510–513, 510t, *510*
    atrial refractory period programmability, *511*, 511–512
    crosstalk in, 515–516, 515t, *515–516*
    lower-rate limit of ventricular stimulation and, 513
    prevention of endless loop tachycardias and, 513–515, *513–514*
    principle problems of, 513–516
    upper-rate limit of ventricular stimulation and, 512, *512–513*
  of rate responsiveness, 516–519, 516t, 517t, *517–518*
  of single-channel pacemakers, 504–513, 505t
    of pacing mode, 510
    of refractory period, 509
    output programmability for, 505–506, *506–507*
    programmability of hysteresis and, 509–510
    rate programmability for, 506–508
      fast rate programming in, *507*, 507–508
      slow rate programming in, 507
    sensitivity programmability of, 508–509
      oversensing and, 509, *509*
      undersensing and, 508, *508*
  programming aids for, 504, 519
Mustard operative procedure, cardiac pacing with, 655–656
Myocardial electrical burns, during electrocautery, 615
Myocardial infarction, acute phase of, bundle branch and bifascicular block in, 163, 165
  clinical variables of risk stratification in, 305
  hemodynamic evaluation of left ventricular function during, 305, 305t
  incidence of sustained ventricular tachycardia (VT) and, 259–260
  sinus node dysfunction and, 116–117
  sustained ventricular tachycardia (VT) and, 247–248
  ventricular arrhythmias in, 57–58
  Wenckebach AV block with, 145, 147
  chronic phase of, 57
  diagnosis of, during ventricular pacing, 576, *577*
  early phase of, 218
  long-QT syndrome and, 277–278, *278*
  multiple and competing risks after, 319–320
  non-Q wave type of, 309–310
  programmed electrical stimulation (PES) results and, 223–224
  risk stratification for, 303
    left ventricular dysfunction with, 303–307
    infarct size and, 303–305
    non-Q wave infarction and mortality, 309–310

Myocardial infarction *(Continued)*
  sudden cardiac death as end point for, 318–320, 319t
  ventricular arrhythmias with, 307–318
    electrophysiologic studies (EPS) after, 311–314, 313t
    exercise testing and, 310–311
    heart rate variability and, 317–318, *318*
    Holter studies of, 307, 308t, *308–309*
    increase in spontaneous arrhythmias and, 310, 310t
    left ventricular dysfunction and, 307–309, 309t, *310*
    signal-averaged electrocardiogram for, 314, 315t, 316–317
  subacute phase of, reentrant ventricular rhythms in, 35–50
  triggered ventricular rhythms during, 24–35
  ventricular arrhythmia after, 96, 96t
  ventricular late potentials in, 379
Myocardial ischemia, acute phase of, arrhythmogenesis during, 60–61, *62*
  electrophysiologic alterations during, 61–69, 63t
    catecholamine release and elevated cAMP levels during, 66
    extracellular potassium accumulation in, 61–66, *63–66*
    free radicals and, 67–68, *67–69*
    intracellular acidosis and lactate accumulation in, 66
    intracellular calcium overload in, 66
    lysophoglycerides, fatty acid esters,
    and free fatty acids in, 66–67
  energy utilization during, 59–60, *60*
  early phase of, ventricular arrhythmias in, 19–24
  post-stress, 84, *85*, 86, 86t
  significance of late potentials and, 398
Myocardial perfusion, influence of sleep on, 87
  neurogenic aspects of, 82–83, *83*
Myocardial revascularization, sudden cardiac death and, 338–339
Myocardial tumors, infantile ventricular tachycardia and, 291
Myopotentials, dual-chamber electrocardiography and, 605, *606*
  pacemaker interference from, 634–642, *635*
    during bipolar pacing, 644–645
    in DDD pacing, 635, *638–641*, 639, 641
    in single-chamber pacemakers, 634–635, *636–638*
    management of, 646–649, *647–648*
    sources of, 642–644
      diaphragmatic myopotential oversensing and, 643–644, *643–644*
      intercostal myopotentials and, 644, *645*
      rectus abdominis muscle and, 642–643
    testing maneuvers for, 645–646, 645t
      electrogram telemetry and, 646, *646*
      Holter recordings, 646
      treadmill exercise testing, 646
    ventricular arrhythmia induction and, 641, *642*

Na⁺ current, inactivation of, with maximum diastolic potential (MDP), 9–10, *9–10*
Na⁺-Ca²⁺ exchange, in vitro studies of triggered activity and, 28, 30, *31*
resting membrane potential and, 6
Na⁺-K⁺ ATPase pump, antiarrhythmic agents and, 401–404
during acute myocardial ischemia, 61–62, 66
energy utilization in ischemic myocardium and, 60
in vitro studies of triggered activity, 27–28
resting membrane potential and, 4–5
torsades de pointes mechanisms and, 275
NASPE specific code, for cardiac pacing, 498–500, 499t
NBG code, for cardiac pacing, 497–500, 499t
Negative hysteresis, in single-chamber pacemakers, 510
Nernst equation, for resting membrane potential, 4
Neurocardiology, research trends in, 87, 88t
tachyarrhythmia prevention with, 761–762
Nodoventricular fibers. See *Mahaim fibers*.
Noise-sampling period (NSP) pacemaker interference and, 609–612, *610*
refractory period extension and, 609, *611*, 611–612, *613–615*
Noninvasive techniques, for antiarrhythmic agents, 101–104, *102*, 102t–103t, *104*
Noninvasive transcutaneous pacing (NTP), 678, 678–679
tachycardia termination with, 708
Nonischemic cardiomyopathy, surgical management of, 447, *447*
Nonparoxysmal AV junctional tachycardia, 175
Non-Q wave, complex ventricular arrhythmia and, 218
infarct size and, 304

Organic heart disease, complex ventricular arrhythmias and sudden death in, 217–219
electrophysiologic studies (EPS) of, 294
programmed electrical stimulation (PES) results and, 223–224
Organophosphorus insecticides, torsades de pointes and, 270–271
Ouabain, ventricular arrhythmia suppression with, 30, 32, *32*
Output circuits, in implantable pacemakers, 496–497
Output programmability, in single-chamber pacemakers, 505–506, *506–507*
Overdrive pacing, corrected sinus node recovery time (SNRTC) and, 125–126
in vitro studies of triggered activity, 24, 26–27, *27*
in vivo triggered activity studies, 34–35
"Overdrive suppression," Na⁺-K⁺ ATPase pump and, 5
Oversensing, AICD discharge and, 754
in DDD mode programmability, 511, *511*
dual-chamber electrocardiography and, *604*, 605
in single-chamber pacemakers, 509, *509*

Oversensing *(Continued)*
in VVI pacemakers, 587
Oxidative metabolism, during myocardial ischemia, 70–71, *70–71*
Oxygen radicals. See *Free radicals*.
Oxygen-derived free radicals. See *Free radicals*.

P wave, AV nodal reentry pattern and, 170–173, *171–173*
in normal AV conduction, 141, *141*
rate-responsive pacing and, 538
sensing abnormalities, in VVI pacemakers, 589, *589*
sinus node dysfunction and, 117, *117*
P-A interval, in normal AV conduction, 141, *141*
Pace-mapping, during catheter ablation, 477–478
Pacemaker escape interval, definition of, 579
Pacemaker pocket, abdominal location for, 566
inspection procedures for, 669
prepectoral location for, 565–566
retromammary location for, 566
Pacemaker syndrome, hemodynamic effects of, *557*, 558
Pacemaker/cardioverter/defibrillator (PCD), development of, 760–761
Pacemakers. See *Cardiac pacing*.
Parasympathetic nervous system, and cardiac arrhythmogenesis, influences on infarcted and ischemic heart from, 81–82, *81–82*, 82t
interactions with sympathetic nervous system, 80–82, *81*
ventricular arrhythmias and, 317–318, *318*
Parasystolic rhythm, in vitro studies of triggered activity in, 24, *26*
Paroxysmal atrial flutter, 709–710
Paroxysmal atrioventricular (AV) block, 156–158, *157–160*
indications for cardiac pacing in, 653–654
Paroxysmal supraventricular tachycardia (PSVT) due to atrioventricular node reentry, 440–442, *441–442*
due to concealed accessary atrioventricular connection, 440
pacing termination of, 709
Passive-fixation electrode, 496
Patch clamp techniques, compartmentalization of metabolism and, 71
during acute myocardial ischemia, 64–65, *65–66*
free radical actions and, 68, *69*
Patch-lead system, effects of automatic implantable cardioverter/defibrillator (AICD) and, 739–740, 747, *748*, 749
Peak paced cycle length, sinus node recovery time and, 123–124
Peptides and cardiac arrhythmias, 88, *88*
Percutaneous Cardiac Mapping and Ablation Registry, 460–462
Percutaneous transluminal coronary angioplasty (PTCA), 338
Perinodal zone of tissue, in sinus node, 126, *127*
Periodicity. See also *Alternate Wenckebach periodicity*.
in late potentials, *368*, 369

"Permanent junctional reciprocating tachycardia," 192–193
pH balance, local anesthetic antiarrhythmics and, 405
rate-responsive pacing and, 527, *527*
P-H interval, His bundle electrocardiography and, 374, *376–377*
Pharmocologic stress, electrophysiologic studies (EPS) of, 296
Phase 4 depolarization, automaticity enhanced by, 99
changes in, with MDP reduction, 10–11
in Purkinje fiber action potential and conduction, 8
sinoatrial node action potential and, 7
sinus node electrogenesis and, 114–115, *115*
Phase shift distortion, in signal-averaged electrocardiography, 352
Phenylephrine, sympathetic nervous system and cardiac arrhythmogenesis, 79, *80*
Phenytoin, disopyramide interaction with, 418
Plasma concentrations of antiarrhythmic agents, 412, 413t
Plateau potential, ventricular action potential and conduction in, 9
Post-Infarction Late Potential (PILP) study, 396–397
Post-repolarization refractoriness, during early myocardial ischemia, 19, *19*
Post-stress ischemia, 84, *85*, 86, 86t
Postventricular atrial refractory period (PVARP), dual-chamber pacemaker timing cycles and, 602
exogenous pacemaker interference and, 609
Potassium, in vitro studies of triggered activity and, 27–28
ischemia-induced increase of, 21–22, 61–66, *63–66*
protective effects of, 65–66
Potassium channels, antiarrhythmic agents and, 401–404
blocking drugs for, 406, 407t
Potassium current, cellular model for, 3
and torsades de pointes mechanisms, 275
time-dependent decay of, 114–115
Power frequency noise, in electrophysiologic signals, 350
P-R interval, in atrioventricular (AV) nodal reentry, 173–174, *173–175*
in first-degree AV block, 142, *143*
in normal AV conduction, 141, *141*
in Wolff-Parkinson-White syndrome, 192, 194–196, 195t, *196–198*
Mahaim fibers and, 193, *193*
with Mobitz II AV block, 148
Practolol, sympathetic nervous system and, 77–78
Pre-atrial activity, high-resolution electrocardiogram of, 372–374, *373*
Pre-ejection interval (PEI), rate-responsive pacing and, 538
Pre-excitation syndrome, accessory pathways for, 205–206, *206*
concealed pathways and, 192
with decremental properties, 192–193
anatomic and developmental aspects of, 191
definition of, 190
future research trends in, 212
historical perspective on, 190–191
incidence and natural history of, 193–194

Pre-excitation syndrome *(Continued)*
  invasive electrophysiology studies of, 199–208
    atrioventricular reentry and, *200*, 200–201, 204–205, *205–206*
    catheter mapping as, 201
    drug therapy evaluation with, 207–208, 208t
    identification of sudden death risk with, 207
    indications for, 199
    retrograde atrial activation patterns and, 202–204, *203–204*
    technical aspects of, 199–200
    ventricular activation patterns and, 201–202, *202*
  Mahaim fibers and, 193, *193*, 206–207, *207*
  management of, 208–212
    acute management of arrhythmias in, 209t, 209–210
    initial evaluation for, 208–209
    long-term management techniques for, 210t, 210–212
  noninvasive evaluation of, 194–199
    electrocardiography as, 194–195, 195t, *196–198*
      with reciprocating tachycardias, 195–196, 198, *199*
    exercise testing as, 198–199
    Wolff-Parkinson-White syndrome and, *191*, 191–192
Premature ventricular beats (PVBs), 60–61
Premature ventricular contractions (PVCs), as risk factor for sudden cardiac death, 334
  ambulatory monitoring of, 335–336
  exercise testing of, 337
Prepectoral pacemaker pocket, 565–566
Prinzmetal's angina, 78
Probability density function (PDF) criteria, 344–345
  defibrillation electrophysiology and, 719–721, *720*
Procainamide, adverse effects of, 417
  clinical pharmacokinetics of, 416
  dosage and plasma concentrations of, 416–417
  drug interactions with, 417
  effect of, with orthodromic SVT, 207–208, 208t, 210–212
  electrophysiologic effects of, 416–417
  hemodynamic effects of, 416
  indications for use of, 417
  long QT–torsades de pointes syndrome and, 273
  role of, in supraventricular tachycardia therapy, 178, *179*
Programmed electrical stimulation (PES), for complex ventricular arrhythmias, 219–229
  clinical variables in, 223–224
  electrocardiographic variables in, 224
  induced tachyarrhythmia specificity in, 221
  left ventricular function indices in, 224
  noninvasive predictors of results, 222–227, 223t
  results of, 221–222, 222t
  signal-averaged ECG and, 224–227, *225–226*, 226t
  stimulation protocols for, 219–221, 220t
  use of, for risk stratification, 227–229, 228t

Programmed electrical stimulation (PES) *(Continued)*
  for management of sudden cardiac arrest, 341
    as prognosis indicator in, 338–339, 343–344
  for reentrant ventricular tachycardia, acceleration with, 690, 693, *697–699*
    prevention of, 693, 700, *702–704*
    termination of, 686, *687*, 688, *688*, 690
  for surgical management of Wolff-Parkinson-White syndrome, 436
  for syncope of unknown origin, 295
  for ventricular arrhythmias, precipitation of fibrillation with, 690, 693, *697–699*
  risk assessment with, 217
  mortality predictions by, 313t, 313–314, *314*
  prognosis assessment with, compared to signal-averaged electrocardiogram, 329
  in ventricular tachyarrhythmias, *325*, 325–327
    end points for, 326
    incidence of inducible arrhythmias, 326, 326t
    inducible arrhythmia characteristics, 327, 327t
    protocols for, 326
    Westmead studies of, 326–327, 326t, 327t
Programming for pacemakers, defibrillation interference with, 620
  electrocautery interference with, 615–616
  follow-up and control of, 663
  reprogramming during pacemaker follow-up, 668
  in single-chamber pacemakers, 506–508
    fast rate programming in, *507*, 507–508
    sensitivity programmability and, 508–509
    slow rate programming in, 507
  testing equipment interference with, 627, *628*, 629
Propafenone, adverse effects of, 424
  clinical pharmacokinetics of, 423–424, *424*
  dosage and plasma concentrations of, 424
  drug interactions with, 424
  electrophysiologic effects of, 423
  hemodynamic effects of, 423
  indications for use of, 424
  prevention of sudden death with, 109
Propanolol, for infantile supraventricular tachycardia, 290
  for repetitive monomorphic ventricular tachycardia, 242, *244*
  impact on cardiac arrhythmogenesis, 77–78
  impact on sinus node recovery time, 125
Protein binding by antiarrhythmic agents, 410–411
  distribution and, 411, *411*
Pseudo Mobitz II atrioventricular (AV) block, characteristics of, 149, *151*
  indications for cardiac pacing in, 654
  similarities with Wenckebach AV block, 144–145, *146*
  distal to His system, *147–148*, 147–148
Pseudofusion beats, in ventricular pacing, *574*, *575*
Psychiatric disturbances, with AICD implantation, 752
Psychotropic drugs, torsades de pointes and, 270

Pulmonary puncture from endomyocardial lead placement, 563
Pulse generators, for temporary cardiac pacing, 708–709
  replacement techniques for, 566
Purkinje fibers, action potential and conduction in, 8, *9*
  antiarrhythmic agents and, 32, *33–34*
  delayed afterdepolarization (DADs) and, 28, *29*
  during acute myocardial ischemia, acidosis and, 66
  in vitro studies of triggered activity and, 24, 26–27, *27*
  reperfusion arrhythmias in, 23–24

Q wave in myocardial infarction, 218
  infarct size and, 304
QRS complex, antitachycardia pacing and, 693, *700–701*
  atrioventricular (AV) reentry pattern and, 170–173, *171–173*
  in atrioventricular (AV) block, acute acquired complete AV block and, 152
    congenital complete AV block and, 152
    first-degree block and, 142, *144*
    high-degree AV block and, 152
    Wenckebach AV block and, *147–148*, 147–148
  in infantile tachycardia, 286–287
  in long QT syndrome, 266
  in nonparoxysmal AV junctional tachycardia, 175
  in normal AV conduction, 141, *141*
  in pre-excitation syndrome, 190
    during exercise testing, 199
  in repetitive monomorphic ventricular tachycardia, 233, *234*
  in supraventricular tachycardia (SVT), 255–256, *256*
    electrocardiographic studies of, 251–253
    in catheter electrophysiologic studies, 253–255, *254–255*
  in time-domain signal-averaged electrocardiograms, 356–359, *357–358*
  in ventricular tachycardia, nonsustained type of, 221
    sustained type of, 250–251, 255–256, *256*
  in Wolff-Parkinson-White syndrome, 192, 194–196, 195t, *196–198*
  Mahaim fibers and, 193, *193*
  pacemaker interference and, during lithotripsy, 625–626
    with AICDs, 622–623
  ventricular late potentials and, 391–392
  ventricular pacing and, 571–576
    fusion and pseudofusion beats and, *574*, *575*
    postpacing ST-T wave changes, *574*, *576*
QRS duration (QRSD), in signal-averaged electrocardiography, 353, *353*
Q-T interval, for rate-responsive pacing, 527–529, *527–529*
Quinidine, adverse effects of, 416
  arrhythmia evaluation with, 101, *102*
  clinical pharmacokinetics of, 414
  dosage and plasma concentrations for, 414–415

Index   777

Quinidine *(Continued)*
   drug interactions with, 415–416
   electrophysiologic effects of, 414
   for repetitive monomorphic ventricular tachycardia, 242, *243*
   hemodynamic effects of, 414
   indications for use of, 415
   long-QT-torsades de pointes syndrome and, 266, *267*, 271–273, *272*
     terminal repolarization and, 268, *269*
   prevention of sudden death with, 107

Radiation therapy, pacemaker interference and, 624
Radio frequency, for catheter ablation, 468–469
   pacemaker interference and, during electrocautery, 614–619
   with magnetic resonance imaging (MRI), 624
Radioactive-plutonium reactors for pacemakers, 495
Radiography, pacemaker follow-up with, 664
Radionuclide imaging, left ventricular function evaluation with, 305–306, *306*
Rapid eye movement (REM) sleep, cardiac arrhythmogenesis and, 86–87
Rate modulation for cardiac pacing, 497, 498t
Rate parameters, of automatic implantable cardioverter/defibrillator (AICD), 738
Rate-responsive cardiac pacing, combined sensors for, 539, *540*
   dual-chamber classification of, 539–540, *540–541*
   implantation techniques for, 566–567
   metabolic demand indicators in, 525–539, 526t
     activity sensing and, 532–534
       Activitrax and, 532–533, *533–534*, 533t
       Sensolog device for, 534–535, *534–535*
     biosensors for, 538
     ideal sensor characteristics for, 525, 526t
     mixed venous oxygen saturation and, 536–538
     dp/dt sensing for, 537–538, *538*
     mixed venous temperature and, 535–536, 536t, *537*
     pH sensing and, 527, *527*
     respiration sensing for, 529–532
       in Biorate device, 529–531, 530t, *530–532*
       in Meta device, 531–532, *532*
     stimulus-evoked T interval and, 527–529, *527–529*
       clinical performance of, 528
       limitations of, 528–529, *528–529*
   patient selection for, 540–542
   philosophy of, 525
   programmability of, 516–519, 516t, 517t, *517–518*
   sensor selection for, 539, 539t
   technical and clinical aspects of, 491, 524–542
     overview of, 524
     terminology of, 524–525
Rate-smoothing option, in DDD mode programmability, 512

Recovery time, modification of spatial pattern of, 47, *48*
Rectus abdominis muscle, as source of pacemaker interference, 642–643
Reentrant arrhythmias, 98–100, *99*
   abnormal impulse conduction and, 14
   anatomic and electrophysiologic substrates of, 35–37, *36, 38*
   atrial flutter and, 185–187, *185–186*
   epicardial activation patterns of, 38–40, *39*
   figure-eight model of, *42, 43*, 686, *686*
   in atrioventricular (AV) node, 170–175, *171–173*
     diagnostic criteria for, 200–201
     drug therapy for, 178, *179, 181,* 182
     hemodynamic effects of, 548, *549–550*
     incessant form of, 204–205, *205–206*
     induction methods for, 201
     intranodal pathways for, 174–175
     pathways for, *171,* 173
     P-R intervals, 173–174, *173–175*
     surgical therapy for, 182
   in sinus node, 118–119, *120*, 176, *177*
   leading circle model of, 686
   pre-excitation syndrome and, 192–193
   recovery time spatial pattern modification and, 47, *48*
   refractoriness and, 43, *44–46*, 47
   ring model of, 685
   "spontaneous" vs. premature stimulation of, 40, *41*
   ventricular arrhythmias as, 35–50
     antiarrhythmic agents and, 47, 50
     continuous arcs of functional conduction and, 47, *49*
     epicardial activation patterns and, 37, 39–40, *39*
     interruption of figure-eight circuit and, *42,* 43
     modification of recovery time spatial pattern and, 47, *48*
     spatial nonhomogeneous lengthening of refractoriness and, 43, *44–46,* 47
     "spontaneous" excitation of, 40, *41*
   ventricular tachycardias as, anatomic and electrophysiologic substrate for, 323–325, *324–325*
     during acute myocardial ischemia, 61, *62*
     high-resolution electrocardiography for, 378–379
     paroxysmal supraventricular tachycardia (SVT) due to, 440–442, *441–442*
     repetitive monomorphic ventricular tachycardia and, 241–242
     sustained ventricular tachycardia (VT) and, 249
     entrainment phenomenon in, 250, *251*
Refractoriness, action potential duration (APD) and, 12
   antiarrhythmic agents as cause of, 413
   ischemic ventricular tachyarrhythmias and, 450
   sinus nodal classification of, 129, 131
   spatial nonhomogeneous lengthening of, 43, *44–46,* 47
   sustained reentry orients around, 47, *49*
Refractory period in pacemakers, 581
   bradycardia and, *594,* 595
   classifications of, 500–501, *501*

Refractory period in pacemakers *(Continued)*
   defibrillation electrophysiology and, 722
   definition of, 609
   interference-induced extension of, *611,* 611–612, *613–615*
   atrial refractory period, 612, *616*
   for full pacing cycle, 612, *618–619*
   partial extension of, 612, *617–618*
   programmability of, in single-chamber pacemakers, 509
Regional action potentials, cardiac electrophysiology and, 7–9
Reperfusion arrhythmias, in early myocardial ischemia, 23–24
Repetitive monomorphic ventricular tachycardia (RMVT), 233–242
   electrocardiographic pattern in, 233–234
     Holter monitoring and, 233–234
     12-lead ECG and, 233, *234*
   electrophysiologic studies (EPS) of, 234–245
   effect of drugs on, 242–245
     beta blockers and, 242, *244*
     calcium antagonists and, 242, 244–245, *245*
     type I drugs and, 242, *243*
   isolated or initial extrasystoles and, 235–238, *236–237*
     adrenergic and rate dependence in, 235–236, *236–237*
     distribution and mechanisms of, *236,* 236–238, *237, 240*
   repetitive activity in, 238–242
     adrenergic dependence and, 238, *239–240*
     coupling interval of initial beat and, *239,* 239, *241,* 241–242
     determinants of, 241, *242*
     possible mechanisms of, 241–242, *242*
     R-R interval and rate dependence in, 238–239, *240–241*
   history and definition of, 233
Repolarization, abnormal, in sudden cardiac death, 277–278, *278*
   torsades de pointes and, 274
   changes in, with MDP reduction, 11
   in Purkinje fiber action potential and conduction, 8
   Na^+-K^+ ATPase pump and, 5
   ventricular muscle action potential and conduction in, 9
Reset phenomenon, defibrillation interference and, 620
   exogenous interference with pacemakers and, 612–614
Resistor-capacitor timers, for cardiac pacing, 485–486, *486*
Respiration sensing for rate-responsive pacing, 529–532
   Biorate device for, 529–531, 530t, *530–532*
Resting heart rate, evaluation of sinus node dysfunction with, 122
Resting membrane potential, 1–7
   basis of, 6–7
   calcium channel and, 5–6
   cation activity values for, 4, 4t
   cellular model of, 2–4, *3*
   during acute myocardial ischemia, 63–65, *64–65*
   Na^+-Ca^{2+} channel and, 6
   Na^+-K^+ ATPase pump and, 4–5
   origin of, 1–2

Retrograde conduction, in pre-excitation syndrome, 202–204, *203–204*
   in pacemakers, hemodynamic effects of, 556, 558
   in sustained ventricular tachycardia (VT), 252–253, *253–255*
Retromammary pacemaker pocket, 566
Risk stratification, 303–320
   after myocardial infarction, 303
     left ventricular dysfunction and, 305–307
     and infarct size, 303–305
     invasive hemodynamic evaluation of, 305, 305t
     noninvasive evaluation of, 305–307
     ventricular arrhythmias with, 307–318
       electrophysiological studies of, 311–314, 313t
       exercise testing and, 310–311
       heart rate variability and, 317–318, *318*
       Holter studies of, 307, 380t, *308–309*
       increase in spontaneous arrhythmias in, 310, 310t
       left ventricular dysfunction and, 307–309, 309t, *310*
       non-Q infarction and, 309–310
       signal-averaged electrocardiography of, 314, 315t, 316–317
   for nonsustained ventricular tachycardia, 229–230, *229*
   sudden cardiac death as end point for, 318–320, 319t
   use of programmed electrical stimulation (PES) for, 227–229, 228t
RMS40 parameter, in signal-averaged electrocardiography, 353
   from Holter monitors, 356
   in time-domain signal-averaged electrocardiograms, 357–358
RMSQRS parameter, in signal-averaged electrocardiography, 353
Romano-Ward syndrome, history of, 265
   torsades de pointes episodes in, 266, *268*
R-R interval, in ventricular tachycardia, repetitive monomorphic form of, 238–239, *240–241*
   sustained form of, 252, *252*
   risk of sudden cardiac death and, 97, 97t
   with automatic junctional tachycardia, 176
RS4-SRT pacing system, rate-responsive pacing and, 538
Runaway pacemaker, defined, 582
Ryanodine, ventricular arrhythmia suppression with, 30, *31*

Safety of exercise testing, 101
Saponin, acute myocardial ischemia and, 68, *69*
Sarcolemmal membrane, during myocardial infarction, 38
Sarcoplasmic reticulum, calcium channel and, 5–6
Selectively permeable channels, resting membrane potential and, 2–4
Sensing. See also *Oversensing; Undersensing.*
   abnormalities of, in VVI pacemakers, 585–592
     apparent failure to sense as, 587, *587–588*

Sensing *(Continued)*
     extrinsic signs as cause of, 587–588, *589*
     intrinsic signs as cause of, 588–591, *589–591*
     oversensing as, 587
     partial sensing as, 591–592, *592*
     undersensing as, 585–587, *586*
   electrodes for cardiac pacing and, 490, *491*
   for rate-responsive pacing, 539, *540*
     ideal characteristics of, 525, 526t
     limits of, 539, 539t
     pH sensing and, 527, *527*
   refractory periods and, 581
   thresholds for, 564–565, 668
Sensolog device, 519
   activity sensing with, 534–535, *534–535*
Series equivalent, cardiac pacing and, 490, *491*
Setpoint, concept of, in cardiac pacing, 491
Sick sinus syndrome, clinical and laboratory evaluation of, 119–132
   definition of, 116
   etiology of, 116–117
   incidence of, 116
   indications for cardiac pacing with, 657
   management of patients with, 133–134
   pacemaker follow-up procedures and, 666–667, 667t
   prognosis for, 134–135, *135*
   sinoatrial conduction time for, 131
   sinus node dysfunction mechanisms and, 119
   reentry tachycardia with, 118–119, *120*
   sinus node recovery time (SNRT) and, 124–125, 131–132
Signal-averaged electrocardiography (SAECG), 351–359
   bandpass filters in, 352–354, *353–354*
   beat-to-beat recording of, 362–364, *365–366*
   for ventricular late potentials, 389–390
     insufficient sensitivity of, 391–392
     specificity of, 392
   frequency-domain analysis of, 359–360, *360–361*
     for ventricular late potentials, 389–390
   from Holter recordings, 354, 356, *356*
   lead systems for, 352
   of sustained ventricular tachycardia (VT), 255
   prognosis assessment with, 327–329, *328*
   programmed electrical stimulation (PES) and, 224–227, *225–226*, 226t, 329
   risk stratification with, 314, 315t, 316–317
   of sudden cardiac death evaluation, 337–338
   signal alignment for, 351–352, *352*
   spectro-temporal analysis of, 360–362, *361–365*
   time-domain techniques for, for ventricular late potentials, 388–389, *389*
   quantitative analysis of, 356–359, *357–358*
Single-chamber pacemakers, 496
   chest wall and esophageal stimulation for, 581, *582*
   electrocardiography of, 568–595
     asynchronous pacemaker (VOO), 576–578, *577–578*
     atrial pacing (AAI) and, 592, 595, *594–595*

Single-chamber pacemakers *(Continued)*
     fusion and pseudofusion beats in, 574, *575*
     Holter monitoring and, 592, *592–594*
     in ventricular (demand) inhibited pacemaker (VVI), 578–581, *579–581*
     in ventricular triggered pacemaker (VVT), 578, *578–579*
     myocardial infarction diagnosis with, 576, *577*
     overview of, 568
     postpacing ST-T wave changes in, 574, *576*
     QRS patterns with ventricular pacing and, 571–576
     refractory periods for, 581
     stimulus artifacts in, 568–571, *569–570*
   malfunction of, 581–592
     exit block as, 583, 585, *585*
     lead displacement, perforation or failure, 582–583, *582–584*
     pacing mode changes as, 585
     rate changes due to battery depletion, 582
     sensing abnormalities in VVI pacemakers and, 585–592
       extrinsic signals as cause of, 587–588, *589*
       failure to sense as, 587, *587–588*
       intrinsic signals as cause of, 588–591, *589–591*
       oversensing as, 587
       partial sensing as, 591–592, *592*
       undersensing as, 585–587, *586*
     stimulus and capture as cause of, 581–585
   multiprogrammability of, 504–513, 505t
   myopotential interference in, 634–635, *636–638*
Sinoatrial conduction time (SACT), atrial premature depolarizations (APD) and, 126–129, *127–128*
   continuous pacing method for, 129, *130*
   in electrophysiologic studies (EPS), 295
   return cycle calculations and, 127–128, *128*
   sinus node dysfunction and, 124
Sinoatrial exit block, first-degree classification of, 117
   response to atrial premature depolarization (APD), 126, *128*
   second-degree classification of, 117–118, *118–119*
   sinus node dysfunction and, 117–118, *118*
   third-degree classification of, 118
Sinoatrial node (SAN), action potential of, 7
   electrogenesis of, 114–115, *115*
Sinus arrhythmia, 117
   in Wolff-Parkinson-White syndrome, *191*, 191–192
Sinus bradycardia, hemodynamic effects of, 546–547, *547*
   torsades de pointes episodes and, 269, *270*
   with myocardial infarction, 116–117
Sinus cycle length, sinus node recovery time and, 123
Sinus node, atrial premature depolarization (APD) and, 126, *127–128*
   conduction time and, 126–129, *127–128*
   interpolation response to, 126, *127–128*
   reentry response to, 126, *127–128*
   reset response to, 126, *127–128*

Sinus node *(Continued)*
  dysfunction of, 116–133
    age of onset of, *116*
    atrial overdrive evaluation and, 122–126, *123*, *125–126*
    autonomic nervous system axis testing, 121
    bradycardia-tachycardia syndrome, 118, *119*
    clinical and laboratory evaluation of, 119–132
    continuous pacing method and, 129, *130*
    definition of, 116
    effects of drugs on, 132–133
    electrocardiogram monitoring of, 117, 117–120
    etiology of, 116–117
    exercise testing evaluation of, 120
    extracellular potential recordings of, 131–132, *132*
    Holter monitoring of, 120–121
    incidence of, 116
    intrinsic heart rate determination of, 121–122
    mechanisms of, in sick sinus syndrome (SSS), 119
    reentry as sign of, 118–119, *120*
    sinoatrial exit block as sign of, 117–118, *118*
    sinus arrest as sign of, 117, *118*
    sinus arrhythmia as sign of, 117
  electrophysiologic characteristics of, 115–116
    autonomic nervous system and, 115
    endocrine system and, 115
    function evaluation of, 295
    hypothermia and, 116
  normal anatomy of, 114
  potentials, high-resolution electrocardiogram of, 372–374, *373*
  reentry and, 176, *177*
  refractoriness and, 129, 131
  sick sinus syndrome and, management of, 133–134
    prognosis for, 134–135, *135*
Sinus node recovery time (SNRT), evaluation of dysfunction with, 122–126, *123*, *125*, *126*
  in electrophysiologic studies (EPS), 295
  limits of, 124–125
  prolongation of SACT and, 129, *130*
Sinus tachycardia, characteristics of, 176
Sleep, cardiac arrhythmias and, 86–87
Slow conduction zone, pacing of, during catheter ablation, 478–479, *479*
Slow wave sleep, cardiac arrhythmogenesis and, 86–87
Sock electrode array, for ventricular tachyarrhythmia evaluation, 445, *446*
Sodium, ventricular arrhythmia suppression with, 30, *31*
Sodium channel, antiarrhythmic agents and, 402, *403*
  defibrillation electrophysiology and, 721–722
  local anesthetic antiarrhythmics and, 404–406, *404*
Source resistance, cardiac pacing and, 490, *491*
Spatial averaging, definition of, 349
  for beat-to-beat recording, 362–364, *365–366*
  for ventricular late potentials, 389

Spectro-temporal analysis, of signal-averaged electrocardiograms, 360–362, *361–365*
ST segment, fast Fourier transform analysis of, 383–384
  influence of, on myocardial perfusion, 87
  ventricular late potentials and, 387–388, *388*
Steady state condition, with antiarrhythmic agents, 410, *410*
Stepwise discriminant function analysis, signal-averaged ECG and, 224–227, *226*
Sticky reed switch, defined, 581
Stimulus artifacts, in pacemakers, 568–571, *569–570*
Stimulus-evoked T interval for rate-responsive pacing, 527–529, *527–529*
Stress. See *Behavioral stress*.
ST-T wave changes, in ventricular pacing, 574, *576*
  in Wolff-Parkinson-White syndrome, 194–195, 195t, *196–198*
Subclavian vein, endomyocardial lead placement
  techniques for, 562–563
  thrombosis of, with AICD implantation, 750, *750*
Subendocardial resection, 343
Sudden cardiac arrest, abnormal repolarization and, 277–278, *278*
  arrhythmias and, 95–98
  complex ventricular arrhythmias and, 217–219
  incidence of, 217
  management of, 334–342
    invasive evaluation of, 338–342
      cardiac catheterization and surgical correction for, 338–339
      electrophysiologic studies (EPS) of, 339–342
    noninvasive evaluation of, 334–338
      ambulatory monitoring techniques for, 334–336
      signal-averaged electrocardiography for, 337–338
      treadmill stress testing for, 336–337
  mobidity and mortality of, 333
  pathophysiology and risk factors in, 333–334
  risk stratification and, 95–98, 318–320, 319t
  significance of late potentials and, 398
  sustained ventricular tachycardia (VT) as cause of, 251
  tachycardia in infants and, 285, *286*
  therapy for, 342–345
    antiarrhythmic agents as, 342–343
    nonpharmacologic techniques for, 343–345
      automatic implantable cardioverter/defibrillator (AICD) and, 344–345
      surgery as, 343–344
Sudden death, prevention of, with antiarrhythmic agents, 413
  with pre-excitation syndrome, 194
  patient identification of, 207
Sudden infant death syndrome (SIDS), incidence of pre-excitation syndrome with, 194
  long QT syndrome and, 278
  near-miss episodes of infantile tachycardia as, 285

Supraventricular arrhythmias, age and prevalence of, 100
  pacing therapy for, 134
Supraventricular premature beats (SPB), 100
Supraventricular tachycardia (SVT). See also *Tachycardia*.
  antidromic, diagnostic criteria for, *200*, 200–201
    electrocardiographic features of, 195–196, 198, *199*
    in Wolff-Parkinson-White syndrome, *191*, 191–192
    multiple accessory pathways and, 205–206, *206*
  atrial origin of, 176–177, *177*, 467
    atrial fibrillation and, 177
    atrial flutter and, 176
    atrial tachycardia and, 176
    sinus node reentry and, 176, *177*
    sinus tachycardia and, 176
  automatic junctional tachycardia and, 176
  AV junctional tachycardias and, 170–176
    AV nodal reentry in, 170–175, *171–173*
    catheter ablation for, 458–462
    nonparoxysmal type of, 175
  cardiomyopathies and, 288, *288*
  catheter ablation techniques for, 182, 453–469
    defibrillators for ablation, 457–458
    direct-current shocks for cellular electrophysiology of, 456–457
    transcatheter biophysics and, 453–454, *453–455*
    electrode catheters for, 457
    for permanent junctional reciprocating tachycardia, 466–467
    laser energy for, 468
    of accessory pathways, 462–467
      experimental background on, 462–463
      indications for, 462
      of free-wall connections, 466
      of posteroseptal AV connections, 464–466, *465*
      technique for, 463–464, *464*
    of atrial tachycardias, 467
    of atrioventricular (AV) junction, 458–462
      complications of, 461–462
      current status of, 462
      experimental background on, 458–459
      indications for, 458
      modification vs. ablation for, 460
      results of, 460–461, *461*
      techniques for, 459–460, *459*
    radiofrequency for, 468–469
    tissue injury mechanisms and, 454–456
    with permanent pacemakers, 467–468
    hemodynamic effects of, 547–548, *549–550*, 550
  in infants, chronic treatment for, 290
    management of, 289–290, *290*
    mechanisms of, 285–287
  orthodromic, retrograde activation patterns and, 202–204, *203–204*
    diagnostic criteria for, 200, *200*
    effect of procainamide on, 207–208, 208t, 210–212
    electrocardiographic features of, 195–196, 198, *199*

Supraventricular tachycardia (SVT) *(Continued)*
  in Wolff-Parkinson-White syndrome, *191*, 191–192
  multiple accessory pathways and, 205–206, *206*
  surgical management of, 182, 436–445
    in Wolff-Parkinson-White syndrome, 436–440
    of atrial flutter/fibrillation, 444–445
    of ectopic (automatic) atrial tachycardia, 442–444, *442–444*
    of paroxysmal supraventricular taachycardia (PSVT) due to atrioventricular node reentry, 440–442, *441–442*
      due to concealed accessory atrioventricular connection, 440
  therapy for, 177–182
    catheter ablation for, 182, 453–469
    drug therapy for, 177–182, *178–181*
    surgical therapy for, 182, 436–445
  termination of, with electrical devices, 761
  with aberrant conduction, differentiation of sustained ventricular tachycardia (VT) from, 255–256, *256*
Surgery, antitachycardia type of, 394–396, *395*
  for ventricular late potentials, 394–396, *395*
  for cardiac arrhythmias, 436–452
    for proxysmal supraventricular tachycardia (PSVT) due to AV nodal reentry, 440–442, *441–442*
      due to concealed accessory AV connection, 440
    for supraventricular tachycardia, 182, 436–445
      atrial flutter/fibrillation as, 444–445
      ectopic (automatic) atrial tachycardia as, 442–444, *442–444*
      in Wolff-Parkinson-White syndrome, 436–440
    for ventricular tachyarrhythmias, 445–452
      in anterior or lateral left ventricle, 450, *450*
      in posterior left ventricle, 450–452, *451*
      indications for surgery with, 445
      intraoperative electrophysiologic mapping of, 445–447, *446–447*
      nonischemic ventricular tachyarrhythmias as, 447–450, *448–449*
      refractory ischemic ventricular tachyarrhythmias as, 450
      sustained tachycardia with, 258–259
    for infantile supraventricular tachycardia, 290–291, 291
    for pre-excitation syndrome patients, 212
  sudden cardiac arrest management with, 343–344
Sympathetic nervous system, automaticity enhanced by, 99
  cardiac arrhythmias and, 77–80, *78*
    adrenergic receptor subtypes and, 77–79, *78*
    alpha-adrenergic receptors and, 79, *80*
    cyclic nucleotides and, 79–80
    parasympathetic interactions and, 80–82, *81*
    torsades de pointes and, 270, *271*
    ventricular arrhythmias and, 317–318, *318*
Syncope, chronic fascicular block and, 656

Syncope *(Continued)*
  of unexplained origin (SUO), 294–301
    definition of, 293
    electrophysiologic studies (EPS) of, clinical and noninvasive predictors of outcome of, 299–300
      diagnostic criteria for, 296–297, 297t, 298t, 299t
      indications for, 294–295
      risk and complications of, 301–302
      technique and study protocols for, 295–296
    initial noninvasive clinical evaluation of, 293–294
    therapy and prognosis for, 300–301, 300t, 301t
  recurrence of, 393
  sustained ventricular tachycardia (VT) and, 250–251

T interval, stimulus-evoked, 527–529, *527–529*
T wave, in ventricular pacing, 574, *576*
  in Wolff-Parkinson-White syndrome, 194–195, 195t, *196–198*
  sensing abnormalities, in VVI pacemakers, 589, *589*
Tachyarrhythmia(s). See also *Tachycardia; specific types of tachycardia*.
  prevention of, electrical devices for, 761–762, *762*
  termination of, with external cardiac pacing, 683
Tachycardia. See also specific types of tachycardia.
  acceleration of, with programmed electrical stimulation (PES), 690, 693, *697–699*
  catheter ablation for, 466–467
  resetting mechanisms of, *689*, 690
  termination of, followed by reinitiation, 690, *691*
    overdrive entrainment and, 690, *694–696*
Tachycardia-dependent paroxysmal AV block, 156, *157–160*
Telemetry, for cardiac pacing, 501–502, 502t
  myopotential interference in pacemaker function and, 646, *646*
Temporal averaging. See *Signal-averaged electrocardiography (SAECG)*.
Tendon of Todaro, 140, *141*
Testing equipment for pacemakers, interference with function from, 626–629
Tetrodotoxin (TTX), in Purkinje fiber action potential and conduction, 8
  release of, during myocardial infarction, 37, *38*
  suppression of delayed afterdepolarization (DADs) with, 30
Thalamic gating system, cardiac arrhythmias and, 88, *88*
Therapeutic AV block, 154
Time-dependent potassium currents, and torsades de pointes mechanisms, 274–275
Time-domain signal-averaged electrocardiography, 356–359, *357–358*
  for ventricular late potentials, 388–389, *389*
Tissue injury from catheter ablation procedures, 454–456

Tocainide, adverse effects of, 419
  clinical pharmacokinetics of, 419
  dosage and plasma concentrations of, 419
  drug interactions with, 419
  electrophysiologic effects of, *418*, 418
  hemodynamic effects of, 418
  indications for, 419
  prevention of sudden death with, 109
Torsades de pointes. See also *Long QT syndrome*.
  clinical features of, 265–273, *267–269*
  definition of, 265, *266*
  etiologies and clinical findings of, 269–273, 271t, *271–272*
  future research trends in, 277–279, *278*
  management of, 273–274
  mechanisms of, 274–277
    action potential prolongation as, 274–275
    in vitro modulation of triggered activity and, 275–276
    models in intact heart of, 276–277
Transcutaneous electrical nerve stimulation (TENS), 626
Transesophageal pacing, tachycardia termination with, 708
Transient outward current (I_{to}), in Purkinje fiber action potential and conduction, 8
Transient reed switch malfunction on pacemakers, magnetic resonance interference (MRI) with, 625
Transmembrane action potential, antiarrhythmic agents and, 402, *402*
  during delayed afterdepolarizations (DADs), 32, *33*
  during early myocardial ischemia, 19, *19*
  during myocardial infarction, 37, *38*
  during normal sinus rhythm, 1, *2*
Transplantation, rejection of, significance of late potentials and, 397
Transtelephonic monitoring system for pacemaker followup, 666, *666*
Transthoracic pacing, impedance, defibrillation and, 731–732
  tachycardia termination with, 708
Transvenous atrial and ventricular leads, 708
  for cardioversion or defibrillation, 711–712
Transvenous catheterization, 131
Treadmill testing. See also *Exercise testing*.
  for myopotential interference in pacemaker function, 646
Triangle of Koch, 440–442, *441–442*
Triboelectric phenomena, *628*, 629
Tricuspid valve, anatomy of, 140, *141*
Tridimensional mapping techniques, for ventricular arrhythmias, 21
Trifascicular block, 163
"Trigger jitter" in signal-averaged electrocardiography, 351–352, *352*
Triggered ventricular rhythms, during subacute myocardial infarction, 24–35
  antiarrhythmic agents and, 30, 32
  dependence on diastolic potentials, 27–28, *28–29*
  in vitro studies of, 24–32, *25–26*, 275–276
  in vivo overdrive pacing, 34–35
  in vivo studies of, 32, 34–35, *36*
  ionic mechanisms for, 28, 30, *31*
  lysophosphatidylcholine, role of, 30
  overdrive pacing effects and, 24, 26–27, *27*

Index 781

Triggered ventricular rhythms *(Continued)*
  in repetitive monomorphic ventricular tachycardia, 241–242
  modulation of, in torsades de pointes and, 275–276
Triggering of pacemakers, from pacemaker testing equipment, 627, *627*
12-lead electrocardiogram, for repetitive monomorphic ventricular tachycardia, 233, *234*

U wave, in long QT syndrome, 266–267
"Uncommitted" ventricular pacing, 501, *501*
Undersensing, atrial type of, 603–605, *604, 606*
  in single-chamber pacemakers, 508, *508*
  in VVI pacemakers, 585–587, *586*
  with defibrillation interference, 620
Unipolar catheters, for catheter ablation, 472, *472–473*
Unipolar pacing, in implantable pacemakers, 495
  obsolescence of, 649
Upper limit of vulnerability, defibrillation electrophysiology and, 715–717, *717*
  critical point hypothesis and, 719, *720*
  threshold correlation with, 716–717, *718*
Upper rate limit in dual-chamber pacemakers, 601–603, *604*
USCI catheters for catheter ablation, 472–474, *472–474*

VA interval, in DVI pacemakers, 600
Vagus nerve activity, and cardiac arrhythmogenesis, behavior stress and, 83–87, *85*, 86t
  in vitro studies of triggered activity and, 24, *26*
  parasympathetic-sympathetic interactions and, 80–82, *81*
  in ischemic and infarcted heart, *81*, 81–82
Variable frequency pacing, 524–525
Vasodepressor carotid sinus hypersensitivity, 132
VDD pacemakers, electrocardiography of, 600
Ventricular arrhythmia(s), after myocardial infarction, 307–318
  electrophysiologic studies (EPS) of, 311–314, 313t
  exercise testing and, 310–311
  heart rate variability and, 317–318, *318*
  Holter studies of, 307, 308t, *308–309*
  incidence of, 96–98, 96t, *97*
  increase in, 310, 310t
  left ventricular dysfunction and, 307–309, 309t, *310*
  non-Q wave infarction and mortality, 309–310
  signal-averaged electrocardiogram and, 314, 315t, 316–317
  analysis of, in pre-excitation syndrome, 201–202, *202*
  complex classification of, 217–229
    incidence of sudden cardiac death and, 217
      in normal heart vs. organic heart disease, 217–219

Ventricular arrhythmia(s) *(Continued)*
  programmed electrical stimulation (PES) in, 219–229
    clinical variables in, 223–224
    electrocardiographic variables in, 224
    left ventricular function indices, 224
    noninvasive predictors of results, 222–227, 223t
    results of, 221–222, 222t
    risk stratification with, 227–229, 228t
    signal-averaged ECG, 224–227, *225–226*, 226t
    specificity of induced tachyarrhythmias and, 221
    stimulation protocols for, 219–221, 220t
  during early myocardial ischemia, 18–24
    amphipathic lipid metabolites and, 22–23
    conduction disorders and, 19–20, *20*
    extracellular potassium increase during, 21–22, *22*
    ionic and metabolic changes with, 21–23
    mapping studies of, 20–21, *21*
    reperfusion arrhythmias and, 23–24
    role of free radicals in, 23
    transmembrane action potential changes and, 19, *19*
  following coronary artery occlusion, 18–19
  incidence of mortality from, 57
  induction of, with myopotential pacemaker interference, 641, *642*
  prevalence of, by population, 93t
  safety of exercise testing and, 100–101
  termination of, with electrical devices, 759–761
Ventricular blanking, in dual-chamber pacemakers, 605, *606*, 607
Ventricular defibrillation, 713–723
  basic concepts of, 713
  electrophysiologic mechanisms of, 713–724
    activation fronts of fibrillation and, 715, *716–717*
    biphasic waveforms and, *722*, 722–723
    critical hypothesis and, 717–721, *719–720*
    defibrillation criteria and, 717
    diphasic waveforms and, *721*, 721–723
      critical point for, 722
      decreased impedance and, 721
      refractory period duration and, 722
      sodium channel reactivation and, 721–722
      strength-duration curves for, *722*, 722–723
    monophasic waveforms and, *722*, 722–723
    probability function of, 719–721, *720*
    subthreshold shock and, 714–715, *714–716*
    upper limit of vulnerability and, 715–717, *717*
      critical hypothesis and, 719, *720*
      threshold correlation with, 716–717, *718*
    very high potential gradients and, 723–724
Ventricular (demand) inhibited (VVI) pacemaker, 490, 578–581, *579–581*
  congestive heart failure and atrial fibrillation in, 761
  defibrillation interference and, 620

Ventricular (demand) inhibited (VVI) *(Continued)*
  diaphragmatic myopotential interference with, 643–644, *643–644*
  electrocautery interference with, 615–616
  exogenous interference with, 612–614
  intercostal myopotential interference in, 644, *645*
  ventricular inhibition in, 605
Ventricular ectopic activity (VEA), as risk factor in sudden cardiac death, 334
  ambulatory monitoring of, 335–336
  exercise testing of, 337
  complex, noninvasive predictors of, in PES studies, 222–223, 223t
  with sustained ventricular tachycardia (VT), 258
Ventricular electrical instability, 296, 296t
Ventricular fibrillation (VF), after myocardial infarction, 323
  as sign of coronary artery disease, 333–334
  clinical implications of, 329–331
  evaluation of antiarrhythmic drug therapy and, 101–102
  failure of AICD and, 755
  in nonsustained ventricular tachycardia, 221
  in sustained ventricular tachycardia (VT), 252, *252*
  inducible, programmed stimulation studies (PES) of, 327, 327t, 690, 693, *697–699*
  with defibrillation interference, 620
  predictive value of, 379–381
  pre-excitation syndrome and, 194
  preoperative evaluation of, 445
  reentrant type of, 323–325, *324–325*
  sudden cardiac death and, 95–98
    ambulatory monitoring of, 335–336
  ventricular late potentials and, 387–388
  ventricular tachycardia (VT), 392
Ventricular flutter, in sustained ventricular tachycardia (VT), 252, *252*
Ventricular late potentials, clinical aspects of, 387–398
  ablation techniques and, 394–396
    antitachycardia surgery for, 394–396, *395*
    catheter ablation for, 396
  antiarrhythmic agents and, 393–394
  detection techniques for, 388–391, *388–389*, 391t
  duration of, 391
  in ventricular tachycardia vs. ventricular fibrillation, 392
  incidence of, with recurrent syncope, 393
  with ventricular tachycardia, 390–391, 391t
  insufficient SAECG sensitivity to, 391–392
  predictability of transplant rejection with, 397
  prognostic significance of, 396–397
  risk stratification with, 397–398
  specificity of SAECG to, 392
  definition of, 387–388, *388*
  high-resolution electrocardiography for, 378–384, *380–383*
Ventricular muscle, action potential and conduction in, 8–9
Ventricular outflow tract obstructions, ventricular late potentials in, 383
Ventricular pacing, for sick sinus syndrome patients, 132

Ventricular pacing *(Continued)*
   myocardial infarction diagnosis in, 576, 577
   QRS patterns with, 571–576
Ventricular passive fixation lead, techniques for, 563–564
Ventricular premature beats (VPBs), aggravation of, with drug therapy, 106
   combined antiarrhythmic therapy and, 105
   evaluation of antiarrhythmic drug therapy for, 102
   prevalence of, in arrhythmias, 94
   risk of sudden cardiac death and, 95–96
Ventricular premature complexes (VPCs), as sudden death indicator, 217–218
   electrophysiologic studies (EPS) of, 295
Ventricular premature contraction (VPC), exogenous pacemaker interference and, 609
   programmability of refractory period and, 509
Ventricular premature depolarization (VPD), after myocardial infarction, 307, 308t, *308–309*
   hemodynamic effects of, 551, *552–553*
   infarct size and, 3040
Ventricular refractory period, dual-chamber pacemaker timing cycles and, 601
Ventricular septal defect, postsurgical AV block with, 655–656
Ventricular stimulation, DDD mode programmability and, 512, *512–513*
Ventricular tachyarrhythmias, surgical management of, 445–452
   arrhythmogenic right ventricular dysplasia and, 448, *448–449*
   cardiomyopathy and, 447, *447*
   idiopathic types of, 447
   in anterior or lateral left ventricle, 450, *450*
   in posterior left ventricle, 450–452, *451*
   indications for surgery for, 445
   intraoperative electrophysiologic mapping for, 445–447, *446–447*
   nonischemic type of, 447–450, *448–449*
   refractory ischemic ventricular tachyarrhythmias and, 450
Ventricular tachycardia (VT), algorithm for management of, 288–289, *289*
   antiarrhythmic drug therapy and, 110
   as risk factor in sudden cardiac death, 110
   ambulatory monitoring of, 335–336
   signal-averaged electrocardiography evaluation of, 337–338
   cardiomyopathies and, 288, *288*
   cardioversion of, 731
   catheter ablation for, 471–482
      activation time measurement equipment for, 476, *477–478*
      analog signal recordings for, 477
      catheter technology and selection in, 471–474, *472, 474–475*
      endocardial mapping for, 477
      fluoroscopic equipment for, 471, *472*
      fulguration and, 474–476, *475, 479, 480*, 481t
      hemodynamic monitoring during, 476
      materials for, 471–477
      pace-mapping for, 477–478
      pacing for slow conduction area, 478–479, *479*
      postoperative surveillance of, 479, 482
      videotape recordings for, 476

Ventricular tachycardia (VT) *(Continued)*
   clinical implications of, 329–331
   definition of, 247
   electrophysiologic studies (EPS) of, 295
   evaluation of antiarrhythmic drug therapy and, 101–102
   failure of AICD and, 755
   hemodynamic effects of, 550–554, *552–554*
   idiopathic type of, 447
   in infants, clinical presentation of, 285, *286–287*
      evaluation of, 287–288
      mechanisms of, 285–287
      treatment of, 288–291
         chronic treatment methods for, 290
         nonpharmacologic therapy for, 290–291
   inducible, after myocardial infarction, 312–313, *313*, 323
      prevalence of, 312
      time course of, 312
      programmed stimulation studies of, 327, 327t
   monomorphic, electrophysiologic study of, 445
   in long QT syndrome, 266, *267*
   nonsustained, noninvasive predictors of, 222–223, 223t
      programmed electrical stimulation (PES) studies of, 219–221, 220t
      risk stratification and management protocol for, 229–230, *229*
      signal-averaged ECG and PES results and, 224–227, *226*
      specificity of induced tachyarrhythmias, 221
      sudden cardiac arrest and, 227, 228t, 341–342
   pacing termination of, 710–711
   polymorphic, electrophysiologic study of, 445
      long QT vs. non-long QT-associated types of, 266, 268t
      mechanisms of, 265, *266*
   predictive value of, 379–381
   reentrant, anatomic and electrophysiologic substrate for, 323–325, *324–325*
      antitachycardia pacing and, 685–686
      prevention of, with programmed electrical stimulation, 693, 700, *702–704*
      termination of, with programmed electrical stimulation (PES), 686, *687*, 688, *688*, 690
   repetitive monomorphic. See *Repetitive monomorphic ventricular tachycardia (RMVT)*.
   sustained, 247–260
      clinical presentation of, 250–251
      definition of, 247
      diagnosis of, 251–256
         with electrocardiogram, 251–253, *252*
      differentiation from supraventricular tachycardia (SVT), 255–256, *256*
      economics of, 259
      electrophysiologic studies (EPS) of, 248–250, 250t
         abnormal automaticity in, 248–249
         reentry in, 249
         triggered automaticity in, 249
      future research trends in, 259–260
      history of, 247

Ventricular tachycardia (VT) *(Continued)*
   invasive electrical recordings and pacing of, 253–255
      catheter studies as, 253–255, *254–255*
      esophageal electrocardiography as, 253
   pathophysiology of, 247–248, 248t
   physical examination for, 253, *254*
   signal-averaged electrocardiography for, 255
   therapy for, 256–259
      implantable devices for, 259, *260*
      long-term procedures for, 257–259
      surgery for, 258–259
      termination procedures for, 256–257
   ventricular late potentials and, 387–388
      incidence of, 390–391, 391t
      vs. ventricular fibrillation, 392
Ventricular-triggered (VVT) pacemaker, 578, *578–579*
   conversion to, with myopotential interference, 646–647, *647–648*
   conversion from VVI, with defibrillator interference, 620
   tachyarrhythmia termination with, 665–665
Ventriculophasic arrhythmia, 117
Verapamil, for infantile supraventricular tachycardia, 290
   for pre-excitation syndrome patients, 210
   for repetitive monomorphic ventricular tachycardia, 242, 244–245, *245*
   in vivo triggered activity studies, 34, *35*
   quinidine interactions with, 415–416
   role of, in supraventricular tachycardia therapy, 178, *180–181*
   ventricular arrhythmia suppression with, 30, *32*
Videotape recording for catheter ablation, 476
Voltage exponential decay curve in pacemakers, 569
Voltage-source pacing, 496
VOO cardiac pacing mode, 490, 576–578, *577–578*
   exogenous pacemaker interference and mode conversion to, 612–614

Warm-up phenomenon, in repetitive monomorphic ventricular tachycardia, 241–242
Wenckebach AV block, 144–149
   distal to His bundle, 147–148, *147–150*
   during early myocardial ischemia, 20, *20*
   in His bundle system, 147, *147*
   in the AV node, 144–147, *145–146*
   reentrant excitation and, 40, *41*
   relationship with Mobitz II AV block and, 148–149
Wenckebach periodicity, alternate, 149–150, *151–152*
Wenckebach response, in dual-chamber pacemakers, 603, *604*
Westmead studies, programmed stimulation protocols in, 326–327, 326t, 327t
   signal-averaged electrocardiograms in, 328–329, 329t
"Window trigger" in signal-averaged electrocardiography, 351–352, *352*
Wolff-Parkinson-White (WPW) syndrome. See also *Pre-excitation syndrome*.
   atrial fibrillation in, 177

Wolff-Parkinson-White (WPW) syndrome *(Continued)*
  AV node reentry tachycardia and, 441
  catheter ablation for, 462
  conduction patterns in, *191*, 191–192
  disopyramide for treatment of, 418
  electrophysiologic studies (EPS) of, 295
  hemodynamic effects of, 547–548, *549*
  incidence of pre-excitation syndrome in, 193–194

Wolff-Parkinson-White (WPW) syndrome *(Continued)*
  surgical management of, 436–440
    indications for surgery for, 436
    intraoperative electrophysiologic mapping for, 436
    preoperative electrophysiologic evaluation for, 436
    surgical techniques in, 437–440, *437–439*

Wolff-Parkinson-White (WPW) syndrome *(Continued)*
  tachycardia in infants and, 285, *287*

Xanthine oxidase, alterations in, during myocardial ischemia, 67–68

Zenner diode, prevention of pacemaker interference with, 619–620

SUNY HEALTH SCIENCE LIB. - SYRACUSE DUPL.
WG 26 C267 1991
Cardiac pacing and electrophysiology

3 2803 00009515 7

#21198738

WG 26 C267 1991

Cardiac pacing and
electrophysiology

DUE DATE

JUN 1 1 1991			
JUL 1 1 1991			
OCT 9 1991			
DEC 5 1991			
FEB 2 5 1992			
SEP 2 0 1993			
APR 2 7 1994			
AUG 0 1 1995			

201-6503   Printed in USA